创伤外科危重症治疗学

Current Therapy of Trauma and Surgical Critical Care

（第2版）

创伤外科危重症治疗学

Current Therapy of Trauma and Surgical Critical Care

（第 2 版）

原　著　Juan A. Asensio

Donald D. Trunkey

主　译　姜保国

译者名单（以姓名汉语拼音为序）

安金刚　陈　彧　都定元　黄　伟　贾　莉　黎檀实

李明武　李　纾　刘　波　刘士军　吕　杰　沈　凯

孙荣距　王传林　王天兵　王志启　魏彦芳　熊　建

易成腊　殷晓峰　郁有来　张大方　张进军　张立红

张　茂　张学民　赵　辉　周　靖　周足力　朱凤雪

北京大学医学出版社

CHUAGNSHANG WAIKE WEIZHONGZHENG ZHILIAOXUE (DI 2 BAN)

图书在版编目（CIP）数据

创伤外科危重症治疗学：第2版 / (美) 涓·阿森西奥 (Juan A. Asensio) , (美) 唐纳德·川基 (Donald D. Trunkey) 著；姜保国主译. -- 北京：北京大学医学出版社, 2019.1

书名原文: Current therapy of trauma and surgical critical care(2nd edition)

ISBN 978-7-5659-1913-8

Ⅰ. ①创… Ⅱ. ①涓… ②唐… ③姜… Ⅲ. ①外科－急性病－诊疗②外科－险症－诊疗 Ⅳ. ①R605.97

中国版本图书馆CIP数据核字(2018)第266387号

北京市版权局著作权合同登记号：图字：01-2017-1635

ELSEVIER

Elsevier (Singapore) Pte Ltd.
3 Killiney Road, #08-01 Winsland House I, Singapore 239519
Tel: (65) 6349-0200; Fax: (65) 6733-1817

创伤外科危重症治疗学（第2版）

主　　译：姜保国
出版发行：北京大学医学出版社
地　　址：（100191）北京市海淀区学院路38号　北京大学医学部院内
电　　话：发行部 010-82802230；图书邮购 010-82802495
网　　址：http：//www.pumpress.com.cn
E-mail：booksale@bjmu.edu.cn
印　　刷：北京信彩瑞禾印刷厂
经　　销：新华书店
责任编辑：刘　燕　靳　奕　　**责任校对**：靳新强　　**责任印制**：李　啸
开　　本：889 mm × 1194 mm　1/16　　**印张**：55.75　　**字数**：1762千字
版　　次：2019年1月第1版　2019年1月第1次印刷
书　　号：ISBN 978-7-5659-1913-8
定　　价：480.00元

译者前言

随着人类社会的快速发展，医疗卫生事业也取得了长足的进步。原本威胁人类生存的重大医疗卫生问题如传染性疾病已得到了很好的控制或消除。现代社会发展带来的心脑血管疾病和肿瘤等慢性疾病，经过多年大量的医疗卫生投入，也取得了诸多突破并建立了稳定、长效的应对体系。在这种情况下，在研究上相对起步晚、发展慢的创伤及外科危重症治疗已越来越凸显出其关键作用。据世界卫生组织（World Health Organization，WHO）报道，在所有疾病中，创伤已经成为40岁以下人群的第一死亡原因，并且创伤导致的残疾不仅严重影响了伤者的工作能力和生活质量，而且给家庭和社会带来了巨大的经济负担。中国是世界上第一人口大国。随着交通建设的高速发展以及汽车保有量的快速增长，以交通伤为首的各种创伤也已经成为威胁我国国民生命健康的重要因素。在未来中国的发展以"健康中国"作为重要目标之一，因此，推动创伤及相关外科危重症治疗的研究就显得意义重大。欧美国家开展创伤及外科危重症的研究时间较长，建立了比较完善的治疗及研究体系，出版了诸多著作，可供我国的研究者借鉴。

《创伤外科危重症治疗学（第2版）》是由美国Juan A. Asensio和Donald D. Trunkey教授组织编写的一部创伤和外科危重症治疗教程。本书在创伤及外科危重症领域既有研究成果的基础上，结合大量最新的研究进展，旨在为读者提供规范的诊疗原则和技术流程，提高创伤及外科危重症的救治效率，降低致死率和致残率。

本书共分为14章，内容包括创伤的院前救护，创伤的初期评估和复苏，以及头部、颌面部、胸部、腹部、脊柱、骨盆及四肢等创伤救治技术。每一章均按照致伤机制、处理原则与步骤及操作技巧等一系列流程进行编写。本书在帮助读者掌握该领域救治理论的同时，也规范了相关操作，是一部理论与实践兼顾的创伤及外科危重症救治经典著作。

鉴于本书在规范创伤及外科危重症救治以及提高救治技术中的重要意义，同时，为了使国内更多的从事创伤及外科危重症救治的同道了解和掌握国际最新、最实用的救治理念、技术和流程，我们组织了国内多位中青年专家翻译了本书，并在北京大学医学出版社的支持下得以出版。参译者大多工作在创伤救治的第一线，对创伤及外科危重症救治有着较为深厚的理论和实践经验，因此对原著理解准确，翻译到位。

科学、规范、合理、有序的救治对降低创伤及外科危重症的危害具有重要意义。近年来，中国的创伤救治取得了一定的进步，建立了包括院前救治、院内多学科团队救治以及专科救治在内的一系列救治规范，并在国家管理部门的支持下，在全国范围内开展了区域性创伤救治体系建设，以期在创伤救治的全过程中提高救治效果。相信本书中文版的出版与推广，必将有助于提升我国创伤及外科危重症的救治水平，使更多的创伤及外科危重症患者和家庭从中获益。

再次向为本书的出版付出辛勤劳动的著者、译者及出版者致敬！

北京大学创伤医学中心主任

姜保国

2019年元旦

原著序

创伤是导致年轻人死亡和残疾的主要原因，严重影响着全世界人民的生命及生活质量。创伤外科综合管理必须着眼于预防，包括对一名伤者或大规模伤亡患者突然到来的直接需求，以及患者的康复和临终关怀。《创伤外科危重症治疗学（第2版）》对所有参与创伤患者护理和治疗的军事人员以及医疗顾问而言都是一笔宝贵的资源。

本书由理论及实践经验丰富的知名专家编写。他们从客观的角度评价各种学术争议。本书以循证医学为指导方针，基于多年的临床和手术经验，讨论并提出了各种最佳实践性意见。本著作中重症治疗的章节写得非常好，把基础生理学和患者的床边评估很好地结合在一起。

本版的新增章节讲述了目前日益重要的领域，包括民用和军用设施的分类、血管损伤、较难处理的复杂创伤，以及与战争伤亡、脑死亡和器官移植相关的最新监护课程。

Juan A. Asensio 和 Donald D. Trunkey 两位主编都是很有远见的专家。他们花费了整个职业生涯来改变我们对创伤监护的认识。他们修订和扩展了《创伤外科危重症治疗学（第2版）》，以帮助创伤系统在日益全球化的社会中迎接新的挑战。

Robert Dunlay，MD
院长
克瑞顿大学医学院

“如果您带着有血压的患者进手术室，那么我会进来。”

我是在芝加哥南部成长和学习的。我清楚地记得在心胸外科做住院医师期间我的导师对我说的这句话。2年后我给他打过两次电话。尽管那时创伤监护已经取得了很大的进展，但许多处理原则都是相同的，而且我们的关注点总是停留在近在手边看得见的损伤。现在我知道这其实是一个不断变化的复杂的“创伤系统”。这需要许多专业人员的努力和协调，务必使患者在血压存在的情况下到达手术台上。

对于从事创伤救治的医护人员来说，《创伤外科危重症治疗学（第2版）》是他们重要的参考书。本版继续对传统的《治疗学》系列进行了更新、修订和扩展。本版还新增了许多章节，包括血管损伤、影像工程学新进展以及通气技术方面的最新信息。Juan A. Asensio 和 Donald D. Trunkey 两位主编都是创伤领域非常有名的专家。他们是全面和权威的代名词。这本书不仅涵盖了完整、统一的监护，而且着重于外科技术尤其是对复杂创伤的处理。

本书的作者都是创伤和危重症监护领域的知名专家。他们力求为读者提供相关方面实用、简明和最新的知识。本书既提供了经过循证医学和临床证实的临床经验和专家观点，也涉及了有争论性的领域和挑战。对于每一位创伤领域的人士来说，这本书都有您感兴趣的部分：创伤救治历史、创伤体系、特殊器官损伤处理、预防、重症监护护理、大规模创伤事件以及姑息治疗。

《创伤外科危重症治疗学（第 2 版）》体现了 Trunkey 和 Asensio 两位医生的无私奉献。他们意在为创伤团体创作一部全面、实用而又简洁的参考书目。我向每一位参与创伤患者监护的医生推荐这本具有阅读和参考价值的著作。

Jeffrey T. Sugimoto，博士
Mrs. Arnold Lempka 外科主任
教授、主席
心胸外科主任
外科病区
克瑞顿大学医学院
克瑞顿大学

原著前言

21 世纪的开端是一个充满动荡慌乱的年代。我非常荣幸地再一次成为《创伤外科危重症治疗学》的主编。实际上这本书已经经过了六次改版。但是由于这部极具价值的教科书增加了外科重症监护内容，因此我们重新将其命名为第 2 版。

有一件事是永恒不变的：现在的世界充满着动荡和危险，而且在未来很长一段时间内将一直存在。无论是通过电视、数字新闻还是印刷文字等传媒信息，我们可以看到这个世界正经历着多种多样的武装冲突。在这些冲突中往往有大量的人员伤亡。我们的职业或许是所有职业中最神圣的，但仍然受到持续的限制。虽然外科医生可以提供最佳的治疗，但经济和市场的某些因素一直侵蚀着医生的能力。我记得人们常说的一句话是“至少还有这些……”意思是说至少还有我们这些可怜的兄弟们。

在所有这些动乱中，外科医生和外科急救专家不但对此应付自如，而且承担着急救手术处理的任务。创伤外科医生再一次成为中流砥柱，成为典型的“兄弟连”。我引用莎士比亚的一段话来形容创伤外科医生：

“如果有谁没有勇气打这一仗，
就随他掉队，我们发给他通行证，
并且把沿途所需的旅费放进他的钱袋。
我们不愿跟这样一个人死在一块儿，
他竟然害怕跟咱们大伙儿一起死。
在这个节日里，
我们也永不会被人们忘记。
我们，是少数几个人，幸运的少数几个人，我们，是一支兄弟的队伍。
今天他跟我一起流着血，
他就是我的好兄弟。”(Henry V, Act IV, Scene 3)

我坚信挽救一个生命的荣誉和特权，不仅可以在手术室，也可以通过患者咨询的方式。这在努力消除创伤性疾病方面的确是一份崇高的工作。我一直怀有这样一个梦想，那就是作为领导者的我们终将看到一个没有战争的世界。在这里会有更多的理解。我们也会有更多的时间及精力致力于改善人类的生活条件。

我们一直相信，所有的奉献和努力一定会带来一些改变。我们希望建立起人与人之间沟通的桥梁，在人际关系和科学研究领域中产生更大的理解和合作。尽管这些理想和目标依然高远，但在与同事交谈时，这种信念仍然强大并持续激励着我们所有人。我深信对于“兄弟连”的精英们，减轻痛苦和拯救生命仍然是其重要的承诺。

我希望并恳求创伤外科所有的同事超越学术界的限制，照顾那些需要照顾的人，通过专业能力体现我们的医德和良知，成为履行人权的领导者和倡导者，医治伤员，教育并指导将来能在创伤外科有所建树的医生。我们必须准备迎接挑战，创造和平，治愈创伤，因为来到我们面前的人都经受着各种创伤，充满着痛苦，而且往往当一个生命结束时，还须要继续拯救其他生命。

如果——

拉迪亚德·吉卜林

如果周围的人毫无理性地向你发难，你仍能镇定自若保持冷静；
如果众人对你心存猜忌，你仍能自信如常并认为他们的猜忌情有可原；
如果你肯耐心等待不急不躁，

或遭人诽谤却不以牙还牙，
或遭人憎恨却不以恶报恶；
既不装腔作势，亦不气盛趾高；

如果你有梦想，而又不为梦主宰；
如果你有神思，而又不走火入魔；
如果你坦然面对胜利和灾难，对虚渺的胜负荣辱心怀旷荡；
如果你能忍受有这样的无赖，歪曲你的口吐真言蒙骗笨汉，
或看着心血铸就的事业崩溃，仍能忍辱负重脚踏实地重新攀登；

如果你敢把取得的一切胜利，为了更崇高的目标孤注一掷，
面临失去，决心从头再来而绝口不提自己的损失；
如果人们早已离你而去，你仍能坚守阵地奋力前驱，
身上已一无所有，唯存意志在高喊“顶住”；

如果你跟平民交谈而不变谦虚之态，
亦或与王侯散步而不露谄媚之颜；
如果敌友都无法对你造成伤害；
如果众人对你信赖有加却不过分依赖；
如果你能惜时如金利用每一分钟不可追回的光阴；
那么，你的修为就会如天地般博大，并拥有了属于自己的世界，
更重要的是：孩子，你成为了真正顶天立地之人！

选自吉卜林诗歌 (1943)
Juan A. Asensio, MD, FACS, FCCM, FRCS, KM

原著人员名单

Kareem R. AbdelFattah, MD
Fellow in Burns, Trauma, and Critical Care, University of Texas Southwestern Medical Center, Dallas, Texas

Michel B. Aboutanos, MD, MPH, FACS
Associate Professor of Surgery, Director, Injury Prevention Program, Director, International Trauma System Development Program, Division of Trauma Critical Care and Emergency General Surgery, Department of Surgery, Virginia Commonwealth University, Richmond, Virginia

Louis A. Aliperti, MD
Department of Surgery, Division of Trauma and Critical Care, Tulane University School of Medicine, New Orleans, Louisiana

John T. Anderson, MD, FACS
Associate Professor, Department of Surgery, Division of Trauma and Emergency Surgery, University of California Davis, Sacramento, California

Devashish J. Anjaria, MD, FACS
Assistant Professor of Surgery, Trauma, Surgical Critical Care and General Surgery, Rutgers New Jersey Medical School, Newark, New Jersey

Juan A. Asensio, MD, FACS, FCCM, FRCS
Professor of Surgery, Chief, Division of Trauma Surgery and Surgical Critical Care, Director, Trauma Center and Trauma Program, Department of Surgery, Creighton University School of Medicine, Creighton University Medical Center, Omaha, Nebraska

Morad Askari, MD
Assistant Professor of Plastic and Reconstructive Surgery, Assistant Professor of Orthopedic Surgery, Division of Hand Surgery, Department of Surgery, Department of Orthopedic Surgery, University of Miami, Miami, Florida

Jeffrey A. Bailey, MD, MPA, FACS
Emeritus Director, Joint Trauma System, Associate Professor of Surgery, Uniformed Services University of the Health Sciences, Bethesda, Maryland

Marcus Balters, MD
Assistant Professor of Surgery, Division of Cardiovascular Surgery, Creighton University School of Medicine, CHI-Health Alegent Creighton Clinic, Omaha, Nebraska

Ron Barbosa, MD
Medical Director, Trauma Intensive Care Unit, Legacy Emanuel Hospital, Portland, Oregon

Philip S. Barie, MD, MBA, MCCM, FIDSA, FACS
Professor of Surgery, Division of Burns, Critical Care and Trauma, Professor of Public Health in Medicine, Division of Medical Ethics, Weill Medical College of Cornell University, New York, New York

Edward J. Bedrick, PhD
Professor of Biostatistics, Department of Mathematics and Statistics, Department of Internal Medicine, University of New Mexico, Albuquerque, New Mexico

John D. Berne, MD, FACS
Clinical Assistant Professor of Surgery, University of Texas at Houston, Houston, Texas

Stepheny D. Berry, MD
Co-Medical Director for Trauma, Assistant Professor of Surgery, The University of Kansas Medical Center,

Kansas City, Kansas

Robert Bertelotti, MD
Resident, General Surgery, Creighton University, Omaha, Nebraska

Pulkesh Bhatia, MBBS
Surgical Resident, Creighton University Medical Center, Omaha, Nebraska

Walter L. Biffl, MD, FACS
Associate Director of Surgery, Denver Health Medical Center, Professor of Surgery, University of Colorado, Denver, Colorado

Brian Biggerstaff, MD
Surgical Resident, Creighton University Medical Center, Omaha, Nebraska

John K. Bini, MD, FACS, LtCol, USAF MC
Assistant Professor of Surgery, Boonshoft School of Medicine, Wright State University; Assistant Professor of Surgery, Uniformed Services University of Health Sciences; Trauma Surgeon, Wright Patterson Medical Center, Dayton, Ohio

F. William Blaisdell, MD, FACS
Professor, Department of Surgery, University of California Davis, Sacramento, California

Matthew C. Bozeman, MD
Assistant Professor, Hiram C. Polk, Jr. Department of Surgery, University of Louisville, Louisville, Kentucky

Steven B. Brandes, MD
Professor of Urologic Surgery, Director of Reconstructive Urology, Division of Urologic Surgery, Washington University School of Medicine, St. Louis, Missouri

Karen J. Brasel, MD, MPH
Oregon Health and Science University, Portland, Oregon

Benjamin M. Braslow, MD
Associate Professor of Clinical Surgery, Division of Traumatology, Surgical Critical Care and Emergency Surgery; Section Chief, Emergency Surgery Service, Department of Surgery, Perelman School of Medicine, University of Pennsylvania, Philadelphia, Pennsylvania

L.D. Britt, MD, MPH, FACS
Henry Ford Professor and Edward J. Brickhouse Chairman, Department of Surgery, Eastern Virginia Medical School, Norfolk, Virginia

Susan I. Brundage, MD, MPH
Section Chief, Acute Care Surgery, Director, Surgical Critical Care, Department of Surgery, New York University School of Medicine; NYU Langone Medical Center, Tisch Hospital; Department of Surgery, Bellevue Hospital, New York, New York

Thomas P. Brush, MD
Resident, Department of Surgery, Creighton University, Omaha, Nebraska

Clay Cothren Burlew, MD, FACS
Director, Surgical Intensive Care Unit, Program Director, SCC and TACS Fellowships, Department of Surgery, Denver Health Medical Center; Professor of Surgery, University of Colorado School of Medicine, Denver, Colorado

Patricia Marie Byers, MD, FACS
Chief, Surgical Nutrition, Division of Trauma and Surgical Critical Care, The DeWitt Daughtry Family Department of Surgery, University of Miami Miller School of Medicine, Miami, Florida

Kim M. Caban, MD
Assistant Professor of Radiology, University of Miami Miller School of Medicine, Jackson Memorial Hospital–Ryder Trauma Center, ER-Trauma Radiology Division, Miami, Florida

Jeremy Cannon, MD, SM, FACS, LtCol, USAF MC
Chief, Trauma and Critical Care, San Antonio Military Medical Center, San Antonio, Texas; Associate Professor of Surgery, Uniformed Services University of the Health Sciences, Bethesda, Maryland

Shawn M. Cantie, MD
Clinical Instructor of Anesthesiology, The University at Buffalo, State University of New York, Erie County Medical Center, Buffalo, New York

José Ceballos Esparragon, MD
Surgical Resident, Creighton University Medical Center, Omaha, Nebraska

Howard R. Champion, FRCS, FACS
Professor of Surgery, Uniformed Services University of the Health Sciences, Bethesda, Maryland

Benjamin Chandler, MD
PGY-4 Resident, Department of Surgery, Rutgers New Jersey Medical School, University of Medicine and Dentistry of New Jersey; Resident, Department of Surgery, University Hospital, Newark, New Jersey

David C. Chang, PhD, MPH, MBA
Associate Professor of Surgery, Massachusetts General Hospital, Harvard Medical School, Boston, Massachusetts

Steven Cheung, MD
Resident, General Surgery, Creighton University Medical Center, Omaha, Nebraska

William C. Chiu, MD, FACS, FCCM
Associate Professor of Surgery, Director, Surgical Critical Care Fellowship Program, R Adams Cowley Shock Trauma Center, University of Maryland School of Medicine, Baltimore, Maryland

A. Britton Christmas, MD, FACS
Associate Professor of Surgery, Trauma, Surgical Critical Care, and Emergency General Surgery, Carolinas Medical Center, Charlotte, North Carolina

David J. Ciesla, MD
Professor of Surgery, Director of Acute Care Surgery Division, University of South Florida Morsani College of Medicine; Medical Director, Regional Trauma Program, Tampa General Hospital, Tampa, Florida

William G. Cioffi, MD, FACS
J. Murray Beardsley Professor and Chairman, Alpert Medical School of Brown University Department of Surgery; Surgeon-in-Chief, Rhode Island Hospital and The Miriam Hospital, Providence, Rhode Island

Christine S. Cocanour, MD, FACS, FCCM
Professor of Surgery, UC Davis Medical Center, Sacramento, California

Mitchell J. Cohen, MD
Assistant Professor in Residence, Department of Surgery, University of California San Francisco, San Francisco, California

Raul Coimbra, MD, PhD, FACS
The Monroe E. Trout Professor of Surgery, Surgeon-in-Chief, Executive Vice-Chairman, Department of Surgery, Chief Division of Trauma, Surgical Critical Care, Burns, and Acute Care Surgery, University of California San Diego Health System, San Diego, California

Peter Collister, MD
Resident, General Surgery, Creighton University, Omaha, Nebraska

Edward E. Cornwell, III, MD, PhD, FACS
Chairman and Professor of Surgery, Howard University, Washington, D.C.

Thomas B. Cox, BS
President, Cox Business Consulting, Inc., Beaverton, Oregon

Martin A. Croce, MD
Professor, Department of Surgery, University of Tennessee Health Science Center; Chief of Trauma and Critical Care, Trauma Division Regional One Health, Memphis, Tennessee

Gary H. Danton, MD, PhD
Medical Director of Radiology, Trauma/ER Radiology, Jackson Memorial Hospital; Director, Radiology Residency Training Program, Assistant Professor of Clinical Radiology, Jackson Health System, Jackson, Florida; Chief, Section of Imaging Informatics, Trauma/ER Radiology, University of Miami, Miami, Florida

Kimberly A. Davis, MD, MBA
Professor of Surgery, Vice Chairman of Clinical Affairs, Chief of the Section of Trauma, Surgical Critical Care, and Surgical Emergencies, Yale University School of Medicine; Trauma Medical Director, Surgical Director, Quality and Performance Improvement, Yale-New Haven Hospital, New Haven, Connecticut

Elias Degiannis, MD, PhD, FRCS (Glasg), FCS (SA), FACS
Professor of Surgery, University of the Witwatersrand; Head, Trauma Directorate, Chris Hani Baragwanath Academic Hospital, Johannesburg, South Africa

Edwin A. Deitch, MD
Professor and Chairman, Rutgers New Jersey Medical School, University of Medicine and Dentistry of New Jersey; Chief of Surgery, University Hospital, Newark, New Jersey

Richard Denney, MD
Chief Resident, General Surgery, Creighton University, Omaha, Nebraska

Christopher J. Dente, MD, FACS
Associate Professor of Surgery, Emory University; Associate Director of Trauma, Grady Memorial Hospital, Atlanta, Georgia

Urmen Desai, MD, MPH
Plastic, Aesthetic, and Cosmetic Surgeon, Desai Plastic Surgery of Beverly Hills, Beverly Hills, California

Rochelle A. Dicker, MD
Associate Professor of Surgery and Anesthesia, University of California San Francisco, San FranciscoGeneralHospital, San Francisco, California

Lawrence N. Diebel, MD, FACS
Professor, Department of Surgery, Wayne State University, Detroit, Michigan

Karev Dimitryi, MD, FACS
Professor, Department of Surgery, Wayne State University, Detroit, Michigan

Andrew R. Doben, MD
Associate Professor of Surgery, Department of Surgery, Tufts University School of Medicine, Boston, Massachusetts; Director, Surgical Intensive Care Unit, Division of Trauma and Acute Care Surgery, Department of Surgery, Baystate Medical Center, Springfield, Massachusetts

Jay Doucet, MD, MSc, FRCSC, FACS, RDMS
Professor of Clinical Surgery, Director, Surgical Intensive Care Unit, Director, Emergency Preparedness and Response, Division of Trauma, Surgical Critical Care, and Burns, Department of Surgery, University of California San Diego Health System, San Diego, California

Therese M. Duane, MD, FACS, FCCM
Vice-Chair, Department of Surgery for Quality and Safety, Medical Director for Acute Care Surgery Research, John Peter Smith Health System, Fort Worth, Texas

Joe DuBose, MD, FACS
Associate Professor of Surgery, Uniformed Services University of the Health Sciences, Baltimore, Maryland; Vascular Fellow, University of Texas Health Sciences Center–Houston, Houston, Texas

Wayne Dubov, MD
Board Certified by the American Board of Physical Medicine and Rehabilitation (ABPMR), Subspecialty–Spinal Cord Injury Medicine, Diplomate of the American Board of Electrodiagnostic Medicine, Lehigh Valley Health Network, Allentown, Pennsylvania; Clinical Assistant Professor, University of South Florida, Morsani College of Medicine, Tampa, Florida

Juan C. Duchesne, MD, FACS, FCCP, FCCM
Trauma Medical Director, GME Medical Director, North Oaks Health System, Hammond, Louisiana; Associate Professor of Surgery, Tulane University, Louisiana State University Health Sciences Center; Chairman, Louisiana Committee of Trauma, New Orleans, Louisiana

Stanley J. Dudrick, MD, FACS, FACN, CNS
Professor of Surgery, The Commonwealth Medical College, Scranton, Pennsylvania; Edward S. Anderson Endowed Chair, Professor and Medical Director of Physician Assistant Studies, School of Arts and Sciences, Misericordia University, Dallas, Pennsylvania; Professor of Surgery, Emeritus, Yale University Medical School, New Haven, Connecticut

Rodney Durham, MD, FACS
Professor of Surgery, University of South Florida, Tampa, Florida

Anthony M. Durso, MD
Assistant Professor of Radiology, University of Miami Miller School of Medicine, Jackson Memorial Hospital, Miami, Florida

Soumitra R. Eachempati, MD, FACS, FCCM
Professor of Surgery, Professor of Medicine, Division of Medical Ethics, Weill Cornell Medical College, New

York, New York

Colonel (Ret.) Brian Eastridge, MD
Trauma and Surgical Critical Care, Director Emeritus, Joint Trauma System Program; Trauma Consultant, U.S. Army Surgeon General, Institute of Surgical Research, Houston, Texas

Aileen Ebadat, MD
Resident, Department of Surgery, University of Texas Southwestern, Austin, University Medical Center Brackenridge, Austin, Texas

David T. Efron, MD, FACS
Associate Professor of Surgery, Anesthesiology and Critical Care Medicine, Emergency Medicine, Chief, Division of Acute Care Surgery: Trauma, Critical Care, Emergency, and General Surgery, Director of Adult Trauma, Department of Surgery, The Johns Hopkins Hospital, Baltimore, Maryland

Eric Elster, MD, FACS, CAPT MC USN
Professor and Chairman, Norman M. Rich Department of Surgery, Uniformed Services University of the Health Sciences, Bethesda, Maryland

Michael Englehart, MD
Billings Clinic, Billings, Montana

Thomas J. Esposito, MD, MPH
Professor, Department of Surgery, Loyola University Chicago, Stritch School of Medicine, Chicago, Illinois; Chief, Division of Trauma, Surgical Critical Care and Burns, Department of Surgery, Loyola University Medical Center, Maywood, Illinois

Glyn Estebanez, MD, MRCS
Surgical Registrar, Wessex School of Surgery, United Kingdom; Trauma Research Fellow, MEDITECH, Neiva, Colombia

Susan Evans, MD, FACS, FCCM
Associate Professor of Surgery, Division of Acute Care Surgery, Carolinas Medical Center, Charlotte, North Carolina

Samir M. Fakhry, MD, FACS
Charles F. Crews Professor and Chief, General Surgery, Medical University of South Carolina, Charleston, South Carolina

Anthony Falvo, DO, FACOS, FACS
Clinical Educator, Wayne State University School of Medicine, Detroit, Michigan

David V. Feliciano, MD
Battersby Professor and Chief, IU Division of General Surgery, Chief of Surgery, Indiana University Hospital, Indianapolis, Indiana

Luis G. Fernández, MD, KHS, FACS, FASAS, FCCP, FCCM, FICS
Assistant Clinical Professor of Surgery/Family Practice, University of Texas Health Science Center, Tyler, Texas; Adjunct Clinical Professor of Medicine and Nursing, University of Texas, Arlington, Texas; Chairman, Division of Trauma Surgery/ Surgical Critical Care, Chief of Trauma Surgical Critical Care Unit, Trinity Mother Frances Health System, Tyler, Texas; Brigadier General, Past Commanding General, TXSG Medical Brigade, (Ret/HR), Austin, Texas

Mitchell Fink, MD
University of Pittsburgh, Pittsburgh, Pennsylvania

Lewis M. Flint, MD, FACS
Editor-in-Chief, Selected Readings in General Surgery, Division of Education, American College of Surgeons, Chicago, Illinois

Donald E. Fry, MD, FACS
Adjunct Professor of Surgery, Northwestern University Feinberg School of Medicine, Chicago, Illinois; Emeritus Professor of Surgery, University of New Mexico School of Medicine, Albuquerque, New Mexico

Takashi Fujita, MD, PhD, FACS
Associate Professor, Trauma and Resuscitation Center, Teikyo University Hospital, Tokyo, Japan

Joseph M. Galante, MD
Associate Professor and Vice Chair, Education, Department of Surgery, University of California, Davis; Division of Trauma, Acute Care Surgery, and Surgical Critical Care, UC Davis, Medical Center, Sacramento, California

Richard L. Gamelli, MD, FACS, FRCSEd (Hon)
Editor-in-Chief, Journal of Burn Care and Research;

Professor Emeritus, Stritch School of Medicine, Loyola University Chicago, Chicago, Illinois

Luis Manuel García-Núñez, MD, FACS, FAMSUS
General and Trauma Surgeon, Chief, Emergency Department, Military Central Hospital, National Defense Department, Mexico City, Mexico

Larry M. Gentilello, MD
Professor of Surgery, Adjunct Professor of Management, Policy, and Community Health, Department of Surgery, University of Texas, Austin, Texas

Ramyar Gilani, MD
Assistant Professor, Michael E. DeBakey Department of Surgery, Division of Vascular Surgery, Baylor College of Medicine; Chief of Vascular Surgery, Ben Taub General Hospital, Houston, Texas

Laurent G. Glance, MD
Vice-Chair for Research, Department of Anesthesiology, Professor of Anesthesiology, Professor of Public Health Sciences, Senior Scientist, RAND (adjunct), University of Rochester School of Medicine, Rochester, New York

Nestor R. Gonzalez, MD
Assistant Professor, Neurological Surgery and Radiological Sciences, UCLA Medical Center, Los Angeles, California

Daniel J. Grabo, MD
Fellow, Division of Traumatology, Surgical Critical Care and Emergency Surgery, Hospital of the University of Pennsylvania, Philadelphia, Pennsylvania

Gerald J. Gracia, MD
Assistant Professor of General Surgery, Trauma, Surgical Critical Care and Minimally Invasive Surgery, Stony Brook University Hospital, State University of New York, Stony Brook New York

Vincente H. Gracias, MD
Interim Dean, CEO, Robert Wood Johnson Medical Group; Professor and Chief, Department of Surgery, Rutgers Robert Wood Johnson Medical School, Robert Wood Johnson University Hospital, New Brunswick, New Jersey

Kirby R. Gross, MD
Colonel, Medical Corps, United States Army; Director, Joint Trauma System, San Antonio Military Medical Center, San Antonio, Texas; Associate Professor, Uniformed Services University of the Health Sciences, Bethesda, Maryland

Ronald I. Gross, MD
Associate Professor of Surgery, Tufts University School of Medicine, Boston, Massachusetts; Chief, Division of Trauma, Acute Care Surgery, and Surgical Critical Care, Baystate Medical Center, Springfield, Massachusetts

Chrissy Guidry, DO
Trauma and Critical Care, Tulane University School of Medicine, New Orleans, Louisiana

Oliver L. Gunter, Jr., MD, MPH, FACS
Vanderbilt University School of Medicine, Section of Surgical Sciences, Department of General Surgery, Division of Trauma and Surgical Critical Care, Nashville, Tennessee

Joseph M. Gutmann, MD
University of South Florida, Tampa, Florida

Erin Hale, MD
Resident, General Surgery, Creighton University, Omaha, Nebraska

S. Morad Hameed, MD, MPH
Associate Professor and Chief, Section of Trauma, Acute Care Surgery, and Surgical Critical Care, Department of Surgery, University of British Columbia Trauma Services VGT, Vancouver, British Columbia

Molly Hartmann, MD
Resident, General Surgery, Creighton University, Omaha, Nebraska

Carl Hauser, MD, FACS, FCCM
Professor of Surgery, Harvard University; Attending Surgeon, New England Deaconess Medical Center, Boston, Massachusetts

Sharon Henry, MD, FACS
Anne Scalea Professor of Trauma Surgery, University of Maryland School of Medicine, University of Maryland Medical Center, R Adams Cowley Shock Trauma

Center, Baltimore, Maryland

Mathilda Horst, MD, FACS, FCCM
Medical Director, Surgical Critical Care; Henry Ford Hospital; Professor of Surgery, Wayne State School of Medicine, Detroit, Michigan

Ari Hoschander, MD
Department of Surgery, Division of Plastic Surgery, University of Miami Hospital, Jackson Memorial Hospital, Miami, Florida

Herman P. Houin, MD
Senior Staff Surgeon, Department of Plastic Surgery, Henry Ford Health System, Detroit, Michigan

David Hoyt, MD, FACS
Executive Director, American College of Surgeons, Chicago, Illinois

Jared M. Huston, MD
Department of Surgery, Division of Trauma and Acute Care Surgery, North Shore University Hospital, North Shore-LIJ Health System, Manhasset, New York

Kyros Ipaktchi, MD
Associate Professor of Orthopedic Surgery, Chief of Hand-Microvascular Surgery, Department of Orthopedic Surgery, Denver Health Medical Center, University of Colorado, Denver, Colorado

D'Andrea Joseph, MD, FACS
Assistant Professor of Surgery, Associate Director of Trauma, Program Director of Acute Care Fellowship, Department of Surgery, Hartford Hospital/University of Connecticut, Hartford, Connecticut

Gregory J. Jurkovich, MD, FACS
Chief of Surgery,DenverHealth and Hospitals; Rockwell Distinguished Professor of Trauma Surgery, University of Colorado, Denver, Colorado

Steven Kalandiak, MD
Assistant Professor of Clinical Orthopedics, University of Miami Miller School of Medicine, Miami, Florida

Riyad Karmy-Jones, MD
Chief of Trauma, Thoracic and Trauma Surgery, Legacy Emanuel Medical Center, Portland, Oregon

Larry T. Khoo, MD
Director of Minimally Invasive Neurological Spinal Surgery, Los Angeles Spine Clinic at Good Samaritan Hospital, The Los Angeles Spine Clinic, Los Angeles, California

Laszlo Kiraly, MD, FACS
Associate Professor, Department of Surgery, Oregon Health and Science University, Portland, Oregon

Orlando C. Kirton, MD, FACS, MCCM, FCCP
Professor of Surgery, Vice Chair, Department of Surgery,University ofConnecticut School of Medicine, Farmington; Ludwig J. Pyrtek, MD Chair in Surgery, Chief, Department of Surgery, Chief, Division of General Surgery, Interim Director, Trauma Service, Hartford Hospital, Hartford, Connecticut

Michael Ksycki, DO
Chief of Surgery, Browning Community Hospital, HIS, Billings, Montana

Anastasia Kunac, MD, FACS
Assistant Professor of Surgery, Division of Trauma Surgery and Surgical Critical Care, Rutgers New Jersey Medical School, Newark, New Jersey

Kulsoom Laeeq, MD
Resident, General Surgery, Creighton University, Omaha, Nebraska

Anna M. Ledgerwood, MD, FACS
Professor, Michael and Marian Ilitch Department of Surgery, Wayne State University, Detroit, Michigan

Benjamin T. Lemelman, MD
University of Chicago Medical Center, Section of Plastic and Reconstructive Surgery, Chicago, Illinois

Ari Leppäniemi, MD, PhD, MDCC
Professor of Surgery, Chief of Emergency Surgery, Meilahti Hospital, University of Helsinki, Finland

David H. Livingston, MD, FACS
Wesley J. Howe Professor and Chief of Trauma and Surgical Critical Care, Rutgers New Jersey Medical School, Newark, New Jersey

Jason Loden, DO
Department of Surgery, Creighton University, Omaha, Nebraska

Gary Lombardo, MD, FACS
Assistant Professor of Surgery, New York Medical College, Westchester Medical Center, New York, New York

Andrew Loukas, MD
Clinical Anesthesiologist, South Miami Hospital/Baptist Health, Miami, Florida

Charles E. Lucas, MD
Professor Michael and Marian Ilitch Department of Surgery, Wayne State University, Detroit, Michigan

Fred A. Luchette, MD, MSc
Chief of Surgical Services, Edward Hines, Jr. VA Medical Center; Vice-Chair, VA Affairs; Professor of Surgery, Stritch School of Medicine, Loyola University of Chicago, Hines, Illinois

Charles D. Mabry, MD, FACS
Associate Professor, Department of Surgery, College of Medicine, University of Arkansas for Medical Sciences, Little Rock, Arkansas

Robert C. Mackersie, MD, FACS
Professor of Surgery, University of California San Francisco; Director of Trauma Services, San Francisco General Hospital and Trauma Center, San Francisco, California

Paul M. Maggio, MD, MBA, FACS
Assistant Professor of Surgery, Co-Director, Critical Care Medicine, Stanford University Medical Center, Stanford, California

Louis J. Magnotti, MD, FACS
Associate Professor, Department of Surgery, University of Tennessee Health Science Center, Memphis, Tennessee

John W. Mah, MD, FACS
Associate Professor, Department of Surgery, University of Connecticut School of Medicine, Farmington, Connecticut; Associate Director, Surgery Critical Care, Hartford Hospital, Hartford, Connecticut

Ajai K. Malhotra, MBBS (MD), MS, DNB, FRCSEd, FACS
Professor of Surgery, Virginia Commonwealth University, Richmond, Virginia

Darren Malinoski, MD, FACS
Assistant Chief of Surgery–Research and Education, Chief, Section of Surgical Critical Care, VA Portland Health Care System; Associate Professor of Surgery, Oregon Health and Science University, Portland, Oregon

Brittney J. Maloley-Lewis, DO, MBA
Surgical Resident, Creighton University Medical Center, Omaha, Nebraska

Corrado Paolo Marini, MD, FACS
Chief of Trauma, Surgical Critical Care and Emergency Surgery; Director of Surgical Critical Care Fellowship, Department of Surgery, Westchester Medical Center, Valhalla, New York

Colonel Matthew J. Martin, MD, FACS
Trauma Medical Director, Madigan Army Medical Center, Tacoma, Washington; Director of Trauma Informatics, Legacy Emanuel Medical Center, Portland, Oregon; Associate Professor of Surgery, Uniformed Services University of the Health Sciences, Bethesda, Maryland

Leonard Mason, MD
PGY-3 General Surgery Resident, Department of Surgery, Rutgers New Jersey Medical School, Newark, New Jersey

Kenneth L. Mattox, MD
Distinguished Service Professor, Michael E. DeBakey Department of Surgery, Baylor College of Medicine; Chief of Staff and Chief of Surgery, Ben Taub General Hospital, Houston, Texas

Kimball Maull, MD, FACS
Adjunct Professor of Surgery, University of Pittsburgh Medical Center, Pittsburgh, Pennsylvania

John C. Mayberry, MD
Professor of Surgery, Division of Acute Care Surgery, Oregon Health and Science University, Portland, Oregon

Dr. Federico N. Mazzini
Trauma and Emergency Surgery Coordinator General Surgery Department Hospital Italiano de Buenos Aires Argentina

Christopher McFarren, MD
Assistant Professor of Medicine, Division of Nephrology and Hypertension, Department of Internal Medicine, University of South Florida College of Medicine, Tampa, Florida

Norman E. McSwain, Jr., MD
Trauma and Critical Care, Tulane University School of Medicine, New Orleans, Louisiana

Mario A. Meallet, MD
A Center for Vison Care, LAC and USC Medical Center, Los Angeles, California

J. Wayne Meredith, MD, FACS
Richard T. Myers Professor and Chair, Department of Surgery, Wake Forest University School of Medicine; Chief of Surgery, Wake Forest University Baptist Medical Center, Winston Salem, North Carolina

Christopher P. Michetti, MD, FACS, FCCM
Medical Director, Trauma ICU, Inova Fairfax Hospital; Associate Professor of Surgery, VCU School of Medicine, Inova Campus, Falls Church, Virginia

Keith R. Miller, MD
Assistant Professor of Surgery, University of Louisville, Louisville, Kentucky

Preston R. Miller, MD
Associate Professor, Department of Surgery, Wake Forest University, Winston-Salem, North Carolina

Richard S. Miller, MD, FACS
Vanderbilt University School of Medicine, Section of Surgical Sciences, Department of General Surgery, Division of Trauma and Surgical Critical Care, Nashville, Tennessee

Joseph P. Minei, MD, MBA
Professor and Chair, Division of Burn, Trauma, and Critical Care, C. James Carrico, MD, Distinguished Chair in Surgery for Trauma and Critical Care, University of Texas Southwestern Medical Center; Surgeon-in-Chief, Parkland Health and Hospital System, Dallas, Texas

Haaris Mir, MD
Plastic and Reconstructive Hand Surgery, Joseph M. Still Burn Center and Burn Centers of Florida, Miami, Florida

Frank L. Mitchell, MD
Medical Director, Trauma and Surgical Critical Care, St. John Medical Center, Tulsa, Oklahoma

Alicia M. Mohr, MD, FACS
Associate Professor of Surgery, Division of Acute Care Surgery, University of Florida, Gainesville, Florida

Ernest E. Moore, MD
Professor and Vice Chairman for Research, Department of Surgery, University of Colorado Denver; Editor, Journal of Trauma and Acute Care Surgery, Denver, Colorado

Anne C. Mosenthal, MD, FACS
Professor and Chair, Department of Surgery, Rutgers New Jersey Medical School, Newark, New Jersey

Felipa Munera, MD
Associate Professor of Radiology, Chief, Department of Radiology, University of Miami Hospital, University of Miami Hospital and Clinics, and Sylvester Comprehensive Cancer Center; ER-Trauma Radiology Division, University of Miami– Miller School of Medicine, Jackson Memorial Hospital–Ryder Trauma Center, Miami, Florida

Alan D. Murdock, MD
Consultant to the Surgeon General for Trauma and Surgical Critical Care, Department of Trauma and General Surgery, University of Pittsburgh Medical Center, Pittsburgh, Pennsylvania; Consultant to the Surgeon General for Surgical Services, Air Force Medical Operations Agency, Lackland-Kelly Air Force Base, Texas

Mamoun Nabri, MD, FRCSI, FACS
Trauma Surgery/Surgical Critical Care Surgeon, Assistant Professor, Department of Surgery, Faculty of Medicine, University of Dammam, Dammam, Saudi Arabia

Lena M. Napolitano, MD, FACS, FCCP, FCCM
Professor of Surgery, Division Chief, Acute Care Surgery (Trauma, Burn, Critical Care, Emergency Surgery), Associate Chair of Surgery, Director, Trauma and Surgical Critical Care, University of Michigan Health System, Ann Arbor, Michigan

Nicholas A. Nash

Scott H. Norwood, MD, FACS
Clinical Professor of Surgery, Morsani College of Medicine, University of South Florida, Tampa, Florida; Trauma Service, Regional Medical Center, Bayonet Point, Hudson, Florida

John Oeltjen, MD, PhD
Associate Professor of Surgery, University of Miami, Miami, Florida

Chris Okwuosa, MD
Surgical Resident, Creighton University Medical Center, Omaha, Nebraska

Turner M. Osler, MD, MSc, FACS
Research Professor, Department of Surgery, University of Vermont, Burlington, Vermont

Angela Osmolak, MD
Surgical Resident, Creighton University Medical Center, Omaha, Nebraska

Yasuhiro Otomo, MD, PhD
Director, Trauma and Acute Critical Care Center, Tokyo Medical and Dental University Hospital of Medicine, Tokyo, Japan

Patrick Owens, MD
Associate Professor of Clinical Orthopedics, Associate Professor of Surgery, University of Miami, Miami, Florida

John T. Owings, MD, FACS
Director of Trauma Services, University Health, Professor of Surgery, Chief of Trauma and Critical Care, Louisiana State University School of Medicine, Shreveport, Louisiana; Professor Emeritus, University of California Davis, School of Medicine, Sacramento, California

H. Leon Pachter, MD, FACS
The George David Stewart Professor and Chair, Department of Surgery, New York University School of Medicine, New York, New York

David Palange, DS
Doctor of Osteopathic Medicine, University Hospital–UMDNJ, Newark, New Jersey

Zubin Jal Panthaki, BEng, MD, CM, FACS
Professor of Clinical Surgery, Division of Plastic Surgery, Professor of Clinical Orthopedics, Director, Hand Surgery Fellowship Program, Associate Director, Plastic Surgery Residency Program, The University of Miami, Leonard M. Miller School of Medicine; Chief of Plastic Surgery, Chief of Hand Surgery, Miami Veterans Administration Hospital; Chief of Plastic Surgery, Sylvester Comprehensive Cancer Center; Chief of Hand Surgery, University of Miami Hospital, Miami, Florida

Manish S. Parikh, MD
Associate Professor of Surgery, New York University School of Medicine, New York, New York

Michael D. Pasquale, MD, FACS, FCCM
Chair, Department of Surgery, Lehigh Valley Health Network, Allentown, Pennsylvania; Professor of Surgery, University of South Florida, Morsani College of Medicine, Tampa, Florida

Andrew B. Peitzman, MD
Distinguished Professor of Surgery, Mark M. Ravitch Professor and Vice-Chair, Vice- President for Trauma and Surgical Services, University of Pittsburgh School of Medicine, Pittsburgh, Pennsylvania

Alejandro Perez-Alonso, MD, PhD
International Doctor in Medicine and Surgery, General and Digestive Surgeon, Master in Tissue Engineering, Master in Trauma Surgery, Assistant Professor of Surgery, Senior Researcher, Department of Experimental Surgery, University of Granada; Attending Physician, Trauma and General Surgery, Hospital Universitario San Cecilio, Granada, Spain

Christopher H. Perkins, MD
Assistant Professor, Orthopedic Trauma, Baylor College of Medicine, Houston, Texas

Austin Person, MD
Resident, General Surgery, Creighton University, Omaha, Nebraska

Patrizio Petrone, MD, MPH, MHA, FACS
Director of Research, Program Director, International Visiting Scholars/Research Fellowship; Division of Trauma Surgery, Surgical Critical Care, and Acute Care Surgery, Department of Surgery, New York Medical College; Westchester Medical Center University Hospital, Valhalla, New York

K. Shad Pharaon, MD
Division of Trauma, Critical Care, and Acute Care Surgery, Department of Surgery, Oregon Health and Science University, Portland, Oregon; Division of Trauma and Acute Care Surgery, Surgical Critical Care, PeaceHealth Southwest Medical Center, Vancouver, Washington

Allan S. Philp, MD, FACS, FCCM
Trauma Medical Director, Allegheny General Hospital; Associate Professor of Surgery, Temple University, Pittsburgh, Pennsylvania

Edgar J. Pierre, MD
Volunteer Associate Professor, Department of Anesthesia and Surgery, University of Miami Miller School of Medicine, Miami, Florida

Greta L. Piper, MD
Assistant Professor of Surgery, NYU Langone Medical Center, New York, New York

Frank Plani, MD, FCS(SA), FRACS, Trauma Surgery (SA)
Principal Specialist and Deputy Head, Chris Hani Baragwanath Academic Hospital Trauma Directorate, Division of Surgery, Soweto; Adjunct Professor, Department of Surgery, Clinical School of Medicine, University of the Witwatersrand, Johannesburg, South Africa

Patricio Polanco, MD
Department of Surgery, University of Pittsburgh Medical Center, Pittsburgh, Pennsylvania

Anthony Policastro, MD, FACS
Department of Surgery, New York Medical College; Associate Professor of Surgery, Westchester Medical Center University Hospital; Division of Trauma and Surgical Critical Care, Associate Director of Surgical Critical Care, Director of Surgical and Trauma Intensive Care Units, Valhalla, New York

Nathan J. Powell, DO, FACOS
Attending Surgeon, Trauma/Acute Care Surgery, St. Francis Trauma Institute, Tulsa, Oklahoma

Riaan Pretorius, MBChB(Pta), FCS (SA), Certificate in trauma surgery (SA)
Trauma Consultant, Chris Hani Baragwanath Academic Hospital; Junior Lecturer, University of Witwatersrand, Johannesburg, South Africa

Brandon Propper, MD

G. Daniel Pust, MD
Assistant Professor of Surgery, Division of Trauma and Surgical Critical Care, The DeWitt Daughtry Family Department of Surgery, Ryder Trauma Center/Jackson Memorial Hospital, University of Miami Miller School of Medicine, Miami, Florida Miami, Florida

Bradley S. Putty, Lt Col, USAF, MC
Assistant Professor, Department of Surgery, Division of Trauma and Critical Care, St. Louis University Hospital, St. Louis, Missouri

Juan Carlos Puyana, MD, FACS
Associate Professor of Surgery and Critical Care Medicine, University of Pittsburgh; Chief Medical Officer, Innovative Medical Information Technologies Center, University of Pittsburgh Medical Center, Pittsburgh, Pennsylvania

Stephen M. Quinnan
University of Miami Miller School of Medicine, Jackson Memorial Hospital, Miami, Florida

David J. Quintana, MD
Emory University School of Medicine, Department of Radiology, Division of Interventional Radiology and Image-Guided Medicine, Atlanta, Georgia

R. Lawrence Reed II, MD, FACS, FCCM
Professor of Surgery, Indiana University; Director of Trauma Services, Indiana University Health Methodist

Hospital, Indianapolis, Indiana

Bibiana J. Reiser, MD, MS
Children's Hospital of Los Angeles, University of Southern California, Los Angeles, California

Peter Rhee, MD, MPH, FACS, FCCM, DMCC
Martin Gluck Professor of Surgery, University of Arizona; Director of Trauma, Critical Care, Burns, and Emergency Surgery, University of Arizona Medical Center, Tucson, Arizona

Michael Rhodes, MD, FACS, FCCM
Professor of Surgery, Thomas Jefferson University; Value Institute Senior Consultant for Advances in Medicine; Chair Emeritus, Department of Surgery, Christiana Care Health Systems, Wilmington, Delaware

Norman M. Rich, MD, FACS, DMCC, COL, MC
Leonard Heaton & David Packard Professor, Senior Advisor to the Chairman, Norman M. Rich Department of Surgery, F. Edward Hebert School of Medicine, Uniformed Services University of the Health Sciences, Bethesda, Maryland

J. David Richardson, MD
Professor of Surgery, University of Louisville, Louisville, Kentucky

Charles M. Richart, MD, FACS
Associate Professor, Department of Surgery, University of Missouri—Kansas City; Associate Director, Trauma Surgical Critical Care, Director, Surgical Critical Care Research and Surgical ANH Program, Saint Luke's Hospital of Kansas City, Kansas City, MO

Luis A. Rivas, MD
Associate Professor of Radiology, Chief, Trauma and Emergency Radiology, University of Miami, Jackson Memorial Medical, Miami, Florida

Jennifer C. Roberts, MD
Marshfield Clinic, Marshfield, Wisconsin

Aurelio Rodríguez, MD, FACS
Trauma and General Surgeon, Associate Director, Division of Trauma, Sinai Hospital, Baltimore, Maryland; Director Emeritus, Allegheny General Hospital, Shock Trauma Center, Pittsburgh, Pennsylvania

Jorge L. Rodríguez, MD
University of Louisville, Louisville, Kentucky

Erwin Rodriguez-García, MD
Department of Surgery, Hospital Militar Central–Universidad Militar Nueva Granada, Bogota, Colombia

Rosaine Roeder, MD, MPH
Lahey Hospital and Medical Center, Burlington, Massachusetts

David Rojas-Tirado, MD
Department of Surgery, Hospital Militar Central–Universidad Militar Nueva Granada, Bogota, Colombia

Michael F. Rotondo, MD, FACS
Chief Executive Officer,University ofRochester Medical Faculty Group; Vice Dean for Clinical Affairs, School of Medicine, Professor of Surgery, Division of Acute Care Surgery, Vice President of Administration, Strong Memorial Hospital, University of Rochester Medical Center, Rochester, New York

Susan Rowell, MD, MCR
Associate Professor of Surgery, Program Director, Surgical Critical Care Fellowship, Department of Surgery, Division of Trauma, Critical Care, and Acute Care Surgery, Oregon Health and Science University, Portland, Oregon

Jerry A. Rubano, MD
Department of Surgery, Division of Trauma, Critical Care, and Burns, State University of New York, Stony Brook University Health Sciences Center, Stony Brook, New York

Andrés M. Rubiano, MD, PhD, FACS
Medical and Research Director, MEDITECH Foundation; Professor of Neurosciences, South Colombian University; Neurosurgeon, Trauma and Emergency Service, Neiva University Hospital, Neiva (Huila), Colombia

Amy Rushing, MD
Assistant Professor of Surgery, Division of Trauma, Critical Care, and Burn, Wexner Medical Center, The Ohio State University, Columbus, Ohio

Irony C. Sade, MD
Resident, 3rd Year, General Surgery, Westchester Medical Center, Valhalla, New York

Christopher Salgado, MD
Professor of Surgery, Division of Plastic Surgery, Section Chief, University of Miami Hospital; Editor in Chief, Journal of Anaplastology, Miami, Florida

Ali Salim, MD, FACS
Professor of Surgery, Harvard Medical School; Chief, Division of Trauma, Burns, and Surgical Critical Care, Boston, Massachusetts

Noelle Salliant, MD
Division of Traumatology, Department of Surgery, Critical Care and Acute Care Surgery, The Trauma Center at Penn, University of Pennsylvania, Philadelphia, Pennsylvania

Jason Salsamendi, MD
Assistant Professor of Clinical Radiology, Department of Radiology, Assistant Professor of Clinical Surgery, Department of Surgery, University of Miami Miller School of Medicine, Miami, Florida

James B. Sampson, MD, FACS
David Grant Medical Center, Travis Air Force Base, Fairfield, California; University of California Davis, Sacramento, California

Juan A. Sanchez, MD, MPA, FACS, FACC
Associate Professor of Surgery, Johns Hopkins University School of Medicine; Chairman, Department of Surgery, Baltimore, Maryland

WilliamSánchezMaldonado,MD, FACS
Department of Surgery, Hospital Militar Central–Universidad Militar Nueva Granada, Bogota, Colombia

Thomas M. Scalea, MD
Physician in Chief, R Adams Cowley Shock Trauma Center, Francis X. Kelly Distinguished Professor of Trauma, University of Maryland School of Medicine, Baltimore, Maryland

William P. Schecter, MD
Professor of Clinical Surgery, University of California San Francisco, San Francisco General Hospital, San Francisco, California

Paul Schipper, MD, FACS, FACCP
Professor of Surgery and Program Director, Cardiothoracic Surgery Residency, Oregon Health and Science University and Portland Veterans Administration Medical Center, Portland, Oregon

Martin Schreiber, MD, FACS
Professor of Surgery, Chief, Division of Trauma Critical Care, and Acute Care Surgery, Department of Surgery, Oregon Health and Science University, Portland, Oregon

John T. Schulz III, MD, PhD
Medical Director, Sumner Redstone Burn Center, Massachusetts General Hospital, Boston, Massachusetts

C. William Schwab, MD, FACS
Professor of Surgery, Perelman School of Medicine, University of Pennsylvania; Division of Traumatology, Surgical Critical Care and Emergency Surgery, Hospital of the University of Pennsylvania, Philadelphia, Pennsylvania

Stephen Serio, MD
Surgical Resident, Creighton University Medical Center, Omaha, Nebraska

Parth Shah, MD
General Surgery Resident, Department of Surgery, CHI Health Alegent Creighton Clinic, Omaha, Nebraska

Marc J. Shapiro, MD
Professor of Surgery and Anesthesiology, Chief of General Surgery, Trauma, Critical Care, and Burns, Department of Surgery, SUNY-Stony Brook, Stony Brook, New York

David Shatz, MD
Professor, Department of Surgery, Division of Trauma and Emergency Surgery, University of California Davis, Sacramento, California

Shreya Shetty, MD
Resident, General Surgery, Creighton University, Omaha, Nebraska

Adam M. Shiroff, MD, FACS
Chief of Trauma, Jersey Shore University Medical

Center, Assistant Professor of Surgery, Rutgers Robert Wood Johnson Medical School, New Brunswick, New Jersey

Ziad C. Sifri, MD
Associate Professor of Surgery, Division of Trauma, Rutgers New Jersey Medical School, Newark, New Jersey

Ronald Sing, DO, FACS, FCCM
Professor of Surgery, Division of Acute Care Surgery, Carolinas Medical Center, Charlotte, North Carolina; Adjunct Professor of Surgery, University of North Carolina School of Medicine at Chapel Hill, Chapel Hill, North Carolina

Amy C. Sisley, MD, MPH
Division Chief, Acute Care Surgery, Department of Surgery, Henry Ford Hospital, Detroit, Michigan

R. Stephen Smith, MD
System Chief, Division of Trauma, Burn, and Acute Care Surgery, West Penn Allegheny Health System; Professor of Surgery, Temple University School of Medicine, Pittsburgh, Pennsylvania

Eduardo Smith-Singares, MD, FACS
Chief, Division of Surgical Critical Care, Department of Surgery,University of Illinois at Chicago College of Medicine; Co-Director SICU, University of Illinois Hospital and Health Sciences System, Chicago, Illinois

David A. Spain, MD, FACS
Carol and Ned Spieker Professor and Chief of Acute Care Surgery, Department of Surgery, Stanford University, Stanford, California

Nicholas Spoerke, MD
Surgical Critical Care Fellow, Oregon Health and Science University, Portland, Oregon

Ananth Srinivasan, MBBS
Creighton University School of Medicine, Omaha, Nebraska

Deborah M. Stein, MD, MPH
Associate Professor of Surgery, University of Maryland School of Medicine; Chief of Trauma, R Adams Cowley Shock Trauma Center, Baltimore, Maryland

Joseph J. Stirparo, MD
Trauma, Surgical Critical Care, Lehigh Valley Health Network, Allentown, Pennsylvania; Assistant Professor of Surgery, University of South Florida, Morsani College of Medicine, Tampa, Florida

Lance E. Stuke, MD, MPH, FACS
Associate Professor of Surgery, Louisiana State University, Spirit of Charity Trauma Center, New Orleans, Lousiana

Mithran Sukumar, MD
Assistant Professor of Surgery, Oregon Health and Science University; Section Head, General Thoracic Surgery, Division of Cardiothoracic Surgery, Portland Veterans Administration Medical Center, Portland, Oregon

Abhishek Sundaram, MD
General Surgery Resident, Department of Surgery, Creighton University, Omaha, Nebraska

Wendy Jo Svetanoff, MD
HO4, Department of Surgery, Creighton University Medical Center, Omaha, Nebraska

***Kenneth G. Swan, MD**
Professor of Surgery, Director, Third Year Surgical Clerkship, Department of Surgery, New Jersey Medical School, University of Medicine and Dentistry of New Jersey, Newark, New Jersey

Vartan S. Tashjian, MD, MS
Resident Surgeon, Division of Neurological Surgery, University of California, Los Angeles, Los Angeles, California

Thomas Templin, MD
Resident Physician, Creighton University School of Medicine, Creighton University Medical Center, Omaha, Nebraska

Erwin Thal, MD, FACS, FRACS (Hon.)
Professor of Surgery, Department of Surgery, University of Texas Southwestern Medical Hospital; Attending Surgeon, Department of Surgery, Parkland Hospital; Attending Surgeon, Department of Surgery, University of Texas Southwestern University Hospital– St. Paul; Attending Surgeon, Department of Surgery, University

of Texas Southwestern University Hospital–Zale Lisphy, Dallas, Texas

Seth R. Thaller, MD, DMD, FACS
Chief and Professor, Division of Plastic Surgery, The DeWitt Daughtry Family Department of Surgery, University Of Miami Health System, Miami, Florida

Gregory Tiesi, MD
Department of General Surgery, Rutgers New Jersey Medical School, Newark, New Jersey

Brandon Tieu, MD, FACS
Assistant Professor of Surgery, Division of Cardiothoracic Surgery, Department of Surgery,Oreg onHealthandScienceUniversity and Portland Veterans Administration Medical Center, Portland, Oregon

Areti Tillou, MD, FACS, MsEd
Associate Professor, Vice Chair for Education, UCLA David Geffen School of Medicine, Los Angeles, California

Glen Tinkoff, MD, FACS, FCCM
Associate Vice Chair, Department of Surgery, Christiana Care Health System, Newark, Delaware; Clinical Professor of Surgery, Jefferson Medical College, Philadelphia, Pennsylvania

Samuel Tisherman, MD, FACS, FCCM
R Adams Cowley Shock Trauma Center, University of Maryland, Director, Surgical Intensive Care Unit, Baltimore, Maryland

S. Rob Todd, MD
Associate Professor of Surgery, New York University Langone Medical Center; Director, Bellevue Emergency Surgery Service, Department of Surgery, Bellevue Hospital Center; Faculty, Department of Surgery, Tisch Hospital, New York, New York

Zachary Torgersen, MD
Surgical Resident, Creighton University Medical Center, Omaha, Nebraska

Peter G. Trafton, MD, FACS
Professor and Vice Chair, Department of Orthopedic Surgery, Brown University School of Medicine, Providence, Rhode Island

Mark Traynham, MD
Creighton University Medical Center, Omaha, Nebraska

L.R. Tres Scherer, MD, FACS
Volunteer Clinical Professor of Surgery, Indiana University School of Medicine, Carmel, Indiana

Donald D. Trunkey, MD, FACS
Professor Emeritus, Department of Surgery, Division of Trauma, Oregon Health and Science University, Portland, Oregon

Peter I. Tsai, MD, MA
Assistant Professor of Surgery, Division of Cardiothoracic Surgery, Michael E. DeBakey Department of Surgery, Baylor College of Medicine/Texas Heart Institute; Medical Director, Department of Cardiothoracic Surgery, Ben Taub General Hospital, Houston, Texas

David W. Tuggle, MD
Associate Trauma Medical Director, Dell Children's Medical Center of Central Texas, Austin, Texas

Anthony M. Udekwu, MD, FRCS(C), FACS

Alex B. Valadka, MD, FAANS, FACS
Chairman and Chief Executive Officer, Seton Brain and Spine Institute, Austin, Texas

Nicole VanDerHeyden, MD, PhD
Trauma Medical Director, Trauma Services, Salem Hospital, Salem, Oregon

Thomas K. Varghese, Jr., MD
Assistant Professor, Associate Program Director–Cardiothoracic Surgery Residency, University of Washington; Director of Thoracic Surgery, Department of Surgery, Harborview Medical Center, Seattle, Washington

Michel Wagner, MD, FACS
Assistant Professor, Division of Trauma, Creighton University School of Medicine, CHI–Creighton University Medical Center, Omaha, Nebraska

Matthew J. Wall, Jr., MD
Professor, Michael E. DeBakey Department of Surgery, Baylor College of Medicine; Deputy Chief of Surgery,

Chief of Cardiothoracic Surgery, Department of Surgery, Ben Taub General Hospital, Houston, Texas

Anthony Watkins, MD
Clinical Instructor in Surgery, Department of Transplantation, Columbia University/ New York Presbyterian Hospital, New York, New York

John Weigelt, MD
Medical College of Wisconsin, Milwaukee, Wisconsin

Leonard J. Weireter, Jr., MD, FACS
Arthur and Marie Kirk Family Professor of Surgery, Department of Surgery, Eastern Virginia Medical School, Norfolk, Virginia

David R. Welling, MD, FACS, FASCRS, DMCC
Professor of Surgery, Uniformed Services University of the Health Sciences, Walter Reed National Military Medical Center, Bethesda, Maryland

Paul W. White, MD, FACS
LTC, Medical Corps, United States Army; Program Director, Vascular Surgery Fellowship, Walter Reed National Military Medical Center; Associate Professor of Surgery, Uniformed Services University of the Health Sciences, Bethesda, Maryland

Lucas R. Wiegand, MD
Assistant Professor of Urology, University of South Florida, Tampa, Florida

Harry E. Wilkins, MD
Associate Professor, Department of Surgery, University of Missouri–Kansas City; Medical Director, Trauma and Surgical Critical Care, Saint Luke's Hospital of Kansas City, Kansas City, Missouri

Robert F. Wilson, MD, FACS, MCCM
Professor of Surgery, Wayne State University School of Medicine; Director, Surgical Intensive Care Unit, Detroit Receiving Hospital, Detroit, Michigan

David H. Wisner, MD
Professor and Vice Chair, Department of Surgery, University of California Davis; Chief of Surgery, UC Davis Medical Center Sacramento, California

D. Dante Yeh, MD, FACS
Massachusetts General Hospital, Harvard Medical School, Boston, Massachusetts

目 录

第1章 创伤系统

创伤系统的发展

Donald D. Trunkey 著
殷晓峰 译

现代创伤救治主要包括三个部分：院前急救、急诊外科救治或住院治疗以及康复。理想状况下，国家（部委、省及地区等）政府应该提供一个确保这三个部分都健全的创伤系统。本章主要介绍创伤系统如何演变，同时讨论该系统是否够起作用，并指出当前存在的问题。

从历史的角度来看，创伤救治和创伤系统与战争有着千丝万缕的联系。人们所不了解的是，创伤系统其实并不是近期才有的概念。它可以追溯到公元前数百年。我们尚不清楚史前人类的创伤主要是由于暴力还是事故造成的。关于战争伤口的第一个有力证据来自在埃及发现的大约建在公元前2000年的大规模坟墓。该坟墓中60名士兵的尸身保存完好，刀剑创伤的开放性伤口清楚可见，箭头仍然存在于身体中。Smith纸草文记录了48例战争创伤的临床治疗，还编写了一本关于如何治疗伤口的教科书，其中大部分是贯穿伤。Majno记载了荷马的伊利亚特中147例创伤，总死亡率为77.6%。其中31名士兵为头部受伤，而且都是致命伤。受伤的希腊士兵接受的外科手术治疗是非常粗暴的。然而，希腊人确实认识到须建立一个战地救护系统。受伤的人员在特别军营或附近的船只上接受救治。当时对伤口的救治是非常原始的，即用刀扩大伤口或将箭头推出伤口的方式来除去弓箭的箭头。通常将植物性药物敷在伤口上。创伤被包扎，但根据荷马的相关记载，止血药物是通过“神化”处理的，也就是说，有人唱了一首歌，或者在伤口上施加魔法。

罗马人进一步完善了战伤救治的运输，并在整个帝国建立了一个创伤中心系统。这些创伤中心被称为医院，建造于公元1－2世纪。目前已经找到了25个这类中心的遗址，但在罗马或其他大城市中都没有发现。有趣的是，罗马的不列颠尼亚有11个创伤中心，超过目前这一区域的医院数量。一些医院处理战斗伤的比例高达10%。有常规医疗的罗马军团内至少有85名军医，主要是因为他们死后有墓志铭而被记载。

来自世界其他地方的证据表明创伤系统是被提供给军方的。印度可能有一个创伤救治体系可与罗马人的相媲美。一本在阿育王统治时期（公元前269－232年）编写的图书记载，印度军队有救护车服务，里面有装备精良的外科医生和妇女以准备食物和饮料。印度医学是专门设立的，是由“shalyarara”（外科医生）治疗伤口。Shalyarara的字面意思是“箭头去除剂”，因为弓箭是印度人的传统武器。

在接下来的1000年中，战争创伤救治在文艺复兴之前没有重大进展。居住地相距250英里的两名法国军队外科医生开创了创伤救治的启蒙时代。

Ambrose Parè医生（1510－1590年）在法国与西班牙民间和宗教战争期间为四名法国国王服务。他对治疗贯通伤的主要贡献包括枪伤疗法。他使用结扎而不是烧灼，并在损伤后期进行营养治疗。Parè对假肢装置很感兴趣，并为一些截肢患者设计了许多假肢。

拿破仑的外科医生Dominique Larrey从系统和组织学的角度来看待创伤。Larrey开创了“飞行救护车”的理念。该救护车的唯一目的是从战场上迅速转送伤员。Larry也提出了把医院设在接近前线的地方，以便尽快对伤员进行手术。他的主要目的是在这段“伤口休克”期进行手术，因为在此期间患者不仅痛觉消失，还能减少截肢术后的感染。

Larrey对战争伤的特性有所了解。他在拿破仑发起的对俄罗斯战争之前所做的努力以及取得的贡献得到了人们极大的认可。Larrey不知道拿破仑计划攻打哪个国家，甚至还有关于入侵英国的猜想。他于1812年2月24日离开巴黎，被分配到德国的明茨（Mentz）。不久之后，他去了马格德堡（Magdeburg），然后到了柏林。在那里他开始为战争做准备，还不知道会被分到哪个法国军队。他自己说：“在离开首都之前，我组织了六辆飞行救护车，每辆车上均有八名外科医生。外科医生每天按照我的指示进行手术操作和使用绷带进行包扎。他们最大限度地学习模仿，遵守最严格的纪律。”

19世纪可能被称为战争外科手术治疗启蒙的世纪。这部分是因为有了更完善的统计报告，也是因为出现了治疗上的重大贡献，包括引入了麻醉。在克里米亚战争期间（1853—1856年），一份英文报告说，腹部发生贯通伤的死亡率为92.7%，法国人的死亡率为91.7%。在美国战争期间，在3717例腹部穿刺伤中死亡人数为3031人，死亡率为81.5%。

克里米亚战争是值得一提的，因为法国人在冲突地区测试了一些消毒剂，发现氯化亚铁对医院相关的坏疽非常有效，但是英国禁止在伤口中使用消毒剂。在克里米亚战争期间，南丁格尔在佛罗伦萨强调对战争伤亡人员进行卫生和人道主义护理。在这一期间，人们创立了两个医学上的重大贡献。

在美国各州之间的战争中人们继续使用消毒剂。在报告的308例患者中，溴的使用将医院坏疽的死亡率降低到了2.6%，而未使用溴的医院的死亡率为43.3%。在医院坏疽中也使用强硝酸作为消毒剂，死亡率为6.6%。联邦军医在8万名患者中使用了麻醉药。悲惨的是，从枪击伤口到四肢伤中死亡率仍然很高，与Parè在16世纪报道的基本一致。肱骨上臂弹创骨折的死亡率为30.7%，前臂弹创骨折的死亡率为21.9%，股骨弹创骨折的死亡率为31.7%，腿部弹创骨折的死亡率为14.4%。在29 980例截肢患者中死亡率为26.3%。

在法国对普鲁士战争（1870—1874年）中，部分外科医生由于不情愿采纳Lister的建议，即在伤口处使用消毒剂而导致战伤死亡率惊人。股骨骨折的死亡率为65.8%，其他创伤造成的死亡率为54.2%～91.7%。在战争后期，外科医生接受了Lister的建议，导致死亡率急剧下降。

在布尔战争（1899—1902年）期间，英国人建议应对所有的穿透性腹部伤口进行切开术。然而，早期的治疗结果是糟糕的。随后，英国军队命令要求保守或择期治疗。

在第一次世界大战初期，腹部受伤患者的死亡率达到难以令人容忍的85%。随着战争的进行，患者被带到清创站接受手术，随后死亡率下降到了56%。当美国参战时，其穿透性腹部伤的总死亡率为45%。第一次世界大战期间对创伤救治最主要的贡献之一是输血。

自第二次世界大战以来，外科手术治疗为死亡率和发病率下降做出了许多贡献。各种战争冲突的死亡率比较如表1所示，手术死亡率比率见表2所示。随着抗生素的引入和麻醉、手术技术的进步、快速院前运输，还有一些创新发现，这些新技术带来了更好的效果。

表1　美国受伤士兵死于战伤的百分比

战争	年份	受伤士兵人数	受伤士兵死于创伤的百分比（%）
墨西哥战争	1846—1848	3 400	15
美国内战	1861—1865	318 200	14
西班牙—美国战争	1898	1 600	7
第一次世界大战（不包括毒气死亡）	1918	153 000	8
第二次世界大战	1942—1945	599 724	4.5
朝鲜战争	1950—1953	77 788	2.5
越南战争	1865—1972	96 811	3.6

表2　美国士兵头部、胸部和腹部伤的外科死亡率

	头部	胸部	腹部
第一次世界大战			
士兵数量	189	104	1816
死亡率（%）	40	37	67
第二次世界大战			
士兵数量	2051	1364	2315
死亡率（%）	14	10	23
朝鲜战争			
士兵数量	673	158	384
死亡率（%）	10	8	9
越南战争			
士兵数量	1171	1176	1209
死亡率（%）	10	7	9

现代创伤系统的发展

在两次世界大战之间，民间创伤救治取得了一些重大进展。1925 年，Lorenz Böhler 在奥地利创建了第一个民间创伤系统。该系统最初只是针对工作相关的受伤，最终扩大到所有事故。第二次世界大战一开始，伯明翰事故医院（Birmingham Accident Hospital）成立。它继续提供区域创伤救治直到最近。到 1975 年，德国建立了一个全国性的创伤体系，使得患者在 15 ~ 20 min 就能到达区域中心。在 Harald Tscherne 等的努力下，这个体系已经持续到现在，死亡率减少了 50%以上（图 1）。

北美正在采用现代创伤系统。1912 年，在蒙特利尔举行的美国外科学会（American Surgical Association）会议上，任命了一个由 5 名委员会组成的关于骨折的管理委员会，并设立了一个常委会。一年之后，美国外科医师学院（American College of Surgeons）成立。1922 年 5 月，美国外科医师学院董事会成立了第一个骨折委员会，Charles Scudder 博士任主席。这个委员会最终成为创伤委员会。从 1918 年开始，该学院的另一个功能是医院标准化计划（Hospital Standardization Program）。该计划发展成为联合医院认可委员会（Joint Commission on Accreditation of Hospitals）。该标准化程序的一个功能是创伤记录的初始开始，从而获取了骨折患者治疗的记录。1926 年，工业医学与创伤外科委员会（Board of Industrial Medicine and Traumatic Surgery）成立。因此，这是美国外科医师学院的标准化计划，由美国外科医师学院任命的骨折委员会和医院标准化计划提供的患者的记录。

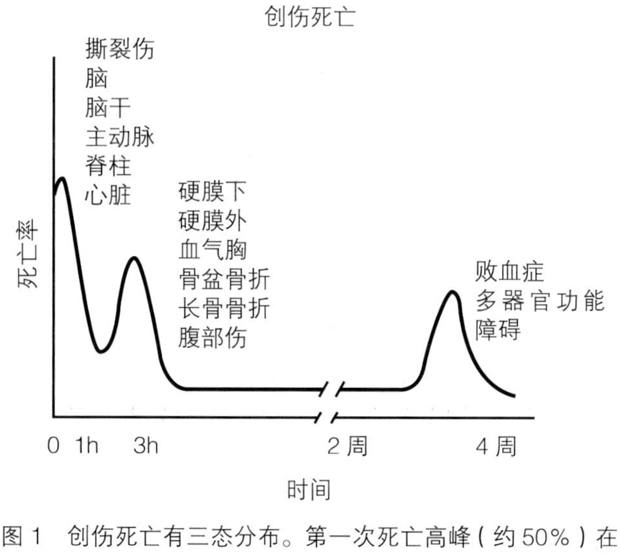

图 1　创伤死亡有三态分布。第一次死亡高峰（约 50%）在受伤的几分钟之内。第二个死亡峰值（约 30%）发生在几小时至 48 h 之内。第三次死亡高峰（约 15%）发生在 1 ~ 4 周内，代表了死于并发症的患者。从公共卫生的角度来看，第一个死亡高峰只能通过预防来解决，这是很难的，因为一部分跟处理者的行为有关。第二个死亡高峰最好由创伤系统解决，第三个死亡高峰须要重要救治和进一步研究

1966 年，第一批两个创伤中心在美国成立：旧金山综合医院的科迪 · 布莱斯德尔中心和芝加哥库克县医院的罗伯特中心。3 年后，RA. Cowley 在马里兰州建立了全州创伤系统。1976 年，美国外科医师学院创伤委员会制订了伤员救治的正式纲要，成为救治患者的最佳标准。随后，美国外科医师学院创伤委员会的工作组大约每 4 年举办一次会议，并更新标准，现已被广泛用于建立区域和国家创伤系统，最近已出口到澳大利亚。美国外科医师学院创伤委员会的其他贡献包括引进高级创伤生命支持课程，建立国家创伤登记处（国家创伤数据库）和国家验证项目。后者类似于旧的医院标准化计划，并通过同行审查程序“验证”医院的创伤中心是否符合美国外科医生指南。

创伤系统真的有效吗?

自 1984 年以来，已发表了超过 15 篇文章报道了创伤系统通过提高患者在特定的中心治疗的生存率从而造福社会。此外，两项研究表明，创伤系统也降低了创伤发病率。1988 年发布了一份关于创伤系统现状和未来挑战的报告。当时，对紧急和创伤计划负责的所有国家紧急医疗服务主管或卫生部门进行了清点。他们于 1987 年 2 月通过电话调查联系，然后被问及有关国家创伤系统的 8 个具体问题。在这 8 项标准中，只有 2 个州——马里兰州和弗吉尼亚州被确定为拥有区域创伤系统的所有 8 个基本组成部分。19 个州和华盛顿特区的全州覆盖面不完整或缺乏必要的组成部分。没有限制该地区创伤中心的数量是最常见的不足之处。

1995 年，美国医学协会杂志（*Journal of the American Medical Association*）又发表了一份报告。这份报告介绍的是自 1988 年报告以来创伤系统发展的最新情况。这是一个更复杂的方法，因为它扩展了原来的 8 项标准，并且更为全面。根据 1995 年的这份报告所描述的，五个州（佛罗里达州、马里兰州、内华达州、纽约州和俄勒冈州）拥有全州系统所需要的所有组成部分，弗吉尼亚州不再限制指

定创伤中心的数量，另有15个州和华盛顿特区拥有创伤系统大部分组成部分。

1995年的报告在1998年的斯卡梅尼亚会议上进行了更新。美国现在有35个州积极参与创伤系统标准的制订。除了报告外，斯卡梅尼亚会议还评估了创伤系统的有效性。搜索医学文献，所有的现有证据分为三类：小组研究报告（尸体解剖研究）、登记比较和基于人群的研究。小组研究受到差异和可靠性的影响，单独的尸体解剖被认为是不充分的。这一发现得到了普遍的共识，即小组研究只是三级证据不足。然而，尽管有这些限制，Mackenzie等的结论是，当所有小组研究被总体考虑时，它们确实提供了一些表观有效性，并支持了非创伤中心相对于创伤中心的不当治疗更少及残疾率更低这种假设。发现注册表评估对于评估创伤系统的整体有效性是有用的。Jurkovich和Mock等认定数据显然不符合Ⅰ类证据。他们对创伤登记的批评有：经常遗漏数据，混乱不堪，可能存在区间可靠性因素，国家规范不是以人口为基础，关于死因的细节缺失，没有考虑到院前死亡。尽管存在这些缺陷，会议参与者仍然达成共识，认为注册研究比小组研究更好，但不如人口研究好。最后，他们对基于人群的研究进行了评估，发现它包含Ⅱ类证据。与注册研究相比，人类研究的优势在于研究和评估创伤护理各个方面的大量人群，包括院前、住院和康复。不幸的是，可用于评估的临床变量有限，难以对损伤和生理功能障碍的严重程度进行调整。尽管这三项研究存在缺陷，但其优点可能适用于各个社区，以帮助影响与创伤系统的启动和评估有关的公共卫生政策。

最近的两项研究报道了创伤系统的有效性。第一项是比较Ⅰ级创伤中心和没有创伤中心的医院之间的死亡率。创伤中心的住院死亡率明显低于非创伤中心（7.6%比9.5%）。损伤后1年存在25%的死亡率差异，与创伤中心相关的死亡率为10.4%，而非创伤中心为13.8%。第二项研究是对佛罗里达州创伤系统状况的评估。这项研究确定了指定的创伤中心中死亡率降低了25%。

目前存在的问题是什么？

在Murray和Lopez的全球疾病负担研究中，世界被分为发达地区和发展中地区。他们还在全球范围内审查各种统计数据。衡量残疾最有用的统计或手段是伤残调整生命年（disability-adjusted life year，DALY）。这是由于过早死亡而导致的生命年损失总数，以及严重程度调整的残疾年数之和。到2020年，道路交通事故将成为全球DALY的第三大成因。这不包括来自战争的DALY（占第8位）。在发达国家，道路交通事故是DALY的第五大原因，也是发展中地区的第二大原因。我们今后几年面临的最困难的问题之一是如何在世界发展中地区提供合理的创伤救治和发展创伤系统。目前大多数这些发展中国家并不存在院前救治。城市地区的创伤中心即使存在也是很少的，那么该国家的农村也没有创伤中心。即使有这样的中心或创伤系统，也几乎完全没有康复，因此，受伤的人在受到严重伤害后很少能够恢复工作或生产力。

如前所述，欧洲在20世纪开创了一些全国性的创伤系统。然而，欧盟没有一致努力为欧盟内部的国家制订创伤制度或协调创伤救治的标准。同样，欧盟也没有院前救治的标准，没有一个具有标准和同行评议的康复设施网络。理论上，在一个欧盟国家接受过培训的外科医生应该能够在不同的欧盟国家内跨国界实施手术，包括创伤救治。关于创伤外科医生并没有制定相关的标准。另外，事实上，创伤手术是一种由不同模式的药物组成的总称。一个典型例子是奥地利。在奥地利，创伤手术是独立的专业。另一种模式是将外伤手术纳入普通外科手术，其中包括法国、意大利、荷兰和土耳其。在第三种模式中，绝大多数的创伤训练都是用矫形外科住院训练模式进行的，比利时和瑞士遵循这种模式。最广的模式是提供特定专业的创伤手术训练，没有任何一个专业对创伤训练负有重大责任，而这种模式在丹麦、德国、葡萄牙、爱沙尼亚、冰岛、英国、挪威、芬兰和瑞典广泛推广。

现在创伤手术中最棘手的一些问题出现在北美，特别是在美国。部分原因在于普通外科手术的变化。预计在未来数年内，美国的普通外科医生将会严重短缺。普通外科医生现在更老了。更重要的是，普通外科医生现在正在专科化。我们现在有肠道、肝胆、血管、乳腺和结直肠外科医生。他们之间有一个共同之处在于他们不想接受外伤的召唤。我们的医疗专业同事的夜班形式现在正在过渡。医院正在招聘所谓的“医院医生”。他们接受家庭医学或内科医学的培训。许多情况下，医院将支付他们的工资，以提供每周7天、每天7 h（24、7 h）的待命，通常是12 h班。在某些情况下，这些医生的数量可能多达 1/3，各种实践组将因这些医院医生在医院接受任务而向其支付费用。影响普通外科手术的另一个趋势是反对性别歧视的迅速过渡。现在至少有 50% 的医学生是女性，但其中只有 7% 的人（约 500 人）致力于做手术。其理由是做手术者的工作时间长，生活方式不良，而这些女性希望将职业与育儿责任相结合。普通外科手术在求职申请中呈总体下降趋势，其原因是复杂且是多方面的。一个重要原因是普通外科医生的收入比一些专科医生的收入要低约 50%。然而，更多的是他们对生活方式的看法。年轻的医学生和医生倾向于不选择外科，是因为时间的投入和相关的生活方式问题，他们特别憎恶外伤手术。另一个可能是美国独有的问题是创伤手术病例的减少。一种转变为从穿透性创伤转变为钝性创伤，或者向非手术治疗的转变，特别是肝和脾损伤。普通外科医生通过将患者转交给专门从事血管外科手术或胸外科手术的外科医生而使问题更加复杂。介入放射科医生也参与某些创伤性损伤的救治。

美国创伤救治中另一个令人头痛的问题是目前专业外科医生对按需付费的需求。在整形外科和神经外科方面尤其如此。在夜里，一个随时待命电话的费用为从 1000 美元到 7000 美元不等。平均来说，一级医院的神经外科医生在一年内只能被叫 33 次。相比之下，整形外科医生在一年中平均约有 275 例紧急病例。显然，这个责任可以在群体之间共同承担。然而，考虑到被呼叫的可能性相对较低，医院被要求向大部分神经外科医生支付报酬。

影响专科外科医生涉足创伤领域的其他因素是外科医生的独立手术中心经常可以规避政府的规定。他们不用接听电话，晚上由医院医生照顾患者。

随着老年人口（65 岁及以上）达到总人口的 30%，未来几年将会加剧这些问题。美国的研究表明，重症监护病房中 65 岁及以上人口的死亡率比年轻人高出 3.5 倍，住院时间更长。不幸的是，这些严重受伤的老年患者大多数在急救后没办法回到独立的生活方式。

有什么解决方案？

纠正发展中国家存在的问题可能是最难的。这些国家大多数完全缺乏提供创伤系统的基础设施，包括院前救治、训练有素的外科医生和康复服务。国际组织，如世界银行（World Bank）和 WHO 必须在院前救治提供经济支持和培训方面发挥主导作用。存在潜在的巨额款项，因为这将须要建立和发展足够的通讯设施、救护车和经过培训的院前救治人员。同样，在培训外科医生上也存在问题。将外科医生送到西方国家进行培训是一个问题，因为其中许多人不会返回原来的国家。在我看来，训练这些人的最佳方法应该是让来自具有成熟创伤系统的国家的外科老师花时间在这些发展中国家合适的医学院校教授外科医生。这也存在问题，因为发展中国家医学院校的水平差异很大。此外，除了外科医生，麻醉医生、重症监护室医生和护士也必须接受培训。创伤系统的第三个组成部分——康复在发展中国家中几乎完全缺乏。这个部分可能不像其他部分那样过度依赖资源或高昂的费用，但它必须与院前和急救同时发展。

发展中地区的根本问题是确定优先事项。如果我们接受 DALY 是制订健康保健政策的合理方法，那么我们可以检查 DALY 的 10 个最常见的原因。发展中国家 10 个最常见的 DALY 的排序是：①单向重性抑郁症，②道路交通事故，③缺血性心脏病，④慢性阻塞性肺病，⑤脑血管病，⑥结核病，⑦下呼吸道感染，⑧战争，⑨腹泻病，⑩人类免疫缺陷病毒感染。我可能带有偏见，但我认为，道路交通事故可能是最费成本的 DALY，因此须要尝试解决。如果美国（包括其他国家）能停止制造和出口香烟，就会在预防慢性阻塞性肺疾病、缺血性心脏病和脑血管疾病中起主要作用。同时我也会认为，随着世界经济全球化的发展，发展中国家为世界经济做出了很大贡献，我们必须及早参与提供一般基础设施建设，特别是创伤救治。

欧洲的解决方案也存在一些问题。可以肯定的是，欧盟没有制订标准来解决什么是最适合的院前救治。我认为，医学教育，特别是外科手术培训在不同的国家之间差别很大。关于重症监护标准也是如此。目前在欧盟内部培训创伤外科医生的方法是不同的，各种专家倾向于提供这种培训。这种方法不一定是消极的，但是应该有一些标准构成最低门槛，以便外科医生越过国界符合这一标准。在欧盟范围内，康复也是多样的。以色列的优秀创伤康复计划是最佳例子之一，可能代表了欧盟的典范。最好的开始是欧盟制订一个类似于美国外科医师学会最佳标准的文件，适用于所有国家。必须将某种形式的审查和核查应用于创伤系统的所有三个组成部分——院前、急救和康复。

与发展中国家相比，美国的解决方案可能更为困难。原因很简单：美国医疗卫生系统已受到破坏。历史上“非盈利”的制度已经“获利”，440 万人没有保险，数千万人没有得到保障，医疗保健费用通货膨胀使美国的医疗支出在国内生产总值的比例比任何其他发达国家都要高。解决这些问题显然要优先于解决创伤救治中的问题，但两者之间可能相关。

从全球的角度来看，美国有很多可行的解决方案来处理美国的医疗保健问题。大多数经济学家认为，医疗保健是一种公共利益，类似于军事、消防和警察服务。通过公益模式，政府可以直接提供支持，也可以与保险公司签约。有人认为，这种安排会花费更多的钱，会使激励机制受损，而且对这个制度的维持是双重的，因为人们仍然可以购买额外的保险或为他们的医疗保健支付额外的费用。另一个解决方案将是公共实用模型，其中医疗保健服务将受到地方州或联邦官员的监管。这个模式最积极的方面是有公众支持。特别是在美国，不利之处在于，鉴于最近与公共事业（例如安然公司）有关的丑闻，这种体系已经显示腐坏迹象。

预计全球经济将有所增长，通过外包给发展中国家可以降低医药成本。多年来，美国引进护士的方式弥补了美国护士培训的不足。引进卫生保健专业人员也可以做出类似的努力，如外科医生。在许多方面，这种模式是完全不切实际的，因为它从最需要他们的国家，特别是资源贫乏的国家抽离了专业人员。

对于公众最合理的模式是用单一付款人或多付款人系统进行普遍保健。这种模式将有一个确定的基本保健水平，灵活地共同付款和进行灾难保障，并且保留选择专业人员和医院的自由。这类系统也会强调预防疾病、患者教育和对保险公司的监督。仲裁裁决将被裁定，过度诊断和过度治疗将被削减。虽然这个最后的解决方案是有价值的，但是需要时间才能实现这种转变。

美国创伤救治中的问题等不及整体卫生保健系统做出转变。最近，美国外科医师创伤委员会（American College of Surgeons Committee on Trauma，ACS-COT）和美国创伤外科协会（American Association for the Surgery of Trauma，AAST）的联合委员会已经为创伤系统提出了一套解决方案。他们建议美国外科委员会（American Board of Surgery，ABS）设立一个名为“美国急救外科手术”的委员会。设置课程将包括 4 年的普通外科手术，接着是 2 年的创伤手术，其中包括一些特定的创伤，像重症监护、血管和非心脏的胸部手术。可能还将包括对可选性矫形外科、神经外科、小型整形手术和一些介入放射学的额外培训。基本上，拟议的课程将设置一个外科住院医生。他将进行转移工作，并提供几乎所有外科紧急情况的全天候覆盖。尚待解决的问题之一是如何提供持续的救治，特别是在换班时。

院前救治和康复也是须要解决的问题。委员会建议我们为院前救治制订最佳标准，包括同行评审和验证。同样，康复护理须要制订经过同行评议的最佳标准。

西半球的创伤救治和创伤系统是世界其他地区的缩影。加拿大有省级创伤系统和中心，但缺乏全国创伤系统。墨西哥、中美洲和南美洲有创伤系统的雏形，包括许多学术医院的创伤中心，但缺乏院前救治、康复和全州创伤系统。对于像哥伦比亚这样的国家来说，这是一个特别的问题。在哥伦比亚，暴力是造成创伤的主要原因。人们可以认为，随着经济的全球化发展，创伤管理和同行审查的全球标准非常重要。我认为这是一个挑战，同时也是一个机会。

哥伦比亚军事创伤的医疗策略结果

William Sánchez Maldonado, Erwin Rodriguez-Garcia, David Rojas Tirado, Juan A. Asensio 著
殷晓峰 译

纵观历史，战争导致了医疗和伤员救治的外科技术的发展。这些技术后来成功地被采用至平民的创伤中。50 多年来，哥伦比亚面临着不规则的武装冲突，因此获得了多种救治经验，尤其是关于复杂创伤的管理。在此介绍我们军事创伤的救治方案及我们项目的结果。

长时间与游击队不规则战争的众多伤员对医疗救治的影响，以及最近的药品商贩和犯罪团伙，促使了医疗救治策略的发展。现代医疗救治策略旨在

以快速、有效和最佳措施确保伤员的生存率最高和满意的康复。

一项在 2000 年初进行的分析发现推动了战略计划，透露了一个令人担忧的数字，战场即时死亡率平均为 32%，并且在创伤性事件发生后没有专业的医疗救治，缺乏医疗运输物流而导致长时间的疏散延误。但与此同时，由于军事中央医院有高级专业医疗救治，因此在这类医院中的生存率更高（死亡率为 6%）。

最初的策略设计是由中校 Lieutenant Colonel Erwin Rodríguez García 博士和少校 David Rojas Tirado 博士在美军南方司令部（US, Army Southern Command）的支持下完成的。这项计划取名 PANTERA，是基于 1970 年 William Haddon 在纽约建造的矩阵模型。当时将其用于分析创伤救治中促进损伤的相关因素——人类、环境和技术，以及事件发生的三个可能阶段——创伤前、创伤期间和创伤后。经过 1 年的策略规划，PANTERA 项目于 2004 年 2 月实施，由行政、军事、培训和医疗领域等多个部门参与。8 年后此项目仍然有效。

七个连续步骤在计划和行动流程图中的描述见图 1。

了解主要敌人

主要敌人（游击队、毒枭和犯罪团伙）的主要特征是他们在犯罪战争中缺乏对国际人道主义法原则的尊重：

1. 这些战士大多数是孩子。他们是被迫挑选的，并在充满暴力的童年和青春期中不正常成长，并成为战士。这使他们承受着严重的心理障碍，这一情况由于社会的排斥进一步恶化。
2. 使用非常规战争元素也是特点之一，包括地雷、生物武器和非传统炸药。
3. 使用敲诈勒索、绑架和酷刑作为社会恐吓动作也是其特点。

因此，主要敌人采取的军事行动有着疯狂的天性。这种非常规战争造成的二级创伤通常是高能量损伤，伴有严重的组织破坏、高比例的截肢和肢解以及高度污染（图 2）。所以，医疗救治计划必须围绕着重伤患者和高概率的发病率及死亡率。

了解次要敌人

在遭受攻击后的瞬间，受害者和医疗团队的敌人发生了改变，出血和感染成为新的敌人。

在战场或者在军事行动中受伤后，控制急性出血成为一项优先的初级救治。所有的医疗措施必须集中于控制持续出血所导致的休克及放血。我们的管理指南包括以下五个连续的步骤：

1. 第一步措施是立即尝试采用外部按压或对受伤肢体应用止血带的方式来控制局部的急性

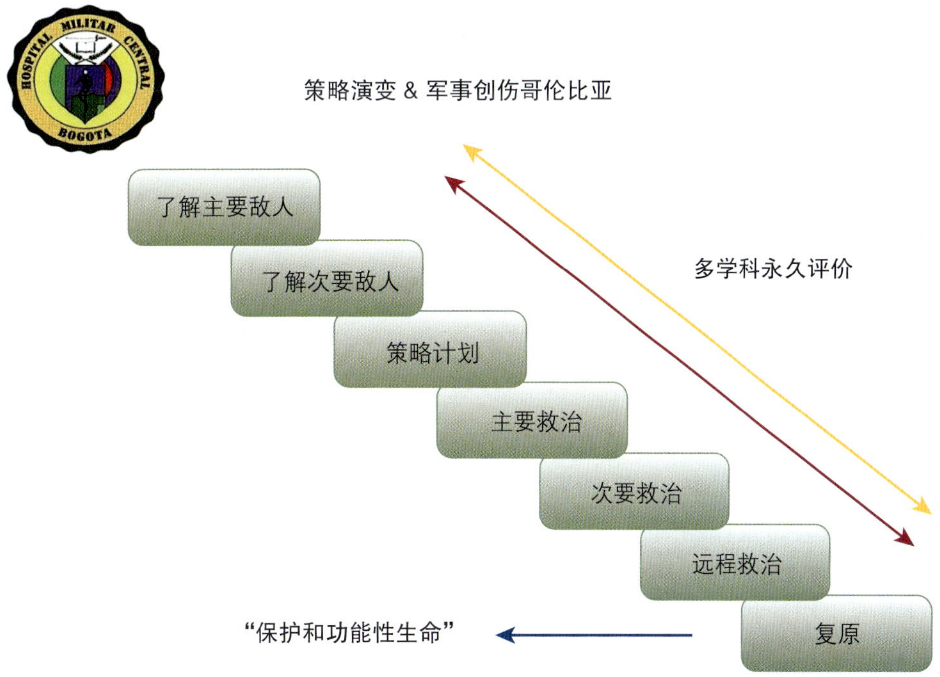

图 1　军事医疗救治计划

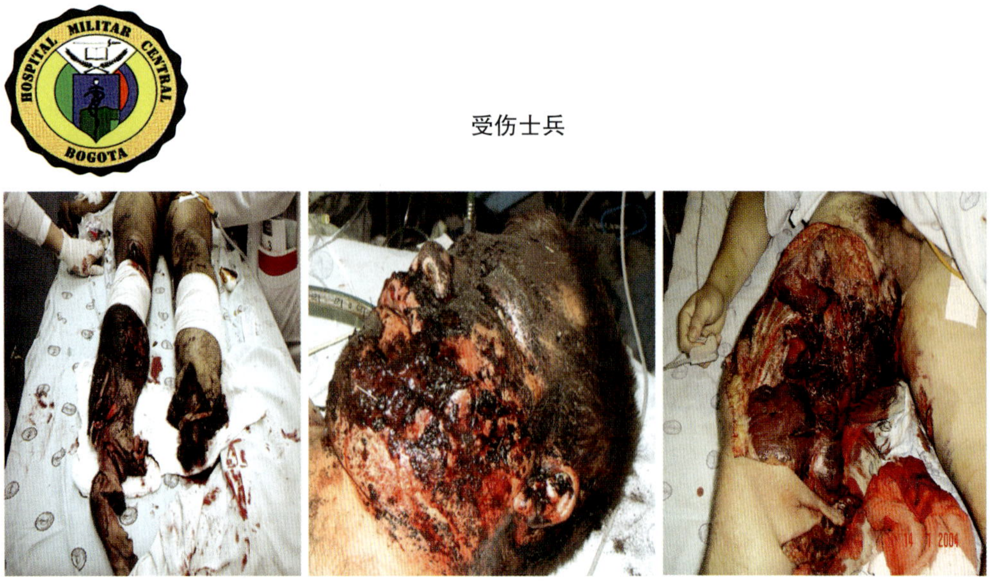

图 2 士兵在战斗中受伤伴有截肢、烧伤和严重的软组织损伤

出血。所有的军事人员均受过急救训练，同时在每次军事行动中均有一组医疗团队随时提供支持和帮助。在一些重要的情况下，拥有良好的医疗判断能力的医生会考虑冒着失去肢体的风险而保全患者的生命。

2. 第二步是由初级救治团队使用局部止血剂，如铸模和热凝聚剂。这些都是急救箱里的组成部分。
3. 第三步是建立安全的静脉通路并进行低血压性液体复苏，最好是使用高渗性液体。
4. 在疏散后，患者会被移送至战地医院（GATRA），在那里可以进行输注全血。必要时，如果患者的病情需要，优先考虑自体输血的可能。
5. 最后，我们为每一个军事单位开发了一个数据库，里面包括了潜在的以及可立即使用的血库捐赠名单。同时，每一个医疗支援队伍必须为全部参与行动的士兵核实是否有合适的血液捐赠。

第二个新的敌人是感染。我们制订的战争受伤感染的管理指南包括如下内容：

1. 在战场上立即用生理盐水直接冲洗与清洁伤口。这一步在控制出血的同时一起完成。

2. 用无菌敷料覆盖和隔离伤口。一些救援队伍和全部战地医院（GATRA）均有封闭式负压引流系统。这对重要组织缺损的伤口管理有非常重要的作用。须要谨记的是，海绵和压力变量的选择要根据患者的个体差异来进行调整。

3. 我们的黄金法则是，认为所有的战争损伤是污染性的或者存在潜在感染。这种想法是基于观察到的游击队的战术作战方案（生物污染武器）和一项我们的前瞻性研究，其中包括了 18 627 份培养，用于明确针对感染患者最常见的细菌。第一个是大肠埃希菌（30%），其次是金黄色葡萄球菌和肺炎克雷伯菌。大肠埃希菌感染占所有的革兰氏阴性感染的 50%（表 1）。因此，抗生素治疗主要是针对治疗革兰阴性细菌的感染。

表 1 军事中央医院 2010–2012 年前十名导致感染的微生物

微生物	年份		
	2012	2011	2010
大肠埃希菌	1869	1769	1868
金黄色葡萄球菌	352	340	434
肺炎克雷伯菌	428	413	412
表皮葡萄球菌	274	271	378
铜绿假单胞杆菌	212	262	319
奇异变形杆菌	253	296	303
肠球菌	300	336	277
白念珠菌	142	165	171
阴沟肠埃希菌	142	165	151
黏质沙雷菌	84	108	116

From Hospital Militar Central, Bogota

医疗救治策略计划

我们的医疗救治计划被命名为PANTERA，它是围绕救治团队等级和类型来建立的(图3)：

第一级：这支团队的西班牙语叫EMEREVAC(作战救援疏散医疗队，Combat Rescue and Evacuation Medical Team)，由一位医生、一位执业护士和两位精通救援的士兵组成。该团队的主要目标是通过控制急性出血、预防感染以及立即撤离的形式提供急救支持，以确保在战场上受伤患者的生存(图4)。

第二级：该级别包含战场医院。西班牙语叫GATRA（空运创伤生命支援队，Air-Transport Trauma Life Support Team），由一位普通外科医生、一位整形外科医生、一位麻醉师、一位医疗助理、一位护士长、一位实验室技术员和四个执业护士组成。该团队在不到1 h内从EMEREVAC接收到伤员，接着执行所有必要的流程来恢复和稳定伤员，其中包括复苏和损伤控制手术。必要时，该团队也可以开始基本的重症监护以及准备将伤员转运至更高级复杂的中心，确保他们在长途中存活并能承受大型重建手术。患者一定不能在GATRA单位停留超过6 h（图5）。每个战场医院所需的GATRA单位数量取决于军事行动的需要。

第三级：在战场医院接受治疗以达到伤害控制后，受伤的患者会被转移至下一个级别，即远距离后方撤离团队，西班牙语为ECCAT（航空运输重症监护团队，Air-Transport Critical Care Team）。该团队的任务是在最佳条件下运输伤员，维持血流动力学的稳定。基本的团队由一位重症救治培训医生、一位护士长、两位执业护士。团队成员数量的增加取决于需要运输的受害者的数量，也同样取决于飞机的数量和类型（图6）。

第四级：最高的一个拥有大学机构救治级别是由军事中央医院提供的，即配备有高技术基础设施和专用于战场伤员的病房。所有的医院工作人员，不管他们的专业如何，都要接受创伤和多学科的综合治疗训练，从修复手术至术后康复，也包括心理康复。大学医院为伤员提供救治，并设置了可持续的集中关于战

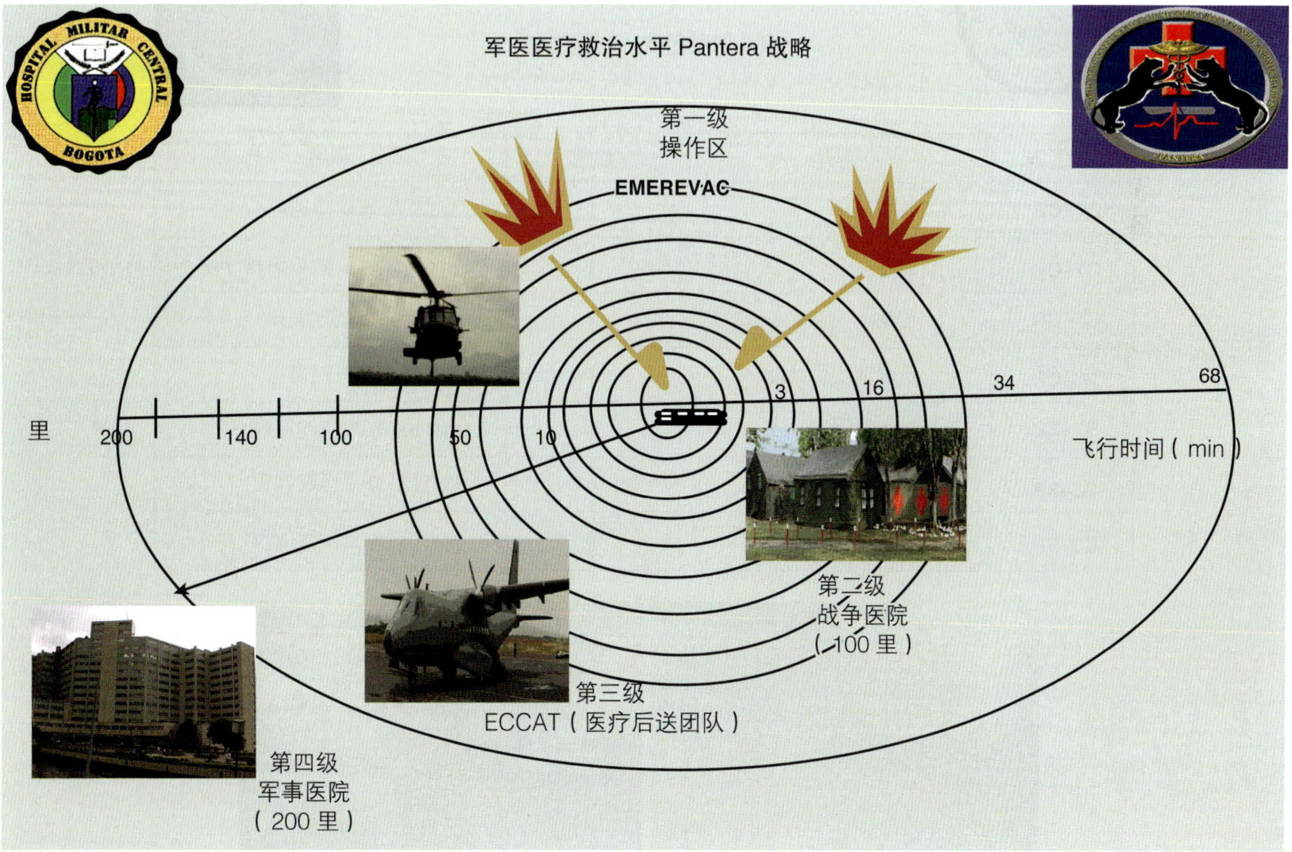

图3 美洲豹(PANTERA)策略——三个手术级别

EMEREVAC 团队

后送——第一级战场团队

分级	简介	数量	训练
TE-CT	医学博士	1	ATLS，军事医院课程
C3-SV	护士	1	PHTLS，军事医院课程
SLP	护理人员	2	CSAR，急求技术 军事医院课程

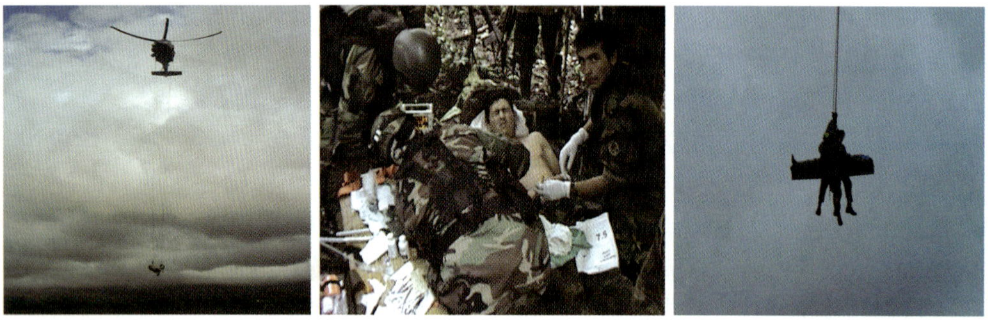

图 4　EMEREVAC 团队 (作战救援及后送医疗团队)——第一级。ATLS, 高级创伤生命支持

GATRA 团队

战斗医院团队——第二级

分级	简介	数量	训练
CT-CR	普通外科	1	ATLS, 军事医院课程
CT-CR	麻醉	1	ATLS, ACLS, 军事医院课程
CT-CR	创伤	1	ATLS, 军事医院课程
TN-CR	医学博士（助理）	1	ATLS, 军事医院课程
ST-TC	护士长	1	PHTLS, 军事医院课程
S3-SP	护士组	2	PHTLS, 军事医院课程
C3-SP	护士	3	PHTLS, 军事医院课程

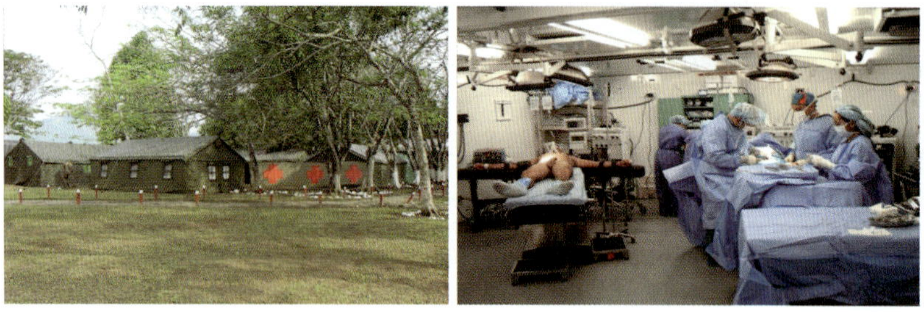

图 5　GATRA 团队 (空运创伤生命支援团队)——第二级。ATLS，高级创伤生命支持；ACLS，高级心脏生命支持；PHTLS，院前创伤生命支持

ECCAT 团队

医疗后送团队——第三级

分级	简介	数目	训练
CT–CR	麻醉，危重护理	1	ATLS, ACLS, 军事医院课程
TN–CR	医学博士（助理）	1	ATLS, 军事医院课程
C3–SP	护士	1	PHTLS, 军事医院课程

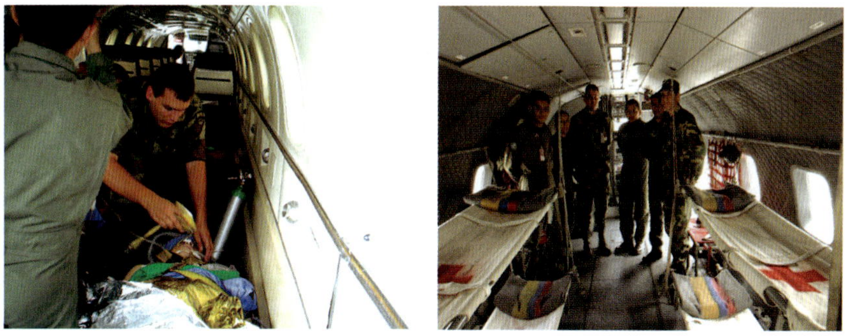

图 6　ECCAT 团队（航空运输重症监护团队）——第三级

争创伤的医疗教育和研究项目，使用当前全部的教育援助（基础和临床研究、模拟以及远程医疗等）。这些措施确保了高标准的创伤培训，最终造福患者。

策略的结果

PANTERA 计划使得在事件发生和士兵在行动中受伤的时刻为其提供高度专业化的医疗救治成为可能。通过对 2000 – 2005 年间非正规战士使用的战争技术的分析显示，80%的军事人员受到大口径高速枪支的伤害，他们在战争中与常规武器作战直接对抗。战争技术发展到了避免人的直接参与。到 2009 – 2010 年，75%的伤亡是非常规爆炸物和地雷造成的结果。这解释了创伤流行病学的变化，伴随的损伤是明显的组织损失、高感染可能以及较高的截肢率和肢体丧失率。

造成战场伤员立即死亡的三个主要原因是胸部伤（34%）、地雷造成的肢解（31%）和头部受伤（17%）。在医疗预防策略中，重点是运用防弹背心、

表 2　与哥伦比亚军事力量战斗中的伤员，2005 – 2010 年死亡率分析

	2005	2006	2007	2008	2009	2010
伤员总数	1543	1538	1419	1248	1355	2500
生存数目	1002	1080	1042	943	999	2075
死亡数目	541 (35%)	458 (30%)	377 (26%)	305 (24%)	356 (26%)	425 (17%)
转移到 HMC	433	290	171	227	297	188

平均年龄：24 岁

战争中伤员总数：8631

死亡：2462 (28.5%)

转移到 HMC, ISS > 15: 1606 (26.3%)

From Hospital Militar Central in Bogota. ISS，创伤严重程度评分（Injury Severity Score）

头盔以及检测和拆除非常规爆炸物的手段。但是，在哥伦比亚发生武装冲突的热带丛林中，这些措施并不容易实施。

这种医疗战略的第一个重要有利成果体现在当士兵受到高素质医疗救援队伍支持，并能确保及时救治，且生存率较高时，这些能助长他们的士气和爱国精神。

从2005年1月至2010年12月期间，哥伦比亚有8631名士兵受伤，在军事行动中死亡人数为2462人（28.5%）。通过他们的行动，EMEREVAC和GATRA团队在战场上大大降低了死亡率。2005年，死亡人数为531人（35%），2010年下降至425人（17%）（表2）。急救和复苏方面的军事人员的培训以及控制急性出血管理指南和预防感染的使用一直对提高伤员的生存概率至关重要。对这些结果有贡献的另一个因素是来自EMEREVAC团队的支持。团队使专业治疗、复苏和撤离时间不超过1.30 h。这是患者生存的关键决定因素。

从1999年1月至2010年12月期间，军事中心医院共接收了伤者4233人，其中严重受伤伤员（ISS>15分）的总人数超过了15 000人。对这组特殊患者三个时期的数据分析显示，医院死亡率逐渐下降，从5.2%降至2.3%。这些结果反映了以多学科方法为创伤患者提供护理，而不会遗忘身体、心理和社会康复过程，并以此作为综合患者护理的基本支柱，体现了高度的专业性（表3）。

除了立即的放血后遗症外，感染是造成患者非急性发病和死亡的主要原因。在我们的机构，战争伤害相关的感染主要是由革兰氏阴性细菌引起的。大肠埃希菌是造成全球感染的主要原因（35%）。须要了解抗生素耐药性的微生物的局部生物学行为，以确定最佳的治疗选择。我们对2010－2012年的资料进行了前瞻性分析，其中包括大肠埃希菌阳性培养的5506例，氨苄西林/舒巴坦、甲氧苄啶-磺胺甲噁唑和环丙沙星的耐药百分比分别为42.9%、37.1%和26%。这意味着抗生素的选择必须排除这些干扰，并且必须基于敏感性和细菌耐药性的结果（表4）。

以下是军事创伤护理中精细伤害控制技术的临床实例：

1. 患有胸腹部穿刺枪伤的患者存在空肠、结肠、脾、隔膜、左肺和胸主动脉损伤。GATRA小组在复苏胸廓切开术下行右心房插管，以恢复血管内容积，然后修复主动脉和肺损伤，并结合剖腹术对腹部损伤进行损伤控制（图7）。
2. 患者的右下肢因手榴弹片而受伤，造成股骨骨折及腘-股动脉损伤。急性出血由EMEREVAC团队的战斗护士使用局部压缩和止血带控制。后来，在救援直升机中，EMEREVAC医生进行外部血管旁路手术，以确保肢体的生存能力，并在医院军事中心进行最后的修复（图8）。

表3 军事中央医院战争创伤——在三个时期的战斗中4233例伤者的院内死亡率分析

年	患者数量	死亡数量	死亡率(%)
1999－2003	1572	82	5.2
2004－2008	1531	49	3.4
2009－2010	1130	27	2.3
总住院死亡率：3.6%			
患者总数为4233人(ISS)>15万			

From Hospital Militar Central, Bogota

表4 5506例大肠埃希菌感染患者的抗生素耐药性分析，2010－2012年

	耐药性(%)					
	2010		2011		2012	
抗生素	数值		数值		数值	
耐药标记	UCI	UCI	UCI	UCI	UCI	UCI
阿米卡星	0.4	1.7	1.6	0	0.8	0
氨苄西林/舒巴坦	31.2	44.8	35.7	41.0	27.6	42.9
β-内酰胺酶(BLEE)	11.7	22.4	12.5	15.4	11.6	17.1
头孢西丁	3.2	0	4.8	5.1	4.2	8.6
环丙沙星	22.9	29.3	30.6	23.1	27.8	25.7
庆大霉素	13.7	19	16.3	23.1	17.6	15.7
亚胺培南	0.4	0	0	0	0.2	0
哌拉西林-他唑巴坦	10.5	24.1	11.3	15.4	6.5	12.9
TMP/SXZ(甲氧苄啶-磺胺甲噁唑)	41.4	42.0	48.0	30.3	39.3	39.2

From Hospital Militar Central in Bogota. UCI, 导尿管感染（Urinary catheter infection）

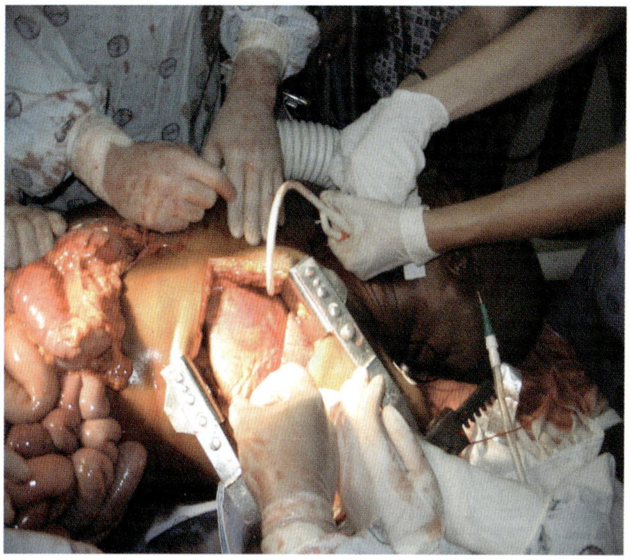

图 7 在战争中受伤的军人，须要采取胸廓切开术来控制损害以及右心房插管来恢复血容量

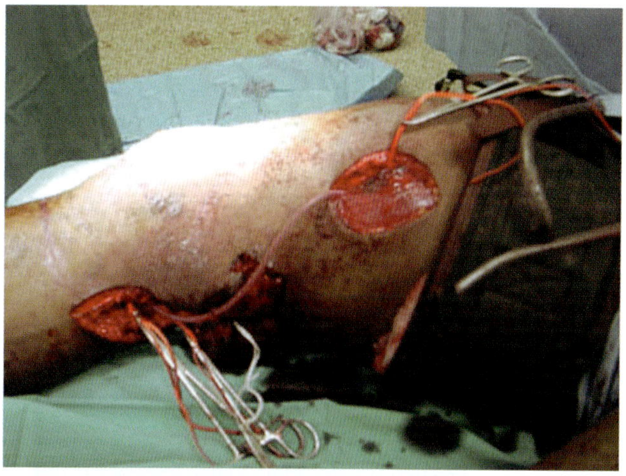

图 8 士兵在战斗中受伤，须要进行股动脉旁路手术作为临时措施，以便下肢保有生存能力

3. 使用现代技术的多学科管理的另一个例子是，一名受到突击步枪手榴弹伤害的患者存在肝、右肾、空肠、结肠、胃、肺和腹壁多次严重受伤。患者须要进行多学科治疗，包括封闭式负压引流（VAC）治疗，以挽救生命并促进其康复（图 9）。

小结

1. 为在行动中受伤的患者制订医疗救治计划的策略时必须考虑将所有可能的变量纳入 Haddon 矩阵分析。
2. 已证明作为哥伦比亚武装力量支柱的“PANTARA 计划”可以成功地提高战争受难者的生存机会。
3. 每一个对创伤和危重患者制订的医疗救治计划，特别是在军医方面，都必须以每一个团队成员的强力、持续的学术培训和教育为基础。

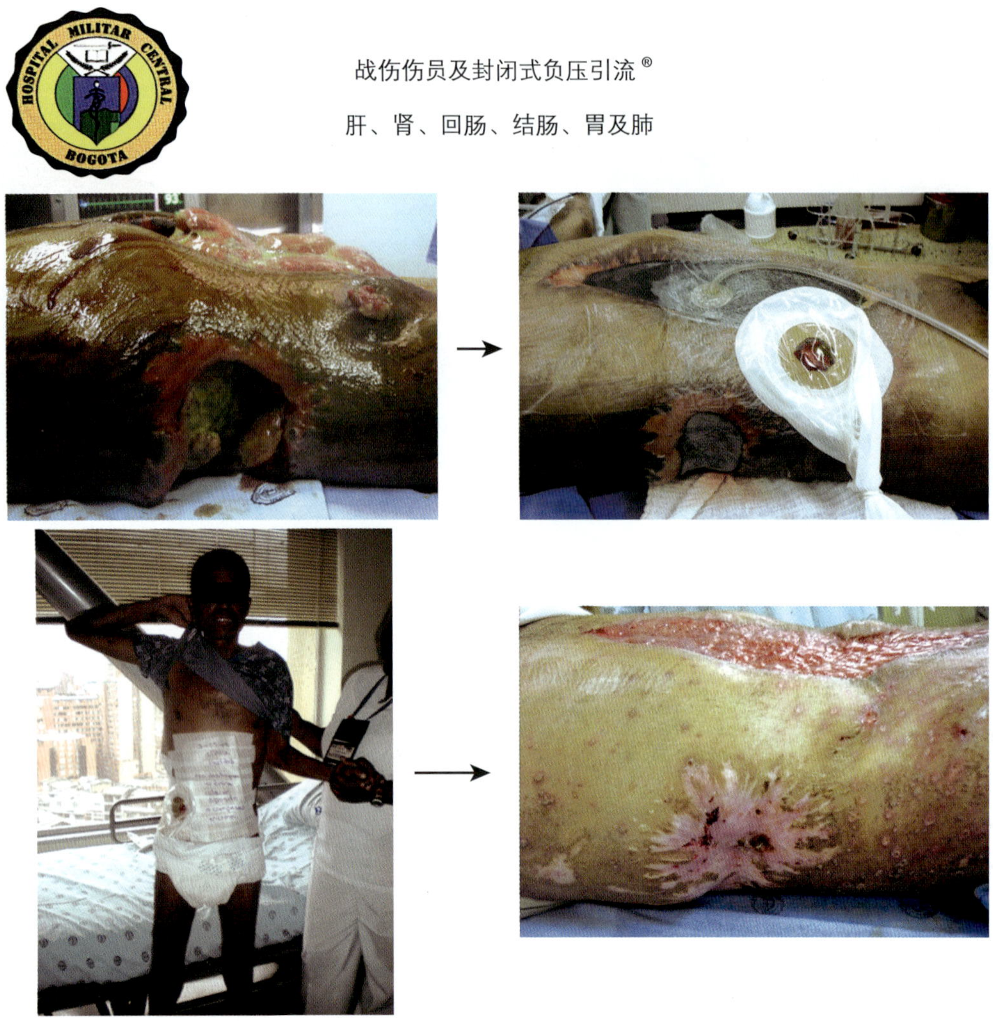

图 9　士兵在战斗中受伤，多个腹内脏器和腹壁受伤。使用封闭式负压引流治疗的治疗顺序

第 2 章 院前创伤救护

紧急医疗服务对创伤中心治疗效果的影响

David Shatz 著
张进军 译

自从创伤系统的有效性在 20 世纪 70 年代得到验证以来，对院前创伤患者的评估、治疗和转运在整个创伤救治管理过程中发挥了重要作用。虽然该创伤系统的作用在某些方面存在争议，但是在快速、有效地转运严重创伤患者方面几乎不存在任何疑问。虽然美国国家急诊医学体系对实践范围的模型（National Emergency Medical Service Scope of Practice Model）已实现标准化，但目前护理人员和急救医务人员的医疗行为在美国范围内存在较大差异，并且在美国交通部（U.S. Department of Transportation）于 20 世纪 70 年代早期制定了相关规定后发生了显著变化。尽管自从早期开展高级生命支持以来，院前救护毫无疑问地改善了创伤的治疗效果，但是有一些实践行为并没有那么有效。

黄金 1 h 还是黄金机会?

1976 年，R. Adams Cowley 医生在接受一个简短的采访时说道："在生存和死亡之间有一个黄金小时。如果您受伤非常严重，那么您将有不超过 60 min 的生存时间。"由此产生了关于创伤黄金 1 h 这个概念，并被大量引用。虽然没有科学证据支持这种观点，但对大多数人来说，很明显这种论述的本质是正确的。但是全面接受这个观念并不是没有成本和风险的，最近的科学对它存在质疑。

我们目前创伤体系的大部分结构是以黄金 1 h 为根据的，并且要尽快地把患者运送到创伤中心，甚至要使用到直升机和地面救护车。在电视、电影和新闻行业的推动下，采用直升机撤离战斗伤亡人员成为朝鲜战争和越南战争的代名词。近几十年来，随着配备直升机的紧急医疗服务（Emergency Medical Service，EMS）的爆炸式增长，使用民用直升机进行救援也变得容易起来。仅在密苏里州，1989 年该州的 500 万居民共配置有 9 架直升机，现在该州的 600 万居民共配置有 33 架直升机。之所以配备这么多的直升机，当然是使用直升机能以更快的速度将创伤患者从事故现场转运到创伤中心。但是直升机转运也导致了一些死亡事件的发生。越南战争期间，直升机在执行无武装医疗转送任务时，2 年内共导致了 39 名机组人员死亡以及 210 人受伤。40 多年后，在 2003 – 2008 年期间，民用的紧急医疗服务直升机共坠毁 85 次，一共导致 77 名患者和机组人员死亡。

通过地面转运患者也不是完全没有风险的。一些研究已经描述了关于患者、救护车急救人员以及与救护车没有直接关联的普通市民的风险情况。意料之中的是，大多数救护车事故发生在执行紧急呼叫任务期间。虽然只有 40% 的致命性碰撞发生在救护车中靠后的患者区域，但其中 72% 的死亡也是发生在这个区域。对于这些致命性伤害，最常见的解释是，急救人员认为在转运途中如果患者系上了安全带，将无法为他们提供有效的治疗和护理措施。虽然已经做了大量工作来研究这个问题，但解决方案不具有普遍性。对于急救人员而言，导致其死亡的最大风险是车祸。然而，并不是所有的救护车车祸只对急救人员造成伤亡。由美国国家职业安全与健康研究所（National Institute for Occupational Safety and Health，NIOSH）开展的一项为期 10 年的研究显示，在300起致命的救护车车祸中，导致了27名急救人员、55名救护车上其他人员、275名社会车辆的乘客以及行人死亡。有趣的是，美国联邦航空管理局（Federal Aviation Administration）提供的数据显示高达80%的飞行事故是由飞行员失误导致的。NIOSH开展的研究显示60%的救护车车祸事故是由驾驶员失误所致。这些研究都没有描述转运患者的原因，但从中可以推断出，在黄金1 h的幌子下，产生了在快速转运创伤患者时的压力和需要问题。

Newgard等进行的研究显示，转运时间和应答人员的专业水平对生理功能严重紊乱的创伤患者的救治结果都不会产生影响。通过空中和地面转运的方式，146家提供紧急医疗服务的机构共将3656名创伤患者转送到美国和加拿大的51家Ⅰ级和Ⅱ级创伤中心。严重创伤患者的入选标准包括收缩压≤90 mmHg，格拉斯哥昏迷评分（Glasgow Coma Scale，GCS）≤12分，呼吸频率<10次/分或>29次/分，或者需要高级气道干预措施。平均响应时间（4.28 min）、到达现场时间（19 min）以及转运时间（10 min）导致总消耗时间为28.4～47 min，平均总耗时36.3 min。在所有不同类型的时间分析中，均没有发现因转运时间而导致死亡率的差异。因此，这些研究证明了创伤救治不仅与院前时间有关，而且与转运方式、最初提供院前急救服务机构的级别、患者的年龄和损伤机制等都有关系。

另一方面，根据以往的经验，对于由于损伤而导致脾、肝或骨盆出血的患者，采用快速转运和明确的治疗方法会有更好的疗效。早期的研究表明，当把60 min以上的时间都消耗在院前急救时，将会增加死亡的发生。1983年，在Trunkey关于创伤导致死亡的早期描述中，确定了死亡的三峰分布。最近已经描述了一种双峰分布，几乎消除了晚期死亡，并改变了早期死亡时间。Gunst等的研究发现，早期死亡发生的平均时间是52 min（Trunkey的研究是120 min），患者受伤后到达创伤中心的平均时间是42 min。24%的患者受伤后具有潜在的存活能力，然而还是在伤后1 h死亡，所以黄金1 h可能确实是真实的。

最后，几乎没有分歧的是，如果一名严重创伤患者越早接受针对性的救护，那么改善治疗效果的可能性就越大。Cowley医生好像十分清楚他所做的是一个在科学上未经证实的论述，但如果他的目的是为了给早期的平民创伤救护提出一个非常重要的教训的话，那么他已经非常成功了。但最重要的是，创伤患者应在没有意外事故发生的情况下被运送到能提供救护的医疗机构，考虑到患者、院前急救人员和无辜旁观者的安全才是最重要的。

院前补液

关于创伤现场卫生保健辅助人员是否应该给患者建立静脉通路进行液体复苏的争论由来已久，并不新鲜。多年来，院前创伤生命支持机构（Prehospital Trauma Life Support）与美国外科医师学院（American College of Surgeons）合作，强调了建立静脉通路和进行液体复苏的重要性，尽管这一概念目前正在发生改变。但是对创伤患者而言，怎么做才是最安全的呢？

长期以来，在对创伤患者的护理中，静脉通路的开放一直被认为是非常重要的一步。并且在血容量严重不足但未影响外周血液循环之前，无论是补液还是给药，都可以开展静脉通路开放。然而，在院前环境中对创伤患者进行治疗时很少使用药物，并且即刻可用的骨髓腔内注射装置使得对于即使是最严重的容量耗尽患者也可以采取药物治疗。建立有效静脉通道的过程不应该延迟将伤者转运到创伤中心。因此问题是，在转运过程中进行液体复苏是否会对伤者的治疗结果产生影响？

20世纪90年代初动物研究表明，尽管生理盐水复苏增加了失血量，但死亡率并没有受到影响。并且高级创伤生命支持（advanced trauma life support，ATLS）的原则是提倡根据须要推注2 L乳酸林格液作为解决方案。这种急救部门的方案随后被应用到院前急救环境，并成为一种常见措施，但只有很少的监测液体复苏是否足够的设备。应关注低灌注包括弥漫性器官缺血的风险，特别是在脑损伤的患者中。另外，是从什么时候开始认为低血容量从可接受变为致命的呢？

尽管存在这些问题，但是当前的普遍共识支持不进行现场液体复苏，即使在急救部门，直到可以对活动性或潜在活动性的出血部位进行控制。对抗血压正常复苏的争论包括稀释凝血因子，增加出血和血红蛋白损失，移除已形成的血块，血管外液体超负荷，以及使用室温液体造成低温恶化的可能性。2011年大型国家创伤数据库（National Trauma Data Bank）回顾资料显示，院前Ⅳ级患者的死亡率明显高于其他患者。虽然有人可能认为存在选择偏倚，但几乎所有的患者亚组都能看到死亡率的增加。这个队列包括钝性伤和穿透性伤，后者导致的死亡率增加更为明显。血压正常患者的死亡率不受影响，但低血压患者的死亡率明显增加，严重脑损伤患者的死亡风险增加了34%。低损伤的严重患者在死亡率方面没有表现出差异。

近年的战斗经验进一步支持放弃对正常血压患者的现场液体复苏。虽然民用与战场环境中的创伤模式不同，但在两者中对出血的控制都是至关重要的。目前推荐合理、有效地使用复苏液，使用晶体液与低容量胶体液仍然存在问题。

如果要让院前人员接受有限液体复苏或容许性低血压的概念，那么这种许可的界限是什么？对于出血已经暂时停止的出血性休克患者，以色列国防军（Israel Defense Force）的指南建议液体复苏旨在恢复桡动脉脉搏，收缩压为80 mmHg。由于考虑到中枢神经系统损伤情况下的脑灌注压，所以建议收缩压为100 mmHg。2009版战术作战伤员救护液体复苏指南（Tactical Combat Casualty Care Fluid Resuscitation Guidelines，2009）现在已经被美国国防部的所有服务部门采用，其中建议不对非休克患者进行静脉输液，对不受控制的出血性休克且明确没有桡动脉搏动的休克患者给予液体复苏。

尽管几十年来相关出版物反驳在院前实施液体复苏，但实践中仍在施行，应该放弃以“正常”生命体征为目标而使用晶体液。虽然越过了允许性低血压的界限而导致患者死亡不是理想的结果，但是有足够的证据表明（尽管不是正常的），复苏应该是期望的终点。在本文中，充分灌注的测量方法包括可触及明显的桡动脉搏动和收缩压为80 mmHg（在疑似创伤性脑损伤患者中收缩压为100 mmHg），这应该是现场复苏的首极终点。这个目标应该通过低容量（250 ml）推注完成，而不是以前所采用的2 L推注方法。

出血还是止血——止血带止血是标准救护吗？

每一位创伤外科医生都目睹过被送到创伤室的肢体损伤患者，有大量敷料覆盖伤口，并且在救护车和创伤室床之间残留血迹。在针对急救人员的紧急医疗救援训练中，提出对大量出血伤口要采用大块敷料进行覆盖并包扎。如果是持续性出血，则使用更大、更多的敷料。然而，显而易见的是，使用大块敷料和采取包扎后都不能达到超动脉压力，那么对于存在动脉损伤的伤者可能会失血更多。公平地说，医务人员常常忙于转运和对其他伤者的救护，并且经常不能全力对出血伤口直接施加压力，此时需要第三只手的帮助，并且须要提供止血带。

Ambrose Paré被认为是世界上第一次使用止血带的人，尽管早在古罗马时代的战场上就已经使用过止血带了。经历过几次调整后，近几十年来在手术室使用充气止血带已经是常见的做法。在战争中已经越来越少地使用止血带，但在最近的武装冲突中又开始重新流行。近些年来对止血带的使用经验主要是从战斗中获得的，现在已将其扩展到了平民院前创伤救护中。

使用止血带的不利因素主要是影响了对组织缺血和出血量增加时的感知与观察。但是十年前的止血带大多是橡胶管或宽橡胶带，这两种止血带都不是为闭塞动脉流入而设计的。相反，这些橡胶止血带被设计为仅用于闭塞静脉流出，辅助静脉导管的放置。结果，毫不意外，随着间质压力的增加，导致出血量增加，随后导致组织缺血。此外，使用橡胶管后，压力被集中在较小的区域内，从而使神经压迫更加严重，这对于伤者而言是非常痛苦的。现在购买到的并且被美国军方广泛使用的止血带更宽一些，并且能使压力更均匀地分布，具有调整阻塞动脉流入所需压力的能力。

在近年来的大规模军事冲突中，已经积累了包括肢体严重创伤等暴力伤害的新经验。虽然大多数现代战争导致的死亡是无法抢救的，但是一项对美国军事特种部队死亡人数的回顾显示，其中13%潜在的可预防的死亡是因为其出血是可以被止血带控制的。在对之后“伊拉克自由行动”伤亡事件开展的研究发现，67例患者使用院前止血带的平均持续时间为70 min，其中超过一半的严重创伤患者出现了可以改善的出血控制。对止血带引起的并发症的关注已经引发了对其使用的争议，但是Beekley等和Kragh等发现，如果正确使用止血带，将很少或几乎没有并发症。这些研究提出的重要警告是，应将止血带放在伤口附近，使用时间应是2 h以内。以色列国防军的经验与之类似，使用止血带20多年后，不良结果主要局限于神经损伤（占5.5%）。其中绝大多数患者之所以造成局部缺血，是因为使用止血带时间超过了150 min。总体而言，军事经验表明在严重出血性肢体创伤患者中使用止血带的作用是挽救生命，并不是因为使用它们而导致了肢体损伤。

尽管现在几乎所有的美国士兵都在个人急救包中装有止血带，但是在民用急救系统中不存在同样广泛的可用性。因此，在民用中止血带的使用是有限的，公布的数据也显示如此。与战争伤害相反，在平民环境中导致致命的单独的肢体损伤非常罕见。然而，这些是可预防的死亡，不应该被忽视。在德克萨斯州休斯敦进行的一项研究显示，14 例这类的患者因所受到的伤害而死亡，但他们并没有使用止血带，尽管在现场所有的病例都存生命迹象。这些创伤一部分是枪伤，另一部分是刀伤和撕裂。所有这些损伤都是可以得到控制和修复的。大多数创伤（占 71%）是损及下肢。波士顿紧急医疗服务系统在 20 世纪 90 年代放宽了对止血带的使用，因为它被认为可以预防肢端损伤导致的死亡。在类似的损伤模式下，他们描述了对 11 名具有穿透性肢体损伤患者使用止血带的情况。只有一名患者存活下来（在事故现场，通过无脉搏搏动判断死亡）。发现所有的患者存在重要的血管损伤。

虽然大多数平民创伤受害者缺乏士兵穿戴的保护性措施，而且幸运的是，爆炸装置是导致平民伤害的罕见来源，然而，这些伤害模式与战争中的模式有很大的区别。尽管因此预计，与军事人员相比，紧急医疗服务急救人员对止血带的使用似乎应该明显减少。但是如果经过正确的培训并在适当的环境下使用，在救生中它们的使用并不会减少。从战场到城市街道，毫无疑问，院前使用止血带挽救了生命。

结论

几十年前城市紧急医疗救护的建立挽救了无数生命。训练有素、技能熟练且有积极性的专业人士把这种关怀带到了事故现场。他们在一些最难以想象的处境中执行救护任务。多年来，他们的急救技能被修正和扩展，大多数技能具有良好的救治疗效。然而，已经证明某些治疗创伤受害者的技能是有害的，应该加以修改，绝对目标就是要将创伤患者迅速转运到确切的创伤救护地点。

院前气道管理：插管术、设备及争议

Raul Coimbra，Jay Doucet，David Hoyt 著
张进军 译

院前创伤气道管理可能是院前急救人员所面临的最大挑战。这些专业人员必须学习并且具有这种必要的急救技能，以便在急救现场以及在将创伤患者转运到创伤中心途中时能充分地管理气道问题。

气管插管术是开展气道管理的明确方法。然而，要学习到这种技能，须要进行大量的培训和实践。虽然针对紧急医疗技术人员（emergency medical technician，EMT）开展的基本课程包含高级气道管理模块，但这些规程的使用频率较低，而使这些专业人员难以熟练掌握。在大多数系统中，辅助医疗人员和飞行护士是唯一被允许进行快速序贯性插管（rapid sequence intubation，RSI）的专业人员。因此，紧急医疗技术人员须要通过更简单的方式来维持气道通畅，直到将患者转运到医院。当气管插管术不容易操作或不具备使用条件时，现在有几种设备可以提供给院前急救人员使用。这些替代的急救方法包括覆盖口腔或鼻咽气道的球囊面罩通气术，或诸如喉罩、引流管 - 通气管双腔管（联合导管）、喉 - 气管气道（主气道）等的声门上气道。还存在可以使紧急医疗技术人员在操作快速序贯性插管时增加其成功可能性的设备，如 Eschmann 气管插管器（Eschmann tracheal tube introducer，ETTI）和视频喉镜。在某些管辖区域和某些状况下，如对战术性实战伤亡人员的救护，可对紧急医疗技术人员训练某些类型的气道手术，如环甲膜穿刺术或切开术。

本章将对院前气道管理的适应证、不同的模式、设备和技术，以及面对的困难和存在的缺陷等展开讨论。

诊断

谁需要气道管理?

在我们界定在院前急救现场谁需要气道管理之前，重要的是须要澄清一个事实：迄今为止，很少有研究显示在送达到创伤中心之前对创伤患者开展高级气道管理是有效的。

作为整个急救复苏工作的一部分，气道管理的目标是为了提供充分的氧合和通气。适应证包括呼吸运动减少或缺失、具有气道阻塞的症状和施行心肺复苏过程中。严重创伤性颅脑损伤（traumatic brain injury，TBI）是院前气管插管术的适应证，这一点将在后面进行讨论。在创伤急救过程中，对濒临死亡的患者进行气道管理是有益的，特别是对于那些在被送到医院时须要施行复苏性胸廓切开术的患者（Durham 等）。

评估气道的状态

在创伤患者，气道阻塞可以是快速地发生，也可以是隐蔽地发生；可以是完全阻塞，也可以是不完全阻塞；可以是进行性的，也可以是间歇性的。气道评估是紧急医疗技术人员须要掌握的一项基本技能。气道管理优先于所有其他针对平民的院前干预措施，因为对呼吸道的治疗失败将会导致无法继续救治患者。可以通过查找直接导致气道创伤的迹象来评估气道状态，如颌面、颈部或喉部的外伤。检查口腔中的异物，如义齿、血液和呕吐物。如存在煤烟、烧焦的鼻毛和炭化痰，则表明对气道造成了热创伤。这些都可能导致进行性气道阻塞。仔细聆听伤者。如果他说话正常，并能表达出气道通畅情况和气道状态良好的相关信息，这就说明其气道状态和精神状态是正常的。糊涂或焦虑的伤者可能患有 TBI、中毒、缺氧或低碳酸血症，并且可能已经发展为气道阻塞。某些异常的声音，如喘鸣、气过水声、喘息或打鼾，可能与气道不完全阻塞有关。

触诊颈部时的捻发音是由皮下空气所致，提示为气道的直接创伤、喉部骨折导致的软骨松动或使气道受压的血肿。

最初的气道维持技术包括抬头举颏法或双手托颌法，对怀疑有钝性创伤的患者应同时固定颈椎。通过这些动作可以打开气道，并显示在仰卧的患者中是否舌头后坠阻塞了气道。对无意识的患者应打开口咽气道以确保上呼吸道通畅。通过患者口咽气道的耐受性通常能够明确其在创伤中心的气道管理方式。对大多数无意识的创伤患者，可使用口咽气道联合球囊面罩进行通气管理。意识清醒和意识半清醒的患者不能忍受口咽气道，但可忍受鼻咽气道。对创伤患者须要补充氧气，即使面罩密封良好，但用在面部有毛发、大脸盘、小下巴或肥胖的患者时，也难以保证能输送 100% 的氧气。可能需要两三个院前急救人员共同努力，从而能保持面罩的良好密封，使其包住患者的面部，并保持颈椎固定。在球囊面罩和口腔或鼻腔气道不能提供足够的氧合和通气时，或者当转运过程妨碍了球囊面罩的最佳操作时，可能须要暴露声门，确认气道。

使用 LEMON 评估表（表 1）进行气管插管困难

表 1　LEMON 气道评估

L 外观	从外部观察患者，查找已知的可导致喉镜检查、气管插管或通气困难的特征。
E 3-3-2 评估规则	为了使咽、喉和口腔三部位做到轴线对准，简易插管术应当遵循以下关系：患者的门牙之间的距离应至少为 3 个手指的宽度（3），舌骨与下颏之间的距离应至少有 3 个手指的宽度（3），甲状软骨切迹和口腔底部之间的距离至少应该有 2 个手指的宽度（2）。
M Mallampati 评分	使咽下部充分可见。传统上通过 Mallampati 评分进行评估（图 1）。患者坐直，完全张开嘴巴并尽可能地伸出舌头。检查者用手电筒查看口腔，以评估咽下部的可见程度。对于仰卧位的患者，可以通过让患者完全张开嘴巴并伸出舌头来评估 Mallampati 评分，并且喉镜的光线可以从上方照射到咽下部。
O 是否存在梗阻?	任何可能导致气道阻塞的情况都会造成喉镜检查困难和通气困难。这些情况可能是会厌炎、扁桃体脓肿和外伤。
N 颈部活动	颈部的活动性是进行成功插管的一个重要要求。可以通过让患者将下颏向下靠到胸部，然后伸直颈部，并看向天花板来进行评估。使用颈部固定器的患者显然不能进行颈部运动，因此更难进行气管插管的操作。

内容选自 From Reed MJ, Dunn MJ, McKeown DW: Can an airway assessment score predict difficulty at intubation in the emergency department? Emerg Med J 22:99–102, 2005

程度的气道评估。第一，是寻找已知的会导致气管插管或通气困难的特征，如小颌畸形、龅牙或大脸盘等。第二，使用 3-3-2 规则评估患者。该规则指患者的门牙之间的距离应当至少有 3 个手指的宽度，舌骨和下颏之间的距离应该有 3 个手指的宽度，并且在甲状软骨切迹和口腔底部之间的距离至少应该有 2 个手指的宽度。第三，Mallampati 评分是评估意识清醒患者的口咽部和咽下部（图 1）。第四，寻找气道阻塞的证据，包括可导致喉镜检查和通气困难的某些状况迹象，例如直接创伤或烧伤。这些迹象有的是可见的，有的是可以听到的。最后，评估颈部的活动性。在戴有颈部固定器的钝器伤患者，由于颈部不能活动，可以预料对其进行气管插管时会更加困难。

对困难气道的识别是为了防止患者的病情恶化以及可能由此造成的死亡。当诊断为气道困难时，应当使用替代设备和应对策略。这些措施包括声门上呼吸道，例如喉罩气道（laryngeal mask airway，LMA）、联合使用导管和 King 气道（主气道）。对困难气道的患者使用具有麻痹作用的 RSI 时，可能导致“不能插管 - 不能通气”的情况而可能须要外科建立呼吸道，或者甚至不能在院前事故现场进行救治。

气道管理

应该使用哪种策略?

这里描述的策略是传统面罩通气的替代方案。

喉罩气道（LMA）

LMA 是气管插管的一种替代方法（图 2）。它对于困难气道的患者和身处“不利环境”中（雨天、光线黑暗或营救时间过长等）的患者显得特别重要。它也可以用作 RSI 失败后的救援策略。此外，由于它是将气管插管通过 LMA 进行操作，因而可以使操作较为方便。

将 LMA 盲插入口咽部，患者通常可以忍受这一操作，无须进行神经肌肉阻滞。将 LMA 置于咽下部声门上的位置。是否能成功放置 LMA 与 Mallampati 评分、是否使用颈托或固定颈椎无关。通过 LMA 有可能自发通气，并且 LMA 的手动通气优于球囊面罩通气，因为后者通常须要用两只手来

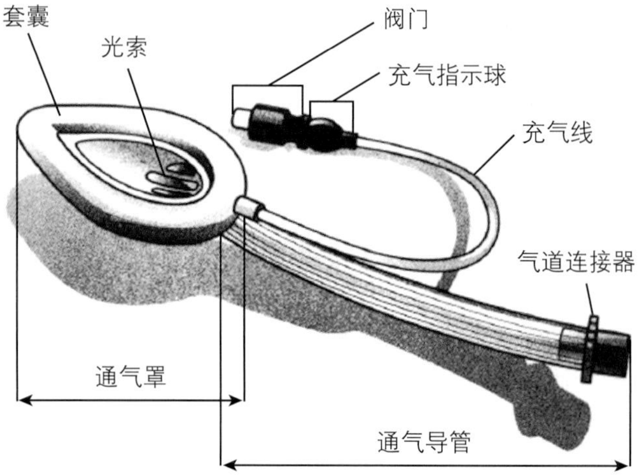

图 2 喉罩气道

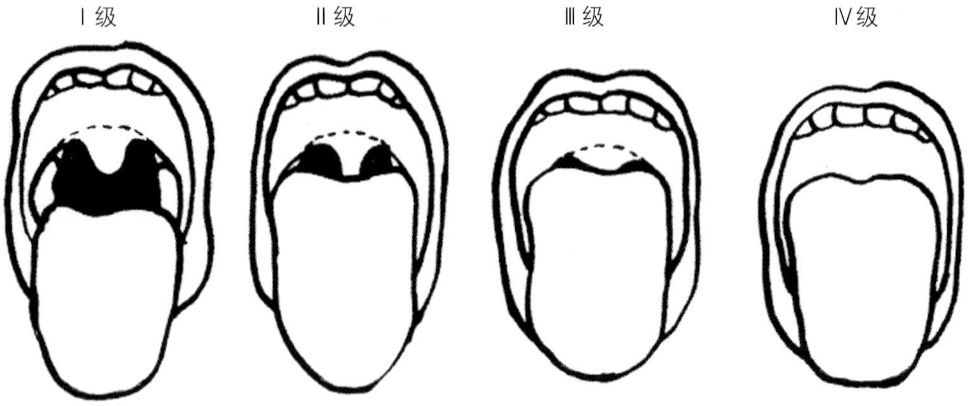

图 1 困难气道——由 Samsoon 和 Young 修改的 Mallampati 评分 (*From Mallampati SR, Gatt SP, Gugino LD, et al: A clinical sign to predict difficult tracheal intubation: a prospective study. Can Anaesth Soc J 32:429–435, 1985.*)

保持良好的密封。对成功率进行比较的研究显示，与气管插管术相比，医务人员放置LMA的成功率较高。LMA可能对气道困难的患者特别有用，因为声门无须直接显示，并且不需要使用神经肌肉阻滞剂。与联合导气管（下文描述）相比，LMA的优点包括发生错位的风险较低，没有食管插管的风险，并且对口咽部造成的创伤较少。LMA的主要缺点是不能避免抽吸，这可能给具有完整气道反射的患者带来了很大的风险。LMA的另一个缺陷是难以产生较高的气道压力，这可能导致无效通气。

联合导气管

联合导气管是由具有两个内腔的装置组成的。其中一个内腔具有类似于气管导管的开放远端，而另一个内腔具有封闭的远端，在其球囊套附近有几个孔。具有较大体积的第二个球囊位于更靠近侧孔的位置，用于将导管固定在适当位置。盲插联合导气管，通过其中的一个内腔进行通气。插入后，其远侧末端通常位于食管内。在使口咽气囊充气后，将食管套囊充气。尝试通过咽腔通气来决定末端是在食管内还是气管内。如果呼气末期二氧化碳检测器显示比色度没有变化，或者呼吸音消失，则提示末端在气管内，应当对患者进行气管腔通气（图3）。

当经过多次尝试后不能获得气道时，或者当被认为是困难气道时，或者当在事故现场通过喉镜不能直接观察到声带时，或者当院前急救人员未接受过气管插管操作的训练时，联合导气管是气管插管的有用替代物。绝大多数使用联合导气管的患者被送入创伤中心后通气和给氧状况良好，无须立即去除食管气管联合导气管。联合导气管也可用于有明显颌面创伤和颈椎损伤的患者。因为食管套管在插入导管后被立即充气，所以联合导气管对防止胃内容物吸入提供了保护。

联合导气管禁用于有完整呕吐反射的患者，或怀疑有上呼吸道梗阻的患者。没有可用于儿科的联合气管导管尺寸。潜在的并发症包括咽和食管损伤，以及未能识别末端的确切位置，并试图通过错误的内腔补氧和通气。

喉－气管气道设备

喉-气管气道也称喉管气道（laryngeal tube airway，LTA）或King气道，在许多地区用于替代联合导气管（图4）。与联合导气管或LMA相似，使用LTA的情况是在不能直接可视声门以及无须对头部或颈部进行重要的操作。由于LTA有一个内腔，并且有研究表明其末端球囊进入食管时是可靠安全的，因此其操作更为简单。与联合导气管不同，它

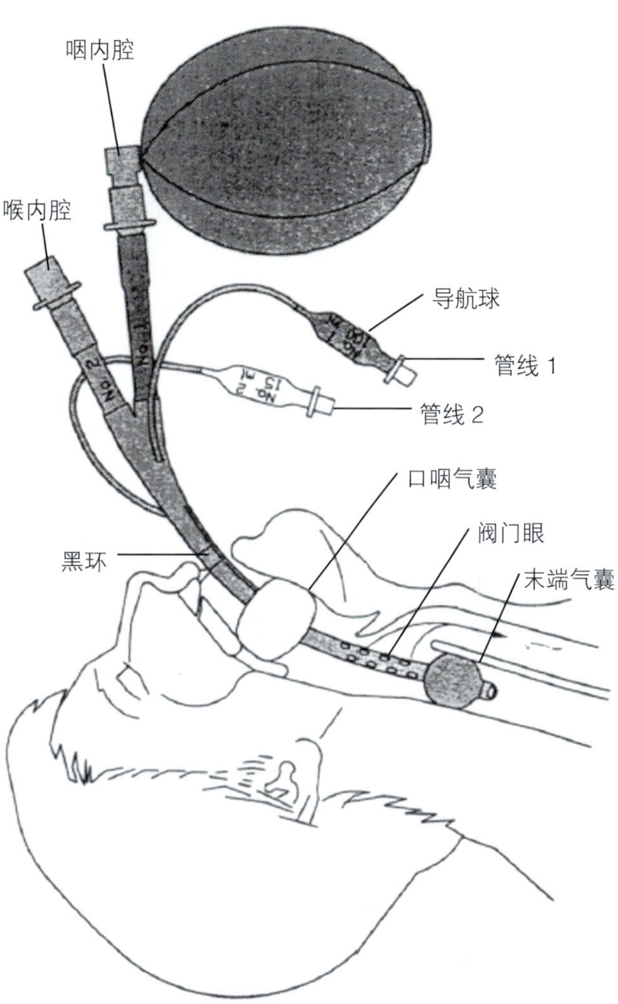

图3 联合导气管，其末端在食管内

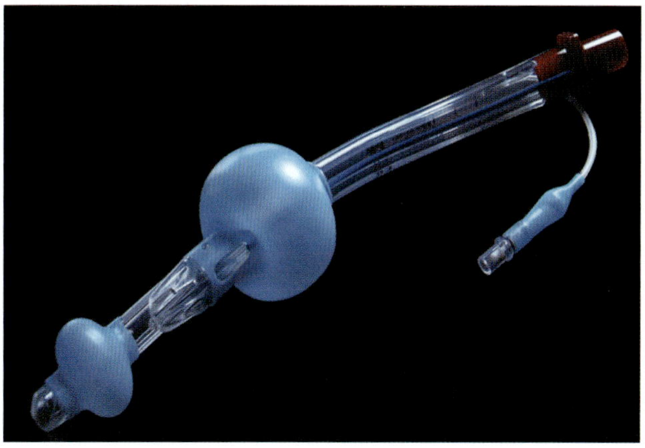

图4 喉管气道（LTA，KingLT ™）（*Reprinted with Permission from Ambu A/S*）

有儿科使用的尺寸。LTA 还有可以让鼻胃管通过的类型，可用于降低胃的压力并减轻反流。在进行模拟训练中，LTA 操作的成功率明显高于联合导气管或气管插管。相对于联合导气管，供应商更推荐使用 LTA。与其他声门上气道相关，它不是确定性的气道，也不提供完全的保护以避免吸入，也不能用在有意识的患者身上，并且须要计划在创伤中心时更换一个确定的气道。长期放置 LTA 可能会导致舌和咽肿大。移除声门气道可能会引起呕吐或反流。在可控的环境中（例如在创伤室或手术室里有创伤外科医生和医疗团队的情况下）由熟练的专业医师更换气管导管才是最安全的操作。

气管插管

气管插管（endotracheal intubation，ETI）是气道管理的金标准。在院前急救环境中，对于不使用镇静剂或神经肌肉阻滞剂的气管插管，只能在深度昏迷或心脏停搏的患者身上操作。因为很少有急救体系允许急救人员进行 RSI，并且由于可能造成预后不良，在这种情况下进行气管插管可能弊大于利。在不理想的条件下，气管插管可能导致较高的并发症，包括低氧血症、食管插管以及主支气管插管，可伴有完全肺塌陷、口咽受伤、反流、加重潜在的脊髓损伤、影响血液循环、使颅内压升高以及延误了将患者转运到创伤中心。这里只是列举出了几个例子。无法识别困难气道可能导致无法进行插管，并且在进行 RSI 之前可能会引发严重的并发症并最终导致患者死亡。气管插管的常见问题将会在以后进行讨论。

改善气管插管成功率的辅助手段

Glidescope、McGrath、Bullard、Storz CMAC 及 Kingvision 等品牌的可视喉镜（video laryngoscopy，VL）设备已有所改进，以适用于院前急救环境。例如，在困难气道中不能使用直接喉镜（direct laryngoscopy，DL）的情况下，可视喉镜能够做到可视声门和声带。可视喉镜需要的提升力比直接喉镜更小，这样可以减少颈椎的运动。可视喉镜能够提供插管失败和意外伤害的报告。这些设备的相对有效性尚未在临床试验中进行评估，而模拟器研究的结果却相互矛盾。在许多急救医学系统中，存在着相对较高的成本和培训负担，这并不合理。这样的设备确实具有记录和传输视频的能力，从而可能引领未来院前气道管理中教育和质量控制领域的应用。

可以首次成功改善气管导管的低成本简易设备是 ETTI，有时其被称为橡胶探条。由于可能存在乳胶过敏，因而现在很少使用真正的乳胶制品。该设备是由软质合成聚合物制成的一个 60 cm、15 F 的插管芯，配有方便使用的折轴尖端。当在直接喉镜上无法方便地看到声带时就使用这种设备。ETTI 通过喉镜的下方，恰好位于会厌的下面，并能反馈其所在的位置信息。当折轴尖端通过气管软骨环时，会感觉到气管通道出现摩擦，随后尖端在大约 50cm 的隆突处会遇到阻力。食管通道并没有这些表现。气管通道成功后将允许气管导管在 ETTI 上通过。有病例报告表明 ETTI 能够对无法采用其他方式插管的院前患者进行插管。

确认插管的位置

有几种因素容易导致气管导管位置不当，包括光线不足、不能充分地接近患者、抽吸不足、困难气道、口腔出血、呕吐、面部创伤和气道肿胀等。

通过声带的导管的直接可视化是用于确认气管导管位置适当的金标准。考虑到急救现场的条件并不理想，这一点显然不是总是可能实现的。在嘈杂和混乱的环境中，在现场听诊呼吸音也可能十分困难。

呼吸末 CO_2 监护仪已被院前急救人员用于确认气管导管的位置。CO_2 浓度较高时，检测器显示颜色将从紫色变为黄色。该设备已被认为是比较可靠的。然而，在心肺骤停的情况下它却缺乏敏感性，原因是肺部血液流动减少了，限制了 CO_2 的传送。因此，即使适合在这种环境下插管，大约有 15% 的患者会因为设备缺少色度改变而会移动气管导管。相反的情况也是存在的，即在摄入大量碳酸液体（啤酒或碳酸饮料等）的患者，使用救囊面罩通气时，导管在食管内或当胃部进入气体时可观察到颜色的变化。

另一种确认气管导管放置正确的方法是注射器抽吸技术。如果导管被正确地放置在气管中，当试图通过安装有 60 ml 注射器或橡胶球气道适配器（Ellick 抽空装置）的气管导管抽吸空气时，急救人员不应该感到有任何阻力。如果导管是在食道内，由注射器产生的负压可导致食管壁塌陷，从而堵塞了气管导管尖端处的开口，急救人员会感觉到抽吸的阻力。

院前有创气道

在美国平民环境中进行院前有创气道操作的概率非常低，在每 10 万例紧急医疗服务救护事件中约有 4 例环甲膜切开术，成功率为 87%。因为没有公开发表的证据支持，所以难以对最佳实践进行定义。因缺乏国家标准，紧急医疗服务医疗主管部门和国家相关条例允许紧急医疗服务人员在执行此类程序的实践时具有相当大的可变性。在其管辖区域内，从不允许实行有创气道，到部分允许实行环甲膜 / 气管穿刺术和环甲膜切开术。紧急医疗服务单位可以配备进行开放手术的装备或经皮肤穿刺使用的 Seldinger 型环甲膜切开术托盘。院前环甲膜切开术的操作在战争救援中更为常见；在“伊拉克自由行动”(Operation Iraqi Freedom) 中，开展环甲膜切开术的比例为 247/10 万，成功率为 77.5%。由于在外科气道操作中缺乏经验以及补救的办法，说明紧急医疗服务机构承担了很大的培训负担。

关于院前气管插管的争议

创伤性脑损伤 (TBI) 的院前气管插管

虽然气管插管等气道管理的积极措施已成为重症 TBI 患者的救护标准，但值得注意的是，并没有证据支持这种方法。事实上，最近的几项研究表明，与院前插管相关的死亡率有所增加。尚不清楚这是否代表具有选择偏倚，或者侵入性气道管理对结果真的产生了不利影响。所谓早期插管的好处包括逆转缺氧和保护气道。然而，与这些继发性损伤相关的发病率和死亡风险在初始损伤后 10 ~ 15min 时，可能无法通过侵入性气道管理进行预防或逆转。此外，近来增加了关于正压通气对结果产生不良影响的认识，特别是过度换气和低碳酸血症。

对早期插管患者的选择显得非常重要，以便使手术达到利益最大化。单独使用格拉斯哥昏迷评分 (GCS) 来选择院前插管的患者存在几个限制。早期 GCS 似乎在鉴定严重 TBI 中仅具有中度特异性。此外，GCS 与误吸之间最好是间接的关系。误气事件可发生在紧急医疗服务人员到达事故现场前或在插管时对喉部操作期间。此外，通过非侵入性的气道操作，低氧血症是可逆的，补氧后的氧饱和度 (SpO_2) 可能是考虑进行院前插管的一个重要因素。虽然没有研究明确界定头部损伤患者中有哪些患者须要进行早期插管，利用创伤登记数据进行神经网络分析后表明，由 GCS 确定的以及存在低血压的危重患者会从院前插管中获益。此外，插管确实对一些患者逆转低氧血症有所裨益。

由谁执行院前快速插管?

圣地亚哥医务人员 RSI 前瞻性试验纳入了没有进行药物治疗的且不能进行插管操作的严重 TBI 患者。主要结果是分析比较了试验患者与没有插管历史的对照受试者在年龄、性别、发病机制、创伤中心部位和身体分区等方面进行匹配比较的受伤量表评分。尽管施行侵入性气道的患者百分比显著增加，但试验患者的死亡率仍较高，预后较好的发生率较低。随后的分析表明，操作程序未达到最佳标准，包括过度通气和深度去饱和化，均导致了死亡率的部分增加。这可能反映了该系统中医护人员在 RSI 方面缺乏经验，以及单个 8 h 培训课程存在的局限性。

对于 RSI，尽管经验掌握与实践操作之间的关系仍不确定，但开展了更多强化训练的其他系统却记录了成功率改善的情况。在圣地亚哥研究中，与以往研究中相匹配的对照受试者相比，由医护人员进行 RSI 以及由航空医务人员进行转运是唯一获得结果改善的亚组。在这个队列中，过度通气的发生率较低，可以解释这个有些意想不到的发现。来自圣地亚哥和宾夕法尼亚州的后续分析的记录显示，与医务人员插管相比，结果更糟。但与急救室紧急插管相比，航空医疗 RSI 的结果显示是得到了改善。综合这些研究结果表明，当由经验丰富、训练有素的医务人员执行院前 RSI 操作时结果可能是有效的。关于初始培训以及正在进行培训的开展范围和频率仍有待定义。

血气监测在院前气管插管中的作用

在对头部损伤患者的处理中定量血气监测有几个优势。首先，血气测量在初始插管和整个院前救治过程中对气管导管的位置提供了准确定位。显然，早期识别出错位的气管导管能避免发病率和死亡率更为严重。将设置定量血气测定作为气管导管放置“金标准”的系统，记录显示未被识别的食管插管发生率接近为零。

对 TBI 患者而言，也许同样重要的是血气监测引导通气的能力。来自圣地亚哥医护人员的RSI试验数据明确了避免过度通气的重要性，并证明了基于达到PCO_2值的定量血气监测具有能够避免过度通气的作用。然而，似乎存在一个经验学习曲线。多年来使用血气监测指导通气的航空医疗人员能比医务人员获得更好的呼气末CO_2值和PCO_2值。一项来自圣地亚哥的注册研究表明，对中度至重度TBI患者进行插管时会表现得更好，但是院前通气过度和通气不足均会导致结果更糟。在院前急救环境中，我们相信定量血气监测应该是针对插管患者的救护标准，特别是对于那些特别容易受到二次伤害的TBI患者。

结论和流程图

院前气道管理是一项艰巨的任务，须要对相关人员进行培训以使其具备技能。气管插管仍然是气道管理的金标准。须要为基础操作部分和高级操作部分提供具体化标准（图5和图6）。如果在使用快速序贯性镇痛和麻痹后再尝试气管插管，成功率将更高。然而，大多数地面医疗单位没有做相应的准备，也不允许使用这种策略。另一方面，大多数航空运输单位都很容易使用RSI，并且采用这种策略后取得了显著的成功。一个成功的RSI项目需要有医疗指导和监督，须要进行培训和继续教育，须要具有用于患者监测的资源，需要进行药物储备和运输，须要确认和监测气管导管的位置，需要制订标准化方案，须要具有备用气道的方法，以及进行持续的质量保证和性能评估。

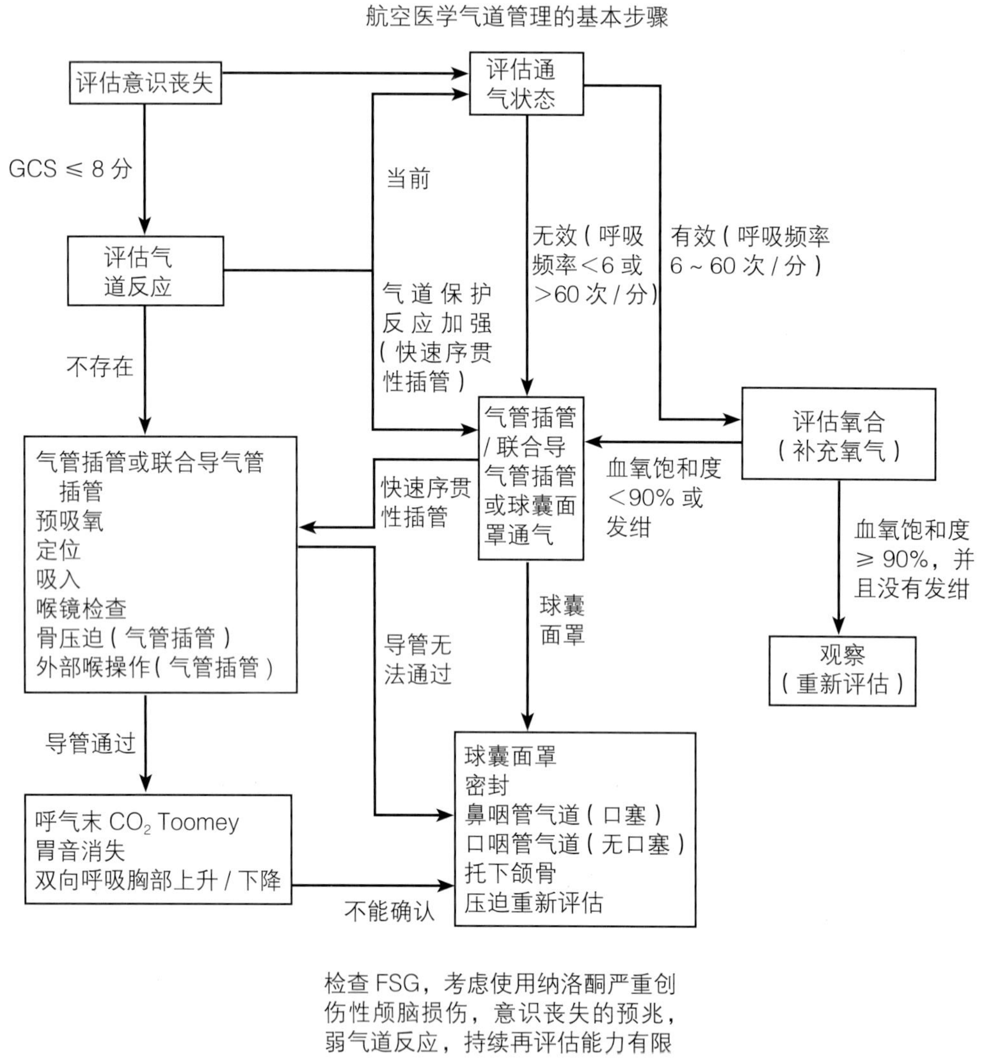

图5 航空医学气道管理的流程图

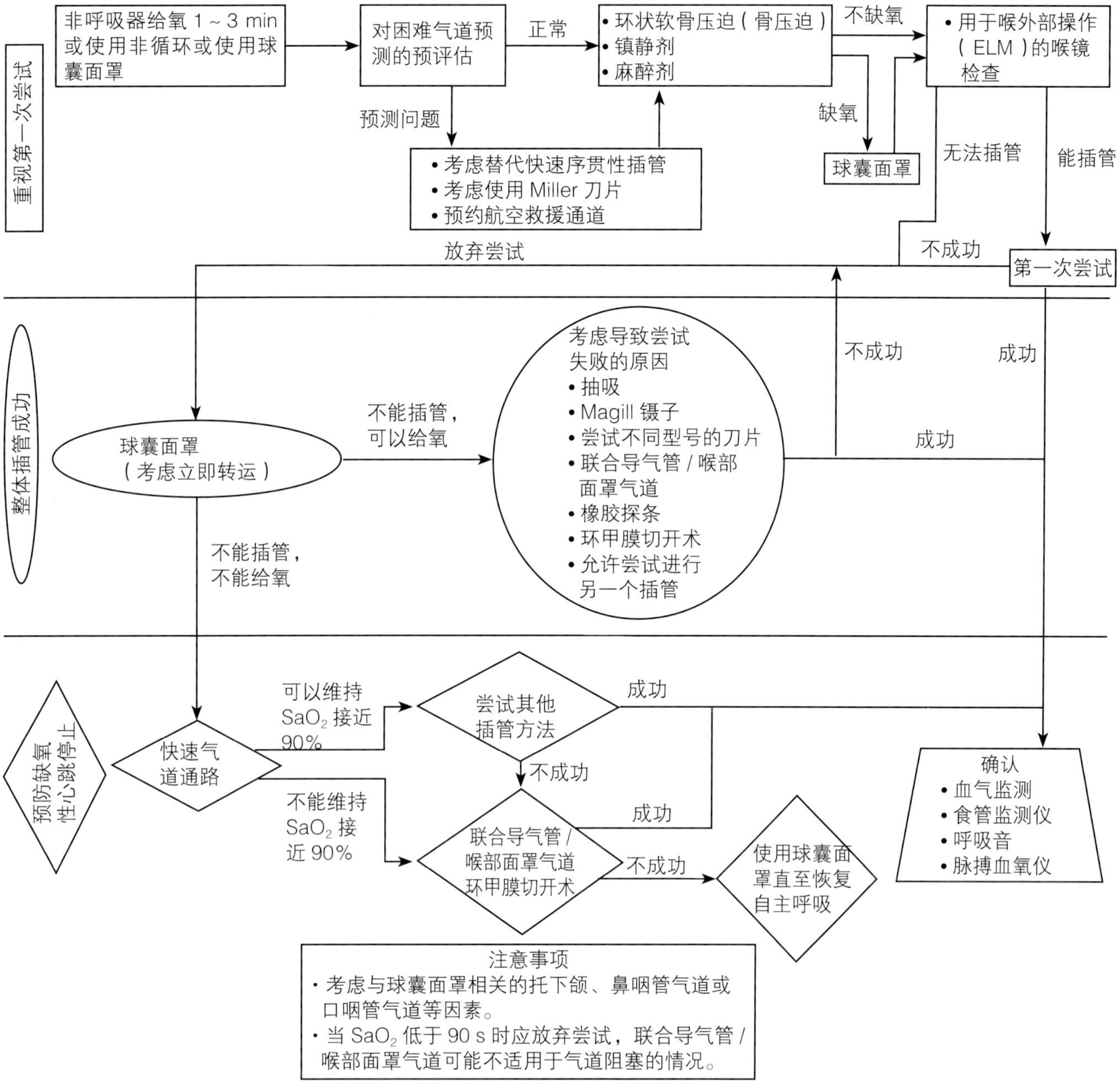

图 6 高级快速序贯性插管（RSI）流程图

院前液体复苏的种类、剂量及争论

Adam. M. Shiroff, Vincente. H. Gracias, Michae lF. Rotondo 著
张进军 译

液体复苏是在低血压创伤患者救护中的重要治疗手段，有效循环血容量的恢复能够改善氧供，从而减少在细胞和器官级别休克造成的不利影响。然而，液体复苏本身并不是灵丹妙药。尽管有效循环血容量的恢复是很关键的，但由于几个混杂因素的复杂影响，供给液体的方法是有争议的。由于不能在现场提供确定性救护，患者群体存在异质性，患者的损伤机制不同以及现场出血控制的水平存在差异，使得对该问题的精确研究具有挑战性。因此，仍然存在关于液体给药的种类、剂量和时机的争论。本章的目的是提供院前环境下对创伤患者使用液体

复苏的借鉴。

流行病学

创伤是造成45岁以下美国人死亡的主要原因，是造成所有年龄段的美国人死亡的第四大原因。出血性休克是导致死亡的主要生理问题。循环血量不足不仅是由失血所致，原因还有广泛的血管内皮损伤以及液体从血管内转移到间质。这些缺陷以及伴随的灌注不足可能导致多器官功能障碍、衰竭和死亡。

大量补液已经是40年来针对创伤患者的主要疗法。据估计，在英国接受院前静脉输液治疗的创伤患者比例从8.6/10万升至65/10万。然而，在过去的15年中，这种估算法已受到质疑，特别是在不受控制出血的情况下。

造成大出血的原因

出血的原因根据损伤的机制有所不同。在钝性创伤中，出血通常来源于实体器官如脾或肝破裂、肠系膜血管撕裂、骨盆和股骨骨折，以及因肺损伤导致的胸部出血或肋骨骨折导致的肋间血管出血，或外部原因如头皮撕裂等。主动脉横断和心脏破裂通常导致现场无法控制的出血。当创伤是继发于穿透性损害时，不受控制的大血管损伤通常是出血的来源。在院前条件下，可以采取直接压迫的方法或止血带控制体外可压迫性出血。然而，空腔或非压缩性出血对于院前急救人员来说是一个明显的诊断和治疗问题。

诊断与评估

在院前环境中，急救医疗技术人员以初级和中级调查的形式对创伤患者进行即时评估。这种评估包括须及时解决的对危及患者生命状况的评估。首先应评估气道的开放度，再听诊呼吸音评估气胸或血胸，随后评估血液循环，包括中心血压和外周血压。控制明显的导致外部出血的原因。测量患者的血压。因为在现场不能提供明确的治疗，所以应该采用“拉起就跑”而不是采用“保持和稳定”的策略。尝试血管内插入套管时不应该延迟将患者转运到创伤中心。在全国各地进行诸如院前创伤生命支持（Prehospital Trauma Life Support）的标准化课程教学，目的是对于急救医疗服务人员而言，在可使用的工具的辅助下，对于存在威胁生命的损伤患者进行检伤分类和治疗时进行标准化。

失血性休克的分级

出血是受伤患者中最常见的休克原因。休克的定义是器官灌注和组织氧合不足。在正常有氧代谢氧不足的情况下，机体经无氧代谢后堆积了大量乳酸。如果这个过程继续，细胞膜将丧失其完整性，导致细胞肿胀、进行性细胞损伤，并最终导致细胞死亡。

出血，即循环血容量的急性损失，是按照血容量损失的百分比来分类的。按照休克程度（表1），会发生特定的血流动力学、呼吸、中枢神经系统以及尿液和皮肤方面的变化。第一类级出血的临床症状很少，并且几乎不需要（如果有的话）补充血容量；第四类级出血会立即引起生命威胁，须输血，并且通常须做外科手术来停止持续出血。

表1　失血性休克的分类

参数	第一类	第二类	第三类	第四类
失血（%）	<15	15~30	30~40	>40
失血量（ml）	<750	700~1500	1500~2000	>2000
收缩压	无变化	正常	减少	非常低
舒张压	无变化	上升	减少	非常低
脉搏	<100	>100	>120	>140

Modified from Advanced Trauma Life Support guidelines

处理

通路

出血性休克的基本处理原则是终止出血并补充缺的血液。首先应该做的是建立具有合适的通气交换和氧合的气道。控制外部出血，同时补充氧气供应。插入两个大口径（最小16 G）静脉外周静脉导管，优选插入肘前静脉。一项回顾性研究显示，即使在低血压患者中，放置第二根静脉导管也没有什么改善。另一种选择是使用骨内导管，可将其可靠地放以下三个位置：肱骨、胫骨和胸骨。应当保留导管，以备用于不能通过常规方式获得静脉通路。复苏液、药物，甚至静脉造影材料都可以通过骨内导管。建立静脉通路时不应当延迟将患者转运到创伤中心。

流体类型

晶体液

晶体液是小的非离子或离子颗粒的溶液。它们可以自由地透过血管膜，并且主要分布在间质中。因此，只有1/3的晶体液分布于血管内。这说明须要提供比血容量损失至少高3倍的晶体液容量。由于胶体渗透压降低是继发于出血、毛细血管渗透和补充晶体液所致的血清蛋白浓度降低，晶体液补充的容量与血容量损失的比例甚至可以接近7：1至10：1。

严重损伤后，组织液容量降低，血管内腔变小。这些可能是使用晶体的原因，可通过液体复苏来补充体液量。通过对动物和人类开展的相关研究表明，与仅仅输血相比，联合使用等渗液和血液的改善效果会更好。将晶体液用于院前液体复苏还有其他优点，包括与其他复苏液相比其成本较低、立即可用以及可长期储存等。

晶体液主要填充于间质空间，组织水肿较为常见，并且可能具有有害作用。在头部受伤的患者中，脑水肿增加可能导致不利后果。若继发于肺水肿，气体交换可能受损。如果内皮和红细胞发生水肿，会损害微循环和组织氧交换，可能导致多脏器功能障碍。

根据高级创伤生命支持（ATLS）指南的内容，对创伤患者进行液体复苏时首先用2 L晶体液，通常是乳酸林格液。乳酸林格液是50：50的L-乳酸盐和D-乳酸盐相混合的等渗液。L-乳酸在肝中代谢为碳酸氢盐，从而提供额外的缓冲液。尽管D-乳酸盐异构体被认为是导致酸中毒的原因，但研究表明，用乳酸林格液复苏不会导致乳酸水平升高。然而，大量使用另一种等渗晶体液——生理盐水会诱导严重的酸中毒，这是由于氯离子浓度升高所致（154 mEq/L）。Healey等建议，在大量出血的动物模型中，与使用生理盐水和血液的动物相比，采用乳酸林格液和血液复苏液体的动物的存活率更高。这种差异被认为是生理盐水/血型中严重酸中毒的结果。

因为乳酸林格液具有比血浆更低的摩尔渗透压浓度（273 mOsm/L vs 285～295 mOsm /L），所以大容量使用乳酸林格液会降低血清渗透压并且导致脑水肿。因此，生理盐水可能是头部受伤患者的首选复苏液。

浓度为3%～7.5%的高渗盐水已被用于治疗低血容量性休克。由于其摩尔渗透压浓度更高（2400 mOsm/L，在7.5%高渗盐水中），高渗盐水在增加血管内容量上远远超过了输注容量（表2）。高渗盐水对心血管的作用包括增强心肌收缩性能，降低全身和肺血管的阻力，促进组织间液回到血管内，并减少静脉容量。然而，这些效应都是短暂的，因此，将高渗盐水与胶体液［右旋糖酐或羟乙基淀粉（hyoroxyethyl starch，HES）］混合以延长其功效，特别是用于小容量复苏液体时。

高渗盐水可降低颅内压（intracranial pressure，ICP），主要是在血脑屏障完整的脑部区域。Cooper等在一项对严重创伤性脑损伤导致低血压患者的随机双盲对照试验中，对在院前复苏使用高渗盐水和乳酸林格液对神经系统的产生的影响和结果进行了比较。研究者发现在3或6个月期间采用格拉斯哥昏迷评分时两组间没有存在显著差异。

关于高渗盐水对免疫调节的作用，是免疫刺激还是免疫抑制取决于其浓度。这一点已有论文进行过阐述。高渗盐水影响细胞核的激活，蛋白质合成和增殖，以及中性粒细胞的功能和细胞骨架的聚合。在动物的出血模型中，这些作用与减轻器官功能障碍和改善存活率有关。

DuBose等描述了在将创伤患者转运到达创伤中心的1 h内对其使用5%高渗盐水，并且发现对格拉斯哥昏迷评分<8分，头部简明创伤分级（Abbreviated Injury Scale，AIS）分数>3分的患者使用高渗盐水后，死亡率会得到改善。

尽管有这些好处，系统定量分析提示高渗盐水与等渗晶体液对创伤患者30天结果的影响却未能显示出生存优势。因此，高渗盐水在院前液体复苏中的作用还有待界定。

胶体液

非生物活性

作为复苏液体，与晶体液相比，胶体液似乎具有许多优点。在有效地增加血容量方面，胶体液要比晶体液强。可使用容量较小的胶体以达到末端复苏，这样做反过来减少了组织水肿。然而，一些研究者认为胶体液会增加组织水肿。在严重损伤后血管内皮细胞出现渗漏，可能使胶体液进入组织间隙并加剧肿胀。

白蛋白是一种天然胶体，在肝中合成，承担了血浆中80%的血浆胶体渗透压。白蛋白的分子量约为69 kDa。输注25%的溶液将使血容量增加为输注容量的4～5倍（表2）。由于白蛋白来自人体血浆库，经过严格的加热和灭菌，因而其传播传染性疾病的风险很低。除了容量替代上的特质，白蛋白还具有药物和内源性物质的转运功能，并且可以对自由基清除及膜渗透性有益。这些理论效应尚未在临床上得到证实。

表2 不同溶液对扩充血容量的作用

解决方法	体积灌注（ml）	扩充血容量（ml）
葡萄糖液（D_5W）	1000	100
乳酸林格液	1000	250
7.5%高渗盐水	250	1000
5%白蛋白	500	375
25%白蛋白	100	450
6%羟乙基淀粉	500	750

修改自 Modified from Rizoli SB: Crystalloids and colloids in trauma resuscitation: a brief overview of the current debate. J Trauma 54:S82–S88, 2003.

白蛋白的缺点包括成本高、供应不足和潜在的疾病传播风险。此外，已证明将白蛋白用于重症患者复苏时会增加甚至显著增加死亡率。因此，不能推荐将白蛋白用于低血压创伤患者的复苏液。

合成胶体包括右旋糖酐、HES以及右旋糖酐和HES与高渗盐水的混合溶液。右旋糖酐是将6%右旋糖酐70（分子量70 kDa）和10%右旋糖酐40（分子量40 kDa）溶液获得的葡萄糖聚合物。输注1000 ml右旋糖酐70后，血容量的增加范围为600～800 ml。右旋糖酐可降低血浆黏稠度，降低血小板的黏附性，并促进纤维蛋白溶解，导致出血倾向增加。也有文献描述了许多严重的、危及生命的过敏反应。当将右旋糖酐作为唯一的复苏液体时，会受到这些副作用的限制。

如前所述，右旋糖酐已经被加入到高渗盐水中以延长其血管内效应。作为复苏液，有学者将其与等渗晶体液进行比较，并针对低血压创伤患者的几项随机对照试验进行了系统的定量分析。虽然高渗盐水较为安全，但是会造成血压升高，并且在早期对复苏液体和血液的需求会降低，对它的使用没有统计学上的显著生存效益。相反，Wade等的研究发现，对于持续穿透性躯干创伤而需要外科干预的患者，使用250 ml高渗盐水作为复苏液后，患者存活出院的概率显著改善。这表明在院前环境中使用高渗盐水，可使部分创伤患者从中受益。

HES溶液是改良的淀粉天然聚合物。每种制剂的药代动力学性质由其分子量、羟乙基化模式和C2∶C6羟乙基化的比率确定。这些性质影响了HES的血容量增加、降解和副作用。

HES相关的副作用包括皮肤瘙痒和出血增加，这是由于Ⅷ因子和von Willebrand因子减少。然而，最新的研究显示现代HES制剂不会导致凝血机制受损或出血倾向增加。

尽管胶体液具有明显的优点，Meta分析表明当它们被用于创伤患者的复苏时，死亡率有增加的趋势。虽然这些研究的方法受到质疑，但直到有设计得更好的临床试验提供无可辩驳的证据表明使用胶体液体会改善复苏结果，这些制剂都不能被推荐使用。

生物活性

在考虑出血性休克的理想复苏液时，其特性应当包括容量增加、携氧能力、普遍相容性、即时可用性、长期储存能力以及没有血管活性和疾病传播。虽然输血能有效地改善容量不足并提供氧的输送，但其在院前环境中使用时会因为费用、保质期较短、供应不足、存在疾病传播的风险以及须交叉匹配而受到限制。同种异体红细胞可能具有不利的免疫炎症反应，因其可增加损伤后多器官功能衰竭（multiple organ failure，MOF）的风险。

因此，基于几种原因，血红蛋白类氧载体（hemoglobin-based oxygen carriers，$HBOC_S$）在院前环境中具有使用吸引力。因为可以对$HBOC_S$进行热处理，使其传播疾病的风险较低。它们的保质期高达3年，具有携氧以及增加容量的特性。它们是普遍兼容的，因此不须要进行交叉匹配。Ⅱ期临床试验以及离体和活体的研究表明用 $HBOC_S$ 代替储存的红细胞进行复苏，减轻了在多器官功能衰竭发病机制中的全身性炎症反应。

对 $HBOC_S$ 开展的临床试验显示出混杂的结果。在一项治疗严重创伤性出血性休克的美国多中心试验研究对双阿司匹林交联血红蛋白（aspirin cross-linked hemoglobin，DCLHb）和生理盐水进行了对比，表明 DCLHb 28 天的死亡率为 46%，而生理盐水为 17%。全身性和肺血管阻力的增加导致心输出量减少被认为是导致死亡率增加的原因。然而，聚合血红蛋白溶液显示更有前途。一项前瞻性随机试验比较了 Poly-Heme 与同种异体红细胞在治疗急性失血中的治疗效果。Poly-Heme 组在输注后表现出与红细胞组类似的总血红蛋白浓度，其中治疗的第一天需须要输较少的 RBC，并且没有由 Poly-Heme 引起的严重或意外的不良后果。在最新的对所有死亡数据分析的研究中，Bernard 等发现 Poly-Heme 受体与对照组相比存活时间更长。这种益处可能是因为这些患者早期进行有氧复苏。这种氧合作用可以在一定的时间内控制出血，否则选定组患者可能会失血而死。今后，可能在出血性休克的复苏中常规使用一种或多种 $HBOC_S$。

复苏目标

延迟

多项研究已经开始审视在不受控制的出血期间升高血压的潜在有害影响。尽管早期关于可控出血模型的工作被用于支持创伤后出血的液体复苏的实践中，这些复苏模型并不模仿实际生活中的不可控出血和同时进行的治疗的情况。在不可控出血的情况下，液体给药可能破坏血栓形成，通过稀释凝血因子引起凝血障碍，并导致出血增加。1918 年，Cannon 观察到因在出血控制之前进行快速补液引起出血增加。最近，在对穿透性躯干创伤的研究中，低血压患者被随机分为立即和延迟进行等渗晶体液复苏，并进行了对比。对立即组开始进行院前液体复苏，但延迟组直到在手术室控制出血后再进行。与延迟组患者相比，立即复苏组的患者死亡率更高，术后并发症的发生率更高。虽然本研究的结果存在争论，但该研究结果重新引起了人们的兴趣，并激发了对于不可控出血治疗方法的思考。

低血压

这种复苏策略试图对重要的器官保持足够的灌注，同时最大限度地减少进一步的出血。将平均动脉压（mean arterial pressure，MAP）为 60 mmHg 作为复苏目标。这一数值被认为是最低的安全水平，因为它是脑血流量自动调节的最低 MAP。然而，低血压复苏的下限没有得到明确。

将血压作为模拟院前场景的一种指南，即血压是唯一的血流动力学参数指标。Dutton 等随机研究了低血压钝挫伤或穿透性创伤患者，收缩压为 70 mm Hg（低血压）或高于 100 mmHg（血压正常）。使用晶体液或血液产品以维持每组的预期收缩压。研究显示两组之间的存活率没有差异性。这部分归因于难以维持目标血压。低血压组和血压正常组的平均收缩压分别为 100 mmHg 和 114 mmHg。这种反应提示是由内在的凝血机制引起的出血减少，并且可以验证在某些不可控出血的情况下使用这种复苏策略的可行性。

正常血压

在出血性休克中，对创伤患者进行复苏的传统方法是使用大容量的晶体液，然后输入血液产品来使血压正常。这种复苏方法是从受控出血的动物模型发展而来的。对重要器官灌注的恢复改善了生存，而未采取治疗的动物出现器官功能障碍和死亡。在不可控出血的情况下，动物研究显示内脏灌注减少以及失血更多。在出血已自然消退的情况下，复苏的标准方法是合理的。然而，难以预测出血是否已自发停止或可能通过积极的复苏而加重。

发病率和并发症

进行院前液体复苏并不是没有并发症。前文已经提到了可导致出血加重、凝血因子稀释和血栓脱出等，还有可能降低出血性休克患者的存活率。此外，须要在复苏不足和复苏过度之间达到平衡，因为这两个问题都会增加患者的发病率和死亡率。院前液体复苏的目的是保持血液流向重要器官（脑和心脏），而不会对其他器官系统（肾或内脏）造成显著的不可逆损伤，过量的晶体液复苏可能导致腹腔间隔室综合征的发展。

发生创伤性休克后常出现低体温，并且因使用冰冷液体而恶化。低体温的不良后果包括凝血功能障碍、氧输送减少和感染率增加。给予温暖的液体可避免低体温的带来的不利影响，这个重要性无论怎样强调都很有必要。

小结

对于大量失血和液体复苏开展的相关临床研究而言，由于数量少、救护紧迫、目标和结果各不相同，以及患者的年龄、患病情况、损伤机制、院前时间和采取的治疗措施以及复苏并发症的异质性而显得复杂化。可以从大量文献中得出一些明确的结论。将创伤患者快速运送至可提供明确救护措施的创伤中心是至关重要的。另外，在进一步液体复苏之前控制出血，这是须一再重要强调的。尽管有许多复苏策略和复苏液体可供选择，但没有单一的选择完全适用于每一个创伤现场。直到人们研究出可以针对特定损伤的特定策略，并且其改善结果得到证实之前，都应该继续实施 ATLS 指南。

地方医院对大规模人员伤亡事件的反应

Rochelle A. Dicker, William P. Schecter 著
张进军 译

2001 年 9 月 11 日，双子塔袭击事件激发了医疗界对常规武器和非常规武器攻击造成的大规模伤亡事件须做好更充分的准备。2004 年南亚地区海啸摧毁了沿海地区，2011 年日本海啸摧毁了沿海地区，2005 年卡特里娜飓风后新奥尔良爆发了洪水。这些都暴露了人们对自然灾害造成的基础设施损失方面的反应不足。因此，一个全面、协调和开展有效演练的灾难计划是至关重要的。东京地铁沙林毒气事件是一个对早期检测释放的毒气和第一批急救人员现场暴露于风险的典型示例。

关键定义

大规模伤亡事件，是指患者数量及其损伤严重程度超出了医疗机构以常规方式提供救护能力的伤亡事件。恰当的第一反应是首先治疗重大创伤患者中具有最大生存机会的人群，这样可以使宝贵的资源没有浪费在受伤轻微的患者或生存希望渺茫的患者身上。

群体伤亡事件是指医疗机构可以通过调动额外资源，以常规方式向大量患者提供救护的伤亡事件。我们的目标是，根据损伤的严重程度，适当地将患者分配送往各家医疗机构，从而将现场的大规模伤亡事件转换为每个接收医院的多人伤亡事件。

检伤分类是指根据患者的治疗需要和可利用的资源对患者进行分类。在大规模伤亡事件中，可能将传统的医疗标准提供给所有的伤者。分诊的目的是优化医疗资源，使最大数量的患者能够得到抢救。

在现场患者被分为四类：轻症、延迟、立即和死亡。在军事检伤分类体系中，还有第五类，即预期救护。他们将可用的稀缺资源用于几乎没有生存机会的患者，这会对其他可救治患者的生存机会产生负面影响。这种类别很少被用于平民，因为调动额外资源通常是可行的。可用数字、颜色或符号来代表分类（表 1）。检伤不足是指将患者分配到不能达到与其损伤程度所需的救护水平。分类过低率大于 5% 是不可接受的，因为可能导致严重创伤患者出现不必要的发病率和死亡率。检伤过度是指将患者分配到大于其损伤程度所需的救护水平。检伤过度率为 50% 被认为是可接受的，以将检伤不足率降至最低。但现场的检伤过度将威胁整个急救系统的反应，因为这会将有限的资源浪费在相对伤害轻微的患者身上。

表 1　检伤分类使用的四种颜色

颜色	描述
轻症—绿色	延迟救护 / 可以延迟长达 3 h
延迟—黄色	紧急救护 / 可以延迟长达 1 h
立即—红色	立即救护 / 危及生命
死亡—黑色	受害者死亡 / 无救护需求

Modified from Los Angeles Community Emergency Response Team

大规模伤亡事件的紧急救援

对大规模伤亡事件的反应须要许多具有不同文化、指挥结构甚至通信设备的救援机构共同协调完成（图 1）。急救机构应当向上级的现场指挥官报告事故状况。事先的联合演练可以打破各个救援部门之间的障碍，提高整体效应。

无论导致事件的原因如何，事件发生区域的安全必须有所保障。在使用常规武器进行恐怖袭击或军事攻击的情况下，必须查明和消灭其他敌方作战人员，以避免受到"第二次攻击"。国内恐怖分子可能会进行第二次攻击，如在格鲁吉亚的流产医院爆炸事件中，第二枚炸弹的设置就是针对急救人员。必须将伤者运出并集中到安全区域，进行检伤分类。对于须要立即救护的患者，应该在控制外部出血、保持气道稳定以及张力性气胸减压（如果存在）之后优先转运。

转运伤者去医院的车辆可能是救护车、公共汽车或私家车。易焦虑的患者和轻伤患者经常会自行来到医院，增加了医院接收的患者数量。

对现场人群的控制是一个重大问题。志愿者们的各种技能可能有所帮助或有所阻碍。最理想的情况是，应确保分诊区是安全和隔离的，由事件现场指挥官来决定其他人员是否能够介入事件并提供帮助。

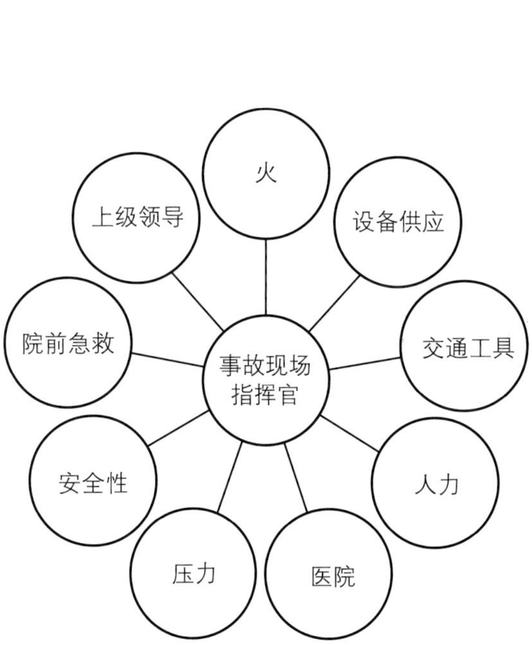

图 1　有关灾害响应的要素

医院检伤分类

在一个真正的大规模伤亡事件中，所有的地方医院都必须参与到对伤者的救护工作中，以避免集中在某一个机构。每家医院应在接到此类事件的通知或有大批伤员意外到达后，启动大规模伤亡事件应急预案。

必须取消所有的择期手术。急诊部门须要快速处置预留的患者。根据事件的大小，可以使适合的住院患者办理出院。并且如果患者需要的话，可以办理院内转移，以确保手术床的最大可用性。

医院最初的检伤分类（图 2）应在急诊部门外面进行。救护车在进入医院之前应通过一个安全检查站进行检查，以识别可能存在于车上的任何恐怖分子或军械。初始检伤分类应由有丰富经验的临床医生完成。如果条件允许，应该通过单独的入口护送可行走的伤员，以避免造成复苏区域过度拥挤。

一旦被担架抬进来的患者进入急诊科，资深外科医生应该将每一位患者分为立即救护或延迟救护（图 3）。应将立即救护区保留给损伤危及生命的需

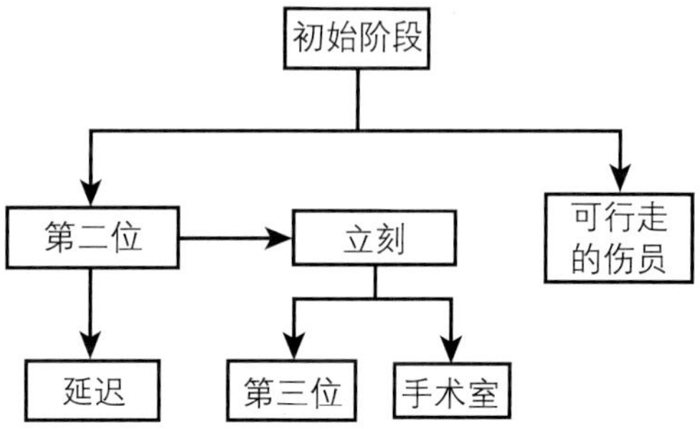

图 2　初始检伤分类站或手术室

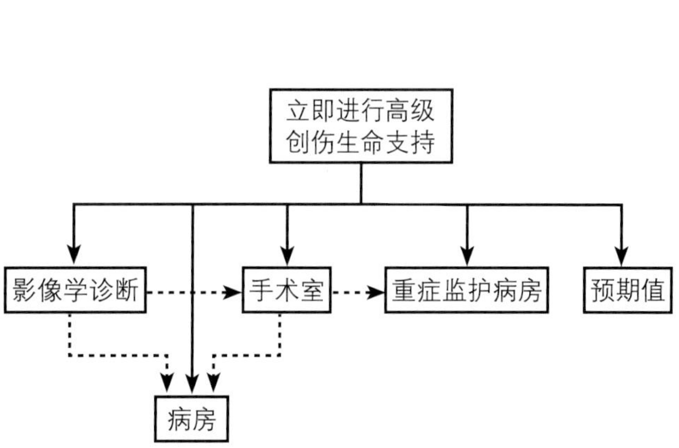

图 3　院内交通流量

要进行抢救的患者。以下人员应出现在立即救护区域中的病床旁：进行决策的资深外科医生，提供气道管理的麻醉师，以及两个急诊科或重症监护室的护士。如有必要的话，还应配备一名能建立血管通路和进行胸腔穿刺术的初级外科医生。

在立即救护区域中开展的治疗是基于高级创伤生命支持的原理。立即救护区域中的治疗目标是终止外部出血、进行气道评估、通气、建立血管通路以及把患者快速转移到下一个合适的治疗站，从而去完成第二次检查和其他的诊断或治疗程序。选择下一个救护场所（手术室、ICU 或放射科）时，是由资深外科医生或事故现场指挥官根据患者的状况和伤亡人数来确定的（图 4）。

应有扩大 ICU 的相关预案。麻醉后的救护区域是扩展 ICU 服务的理想选择。因为无须将大多数伤者立即进入手术室（除非他们由于弹片或创伤性截肢而具有穿透性创伤），甚至闲置的手术室也可被临时管理，以用于突发情况下的危重患者。

病情严重但没有危及生命的患者被分到延迟救护区，并且应该为这些患者分配一名初级外科医生和护士。然而，资深外科医生也应该对延迟救护区进行指导，并纠正分诊错误。

护士和医生应在医院的一个独立区域内对可行走的伤者进行处理。如果可能，外科医生或急诊医生应指挥这个区域。大多数可行走的患者在接受心理创伤筛查后就可以从急诊部门离开医院。

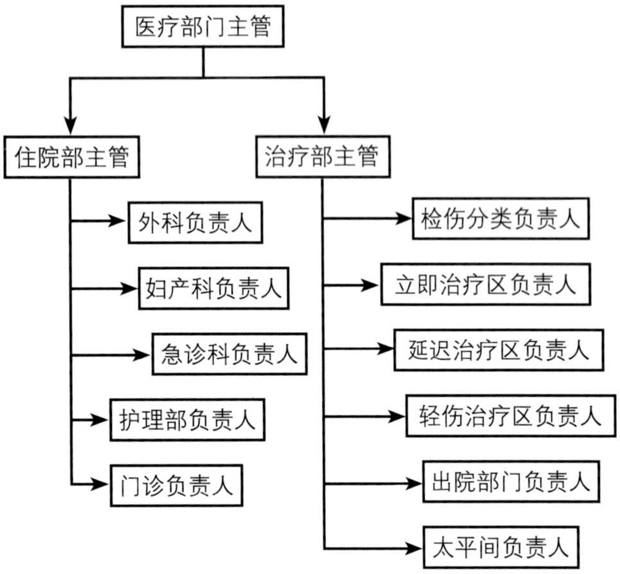

图 4　医院突发事件指挥系统的简化模型

医院紧急事件指挥系统

医院紧急事件指挥系统（Hospital Emergency Incident Command System）秉持的基本原则是，一个人所管理的人数不能超过五人，并且只向一个人汇报。资深外科医生是理想的事故现场指挥官。该系统要求具备有效的沟通渠道和直接问责制。有四个主要部门负责人：规划、后勤、财务和运营。运营主管全面负责对伤者进行检伤分类、临床救护工作以及与其他医院的沟通协调（图 5）。

在区域性灾难响应协调机制中，每家医院都必须发挥其作用。

例如，洛杉矶有 13 家具有确定级别的 Ⅰ 级和 Ⅱ 级创伤中心。然而，当发生大规模伤亡或群体伤害事件时，医疗警报中心（Medical Alert Center）将协调创伤中心和社区医院之间的伤亡分布情况，为受伤最严重的人提供 Ⅰ 级创伤救护，而不会使任何一个中心的救治负担过重。

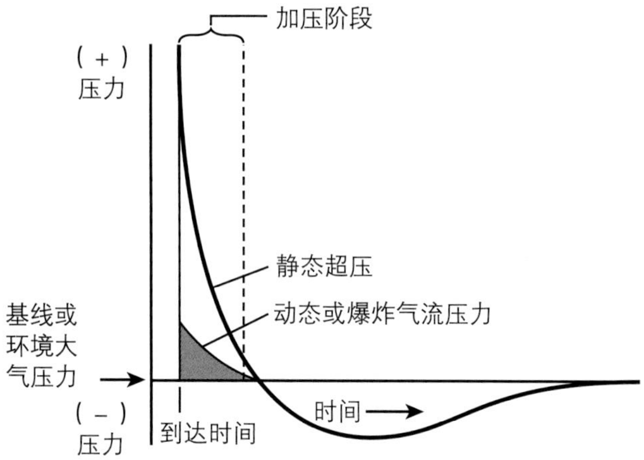

图 5　物理冲击波

发生大规模伤亡事件的原因

常规武器 / 爆炸伤

1980–2001 年，美国及其领土上几乎 70% 的恐怖袭击都属于炸弹伤害。许多恐怖炸弹包含各种弹片，如钉子和螺栓，这是能造成最大化伤亡人数的设计。

爆炸造成的伤害程度取决于几个因素：所用材

料、周围环境（开放空间或者封闭空间）、受害者与爆炸的距离以及是否存在防护屏障等。

当冲击波直接撞击身体表面时，会导致原发性爆炸伤。具有空气 - 流体界面的器官特别容易受到损伤（如肺、肠和耳朵），也可能发生对眼睛和大脑的损害。相关伤害的总结详见表 2。第二次爆炸伤害是由于飞行碎片造成的，它可以导致钝伤和穿透伤。第三次爆炸伤害发生时，受害者被爆炸波扔向固体物。第四次爆炸伤包括烧伤和挤压伤等其他损伤。可以将与爆炸直接有关的疾病，如创伤后应激障碍、支气管痉挛、心绞痛或吸入有毒气体，划分为第四次冲击伤。

爆炸性肺损伤是气压对肺实质的直接损伤，其临床表现类似于肺挫伤。最常见的症状和体征是咯血和缺氧而导致的呼吸困难、呼吸急促和顺应性差。与肺挫伤不同的是，肺损伤通常不伴有肋骨骨折。典型的胸部 X 线检查结果包括浸润、纵隔气肿、血胸和气胸的“蝴蝶”模式（图 6）。

如果需要机械通气，则应将潮气量、峰值吸气压力和呼气末正压水平保持在尽量低的水平，以降低与呼吸机相关的气压性肺炎的风险。有时，患者还会由于肺泡毛细血管膜破裂而导致神经系统症状或出现冠状动脉闭塞的双侧空气栓塞。

表 2　爆炸导致相关伤害的范围

器官 / 系统	影响
听觉	鼓膜破裂（常与肺爆炸性肺损伤同时出现）、耳穿孔、异物
眼睛、眼眶和面部	眼球破裂、异物、骨折、空气栓塞
呼吸系统	肺震伤、肺挫伤、左侧气胸、空气栓塞、穿刺
循环系统	心肌挫伤、心肌梗死（空气栓塞）、失血性休克
神经系统	闭合性或开放性颅脑损伤、脑卒中或脊髓损伤、空气栓塞、闭合性脊髓损伤
肾	挫伤、裂伤、低血压或横纹肌溶解症导致的急性肾衰竭
胃肠道	肠穿孔、出血、实体器官损伤，肠系膜缺血（空气栓塞）
肢体*	截肢、粉碎、骨折、筋膜室综合征、烧伤、血管损伤

* 最常见的需要手术干预的系统

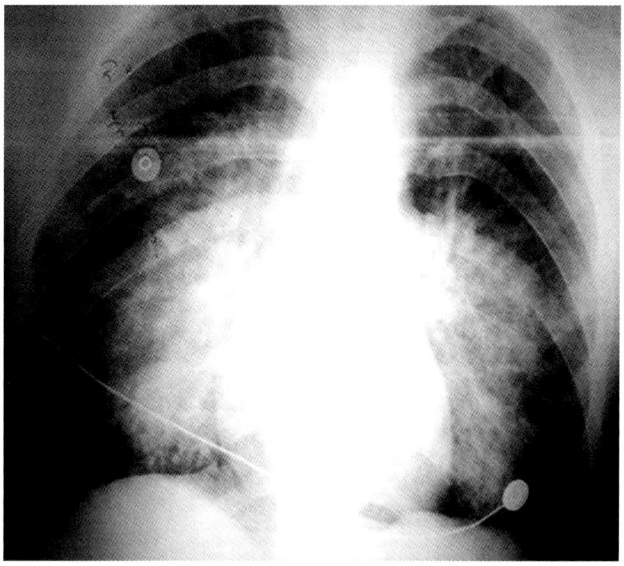

图 6　爆炸性肺损伤

生物制剂

与传统的大规模伤亡事件不同，生物恐怖袭击的破坏程度在一段时间内可能是未知的。许多受害者最初可能不知道他们已经被感染并且具有传染性。在确认攻击发生之前卫生保健机构可能就已经受到了污染。

根据对人群造成的风险程度，美国对生物制剂进行了分类。A 类制剂易于传播，具有较高的致死率，会引起大众恐慌，并且需要大量的公共卫生方面的努力才能控制疾病的传播。表 3 列出了四种主要 A 类制剂的携带主体、特点和管理方法。

B 类制剂具有中等传播性，在导致发病和死亡上具有中度风险。B 类疾病 / 制剂包括布鲁菌病、产气荚膜梭菌、沙门菌、大肠埃希菌、志贺菌、鼻疽、蓖麻毒素、斑疹伤寒、链球菌肠毒素 B、Q 热、鹦鹉热、水安全威胁和病毒性脑炎。

C 类制剂是新出现的病原体，未来可以被设计为生物武器。它们会导致很高的发病率和死亡率。

医疗卫生机构和医院对生物恐怖袭击的反应

在使用 A 类生物武器的袭击中，可能没有明显的初始场景。患者与医疗卫生机构间的第一次接触可以是在医生的办公室、独立诊所或急诊室。多家公共卫生机构将暴露在病原体下，包括医院及其工作人员。

对生物袭击的处理原则与对流行病的处理原则

表 3 A 类疾病 / 制剂*

疾病	携带主体	潜伏期	传播途径	演变	治疗	预防
炭疽†	炭疽芽孢杆菌	1 天至 8 周	吸入，皮肤接触，摄入	症状类似流感，并有呼吸衰竭，X 线胸片显示纵隔增宽	氟喹诺酮或多西环素	灭活疫苗，有限的可用性
肉毒杆菌中毒	肉毒梭菌产生的 7 种毒素	12~72 h	摄入，吸入孢子（没有人传人）	对称的脑神经病变从近端到远端肌肉逐渐衰弱，呼吸功能不全	通过机械通气可以持续 2~3 个月，同时神经功能恢复	研究五价疫苗
瘟疫	鼠疫耶尔森菌	2~8 天（如果吸入，可能时间更短）	感染的跳蚤，生物恐怖袭击，可能雾化	发热、咳嗽、咯血、胸痛	多西环素，第二选择是环丙沙星	在美国不可用
天花	天花病毒	7~17 天	吸入，可人传人，或与损伤的皮肤接触	发热及肌痛，主要是面部和四肢的皮疹	接种疫苗，除外怀孕或免疫功能低下者	活病毒疫苗，不得终身免疫

* 病毒性出血热，例如，现在丝状病毒和沙粒病毒也被认为是一种潜在威胁的类别

类似：①快速检测和严格隔离患者。②识别和治疗接触者。③严格进行医院感染控制，可能包括封锁医院。④避免葬礼上与尸体密切接触。这些公共卫生措施十分重要，但是很难实现。

在生物袭击中受伤的患者很可能是通过吸入途径而被感染的。常规隔离对所有这些患者都已足够。那些具有高度传染性的病毒性出血的患者除外，须由穿戴 A 级防护服的专业人员对他们进行严格的隔离和治疗。

化学制剂

有四种类型的化学武器可能被用于恐怖袭击——神经性毒剂、氰化物、糜烂性毒剂及窒息性毒剂。其中最有可能使用的化学武器是神经性毒剂和氰化物。

神经性毒剂

神经毒剂是有机磷化合物，能抑制突触和神经肌肉连接处的胆碱酯酶，导致乙酰胆碱过量引起胆碱能危象。已经有五种神经毒剂被用作武器：沙林、梭曼、塔崩、GF 和 VX。

胆碱能危象的症状和体征

乙酰胆碱与突触后细胞膜上的受体、平滑肌终端和分泌腺体结合，导致乙酰胆碱的毒蕈碱效应。这些影响包括支气管痉挛、肺顺应性低、恶心、呕吐、腹泻、瞳孔缩小、视力模糊、心动过缓，以及口咽、结膜、支气管和胃肠道的过度分泌。

乙酰胆碱也能结合骨骼肌终板和突触神经节，引起烟碱效应。乙酰胆碱的烟碱效应包括肌束震颤、松弛性麻痹、心动过速和高血压。由于烟碱效应和毒蕈碱效应的作用相反，所以在胆碱能危象期间心率是变化的。当胆碱能危象的严重程度增加时，患者可能经历初始的心动过速及后续的心动过缓。

神经性毒剂损伤的治疗

有两种独立的用于胆碱能危象的解毒剂。阿托品是毒蕈碱效应非常有效的解毒剂，但对烟碱效应没有效果。阿托品通过竞争性地结合突触后毒蕈碱受体，从而置换乙酰胆碱。临床上给予阿托品，直至分泌物减少，肺顺应性改善。

乙酰胆碱的烟碱效应的解毒剂是一类称为肟类化合物的药物。在美国，氯化吡啶肟是选定的肟类化合物。肟作为“分子撬棍”，将神经剂与胆碱酯酶分开，从而使乙酰胆碱在烟碱受体处分解。不幸的是，必须在神经剂和胆碱酯酶发生不可逆结合之前使用肟类化合物，这种现象被称为衰老。持续时间在 2 min 到几个小时之间发生变化。

治疗轻度至中度神经性毒剂损伤的初始推荐药物是肌内注射 2 mg 阿托品和肌内注射 600 mg 氯普胺氯化物。对于严重的损伤，可肌内注射 6 mg 阿托

品和肌内注射 1200 mg 氯普胺氯化物。

氰化物

第二次世界大战期间，纳粹集中营毒气室的犯罪效率证明了氰化物是一种非常有效的化学武器。氰化物的挥发性很高，从而使其在开放空间中由于快速传播而成为无效的武器。

中度地暴露于氰化物会导致皮肤和静脉血液呈现出鲜红的外观及代谢性酸中毒，并发出苦杏仁的气味。严重的暴露会导致昏迷、呼吸暂停和心搏骤停。

最新出现的氰化物中毒的解毒剂包括“溶液 A 和 B”，即溶解于柠檬酸和碳酸钠中的硫酸亚铁，两者都是口服药。它们仅对减少吞入氰化物的吸收有效。对于硝酸戊酯，可以通过吸入给药，但其在安全性和有效性记录方面存在问题。存在中毒严重的人可以静脉内给予二钴，但它本身也是有毒的。

糜烂性毒剂

芥子气是液态化学武器，其引起对皮肤和黏膜的烧伤并诱导骨髓抑制。对它的治疗涉及去污、烧伤创面的处理和血液学异常的治疗。20 世纪 80 年代，伊拉克在两伊战争期间使用了芥子气，至少造成 4 万名伊朗人受到了严重伤害。

窒息性毒剂

在第一次世界大战期间，氯气和光气等是引起肺水肿和呼吸功能不全的化学武器。暴露于这些毒剂下的患者会出现胸闷，并在 2 ~ 4 h 内发展成咳嗽、声音嘶哑、肺扩张和缺氧，取决于暴露的程度。实质上肺损伤类似于暴露于烟和燃烧的塑料而引起的吸入性损伤。

化学武器袭击对事故现场管理和医院灾害事件应急计划的作用和影响

如果怀疑现场有化学制剂，那么在现场提供救援的每个人都应穿防护服。条件准许的话，在将伤者转送到医院之前应在现场对其进行消毒（图 7）。

Aum Shinrikyo 日本沙林恐怖袭击事件的经验表明，神经性毒剂更像是一种“大规模歇斯底里”性武器，而不是“大规模毁灭性”武器。大多数严重的患者在现场死亡，大量忧心忡忡的人群或轻度暴露的患者会涌入医院。正如东京沙林毒气袭击事件，保证医院安全和早期封锁对防止医疗机构和人员被污染是必要的措施。但在第一位患者到达之前可能没有时间去部署去污设备。旧金山总医院（San Francisco General Hospital）在预先安排的白天演练期间，在主要参演人员集合之前，需要至少 1 h 来架设去污帐篷。

去污是处理的关键部分。早期的去污措施能保护患者免于被进一步暴露，后期的去污能保护医疗队。脱掉衣物可以简单地去掉约 80% 的液体神经制剂造成的污染。在恐怖主义神经性毒剂袭击的情况下，去污淋浴应该是医院大规模伤亡事件应急计划的一部分。当然，在寒冷气的天气进行去污时，遇到的低温问题还有待解决。

对于有严重胆碱能危象的患者，需要医护人员在去污区佩戴个人防护装备后才能进行复苏。由未经培训、穿着厚重防护服的工作人员对大量神经中毒导致的大量胆碱能危象的患者进行高效复苏，这种想法十分天真。外科医生和麻醉师应该知道神经

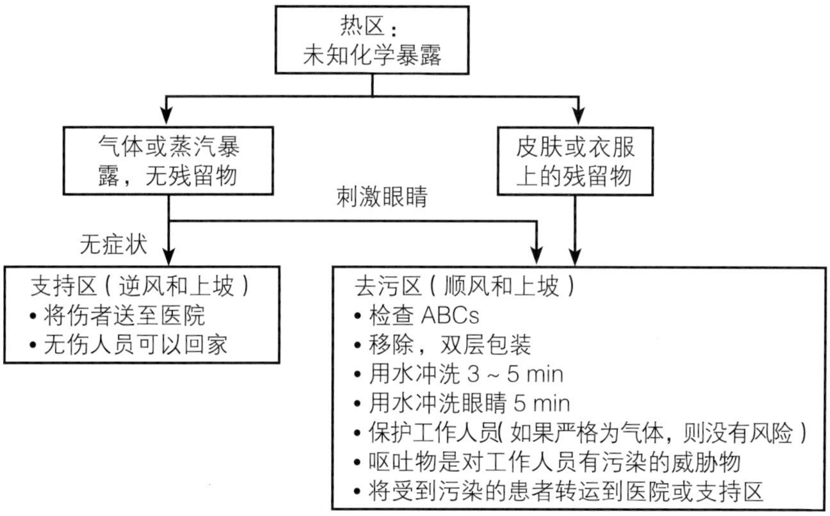

图 7　现场化学污染清除的流程图。ABCs，气道、呼吸和循环（*firway，breathing and circulation*）

性毒剂对神经肌肉阻滞的增强作用以及过度分泌和支气管痉挛对全身麻醉的影响，在神经性毒剂中受到损害的患者须进行手术治疗。

辐射损伤

有三种不同类型的可能的辐射暴露。第一种暴露是由辐射扩散装置（脏弹）造成的常规爆炸伤害引起的，辐射水平通常不足以高到引起急性综合征（见后文）。因为85%的发射性物质在去除衣物时就已被去除，因而对医护人员的辐射暴露是很小的。第二种暴露发生在无意或故意损害核电厂反应堆之后，受害者受到爆炸和辐射伤害。首先接触的人将面临严重辐射的风险，并且可能污染周围地区。第三种暴露是核爆炸在现场造成大规模破坏和大量人员伤亡。

严重的辐射暴露会导致脱发、烧伤、急性放射病（acute radiation sickness，ARS）和死亡。有三种综合征与大量暴露相关：造血系统综合征、胃肠道综合征和神经系统/心血管综合征。造血系统综合征的初始症状是恶心、呕吐和厌食。在潜伏期，骨髓中的干细胞死亡。直接暴露（超过120 rad）的患者可能在几个月内死亡，不太严重的患者可能完全康复。

胃肠道综合征的初始症状类似于造血系统综合征并伴有腹泻的症状。该综合征的 LD_{100}（完全致死剂量）大约为1000 rad，伤者会死于感染和脱水。在暴露量>2000 rad时能观察到心血管/中枢神经系统综合征。其初始症状与胃肠道综合征的症状类似，伴有精神状态改变，也可在数小时内发生惊厥和昏迷。

第一急救者应穿戴个人防护装备。应将应急设备和去污区置于受污染区域的上风处。在将无生命危险的爆炸伤患者运送到医院之前应在现场进行消毒。

医院应配备辐射测量装置，并应在急诊室外设立独立的去污区。与化学暴露一样，去污时应包括去除所有衣物并用水彻底洗涤；应先清洗明显的伤口；对符合急性放射病症状的患者应进行对症治疗。在患者去污之后，卫生保健工作者就不会有遭受辐射损伤的风险。患者虽然受到辐射照射的影响，但并不是放射性的。可从辐射紧急援助中心（Radiation Emergency Assistance Center）和培训机构以及医疗放射生物学咨询小组（Medical Radiobiology Advisory Team）等处获得更多的帮助。

大规模伤亡期间的通讯系统

有关当局可能关闭手机系统，以防止第二次袭击再次导致大规模伤亡事件或者由于家庭成员出于担心而大量通话，这些都可能使通信系统不堪重负。所以在大规模伤亡事件后，立即使用标准通讯设备是不明智的。发生大规模伤亡事件时，以色列的区域防御弹药（Area Defense Anti-Munitions，ADAM）系统要求以色列医院开放通讯中心。市政官员、卫生部、法医研究所和警察都可以通过ADAM轻松地获取所需信息。

结论

外科医生应该在应对灾难和大规模伤亡事件方面发挥积极作用。制订周密的计划并且进行有效的检伤分类和资源分配对于最大限度地保护生命是至关重要的。除了恐怖袭击外，大规模伤亡事件很可能涉及常规的爆炸装置。但是，如果发生化学、生物或辐射攻击，医疗机构应制订灾难应急方案。

爆炸伤

Howard R. Champion 著
张进军 译

炸药已被用于美国参与的每一次重大冲突，如今是导致美国战斗人员受伤的主要原因（图1）。炸药中最著名的是简易爆炸装置（improvised explosive devices，IEDs），也常被用于平民目标。在发生针对平民的炸弹袭击后，现场救援人员负责检伤分类和转运，然后医院人员必须重新进行检伤分类并重新评估所有送达的患者。大多数爆炸事件都是大规模伤亡事件，因此，在混乱的、患者激增的情况下，早期识别症状，找出更为严重的伤害症状是优化患者治疗结果的关键。

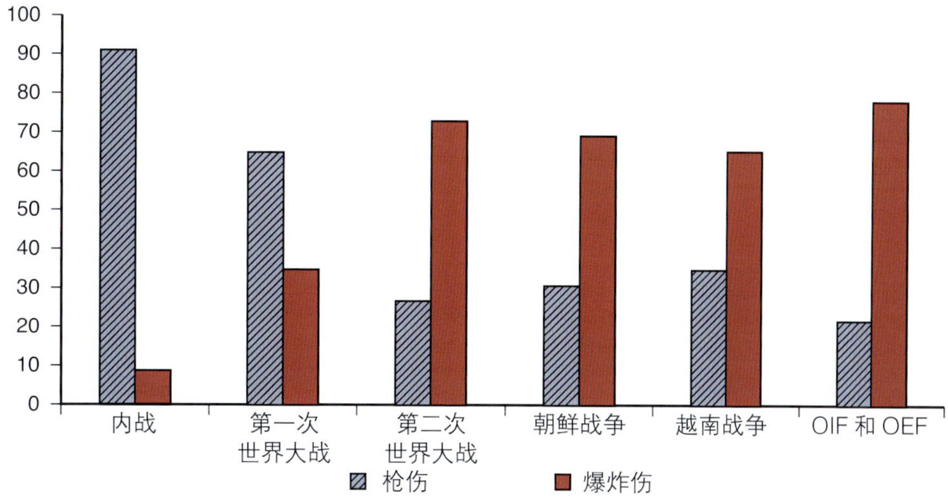

图 1 美国军队从内战开始到目前冲突的爆炸和枪伤的伤害和致死机制。OEF (Operation Enduirg Freedom)，持久自由行动（阿富汗）；OIF (Operation Iraqi Freedom)，伊拉克自由行动（伊拉克）(*数据来自 Data from Bellamy RF, Zajtchuk R: Assessing the effectiveness of conventional weapons. In Conventional warfare: ballistic, blast, and burn injuries. Washington, D.C., Office of the Surgeon General, 1991, pp 53–82; Beebe GW, DeBakey ME: Death from wounding. In Battle casualties, Springfield, Ill., Charles C Thomas, 1952, pp 74–147; Reister FA: Battle casualties and medical statistics: U.S. Army experience in the Korean war.Washington, D.C., The Surgeon General, Department of the Army, 1973; HardawayRM: Viet Nam wound analysis. J Trauma 18:635–643, 1978; GlobalWar on Terrorismby Reason, October 7, 2001 through April 4, 2011. Available at http://siadapp.dmdc.osd.mil/personnel/CASUALTY/gwot_reason.pdf. ; Gawande A: Casualties of war—Military care for the wounded from Iraq and Afghanistan. N Engl J Med 351:2471–2475, 2004.*)

发病率

炸药是在战斗中恐怖分子最常使用的武器。在阿富汗和伊拉克，在 5 万名伤亡的美国部队中几乎 3/4 是由爆炸装置（常常是简易爆炸装置 * ）造成的。在世界各地的民众中，从 1990 年 1 月至 2011 年 4 月间，发生了 77 134 起恐怖袭击事件，共造成近 50 万人（分别为 317 029 人和 157 023 人）受伤和死亡，其中有 60% 的人是由炸药造成的 †。

损伤机制和诊断

炸弹内装有爆炸材料，是由时钟或其他装置引发爆炸。恐怖分子使用的炸弹主要是简易爆炸装置，可能有多种设计或爆炸物，有两种类型：①常规性（装有含氢、氧、氮和碳的化学类炸药）。②分散性（装有化学药品或投射物如钉子、钢丸、螺钉和螺母）。核装置（在本章范围之外）依赖于核裂变或融合。术语“爆炸损伤”是指当活体暴露于爆炸时发生的生物物理学和病理生理事件以及临床综合征。

爆炸伤是独特的，因为它们具有多种损伤机制，包括钝性的、穿透性和热的损伤机制。因此，了解爆炸效应机制的相关知识以及早期识别潜在损伤在爆炸伤患者的管理中是至关重要的。根据基本机制可将爆炸伤分为五类（表 1）。

一级爆炸伤

一级爆炸伤是由压力差（高压和低压交替）的影响造成的。最容易发生原发性损伤的是具有密度界面的器官，即耳、肺和胃肠道。压力的影响具体见表 2。

* 为从 2001 年 10 月 7 日至 2011 年 4 月 4 日之间的数据。这个军事数据集中的爆炸类别包括：武器装备，火炮 / 迫击炮 / 火箭；武器装备，炸弹；武器装备，手榴弹；武器装备，火箭推进手榴弹。“武器装备，炸弹”是迄今为止最大的类别，86% 的爆炸伤害和死亡与其相关。

† 民用数据集中的爆炸类别包括以下内容：纵火 / 燃烧弹、轰炸和自杀式事件。“轰炸”类别包括了几乎 70% 的爆炸伤害和死亡与其相关。

表 1　爆炸：相互作用和损伤、分类、典型伤害以及受到影响的身体部位的关系链

爆炸的相互作用	损伤分类	典型伤害
爆炸 ↓ 爆炸所产生的冲击波 ↓ 冲击波消散 ↓ 爆炸气浪 ↓ 爆炸气浪推动物体、爆炸碎片、人 ↓ 产生热、火焰、气体和烟雾，也可能释放细菌或辐射	**一级爆炸伤**	
	由压力引起的直接组织损伤	伤及主要有密度界面的器官，例如：鼓膜破裂、肺爆炸伤、眼睛损伤、腹部出血、脑震荡，也可炸裂组织和四肢
	二级爆炸伤	
	由来自爆炸装置的一级碎片（套管以及被装入的成分）和二级碎片（来自环境的投射物，如碎片、玻璃和车辆金属等）	任何 / 所有的身体部位 穿透性损伤、创伤性截肢、眼睛损伤、撕裂伤、脑震荡和多发伤是最常见的损伤类型
	三极爆炸伤	
	由爆炸冲击波产生的损伤，是将人推进硬物内或将硬物推到人的身上。包括由建筑物的结构损坏和坍塌所造成的损伤	任何 / 所有的身体区域 钝性损伤、挤压和隔室综合征、骨折、外伤性损伤和截肢、脑损伤、脑震荡
	四级爆炸伤	
	其他爆炸影响造成的伤害，包括热、有毒气体和环境污染	任何 / 所有的身体区域 烧伤、吸入性损伤、环境污染造成的伤害、窒息
	五级爆炸伤	
	由加入到爆炸装置中的成分导致的损伤带来的伤害，如辐射或细菌；包括由推进性生物材料如骨折碎片引起的疾病传播	任何 / 所有的身体区域 辐射病，增加疾病发生的风险

数据来自 Data from Federal Emergency Management Agency: Explosive blast. In Primer to design safe schools projects in case of terrorist attacks, Washington, D.C., Federal Emergency Management Agency, 2003, 4-1–4-13; Department of Defense Directive. Medical Research for Prevention, Mitigation, and Treatment of Blast Injuries. Number 6025.21E. July 5, 2006 (Defense Technical Information Center website). Available at http://www.dtic.mil/whs/directives/corres/pdf/602521p.pdf. Accessed May 25, 2011; DePalma RG, Burris DG, Champion HR, et al: Blast injuries.N Engl J Med 352:1335–1342, 2005; Explosions and blast injuries: A primer for clinicians. CDC Mass Casualties. Reviewed June 14, 2006. Available at http://www.bt.cdc.gov/masscasualties/explosions.asp

表 2　对无任何保护的人员短时间压力产生的影响

压力（psi）	影响
5	可能导致耳膜破裂
15	发生鼓膜破裂的概率为 50%
30~40	轻微肺损伤
80	发生肺损伤的概率为 50%
100~200	死亡的可能性不大
130~180	死亡的可能性为 50%
200~250	极可能死亡

Table reproduced from Nursing Mirror with kind permission of EMAP. psi，磅 / 每平方英寸

诊断和管理

患者在如下情况时发生一级爆炸伤的风险更大：接近爆炸点时，在封闭的空间时（无论爆炸发生在封闭空间的内部还是外部），接近能够反射和放大冲击波的固体表面如墙面时。对一级爆炸伤的诊断较为复杂，因为它可能很少或没有外部损伤的迹象，并且症状可能不是立即显现的。

耳朵

出现如下情况时应怀疑有耳外伤：有耳出血或渗出物，耳痛、耳鸣或眩晕，直接听力丧失或偶尔出现短暂听力丧失。鼓膜破裂是耳朵最常见的损伤，但高压可能引起更显著的损伤，如听小骨的脱臼和断裂、耳蜗损伤、卵圆形或圆窗的创伤性破坏以及随后的永久性听力损失。疾病预防控制中心（Centers for Disease Control and Prevention，CDC）建议，暴露在爆炸事件下的患者应接受耳科的专业评估和听力测量。

鼓膜损伤发生在低压情况下，需要压力更大才能对其他结构造成损害。这一事实表明，鼓膜穿孔

是一级爆炸伤的指标。然而，最近的研究表明鼓膜穿孔是不可靠的指标。因此，应对所有爆炸的伤者评估一级爆炸伤，无论其鼓膜是否穿孔。

在治疗鼓膜破裂时，不应将异物从耳朵中除去，也不应注入水或其他非无菌物质。既不能注入预防性抗生素，也不能注入耳科悬浮液，但可以使用眼科的庆大霉素。治疗原则主要包括对疼痛的处理。如果存在明显的碎片或持续性症状，应转给耳鼻喉专家诊治。

肺

肺的一级爆炸伤（通常称为“爆炸肺”）发生在56～76磅/每平方英寸（psi）的空气压力下，有时伴有呼吸暂停、心动过缓和低血压。患者可在一开始就出现明显的体征和症状，也可以在最初事故发生后48 h内出现。爆炸性肺损伤的潜在特征包括初始体征和症状容易被低估或遗漏，并且患者的状况可能快速恶化到需要机械通气。对临床医生而言，警告症状可分为大出血或空气逃逸两类。常见的原发性损伤的非特异性症状有胸痛和呼吸困难，可通过发绀和呼吸急促等进行确认。

CDC建议对暴露于爆炸下的所有人进行胸部X线片检查，以排除爆炸肺。可以通过特征性的“蝴蝶”模式来识别爆炸肺。如果不会引起治疗延迟，也可以使用CT、多普勒扫描以及动脉血气分析以帮助做出诊断。当怀疑有爆炸肺时，CDC还建议在行空运后送或全身麻醉之前进行胸腔穿刺术。

对爆炸性肺损伤的治疗与肺挫伤的治疗类似。治疗方式包括液体管理（无容量超负荷）和给予高流量氧，必要时治疗气道损伤，存在血胸或气胸时要及时减压和插管（要小心，以免发生肺泡破裂和空气栓塞）。

腹部

腹部的一级爆炸伤是高度致死性的，并且可以几乎没有初始迹象。临床检查可能显示腹膜炎、无肠鸣音、休克、腹部压痛和随后出现败血症。直接损伤可包括肠系膜损伤、实体器官撕裂、睾丸破裂、出血（血肿和随后的阻塞、胃肠道出血和腹腔积血）或内容物的脱出（纵隔炎或腹膜炎）。症状可能包括腹部、直肠或睾丸疼痛、恶心、呕吐、呕血、里急后重以及不明原因的血容量减少或任何急腹症征象。肠穿孔可立即显现或者数小时都不明显。隐性症状及其他危及生命的伤害往往使腹部损伤难以识别，因此，有必要进行反复的临床检查。

头部

由一级爆炸效应引起的其他损伤包括面部骨折、脑震荡、脑空气栓塞和眼睛创伤。轻度创伤性脑损伤已经成为过去十年中的主要问题。大量研究正努力探索其发生的机制、可能影响性能的症状和认知减退，诊断方法包括生物测定、治疗方式和长期后果的研究。伴随脑震荡的创伤性脑损伤可能是由一级爆炸（如在伊拉克和阿富汗）引起的，特别是患者接近引爆点并且当他们出现头痛、疲劳、注意力无法集中、抑郁、焦虑或昏睡等症状时。研究人员目前正在探索由爆炸冲击波造成的脑损伤的机制在军事作战和平民条件下是否有所不同，以及多次暴露于低水平爆炸是否会导致长期后遗症。

四肢

当一级爆炸冲击波向长骨延伸时，它们产生强大的剪切力，可以撕裂软组织并导致粉碎性骨折或创伤性截肢（尽管对于冲击波是否是造成该结果的唯一原因还存在某些不确定性）。后者发生在违反直觉的位置，即沿着轴与通过关节的路径的1/3。创伤性截肢也可能是由三级爆炸效应所致，具有较高的死亡率（在病例中占50%～99%）。对于所有患有爆炸相关损伤的患者，应始终考虑进行筋膜室综合征四室切开减压术。

二级爆炸伤

炸药产生的最常见的影响是由一级和二级碎片的高速扩散引起的。碎片投射物能以每秒2700英尺的速度移动，这是穿透皮肤所需速度的50倍，并且几乎是进入和损坏所有主要体腔所需速度的7倍。它们比典型的简易爆炸装置超压爆炸效应更强，从而导致更多的伤害。主要碎片包括由炸弹壳体的破坏和炸弹壳体内的尖锐物（为增加伤害潜力而添加）产生的射弹。二级碎片通常包括投射物和破碎的周围环境的碎片，包括玻璃。

二级爆炸伤是与爆炸事件相关的最常见的损伤类型，不管是发生在平民还是战斗人员中。目前大多数战争伤亡具有继发性/碎片性损伤（有些伴有一级爆炸伤）。由于战斗员身着防弹衣，肢体损伤是最常见的与爆炸有关的战争伤害。这些通常包括大撕裂、多个小伤口（“胡椒刀”）和受伤的四肢。高爆导弹引起的细碎射弹路径迫使外来物体和污染物深入组织内。

诊断和管理

与一级爆炸伤不同，由碎片引起的二级爆炸伤的诊断和治疗方式与其他穿透性损伤相同。虽然这些损伤中很多是不重要的软组织和骨骼损伤，然而这些损伤可能数量较多，并且广泛，处理上也较为耗时。需要记住的重要事项包括：

- 看似无关紧要的伤口可能预示存在潜在胸部、腹部或血管损伤。小伤口可能会掩盖大碎片的入口伤口。
- 在穿透性肢体损伤患者中，应评估血管的完整性以排除延迟性血管闭塞。
- 应该尽可能快地冲洗贯通的伤口，并将其造成的危险最小化，包括去除坏死组织和容易深入的碎片。
- 通常须要延迟闭合创面，特别是伤口涉及肌肉、臀部或大腿时。对于不易立即采取措施或不容易发现的碎片可以随后去除。
- 在爆炸的幸存者中，由于碎片所致的穿透性眼损伤很常见，所以应该进行眼部检查。如果怀疑存在任何眼部损伤，应该将眼睛遮住。
- 当存在多个穿透性伤口时，应优先排除心脏或血管损伤。

三级爆炸伤

三级爆炸伤是由于建筑物、车辆和其他物体的倒塌和破碎引起的，包括大型物体（如混凝土块）和钝力碰撞引起挤压造成的截肢。在炸弹爆炸现场，建筑物倒塌是导致大量人员死亡的常见原因，也是影响伤者预后的主要因素。在比较爆炸类型的结果时，结构性崩塌所致的立即死亡率占25%，而没有发生结构性崩塌所占的立即死亡率占4%。

当受害者自身被冲击波炸飞并与附近的物体发生碰撞时，也可能发生三级爆炸伤。这些爆炸伤者通常非常接近爆炸点，因此经常有多种损伤，如脊髓、骨、头部以及实体和空腔器官受伤。任何身体部位都可能受到伤害，并且开放性骨折、创伤性肢体损伤和脑损伤也并不罕见。

诊断和管理

三级爆炸伤可遵循任何钝性创伤的典型模式，因此本身没有特殊的治疗参考。复杂性的因素与其他损伤的并发症或与大规模伤亡事故相关。

身陷倒塌的建筑物瓦砾下可以导致挤压综合征，从而可能导致肾衰竭、酸中毒和代谢紊乱而死亡。在被长时间埋压的患者中，发生横纹肌溶解的风险较高，具有与再灌注一致的损伤以及深色尿液（如果有的话）。可以通过血清肌酐激酶或尿肌红蛋白升高来确认诊断，并且用强化水合作用、尿碱化、甘露醇利尿、肾替代疗法以及调整电解质作为治疗方法。

在被困的情况下，发生筋膜室综合征的风险也升高。因此，临床医生应该注意早期症状，包括与损伤成正比的疼痛、被动拉伸的疼痛以及隔室紧张和肿胀。晚期症状包括感觉异常、无力、苍白和麻痹。可采用压力监测以确认临床诊断，但只有当怀疑指数较高且不延迟治疗时才适用。如果不执行筋膜切开术以减轻隔室压力，则筋膜室综合征可能导致肢体截肢甚至患者死亡。

四级爆炸伤

四级爆炸伤包括灼伤、吸入性损伤、辐射暴露或诸如一氧化碳、氰化物、有毒粉尘或气体等物质吸入引起的窒息。四级爆炸伤可能加重慢性疾病，如哮喘、糖尿病、高血压、冠状动脉疾病、精神健康问题和药物滥用，并引发行为问题。

烧伤可能是由爆炸、火球引起的闪光烧伤/皮肤烧伤，可以是全部，也可以是部分烧伤。燃烧弹中的材料可能导致严重烧伤。比起露天空间，封闭空间中的爆炸会对更大面积的体表造成影响。烧伤在爆炸事件中比在其他类型的创伤中更常见。烧伤患者经常并发其他钝挫伤或穿透伤，这将给临床治疗带来一定的困难。例如，在需要液体给药的烧伤患者和需要液体限制的爆炸肺患者，需要复杂的侵入性监测来用于液体管理。

在船舶上，吸入性伤害可能是由气体或颗粒成分引起的，而额外的伤害可能是由组织剂如哈龙引起的，这可能导致缺氧。哈龙比空气重，因此，其碳释放增加了在较低的位置造成吸入伤害的危险因素。在最近的一个例子中，一位伤员被放置在已经着火的后送直升机的地板上，因吸入哈龙而导致呼吸窘迫。

诊断和管理

如果从爆炸装置本身或爆炸所点燃材料的烟雾中吸入了化学品或毒素，则可能引起吸入性损伤。有许多变量可影响诊断和治疗，如吸入的物质的类型和数量，暴露的持续时间和患者患有的其他疾病（如高龄或心肺疾病等）。

五级爆炸伤

五级爆炸伤是指由于皮肤和黏膜吸入爆炸物释放的有毒物质引起的损伤。这些伤害通常发生在燃烧装置炸弹袭击后。与四级爆炸的吸入损伤不同，它们是由于吸收具有血管扩张性质的爆炸物（例如 Detasheet 或季戊四醇四硝酸酯）引起的，并且其特征在于类似全身性炎症反应综合征的“高炎症状态”，表现为心动过速、发热、低中心静脉压和过多的液体复苏需求以维持足够的组织灌注。另一种类型的异常性爆炸伤是生物异物损伤，主要是由自杀式爆炸袭击人员的骨碎片嵌入引起的，这使受害者具有发生血源性疾病如人类免疫缺陷病毒（human immunodeficiency virus，HIV）感染和乙型肝炎的风险。

创伤的解剖位置

简易爆炸装置造成的 100 名伊拉克伤员的解剖模式见图 2 所示。所有幸存者和非幸存者都有开放性伤口。其他创伤分类如下（分别为幸存者和非幸存者）：骨折（39% 和 100%）、烧伤（15% 和 16%）、截肢（7% 和 50%）、颅内损伤（2% 和 75%），以及胸内、腹部或盆腔损伤（0 和 67%）。末端和头 / 面 / 颈部伤口的高百分比可能与以下因素有关：士兵通常佩戴一些能提供胸部保护的个人防护装备（personal protective equipment，PPE）。

发病率和死亡率

在一项涉及 4765 名美国军事人员的发病率和死亡率的回顾性调查中，在伊拉克和阿富汗的军事人员伤亡中，爆炸造成的伤害占 78%，死亡占 77%。当比较 2003 — 2004 年和 2005 — 2006 年的数据时，简易爆炸装置有较高比例的爆炸相关损伤，损伤严重程度与一级爆炸伤的发生率相比显著增加。虽然与爆炸相关的死亡率仍然很低（1.4% 和 1.5%），但受伤的严重程度表现为治疗后的回报率下降（18%），比先前的一半还低（40%）。

恐怖分子将炸弹袭击的伤害效应通过各种策略加以最大化，例如制造二次爆炸（例如集束炸弹），部署第二枚炸弹；将炸药部署在封闭空间中，以使爆炸冲击波的伤害潜能达到最大化，以及在近距离处产生和推进碎片；引起建筑物结构崩塌；添加化学、生物或放射性活性材料以导致五级爆炸伤。

对于封闭空间的爆炸（例如，在建筑物或车辆中）须要值得特别注意，原因在于它们与一级爆炸伤的发生率相关，并且比在露天的爆炸会更易致命。虽然在军事背景下开放空间爆炸占主导地位，但在针对平民的恐怖主义炸弹袭击中，封闭空间爆炸和

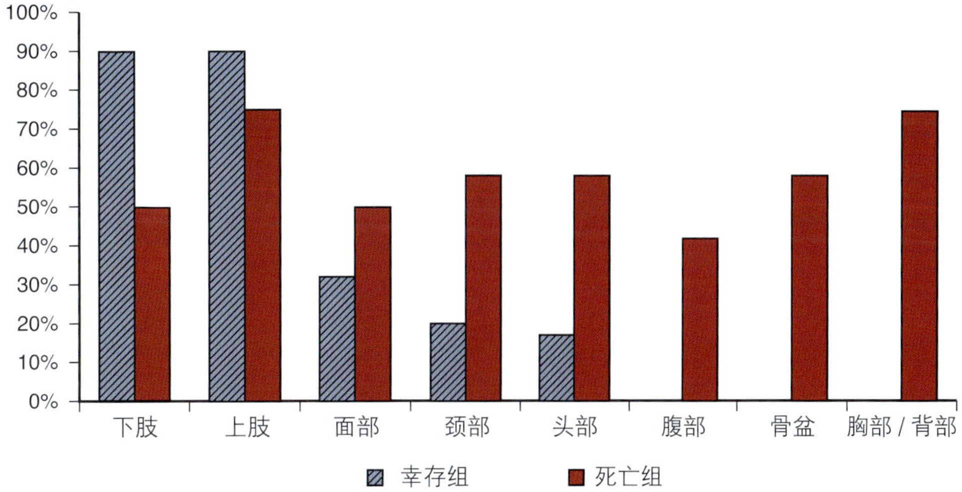

图 2　2006 年在伊拉克路边简易爆炸装置爆炸造成的幸存患者和死亡者的伤口解剖模式。图中所列数字是占总数的百分比。数字之所以重叠，是因为大多数伤员有多处受伤（在幸存者中平均有 2.6 个解剖位置受到影响，在死亡者中有 4.7 个解剖部位受到影响）（*Modified from Ramasamy A, Harrisson SE, Clasper JC, et al: Injuries from roadside improvised explosive devices. J Trauma 65:910–914, 2008.*）

建筑物崩塌占据主导地位。因为恐怖分子一般会针对人口稠密地区，以获得最大的效果。与露天爆炸相比，在受限的空间（例如公共汽车）中的爆炸造成的损伤严重性更高［平均损伤严重程度评分（injury severity score，ISS）18 vs 4］，死亡率也更高（49% vs 8%）。

手术管理

比起普通创伤手术，管理爆炸伤患者的外科手术在技术上的难度不会更高。区别在于爆炸伤害的多机制和多系统性质。应充分了解每一位患者的创伤机制和动力学，最好还包括距离和损伤场景等，这将大大有助于治疗的优先级和对资源的管理。具体问题包括：

- 早期识别和积极管理对肺和脑的超压力创伤。
- 诊断重大隐匿性躯干创伤，特别是伴有出血或血管损害者。
- 充分修复可能发生的广泛性软组织损伤，特别是佩戴个人防护装备的伤员，其暴露的肢体会受到简易爆炸装置的伤害。
- 当存在超压、多个碎片或碾压而造成任何肢体筋膜室受到损伤时，应尽早使用筋膜切开术。

当向患者或院前救急人员询问病史时，重要的是要尽可能多地得到以下问题的答案：

- 爆炸是发生在自由空间还是封闭空间中？（后者的风险较大。）
- 伤者是车辆上的乘客吗？（如果是，则风险较低，但是可能具有来自车辆移动造成的次生钝性损伤。）
- 伤员与爆炸源的距离是多少（他或她离爆炸点有多远）？（距离越远，则在爆炸超压下的暴露就越少。）
- 事件的总体严重性如何（即伤员离其他死者的相对位置有多远）？
- 伤员是否有遭受挤压伤的风险？

这些数据对于了解病理生理学、优先诊断和手术方式来说是必要的。后者是由美国外科医师学会（American College of Surgeons Committe on Trauma）关于创伤的战术伤亡和高级创伤生命支持委员会提出的。

伤害严重程度评分

创伤严重程度评分对于描述和分类损伤是必要的。精确的损伤编码是损伤数据库的基石。其储存库经常作为增强下述方面研究的基础：患者救护和保护设备设计、救护评估、临床研究、质量保证和资源分配。

国际疾病分类（International Classification of Disease）是广泛用于描述创伤的一种分类法。然而，它不是被设计用于解剖损伤评分系统，不是专门为创伤而开发的，不代表损伤严重程度，也不能预测结果。另一种评分系统是器官创伤度量表（Organ Injury Scale），根据其重要性被开发用作对单个器官的损伤进行分类。然而，简明创伤量表（AIS）是最常用的解剖学评分系统。AIS 在 20 世纪 70 年代早期被开发以作为平民创伤（主要是汽车碰撞）的评分系统，已经成为描述解剖学创伤的国际标准。然而，没有证明 AIS 能够完成准确地描述平民穿透性创伤和战斗创伤的任务，在当前的冲突场景中主要包括与爆炸相关的创伤。

尽管为了更好地描述战斗 / 爆炸相关伤害 AIS 做了一些努力，但由于 AIS 的代码（包括 ISS）仍然不足以描述这些创伤类型，因此，已开发出来新的替换工具，包括创伤专用语。其能准确地描述战斗解剖创伤，特别是来自爆炸的伤害，并且还能标示即时战术和功能障碍。这种军事作战伤害度量指标能够与军事和民用历史数据库进行比较；将链接测试、伤害和军事车辆安全标准，以用于未来军用车辆的开发；并将纳入多种创伤机制以增强对战斗创伤结果的预测。这将增加我们对爆炸相关创伤的理解，并帮助量化相关的发病和死亡风险。

小结

与爆炸相关的创伤和伤亡人数不断增加。它们具有破坏性的后果，并且可以压垮医疗资源。其造成的多重和复杂的创伤，并同时具有多处身体部位和大规模伤亡情况，对院前急救人员、急诊医生和外科医生均具有挑战性。了解发病机制、临床方面和检伤分类，对创伤外科医生和涉及对爆炸伤患者进行管理的所有人员来说都是非常重要的。

生物制剂引发创伤的院前救治

Kenneth G. Swan，Charles D. Mabry, Juan A. Asensio 著
张进军 译

在巴格达一座横跨伟大的底格里斯河的拥挤的桥面上，从伊拉克的北部到南部，一群人混杂在双向人流中。在大桥下面河流的东边，大多数人匆忙地来往于附近的市场。有些人携带包裹，怀抱或肩背婴儿，有人在高声叫喊着什么；尽管无法确定任何人或事，但听到的人将报警当成警告，有可能是由被放置在桥上的简易爆炸装置引起的。本就担心不已的民众十分恐慌，迅速扩散到了四面八方。有些人试图跑到河对岸，其他人试图从其前进的地方撤退，另一些人跳入水中。从众心理破坏了所有的平衡，假定的逃跑心理主导了恐惧人群的思维。事件发生后，造成将近1000人死亡，并有更多的人受伤。死亡的原因包括窒息、躯干创伤、头部创伤和多发性长骨骨折出血，还淹死了很多人。但所谓的简易爆炸装置从未引爆，也没有被发现。事件的发生日期是2005年8月31日。这是一起煽动性事件，但是它验证了与创伤外科医生有关的两个现象。

针对平民的恐怖主义行为可能源于多种机制或未知的原因。同样重要的是，如果在高度焦虑或忧虑的情况下发生，人们会产生恐慌，进而造成踩踏和创伤的灾难性后果。煽动事件的起因不一定是爆炸装置，只要存在一个或任何数量的对人身安全有危害和有威胁的替代品，都有可能导致相同的结果。这些替代物包括与恐怖主义有关的生物制剂。当怀疑存在威胁时，无知和迷信（主要是前者）会迷失群众的理性。因此，在这种情况下，院前急救人员必须考虑两种形式的创伤：生物危害本身以及由其产生的恐慌而导致的创伤。

院前急救是由现场和去往医疗治疗区途中最资深的医疗人员提供的。这样的医疗人员可以是急诊医疗技术人员（emergency medical technicians，EMTs）、护理人员，甚至医生。必要时，他们须对患者进行评估，包括威胁评估、检伤分类和现场急救，直到其他的援助到达。对患者的评估是根据美国外科医师学会及其高级创伤生命支持计划建立的标准化准则进行的，并对其进行了修改以补充不同的技能水平的标准，例如与护士、医护人员和EMTs（院前创伤生命支持）相关内容。威胁评估应包括在对患者的评估中。是什么原因导致恐慌？是爆炸、放射性、化学性还是生物制剂？它是否仍然构成威胁？最初，这些问题的答案可能不是十分明显，然而，答案对成功地进行检伤分类、患者复苏、稳定和转运以及通知和保护那些尚未暴露于危险的人而言是十分关键的。

对患者的检伤分类取决于其位置。生物制剂引起的创伤可能在事故现场或在制剂暴露的现场中遇到。在这个层次上，术语“现场分类”是适当的，以有别于“医院分类”。“分类”（triage）这个词汇来源于法国动词“trier”，意思是排序，可追溯到15世纪的欧洲市场，当时对毛皮和纤维根据质量和价格进行分类。分类时可以指定任意数量的类别，但也许最简单的安排包括三个级别。大多数“患者”感到很恐惧，接近歇斯底里。应该让少数急救人员对他们重新安置和安慰。这个类别可能包括现场最大百分比的患者。其余的一小部分是极端情况或濒死的患者，他们被称为“姑息治疗者”。对于他们而言，除了被允许以最少的痛苦和在这种情况下所能提供的尽可能多的尊严死去之外，我们别无选择。其余的分类为“优先”，并且须要将他们运送到医疗治疗区。这些患者可能有出血、气道问题、头部创伤、烧伤、胸部或腹部疼痛或脊柱或长骨骨折的迹象。后一类别可能只占伤亡人数的20%，但这一类别是最重要的。

必须理解的检伤分类原则包括：不仅在所有级别的救护中，而且在救护级别的内部，都须要对患者进行检伤分类和重新检伤分类。假设有一个或一个以上的急救人员在场，分诊员则不负责治疗。分类员只须根据受伤程度和可能造成的后果对患者进行分类，它们取决于可用的资源（时间、人员和设备），以及对它们的有效使用情况。天气、通信和可用的交通工具将在确定预期后果中发挥关键作用。假设爆炸性弹药、辐射和化学制剂的威胁已被消除，但是生物制剂的威胁仍然存在，那么急救人员或看护人员在平民恐怖主义行为现场中应该采取什么步骤？

不同级别的医疗人员之间必须建立沟通，确认

附近地区存在额外威胁的风险。除了向最需要的人提供急救外，还要努力确定会造成大规模伤亡的生物制剂和可能发生的时间。

目前存在五种被认为是恐怖主义的生物制剂。它们具有以下几个方面的特征，这使得它们比其他生物制剂更易用于恐怖袭击。这些特征包括：相对容易制造、包装、运输和递送，不仅致命，而且具有较高的发病率。与那些导致大量患者在长时间内产生极严重病情的药物相比，能导致人迅速死亡的药物引起的恐慌和恐惧可能更小。它们显然是可传染的。最常使用的具有潜在威胁的五种制剂是炭疽、天花、肉毒杆菌中毒、鼠疫和兔热病相关的病原。对每种疾病及其制剂的特点的讲述将重点放在检测、诊断、治疗、预防、检疫、去污染和坏死（表1至3）。其他制剂，如引起脑炎和埃博拉病毒的生物制剂，将只简要提及，因为遭遇它们的可能性要低得多。

表1 五种最常使用的生物恐怖制剂及相关疾病：特征、识别和检测

疾病	生物	气雾剂	开始时间	症状	特征	检测
炭疽	炭疽芽孢杆菌	孢子	2 天	急性发作，流感样疾病	纵隔扩大	较大的革兰氏阳性杆菌，血液
天花	正痘病毒	病毒	12~14 天	严重发热性疾病	皮疹	病毒，脓液
鼠疫	鼠疫耶尔森菌	细菌	1~6 天	严重肺炎，败血症	血液渗出	双极（"安全销"）革兰氏阴性杆菌，痰液
肉毒杆菌	肉毒梭菌，菌毒素	毒素	数小时或数天	麻痹	没有发热	小鼠生物测定，血液
兔热病	土拉热弗朗西斯菌	细菌	3~5 天	急性发作，发热性疾病，非特异性	进展较慢	小革兰氏阴性杆菌，痰液

表2 五种最常使用的生物恐怖制剂及相关疾病：治疗、预防、死亡原因及死后情况

	治疗				
疾病	肠外	口服	预防	死亡原因	死后情况
炭疽	环丙沙星 400 mg	环丙沙星 500 mg	疫苗，6 剂量系列，美国军队	呼吸衰竭，败血症	土葬，火葬
天花	继发性感染		无可用	脓毒症	火葬
鼠疫	链霉素 1.0 g，庆大霉素	多西环素 100 mg，环丙沙星	无可用	脓毒症	土葬
肉毒杆菌	继发性感染		抗毒素	呼吸衰竭	土葬
兔热病	链霉素 1.0 g，庆大霉素	多西环素 100 mg，环丙沙星	无可用	脓毒症	土葬

*抗生素（q12h）

表3 5种最常使用的生物恐怖制剂及相关疾病：预防、感染控制和去污染

疾病	预防	感染控制	去污染
炭疽	同治疗，60 天	无人对人传播，标准预防措施	初次，二次雾化，无直接接触，肥皂和水
天花	疫苗接种	对所有患者及接触者进行隔离和接种	自发，6 ~ 24 h
鼠疫	相同的治疗，所有的接触者加上任何有发热或咳嗽的人	呼吸滴剂预防（戴面罩）直到48 h 抗生素治疗	自发，1 h
肉毒杆菌	密切观察，抗毒素稀缺	服务提供商	毒素容易被破坏，漂白 1 ∶ 10 稀释，肥皂和水
兔热病	同治疗相同，任何暴露	无人对人传播，标准预防措施	半衰期短，肥皂和水，漂白 1:10 稀释，乙醇 70%

炭疽

炭疽是一种历史悠久的动物性疾病，但是在人类中很少遇到。炭疽杆菌的孢子已经被许多国家政府制成了武器。有人在俄罗斯意外暴露于炭疽，并且其在日本和最近的美国攻击事件中出现。虽然这些暴露造成的死亡人数相对较少，但其破坏潜力令人印象深刻。根据世界卫生组织（World Health Organization，WHO）预计，在500万人口的城市上空释放50 kg炭疽孢子会造成25万人伤亡，其中几乎有一半人将在没有接受治疗的情况下死亡。目前已将炭疽孢子的雾化攻击与大城市的氢弹攻击的效果进行了比较。

在人类中有三种暴露于炭疽的传染途径：呼吸吸入、皮肤和胃肠道（图1）。炭疽孢子的直径仅为1.0 μm，非常坚硬，当雾化时会无色、无味且不可见（图2）。显然，恐怖分子很可能通过从飞机喷雾释放孢子而让人们吸入。炭疽有两个发病阶段。在持续数小时至数天的主要阶段中，受害者在几天至几周内经历发热、呼吸困难、咳嗽、头痛、恶心、

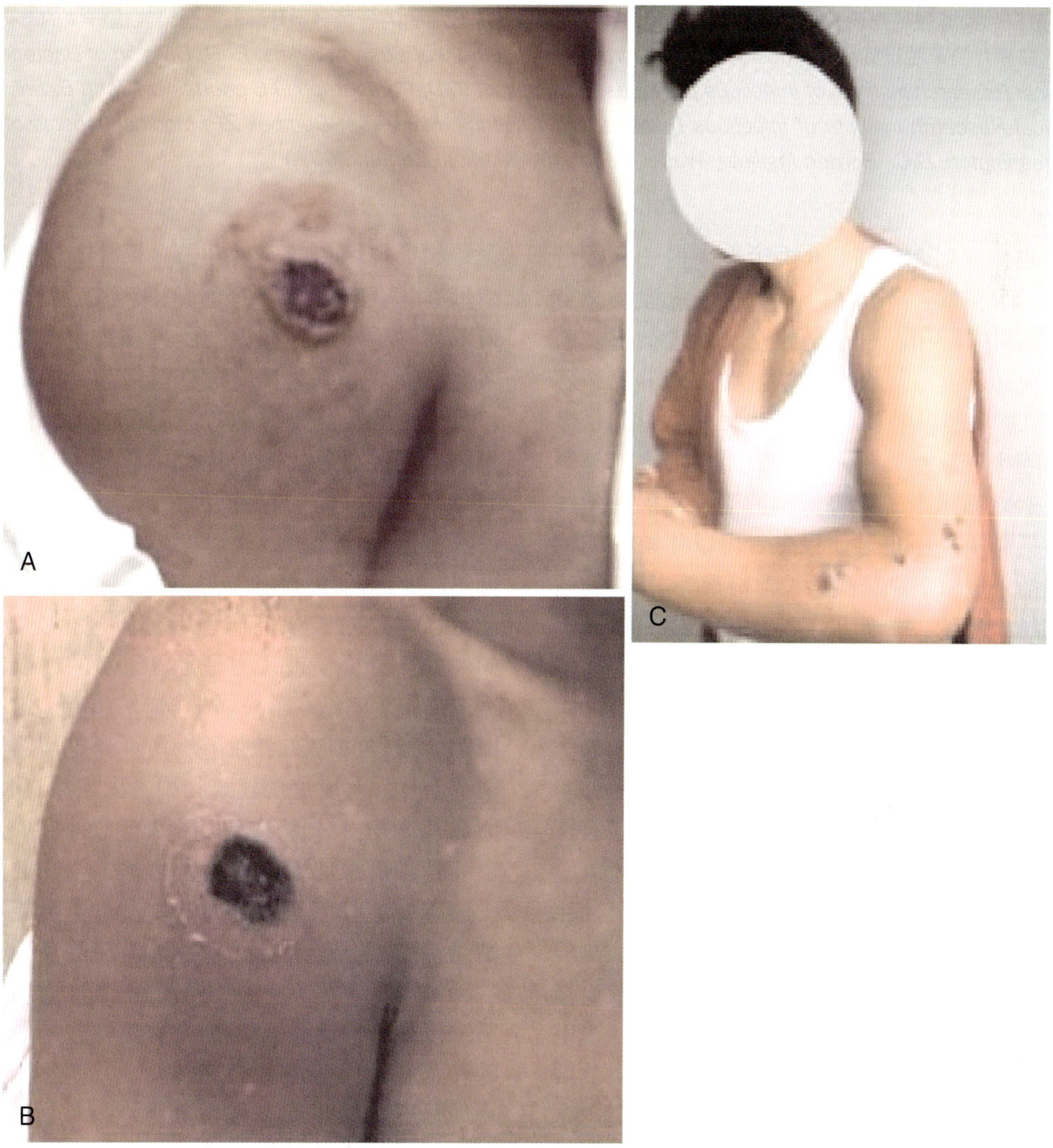

图1　皮肤的炭疽病变。**A**，具有囊泡环的溃疡。**B**，周围有红斑的焦痂。**C**，继发于炭疽水肿毒素的显著末端肢体水肿，伴有多个焦痂（*Photographs courtesy of the Centers for Disease Control and Prevention, Atlanta, Ga. Available at www.bt.cdc.gov/agent/anthrax/anthraximages/cutaneous. asp. From Dembek ZF: Medical aspects of biological warfare. Washington, D.C., Borden Institute, Walter Reed Army Medical Center, 2007.*）

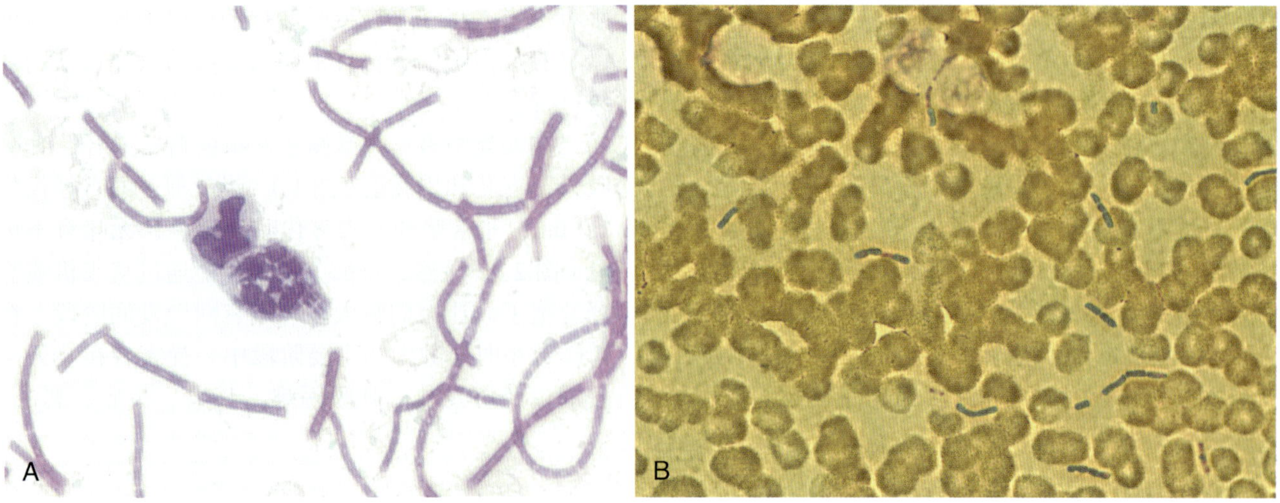

图 2 **A**，来自感染豚鼠的血涂片的革兰氏染色，显示多核粒细胞内的细胞内杆菌链。**B**，来自感染炭疽杆菌的非人的灵长类动物的外周血涂片的革兰氏染色，Ames 菌株 (*Photograph in A courtesy of Susan Welkos, PhD, Division of Bacteriology, U.S. Army Medical Research Institute of Infectious Diseases, Fort Detrick, MD; Photograph in B courtesy of John Ezzell, PhD, U.S. Army Medical Research Institute of Infectious Diseases, Fort Detrick, MD. From Dembek ZF: Medical aspects of biological warfare. Washington, D.C., Borden Institute, Walter Reed Army Medical Center, 2007.*)

呕吐、寒战、虚弱和疼痛（取决于吸入孢子的数量和大小）。第二阶段开始时，症状的严重程度会突然增加。如果未经治疗，会导致全身淋巴结病、菌血症、低血压和死亡。在放射学上大肺门淋巴结病被看作是“扩大的纵隔”。在第二阶段中常见的是纵隔炎、脑膜炎和发绀。诊断的线索是很多之前健康的市民突然之间患上了来势汹汹的流感样疾病。鉴别诊断包括肺炎性鼠疫。如果患者可以住院，则治疗方式包括采取胃肠外抗生素（青霉素等）、辅助通气和采用压迫感受器。如果不能住院，则要口服抗生素。抗生素治疗前的血液培养是验证性的，大多数受害者在出现症状的前 2 天内会被病痛击垮，且病死率接近 80%。潜在的对策包括最近开发的人类 IgG1 单克隆抗体，其与炭疽毒素直接相互作用并将其中和。抗体瑞西巴库在对兔和猴的实验中是有保护性的，但其在人类中的功效尚未经过测试。

预防方式包括已经对所有的美国军事人员使用的疫苗接种（六剂疫苗系列）。然而，最近对大规模军事人员的评价显示，一半以上的疫苗具有低血清水平的体外毒素中和能力。

因为患者与患者之间不存在相互传播炭疽的威胁，所以接触过患者的人无须治疗。然而，由于孢子坚硬，患者死后应该将其火化。对所有可能吸入炭疽杆菌的受害者进行去污染是有必要的，以避免残留在衣服和其他表面上的孢子出现二次烟雾化。同理，医护人员在接触炭疽受害者后必须洗手。

如果现场急救人员和卫生医疗人员怀疑炭疽杆菌烟雾化会导致随后的恐惧和恐慌，那么须要立即采取几种重要的措施。与所有涉嫌生物恐怖主义的案件一样，必须将情况通知给适当的地方、州和联邦报告中心。此外，地方医院还需要警惕并采取适当的措施，以最大限度地提供通气机的可用性，因为吸入炭疽杆菌的患者可能需要气管插管和呼吸支持。在这种情况下，患者的数量可能会超过资源的可用性，因而须要实施分流。

当需要对大量烧伤患者分流进行资源管理时，50% 的全身烧伤被认为是足以致命的，以在这种情况下指定为“姑息治疗者”。烧伤患者经常有相关的损伤，额外的创伤增加了烧伤百分比。例如，如果某个人从一幢燃烧的建筑物中逃出来并有股骨骨折，那么其烧伤百分比（50%）将增加到 55%（对于每个长骨骨折添加了 5%）。类似地，受伤的患者在试图逃离使其吸入炭疽制剂的攻击时更可能被宣布为姑息治疗者，因为会导致不可避免的预后不良。在这种情况下，发病时机的不可预测性对检伤分类人员来说是一种挑战。

天花

在前五名恐怖主义生物制剂中，也许最可怕的就是天花病毒。它能成为特别严重的威胁是有一些原因的。由于近30年前宣布通过疫苗接种而使天花在全球得到根除，疫苗接种被终止。因此，今天没有人能免受于天花的袭击。已知的唯一来源的病毒（天花病毒，Orthopoxvirus, variola）被保存于美国和俄罗斯的国家实验室。另外，没有已知的天花治疗方法。人与人的接触可能会造成身体分泌物通过空气传播。受污染的衣物和床上用品很容易保存病毒，并将病毒从患者传移到接触者。极少量病毒就可以造成病毒血症，并持续好几天。患者的造血系统和网状内皮系统被感染，并在8天内导致更重的病毒血症。受害者表现出高热、不适、头痛、虚脱、背痛和腹痛。典型的水疱性皮疹累及手掌和脚底，可将天花和水痘区别开来（图3）。前者的病变符合单一阶段，而水痘则是分批出现的，并且是离心发作。

天花的治疗包括支持性措施，含抗生素，但病死率超过30%。接触者须接种疫苗，这当然不仅包括所有暴露的医护人员，而且包括所有与受害者有接触的人。必须隔离患者。他们可以被限制在指定的医院，甚至可能是自己的家中。天花的潜伏期为12～14天，随后的病毒血症的进展过程如前所述。即使患者死亡，因为其仍然具有高度感染性，将尸体火化是必要的，同炭疽受害者一样。

虽然天花病毒可能是最可怕的生物恐怖主义的代名词，但这是被全世界所谴责的，再加上执行起来非常困难，几乎不可能获得足够的病毒，所以天花病毒的使用是非常不切实际和不可能的。尽管如此，由于对俄罗斯而言仍然有些不可预测性，而且由于俄罗斯和美国可能不是唯一的病毒库，所以天花病毒的威胁仍然存在。必须将天花病毒囊括在美国和其他地方的所有反生物恐怖主义培训计划中。

瘟疫

瘟疫在生物恐怖主义的使用史上早有记载，在死亡人数方面（按照占世界人口的百分比），它超过任何其他生物制剂引起的疾病，包括1918年的大流感。瘟疫在生物恐怖主义分子的选择列表上位于优先地位，因为它们比较容易获得，并且易于生产和适于雾化。据估计，将50 kg的鼠疫耶尔森菌这种致病微生物在超过500万人口城市的空中投放，可导致15万人感染肺鼠疫，3.6万人死亡。该菌将在该区域内存活1 h，并且在这段时间内都具有威胁性。因为肺炎性鼠疫可以从一个人传播到另一个人，

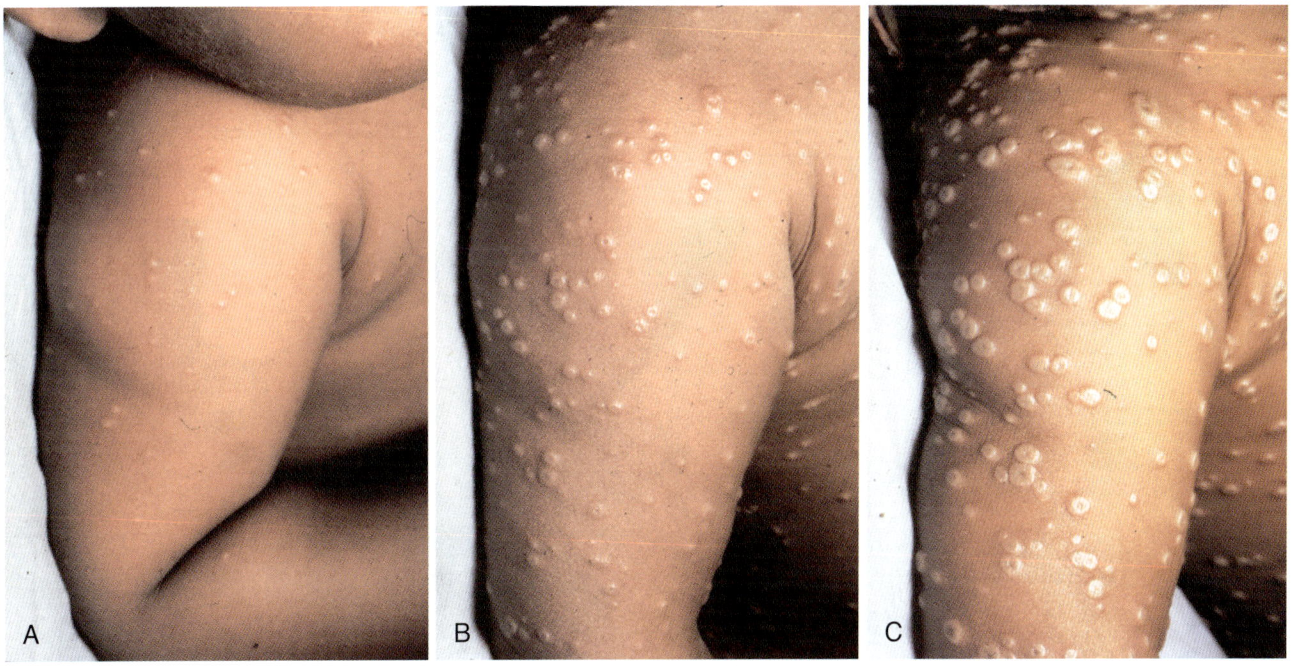

图3 这一系列照片显示了在未接种疫苗婴儿其皮肤损伤的进展情况，具有经典形式的天花。**A**，第三天皮疹同步暴发，一些皮疹正在变成脓疱疹。**B**，第五天的皮疹，几乎所有的乳头都是水泡或脓疱。**C**，皮疹的第七天，许多病变形成脐形，并且所有病变处于相同的发展阶段（*From Fenner F, Henderson DA, Arita I, et al: Smallpox and its eradication. Geneva, Switzerland, World Health Organization, 1988, pp 10–14. Photographs by I. Arita. As printed in Dembek ZF: Medical aspects of biological warfare. Washington, D.C., Borden Institute, Walter Reed Army Medical Center, 2007.*）

并且初始感染源可以更容易传播恐慌情绪。该疾病在暴露后 1～6 天表现为严重的呼吸道疾病（图 4）。由于实际暴露可能是未知的，对于肺鼠疫可通过同期发现大量既往健康、无其他疾病的个体也均患上该疾病来进行识别。历史上，在城市中出现大量死老鼠后，便预计会有瘟疫发生，从而导致携带杆菌的跳蚤转向人类作为宿主。然而，在恐怖袭击中，这一阶段的生命周期是缺失的。

这种疾病如发生在人类身上则被称为“黑死病”，是与手指血管痉挛和坏疽性瘟疫有关的急性发病，这是任何形式的鼠疫耶尔森菌感染的并发症。有些人将该术语归因于严重的全身发绀。这与肺鼠疫及其导致的低氧血症同时发生的。因为肺炎瘟疫的前驱症状包括鼻炎，因而在 14 世纪，某人打一个喷嚏便会被共同出席者称为“上帝保佑你”，然后他们就会迅速离开。因为大家假设认为打喷嚏的人即将感染瘟疫，而且没有治疗方法，几乎必死无疑。

由于肺炎与炭疽具有相似性，这里提及几个区别特征。与炭疽引起的肺炎相比，咯血更提示为瘟疫肺炎而不是肺炎（图 5）。瘟疫患者的痰液显示为革兰氏阴性球菌。由于它们具有双极核，因此在外观上被比作“安全别针”（图 6）。治疗优先使用胃肠外抗生素（四环素和庆大霉素）。但面对大量的患者和有限的医院空间时，建议口服四环素、多西环素或环丙沙星。有一种疫苗被开发用于预防黑死病，

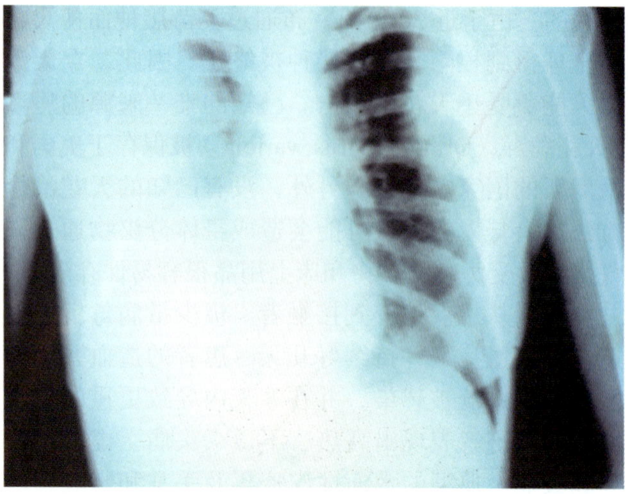

图 5　这种胸部 X 线片显示的是患有肺炎性鼠疫患者的右肺中叶和下叶 (*Photograph courtesy of Kenneth L. Gage, PhD, Centers for Disease Control and Prevention Laboratory, Fort Collins, Colo. From Dembek ZF: Medical aspects of biological warfare. Washington, D.C., Borden Institute, Walter Reed Army Medical Center, 2007.*)

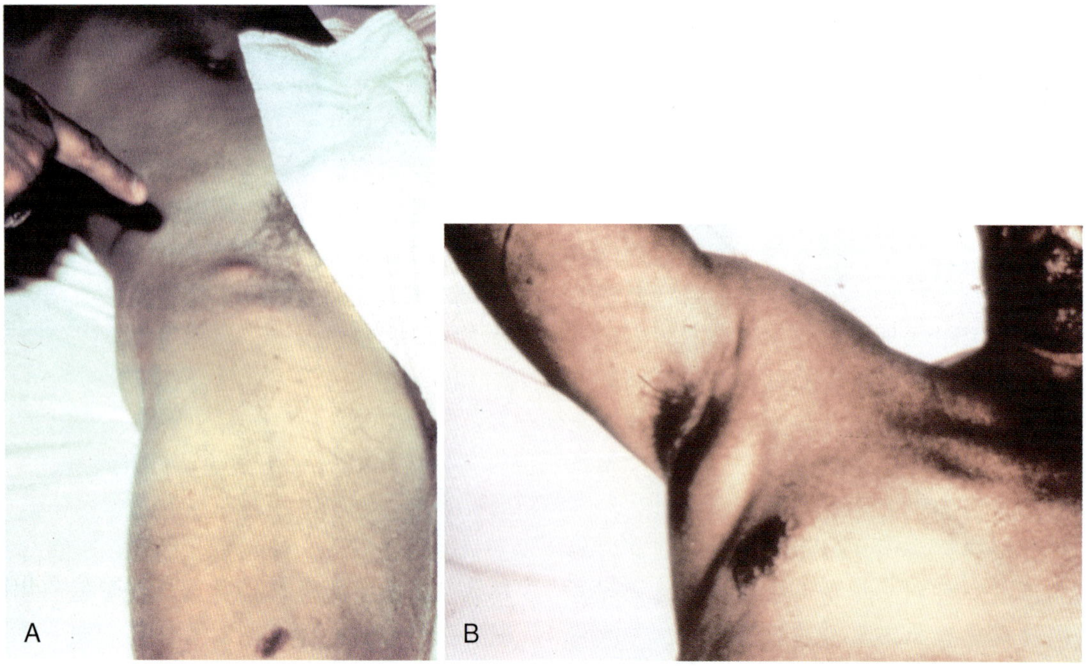

图 4　在患有瘟疫的患者中，腹股沟淋巴结炎（A）是最常见的淋巴结累及部位，表现为红斑、柔软及肿大的淋巴结。对于这种疼痛性病变，可以以无菌方式吸出，以减轻疼痛和压力。不应将其切开和引流。接下来最常见的淋巴结区域是腹股沟、腋窝（B）和颈部区域。腹股沟位置是携带鼠疫耶尔森菌的跳蚤容易感染的身体部位 (*Photographs courtesy of Kenneth L. Gage, PhD, Centers for Disease Control and Prevention Laboratory, Fort Collins, Colo. From Dembek ZF: Medical aspects of biological warfare. Washington, D.C., Borden Institute, Walter Reed Army Medical Center, 2007.*)

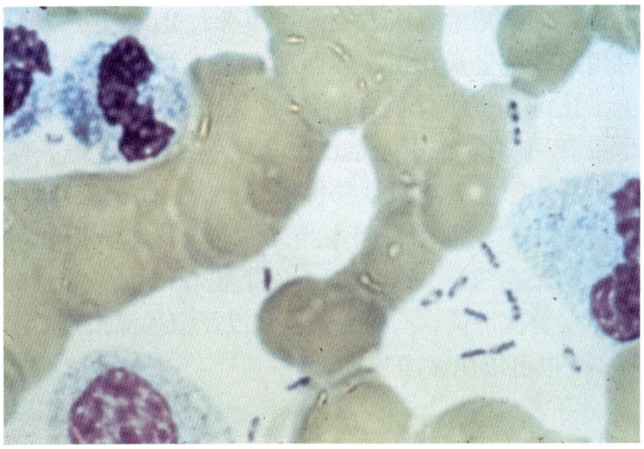

图 6 该图片来自患有败血病性瘟疫的患者，其外周血涂片的 Wright-Giemsa 染色证实了鼠疫耶尔森菌的双极、安全针样外观。革兰氏和 Wayson 染色也可以证明这种形式 (*Photograph courtesy of Kenneth L. Gage, PhD, Centers for Disease Control and Prevention Laboratory, Fort Collins, Colo. From Dembek ZF: Medical aspects of biological warfare. Washington, D.C., Borden Institute, Walter Reed Army Medical Center, 2007.*)

但它对气雾化收缩引发的肺炎鼠疫只能提供很少的保护。事实上，它已经不再被制造。一旦确定了病菌，卫生保健人员应该隔离患者。因为他们仍然有感染性。接触者应该实施标准的呼吸道飞沫预防措施，其中包括穿长袍和戴手套，还有戴面具和戴眼罩。对于不能存活的患者可以将其埋葬，因为病菌将不能存活。环境预防措施通常不是关注点，因为病菌在释放后的预期寿命较为有限（1 h）。

肉毒杆菌中毒

生物恐怖主义的第四种制剂是肉毒杆菌。肉毒杆菌是产生肉毒杆菌毒素的细菌，被认为是人类已知的最有毒的物质。雾化 1 g 肉毒杆菌毒素后，如果充分弥散并且被暴露者充分吸入，可以杀死 100 万人。静脉给药 1 μg 的 1/10（0.1μg）剂量就足以杀死成年人。该毒素阻断了乙酰胆碱在神经 - 肌肉接头处的释放，并且通过不可逆的与胆碱能突触结合而发生作用。本病在临床上是一个典型的三合一症状：①对称的、下行松弛性麻痹与突出的延髓麻痹。②患者无热。③有清晰的感觉中枢。延髓麻痹常常被称为“4D”：复视（diplopia）、烦躁（dysphoria）、情绪失调（dysarthria）和吞咽困难（dysphagia）。吸入肉毒杆菌后须对患者全面开展救护、通气和营养支持，这可能需要持续几周至几个月，因为需要神经再生来置换先前在神经 - 肌肉接头处的突触。仅仅因为此，就会造成许多受害者长期残疾和延迟康复，因此，该毒素是非常有破坏性的生物恐怖制剂。事实上，在 1991 年海湾战争爆发之前，据说伊拉克储存了足以杀死世界人口 3 倍的肉毒杆菌毒素。该毒素易于生产、储存、运输和释放。

在反恐怖袭击时如果还没有识别肉毒杆菌毒素的经验，对此应高度怀疑。如果没有其他形式疾病（如食物中毒或伤口脓肿）的健康个体，存在之前提到的神经系统症状，并有从先上肢继而发展至下肢的对称趋势，则对此情况必须怀疑。必须启动适当的警示，同时在吸入肉毒杆菌的情况下，从生物血清测定寻求确实性证据，在肠道肉毒杆菌病的情况下寻求大便样品的确实性证据。由于需要通气支持以避免呼吸麻痹导致的死亡，医院良好的准备措施对于成功处理大量受到该攻击的受害者来说是至关重要的。大量长期依赖呼吸机的患者可能消耗掉很大的医疗和社会资源。因此，可以改善麻痹状态以及缩短恢复时间的抗毒素的价值有所增强。目前，通过位于佐治亚州亚特兰大 CDC 可以获得这种治疗，但供应量有限，并且抗毒素仅在个案基础上供临床使用。

2006 年泰国爆发了肉毒杆菌中毒事件。人们是从竹笋中摄入的。有 209 人受到了影响，其中 42 人发生呼吸衰竭，25 人须住院进行通气支持。在疾病第 4 天接受肉毒杆菌抗毒素（抗 BoNT，CDC）的患者比在第 6 天接受抗毒素的患者恢复得更快。

在使用雾化的肉毒杆菌毒素的生物恐怖袭击时，在院前阶段能预估到会发生什么吗？如炭疽的芽孢一样，该制剂甚至在大体积和大浓度下，也是无色、无味且不可见。因此，至少在最初对其检测时易被忽视。1 h 内症状可能不会出现。肉毒杆菌吸入后相关的治疗经验非常有限。在 20 世纪 90 年代初期，日本恐怖分子在针对平民的唯一尝试中失败了（在三个场所），可能是出于技术原因而导致了失败。然而，“攻击”这一字眼确实吓坏了很多人。许多逃离现场的人受伤，但最后报告得出的结论是“非毒素攻击的轻微伤亡事件”。如果人们提前得到可能会发生攻击的警告，或像之前提到的几年前巴格达桥上的伊拉克平民一样，随之而来的恐慌可能会造成更大的伤害。加上这种可能性，症状的出现可能非常迅速，恐慌情绪在人群中传播，除非受害者能够到达重要的治疗区，否则会迅速死亡。随后将发生骚乱，附近的医院将在几分钟内被人群所淹没。这样的例子表明，须对民众、现场急救人员和医院医务人员开展培训。对于民众，他们须知道应该避免恐慌，等待指示，离开现场，并听从收音机和其他媒体传达的进一步信息和指示。同样，现场和医院的工作人员必须得到通知，知道患者及病菌可能会激增，以及最新的诊断、治疗和报告程序。院前团队、EMTs、医护人员和急救人员应该对须运送到医疗治疗机构的有症状的受害者进行快速的现场评估。

肉毒杆菌毒素很容易被各种溶液净化，包括肥皂水或0.1%次氯酸盐漂白剂。无须特别关注的是，该毒素在中性环境中即可以每分钟1%的速率衰变。

兔热病

土拉热弗朗西斯菌（*Francisella tularensis*）是一种小的、无活动力的、需氧的革兰氏阴性球杆菌，会造成人类兔热病，是人类已知的最具感染性的致病菌之一。接种或吸入最少10个病菌就足以引起疾病。由于其极端的感染性，以及易传播性和引起严重疾病甚至死亡的能力，土拉热弗朗西斯菌是一种可能被用于生物恐怖主义的制剂。WHO估计，若在500万城市人口中心气雾化50 kg活体，将会造成25万人伤亡，包括1.9万人死亡。

该病菌普遍存在。它的载体是节肢动物，可贮存寄生在小型哺乳动物身上。它可以通过昆虫叮咬、与动物尸体或土壤直接接触、摄取污染的水或食物以及吸入而传播给人类。后者将是恐怖分子的首选方法。本病不发生人与人传播，因此，人类感染不会像天花一样流行。

该病菌通过气雾化释放后的影响范围较大，会在吸入3～5天后造成大量患有不寻常呼吸道疾病的患者。还须采用高度怀疑的指标来区分兔热病和社区获得性感染，如流感或非典型性肺炎。如果怀疑出现生物恐怖袭击，须与其他相关疾病进行鉴别诊断，如瘟疫、炭疽以及尚待讨论的Q热。兔热病通常症状进展较慢，病死率较低。瘟疫可进展为咯血、呼吸衰竭、败血症和休克，但在兔热病中并不常见。炭疽病具有特征性影像学表现外观（纵隔扩大），在兔热病中是不可见的。虽然对痰液进行光学显微镜检查可能揭示存在革兰氏阴性杆菌，但痰液培养是确定性诊断。治疗方法包括理想条件下的胃肠外抗生素，如链霉素或庆大霉素。当有大量群众伤亡时，可用肠外抗生素，口服多西环素或环丙沙星来替代。由于该菌在人类体内的潜伏期很短，所以接种疫苗是没有用的。无须隔离患者，因为没有发生过人与人传播。医务人员只须要提供标准的预防措施即可。环境净化是小问题，因为当暴露于干燥和太阳辐射时，病菌会进入短半衰期。如果担心设备或其他材料存在潜在污染，乙醇、肥皂水以及家用漂白剂（稀释剂）也可以用做净化剂。

其他制剂

其他可利用制剂的可能性是较广泛的。如前所述，我们将简要地介绍经常提到的其他制剂，但不会像前面的“五大”那样详细论述。这里包括的制剂是柯克斯体（Q热）、葡萄球菌（葡萄球菌肠毒素B）、马脑炎病毒和出血热病毒。每种病菌都对生物恐怖分子有特殊的吸引力，因在使用上比“五大”更容易。

Q热是由吸入致病剂——贝纳柯克斯体（*Coxiella burnetii*）引起的流行病。一些人称为立克次体，另一些人称为细菌。从这个冲突可看出，其名称由疾病得来。“Q”代表“疑问”，表示其定义之谜。该菌对恐怖分子的吸引力与其高度传染性有关。这种“资产”是相对于较低的杀伤力和自我限制的临床过程。确诊疾病须要采取血清学测试。如果必要，要用到抗生素（多西环素）进行治疗。

葡萄球菌肠毒素B是可以雾化的毒素，吸入后会导致败血症。它的吸引力在于能够造成一种无法行动的疾病。这种疾病将持续足够长的时间，以在大量（基本上所有）暴露者中传播恐怖甚至恐慌的情绪。从理论上讲，生者比死者更易于传递威胁情绪，因为他们仍能发出自己的声音。虽然生物恐怖主义的“缺点”是杀伤力非常低和易于治疗，这在很大程度上得到了认证。诊断取决于高度怀疑，确诊则基于血清学检查。但令人担心的是气雾剂的潜在混合物，这将导致医务人员造成明显混淆，并加剧了恐怖和恐慌情绪。

马脑炎是由三种病毒引起的病毒。生物恐怖主义者对其特别感兴趣。这些RNA病毒具有高度致命性，东部马脑炎尤其致命，可造成人与人之间的传播的重大风险。诊断基于病毒性疾病的进展。可采用支持性治疗。确诊是从咽喉拭子或血液样品中找到生物体。

出血热病毒包括一种生物恐怖主义者可能感兴趣的终极制剂，即埃博拉病毒。后者是一种最常被提及的制剂，因为它的病死率接近100％。这组病毒还包括造成登革热和黄热病的某些病毒。由于这些病毒攻击内皮细胞，因而在各种症状中出血障碍是其特征。本病不可能造成人与人之间的传播，所以显然生物恐怖主义者还没有尝试使用它。最可能的是，把所有这些制剂通过雾化递送。

小结

由于生物恐怖主义的受害者可能求助于不同的医疗单位，并且由于症状的发作可能不总是同步的，医护人员必须具有监视系统，使能将任何数量或呈现不寻常的“流感样疾病”报告给所有区域的卫生保健机构。这种做法对于早期发现生物恐怖袭击至关重要。在准备这样的活动时还能做些什么？目前疫苗可用于预防炭疽、霍乱、瘟疫、Q热和天花，但没有可用于预防肉毒杆菌中毒或病毒性脑炎的疫苗。人们对伦理、经济和政治等重要因素提出了关注，目前限制了针对生物恐怖主义制剂的所需疫苗的开发。抗生素是炭疽、瘟疫和Q热的推荐治疗方法，抗毒素和抗病毒剂分别被用于治疗肉毒杆菌中毒和天花。

创伤弹道学：每一位创伤外科医生应该知道的

Laszlo Kiraly，John C. Mayberry, Donald D. Trunkey 著
张进军 译

在经历早前的下降趋势后，过去十年间美国枪支受伤和死亡的发生率保持相对稳定的状态。枪械造成的伤害不仅会在城市“高犯罪”地区出现，而且也会发生在狩猎事故的郊区。在军事环境中出现的伤口具有临床上重要的独特特征，并且与在民事环境中看到的有所不同。伊拉克自由行动（Operation Iraqi Freedom，OIF）和持久自由行动（阿富汗）（Operation Enduring Freedom，OEF）在处理军事射弹伤害方面提供了重要参考。创伤弹道学的研究是普通医生和创伤外科医生培训内容的重要部分。

表1　参与伤口弹道的因素

子弹设计
口径（直径）
质量
形状（轮廓）
夹套
弹丸
粉末（数量和类型）
武器的设计
枪管长度
膛线
单镜头
自动化机器或设备
半自动
便携性（重量和尺寸）
受害者
位置
与武器的距离
伤口的位置
组织特性（骨骼、肌肉、血管或器官）

弹道理论

虽然有许多变量，然而，枪口速度（子弹离开枪管时的速度）和子弹特性（如质量和变形性）是特定武器产生伤口的最重要的决定性因素（表1）。枪口速度是由子弹的口径（直径）、套管的容量（火药粉的量）和枪管长度决定的。子弹的速度随着其沿枪管向前运动而快速增加，但是当它已经离开枪膛遇到空气阻力时就会逐渐减慢。通常手枪的子弹更

小，并且枪管比步枪更短，因此会产生速度明显较慢的射弹（表 2）。

在射弹撞击其目标后，子弹和组织之间发生两种明显的相互作用。首先，快速移动的子弹产生直接组织破坏的路径。这种破坏性的相互作用通常被称为“永久空腔”。沿着子弹的路径，也形成“临时空腔”。这个“临时空腔”是由子弹被迫通过身体时与相邻组织的横向移位组成的。这些力可以影响比子弹直径本身大出许多倍的区域。根据不同的组织部位和弹性，临时空腔在临床上的重要性表现不同。例如，胸部组织的快速移位可导致严重的肺挫伤。

由于铅的质量更重，因此能使给定速度的能量增加，所以铅是大多数子弹的主要组成元素。然而，铅是相对较软的金属，在高速飞行期间容易变形。“夹套”子弹的主体为铅，具有合金覆盖的引线体，防止飞行期间变形，因此能帮助子弹保持长距离的速度和精度。通常，夹套子弹在撞击致密组织时将变形，但是具有更厚夹套的子弹可保持其形状，从而更深地穿入大型动物（如大象）（图 1）。在击向身体时，与不可变形子弹相比，变形子弹通过直接接触、气蚀和冲击波会引起更多的附带组织损伤。当子弹撞击骨骼时，会发生子弹分裂，并通过破坏周围组织而增加损伤（图 2）。动物模型已经证明，可变形的空心子弹能造成更多的组织破坏和更大的损伤区域。然而，夹套子弹更容易穿透受害者，从而不会将所有的动力损伤转移到身体中。

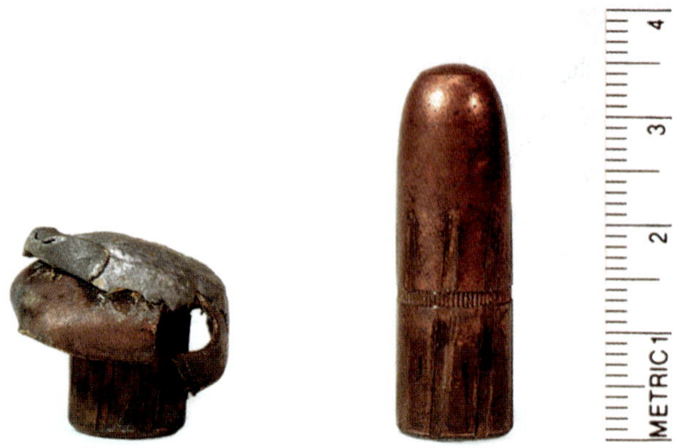

图 1　全金属外套 308 口径步枪子弹在动物游戏（左）中撞击打开。与相同口径的子弹相比，有较厚外套的子弹穿过动物时未变形（右）。注意由枪管的内部膛线引起的每个子弹基部上的凹槽（Bullets courtesy of Gerald Warnock, MD, Portland, Ore）

表 2　枪口速度、枪与子弹类型

手枪	速度（m/s）
.特种 38	290
.44	305
9mm	315
.44 马格南	420
步枪	
.22 长	380
30.06	890
.308（7.62mm）	860
军事	
.223 (M-16)	950
.30 (AK-47)	720
.50（布朗宁）	850

根据 1899 年的《海牙宣言》（The Hague Declarations），军事步枪子弹因“在人体内容易扩张或变平，如具有不完全覆盖核心的硬包壳的子弹”而被禁止。这项禁令旨在减少伤口的严重程度，从而减少士兵在战场上的痛苦，但不适用于非接触组织的战斗人员，并且不适用于通常用于狩猎的子弹。事实上，在许多法律管辖区，用于游戏狩猎的“全金属外套”（full-metal-jacket，FMJ）子弹是被禁止的。为此，狩猎步枪伤口可能比由同等的军用步枪产生的伤口更加严重。这一原则的例外是突击步枪，虽然它使用夹套子弹，但可以因子弹在组织中的翻滚倾向而引起严重的伤口。

手枪

手枪通常被用于城区，因为它们的重量较轻并且可以被隐藏。幸运的是，手枪不能产生像步枪那样高度加速和准确的射弹。必须限制包装在手枪子弹壳体中的火药量，以避免损坏枪管，并允许射手仅通过手臂支撑来射击。经验丰富的射击者可以在受控的情况下掌握手枪，但是，警察和罪犯射中目标的机会可能不到一半。射击距离越长，则射击精度急剧下降，因此，大多数手枪伤口是在 10 码或更近的距离内造成的。

手枪伤口的直接危险来自对头部、颈部或胸腔内重要器官的直接伤害。手枪伤口对脉管系统的造

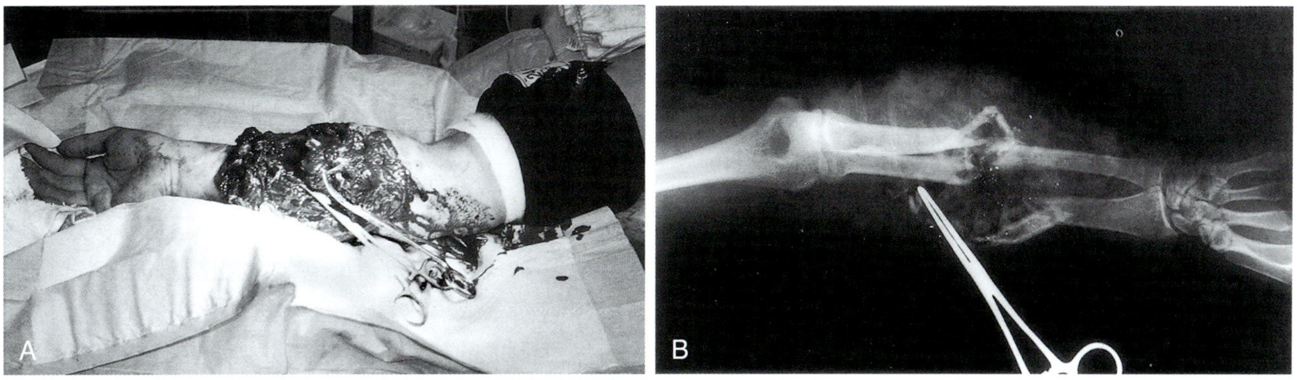

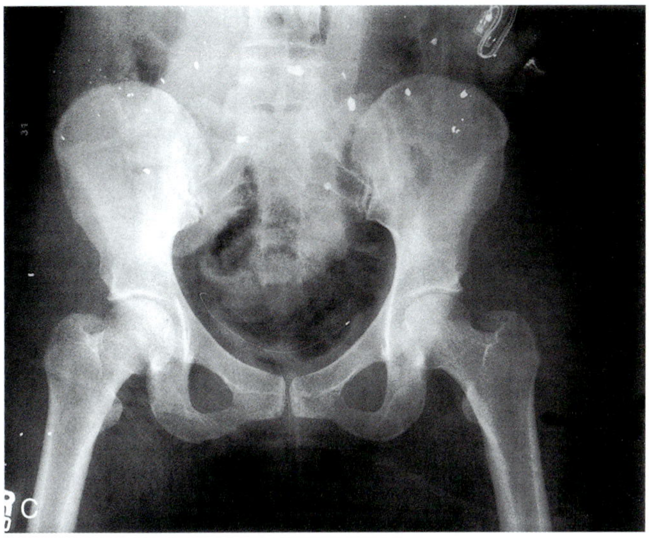

图 2　**A**，右前臂近距离 30-06 狩猎步枪伤。**B**，同样损伤的放射照片显示有广泛的骨粉碎和子弹碎片。**C**，在同一患者的骨盆射线片上可见广泛的子弹碎片。对该患者须进行要较低的腹壁重建

成的邻近损伤的概率低于用步枪或自动武器伤害的概率，但是仍应予以考虑。因为当子弹撞击组织时，手枪子弹的速度较小，不太可能变形或碎裂，组织空腔化可能很轻微。比起非夹套子弹，夹套手枪子弹甚至会导致更小的附带损害，在某些情况下可能穿透组织并随后离开人体，此时其仍有较大的破坏性潜力。

尽管如此，仍可能遇到一些用来增加伤害潜力或“停滞力”的措施。这些措施包括被设计于膨胀的“中空点”子弹（图 3）以及被设计成在冲击后分解成微小颗粒的子弹。这些子弹被执法和安全人员所青睐，用于在拥挤的环境（例如机场或飞机上）中确定罪犯目标，而不用担心过度穿透或弹片跳到无辜的旁观者身上。“马格南”手枪有更多的火药和更长的枪管，能在近距离产生毁灭性的伤口。幸运的是，马格南手枪并不像常规手枪一样常见，因为它们昂贵、重并且难以掌握。

对颈部、胸部和腹部手枪创伤进行手术的适应证，包括强制性探索Ⅱ区颈部创伤，因出血而选择

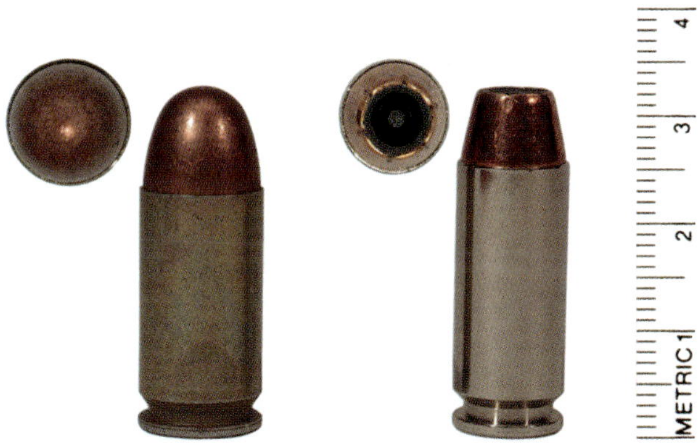

图 3　A.45 口径全金属外壳手枪子弹（左）和 10mm “空心点”，部分包壳弹（右）(*Bullets courtesy of Bruce Ham, MD and Gerald Warnock, MD, Portland, Ore.*)

性探查胸部，并强制探查除了不穿透筋膜的切向损伤和选择性肝损伤的所有腹部穿透性损伤。如果存在腹部疼痛，可用诊断性腹膜灌洗液来确认所怀疑的问题，否则在 X 线片上不能很好地显示胸膜。对于胸部乳头下方子弹入口部位的患者须要进行腹部

探查。对于具有右上象限伤口的稳定的患者，如果明确子弹仅损伤了肝，则可以通过 CT 检查进行选择性评估和手术治疗。

猎枪

平民步枪创伤，例如由狩猎事故造成的伤口，是外科医生能看到的最具有破坏性的伤害。子弹壳中的火药大，枪管更长（可使子弹暴露于火药爆炸力的长度增加），因而射弹加速度会比手枪（图 4）更为显著。步枪枪管的内部螺旋槽使子弹旋转，从而提高距离和精度。30-06 猎枪的平均枪口速度为 890 m/s，并且可以在 100 m 处保持高达其动能的 90%。无论是近距离还是远距离，步枪伤到肢端都将破坏软组织、骨骼和血管，并导致严重的出血，对此可能须采取直接压力或止血带在现场进行救治（图 2）。

由于步枪子弹可能对击中的肢体造成广泛损伤，因此强烈建议拍片寻找骨折部位，探查手术伤口以及进行术中血管造影。即使上层皮肤没有受伤，隐藏在下面的软组织也可能受到不可逆的损坏。应该去掉所有的脱血管组织和衣服，每天进行的一系列清创可能是鉴定所有不能存活的组织所必需的。对于由狩猎步枪造成的腹部枪伤，如果几个器官同时受伤，最好的救治方法是进行开腹手术与后视操作。

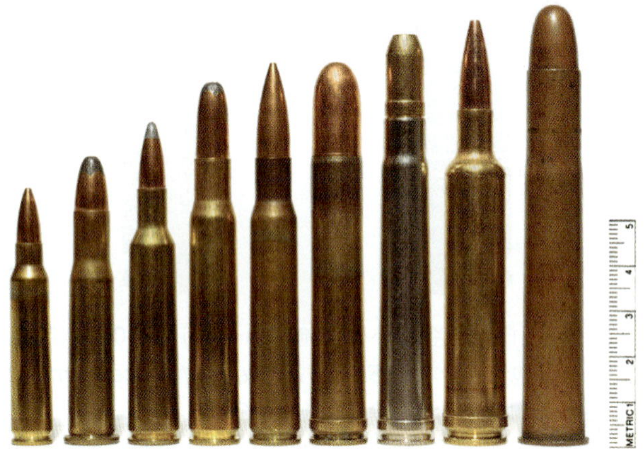

图 4　各种步枪子弹比较。从左到右，.223 口径 FMJ（M-16 突击步枪），30-30 软尖弹，6 mm 软尖弹，30-06 软尖弹，.308 口径军用式 FMJ（7.62 mmNATO），.458 口径 FMJ，.375 口径 FMJ 大号，.378 口径 FMJ 空心尖，第二次世界大战 .47 口径 FMJ。FMJ: 全金属外壳（full metal jacket）。(*Bullets courtesy of Bruce Ham, MD and Gerald Warnock, MD, Portland, Ore.*)

突击步枪

M-16（美国），AK-47 和 AK-74（俄罗斯），Uzi 和 Galil（以色列），Fal（比利时）以及它们的改造型均是相对轻量级的短桶军用步枪，能够快速、连续地发射高速子弹，且子弹在撞击组织后会进行翻滚和侧偏。依靠这些武器开展的军事行动的目标是使尽可能多的战斗人员快速残废。虽然这些步枪及其弹药不再在大多数西方国家的民用市场上销售，但在 1994 年之前拥有的步枪可以在美国合法使用，例如在打靶训练中。这些是军事行动中最常见的突击步枪。据估计，全世界已经制造和分发了数以千万计的 AK 和 Uzis。用于突击步枪的子弹口径范围从较小的 5.45 mm（0.21 英寸）AK-74，到 0.223 英寸的 M-16，到 7.62 mm（0.3 英寸）的 AK-47，再到 9 mm（0.35 英寸）的 Uzi。

一般来说，这些子弹会产生严重的伤口，须要进行软组织修复。然而，在外科医生对因突击步枪而受伤的患者进行治疗时，偶尔也会注意到他们的伤势并不明显。这是因为 M-16 和 AK-74 使用的 FMJ 子弹不会比 22 小口径的步枪大得多。如果一颗子弹迅速穿过肢体，那么周围的组织损伤就不会像一个变形的大口径猎枪子弹所造成的那样夸张。因此，对其余组织进行清创的决定应由操作外科医生自行判断，而不应仅仅基于武器或弹药的类型。

突击步枪的另一个特点是，在打击受害者之后，可能难以确定子弹的轨迹。腹部伤口可能包括几个区域的肠损伤以及实体器官破坏。如果选择非手术方法治疗胸腔穿透，须得到将心包和食管对比放射照相的可视化超声。肢体伤口可能需要手术探查和清创，如果踝肱指数（ankle-brachial index，ABI）为 0.9 或更小，则需要血管造影。

霰弹枪

霰弹枪和弹壳主要有四个尺寸：410 小尺寸、20 标准尺寸、12 标准尺寸以及 10 标准尺寸。标准尺寸与 1 磅铅球的直径相等。例如，一个 10 标准尺寸的霰弹枪能使一个 1/10 磅的铅球进入桶孔。颗粒大小不等，用铅或钢制造。较小的颗粒被称为霰弹枪，直径小于 0.11 英寸（6 号子弹）。霰弹枪的射程较小，但比起更重更大的铅弹而言，更加分散。较重的铅颗粒没有钢颗粒分散，用其射击水鸟是非法的。铅弹也可用于猎枪，并且通常用于某些州（例如新泽西州）中的游戏狩猎（图 5）。霰弹枪，特别是鸟弹，在距离大于 10 或 15 码（30～45 ft）时是没有影响的，但是对胸部或腹部的近距离（<4 ft）爆炸是致命的（死亡率高达 85%）。霰弹枪具有相对较低的枪口速度，但是它们的伤口是极度病态的，并且通常需要多种操作和多学科治疗。射弹在各个方向上蔓延并撞击多种类型的组织。但幸运的是，由于它们的质量较小，射击的损伤潜能可以快速消散。颗粒可能进入动脉和静脉，并在外围或中心造成栓塞（图 6）。在近距离损害造成的创伤中，建议寻找壳体中的塑料插入物或填塞物，以及隐藏在伤口中的患者衣物碎片（图 7）。没有必要去除所有的铅弹，永久地留在人体组织中的颗粒或子弹也不会导致铅中毒。

如果出现胸壁创伤（膈肌移位或紧急肌皮瓣），那么治疗近距离猎枪爆炸创伤可能是具有挑战性的。爆炸效应可导致缺血和损伤，可能在初次检查时不表现出来。但是由此造成的开放性腹部创伤可以用真空或其他临时敷料采取救治。对霰弹枪爆破导致的肢端创伤通常须要进行伤口探查和手术血管造影术。

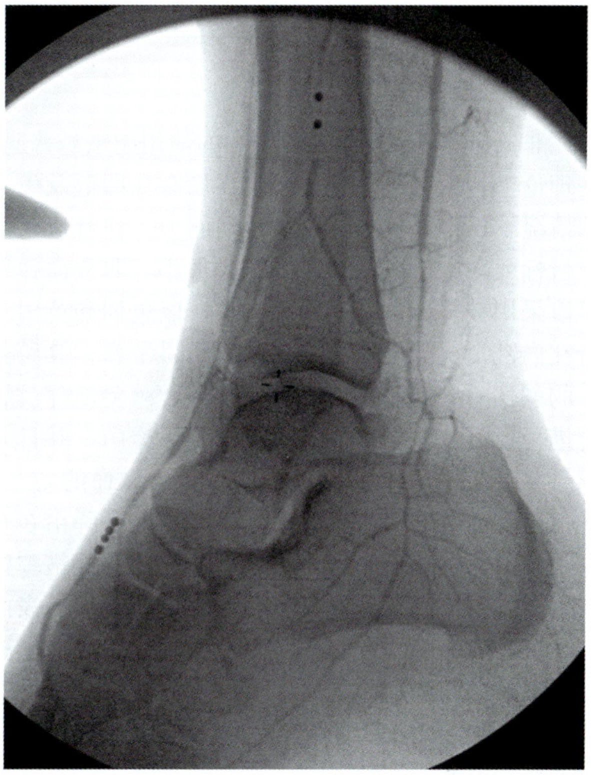

图 6　血管造影显示被霰弹枪击中的患者的右侧股骨，股动脉损伤造成动脉栓塞。进行股动脉重建和胫前动脉栓塞的切除术

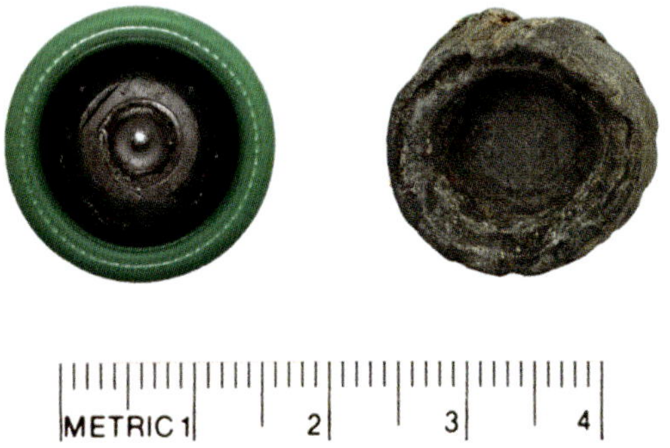

图 5　霰弹枪炮弹装有铅芯而不是铅弹（左）。从动物中取出的相同类型的铅芯。注意由飞行和接触造成的中心区的畸形 (*Bullets courtesy of Gerald Warnock, MD, Portland, Ore.*)

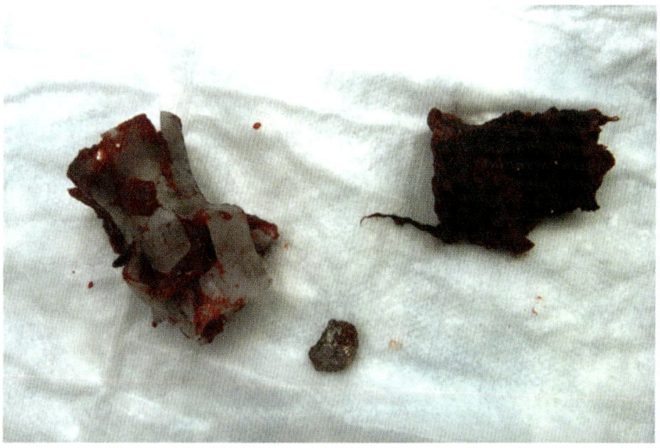

图 7　从肢端伤口取出的霰弹枪炮弹的各种部件

非致命性弹药

非致命性弹药在执法机构中的使用越来越普遍。在理论上，这种子弹允许警察在没有立即危及生命的情况下，使怀疑目标失去行动能力，并且造成怀疑目标死亡或永久性残疾的风险很小。非致命弹药可以采用较软、较轻的子弹形式。以色列和英国政府在内乱情况下广泛使用橡胶或塑料子弹，其所产生的创伤不一定是良性的，并且经常须要治疗。尽管进行了设计，但确实发生了皮肤穿透伤，并且人们已经注意到面部和头部的损伤是能够致命的。

豆袋弹也被用作非致命弹药。这些子弹由在布壳中的铅弹组成，并且由标准的 12 号规格的霰弹枪发射。在理论上这些子弹将冲击扩散到较大的表面上，并且含有布以防止渗透。然而，伤害本身取决于距离和撞击部位。已经发现了数起严重的钝性腹部创伤以及穿透性创伤。当治疗这些创伤患者时，须要进行彻底的评估以排除更深的损伤。

防护衣

有许多种类的“防弹”背心，是由连续的合成材料层制成的，例如 Kevlar（DuPont）。其具有极高拉伸强度的轻质芳族聚酰胺纤维。将这些背心根据其防护等级进行分类：Ⅰ级将保护穿戴者免受 259 m/s 的 .38 手枪伤害，Ⅱ级将免受 332 m/s 的 9 mm FMJ 伤害，Ⅲ级将免受 9 mm FMJ（突击步枪），速度为 427 m/s。为了防备较高速度的步枪子弹，须要向背心添加陶瓷板来进行保护。但是，背心不能保证 100%是有效的。即使子弹无法穿透，胸壁和肺部挫伤也可由弥散到背心和胸壁上的钝力所致。高保真模型研究了子弹袭击防弹衣后随后产生的压力效应。强大的压力波会影响中空器官和实体器官。尽管没有明显的进入或出去的伤口，但应该注意排除创伤。许多品种的“穿甲”子弹是为手枪和步枪制造的，并且在军事和非军事情况下都可能遇到，虽然将它们用于民用是非法的。这些子弹是夹套的并且具有铅内壳和硬化的钢或钨内芯。子弹的常规部分撞击背心，它变形并“软化”障碍物。这些子弹的硬化核穿过较软的壳体以穿透身体和车辆装甲，甚至在某些情况下能够穿透混凝土墙。

地雷和简易爆炸装置

简易爆炸装置在 OIF 和 OEF 期间已经变得臭名昭著。简易爆炸装置是美国和联军在目前冲突中造成死亡的主要原因。这些装置包括从较小的常规爆炸物到复杂的强大的成形炸药，简易爆炸装置在其复杂性和结构上是高度可变的。爆炸具有潜在的能造成立刻致死的伤害。隐藏的爆炸装置如常规地雷或简易爆炸装置的直接爆炸通常导致对触发肢体的立即截肢或至少部分截肢。大血管可能受到损伤，因此可能需要大静脉止血带。金属和碎片也会损害对侧肢体、会阴、躯干和面部。腹部创伤通常具有须要开腹进行多次探查的弥漫性损伤。来自爆炸效应的额外损害可导致在最初剖腹时不能立即显现出的损伤。现行的关于手术治疗的军用标准是损伤控制。建议对出血组织应反复清创和使用外部固定物体稳定骨骼。如果情况严重，对血管损伤可以通过使用分流器来暂时稳定。由脚触发的常规地雷将引起伞状效应，伤害下肢的皮肤和皮下组织，同时破坏肌肉和骨骼（图 8A），表面覆盖的皮肤可能会掩盖了更严重的摧毁部分和皮肤下面的污染（图 8B）。应积极进行清创，以预防血管和神经鞘的感染。来自国际红十字会（International Red Cross）的 Robin Coupland 提出了一个论点，即保护部分腓肠肌以用于重建。

创伤探查和子弹清除

并不是所有的枪伤都须要探查或清创，通常这些创伤没有明显的组织破坏或骨折。可以观察到由子弹穿过软组织和肌肉，而没有血管损伤或明显血肿的简单伤口。应对创伤进行评估，基本灌注应在 6 h 内进行，因为造成感染最重要的风险因素是治疗延迟。没有必要用静脉内抗生素，因为感染的风险低于 2%。无论在简单创伤还是复杂创伤中，医务人员都应该处理伤者的破伤风状态。

通常取出子弹也不是必要的，理想的情况下其不能作为外科手术的唯一理由。偶尔伤者的症状严重，促使外科医生尝试取出子弹。然而，许多外科医生只是徒劳地在皮下组织寻找一个似乎存在皮肤下面的异物。此时有必要行 X 线检查定位。

造成铅中毒的唯一风险似乎是来自与滑液或骨髓液接触的子弹。穿过结肠并随后陷入骨中的子弹

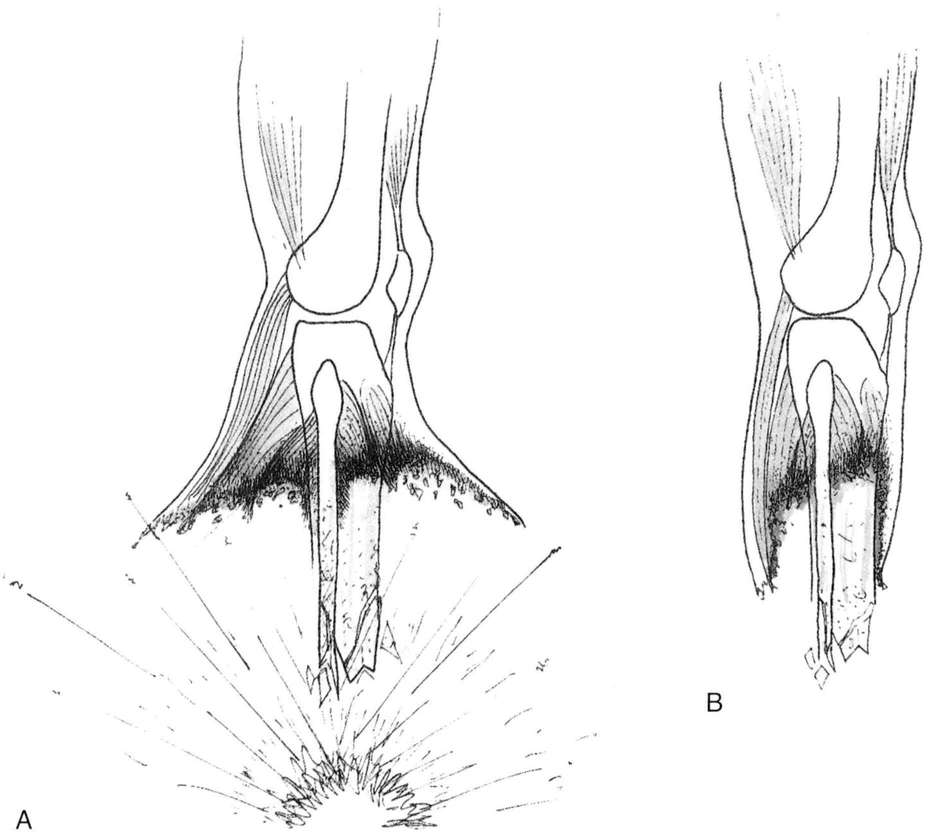

A

B

图 8　**A**，由脚触发的地雷引起的“伞状”效应作用在小腿上。**B**，小腿隔室的严重损伤可以被覆盖的皮肤所隐藏 (*From Coupland RM: War wounds of limbs: surgical management. Oxford, Butterworth-Heinemann, 1993*.)

有引起骨髓炎的风险。目前有一些关于风险程度的争论，但在我们的治疗中心，我们倾向于按照取出子弹的可能性而将其取出。替代方案是灌注管道和至少静脉注射 10 天广谱抗生素。须要去除子弹的其他适应证包括：动脉和静脉中的子弹栓塞，以及心室中的子弹。

院前常见的并发症和创伤患者救治中的陷阱

Frank L. Mitchell, Charles M. Richart, Harry E. Wilkins 著
张进军 译

美国的院前救护的发展较为有趣，并且是不断发展的。虽然早在公元 900 年就有了用于运送患者的货车和手推车的记录，但直到在其被西班牙 Isabella 女王于 15 世纪初引入之后，才出现了术语“救护车”(ambulance)。即使当时，该术语更多地是指军事野战医院和伤员帐篷，而不是从战场运送伤员和死者。一直到 Larrey 男爵的时候，“救护车”这一术语才具有其现代意义：“用于运送患者或伤者去医院的特别装备的机动车辆、飞机或船”。

Dominique-Jean Larrey 男爵是拿破仑的外科医生，他开发了所谓的“飞行救护车”。1792 年之前，几乎没有开展有组织地从战场运送伤员的行动。与大多数医疗进展的情况一样，采用救护车运送的进展是军事冲突的结果。在 19 世纪和 20 世纪初的一系列军事冲突中，人们已经开始使用救护车和其他运输手段从战场上运送伤员。

20 世纪 50 — 70 年代，在韩国军事和越南的军事冲突中，人们将直升机用于将战场上的伤者运送到流动军队手术医院 (mobile army surgical hospital, MASH)，且效率较高。在 20 世纪的前几十年，针对伤者的民用运输持续落后于军用运输的发展。

战场伤亡率从第一次世界大战中的8%持续下降到越南战争中不到2%，主要原因之一是缩短了从受伤到开始医疗救护的时间。在这种背景下，从20世纪60年代中期和70年代初期，人们开始寻求改善院前救护、教育、设备和流程。20世纪60年代初，人们将基础和高级急救培训扩大到更多的普通人群，并在全国范围内准备课本、培训材料以及针对救援队人员、警察、消防队员和救护车急救人员的指导课程。20世纪60年代，救护车急救服务十分零散，充其量只是数量足够。在少数几个大城市，已专门配备救护车以照顾伤者和患者，并且由训练有素的专业人员进行有效的院前急救。然而，在当时约50%的救护车服务是由12 000多名殡仪工人提供的，主要是因为他们的车辆更能够适应将患者置于轮床或担架上进行运输。

20世纪60年代中期，《国家交通和汽车安全法》（National Traffic and Motor Safety）及《公路安全法》（Highway Safety Act）制定了二手机动车、机动车辆检查和紧急服务的国家标准。另外，通讯也存在问题。当时美国刚把人类送上月球。在大多数情况下，与地球外的人进行通信比院前急救人员与即将前往的急诊部门进行通信显得更为容易。

在接下来的几十年里，对特种车辆的培训和规定也取得了进步。20世纪80年代中期，报告《损伤在美国：一种持续的公共健康问题》（Injury in American: A Continuing Public Health Problem）发表。虽然该报告发现在院前急救人员的证书和教育方面取得了重大进展，但是超过250万美国人在1966—1985年死于受伤。这促使支出更多的联邦资金来持续研究公共卫生问题。该报告呼吁建立更多的通信和运输系统，将伤员送到具有专业设备以及能够救治重伤患者的医疗机构。

1992年，由1990年《创伤系统规划和发展法办公室》（Authority of the Trauma Systems Planning and Development Act）管理下的卫生资源和服务管理局（Health Resources and Services Administration）制定了“创伤救护系统计划模型”（Model of Trauma Care Systems Plan）。这是与创伤救护有关的卫生政策发展中的下一个重要步骤。该计划强调需要一个全面包容性创伤救护系统，不仅包括创伤中心，而且还包括根据创伤资源（包括院前急救人员）提供的所有医疗机构。该计划使专业的创伤中心和国家创伤系统的数量增加了，尽管仍然不够完美。创伤中心成为紧急医疗应急机构的资源机构。同时开发了诸如院前创伤生命支持、基础创伤生命支持及其他教育培训计划，各州有权授权及提供各级证书。

今天，针对伤者的最初救护继续由受过专业训练的院前急救人员提供。急救医疗技术人员应具备有基础、中级和辅助医疗的教育水平。警察和消防部门人员也接受了基础生存支持的培训，并增加了与公众的交流以及对他们的教育，内容包括心脏停搏、安全带的使用以及头盔和其他预防措施等，以继续努力消灭由于蓄意和无意伤害造成的不可接受的高死亡率和残疾率。

随着院前急救人员急救技术的不断发展，使用这些设备和流程可能伴有一些意外风险。本章讨论了一些更常见的院前并发症。

发病率

根据国家高速公路交通安全管理局（National Highway Traffic Safety Administration）的数据显示，2002年美国4～34岁人口死亡的主要原因是机动车辆交通事故（表1）。从寿命损失的角度来看，机动车辆撞车的排名在恶性肿瘤和心脏病之后名列第三，占整个人口总寿命的5%。

共有37%的创伤死亡是由机动车辆碰撞和摩托车碰撞引起的。造成创伤死亡的其他重要原因是枪伤、刺伤和跌倒。如今在绝大多数情况下，院前急救人员能够成为这些伤害发生时或之后不久的第一响应者。

造成院前死亡的主要原因是继发于严重的头部创伤、呼吸道损伤和大出血。最初和紧急的院前急救集中在治疗和预防这些创伤。

美国外科医师学院（American College of Surgeons）的高级创伤生命支持（ATLS）基础强调ABC［气道（airway）、呼吸（breathing）和循环（circulation）］方法。重点强调院前急救和随后的创伤护理，包括合适的气道管理，通过呼吸为患者提供通气，以及控制出血和恢复循环血容量。毫无疑问，最常见的院前并发症就发生在这三个领域。

气道

确保创伤患者拥有可通气的气道是最高优先级的创伤急救管理。如果手动操作（清除气道异物、

别须要医疗抗凝的患者可能会导致延迟识别严重的颅内、胸内或腹内出血。另外，对医学上抗凝状态的识别可使院前急救人员更加怀疑有严重创伤的可能性，尽管可能看起来只是轻微的创伤。

必须考虑的慢性医学病症包括涉及心肺、肾、肝和内分泌系统的疾病。

慢性充血性心力衰竭患者常常服用多种药物，这可能削弱了他们对创伤反应的能力。例如，β 受体阻滞剂可以防止这些患者对急性出血产生心动过速反应。长期慢性利尿剂的使用可能导致这些患者血液的消耗。这些患者通常会有严重的呼吸困难，无法仰卧在运输担架车上。慢性充血性心力衰竭可能使他们容易出现液体超负荷，因而要进行相对最小量的静脉液体复苏治疗。

可能难以对患有慢性阻塞性肺病（COPD）的患者进行评估，因为听诊时可以听到长期减弱的呼吸音。这使得很难在临床检测诸如气胸、胸廓和心包压塞的病症，虽然不是不可能。此外，重症 COPD 患者可能依赖于相对低的血氧来促进呼吸能力，补充太多的氧会急剧钝化这种驱动，导致急性的呼吸停止。

慢性肾功能不全和肝功能不全的患者在院前环境中可能须要减少静脉给药。苯二氮䓬类药物和阿片类药物的选择和剂量必须仔细考虑患者的肌酐清除率。

糖尿病、肾上腺功能不全和甲状腺疾病的患者也会表现出对急性创伤的不同生理反应，从患者本人或其监护人那里掌握该患者的病史，可能有助于对这些患者的急救和随后的治疗。检查患者所服用的药物可明确这些疾病。从家庭成员、看护人员或患者本人获取病史资料，对于在院前环境中帮助和进一步救治患者来说是非常有用的。

小结

对创伤患者的初始管理是一项具有挑战性的工作，其将有助于采取有序的救治方法。遵循 ABCs 原则，对患者出现的创伤进行优先排序，以及快速将患者转运到确定的医疗场所，能为患者带来最好的结果。院前环境中容易犯的错误，如同其他领域一样，包括疏漏和刻板化的错误。通过仔细注意、细心照顾患者的方法和原则，这两种类型的错误都可以避免。

第3章 最初评估和复苏

气道管理：每一位创伤外科医生必备的气管插管和环甲软骨切开术知识

Andrew R. Doben 和 Ronald I. Gross 著
易成腊 译

医学的所有学科都涵盖立即和适当的气道管理概念。开放、保护和维护气道已被公认为严重疾病或创伤患者复苏的初始必要步骤。开展高级创伤生命支持（ATLS）的基本前提是遵循ABCDE复苏顺序：气道（Airway）、呼吸(Breathing)、循环（Circulation）、残疾（Disability）和暴露（Exposure）。根据ATLS的要求，对所有受伤患者在评估和处理的过程都应该遵循ABCDE顺序。

最佳的气道是清醒患者可以自主呼吸的气道，最差的情况是只能通过外科干预的“不能插管、不能通气”的危急情况。开放并维护适当的气道取决于很多因素。临床医生开放气道的技术从易到难。气管插管不是一个新的概念。事实上，首次报道的气管插管可追溯到1543年，实际上当时是指气管切开术。文艺复兴时期的解剖学家Andreas Vesalius在《人体构造图谱》（*On the Fabric of the human Body*）中写道：“从某种意义上说，生命可以恢复。必须在气管上做一个开口，然后插入一根芦苇或藤条，之后用它吹气，这样肺就可以再次扩张。”

从临床医生的角度来看，合适的气道管理是患者最初护理中最困难的部分。本章将从头颈和呼吸系统的解剖方面来帮助临床医生成功地管理气道，同时还会指出解剖结构变化和临床情况是如何影响临床医生的气道管理的选择。本章将会描述一些可以用来开放和维护安全气道的技术。

气道解剖

任何程序的成功执行都须要对程序进行彻底的了解：适应证、技术要求以及完成任务所需的设备。此外，操作者必须知道潜在的并发症以及对其的处理。无论是通过常规手段还是手术来开放气道，与其他程序相比没有什么不同。由于构成上呼吸道的结构的解剖与正常功能较为复杂，所以为了有效管理气道，外科医生必须对必要的解剖结构有所了解。

鼻子和嘴是气道两个天然的外部开口。鼻腔由鼻中隔分为两个含有骨、软骨和窦孔的锥体。鼻腔顶由鼻骨、额骨、筛骨和蝶骨体构成。鼻腔底由颌骨和腭骨构成。鼻中隔软骨、犁骨和筛骨垂直板构成了鼻腔内侧壁。在侧面，内侧壁包含一部分筛骨，以及上、中、下鼻甲。此外，它包含鼻旁窦和鼻泪管的开口（图1）。鼻腔神经来自嗅觉和三叉神经（分别为第Ⅰ和Ⅴ对脑神经）。血供来源于眼动脉的前、后支，以及上颌骨和面动脉的分支。

外表上，嘴由嘴唇和脸颊构成的，在上方有牙龈、牙齿和腭，在下方有黏膜和舌。腭既是口腔的顶，也是鼻腔的底。腭的前4/5是硬腭。它是一个有黏膜覆盖的骨框架。腭的后1/5是软腭。它是一个肌纤维褶皱。当吞咽或说话时软腭向后移动关闭口咽腔。

虽然嘴和鼻被腭在前部分隔开，但是在软腭后方两者又相连形成了咽。咽分为鼻咽和口咽。咽从环状软骨下缘延伸到第6胸椎椎体下缘。咽壁由两层咽肌构成：外圆层由括约肌组成，内纵层的肌肉在吞咽和说话时抬高咽喉。鼻咽与鼻腔同在软腭水平，并且通过鼻后孔与鼻腔相连，通过咽鼓管与鼓

咽

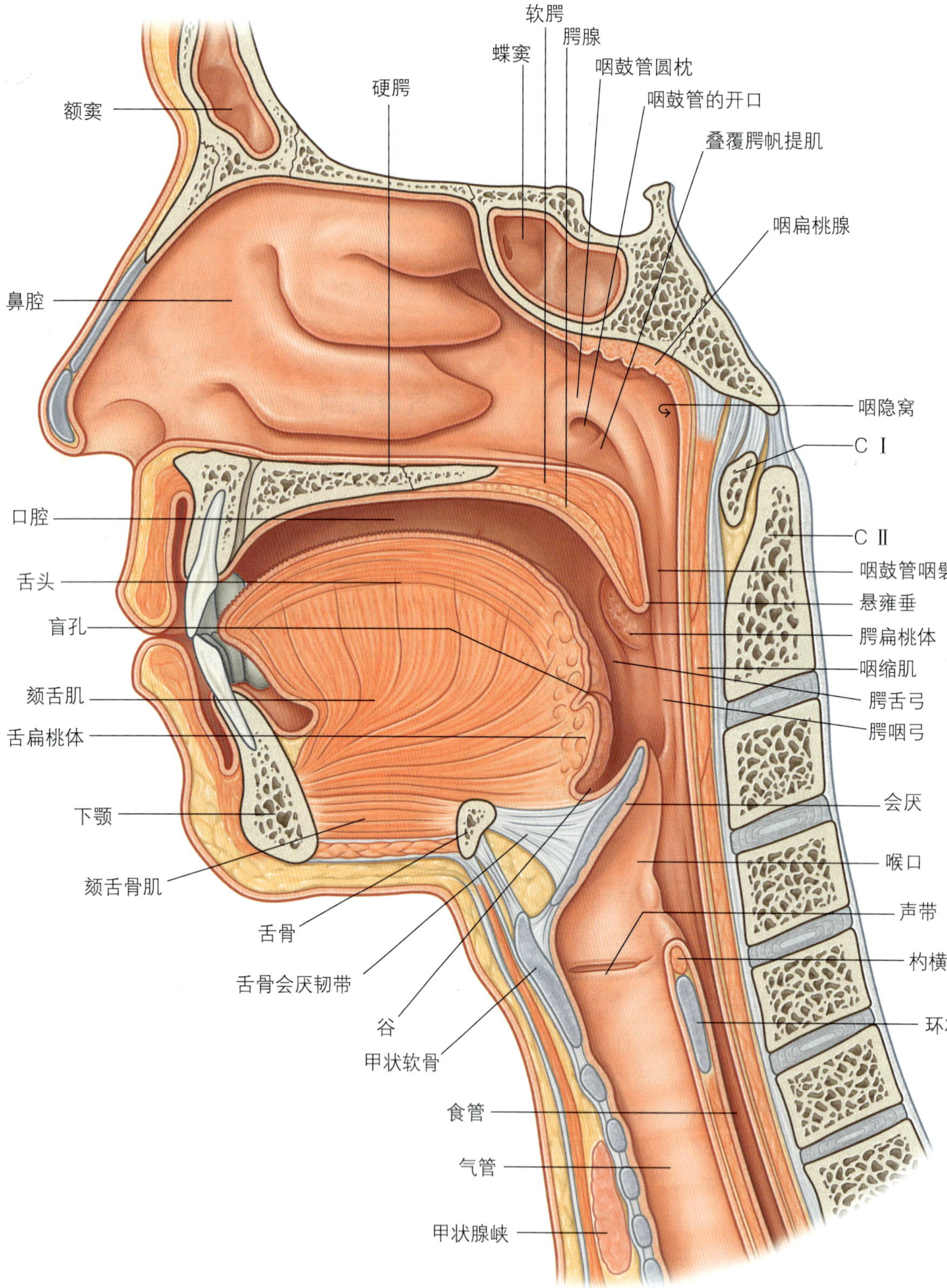

图 1　咽部侧视图（鼻、口和喉）(*From Drake RJ, Vogl AW, Mitchell AWM, et al, editors: Gray`s atlas of human anatomy. Philadelphia, Churchill Livingstone, 2008.*)

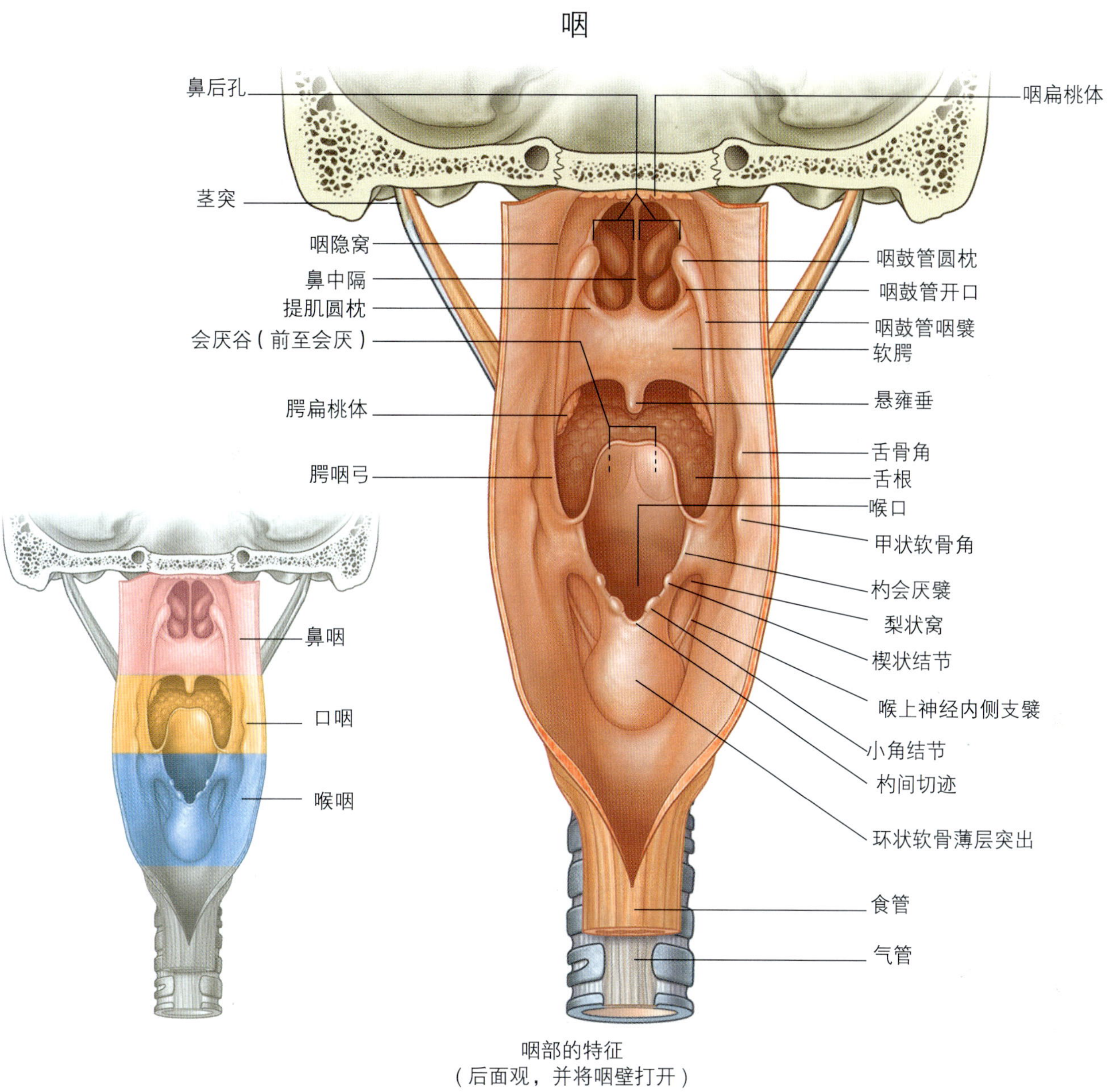

图 2　咽部的后视图（鼻、口、喉）(*From Drake RJ, Vogl AW, Mitchell AWM, et al, editors: Gray`s atlas of human anatomy. Philadelphia, Churchill Livingstone, 2008.*)

室相连。它的后壁有咽扁桃体。口咽始于软腭，一直延续到会厌的顶端（图 2）。它包括腭扁桃体，这是 Mallampati 气道分类法的重要标志。

会厌是在舌后的勺形弹性软骨。吞咽时，它通过关闭声门，打开喉来防止发生吸入。喉咽从会厌上缘延伸到环状软骨下缘。会厌与喉在杓会厌襞的侧面分离，该处有梨状隐窝。喉口两侧各有一个梨状隐窝，这里有喉下神经并且异物常滞留于此。

喉的骨架是一些连接着韧带和肌肉的软骨，包括甲状软骨、环状软骨、会厌软骨和成对的勺状软骨。喉的作用就像括约肌，在吞咽时防止食物和饮料进入气管和肺部。它还通过声带和调节进出肺的气流来发音。在气管插管时，气管导管通过时使声带外展才能前进（图 3）。

甲状软骨由左软骨板和右软骨板在中线相连构成，并形成甲状腺切迹与甲状腺隆起。甲状软骨的左、右上角与舌骨相连，下角通过环甲膜与环状软骨相连。在气管切开术中后者的解剖位置是十分重要的（图 4）。

不同于甲状软骨，环状软骨是一个完整的软骨环，它与甲状软骨和第一个气管软骨都相连。利用这种解剖关系，Sellick 提出的在全身麻醉时通过对环状软骨加压来预防胃内容物反流已经成为了一种

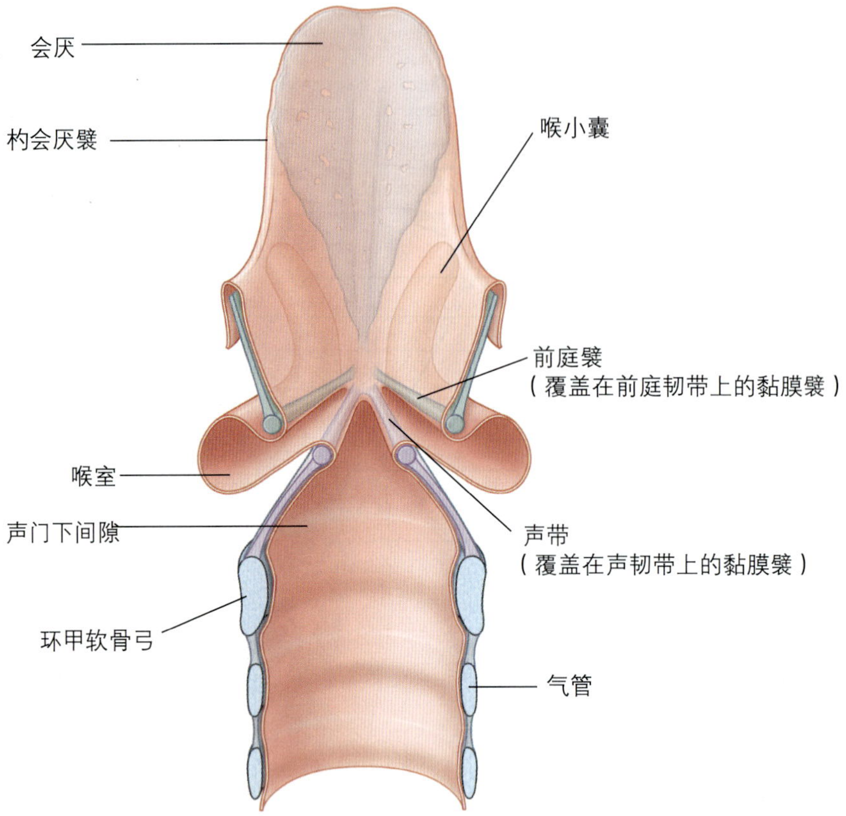

后面观（下摆）

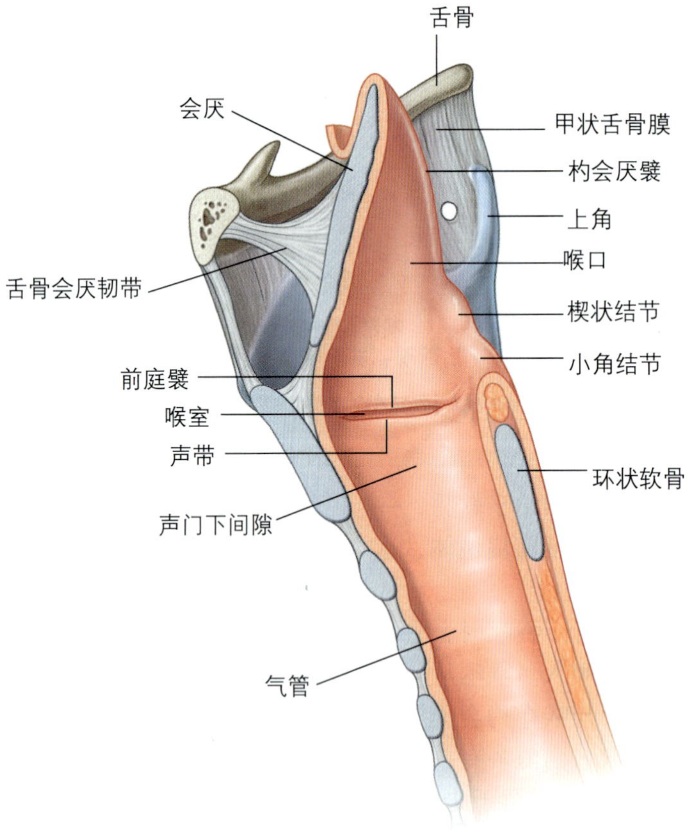

喉的矢状面

图 3　喉腔前侧面观 (*From Drake RJ, Vogl AW, Mitchell AWM, et al, editors: Gray's atlas of human anatomy. Philadelphia, Churchill Livingstone, 2008.*)

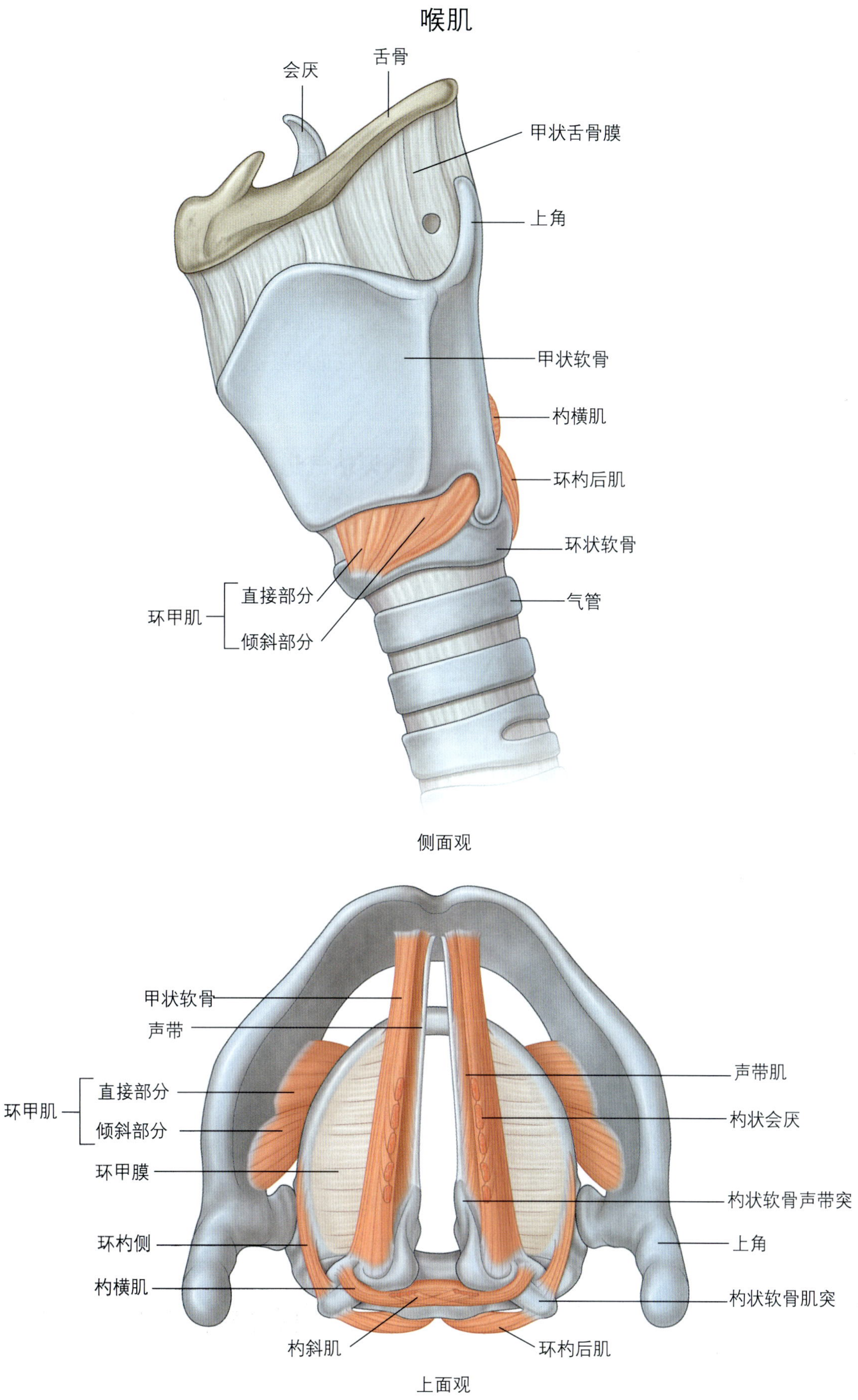

图 4　喉的肌肉和骨的标志 (*From Drake RJ, Vogl AW, Mitchell AWM, et al, editors: Gray`s atlas of human anatomy. Philadelphia, Churchill Livingstone, 2008.*)

公认的治疗标准。

会厌是覆盖着黏膜的弹性软骨。黏膜表面有一个轻微的凹陷，称为“谷”。为了抬高会厌和看到声带，要将喉镜叶片尖端放置在这一点上。会厌的前部通过会厌韧带与舌骨相连，下部通过甲状会厌韧带与甲状软骨相连。方形膜延伸在会厌软骨与杓状软骨之间的侧面。其下缘游离，称为前庭韧带，表面覆盖着黏膜，并在声带上方形成了从甲状软骨延伸到杓状软骨的前庭襞。勺状软骨与环状软骨侧上方相连，在每一侧都通过声韧带与声带相连。其下缘游离形成杓会厌韧带，表面覆盖黏膜形成杓状会厌襞。在杓状会厌襞后方可以看到有角的楔状软骨。这些软骨结构位于杓状软骨突起上。杓状软骨的弹性能力可以使其在外展结束后回到正常的解剖位置。通常可以在直接喉镜检查下看到。因此，在气管开放难以看到声带时，可以用它作为标志（图 5）。

声门包含在喉内，也是在成人呼吸道最窄的地方。声门由声带（或襞）构成，它们之间的空隙称为声门裂。因为声带表面覆盖着复层上皮，所以用光照射时可以看到特殊的珍珠白色。喉返神经控制着声带，喉肌则被迷走神经的分支（第 X 对脑神经）支配。喉包含了之前提到过的所有结构。

气管从环状软骨下缘开始延伸一段长度后，在胸骨角平面第 4 — 5 胸椎椎体处分成左、右主支气管。与甲状软骨一样，气管是由 16 ~ 20 个不完整的 C 形软骨环构成的，随着气道通气量的改变依次开放不同的直径。气管直接与后面的食管相连。这可能对有食管肿瘤或者纵隔血肿（创伤或者手术后）或者吞咽了异物的患者有重要意义。这些都会导致上（气管）气道的阻塞。

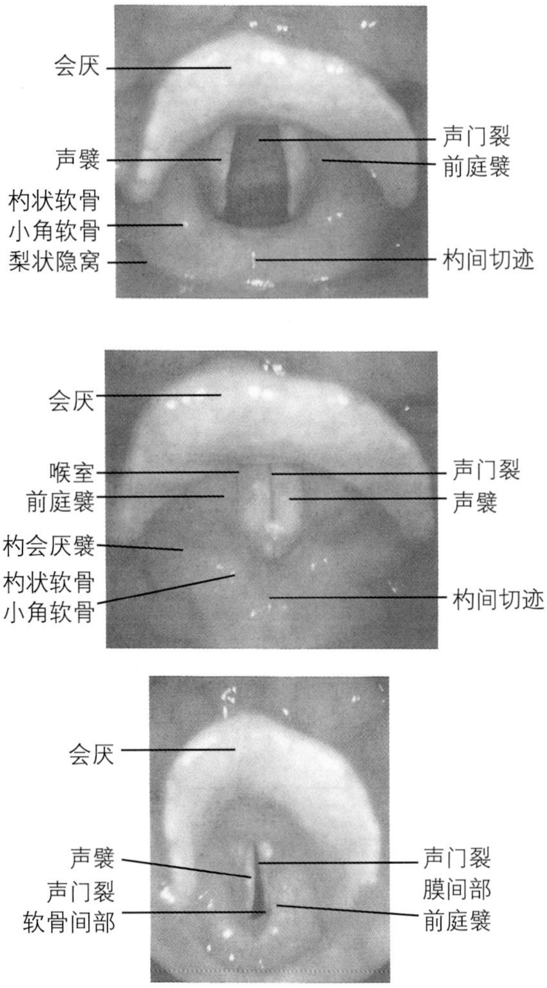

图 5 气管开放的标志 (*From Putz R, Pabst R, editors: Sobatta atlas of human anatomy, 13th ed. Baltimore, Williams & Wilkins, 2001.*)

评估气道

对创伤患者的气道和呼吸进行彻底而迅速的初步评估是首要任务。这一步必须完成，除非患者已被明确地诊断为颈椎损伤。如果没有完好的呼吸道，则患者不可能呼吸或说话。简单地询问患者的名字会有作用。显而易见，声音缺乏反应和改变是因为气道受损，这提示我们须要保护气道。

对于所有格拉斯格评分（GCS）为 8 分或以下的患者，无论是什么原因，都要进行气管插管来保护和固定气道。中毒和非法物质的使用是导致精神状态改变的常见原因，如闭合性头部损伤和缺氧。因此我们必须谨慎行事，始终假设 GCS 下降与损伤有关，然后进行气管插管来保护气道。声音嘶哑、呼吸急促、炭化痰或鼻孔和口腔外部有烧伤痕迹都可以提示临床医生气道可能处于危险状态，即使患者能做出适当的反应。对这些患者必须进行仔细、频繁地间断的评估，并且要降低气管插管的标准。此外，对这些患者进行气管插管可能会特别困难，所以在这种情况下，必须强调要对每个单独的气道进行快速、仔细的评估。

患者的解剖，无论是先天的还是由损伤所致，都须要临床医生在明确气道管理之前进行认真的评估。对于创伤患者，临床医生必须始终考虑到潜在的颈椎损伤。这一点对于存在精神状态改变的患者特别重要，无论是什么原因导致。在决定固定和保护气道的最佳方式时，也必须考虑到颌面部创伤和颈部软组织损伤。在没有损伤或病理的条件下，通气和控制声门气道是一种气道的大小和上喉组织的顺应性功能。应该记住的是，在正常情况下，气流通过鼻腔通常不是问题，因为这部分气道通常是由骨性鼻中隔支持。相反，因为咽没有一个刚性支撑系统，所以它更容易崩溃。导致上喉梗阻最常见的原因是反应迟钝或患者昏迷后舌头所致。通常这个问题可以在最初通过有效地使用口腔气道来解决。

更差的情况是，在喉的入口处因为舌根或者会厌的尺寸而导致呼吸道阻塞。这个区域的气流与这些结构的大小以及喉周的组织情况成反比。某些原因可以限制气流到这些区域，常见的有造成解剖中断或组织水肿的颈部外伤、照射前颈部、头颈部肿瘤以及因中等肥胖间接导致喉周多余脂肪组织堆积。这些因素可能导致上述的“不能通风、无法插管”的情况。这是一个潜在的致命情况，即便是对最熟练的气道管理人员而言也是如此。

与其他医疗程序一样，要谨慎地对病情进行有条理的评估，然后确定更有效地执行任务所需的方法和设备。除了先前讨论的因素外，还必须评估气道和周围组织的瘢痕和纤维化、气管损伤、先天性异常、急性炎症或气道肿瘤性疾病。最后，也要考虑牙龈、下颌和牙的畸形或疾病。对于个子矮小、肌肉发达的脖子较短的患者和肥胖的患者插管都比较困难。病态肥胖患者可能在扁桃体旁和声门旁区域因为多余组织阻挡气道，而使在进行喉镜检查时看不到声门。应该评估的解剖学因素包括颞下颌关节的下颌移动性、寰枕关节头的移动性（当已排除颈椎损伤时）、脖子的长短粗细及强壮程度、腭的大小和形态、下颌骨相对于面部的比例以及上颌牙齿的咬合。有两种相当实用的方法可以快速评估这些因素。当下颌与舌骨间的距离不到 3 指宽时采用面罩通气十分困难。另外，麻醉科采用的 Mallampati 评分（见第二部分的“院前气道管理”图 1）也表明很难直接进行喉镜检查。

为了对 Mallampati 评分进行分类，要求患者在坐着时将头摆正，并尽量张大嘴巴和伸舌。这对创伤患者来说是不可能完成的。然而，熟悉 Mallampati 分类的临床医生可以通过用压舌板或喉镜口咽进行粗略的评价。这为临床医生提供了某些困难插管的潜在思路。这也可以显示出口咽受伤的证据以及异物、出血和呕吐物。

因为不能总是依靠麻醉医生来保护气道，所以所有治疗创伤患者的临床医生必须有能够提供即时、有效的气道保护和通气的能力。因此，临床医生必须能够认识到限制气道通路的原因，还必须具备解决这些问题的技术。许多工具和技术在麻醉师的选修课中可以找到，尽管许多麻醉师可能在紧急创伤救治中不会应用，也许只会用几个。这些将是本次讨论的其余的重点。

控制气道

最好的气道是患者在没有任何外部干预的情况下可以安全地维持气道。创伤外科东部学会（Eastern Association for the Surgery of Trauma）已经提出对有气道阻塞和通气不足的创伤患者须要进行紧急气管插管，而不管是否存在严重缺氧、严重认知障碍（GCS 评分<8 分）、心搏骤停和严重的出血性休克。一旦患者的气道通气不够，或者患者不能保护呼吸道，那就必须以快速、高效和安全的方式完成气管插管。须要记住的是，所有创伤患者在插管时要保持颈部固定，以用来保护可能受伤的颈椎。

与所有其他程序一样，成功的结果取决于操作者的经验以及能够立刻使用所有正确的设备。大多数急诊部门配有装备了所有设备的气道推车，里面有紧急插管所需要的常规设备，还有专门为“困难插管”准备的推车。虽然这些推车的物品在不同的机构有所区别，但是它们通常在每个医院都会标准化。

一旦决定插管，所有的患者都应该吸入纯氧。双手托颌法和抬头举颏法可以做到不伤及颈椎，也可以尝试打开昏迷患者被舌头阻塞的呼吸道。抬头举颏法要将手指放置在患者的下颌，然后轻轻地向上抬起下颌，用同一只手的拇指压低下嘴唇来张开患者的嘴巴。必须注意，在使用抬头举颏法时不要过度伸展脖子。对于昏迷的患者，可以单独使用双手托颌法，也可以联合球囊面罩（BVM）通气使用。对于有呼吸的患者或者呼吸费力的患者，可以联合使用压缩袋。抓住两个下颌角并将下颌骨推向前，一方面是能够同时打开气道，另一方面是获得并保持有效的密封性来配合使用面罩期间辅助袋面罩通气。虽然这一技术是可以由一个操作者来完成，但最有效的方式还是由两名熟练的操作者配合完成。

口咽和鼻咽部的气道（图 6）是有用的，但是插管时必须谨慎，并且有严重面部创伤和筛骨板骨折的患者禁止插管。虽然没有一种办法是清醒患者可以很好耐受的，但是对于反应迟钝的患者来说鼻咽气道可以更好地耐受，可能是因为更不容易刺激患者作呕和呕吐。它们都可以用来维持迟钝患者的上呼吸道。对于成人，刚插入口腔气道时凸面朝下。必须小心轻放，使其不将舌头向后推移，相反，它要位于舌后的位置并将舌头向前推动。对于儿童，必须始终保持口腔气道凸面对着头部，以避免损伤口腔及咽部的软组织。重要的是要记住，对于有持续性（完整）上呼吸道咽反射的患者，口腔气道插入可能诱发喉痉挛、支气管痉挛，以及咳嗽、窒息、呕吐，最终吸气。

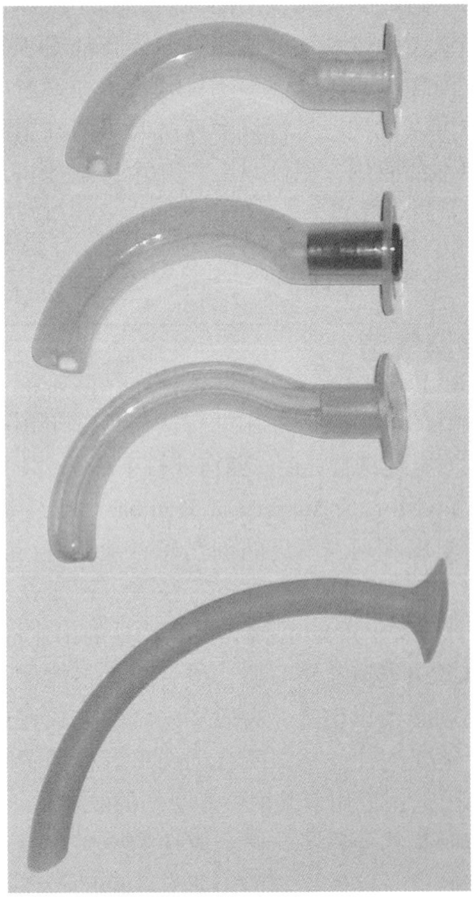

图 6　口腔气道（上面 3 个）和 鼻气道

记录气管导管的正确位置

无论使用何种技术保护呼吸道，一旦确定要获得气道，那么当务之急是确认和记录正确的管道位置。确认适当的导管位置最好的方法是在喉镜检查中看到导管穿过声带。因为并不是总是看到，所以通过体格检查可以迅速、暂时地确定导管的位置。胸部的视诊和听诊是可用的临床手段。对于没有胸壁破裂的肋骨骨折，将导管放在适当位置通气后临床医生可以看到对称的胸壁运动。

在前部和腋侧听诊胸部，当在双侧同等位置上听诊听到呼吸声相等时表明有作用。当创伤患者有气胸或血胸时，即使导管的位置适当，情况并不总是如此。临床医生应该立即治疗气胸或者血胸，然后通过物理检查和 X 线胸片来确认胸膜腔造口术中导放置的位置。听诊腹部的左上象限是十分重要的。将气管导管放置在适当位置时，通气时在胃部听不到淙淙声。

发绀是氧浓度下降的一个晚期表现，并受到诸如房间照明、贫血和血红蛋白异常的影响。解决了缺氧是将管道放置得合适的可靠迹象，但可能须要经过一段时间颜色才会变淡，特别是对于已经历过预充氧法的患者。测定呼气体中的 CO_2 已成为紧急情况下正确放置气管导管的标准。这可以通过 CO_2 分析仪来检测。由于使用方便、快速，比色 CO_2 探测器已经成为大多数机构的标准。通常将比色 CO_2 探测器插入气管内管的一端与通气管或气囊之间的呼吸回路，并在插管通气后就开始检测 CO_2。颜色的变化意味着在呼气中存在 CO_2。必须记住，尽管该方法很有用，但是 CO_2 的存在与否并不是将管道放在合适位置的绝对保证。当没有将气管导管放置在主支气管时也可以检测到 CO_2。在心搏骤停的患

者中不能检测到 CO_2。在气管插管前进行通气的患者，当误将气管导管放置在食管内时，在胃内可检测到 CO_2。通过几次呼吸就可以明确这一点，并提示临床医生管道位置放置得不对。

气管导管的弯曲部分至少要在声带下 1 ~ 2 cm。对于普通患者，气管导管进入 21 ~ 23 cm 后系将其紧并固定在牙齿上。在气管插管结束后，应该拍一张胸片来确定导管放置的位置。对于一般成年人来说，放置适当时，气管导管的尖端应该在胸片上可见，应在气管隆嵴上方 5 cm。

尽管所有的设备和技术都在不断进步，但是在气道管理中，临床医生、临床判断、体格检查和关注的细节都是必不可少的。

联合管

因为无法插管引起的通气不足可以导致缺氧而致命，因此，要对生命垂危或受到损伤的患者提供氧气。有一些技术可以解决这一问题，如联合管的双腔气管食管导管（Tyco Healthcare Group LP, 2001）。这种管子有常规尺寸和小号的成人尺寸。其已经把使用食管闭孔气道作为气道抢救技术出现的问题最小化了。虽然 Wissler 建议使用喉镜在直视下置管，但是对这种管子可以从口腔盲插。

虽然该管的顶端可以终止于气管，但其进入食管的可能性为 99%。一旦成功置管，向气囊内充入空气，向咽部气囊充入 100 ml 空气用于阻塞咽部，并在远端球囊充入 15 ml 空气用于闭塞食管或气管。开始用 1 号管道通气。如果管尖位于食管内（首选位置），可听到两侧的呼吸音，CO_2 描记仪将显示 CO_2 为阳性。胃胀气时，听诊腹部左上象限将为阴性。此时，胃管可以通过 2 号管放置（图 7）。

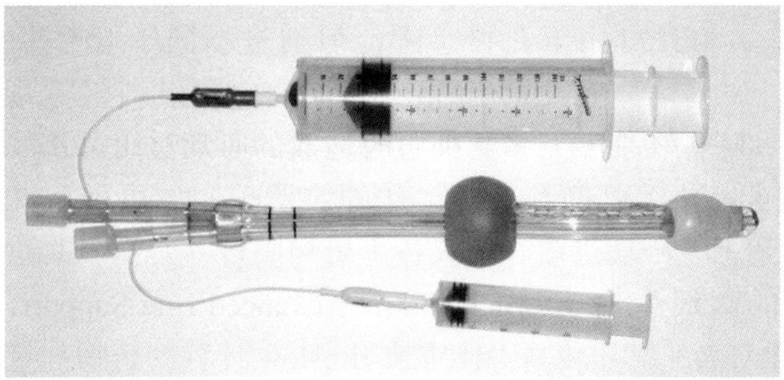

图 7 联合管的两个气囊都充气。用较大的注射器给蓝色管（1 号）气囊充气

如果导管的尖端在气管内，则在胸部不会听到呼吸音，并且 CO_2 描记仪将显示 CO_2 为阴性。应立即将通气切换到 2 号管，并反复通过听诊来检查确认呼吸音，并通过 CO_2 描记仪检查 CO_2。

临床已显示，对于具有严重颌面创伤的患者，在快速顺序插管（RSI）失败后，联合管是院前急救环甲膜切开术的一种有效替代方法。实际上，Blostein 等研究了 10 例气管插管失败的患者，有 7 例成功地使用联合管取代口腔气管，只有 3 例需要手术气道。必须记住，在临床情况允许时必须尽快用一个明确的气道更换联合管。此外，还要记住使用联合管的禁忌证：①年龄小于 16 岁。②具有完整的咽反射。③已知患有食管疾病。④有已知摄入腐蚀物质。虽然联合管是气管插管的重要辅助手段，但是在创伤中的使用仍然有限。

气管内插管

对于成人来说，在气管管腔中放置气管导管被认为是一种安全的气道。可以通过鼻腔、口腔或者手术（环甲软骨切开术或气管造口术）来完成这种气道。气道控制的紧迫性和临床医生的能力将决定如何选择这些技术。

鼻插管

鼻插管是一种公认的用于反应迟钝的患者的插管技术，但患者必须有自主呼吸且不能在紧急情况下。大多数创伤患者都有鼻插管的禁忌证。因为受伤的患者往往情况紧急，且伴有精神状况差，还有可能存在潜在的没有发现的面部骨折，所以鼻插管极少被用于多发伤的患者。此外，因为大多数创伤患者没有禁食，有发生呕吐和抽吸的风险，所以最常使用 RSI 技术进行插管。RSI 技术会使患者窒息，所以鼻插管是禁忌的。

经口气管插管

经口气管插管主要是在紧急情况下用来明确气道控制。当麻醉师在选修课上演示操作时，要伸展患者的头部才能完成经口气管插管，这就是所谓的“监听位置”。在有潜在颈椎损伤的创伤患者中，禁忌行颈部伸展。重要的是要记住，对于创伤患者，经口气管插管是一个两人操作，即一个人插管，而另外一个人固定颈椎。

须要插管的创伤患者通常有各种解剖和生理上的紊乱，这使得插管变得更加困难。这些患者经常有不同程度的缺氧、酸中毒和血流动力学不稳定。在合并有心脏或肺功能受损的患者，尤其是老年患者，延长气管插管的时间将会进一步增加心肌缺血或脑缺血的风险。实际上，对患者进行经口气管插管会加重与创伤性事件有关的症状，如颅内压增高、心肌功能障碍、上气道出血、吸入性损伤和呕吐。当有必要行紧急插管时，对这些因素须要制订一个标准化的方案。RSI 提供了这种标准化方案，以照顾那些危重患者。

在进行 RSI 的同时可使用一种诱导剂（镇静、抗焦虑、失忆）和一种神经肌肉阻断剂（NMBA）。RSI 的目标是获得安全气道，同时避免呕吐和吸入、心律失常或喉镜引起的交感反射性反应等并发症。相对禁忌证包括使用球囊通气将最有可能是无效的或不可能的情况。适当使用时，已证明 RSI 可以减少插管相关的并发症，同时使插管的成功率增至 98%。最常用的 RSI 药物包括利多卡因，诱导剂咪达唑仑或依托咪酯，还有 NMBA 琥珀胆碱和罗库溴铵，详见表 1 去极化和非去极化神经肌肉麻痹剂的总结。

表 1　去极化和非去极化神经肌肉麻痹剂

药物	剂量
去极化剂	
极短（<10~12 min）	
琥珀酰胆碱	1.5 mg/kg
非去极化剂	
短效（15 ~ 20 min）	
米库氯铵	0.2 mg/kg
中效（20 ~ 50 min）	
维库溴铵	0.08 ~ 0.1 mg/kg
罗库溴铵	0.6 ~ 1.2 mg/kg
阿曲库铵	0.5 ~ 0.5 mg/kg
顺式阿曲库铵	0.15 ~ 0.2 mg/kg
长效（>50 min）	
泮库溴铵	0.06 ~ 0.1 mg/kg
哌库溴铵	0.07 ~ 0.1 mg/kg
甲筒箭毒	0.2 ~ 0.4 mg/kg
多沙氯铵	0.05 mg/kg
加拉	1 mg/kg（最大量 100 mg）
双烯丙毒马钱碱	0.2 ~ 0.3 mg/kg
筒箭毒碱	0.5 ~ 0.6 mg/kg

Modified from Miller RD: Miller' s Anesthesia, 7th ed. Philadelphia, Elsevier, 2010, and consulting editors, Micromedex 2.0 5/2/2012

利多卡因常被用于降低高血压反应和喉镜检查气道时的反应性，降低颅内压增高，并减少插管时心律失常的发生率。为了达到效果，可在经口气管插管前 3 min 静脉给药 1.5 mg/kg。

诱导剂可使患者昏迷，从而方便迅速插管。咪达唑仑和依托咪酯均迅速、有效，并且具有相似的清除半衰期。肠外给药时，咪达唑仑（1 ~ 2.5 mg/kg）更有可能引发低血压与心肌抑制。相反，依托咪酯（0.15 ~ 0.3 mg/kg）不影响血压，通过降低脑血流量和脑部氧吸收的吸收具有脑保护作用。因此，它是低血压创伤患者的首选诱导剂。

琥珀酰胆碱是去极化剂中最常使用的 NMBA。它有一个快速发作（30 ~ 60 s）和相对较短的生效时间（5 ~ 15 min），9 ~ 10 min 后就可以恢复正常的通气状态。给予琥珀胆碱后 10 ~ 15 s 可发生肌束震颤，可能与颅内、眼内和胃内压力短暂的增加有关。然而，颅内压增加得很小，以至于其产生的影响被通过提高插管成功率从而避免缺氧所抵消。不能将琥珀酰胆碱用于治疗贯通伤、胆碱酯酶缺乏、肌病或肌营养不良症。此外，在有高钾血症或有发生高钾血症风险的患者，如热（烧）伤在 24 h 以上，或存在挤压综合征伴心肌坏死 / 横纹肌溶解，或不能透析，此类患者不能使用琥珀胆碱。罗库溴铵是一种去极化 NMBA，生效时间也很快（30 ~ 60 s），剂量为 1 mg/kg。但与琥珀胆碱相比，其恢复自主呼吸需要更长的时间（45 ~ 60 min）。它没有任何琥珀酰胆碱具有的有害的副作用。并且根据 Perry 等的研究，在任何试验条件下使用罗库溴铵或琥珀胆碱插管的成功率是相似的。

RSI 可用于儿科患者，但剂量不同于 10 岁以上的患者。在儿科患者使用时会增加迷走神经紧张和降低功能残气量。插管时造成的心动过缓可诱发迷走神经刺激和缺氧。此外，琥珀胆碱可引起儿童患者心动过缓。建议各个机构制订一套基于儿童的高级生命支持（Pediatric Advanced Life Support，PALS）课程和基于体重或 Breslow 计算的药物剂量的 PSI 方案。

理论上，在插管之前，要用 100% 氧气面罩吸氧，直到脉搏血氧仪的 SO_2 在 100% 或达到最大水平。球囊面罩通气可用于协助患者的呼吸，也可以用于对窒息患者插管前控制气道。当要减少吸入的可能性时可以直接压迫患者的环状软骨，这被称作 Sellick 动作。在采取球囊面罩通气时胃内可能进入空气，所以插管成功后应立即插入一根鼻胃管。

对于昏迷和窒息的患者，无须使用药物，可以直接在喉镜下看到声带后进行插管。有几种不同的喉镜叶片可用（图 8）。插管时应选择合适的形状和大小。将喉镜插入口腔，注意不要损伤嘴唇或牙齿。将喉镜的叶片先推向后方，然后卷动舌头向上和左方移动。一旦见到扁桃弓，将叶片的尖端置于谷部，然后暴露喉和由声带环绕形成的声门裂。如果看到会厌悬于喉上，要将叶片更进一步推进谷部，以暴露声带。一旦看到声带，就将气管导管轻柔地穿过声带进入气管。使用气管插管内半金属管是很普遍的，但不是强制性的。气管导管根据不同的患者可选择大小不同的型号。从历史上看，儿童气管插管使用胶管气管导管，但据儿童高级生命支持（PALS）新的推荐，对住院的儿童应该放置通气管。对于成人，气管导管的大小由两侧声带间的间隙大小决定。大多数成年人可以容忍在气管内放置内径为 7 mm、7.5 mm 或 8 mm 的管子，其长度距离嘴唇 21～24 cm。对于孩子来说，气管导管应该是通气管，大小相当于孩子的鼻孔或小手指（第五指），位置不超过声带 2 cm。绝对不能使气管导管强行通过声带，而是应该轻柔地引导其通过声门（图 9）。

保护困难的气道可能存在巨大的障碍。已证明，血流动力学改变、氧合和通气困难相关的并发症是

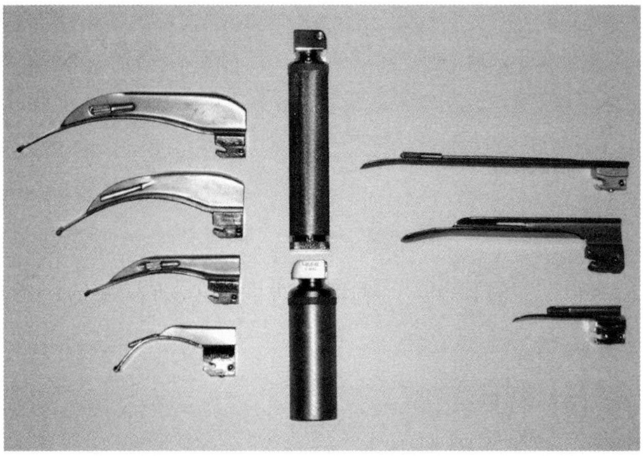

图 8　左侧，Macintosh 弯曲叶片（从上到下，编号为 4、3、2、1）；中间，喉镜手柄；右侧，Miller 直叶片（从上到下，编号为 3、2、0）

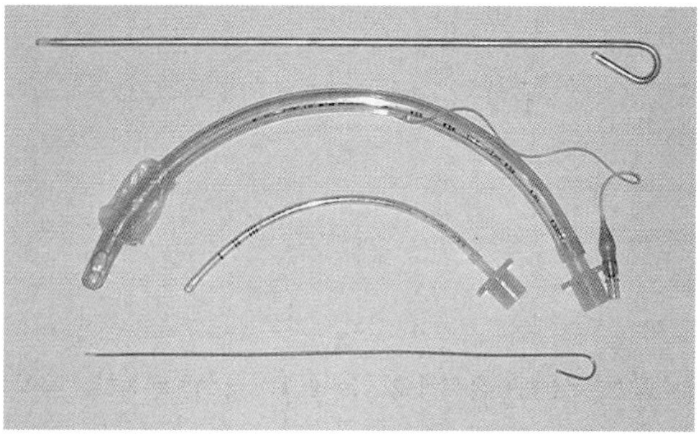

图 9　成人和儿科型号以及气管内管

须要在手术室外进行紧急气管插管的患者存在的严重问题。一项研究表明，在所有须要尝试三次以上的气管插管中，困难气管插管占了 10%，并且气道相关和血流动力学相关的并发症是“比较常见的”。这表明，无论是谁，在进行紧急气管插管时，都需要有一个备用的方案。这些备用方案应包括联合导管（前面讨论过）、弹性探条、喉罩气道（LMA）、插管性 LMA、Glidescope 视频喉镜（glide- scope video laryngoscopy，GVL），最后是紧急环甲膜切开术。此外，只要有可能，为了避免处理困难气道时可能出现包括死亡在内的并发症，必须具有能熟练插管的帮手。

经口气管插管的附件

在过去的几年里，在紧急气道中 GVL 已成为主角。这种间接视频喉镜通过使用喉镜增加了经口气管插管的成功率（图 10）。有研究表明，GVL 已经将插管成功率提升到了 94%～97%，即使将其作为直接喉镜失败的抢救技术。虽然没有研究显示 GVL 增加了颈椎制动患者气管插管的成功率，但是它可以制造一个良好的喉镜视野。

虽然 GVL 是一种将气管导管穿过声带放置的“两手操作”的技术，但是它也允许用第二只手进行吸气和疏通后咽。此外，该设备可以设置速度，从而使这种技术在创伤情况下比柔韧的纤维支气管镜更有效。虽然 GVL 明显地提供了更好的视野和额外的工具以进行插管，但是有显著流血或者液体的大面积颌面部创伤是其禁忌证，因为血液或液体会使摄像头模糊而变得无效。

探条是尖端弯曲的半刚性、弹性胶样导丝状设备。它应该是任何困难气道推车上的标准设备，而

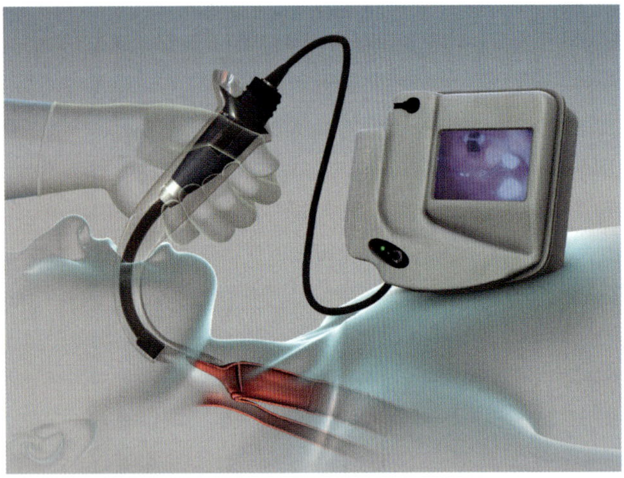

图 10 使用 Glidescope 视频喉镜气管插管的应用实例 (*Used with permission © Verathor Inc.*)

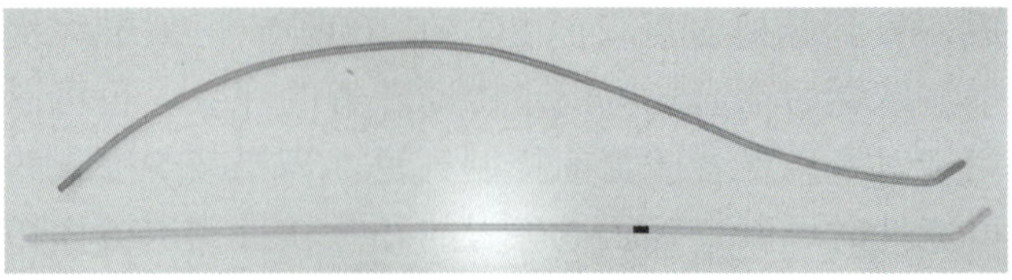

图 11 半刚性弹性树胶探条

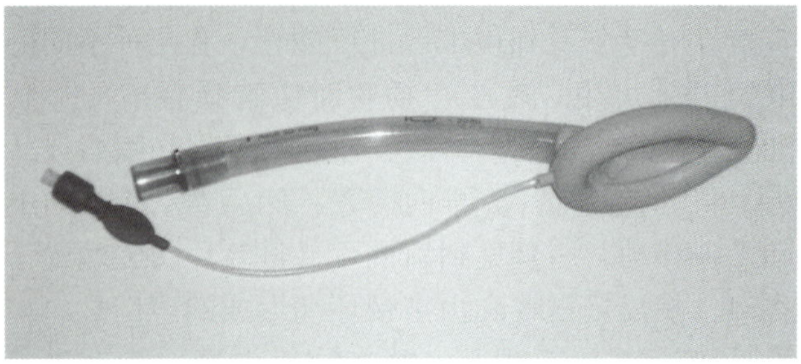

图 12 喉罩气道

且要保证，无论何时出现困难气道，都能立即使用。通常只有在杓状软骨或者会厌可见时才使用探条。使用喉镜或 GVL 时，使探条先进入喉，然后通过声带，最后进入气管。当探条进入气管后，其尖端摩擦气管环。操作者可以体验到“搓板效应”。必须小心，以避免探条进入过深，否则可能造成支气管损伤。一旦探条到达合适的位置，由一个临床医生维持探条位置不动，另一个临床医生把已经润滑过的气管导管向前推进，通过声带，并进入喉镜下可见的气管位置（尽可能）。然后移出探条，并按照之前提到过的步骤来确认气管导管的位置（图 11）。

LMA 最初是在 1983 年由 Brain 提出的，但是现在常用于择期行全麻手术处置的患者的呼吸道管理。LMA（Laryngeal Mask Company，Ltd.）和 LMA Fastrach 现在成为紧急气道管理的医疗设备的有价值的补充，虽然不太常用（图 12）。

喉罩是一种连接着一个卵圆形或椭圆形硅胶套的大口径管，只要润滑好，就可以尽可能深入地盲插进气管。一旦安置恰当，向导管充入 20 ~ 30 ml 空气，导管的前缘或尖端将阻塞食管腔，并且还能在喉的入口处提供低压密封。它能在紧急情况下允许通气。须要记住，存在咽反射的患者不能很好地耐受 LMA，因为会引起患者呕吐和吸入。LMA 有多种型号，被用于成人和儿童。作为气管插管，要想成功地插入须要选择适当的型号。对创伤患者而言，紧急置入 LMA 的适应证包括在快速序列给药后 GCS 评分为 3 分或者经口气管插管失败。一旦建立了通气，就须要获得更加明确的气道。

虽然 LMA 已经被用于保护创伤患者的气道，但它确实更适合用于择期气道管理的情况。另一方面，当在创伤环境中使用时，已证明 LMA Fastrach（图 13）或气管插管喉罩是有效的。LMA Fastrach 的咽口和普通 LMA 有所不同（图 13 和 14）。它有一个专门设计的通道和兼容的气管导管。LMA Fastrach 允许的气管导管的最大直径为 8 mm。与 LMA 一样，放置 LMA Fastrach 的适应证是 GCS 评分为 3 分并须要立即控制气道。放置气管插管喉罩的方式与 LMA 一样，但是气管导管的通道是“两人操作”技术，其中一个人控制 LMA，另外一个人充分润滑气管导管。一旦确认了放置气管导管的快速序列给药后位置，就要小心地移除 LMA，同时维持住气管导管的位置。

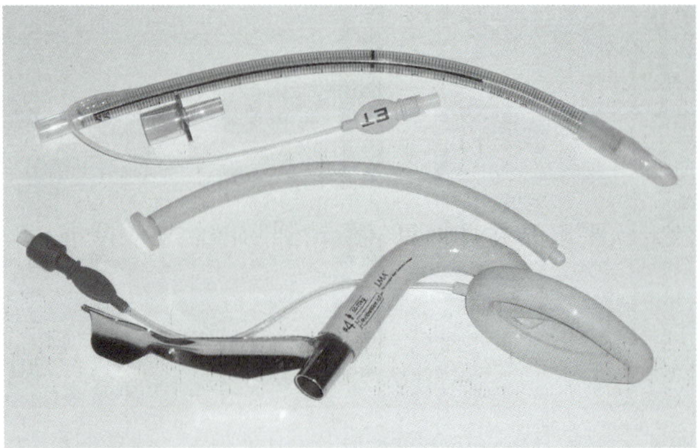

图 13 插管型喉罩气道（LMA）。特制的气管内管 LMA（上）、探针（中）、插管型 LMA 和插管手柄

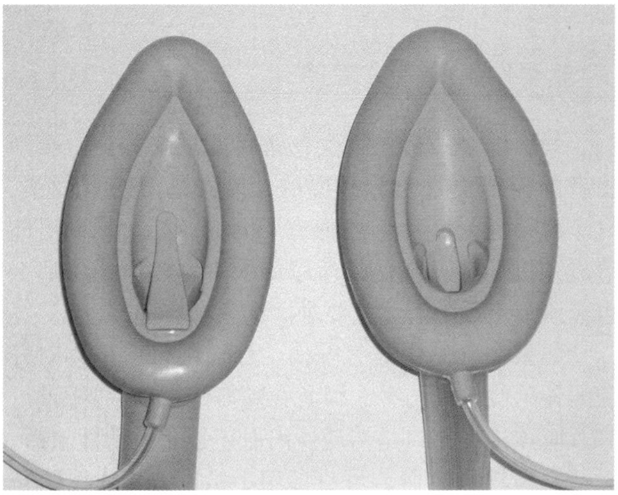

图 14 咽孔喉罩气道（LMA）（左）和普通喉罩（右）

手术气道

首选的气道管理方法是由患者执行，医生仅给予较少的帮助。临床医生可以监测空气进入气道以及观察通气中的所有困难。不幸的是，这种方法并不经常使用。

一旦上述任何气道措施宣告患者的气道未受保护并且不能通气，那么就提示可用手术气道。

环甲膜穿刺

环甲膜穿刺是一种快速、有效而安全的通过环甲膜进入气道的方法。此操作的优点在于操作简单而且需要很少的设备。绕过声带水平的障碍，然后使空气直接进入支气管树。

这种方法的缺点是，即便是大口径的针也不能充分地维持患者的通气超过几分钟。这种气道控制方法旨在为不能通气的患者提供氧气，直到获得更为正式的手术气道。

不幸的是，即使通过使用 14 G 或更大的针获得高流量的氧气，但患者的呼气能力较弱。患者的 CO_2 水平上升并且将氧气运输到肺泡的功能受损。

步骤

需要一个连有 14 G 针头的注射器。取一个 Y 形连接器，将氧气连接于 Y 形连接器的一侧。另一侧可以用手指堵住，使氧气流入气管。然后可以看到胸壁随着吸气上抬。移开堵住的手指可以影响呼气。触诊喉并确定喉下缘。然后确定环甲软骨，其为喉下第一个软骨结构。环甲软骨和喉间的间隙是环甲软骨膜（图 4）。用手指触诊后，用连接着装有 2 ml 液体注射器的针头，先以 45° 的角度进针穿过皮肤和环甲软骨膜，然后进入气管腔内。当插入针头后，轻轻回抽注射器。当针头“啪啪”地穿透环甲软骨膜时，立刻可以看到注射器中的 2 ml 液体里有气泡。空气是很容易流入注射器内的。然后抽回针头，将插管固定在正确的位置。然后将氧气供应管道连接 Y 形连接器，然后再与插管的圆筒相连。然后氧气就可以从插管直接流进气管。移开堵住 Y 形连接器的手指，CO_2 就可以从支气管树中流出。应将氧气保持较高的流量，为 10 ~ 12 L/min。氧合和通气只能维持几分钟，直到获得更加明确且大范围的气道。

环甲软骨切开术

正式的环甲软骨切开术比环甲膜穿刺有明显的优势。因为可以用更大的插管穿过环甲膜，并且有更足量的通气。其优点与环甲膜穿刺类似，既便于识别解剖结构，操作也简单。其缺点是这种切开的位置在颈部太靠近上方，以至于难以维持长期气道。出于这个原因，环甲软骨切开术被当做一种临时措施，直到可以在可控的情况下做气管切开术。

步骤

可以在颈部中线辨认出喉，也可以辨认出环甲软骨环。在这些结构之间可以触诊到菱形的环甲膜。使环甲膜处于中线是十分重要的，因为中线处没有血管。当操作者向侧方移动时，可能会碰到颈静脉与颈部的主要血管和神经。内侧带状肌正好在中线的侧方。虽然认为做一个水平切口直接穿过环甲膜是最佳选择，但是在紧急状况下这可能会造成严重的静脉损伤和大出血，导致切口视野模糊。因此，在紧急状况下进行环甲软骨切开术选择垂直切口是更合适的方案。切口长度为 1 ~ 2 cm，依次通过皮肤、皮下组织和颈阔肌。一旦进入颈阔肌，伸入一根手指确认环甲膜（图 4）。用手术刀做一横行切口穿过环甲膜进入气管。用手术刀片在中线处对环甲膜做一小缺口。然后将手术刀的手柄垂直于垂直切口，并通过在上述步骤中环甲膜上的小缺口进入气管。然后将手柄旋转 90°。另外，也可以用 Halsted 蚊式血管钳来分离环甲膜，先横向，然后纵向。这样就有了一个直接进入气管的较大切口。这种使用手术刀柄的技术是十分有用的。因为在横向水平上，环甲膜的任何一侧都有血管，所以选择钝性分离环甲膜是更适合的方式。选择 4 号，最大不能超过 6 号气管切开管，可以直接通过环甲膜进入气管。如果没有气管切开管，那么就可以选择 6 号气管导管。

如果该区域的解剖结构变形，或者有严重损伤并伴有血肿，那么最适合的选择是将 Robinson 红色橡胶管穿过环甲膜进入气管。然后把气管切开管从红色橡胶管中穿过。这样就避免了制造一个假通道和损伤气管。一旦气管切开管位于气管内，那么患者就可以通过管子通气。用缝线来固定管道是十分必要的。然后用本章所描述的气管插管后确认管道位置的方法来检查管道的位置。

急救外科气管切开术

该操作只有在危及生命时才会做。这种情况很少发生。它的一个适应证经常是由晾衣绳导致的罕见的环状软骨气管的分离。在进行气管切开术之前，最好使用上述任何一种方法来控制患者的气道并保证足够的氧气。对于所有紧急的危及生命的气管切开术，都应该做垂直切口。

步骤

确认甲状软骨以下的气管，并用一只手控制住。做一个切口并向下延伸通过皮肤和颈阔肌。当打开颈阔肌后，那么所有的切开都应该在中线进行。这一点十分重要。这样就可以避开颈前静脉和内侧带状肌。应该在直视下切开气管。最好选择钝性分离，并用指尖确定气管环。如果在气管表面触诊到甲状腺峡部，那么就应该向头侧移动，然后再确认气管。应在气管环之间的膜上做一个距离约为 1 cm 的十字切口。选择一根 2.0 聚丙烯缝线放在气管的侧面，用来作为长牵引线。确认气管腔，并将一根红色橡胶导管进入气管腔，以确保没有假腔。当气管受到损失并且气管出血或黏膜出血时，这样做就特别重要了。在气管切开术中要使用气管切开管，然后将闭塞物移开并用内部的套管替代。然后就可以通气了。之后要固定气管切开管，应使聚丙烯缝线穿过切口的上面，然后留在原来的位置。这项技术在防止气管切开管脱离上是极其有用的。

颈部受伤时的气道管理

颈部前部或者侧面受伤都可能损伤气道。获知患者的受伤史是十分必要的。损伤是刀伤、刺伤、汽车碰撞还是坠落伤，都有不同的意义。刺伤可能造成颈椎和脊髓损伤，所以如果有脊柱损伤，那么也应该治疗颈部。这就要求固定颈部。

如果在袭击中被刀割伤，那么很可能不会对脊髓的骨单位造成伤害，因此脊髓损伤不是主要因素。

应该检查伤口是活动性出血还是非活动性出血。对活动性动脉出血，可直接用手指压迫止血以防止发生大出血。如果出血是非活动性的深静脉血，那么就有必要记住，在大静脉损伤时，可以通过吸气导致空气栓塞进入深静脉或者心脏。这会导致空气栓塞进入主要的肺动脉。然后产生气塞，并且使肺灌注显著受损。

因为颈部有重要的神经和血管结构，所以要避免盲目地把夹子放入伤口。出血控制应该在直视下进行或者使用非止血钳。

应触诊伤口以发现捻发音。伤口中有空气可能是气道或食管损伤的征兆。须要检查气道或食管，任何损伤都须要在手术室中处理。对气道应该用气管导管或外科气道进行控制。一旦气道充分控制并且患者能够有效通气，即应将患者转移到手术室，以对出血进行确切的控制，还要通过外部直视、内镜或两者结合使用对消化道进行评估，然后应进行适当的修复。

小结

在管理多发伤和垂危的患者时，对创伤患者的气道管理仍然是最重要的救生事件。所有的外科医生都有必要知道侵入性和非侵入性气道管理方式。发现那些不能通过常用气道管理方式来处理的患者是至关重要的。确定何时进行手术气道，并且知道获得急救手术气道的标志和潜在的困难是十分重要的。掌握这些技术和操作有助于对多发伤患者的气道进行紧急管理。

液体复苏

Ron Barbosa, Brandon Tieu, Laszlo Kiraly, Michael Englehart, Martin Schreiber, Susan Rowell 著
易成腊 译

静脉输液开始于 17 世纪。自从 1638 年 William Harley 提出现代循环系统后，静脉输液进展缓慢。William O' Shaughnessy 提出以下理论：患者继发于霍乱的容量损失会从血液中恢复到原来的比重，而取代缺乏盐分的状态。这成为当代静脉注射液体疗法的第一个概念。1832 年，Thomas Latta 被认为是运用 O' Shaughnessy 理论来治疗霍乱患者的医生。之后在 19 世纪，Sydney Ringer 在其动物模型上描述了一种主要含有电解质的生理溶液。Hartman 通过加入乳汁作为缓冲剂来修正这种生理溶液。大多数概念受到了批评并且大部分被遗忘，这种情况一直延续到 20 世纪。现代手术的出现提高了对维持血容量的重要性的认知，因此导致了对静脉输液的使用的研究。

第一次世界大战提供了大量的失血性休克复苏经验。Walter Cannon 的研究很好地描述了自然历史并且提出了休克是导致战场牺牲最主要的原因。他的研究表明，术中延迟控制出血会大幅度地增加死亡率。此外他表示，不进行手术干预的积极复苏会加重失血性休克。他还表示，生理盐水复苏可能会加重现有的酸中毒。然而，在随后的几十年里，他的许多研究被遗忘或忽略了。之后，在第二次世界大战和朝鲜战争中，转向使用血浆和血液进行复苏。在对狗的实验基础上，Blalock 指出晶体液会快速地从血管内流失。1963 年，Shires 表示休克时会伴有细胞间液转移进入血管。这一发现给盐溶液治疗带来了新的方向（表 1）。在随后的几十年里，积极的复苏进一步被优化。在重症监护、监测、静脉输液和复苏终点等领域已经有了明显的获益。尽管有这些进步，但仍然存在许多争议和问题。液体的选择仍然存在争议。对休克机制的研究已经提供了大量细胞和分子水平的信息，但是还没有转化成可以直接适用于临床的治疗。更重要的是，现代复苏的并发症常见于创伤重症监护病房（ICU）。

液体选择

关于晶体液和胶体液的使用已经持续争论了数十年（图 1）。在越南战争中，等渗晶体溶液被使用，因为从 19 世纪 70 年代开始，Shires 等开展的实验室研究都表明大量使用等渗晶体溶液进行复苏会提高生存率。他们注意到，在休克时细胞外液会重新分配到血管内和细胞内，要想快速纠正这种细胞外液的亏损，就须要输入晶体液。晶体液与失血量之比为 3：1。采用此复苏方法后，总死亡率和急性肾衰竭的发生率降低，但出现了休克肺这个新的问题。休克肺现在被称作“急性呼吸窘迫综合征”。

理论上使用胶体液复苏存在很多优点。在给予

表 1　平衡盐溶液的构成（mEq/L）

溶液	糖 (g/L)	Na^+	Cl^-	NCO_3^-	K^+	Ca^{2+}	Mg^{2+}	HPO_4^-	NH_4^+
细胞外液	1000	140	102	27	4.2	5	3	3	0.3
5% 右旋糖酐和水	50								
0.21% 氯化钠 (0.25 NS)		34	34						
0.45% 氯化钠 (0.5 NS)		77	77						
0.9% 氯化钠 (NS)		154	154						
3% 氯化钠 (HS)		513	513						
7.5% 氯化钠 (HS)		1283	1283						
乳酸林格液（LR）		130	109	28*	4	2.7			

HS, 高渗盐水（hypertonic saline）; NS, 普通盐水（normal saline）
* 在溶液中表现为乳酸盐，但是代谢为碳酸氢盐

图 1 晶体液和胶体液对细胞外液容量的影响的比较 (*Data from Imm A, Carlson RW: Fluid resuscitation in circulatory shock. Crit Care Clin 9:313, 1993.*)

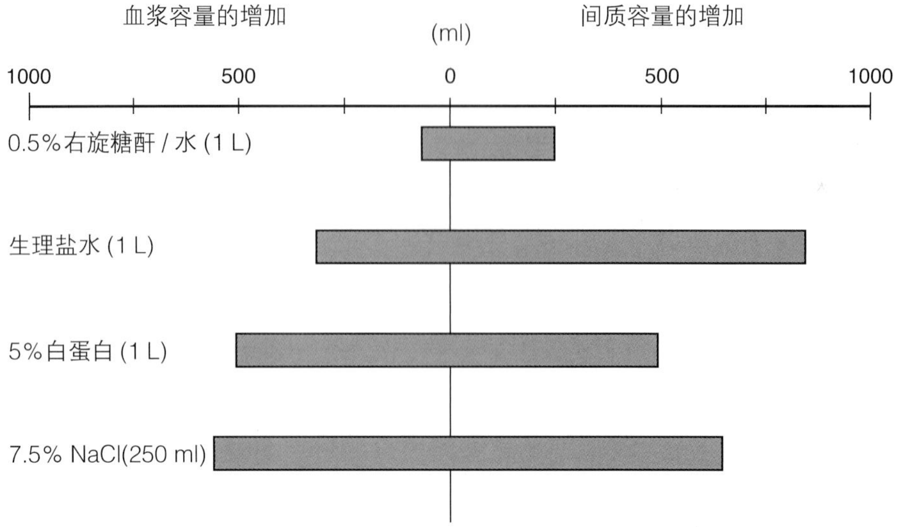

胶体液后，血容量和胶体渗透压立刻增加。曾经普遍认为这种效应可以持续很长时间，但是最近的动物研究表明这种效应只能短时间存在，而胶体分子在几秒钟内就会扩散到血管外。曾经也普遍认为使用胶体液比晶体液更不容易出现组织水肿。这一点从来没有在临床上被证明过，并且最近的临床试验表明，在使用胶体液或者晶体液后，血管外液容量和对机械通气的需求是一样的。

在过去的几十年里，对大量不同的患者进行了使用胶体液和晶体液效果对比的临床研究。许多研究因为数量小或者方法学上存在缺陷而难以解释。然而，在过去几年里，已经完成了这个方面的一些高质量随机对照试验和 Mata 分析。生理盐水和白蛋白对比评估（Saline verus Albumin Fluid Evaluation，SAFE）研究随机选取了 6997 例 ICU 患者接受 4% 白蛋白或者生理盐水。这项研究的人群是各种各样的，其中包括 43% 的手术患者和 17.4% 的创伤患者。医生选用盲法，并且只允许根据临床情况来决定输液的速度和数量。结果显示，在病死率、ICU 住院天数、机械通气天数和肾替代治疗天数上都无显著差异。SAFE 的研究人员随后对原始队列中的创伤性脑损伤（TBI）患者进行了事后分析，发现使用白蛋白会显著增加死亡率。在严重的 TBI 患者中，白蛋白组有 41.8% 的患者死亡，而生理盐水组中的死亡率为 22.2%。因为组间的复苏终点没有明显差异，所以假设，使用白蛋白可能加剧了血管源性或细胞毒性脑水肿。

最近的一项 Cochrane 协作的 Meta 分析审查了在危重患者中使用胶体液或晶体液复苏的随机对照试验，并没有发现使用胶体液复苏存在优势。将白蛋白、羟乙基淀粉、改良的凝胶和右旋糖酐单独分开检测，在每一种情况下接受胶体液复苏的患者相对死亡率为 0.91 ~ 1.24。其他的 Meta 分析也表明使用胶体液复苏并没有益处，甚至有些患者的情况会恶化。其他可能的缺点是过敏反应和肾衰竭（右旋糖酐）的发生率增加、血小板功能改变（右旋糖酐、羟乙基淀粉）、高氯性酸中毒（羟乙基淀粉）和费用高昂。总之，没有临床证据支持在液体复苏时使用胶体液多过晶体液。

类晶体的选择是争论多年的原因。生理盐水已经普遍地被用于创伤患者的液体复苏。生理盐水是由 154 mEq/L 钠和 154 mEq/L 氯组成的。它已经被一些创伤系统所选择，某种程度上是因为担心同时输注乳酸林格液和血红细胞会导致凝血。生理盐水的渗透压也比乳酸林格液高，所以对于重度颅脑损伤患者可能会有潜在的好处。然而，大量使用生理盐水进行液体复苏可能会导致高氯性代谢酸中毒。对择期手术患者开展的研究表明，接受生理盐水的患者比接受乳酸林格液的患者在术后需要更多的碳酸氢盐和更低的 pH。

林格液最初是由 Sydney Ringer 发明的。他在某次实验中把分离出来的青蛙的心脏悬浮在被无机盐污染的氯化钠溶液中，之后他发现钾和钙可以增加心脏收缩性。这种溶液后来被 Hartman 通过加入乳酸而得到改良，即现在所称的乳酸林格液。使用乳酸林格液复苏可以避免出现像使用生理盐水导致的高氯性代谢性酸中毒。对择期手术患者开展的临床试验表明，与使用乳酸林格液溶液相比，使用生理盐水后血液流失会减少。未控制的失血性休克动物模型表明，与使用生理盐水进行液体复苏相比，使用乳酸林格液可以减少血液流失并且在血管外肺水指数方面更有效。

美国血库尚未批准将乳酸林格液联合袋装红细胞一起输注，因为担心液体中的钙可能被血液中的柠檬酸盐螯合，从而导致过滤器凝结。其临床意义目前尚不清楚，最近的研究表明，同时使用乳酸林格液复苏和快速输注红细胞并不会导致凝血增加。在 19 世纪 80 年代，乳酸林格液被发现可以活化中性粒细胞，并且随后的研究表明非人类正常代谢产生的乳酸右旋体是导致中性粒细胞活化的原因。这表明乳酸林格液中只有左旋体是用来液体复苏的。

血浆电解质作为一种平衡的晶体溶液，其在全球贩卖的配方种类各有不同。它被设计成平衡的溶液，并且大多数配方里都有钠、钾、镁、氯，但是没有钙。醋酸盐、葡萄糖酸盐或乳酸作为碳酸氢盐的初期形式存在。它不会导致高氯性酸中毒，并且可以安全地与药物或血制品一起使用。大多数临床研究涉及血浆电解质在心脏手术或移植患者中的使用，但是没有充分研究其在低血容量性休克时的使用。目前还没有证据表明对于创伤患者来说，使用血浆电解质比使用其他晶体液有理论上的优势。

在过去的几十年里，作为复苏液，人们已经广泛地研究高渗盐水。它提高了血浆胶体渗透压，通过把细胞间隙的液体吸收进入血管内，导致血压升高，改善循环血流量。与等渗晶体相比，它的液体量更少。渗透效应也会降低严重脑损伤患者的颅内压，还可能调节损伤后全身炎症反应。已经完成了许多使用 3% 或 5% 高渗盐水的动物研究，但仍缺乏失血性休克患者使用高渗盐水的临床数据。一项研究表明低血压创伤患者输注 3% 高渗盐水后，恢复到了正常的血压和尿量。另一项小型研究表明，对严重脑损伤的患者使用 5% 高渗盐水后死亡率有下降的趋势。最近几年这两种溶液都没有在随机对照试验中进行评估。

在临床试验中，高渗盐糖右旋糖酐液（HSD）被研究得更加广泛。它是 7.5% NaCl 和 6% 右旋糖酐 -70 的混合物。加入右旋糖酐是为了尝试延长高渗对血流动力学的影响。大量院前使用 HSD 的试验表明其有增加生存率的趋势，但是没有达到统计学意义。后来 Wade 等进行了三篇 Meta 分析。有一篇分析表明 HSD 组的患者总体生存率提高，其他分析表明有创伤性脑损伤的低血压患者 HSD 组的生存率提高。2003 年，一项随机试验对失血性休克患者的院前处置中分别使用 HSD 和乳酸林格液进行了比较。在第二次中期分析无效后，该试验于 2005 年停止。据猜测，结果无明显改善的可能原因是部分登记患者只是暂时的低血压，而不是真正的失血性休克。后来一项由复苏预后协会（Resuscitation Outcomes Consortium）开展的试验随机分配患者，无论其是低血压还是创伤性脑损伤，都随机地在院前处置时输注 HSD、乳酸林格液或生理盐水。因为参与高渗组的无效和安全问题，登记休克的队列暂时停止。后来创伤性脑损伤组也因为无效而暂停。目前，在处置平民创伤时，使用 HSD 进行液体复苏并没有显著的临床意义。

复苏策略

传统的复苏策略是针对恢复正常的血管内液体量和动脉血压，从而维持对重要器官的灌注。从 20 世纪 90 年代以来，这种方案已经被再次审视。在延迟复苏时，是不进行液体复苏的，直到出血已被控制。这不是新的概念。Cannon 说过早期控制出血是最重要的，如果在此之前尝试液体复苏，那么就会增加出血和死亡的风险。快速复苏会加重出血，其机制是冲走脆弱的血凝块、降低血液黏滞度。快速复苏还会导致颅顶、腹部及四肢骨筋膜室综合征。它还会加重“死亡三联征”——低温、酸中毒和凝血功能障碍。在低血压复苏中，以较低的速率（或完全停止）和以较低的收缩压为目标输注液体。局部低灌注导致的组织损伤是这些策略的风险。尚未确定一种单一的准确的方法来评估区域性低灌注。

以前的动物研究采用控制出血模型，通过早期止血，使其快速恢复血容量正常。不幸的是，在临床处置时，可能不会立即知道并控制出血源。已经开发了许多失控出血的动物模型。在猪的主动脉切开模型中，Sondeen 注意到，随着失控性出血性休克和自发性凝血导致的再次出血，其平均动脉压（mean arterial pressure，MAP）只有 64 mmHg。这与复苏时间无关。Bickell 等发现，在用幼猪建立主动脉切开模型中，使用乳酸林格液或者 HSD 复苏的猪比没有用液体复苏的猪结果要差。

临床上也对此问题进行了研究。在一项前瞻性随机对照研究中，Bickell 等对低血压（收缩压 $<$ 90mmHg）伴有躯干穿透伤的患者进行了即时和

延迟液体复苏比较。两组的生存率有着显著的统计学差异，分别为 62% 和 70%（ $P=0.04$ ）。这表明延迟复苏对躯干贯通伤有改善效果。这项研究后来受到了批评，原因是患者以年轻男性患者为主，并且转移到城市所需要的时间较短。随后的亚组分析显示，只有心脏损伤患者的存活率有所改善。将死亡分为术前、术中和术后时间段时，生存率无显著差异。Dutton 等比较了收缩压为 70 mmHg 和收缩压 >100 mmHg 的活动性出血患者的液体复苏。对低收缩压患者进行液体复苏时不影响总体死亡率。钝性和穿透性创伤患者被纳入了本研究。

要确定低血压患者的液体复苏策略，须进行进一步的随机对照试验。目前，对钝性损伤患者应采用传统的策略管理。虽然理想的目标血压仍然难以捉摸，但对穿透伤而言，收缩压在 80 ~ 90 mmHg 可能是足够的。对于创伤性脑损伤患者来说，院前低血压（收缩压 <90 mmHg ）与预后差有着显著的联系。对于头部受伤的患者来说，尝试维持收缩压 >90 mmHg 可能会降低不良后果，虽然没有 I 类证据可以证实这一点。

不能将目前的对低血压复苏的文献外推到所有的创伤患者，但它强调了快速诊断和治疗的重要性。早期识别出血源和控制出血会使血容量快速恢复，并降低死亡率和死亡风险。

输血

自从在第一次和第二次世界大战中开始使用输血后，在复苏中输血这个问题一直存在争论，而现在这已经成为了一种常规治疗方法。尽管早期存活率增加，但后期有很多人死于肾衰竭。人们普遍认为，如果对休克患者输注了 2 L 晶体液之后仍没有反应，那么就需要输血。对于有活动性出血或者失血性休克的患者，应该立刻给予输血。当大量输注晶体液和红细胞后，或许也须要输注新鲜冰冻血浆、血小板和冷沉淀来逆转相关的稀释性凝血功能障碍。还必须考虑输血的内在风险，例如输血反应、输血相关性急性肺损伤、感染和免疫抑制。已经发现，输血包含了激活中性粒细胞的促炎介质。这已被提出是多器官功能衰竭发展的重要机制。存储的红细胞也发生极大的形状变化，并且从存储的第 2 周开始变形能力受损。这种畸形的减少可能导致微血管阻塞，并已经发现与内脏缺血的发展有关。Malone 等报道，在入院前 24 h 内输血的创伤患者，无论休克严重程度如何，死亡的概率都是那些未输血患者的 3 倍。早期临床研究得出血红蛋白（ hemoglobin，Hb ）水平在 100 g/dl 对休克复苏来说是最理想的。但最近的共识指出，浓度低一点就足够了。一项前瞻性随机试验表明，对 ICU 患者输血使血红蛋白低于 70 g/dl 或者维持在 70 ~ 90 g/dl，比那些输血不受限制的使血红蛋白低于 100 g/dl 甚至维持在 100 ~ 120 g/dl 的效果更好。所有患者均无持续出血、急性心肌梗死或不稳定型心绞痛。对创伤患者限制性红细胞输注策略的亚组分析表明，相对于那些自由输注红细胞的患者来说，其死亡率、多器官功能衰竭发生率和住院天数都没有显著的统计学差异。随机对照研究须要旨在提供证据来帮助指导危重创伤患者的输血。

人工携氧血液代用品

虽然晶体液和胶体液都可以代替血管内容量，但这两种产品在丢失了红细胞后都失去了携氧能力。人工血红蛋白产品可以提高携氧能力，却没有存储、可用性、免疫抑制、输血反应、兼容性或传播疾病等与输血相关的问题。不幸的是，这些产品也不能恢复凝血因子，并且会阻碍止血，因为细胞因子的丢失，血液黏滞度低。尚未充分开展大量人工携氧溶液在严重出血中的应用的研究。

通过人血、牛血和重组 DNA 技术得到基于血红蛋白类氧载体（ hemoglobin-based oxygen carriers，HBOCs ）可以追溯到 1933 年。运载溶液需要无基质聚合或交联血红蛋白四聚体，它的携氧能力必须在血管中保持一段时间。因为 2, 3- 二磷酸甘油酸的损失，早期血红蛋白替代品有更大的氧亲和力。然而，随着血红蛋白四聚体吡哆酰基化后，这个问题已经解决了。HBOCs 也可以引起血管收缩，因为四聚体血红蛋白可以结合血管壁中的一氧化氮，拮抗一氧化氮的扩张血管作用。由于这种现象，血压可能高于预期的血管内容量置换失血性休克患者的水平。对这些人造产品的初步研究是令人失望的。由于治疗组意外的高死亡率（ 46% vs 17% ），一项双阿司匹林交联血红蛋白的Ⅲ期临床试验提前停止了。多聚血红蛋白，即聚集的戊二醛吡啶甲酸盐人血红蛋白，在Ⅰ期和Ⅱ期实验中作为血液替代品显现出希望。然而，在Ⅲ期试验中，并没有发现患者有生存益处，并且有发生不良事件增多的趋势，特别是心肌缺血不良事件。FDA 没有授权，目前血红蛋白没有被积极地应用于临床。

另一种血液替代品——HBOC-201 在动物模型上升高 MAP 的程度大于晶体液或胶体液，还在其他临床前研究中显示具有免疫调节的效果。研究证明在军事情况下它不比 6% 高渗盐水差。然而，在针对平民开展的阶段性Ⅲ期临床试验中，输注 HBOC-201 比输注红细胞造成的不良反应更多。据认为，导致这些不良反应的原因可能是因为 HBOC-201 清除了一氧化氮而导致血管活性继发性降低，防止这一过程的基础科学工作正在进行中。由于这一原因，HBOC-201 的临床试验正在进行。

全氟化碳是化学和生物惰性液体，它可以溶解大量气体。它们须要弥散在血浆状的水溶液，如白蛋白或生理电解质溶液，以提供足够的携氧替代物。它们的携氧能力比正常血液低，并且须要 FIO_2 高于 70% 才能运载满足生理功能需求的氧气。吸收、分布、代谢和排泄的长期生物学效应以及对网状内皮系统（reticuloendothelial system，RES）的效应须要进一步评估。考虑到对 RES 的毒性和较高的 FIO_2 的需求，在严重出血时这些可能会限制它们的使用。

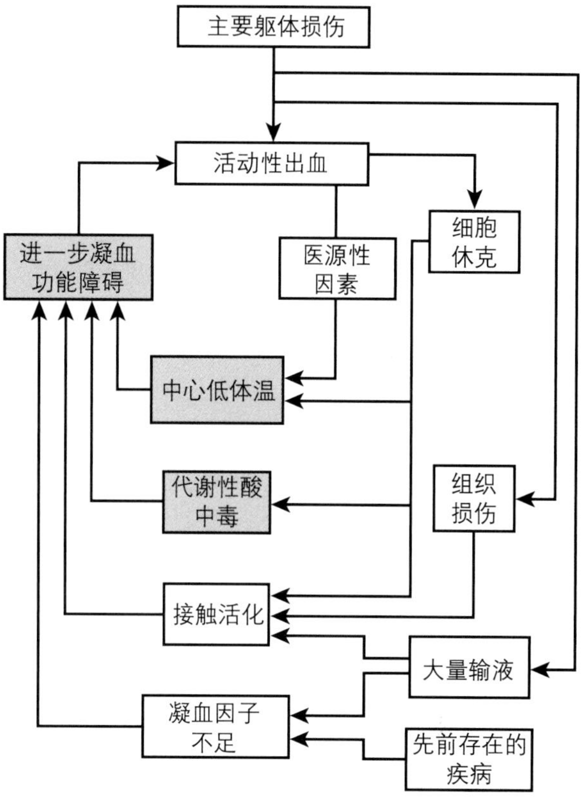

图 2 致死三联征 (*Modified from Moore EE: Staged laparotomy for the hypothermia, acidosis, coagulopathy syndrome. Am J Surg 172:405–410, 1996.*)

复苏的并发症

在 20 世纪 80 年代和 90 年代，有一个改变就是使用大量液体用来复苏急性受伤的患者。重症监护的进展和损伤控制技术的应用导致越来越多的危重患者在即时伤后阶段得到存活。然而，大量使用晶体液复苏导致复苏的并发症增加，例如酸中毒、低体温、凝血功能障碍和腹部及四肢筋膜室综合征。这可能会导致一个正反馈循环，使酸中毒、低体温和凝血功能障碍加重（图 2）。

低体温

低体温的定义为中心体温低于 35℃。内部中心体温是产热和散热的最终结果。热损失是蒸发、辐射、传导或对流的结果。产热主要是细胞代谢的结果。在急性损伤患者有大量潜在的导致热损失的原因。在野外暴露可导致患者入院时体温过低。开展高级创伤生命支持（ATLS）的各项举措会造成进一步热量损失。通过蒸发和传导，接触暴露部位的操作会造成明显的热量散失。静脉输注液导致的热损失的潜力最大。这可以通过以下方程量化。

热量 = 质量 × 比热容 ×（身体体温 - 液体体温）

假定水的比热容是 4.19 kJ/（kg · ℃），将 1 L 25℃的晶体溶液注入体温正常的患者，会导致患者散失 50.3 kJ 的热量。这种损失的热量超过了 1 h 内通过传统方法恢复的热量。血制品通常被保持在 4℃，大量使用不温暖的血制品会导致大量热量丢失。通过使用血液或液体加热器可以使热损失最小。复温是一个渐进的过程，因为它需要大约 12 L 温液体，才能使核心温度提高 1℃。

创伤患者在复苏期间亚低温的发生率可高达 66%。虽然 Gregory 等发现，在到达急诊室的患者中只有 12% 的人体温过低，46% 的患者在到达手术室时体温过低，57% 的患者在离开手术室时体温过低。这表明大部分热损失发生在复苏过程，而且目前的辅助措施不能完全阻止术中热量的丢失。

在创伤患者体温过低是预后不良的指标，已证明其是可以独立预测死亡率的因素。意外暴露的中度低温患者的死亡率通常约为 20%，然而，类似中心体温（<32℃）的创伤患者死亡率基本上是 100%。关于这种差异有好几种解释。创伤患者有类似于继发于暴露导致的热损失，然而，在这些患者

中因为出血和身体腔隙暴露丢失的热量更多。除此之外，由于失血和休克导致的心输出量减少和耗氧量减少可导致产热量的降低。考虑到这些机制，死亡率较高可能不只是因为低体温，也是损伤严重程度的一种表现。

由于低体温与死亡风险强烈有关，还有“致死三联征”的其他因素，因而应将复温及预防持续的热损失列于复苏之前（表2）。第一步是获得准确的中心温度。已证明测量食管或膀胱的温度比直肠或腋窝的温度更可靠。鉴于输液会丢失大量热量，所以应加温所有的复苏液体。应提高手术室的温度，使通过热传导和热辐射散失的热量降到最低。一旦完成进一步评估，应将患者盖好。头皮可以发生显著的热损失，并且会经常忘记盖住头部。可以使用加温器或者类似的装备积极地温暖患者。对于深低体温，可以采用积极的内部升温。这是通过灌洗体腔（胸腔或腹腔）升温或者血管内升温。血管内升温包括静脉升温、动静脉升温或者心肺旁路升温。已证明持续动静脉升温（图3）可以降低危重的低体温创伤患者的死亡率。

表2　现有的复温方法的传热近似率

复温技术	传热率 (kcal/h)
气道复温	8 ~ 12
高架暖气	17
电热毯	20
对流取暖器	15 ~ 26
体腔灌洗	36
连续动静脉复温	92 ~ 139
体外循环	710

Modified from Gentilello LM: Practical approaches to hypothermia. In Maull KI, Cleveland HC, Feliciano DV, et al, editors: Advances in Trauma and Critical Care, Vol. 9. St. Louis, Mosby, 1994, pp 39–79

凝血功能障碍

失血是导致创伤早期死亡的主要原因。在创伤患者凝血功能障碍主要发生在大复苏过程中。其机制被认为与体温过低、代谢紊乱、稀释和弥散性血管内凝血有关。其中的大多数机制都可以追溯到某种复苏方式上。

稀释是创伤患者在复苏中发生凝血功能障碍的主要原因。含有凝血因子的血管内液丢失，并且被缺乏这些凝血因子的溶液所替代。实际上不好预测凝血功能障碍的严重程度，因为血浆物质交换太过复杂。在创伤后的治疗过程中凝血因子不断产生和消耗。在将大约1个血容量（70ml/kg）单位的替代溶液输注到体内前稀释性凝血功能障碍并不是特别重要。因此，在没有临床出血的证据或实验室数据时一般不推荐给予预防性制品。然而，越来越多的证据表明在失血性休克时应该早期使用凝血因子。

低体温对凝血活性有深远的影响。Reed和Rohre在不同的实验中，都表明低体温延长部分凝血活酶时间（partial thromboplastin time，PTT）和凝血酶原时间，并且与酶的实际水平并没有关系。Gubler等表明血液稀释与低体温的作用是相辅相成的（图4）。除了这些酶的作用外，体温过低还会增加纤维蛋白溶解。动物研究表明，在低温时，血小板被脾隔离，血小板的黏附也减弱。临床研究表明，在代谢性酸中毒和低体温患者，即便有充足的血液、血浆和血小板替代，仍然会有明显出血。

对于任何疾病，对凝血功能障碍的治疗都始于对这个问题的认识。对于任何有明显的组织损伤或者活动性出血的创伤患者，都应该筛查一遍国际标准化比值（international normalized ration，INR）、PTT、血小板计数和纤维蛋白原水平。在积极创伤性出血的救治中，血小板计数应保持在500×10^9 L，INR＜2，纤维蛋白原＞100 mg/dl，PTT小于正常的1.5倍。最后，推荐密切监测这些参数，因为经验性治疗往往会产生不可预见的后果。当没有实验室检查结果时，可以开始经验性治疗。

凝血功能障碍与脑损伤也有特别的关联。从受伤的脑组织中释放的促凝血酶原激酶被认为会导致严重的消耗性凝血病，从而造成弥散性血管内凝血。处理头部创伤的患者时应该有更加广泛的凝血功能检测。出于这个目的，目前，血栓弹力图（thrombelastography，TEG）正在被研究，因为研究表明TEG可以比标准试验更早地检测到有临床意义的异常凝血。

酸中毒

代谢性酸中毒通常发生在创伤失血性休克患者中，并且认为继发于在心输出量降低和携氧能力降低的情况下组织的灌注不足。这一连串的事件最终导致无氧代谢和乳酸的生产。大规模使用晶体液复苏与代谢性酸中毒的恶化有关。按照Stewart的酸

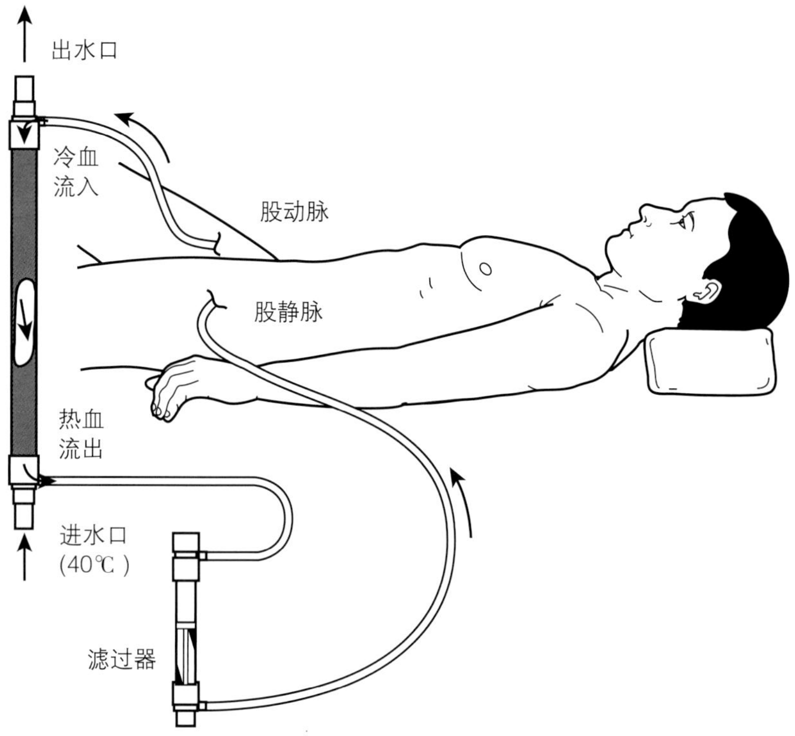

图 3　连续动静脉升温 (*From Gentilello LM, Jurkovich GJ, Stark MS, et al: Continuous arteriovenous rewarming: rapid reversal of hypothermia in critically ill patients. J Trauma 32:316–327, 1992.*)

碱平衡模型，使用相对于钠而言超过生理水平的氯的溶液会导致强离子差值（strong iron difference，SID）（Na+K+Ca+Mg-Cl- 乳酸）下降。SID 的降低导致进一步从 H_2O 解离 H^+ 来保持电荷中性，从而导致 pH 下降。因为晶体液的阳离子和阴离子浓度不一样，所以对 SID 的改变也不一样。乳酸林格溶液比生理盐水有更高的 SID。因为这种差异，大量使用乳酸林格溶液不会导致像生理盐水溶液那种程度的代谢酸中毒。

尽管没有高氯性酸中毒和增加死亡风险直接相关的证据，但严重的酸中毒还是有很多潜在的危险。酸中毒对心肌有抑制作用，还会增加室性心律失常。发生酸中毒时交感神经 - 肾上腺轴受到刺激。然而，心肌对血液循环中的儿茶酚胺的反应性降低。长时间的酸中毒也会增加呼吸动力，使脑损伤患者的颅内压增高，还会加重凝血功能障碍。一个更常见的危险在于持续的低灌注和休克导致误认为是高氯性酸中毒而无须治疗。

为了避免高氯性酸中毒，应避免与超生理浓度的氯液。与生理盐水相比（154 mEq/L），乳酸林格液中含有更多的生理浓度的氯（109 mEq/L）。一些临床试验和动物研究证明，在使用大容量的生理盐水溶液情况下，会发生严重的酸中毒。尽管可能性很小，但是使用乳酸林格液也可能出现酸中毒，是因为乳酸林格液的 SID 比血浆的 SID 低。仔细监测电解质与阴离子间隙可以辅助指导治疗。在独立的高氯性代谢性酸中毒情况下，可以发现阴离子间隙正常或者缩小，与之相反，在乳酸性酸中毒中该间隙扩大。改用少氯溶液（乳酸林格液或者血浆电解质）或者无氯溶液（醋酸钠溶液）可以解决高氯性酸中毒。

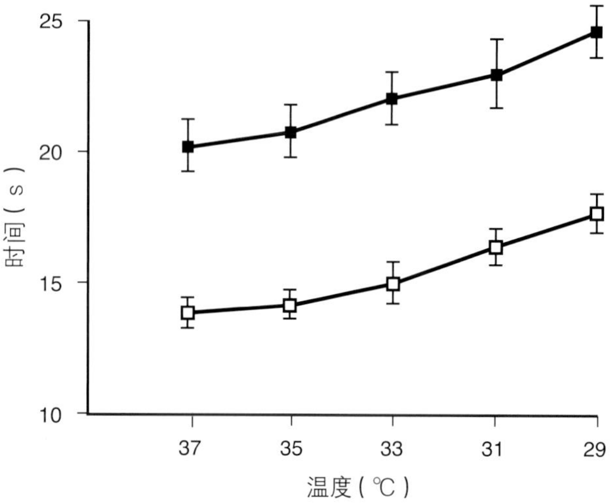

图 4　低温和稀释对凝血酶原时间的影响。空心区，稀释样品；实心区，非稀释样品 (*From Gubler KD, Gentilello LM, Hassantash SA, Maier RV: The impact of hypothermia on dilutional coagulopathy. J Trauma 36:847–851, 1994.*)

对酸中毒患者凝血功能的研究仍然是一个热门

问题。体外实验表明活性因子Ⅶa和组织因子Xa VA复合物减少。体内动物实验表明，酸中毒独立地降低纤维蛋白原和血小板计数，增加PTT，并延长临床出血时间。一份对大量输血患者开展的研究表明，pH不高于7.10可以独立预示凝血功能障碍。

筋膜间隔综合征

组织水肿是休克时使用大量液体复苏常见的结果。在大多数情况下，这种水肿不会产生立即明显的害处。然而，在有限的身体间隔里，压力增加可能导致缺血和随后的组织坏死。三个受到影响的部位是四肢、腹部和颅穹窿。

肢体间隔综合征大多继发于创伤性损伤，可伴或不伴骨折。虽然筋膜间室综合征较为罕见，但是已经有报道对创伤患者使用大量液体复苏时可出现此症。认为其本质为继发性肢体筋膜间隔综合征。这个过程可能是严重休克后一段时间缺血再灌注导致的。随后释放的炎症介质会导致毛细管渗漏现象。当这种情况伴有大量血液和液体时，水肿会对筋膜室造成损害，导致肢体或肌肉缺血。不管是何种筋膜间隔综合征，早期识别诊断和治疗对保肢都是最重要的。

腹腔间隔室综合征（abodominal compartment syndrome，ACS）已被发现了一个多世纪，但是对其明确识别和定义还是在20世纪90年代。它是指继发于腹腔内高压的器官功能障碍。ACS最初被发现于有腹部手术或腹部创伤的患者。从那时以来，ACS可以进一步分为有腹腔内脏器损伤的原发性ACS，以及因为休克或者大面积创伤导致的继发性ACS。理论上继发性ACS有几种发生机制。静脉输液越多，则间质性水肿越严重。浆蛋白也可能进一步稀释，导致血管内胶体渗透压降低。水肿的形成增加了腹内压，并减少了内脏静脉回流。这一过程最终导致中心静脉回流减少，并使输液量增加。最终就形成了一个复苏的恶性循环。

一些研究调查了继发性ACS的死亡率和危险因素。所有的研究都表明，严重休克和大规模复苏是诱发因素。一项回顾性病例研究表明液体复苏的晶体平均从16 L到38 L，血液从13到29个单位。Balogh等认为如果创伤患者通过超常的复苏（DO_2 >600）获得了更多的晶体液，则有较高的概率发生ACS（16% vs 8%）。与标准复苏组的7 L溶液相比，使用乳酸林格液可以用到13 L。继发性ACS患者的死亡率为38%~76%。这表明可以通过正确地使用液体和避免容量过量来避免继发性ACS。

对于有ACS临床症状的患者或者正在接受大量液体复苏的休克患者，都应该监测膀胱压力。如腹肌紧张并伴有低尿量、高气道压和低血压，则可以诊断为ACS。Maxwell的一系列研究表明，继发性ACS死亡组的患者去手术室用了25 h，而生存组只用了3 h。这表明继发性ACS发生在复苏的很早期。此外，及时诊断和治疗也有助于生存。

颅内压增高是创伤性脑损伤和颅内出血的常见结果。颅内总容积大约为1600 ml。一般脑组织占80%，血液占10%，脑脊液占10%。直接脑损伤和毛细血管渗漏导致的脑水肿与其他的筋膜室综合征相似。进行太多的静脉输液复苏会恶化这个过程。使用高渗盐水可以减轻脑水肿，但是其在脑损伤患者的液体复苏中的作用仍存在争议。鉴于颅穹窿的结构，一旦出现病理性颅内压增高，那么能够提供的治疗是有限的。更具侵入性的方法，如脑室造瘘术或颅骨切除术，应在药物治疗无效时及时使用。

开胸复苏

Juan A. Asensio, Patrizio Petrone, Alejandro Perez-Alonso, Wendy Jo Svetanoff, Molly Hartmann, Eric Elster, Gerd Daniel Pust, Michel Wagner 著
易成腊 译

急诊胸廓切开术（emergency department thoracotomy，EDT）仍然是创伤外科医生手术中的强大工具。自从20世纪60年代开展该手术以来，其使用的范围逐渐扩大。在很多城市的创伤中心，这个操作成为了复苏程序的一部分。由于急救医疗服务系统的改进，许多危重患者在被送到医院救治时处于垂危状况。这提示创伤外科医生要执行EDT来挽救他们的生命。这种复杂的手术只能由熟悉穿透性胸部损伤管理的外科医生执行。文献中提到的使用EDT的指征从模糊逐渐演化成相当具体。EDT

已被用于各种情况，包括穿透性和钝性胸部损伤、胸腹联合伤、心脏损伤，以及为腹部血管损伤抽血。它也偶尔对心肺骤停或者小儿创伤患者的外周血管损伤抽血。许多文献报道当发生了继发于钝挫伤的心肺骤停时使用 EDT。

历史回顾

1874 年，Schiff 率先推广开放式心脏按压理念。1896 年，Rehn 报道了第一例成功修复右心室损伤手术。1897 年，Duval 描述了现在广泛使用的经胸骨正中切口。1901 年，Igelsrud 第一次报道了通过胸廓切开术和开放式心脏按压成功地复苏一例创伤后心脏停搏的患者。Spangaro 在 1906 年描述了左前外侧开胸术，现在作为一种肋间开胸术而被广泛地应用于复苏。Zoll 在 1956 年第一个提出了外部心脏除颤理念。Kouwenhoven 在 1960 年描述了心肺复苏（cardiopulmonary resuscitation，CPR）。Beall 等于 1961 年率先提出应该直接对心脏停搏的患者进行开胸复苏，无论是在急诊室、手术室还是康复病房，并且 Beall 也是第一个尝试这个操作的医生。类似的，1966 年，他主张在急诊室中立即进行心脏修补术和安装仪器，同时他也是第一个成功地完成该操作的人。

目标

EDT 操作的目标包括如下内容：

- 复苏心胸贯通伤的患者（图 1 至 6）。
- 排空心包积血和血凝块来缓解心包压塞（图 7 至 8）。
- 控制胸廓出血。
- 修复心脏损伤（图 9 至 11）
- 十字钳闭降主动脉（图 12 至 14）
- 进行开放式心脏按压。该操作可以产生 60% 的正常心脏射血分数（图 15 至 16）。

生理学

胸主动脉十字钳闭的生理学效应有正面的，也有负面的，还有一些其他未知的效应。

正面效应

- 保存剩余血容量和进行再分配，用于改善冠状动脉 / 颈动脉灌注。
- 减少膈下血液流失。
- 提高左心室每搏做功指数。
- 增强心肌收缩力。

负面效应

- 减少约 10% 的正常腹腔脏器的血流量。
- 减少约 10% 的正常肾灌注。
- 将脊髓的血流量降至 10%。
- 导致无氧代谢。
- 导致缺氧或乳酸酸中毒。
- 极大增加了左心室后负荷。
- 未知因素。
- 延长安全十字钳闭的时间。
- 提高了再灌注损伤的发生率。

适应证

EDT 的适应证可以分为三类：①接受；②选择；③罕见。

接受性适应证

EDT 最适合用于那些经过较短的现场和运送时间后被送到创伤中心的持续性穿透性心脏损伤患者。应已对这些患者监测或者客观测量过生理参数（生

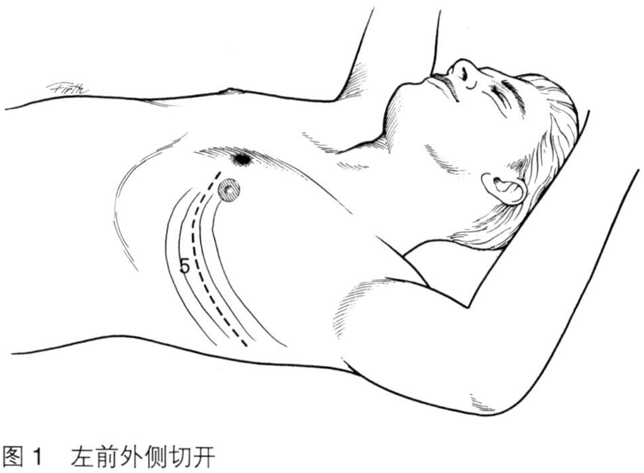

图 1　左前外侧切开

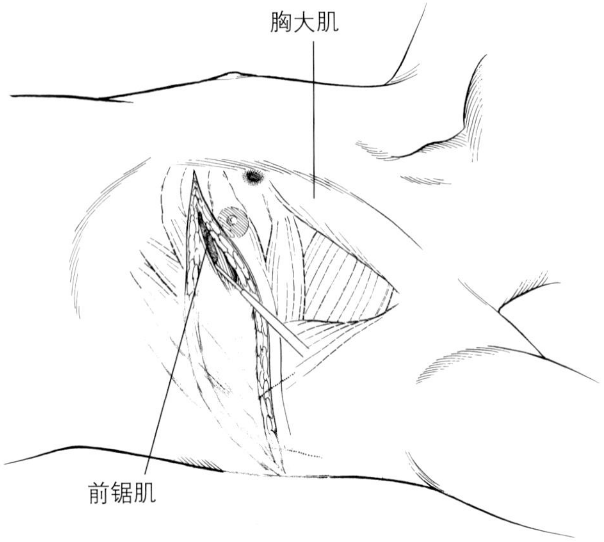

图 2 横断左侧胸部肌肉进入胸腔

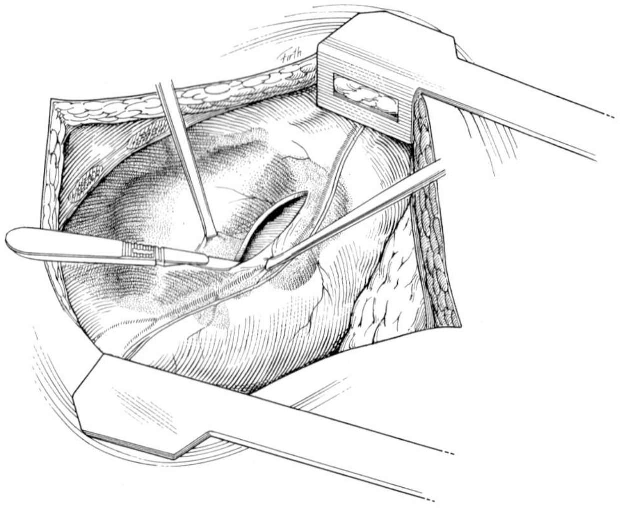

图 5 用 Allis 钳拉紧心包膜，然后用手术刀做一小切口

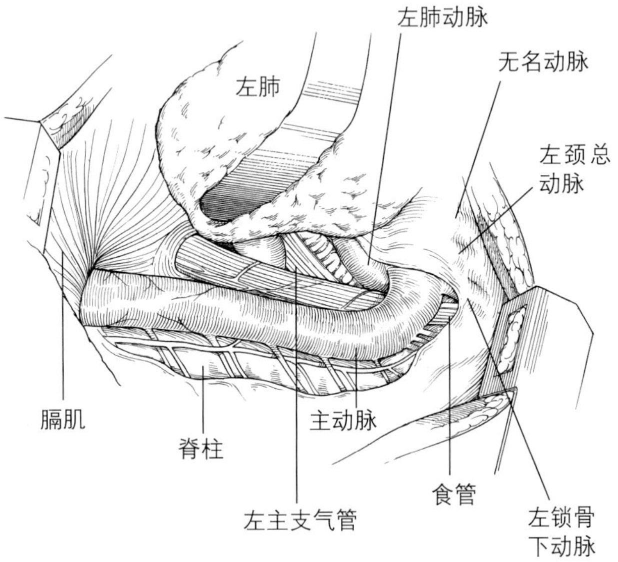

图 3 左侧胸腔的解剖。注意食管和胸主动脉的位置关系

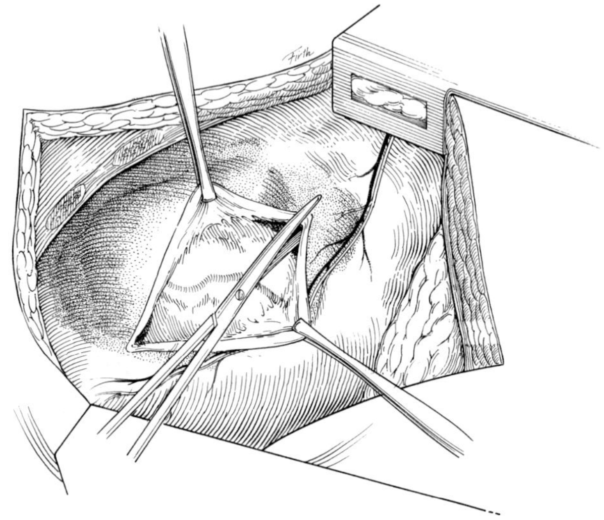

图 6 用 Metzenbaum 剪刀沿着头尾方向将切口锐性分离

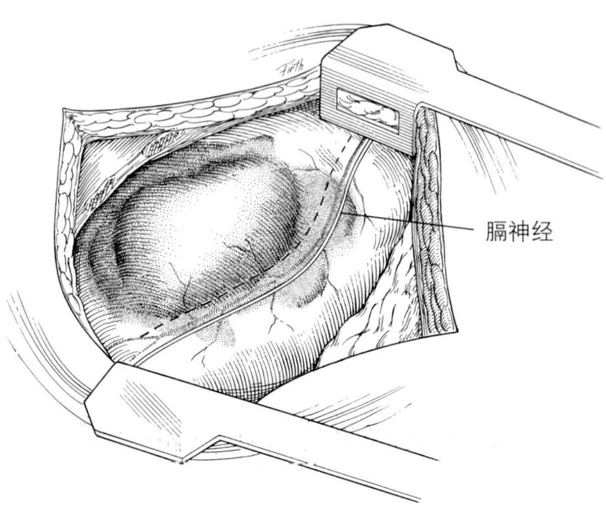

图 4 紧张的心包积血。在膈神经左前侧做切开

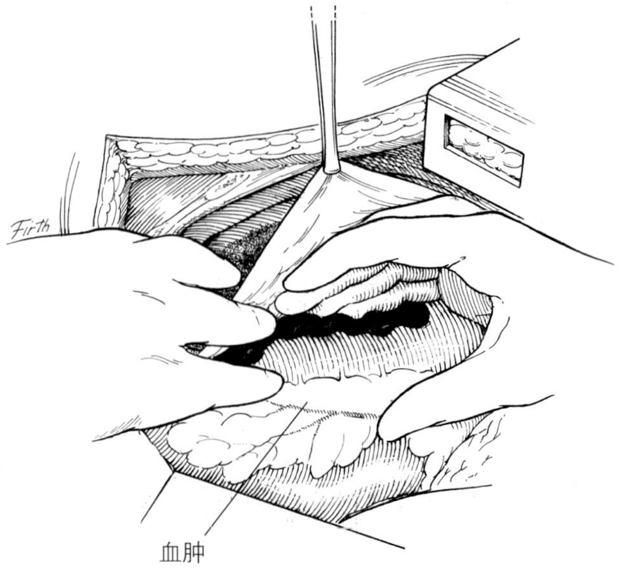

图 7 手动清除心包血块

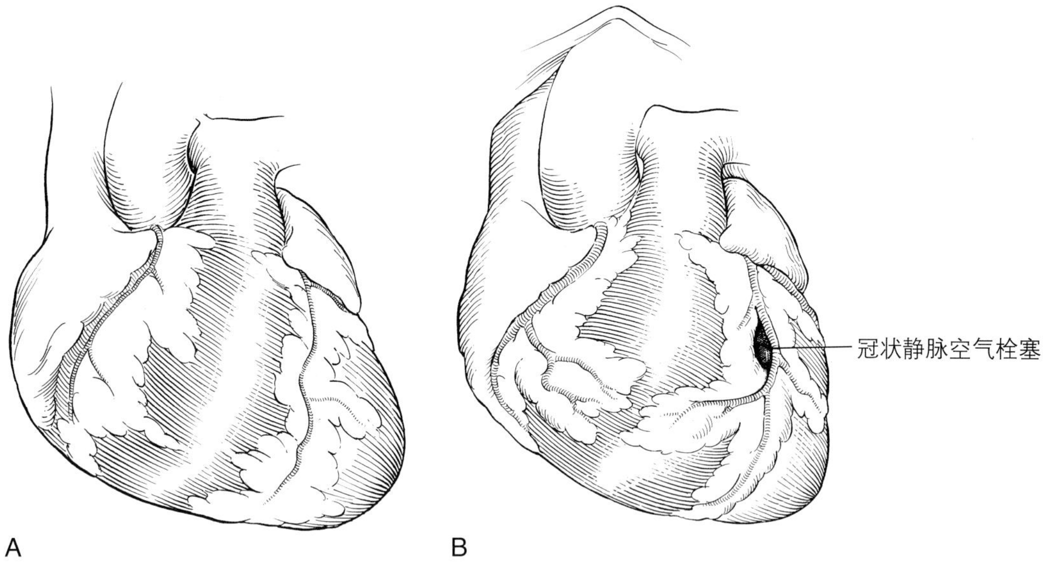

图 8 打开心包后所见。**A**，因为灌注不足导致冠状动脉血管收缩；**B**，在冠状静脉内发现空气栓塞。空气栓塞造成冠状动脉血流暂时阻断，但由于壁厚而不能看到。检查时，应对心室使用针头排气。空气栓塞是预后不良的有力预测因子

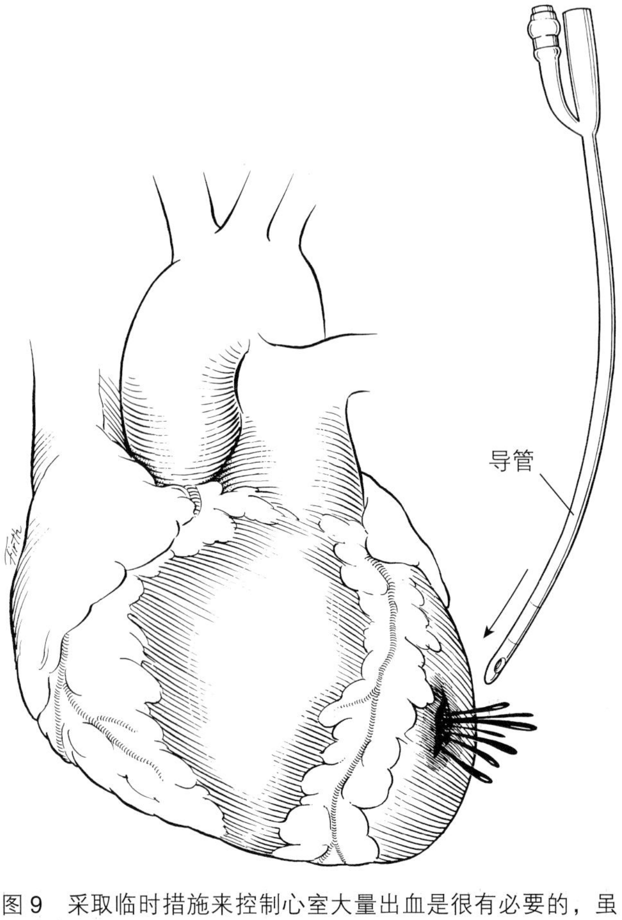

图 9 采取临时措施来控制心室大量出血是很有必要的，虽然其较为罕见

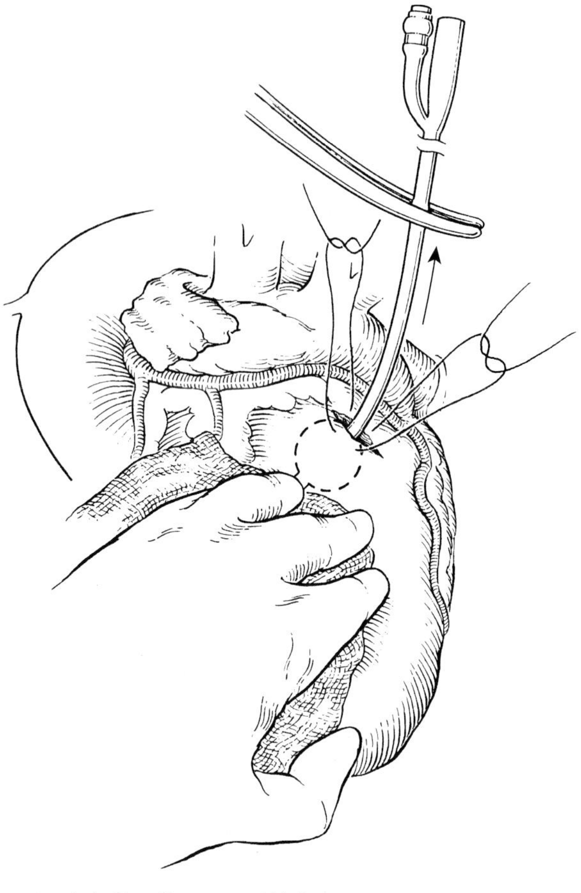

图 10 缝合插入的 Foley 导管来止血

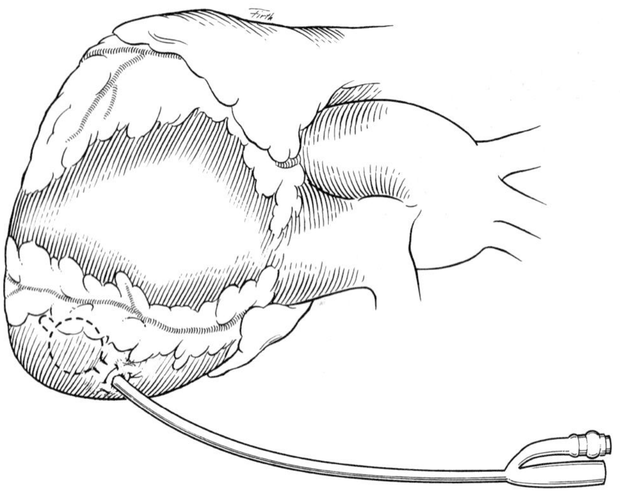

图 11　给心室内的 Foley 导管球囊充气

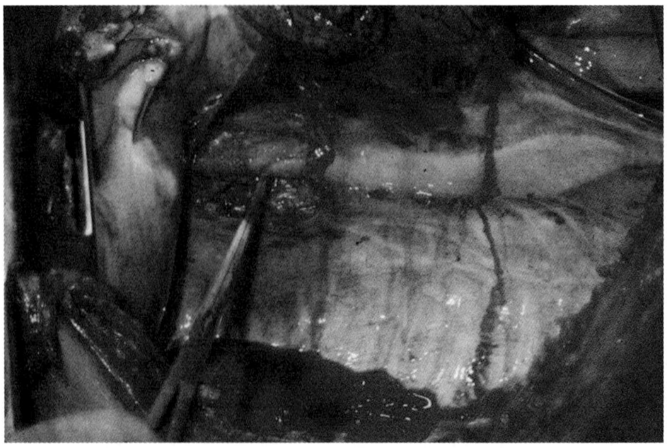

图 13　降主动脉进入主动脉裂孔。在夹闭之前分离动脉。注意上方的食管

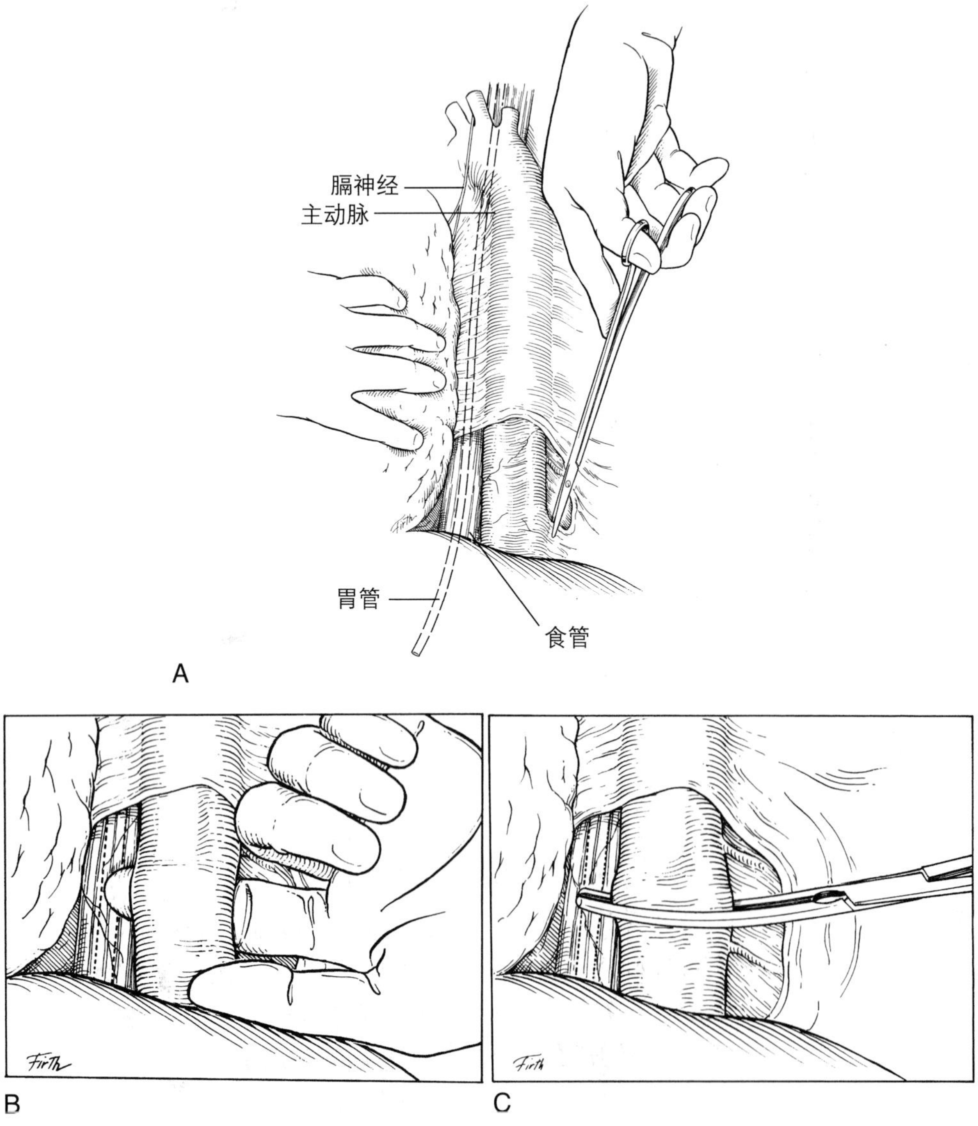

图 12　**A**，锐性分离降主动脉。将左肺前移。注意食管恰位于降主动脉的下方。**B**，用手指抬起降主动脉。**C**，在 Crafoord-DeBakey 主动脉处十字钳闭

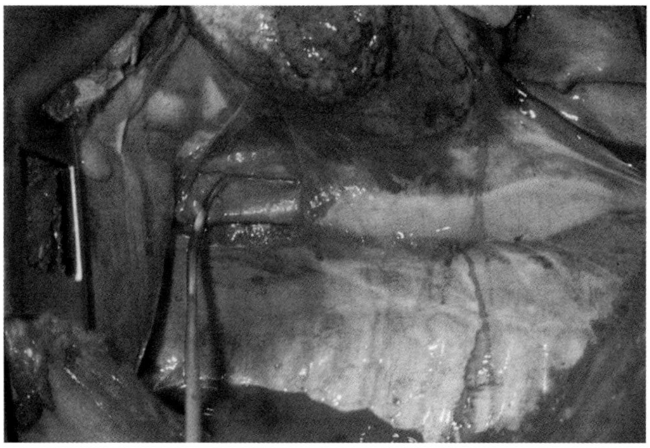

图 14　在此位置十字钳闭主动脉。注意左侧胸腔的大小，它需要容纳放血过程中患者所有的血液

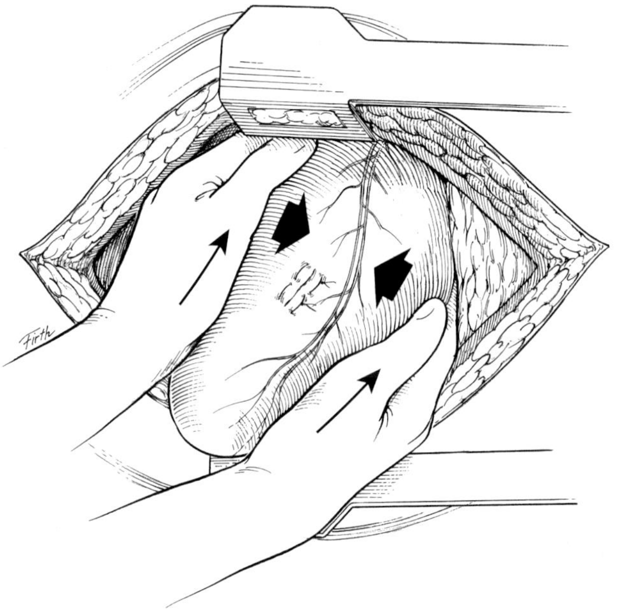

图 15　记录心室心动图后，通常须要用双手手掌进行开放式心肺复苏

命体征）、瞳孔反应、自主呼吸（即便是濒死）、颈动脉搏动存在、可测量的血压或可触及的脉搏、肢体运动以及心脏电活动。

选择性适应证

应该选择性地将 EDT 用于持续性穿透性的非心胸损伤患者，因为这类患者的存活率很低。由于很难确定损伤是否是心胸性的，所以可用操作进行诊断。

应该选择性地将 EDT 用于持续性腹部血管损伤导致出血的患者，因为这类患者的存活率很低。应该谨慎选择患者。应将此过程作为明确的修复腹部血管损伤的一部分。

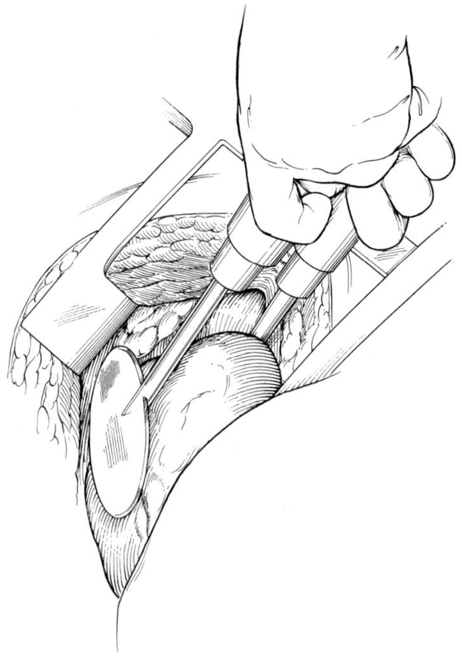

图 16　如果检测到心室纤颤，除了药物治疗外，还要用 50 J 的除颤仪处理

罕见适应证

很少将 EDT 用于继发于钝性创伤的持续性心肺骤停患者，因为这类患者的存活率很低，而且神经系统预后不良。选择患者时应该特别谨慎。应该严格限制在到达创伤中心后生命体征正常或者经历过一次心肺骤停的患者中使用 EDT。大多数作者都会警示这些适应证。

心脏损伤的修补技术

切口

用于心脏贯通伤的切口主要有两种。创伤外科医生应该明白导弹造成的创伤是不可预测的，因为其弹道以及导弹穿透一侧胸腔时可能不限于入口区域，也可能会损伤对侧胸腔。所以这就要求医生须要检查对侧胸腔。

Duval 所描述的胸骨正中切口适用于有一定程度的血流动力学不稳定的心前区贯通伤的患者，并且已进行过术前检查（FAST 或者 X 线胸片）。也可以将该切口用于被认为有隐匿性心脏损伤的患者。左前外侧切口适用于紧急情况下的患者的处理。该切口被用于紧急情况下的复苏。

可将 Spangaro 所描述的左前外侧切口延伸越过胸骨，以进行双侧前外侧开胸术，如果在复苏期间确定了损伤延至右侧胸腔的话（表 1）。延伸到双侧前外侧开胸术的切口适用于纵隔损伤后血流动力学不稳定的患者。通过这个切口可以充分地暴露前纵隔、心包膜和两侧胸腔。须要注意的是，当横断胸骨时，也会横断两侧的乳房动脉，并且在灌注压恢复后必须要将其结扎。如果未对其进行控制，它们可以成为一个重要的失血源。在损伤控制时这可能是一个常见的陷阱，因为创伤外科医生可能忘记结扎这些血管，导致那些无法承受这种损害的患者再次回到手术室做手术。在手术室对胸腹联合损伤的患者进行剖腹探查时，如果情况恶化，那么左前外侧切口也是一种选择。

表 1　急诊开胸手术的手法

术者	熟练的外科医师
初步评估与复苏	气管插管 立即建立静通道 快速补液
体位	左臂抬高并取仰卧位
切口	左前外侧切口 从左胸肋沿第五肋间间隙至背阔肌
手术经过	如上述切口 切开肋间肌 打开胸膜 放置牵开器 打开心包 抬高左肺 定位并分离降主动脉 用 Crafoord Debakey 钳交叉钳夹主动脉
如心脏损伤（蓝色紧张心包）	纵向打开心包，注意保护膈神经 清除积血 修复心脏损伤
如肺门活动性出血	用 Crafoord Debakey 钳交叉钳夹肺门
如肺挫裂伤	用 Duval 钳钳夹
如对侧胸腔损伤	延长切口至对侧 横断胸骨 转为双侧前外侧开胸
如怀疑有空气栓塞（空气进入冠状静脉）	从左心室吸出
其他	结扎乳内动脉全身或室内用肾上腺素 体内电除颤 10–50 J 临时起搏器
复苏成功后迅速转移至手术室	

辅助手法

创伤外科医生必须具备几种用来处理穿透性心胸损伤的手法。第一种处理这些损伤的辅助手法是由 Sauerbuch 在 1907 年提出的，并被 Brantigan 使用。这种手法须要通过压迫根部来控制血液流向心脏。这种手法很难通过左前外侧开胸术进行，所以已被废弃，仅是出于历史原因在此处提起。

闭塞所有流向心脏的血流是一个复杂的策略，这须要同时十字钳闭上腔静脉和下腔静脉（IVC）在心包内的位置，以此来止住所有流向心脏的血流。使用 Crafoord-DeBakey 十字钳可使心脏立刻清空。创伤外科医生必须认识到，十字钳闭下腔静脉在心包内的 Gibbons 点是相当危险的，因为下腔静脉往往与心包后方融合。缺乏经验的创伤外科医生经常为了试图迅速达到全部闭塞而大力使用十字钳，从而对心包内的下腔静脉造成医源性损伤。同样，环形解剖这个纤细的血管也可以导致医源性损伤。为了完全阻塞心包内的下腔静脉，必须小心地放置钳子，有时还要成角度放置。

处理右心房最侧面的损伤和上下房腔交界处损伤是闭塞所有流向心脏的血流的适应证。闭塞所有流向心脏的血流可导致心脏直接清空，使损伤部位可见并对其进行修补。通常患者是可以耐受这个操作导致的心肺骤停，但是患者对酸中毒、低体温和心肌缺血的耐受是有限的。目前还不知这种策略的安全期，尽管很多文献提出闭塞 1 ~ 3 min 就要松开钳子。当松开钳子时，静脉回流并充满了右侧心腔，并且心脏泵运动将重新开始。心脏经常会发生颤动，这时须要立即用药物来除颤。这可能是不会成功的，特别是如果时间超过了 3 min。通常不可能恢复正常的窦性心律。

对于肺相关损伤的患者来说，特别是肺门中心有血肿或者活动性出血的患者，对肺门进行十字钳闭是另一种有意义的手法。这种手法阻止了肺出血，并防止空气栓子到达全身循环。然而，其造成的一个负面影响是显著增加了右心室的后负荷，因为一半肺循环将不再用于灌注。在酸中毒、低体温和缺血的情况下，右心室可能无法耐受这种手法，因为可能导致心室颤动或者心室骤停。

最近 Grabowski 描述了一种方便暴露心脏后方损伤的方法，通过在右心室角处放一把 Satinsky 钳。这一角度是在右心室的前下缘急性形成的，因为它反映出右侧膈肌。Grabowski 建议钳子只抓住右心室的一部分。他建议用这种方法把心脏抬离心包，以修复心脏后部的损伤。我们没有使用这种方法的经验，因而不能推荐。我们有一种强烈的感觉，如果操作不当，该操作会引起严重的心律失常。

在心脏修补术后向心脏的左、右心室通气的方法是被推荐的，因为这一方法给陷在这些心腔里的空气栓塞提供了外出的通道。通常是通过 16 G 静脉导管完成这一操作。理论上来说，应该从修补的心腔里喷出空气，这样才能防止空气栓塞。尽管很多学者很成功地使用了这种方法，但是把结果写进文献里的却很少。

有时，创伤外科医生须要将心脏抬离心包以修复某些损伤。快速和不当的心脏操作可能会导致复杂的心律失常，包括心室颤动甚至心肺骤停。有时，根据活动性出血的程度，必须迅速地将心脏从心包取出以进行心脏修补术。无论何时进行该操作，创伤科医生都要与麻醉医生进行沟通。如果可以用手指控制出血，可通过逐步放几个剖腹手术包来抬高心脏。此举提高了患者对这种方法的耐受性，并且降低了发生心律失常的风险。

最近提出的心脏机械稳定系统已经在常规的冠状动脉旁路移植中被使用。它使用的是传统的体外循环，从而让心脏外科医生可以对泡在心脏停搏液中的停跳心脏进行操作。通过心肺泵的体外循环清除血液有害炎症的作用，促进基线稳定剂系统的功能。

Waterworth 最近报道了第一例将 Octopus 四号机械心脏稳定器（Octopus Iv Mechaniceal Cardiac Stabilizer）用于一名 20 岁的患者。在肺动脉瓣下方约 1 cm 的右心室流出道中有一个连续 2 cm 的刺伤。据笔者介绍，由于患者有持续的心动过速，并且该区域较为脆弱，难以在缝合该区域时不引起进一步的撕裂。在采用直接压力控制出血后，放置 Octopus 四号机械心脏稳定器，以保证这部分心脏区域静止，从而促进修复。在这种病例报告中，笔者描述了该装置的使用，表明可将具有可调吸力足部金属板的心脏稳定装置用于控制出血以及促进修复，特别是在手动处理困难或危险的区域。推荐其位置与伤口方向平行，足部金属板可能导致伤口闭合，并为修复提供了一个干净的区域。Waterworth 的病例报告似乎是第一个也是唯一的在文献中报道利用机械性心脏稳定器治疗穿透性心脏损伤的报告。未来稳定器是否会常规被用于治疗穿透性心脏损伤有待观察。

修复心房损伤

通常可以通过放置 Satinsky 部分闭塞血管夹来控制心房损伤。控制伤口时创伤外科医生可以开展心脏修补术。我们建议以跳跃或者间断的方式在 MH 针上使用 2-0 或 3-0 聚丙烯单丝缝合线。重要的是可以看到两侧心房损伤，特别是导弹引起的损伤。导弹损伤通常会导致大量组织破坏，可能须要在关闭之前进行细致的清创。类似地，在一部分心房切除或者心脏修补术中可以使用 2-0 或 3-0 聚丙烯单丝缝合线进行跳跃缝合。创伤外科医生必须意识到，心房壁是相当薄弱的，并且在心脏修补术中容易受到损伤，因为它们很容易撕裂和扩大原来的损伤。不建议使用特氟隆材料的生物仿制材料来处理这些损伤。

修复心室损伤

心室损伤通常会引起明显的出血。对于这种情况，应该先用手指压迫止血。与此同时，使用单纯间断缝合或者 Halsted 水平褥式缝合来修补。心室修补术也可以通过在 MH 针上使用 2-0 聚丙烯的跳跃单丝缝合来完成。心室刺伤时进行心脏修补术通常比枪伤的挑战性更小。导弹伤害往往会产生一定程度的引起心肌纤维退缩的爆炸效应。通常，对导弹造成的伤害成功缝合和控制后会随着受损的心肌缩回而变得十分脆弱。通常情况下，对这些损伤须要多次缝合才可以控制显著的出血。在这种情况下，通常须要使用生物仿制材料来支撑缝合线，如特氟龙带或纱布。通常使用长度为 1 ~ 5 cm 的特氟龙带（图 17 和 18）。这条带由助手用 2 把直 Crile 钳夹住。同时，创伤外科医生可以将双臂 2-0 聚丙烯单丝缝线放在 MH 针上。先穿过条带，然后再通过两侧伤口。然后以类似的方式保持第二条特氟龙带，使创伤外科医生将两根针头通过第二条特氟龙带。然后将缝合线轻轻地绑在特氟龙带或纱布上，从而支撑和加固缝合线。必须重复此操作，直到完全控制住心室出血。笔者最近使用商业化的纤维蛋白密封剂来密封复杂的心室损伤。

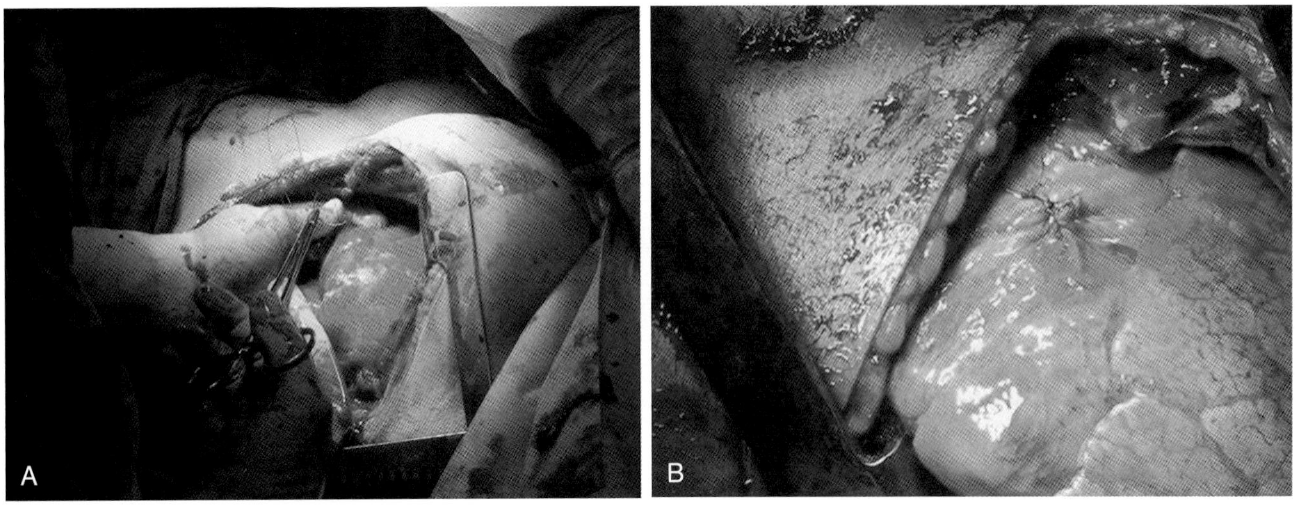

图 17 **A**，在急诊室开胸后，修复刺伤的心脏。**B**，缝合完成

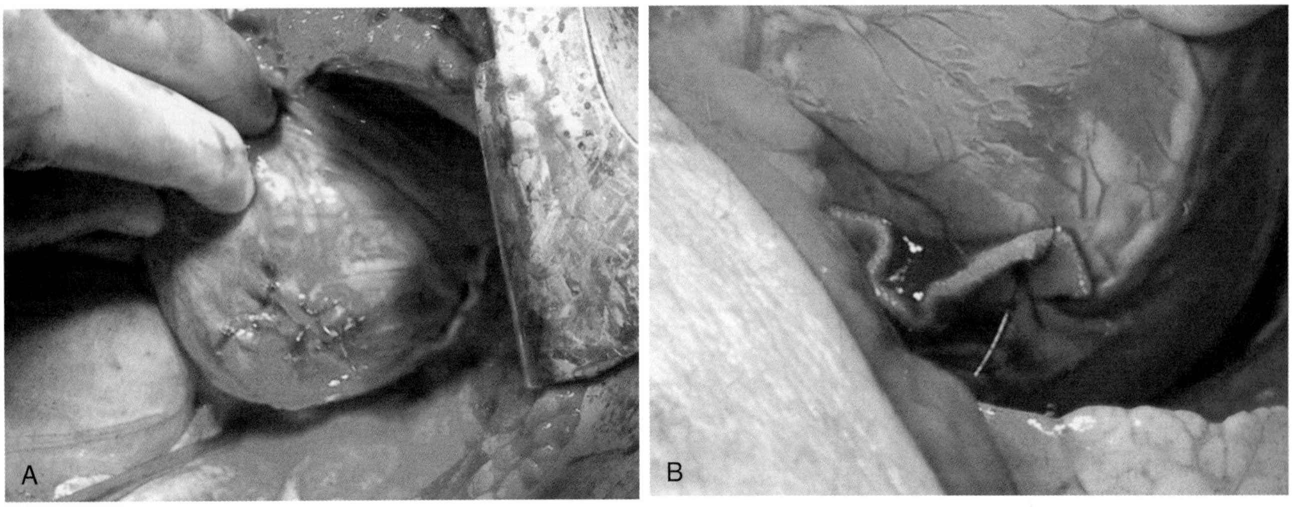

图 18 **A**，患者的心脏最高点存在持续穿透伤害。**B**，用特氟龙贴片加强缝合线

冠状动脉损伤

对与冠状动脉相邻的心室损伤进行修复可能是非常具有挑战性的。在心脏修补术期间，不正确或不适当地放置缝线可能会造成冠状动脉或一条分支狭窄或阻塞。因此，建议将缝线放置在冠状动脉床的下方。冠状动脉通常分为三个部分：近端、中段和远端。如果冠状动脉近端受伤，通常须要进行体外循环以进行修复，尽管通常是非必要的。冠状动脉中段损伤也可能需要体外循环。如果不顾一切地结扎，可能在手术台上会立即发生心肌梗死。先建立主动脉内气囊反搏，然后建立主动脉冠状动脉旁路，可能会使这些患者受益。特别是对于在冠状动脉最远端的 1/3 远侧段的血管撕裂，须要结扎处理。

生物材料和自体材料的使用

创伤外科医生对使用铁氟龙纱布或条带在易碎的心肌组织上支撑缝合线十分熟悉。Mattox 首次在其文献中暗示了使用这种材料。笔者强烈地相信，在有指征时使用特氟龙纱布来支撑复杂的缝合线是有必要的。然而，没有进行任何研究来确定使用特氟龙纱布是否增加了修复的抗拉强度。使用诸如心包膜之类的自体材料来加强缝合线也是众所周知的。有一种由心包膜分离和制作的小瓣膜，以类似特氟龙纱布的方式来使用。经验不足的创伤外科医生常常将心包膜和心室损伤一起缝合，使得腔室被固定，这会造成心律失常。之所以提到这一点，是因为这是一个无论如何都应该避免的陷阱。

复杂和联合损伤

尽管创伤外科医生和创伤中心关于处理穿透性心脏损伤的专业知识仍在不断发展，但是在城市战区中的伤者遭受到了更大程度的暴力。除了心脏穿透外，许多伤者还有多种联合损伤。复杂和联合的心脏损伤可以定义为穿透性心脏损伤加上相关的颈部、胸部、胸部血管、腹部、腹部血管或外周血管损伤。这些损伤很难处理，应该优先考虑造成最大失血或威胁患者生命的损伤。

Wall 和 Mattox 描述了 60 例复杂心脏损伤的患者，认为他们的严重程度超过了心肌撕裂。这些损伤定义为伴有冠状动脉损伤、心脏瓣膜损伤及心脏内瘘等异常损伤。在这一系列患者中，包括了 39 例冠状动脉损伤；2 例瓣膜损伤；14 例心包内瘘，其中包括室间隔缺损和心内膜缺损，以及另外 10 例从室性假性动脉瘤至冠状窦损伤的不常见损伤和 2 例发生导管栓塞的心脏病患者。这些类型的损伤也可以被认为是复杂和联合损伤。

结果

描述EDT的回顾性研究在文献中有很多。然而，在评估这些案例的结果时存在很大的困难。如果仔细观察，则可以发现这些研究存在几个缺陷。大多数案例都是回顾性评论，而且许多案例来自于不经常使用这种技术的机构。此外，许多机构报告了很多涵盖多年经验的重叠研究。许多案例选择将生理参数作为结果的预测因子，但没有一个在统计学上验证了其预测价值。这些案例总是省略了与患者生理状态有关的初始数据。据我们所知，只有一篇前瞻性研究文献。因此，还有很多问题须要回答。

哪些患者应该接受这个手术？是否有前瞻性验证的生理预测因素，可以安全、准确地识别从手术中受益的患者，并且安全地排除那些不受益的患者？这个手术的真实存活率是多少？在幸存的患者中，有多少是伴有严重的神经损伤或维持在持续的植物人状态？我们如何确保实施手术的人员是合格的？

众所周知，预测不良结局的生理因素包括院前和急诊室无生命体征，瞳孔固定和扩大，存在心律失常，无四肢运动以及濒死呼吸。同样，在心肺骤停的情况下，如果脉搏可触及，也预示着不好的结果。这些因素已由 Asensio 等进行了验证。他们在两项关于穿透性心脏损伤的前瞻性研究中，现场追踪交通转运过程直至抵达急诊科。有趣的是，在许多研究中，这些预测结果的生理因素，以及在 EDT 之前描述患者生理状况的数据通常并不存在。

Buckman 等和 Asensio 等之前的工作应用和验证了创伤评分（TS）中的心血管呼吸评分（cardiovascular respiratory score，CVRS）。TS 的心血管呼吸评分反映出个体血压、呼吸频率、呼吸力和毛细血管再灌注。CVRS 的最高值为 11 分，表示收缩压＞90 mmHg，呼吸频率在 10～24 次 / 分之间波动，具有正常的呼吸力和毛细血管再灌注。CVRS 评分最低为零分，表明血压不足，颈动脉搏动不明显，呼吸困难，毛细血管再灌注不足。CVRS 已经被统计学所验证，并在仅有的三篇穿透性心脏损伤案例文献中应用。

Asensio 等在其唯一使用 EDT 的前瞻性研究文献中，分析了在将心肺骤停患者从现场至创伤中心的转运过程中测量的生理状况参数。对 CVRS、损伤机制和损伤解剖部位以及血压恢复进行了追踪，目的是确定一组可以可靠地预测死亡风险的参数，并使患者免于在急诊科治疗。这项为期 2 年的前瞻性研究只有一项纳入标准——继发于创伤性损伤的心肺骤停，这同样也是 EDT 复苏的单一变量。这项研究的主要结果是 1 h 存活以及存活出院。

该研究对 215 名持续心肺骤停的患者进行了前瞻性研究。其中 167 人（78%）存在持续性穿透伤，包括 142 人（66%）枪伤，21 人（10%）刺伤和 4 人（2%）霰弹枪伤。此外，有 48 人（22%）存在持续性钝性伤。平均修复创伤评分（revised trauma score，RTS）为 0.6 分，平均伤害严重程度评分为 42 分，平均 CVRS 为 1 分，表示为存在严重受伤和生理损伤的患者人群。在到达创伤中心前的 CPR 平均持续时间为 12 min。

共有 162 名患者（75%）在急诊科死亡。53 名患者（25%）存活达 1 h。在成功的急诊复苏恢复生命体征后，可以将患者立即运至手术室。在 215 例心脏损伤患者中，只有 6 例（3%）存活，8 例钝性创伤患者均未存活。在急诊中死亡的患者与至少存活 1 h 的患者相比较，所有的生理参数预测结局（$P<0.001$）。与存活 1 h 的患者与总体幸存者相比，没有生理参数预测出结局。CPR 的持续时间（$P=0.04$）、损伤的穿透机制（$P<0.001$）和出血（$P<0.006$）是结果的预测因子。CVRS 显示出

生存预测的趋势（P=0.07）。当将死亡患者与幸存者进行比较时，恢复血压是结局的重要预测因素（P<0.001）。

作者从这些数据得出结论，生理参数和CVRS评分可以预测EDT患者的生存率。根据这些标准，作者估计，其中有75%的患者可以不必做该手术，这可以为相关机构节省超过50万美元的成本，同时建议EDT应限于持续穿透性心脏损伤的患者，而不是继发于钝性创伤的心肺骤停的患者。

正是由于文献报道的报告过程缺乏一致性，美国创伤外科医师委员会结局特设小组（Ad Hoc Subcommittee on Outcomes of American College of Surgeons Committee on Trauma）中的Asensio等紧紧围绕文献制定了EDT的实践管理指南。

在广泛的文献检索中，研究分为三类。第一类包括前瞻性随机对照试验，这仍然是所有临床试验的黄金标准。在这一类中，由于研究的设计不佳，数量不足，或者方法学上的不足而使其没有明显的临床意义。在这个类别中，没有建立前瞻性随机对照试验。第二类研究包括前瞻性收集数据的临床研究，以及基于清晰、可靠数据的回顾性分析。这里包括观察法、队列研究、流行率和病例对照研究。作者发现有29项研究属于第二类，其中3项是前瞻性的。最后，第三类为回顾性收集数据，从临床案例、数据库或注册管理机构、案例审查、病例报告和专家意见中，作者找到了63项研究。

作者通过将案例分为经历EDT的案例、报告神经学结果的EDT案例、专门针对穿透性心脏损伤的案例以及处理儿科患者的案例来进行数据分析。在经历EDT的42个案例（表2）中，有7035个EDT患者和551个幸存者，存活率为7.83%。当根据损伤机制分类数据时，有4482例穿透伤患者进行了开胸手术。其中500例患者存活，生存率为11.16%。有2193例钝性损伤患者进行了开胸手术。其中只有35例患者存活，存活率为1.60%。

在14项报告神经病学结局的病例研究中，共有4520例患者接受了EDT，其中有226名幸存者，存活率为5%。在这226名幸存者中，34名（15%）患有神经功能障碍。在专门针对修复穿透性心脏损伤的EDT的病例中（表3），共有1165例EDT，363例患者存活，生存率为31.1%。发现只有4个病例研究是专门针对儿科患者（表4）。总共执行了142次EDT。对57例穿透性损伤患者进行了胸廓切开术，其中7例患者存活，生存率为12.2%。对5例钝性损伤患者进行了胸廓切开术，其中2例存活，存活率为2.3%。

尽管EDT并没有进行前瞻性随机对照试验研究，但作者提出了以下建议：

1. 由于存活率非常低且神经学预后较差，因此，对继发于钝性损伤的心肺骤停患者不应进行EDT。应限用于那些到达创伤中心时有生命体征或者突然发生心肺骤停的患者。
2. EDT最适用于存在于持续穿透性心脏损伤的患者，如在短暂的现场和运输时间之后到达创伤中心，有目测或客观测量的生理参数（生命迹象），如瞳孔反应、自发性通气、颈动脉脉搏的存在、可测量或明显的血压、肢体运动或心脏电活动。
3. 对穿透性非心脏胸部损伤的患者应行EDT，但这些患者的生存率通常较低。因为难以确定伤口是否位于心脏，EDT可用于确定诊断。
4. 对于持续性腹部血管损伤出血的患者应行EDT，但这些患者的生存率通常较低。应慎重选择患者。这个手术应该作为明确的腹部血管损伤修复的辅助手段。
5. 对于儿科患者，准则1—4可用。
6. 总之，在外科医生的手术中EDT仍然十分重要。应明确严格地遵守适应证，并且只能由经过适当训练的创伤科医生和外科医生来操作。只有通过明智的科学探究，我们才能挑战极限，拯救生命，推进科学发展。

表 2 42 例急诊开胸手术数据分析

主要作者 *	年份	研究类型	生存者 / 总人数	神经功能障碍（n）	生存者 / 穿透性创伤	生存者 / 钝性伤
Mattox	1974	R	11/106	0	8/87	3/19
McDonald	1978	R	3/28	0	3/26	0/2
Moore	1979	R	12/146	4	11/98	1/48
Baker	1980	R	32/168	2	31/108	1/60
Hamar	1981	R	5/64	0	—	—
Ivatury	1981	R	8/22	1	8/22	—
Flynn	1982	R	4/33	0	4/13	0/20
Bodai	1982	R	0/38	0	—	0/38
Rohman	1983	R	24/91	0	24/91	—
Vij	1983	R	5/63	1	5/57	0/6
Cogbill	1983	R	16/400	4	15/205	1/195
Shimazu	1983	R	6/267	2	4/50	4/217
Danne	1984	R	10/89	1	10/60	0/29
Tavares	1984	R	21/37	0	21/37	—
Washington	1984	R	6/23	0	6/23	0
Washington	1985	R	8/55	0	8/55	—
Brantigan	1985	R	6/32	1	6/32	
Feliciano	1986	R	28/335	1	25/280	3/53
Roberge	1986	R	7/44	0	7/44	—
Schwab	1986	R	14/51	0	14/36	0/15
Moreno	1986	R	4/69	0	4/69	—
Ordog	1987	R	6/80	1	5/64	2/16
Demetriades	1987	R	5/73	0	5/73	—
Baxter	1988	R	29/632	0	22/313	7/319
Clevenger	1988	R	3/72	0	3/41	0/31
Hoyt	1989	R	33/113	0	33/74	0/39
Mandal	1989	R	7/23	0	—	0
Esposito	1991	R	2/112	1	1/24	1/88
Ivatury	1991	R	16/163	0	16/134	0/29
Lewis	1991	R	8/45	0	8/32	0/13
Durham	1992	R	32/389	0	32/318	0/69
Lorenz	1992	R	41/424	4	37/231	3/193
Blake	1992	R	5/22	0	5/22	—
Bond	1992	R	2/28	0	2/11	0/17
Millham	1993	R	13/290	4	13/290	—
Mazzorana	1994	R	10/273	0	10/252	0/21
Velmahos	1995	R	43/855	0	42/679	1/176

表 2 42 例急诊开胸手术数据分析（续表）

主要作者 *	年份	研究类型	生存者 / 总人数	神经功能障碍（n）	生存者 / 穿透性创伤	生存者 / 钝性伤
Jahangiri	1996	R	1/16	0	1/4	0/12
Brown	1996	R	4/160	0	4/149	0/11
Bleetman	1996	R	8/25	0	8/24	0/1
Branncy	1998	R	41/868	7	33/483	8/385
Asensio	1998	P	6/215	0	6/167	0/48

Modified from Working Group, Ad Hoc Subcommittee on Outcomes, American College of Surgeons, Committee on Trauma: Practice management guidelines for emergency department thoracotomy. J Am Coll Surg 193(3):303–309, 2001

EDT, 急诊胸廓切开术（Emergency department thoracotomy）; P, 前瞻性（prospective）; R, 回顾性（retrospective）

表 3 急诊开胸手术治疗心脏损伤 46 例分析

主要作者 *	年份	研究类型	生存者 / 总数 EDT	生存者 / 穿透性创伤
Boyd	1965	R	0/0	17/25
Beall	1966	R	3/16	42/197
Sauer	1967	R	12/0	12/13
Sugg	1968	R	0/0	63/459
Yao	1968	R	0/0	61/80
Steichen	1971	R	7/21	35/58
Beall	1971	R	29/52	42/66
Borja	1971	R	0/0	24/145
Carrasquilla	1972	R	8/30	20/245
Beall	1972	R	0/0	67/269
Bolanowski	1973	R	0/0	33/44
Trinkle	1974	R	0/0	38/45
Mattox	1974	R	25/37	31/62
Harvey	1975	R	0/0	22/28
Symbas	1976	R	0/0	50/98
Beach	1976	R	0/4	26/34
Asfaw	1977	R	0/0	277/323
Sherman	1978	R	32/41	37/92
Trinkle	1978	R	0/0	89/100
Evans	1979	R	0/4	29/46
Breaux	1979	R	39/44	78/197
Mandal	1979	R	/38	26/55
Gervin	1982	R	4/21	4/21
Demetriades	1983	R	2/16	40/125
Demetriades	1984	R	1/11	45
Tavares	1984	R	21/37	64
Feliciano	1984	R	5/15	3/2

表 3　急诊开胸手术治疗心脏损伤 46 例分析（续表）

主要作者 *	年份	研究类型	生存者 / 总数 EDT	生存者 / 穿透性创伤
Mattox	1985	R	50/119	204
Demetriades	1986	R	1/18	70
Moreno	1986	R	4/69	100
Ivatury	1987	R	28/91	—
Jebara	1989	R	4/17	—
Attar	1991	R	21/55	—
Knott-Craig	1992	R	5/13	—
Buchman	1992	R	1/2	23
Benyan	1992	R	1/13	—
Macho	1993	R	12/24	—
Mitchell	1993	R	7/47	—
Kaplan	1993	R	2/23	
Henderson	1994	R	6/122	215
Coimbra	1995	R	0/20	
Arreola-Risa	1995	R	11/40	
Karmy-Jones	1997	R	3/6	16
Rhee	1998	R	15/58	41/96
Asensio	1998	P	6/37	6/37
Asensio	1998	P	10/71	10/71

Modified from Working Group, Ad Hoc Subcommittee on Outcomes, American College of Surgeons, Committee on Trauma: Practice management guidelines for emergency department thoracotomy. J Am Coll Surg 193(3):303–309, 2001

注意：该表格没有钝性伤生存者

EDT, 急诊胸廓切开术（emergency department thoracotomy）; P, 前瞻性（prospective）; R, 回顾性（retrospective）

表 4　儿科急诊开胸手术

主要作者 *	年份	研究类型	生存者 / 总数 EDT	生存者 / 穿透性创伤	生存者 / 穿透性创伤
Beaver	1987	R	0/17	0/2	0/15
Powell	1988	R	5/19	4/11	1/8
Rothenberg	1989	R	3/83	2/36	1/47
Sheikh	1993	R	1/23	1/8	0/15

Modified from Working Group, Ad Hoc Subcommittee on Outcomes, American College of Surgeons, Committee on Trauma: Practice management guidelines for emergency department thoracotomy. J Am Coll Surg 193(3):303–309, 2001

注意：该表格没有钝性伤生存者

EDT, 急诊胸廓切开术（emergency department thoracotomy）; P, 前瞻性（prospective）; R, 回顾性（retrospective）

创伤重点超声评估

Andrés M. Rubiano, Glyn Estebanez, Aurelio Rodríguez 著
易成腊 译

在过去的二十年里，在对创伤患者的管理中使用创伤重点超声评估（focused assessment with sonography in trauma，FAST）越来越普遍。随着超声技术的连续改进，其可移植性和图像质量使得在急诊室初始复苏期间可以得到快速、可靠的诊断图像。由于其使用的接受程度和重要性，美国外科医师学院（ACS）将 FAST 纳入了 1997 年高级创伤生命支持（ATLS）课程。目前，多学科团队在世界范围内开展了 FAST，包括创伤外科医师、急诊医师和院前急救提供者。在不同的环境中关于 FAST 有几个准则和循证评论，包括战区的操作和战术场景。目前已推广了提出的经典技术，并开发了无线设备。本章的目的是描述技术、适应证、争议和过程演变。

超声的简要历史

1917 年，第一台压电发电机被用于开发超声波。发生器的晶体也被用作接收器，其在检测到反射的机械振动或声波时产生电信号。在第二次世界大战期间，超声技术因具有较大的潜力开始被认可，在声音导航和测距（Sound Navigation and Ranging，SONAR）系统中使用，能够检测潜艇，从而挽救无数生命。1959 年，在超声检查期间使用多普勒效应能够检测到外周动脉的流动。然而，1971 年引入了灰度级标准，标志着开始广泛接受将超声作为诊断工具。

20 世纪 80 年代，德国医师率先在创伤中利用超声，并于 1988 年为外科手术人员引入了标准化的超声训练计划。1992 年，北美认识到了超声在患者护理中的潜在作用，并开始实施其在创伤患者评估中的教学，如 Hoffman TSO 和 Rodriguez 的论文所述。在出版了几篇案例系列证明超声在创伤患者中的成功使用后，ACS 将 FAST 纳入了其 1995 年处理腹部创伤的原则中。最初，该技术集中于腹部区域。1996 年，Rodriguez 和 Rozycki 等发表的论文描述了 FAST（创伤重点腹部超声图，focused abdominal sonogram for trauma）的内容。同年晚些时候，该方法已被纳入 ATLS 培训计划，并且 FAST 的定义改为对创伤患者超声检查的重点评估。1997 年，当被列入 ATLS 课程时，FAST 被认为是创伤患者护理中的基本且有价值的工具。

FAST 培训的演变

该技术最初在外科医师和手术人员中普遍使用。但实际上，其他涉及创伤护理的专业也参加了培训过程，包括急诊医师、重症监护医师和院前医师。FAST 培训计划的目的仅仅是提高准确诊断存在自由液体的能力。FAST 是一种快速、准确、无创和易于重复的方法，用于检测在初次测量期间以及在初始复苏期间在不稳定患者中的自由液体。已经在几项共识中制订了适用于 FAST 的准则，包括以下建议：

- 必须保证复苏室的床边超声评估每天 24 h 可用。
- 执行 FAST 的创伤外科医师必须接受适度的正确执行和解释扫描的训练。
- 每个医院必须对医师进行培训和评估，以确保有效地利用资源，并利用不同的专家来帮助医师提高其解释和决策能力。
- FAST 培训必须成为外科住院课程的一部分（图 1）。
- 在对创伤患者的管理过程中，FAST 在决策中的价值取决于操作者。因此，开展有效的教学和持续的培训是医生正确开展 FAST 并解读其结果的重中之重。

超声原理

通过记录定向到组织中的超声脉冲的回波并对密度变化的组织进行平面反映，可以将超声波定义为深体结构的成像。可听声波的频率范围在 15 kHz 和 20 Hz 之间；次声波的频率低于 15 Hz，医疗成像中使用的超声波范围从 1 MHz 到 60 MHz。用于医学成像的超声波是可以通过液体和软组织的纵波，

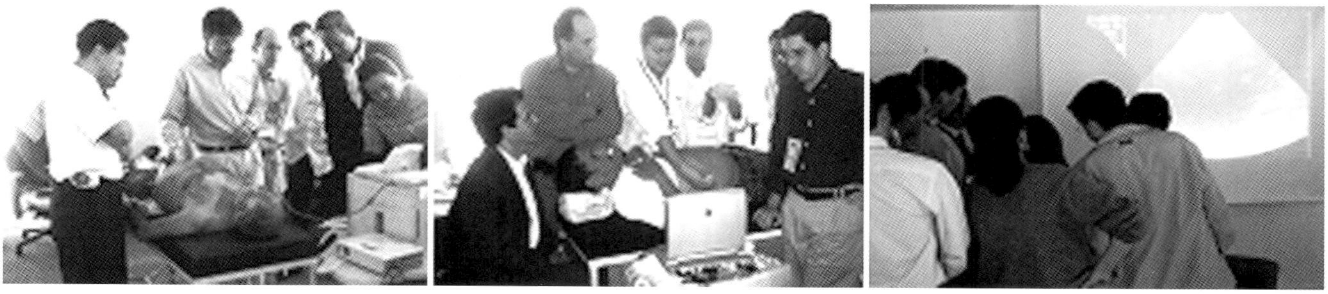

图 1　为外科和急诊科医师开展的 FAST 培训。创伤和急诊室超声培训项目是拉美国家开展 FAST 培训的泛美创伤学会（Pan-American Trauma Society）课程 (Courtesy Dr. Andres Rubiano [USET instructors group].)

但是在没有这些物质的情况下不容易传播。因此，当超声通过诸如肺之类的空气填充结构时显示不良。一旦超声波遇到具有不同密度或声阻抗的材料时，一部分声波被换能器反射和检测。组织或结构的密度越大，则反射或回波就越大，因此，较高密度的组织在显示器上显示为较亮的图像。换能器既是发射器，也是接收器。超声波是由电脉冲压电效应激发的晶体的机械运动或振荡产生的。在传播到患者体内的声波中，一小部分声波被反射回到换能器内的晶体，并且这些反射的声波在接收后产生电脉冲，然后这些电脉冲被处理成图像。

作用于换能器内的晶体的电脉冲的强度允许一段时间的静默，从而足以在产生下一个传递的声波之前接收到较浅以及较深反射的声波或回波。一个脉冲由三个阶段组成：①发射相位。②平衡相位。③接收相位。当产生超声波时为发射相位。接收相位是发生反射声波的接收的周期。而平衡相位是既没有接收也不发射超声波的时期。

大多数超声波扫描仪的最大检测深度为 20 cm，有时重要的是要从不同的角度分析该区域，以获得最佳图像。声波具有 1540 m/s 的恒定速度，因此，如果某个声波的“发射和接收”到换能器的持续时间缩短，即表明这是一种软组织，如果某种组织反射声波，那么就是密度更大的组织。当软组织不反映声波，并且没有获得信号时，则通常表示是囊性的。

换能器

换能器由几个基本部件组成。换能器的晶体是由压电材料制成的，通常为单晶石英或锆酸铅。晶体的目的是将电脉冲转换为透射声波，反之亦然。绝缘材料（最常用的是橡胶）被用于换能器的“鼻子”，并增加了声波的聚焦传播，从而增加了声波穿透的轴向分辨率和深度。使用外部保护器或隔声器来包围换能器，并将其与任何不需要的声波干扰隔离。换能器通过电子电缆连接到外部显示器，从而使电压脉冲朝向和远离压电晶体传输。

换能器的类型及使用

使用特定换能器的适用性取决于扫描的目的以及视野所需的深度。常用于医学成像的频率范围为 2 ~ 20 MHz，较高的频率是对表面结构观察的最佳频率。这是因为较高的频率的波长较短。与较低的频率相比，这些波长在更短的距离内会受到更大程度的衰减。用于观察表面组织的换能器倾向于使用 7 ~ 12 MHz 的频率，并且最大成像深度为 4 cm。使用 3 ~ 5 MHz 的较低频率的换能器可以将声波传到更高的位置，因此适用于腹部和盆腔区域成像，因此被用于 FAST。

换能器的形状是“鼻子”形的，这是在适当使用换能器时的重要因素。线性扫描器允许彼此平行延伸的声波的传输，并保持相同的距离，而不管传播的深度如何，因此，最好将线性扫描器用于直视表面结构和软组织。弯曲的表面扫描仪以扇形方式传输超声波，从而增加了感知视野的宽度。当与更好的穿透低频声波联合使用时，弯曲扫描仪提供了可以精确进行 FAST 检查的最合适的视图（图 2）。

超声设备

现代超声机器在扫描身体的不同部位时已将不同形状的换能器和波长频率进行了优化组合（图 3）。因此，操作员经常只须要在机器上选择适当的观看设置，然后在进行扫描之前选择适当的换能器。在执行 FAST 时，可能须要对超声设备的设置进行实

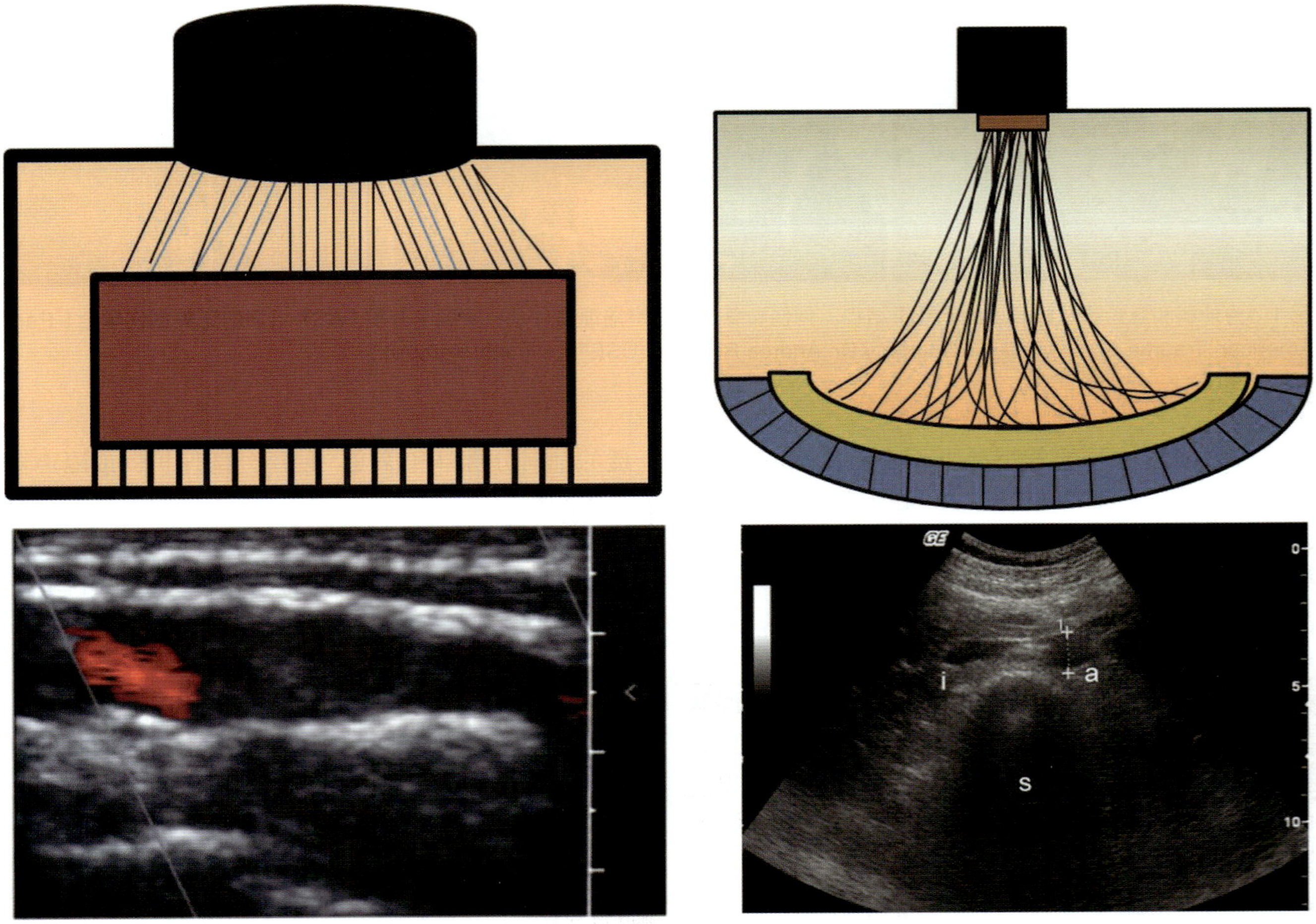

图 2　7.5 MHz 线性（左）和 3.5 MHz 凸（右）换能器样式。第一张图像是一种典型的经常用于血管扫描的方形盒子。梯形视图形式是凸形传感器的特征，被用于 FAST

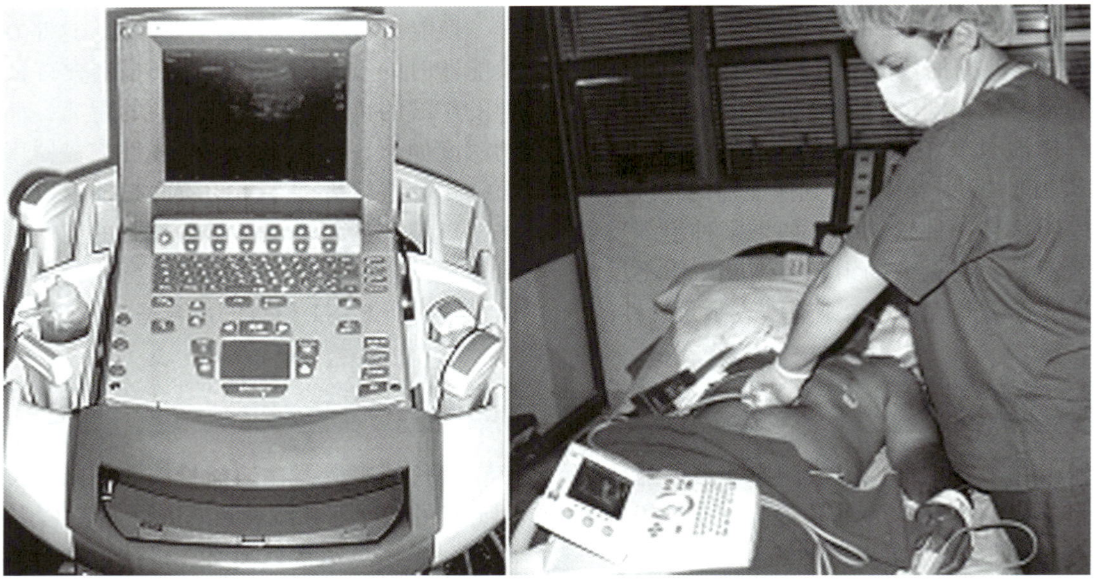

图 3　现代便携式超声波设备可短时间内在床边进行超声检查以进行创伤程序的重点评估。预设传感器通常节省时间，并能最大限度地减少操作者造成的错误

时调整，以便微调所获得的图像的质量。

详细了解提高超声波图像质量的各种手段，可增加在这些手段上制订的治疗决策的准确性，并且潜在地避免了诊断中的错误。

- 声功率 / 输出：其控制了施加到压电晶体的电压，增加输出功率会增加产生的声波的强度。通常，通过最低级别的输出功率可获得适合解读的图像。
- 回放：将图像序列以数字形式存储，这可以在检查完成后进行审查。
- 深度：深度决定了在显示屏幕上可以看到的穿透程度。根据所使用的换能器的类型最大深度而有所变化。频率越高，则深度（>5 MHz<深度）越小；频率越低，则深度越大（<5 MHz>深度）。
- 聚焦：聚焦可使其在扫描期间在所选择的目标深度上获得更高的图像清晰度。焦点可以根据检查期间的目标而变化。
- 增益：增益可调节返回到换能器的所有超声波的放大程度。增益太多或太少都会影响所获得图像的质量。如果将增益设置得太高，则所获取的图像将会随着伪影噪声而变形。另外，由于所有反射回波逐渐变亮，所以不同结构之间的对比度将会有所损失。如果将增益设置得太低，将会丢失一些真实回波的感知，从而降低了图像的质量。
- 近场增益：近场增益控制了表面场内回波的放大。
- 远场增益：远场增益控制了深场中回波的放大。
- 变焦镜头：变焦镜头允许我们放大图像以更好地观察较小的结构。然而，放大可能导致图像的失真以及随后的图像质量损失。

FAST 的使用

FAST 成像中的伪像

- 噪声：由于其他电气设备的存在而引起的图像干扰。
- 遮盖：指当同时使用几个焦点区域时，在某些深度处可观察到的回波性增加的带。应该适当减少使用焦点区域。
- 回响：在存在声波多重反射的情况下，当波从皮肤换能器界面反射到身体中时产生的伪影。
- 镜像：复制可视化的结构的图像。选择身体不同的角度或者位置来重新观察目标点可能会有所改善。
- 增强：指在流体之下亮度增加的区域。这是因为流体的声波阻抗远小于其后较大的反射组织。

FAST 中使用的词汇

- 无回声的：不会引起声波反射并因此在超声波图像上呈黑色。
- 衰减：声波的振幅降低，就像是通过组织或介质的距离的函数。声波的进一步弱点通常是由于各种组织的吸收所致。
- 回声：指组织回声超声波的程度（通常在超声图像中表现为亮度的程度）。
- 低回声：比周围组织回声少（较暗）。
- 强回声：比周围组织回声多（较亮）。
- 等回声：与周围组织有相似的外观。

FAST 技术

FAST 的吸引力在于它提供了一种快速、安全、无创且易于重复的方法，可准确地识别腹膜或心包膜内游离液体的存在。与诊断性腹膜灌洗（diagnostic peritoneal lavage, DPL）不同，FAST 是一项非侵入性检查手段，相对容易进行，无禁忌证，并且在怀孕的创伤患者中也可以安全地进行。

在 FAST 中获得的四个窗口或视图可用“四 P”来表示：①心包（Pericardial），②肝周（Perihepatic），③脾周（Perisplenic），④盆腔（Pelvic）。这些视图能够更容易地识别自由液体存在的位置，从而更好地对其进行评估。在 FAST 检查中获得的视图序列可以变化。有些医疗机构是从心包的视图开始的，特别是如果患者的血流动力学不稳定时，可以通过这一举措来排除心包压塞。最常见的是，序列是从正确的象限开始的——Morison 陷凹视图（肝周），因为在统计学上它是找到自由液体最常见的位置（图 4）。还有的人是从盆腔窗口开

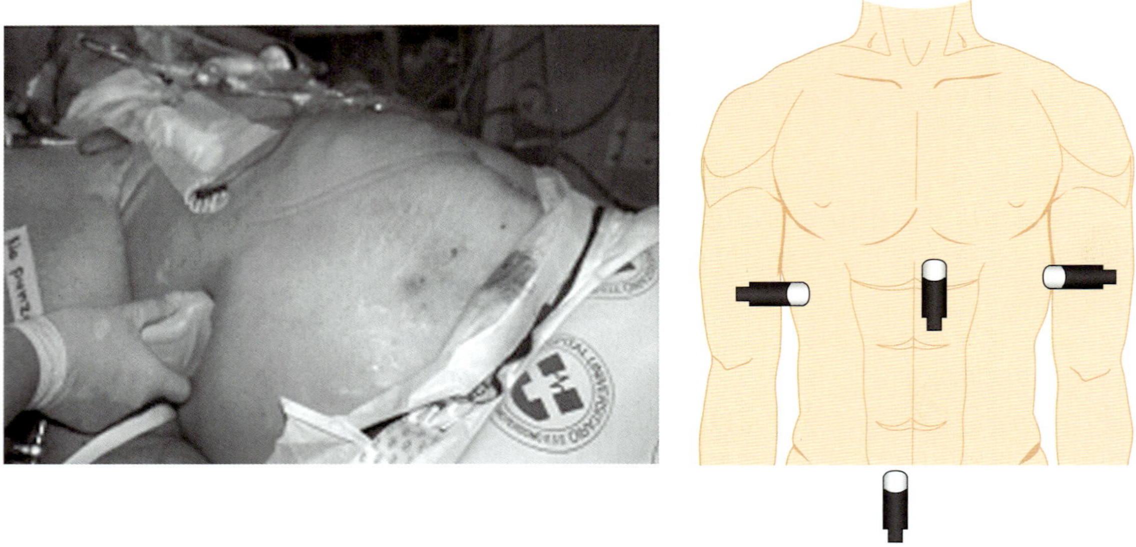

图 4 采用超声检查对创伤序列的重点评估时有不同的开始。最右边的象限是统计学上发现自由液体最常见的区域（Morison 陷凹）

始的，以获得膀胱中液体的适当视图，然后将该图像保留在内存中，以便与其他视图进行比较。当操作者的经验不足时，这个技术很有用。

已经开发了经典 FAST 检查的扩展版本——E-FAST，其中还包括两侧胸腔的视图，可以用之确认气胸或血胸的存在。虽然这种扩展检查有可能提供额外的有用的信息，但其尚未被正式纳入对创伤患者的常规超声评估。当由经验丰富的创伤临床医师操作时，已证实 FAST 可以确定存在少至 250ml 游离的腹膜内液体。然而，与 CT 不同，FAST 的灵敏度和特异性在很大程度上取决于操作者的经验和技巧。几项研究表明，FAST 在“排除”自由腹膜内血液或心包血液方面的准确性随着检查者先前进行的扫描次数的增加而提高。

该检查被专门用于检测自由液体和心脏阻塞。这种技术很难评估实体器官、中空内脏和腹膜后损伤。传感器的类型（在便携式设备中更多）有 2.5 MHz（肥胖患者）、3.5 MHz（凸）和 5 MHz（儿科患者）。凝胶被应用于四个区域，并且依次按以下顺序使用：右上象限、心包、左上象限和盆腔视图。

- 肝周窗：将传感器置于右侧腋中线，在第 11 至第 12 肋之间。检查 Morison 陷凹，并识别肝、肾和隔膜。通过检查这些结构中的平面来检查自由液体。在统计学上，这是自由液体最常见的位置（图 5 和图 6）。
- 心包窗：其经典位置是靠近剑突下。将传感器置于指向左肩的剑突上。检查心包膜是否有自由液体。在一些患者，特别是肥胖患者中，这种方法很困难。另一种方法是平行于左侧胸骨边缘的第 4 肋骨和第 5 肋骨之间。这种方法经常被心脏科医师用来进行超声心动图检查。使用这种方法时，微凸的传感器比常规凸的传感器要好（图 7）。
- 脾周窗：将传感器置于左侧腋后线第 10 至第 11 肋骨间。检查肾 - 脾窝，并识别脾、肾和膈肌。通过检查其中的平面来检查自由液体（图 8）。
- 盆腔窗：将传感器置于耻骨上方约 4 cm 处。很容易识别膀胱，特别是充满尿液的话。如果没有尿液，并且 Foley 导管已就位，可以注射盐水以充满膀胱。检查直肠和直肠间隙（道格拉斯陷凹）以发现自由液体。在几项研究中，这是自由液体第二个最常见的位置（图 9 和图 10）。

FAST 在胸部创伤超声中的拓展

Lichtenstein 等首次描述了使用超声诊断 ICU 患者气胸的情况。随后，已证明在急诊科可使用超声诊断 ICU 患者的气胸。2004 年，Kirkpatrick 等提出将 FAST 拓展，至检查胸部，称为 E-FAST。与胸部 X 线片或 CT 扫描不同，采用胸腔超声评估气胸或血胸更为快速，可在检查时立即提供诊断，还可在

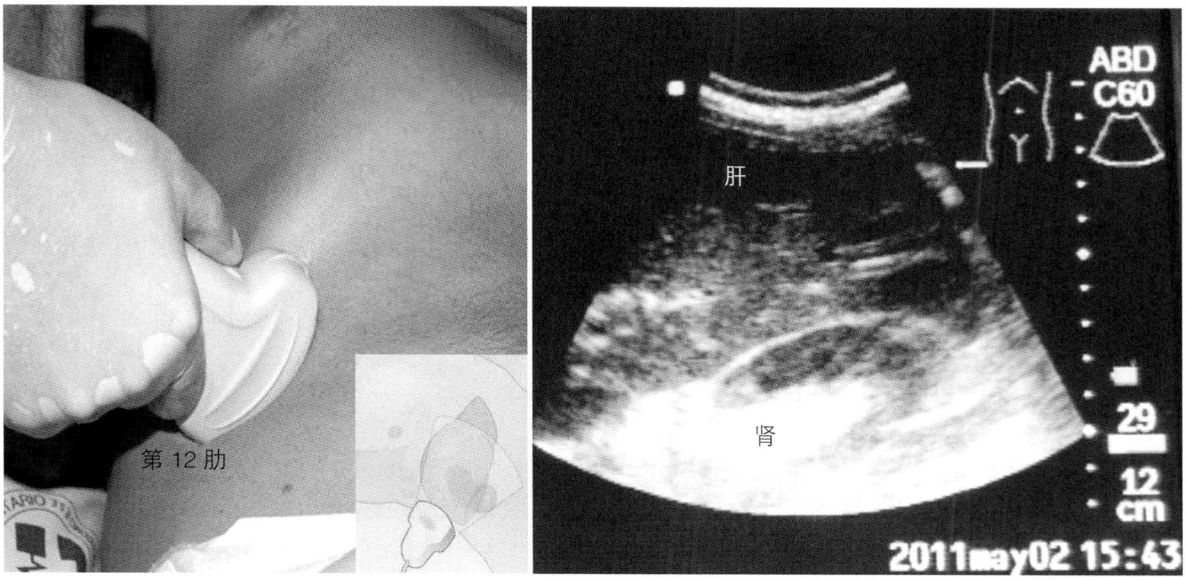

图 5　肝周窗位于右侧腋中线，在第 11 至第 12 肋之间。识别肝和肾，在两者之间没有自由液体。正常视图

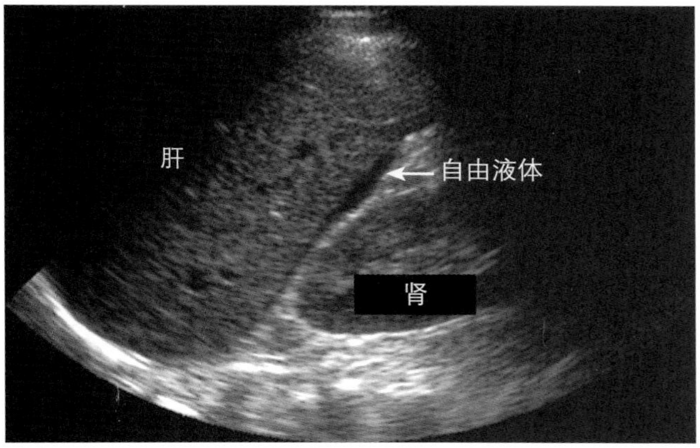

图 6　肝周窗在右侧腋中线第 11 至第 12 肋之间。识别肝和肾在两者之间可见的自由液体。不正常视图。(*Courtesy of M. Perdomo, USET Instructors Group.*)

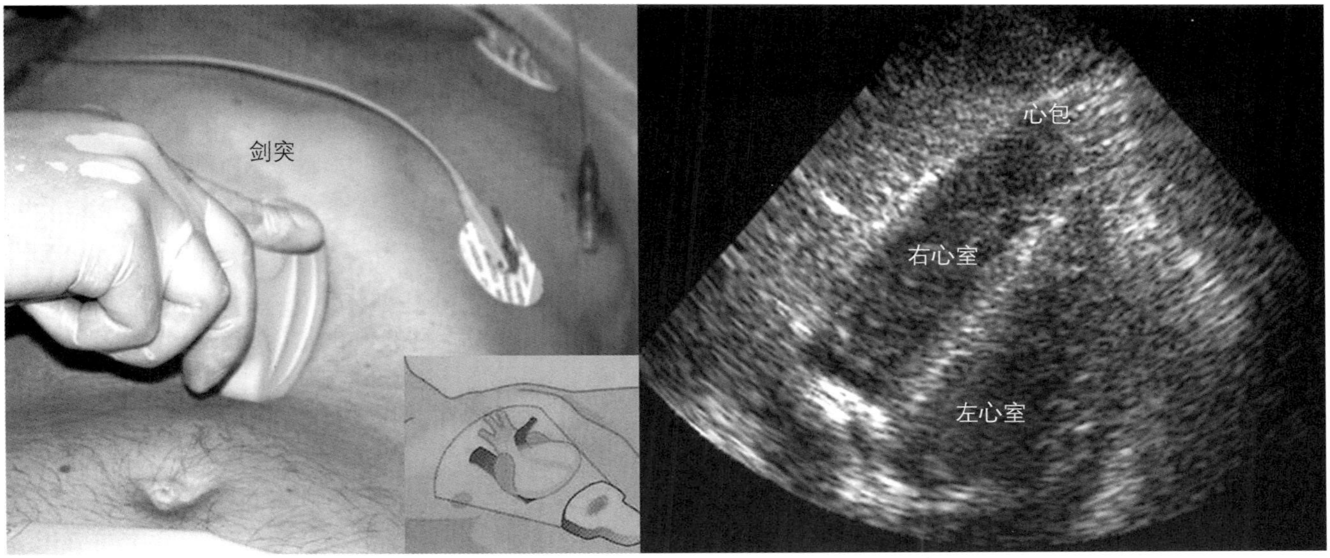

图 7　靠近剑突下的心包窗。识别心室，并且在周围的心包没有自由液体。正常视图

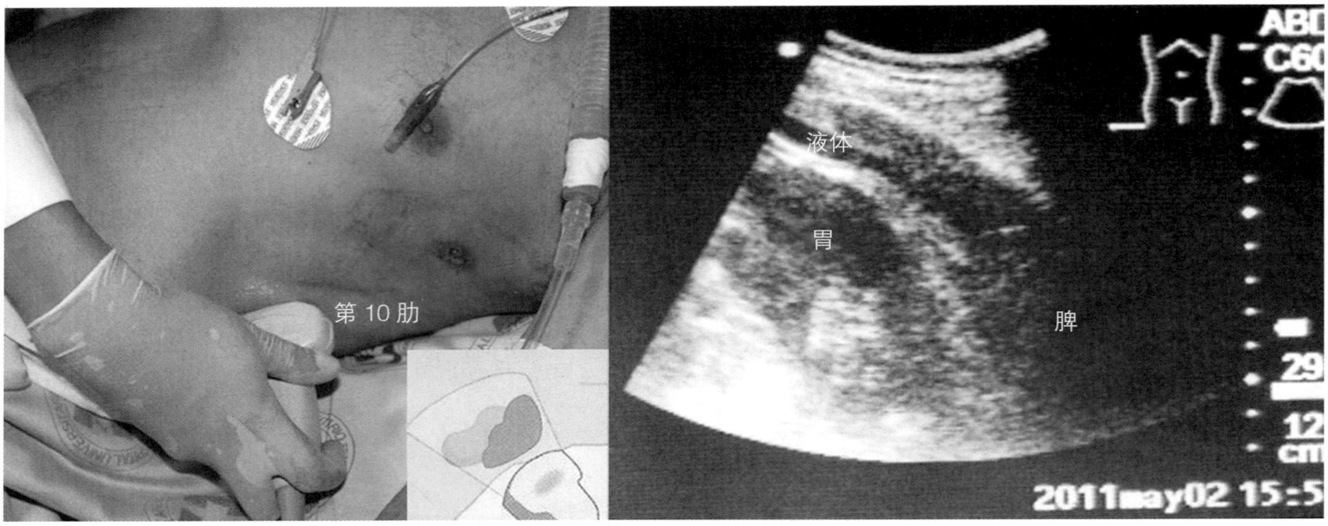

图 8 脾周窗。在左侧腋后线第 10 肋下识别脾和肾。该患者有贯通伤，在两个器官之间有自由液体。不正常视图

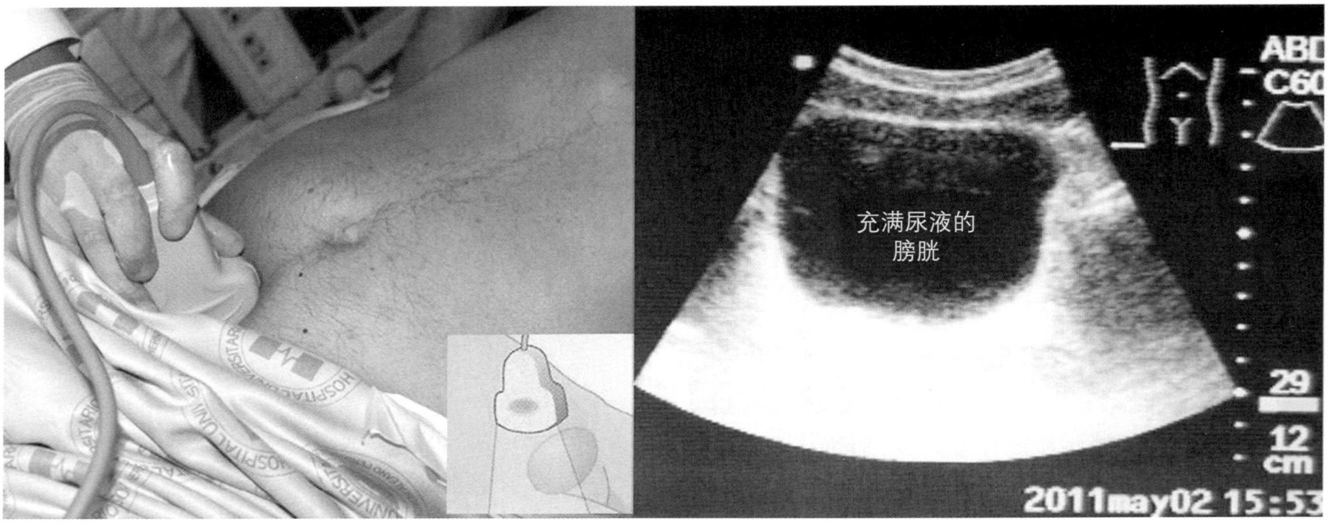

图 9 盆腔窗。在耻骨上方约 4 cm 识别膀胱。在器官周围没有自由液体。膀胱后方有增强高回声。正常视图和正常的人工制品（增强）与其后面较大的反射组织相比，液体的声波阻抗不足

患者复苏期间进行，并且避免有害辐射。此外，与当前确定的诊断方法相比，超声诊断气胸和血胸具有相当甚至更高的准确度。1997 年，Ma 和 Mateer 证实在使用超声检测创伤性血胸中具有与胸部 X 线片同等的精度，并且比 X 线片更为快捷。在对外伤性气胸的检查中，与仰卧位 X 线胸片相比，超声检查具有较好的灵敏度（21% vs. 49%；75.5% vs. 98%），并且具有与 CT 扫描同样的准确性。

E-FAST 技术

使用更高频率传感器（7.5 MHz）的超声可以发现气胸，因为涉及的可视化深度减少。当患者处于仰卧位时，将传感器放在腋中线的第 3 至第 4 肋水平，并在肋间的矢状面和横断面上缓慢地向中间和外侧移动换能器，以检查每一个血胸。检查肺胸膜，以评估是否存在“胸膜滑动”和“彗尾”伪影。正常的胸部检查应该常规包括这两项（图 11）。可采用实时运动模式评估“平流层征”。如果不存在空气，则

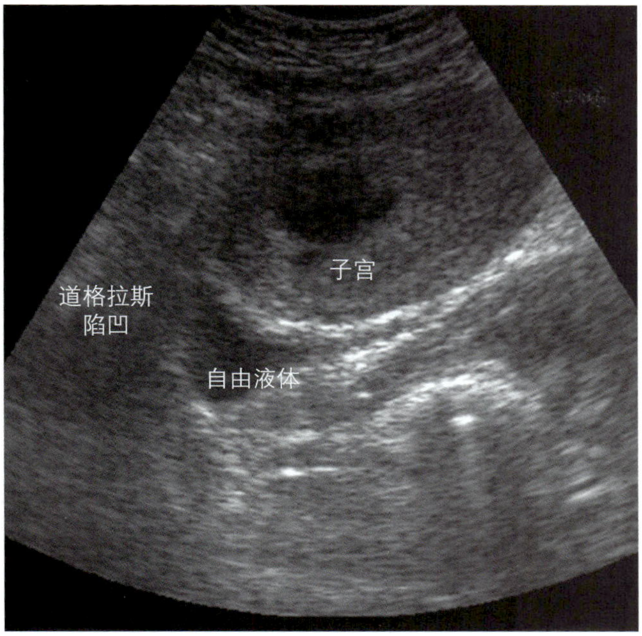

图 10　在盆腔视图上可见自由液体。在子宫周围道格拉斯陷凹内有自由液体。该视图中有一些流动的液体是正常的 (*Courtesy of M. Perdomo, USET Instructors Group.*)

可区别软组织图像（平流层线）与肺组织图像（沙滩沙线）之间的差异。如果存在空气，整个图像将显示没有沙滩沙线的"平流层"图（图 12）。

胸膜滑动提示在内脏和顶叶胸膜之间存在高回声线，代表这些层在整个吸气和呼气运动期间连续并列。存在气胸时，空气分离胸膜层，随后阻碍了超声波的传播，从而看不到内脏胸膜，并且不能看到胸膜滑动。当超声波在两个密切相关的组织界面之间混响时，可出现彗尾伪像，导致出现多个混响并形成明亮的垂直线，即"彗尾"。在正常的半侧胸腔，超声被肺组织强烈反射，因此，在脏胸膜深处可见高回声渐变的彗星尾巴。在存在气胸的情况下，超声波的传播受到胸膜空间内空气的阻碍，不显示该伪像。

FAST 算法

FAST 提供了一种快速、准确的手段，将创伤患者（通常在复苏室内）分类到手术室、CT 扫描室或血管造影室。FAST 在评估钝性腹部创伤患者时

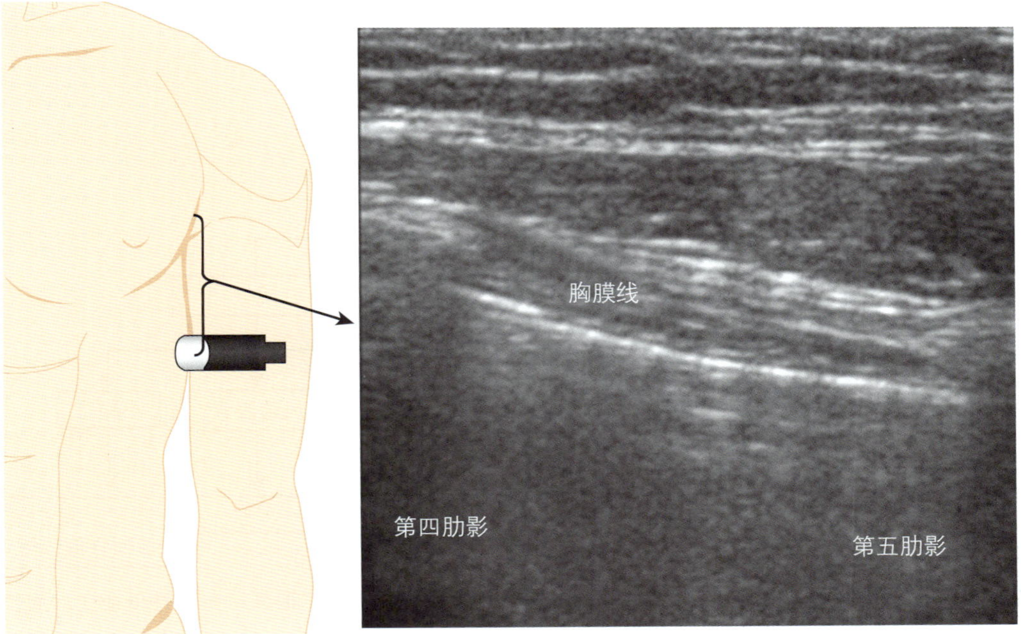

图 11　E-FAST。在第 4 肋和第 5 肋之间确定胸膜线。识别滑动运动，"彗尾"伪像为正常发现。该照片显示了正常的胸膜间隙 (*Photograph courtesy of M. Perdomo, USET Instructors Group.*)

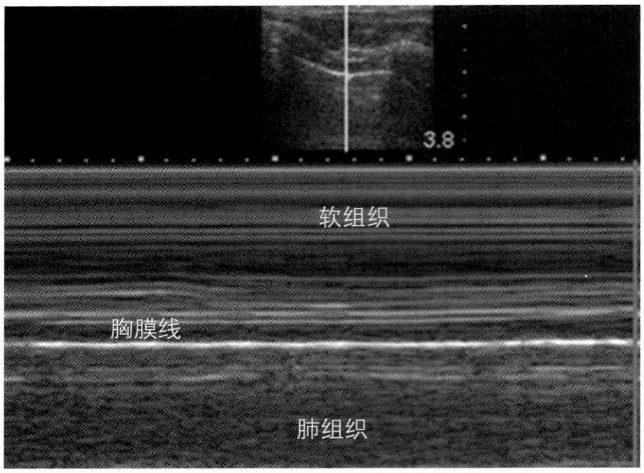

图12 E-FAST，M模式（使用的是运动模式）。在软组织（平流层线）和肺组织（海滩沙线）之间识别胸膜线。不存在空气。如果存在空气，整个图像将显示为软组织。该照片显示了正常的胸膜间隙（*Courtesy of M. Perdomo, USET Instructors Group.*）

尤其重要。在血流动力学稳定的钝性腹部创伤患者，如果FAST检查发现腹膜内液体，应进行CT扫描以查找出血的潜在来源。在血流动力学不稳定的钝性腹部创伤患者，FAST检查显示腹膜内液体通常提示有必要进行急诊剖腹术。虽然FAST在检测腹部内脏损伤时的灵敏度低于CT，但在不能安全或不适合进行CT的患者，它确实提供了一种快速、准确的评估不稳定患者的方法。作为快速分类创伤患者的手段，FAST的作用已经被几项研究所强调。这些研究表明，使用FAST与从急诊室到达手术室的时间显著减少相关（图13和14）。

FAST 评分系统

一些组织提出量化FAST系统，以根据液体量来识别具有手术指征的患者。Huang等开发了一个评分系统，在每个腹部区域，血液阳性计为1分，自由肠浮动计为1分。在肝周或脾周如有大于2 mm的液性暗区则计2分（表1）。他们发现，96%的3分以上的患者须要进行剖腹手术。然而，38%的评分小于3的患者仍然须要进行剖腹术。剖腹手术中积液大于1 L的灵敏度和特异性分别为84%和71%。

McKenney等开发了第二个评分系统。定义为最深的液性腔隙深度，加上发现液性区域的数量。他们发现85%的患者得分≥3分，只有15%的评分<3分的患者须要剖腹术。该评分系统的灵敏度、特异性和准确度分别为83%、87%和85%。这两个评分都比较有用，但仍然没有达成广泛的共识。

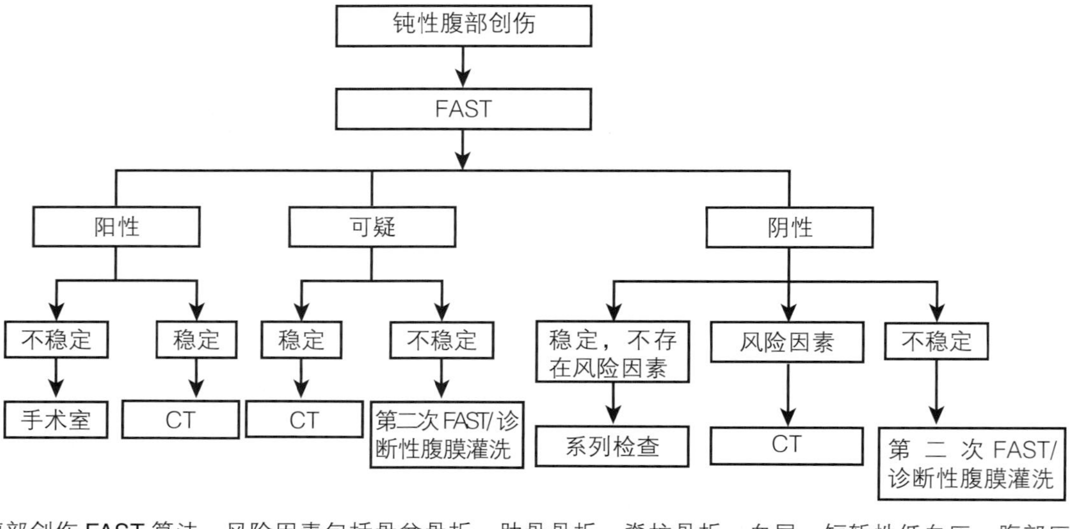

图13 钝腹部创伤FAST算法。风险因素包括骨盆骨折、肋骨骨折、脊柱骨折、血尿、短暂性低血压、腹部压痛、头部损伤、中毒和持续性碱缺失（*Dunhan M, McKenney M, Shatz D: The role of focused assessment with sonography for trauma: indications, limitations, and controversies. In Asensio JA, Trunkey DD, editors: Current therapy of trauma and surgical critical care. St. Louis, Mosby Elsevier, 2008, pp 121–135.*）

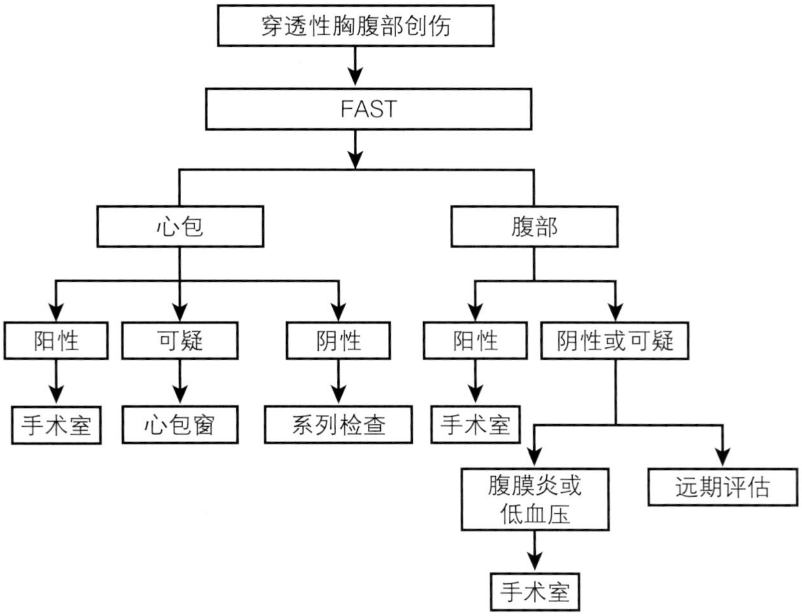

图 14　穿透性胸腹部创伤 FAST 算法 (*Dunhan M, McKenney M, Shatz D: The role of focused assessment with sonography for trauma: indications, limitations, and controversies. In Asensio JA, Trunkey DD, editors: Current therapy of trauma and surgical critical care. St. Louis, Mosby Elsevier, 2008, pp 121–135.*)

表 1　Huang FAST 评分系统

窗口	大小	评分 *
陷凹	>2 mm	2
	<2 mm	1
陷凹	>2 mm	2
	<2 mm	1
脾周影像		1
肝周影像		1
自由肠漂浮		2

Modified from Huang M, Liu M, Wu JK, et al: Ultrasonography for the evaluation of hemoperitoneum during resuscitation: a simple scoring system. J Trauma 36:173, 1994

*3 分或 3 分以上的患者中有 96% 的人须要剖腹手术

儿科 FAST

20 多年来，FAST 已被常规用于检查儿科创伤患者，用于发现腹腔内或心包腔内的液体，并根据血流动力学稳定性确定是否须要紧急手术。儿童 FAST 的表现与成年人相同。用于进行儿童检查的技术也与成人评估中使用的技术相同，只是通常使用 5 MHz 传感器来改善可视化。

儿童更适合采取 FAST 检查，因为他们的腹腔较小，并且获取的图像质量很少被脂肪或病态肥胖干扰，从而有别于成年人。FAST 也可以使儿童避免受到不必要的 CT 辐射诱发的恶性肿瘤相关风险。在青少年，每做 500 次 CT 检查就可出现 1 例致死性放射诱导的恶性肿瘤和 3 例非致死性恶性肿瘤。

在小儿钝性腹部创伤，FAST 的评估准确性与成人中的准确性相当。对 196 例儿科创伤患者开展的一项研究发现，FAST 具有 80% 的灵敏度和 100% 的特异性，并且显示 FAST 在 5.3% 的患者中为阳性，反映了在小儿腹腔出血的发病率较低。对 224 例血流动力学稳定和不稳定的儿科患者开展的 FAST 研究发现，灵敏度和特异性分别为 82% 的 95%，并且发现所有 7 例不稳定且 FAST 阳性的患者在紧急剖腹术后发现腹膜内损伤。在儿科患者中，剖腹探查术是例外情况，而不是常规对大多数 FAST 阳性的血流动力学稳定的患者随后进行 CT 检查或预期观察。在血流动力学不稳定的儿科创伤患者中，已证明阳性 FAST 与紧急剖腹探查术密切相关。

FASTER：小儿 FAST

除了在儿科创伤患者中评估腹膜内、心包和胸腔内的损伤外，还提倡采用超声检查肢端骨折。Dulchavsky 等建议将对骨折端的评估增加到 E-FAST 检查中，从而出现了另一个缩写，即 FASTER 检查。几项研究已经显示超声检查儿科患者长骨骨折的特异性超过 90%，在排除骨折时的敏感度为 78% ~ 97%。超声已被用于对伴有血管损伤的严重移位长骨骨折复位后的立即评估。与放射片或 CT 扫描不同，超声波不会使儿科患者暴露于有害辐射。另外，由于其便携性，可能会在院前环境中使用，以帮助迅速完成潜在的危及肢体损伤的紧急治疗。

FAST：事实和证据

培训

FAST 的准确性在很大程度上取决于操作人员的经验和能力。一个国际共识认为，操作经验对 FAST 的灵敏度和特异性很重要，建议操作员在获得认证之前开展 200 次监督下的扫描。相反，其他研究得出结论，仅进行 10 次监督下的检查后就能达到令人满意的准确性水平。这种观点强调 FAST 的认证应基于个人开展技能的能力而不是开展的次数。目前，关于临床医师在获得检查前须要开展的监督下的 FAST 检查的次数尚未达成共识。国际共识认为需开展 50 ~ 200 次监督下的 FAST 检查，以达到适当的专业水平。在我们自己的经验中，通过泛美创伤学会课程，包括创伤和急诊室超声（USET）在内的拉丁美洲国家的居民和小学和专业医师（包括 9 个以上国家的近 600 名学员）一个 8 h 的理论课程，我们建议受训人员在没有独立扫描前进行 50 次的监督下的扫描。我们鼓励发展中国家的卫生机构根据当地的资源，并根据国际协商一致的地方议会或科学协会认证培训水平，以适当的方式制定指导方针。世界超声协商会议（World Consensus Conference on Ultrasound）FAST 委员会是一个不同专业的国际专家小组。1997 年，其建议开展为期 1 天的培训课程，包括 4 h 教学部分、4 h 实践部分和 200 个监督下的扫描。

Thomas 等开展的一项有趣研究显示了研究的数量如何提高灵敏度，并最大限度地缩短开展技术所需的时间（表 2）（图 15 和 16）。

与没有使用 FAST 的组相比，已证明使用 FAST 作为快速分析工具具有显著的益处。Melniker 等发现与接受标准创伤护理的患者相比，FAST 的使用与持续时间缩短有关，直到在须要开展外伤创伤手术的患者中进行手术护理（57 min vs 166 min）。该研究还显示，FAST 组患者的住院时间（6 天 vs 10.2 天）缩短，使用的资源减少（10 600 vs 16 400），需要 CT 扫描的概率降低（53% vs 85 %）。Rose 等也证实了 FAST 检查后 CT 使用的减少。其对 208 名患

表 2　医生队伍中 FAST 检查的准确性

检查的准确性	腹腔积血 (%)	手术需要 (%)
敏感度	81.0	73.9
特异性	99.3	99.3
阳性预测值	89.5	89.5
预测价值	98.0	97.9
最终准确性	98.0	97.3

Modified from Thomas B, Falcone RE, Vasquez D, et al: Ultrasound evaluation of blunt abdominal trauma: program implementation, initial experience and learning curve. J Trauma 42:384-390, 1997

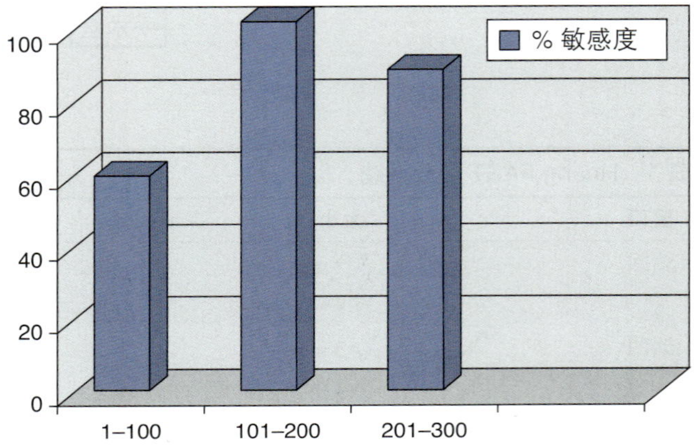

图 15　根据研究次数评估 FAST 的敏感度曲线。经过 100 次研究后获得了最佳的敏感度，并在 200 次检查后稍微降低

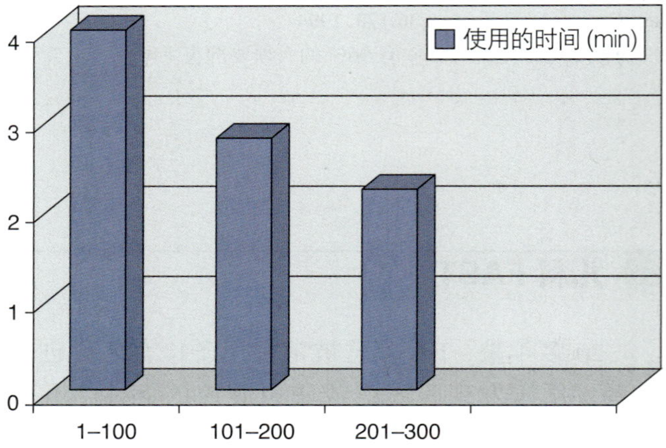

图 16　FAST 的时间。100 次研究后，时间开始减少，在 200 次检查后达到最佳表现

者开展的随机对照试验显示，FAST 组中有 36% 的患者接受 CT 治疗，而标准创伤护理组为 52%。

2008 年，一项 Cochrane 系统评估根据对钝性腹膜创伤的诊断和治疗的影响分析了紧急超声，显示在 FAST 评估的患者组中 CT 扫描的使用减少了 50%。尽管如此，报告的总体结论是，在随机临床试验中没有足够的证据支持基于超声的临床路径用于诊断钝性腹膜创伤患者。因此，目前尽管提供了一种安全、无创、快速和容易重复的准确评估和分类创伤患者的手段，但仍然须要进行更多的大规模研究来评估 FAST 在创伤患者治疗中的重要性。

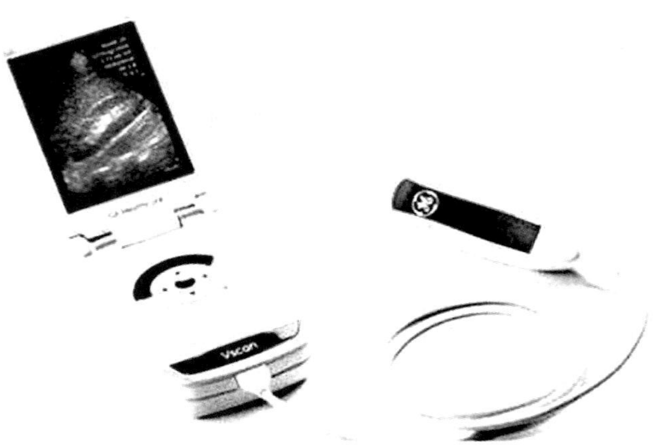

图 17　通用电动 V 扫描手持式超声波。可将这种小型装置用于超声心检查的重点评估，在几英里外无线传播创伤信息。图像的分辨率对于远程协助来说尚可 (*Courtesy of General Electric Company.*)

FAST 的前景

虽然关于 FAST 技术的未来仍然存在很多争议，但是新的研究侧重于便携式设备对院前急救人员的作用和下述情况的优势，如大量伤亡的检伤分类、严酷的环境（战区）以及新入院患者（图 17）。最近对 FAST 在院前护理中应用的系统评估显示了该技术的益处，但是在该领域缺乏研究。在将手持设备和便携式设备用于伊拉克战争之前，人们也进行了少量研究。执行检查的非医疗院内人员使用无线设备将图像发送给急诊内科医师，并由急诊科医师决定如何对扫描的患者进行检伤分类。

最近已发表了关于使用静脉超声造影剂来增强超声成像在实体器官损伤评估方面的研究。造影增强超声成像的诊断测试性能可能接近于腹部 CT 扫描对腹部创伤中实体器官损伤的灵敏度和特异性。如果 CT 扫描放射性恶性肿瘤带来的风险在将来变得不可接受，那么避免不必要的 CT 扫描的方法将成为关注焦点。已经存在将超声与儿科创伤腹部 CT 扫描相结合的临床决策规则中的研究。

FAST 中的要点

- 腹腔游离液体不代表一定是血液。游离液体也可能来自破裂的卵巢囊肿、腹水或破裂的膀胱。这些可能是造成 FAST 检查假阳性结果的来源。
- 即使 FAST 检查为阴性，也可能存在腹内损伤。超声检查可能无法检测到有轻微出血的实体器官、肠道和膈肌损伤。
- 只有在气胸位于探头下方时才能通过胸腔超声检测到气胸（缺少肺部滑动）。可能须要检查胸壁上的多个部位，特别是锁骨上窝，以便在肺顶点，特别是直坐的患者中观察小气道。
- 在骨的末端或近关节部位检测骨折时，由于轮廓弯曲和不规则而使检测较为困难，因而导致诊断的准确性降低。与对侧正常肢体相对比有助于区分正常与异常。

放射学在创伤的初步评估中的作用

Kim M. Caban, Gary H. Danton, Anthony M. Durso, Felipa Munera, Luis A. Rivas 著
易成腊 译

过去十年关于放射学使用的研究在急诊室和创伤情况下大大增加，包括X线、荧光透视、超声、CT和MRI。使用CT的主要问题是费用和辐射剂量，1996－2007年期间CT的使用增加了330%，其中急诊科占全部CT扫描的1/3。在此期间，急诊室护理总人数的增加只有30%。卫生保健系统的大量成本和患者安全问题源自对成像资源的过度利用。安全问题包括理论上暴露于辐射的患者发生癌症的风险，造影剂引起的肾衰竭或过敏反应的风险，以及MRI造影剂造成的肾源性全身性纤维化。虽然诊断的益处往往超过了这些风险可能的坏处，但全国各地的放射科医师报告在对有问题的适应证进行检查时出现的阴性结果过多。虽然医疗法律问题经常是进行成像的原因，但在不太遥远的将来，可能会对进行过度辐射检查的医师提出诉讼。尽管有这些担忧，成像仍将是创伤医师诊断手段中的重要工具。确定对某一种特定适应证最佳研究须要了解每种模式的用途和风险，以及了解预测试概率和证据是如何影响诊断决策的。

X线片

普通放射片（也称为平片或“X线”）是通过电离辐射（是潜在致癌的原因）在组织的相对密度基础上产生图像。金属（密度最高）呈现的颜色最白，空气（密度最低）呈黑色，其他所有的组织介于两者之间。平片的空间分辨率极佳，并且有便携式器械，对患者的转移要求最低。在CT普及之前，X线片是对肌肉骨骼损伤和胸部评估最可靠的检查。它仍然常被用于创伤患者，以快速评估胸部、骨盆和四肢。

胸部和骨盆的初始放射片可用做快速筛查工具，以评估创伤性损伤的程度，尽管如果患者的位置不是最佳的，则对软组织和骨骼损伤检查的敏感度最多视为低度或中度。灵敏度还部分取决于射线片的质量（图1）。上覆的结构（如背板和心电图线）限制了对软组织的评估，并掩盖了可能存在小气孔的肺顶点。因为肺容积通常较低，所以心脏和纵隔通常显得较宽或扩大。很难发现提示主动脉损伤（如椎旁条纹增厚或遮蔽）的微小表现。由于在呼吸的呼气阶段在仰卧位患者中常见肺不张，心后组织可能会遮挡降主动脉和左隔膜。外侧肋骨骨折尤其容易被忽视。骨盆X线片也可能会遗漏微小的损伤，通过身体检查证明骨盆创伤是解决这些检查相对于预测试概率的关键（图2）。

荧光透视法与X线平片方式相似，都是使用X线，但是通常会使用造影剂并实时观察图像。在荧光检查期间产生的放射剂量通常小于常规放射片。然而，由于在标准步骤中包括多次荧光透视，因而累积辐射剂量可以迅速增加。诊断性荧光检查程序可用于评估空腔脏器或任何可以使用造影剂的结构。其图像是一个管腔图，可用于识别肠泄漏（图3）、膀胱泄漏或血管造影时的外渗。骨外科医师经常使用荧光透视来检查骨骼。使用荧光检查的手术者应穿铅衣、甲状腺防护装置和并佩戴放射徽章。

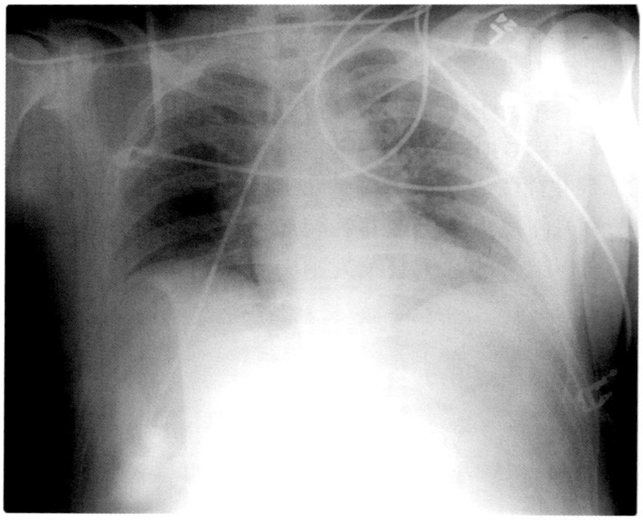

图1　创伤患者的典型胸片显示在评估胸部时灵敏度有限的特征。除了陈旧性锁骨骨折外，该患者的胸部正常。肺容积低，从而使肺显得模糊。可以将其认为是挫伤的假阳性表现。背板和上覆线掩盖了骨骼和胸部的部分，改变了正常的密度。由于处于仰卧位且体积小，心脏和纵隔显得较宽。这些对于这种检查方法而言是正常的，但可能导致漏诊纵隔损伤

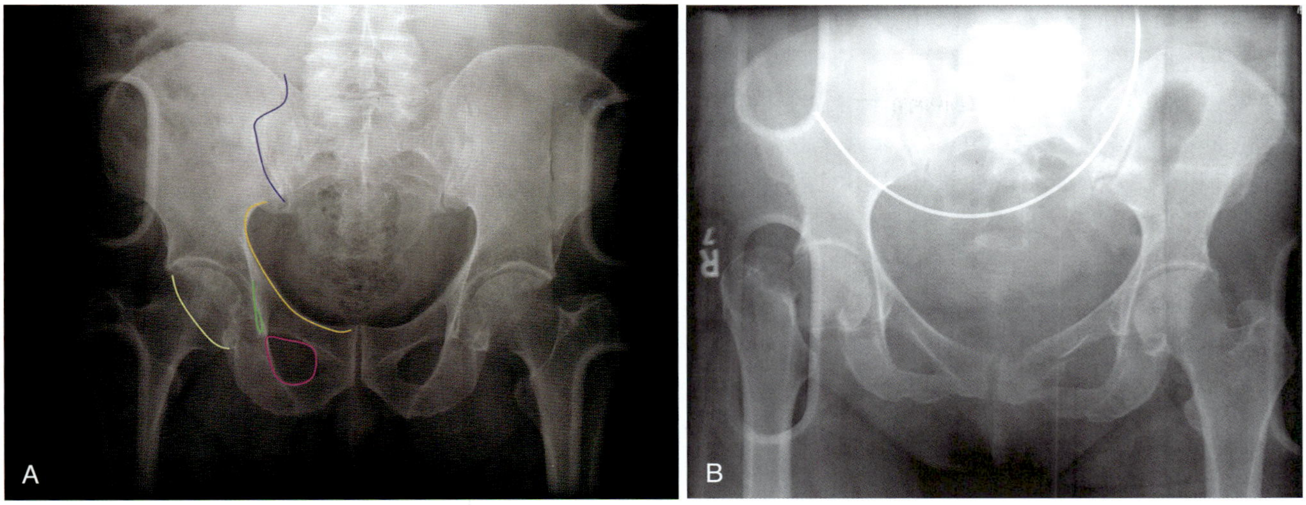

图2 两个不同患者的正常（**A**）和骨折（**B**）骨盆的放射片。在两张X线片中，背板干扰了图像质量，降低了骨折检查的灵敏度。在图A中，沿着左髂骨走行的黑线是一件人造物。在阅读这些有限制的检查时医师应该谨慎。至少应该看到以下几条线，并确保它们是光滑和规则的：反映前柱的髂耻线（橙色），骶髂关节（蓝色），评估耻骨的闭孔环（粉红色），反映内侧髋臼壁、髋臼切迹和四边体前部的泪滴（绿色），以及髋臼后缘（黄色）。图B显示了右股骨颈、耻骨右下支、左上左下支和左耻骨的骨折。左侧的骶髂关节略宽

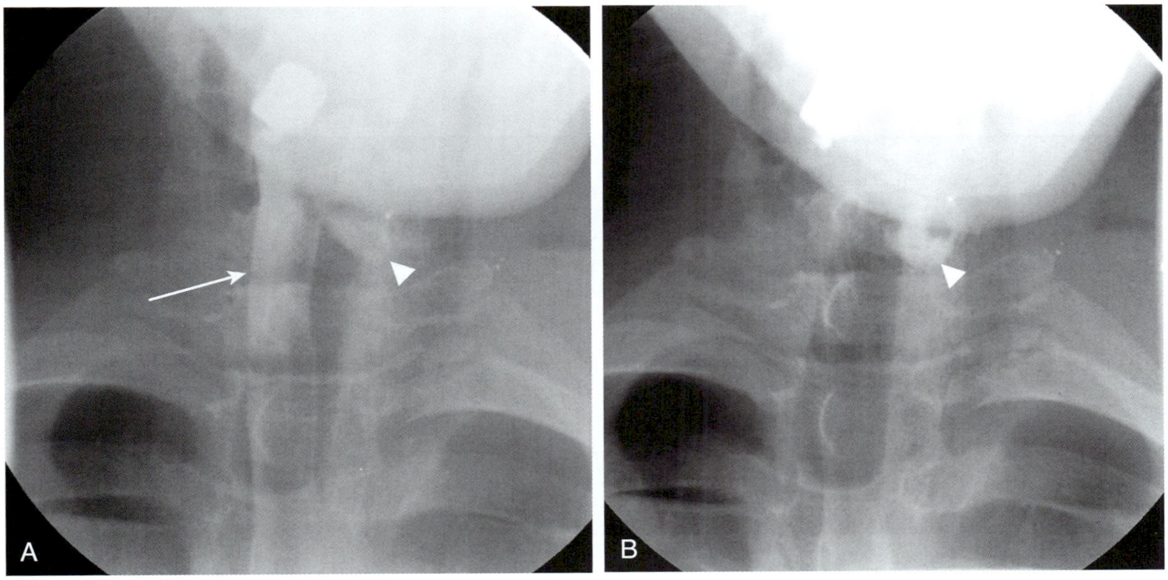

图3 吞咽造影剂期间（**A**）和之后（**B**）的食管造影图。在图**A**中，在食管（箭头）中可看到造影剂柱，并且造影剂有少量外漏（箭头）。清理食管后，造影剂仍然存在（**B**），提示已经泄漏。在枪伤情景下可见到金属弹片，这最有可能是创伤后的

超声

超声通过传感器产生声波。声波传入身体并被能够反射声波的组织反射。反射的声波返回并由传感器检测。知道返回到传感器的声音多少以及声波持续时间后，计算机就可以计算组织的深度和相对亮度。因此，其图像不是密度图，相反，其图像是基于各种组织反射声音的能力。因此，明亮的物质被称为回声或反射回声（许多回声），比周围组织更深的物质属于低回声（较少回声），而完全黑色的消息则是无回声。因为水可以传导声音，所以看起来很黑，因为没有声波被反射出来。相比之下，空气是强烈的声波反射物质，所以大部分声波被反射到换能器。因此，空气以“脏阴影”或其下方的模糊外

观表现出白线，掩盖了比空气深的组织的特征。有时放射学技术专家会说，胰腺这样的结构是因“气体遮挡”造成的，意味着肠道的气体遮盖了这种结构。如果气体影响了检查，可以要求患者喝水，使水充满胃和十二指肠，则能更好地显示上腹部结构的图像。当结构被气体或骨骼遮挡时，则认为患者具有“不良窗口”，并且喝水后可以改善这些“窗口”（图 4）。

超声具有优异的时间分辨率，并可以得到身体的实时成像，特别适用于在创伤环境下检测液体或液体的特征，如腹腔积液。超声也适用于检测实体器官的损伤，通过多普勒技术确认脉管系统的通畅性。重要的是，由于超声使用声波，因而没有电离辐射。因为通常在创伤情况下不会使用超声造影剂，所以不会有发生造影剂反应或过敏反应的风险，因而超声的安全性极好。然而，在检测实体器官损伤等时超声的敏感性低于其他方式，如 CT。

CT

由于可用性的提高和获取图像所需的时间较短，CT 已经成为创伤下的常用检查手段。CT 使用的是 X 线。这是其具有潜在致癌的电离辐射。通过使用各种投影来测量身体中特定位点的 X 线的衰减，计算机根据 Hounsfield 标准为该区域分配值，其中水被分配为 0，空气被分配为 –1000。然后将所有其他密度分配为反映其相对密度的 HU 值（图 5）。CT 具有优异的空间分辨率和良好的对比度分辨率。CT 的空间分辨率是指区分间隔极短的两条线的能力。空间分辨率使检查者能够看到较小的结构。CT 的对比度分辨率是指区分密度变化较低的两个相邻组织的能力。CT 检查肝挫伤的能力非常依赖于对比度分辨率和图像噪声。对检查者而言，嘈杂的图像看来为颗粒状，并且可以通过降低对比度分辨率来掩盖发

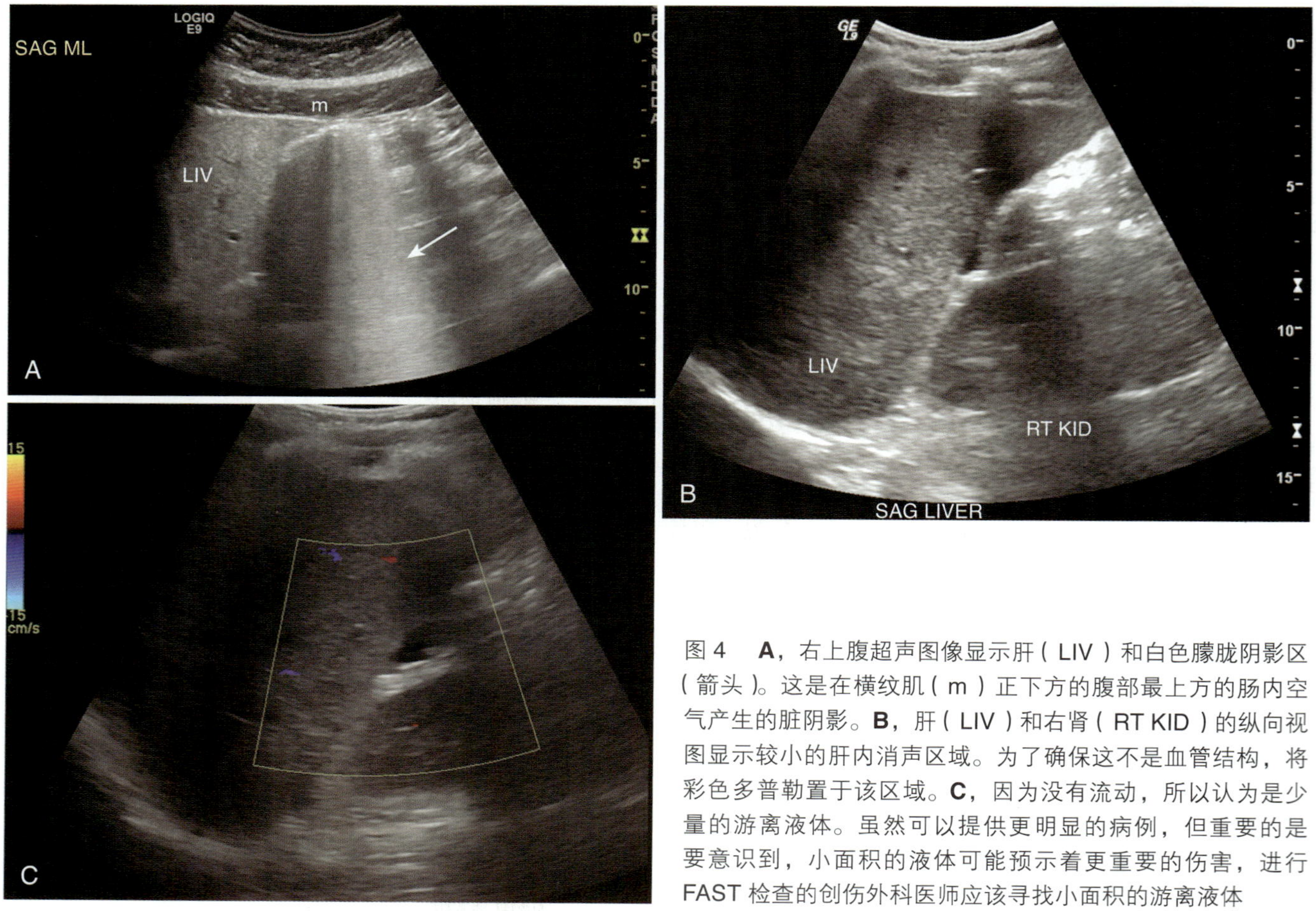

图 4　**A**，右上腹超声图像显示肝（LIV）和白色朦胧阴影区（箭头）。这是在横纹肌（m）正下方的腹部最上方的肠内空气产生的脏阴影。**B**，肝（LIV）和右肾（RT KID）的纵向视图显示较小的肝内消声区域。为了确保这不是血管结构，将彩色多普勒置于该区域。**C**，因为没有流动，所以认为是少量的游离液体。虽然可以提供更明显的病例，但重要的是要意识到，小面积的液体可能预示着更重要的伤害，进行 FAST 检查的创伤外科医师应该寻找小面积的游离液体

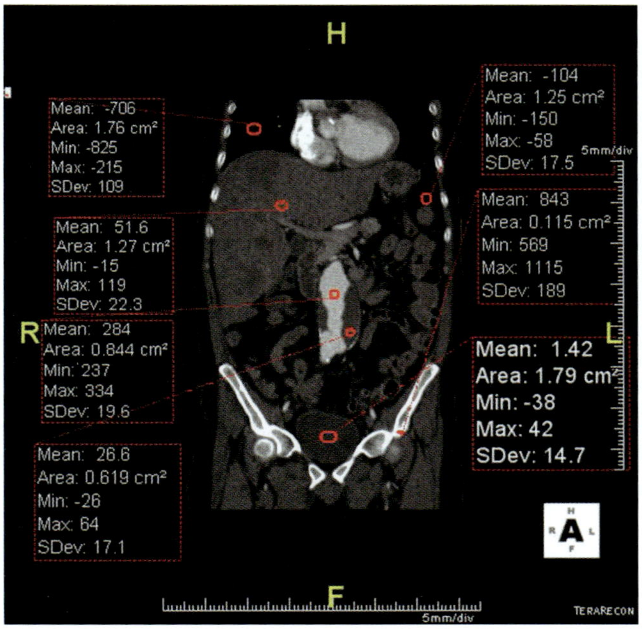

图 5　腹部和骨盆的冠状视图显示圆圈组织的 Hounsfield 单位（HU）不同。注意，是基于圆圈区域中的所有像素计算平均 HU 值，并计算最小值、最大值和标准偏差。该患者的平均 HU 值如下：肺 706，肝 51.6，增强主动脉 284，主动脉血栓 26.6，脂肪 104，皮质骨 843，尿 1.42

现。通常，使用的辐射剂量越多，噪声越小，整体图像质量就越好。提高对比度分辨率的另一种方法是静脉注射 CT 造影剂。用于 CT 的静脉造影剂由碘化分子组成，其能够衰减 X 线并且在图像上表现得很明亮。

静脉注射造影剂反映了组织的血管分布或组织内的病理特征。造影剂显示的时间很重要，因为对比度的不同阶段影响了图像中可以看到的内容。这很重要，因为它解释了为什么放射科医师必须多次扫描患者，以及让放射科医师在进行检查之前就明确扫描的目的。注射造影剂后 15 ~ 30 s 获得动脉期，取决于正在扫描身体的哪一部分以及 CT 扫描仪的快速程度。在动脉期获得的 CT 扫描称为 CT 血管造影或 CTA。动脉期仅显示动脉供血，对于造影剂未达到的组织背景，观察到腔外对比（活动性外渗）是能确诊的征象（图 6）。不幸的是，有时难以确定在图像上看到的特定对比线是小血管的一部分还是造影剂外渗。为此，须要获取更延迟的对比图像。在动脉期观察脾实质也特别困难，因为变异的血液供应导致可能被误认为是脾损伤的混合模式图像。

"门静脉"期通常在注射造影剂后 60 ~ 75 s 获得。在此期间，应优化增强门静脉以及包括肝、肾、胰和脾在内的实体器官，以评估实质。这是检查微小的挫伤或裂伤的理想方法。但是由于固体器官的实质增强，动脉仍然增强，因而可能难以评估外渗。在这个阶段，大静脉也增强，可能会发现静脉损伤。延迟期在造影剂注射后 5 min 获得，最适合评估肾集合系统和膀胱，因为它们会发生造影剂填充。5 min 后，实体器官的大部分实质增强消失。由于在延迟检查期间动脉确实没有增强，所以外渗对比度比在动脉期观察到的外渗对比度更大，将会显现为更广泛的对比度增强（腮红）面积。通过将延迟期或甚至是门静脉期与动脉期比较，可以诊断活动性外渗。获得多个对比度的不利之处在于放射剂量可达到 2 倍或 3 倍。为了减少获得不必要的扫描的可能性，放射科医师可以在延迟阶段之前查看图像，然后决定是否须要附加的相位。

CT 技术在过去 15 年中发生了巨大变化。传统的 CT 扫描仪获得了一个给定厚度的图像（切片）。获取图像后，台面将患者移动到下一个位置，并获得另一个图像。这被称为移动和拍摄。由于各种原因，重建图像受到限制，扫描速度相对较慢。使用螺旋或螺旋 CT，当台架围绕患者旋转时，桌子以整个图像采集的速度移动。软件将图像重建成可在任何平面中重建的体积数据集。多检测计算机断层扫描（multidetector computed tomography，MDCT）使用多行检测器来扫描身体的每个旋转的更宽的区域。因为扫描覆盖较大的区域，所以台面速度可以增加，总时间减少。这在创伤情况下特别有帮助，因为精神状态改变的患者可能不能保持静止，运动降低了图像质量，而使诊断困难。在对检查期间试图站在 CT 检查台上的儿童进行扫描时，一些最新和最快的方式已经获得了诊断图像。所有新的 CT 单元都是 MDCT，检测器行数为 64、128 和 320，得出具有革命性的 CT 成像。

CT 图像处理

随着螺旋 CT 和各向同性数据集的出现（每个体素或图像的一部分构成等边的立方体），可将图像重建成任何平面。通过改变分配特定浓度的颜色或亮度，可以生成各种图像。通过将颜色分配给体积数据集中的各种密度来生成三维（3D）图像。最大强度投影（maximum intensity projected，MIP）图像强调高密度结构，如对比度增强的血管和骨骼。低密度结构被抑制。MIP 图像对于评估创伤患者的动脉

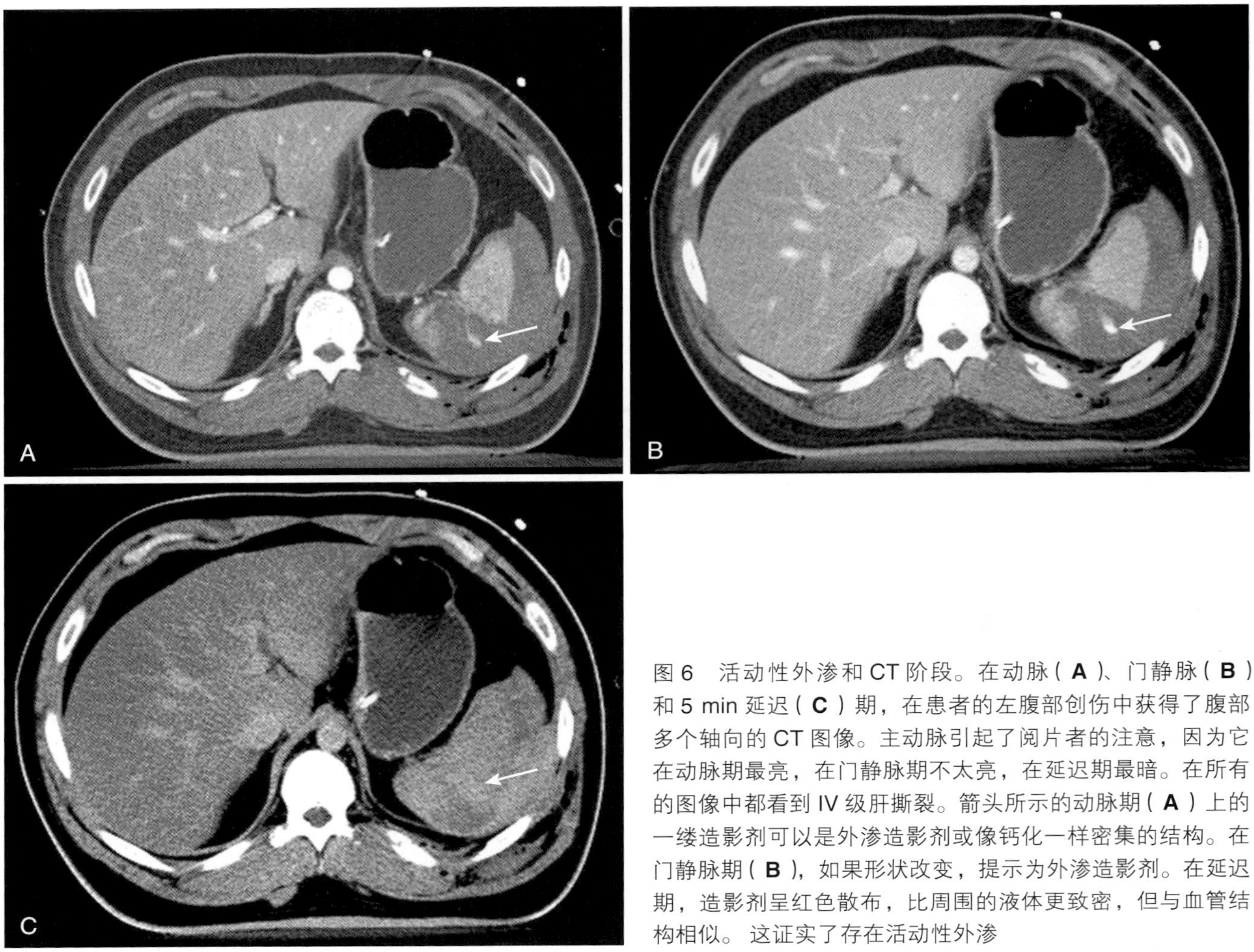

图 6　活动性外渗和 CT 阶段。在动脉（**A**）、门静脉（**B**）和 5 min 延迟（**C**）期，在患者的左腹部创伤中获得了腹部多个轴向的 CT 图像。主动脉引起了阅片者的注意，因为它在动脉期最亮，在门静脉期不太亮，在延迟期最暗。在所有的图像中都看到 IV 级肝撕裂。箭头所示的动脉期（**A**）上的一缕造影剂可以是外渗造影剂或像钙化一样密集的结构。在门静脉期（**B**），如果形状改变，提示为外渗造影剂。在延迟期，造影剂呈红色散布，比周围的液体更致密，但与血管结构相似。这证实了存在活动性外渗

非常有用。这些图像处理技术有助于显示损伤、解剖学和异物之间的空间关系（图 7）。

MRI

因为其他专业的过度使用和有限的可用性，MRI 在早期创伤情况中的用途有限。获取图像需要相当较长的时间，且患者体内必须没有金属异物。MRI 具有优异的对比度分辨率，但 CT 的空间分辨率更高。CT 能够提供大部分诊断，这对稳定患者的病情至关重要。可以通过 MRI 改善对脊髓的详细评估或微小弥漫性轴索损伤（diffuse axonal injury，DAI）的评估。

碘制剂过敏的管理

如果已知患者有对碘化造影剂的严重变态反应，则可以在不使用静脉注射造影剂的情况下进行 CT 检查，尽管对血管、实体器官和空腔脏器损伤的评估将受到显著限制。另一个选择是预先给予患者糖皮质激素和苯海拉明。然而，在签署同意书之后，最快也需要 6 h 的准备时间。只有在报告有对静脉注射造影剂有轻微反应，存在中度至重度哮喘病史，对一种物质存在严重反应，或对多种已知食物、药物或其他物质过敏的患者中，才进行预处理后的静脉注射造影剂给药。与以前的观点相反，研究表明，

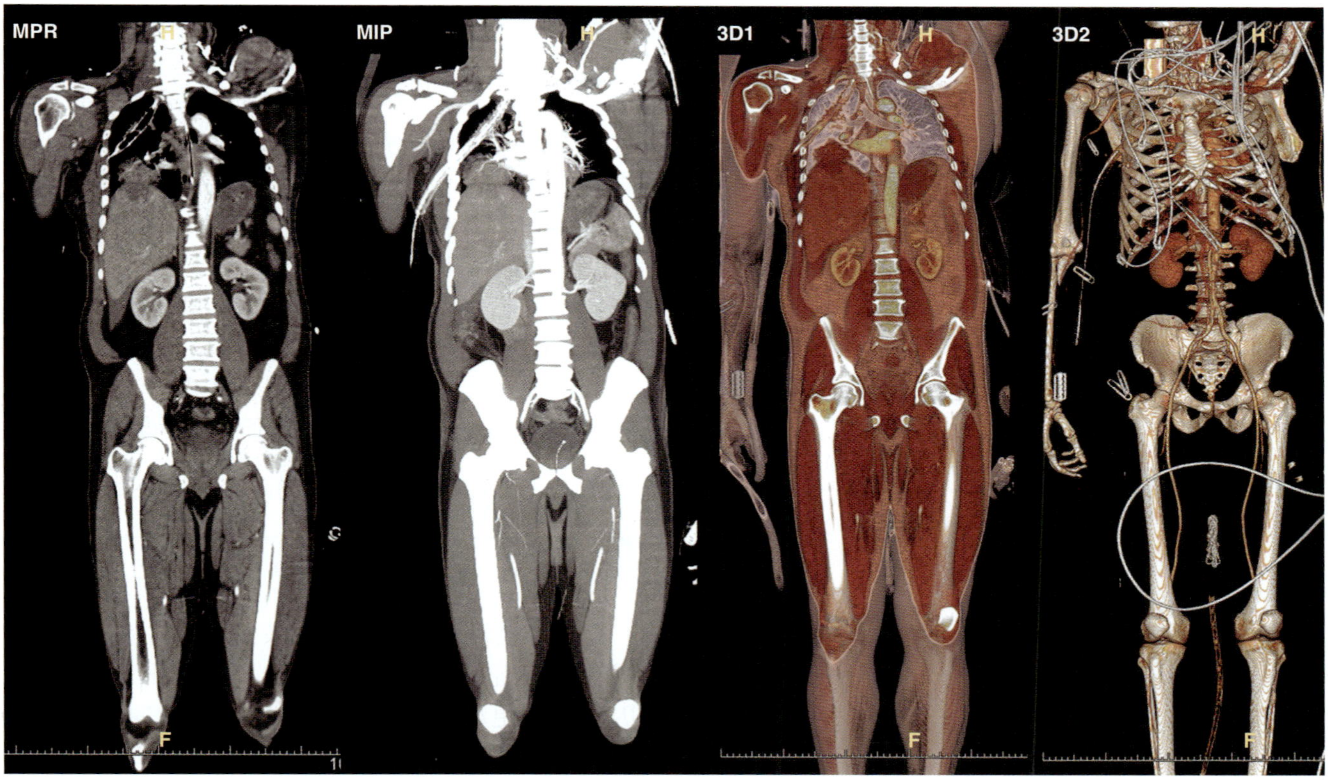

图 7 多探头计算机断层扫描：创伤患者的冠状图像，在横膈受到枪击损伤后有肝撕裂。这些图像是在标准轴向平面上获得的。但由于它们具有各向同性，所以它们被重构成冠状平面。多平面重新格式（MPR）是典型的计算机断层摄影图像，具有 1.5 mm 的切片厚度，灰度显示在软组织窗口上。肝穹窿和肝边界以下的撕裂容易被发现。该实例的最大强度投影（maximum intensity projection，MIP）图像具有 90 mm 的组织切片厚度，并且显示像骨骼一样的更高密度结构，对比度增强的血管，比低密度结构更亮的肾。通过将颜色代替灰度分配给 90 mm 厚度的组织（3D1），或查看整个组织的整个厚度（3D2），可以创建三维体积渲染。在 3D2 中，软组织没有颜色，因此这些结构不包括在图像中

对贝类有过敏病史的患者不会对造影剂产生反应。如果有暴露于静脉注射造影剂后过敏反应或支气管痉挛史，则不应给予药物。对于采用慢性糖皮质激素治疗的患者，对任何一种物质都有严重过敏反应的患者，以及严重过敏者，都应慎重使用造影剂。请注意，即使进行过预处理，患者仍可能对静脉注射造影剂产生不利的影响。目前没有根据情况的预处理协议。表 1 和表 2 列出了广泛接受的预处理协议。

颅骨和脑

创伤性脑损伤（TBI）的患者有显著的发病率和死亡风险。脑的 CT 平扫评估是常规检查，应该是排除 TBI 的第一步。检查的候选者包括存在意识丧失、精神状态改变、神经功能缺陷、中毒、Battle 征（乳突瘀斑）、液体或血性渗出，以及疑似脑脊液漏和面部创伤。

蛛网膜下腔出血表现为大脑脚间池的高密度外轴波形影，脑沟和小脑叶中的局灶性高密度影，以及沿着半球体裂缝或沿着透壁的高密度影（图 8）。急性硬膜下出血通常表现为外轴新月形密度影，但也可能呈现沿小脑幕的血液层或半球裂隙间的致密厚层。急性硬膜外出血呈斑状或凸形的轴外密度影，通常有邻近颅骨骨折。出血性皮质挫伤表现为大脑皮质内的高密度灶。白质束的 DAI 很难诊断。在识别这些病变时，MRI 比 CT 更敏感，因此应首选 MRI。MRI 梯度回波序列和扩散张量成像是识别这些病变的最佳序列。在 MRI 上，白质区可见 1 ~ 15 mm 水肿或出血灶。DAI 显示为出血灶（高密度），可能出现在 CT 上的灰白色物质交界处、胼胝体内、丘脑、大脑脚和基底神经节内。DAI 是创伤患者持续无意识和植物状态以及持续性神经损伤的主要原因。在

表 1　标准预处理方案

药物	剂量	给药
泼尼松	50 mg PO	在 IV造影剂给药前 13 h、7 h和 1 h 施用
甲泼尼龙	32 mg PO	在 IV 造影剂给药前 12 h 和 2 h 施用
氢化可的松	200 mg IV	在 IV造影剂给药前 13 h、7 h和 1 h 施用
苯海拉明	50 mg PO，IV，or IM	在 IV 造影剂给药前 1h 施用

IM，肌内注射；IV，静脉注射；PO，口服

表 2　紧急预处理协议

药物	剂量	给药
氢化可的松	200 mg IV	在 IV 造影剂给药前 6 h 施用
苯海拉明	50 mg IV	在 IV 造影剂给药前 1 h 施用

持续昏迷和阴性 CT 的患者中，应进行 MRI 检查以评估 DAI。

头部和颈部的穿透性损伤和钝性创伤都可能导致血管损伤。如果存在血管闭塞、切割、横断、血管外渗或颈动脉海绵窦瘘的可能（图 9），则应进行头颈部的 CTA 检查。CTA 应该在非增强脑 CT 后进行，因为造影剂通常会掩盖出血（图 8B）。

如果患者出现颅底损伤迹象，则应进行专门的颞骨 CT 检查。通过颞骨获得轴向 1 ~ 2 mm 剖面 CT 图像。对矢状和冠状图像应重新格式化，以帮助检查微小的非移位骨折，并评估损伤的程度和路径。

脊柱

传统上，脊柱的 X 线片被用于评估骨折和韧带损伤。随着 CT 的出现，X 线片的使用已经减少，因为人们更好地意识到了常规 X 线片的限制。CT 不仅速度更快，而且被证明在脊柱损伤评估中更为准确。脊柱现在被常规地纳入全身 CT 协议。矢状面和冠状面重新格式化的图像有助于评估脊柱损伤（图 10）。MRI 仍然是评估韧带损伤、脊髓损伤和硬膜外血肿的最佳方式。

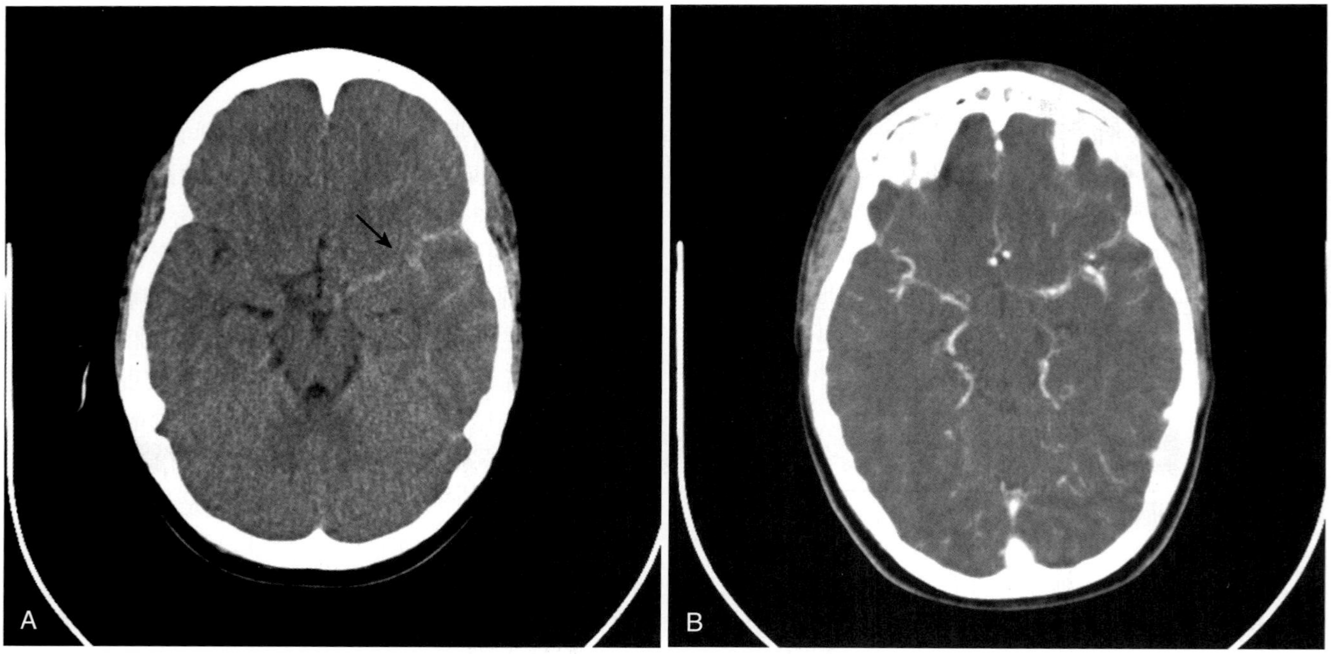

图 8　**A**，大脑的非对比 CT 检查，显示左侧大脑侧裂和颞叶蛛网膜下腔出血（箭头）。**B**，同一患者的脑 CT 图像。注意造影剂是如何掩盖蛛网膜下腔出血的

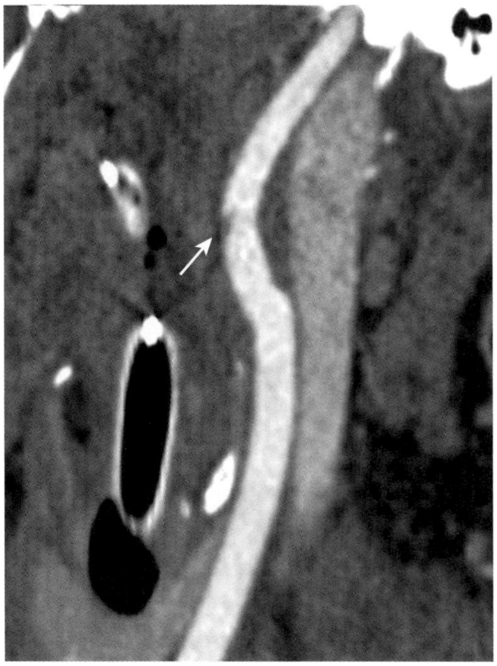

图 9　颈内动脉的 CTA 冠状重建图像显示内膜瓣（箭头）

面部

任何有面部创伤、磨损、肿胀、严重畸形和裂伤的患者都应接受面部 CT 检查。冠状面和矢状面的面部重建图像有助于诊断微小和非移位的骨折。3D 图像也被证明对手术计划有益。面部 CT 检查可以识别眼球的损伤、眼球后血肿、眶外血肿、肌肉夹带和异物的存在。

血管损伤

CTA 已经取代数字减影血管造影（DSA）用以识别血管损伤（图 11）。CT 对患者的风险最小，可以快速识别出血区域。通过利用多相成像，CT 不仅可以识别出血的位置，而且可以鉴别其严重程度，并且可以区分动脉出血与静脉出血。因此，CTA 被用于指导患者治疗，无论是观察、经导管栓塞、其他血管内治疗，还是外科手术。研究表明，多达 40% 的骨盆骨折患者有潜在的活动性出血，20% 的患者须要经导管栓塞。

损伤血管可能导致闭塞、假性动脉瘤形成、动静脉瘘（arteriovenous fistula，AVF）形成、内膜损伤、切割、痉挛、活动性出血和横断。闭塞可能由直接钝性损伤、痉挛或栓塞引起。闭塞表现为血管的突然中断。可以通过伴行或分支血管重建损伤血管（图 12）。内膜损伤或切割在血管腔内表现为偏心的填充缺损（图 13）。AVF 表现为静脉的早期造影

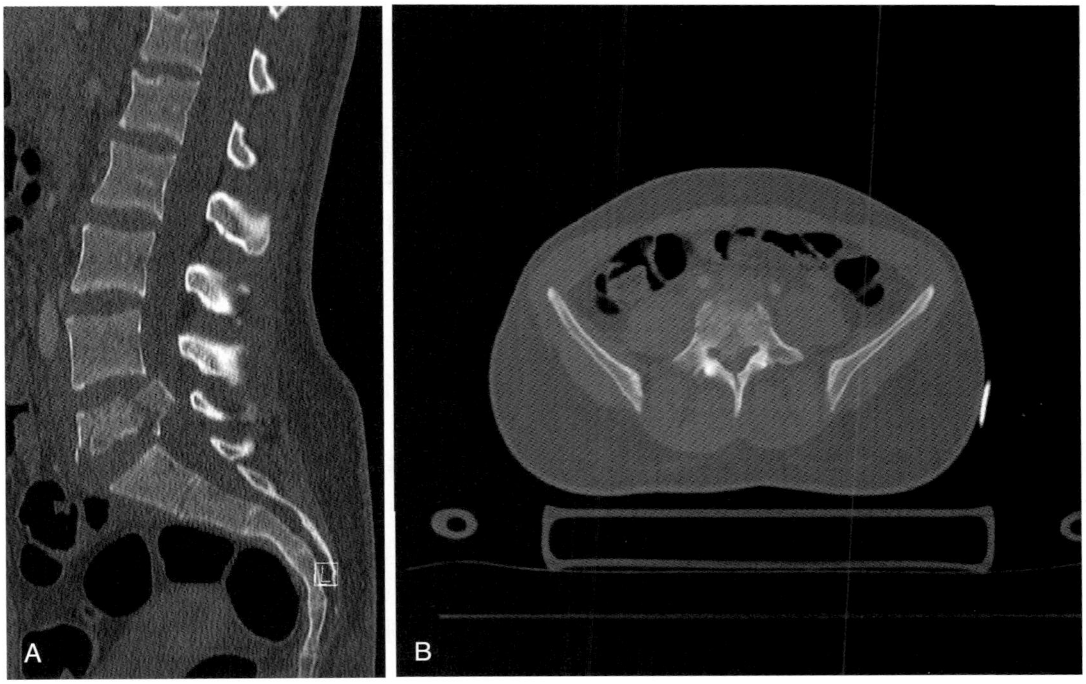

图 10　**A**，CTA，矢状重建图像。**B**，腰椎的轴向图像。注意 L5 爆裂性骨折，伴骨质向后进入椎管

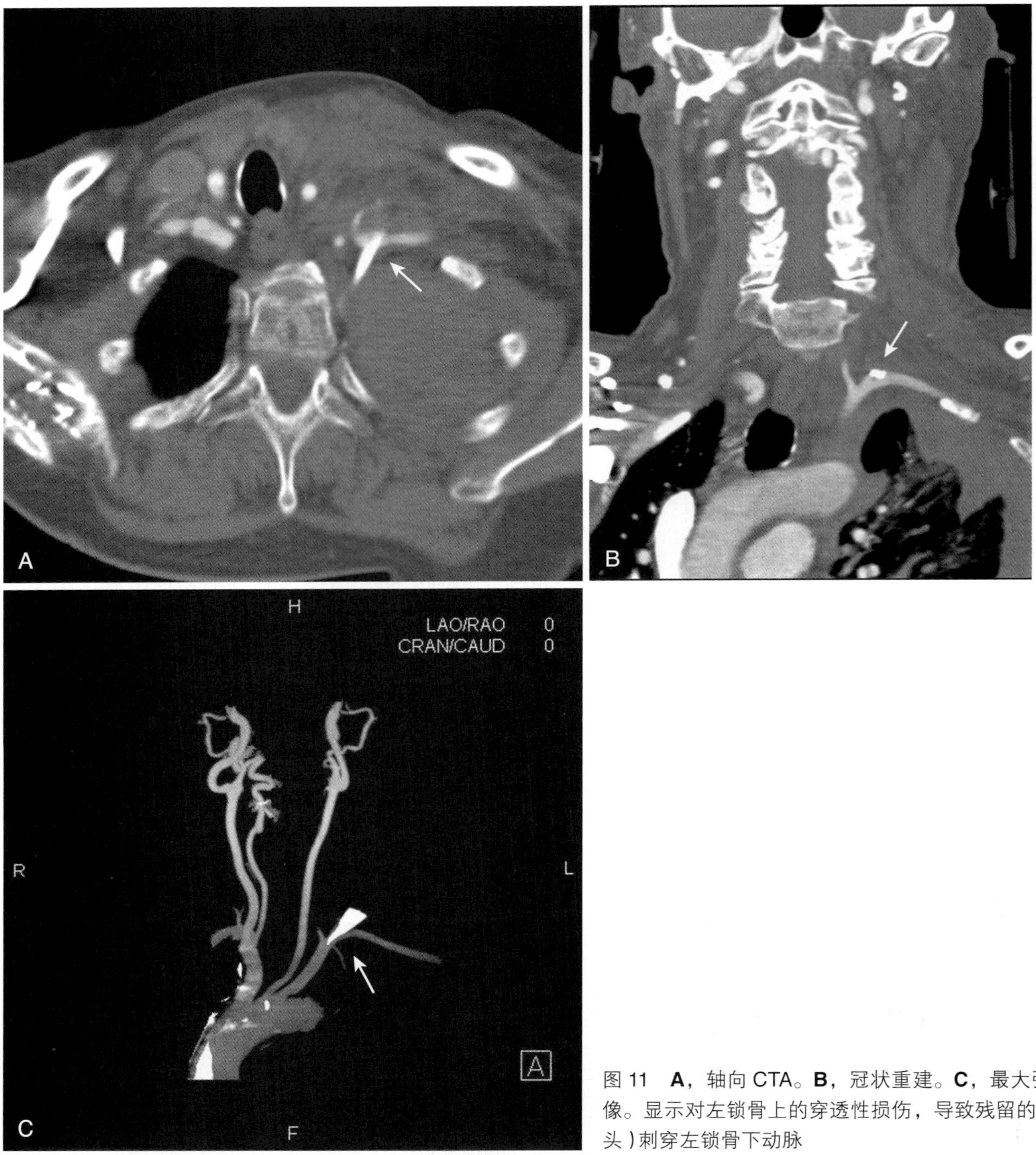

图 11 **A**，轴向 CTA。**B**，冠状重建。**C**，最大强度投影图像。显示对左锁骨上的穿透性损伤，导致残留的玻璃片（箭头）刺穿左锁骨下动脉

剂不对称不透明。当血管壁被破坏，并且血液被外膜或相邻的软组织包含时，则形成假性动脉瘤。假性动脉瘤显示为对比度不透明的血管腔的焦点小叶状外翻。在图像的所有相位上，假性动脉瘤的衰减应保持与起始血管的衰减相等（图 14）。延迟 CT 图像可以将假性动脉瘤与活动性外渗区域区分开，因为前者不会在大小或形状上发生变化。

血管的横断可导致闭塞或主活动性出血。与活动性出血一致的表现对比外渗区域通常显示为成像过程中每个时像大小都增加的腔外超衰竭区域（图 15）。使用动脉源，这些区域的衰减值等于或大于成像早期动脉期的主动脉衰减，并且大于后续门静脉和延迟期的主动脉衰减。对于静脉来源的造影剂溢出，腔外腮红对比仅在门静脉或成像延迟阶段才能确定。有时只能在门静脉期图像上看到动脉外渗或间歇性动脉出血的微小区域。

人造物，如相邻金属异物、上覆线和监测引线、脊柱或矫形硬件、假体、造影剂填充的膀胱和骨碎

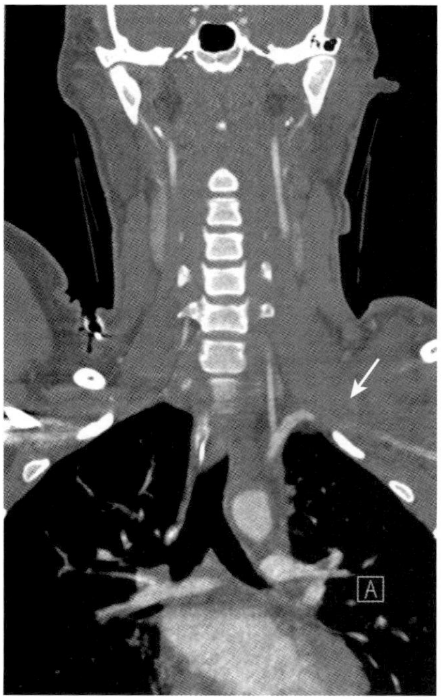

图 12 左锁骨下动脉的 CTA 冠状重建图像，显示继发于钝性创伤性损伤的伴远端重建（箭头）的节段闭塞

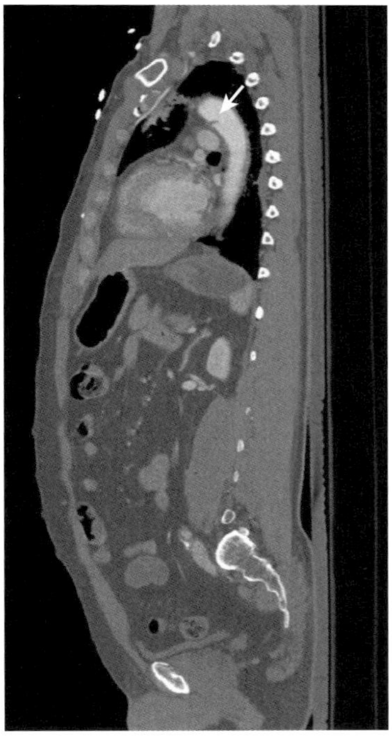

图 13 下行胸主动脉的 CTA 矢状位重建图像，显示主动脉峡部的内膜瓣（箭头）

片，可能会掩盖或类似血管外渗（图 16）。检查不同阶段的 CT 图像有助于区分骨碎片与造影剂外渗区域，因为骨碎片不会发生尺寸变化或衰减。来自相邻软组织血肿或水肿的脉管系统压迫也可能类似血管损伤。患者移动和呼吸运动也可能会限制对受伤的评估。

如果初始胸部 X 线片显示纵隔扩大、左胸膜积液、不明显的主动脉闭锁、左侧气管旁条纹扩大或左侧脊柱旁线扩大，应进行 CTA 检查，以进一步评估胸廓以排除胸主动脉的损伤（图 17）。在钝性损伤，胸主动脉最常受累的部位为主动脉根部、主动脉弓、主动脉峡部（胸主动脉近端降部）和主动脉膈裂孔（图 18）。在临床实践中，90％的受伤发生在主动脉峡部。大多数主动脉损伤表现为主动脉旁血肿。CTA 可显示主动脉内膜瓣 / 裂伤、内膜血栓、假性动脉瘤、轮廓异常、横断和活动性出血部位。推荐对近端主动脉损伤的评估采用心脏门控的 CTA，因为该区域的常规CTA对主动脉搏动评估存在限制。主动脉损伤通常与其分支的栓塞相关，可导致实质性梗死。CTA 也显示主动脉分支受伤。如果出现围绕大血管的血管周围血肿，应怀疑血管损伤。

纵隔血肿可能源于主动脉、胸廓内动脉、胸廓内静脉、头臂动脉 / 静脉、颈动脉、锁骨下动脉或纵隔静脉损伤。心包积血可能由近端主动脉、肺动脉、肺静脉、上腔静脉、下腔静脉、心包和心脏的损伤引起。

非血管性胸部 / 胸腔

前后仰卧位胸片是创伤患者的标准初始成像，用于快速诊断须要立即注意或治疗的病症。X 线胸片可以较好地显示张力性气胸、胸膜积液、纵隔扩大、膈损伤和生命支持线定位。张力性气胸经典地表现为对侧纵隔移位、同侧肺强烈充气、同侧隔膜倒置或扁平。胸膜积液表现为肋骨角变钝、出现半月征以及半侧胸部密度不对称增加。

CT 用于确认和评估胸部 X 线片提示的肺挫伤、肺裂伤、纵隔气肿、气胸、肋骨骨折、纵隔血肿、主动脉损伤、心包积液和胸膜积液的亚型。CT 检查能较好地显示胸膜积液。血胸（血液）的 CT HU 衰减值≥35 HU，普通胸膜液小于这个值，普通液体为 20 HU 或更小。

建议采用胸部 CTA 评估创伤患者。最好在动脉期获得胸部图像，以评估脉管系统和心脏。应在轴向平面进行薄截面成像，以便获得 CTA 和多平面重建（冠状面和矢状面）。

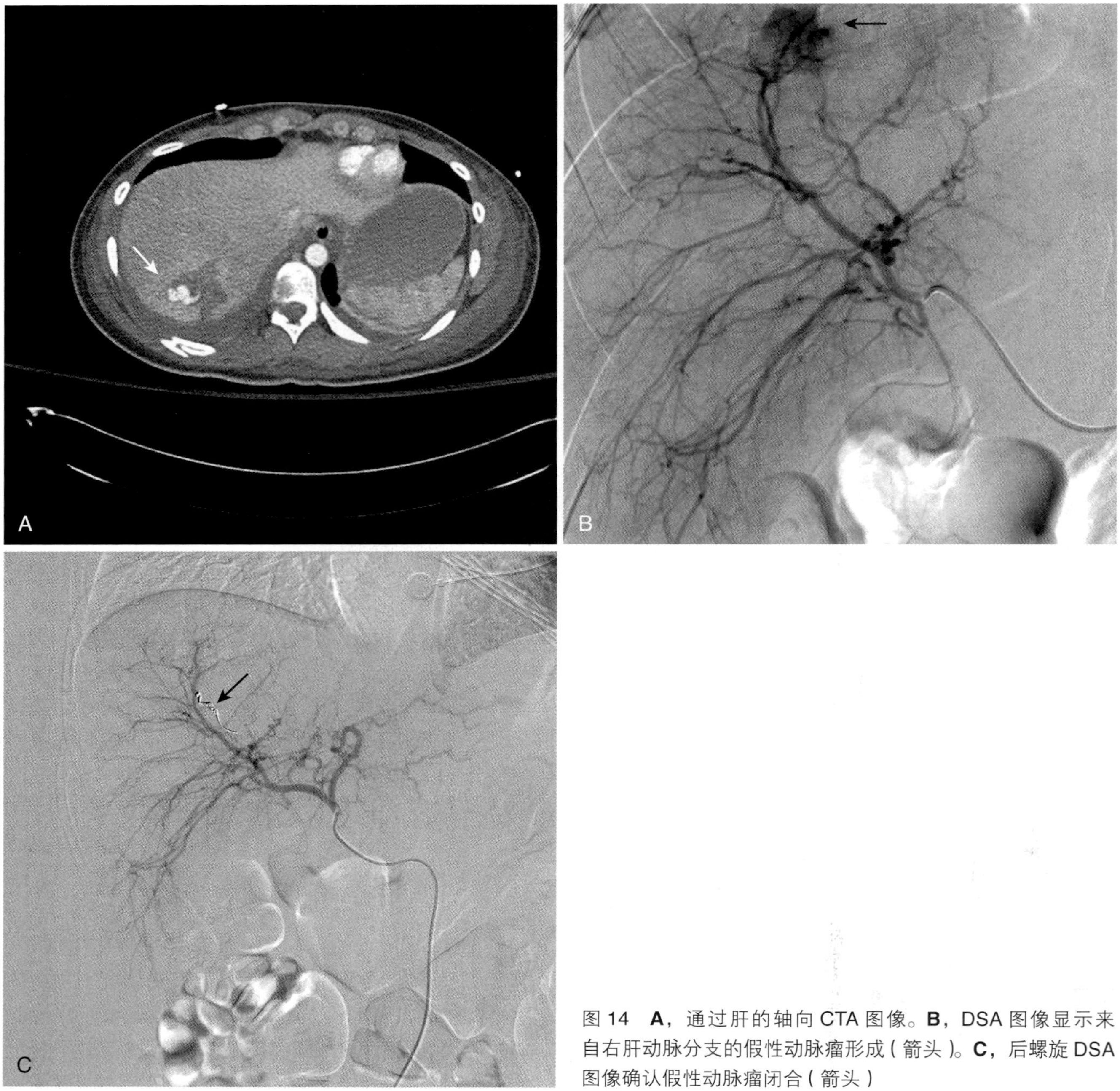

图 14 **A**，通过肝的轴向 CTA 图像。**B**，DSA 图像显示来自右肝动脉分支的假性动脉瘤形成（箭头）。**C**，后螺旋 DSA 图像确认假性动脉瘤闭合（箭头）

CT 也可以识别胸部 X 线片上微小和隐蔽的损伤。重要的是，当患者仰卧时，气胸往往会积聚在前、下和内侧胸膜间隙中，因此，可能会在初次仰卧位胸部 X 线片上表现隐蔽。胸部 X 线片上有几个迹象可以表明气胸的存在：深沟征、纵隔轮廓边界清楚、肺底边界清楚和双隔膜征。

肺实质性损伤很常见，包括肺挫伤和裂伤。胸部钝伤损伤最常导致挫伤，表现为块状的非节段空间不透明或边界不清的整体，并且一般不涉及胸膜下间隙（图 19）。在 24～48 h 内，挫伤开始清除，完全清除发生在 3～10 天。肺实质裂伤表现为可能充满空气或血液的腔。肺内的这些裂伤可能持续数月。通过损伤机制将裂伤分级，与肋骨骨折相关，并表现在 CT 上。

纵隔气肿可由气胸、食管或气道损伤发展而来。伴随气胸和肺泡损伤，空气可以通过支气管血管束进入纵隔。也可能发生气管和支气管的裂伤，导致纵隔气肿。当支气管出现完全横断或破裂时出现“肺陷征”（塌陷的肺处于分离的位置，悬挂于半侧胸腔肺门血管蒂的后外侧）。气管损伤表现为纵隔气肿，

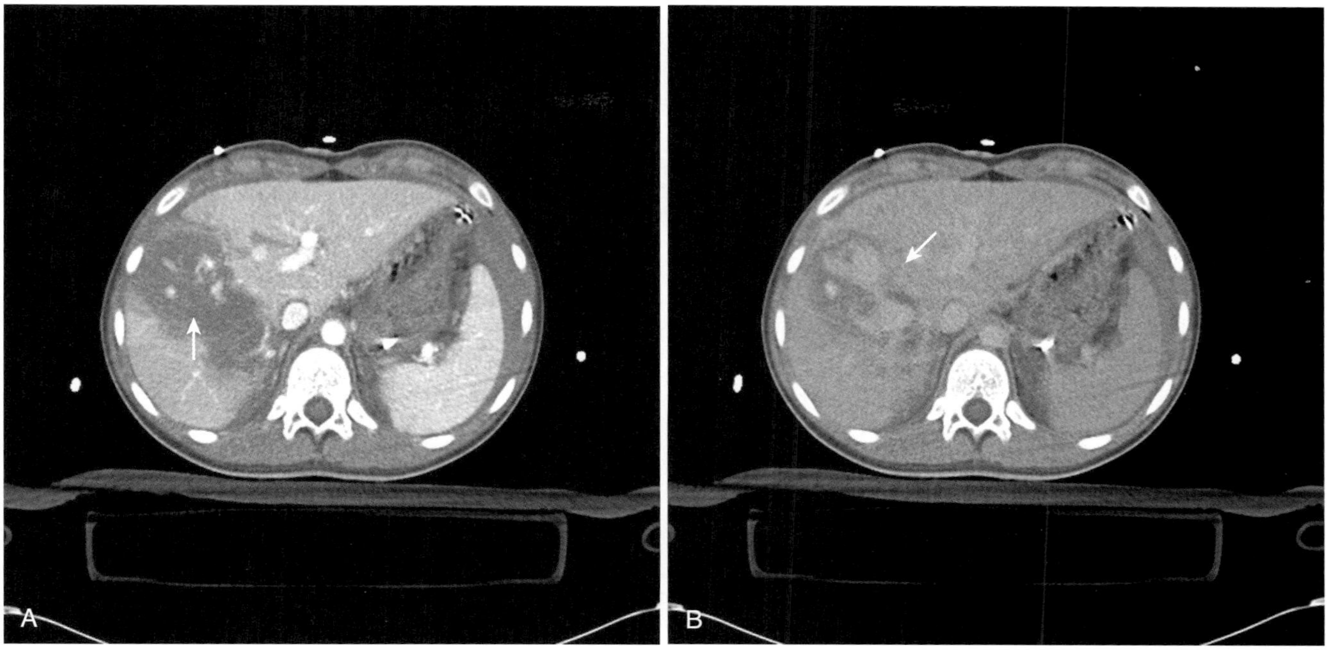

图 15　动脉期（A）和门静脉期（B）的肝 CT 图像。在动脉期内，在肝右叶中看到腔外对比（箭头）的腮红。在门静脉期，这种腔外对比区域的大小（箭头）增加，与活动性动脉造影外渗一致

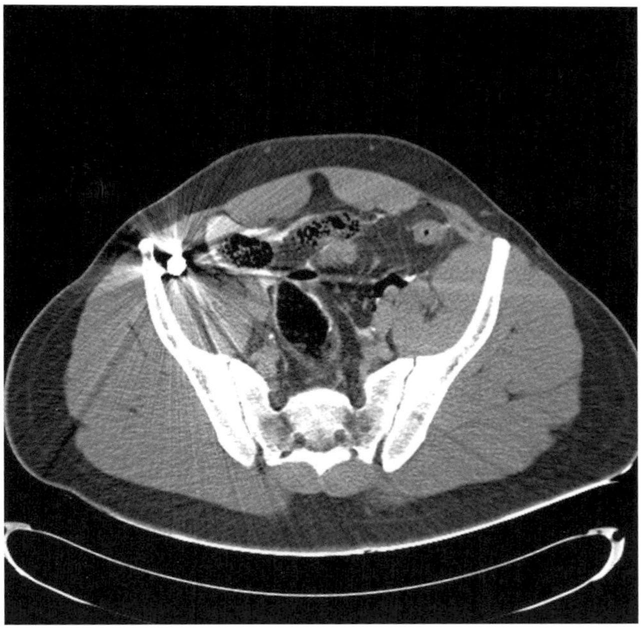

图 16　骨盆的轴向 CTA 图像。注意子弹如何导致条纹伪影，进而限制了对周围结构的评估

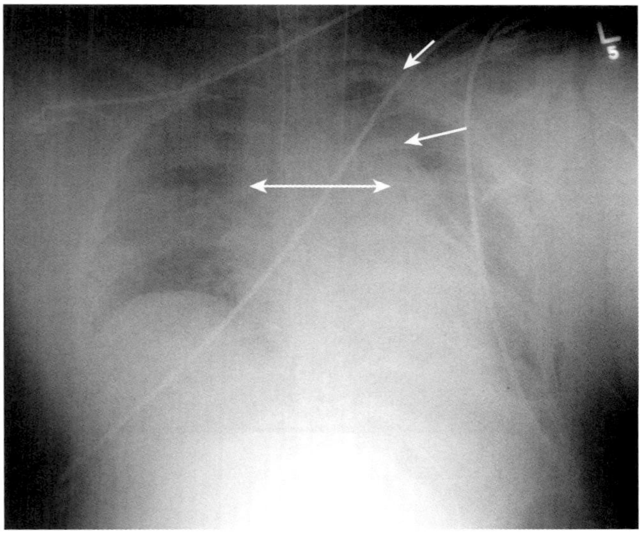

图 17　便携式前后胸部放射照片显示扩大的纵隔（双箭头）、左顶盖（顶部箭头）、左胸膜腔积液（中间箭头）和不明显的主动脉结节。出现这一现象时应该提高对主动脉损伤的怀疑

延伸到颈部的皮下气肿，以及过度膨胀或突出的气管内气球，投射在气管的范围之外。

食管的近端和远端部分是最常见的受伤部位。食管损伤在穿透伤后更常见，很少见于钝性创伤。临床上食管损伤的患者出现食欲不振或吞咽困难。内镜检查时可见食管内血肿或出血。如果怀疑食管损伤，可以在进行胸部 CT 前口服造影剂。CT 检查结果表明食管损伤由纵隔气肿、食管周围的液体、

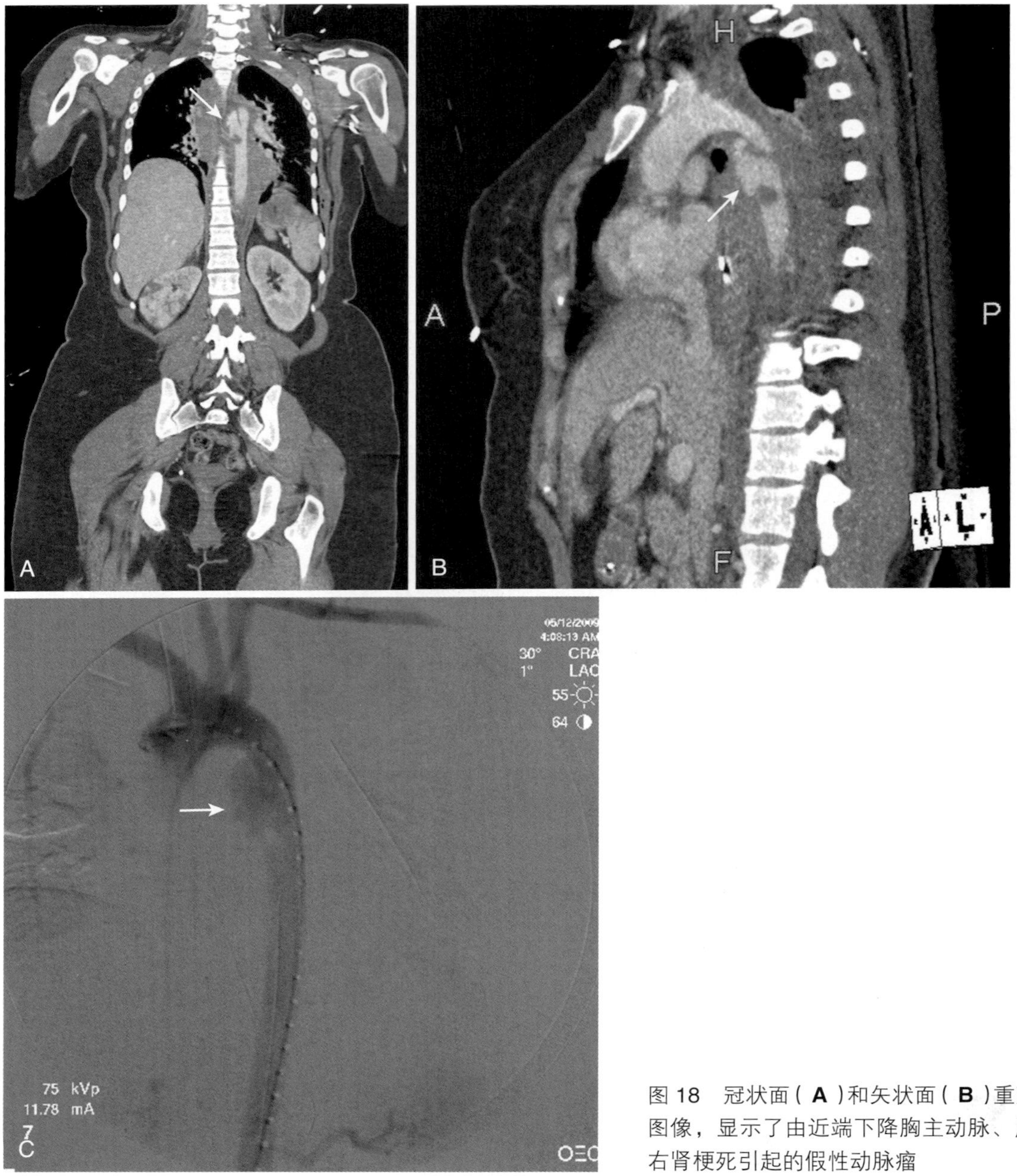

图 18 冠状面（**A**）和矢状面（**B**）重建的 CTA 和 DSA（**C**）图像，显示了由近端下降胸主动脉、周围纵隔血肿和伴随的右肾梗死引起的假性动脉瘤

气体或脂肪、增厚的食管壁、纵隔炎、外渗的口服造影剂和气胸组成。如果 CT 不能排除或征象不明确，应利用水溶性造影剂的食管造影和内镜检查评估食管损伤。

心脏损伤

超声和 CT 均可用于评估心脏损伤。超声心动图可以评估心包液、瓣膜功能、室壁运动异常、动脉瘤、心肌血肿和腔内血栓。CT 检查表明存在心脏损伤的征象包括心脏移位、心包积血、心包积气，心肌血肿、腔内血栓和动脉瘤，以及静脉注射造影剂外渗入心包空间或纵隔。

横隔损伤

穿透性和钝性创伤性损伤可能导致膈肌损伤和随后的疝气。横隔的穿透性损伤更常见，并且倾向于表现为小的损伤，难以发现。钝性创伤导致的膈肌损伤最常见于后外侧，但可能发生在其表面的任

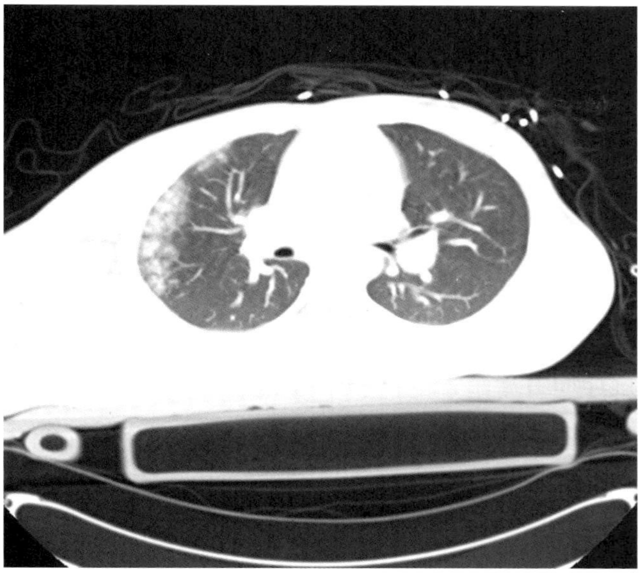

图 19　肺的轴向 CT 图像显示肺挫伤的典型外观

何地方。左侧膈肌最常受到钝性损伤，因为肝被认为对右侧膈肌起到加强作用。膈肌裂伤可导致脂肪和器官进入胸腔，导致这些组织出现穿孔、不能回缩和发生绞窄的风险。疝气可能立即出现或在几年后出现。最初的前后位仰卧位胸部 X 线片可能会显示半侧胸腔的块状不透明影，不明确或一侧的膈肌升高，或者甚至在胸腔中出现胃的投影（图 20）。在胸部 X 线片上通常会看到邻近肺和胸膜积液的后续损伤。MDCT 可以显示膈肌裂伤，突出内容物的位置和大小，以及其对肺和心脏的影响。在 CT 上有许多迹象表明有膈肌疝："驼峰征、衣领征和内脏坠落征"。在穿透性损伤，如果损伤轨迹穿过隔膜，或隔膜两侧均有相邻的损伤，则应怀疑裂伤。如果隔膜两侧出现液体或血液，也应怀疑膈肌损伤。请记住，这种发现在多部位穿透伤中没有特异性。

超声检查在创伤中的焦点评估

超声如同前后位胸片和盆腔 X 线片，可用于不稳定创伤患者的初步评估。超声可以快速指导不稳定患者的治疗，并避免风险。FAST 可评估五个空间的液体，并且可以检查空腔或实体器官损伤。这五个空间包括：①心包。②脾、肾。③肝、肾。④两侧结肠旁沟。⑤道格拉斯隐凹。有时超声也可以区分单纯液体与腹腔积血，因为血液回声更强，并且可以看到血凝块。超声不能区分尿液和普通液体，在评估腹膜后间隙时功能有限。

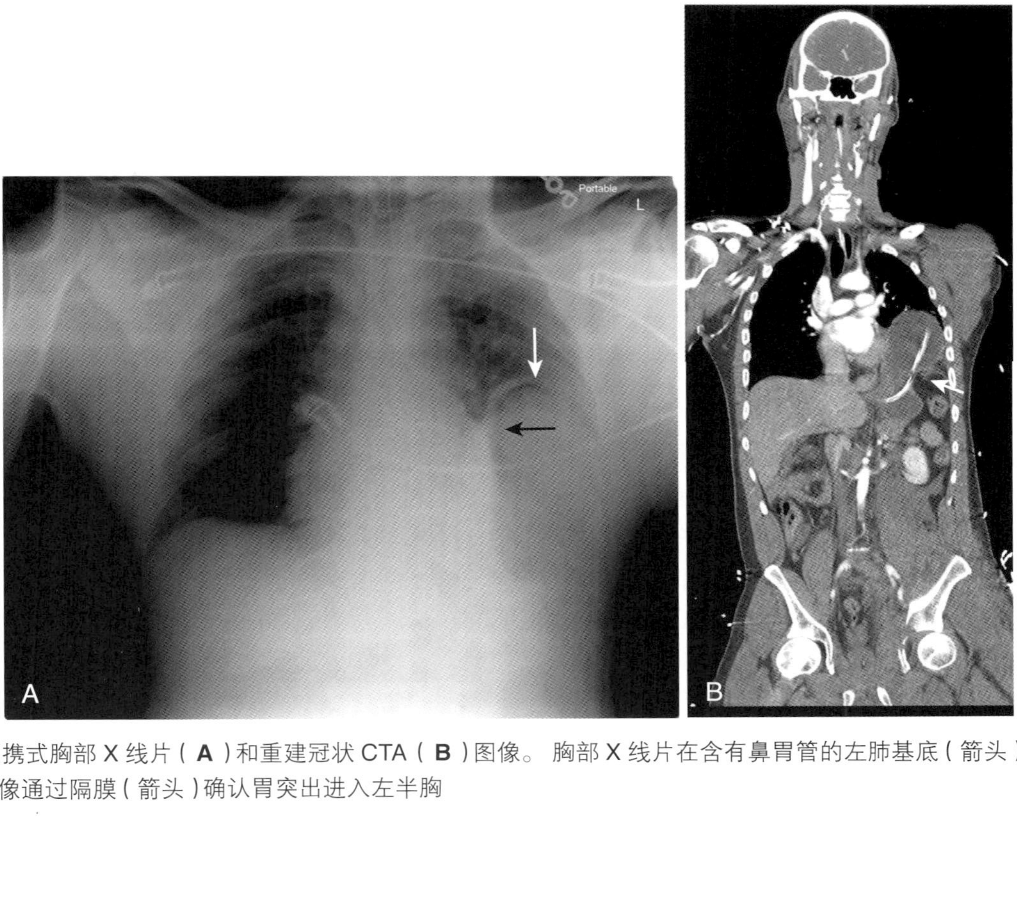

图 20　前后便携式胸部 X 线片（**A**）和重建冠状 CTA（**B**）图像。胸部 X 线片在含有鼻胃管的左肺基底（箭头）中显示块状不透明。CTA 图像通过隔膜（箭头）确认胃突出进入左半胸

游离液体

有多种诊断方式来评估腹部游离液体的存在和类型：DPL、FAST 或 CT。如果存在腹膜内游离液体，应怀疑实质或空腔器官损伤。在 Brofman 等进行的肠和肠系膜钝性创伤的 MDCT 研究中，在 54 例肠或肠系膜损伤患者中有 50 例（93%）存在腹膜内液体。液体通常位于受伤部位或附近，但也可能远离损伤部位或遍及腹部和骨盆。

请注意，在绝经前的女性中预计可见少量的游离液体，在绝经后的女性中也可以看到。也有人认为，在男性中少量普通的无衰减盆腔液可能属于正常。腹膜内和腹膜后的游离液体也可以由激进的补水引起，但通常伴有其他支持体征，包括门静脉周围水肿、IVC 充盈、肝静脉充盈和弥漫性肠壁水肿。此外，DPL 可能会导致游离气体和液体，从而难以辨别结果的来源。

游离气体

肠外游离气体常见于前腹壁腹膜壁层深处、肠系膜内、肠系膜静脉和门静脉内以及肝门区域。如果存在腹膜后游离气体，应怀疑十二指肠、升或降结肠损伤。

必须牢记，除了肠穿孔或损伤以外，外伤患者有许多原因可以导致游离气体。腹腔游离气体可见于以下情况：气胸或纵隔气肿的气体进入腹腔，DPL 后，机械通气引起的气压伤，腹壁和胸壁穿透性损伤，以及腹膜内膀胱穿孔后放置 Foley 导尿管。

胃肠道

穿透性损伤和钝性创伤都可能导致空腔脏器损伤。由于减速作用力，肠道可能会被撕裂，并且可能被直接作用力而压碎或破裂。已经表明，MDCT 比 FAST 和 DPL 的特异性和灵敏度更好。如果患者稳定，建议使用“三重对比”来评估腹部和骨盆的穿透性损伤。三重对比是指同时使用静脉注射、口服和直肠给予造影剂后进行 CT 检查。如存在游离气体和液体则表明腹膜受到累及，但不能诊断空腔或实质器官损伤。在没有口服造影剂的情况下，如果在初始 CT 上不能确定游离气体或液体的来源，可以在 6 ~ 8 h 后给予口服造影剂并重复检查 CT。

肠道损伤可能表现为周围出现游离液体、周围脂肪绞合、肠系膜血肿、肠壁增厚、肠壁不连续、游离气体、肠壁不连续和不规则的急剧增强、继发于血流阻断的肠壁增强减弱、腹壁损伤和口服造影剂外渗。最具有特异性的肠损伤迹象包括肠壁中断、活动性口服造影剂外渗以及游离气体。空腔脏器损伤的唯一明确标志是出现腔外胃肠造影剂（图 21）。

最常见的是，小肠损伤位于固定或附着位置，例如回盲瓣附近的回肠末端和 Treitz 韧带附近的近端空肠。注意，十二指肠的第二、第三和第四部分位于腹膜后，因此，若存在腹膜后的游离气体或液体，应怀疑十二指肠损伤。此外，如存在右前方肾周间隙的游离液体，应怀疑十二指肠损伤。

穿透性损伤是造成直肠损伤的最常见原因。钝性损伤引起的直肠损伤是罕见的，通常由会阴骑跨伤导致。直肠损伤的患者通常直肠有鲜红色血液。CT 检查可能会显示直肠周围脂肪绞合、直肠周围血肿、直肠周围游离气体、骶骨前液体或血肿和局灶性直肠壁增厚。

肠系膜损伤

区分肠系膜损伤与肠损伤常常很困难，因为两者在特异性和灵敏度不强的成像结果上表现相似。虽然肠和肠系膜损伤的影像学检查结果可能重叠，

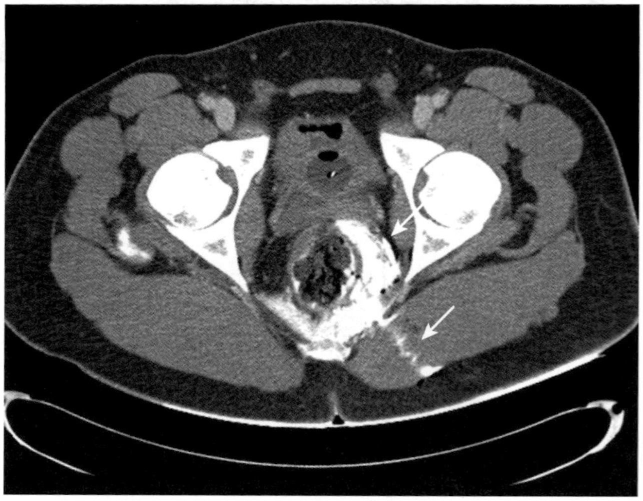

图 21　轴向 CTA 三维对比图像通过骨盆后枪伤伤口到左臀部区域。请注意，直肠造影剂已经从直肠腔外渗到直肠周围和子弹弹道（箭头）

肠系膜血肿、肠系膜的静脉注射造影剂外渗、肠系膜血管闭塞以及肠系膜血管的珠状外观对肠系膜损伤具有特异性（图 22）。肠系膜损伤可导致相邻肠环的血流阻断，表现为肠壁增厚和不规则增强。肠系膜损伤的其他非特异性检查结果包括肠系膜脂肪绞合、腹壁损伤和清楚的肠系膜血肿。

实质器官损伤（肝、脾、肾）

尽管器官不同，但肝、脾、肾和胰腺的损伤表现类似。除了对器官周围的游离液体、腹腔积血及包膜下血肿的评估外，超声局限于对实质器官实质损伤的评估。在超声上，局灶性裂伤、挫伤和血肿可能表现为器官实质内的高回声、低回声、不均匀扩散或地图样表现。在超声上，裂伤也可以表现为垂直于器官表面的低回声线性和分支区域。

在 CT 成像门静脉期，实质器官的损伤表现最为明显。微小和不太严重的损伤表现为不同程度的器官周围脂肪绞合或游离液体。包膜下血肿通常表现为符合器官包膜限制的低密度器官周围积液。当器官包膜受到裂伤时，包膜下血肿可能是高密度的，并且显示静脉注射造影剂活动性外渗的区域与活动性出血的区域一致（图 23）。挫伤表现为器官实质内的低衰减或增强减弱区域。非增强 CT 上的血肿可能表现为强衰减实质区域。裂伤显示为线性不增强，有时为分支或甚至复杂表现，贯穿器官实质的低衰减缺损（图 24）。确定损伤是否累及器官的门是重要的。CT 还用于识别实质器官血管损伤。梗死表现为外围楔形低衰减或低增强区域。梗死可源于血管损伤，也可能继发于大动脉损伤后的血栓栓塞性疾病。

美国创伤外科协会（AAST）实质器官损伤分类考虑了裂伤的大小、实质和包膜下血肿的大小以及血管损伤。肾的 AAST 分级标准也考虑到了集合系统的损伤。

集合系统

肾裂伤可以延伸到集合系统（图 25）。无论是肉眼血尿还是镜下血尿，如果伴有损伤机制和休克征象，应该评估肾集合系统损伤。注意，如果输尿管 - 肾盂连接部或输尿管完全被切断，可能不出现血尿。在初始静脉注射造影剂给药后 5 min，延迟的 CT 图像在评估尿路损伤和尿液外渗中很重要（图 26）。尿外渗可以是受限或游离的。如果在远离外渗位置的集合系统看到造影剂，则可能为部分裂伤。

对于膀胱损伤，应怀疑有骨盆骨折和已知的后尿道损伤。常规的透视或 CT 膀胱造影可以识别膀胱损伤。在大型创伤中心，CT 替代了常规膀胱造影。通过 Foley 或耻骨上导管，将膀胱用包含 50% 盐水和 50% 静脉注射造影剂组成的 300 ml 混合物滴注，

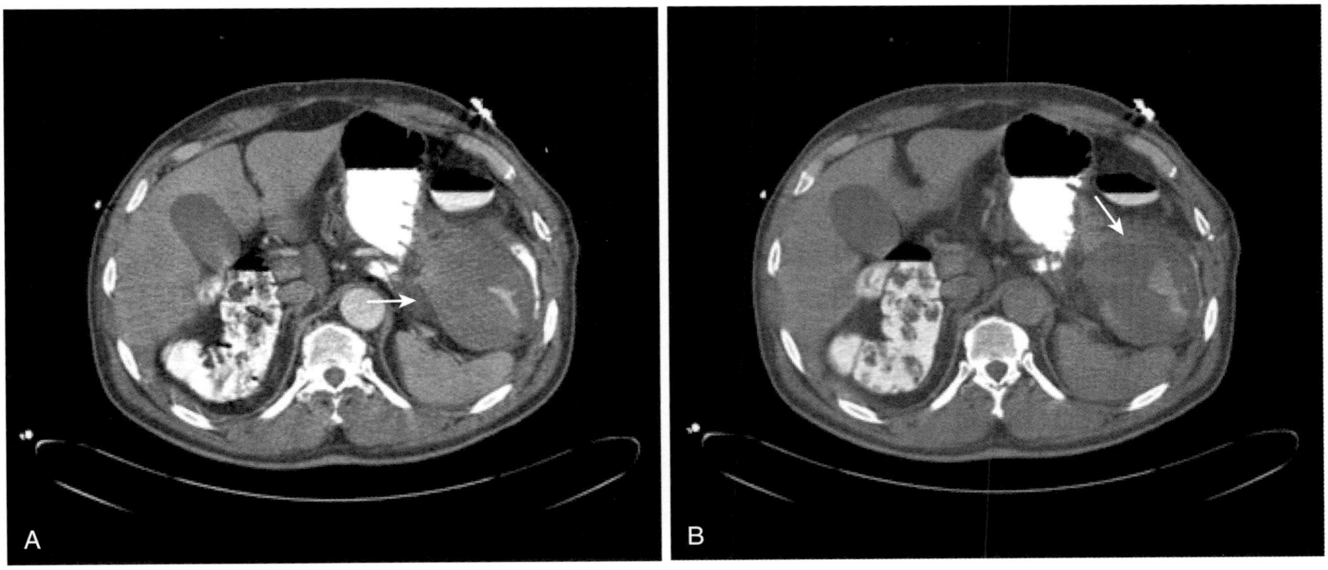

图 22　上腹部轴向 CT 图像的动脉期（A）和延迟期（B）成像。肠系膜血肿（箭头）在图 A 的左上象限中注明。在图 B 中，成像延迟期放大的对比度表现（箭头）与活动性出血一致

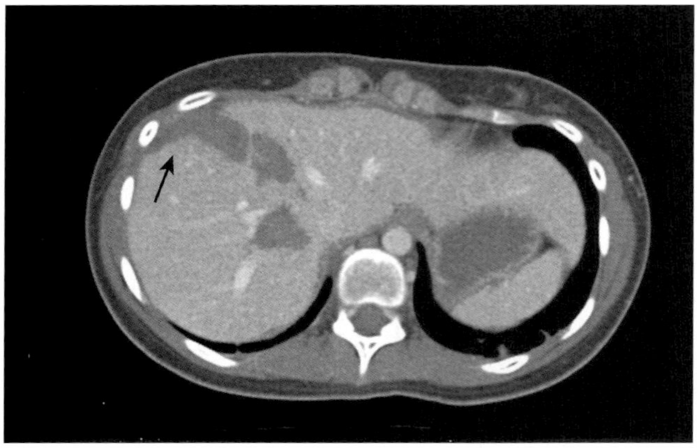

图 23　肝的轴向 CTA 图像显示肝和包膜下血肿的撕裂（箭头）

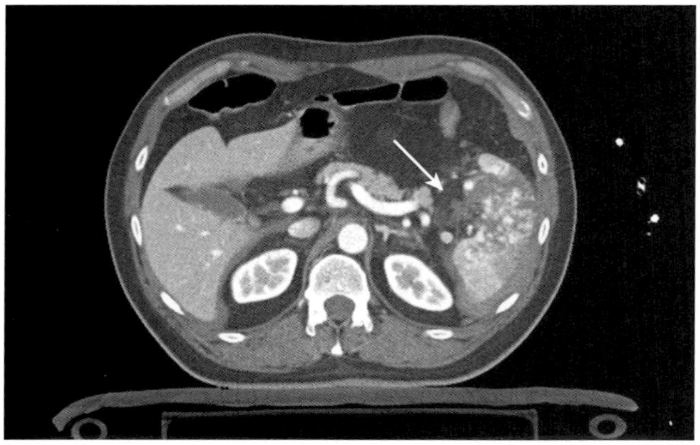

图 24　脾的轴向 CTA 图像，显示脾周血肿、活动性动脉造影外渗和有多个小假性动脉瘤（箭头）的破碎脾

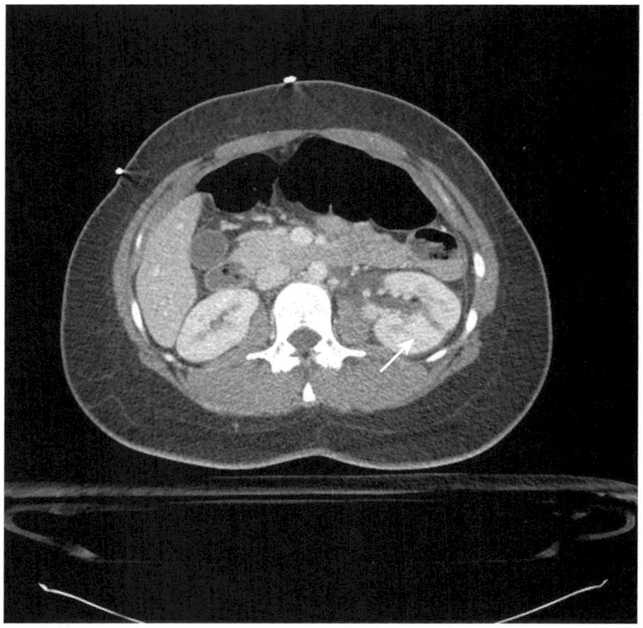

图 25　肾的轴向 CT 图像门静脉期，显示左肾裂伤（箭头）延伸到集合系统伴肾周积液（血肿和尿液）

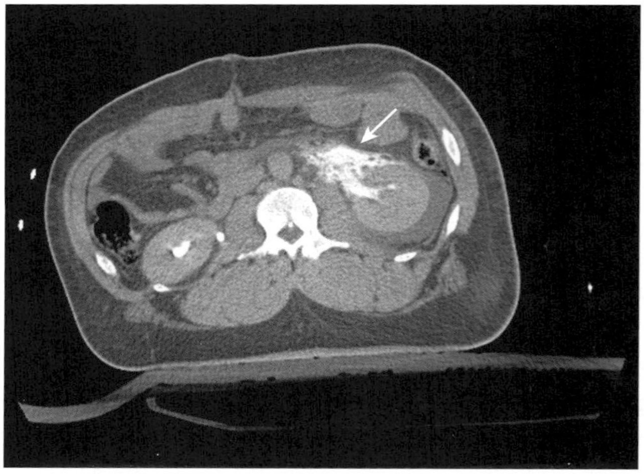

图 26　肾的轴向 CT 图像延迟期，显示左侧近端集合系统和肾周血肿的外渗（箭头）

然后进行骨盆的有限 CT 扫描。对于儿科患者，应将 100 ~ 150 ml 盐水或造影剂混合物滴入膀胱。直到全膀胱膨胀前是无法确定膀胱的完整性的。应在最后进行 CT 膀胱造影，因为造影剂充填的膀胱以及受伤或破裂的膀胱可能会掩盖邻近的血管或胃肠道造影剂外渗。

70% 的膀胱损伤发生在腹膜外，大多数与骨盆骨折有关。在腹膜外膀胱破裂时，液体（尿）或膀胱造影剂将积聚在膀胱周围或膀胱前（图 27）。膀胱前腹膜间隙也称为 Retzius 间隙，从耻骨联合延伸到脐部。外渗的造影剂可呈现“火焰”状外观。如果泌尿生殖器膈肌破裂，尿液或造影剂会渗出阴囊、大腿和阴茎。

20% 的膀胱损伤发生在腹膜内。腹膜覆盖顶部是膀胱的最薄弱处。在腹膜内膀胱损伤中，尿液或造影材料将外渗到腹膜内，并且可以在腹膜内肠管和实质器官周围、结肠旁沟内、道格拉斯凹内和膈下空间中看到。

10% 的膀胱损伤合并腹膜内和腹膜外损伤，通常由穿透性损伤引起。

尿道

如果存在尿道附近渗透性损伤病史或已知的骑跨伤，应该怀疑尿道损伤伴有骨盆骨折。患者可能表现为尿道口滴血、血尿或不能排尿。进行直肠检

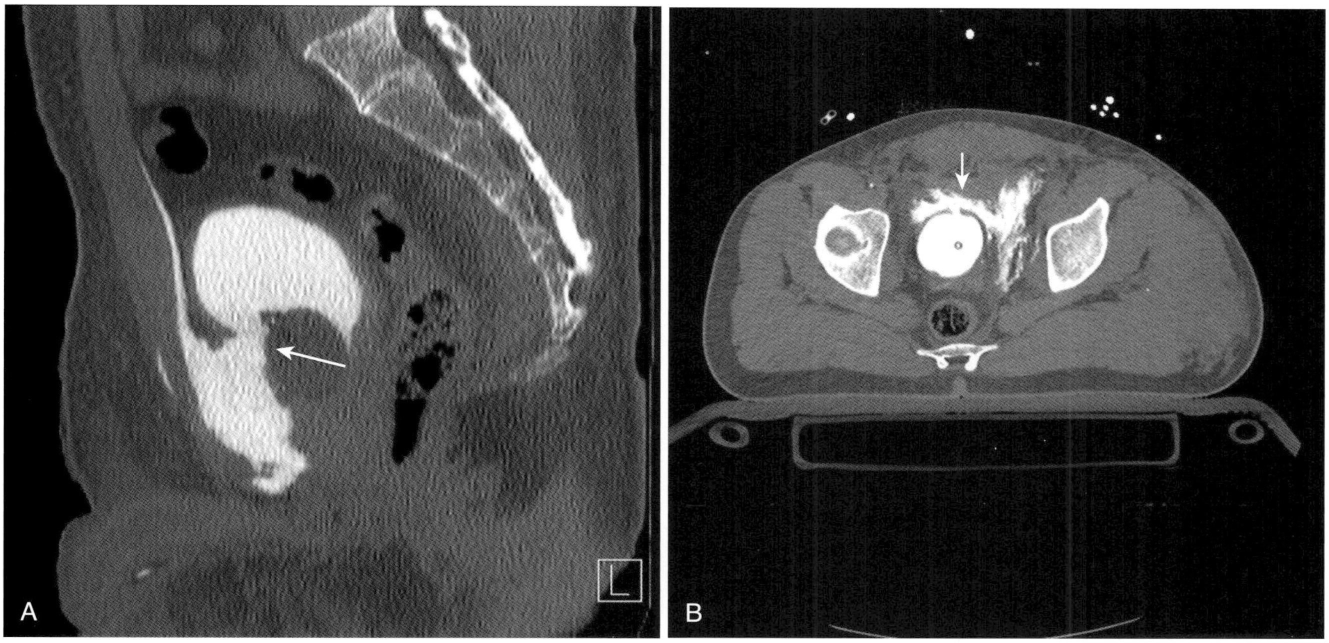

图 27 膀胱计算机断层扫描矢状（A）和轴向（B）重建图像。注意造影剂通过腹膜外缺损渗入膀胱（箭头）

查时可发现前列腺处于高位。当存在尿道损伤时，放置 Foley 导管可能会加重损伤。如果怀疑尿道损伤，则应在置入 Foley 导管前进行逆行尿道造影。尿道造影可以定位损伤的部位（前尿道与后尿道），并确定是完整损伤还是部分损伤。在后尿道损伤，造影剂将积累在耻骨后空间。请注意，后尿道损伤患者也可能有膀胱损伤。发生前尿道损伤时，造影剂会渗透到阴茎海绵体或海绵体，并可能回流到阴茎的引流静脉。当损伤累及泌尿生殖膈时，造影剂会积聚在会阴。部分尿道破裂可见膀胱部分充盈。有时，即使放置了 Foley 导管，也可以在延迟期 CT 检测到尿道损伤。

腹膜后损伤

体格检查、实验室检验以及 DPL 和 FAST US 都难以对腹膜后损伤进行评估。

胰腺

大多数胰腺损伤的原因是钝性伤或减速伤。在机动车辆事故、自行车事故和摩托车碰撞中，方向盘或手柄杆的直接冲击导致胰腺受伤。通过对比增强 CT 可以发现胰腺损伤。胰腺损伤可能呈现微小的变化，如胰周脂肪绞合或液体。挫伤出现在实质的低衰减或增强区域，并且可能伴随着周围的脂肪绞合和流体。裂伤表现为贯穿胰腺实质的线性低衰减非增强性缺损。横断损伤指 >50% 腺体厚度并涉及胰管的裂伤。大多数横断损伤发生在胰腺颈部。MRI 胰胆管造影可进一步评估胰管损伤。胰腺损伤通常与十二指肠损伤有关。

肾上腺

通过平扫 CT 和增强 CT 都可以很容易地检测到肾上腺损伤，结果包括肾上腺脂肪绞合至放大的低衰减腺体（图 28）。出血可能由上肾上腺动脉引起。肾上腺损伤与肝裂伤和 IVC 损伤有关。

脊柱以外的骨

MDCT 还可以在 X 线片上显示隐匿性骨折，并进一步评估 X 线上显示的骨折范围。骶髂关节的轻微扩大、耻骨联合的分离、关节内骨折延伸、关节内松动和关节半脱位均在 CT 上得到很好的显示（图 29）。轴向平面上的骨折可能隐藏在轴向 CT 图像上，

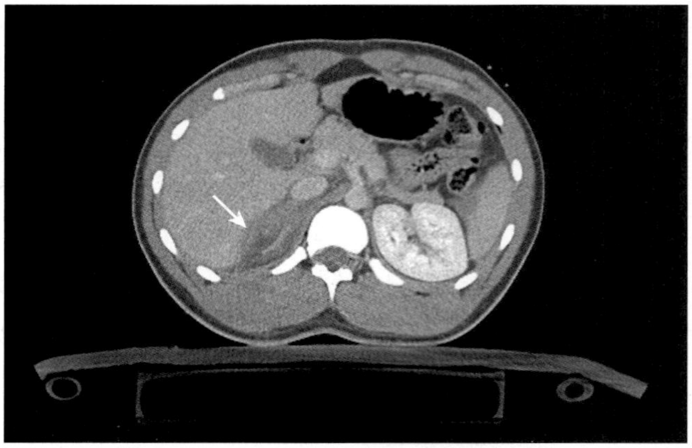

图 28 CTA 照片轴图像显示右肾上腺血肿（箭头）

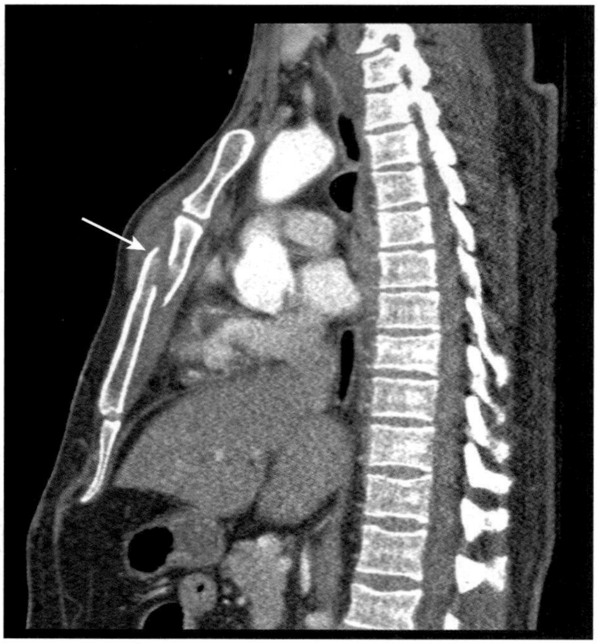

图 29 胸部的 CTA 矢状重建图像显示斜胸骨骨折（箭头）和胸后血肿

图像上，但通常在矢状面和冠状面重新格式化图像上可得到很好的显示。

休克

可见低血容量性休克的几种 CT 征象，如肾上腺和肠壁剧烈增强、IVC 扁平、动脉口径变小、胰腺水肿、腹膜后水肿和弥漫性小肠壁水肿或增厚。

复苏效果

CT 检查结果包括 IVC 和肝静脉充盈、门静脉周围水肿，以及骨盆和腹膜后相关部位的低衰减的游离液体。CT 上的门静脉水肿表现为肝内门静脉分支两侧的管状低衰减平行影。

腹腔间隔室综合征

CT 检查发现包括腹部膨隆、液体压迫 IVC、腹膜后密集浸润、肾压迫、腹股沟疝、肠壁增厚和肠壁剧烈增强。

介入放射学：诊断和治疗作用

David J. Quintana, Jason Salsamendi 和 Felipa Munera 著
易成腊 译

在腹部和盆腔创伤中最可预防的死亡原因之一是未经治疗或无法识别的动脉出血。在过去十年中，放射学已经取得许多进展，特别是非侵入性成像和介入血管造影，使临床上的动脉出血能更快地被识别和治疗，从而常常挽救患者的生命。然而，正如我们将要看到的，介入放射学除了血管造影术外，CT 引导的经皮介入和其他成像引导技术也在创伤患者的紧急治疗中发挥重要的作用。

动脉止血的基石是早期干预，包括对受伤血管的直接止血、血管内技术、开胸手术、开放式剖腹术或干预措施及其组合。早期干预需要高灵敏度和特异性的诊断研究，可以快速进行和得出结果。在过去，主要通过诊断性血管造影确定动脉损伤。这种方法时间急迫，并具有侵入性。然而，随着 CT 技术的进步，CTA 已经基本上取代了传统的诊断性

血管造影术，用来评估血管损伤。血流动力学稳定的患者传统上不采取剖腹术，采用CTA评估，并接受非手术治疗（non-operative management，NOM）。这些NOM患者保留做血管造影的可能性。但随着介入技术在过去十年的不断发展，栓塞已被纳入对非手术患者和手术患者的治疗。血管内技术的进一步发展在不稳定患者的治疗中取得了巨大进步。在适当的临床环境中，许多领先的创伤中心已经将动脉栓塞用做原发性复苏的一个组成部分，特别是在骨盆创伤。

简而言之，介入放射学在创伤患者的诊断、治疗和管理中起着重要作用。介入放射学需要多学科的融合，创伤外科医师和介入医师须要了解其适应证和局限性。

CTA

CTA通常被用于血流动力学稳定的创伤患者。血流动力学不稳定的患者经历复苏，一旦生命体征稳定，就进行CTA。然而，CT技术的发展已经扩大了适应证，CTA正在被用于较不稳定的患者。这主要是由于多探头CT（MDCT）技术的进步减少了检查时间，并且能更快地定位活动性出血。最先进的多层扫描仪不仅在时间和空间分辨率上得到了改进，而且可以在不到1.5 s内获取全身图像，这比传统的胸部平片和骨盆X线片要快。MDCT获取等容数据，从而可以在无限个平面上重建图像。多平面重建和最大密度投影有助于确认疑似血管病变，并发现可能被相邻的高衰减骨骼或异物掩盖的血管损伤。

在20世纪80年代，已经发现50%～70%的肝和脾损伤在手术时已经停止出血。只要患者的血流动力学状态不受影响，就可以保守治疗。然而，血管损伤已经成为CTA评估的焦点，因为其存在与NOM的失败相关。对实质器官损伤也用CTA评估，历史上已经使用美国外伤外科协会（AAST）标准进行了定义和分级。然而，这些分级量表是基于解剖学发现，并没有被证明可以精确地分辨不能进行非手术治疗或延迟性出血失代偿的患者。事实上，Durham将CT扫描结果与手术结果进行比较并得出结论，CT可能实际上低估了肝损伤的程度。随后，有许多研究尝试定义临床相关的CT成像结果。虽然目前没有普遍接受的标准，但本节的目标是将这些CT发现定义为高风险，这些情况可能受益于早期干预。

造影剂外渗是血管损伤最可靠的CTA征象之一，具有99%的特异性和80%～97%的灵敏性，用于鉴定须要栓塞的患者。1993年，Shanmuganathan发现在CT上可以区分凝血和活动性出血。持续性出血在CT上表现为高衰减，平均130 HU，凝固血液的测量值为40～70 HU。因此，对大于100 HU的衰减应怀疑有活动性出血。使用造影剂可以看到对比度腮红，经常褪色成实质性血肿或腹膜内液体。造影剂外渗的衰减通常在邻近注射动脉源的10 HU以内。活动性外渗通常边界不清，表现为低衰减的线性或聚焦区域。在延迟CTA成像中，血肿尺寸扩大或衰减值变化提示活动性出血。总体来说，对于活动性外渗诊断的关键是一个高衰减的实体，其延迟成像发生变化。

区分实质内血肿的活动性出血和裂伤至关重要。如果怀疑血管损伤，尽管没有活动性外渗的证据，连续的CTA可能有助于监测患者的病情进展。延迟性出血可以表现为血肿增大，中央性实体器官血肿破裂，或与积液接触的假性动脉瘤（如胆汁瘤或血肿）破裂。如临床状况突然改变或疼痛增加，应怀疑延迟出血。此外，涉及三个以上肝段的肝撕裂和延伸到肝门的撕裂与血管损伤有关，应及时干预。应注意肝门范围内的撕裂，因为可能是累及门静脉或下腔静脉的不稳定性病变，最好采取手术治疗。

实质内血肿的位置同样重要。某些位置可能与较大的腔室相同。由于缺乏支撑结构填塞，具有较高的排血风险。累及Ⅶ肝段的肝血肿可延伸到肝的裸露区域，导致腹膜后排血。中央性肝血肿与血管周围空间相通，并可能排血到肝门。最后，肝或脾实质性血肿可能延伸到囊内。如果囊受损，血肿可能扩大到腹膜腔。实际上，含有游离液体的象限越多，CTA对血管损伤的特异性就越高。对结肠旁沟和盆腔陷凹存在游离液体的患者采用NOM更容易失败，并且须要栓塞，但是莫里森陷凹和脾周区域的游离液体一般无须栓塞。尽管腹腔积血不是单独的CT检查结果，超过三个象限的造影剂外渗或哨兵凝块会增加血管损伤的特异性，须要早期干预。如果在多于一个象限中发现腹腔积血，应进行流体衰减的比较。最靠近损伤部位的血液有更多的时间回缩，形成更高密度的凝血，即所谓的“哨兵凝块征”。这对于多发性实质器官损伤患者的介入医师而言很重要，因为它可能有助于决定首先应选择性动脉造影的部位。

CT 上观察到的血管损伤的其他迹象包括包含造影剂的血管损伤和内膜损伤。假性动脉瘤和动静脉瘘（arteriovenous fistula，AVF）被分类为单独的动脉病变。与活动外渗相比，假性动脉瘤在 CT 上表现出不同的特征。它们通常表现出类似于邻近注射动脉的衰减，但在圆形配置中显示明确的边缘。假性动脉瘤在延迟成像中也不太明显。如果存在相邻的血肿，其尺寸或衰减不会改变。取决于位置，假性动脉瘤可以容易地在多普勒超声上分辨（图 1）。单独的 AVF 在 CT 上难以诊断，因为 CTA 需要长时间的静脉注射时间，导致脉管系统非选择性地不透明。最后，可能在 CTA 上检测到外伤性内脏内膜损伤，最常见于肾动脉。由于存在血栓形成、实质功能障碍甚至肾衰竭的风险，钝性肾动脉损伤被认为是高危病变。

诊断性 CTA 确实有其局限性。重要的是要了解当前的 CTA 成像只反映某一个时间的状况，并且它可能无法检测到存在的所有血管病变。此外，CTA 无法准确地预测迟发性出血。如前所述，CTA 潜在地低估了实质器官损伤，因此临床表现至关重要。然而，毫无疑问，CTA 是一种强大的工具，能可靠地帮助创伤患者的治疗决策。

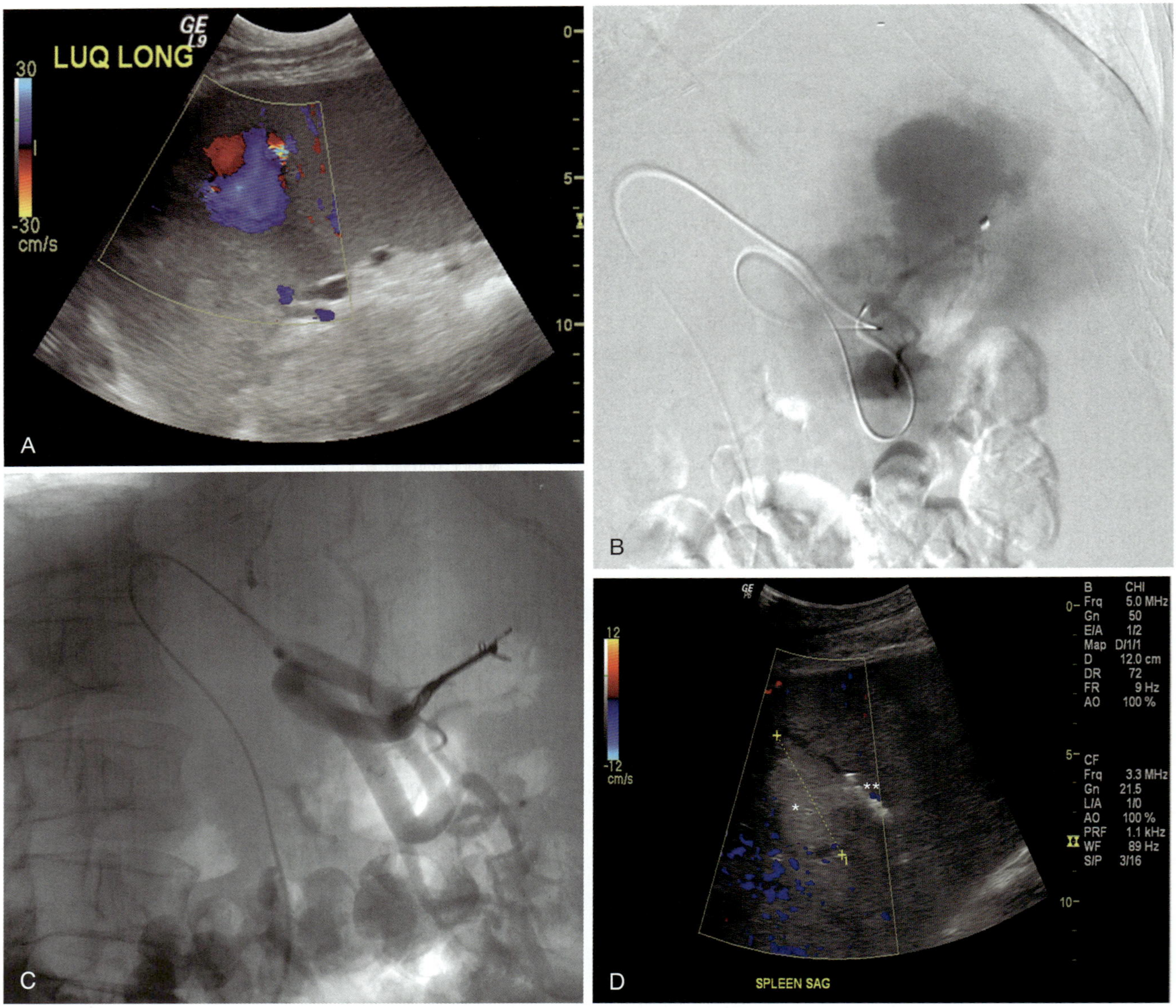

图 1　矢状彩色多普勒超声（A）显示通过超选择脾血管造影（B）证实的 4.5 cm 脾上的极假性动脉瘤。在先前的对比增强 CT 观察到的脾损伤确认部位，假性动脉瘤扩展到包膜附近。对实质内假性动脉瘤用超选择性栓塞治疗，使用可分离的微线圈和液体栓塞（玛瑙）（C）。栓塞后多普勒超声显示栓塞的假性动脉瘤（单星号）以及主体脾动脉分支（D）中的回声物质（双星号）没有流动

经导管血管造影

诊断性血管造影

血管造影可证实 80%～90%的 CTA 发现的可疑动脉损伤，但呈现持续的诊断挑战。活动性出血和血管损伤可能很微小。这些病变在 CTA 和血管造影上的表现不同。血管造影术的造影剂外渗表现为持续腮红，其出现早于静脉期，并且在延迟期不能洗出。假性动脉瘤被诊断为独立的囊性突出，其密度与相邻的血管相同，并且没有外渗证据。突然的动脉中断表示血管的横断和闭塞。

当 CTA 与血管造影术之间出现差异时，重要的是确定差异是否源于动脉出血停止或血管痉挛，血流动力学不稳定的生理反应是否掩盖了血管损伤。如果高度怀疑活动性出血，并且初始诊断性血管造影术并不能定位病变，那么有必要采取激进性血管造影揭示造影剂外渗。最常用的药物是硝酸甘油、肝素或组织纤溶酶原激活剂。硝酸甘油在创伤情况中是最安全的，因为它的半衰期为 3min。硝酸甘油帮助介入医师确定潜在的危及生命的出血，并且作用时间足够短暂，通常不会引起进一步的血流动力学性死亡。如果在激进性血管造影术之后存在差异，或者在没有 CTA 的情况下临床上高度怀疑出血，则可以进行预防性栓塞。然而，重要的是考虑动脉出血的自发停止，或出血可能来自静脉。

在执行诊断和治疗性血管造影术之前，建立动脉通路非常重要。在创伤情况中最常见的动脉通路部位是正常的股动脉（common femoral artery，CFA），因为其位置表浅。如果不能建立 CFA 通路，可以建立对侧通路或肱动脉通路。在股骨头下 1/3 建立 CFA 通路，以便在操作终止时进行按压。触诊后，微穿刺针穿过动脉前壁以 45° 进针，直到出现血液回流。如果在 CFA 的分叉远端建立通路，按压可能变得困难。此外，医源性动静脉瘘（AVF）可以使 CFA 通路复杂化，因为在该水平股静脉位于动脉后面。如果不能建立 CFA 通路，可以建立肱动脉通路。由于必须通过椎动脉和颈动脉，所以肱动脉通路具有确定的卒中风险（0.5%）。此外，血肿的风险略有增加，这在上肢有潜在的不利后果。压迫性血肿有发生内侧肱间隔综合征和周围神经损伤的风险。最后，左侧肱动脉应优先于右侧，因为只有一条脑血管与此通路相交。

血管造影在很大程度上取决于 CTA 的预评估结果。如果已经进行 CTA，则可以首先进行选择性血管造影，以鉴定 CTA 诊断的已知或疑似血管损伤。选择性血管造影后，应始终执行非选择性血管造影以识别未确诊的血管病变，并确保没有其他活动性出血部位。在不稳定的骨盆创伤患者，CTA 常常无法使用，应首先实施非选择性血管造影，为更有选择性的动脉造影提供走行图。

非选择性主动脉造影不仅为内脏脉管系统提供了走行图，还可能显示潜在的对于栓塞有重要意义的解剖学侧支通路。这些侧支通路虽然罕见，但可能会为活动性出血提供持续的血流，因此对其识别很重要。另外，在随后可能进行的手术中，这些侧支通路在创伤患者的手术中可能是重要的。Buhler 动脉弓是腹主动脉和肠系膜上动脉（superior mesenteric artery，SMA）之间的胚胎期交通，其通过背侧胰动脉延续。Barkow 动脉弓代表腹主动脉和 SMA 通过网膜动脉的交通。来自胃十二指肠和脾动脉的右和左胃网膜动脉分别给大网膜导入侧支血流。另外，横向胰腺和中间结肠动脉（来自 SMA）的后部网膜动脉给大网膜供血，并与胃网膜动脉连接，从而形成动脉 Barkow 弓。虽然在创伤情况下不太重要，但是 Riolan 动脉弓代表 SMA 通过近端中部结肠动脉和近端左侧结肠动脉的中心连接与肠系膜下动脉交通。

治疗性血管造影

当怀疑血管损伤时，可以使用大量的手段，需要良好的血管造影技术基础。本章讨论的主要装置是支架移植物、闭塞气囊和栓塞剂（液体和固体）。支架移植物可用于动脉止血以及恢复远端器官和组织的天然动脉血流。成功利用支架移植物需要合适的动脉，因此不能用于所有的血管病变。血管至少为 5 mm 或更大，并且走行相对较直。由于存在发生移位的风险，弯曲血管不适合做支架移植。此外，由于类似的原因和分支闭塞的风险，支架移植不适合于分叉血管。由于新生内膜增生可导致支架内狭窄，故也应避免应用于年轻患者。支架移植的理想动脉包括髂外和浅表股动脉。闭塞气囊通常用做手术的临时辅助措施或作为快速失血的确定性血管内治疗。

对栓塞可以使用线圈、血管塞、明胶海绵脱脂棉、颗粒、液体栓塞剂或上述器材的组合。线圈通过诱发血栓形成而不是机械阻塞进行栓塞，通过掺入线圈中的涤纶羊毛尾巴增强血栓形成作用。这些器材在近端栓塞中非常有效，也可用于三明治技术。三明治技术通常用于可能存在侧支的区域，如肝动脉或脾动脉损伤。在肝动脉破裂或脾动脉孤立性假性动脉瘤的不连续流动情况下，三明治技术很有用。线圈和血管塞也可用于其他栓塞剂难以治疗的 AVF 或出血病例。可分离的微线圈可允许准确的针尖栓塞，这是治疗潜在的血管损伤同时保持正常组织灌注的关键，特别是在终末血管器官的损伤，例如肾损伤的情况下（图 2）。线栓 / 血管塞的主要缺点是，一旦进行近端栓塞，进入血管的远端血流就被阻止，

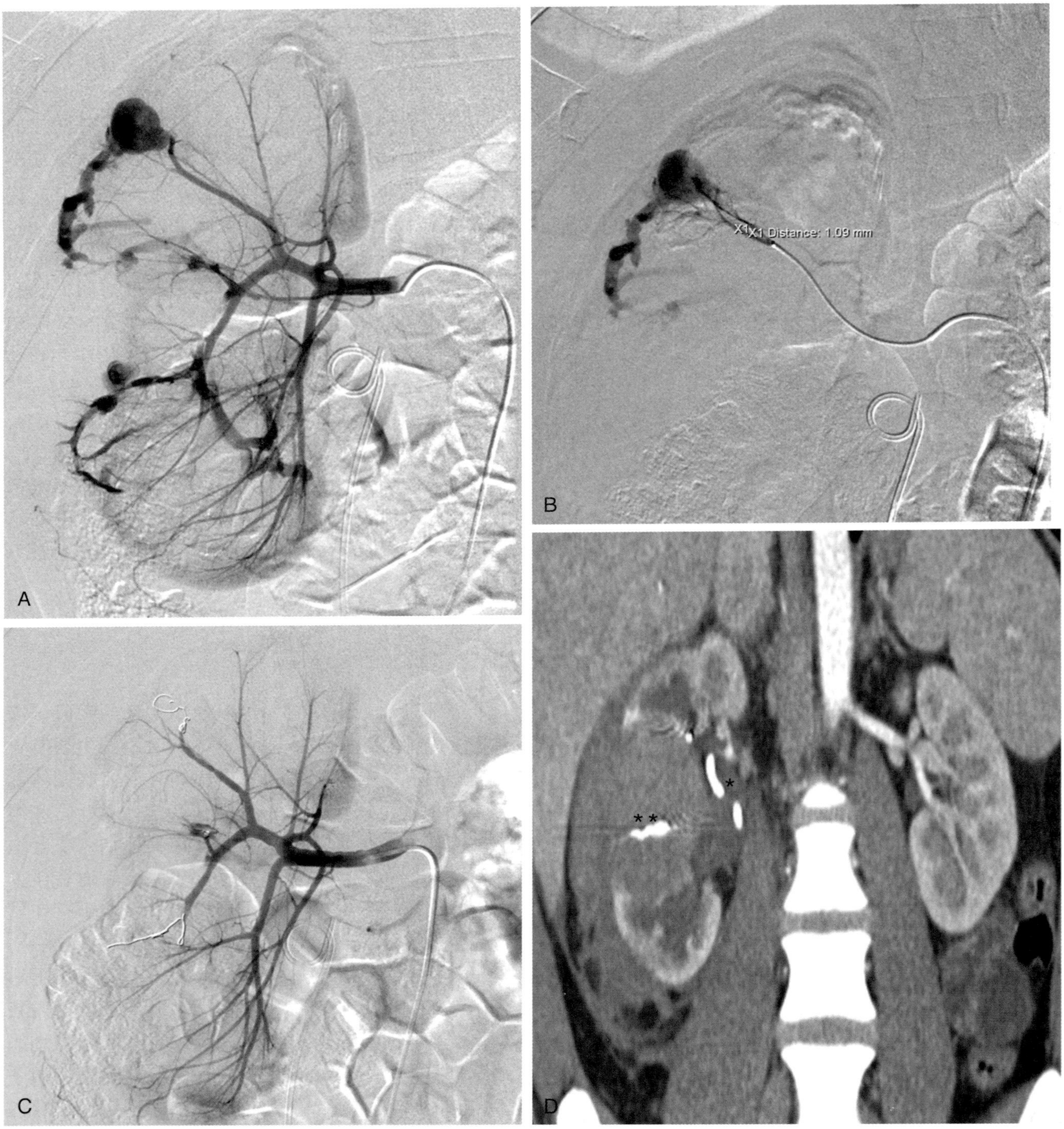

图 2 **A**，选择性右肾血管造影显示多个动静脉瘘和胸膜内假性动脉瘤。**B**，超选择性间质动脉造影显示了一个明确的假性动脉瘤和相通的动静脉瘘。**C**，可分离的微线圈超选择性栓塞后右侧肾血管造影显示，先前的假性动脉瘤和动静脉瘘已经解决。**D**，随访对比 CT 显示未涉及的肾实质和两极间实质内血肿维持灌注。注意输尿管支架（单星号）和微孔（双星号）

因此不可能重复血管内介入。

明胶海绵是另一种栓塞剂，具有水溶性并且可以快速备用。它是临时栓塞剂，可以被身体完全吸收。动脉血管通常在 2 ~ 3 周内再通。它在多个假性血管瘤区域被有效使用，被广泛应用于盆腔创伤，沿着动脉血流远端快速封闭活动性出血。

有时将栓塞颗粒用于创伤。颗粒有许多不同的尺寸，然而，创伤中使用的尺寸范围为 500 ~ 700 μm 和 700 ~ 900 μm。虽然不经常使用，液体剂也是非常有效的栓塞材料。氰基丙烯酸丁酯或 NBCA 通常称为液体黏合剂或胶水，在与离子化流体如血液接触时立即聚合。放热反应导致胶体形成，从而破坏了血管壁，因此不适用于能用微导管进入的较小血管。一旦注射了胶水，必须迅速将导管从血管腔移开，以防止导管与血管壁粘连。颗粒和液体栓塞是永久性远端栓塞剂，并且存在组织缺血的潜在风险，特别是如果存在毛细血管床闭塞。一般避免在脾和下臀动脉中使用液体和颗粒状栓塞剂，以降低脓肿和坐骨神经损伤的发生率。

表 1 内脏动脉血管

血管	动脉变异	频率
	腹部来源的左胃动脉、普通肝动脉和脾动脉	70%
腹部的	左胃动脉，普通肝动脉常见，背侧胰腺动脉，腹腔来源的脾动脉	10%
	主动脉起源的左胃动脉	2%
	腹部来源的左胃动脉和脾动脉	3%
	普通肝动脉来源的右肝动脉和左肝动脉	55%
	替代的右肝动脉	12%
肝的	右肝动脉属支	6%
	替代的左肝动脉	11%
	左肝动脉属支	11%
	右肝动脉起源于肠系膜上动脉，左肝动脉源自左胃动脉	2%

Modified from kaufman JA. Kaufman JA: Fundamentals of angiography. In Kaufman JA, Michael JL, editors: The requisites: vascular and interventional radiology, Philadephia, Mosby, 2004, pp 31 - 66

介入医师的陷阱

即使是最有经验的介入放射科医师也可能遇到陷阱。理解正常内脏和盆腔脉管系统的潜在变异对于掌握并可能防止治疗失败至关重要。只有 70%的患者表现为腹主动脉的传统解剖。虽然在 95%的患者中，肝动脉来自腹主动脉，然而仅有 55%的人肝的动脉脉管系统没有解剖变异。虽然内脏和盆腔脉管系统存在许多变化，但是在寻找血管造影外渗时，三个主要的异常最重要（表 1）。首先，10%的患者背侧胰腺动脉来源于腹主动脉，不应将其误认为是出血。其次，12%患者的右肝叶由替代的右肝动脉供血，来源于 SMA。在这种情况下，须要对 SMA 进行选择性动脉造影来排除右肝叶的出血。最后，在盆腔血管造影术中，多数情况下闭孔动脉来源于股动脉，在 20%的患者来源于腹壁下动脉，须要对髂外动脉进行选择性血管造影。初步的非选择性血管造影或先前的 CTA 成像通常足以诊断这些异常。

对血管造影的解释也是潜在的问题根源。在男性患者的盆腔血管造影中，重要的是区分活动性外渗和海绵体的干扰。差异可能是微小的，但阴茎动脉栓塞造成的后果很严重，尤其是在年轻患者。重要的是，海绵体的干扰通常在耻骨联合或低于耻骨联合的中线，来自阴部内动脉，并完全洗出，但活动性外渗将持续整个延迟期。另一个潜在的陷阱是小动脉被阻塞性血栓的阻断。这些病变也可能非常微小，然而，如果不仔细检查血管造影，可能容易错过动脉阻断。最终，了解血管造影的局限性以及可能发生的假阴性结果至关重要。如前所述，患者的血流动力学状态显著影响诊断性血管造影的表现。血管痉挛可能暂时使活动性出血停止，如果没有发现外渗，延迟出血可能在远期导致患者死亡。

实质脏器损伤

脾损伤

脾是钝性腹部创伤中最常受伤的腹部器官。事实上，97%的创伤外科医师认为血流动力学不稳定可能是钝性脾损伤的脾切除术适应证。然而，现行的对血流动力学稳定脾损伤患者的标准是采取非手术治疗。非手术治疗失败发生于 12% ~ 15%的脾创伤，已经表明早期栓塞可以降低这个发生率。栓塞对脾挽救有额外的益处，报告显示挽救率在 85%以上。然而，脾损伤的血管造影或栓塞的适应证并不统一。有人主张为所有的脾损伤提供血管造影，但其他人认为血管造影适用于高分级实质器官损伤、CTA 提示的血管损伤和大量腹腔积血。

可以在脾动脉或实质内分支远端进行脾栓塞，或将两者相结合。许多介入治疗者偏向于近端栓塞，尽管近端栓塞和远端栓塞的结果相似。近端技术通过阻塞入脾血流，降低脾的动脉压来进行止血。由于保护侧支血流，其发生梗死的风险降低，然而，栓塞后脾的整体功能受到担忧，因为脾整体缺血。近端技术用于多种血管损伤或高分级实质损伤。线圈或血管塞通常部署在远离胰血管的脾动脉中。远端栓塞用于孤立性血管损伤或低分级脾损伤患者。远端技术的主要优点是保留脾功能。通常使用明胶海绵浆液，因为理论上临时药物的脓肿形成风险低于永久性栓塞剂（如颗粒）的风险。

脾干预不是没有风险的，包括远端和近端技术的并发症的发生率高达 35%。虽然并发症比较常见，但对脾补救成功率没有不利影响。脾梗死的定义为去血管化大于 25%，是最常见的并发症，发生在 20%的患者中，并且在远端栓塞中更常见。大多数脾梗死是无症状的，可以采取非手术治疗，无后遗症。最常见的主要并发症是出血（11%），经常须要重新栓塞或脾切除术。另一个较为常见的并发症是脓肿形成。如果早期发现，脓肿腔可以经皮排出或可能须要手术修复。联合栓塞技术和使用颗粒时，常常遇到脓肿并发症。近端栓塞技术具有的独特的晚期后遗症不见于远端栓塞，胃黏膜的 Dieulafoy 型病变可能导致肥厚的短胃血管。这是由脾动脉侧支引起的慢性并发症，不见于急性情况。胰腺和胃壁梗死是非常罕见的，因为内脏脉管系统具有极大的储备能力，通过短的胃动脉和周围脉管系统提供侧支血流。

肝损伤

肝是钝性伤中第二个容易受伤的腹部器官。由于肝的外分泌功能及其解剖复杂性，存在发生并发症的重大风险，因为创伤可引起静脉、动脉甚至胆管损伤。因此，超过 85%的创伤相关肝损伤受到某种干预治疗。大多数肝出血来自低压静脉出血，但是动脉和胆管损伤对介入医师来说是最重要的。Asensio 等描述了治疗复杂肝损伤 AAST Ⅳ和Ⅵ分级法，这是一种多学科方法。众所周知，AAST 分级损伤增加了动脉和胆管损伤的风险，提示有必要早期干预。此外，高分级肝损伤和血流动力学不稳定通常须要多学科手术和血管内干预，首先进行手术治疗，术后辅助栓塞治疗剩余的动脉出血。

因为与创伤相关的并发症有重叠，尚不清楚栓塞和随后的肝相关并发症的发病率。然而，栓塞对严重肝损伤的疗效显著，成功率为 85% ~100%，死亡率显著改善。此外，最近的研究已经证明，使用或不使用栓塞的肝发病率没有显著差异。用于肝创伤的栓塞技术与用于脾创伤的技术相似。由于肝动脉系统有丰富的侧支网络，夹心技术（见治疗性血管造影）在肝创伤中更频繁地使用。线圈栓塞和液体栓塞剂也常被用于肝。

与肝创伤相关的并发症可分为早期和晚期表现。持续性出血是最常见的早期并发症，可发生于高达 9%的保守治疗患者。在患者的复查 CTA（参考以前的 CTA）中区分活动性出血和延迟出血很重要。对主动脉出血可以采取栓塞治疗，但延迟出血可能须要手术治疗。肝创伤的晚期表现包括胆道瘘、脓肿形成和胆道出血。导致胆汁漏出或胆汁瘤的胆管损伤发生在 14%的高度肝损伤患者。经皮成像引流引流对胆管瘘治疗至关重要，是首选的治疗方法。内镜逆行胰胆管造影（ERCP）下胆管支架置入通常用于难以经皮治疗或胆汁渗漏明显的患者。最终目标是减少相邻组织的压力，以防止坏死并允许胆汁充分引流。通常情况下，患者平均需要 4 周才能完全修复胆道。每天监测引流管，引流量一般会在几周内下降。引流量很少提示胆汁流入十二指肠，并表明胆管已完全愈合。这时可以拔出引流管。在胆汁引流时间超过 6 周的患者中应考虑使用 ERCP 双重引流。脓肿形成也可能使肝创伤复杂化。脓肿代表周围组织高压力的实质内积液后遗症，导致坏死，最终导致脓肿。成像引导经皮引流是治疗脓肿形成的首选。

胆道出血患者的严重并发症通常发生的病程较晚。这是深部动脉损伤的结果，通常是假性动脉瘤连通或破裂到胆道中，导致大量凝块负荷、阻塞性胆管炎和可能的放血。未经治疗的胆道出血的死亡率达 60%，因此须要进行紧急血管造影和栓塞。最后，胆囊和胆道坏死在创伤情况中很少见，与肝细胞癌（hepatocellular carcinoma，HCC）的肝动脉栓塞不同。可能是由于多数创伤患者肝实质正常并保留侧支循环。有肝硬化或肝硬化史的创伤患者发生胆囊坏死的风险可能会增加，应予以高度关注。

肾损伤

在钝性创伤中肾损伤的发生率约为2%，钝性肾动脉损伤更少，见于不足于1%的钝性创伤患者。肾损伤几乎从来不单发于钝性创伤，一般是脾和肝先受伤。大多数肾损伤较轻。超过80%的肾损伤是小血肿或具有包膜完整的撕裂，可以保守治疗。在肾撕裂的患者中，17%的患者损伤超过包膜，其中7%与集合系统连通，可能须要干预。高危人群患有肾功能异常、肾血管性高血压甚至肾衰竭。因此，虽然对肾损伤的治疗没有达成共识，但高分级肾损伤通常需要干预。对Ⅱ级至Ⅳ级实质性损伤采取以血管造影或手术的多学科方法进行治疗，力图保留肾，对Ⅴ级实质损伤多采取手术，多为肾切除术。

肾血管系统与肝或脾不同。肾由于侧支循环不丰富，依靠末端动脉供应血液。虽然近端栓塞和三明治技术在肝和脾中有利，但在肾中需要其他方法来保护肾功能。随后开发了周围栓塞技术，尽可能选择性地进行远端栓塞。这些技术通常需要微型导管同轴方法，以获得尽可能高的选择性，并将发生实质性梗死的风险降至最低。微血管和液体栓塞，如NBCA，通常用于这些实质内动脉损伤。近十年的检查显示，当作为主要治疗时，栓塞的成功率为94%。与栓塞相关的严重并发症很少见。肾梗死是一种比较常见的现象，但一般没有不良后遗症。由梗死发展而来的肾脓肿不足5%。

主要肾动脉的外伤性损伤可导致肾动脉撕裂、内膜夹层，甚至血栓形成而导致急性动脉血流中断。内膜夹层可以进展为非闭塞性撕脱，进一步进展到闭塞性撕脱和血栓形成，导致实质细胞死亡。因此，在肾动脉内膜损伤/撕脱患者中，肾动脉支架置入术是一个合理的选择，特别是在存在压力梯度或者血管性高血压的患者。通常，涂覆或裸金属支架具有良好的1年主要通畅率。肾动脉截断表明动脉横断和阻塞性血栓形成，对这些病变应该单独对待，因为不稳定的血栓可能移位，而导致腹膜后出血。虽然一些介入医师可能会采用激进性血管造影术，但在我们的经验中，对这些病变最好采取保守治疗。一旦患者的状况稳定下来，可以对梗死的肾进行肾切除术。在某些情况下，一旦临床状况改善，多发伤患者或手术风险较高的患者可能须要进行主要肾动脉栓塞，作为确定性治疗或间隔肾切除术的后续治疗。

最后，活动性出血和实质血肿可能导致尿路集合系统明显的凝块负担，随后可能引起尿路阻塞。通常须要置入Foley导管和持续膀胱冲洗，可以使用或不使用膀胱镜支架置入，成功率良好。在输尿管有严重凝块负担的复杂病例，可能须要经皮肾造瘘以对集合系统减压。此外，肾周血肿可引起外源性肾压迫，即所谓的肾周间隔综合征，可在超声引导下经皮引流治疗。

骨盆创伤

由于骨盆带的解剖限制和邻近骨结构，血管损伤在盆腔创伤中相对较为常见，并且是导致该组患者死亡率高达25%以上的原因。骨盆出血大部分是由静脉、骨质和动脉出血引起的。骨盆固定可以成功地控制静脉和骨出血，然而，危及生命的动脉出血不能被压迫止血。事实上，据报道，10%～15%的骨盆出血是由于动脉损伤引起的。一旦发现动脉出血，死亡率就会大大增加。由于骨盆容积的潜在增加特性，骨盆骨折导致高达20%患者的血流动力学不稳定。

骨盆骨折是由横向压迫、前后压迫、垂直剪切或组合机制造成的。对前后压迫、垂直剪切力和组合机制单独采用骨盆固定的失败率更高，通常须要血管造影。此外，盆腔创伤栓塞的成功率超过87%。因此，栓塞已经发展成为盆腔创伤初次止血的先锋，已成为许多机构的治疗标准。活动性外渗或血流动力学不稳定的骨盆骨折患者是血管造影栓塞的候选者。

髂内动脉（internal iliac artery，ⅡA）的分支是盆腔创伤中最常受损的动脉血管（图3）。来自ⅡA后分支的臀上动脉的损伤最为常见，其次是来自前分支的阴部内动脉。对栓塞通常用明胶海绵浆液或线圈控制出血。由于存在大肠神经损伤和黏膜剥落的风险，通常在骨盆中避免使用脱水乙醇。在血流动力学不稳定的患者中，由于深度血管痉挛，可能难以识别血管造影对比剂外渗。如果没有发现外渗，并且没有激进性血管造影的指征，可以进行预防性近端IIA栓塞。确定骨盆骨折的一侧，随后用明胶海绵或线圈进行同侧IIA栓塞。在某些临床情况下可能须要双侧预防性IIA栓塞。这能有效地治疗动脉出血，并间接停止骨盆静脉和骨源的出血。在这种方法中，发生臀部跛行和坏死的风险显著增加，

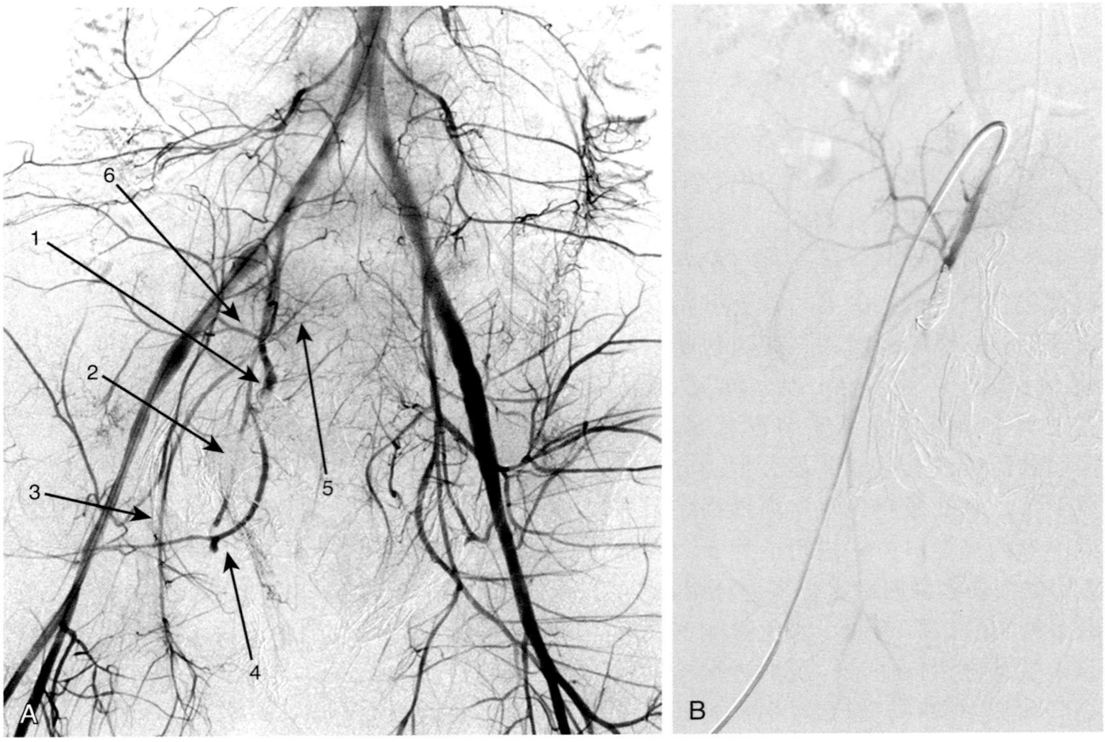

图 3 **A**，盆腔血管造影显示主要是右侧盆腔血管损伤（按伤害发生率减少编号）：①右臀上（后），被截断；②右阴部内（前），表现为截断和痉挛；③右闭孔（前）；④臀下（前），表现为小的假性动脉瘤；⑤右侧骶骨（后）；⑥右髂腰（后）。**B**，选择性右髂内栓塞血管造影显示臀下、阴部内及臀大动脉的微线圈闭塞，以及闭孔、侧骶骨和髂腰动脉

因而只能在特定情况下采用。

髂外动脉（external iliac artery，EIA）也可能在盆腔创伤中受伤。最常见的损伤类型是内膜损伤导致撕脱，透壁性损伤导致活动性外渗。对 EIA 撕脱采用裸金属支架治疗。最关键的是确保支架置入后涵盖入口和再入口。在再入口位置的支架可导致进一步的撕脱甚至破裂，因为这是动脉壁最薄弱的地方。如果病变可以穿过，可以用涂覆支架移植物治疗 EIA 出血。 EIA 支架的 1 年通畅率超过 90%。这些患者的预后通常遵循简单过程。在 EIA 横断的特殊临床情况下，临时血管内气囊可以是手术血管重建之前的抢救手段。

考虑到盆腔创伤有较高的死亡率，血管造影栓塞的并发症通常可以接受。此外，与肝一样，大多数并发症难以与实际创伤相关的并发症区分开来。臀部坏死可以在单侧 IIA 栓塞中看到，并且在 IIA 的双侧栓塞中更经常遇到。约 10% 的骨盆创伤可见皮肤溃疡和坏死。最近的研究表明，栓塞和非栓塞患者之间在皮肤坏死、脱落或会阴感染率上无明显差异。阳痿和不育也是阴部内动脉栓塞的潜在风险，尽管没有长期的研究来评估这一点。必须注意不要将腮红误认为外渗，因为如果发生栓塞，可能会增加阳痿和不孕的风险。

下腔静脉过滤器预防栓塞

肺栓塞（PE）和深静脉血栓形成（DVT）在创伤人群中的发病率高，报道高达 15%。Virchow 的静脉淤滞、血管壁损伤和凝血功能增加三联征，使患者发生 DVT 和 PE 的风险增加，创伤患者表现为这些特征性症状。IVC 过滤器对肺栓塞的治疗无效，不防止 DVT，在复发性肺栓塞时中断静脉血流。传统上，IVC 过滤器放置通常在诊断为肺栓塞和抗凝禁忌证的患者中使用。由于创伤和 DVT / PE 的高度关联，预防性 IVC 过滤器被放置的频率越来越高。目前，预防性 IVC 过滤器有两种适应证：①发生肺栓塞风险高的多发性损伤患者。②有 PE / DVT 病史和 DVT 术后风险大的外科手术患者。

通常将 IVC 滤器放置在肾静脉的最下方，通常在 L3 椎体水平。在放置过滤器之前，通常获得下腔静脉图，以确保 IVC 的通畅并筛选解剖变体。虽然静脉异常罕见，但介入医师必须认识包括环主动脉左肾静脉、主动脉后左肾静脉、重复IVC、左侧IVC和巨型腔静脉。在环主动脉左肾静脉的情况下，必须在上面放置IVC过滤器。通常在下腔静脉插入主动脉后肾静脉，这也影响过滤器的置入。重复的IVC须要在每个IVC中安装双重过滤器。左侧IVC是重要的，因为血管造影显示不同，并且于荧光透视下在技术上可能更难置入。最后，直径超过30mm的IVC的定义为巨腔静脉，须要放置较大的鸟巢过滤器，或者在双侧髂总静脉放置过滤器。通过超声技术的最新进展，通过血管内超声引导，使执行床旁IVC滤器变得更加可行。

应该仔细考虑过滤器的类型和未来管理，因为IVC过滤器促进血栓形成。创伤患者仅暂时处于高凝状态，急性期外不需要血栓栓塞的保护。此外，创伤患者总的来说是一个年轻的患者群体，其中栓子导致的IVC阻塞可导致显著的发病率。随后，在创伤情况中优选可撤出的IVC过滤器，在3～6个月内撤出以防止内膜融合。

小结

总之，介入放射学在腹部和盆腔创伤的诊断、治疗和治疗中具有关键作用。对创伤患者评估的主要目标是快速鉴定潜在危及生命的出血和早期干预。在非手术和手术治疗方案中使用介入技术，用于血流动力学稳定和不稳定的患者。血液造影术和手术在提供止血方面效果好，通常需要多学科的方法。在某些临床情况下，血管造影甚至可以被认为是手术的替代方法。

鉴于许多创伤性损伤的复杂性，往往是多重损伤，因此必须了解这种介入技术的适应证，并且必须对可能需要进一步干预的不可避免的创伤相关并发症做好防备。在介入放射学中，应重视设计更新的血管造影套件。这些套件正在集成到急诊室布局中，以便更容易置入。此外，一些领先机构正在将CT机器与血管造影术套件相结合，以减少诊断与干预之间的延误。最终，随着介入放射学领域的进展，须要对针对创伤患者的技术进行进一步的研究和调查，不仅允许早期干预，而且可以推进患者护理，并提供最安全、最有效的治疗方法。

复苏的终点

Susan Rowell, Ronald Barbosa, Michael Englehart, Brandon Tieu, Martin Schreiber 著
易成腊 译

自20世纪初以来，Walter Cannon医师提出了有限体积复苏的争议观点，复苏的最佳终点一直存在争论，仍然是一个讨论和研究的话题。复苏的理想终点应该容易获得、易于解释并与临床结果直接相关。目标是提供足够的氧气输送（DO_2）和组织灌注，而不会产生过度复苏的并发症。这主要是通过增加前负荷（体积负荷）或血管活性药物来增加心输出量。已经使用多重诊断标准来确定最佳心脏性能和足够的组织灌注。尽管不能单独使用任何检验结果，但是在比较复苏的充分性时，可以进行多种测量。这些值提供了随着时间的推移来确定患者是否被正确复苏的能力。它们可以分为血流动力学参数、代谢参数和区域灌注终点。

临床和血流动力学终点

休克有多种定义方式，但最好描述为缺乏足够的组织灌注、氧气输送和废物的清除受损。用于识别休克的六项基本高级创伤生命支持生理参数是心率、呼吸频率、血压、尿量、意识状况和脉压。尿液输出和意识水平与组织灌注直接相关，包含在每一类休克的定义中。肾血流量与动脉压有关，但在灌注不足期间可能会出现明显的自体调节作用。受中毒、中枢神经系统损伤和药物治疗影响时，意识水平较低。众所周知，心率和呼吸频率容易误导（表1）。焦虑、疼痛和继发于创伤的情绪影响可能会错误地提高这些生理参数。这可能会混淆表现并掩盖潜在的休克严重性。临床研究和动物模型均表明，经常存在系统循环与微循环之间的某种程度的分离。生命体征相对正常并不能保证区域灌注足够。最好通过观察身体的主要补偿机制诊断休克：血流的再分配。

表 1 休克程度与脉率的关系（106 例）

脉搏频率	休克程度 * 没有 (n513)	轻度 (n524)	中度 (n534)	重度 (n535)
最小值	70	88	80	60
最大值	140	150	160	144
平均值	1037.2	1113.4	1133.6	1163.3

Modified from The Physiologic Effect of Wounds. Washington, DC, Office of the Surgeon General, 1952.

*这些数据在第二次世界大战期间在北非 - 地中海区域收集。尽管休克的严重程度有明显差异，但组间差异无显著性。轻度休克为占正常血容量的 80%，中度休克占正常血容量的 70%，严重休克占正常血容量的 55%

由于条件严峻及无法测量血压，美国在伊拉克自由行动和持续自由行动中的作战医疗已经接受了培训，使患者复苏直到有意识，或者无法评估意识时，直到可触及桡动脉脉搏。目前的英国陆军指南还包括复苏直到可触及桡动脉搏动。在第一次世界大战期间，Cannon 指出，75 mmHg 是维持生命的关键收缩压。然而，许多人主张避免严重脑损伤患者的血压过低，以确保足够的脑灌注压力。低血压的存在预示着头部受伤后更糟糕的结果。此外，尽管有“正常”的平均动脉压（MAP），但先前高血压的患者可能会出现器官灌注不足的症状。由于患者预先存在的疾病状态与损伤严重程度的复杂相互作用，不幸的是，没有统一的“目标”MAP 来确定充分的复苏。

氧气输送是血红蛋白浓度、氧饱和度和心输出量的功能参数。血红蛋白浓度和氧浓度相对容易操作和监测，但心输出量可能更有问题。足够的心脏性能主要是前负荷。已经设计了多种方法，通过评估心脏的静脉回流来间接地估计患者的血容量状态。随着中心静脉和肺动脉导管（PAC）的引入，中心静脉压（CVP）和肺动脉闭塞压力（PAOP）已被用作容量状态的测量。虽然这些测量值用于指导复苏，但对绝对值应谨慎地解释。瓣膜性或全身心脏功能障碍以及限制性肺部疾病可以显著地改变这些数值。使用机械通气，特别是当将压力设置得很高时，也会使 CVP 和 PAOP 更难解读。由于传感器归零的差异或测量呼吸和心脏周期中相同参考点压力的失败，也可能在观察者之间引入相当大的变异性。

较新的容量或血氧 PAC 具有动态测量先前无法获得的额外血流动力学参数的能力。由于使用加热细丝的导管的发展来获得测量值，可以连续监测心输出量。可以使用心室功能和舒张末期容积指数来评估心脏功能。最近的一项研究表明，右心室舒张末期容积指数（RVEDVI）是比 CVP 或 PAOP 更敏感的前负荷数值，特别是在机械通气患者。Cheatham 等证实，相比 PAOP，心脏指数（CI）与 RVEDVI 的相关性更好，即使处于极高的呼气末正压水平。在 RVEDVI 与创伤患者内脏灌注的比较中，Miller 等和 Chang 等发现，休克期间 RVEDVI>120 ml/m^2 的复苏与更好的预后相关。其他研究也显示出类似的优点。然而，使用这些技术需要重大的机构承诺，可能因为仅少数患者受益于这种监测而被禁止。

尽管 PAC 取得了进展，但自 20 世纪 90 年代中期以来，其效用一直存在疑问。Connors 等发表了一项观察性研究，表明 PAC 与死亡率增加和资源利用率相关。尽管有研究的局限性，置入 PAC 的危重患者在 30 天、60 天和 180 天的死亡率更高，医院成本增加，在重症监护病房（ICU）的停留时间更长。在最近包括 5051 名医学和外科 ICU 患者的 Meta 分析，13 项评估 PAC 的随机对照试验显示，PAC 的使用并不能改善住院时间或减少住院时间。在放置 PAC 的患者中没有显示出死亡风险增加。最近的研究表明，PAC 的使用在美国普遍下降，特别是在创伤患者中。总体而言，这些数据表明 PAC 不应该在外科 ICU 患者中常规使用，除非可以发现在与该诊断工具结合使用时可以改善结果的有效疗法。

脉冲轮廓导出的 CO 测量（pulse contour-derived CO measurement，PCCO）还可以连续测量心输出

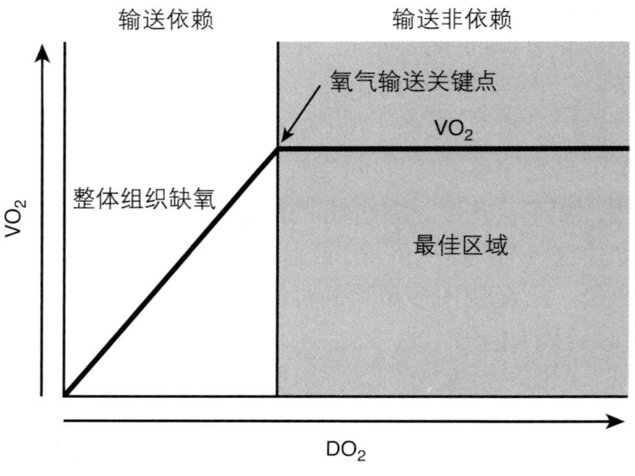

图 1 氧气输送（DO_2）和氧气提取（VO_2）之间的关系

量，并与热稀释测量结果良好相关。PCCO 须要在隔膜的对侧放置动脉导管和中心静脉导管。它可能比 CVP 或 PAOP 能更准确地反映心脏前负荷。不幸的是，血流动力学状态的快速变化可能改变监测，有必要重新校准。

许多人试图定义氧气消耗 / 输送终点本身，但没有明确的结果。Fick 方程式表明 DO_2 和 VO_2 是 CI、血红蛋白（Hb）以及动脉和静脉血氧饱和度（SaO_2 和 SvO_2）的函数。

$$Do_2 = CI \times 13.4 \times Hb \times Sao_2$$
$$Vo_2 = CI \times 13.4 \times Hb \times (Sao_2 - Svo_2)$$

不幸的是，DO_2 和 VO_2 均来自心输出量，实际上图 1 中描述的稳定平台不可能获得。目标导向治疗旨在确保 CI＞4.5 L/（min · m^2），DO_2 指数＞600 ml/（min · m^2），VO_2 指数大于 170 ml/（min · m^2）。这是由 Shoemaker 等提出的，证明与重症患者的发病率和死亡率降低有关。然而，Gattinoni 的多中心随机对照试验以及 Heyland 的 Meta 分析显示没有这样的益处。此外，Velmahos 的一项前瞻性随机对照试验比较了常规与超常规终点，显示尽管做出所有的努力，只有 70％的患者能够达到这些终点。他们得出结论，无论是什么复苏策略，患者实现“最佳血流动力学值”的能力都显著影响了结果。McKinley 等单独关注 O_2 输送，发现复苏至 600 ml/（min · m^2）的 O_2 输送与 500 ml/（min · m^2）的 O_2 输送之间无差异。

复苏至超常终点与许多并发症有关。Shoemaker 方案包括使用晶体和血液的容量负荷，以及使用多巴酚丁胺增强心输出量。由于减少组织灌注，通过血管活性药物改善血压和心脏功能可以产生负面效果，常常导致组织缺血。Hayes 等在医疗和外科危重患者中发现，使用多巴酚丁胺来增加氧气输送可能会增加死亡风险。晶体溶液过度复苏可导致心脏病患者发生室间综合征、凝血病和高血酸性酸中毒，以及发生其他医源性并发症如充血性心力衰竭。

已经开发了用于测量心脏性能的微创技术。胸部电生物阻抗测量胸部对低电压电流的阻力。它与胸腔液含量成反比，从而可以计算心输出量。几项研究表明，该方法与心输出量的热稀释测量值相关。然而，Meta 分析显示其在趋势分析中有临床效用，但用于诊断解释并不准确。这些方法在心动过速或病理性积液（如胸腔积液）中也有显著的不精确性。

经食管超声心动图可以评估前负荷和峰值速度，并进行连续心输出量监测，已经用热稀释技术进行了验证。在出血性休克的动物模型中，它准确反映了心输出量变化的幅度。Gunst 等最近还研究了床旁经胸超声心动图（TTE）。在这项研究中，进行过适度数量的超声心动图训练的创伤外科医师能够获得与 PAC 相似的 CI 的估计值。然而，TTE 的效用受到观察者间变异性和技术困难的限制，难以获得足够高质量的图像，特别是在仰卧位。Ferrada 等也使用 TTE 来测量下腔静脉直径和呼吸变化作为危重患者流体状态的量度。虽然在技术上可行，但是基于这些数据的干预措施还没有被证明有直接的临床益处。

在危重患者中研究了心率变异性（HRV），试图在标准血流动力学参数之前确定其有临床恶化风险的患者。HRV 基于以下观察：危重患者具有一定程度的自主神经功能障碍，其中除了其他因素外，还显示了心律减少的变化，无论是在几分钟还是在一小时的时间内。临床研究表明，HRV 降低的创伤患者死亡风险增加。心脏复杂度（heart rate complexity，HRC）也在创伤人群中进行了研究。HRC 是分析心率数据的不同方法，可以分析信号中的不规则度和随机程度。在 Cancio 等最近的一项研究中，HRC 增加与住院前插管的需求增加相关。虽然有些作者认为 HRV 和 HRC 可能被用做复苏的新生命体征，但由于多种原因尚未被广泛接受。首先，没有用于衡量或报告 HRV 和 HRC 的标准方法，并且大多数研究这些方法的机构都设计了自己的定制算法。此外，对数学观察背后的潜在生理机制了解甚少。另外，还不清楚 HRV 和 HRC 是否可以用做真正的复苏终点（即复苏后恢复正常 HRV 或 HRC 会获得更好的结果）。

代谢终点

可测量的代谢终点使得临床医师可有效地评估微循环。由于厌氧条件下可发生乳酸的积累，因此，乳酸是微循环氧输送不足的标志物，所以乳酸盐水平可以提供休克程度的量度。虽然乳酸水平升高提示休克程度恶化，但没有明确的临界值来确定“令人满意”的复苏和足够的氧气输送到组织。Manikas 等发现，乳酸盐初始和最高峰值以及高乳酸症持续时间与创伤后多器官功能障碍综合征的发展相关。随着时间的推移，乳酸盐清除率可能比数值更能预测死亡率。在 24 h 内清除（乳酸水平 <2 mmol/L）时，外伤患者的连续乳酸水平与 0～10%死亡率相关，如果在 24～48 h 内清除，死亡率为 25%，如果超过 48 h 清除，死亡率为 80% ～86%。

已经提出碱缺失是评估组织灌注减少的临床标志物，作为乳酸水平升高的方便的标志物。其定义为将 1 L 全血提升至正常 pH 所需的碱（mmol）量。Davis 首先按照严重程度划分碱缺失：轻度（2～5 mmol/L）、中度（6～14 mmol/L）和严重（>15 mmol/L）。缺失的严重程度与前 24 h 内需要的晶体和血液体积直接相关。已经表明，可能更容易测得的血清碳酸氢盐水平与碱缺失相关，但是受到患者通气状态的影响。与乳酸盐类似，通过绝对碱缺失可以估计休克的严重程度，但不能将单一值用做终点。持续高值或恶化的碱缺失可能是并发症的指标，如腹腔间隔综合征或活动性出血。已经证明更严重的碱缺失可预测氧消耗减少、多器官功能障碍综合征风险增加及死亡风险增加。然而，Brill 等（表 2）表明，继发于高氯酸中毒的碱缺失与死亡风险或并发症增加无关。对与高氯酸中毒真正相关的碱缺失升高的不准确判断可能导致不必要的干预措施，例如持续的液体复苏、输血或甚至手术干预。与乳酸盐一样，随着时间的推移，碱缺失的趋势在预测预后方面更有用。

表 2　高氯组 vs. 高及混合性负离子间隙

	高氯组	混合	
参数	组	组	*P* 值
患者数量	37	38	
平均年龄	53.9 ± 19.8	54.8 ± 22.9	0.85
男性 (%)	54	60	0.71
APACHE Ⅱ	12.2 ± 6.01	15 ± 7.5	0.10
平均SICU住院日	7.8 ± 6.9	10.4 ± 9.9	0.19
平均失血量估计 (ml)	1088 ± 1835	1343 ± 1930	0.61
平均复苏 (ml)	5598 ± 3950	6500 ± 5227	0.41
平均乳酸盐 (mg/dl)	1.5 ± 0.29	3.9 ± 2.2	<0.001
平均碱缺失 (mEq/l)	5.3 ± 2.5	7.8 ± 5.4	0.01
死亡	4	13	0.03

Modified from Brill SA, Stewart TR, Brundage SI, Schreiber MA: Base deficit does not predict mortality when secondary to hyperchloremic acidosis. Shock 17:459–462, 2002

注意：死亡率在 SICU 患者中显著下降，此时酰中毒是抗乳酸酰中毒的高氯性酸中毒 的继发性表现

混合静脉血氧饱和度（$S\bar{v}O_2$）已被用做复苏的终点，因为它随着 SaO_2、心输出量和血红蛋白的变化而直接变化。如数值下降表明组织缺氧。目前应用的脓毒症指南推荐 $S\bar{v}O_2$ 达到 70%或更高。尚不清楚出血性休克复苏的理想 SO_2。SO_2 的测量也须要放置 PAC。有学者研究了中心静脉血氧饱和度（$ScvO_2$），因为它仅须要放置中心静脉导线。测量的 $ScvO_2$ 值反映了上半身的静脉血氧饱和度，但被认为与 SO_2 值直接相关。然而，$S\bar{v}O_2$ 和 $ScvO_2$ 值的互换性仍然有争议。

区域灌注终点

已经开发了许多直接测量组织微循环的技术。它们包括胃黏膜测量、舌下二氧化碳监测和近红外光谱（near infrared spectroscopy，NIRS）。胃黏膜测量法通过测量组织 PCO_2 水平来监测胃黏膜内 pH（pHi）。内脏灌注降低时，pHi 降低。为了使该测试准确，须要禁止胃饲，抑制胃酸分泌。不幸的是，它与乳酸盐和碱缺乏相关性，并且校准时间延长。在研究中已经提出，较低的 pHi 与多器官功能障碍综合征的发展和死亡风险增加相关。舌下二氧化碳监测的前提是，整体组织低灌注引起全身性高碳酸血症。已经显示其与乳酸盐水平以及休克的严重程度相关，并已被用做死亡率的预测因子。

最后，NIRS 可用根据血红蛋白对红外线的吸收来确定外周组织氧饱和度（StO_2）（图 2）。NIRS 技术允许同时测量组织 PO_2、PCO_2 和 pH。在出血性休克的动物模型中，StO_2 与测量的氧气输送密切相关，并且与乳酸、碱剩余或 $S\bar{v}O_2$ 相比，能更好地衡量休克。McKinley 等发现，StO_2 与严重受伤创伤患者的氧气输送、碱缺失和乳酸盐水平相关。NIRS 还可以通过监测细胞色素 aa3 的氧化还原状态来监测线粒体功能，这反映了线粒体氧消耗。在正常条件下，组织氧合血红蛋白水平和细胞色素 aa3 水平紧密耦合。Cairns 等在 24 名严重受伤的创伤患者的研究中指出，多器官功能衰竭患者更容易去耦合。已经显示，StO_2 监测应用于院前环境在技术上可行，尽管其潜在作用尚不清楚。目前的 StO_2 装置还没有

得到广泛的应用，还没有建立起复苏的参数。

小结

总之，复苏的目标应该是优化前负荷、心脏功能、血压、氧气输送和终末器官灌注。不幸的是，没有单一的血流动力学指标或实验室测试普遍适用。最好的方法是整合和优化这些终点。鉴于休克仍然是临床诊断，最好在床边进行复苏评估，依靠体征和症状进行准确评估。

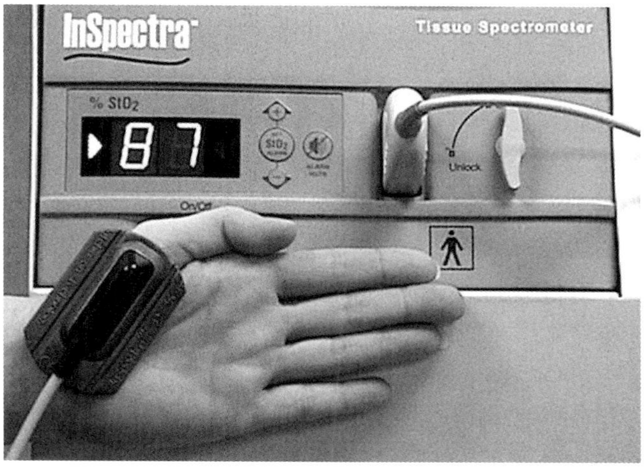

图 2　用近红外光谱测量仪检测组织氧饱和度。InSpectra 组织光谱仪可以用大鱼际遮挡，也可用三角肌遮挡

第 4 章　头部与中枢神经系统损伤

创伤性脑损伤：病理生理学、临床诊断及院前和急救中心的处置

Aileen Ebadat, Alex B. Valadka 著
魏颜芳 译

死亡、长期甚至永久性功能丧失使很多创伤性脑损伤（TBI）患者及其家庭不堪重负。即使初期根据临床及影像学诊断标准为损伤较轻的患者，也可能面临神经功能永久性缺陷，从而阻碍其恢复工作能力，以及重返丈夫或妻子、父母及经济支柱等家庭角色。

急诊开颅手术和颅内监护仪置入是治疗 TBI 患者最引人关注的方向。由于受损大脑较为脆弱，轻微一过性代谢紊乱也可能对 TBI 系统监测参数产生显著的影响。因此，在某些情况下，非神经外科医师对患者的处置方式比神经外科医师干预更为重要。

本节将讨论关于基础病理生理学、初期评估、院前和急诊中心对 TBI 患者处置的一些原则。下一节主讲述急性入院的相关课题，侧重于重度 TBI，但很多基本原则同样适用于轻中度 TBI 患者。

发生率

在多发伤患者中，头部是身体最常见的损伤部位。与其他器官系统损伤相比，多发伤的预后更多地取决于脑损伤程度。脑损伤的医疗和康复护理费用占全部治疗费用的 1/3 左右，并造成患者收入和社会生产力的损失。

根据 20 世纪 90 年代 CDC 的数据，每年 150 万美国人中就有 1 例 TBI 患者。据此推算，每年入院最终存活的患者约有 230 000 人，死亡 50 000 人。长期残疾 80 000 ~ 90 000 人。据估计，在美国已有超过 500 万男性、女性和小孩伴有永久性 TBI 相关性残疾生存。

车祸是导致 TBI 住院最常见的原因，然而暴力是导致 TBI 相关死亡的主要原因。跌倒是导致老年人 TBI 的主要原因。1990 年，在美国，头部枪伤超过跌倒致伤成为 TBI 相关死亡最常见的原因。

在美国，TBI 的死亡率大约为 20/100 000。在所有年龄组中，男性的死亡率高于女性，TBI 相关死亡发生率高峰在十几岁到二十几岁，在随后的几十年里递减，直到退休年龄呈指数飙升。

损伤机制

虽然硬膜外、硬膜下或者脑实质内血肿在 CT 扫描中有显著表现，但临床医师必须记住，这些表现与临床患者的实际神经功能损伤并不完全一致。在发生弥漫性脑实质功能障碍时应最先考虑到 TBI，而不是脑血栓和脑挫伤。弥漫性脑功能障碍可于随其他脑外伤同时出现，也可独立出现，并且多数可发展为占位性脑损伤。

硬脑膜下血肿

一般来说，硬膜下血肿被认为是桥静脉（即，直接穿过皮质到上覆硬脑膜的静脉）撕裂后发展而成。创伤的机械力会导致这些静脉发生撕裂而造成出血。最新的证据表明，实际上有些血肿形成是硬脑膜内层和外层的分离，因此，它们实际上是“硬膜内血肿”。此外，一些硬膜下血肿是由于脑实质

上血肿或受损的皮质动脉或静脉直接进入硬膜下引起的。

硬脑膜外血肿

硬膜外血肿通常出现在头部一侧受到打击后，薄弱的颞骨骨折导致脑膜中动脉瞬间撕裂所致。患者在遭受打击初期可能出现短暂的意识障碍，但很快恢复自主意识，因此脑损伤较轻。但不幸的是，颅骨骨折及可能撕裂脑膜中动脉。断裂的脑膜中动脉持续出血，产生不断增大的硬膜下血肿，从而表现为进行性加重的头痛以及意识障碍等症状。

从出现脑震荡到随后陷入昏迷，中间意识好转的时期一直被描述为“中间清醒期”。但颅骨骨折后不一定都会发生意识丧失（loss of consciousness，LOC），许多巨大硬膜外血肿的患者在最终昏迷之前始终保持清醒，而且很多硬膜外血肿与脑膜中动脉出血无关，而是颅骨骨折处的渗血。

因此，根据其损伤情况分析认为，在出血量大小相似的情况下，硬膜外血肿患者的症状比硬膜下血肿患者要轻。之所以出现这种情况，是因为单纯的硬膜外血肿在本质上是没有脑实质损伤的颅骨骨折渗血或脑膜动脉出血所致；而桥静脉撕裂被认为是导致硬膜下血肿的重要因素。在这种损伤机制中，剪切力的损害也可能引起弥漫性脑功能损伤，后文有论述。因此，硬膜下血肿与脑实质损伤更为密切相关，这就解释了硬膜下血肿预后更差的原因。当然，这个解释只适用于硬膜外血肿及硬膜下血肿在病理生理学范围内的结局，因为临床上有很多硬膜外血肿患者的情况很差，但一些硬膜下血肿患者往往可能伤后恢复良好。无论怎样，这是一种解释颅内占位性病变和弥漫性脑损伤之间相互作用的有效说法。

蛛网膜下腔出血

最常见的外伤性颅内出血不是占位性病变，而是弥漫性蛛网膜下腔出血（图1）。一些回顾性报道指出，创伤后蛛网膜下腔出血与较差的预后独立相关，但关联机制尚不明确。在急性期，蛛网膜下腔出血似乎对患者没有太大的影响，而临床上更关注脑实质本身的损伤问题。

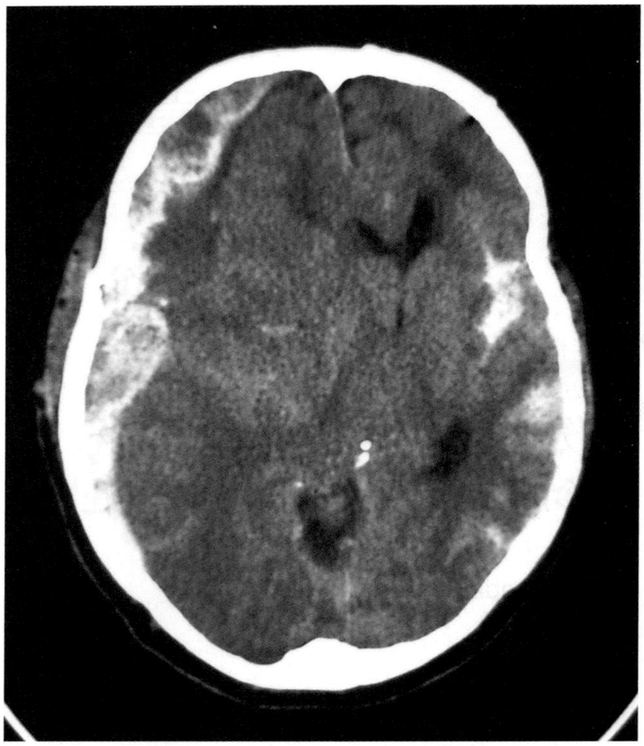

图1 较大的急性硬膜下血肿伴随中线移位。对侧蛛网膜下腔出血明显

脑实质损伤

挫伤通常发生在创伤性脑损伤之后，特别是额叶底部和颞叶前缘。在头部遭受暴力打击或快速旋转运动并突然停止时，该区域脑组织会持续向颅底方向移动并撞击颅底。幸运的是，这些挫伤很小，往往无须手术治疗。但当病变严重时或轻度损伤加重时，可能须要急诊手术。

脑内血肿不同于脑挫裂伤，是由固化血块和自身脑组织混合，发生率比挫伤小，但分布上往往更广泛。

缺血

弥漫性脑损伤可分为几种类型。缺血是弥漫性损伤的常见形式。在一些情况下，外伤性血肿的占位效应会引起颅内压增高和局部组织压迫，并导致脑血流灌注量全部和局部减少。特别是在受伤早期，没有占位病变时，创伤后脑缺血也会发生。在这些情况下，虽然CT扫描表现得较不明显，但患者很可能受这种继发性损伤如低血压和缺氧的影响。在随后的几小时和几天，脑灌注量通常增加，但是早期缺血性损害在脑灌注量增加之前就已经形成（图2）。一些研究中心已经利用氙CT或灌注CT来测量脑灌注量和识别损伤后立即缺血。

弥散性轴索损伤

弥漫性轴索损伤是大脑弥漫性损伤的另一种常见类型。虽然最具弥漫性轴索损伤特点的轴索断裂通常被认为发生在损伤时，但是只有当损伤产生严重的脑实质损伤时，这种轴突断裂才可能发生。相反，似乎更可能的是，在创伤过程中产生的旋转和机械力产生轴质流动造成局灶性损伤，进而在损伤后数小时内导致轴突断裂。由于这种短时间的损伤延迟产生，因而可能存在治疗时间窗，并给我们在研究保持轴索解剖和功能的完整上提供了希望。

当然，轴索损伤在CT扫描下无法看到。然而，弥漫性轴索损伤经常与剪应力伤所致的较小的散在脑实质出血一起出现。可能是因为脑内不同深度的组织以不同速度旋转所致。脑内各组织间进行相互剪切，致使出现小的点状出血。不管这种解释是否成立，散在小的出血灶可以提示弥漫性轴索损伤的存在。

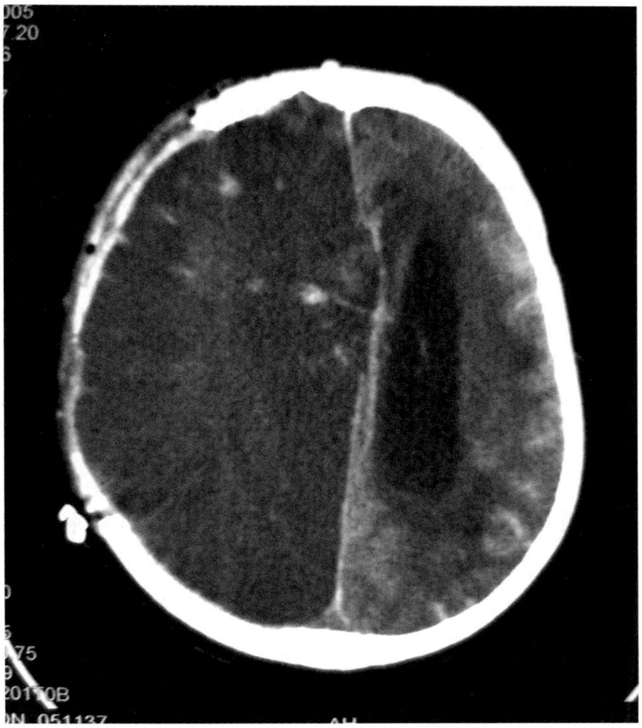

图2 CT扫描可见右侧整个大脑半球梗死

细胞和分子因素

在细胞水平，发生脑损伤后引起的分子水平变化异常复杂。谷氨酸和其他兴奋性神经递质的释放可导致神经元过度去极化和钙离子细胞内流，伴随蛋白酶的激活和导致细胞死亡的其他过程。血液灌注不足可导致从有氧代谢转化为无氧代谢。乳酸的产生进一步降低了局部组织的pH，继而酸中毒加剧了组织损伤和死亡。创伤诱导细胞凋亡进一步促进（神经）细胞死亡。这些变化以及其他生物化学和细胞过程在个体化患者的遗传构成的背景下发生。各种基因的特异性等位基因的存在可以使个体对于各种病理生理过程的损伤作用或多或少地易感。

临床诊断

临床检查

理想状态下，可通过神经系统检查来确定脑损伤的严重程度。在影像学检查研究中发现，占位性病变的大小和外观不如病变本身对患者的神经功能和觉醒水平具有的影响那么重要。

对一个具有潜在头部受伤的患者而言，其是否遵从简单的单一指令是最重要的一个问题。昏迷的简单定义是当一个人被要求做伸出2个手指或伸出舌头时，这个人不能做出这些动作。遵嘱动作的失败被广泛用于判断严重脑损伤的指标。其他简单、重要的方式是观察患者的运动类型（局部疼痛刺激定位、躲避、屈曲和过伸等）；是否左右对称；言语类型；睁眼运动存在或缺失；瞳孔大小、对光反射和双侧对称性。

调节瞳孔收缩的神经纤维位于第三对脑神经的表面上。占位性病变可导致脑疝形成，压迫该神经而导致瞳孔调节纤维的失活。结果是导致瞳孔散大，在强光照射下不能缩小。在昏迷的TBI患者，出现这种体征表明须要对其立即进行CT检查来明确较大的急性（颅内）血肿。

但是，散大、固定的瞳孔也可能是脑干缺血或直接的眼外伤所致。

已经开发了很多用于评估损伤后的意识或神经状态的评分，其中被应用得最广泛的是格拉斯哥昏迷评分（GCS）（表1）。结合诸如瞳孔反应性状态和患者的神经系统疾病的发展速度或变化率的信息，

GCS 对评估患者的基础状况及随后的病情进展是一个非常有用的工具。

表 1 Glasgow 昏迷评分

分数	运动	言语	睁眼
6	遵从命令	–	–
5	刺激定位	回答正确	–
4	刺激躲避	回答含糊不清	自主睁眼
3	刺激肢体屈曲	仅能说单词和短句	呼唤睁眼
2	刺激肢体过伸	仅能发声	刺痛睁眼
1	没有反应	没有反应	无反应

血清标志物

目前人们对脑损伤血清标志物的检测存在浓厚的兴趣，适用于在院前或战场情景下对患者进行更精准的病情评估；在急诊更全面地评价明显轻度的脑外伤患者；在重症监护室进行连续监测。很多化合物被发现对揭示 TBI 的存在是敏感的，但特异性很差。鉴于这样的标志物具有迫切的临床需要以及其存在潜在的商业利益，其可能在不久的将来被广泛应用。

早期临床干预：院前及急救中心救护

近几十年来救治 TBI 的基本原则是维持机体内环境稳定，预防和迅速处理二次伤害。发生急性创伤后脑组织变得非常脆弱，甚至无法耐受一过性低血压或缺氧。有证据表明，发热、癫痫发作和高血糖等情况均可能导致病情加重。通常短暂、不良的刺激可被正常脑组织较好地耐受，但对创伤后脑组织则会产生严重的危害。

TBI 救护的基本内容围绕着 A、B、C 方案，即气道、呼吸和循环。虽然一些参数管理的细节在院前环境下与 ICU 之间不同，重要的是，应将 ABC 的管理作为疾病的整个急性期恒定的目标。因为这种连续性，以下讨论气道、呼吸和循环与院前环境的关系，然后是转入 ICU 的注意事项。

气道

在气道控制方面，在重度 TBI 或可能存在气道损害或应激性气道保护等其他问题的患者，应考虑院前给予患者气管插管。但最近在创伤文献中报道，严重 TBI 患者的院前气管插管的预后更差。一个可能的原因是难以在院前状态下进行成功的气管插管，特别是院前急救人员会很少这样做。而对于没有经验的救援者，其可能反复尝试直到成功地放置气管插管。这个过程可能造成患者严重缺氧。另一个原因可能是气管插管后导致过度通气（$Paco_2$ 降低到危险的低水平）。

呼吸

在呼吸方面，标准的建议提倡能够维持充足氧合的最低吸氧浓度。尽管在氧合血红蛋白解离曲线基础上可接受的 Pao_2 最低限为 60 mmHg，但是大多数医师在 TBI 患者中设定的目标最小值范围为 80 ~ 100 mmHg，以保证脑组织供氧。

不再推荐使用过度通气作为预防颅内压增高的措施。目前已知过度换气可导致大脑血管收缩，并且由此导致的脑血容量的减少可以急剧降低颅内压。然而，脑动脉的收缩可能导致脑血流量下降到临界水平。另外，在过度通气开始的 24 h 内，脑动脉可能扩张回其原始直径。随后使 $Paco_2$ 增加的尝试可导致动脉扩张超过其原始基线，可能增高颅内压。

大多数临床医师的目标是 $Paco_2$ 低于正常范围，目标值为 35 ~ 40 mmHg。保持 $Paco_2$ 维持在正常范围的低值可优化脑血管系统的自我调节能力。

过度换气应用于伴有占位性病变迹象的急性恶化，例如具有双侧瞳孔不等大或查体不对称活动的颅内压增高。在这种情况下，假设须要对患者采取紧急手术以解除占位。过度通气和其他措施，如给予甘露醇，仅意在争取几分钟以在进行手术之前获得紧急 CT 扫描。如果扫描显示没有手术指征，应尝试通过使用下一节（创伤性脑损伤：影像学、手术治疗及非手术治疗和并发症）中阐述的一些步骤来处理无过度换气的颅内压增高。

循环

字母“C”代表循环。对于脑损伤患者，可以认为是对血压和静脉输液的管理。

在过去的几年中，常见的做法是使患者脱水以“防止脑水肿”。20 世纪 90 年代，人们倾向于对 TBI 患者积极地使用静脉输液（扩容补液）和升压药物，以人为地升高血压。然而，随后的研究表明，通过扩容补液和升压药进行血压升高的患者并未显示出在神经功能上有所改善。事实上，发生急性呼吸窘迫综合征的可能性提高了 5 倍。

当前的治疗策略须要维持正常的血压，其中临床或生理监测表明须对采取这种治疗的患者积极地进行升压治疗，如治疗脑缺氧或逆转神经病变的恶化。

目前直接监测脑组织压 $PbtO_2$ 可通过脑实质内导管实现。有一些临床医师通过增加吸氧浓度治疗低 $PbtO_2$。我们首选通过升高血压来治疗脑组织低 PO_2，以改善受影响脑组织的灌注。难以精确界定脑组织的缺血阈值。低于 15 ~ 20 mmHg 的 $PbtO_2$ 通常被认为是低的，而低于 8 ~ 10 mmHg 则可能建议须要进一步的评估和干预。

影像学方式：内容、时机及目的？

CT 扫描

在对 TBI 患者进行初步评估和稳定后，下一个任务是进行影像学检查。用于评估急性 TBI 最重要的检查是 CT 扫描。这种成像模式可精确地显示急性出血、脑水肿和占位效应。这是在初步评估期间最直接而明显的特征，通过骨窗也可以检测颅骨和颅底骨折。另一个优点是，CT 扫描是一种快速成像，至少在大多数发达国家被广泛使用。为了解决院前插管以及在这些患者中频繁使用镇静药所带来的影响（这使准确的临床评估变得更复杂），Marshall 基于 CT 扫描发现设计了 TBI 分类方案（表 2）。

表 2　Marshall CT 分级方案

分类	定义解释
Ⅰ级弥漫性损伤（正常）	在 CT 扫描上没有可见的颅内损伤
Ⅱ级弥漫性损伤	中线结构偏移在 0 ~ 5 mm，和（或）高密度或混合密度影体积不超过 25 cm^3，可能会有骨碎片或异物
Ⅲ级弥漫性损伤（水肿）	脑池受压或消失，中线移位 0 ~ 5 mm，高密度或混合密度病变不超过 25 cm^3
Ⅳ级弥漫性损伤（移位）	中线移位 >5 mm，高密度或混合密度病变不超过 25 cm^3
Ⅴ级局灶性损伤	无外科手术处理的指征
Ⅵ级局灶性损伤	高密度或混合密度病变超过 25 cm^3，须要手术治疗

MRI

历史上 MRI 在急性状态下的应用有限，原因有：获得结果需要相当长的时间；在检查期间对患者的评估有限；并且在患者进入检查室之前必须移除含有金属或铁磁的监测和复苏设备。然而，在患者稳定之后，MRI 可以发现细微的实质损伤，这可能发现一些无法获得改善的患者的原因。在评估轻度 TBI 患者时，MRI 也有作用，特别是当其症状与 CT 扫描的情况严重不符时。

值得强调的是，这种广泛使用的 TBI 分类方案是基于功能性而不是解剖学标准。这种方法与大多数一般创伤文献中使用的方法形成对比，其中解剖学标准用作分类损伤的主要手段。

血管造影

血管造影在脑损伤初期伤情评估中的作用仍不明确。在 20 世纪 70 年代 CT 扫描技术发展之前，神经外科医师仅将气脑造影术和血管造影技术用于发现中线偏移或其他占位性病变。应用颅骨 X 线照相技术可显示钙化松果体的位移。

自从 CT 出现以来，脑血管造影术通常用于治疗高度怀疑颅内血管病变的情况，如假性动脉瘤或大脑动脉夹层。然而，其治疗结果尚不明确。介入性放射疗法通常予以患者使用抗凝药物，但绝大多数急性脑损伤的患者却不宜应用肝素或华法林。同时，许多重度 TBI 患者的脑灌注量急剧下降，对缺血脑组织实施动脉闭塞是有待商榷的。

许多情况下，CT 血管造影术和 MR 血管造影术的持续发展使得这些技术与用于检测血管损伤的常规血管造影术水平相当。因此，血管造影技术在对 TBI 患者的急性评估中的使用率呈下降的历史趋势。

损伤分级

Glasgow 昏迷评分（GCS）

已经提出了许多不同的方案用于脑损伤分级和分类。如前所述，最著名的是 GCS。作为脑损伤患者的评估和分类的一部分，该评分的引入加强了对精准神经学查体的需要。这一点与最初描述 GSC 时一样重要。因为这种评分使得对患者进行更客观的评估成为可能，观察者之间和国际研究之间的变异性可以减少，从而有助于创建多中心甚至多国研究。

然而，在酒精或其他药物中毒的患者中，或因外伤导致广泛的眶周水肿而使眼睛肿胀不能睁开的患者，准确测定 GCS 通常是困难的，从而不能做睁眼评分。使 GCS 复杂化的其他因素反映了 30 年前的 GCS 初始类型已在院前急救的实践中发生变化。目前，许多患者在院前环境中被进行气管插管，并且通常在进行准确和彻底的神经学评估之前使用麻痹剂和镇静剂。这些问题导致了其他评估工具的创建，如基于 CT 结果的那些工具。避免不准确的神经学检查问题的另一种方式是使用血清学标记来鉴定可能具有严重的中枢神经系统损伤的创伤患者，类似于在诊断中使用心肌酶谱的血清水平方式诊断急性心肌损伤。这是一个迅速发展的有趣领域。

通常的做法是根据 GCS 将脑损伤分为轻度、中度或重度。轻度 TBI 传统上等于 GCS 得分为 13～15 分，而中等 TBI 是指 GCS 得分为 9～12 分。然而，一些研究表明，13 分的评分更能表明中度损伤。严重 TBI 是指 GCS 评分为 8 分或更低的患者。

表 3　简易脑损伤分级量表

AIS 分数	创伤严重度	脑损伤的举例
1	较小	轻微的头皮损伤
2	中度	更严重的头皮损伤 脑神经损伤 单纯颅骨骨折 意识丧失 <1 h 创伤后遗忘
3	严重	严重的头皮损伤 脑血管损伤 颅底骨折 粉碎性颅骨骨折 小实质挫伤 创伤性蛛网膜下腔出血 意识丧失 1～6 h
4	特重	脑血管损伤加重 严重的颅骨骨折 颅内血肿 意识丧失 6～24 h
5	危重	最严重的脑血管损伤 更大的颅内血肿 意识丧失 >24 h
6	致命	大面积（脑组织）破坏 挤压伤

Marshall CT 扫描

Marshall 等使用来自创伤性昏迷数据库（Traumatic Coma Data Bank）的数据开发了基于 CT 的分类方案（表 2）。该系统通常称为 Maeshall 量表或 TCDB 量表，根据诸如脑脊液池的中线移位和压缩的因素对 CT 扫描进行分类。虽然这种量表在某些情况下是有用的，但它不应该被认为是准确的神经学检查的替代品。

简易创伤分级量表

简易脑损伤分级量表（表 3）为轻微头皮损伤（如擦伤和撕裂）指定 1 分，较长和较深的撕裂得分为 2 分，而伴有明显失血或以总头皮缺失为特征的头皮损伤评分为 3 分。脑神经损伤编码为 2 分。

主要脑血管的损伤通常编码为 3 分或 4 分用于血栓形成或创伤性动脉瘤形成，4 分或 5 分用于血管撕裂。

颅骨骨折的分数范围从穹窿部的简单骨折为 2 分，到颅骨基底骨折或粉碎性穹窿部骨折为 3 分，最复杂的开放性骨折与暴露脑组织或显著的闭合性凹陷骨折为 4 分。

脑实质损伤的评分范围为 3～5 分。小的单个或多发性挫伤为 3 分，如蛛网膜下腔出血、水肿或与创伤直接相关的梗死。根据其大小，血肿被评分为 4 分或 5 分。

大面积毁灭伤或挤压伤的得分为 6 分。

如果这些分数超过基于解剖损伤的分数，意识丧失的持续时间和相关神经缺陷的存在可以用于评估损伤的严重性。这样分数范围为从 2～5 分。

美国创伤器官损伤量表协会（American Association for the Surgery of Trauma）并没有针对脑损伤进行说明。

其他分类方法

GCS 的局限性影响了临床研究试验以及对患者的护理。美国政府为 TBI 临床试验提供资金的主要机构已经召开了临床试验者研讨会，开始重新思考

TBI 的分类方法，特别是促进针对 TBI 病理生理学特定方面的治疗的开发。

轻度和中度创伤性脑损伤

本章重点关注的是重度 TBI 患者。而对于中度脑损伤患者，其 GCS 为 9～12 分，通常具有显著的颅内损伤，但仍然服从命指令。对他们的治疗类似于重度脑损伤患者，均应密切观察病情并着重预防二次损伤。然而，这些患者中可能很多并不需要颅内压监护仪，并且它们可能不需要与严重 TBI 患者相同程度的护理。

在脑损伤后就诊的患者中绝大多数有轻度创伤性脑损伤。他们经常被诊断为有脑震荡。重要的是，轻度创伤性脑损伤的诊断（或脑震荡）不要求患者意识丧失。一些数据表明，轻度 TBI 的大多数患者从未失去自主意识，但他们可能主诉有各种症状，如头痛、创伤后遗忘、注意力难以集中、耳鸣和步态失稳。

与严重 TBI 患者的情况不同，对轻度 TBI 患者的主要关注点并不在于患者是否将存活或死亡，或患者是否成为植物人或有严重残疾。几乎所有的患者都能生存下来。相反，主要的发病率与记忆、认知、注意力、情绪稳定性和类似区域的干扰有关。由于缺乏神经学损伤的“硬”证据，导致许多医师并未重视这些症状的意义。然而，这些患者往往会失去工作、辍学或离婚，或者在生活中经历其他重大动荡。最终，绝大多数人恢复，但这样的过程可能需要几个月。使患者和家人安心可能是有所需要的。事实上，这些可能都可以提供。如果须要客观记录损伤，或者如果医师怀疑诈病或症状增益放大，那么咨询和正式测试可能是恰当的。

小结和算法

图 3 总结了对 TBI 患者评估和处置的优先级别。精确的神经系统评分和对 ABC（气道、呼吸和循环）的关注是至关重要的。在患者转院途中、复苏过程中以及被送去做 CT 扫描时，都应持续监测。

图 3　创伤性脑损伤（TBI）患者的基本初始评估和管理

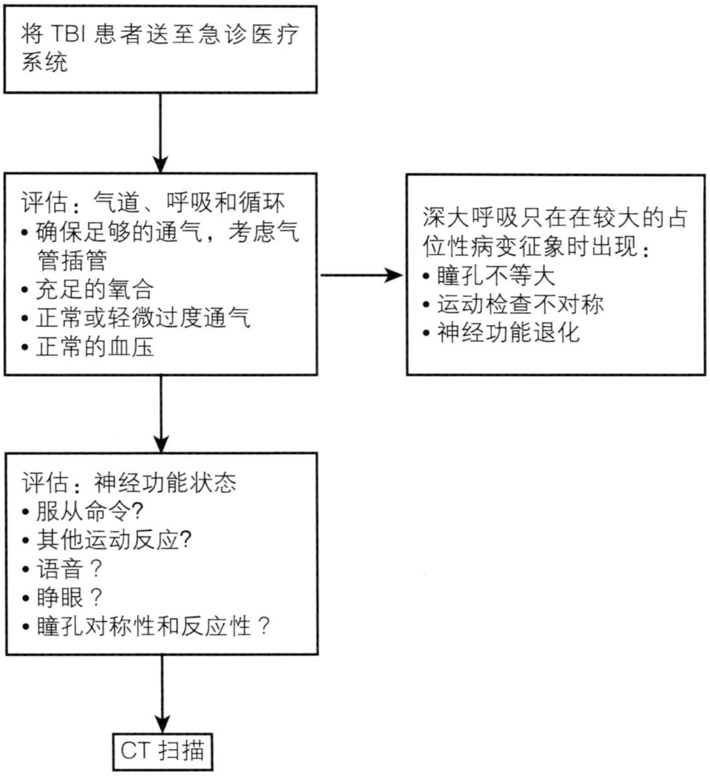

创伤性脑损伤：影像学、手术治疗及非手术治疗和并发症

Aileen Ebadat, Alex B. Valadka 著
刘波 译

以前的章节描述了TBI患者的病理生理学以及最初的治疗。本节将对有关TBI的一些特定的方面，如手术治疗及非手术治疗、并发症以及预后进行综述。

手术治疗

因为颅骨较为坚硬和牢固，并且表面覆盖着具有丰富血供的头皮和需要处理的头发，因此使得脑部手术比全身大多数器官更难操作。因此，在进行开颅手术前，尤其是在急诊的情况下，外科医师一定要仔细准备。如果在处理损伤前体位摆放和暴露不当的话，可能产生严重的后果。而且平时极少出现的意外事件在紧急开颅手术中似乎会出现得极其频繁。如果在术中忽然出现必要的额外暴露，将会付出诸如出现大量失血、脑肿胀或其他并发症之类的代价。

体位摆放

在大多数情况下，可通过将患者摆放为仰卧位，同时将头部转向病灶对侧来抵达病灶（比如，对于左侧开颅术选择头偏向右侧）。在一侧肩胛及上胸部下方放置卷筒或其他支持物可以使头部的旋转角度更大。对于大多数创伤手术来说，使用头钉严格固定头部是没必要的。在这种情况下通常使用的是普通的头圈、泡沫头垫或其他装置。在大多数颅脑损伤病例中，目的是使头部中线与地面或多或少地保持平行。

对于有硬质颈托的患者，可以将上述体位进行调整，使患者处于侧卧位。将患者摆放至这样的体位须要手术团队中的所有人员付出更多的工作，但是一个有经验的团队须要迅速地将患者摆放至这种体位。

头部受伤的患者可出现的解剖上的病变位置看似是无限的，这就要求外科医生应该知道如何抵达脑部和颅骨的任何位置。在治疗枕部、颞部后方、顶部后方以及颅后窝的损伤时，需要患者呈俯卧位。对于颅底前方中线处的损伤，比如凹陷的额窦骨折，通常采用的体位是头部处于中立位置，而颈部略伸展。对神经外科所使用的各种体位和入路的详细讨论将超出本书的范围。在处理颅脑损伤时熟悉并且灵活地采取不同手术入路才是问题的关键。

骨瓣

对于TBI患者的另一项手术基本原则是建立一个大骨瓣。对于急性硬膜下血肿（SDH）来说更是如此。在这种病变中，血肿有时累及相当大部分的大脑半球范围。清除距离较小的骨窗边缘很远的血肿会使手术医师很受挫，而且可能会对患者造成危险。另外，与硬膜下血肿伴发的硬膜下出血可能会在任何部位出现：来自靠近中线的上矢状窦的回流静脉，来自颅前窝或颅中窝的底部，来自额极下方或内侧，或者来自横窦。这些只是一些常见的出血来源。一个大骨瓣是确保能够抵达尽可能多的出血部位的最好方式。

大多数创伤的手术切口是从颧弓后根部开始的，就在外耳屏稍前方的部位，然后向后方拐弯，到达耳的上方和后方。在创伤病例中，这种向后方的外延应该尽可能地远。然后，使切口向内侧和上方弯曲。使皮肤切口到达中线是明智的，因为这样可暴露上矢状窦，以免有来自中线的棘手的出血。

虽然皮瓣可能接近或到达中线，然而使骨瓣内侧边缘与中线保持几厘米的距离将会是明智的。将中线上方或紧挨中线的骨头移除时可能会导致来自瞬间的蛛网膜颗粒硬膜外出血或是来自硬膜静脉池的硬膜出血。虽然这种出血可用轻柔的压迫填塞来控制，但是这种额外动作会延误快速清除硬膜下血肿的速度并分散注意力。同样，当外科医师专注于清除血肿时，也可能会忽略此处位置复发的出血。如果骨窗内侧边缘下方出现了快速出血，最好的处理方式是使用可吸收的止血材料填塞，并且多挂几针进行硬膜悬吊。

清除硬膜外血肿所需的骨瓣大小通常比硬膜下血肿的要小，因为硬膜与上方覆盖的颅骨连接紧密。这通常可以限制血肿的扩散。也正因此，硬膜外血肿病变在CT上看来通常显得“又短又胖”，但是硬膜下血肿通常扩散开来，看上去“又长又瘦”。这就是因为硬膜下血肿可以在大脑半球表面无障碍地扩散。然而，还是应该注意，在清除硬膜外血肿时不应把骨窗开得过小。

对于脑实质内的病变如血肿和挫伤，通常使用较小的开口即可清除。事实上，甚至巨大的实质内出血都可通过脑皮质上的小口进行清除。当血肿被清除后就有了空间，脑皮质边缘回缩变得更加容易。

脑肿胀

脑的快速肿胀是急性硬膜下出血清除后的关注重点。这种现象的出现速度表示受损的自动调节能力可能起到重要作用。目前一种流行的做法是保持硬膜为开放的状态（但是用一层人工硬膜松散地覆盖在脑组织上），并且去除骨瓣。一些神经外科医师强烈推荐这种方法，而且它确实在降低颅内压方面很有效。然而，这种方法对预后的影响至今仍不清楚。几十年前的文献报告很多存活者都是以持续植物状态生存。最近的数据显示对弥漫性脑肿胀进行减压不会改善预后，甚至可能是有害的。另一些研究则是担心去骨瓣减压术可能进行得过于频繁，从而可能在适应证不足或不当的情况下实施。经常的情况是，由于骨窗过小，导致膨胀的脑组织疝出坏死，引起水肿向内产生压迫，进一步加重了颅内压增高。

虽然术者经常别无选择，只能将骨瓣去除，但更好的策略则是采取一些措施，使陷入这种境地的可能性降到最小。硬膜的切口不宜宽大，应该在位于暴露区域硬膜的四个不同象限处切出缝隙，并从缝隙中仔细地吸出血凝块。应该缓慢地清除血肿。这样做比起迅速清除整个血凝块可防止脑组织瞬间大面积肿胀。如果大多数血肿已被清除，而且没有证据表明正在出现硬膜内出血时，若脑组织开始肿胀了，可以迅速关闭先前切开的缝隙。然而，如果仍然存在持续的硬膜内出血，则必须将之前切开的缝隙连接起来形成一个更宽大的硬膜开口，从而寻找并控制出血的来源。这种措施必须全速进行，才能在脑组织开始肿胀之前关闭硬膜切口。

可是在先前的讨论中隐含的是在脑组织发生肿胀之前关闭硬膜是不可行的。因为前文曾提到过，目前流行的治疗方式是简单地不再将骨瓣放回原处，这使得这种治疗方式显得陈旧。但是，上述治疗方式的使用者在应用这套措施时鲜少遇到问题，就算是须要用牵开器来温和地将肿胀的脑组织压迫回去，以便使用钳子迫使硬膜边缘对位从而进行缝合。上述术式之所以可行，是因为实际上有实验室数据提出去骨瓣减压术可使脑水肿加重。

硬膜外血肿

硬膜外手术通常更加简单。有时术者可能感到有必要在硬膜上做一个小口，以辨别是否存在硬膜下出血。此时见到一薄层的硬膜下出血是很普遍的情况，不过这些血液通常可被轻松地清除。另一种常见问题是，硬膜外的区域出现持续性出血，出血来源可能是脑膜静脉或脑膜静脉窦，或是来自骨瓣边缘的下方。如果硬膜外静脉出血不能通过烧灼进行止血，使用市场上任何一种神外止血材料进行轻柔压迫都是有效的。在大多数病例中，在适当位置留置这些自体吸收材料比试图将这些材料取出更好。注意，脑膜中动脉出血的发生概率并不像某些书籍所说的那样频繁，但是如果真的出现了，那么直接将出血的动脉进行烧灼通常是有效的。

脑实质损伤

对脑实质血肿和挫裂伤的清除通常可利用较小的皮质切口进行。值得庆幸的是，一旦某处损伤被清除以后，脑组织的张力将会松弛下来。在此类病例中，主要的难点是确保损伤得到彻底的清除，并止血充分。如果血肿腔巨大的话，则会较难达成上述目标。有时在处理巨大挫裂伤或血肿时，可以在另外一处进行皮质切开，这样可以到达那些初始皮质切口不可及的部位，从而进行清除和止血。

颅内压监测

对于患者术后是否有必要接受颅内压监测的问题经常是难以回答的。一般来讲，如果医师并不认为某位患者在术后能醒转过来的话（例如，不认为患者能遵嘱活动或是格拉斯哥昏迷评分 >8 分），则强烈建议对其进行监测装置置入。推荐进行脑室穿刺术，因为这样可以在颅内压升高时对脑脊液进行治疗性引流，通常可在初始的开颅术中置入这种装置。但是一些术者倾向于等开颅术结束后再在术间或重症监护病房进行脑室穿刺术。如果脑室穿刺失败，也可使用脑实质内监测装置。

凝血功能障碍

如果患者有凝血障碍，应提早告知血库在手术室紧急使用血小板和冰冻血浆。发生严重的弥漫性渗血时则须要使用重组凝血因子Ⅶa。术中可进行实验室检查，从而判断上述措施对于改善凝血分析和血小板计数情况是否有效。但是，还有一个更简单的方法来估计凝血状态，即观察滴入术区的血是否能够形成凝血块。

小结

综上所述，提早想好可能存在的障碍和解决方案可帮助术者避免陷入不利境地。恰当地暴露从而充分清除凝血块是极其关键的。轻微抬高床头可减轻静脉出血情况。在出现横跨硬膜上主要静脉窦的凹陷性骨折时，应预计到大出血的可能。清除急性硬膜下血肿时缓慢地切开硬膜可能对最大化减轻脑组织广泛水肿起到帮助。

非手术治疗方式

治疗地点

TBI治疗的复杂性和TBI对于远期预后的巨大影响使得TBI患者在入院伊始便应入住ICU病房，并接受对TBI患者有丰富经验的医师和护士的治疗。对于TBI有专门经验比仅在一般外伤或危重护理方面精通更加重要。在受伤后的头几天，TBI患者须要接受血压监测、血红蛋白浓度检验、复杂通气管理等以及那些没有头部损伤的患者所需要的相同常规干预措施。但在这些基础措施之外，也要对脑损伤进行仔细评估和管理，并且整合全身治疗和针对脑损伤的治疗。虽然很多普通ICU以及创伤ICU在TBI的细微差别管理上不擅长，但大多数神经外科ICU很擅长处理重大全身性疾病的患者。

如果TBI患者在几天内好转或保持神经功能稳定，那么就可以将其转入其他ICU，或过渡到监护治疗病房，或是普通病房。这种方案与目前所主张的观点不同，目前认为患者应该先被送入标准外伤病房，而不是直接进入神经外科ICU。在很多标准外科ICU中，是基于患者的全身监测指标进行管理，但这些指标对TBI患者的最佳方案而言不是必要的。在实际操作中，每个机构对上述差异的对待都是不同的，因为治疗方案是根据那些照看这些患者的不同团队所制订的。

继发性损害

入院前所强调的对继发性损害的预防和早期治疗在患者进入ICU后应继续进行，而且，实际上，这应是对他们治疗的基础。应额外关注他们的基础代谢和生理参数，包括血压、氧饱和度、血红蛋白浓度和血钠浓度。最好推后对那些不必要采取紧急处理的损伤部位的手术，因为这时遭到损伤的脑对于可能的术中代谢障碍还很脆弱。此类手术的例子有面部骨折，手或足的损伤，甚至包括大多数长骨骨折。

撤呼吸机和气管切开

撤机和最终拔管是由患者的临床表现所决定的。很多特护医师推荐对这类患者早期进行气管切开。然而，如果患者有逐步恢复意识的迹象，那么逐步降低间歇指令通气频率，甚至增加尝试持续正压气道通气对患者几乎没有害处。在大多数TBI患者中，导致持续插管状态的原因是脑损伤，而非原发的肺部疾病。因此，拔管的决定是根据意识状态的好转而做出的。甚至对于那些显然不会很快醒来的患者而言，持续的气管插管状态也是有必要的。因为当患者的颅内压仍处于频繁或持续升高状态时进行气管切开会出现潜在的颅内压增高加重的风险。

镇静

在很多ICU中，医师会习惯性地将患者深度镇静，并且通过同时向静脉中注入多种药物形成药物致瘫。几乎没有人质疑对患者进行如此大量用药的原因。如果一名TBI患者的颅内压不高或没有发生躁动，那么可能无须超量应用止痛药物进行深度镇静。在这种理念的指导下，可以准确地评估神经功能状态，而且可以更容易地快速脱离呼吸机。这也是我们不像其他机构那样积极地对这类患者进行气管切开的另一部分原因。我们更倾向于给他们机会，让他们恢复到可拔管的状态，如果他们出现了朝向这一目标的早期恢复迹象的话。

脑部监测

监测大脑的生理功能可提供可用于修正治疗的重要信息，以防止和及时治疗继发性损害。

颅内压监测在几十年内都应用广泛。在任何可能的时候，推荐使用脑室内置管，因为它相对费用不高，在引流脑脊液时可用做治疗工具，而且在必要的时候可以为监测器调零。抗生素浸渍导管的开发似乎降低了脑室穿刺术感染的风险。

额外的脑监测装置可在市场上购买到。颈静脉氧饱和度可由血氧导管连续监测，将血氧导管以逆行的方式向上插入颈静脉并进入颈静脉球。颈静脉球血氧浓度的下降意味着由于缺血或其他病理过程导致的脑氧消耗增加。

脑组织氧分压监测（$PbtO_2$）引起了人们相当大的兴趣，因为 $PbtO_2$ 和脑血流量之间存在良好的相关性。关键问题是，解读数据前须要了解导管测量的是正常脑组织还是遭到挫伤或是受损的脑组织。导管位置的不同代表着所监测的是脑整体代谢水平或是探针附近局部脑组织的代谢水平。如果仅仅使用了一个整体监测器，代谢明显异常的大范围区域可能会在背景中丢失而且不被监测到。我们的习惯是使用如 $PbtO_2$ 导管这样的局部监测器，以监测挫伤或其他受损部位附近的脑组织。

还有一些其他监测器，可以追踪脑血流量，进行脑微透析，追踪脑电活动，以及测量其他生理参数。这些都可以提供有价值的信息，为仔细的神经功能评估和 CT 检查做补充。但是如果想进行随机前瞻对照研究以展现这些设备的实用性（或缺乏实用性）则是困难的。现在人们对于建设国际性的前瞻性数据库的兴趣日益增加，包括收集神经心理学和其他预先指定的结果指标，以便能够进行那些比较有效性的研究。这些分析可以提供各种干预措施价值的重要数据，并对监测技术给予合理的指导，以便促进目标患者管理。

营养

应尽早进行营养补充，通常是经肠内给予营养。如果在尝试几天后仍不能建立肠内营养通路，则应该考虑进行肠外营养。较差的预后与升高的血糖之间的联系得到了越来越多的关注，因此要多进行监测，如有必要，则应对血糖浓度进行处理。

水与电解质

其他一些基本原则包括维持正常的血容量以避免脱水或水潴留。我们建议血钠浓度在正常范围内，而且不要故意使血钠浓度升至超过正常高值。然而，我们更为关注的是低钠血症可能会加剧脑水肿并使颅内压增高。因此，我们在对待 120 s 甚至低 130 s 的血清钠浓值（mEq/L）时可以更加不必顾虑地使用高渗盐水进行处理，从而在脑和血管之间建立更理想的渗透梯度。

理疗、职业治疗与言语障碍矫正

早期应用理疗和职业治疗可以非常有帮助。这体现在肢体远端活动功能的保留和随后在患者的康复过程中，加快坐起和下床活动的进程。言语障碍矫正在一些患者中也是有效的。

发热

体温过高是一种使神经损伤患者预后不良的促进因素，正受到越来越多的关注。如果对患者使用解热药、外部降温并对已知的各种发热病因进行治疗却仍然发热，这时就可以考虑使用各种类型的降温装置了。

深静脉血栓

对可能长期卧床的昏迷患者进行深静脉血栓的预防是重要的。在我们的病房，患者入住 ICU 后便立即使用连续压迫装置是有效的。患者受伤后我们不会立即常规使用药物预防，因为担心这样做会加重潜在的凝血障碍，而且可能会导致迟发或复发的颅内出血。我们通常的策略是在伤后 72 h 使用低分子肝素（low-molecular-weight heparin，LMWH）进行预防。但有时，对那些可能有高风险的患者，我们的间隔时间会缩短。当发生深静脉血栓时我们也会用 LMWH 来进行治疗。我们不常规放置下腔静脉（inferior vena cava，IVC）滤网进行预防。相反，对于那些有 DVT 病史的 TBI 患者，我们通常保留下腔静脉滤网。我们对那些有脊髓损伤的瘫痪患者则更积极些。

输血阈值

关于何时进行输血一直是有争议的。对于 TBI 患者或者动脉瘤性蛛网膜下腔出血患者，神经外科医师一直以来的观点是推荐将血红蛋白水平保持在大约 10 mg/dl。虽然在这种亚正常状态下血携氧能力会下降，但是携氧能力与血液黏稠度之间的非线性关系使得在上述血红蛋白浓度条件下，血液黏稠度较携氧能力的下降程度更多。由于血黏稠度下降对血流量的改善感觉上可以抵消携氧能力的降低，因此，在一些研究中论证到输血反而会增加死亡的风险，而且将输血条件放宽至血红蛋白不低于 7 mg/dl 以后对患者更有利。然而，另一些数据显示将心肌缺血患者的血红蛋白维持在 10 mg/dl 比维持在 7 mg/dl 表现更佳。争论的焦点则是上述发现是否适用于 TBI、脑卒中和罹患其他神经性疾病的患者。目前，我们推荐的是传统观点，即在脑严重外伤后最初几天将目标血红蛋白浓度维持在 10 mg/dl 附近。

颅内压增高的治疗

对于颅内压增高的治疗流程有很多步骤（图 1）。通常是从安全、无创的治疗方法开始的。如果颅内压持续性升高，则逐步采用更积极的疗法。可选用的治疗流程的多样化反映了各个中心在处理每一个个体时的不同，正是这些不同之处组成了这些治疗流程的步骤。值得注意的是，不推荐使用激素类药物治疗 TBI 患者。

CT 扫描

如果怀疑造成颅内压增高的原因可能是延迟或复发的血肿、脑水肿或失败的脑室外引流术或是大范围缺血，则应该予以重复的 CT 扫描检查（图 2）。

镇静和麻痹

镇静剂和止痛剂可能会有助于降低颅内压，在需要神经肌肉阻断时应补充这种药物的治疗。

脑脊液引流

如果事先做过脑室外引流术，脑脊液引流对持续性升高的颅内压是有效的。既往的观点认为应每过 5 ~ 7 天即对脑室外引流管进行更换，以免发生感染。这一点似乎没有被更近期的研究证实。一些中心报告，留置引流管 2 周或更久不会导致感染率增加。随后开发的抗生素浸渍导管似乎对降低脑室外引流术相关感染的风险产生了相当大的影响。

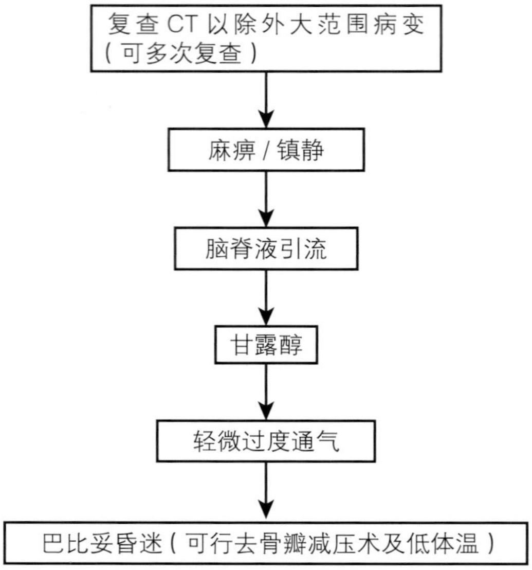

图 1　颅内压增高的治疗流程的基础步骤

渗透性利尿剂

应用甘露醇通常是有效的。甘露醇的渗透性效果可促使液体从脑组织流入血管间隙。这也可以降低血黏稠度，从而促使大脑动脉进行收缩（从而也降低脑内血容量），同时不影响脑血流量。血黏稠度的降低使得较细的动脉更易获得充足的血流。高张盐水作为一种甘露醇的潜在替代或补充很受关注。小儿特护医师对于它的使用更为广泛。虽然初期的结果令人鼓舞，但是对于最佳的治疗方法仍需要更有力的数据来证实，包括相关的适应证、禁忌证和不良事件。

过度通气

颅内压的持续增高可能会对轻微的过度通气起反应。只要有可能，我们会尝试使用脑氧合监护仪来避免出现由超出脑组织承受范围的过度通气所导致的脑缺血。

巴比妥昏迷

持续性颅内压增高可能会对苯巴比妥导致的昏

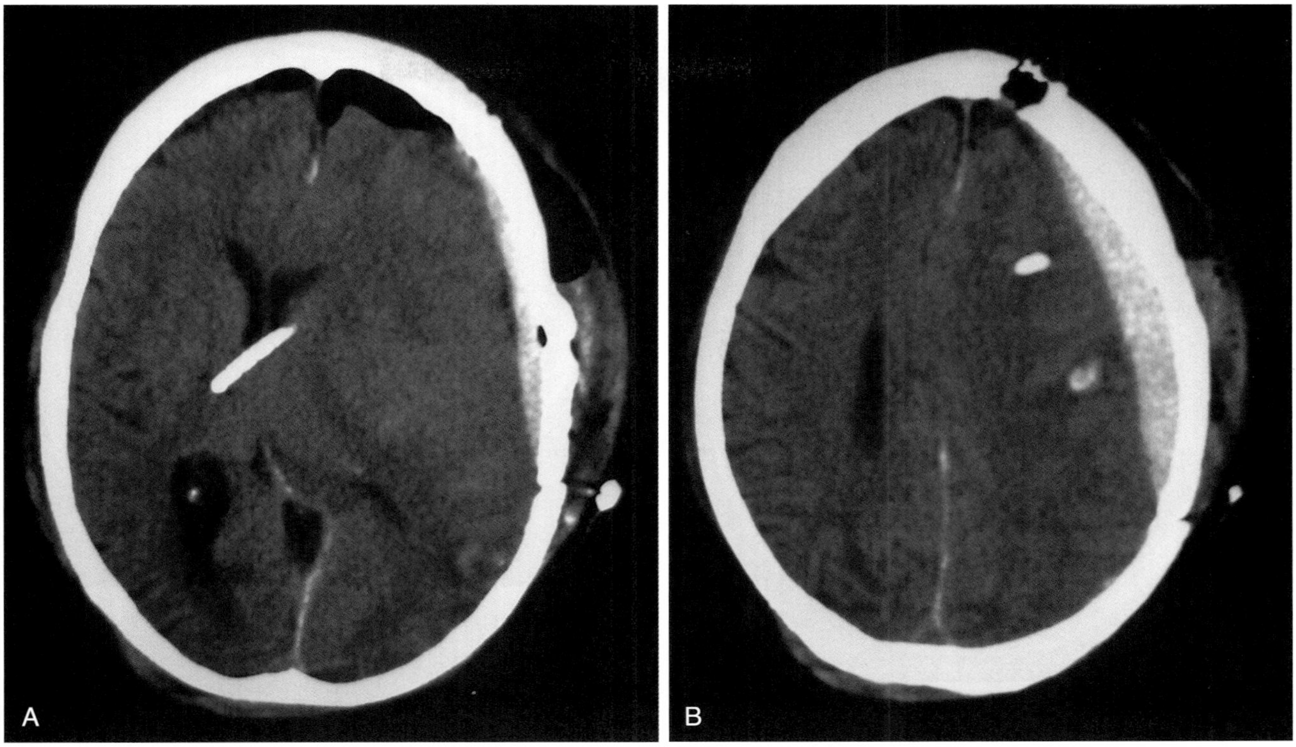

图 2 急性硬膜下血肿清除术后 CT 复查，术后显示依旧存在颅内压增高，CT 检查显示术后硬膜外血肿，患者将接受再次手术

迷起反应。这种治疗方式可有效地降低颅内压，但是低血压却是一个主要问题。在使用巴比妥类药物之前，我们应先准备好可立即输注的升压药物，以免血压出现下降。

去骨瓣减压术

即使实施了图 1 所列的各种治疗方法也不能控制的持续性颅内压增高是一个严峻的问题。去骨瓣减压术是暂时去除一大块颅骨，从而为损伤的脑组织提供肿胀空间的手术。这是目前所普遍采用的治疗措施。去除一大块骨头看起来可以明显地降低颅内压，但是这种做法是否可以改善患者的预后却仍然不得而知。有可能的是很多的这类手术都进行得过早，或者没有恰当地去除骨头（图 3）。去骨瓣减压术的并发症也会很麻烦，包括出现对侧硬膜下积液以及脑组织自骨瓣去除处疝出（图 4）。

低温

另一个潜在的治疗方法是低温。第一次全国急性脑损伤研究：低温（National Acute Brain Injury Study: Hypothermia, NABIS: H）研究结果显示，当低温被不加选择地应用到所有脑损伤患者时并未取得效果。同样的结果在第二次 NABIS: H 研究中也可看到，该研究旨在让年轻患者更快地降温。然而，其与去骨瓣减压等其他干预手段的效果类似，低温仅使部分脑损伤患者获益。此外，立即开始对所有患者进行低温治疗与有选择性地在存在难治性颅内压增高的患者进行低温治疗，效果也不相同。对于研究者和临床医师来说，困难在于如何选择适合低温治疗的患者，以达到最大的效益风险比。

个体化治疗

虽然大多数研究建议患者按照相同的干预措施接受治疗，实际上患者的情况各不相同，应该根据患者的不同情况选择不同的有针对性的治疗措施。在颅内压增高的治疗中，存在严重脑水肿时应考虑渗透性利尿剂；存在脑脊液梗阻时应该行脑室外引流；存在脑血流量增加时，早期应用温和的过度换气可能使患者获益。

最有可能的是，每种特定的降低颅内压的治疗方法都仅在针对某类型特定的患者时才是最佳的治

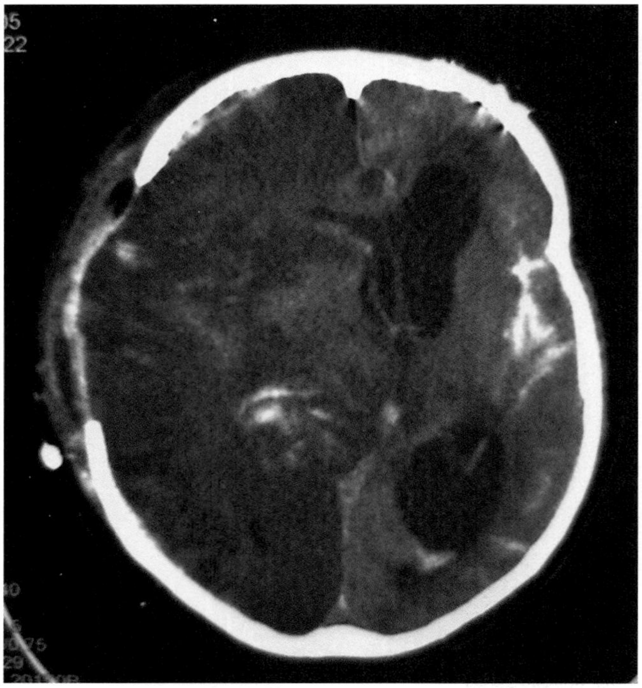

图 3 术后 CT 检查。术前 CT 检查见以前章节（TBI：病理学、临床诊断及院前急救处理）的图 1。尽管没有放回骨瓣，但去骨瓣的范围太小，不能起到充分的减压效果

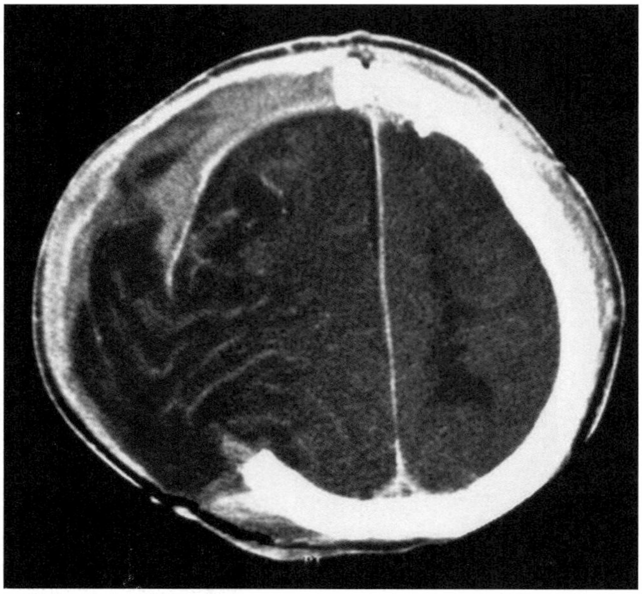

图 4 巨大的坏死脑组织从骨缺损处疝出

疗方法。我们的问题在于在针对某个指定的患者时，在针对特定的病情发展阶段时，无法鉴别哪种治疗方法为最佳。造成这一问题的部分原因是针对严重 TBI 的临床试验。该研究囊括了所有的 TBI 患者，而没有考虑每个患者在具体病理生理机制上的不同。当一种治疗方法在治疗特定类型的患者有效而在其他患者无效时，不能说它就一定是有效的。有针对性的试验更难以操作，但是却可以提供所需要的各个种类的不同的信息。

预防性颅内压增高治疗的失败

另一个我们一次又一次得到的教训是对颅内压增高的治疗不能预防性地实施。这么做不仅不能使患者获益，对许多病例还是有害的。作为临床医师，我们自然地倾向于从一开始就采取某种治疗手段以阻止颅内压增高。我们担心出现颅内压增高会使患者处于风险之中。然而，很多年来，预防性过度换气、巴比妥类药物昏迷、药物性麻痹、低温或升高血压治疗均已在Ⅰ类或Ⅱ类研究中并没有显示出益处。而且，在许多情况下，这些治疗方式存在重大风险。因此，在这个时候我们能做得最好的是严密观察患者的病情变化，专注于 ABC（气道、呼吸与循环），预防继发性损害的发生，以及在颅内压升高到一定程度或在其他不良事件发生时及时干预。

指南

关于颅脑损伤患者管理的各种指南被广泛传读。对不同的文献进行回顾综述并按照一定的权重进行总结形成合理的指南内容，而这些文献的权重也是根据文献本身质量以及对回顾性研究的严格评价决定的。例如论证方法完善的文献级别要高于存在缺陷的研究，最终的推荐级别也是根据不同的权重来决定的。

毫不奇怪，大多数临床决定很少具备具有随机性和前瞻性，并且有对照试验的方法来支持他们。同时，这种建构良好的试验通常是为了回答在特定人群中设计的特定问题，同时具备特定的观察指标。在大量人群中具有普遍性的发现常常是不可靠的。

指南的局限性决定了盲目地遵循指南推荐是不明智的。相反，更加合理的方法是将循证指南与医师的经验与判断、患者的具体情况、护理环境的特定方面整合起来。这种方法既不能是对指南的盲目遵循，同时又要保证指南受到严肃、合理的重视。

临床试验的失败

人们已经投入了数百万美元和无数小时的努力

来进行临床试验，以测试旨在改善TBI预后的药物和其他治疗方法，包括高渗盐水和羟乙基淀粉，但均以失败告终。分析这些试验和建议以改善未来试验的设计已经成为研究的不断变化的领域，但这样的考虑超出了本章的范围。从这些失败中学到的教训是，目前我们必须继续关注患者治疗的基础，而不是仅仅因为某个针对TBI的单纯药理学上的“治愈”产生不正确的乐观。

致残率及并发症

TBI患者与其他部位外伤患者的并发症类似。这些并发症包括呼吸道、泌尿系统及身体其他系统的感染，以及治疗操作所引发的感染，如外周和中心静脉以及动脉置管所引起的感染。在危重患者中，DVT、褥疮溃疡、心肌梗死及体重减轻等负性事件的发生将延长患者在ICU的住院时间。

在很大程度上，对这些并发症的治疗与没有脑外伤的患者发生此类并发症时的治疗并无区别。一个常见的诱惑是将这些并发症的出现归咎于脑损伤的异常发展，即“中枢性”的，但是只有经过彻底的检查排除其他可能的原因以后，这种结论才可能是正确的。

一些并发症是脑损伤患者所独有的。颅内压增高及其治疗已经被讨论。过分的以及不适当的镇静不仅会影响对患者神经系统状况的精确评估，同时也不必要地使患者增加了因为镇静所引起风险的可能性，并延长了患者在ICU的住院时间。

目前一般推荐在脑损伤后第一周进行预防性抗癫痫治疗。一周后如患者无癫痫发作可以停药。已接受抗癫痫治疗的患者如出现癫痫发作，则应检测血清药物浓度，可给予抗癫痫药静脉注射并增加药物的维持量，或者增加另一种药物。最理想的抗癫痫治疗的维持时间依旧不清楚，比较合理的时间应该是几个月或者可能更长。

再出现颅内出血或迟发性颅内出血可以是灾难性的（图2）。部分原因可能与手术技术有关，如止血时间不够则不能保证充分止血。然而，更加常见的情况是患者本身有肝疾病病史，而且创伤本身容易诱发凝血功能障碍。积极使用新鲜冷冻血浆和血小板可能有助于对持续弥漫性渗血患者的止血。最近的报告显示在这些病例中使应用重组因子Ⅶa取得了显著的效果。

死亡率

许多创伤研究文献报道的疾病结局中就有关于出院死亡率方面的内容。之所以选择这种结局测算方法，通常是由医院创伤注册数据所推动的。对于胸部和腹部外伤或因并发症入院的患者，选择这样的终点事件是易于理解的。因为在这样的观察终点，患者要么趋于健康恢复，要么死亡。

表1　格拉斯哥结局量表（GOS）

得分	分类	描述
5	预后良好	尽管有轻微的功能障碍，能够独立地生活和工作
4	中度功能障碍	尽管有功能障碍，能够独立生活。可以使用公共交通工具。工作须要辅助/监护，等。
3	严重功能障碍	神志清醒，生活不能自理，常须要相应的看护机构照料
2	持续植物生存状态	无意识或“醒状昏迷”
1	死亡	—

不幸的是，出院死亡率对于衡量TBI患者的预后并不是一个好的结局评价方法。如果当患者仍处于持续植物生存状态，生存也不能被认为是理想的结局。多数TBI研究把死亡、持续植物生存状态或严重功能缺失作为不良结局，而将恢复良好或中度功能缺失作为良好结局。这些疾病结局分类方法依据的是格拉斯哥结局量表（Glasgow Outcome Scale，GOS）（表1）。作为GOS的补充或是替代，有些研究使用了更为细致的研究工具以评估疾病结局，尤其是对难以进行测量的疾病数据，比如对神经心理功能数据的测量。

结局评价的时机也很重要。当某个患者在受伤后1～2周开始快速康复，那么他从急救医院（acute care hospital）出院时功能等级的评价就会很高。而当一个患者在较早的时候，转院到长期护理机构或是康复医院，那么他在急救医院出院时的功能等级评价就会比较低。即便后一个患者恢复得比较慢，在伤后6个月这两个患者的功能等级就具有可比性。脑外伤的恢复可能持续若干年。从实际考虑，多数TBI研究结局数据应该在伤后6个月收集。

近期的一些研究报告TBI会有非常好的结局，

死亡率接近 20% 甚至更低。然而，这些研究中很多都没有把 GCS 评分 3 分、瞳孔散大固定或是其他出现预示结局不良征象的患者纳入其中。创伤昏迷数据库纳入了四个学术中心的全部患者，共 753 例。TBI 患者的总体结局是，27% 的患者结局良好，16% 的患者中度功能障碍，16% 的患者严重功能障碍，5% 的患者持续植物生存状态，36% 的患者死亡。依据现有的经验，尽管这些百分比数据是在 20 世纪 80 年代收集的，但在今天依旧有用。随着急诊医疗服务系统和神经重症监护的不断进步，重新收集这些数据可用于研究这些进步是否能够实质性地改善患者的结局，仍显得很有意义。

脑穿通伤

造成脑穿通伤的主要原因是头部遭受火器打击。绝大多数患者在到达医院之前就已经死亡。许多研究也表明，活着到达医院的患者大多数也会死亡。另一方面，生存下来的患者依然会有恰当的比例预后良好。

有的学者认为对于 GCS 3～4 分，甚至是 5 分的患者，不建议进行特别积极的治疗手段。但也有研究表明，初始神经系统评价非常低的患者偶尔也能获得良好的预后。不过这些学者一致认为对此类患者须要进行积极的复苏救治以稳定其生命指标。外科手术干预的范围因需要而定，可以涵盖广泛的开颅重建到床旁简单清创手术。

须要注意的是，那些结局预后很差的患者进行器官捐赠可能是唯一有意义的事情。

小结和准则

图 5 列举了救治 TBI 患者的一些基本准则和目标。一如既往，其主要目标依旧是避免二次损伤。最佳的监护是可靠的、反复的、有规律的、间断的神经系统检查。当患者不能遵从指令配合检查，则须要进行颅内压监测以及其他指标的监测，以帮助及时发现不良代谢事件的发生。颅内压增高的一般治疗准则见图 1。当患者的监测数据提示存在特殊的病理生理学变化时，个体化的治疗干预措施可能会增补或替代这些治疗准则。

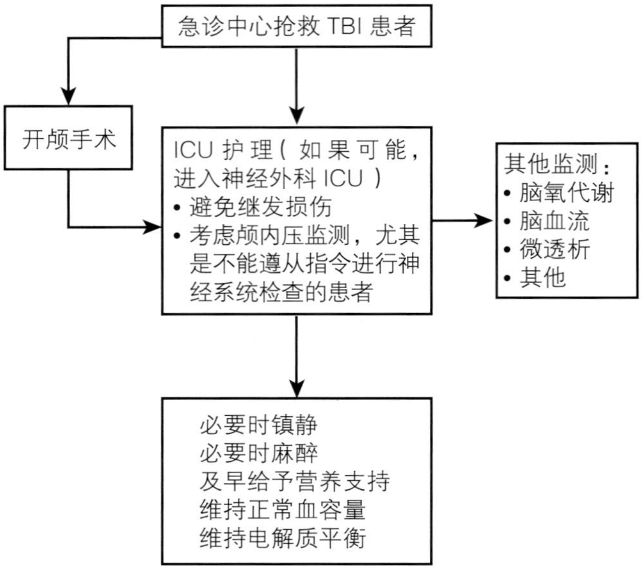

图 5　TBI 患者的住院处理

要点

- 术前体位摆放要考虑周全。
- 使用大骨瓣。
- 要预计到在巨大硬膜下血肿吸出过程中可能出现脑肿胀，要意识到逐步通过硬膜裂孔减压。
- 关颅前一定要确切止血。
- 如对病情存在疑问，留置颅内压监测。
- 术后 ICU 监护的重点是防范继发损伤。
- 不要进行不必要的镇静治疗。

脊柱：脊髓损伤、钝击伤和穿透伤、神经源性和脊髓休克

Vartan S. Tashjian, Nestor R. Gonzalez, Larry T. Khoo 著
熊　建 译

在紧急的情况下，脊髓损伤会面临一系列复杂的处理问题，包括如何能执行流畅的诊断、治疗干预方式以达到对患者最好的治疗，这包括在医疗领域内许多不同的原则。这些包括急救医疗服务（EMS）人员、急诊科团队、放射学专家、骨科及神经外科医师、重症护理人员以及理疗师。而对于所有这些来说，损伤后几小时内采取的快速干预经常决定了整体的预后，并给患者提供了获得远期功能结果的最好机会。由于这个原因，充分的脊柱固定、快速的诊断以及早期会诊决定了采取适当的外科干预方式，所有这些方式都是每一个急诊科医师应该在评估每个创伤患者时同时做的。本节主要描述脊髓损伤的流行病学、分型、处理，以及急、慢性脊柱损伤患者常见的并发症。我们通过对脊髓损伤诊断、治疗的指南和推荐的理解，知道了与之相关的发病率和死亡率在过去的30年里在持续地下降。

发病率

整体而言，脊髓损伤最经常累及年龄在16～30岁的年轻人。平均年龄29.7岁，分布不均，其中82%的患者为男性，这可能反映出年轻男性从事危险相关活动的更大的趋势。损伤经常出现在更温暖的夏天，特别是在周末。53%的脊髓损伤发生于在周五到周日间。关于脊髓损伤的特殊原因，每个创伤中心经常不尽相同，这在很大程度上取决于各个机构所处的社会经济背景。作为脊髓损伤的头等致病原因，交通伤不论是在乡村还是在城市的医疗机构都是很常见的。近些年，包括强制的安全带法律和汽车安全性的不断革新在内的预防措施显著地降低了机动车事故带来的脊髓损伤的发生率。在1980—1990年这10年间，交通事故创伤导致的脊髓损伤的发生率从47.2%降到了38.1%。在乡村中心，坠落为造成脊髓损伤的第二大致病原因，反而在城镇中心，暴力与交通伤不相上下，成为脊髓损伤的首要致病原因。特别是手枪带来的枪伤占城镇中心暴力引起的脊髓损伤的90%。在这些特殊的病例中，少数民族非常常见。不考虑社会经济因素，运动相关的脊髓损伤一直在所有脊髓损伤中持续扮演着重要的角色。在一项对伯明翰Alabama大学运动相关脊髓损伤的研究中，以下这些体育项目的脊髓损伤发生率从高到低排序为：跳水/冲浪、美式足球、冬季运动、体操、摔跤和骑马。随着老龄化人口的增加，年轻人暴力发生率的上升，跌倒和穿透伤导致的脊髓损伤在今后会在所有脊髓损伤病例中占有越来越高的比例。

脊髓损伤由于各种原因表现为对卫生事业的巨大的经济负担。事实的核心问题是，脊髓损伤的患者不但在早期处理上面临巨大挑战，根据不同的神经损伤程度，在伤后第一年的平均花费从123 000美元到417 000美元不等，而且有着各种长期的直接和间接的经济负担。直接损失是明显的，是由损伤直接带来的，包括再入院、家庭护理、持续使用装备及护理人员照顾。间接的花费更加隐秘，包括未来薪水、附加福利和工作能力的损失。虽然在初次住院的脊髓损伤患者中有95%的人能够存活是现代医学和危重患者护理的巨大成功，但随着普通人整体寿命的延长，这些因素也只不过会进一步增加脊髓损伤患者毕生护理的直接和间接花费。脊髓损伤患者出现损伤时的平均年龄较为年轻，这会进一步影响脊髓损伤的经济因素，对于高位脊髓损伤患者（C1～C4），按预估寿命的直接和间接经济损失会多出250万美元。

解剖学和生物力学

脊柱解剖

Denis首先描述了脊柱解剖的三柱模型，将脊柱分为纵向的三个柱（图1）。前柱包括前纵韧带（anterior longitudinal ligament，ALL）、椎体以及椎间盘前1/2。中柱包括椎体/椎间盘的后1/2和后纵韧带（posterior longitudinal ligament，PLL）。最后，

图 1 本图显示了脊柱的三柱模型。前柱包括前纵韧带（ALL）和椎体 / 椎间盘复合体的前 1/2。中柱包括椎体 / 椎间盘复合体的后 1/2 和后纵韧带（PLL）。后柱包括完整的椎弓和相关的韧带结构

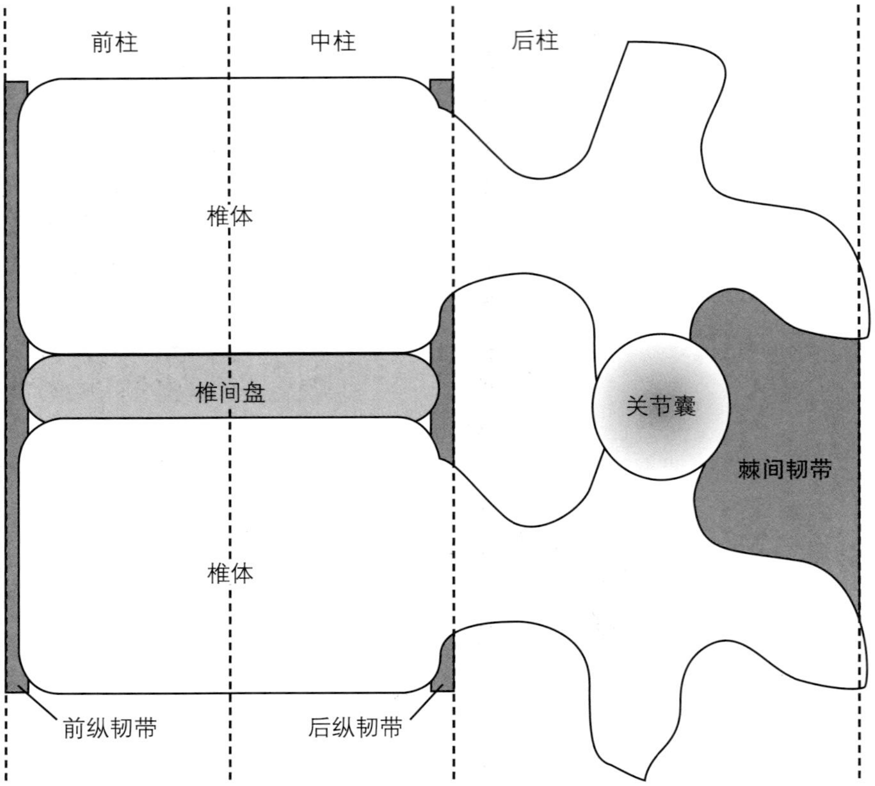

后柱包括所有后纵韧带后方的骨 / 韧带结构（椎弓根、椎板、棘突、黄韧带和棘间韧带）。根据定义，三柱中至少有两柱断裂导致的脊髓损伤被认为是不稳定损伤。这种对脊柱解剖多少简单化的描述有助于对分析脊柱的生物力学以及钝性和穿透力造成的潜在损伤提供脑海里的框架。

脊柱的生物力学

在探究脊髓损伤的潜在机制之前，对脊柱的生物力学有正确的理解是十分必要的。在分析病例时经常会出现的情况是，在脊柱致畸损伤的实际程度和实际的影像学发现及损伤相关神经障碍之间总是会存在一定的偏差。多种机制同时作用而产生脊髓损伤。其中有四种损伤作用力会传递到正常的脊柱：①屈曲和伸直（侧弯）损伤，②垂直压缩和纵向牵张创伤，③旋转损伤，和④复合机制损伤。

对于脊柱的屈 - 伸损伤，脊髓经常被压迫、横向 / 纵向剪切以及捻搓和旋转力所损伤。这些损伤一般会累及颈椎，经常导致椎间盘突出，也可能包括棘突间、前柱或后柱韧带撕裂。当一个相关的椎间盘出现突出或半脱位时，局部脊髓损伤的发生率很高，而且主要可看到脊髓中央坏死和出血。在 8 岁以下的儿童，极度过伸伤经常会与完全脊髓横断有关，这主要与儿童正常情况下颈椎韧带生理性过度松弛有关。

过伸（反屈）损伤经常导致 C5 ~ C6 节段的脊髓损伤，因为从生物力学的角度讲，伸直的角度在这个特殊节段是最大的。这些损伤经常与骨性脱位、腹侧骨折脱位、关节突撕脱、椎间盘破裂 / 移位以及前纵韧带 / 后纵韧带撕裂有关。所有这些都会导致椎管的前后径变小而带来继发的脊髓中央损伤。

压缩和纵向牵张损伤最经常见于继发于头部、臀部或颈部坠落带来对脊柱的垂直应力。它们经常出现在机动车事故中的急性增加的轴向负荷力。在影像学上，这些损伤典型地表现为椎体变扁、终板骨折和急性椎间盘突出，通常也会有骨块和椎间盘组织向后突入椎管而造成不同程度的脊髓压迫。当损伤机制为坠落伤时，这些损伤主要出现在脊柱活动性最大的胸腰椎结合部。相反地，在脊柱受到垂直轴向负荷力的病例中下颈椎更常受累及。

与压缩 / 纵向牵张损伤类似，脊柱的旋转损伤也最常累及胸腰结合部和上腰椎。根据定义，它们可能会累及椎体的每个部分，还包括椎弓根、小关

节和韧带复合体。这些损伤由于椎体的交锁及椎间盘的分离，经常会导致单侧或双侧脱位或稳定 / 不稳定骨折脱位。

损伤机制

脊髓创伤是一个广义的名词，它描述了一个在特定节段导致脊髓功能或解剖完整性受损的事件。虽然单独的腰椎损伤占脊髓损伤的绝大部分，但是大量较轻的脊髓损伤主要发生在颈、胸椎创伤中。因此，讨论的焦点将是从颈椎到胸腰椎结合部的脊柱损伤。考虑到总的损伤机制，所有的脊髓损伤都能够归入下面三个亚组中的一个：①直接（穿透）脊髓损伤。②间接（钝性）脊髓损伤。③联合的直接 / 间接脊髓损伤。根据损伤相关的潜在机制，对脊髓损伤的发病机制可以进一步再分类。原发性损伤是针对脊髓实质的直接机械损伤，有代表性地是出现在最初损伤时。继发性（反应性）损伤并不是由损伤刺激直接引起的，而是由一系列损伤相关因素发展而来的，包括水肿、缺血以及不正当固定带来的继发性机械损伤和其他生化异常因素。最终，原发性和继发性损伤共有的是都可能会引起迟发的神经后遗症，包括瘢痕形成、继发性变性或再生现象。

脊髓穿通伤

历史上，对穿透性脊髓损伤（penetrating spinal cord injury，PSI）的处理是归入到军医的处理任务里的，因为这类损伤绝大多数出现在战斗中。不幸的是，在过去的 20 年里，在许多城镇中心，暴力作为脊髓损伤首要原因的出现强调了急诊室医师在处理群众操作中掌握这些损伤急性处理方法的重要性。总的说来，穿透性脊髓损伤可以被分为枪伤相关或穿刺（非枪伤）性穿透性脊髓损伤。这两种类型最经常累及胸椎，累及范围很少超过一个椎体节段。因此，所有穿透性脊髓损伤中有 52%～57% 的患者会出现完全性脊髓损伤（骶部会阴区无感觉运动保留），虽然穿刺伤经常会导致不完全脊髓损伤。虽然根据定义，穿透性脊髓损伤意味着硬膜或实质的直接损伤，但在一些病例，损伤机制更类似于震荡损伤。大量军事相关研究已经证明，在许多病例行椎板切除术后发现硬膜是正常的。

钝性脊髓损伤

在临床中，脊柱闭合性损伤是引起脊髓损伤最常见的类型。它们经常出现于交通事故、工业事故、坠落伤以及体育活动中。在这些病例中，潜在损伤脊髓的脊柱骨折脱位和半脱位可能伴发或不伴发软组织损伤。损伤的生物力学和发病机制对脊髓损伤的类型和范围起着最核心的作用。为了能够预期在初发损伤后继发反应损伤的进展，对在损伤时分布在脊柱各部的机械力的潜在分型有一个彻底的了解是十分重要的。总的说来，闭合性脊髓损伤能够被归纳为两大类。第一种包括由于钝性创伤引起的间接脊髓损伤，椎管没有被侵占或没有穿透伤。这种损伤病例通常可以在损伤机制包括纵向剪切 / 牵张、屈曲、旋转、旋转 - 屈曲或前后加速的患者中观察到。闭合性脊髓损伤的第二种类型包括继发于钝性或穿透性力量导致的多种原因的椎管压迫带来的脊髓损伤。这些包括骨骼 / 韧带损伤、骨折脱位或半脱位。值得注意的是，脊髓损伤很少只限于解剖上的直接损伤点。在将近 15% 的脊髓损伤病例中，由于原发性和继发性创伤改变，损伤可以出现在多个节段。

脊髓损伤的严重性 / 分级

神经损伤平面（neurologic level of injury，NLI）是一个特殊的名词，指脊髓损伤后残留正常运动 / 感觉功能的最尾端的脊髓平面。虽然在损伤的解剖和神经平面间存在一定程度的相关性，但这种关系并不总是一致的。一旦证明有继发性损伤，许多因素如累及脊髓节段和损伤潜在机制都会对最终的神经损伤平面有影响。总体上，根据美国脊柱损伤协会（American Spine Injury Association，ASIA）的数据，将近 53% 的脊髓损伤患者为四肢瘫，46% 的患者为截瘫，而剩余的 1% 患者在出院时可完全恢复。脊髓损伤可进一步分为完全性或不完全性损伤，这主要取决于骶部会阴区是否有感觉 / 运动的残留。最常见的类别是不完全性四肢瘫（31.2%），接下来是完全性截瘫（26%）、完全性四肢瘫（21.9%）及不完全性截瘫（20%）。

神经和功能结果的评价

在过去的这些年，大量的分型方法被用来描述脊髓损伤患者。总的说来，存在两种评价方法，即神经检查方法和功能结果方法。现在公认的最有意义的对脊髓损伤的描述，是在急性期联合应用神经评价和功能结果评价表，以给这种患者提供评估每日神经功能恢复显著性的方法。第一个标准的脊髓损伤神经评价方法是由 Frankel 等在 1969 年提出的。在这个评价表中，根据损伤后保留的不同级别的运动 / 感觉功能，用五级（A 到 E）用来评价脊髓损伤患者。Frankel A 级是指完全运动和感觉损伤的患者。B 级是指损伤平面以下只有感觉功能的患者。C 级指是在损伤平面以下有一定程度运动和感觉功能的患者，但是残留或恢复的运动功能是无效的。D 级指是在损伤平面以下存在有用但异常的运动功能的患者，E 级是指在出院前足够幸运地运动和感觉完全恢复的患者。Frankel 分级的主要局限性是很难区分 C 级和 D 级损伤，以及在实际应用时观察者间的可信度较差。尽管有这些缺陷，Frankel 分级法仍然优于同期的许多其他分类方法，能够提供一个重要的分类框架。实际上，ASIA 损伤分类法很大程度上被视为最科学和有用的脊髓损伤神经分类方法，它是对最初的 Frankel 法的一个主要变更，它提供的一系列客观参数可以更好地评价 C 级和 D 级患者的残留的运动功能。与 Frankel 法类似的脊髓损伤神经检查工具是作为功能结果评价的功能独立自主量表（Functional Independence Measure，FIM）。它是一个包括 18 项、7 个级别的被设计用来评价患者残疾严重程度、护理负担、医疗康复预后及整体功能结果的量表。特别指出的是，FIM 补充了神经功能评价，可以对整理家务、洗澡、吃饭、上身穿衣、下身穿衣及如厕等活动提供评分。对急性脊髓损伤患者在整体评价损伤的影响时要同时做神经和功能缺陷的评估。此外，这些独立量表间的联系能够使医师评估那些能够提高神经评分的治疗方法是否也能够增强患者的功能恢复。不同治疗方法的总体有效性都要以功能结果作为基础，才能够被真实地评价。对急性脊髓损伤患者急性期用甲泼尼龙治疗的获益进行评价的国家急性脊髓损伤研究（National Acute Spinal Cord Injury Study，NASCIS）Ⅰ和Ⅱ的临床研究忽略了这样一种功能结果评价。它经常作为一种研究设计的缺陷被引用，只描绘了本质上不可能的神经结果的改善。一项对于现有的关于脊髓损伤分类文献的最新 Meta 分析指出，对于脊柱和周围神经损伤部分，美国神经外科协会（Association of Neurological Surgeons，AANS）和神经外科会议（Congress of Neurological Surgeons，CNS）推荐将脊髓损伤神经和功能分类的 ASIA 标准作为临床医师在评价和处理急性脊髓损伤时首选的神经检查方法。这个推荐很大程度上是基于发现 ASIA 评分能够对于复杂损伤中的脊髓损伤分类提供最大的组间分辨度，并有相当高度的观察者间可信度。与其他脊髓损伤分类方法类似，ASIA 评分从 1984 年最初提出到现在经历了许多次修改。现在，这个评分由许多组成部分组成，包括 ASIA 损伤评分、ASIA 运动指数评分、ASIA 感觉评分和 FIM（图 2）。

脊髓综合征

对于急性脊髓损伤的描述有多种脊髓损伤综合征。典型的脊髓中央综合征出现在颈段，表现为上肢无力较下肢明显，同时骶尾区感觉运动保留。典型的 Brown-Séquard 综合征见于穿透性脊髓损伤，导致脊髓的半切损伤。它主要表现为损伤平面以下同侧的本体感觉和运动丧失及对侧的痛温觉丧失。相反，脊髓前角综合征表现为运动功能和痛温觉的不同程度的丧失，而管理本体感觉的后束是完好的。脊髓圆锥综合征表现为骶髓和腰部神经根损伤，会导致膀胱、肠和下肢无反射，骶尾段偶尔保留反射。最后，马尾综合征是由于损伤累及椎管内的腰骶神经根，导致膀胱、肠和下肢无反射。与不同的脑干血管综合征类似（如 Wallenberg 综合征），脊髓综合征经常不会表现出典型的教科书上描述的一系列症状和体征。然而，就像脑干血管综合征的病例，对于脊髓本质上复杂的结构组织来说，对不同的脊髓综合征的理解可以提供一个大概的神经解剖框架。

诊断

中枢神经系统的组织结构可以使医师有机会只通过仔细的神经系统体格检查对脊髓的损伤部位进行定位，并有相对较高的精确性。然而，充分的术前准备及理想的手术计划都要仰仗于对脊柱精确的影像检查。几十年来，脊柱的 X 线照相一直是各种原因导致脊髓损伤的非常重要的定位诊断工具。首先，与其他更高端的影像手段不同，这项技术和需要的资源明显不是一个限制因素。其次，X 线技术的便携性和获取相对简单性也使医师有机会快速地获得重要的解剖信息，甚至在最忙碌的情况下。最后，脊柱平片可以对潜在脊髓损伤患者提供整体的信息，包括是否有骨折、半脱位 / 脱位以及椎管是否通畅（图 3）。虽然标准 X 线技术不能够很好地显示软组织结构，但平片上显示的脊柱序列 / 成角可能会提示存在潜在的急性韧带或椎间盘损伤。从 2000 年至今，大多数创伤中心越来越多地使用 CT，已经使急性脊髓损伤的诊断发生了重大变革。在许多中心，CT 已经取代了 X 线平片作为创伤患者脊柱紧急评价的方法，这在很大程度上是由于这项技术越来越高的可行性。CT 在很多方面优于 X 线平片，它对骨性结构比任何其他影像学手段都有着更优异的显示。另外，三维重建软件的出现现在可以在轴向、冠状面和矢状面上更好地观察相关解剖（图 4）。基于这些原因，CT 对观察椎体骨折总是比单独行 X 线片有更好的灵敏度和特异性。虽然对相关的软组织损伤的观察远远不如 MRI 技术，但 CT 也能够提供一定的软组织分辨，包括棘突旁出血。这进一步提示潜在不稳定韧带损伤的可能性。结合脊髓造影术，CT 技术可用于诊断椎管内占位性损伤，能够观察椎管内解剖并能够有与 MRI 相似的特异性。

从 1971 年 Raymond Damadian 将 MRI 作为医学检查手段到现在，其已不断进步成今天的诊断工具。这种技术上的发展反映出它的应用越来越广泛。虽然对于骨性结构的分辨和观察不如 CT，但 MRI 毫无疑问为软组织结构损伤提供了最多的信息，特别是对于脊髓本身。特别是 T2 加权相为实际损伤平面提供了有价值的信息。一旦出现继发性损伤，如脊髓水肿，它也能清楚地显示（图 5）。最重要的是，

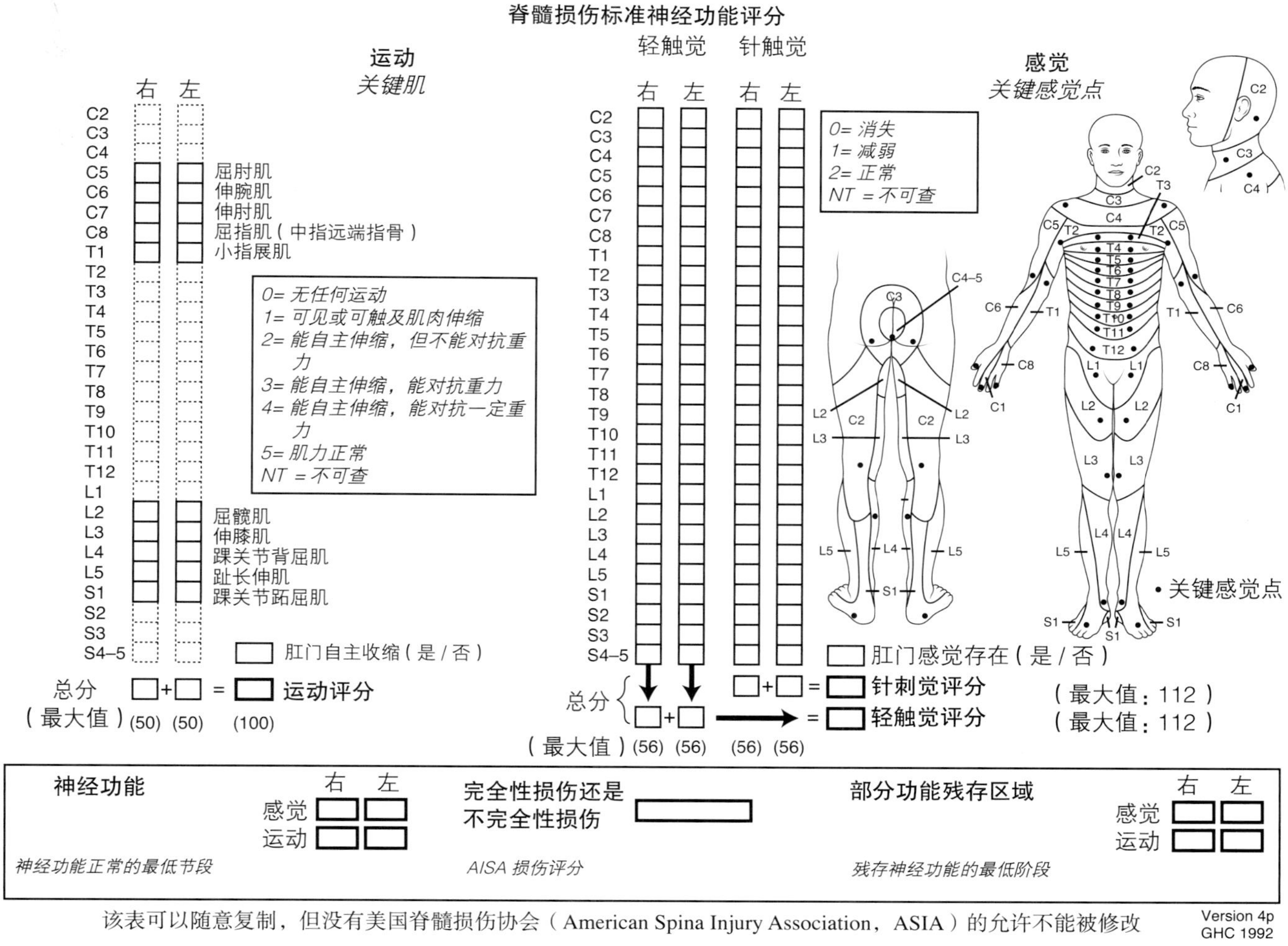

图 2 美国脊柱损伤协会（ASIA）损伤评分和对于脊髓损伤（SCI）的 ASIA 神经分类表。损伤评分是对于最初的脊髓损伤的 Frankel 评分的变更。实际的 ASIA 分类表包括 ASIA 损伤评分、ASIA 运动 / 感觉指数以及功能独立自主量表（并未显示）。（Courtesy of The American Spinal Cond Injury Association and The International Medical Society of Paraplegia.）

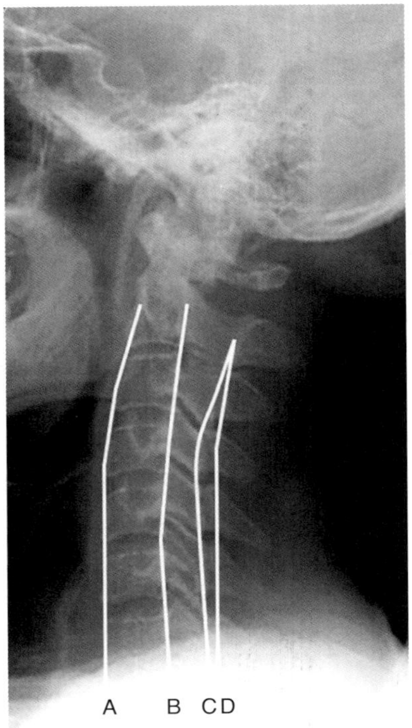

图 3　正常颈椎的侧位片，显示椎体前缘（A）、椎体后缘（B）、椎板 - 关节线（C）和棘突椎板线（D）的正常序列

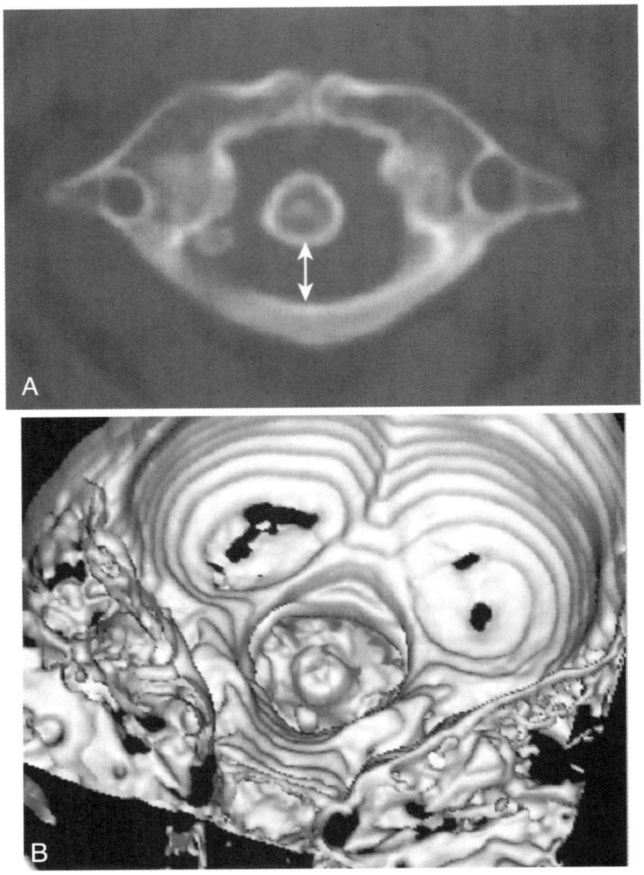

图 4　1 例创伤后寰枢椎半脱位的 35 岁唐氏综合征患者。A，显示寰椎 - 齿突间隙增大，同时椎管前后径明显缩小（双箭头），三维重建可以更清楚地显示（B）

明显的脊髓机械性压迫和脊髓的直接实质损伤能够直接地被 MRI 查明，从而为外科减压 / 固定的整体时间表提供了参考。

急性脊髓损伤的处理

对急性脊髓损伤最佳的处理是一项非常具有挑战性的任务，亟须多学科合作，以能够提供给患者最大的神经恢复的机会。从广义上来说，急性脊髓损伤的处理能够被分为很多重要的阶段，从最开始的急救医疗服务人员就地的照顾处理，到最终急性期住院后的加强脊髓康复。在这两者之间，急诊人员、放射学家、外科医师、重症护理人员和理疗师之间对患者照顾的精诚合作对于脊髓损伤患者的整体预后和结果是非常关键的，而且他们都起着相同重要的作用。总体说来，脊髓损伤处理的阶段包括：①院前处理。②紧急急诊室评估 / 急救。③亚急性期护理。④出院后护理 / 康复。处理的各方面都说明，特殊阶段的治疗可能会与接下来的处理过程重合。例如，药物治疗从在急诊室的急性评估时就开始了，经常持续到治疗的亚急性期。另外，一些治疗选择，如外科手术，也可能在不同的治疗点开展（例如急性或亚急性外科干预）。

院前救治

脊髓损伤院前救治的主要原则一直是快速和有效的脊柱固定，以防止继发于不稳定脊柱的病理性活动造成的进一步的神经损伤加重。在最初的创伤发生后，3% ~ 25% 的患者存在脊髓损伤，可能发生在转运或早期处理的过程中。因此，对所有存在可能发生脊髓损伤的创伤机制的创伤患者推荐使用硬颈围，要正确地使用脊柱固定器，并快速、间断地进行调整。一旦提出最终的评估和治疗，要注意制动装置相关疾病的发病率。特别是颅内压增高，受压溃疡的发生，患者明显不适或痛苦、跌落以及呼吸的危险性升高，所有这些都与脊柱固定装置有关。一旦患者被安全地救出并固定，及时将其转运至有

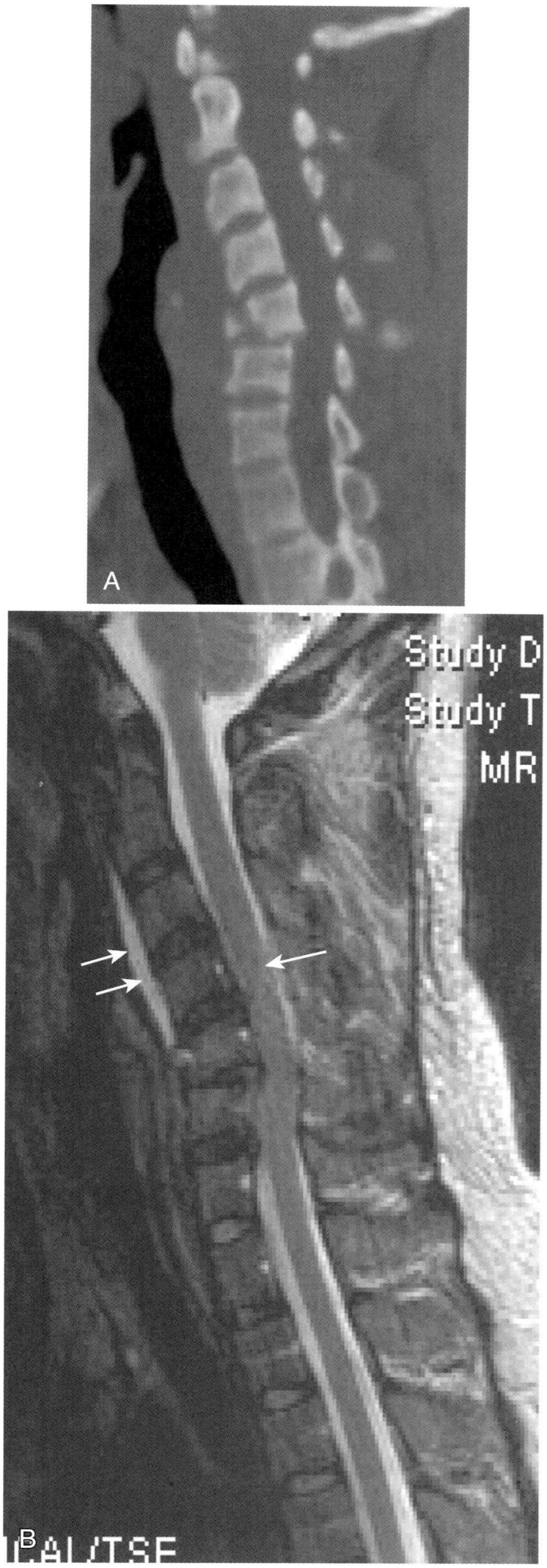

图 5 同时使用 CT 和 MRI 技术评估脊髓损伤能够提供更加详细的信息。对于这个特殊病例，从 CT（**A**）中可明显看到 C5 前缘的泪滴样骨折和局部后凸畸形，MRI（**B**）可以更清晰地分辨脊髓水肿（单箭头）和椎体前出血（双箭头）

能力评估和治疗急性脊髓损伤的区域医疗机构是最重要的。

急性期急诊室评估 / 处理

一旦患者进入急诊室，快速地对患者处理的责任就落在了急诊接诊医师的身上。对创伤患者进行早期评估时，急诊室医师的重要责任是确保就地对脊柱进行合适的预防措施，并在初期和后期的处理过程中一直保持。要仔细、充分触诊整个脊柱，以评估是否有潜在的骨性序列分离，以及相关的软组织肿胀或损伤。在最初的处理过程中应进行完整的神经系统和体格检查，发现任何明显的神经功能障碍后，如果可能，都应该尽早咨询相应的外科部门（神经外科或骨科）。接下来应根据放射学同事的建议尽快进行相应的放射学检查。如存在提示潜在急性脊柱损伤的任何影像学结构异常，都应该进一步咨询外科。如果是在一个神经外科或骨科不能会诊的医疗机构，那么就要在最早发现患者有神经损伤体征或放射学异常时把患者转运到最近的有相应处理能力的外科的医疗机构。只有对那些血流动力学不稳定，须要在转运前复苏的患者，才应该延迟转运。

依靠机构，在神经外科或骨科的范畴对急性脊髓损伤患者进行评估。外科医师干预的最重要的方面其实在急诊就已开始了。快速处理许多不同的信息是外科医师的责任，包括神经检查结果、放射学发现及其他转移损伤的出现，目的是为了到达脊柱损伤患者早期处理的主要分支点：尽早采取外科手术还是保守治疗并可能延迟手术。是否须要采取外科手术治疗的决定要根据每一个具体病例而定，因为每一个病例都会有独一无二的情况去考虑，以及须要克服的诊断 / 治疗障碍。总的说来，急性期手术的决定主要由特殊的类型所影响，包括损伤的放射学表现、患者神经查体的发现以及相对于其他潜在即刻威胁生命损伤的患者的整体稳定性。在脊髓损伤患者中多发创伤很常见，以下损伤的出现率逐渐递减：躯干骨折（17.2%）、长骨骨折（13.9%）、头面部创伤（13.8%）、气胸和胸部损伤（8.8%）以及腹部损伤（8.6%）。对于这些病例，应延迟手术，直到患者首先被充分的复苏，包括治疗即刻威胁生命的损伤，保持适当的血压参数，以及在认为合适的情况下使用颈椎牵引和糖皮质激素治疗。

外科手术

关于脊髓损伤的手术治疗，AANS 和 CNS 在脊柱和周围神经疾病的章节中从事了一项巨大的任务，就是对相关文献进行了系统回顾，以对不同类型的颈椎损伤的手术提供推荐依据。这部分外科选择是他们推荐的反映，虽然是以一种更加浓缩的形式。

对创伤性寰枕（C1- 枕骨）脱位损伤最好采用内固定和关节融合术治疗，采用各种各样的颅颈融合技术。虽然牵引和外固定也用来治疗一小部分这种损伤，但是相比于手术治疗病例，这些病例更容易出现短暂或持久的神经功能恶化，或迟发性不稳定。枕骨髁骨折最理想的治疗是颈椎外固定。如果出现特别的寰椎骨折，则须要对单独的寰椎（C1）骨折进行处理。对所有横韧带完好的单独的寰椎骨折推荐只用制动治疗。对于单独的寰椎骨折同时合并横韧带断裂，应该单独用颈椎外固定治疗或采取手术内固定治疗。在 Spence 对于寰椎骨折治疗的原则中，他提到，在开口位 X 线片上，当 C1 相对于 C2 侧块移位距离总和超过 8 mm 时，发生横韧带断裂的可能性特别高，这时可能须要进行 MRI 检查以进一步评估。

对枢椎（C2）骨折的处理取决于骨折的类型。对Ⅰ型（齿突尖）、Ⅱ型（齿突基底）和Ⅲ型（累及齿突并延伸至 C2 椎体）齿状突骨折，最初都可能采取外固定保守治疗（图 6）。然而，对于Ⅱ / Ⅲ型齿状突骨折的病例，当齿突移位超过 5 mm 时，齿突粉碎骨折（Ⅱ A 型）或骨折序列很难只通过外固定保持时，应考虑手术内固定治疗。此外，对于超过 50 岁的Ⅱ型齿突骨折应该考虑手术内固定，因为这类患者的骨折会有相对较高的不愈合率。虽然要重点平衡考虑使用 halo 架的副作用，但对于大多数的 C2 Hangman 骨折（创伤性枢椎滑脱）病例，是可以用外固定方法治疗的。对于严重的 C2 ~ C3 成角、C2 ~ C3 椎间盘间隙断裂或通过外固定不能维持序列时，应考虑手术固定治疗。对单独的枢椎椎体骨折可以只采用外固定治疗。对于寰枢椎联合骨折的处理最初应该基于潜在的枢椎骨折的特征。大多数 C1 ~ C2 联合骨折可以用外固定治疗，除了 C1 Ⅱ型齿突联合骨折同时寰椎 - 齿突间隙≥5mm，以及 C1 Hangman 联合骨折同时 C2 ~ C3 成角≥11°。采用的外科技术必须改良，以适应任何寰椎环完整性的丢失。

对下颈椎关节脱位及骨折 / 脱位损伤的处理要进行闭合或开放复位，并进行严格外固定、前路融合钢板内固定或后路融合钢板，钉棒或椎板间钳内固定。

胸腰椎骨折

在评估胸腰椎损伤时，脊柱解剖的三柱模型特别有帮助。总体上，累及胸腰椎有 4 种主要的钝性损伤：压缩骨折、爆裂骨折、屈曲牵张及骨折脱

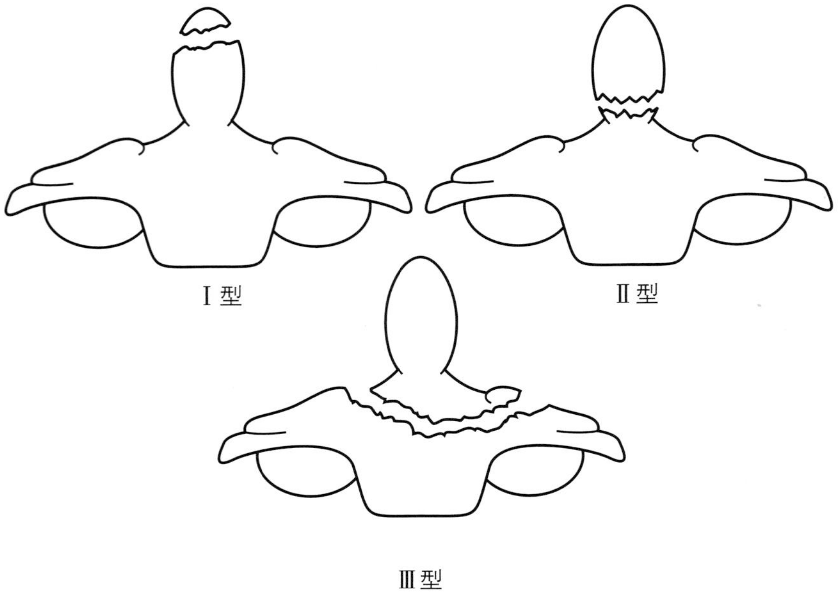

图 6　图示为齿状突骨折的类型。Ⅰ型骨折累及齿突尖。Ⅱ型骨折累及齿突基底。Ⅲ型骨折累及齿突基底并延伸至 C2 椎体

位。压缩骨折的特点是中后柱完整，前柱压缩伴高度丢失。相反，典型的爆裂骨折累及前柱和中柱，最常是由单纯的轴向负荷损伤引起的。它最常见于T10～L2。根据定义，它合并有骨/韧带复合体后凸入椎管，并经常引起明显的脊髓压迫（图7）。屈曲牵张损伤典型地包括水平骨折，可只经过骨（Ⅰ型），通过骨和韧带（Ⅱ型），通过椎间盘、关节囊和棘间韧带（Ⅲ型）。因为骨折为水平走向，因此这些损伤可能在传统的轴向CT上不易被发现。典型的骨折脱位是由剪力造成的，属于高度不稳定损伤，并经常与明显的椎管压迫有关（图8）。

脊髓损伤手术治疗的理想时间

急性脊髓损伤外科减压的作用一直是大量争论的话题。然而，根据动物模型进行早期减压的试验数据一直证明神经减压可促进神经恢复，但这些结果很难在实际脊髓损伤患者的身上证实，主要是因为缺乏说明早期外科减压治疗脊髓损伤有确定及明确获益的临床试验。文献中关于外科减压的大量研究提供了大量历史对照的回顾性病例序列。总体说来，大多数比较减压手术和保守治疗的研究实际上不能明确地说明手术治疗的效果更好。有趣的是，在最近La Rosa等做的一项Meta分析中，伤后24 h内行早期外科减压可以比延迟手术（伤后超过24 h）和保守治疗获得更加满意和显著的神经功能恢复，特别是对于那些最初不完全损伤的患者。然而，尽管缺乏不可反驳的支持性证据，对于急性脊髓压迫的患者而言，早期外科减压仍然是推荐的治疗。

穿透性脊髓损伤

与早期手术治疗钝性（非穿透性）脊髓损伤相似，早期手术治疗穿透性脊髓损伤的价值一直保有争议。典型的穿透性脊髓损伤的回顾性分析说明早期手术不会对结果有任何提升。此外，穿透性脊髓损伤患者在急性期行椎板切除术治疗有更高的并发症发生率。因此，对于急性穿透性脊髓损伤的患者进行早期手术治疗时，只推荐在那些进行性神经功能恶化的患者身上实施。然而，开放性伤口或怀疑有脑脊液漏的伤口可能须要外科清创/探查和硬膜修复。

急性期的非手术干预

当患者还在急诊室时，除了可能的急性期手术评估外，还有其他的干预方法。这些方法包括颈椎脱位的闭合复位、药物治疗干预和低血压的纠正/预防。只有对颈椎骨折脱位的清醒患者应该早期用颅骨颈椎牵引行颈椎的闭合复位，以达到保持脊柱的解剖序列的目的。与闭合复位相关的暂时的和永久的神经并发症发生率分别为2%～4%和1%。如果患者是警觉的，可以配合检查，那么虽然没有做MRI，但复位/牵引的危险性是较低的。因此，一旦放射学检查确认诊断，应尽可能早地行颈椎外复位。只有对那些复位过程中不能检查的患者推荐行复位前MRI检查。在这种情况下，如果出现明显的椎间盘突出，在复位前行腹侧开放减压是相对的手术指征。此外，对那些初次尝试闭合复位失败的病例推荐行MRI检查。创伤患者颈椎检查的流程图见图9。

药物治疗与脊髓损伤

与颈椎脱位闭合复位的病例不同，采用药物治疗急性脊髓损伤的作用很少明确。关于治疗急性脊髓损伤可用的各种药物，人们对糖皮质激素进行了最为深入、广泛的研究。在对于急性脊髓损伤早期用糖皮质激素激素治疗可获得潜在获益的热情退去后，最近的研究以及对NASCIS的原始临床试验的参数和数据分析减少了对于糖皮质激素治疗脊髓损伤可以带来功能结果显著提高的争论。对NASCIS的试验的主要批评一直与决定治疗的理想时间、运动评价方法以及在运动恢复评分与功能结果评估之间的相关性缺乏这些因素有关。这些缺点，加上在许多独立研究中不能够证明糖皮质激素治疗对脊髓损伤结果有明确的治疗效果，都促使AANS和CNS推荐糖皮质激素作为唯一的治疗选择，这要在充分了解除了临床获益及不良反应之后才能够应用。糖皮质激素治疗的不良反应包括肺炎、败血症、高血糖症、胃肠道溃疡/出血和股骨头缺血坏死。所有这些在NASCIS Ⅱ/Ⅲ方案糖皮质激素治疗脊髓损伤的患者中有着明显更高的发生率。相似地，一直证明GM1神经节苷脂可以增强急性脊髓损伤的神经恢复。然而，现有的医学证据并不支持这种结果。因此，对急性脊髓损伤时GM1神经节苷脂的管理只允许它作为一种可能的治疗选择时推荐使用。尼莫地平、纳洛酮和替拉扎特是脊髓损伤后潜在的神经保护剂也是现在进行的临床试验重点关注的地方。

血压参数的建立

然而，另一个在急性脊髓损伤患者相对早期应

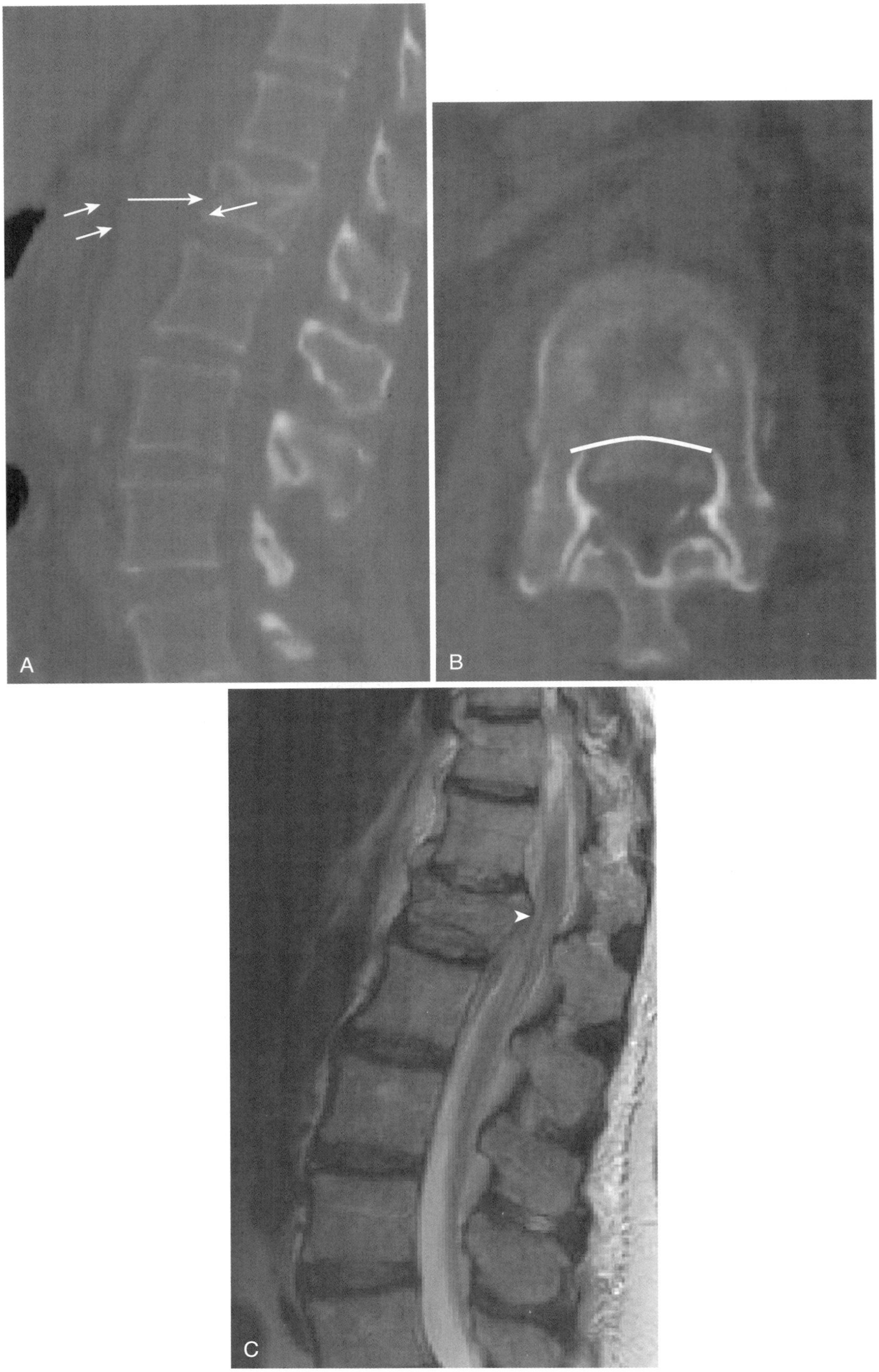

图 7　**A**，矢状位 CT 重建显示 L1 爆裂骨折（箭头），轴位相显示（**B**）继发于骨块后凸导致明显的椎管狭窄。图 **B** 中，白线显示的是正常的椎体后缘。**C**，MRI 扫面显示继发于后凸骨块（箭头）的对脊髓圆锥明显的压迫

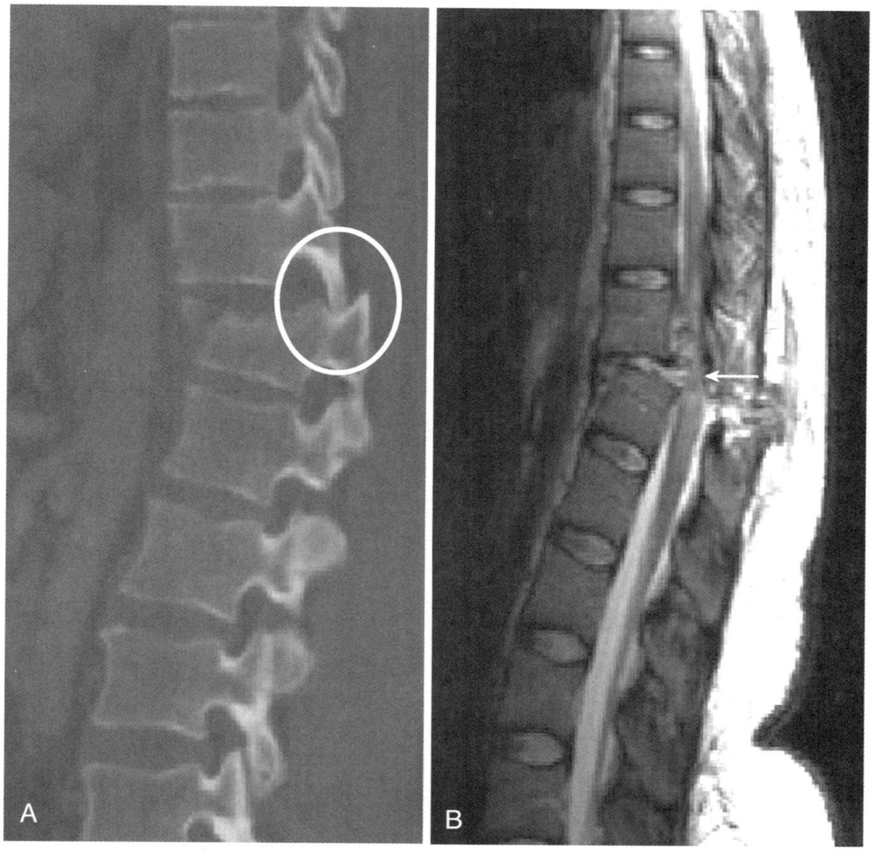

图 8 矢状位重建 CT 显示 T12-L1 骨折脱位（**A**），合并小关节完全脱位（圆圈），MRI（**B**）显示圆锥在 T2 相上信号改变并有明显的压迫

图 9 创伤患者颈椎筛查流程图

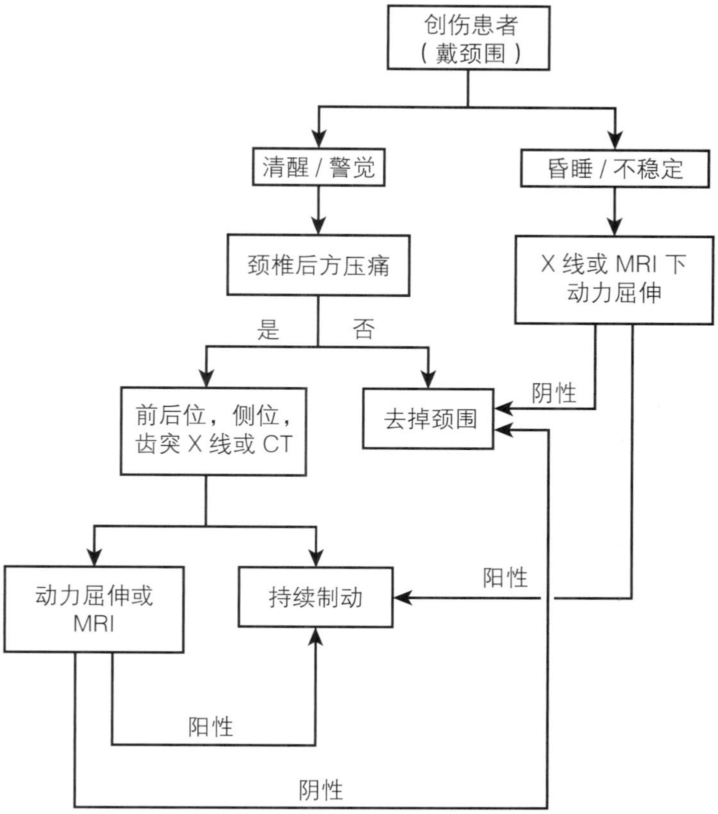

采取的干预措施是保持充分的血压参数。低血压在急性脊髓损伤中常见，通常是由于存在导致低血容量的相关性损伤及脊髓/神经休克。无论是何种潜在机制在作用，都应该避免急性脊髓损伤中的低血压，因为这会导致潜在的脊髓低灌注、缺血以及继发性创伤损伤加重。由于伦理学问题，关于脊髓损伤患者早期住院时低血压发作可提供的关于神经结果的文献只有回顾性（Ⅲ级）的证据。根据现有的证据，AANS 和 CNS 的主流推荐是急性脊髓损伤患者应避免收缩压低于 90 mmHg，目标是在受伤后的头 7 天保持平均动脉压（MAP）>85 mmHg。这经常须要放置中心静脉导管和使用静脉升压药。

脊髓损伤的亚急性期处理

在初步复苏和手术后，脊髓损伤患者进入其初次住院的亚急性期。对文献的回顾发现，在损伤后的第一个 7～14 天，严重的脊髓损伤患者很容易出现威胁生命的心血管不稳定和呼吸功能不全。这对于严重颈髓损伤患者特别明显。因此，强烈推荐将严重的颈髓损伤患者在重症监护室（ICU）内处理，在 ICU 可以应用心脏、血流动力学及呼吸监护设备以发现任何心、肺功能异常。有时甚至对相对稳定的患者，持续输注升压药以维持平均动脉压参数也需要 ICU 的护理。在 ICU 以及以后在普通病房内，物理治疗和职业治疗科的快速评估以及患者尽早参加相关的康复活动都会使其受益。要注意预防压疮及肢体挛缩，因为这些因素总体上会潜在地对神经恢复和结果造成负面影响。一旦患者转出 ICU，为了给脊髓损伤患者提供重获神经功能和提高总体功能结果的最大机会，应该将他们优先、及时地转到合适的康复中心。

脊髓损伤的发病率和并发症的处理

讨论脊髓损伤相关的各种并发症时，根据初次损伤后这些并发症出现的典型时间线进行分类是非常有帮助的。急性并发症出现在脊髓损伤后的头几个小时至几个星期内，经常出现在急性期住院时。这些并发症包括血流动力学不稳、心肺功能事件、肺炎、泌尿系感染、败血症和血栓栓塞现象。相反，慢性并发症出现在最初损伤后的几个星期后至几年，包括呼吸、泌尿生殖、精神、血栓栓塞、骨骼肌肉、胃肠道、感染和皮肤护理等方面的问题。在脊髓损伤急性期须要处理面临的很多并发症包括肺部并发症。对于生殖泌尿问题和血栓栓塞，须要采用积极的预防措施以降低它们在慢性期出现的风险。

神经源性休克

急性脊髓损伤患者经常面临的很多潜在并发症。这些并发症预示着血流动力损害在发展，并在这些患者的早期发病率与死亡率上占有重要的比例。典型的神经源性休克一般发生在急性脊髓损伤的平面位于 T6 或更高，表现为低血压、心动过缓和核心体温低三联征。胸交感神经链的损伤可引起不可抑制的明显的迷走神经紧张，从而影响效应器官的功能，包括外周血管阻力下降、体温调节受损和心动过缓。血管紧张度减小，同时合并继发于心动过缓的心搏出量减少，经常会导致明显的低血压，从而产生对晶体/胶体复苏的抵抗。如果不处理，全身性的低血压会导致脊髓缺血，更容易加重二次损伤严重度和进展。对急性脊髓损伤患者进行治疗的前提是要强调维持目标平均动脉压的原理。代表性的措施是通过晶体/胶体复苏，使用升压药，或两者联合使用。用内源性 β_1 激动剂的变时性活性升压是特别有效的，包括多巴酚丁胺和多巴胺，因为它们同时从血管源性和心源性两方面治疗神经源性休克。对持续的心动过缓可以间断地使阿托品治疗，但同时要了解到阿托品可由于增加分泌物而加重肺部功能障碍。总体说来，交感神经紧张在 3～7 天开始恢复。然而，在这期间脊髓损伤患者存在发生心肺并发症的风险是最大的，因此，在损伤后 1～2 周强烈推荐对这些患者进行持续的 ICU 监护。

脊髓休克

与神经源性休克不同，脊髓休克是在损伤平面以下一种短暂的脊髓生理反射功能的抑制状态，表现为所有感觉/运动功能消失。最初由于儿茶酚胺的释放表现为血压升高，接下来则表现为典型的顽固性低血压，包括肠和膀胱在内的迟缓性瘫痪是脊髓休克的标志性特点。也能够在许多病例中观察到阴茎的持续性异常勃起。这些典型的异常表现可以在伤后持续数小时至数天，直到损伤平面以下的反射弧恢复功能。球海绵体肌反射是指在挤压龟头或牵拉尿管时引起的肛门收缩。这个反射包含S1、S2和S3神经根，是脊髓介导的反射弧。脊髓受到创伤后，这个反射的出现与否明显提示预后。特别是对颈髓或胸髓损伤的病例，这个反射的消失说明存在脊髓休克或在反射弧水平存在损伤。脊髓休克持续的时间通常在48h内，球海绵体肌反射的恢复是脊髓休克终止的信号。远端的运动或感觉功能或肛周感觉完全消失，合并球海绵体肌反射的恢复，提示是完全性脊髓损伤。这些患者神经功能恢复的可能性极小。因此，如果在损伤平面下没有运动或感觉恢复，说明患者是完全性脊髓损伤并且没有进一步运动功能恢复的可能。另外，损伤平面下残留有运动或感觉功能说明是不完全脊髓损伤。在急性期，由于其他损伤的出现从而使休克的类型很难分辨。因此，必要时可使用侵入性肺动脉压监测以区分是神经源性、低血容量性还是心源性休克。

肺部并发症

对于脊髓损伤患者，不论是在急性期还是慢性期，肺部并发症是造成死亡的常见原因。颈髓和中胸段脊髓损伤经常导致呼吸功能障碍，也增加了肺部感染的概率。C4水平以上的脊髓损伤经常会损伤膈神经的功能，导致继发的膈肌功能障碍。因此，大多数高位颈髓损伤患者需要长期的机械通气，并经常被迫行气管造口术，以避免因长期气管插管造成的喉气管软化。低位颈髓或上胸段脊髓损伤会损伤辅助呼吸肌肉的神经支配，包括肋间肌，从而导致肺活量、潮气量和负压吸气功能的进行性丧失。这会明显降低肺容量，因肺内分流而导致通气灌注不匹配，并降低动脉血氧饱和度。充分咳嗽和正常叹气机制的丧失会导致不能清除分泌物的蓄积，从而导致终末肺段的阻塞和塌陷。这会促使理想的肺泡内环境变为反复发作的肺炎，甚至在许多病例是致死的肺炎。止痛药和镇静药的过度使用会进一步抑制呼吸功能。为了降低肺部并发症的风险，立刻制订积极的肺部护理计划是非常紧要的，包括雾化治疗、胸部理疗、间断正压通气以及插管患者的经常机械性吸痰。对于慢性重症患者，支气管镜一直是清除黏性气道分泌物的有价值的工具。此外，尽可能地早活动也会有助于提高整体肺功能。

血栓栓塞

血栓栓塞现象，包括深静脉血栓和肺栓塞，在脊髓损伤人群中是明显和致命的并发症。DeVivo等报道在脊髓损伤后的第一个月因肺栓塞死亡的危险性比同年龄性别的人高500倍。虽然深静脉血栓和肺栓塞的风险看似随着时间的推移相应地下降，但特别是对于那些完全性脊髓损伤的患者，他们由于制动而存在终身血栓栓塞的高风险。因此，损伤后预防至少3个月成为脊髓损伤患者的推荐标准治疗。可使用多种方法，包括低分子肝素、下腔静脉滤器、翻身床、调整剂量肝素、小剂量华法林、弹力袜、充气加压袜和电刺激器。对于所有这些方法中，尽管缺乏协同作用的直接证据，低剂量肝素联合使用充气加压袜仍是大多数中心选择的预防标准。使用预防方法可以使脊髓损伤患者深静脉血栓的风险从27.3%降到10.3%。如果发生了深静脉血栓或肺栓塞，要保证4～6个月以上周期的足量抗凝治疗。对于那些尽管抗凝但仍有顽固的血栓栓塞，以及有抗凝禁忌证（如最近或即将手术）的脊髓损伤患者，推荐使用腔静脉滤网。用多普勒超声诊断深静脉血栓的敏感度将近90%。对于那些尽管超声检查阴性，但仍高度怀疑有深静脉血栓的患者，应采取有创的诊断技术如静脉造影。同样，对于那些尽管通气灌注或螺旋肺CT血管造影检查阴性，但仍高度怀疑肺栓塞的患者，应采取有创的诊断设备来诊断肺栓塞如经股肺血管造影。

生殖泌尿并发症

由于膀胱压力升高、感染和膀胱/肾结石而产生的泌尿系并发症一直在脊髓损伤患者中保持着很高的发病率。逼尿肌运动功能和膀胱感觉的改变，以及括约肌异常，都导致膀胱不能完全排空、膀胱内压力升高和继发的泌尿生殖器损伤。慢性的膀胱压力升高会导致输尿管积水性肾病和膀胱输尿管反流的严重后遗症。此外，尿停滞也增加了脊髓损伤中发病率很高的泌尿系感染的风险，如尿脓毒症。为了控制这些并发症，推荐使用严格的膀胱护理计划。应该只限于在ICU内留置尿管。对尿潴留或尿失禁应该每4～6h进行间歇性清洁导尿，目标是随时保持膀胱容量在500ml以下。不推荐使用预防性抗生素。然而，对任何可能的泌尿系感染都应该迅速地诊断和治疗。

胃肠道并发症

在急性期，脊髓损伤患者有发生上胃肠道应激性溃疡的风险，可能与胃的毛细血管缺血有关，这会导致胃内黏膜层对胃分泌的正常的消化液的抵抗力降低。使用高剂量的糖皮质激素治疗急性脊髓损伤也会使这些患者发生应激性溃疡的危险性升高。近年来，脊髓损伤患者的消化性溃疡出血的发生率下降了，这被认为是大部分应用应激性溃疡预防的结果，包括组胺受体2阻滞剂、硫糖铝或质子泵抑制剂。对于神经损伤，制订肠道护理计划对于治疗相关的无动力肠梗阻是非常重要的。健康的肠道护理计划包括联合使用大便软化剂、高纤维饮食、手指刺激、栓剂、灌肠剂和人工通便。

皮肤护理

在神经损伤的情况下，出现压力性溃疡会带来明显的不适，而且这些溃疡会带来潜在的感染。骶尾部隆起部、股骨大转子、坐骨结节和足跟特别容易形成压疮。如脊髓损伤发生时间在2年内，须要外科清创的压力性坏死的发病率将近4%。预防是最重要的，典型的包括患者早期活动，使用气褥垫，限制使用支架/矫形器，积极的皮肤检查和伤口护理。

创伤后脊髓空洞症

创伤后脊髓空洞症（post-traumatic syringomyelia，PTS）通常发生缓慢。然而在过去的20年中，它越来越频繁地出现在脊髓损伤患者中，这可能由于多种因素包括脊髓损伤患者的预期寿命增加，以及MRI技术作为一种高度敏感的诊断工具的出现。根据定义，创伤后脊髓空洞症是在脊髓中央形成腔隙，典型地出现在伤后几个月至几年。虽然根据病变的位置和严重程度患者表现出不同的症状，但常常出现的是持续的局部或放射性疼痛、肌力下降、痉挛状态、感觉分离减退、自主反射障碍、括约肌障碍、性功能障碍、霍纳综合征和呼吸功能障碍。颈髓的空洞延伸进入延髓叫做延髓空洞症，表现为皮质延髓功能障碍。虽然有关空洞形成的确切病理机制并未被最终解释清楚，但流行的假说是由创伤后囊性脊髓病进展而造成的。继发于创伤后蛛网膜炎的脊柱蛛网膜下脑脊液流动力学的改变也可能发挥作用。创伤后脊髓空洞症的发生率从1.1%到超过50%，从发生创伤到诊断空洞的时间为2个月到33年不等。脊髓空洞症症状的发展预示着预后不良。虽然采用包括放置囊腹膜腔及囊胸膜腔分流在内的许多手术方法治疗，但这些手术的总体成功率普遍很低。

死亡率

尽管第一抢救者对脊髓损伤的处理已取得了显著的进步，但还是有10%～20%的急性脊髓损伤患者不能活着抵达医院，而3%的患者在急性期住院时死亡。对于那些急性期住院而存活下来的患者，死亡的主要原因是肺炎和其他呼吸系统并发症，然后是心脏病、并发创伤和败血症。不全截瘫患者死亡的主要原因是癌症和自杀。自杀也是完全截瘫患者死亡的主要原因，其次是心脏病。一般来说，自杀率在25岁以下的脊髓损伤的人群中更高。就生命预期而言，对于20岁受伤的个体来说，四肢瘫的预期寿命大约为33年，低位四肢瘫为39年，截瘫为44年。

小结

对于急性脊髓损伤，在很大程度上要感谢第一抢救者和急诊在处理上的显著进步，使在过去30年内这类患者的总体发病率和死亡率大大下降。同样，对包括血栓栓塞、泌尿系感染、肺部感染及压疮在内的许多脊髓损伤常见并发症的积极预防的实施/预防措施进一步改善了患者的生活质量。随着脊髓损伤患者的平均寿命接近普通民众，终身治疗这些患者相关的经济负担在未来将无疑继续增加。在急性期适时诊断并结合使用适当的治疗指南/推荐，可以为患者提供神经功能恢复的最好机会。一些特定的干预措施，包括脊柱固定、颈椎脱位闭合复位、维持血压参数稳定也在脊髓损伤的处理中获得了普遍接受，而包括糖皮质激素治疗和急性手术减压在内的其他措施，还有更加广泛的讨论和多种理解、解释。

第 5 章 颌面损伤和眼部损伤

颌面创伤

Urmen Desai，Rosaine Roeder，Benjamin T. Lemelman，Seth R. Thaller 著
安金刚 译

颌面创伤患者常由创伤科和整形科医师接诊，其伤情一般并不致命。当患者首次来到急诊室时，颌面创伤通常很容易被发现。在对患者进行初步评估和复苏的过程中，颌面创伤不应对外科医师造成干扰，但患者需要保证安全气道的情况属于例外。作为标准程序的一部分，其治疗过程须要严格遵守高级创伤生命支持（ATLS）的指令。

气道和呼吸

在创伤的救治中，第一要务是保证上呼吸道的安全，然后是确保充分换气和防止误吸。颌面损伤可以从几个方面对呼吸道造成损伤，包括组织移位、水肿和出血。下颌骨、鼻骨或上颌骨的多发骨折也可造成呼吸道损伤。从解剖学角度来说，舌体被下颌骨固定于口腔内，任何损伤两者关系的创伤都可能造成舌体移位至口咽部，从而出现气道梗阻。由损伤引起的周围组织水肿和局部血肿也可能造成呼吸道狭窄。另外，出血、呕吐物、脱落的牙齿或义齿以及异物均可能阻塞呼吸道。呼吸道梗阻的体征包括喘鸣音、发绀和流涎。由于酒精的作用、药物中毒或合并创伤性脑损伤，患者可能丧失保护性咽反射。对于这些患者，适合选择气管内插管或环甲膜切开。经鼻气管插管从技术上来说更为困难，更易造成并发症，并需要明确的鼻腔通道。

循环和止血

面部的动脉血供来源于颈外动脉的多个分支，其广泛的吻合形成丰富的血管网。许多动脉向浅表走行并进入颌面骨骼，其结果是容易出现损伤。但是，绝大部分浅表动脉出血可由压迫和血管修复（极少情况下）加以止血。还有，由于侧支循环丰富，结扎浅表血管并不会损伤相邻面部结构的血供。动脉修复只适用于管径较大的动脉损伤，并应该在手术室进行。

在面部外伤中，静脉由于比动脉更表浅，且无动脉瓣，因此更容易出现损伤，并且更容易出现失血过多。静脉出血可由压迫和结扎进行止血。

应优先处理由出血导致的呼吸道梗阻，因为出血可以妨碍对上消化和呼吸道的观察。对声带结构的观察不清经常使经口气管插管变得困难。在这种情况下，就要考虑采用外科手术的方法建立呼吸道。软组织伤口出血在患者的情况稳定后应加以处理。软组织损伤的外科治疗在本章的后部加以叙述。对面部骨折的出血一般采用骨折复位固定进行止血。

鼻出血

鼻出血常发生在面部创伤后，一般有自限性。它可能合并鼻骨骨折。出血可能来自鼻腔前部或后部，明确出血的部位对最终的止血来说很重要。鼻出血经常采用直接压迫最少 30 min 进行止血。如果出血持续不止，应进行鼻腔填塞止血。一般采用凡士林油纱条进行填塞。如果是鼻腔前部出血，用鼻

镜撑开鼻道，在直视下用枪状镊将油纱条逐层填入鼻腔，将油纱条逐层压紧充分填塞，要足够紧以达到止血的目的，同时又不能造成鼻腔黏膜和鼻中隔坏死。如果局部出血点很明确，用硝酸银直接烧灼止血也很有效。

鼻腔后部出血可由后鼻孔填塞加以止血。可采用导管辅助将填塞物通过鼻孔引入鼻咽部，也可通过口腔引入。采用鼻腔球囊导管可能更简单。如果鼻腔球囊止血不起作用，也可用一根 10-14Fr 的带气囊的导尿管来进行鼻腔后部止血。将其插入口咽部后，充气 10ml，然后小心地将导管向前牵引进入鼻腔，直至出血停止。必须避免气囊过度充气，以免造成组织压迫性坏死。如果可以看见出血部位，可用双极或电刀进行电凝止血或采用化学方法烧灼止血。

病史和物理检查

一旦初步评估完成，即开始二次评估，进行简要的病史采集和全面的物理检查。对于创伤患者，可以采用首字母缩略词 AMPLE 来记忆病史采集相关的内容：过敏史（A, allergies）、药物治疗史（medications, M）、既往史（past medical history, P）、最后一餐情况（last meal, L）以及受伤相关情况灶（events of the injury, E）。对于存在明显面部创伤的患者来说，损伤的机制非常重要。这一信息可以帮助临床医师预估损伤的范围和严重程度，以及推测是否可能合并某些隐匿性损伤。如果患者的损伤原因为机动车事故或枪弹伤，提示患者可能存在全面部骨折。运动损伤常导致单发的面中部上方骨折。暴力伤害常导致单侧下颌骨骨折。与由暴力、摔跌或运动造成的面部创伤相比，由枪击或机动车事故导致的面部创伤常更加严重。

为了防止遗漏任何损伤，必须从上到下以一定的顺序进行物理检查，并应记录检查时发现的任何不对称或明显的面部畸形。从头皮开始向下，检查软组织是否存在肿胀、裂伤、擦伤和钝挫伤。评价上、下颌骨，明确是否有缺失或碎裂的牙齿，以及是否存在错䏲畸形。触诊面部骨骼，看是否存在骨擦音、台阶感或明确的触痛部位。正常情况下，大张口时测量上下中切牙切缘之间的距离为 4～5cm，下颌侧方运动的范围正常大约为 1cm。这些检查结果都要记录。除了要检查鼻腔和口腔之外，还要用耳镜检查外耳道，以除外这些部位是否存在隐匿性损伤。脑神经的状况也须要检查，以明确是否有局灶性神经功能缺陷。

对患者进行重新评价很重要。在初次检查中，许多致病和后续致死的原因不能被发现。例如，患者可能在任何特定的时间发生呕吐，而出现误吸的危险。随着时间的推移，出血和水肿可以逐渐累积，最终造成呼吸困难。

影像学检查

对于面部创伤最好采用 CT 进行检查，并联合曲面体层片以评价牙齿的情况以及是否存在下颌骨骨折。应选择轴位、冠状位及矢状位 CT 图像以及 1～2mm 的扫描层厚来显示面部解剖，并明确是否存在骨折及移位。对全面部骨折和骨缺损应采用三维重建进一步评价。曲面体层片可以显示上下颌骨的解剖结构，并对所合并的牙源性损伤提供最好的评价效果。目前来说，急诊室可能会选择平片检查，但是，对于面部创伤的最终治疗，平片的作用有限。

软组织损伤

对于前来就诊的创伤患者来说，面部软组织损伤的评价和诊断是所有检查中不可分割的一部分。但是，绝大多数软组织损伤并没有生命危险，最初的处理主要是清洁伤口、去除异物、手术清创和控制出血。一旦患者的情况稳定，手术修复大的面部外伤应在手术室进行。

局部麻醉

面部裂伤可以在局麻下进行缝合修复，在此过程中可以配合静脉镇静。利多卡因和丁哌卡因是最常用的麻醉剂。如果使用 1% 利多卡因溶液，建议采用的剂量为 4.5 mg/kg，如果联合肾上腺素，剂量可以增加为 7 mg/kg。利多卡因的麻醉效果可以持续 30～60 min。丁哌卡因比利多卡因更加长效，可以持续 2～4 h。联合使用肾上腺素可以适当加大麻醉药的使用剂量，还可以促进血管收缩。表面麻醉药膏，例如 EMLA（含丙胺卡因和利多卡因），尤其对于儿童患者来说，可以减轻伤口的疼痛，并避免了注射麻药所产生的疼痛。

抗菌药物

可以选择第一代头孢菌素，在手术开始前 30 min 使用。如果患者对青霉素过敏，可以选择克林霉素。对于口内伤口，常须要对厌氧菌加以覆盖。如果是动物咬伤，还要针对革兰氏阴性细菌和厌氧菌进行更广泛的抗菌覆盖。所有患者均要接受预防破伤风的措施。

擦伤

所有的擦伤均应用温和的皂液清洗，去除异物，并用干净、无菌的敷料覆盖。对这类损伤患者应每天复查，以防出现感染或延迟愈合。

裂伤修复的一般概念

所有的裂伤均应在无菌的环境下进行缝合修复，并配合充分的照明以及相关设施和器械。理想的情况下，裂伤应在伤后 6～8 h 内进行关闭，但是，可以延迟至 24 h 之内进行缝合，然后严密观察是否出现感染征象。应尽早使用抗菌药物以预防感染。所有裂伤均应分层关闭，但是，对于简单、表浅的裂伤，采用组织黏合剂关闭伤口也比较安全。

头皮裂伤

头皮裂伤可造成大量失血。对这类伤口须要彻底冲洗，并仔细取出异物。可以采用订皮器快速关闭伤口进行止血。如果需要，还可以使用电凝止血。正规的手术应分层进行缝合。

口内伤口

在面部创伤的患者牙齿损伤非常常见。对牙齿 - 牙槽骨损伤处理时应去除所有松动的牙齿。对黏膜或牙龈裂伤可以压迫或采用细的可吸收铬肠线进行缝合。患者使用含氯己或过氧化氢的含漱液进行含漱，以保持口腔卫生。骨折合并口内损伤的情况将在本章后部加以讨论。

舌体裂伤

轻微裂伤一般不用处理，可以自行愈合。但是，如果裂伤很深，可能会波及舌动脉，有出血造成呼吸道梗阻的危险。处理过程中应吸干净伤口中的血液和口腔分泌物，明确出血的来源。如果舌动脉已经横断，在较大的创伤治疗过程中要及时修复。

唇部裂伤

唇部裂伤修复的难度与损伤部位的肿胀程度相关。在唇部裂伤的缝合过程中，其前部要对齐唇红缘，并间断分层缝合裂伤，向后达口内黏膜。对肌肉断端应采用可吸收编织缝合线缝合，对唇红部和黏膜伤口应采用可吸收铬肠线缝合，对皮肤用不可吸收缝线进行关闭。在缝合之前经常采用阻滞麻醉，以免使关键的解剖标志发生扭曲变形。在缝合之前，应描画出手术标志点，以便更好地对位缝合。

鼻部裂伤

鼻部简单的裂伤可用细的尼龙线间断缝合或进行组织黏合。但是，如果鼻软骨断裂或鼻黏膜裂伤，应请专科医师会诊。对软骨和黏膜表面应采用细的快速吸收的铬肠线缝合。

耳部裂伤

耳郭损伤应在伤后 12 h 内进行修复缝合。在此过程中应彻底冲洗伤口并清创取出异物。缝合应采用快速吸收的铬肠线。要对断裂的软骨进行对位，但无须缝合。缝合后用油纱垫对耳郭进行支撑。对耳郭撕脱性损伤应进行重建修复和再植。对于耳郭的部分撕脱损伤，可以选择复合组织移植和局部皮瓣进行修复，而完全性撕脱，常须要多阶段修复。

眶周裂伤

涉及眼部的损伤须要眼科会诊。在损伤修复之前应进行详细的眼科检查，并应记录在案。必须明确眼球是否存在明显的损伤。在修复之前应对眼周区域进行冲洗。涉及眉毛和眼睑的简单裂伤可以采用组织黏合或用细线间断进行缝合。复杂的裂伤应分层进行缝合。缝合过程中应注意对齐睑缘。眶周损伤可能合并泪小管损伤，尤其在内眦部位损伤的情况下。该类损伤的后遗症是持续溢泪。泪小管损伤应等待至症状持续存在后再进行修复。

腮腺损伤

腮腺损伤并不常见，但可以造成严重的并发症。对于腮腺损伤，鉴别并及时诊断很重要。Lewlowicz等提出了一种处理腮腺损伤的流程。首先，应将损伤的腮腺插入导管，注入生理盐水或亚甲蓝来评价损伤情况。如果结果为阴性，导管应留置1周，并关闭裂伤。如果结果为阳性，应探查寻找导管的两个断端，并决定是否须要延长伤口。如果导管断端均找到，则一期进行吻合，外部加压48 h，口内引流1周，插管留置14天。

面神经损伤

面神经的分支位于面部表情肌深方。对于轻微的面部损伤，一般不会波及面神经。但是，对于可疑面神经损伤，医生应佩戴放大镜仔细检查。如果面神经明确损伤或可疑损伤，应在手术室及时探查伤口，寻找断端，在显微镜下进行吻合修复。

面部骨折

鼻骨骨折

骨性鼻支架是由成对的鼻骨和上颌骨额突构成的锥体结构。在鼻腔内表面，鼻骨和筛骨的垂直板相融合，为鼻支架提供额外的支撑。由于鼻支架的位置较突出，并且构成的骨骼较脆弱，外鼻是最易损伤的面部结构。因此，鼻骨骨折是最常见的面部骨折。了解损伤相关的细节对于明确损伤的类型和严重性非常重要。体育运动、机动车事故、暴力以及由站立位摔倒是鼻骨骨折最常见的发生机制。打击力的方向、速度、打击物体的特点以及患者的年龄则是进一步影响鼻骨损伤程度的几个因素。对于鼻骨来说，侧面撞击造成的损伤更加常见。与正面撞击造成的鼻骨骨折相比，侧面撞击造成的损伤手术效果较好。在鼻骨损伤中男性是女性的2倍，最常发生在10～20岁或20～30岁。老年患者由于其骨骼变脆以及出现骨质疏松改变，鼻骨骨折多为粉碎性。年轻成人患者更易发生鼻支架主要骨段的脱位。与之相反，儿童患者由于其骨骼中软骨成分较多以及鼻骨的不完全骨化，青枝骨折更为常见。另外，侧面撞击造成的鼻骨骨折更加常见，但其治疗效果较好。鼻骨骨折可以分为单侧、双侧、粉碎性、凹陷性、压缩性、嵌入性或者青枝骨折。另外，鼻骨骨折还可以累及相邻的骨性结构，包括上颌骨、泪骨、筛骨或额窦。

鼻骨骨折典型的表现为鼻畸形、外鼻和鼻腔内部结构水肿、鼻出血以及眶周瘀斑。详细的病史还可以提示存在鼻腔呼吸功能的改变、嗅觉改变、鼻出血，以及鼻腔内有清亮的水样液体流出或有甜咸味道的液体，须要进一步检查，以排除脑脊液漏的可能性。还应该询问患者的病史，以前是否有过外鼻损伤、鼻骨骨折、过敏或鼻旁窦疾病。

通过详细询问病史以及仔细的物理检查，可以对鼻骨骨折进行诊断。如果鼻梁扭曲或不对称，则可能存在创伤性损伤。另外，其他的一些表现，例如鼻出血、眶周瘀斑和鼻腔内部水肿也支持可能存在外鼻损伤。此时应详细检查外鼻以及鼻腔内部，明确外鼻支架是否扭曲，鼻骨是否塌陷并向内侧移位，上部外侧软骨是否有内侧移位，或是否存在鼻梁增宽。检查过程中如果发现鼻中隔血肿，应立即切开引流。如果没有及时发现并治疗鼻中隔血肿，则会出现鼻中隔坏死和穿孔，最终可能会造成鞍鼻畸形。对于鼻骨骨折来说，平片或CT影像学检查的意义不大。对于区分陈旧性骨折还是新鲜骨折也存在困难。影像学检查也不能发现软骨损伤，而软骨损伤对于儿童患者来说更为常见。

合适的治疗时机对于理想的复位效果和满意的术后效果都很重要。对于鼻骨骨折，存在两个理想的治疗窗口。第一个治疗窗口为损伤后前3 h，在软组织开始肿胀之前，而软组织肿胀常会掩盖其深面的骨性结构损伤。第二个窗口位于伤后3～10天，在肿胀基本消除以后。在这一时期之后，骨折线周围开始出现纤维结缔组织，可能会限制骨折的充分复位。对于简单的鼻骨骨折，例如简单的单侧鼻骨骨折，常采用闭合性复位的方式。相反，对于严重的鼻骨创伤或超过4周的陈旧性骨折，则须要开放性复位骨折的鼻骨。

鼻骨骨折并不致命。但是骨折如果没有充分复位，则可以导致鼻外形长期明显的改变，包括鼻突度减小和鞍鼻畸形，以及鼻通气的持续性损伤。另外，儿童鼻骨骨折可能会造成外鼻支架和面中部骨性结构的发育不良。

颧骨骨折

颧弓的前突度对于维持面部外形来说有重要的美学意义。由于其位置和显著性，颧骨容易出现创伤性损伤和骨折。在后方，在颧骨和颞骨交汇处，咬肌附着于该部位。在内侧，颧骨对眶外缘和下缘以及眶外下壁提供结构支持。颧骨向下和向内扩展的部分形成面中部的外侧支柱，在这一部位颧骨和上颌骨相连接。颧骨是位于上颌骨和颅骨之间重要的支柱结构，并形成面中部骨骼的外侧支柱。颧骨周围4条骨缝（颧额缝、颧颞缝、颧颌缝和颧蝶缝）同时发生骨折时被称为四点骨折或颧上颌复合体（zygomatico maxillary complex，ZMC）骨折。与颧骨相连接的骨骼常吸收强大的撞击力，而出现骨折。在这种情况下，眶底常发生骨折并塌陷进入上颌窦。颧弓单一部位骨折常发生在其中点部位，或发生两处骨折而造成中央骨段松动游离。与上颌骨骨折相似，骨折移位的程度与损伤的严重性直接相关。这决定了骨折修复的复杂程度。ZMC骨折的患者常可在颧骨或眶下缘触及台阶感，另外，由于颧弓内侧移位，还会出现颧骨区域扁平。在初步检查时，这些表现可能不明显，而在损伤发生几天后，骨折表面软组织水肿消退后才能显现出来。由于喙突和颞肌被塌陷的ZMC所压迫，患者还会出现张口受限。由于眶下神经受损，患者还可能会出现相应区域感觉减退或麻木。

评价和诊断ZMC骨折的影像学检查的金标准是轴位CT图像。创伤患者在正常治疗过程中，一般应进行颅脑的影像学检查以除外颅内损伤。做颅脑CT检查时应向下扫描，范围包括面中上1/3部分，观察是否存在ZMC骨折。这些影像对于辅助制订手术计划很关键。骨折移位和粉碎的程度决定了创伤的复杂程度和手术修复的范围。

手术修复颧弓的水平部将恢复面颊的前方及侧方突度。手术修复颧弓的垂直部骨折将恢复与面中1/3相关的颧突的高度。向外下移位的ZMC骨折应引起重视。这类骨折常合并眼眶骨折，后者可导致眼眶体积增大。骨折可能导致眶内脂肪疝入上颌窦或筛窦。所以治疗ZMC骨折时，有必要考虑对合并的眼眶骨折的诊治。复位眶缘骨折的同时应恢复眼眶的体积，这一点很关键。术中，手术医师应取出可能造成重要神经和肌肉结构损伤的骨片。进行颧骨复位以后，再依靠稳定的骨支架来修复眶壁骨折。

手术治疗ZMC骨折最常见的并发症是骨折复位不理想。这可导致错𬌗畸形、骨折错位愈合或不愈合，后者可造成骨折部位异常动度、面部不对称，甚至可能出现骨髓炎。骨折错位可能造成眼球内陷或眼球下移位畸形。还可能发生多个软组织并发症，包括瘢痕或下睑外翻。

眼眶骨折

对眼眶相关的软硬组织解剖进行深入、透彻的理解对于眼眶创伤的治疗非常重要。眼球的位置由其周围悬吊它的韧带以及眶壁的完整性决定。眼眶是一个复杂的骨性结构，由多个面部骨骼共同构成。视神经管位于眶内壁的后方并向后内走行。除了最严重的眼眶骨折外，一般情况下视神经管都会被保护而不受损伤。撞击力可通过内侧眶突传递至眶下缘和眶底。上颌窦前壁和眶下缘损伤常造成颧上颌骨骨缝和泪囊窝之间骨性结构的粉碎性骨折。撞击力量的大小总是与损伤的严重程度相关联。发生眼眶骨折时，眼眶中部凹下的部分常被累及。来自诸如网球或棒球的眶周高速撞击损伤可向深方传递至眶底后部凸起的部分以及眶内壁，结果会造成显著的骨折移位。尽管眼球位于眶壁后方凸起部位的前方，在伤后最初评价和手术修复骨折的过程中，眼眶后方凸起的部位都是重点考虑的关键部位。损伤可以造成眼眶的一个或一个以上眶壁骨折，并向外移位，从而导致眼眶体积增大。还可以造成眼周悬吊韧带所构成的网络结构的破坏，导致眼球向后移位（即眼球内陷）和眼球位置降低（眼球下移位）。最终，由于重力的作用，眶内软组织发生移位，同时纤维性瘢痕开始收缩。

对于面上1/3遭受损伤的每一位颌面创伤患者，都应进行全面的眼科检查。检查项目应包括视力、瞳孔反应和眼球动度，检查前房是否有积血，并进行全面的眼底镜检查。在初步评估时，必须尽早检查视力情况。视力进行性下降提示存在眶内压增大或视神经损伤，必须进行早期手术干预。球结膜水肿、结膜下出血以及眶周瘀斑都是眼眶损伤典型的临床体征。在眼眶骨折的患者在其眶下缘可能触及台阶感，但由于表面的软组织肿胀和水肿程度的逐渐加重，台阶感可能不明显甚至很难触到。另外，由于邻近的眶下神经损伤，患者可能存在一定程度的感觉减退。应对眼球运动进行全面的检查。眼球向上运动受限以及主观存在复视可以帮助检查者确定下直肌是否存在嵌顿。被动牵拉试验可以帮助明确所有的眼外肌是否存在嵌顿。最后，还应从水平方向和垂直方向评价眼球的位置，并记录眼球内陷和眼球向下移位的程度。

在手术重建骨折的眼眶之前，应进行详细的术前 CT 检查，并根据 CT 检查制订治疗计划。针对任何类型的眼眶骨折，轴位和冠状位 CT 被认为是影像学检查的金标准，矢状位影像也可以为手术计划的制订提供有用的信息（图 1 至 4）。轴位 CT 图像主要针对眼眶的内外壁骨折的诊断。冠状位图像则用于评价眶底损伤的情况，对于眶底后部凸出的部位尤其有用。爆裂性骨折（blowout fracture）是指眶缘完整而一个或多个眶壁发生骨折的情况。这一名词还提示创伤发生的机制是钝性打击力作用于眼球，然后传导到周围的骨壁，导致眶壁发生骨折。由于眶下神经行经眶底，眶底骨折可以损伤眶下神经。

由于颌面骨骼为眼球、眼眶和面颊软组织提供支撑，因此，在骨折后必须得到彻底评估和积极治

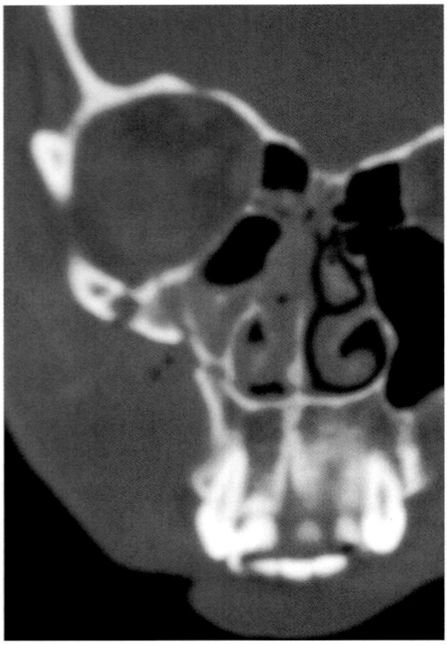

图 1 冠状位 CT 图像显示右眶下缘骨折波及眶下孔（*Courtesy of Seth Thaller, MD, DMD, FACS*）

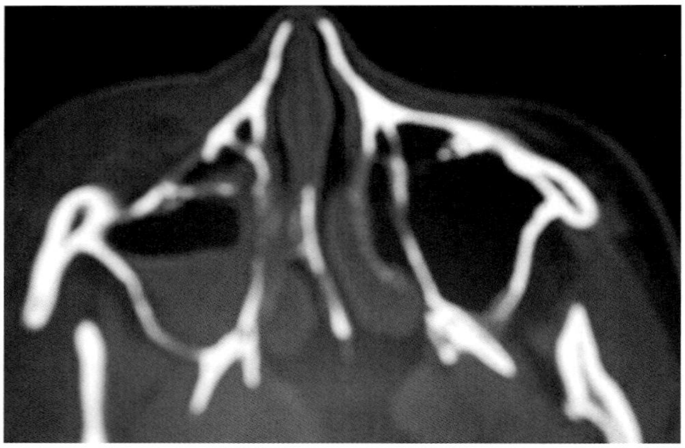

图 2 轴位 CT 图像显示右眶下缘骨折，右上颌窦窦腔内积血，骨折前部软组织肿胀（*Courtesy of Seth Thaller, MD, DMD, FACS*）

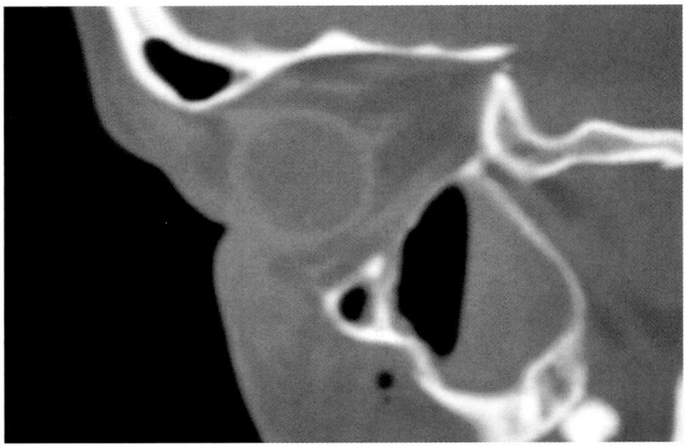

图 3 矢状位 CT 图像显示右眶下缘骨折波及眶底，右上颌窦内存在积血（*Courtesy of Seth Thaller, MD, DMD, FACS*）

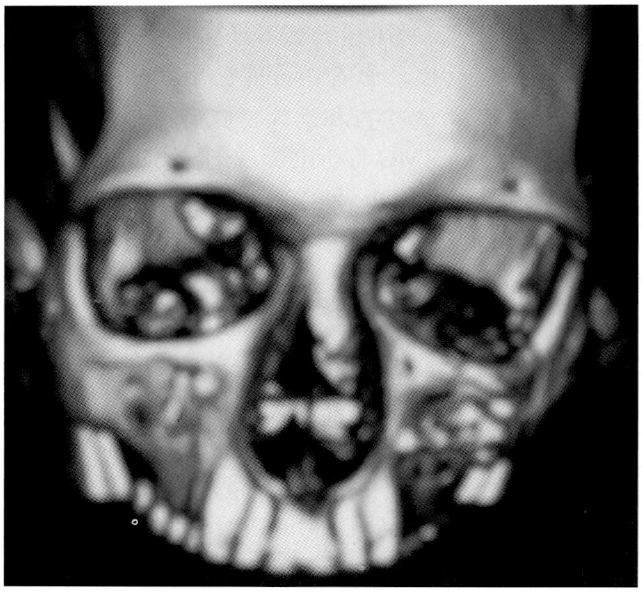

图 4 三维重建图像显示右眶下缘骨折波及眶下孔（*Courtesy of Seth Thaller, MD, DMD, FACS*）

疗。手术时，应将眼眶作为一个独立的单元，逐步复位和固定每一条骨折线。正常眶底前部外形向下凹陷，重建这一部位可以应用多种人工材料或自体组织。应将眶底完全暴露，以便获得缺损畸形的两个稳定的骨边缘来支撑植入材料。目前有很多种人工材料可供选择，不但容易获得，植入后很少移动，术中还容易塑形以及进行个性化的修整，以达到理想的匹配效果。另外，对颅骨也成功地应用眼眶重建。

眼眶骨折一个最常见的并发症是复视。这种视觉缺陷常在向上和向外侧凝视时出现。它可由眶内容物嵌顿、神经失用症或眼外肌挫伤造成。睑外翻主要由下睑下缘切口愈合过程中眼睑前层（包括皮肤和眼轮匝肌——译者注）瘢痕形成所致，可表现为巩膜过度暴露或角膜干燥，可导致角膜溃疡。睑内翻由眼睑后层（包括睑板和结膜——译者注）形成瘢痕所致，常由经结膜切口瘢痕愈合造成，可由于倒睫和角膜暴露而造成角膜擦伤。眼球内陷也是一种常见的并发症，由眶底和眶内壁重建不充分所致。另一个并发症是术后眼球内陷，其原因是眶底后部凸出部分的缺损重建不充分，或者没有正确诊断和修复眶内壁骨折。最后，钛板相关的并发症包括软组织刺激、对寒冷敏感以及钛板暴露。如果出现这些并发症，应等骨折线完全愈合后，及时取出固定的板钉。

有关眼眶筋膜室综合征和外眦切开术的内容见第 6 章。

下颌骨骨折

下颌骨骨折的检查和治疗常具有挑战性。其治疗的基本原则是恢复上下颌牙齿精确的咬殆关系。这使得手术治疗成为唯一的选择。但是，骨折复位、坚固内固定和骨折愈合的一般原则与长骨的相关原则相同。下颌骨是一个弓形结构，包含两侧的水平部分和垂直部分。其外侧面和内侧面由坚硬的皮质骨构成。其内部是松质骨，其内存在神经血管束和淋巴引流系统，为下颌骨和牙齿提供营养支持。其中一个重要的解剖结构是下牙槽动脉（下颌动脉的分支）。它通过位于下颌骨舌侧的下颌孔进入下颌骨。在下颌骨内与下牙槽动脉平行走行的是下牙槽神经（第三对脑神经的分支），并发出分支——颏神经，由下颌骨前部的颏孔出下颌骨。对于完全发育的下颌骨来说，其上共有 16 颗牙齿。下颌骨的水平部可以分为两个主要的区域。上部或牙槽部由围绕和支持牙根的松质骨构成，而下部或基底部是血管神经束走行的区域。下颌骨最前部和最中央的部位称为正中联合，其侧方为正中联合旁。下颌骨正中联合旁远中的区域为下颌体。下颌骨水平部和垂直部相连接，垂直部为下颌支。下颌支上行并逐渐变细，移行为髁突颈部和喙突。髁突颈部向上逐渐增粗形成髁头。髁头和位于颅底由颞骨构成的关节窝一起形成颞下颌关节（图 5）。该关节包含一个纤维软骨结构，构成关节的关节盘。该关节是一个铰链 - 滑动关节，也就是说该关节不但可以进行铰链和转动，还可以完成滑行的动作。尽管下颌骨能够耐受相当大的撞击力，但它存在几个先天的薄弱区域。髁颈区域向下至下颌角区域被认为是容易发生骨折的部位。第三磨牙的存在使下颌角区域变得更加薄弱。髁颈比较狭窄，作用于正中联合的力传导至该部位，从而累及髁颈。如果打击力超出了髁颈的耐受程度，则最终导致骨折。与下颌角部位的特点相似，正中联合旁区域由于尖牙牙根和颏孔的存在，使得该区域在下颌骨遭受创伤时常发生骨折。因此，基于下颌骨的结构特点，下颌骨骨折最常发生的部位为髁颈、下颌角和正中联合旁。

绝大部分下颌骨骨折是由钝性损伤、暴力、摔倒和机动车事故造成的，它们是造成下颌骨骨折的主要原因。对于成人来说，下颌骨是头颈部最突出

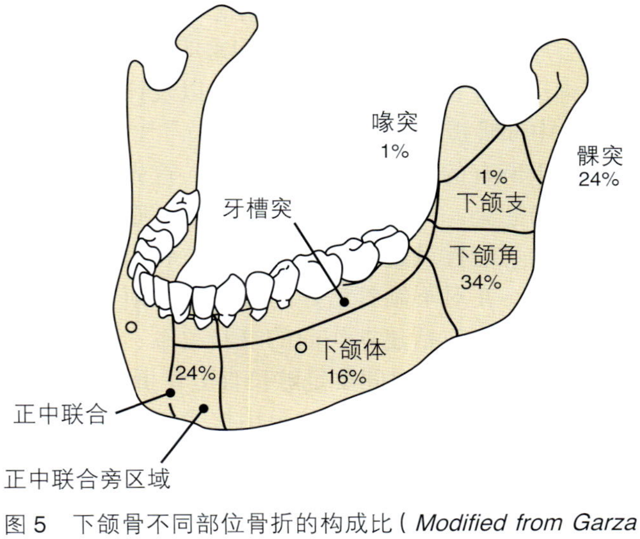

图 5 下颌骨不同部位骨折的构成比（*Modified from Garza JR: Mandible fractures. In Papel I, editor: Facial plastic and reconstructive surgery, 3rd ed. New York, Thieme Medical Publishers, 2009,Chap. 72, p. 1001.*）

的部位，较之儿童的下颌骨更容易发生骨折。当下颌骨发生骨折时，由于升颌肌群（咬肌、颞肌和翼内肌）或降颌肌群（舌骨上肌群和翼外肌）的牵拉，骨折段将发生错位。

如前面所讨论的，对下颌骨骨折也可以采用与长骨相似的分类方法进行分类，可以分为开放性、闭合性、简单、复杂或粉碎性骨折。如果下颌骨骨折部位通过牙根周围的牙周膜和口腔相通，则为开放性骨折。还可以把下颌骨骨折分为有利型骨折和不利型骨折。作用在骨折段上的肌肉的力量可以将骨折段保持在一个有利于骨折愈合的位置上，这种下颌骨骨折为有利型骨折。如果肌肉的力量使骨折段之间发生错位，阻碍骨折段接触并愈合，则这种骨折即为不利型骨折。一般来说，如果骨折线向下向后走行，则骨折为水平不利型骨折；如果骨折线向下向前走行，则骨折为水平有利型骨折。

常通过临床检查来对下颌骨骨折进行诊断。下颌骨骨折的症状和体征包括疼痛、肿胀、张口受限、错狢畸形、口内出血以及开口偏斜。触诊骨折部位可以触及骨折台阶并引发疼痛。在开放性骨折，其骨折部位邻近的口底黏膜有瘀斑并有裂伤。可以采用下颌骨压力试验来证实是否存在下颌骨骨折。将两个大拇指置于双侧下颌骨的舌侧，并向外推。如果能感知双侧骨段有轻微的动度，患者有痛感，则可以证实存在下颌骨骨折。

通过影像学检查可以明确骨折的部位和特点。曲面体层片可以将下颌骨复杂的三维结构显示为两维图像并进行全面的检查。下颌骨系列平片可以帮助进一步评价髁突部位损伤的情况，髁突骨折在曲面体层片上显示不清。CT也常用来明确是否存在下颌骨骨折，并帮助制订治疗计划，以及评估是否合并有面中部骨折。

对于所有的下颌骨开放性骨折，首先要应用抗生素预防感染。对骨折越早手术治疗，则术后发生并发症的可能性就越小，骨折的复位和固定的效果也就越好。在对下颌骨治疗的过程中，须要考虑几个治疗原则。包括建立伤前的咬狢关系；解剖复位骨折；骨折固定的时间要足够长直至骨折完全愈合。这些可以通过切开复位，并采用接骨板钉进行坚固内固定加以实现。对于下颌骨粉碎性骨折，可以放置外固定支架装置进行固定。对于颌间结扎固定的时间以及骨折线上牙齿的处理问题，持续存在很多争议。

下颌骨骨折相关的并发症常与以下因素相关：不正确的手术操作，患者的依从性差，或者骨折的愈合出现问题。骨折部位的感染常见于骨折线部位的牙根损伤或感染、口腔卫生差或者手术复位固定技术差而导致骨折部位有明显的动度。手术复位固定后出现动度的原因有钛板尺寸选择错误、钛板放置不正确以及螺钉的数量错误。这些均能导致骨折部位出现异常动度，并出现钛板折断、钛板外露以及骨折不愈合。骨折不愈合可造成骨折部位骨坏死，骨折间隙内充满纤维组织，而不是新生的骨质。当骨折复位固定不充分，骨折愈合欠佳时，也可发生错位愈合。在骨折治疗过程中还应考虑避免损伤周围的神经和血管，在骨折暴露和固定过程中，下牙槽神经很容易被过度牵拉、挫伤甚至直接离断。

Le Fort 骨折

上颌骨内有两个大的充满空气的上颌窦。与相邻部位的面部骨骼相比，需要较小的力量就可以使上颌骨发生骨折。面中部结构的复杂性就表现在它由水平和垂直支柱交互构成。这一特点有利于力量向颌面部其他区域和颅底传递和扩散。一般认为，人类进化出这种精细复杂的结构是为了很好地吸收作用力，以避免眼眶和颅腔内容物的损伤。因此，某些对面中部的撞击力量常常造成的损伤比预计的要小很多。

1901 年，Rene Le Fort 通过将尸颅从不同的高度抛下，首次描述了一系列经典的面中部骨折模式（图 6）。尽管在临床上，孤立的和单纯的 Le Fort 类型的骨折非常少见，但是他的这一研究工作还是对于明确骨折的高度和严重性有所帮助。Le Fort I 型骨折为沿上颌骨和腭骨水平扩展的低位水平骨折，

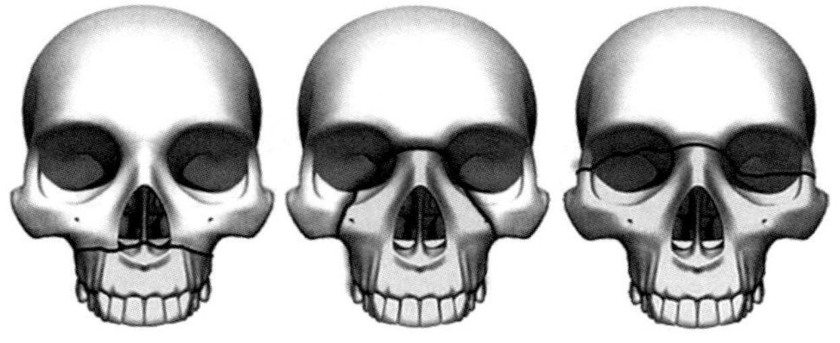

图 6　Le Fort I、II、III 型骨折的骨折方式（*Orloff G: Management of facial fractures. In Thaller S, Garri JI, Bradley JP, editors: Craniofacial surgery. New York, Informa Healthcare USA, 2007, p 305*）

位于上颌牙列上方，将上颌牙齿和其他颅面骨骼分开。骨折线横过鼻中隔，向后通过上颌窦后壁以及翼板。这一类型的骨折大约占所有 Le Fort 骨折的 30%。它常是由作用于面中部下方的前后向打击力造成的，使得面中部的垂直和水平支柱发生骨折。

Le Fort Ⅱ型骨折常由作用于面中部的水平向打击力或由下颌前部传导至面中部的力量所导致。该类型骨折始于鼻骨，然后横过上颌骨额突和泪骨，然后向下通过眶底、眶下缘和上颌窦外侧壁，向后扩展至翼板。结果造成骨折线下方骨段形似锥形的骨折，并与其他颅面骨骼分离。与 Le Fort I 型骨折相似，该类骨折也横过鼻中隔、上颌窦后壁和翼板。这一类型的骨折是最常见的 Le Fort 骨折，占所有病例的 60%。

Le Fort Ⅲ型骨折发生于颅底水平，骨折线将颧骨和上方的颞骨和额骨分开，横过内外侧眼眶并在鼻额缝处到达中线。与 Le Fort Ⅰ、Ⅱ型骨折类似，这类型骨折也横过鼻中隔、上颌窦后壁和翼板。骨折导致颅面完全分离。这种骨折常由斜向的打击力作用于面中部垂直支柱上造成，是所有这三种类型骨折中最为少见的一种。该类骨折常为高速撞击伤，存在严重的粉碎性骨折和颅内损伤。实际上不是所有的面中部骨折都严格遵从这一分类方案，但它确实提供了一个有用的工具来帮助医师就患者骨折的诊断和手术治疗进行沟通和交流。绝大部分面中部骨折较上述三种骨折类型更加复杂。骨折经常表现为多个不同的 Le Fort 骨折类型分别出现在面部骨骼两侧。

对于所有的面部骨折，Le Fort 类型的骨折占其中的 10%～20%。该类型骨折最常见于机动车事故、暴力或高坠损伤中。骨折最常发生于年龄为 40～50 岁的男性。随着人口老龄化的加剧，预计 Le Fort 骨折的人数也会有所增加。与之相反，儿童很少发生 Le Fort 类型的骨折。儿童的下颌骨和额骨相对较大，再加上面部骨骼更具有弹性，上颌窦未发育以及牙齿还未完全萌出，这些解剖特点均阻止儿童发生 Le Fort 骨折。Le Fort 骨折常合并其他类型的头颈部损伤，包括颅内损伤、眼外伤以及颈部损伤。因此，对于 Le Fort 骨折患者，在其最初的检查评估中，应对头面部进行全面检查。

在急诊室环境下，尽管非常困难，外科或急诊科医师也应该在充分执行生命复苏措施以后，对面部创伤进行全面的评估。出血常使得面中部损伤的评价变得困难和复杂化。出血常继发于鼻中隔、鼻腔以及鼻旁窦黏膜撕裂。患者的情况一旦稳定，应及时了解患者伤前牙齿咬合的情况以及是否有牙齿损伤的病史。对于视力发生明显变化的患者，还应详细询问其眼科病史。检查应包括对整个面部骨骼的视诊和触诊，以评价面部结构的损伤情况。面中部创伤后常出现严重的软组织水肿，可使面部变形，并掩盖深面的骨折塌陷。移位的上颌骨常造成错𬌗畸形，表现为牙齿早接触或开𬌗畸形。面中部创伤后常沿着颅底向后发生移位，使得面部表现为扁平和变长。如果损伤扩展至骨性眼眶，可出现眶周瘀斑或眼球位置出现异常。对于所有的 Le Fort 类型的骨折，均会出现面中部不稳定。可以用一只手的拇指和示指抓住患者的前颌骨，另一只手稳定眶下缘，检查上颌骨是否有整体松动。Le Fort Ⅰ型骨折只有前颌骨出现动度。对于 Le Fort Ⅱ型骨折，摇动上颌骨时，眶下缘可以出现动度。而对于 Le Fort Ⅲ型骨折，前颌骨、颧骨以及其他面骨均在鼻额缝和颧额缝部位出现动度。发生 Le Fort Ⅱ型骨折时，可出现皮下瘀斑和眶下缘出现骨折台阶以及眶下神经分布区域麻木。

对于 Le fort 骨折患者，CT 是可供选择的影像学检查手段。应注意观察涉及眼眶和颅底的影像，因为颅内损伤可能会改变外科治疗的顺序。

Le Fort 骨折的手术治疗主要集中在恢复面部的功能以及美观方面。手术修复的主要目标是重建面部的高度和前突度，并将患者的咬𬌗恢复至伤前状态。以前曾认为，Le Fort 骨折的治疗应等待至面部肿胀消退后，这样才能更好地评价手术标志，术后才能更好地加以恢复。但现在的观点是早期手术干预，切开复位内固定，可以在延迟手术所造成的骨折断端吸收和纤维长入骨折间隙之前更精确地修复骨折。一些作者报告，伤后及时手术修复骨折可以早期恢复功能，降低感染率，减少术后瘢痕和降低术后并发症。对面中部骨骼可以通过联合一些隐蔽的切口，例如口内切口、经结膜切口、冠状切口或面中部脱套入路来进行暴露，以便复位所有的骨折支柱。切口的选择由骨折的部位和范围决定。一旦骨折得以充分复位，须用微型和小型接骨板进行坚固内固定。术中患者须要利用牙弓夹板和钢丝结扎进行颌间固定，以限制骨折移动，并保持骨折线处于复位状态。

面中部骨折的并发症常可分为骨性和软组织缺陷，给患者带来功能和美观的问题。骨性并发症包括继发于骨折延迟愈合、错位愈合、不愈合或纤维愈合的错殆畸形。当发生真性骨折不愈合或纤维愈合时，必须将所有的死骨和纤维组织彻底清除干净，并用自体骨移植来修复缺损。与之相反，软组织并发症更容易处理，例如伤口感染、感觉异常或感觉迟钝、颧骨区或颞区凹陷以及眼睑错位。

额窦骨折

出生时，额窦还不存在。从6岁开始，额窦才开始发育，到15岁时，达到成人额窦大小。额窦的窦底形成眶顶的内侧，额窦的后壁形成颅前窝的前壁。尽管成人额窦在大小和形状方面变异较大，但额窦一般为左右两个，被窦内的分隔分开。鼻额隐窝位于额窦窦底，作为额窦的引流通道，将分泌物引流入鼻腔。额窦的前后壁可以抵抗较大的撞击力。额窦窦壁存在较厚的皮质骨，使之成为面部骨骼中最坚固的部分，对额骨起到保护的作用。由于这一特点，较少发生额窦骨折，其只占颌面损伤的5%～15%。这类损伤常由机动车事故、运动损伤和暴击袭击造成。

对额窦骨折做出准确的诊断是快速制订治疗计划并及时手术的关键。额窦骨折患者常主诉前额区疼痛和头痛。应进行详细的病史采集，明确骨折的原因，并检查是否存在其他临床表现，例如鼻腔是否有清亮的液体流出，或者口腔内是否存在有咸味的液体，此时须明确是否存在脑脊液漏。如果怀疑有脑脊液漏，应采集液体进行 β_2 转铁蛋白实验以明确诊断。在临床检查中，额窦表面软组织水肿和瘀斑明显。其他表现还有眶上和滑车上神经分布区域感觉异常、复视和鼻出血。

诊断额窦骨折时须要进行CT检查。轴位CT图像可以显示前壁骨折、后壁骨折以及颅腔积气（图7）。冠状位CT图像可以显示额窦窦底骨折和眶顶骨折。

额窦手术治疗的目标包括：发生后壁骨折时要保护脑部不受损伤，治疗和预防脑脊液漏，预防黏液囊肿和黏液脓囊肿，恢复前额区域的外形以及额窦的正常功能。目前，有一个很好的额窦骨折治疗流程图可供参考。该流程主要的依据是骨折的部位（前壁、后壁、前壁和后壁联合）、骨折的范围、骨折粉碎的程度、鼻额引流系统损伤情况以及持续脑脊液漏（图8）。治疗方法包括观察、切开复位内固定、内镜辅助下骨折复位、窦腔填塞、窦腔切除和额窦颅腔化。

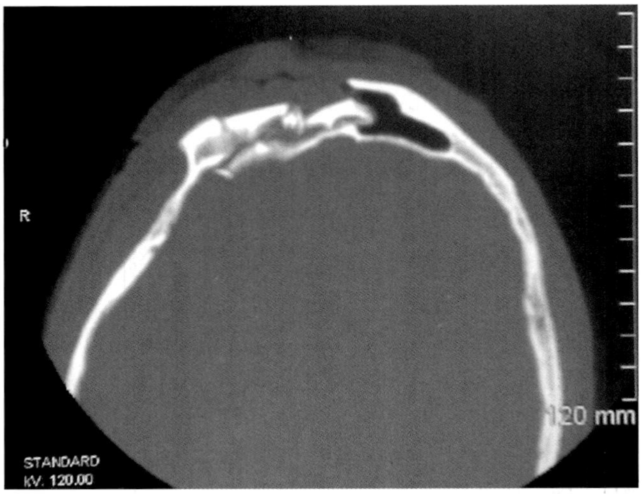

图7 轴位CT图像显示双侧额窦前后壁联合骨折，未见颅腔积气

额窦骨折的并发症常是由不正确的手术治疗造成的，可出现畸形、慢性额窦炎、颅腔积气、黏液脓囊肿、脑膜炎和脑内脓肿。当窦腔黏膜撕裂或损伤时，可能后期会出现黏液囊肿，囊肿可以缓慢发展和生长，在原发损伤后很多年才被发现，而很多创伤患者并没有进行长期随访。

鼻眶筛骨折

鼻眶筛（naso-orbital-ethmoid，NOE）复合体是一个复杂的解剖区域，由多个重要的骨性结构构成，包括鼻骨、泪骨、筛骨、上颌骨和额骨。其中鼻骨侧方与上颌骨额突相连，上方与额骨相连。筛窦位于成对的鼻骨之后，将眼眶和鼻腔隔开。该区域主要的水平支柱是眶上缘，主要的垂直支柱是上颌骨额突。如果任何一个支柱发生骨折断裂，那么整个鼻眶筛复合体就会塌陷变形。

内眦韧带是鼻眶筛区域的一个关键结构，主要功能是维持正常的内眦间距。正常的内眦间距是30～35 mm，相当于瞳孔间距的一半或与鼻翼基底宽度相同。内眦韧带附着于前后泪嵴和上颌骨额突上。

鼻眶筛复合体骨折可以通过临床检查进行诊断。内眦韧带的完整性可以通过侧方牵拉下眼睑进行检查。如果内眦韧带没有足够的张力，或者眶内壁存在明显的动度，这些特点均支持鼻眶筛复合体骨折。其他一些临床表现有远内眦畸形、眼球内陷、面中

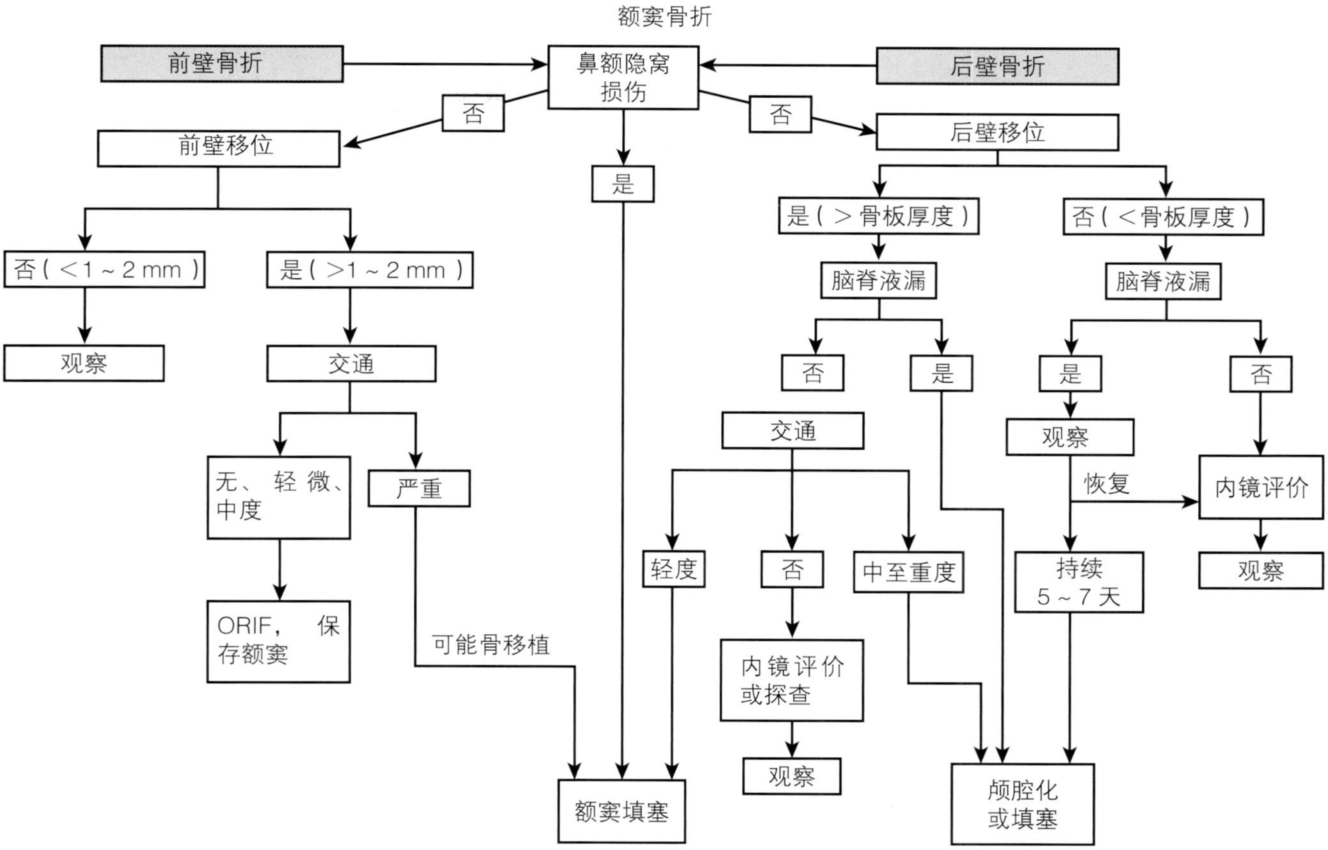

图 8　额窦治疗流程图，ORIF：切开复位内固定（引自 Strong BE: Frontal sinus and naso-orbital-ethmoid complex fractures. In Papel I, editor: Facial plastic and reconstructive surgery, 3rd ed, New York, 2009, Thieme MedicalPublishers, p 980）

部塌陷、瞳孔反应和眼球运动异常。

薄断层 CT 影像以及三维重建影像有助于明确骨折的特点，并辅助制订手术计划。CT 检查时应注意的区域包括筛状板、额隐窝、眼眶以及鼻眶筛复合体粉碎的程度以及是否合并其他面部骨折。

有人提出了鼻眶筛骨折的分类方法，以便进一步描述骨性损伤的程度。实践证明该分类系统对明确骨折的类型很有帮助，并能辅助制订手术计划（图 9）。对于鼻眶筛复合体骨折的治疗来说，内眦韧带附着的中央骨段是鼻眶筛复合体重建的解剖关键点。Ⅰ型骨折是指附着内眦韧带的中央骨段骨折，与周围骨骼分离。Ⅱ型骨折是指附着内眦韧带的中央骨段粉碎性骨折。Ⅲ型骨折是指附着内眦韧带的中央骨段粉碎性骨折，且内眦韧带从骨折的骨片上脱离。这些骨折很少见。

绝大多数专家都承认，在所有面部骨折的手术治疗中，鼻眶筛骨折的治疗最具有挑战性。如果在手术过程中暴露不佳、骨折复位不精确或者内眦韧带修复效果较差，都会导致骨折治疗效果不满意。通过冠状切口、面中部脱套入路、眉间切口或开窗入路，可以获得理想的手术视野。一旦骨折线被充分暴露，根据骨折粉碎的程度，可以联合穿鼻钢丝和微型钛板进行固定。

失明、内眦间距过宽、眼球内陷、脑脊液漏和嗅觉丧失是鼻眶筛复合体损伤的潜在并发症。另外，还可出现一些良性的并发症，包括鼻窦炎、溢泪和鼻畸形。

小结

对颌面骨骼的创伤性损伤的诊治须要临床医师具备面部三维解剖结构方面广泛的知识。然后，对面部创伤患者应进行全身系统性的评价，并制订特殊的治疗流程。对于颌面创伤的治疗，骨折的愈合原则很重要。通过上述准备，对骨折实施切开复位，

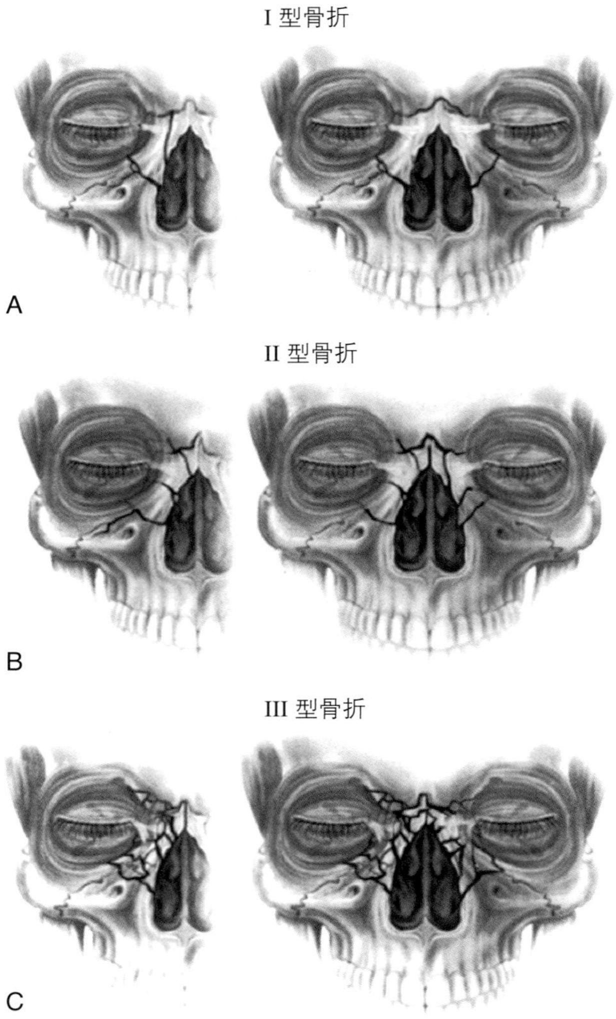

图 9　鼻眶筛 I 型（**A**）、II 型（**B**）、III 型（**C**）骨折的方式（*From Strong BE: Frontal sinus and naso-orbital-ethmoid complex fractures. In Papel I, editor: Facial plastic and reconstructive surgery, 3rd ed, New York, 2009, Thieme Medical Publishers, p 989.*）

并使用接骨板对骨折进行内固定，最终可以达到良好的功能和美观效果。检查诊断和手术治疗最终的目标是恢复伤前的功能，以及获得良好的美观效果。但是，面部创伤常与其他威胁生命的创伤联合发生，这一点不能忽视。面部损伤尽管多由创伤造成，但很少致命。为了避免患者出现严重问题，尽早进行初步评估和治疗非常重要。

眼和眶创伤

Mario A. Meallet, Bibiana J.Reise 著
李明武 译

作为创伤中心和急诊的医师，常常须要对严重的眼外伤进行评估及处理，其中多数情况须要立即会诊和向眼科转诊。我们希望讲述几种急诊及创伤科医师可以处理的眼部急诊，并且把相关技术描述清晰。当面部骨折仅局限于眶骨时，眼科的评估就足以拟定治疗方案了。在涉及更大范围的鼻咽部、颅骨、上颌骨和下颌骨的骨折中，就须要包括整形外科、眼科、头颈部外科和口腔颌面外科等多科室的合作诊治。在急诊室内就要做出恰当的分诊决定，而我们所希望的就是为急救室做出决定提供有用的临床指南（图 1）。

眼部的直接外伤须要能提供眼部治疗的人员（眼科医师、验光师以及经过眼部诊疗培训的人员）立即的参与，严重的外伤患者常常不能配合全面的眼科检查，须要通过眼部客观所见来决定治疗方案。在明显的开放性眼外伤中，急诊医师和创伤外科医师可以通过明确的外伤病史进行急救，并及时决定进行放射学检查。当怀疑有眼内异物，或者不能获取详尽的病史时，则应立即进行 CT 扫描检查，同时可以使用 Fox 防护眼罩来保护伤眼，而将剩下的评估及治疗工作交给专业的眼科医师来做。急诊科医师尤其不要立即进行裂隙灯检查，而且要绝对避免进行眼压测量。同时应该告知患者注意避免一些会造成眼内出血的动作，比如咳嗽或者 Valsalva 动

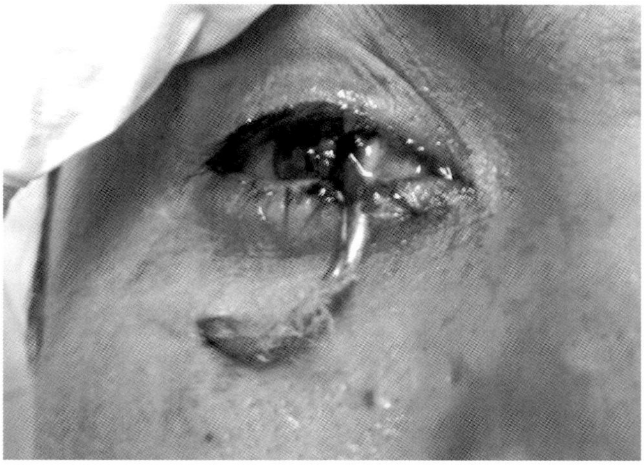

图 1　射钉枪造成的眼外伤

作（深吸气后紧闭声门，再用力做呼气动作），而且力劝患者要安静地休息直到创伤被修复。

当眼部开放性外伤并不是很明确时，要从肉眼检查以及对双眼分别的进行视力检查开始，进行全面、有条不紊的眼部检查。通过检查是否有相对性瞳孔传导障碍来判断视神经的功能。如果条件允许，要进行眼压的测量以及小心地进行裂隙灯检查。散瞳下的眼底检查只能交给接受过培训的人员或者留给眼科医师来做。如果综合临床所见和辅助的测试不足以明确开放性眼外伤，但仍然高度怀疑时，则推荐麻醉下探查。任何时候只要条件允许，都建议留下照相的资料。急诊和创伤医师最初的及时处理对患者的最终视力预后有着极其重要的影响，而且对于各种类型的急性眼外伤的熟悉可以形成更完善的分诊系统（图 2）。

发病率

在美国，眼部创伤的发生率为每年 200 万只眼（每 1000 人中有 7 个人）。McGwin 等的从国家门诊护理调查以及医院出院记录的资料中发现美国的眼外伤患者最主要是在急诊进行治疗（50.7%），其次是私人诊所（38.7%），接下来是门诊（8.1%）和住院治疗（2.5%）。人口学分析发现眼外伤发生率最高的是 20～30 岁的男性，没有明显的种族差异。

眼外伤的发生率从童年的末期开始攀升，在 30 岁时达到高峰，之后是缓慢地降低。第二个高峰出

图 2　眼的解剖（Narina Sokolova 绘制）

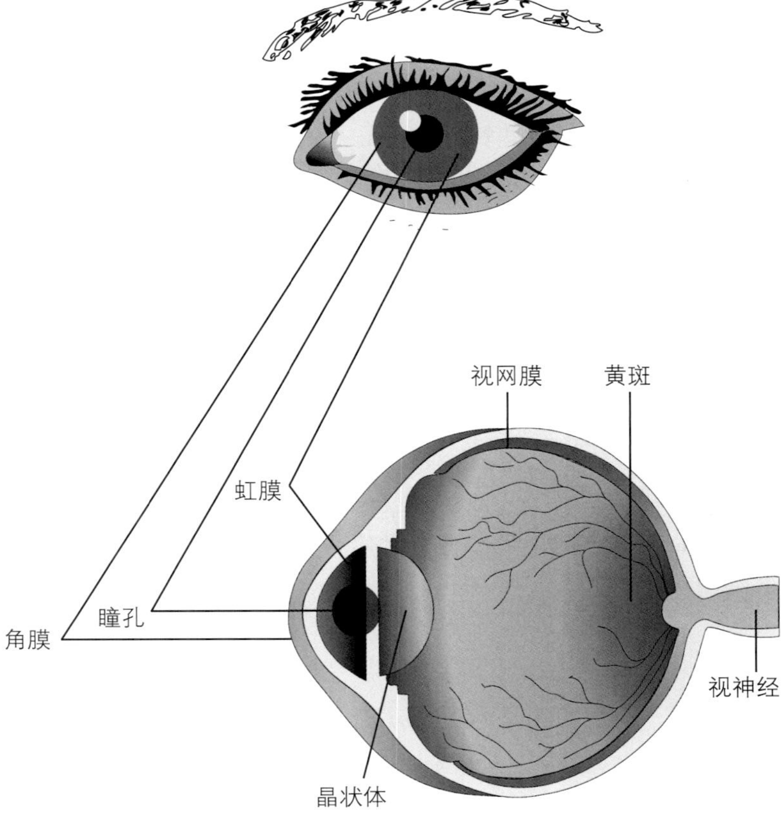

现在很高龄的时候。这种出现在青年和老年发病率的双峰以及男性的高发是青年男性参加一些高危活动以及老年人容易出现外伤和摔伤的反映。正是这种趋势导致了外伤主要发生在这些人群中。

受伤的情形对外伤的严重程度以及视觉预后有明显的影响。一项针对工作场所中眼外伤发生率的研究报道发现，开放性眼外伤最为常见（46%），接下来是眼附属器的外伤（20%）、眼眶骨折（11%）以及创伤性前房积血（11%）。耐人寻味的是，护目镜对绝大多数眼外伤（约 90%）有着重要的防护作用（例如工作场所，体育运动如篮球、真人射击和气枪）。实际上，这些活动按法规的要求是须要佩戴护目镜的，但多数外伤发生时患者恰恰没有佩戴护目镜。所以据估算，在参加这些活动时如果按要求佩戴了护目镜，有接近 90% 的眼外伤是可以避免的。

在少数车祸造成的眼外伤中（在美国约占所有眼外伤的 1.8%），很少出现开放性眼外伤。强制系安全带使眼外伤患者减少了一半。奇怪的是，减少的这一半眼外伤患者却因为安全气囊的弹出造成的眼外伤成倍增加而被抵消掉了。造成车祸的眼外伤的最主要原因是挡风玻璃，接下来是安全气囊、方向盘和飞溅的玻璃。当然，这些数据必须在安全气囊以及安全带的使用带来的车祸死亡人数减少这个背景下来进行解读。

总的来说，在急诊只有很小比例（2.3%）的眼外伤表现为裂伤或者穿通伤（表 1 和图 3）。最常见的眼外伤原因是异物伤（44.6%）和钝挫伤（33.0%）（表 2 和图 4）。在一些钝挫伤中，存在着非常不明显且检查者很难发现的巩膜裂伤。在这些病例中，检查者就必须依赖与隐匿性巩膜裂伤相关的关键的临床表现了，这将在随后讲述诊断的部分中叙述。

表 1　急诊的眼创伤所见

眼外伤类型	频率（%）
挫伤 / 擦伤	44.6
异物	30.8
结膜炎	10.2
出血	9.9
裂伤	1.8
穿通伤	0.5

Modified from McGwin G Jr, Owsley C: Incidence of emergency departmenttreated eye injury in the United States. Arch Ophthalmol 123:662–666, 2005

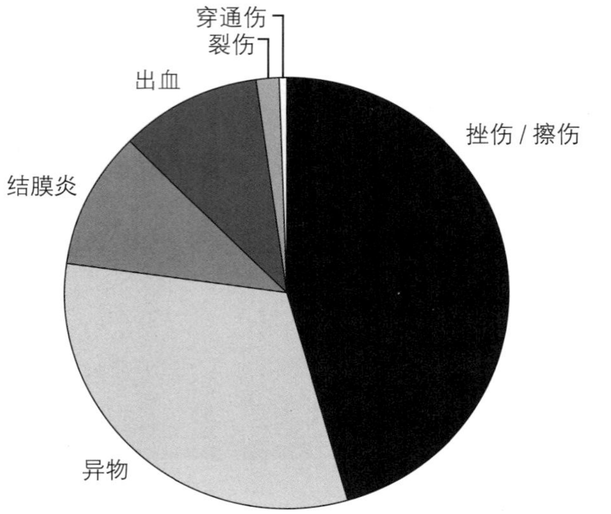

图 3　急诊的眼创伤后的表现（*Data from McGwin G Jr, Owsley C: Incidence of emergency department-treated eye injury in the United States. Arch Ophthalmol 123:662–666, 2005.*）

Werner 等报道在所有潜在的眼球破裂的患者中，隐匿性巩膜裂伤可以占到接近 25% 的比例。在可疑隐匿性破裂伤的患者中，粗略估计有 1/3 可以在手术探查中发现确凿的裂伤。

眼眶的骨折与头部的创伤有显著的相关性。在一项涉及 4426 名出现面部和眼眶骨折的美国军人的研究中发现，有 26% 的人出现了眶底骨折。同样在这组研究中，有 30% 的人出现了眼球的损伤，还有 70% 的概率合并全身损伤。眼眶骨折的绝大部分是眶底骨折和眶内侧壁骨折，排第三位的是眶外侧壁的骨折，而只有一小部分为眶顶部骨折（图 5）。眶

表 2　急诊的眼外伤关键机制

眼外伤机制	频率（%）
异物	44.6
钝挫伤	33.0
烧伤	12.0
机械伤	3.1
车祸伤	2.3
摔倒	1.8
枪伤	<1.0

Modified from McGwin G Jr, Owsley C: Incidence of emergency department-treated eye injury in the United States. Arch Ophthalmol 123:662–666, 2005

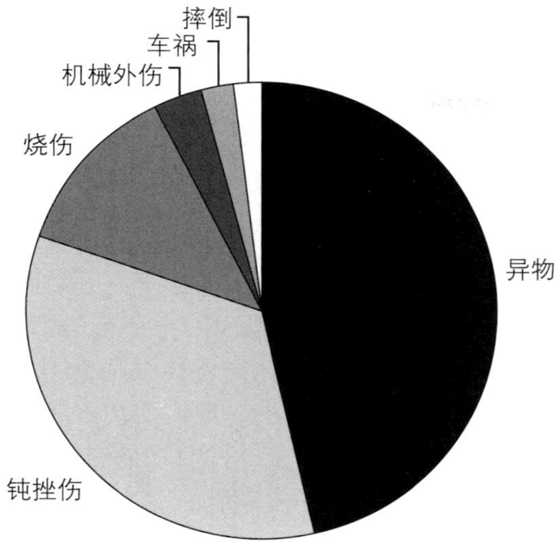

图 4　急诊的眼外伤关键机制（*Data from McGwin G Jr, Owsley C: Incidence of emergency department-treated eye injury in the United States. Arch Ophthalmol 123:662–666, 2005.*）

底内侧紧靠眶下沟处最容易受损，而眶内壁最容易骨折的部位是筛板——仅如纸一样厚度的骨性薄膜。

损伤机制

造成眼及周围结构损伤的机制主要是异物、钝性创伤和热与化学烧伤。机器的、机动车的以及枪伤是相对少见的原因（表 2 和图 4）。各种原因有着相当比例的重叠，所以医师必须综合考虑各种因素的影响，同时根据损伤情况进行个体化处理。例如，如果钝性创伤所致的眼球裂伤出现传入性瞳孔障碍，可能因创伤性的视神经病变而需要短期的全身激素治疗。作用于眼的钝性外力也可以被描述为冲击伤 - 对冲伤，或与脑外伤类似的压缩力。角膜擦伤、结膜下出血、脉络膜出血和视网膜坏死都是冲击伤的例子。另外，由彩弹或气枪子弹造成的虹膜根部离断或虹膜损伤所致的前房积血也是冲击伤的例子（图 6）。对冲伤最好的例子是视网膜震荡，前部的作用力被传导至视网膜并造成视网膜各层的剪切作用。另外，眼球的压缩常常会造成巩膜的裂伤。开放性眼外伤将在后面再叙述。

眼眶骨折可以是钝性外力造成眶内压升高并导致眶内壁和眶底爆裂性骨折，也可以是对面骨直接的外伤造成的眼眶任何一面的骨折。由于眼眶外侧壁和眶顶壁最不容易发生骨折，所以这两处的骨折也提示了可能是由对面部和眼部的直接作用力造成的，对所伴随出现的眼球外伤也应该谨慎地进行评估。异物穿通眼眶可以直接波及眼及周围任何结构。

对于眼睑和眼球附属器的化学和热损伤必须进行长期的评估，要远远长于表层组织的修复时间。眼睑及皮肤的烧伤会造成局部的瘢痕及瘢痕收缩，

图 5　眶骨、眶骨折发病率的示意图

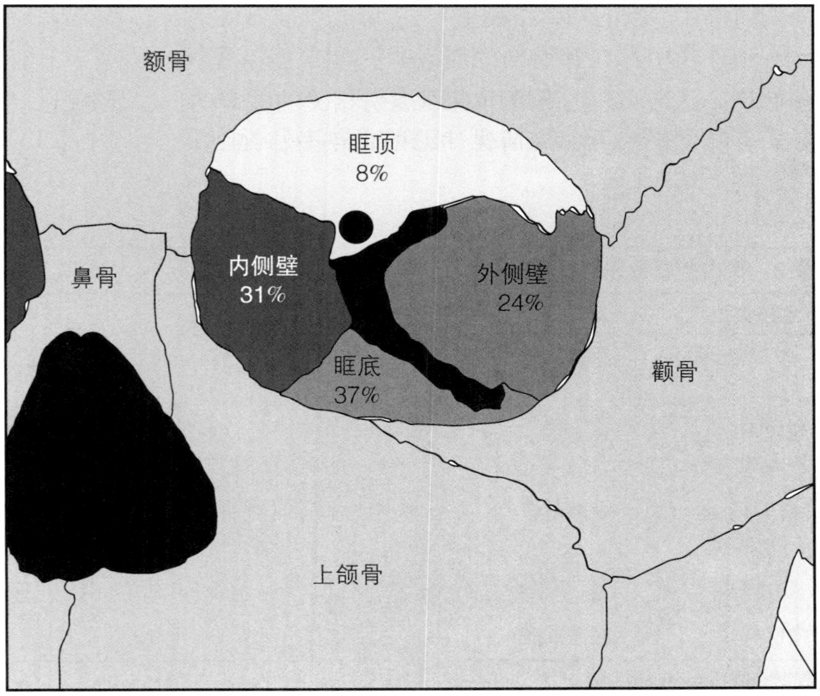

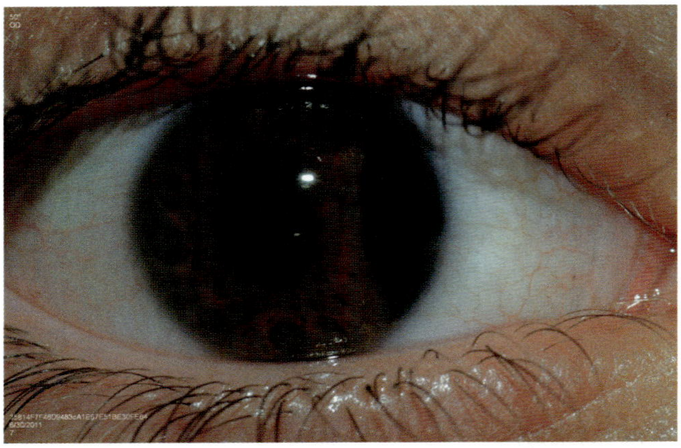

图 6 气枪子弹伤造成该青年男性右眼虹膜解离。起病时，厚厚的前房积血导致无法看到虹膜

导致眼睑退缩，角膜和眼表组织的暴露。所以对于这类患者，长期的观察非常重要，尤其是患者在危重病房时。对这些患者要积极地使用眼部润滑剂，直至患者可以自由地通过眨眼来保护自己的眼睛。强烈建议所有的重症监护室和创伤病房把对于这些患者的眼部治疗处理流程写好。

开放性眼外伤分为穿通伤和非穿通伤。后者是因为钝性外力造成眼球的压缩从而导致眼球壁的破裂。破裂伤的位置多数在眼球壁最薄弱的区域，即角巩膜连接部（角巩膜缘）、眼外肌附着点以及视神经附着部位。可能难以判断角巩膜缘后的破裂伤，所以所有的医师必须熟悉隐匿性破裂伤的体征，这些我们将在诊断的章节中叙述。

当外伤中存在穿通伤的因素时，常常可以看到穿通口，这时可以直接决定需要外科干预。判断穿通伤有三个须要考虑的情况：①穿通异物是否已不在眼球上了。②异物是否在眼球内。③异物是否已经穿透整个眼球了（贯通伤），这时异物可能已从眼球后部穿出到达眼眶里了。

如果存在眼球内或眶内异物的证据，异物的材质也会提示其对眼的毒性大小，以及眼球或眶内感染的风险有多大（表 3）。如果提示外伤的类型的病史不明确，则应尽快行眼眶 CT 检查，并且将防护眼罩罩在眼外。即使异物露在眼球或周围组织外面并很容易接触到，急诊或创伤外科医师也不要做任何操作去试图取出异物。小心地将防护眼罩覆盖于患眼外，可在外科干预修复的同时评估损伤的程度。

诊断

眼眶外伤

需要紧急处理的眼眶外伤的主要临床特征包括：①明显的眼球运动受限，②出现传入性瞳孔障碍，③出现眼球突出（眼球异常向前鼓出），④出现眼球凹陷（眼球异常向后移位）。如果出现这些特征中的任何一项，都须要立即进行眼眶 CT 扫描、眼科的专业评估并考虑外科干预。在一项 Lee 等报道的 CT 检查在眼眶外伤中作用的研究中，眼眶损伤继发视力下降的病因按频率从大到小顺序排列分别为球后出血、视神经变厚（推测继发于水肿）、眶内气肿、视神经挫伤、视网膜脱离和眼球破裂。另外，要评估上述情况，医生须要触诊眶缘是否有骨折（错位），同时检查眼下方是否有眶下神经异常造成的感觉减退，并且记录是否存在眼球下陷（眼球向下方移位）。感觉减退提示累及眶下管及眶下神经的爆裂

表 3 球内金属毒性的表现形式

金属类型	角膜	虹膜	晶状体	玻璃体	视网膜	体征 / 症状
铁（铁锈症）	角膜基质锈染	瞳孔不等大 / 虹膜异色	花样白内障	棕色浑浊	弥漫性视网膜色素	夜盲，视野缺损
铜（<85%）（慢性铜锈症）	Fleischer 环	虹膜变或绿色	向日葵样白内障	棕红色浑浊	血管和黄斑微颗粒	进行性视力和视野丧失
铜（>85%）（急性铜锈症）	重度炎症	虹膜变或绿色	向日葵样白内障	弥漫性玻璃体炎	血管和黄斑微颗粒	爆发性炎症 / 眼球丧失
金	—	—	前囊沉积物	—	—	—
铝 / 锌	轻微炎症	—	—	—	—	—

数据来自 Yanoff M, Duker JS: Ophthalmology, 2nd ed, St. Louis, 2004, Mosby

性骨折，但这本身并没有急迫的意义。

评估眼球运动包括评估眼球运动是否受限和眼球运动减弱所诱发的症状。患者常主诉为视物成双，但遮挡一眼后重影消失。确定复视相的方向（水平、垂直或倾斜）对于下一步检查定位很有帮助。在急性炎症期，眼球运动常常因眶内的拥挤或肌肉的挫伤而受到影响，进一步检查以区分肌肉麻痹和肌肉受限或嵌顿。在牵拉试验中，当用镊子夹住眼肌移动时，可以分辨出是否有机械性的限制因素。另外，在局部用麻醉滴眼剂后，要求患者向眼球活动受限的方向看，然后向相同方向牵拉眼球，感觉眼球是否有被东西“拴住”的感觉（图 7）。如果存在明显的牵拉受限，须要怀疑可能有肌肉的嵌顿，须要立即行眼眶 CT 检查。如果影像学有证据提示嵌顿，就须要立即考虑手术干预以防止肌肉的缺血和坏死。

如果发现创伤后的眼球突出，就须要立即测量眼内压并且评估有无球后出血。眼球突出和眼内压的升高提示了眶骨筋膜室综合征，须要立即行轴位和冠状位的眼眶 CT 检查（图 8）。进一步检查还可以发现将眼球往后推存在阻力，弥漫性结膜下出血，

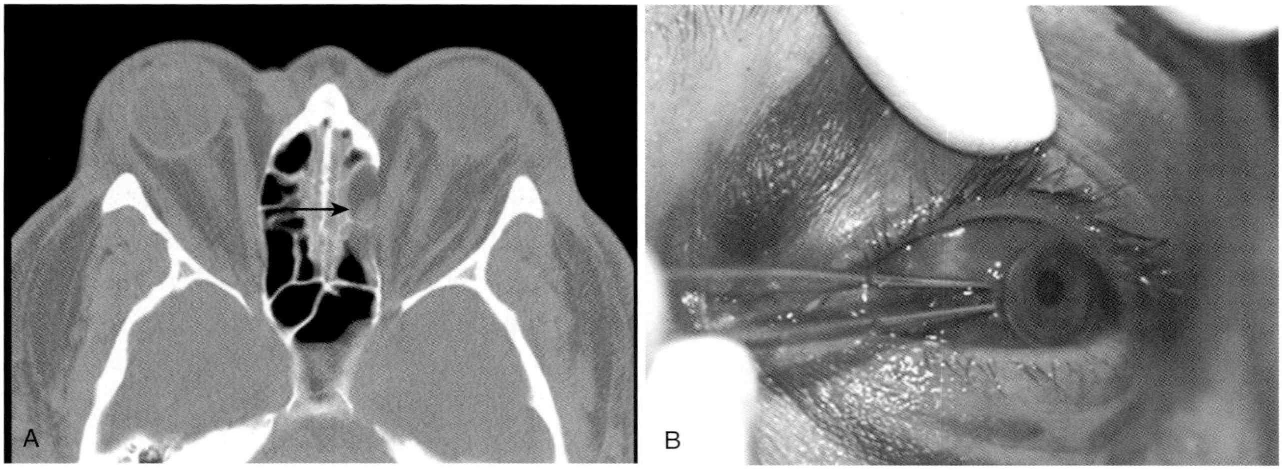

图 7　青年男性左眼钝挫伤后。**A**，患者向左看时眼球活动受限，从 CT 上看可能存在眶内的限制因素（箭头）。**B**，牵拉试验显示可以充分外展，限制因素被排除

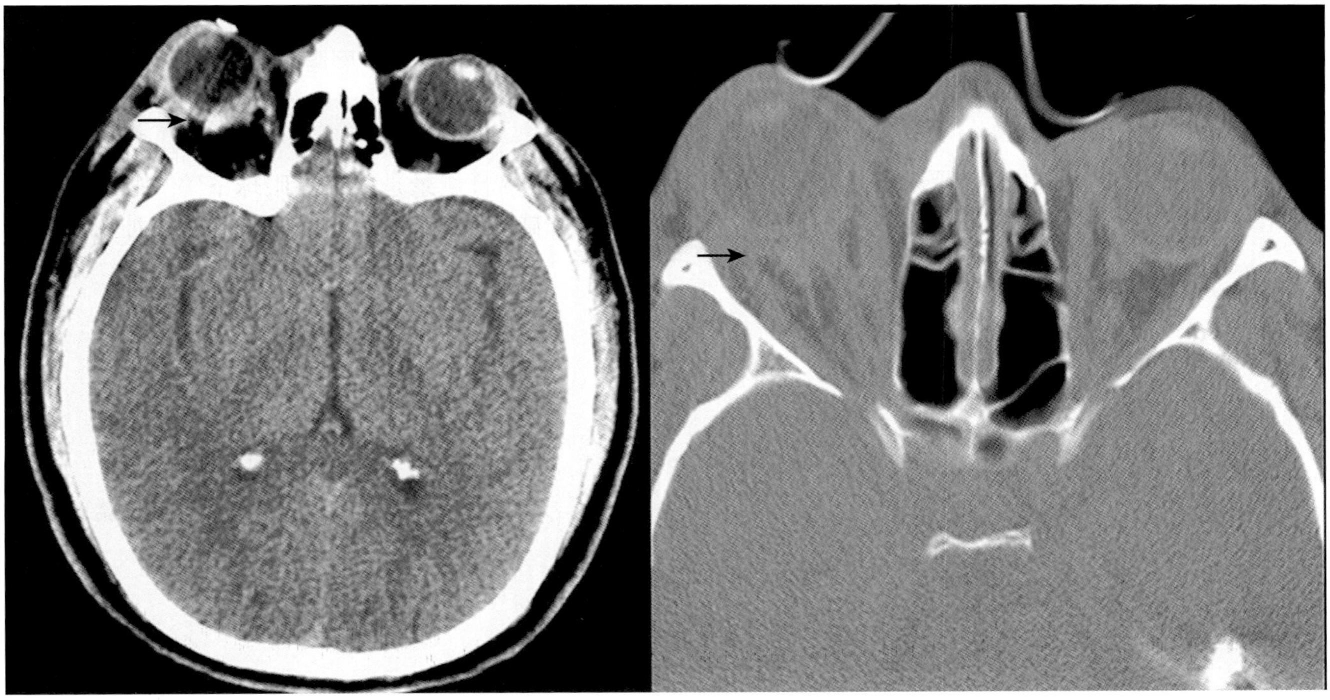

图 8　男性受右眼钝挫伤后出现明显的眼球突出以及 CT 上右眼球后的放射线遮挡（球后出血，箭头）。其眼压达到 40 mmHg。在切开外眦后，眼压迅速降到 20 mmHg

紧绷的眼睑和眼眶，视力下降，传入性瞳孔障碍和色觉的减弱。药物治疗首先须要立即给予降低眼压的药物（将在本章节后面治疗的段落叙述），并且要多次测量眼压确认药物治疗的效果。如果眼压非常高（>30 mmHg）或者药物治疗无效，则应进行外眦切开（在药物和手术治疗的段落再叙述）。如果有眼压明显升高和传入性瞳孔障碍的征象，可以在做眶CT扫描之前就进行外眦切开。如果存在传入性瞳孔障碍，就须要立即进行眼眶CT检查以排除骨片或者异物在眶内影响视神经。只要有对视神经产生挤压的证据，就应立即行外科手术来解除对神经的压力。如果没有对视神经的侵犯和前部视路的明显病变，对传入性瞳孔障碍要高度怀疑创伤性视神经病变，就应进行3天静脉注射糖皮质激素的治疗。

目前有非常多种的影像学方法可以用于观察眼眶和其周围骨性结构。急诊科进行4 mm断层的标准头颅CT对于眼眶创伤的评估常常就已经足够了。对于创伤眼眶和眼的精细的检查须要使用2 mm轴位和冠状位的断层扫描，并且把扫描部位扩展到从眼睑到视交叉。常规头颅CT中提示眶骨折的征象包括鼻窦的混浊、眶周皮下气肿和周围软组织水肿。如果出现这些征象，须要及时进行全眶序列的扫描。各种重要的CT检查的关键征象在图9到图11中被着重描述。

眼创伤

评估直接眼外伤的最关键点就是判断是否有开放性眼外伤。在穿通伤中，穿通的位置常因有暗色的色素膜组织（虹膜和脉络膜）露出而非常明显（图12）。这也常常能在床旁通过笔形电筒看到。如果有非常可信的病史证明穿通物已从眼部离开，影像学检查可以暂缓做，但如果有明确的异物在眼内的病史，应立即做包含2 mm轴位和冠状位的CT断层扫描。在这种情况下，不推荐进行MRI检查，因为它会造成金属异物的移动。眼部要立即盖上防护眼罩，并且把剩下的检查留给眼科医师，如果可能在全麻下进行外科修复时再做。眼球破裂不能仅有CT检查就下判断，虽然通过CT的表现常常就能评估眼部的情况（图13）。及时的诊断和修复被证实可以减少感染的发生。所有眼球破裂伤后都要考虑交感性眼炎发生的可能。在眼球破裂伤的情况下，外伤会激发眼部抗体的产生，并攻击非外伤眼——交感眼，并且造成健康眼发生严重的威胁视力的炎症反应。在开放性眼外伤中发生交感性眼炎的比例高达1 ：500。

眼球顿挫性外伤最容易发生破裂的部位就是眼球壁最薄弱的部位，包括角巩膜连接部（角巩膜缘）、直肌的止端以及视神经附着部位（图14）。尽管如

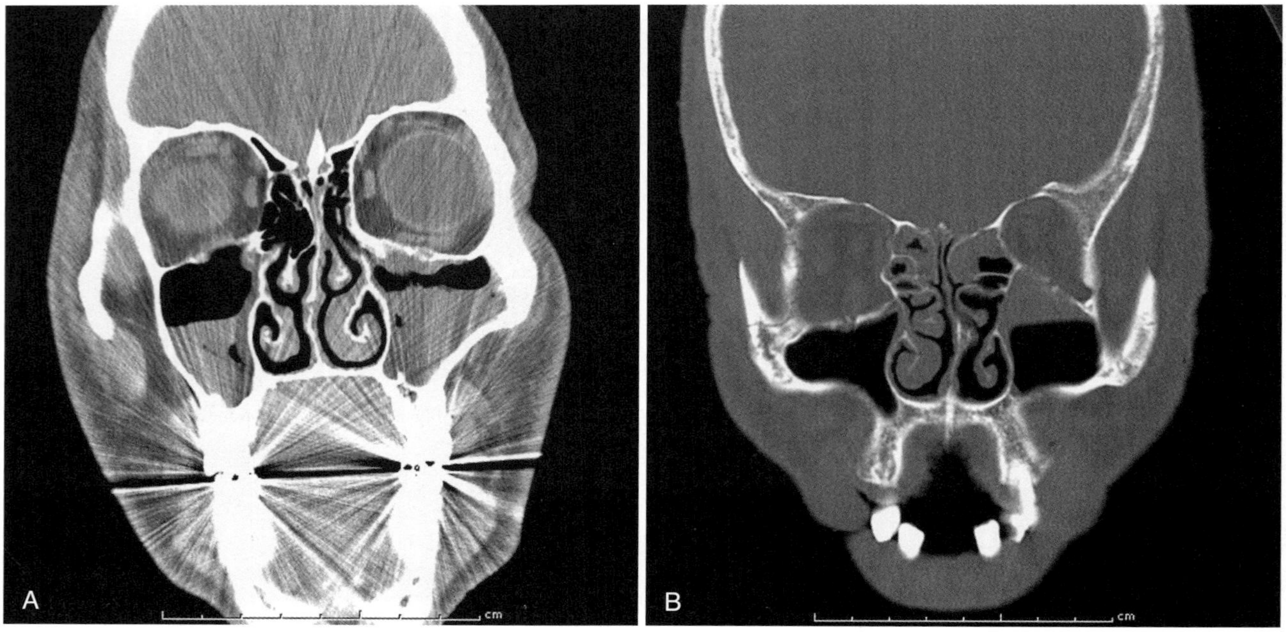

图9 双侧眶骨折。**A**，可见上颌窦气液平面，以及左眶软组织脱垂。**B**，左眶骨折伴眶脂肪脱垂

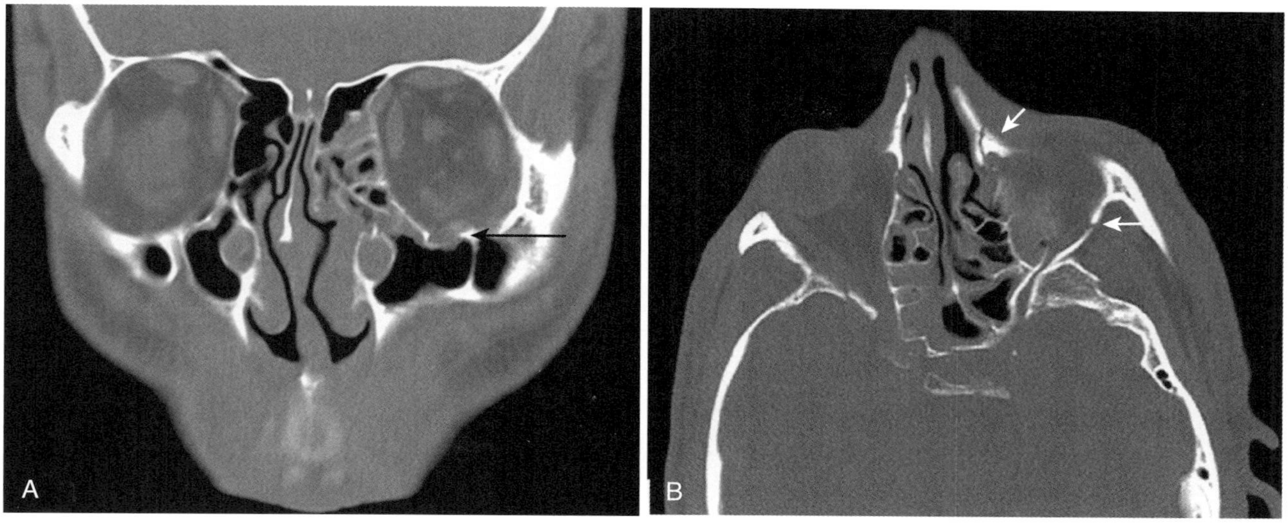

图 10 左眶骨折伴肌肉受限。**A**，表现为遮挡放射线的肌肉向骨折“天窗”突出（箭头）。**B**，鼻骨和眶外侧壁骨折。此病例眼球完好无损

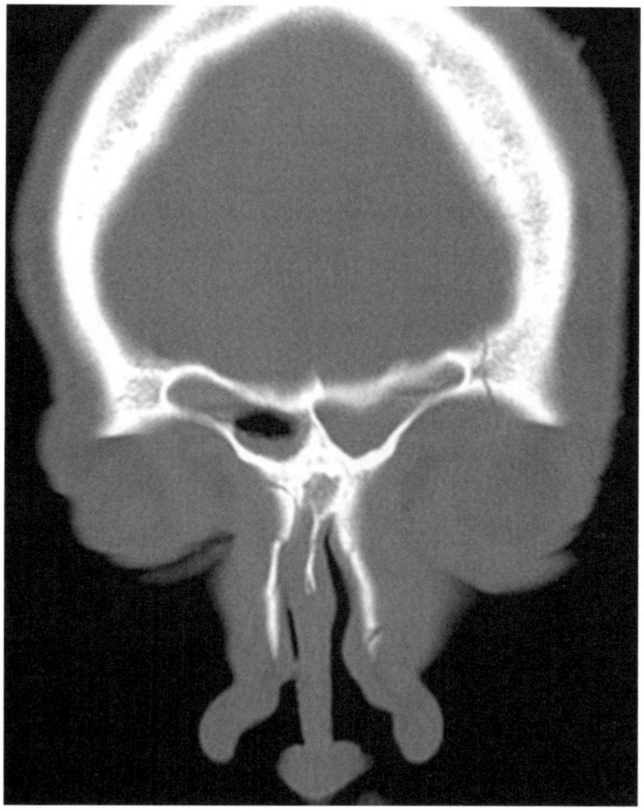

图 11 左侧眶顶骨折的冠状位片

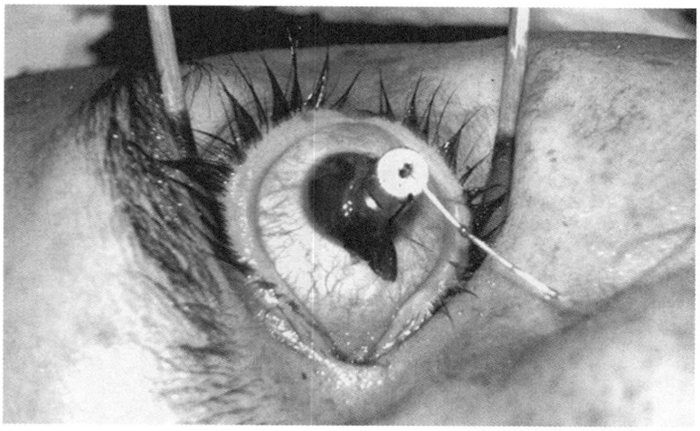

图 12 左眼电击枪探针伤，深色的葡萄膜组织突出于角膜。将患者的左眼立即用眼罩盖住后转入眼科门诊进行进一步治疗

此，巩膜的破裂仍然可能发生在角巩膜缘后，并且在标准的裂隙灯检查下并不明显清晰。在这些很难诊断的病例中，检查者必须依赖判断隐匿性巩膜裂伤的最重要特征来决定是否须要外科进一步的探查。Werner 等报道了 49 只怀疑巩膜裂伤并找到真正能提示裂伤的因素的眼睛，来决定是否需要外科探查。这些因素包括：视力低于 20/400，创伤眼眼压低，出现前房积血、传入性瞳孔障碍以及玻璃体积血。使用这个标准，49 个患者中有 17 个在外科探查中发现了真正的破裂伤。结膜下血肿合并尖型瞳孔同样对判断是否有隐匿性巩膜破裂很敏感。这些数据与 Kylstra 等的很相似。玻璃体积血只能让有经验的眼科医师来确认，通常须要超声检查。这一点对于判断之后是否可能发展成增殖性玻璃体视网膜病变非常重要。所谓的增殖性玻璃体视网膜病变最早被 Cleary 和 Ryan 描述成玻璃体的纤维增殖造成对视网膜的牵拉，有并发视网膜脱离倾向的一类病变。当这些表现同时出现时，对于外科探查和修补可能存

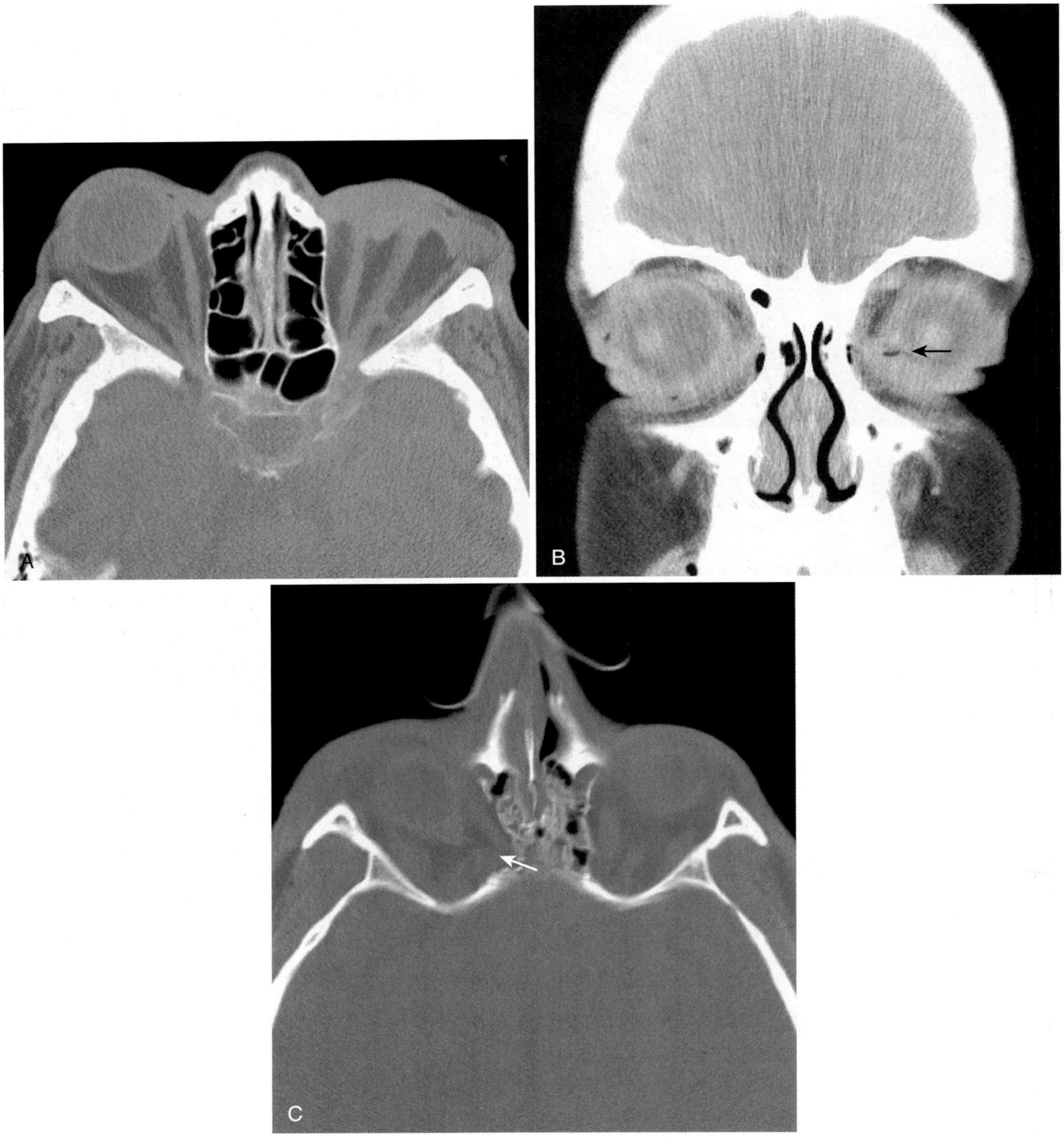

图 13 眼球外伤的 CT 扫描。**A**，左眼变扁平。**B**，左眼巩膜裂伤（箭头）。**C**，右眼视神经撕脱（箭头）

在的巩膜裂伤是非常有帮助的。图 15 和 16 展示了三个关键的表现。现将它们的敏感性和特异性总结在表 4 里。

开放性眼外伤有两个特别重要的亚类就是球内异物和感染性开放性外伤。异物在眼内的存在会带来更大的感染风险以及异物本身对眼内的毒性，常常须要立即进行玻璃体视网膜手术以挽救眼球。异物可以是金属、木质以及其他有机物质。眼眶 CT 检查是非常敏感的探测金属异物的方法（图 17）。尽管如此，对怀疑眼内异物的眼仍应进行超声检查。如果有明显的角膜伤口，同时有小的硬质异物入眼的病史，则须要使用房角镜谨慎地检查前房角。

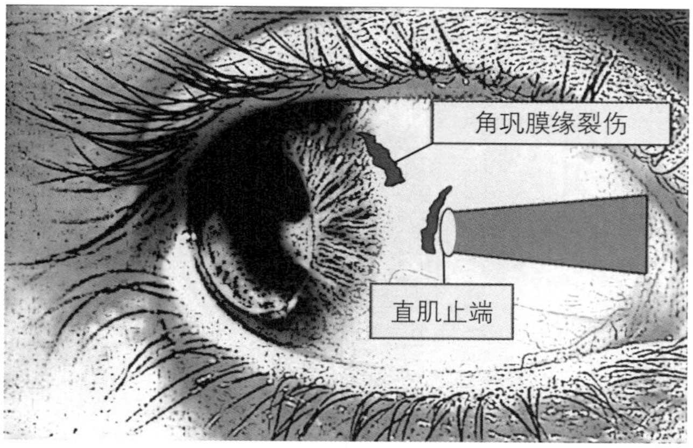

图 14 眼钝挫伤最容易出现破裂的位置 (*Artistic rending by Narina Sokolova*)

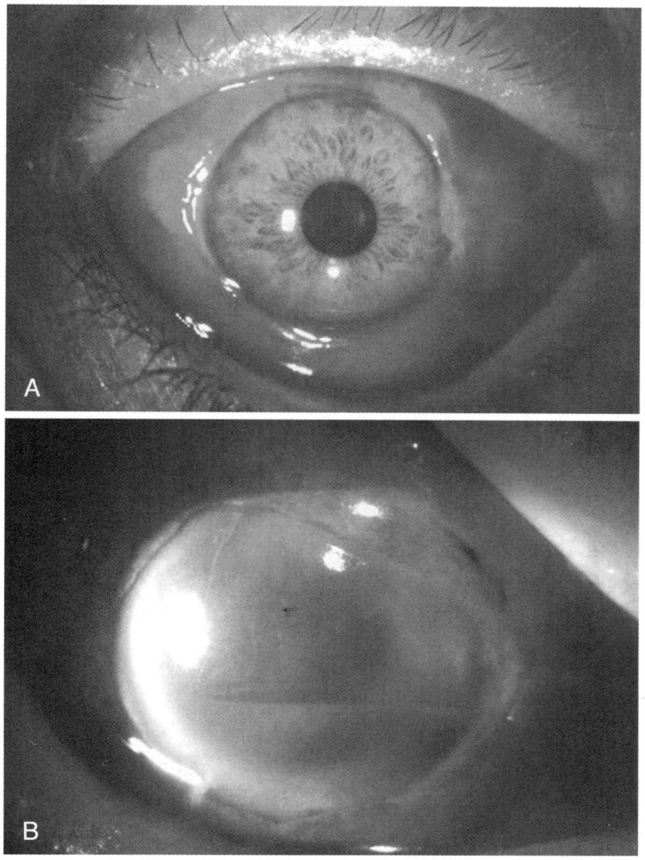

图 15 **A**，血肿。结膜弥漫隆起，与良性球结膜下出血时结膜平平的表现不同。**B**，45% 水平的前房积血。两者都提示可能存在隐匿性的巩膜破裂

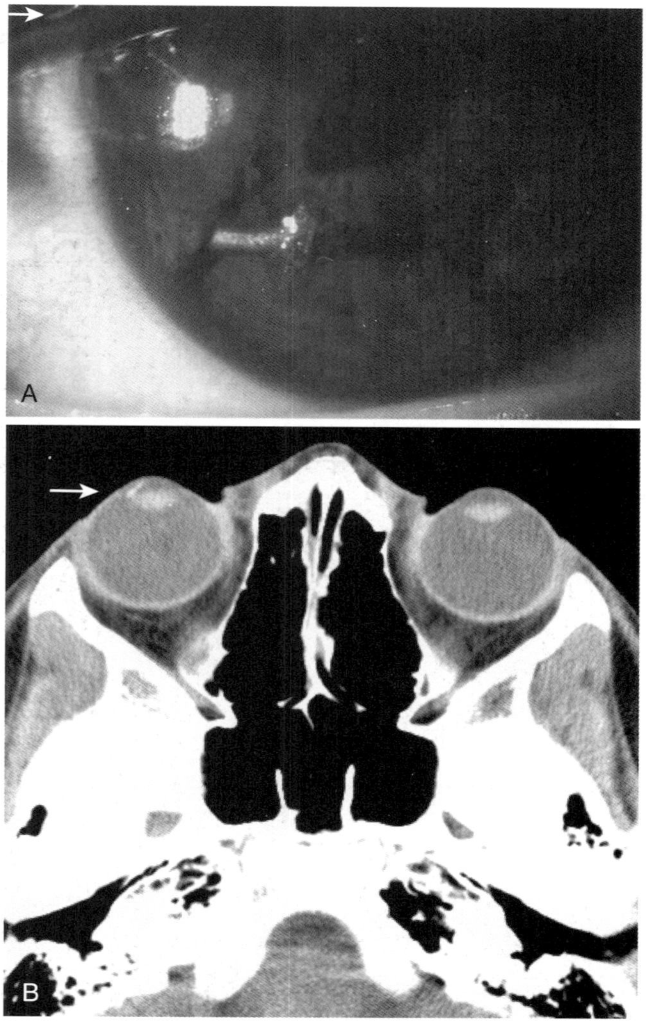

图 16 **A** 和 **B**，患者为铅笔导致的眼球穿通伤 (注意瞳孔的尖部)。眶部 CT 扫描显示异物未超出前房的范围 (箭头)

表 4 判断眼球破裂的特殊体征的敏感度和特异度

发现	敏感度	特异度
视力低于 20/400		
健眼眼压高于外伤眼		
前房积血		
传入性瞳孔障碍		
玻璃体积血		

Modified from Werner MS, Dana MR, Viana MA, Shapiro M: Predictors of occult scleral rupture. Ophthalmology 101:1941–1944, 1994.

如果检查有伤口污染的证据 (例如植物性外伤)，须要高度警惕是否存在感染，并且要积极地处理。开放性眼外伤后眼内炎的发生为 4%～8%，但如果在乡村环境出现外伤，感染的概率可增加到 30%。感染眼出现前房积脓是非常经典的表现，但是常常因为前节出血遮盖而变得不清，无法看到前房积脓。对于所有的开放性创伤，创伤科医师和急

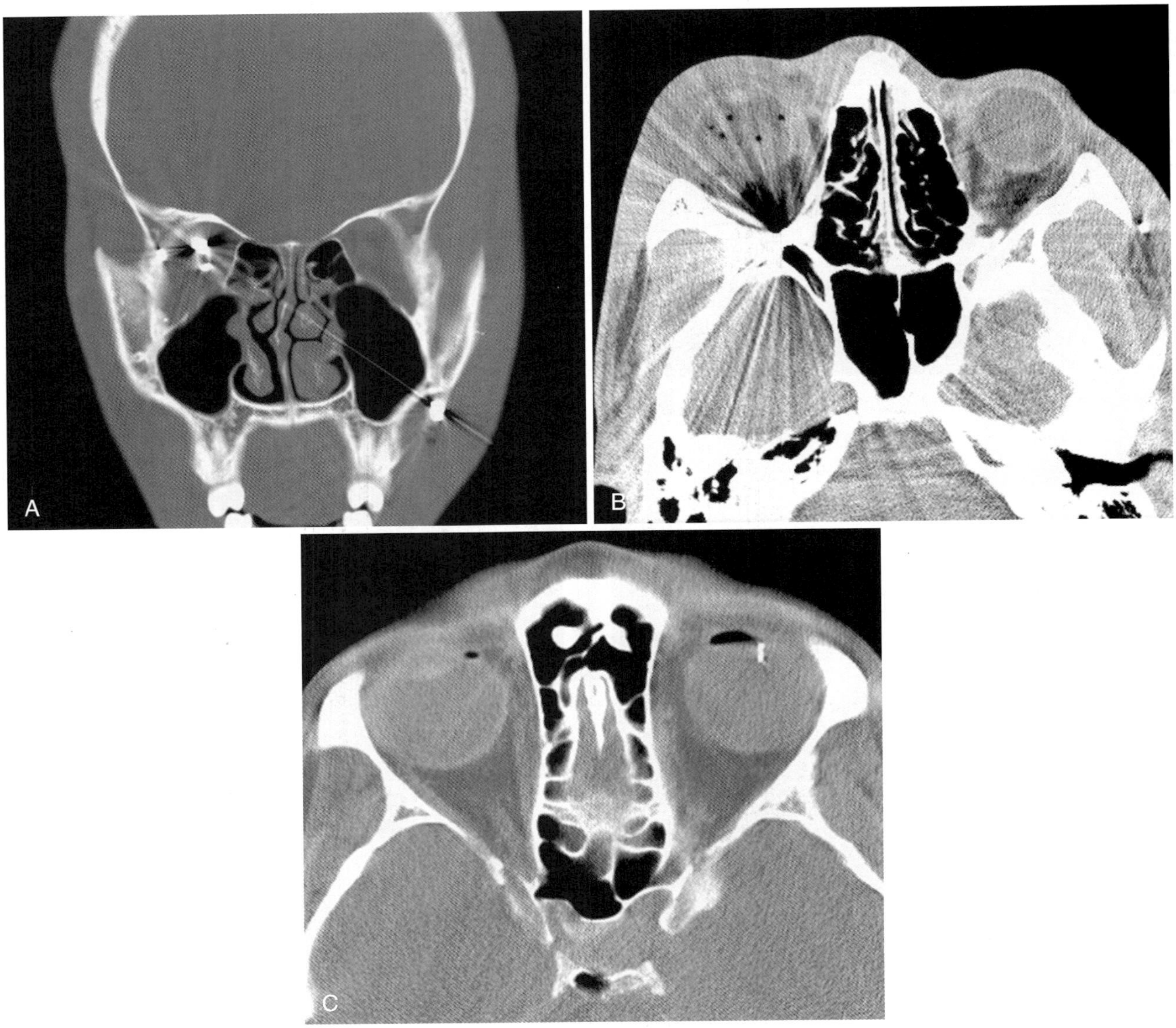

图 17 **A**、**B**，右眼内猎枪子弹。**C**，左眼前房内金属异物和气体

诊科医师的作用就是立即联系眼科会诊，并且立即进行眼眶 CT 检查。进一步的治疗则需要专业的眼部治疗人员的参与。

评价眼球裂伤最有效的方式之一就是超声检查。眼睑明显的水肿以及患者的不适感常会造成眼部创伤评估非常难以进行，而且检查者须要最大程度地不去骚扰开放性外伤眼。熟练地应用超声可以获得充足的信息用以判断眼内容物的状态以及是否存在球内异物。进行超声检查时，即使闭着眼，而且不对眼球施加任何压力，仍然可以检查从角膜到视神经的全部眼组织。当存在前房积血或玻璃体积血时，可能非常难观察到眼后极部，但超声检查仍可以很好地进行评估。后部巩膜破裂常常表现为明显的结膜血肿以及玻璃体积血（图 18 和 19）。这些病例都是隐匿性的，看不到巩膜的破裂，而且眼压是正常的。寻找球内异物进入的轨迹并最终定位异物的线索就是靠超声检查去寻找血性的伤道。通过追踪这条伤道，异物可以被定位并且确认（图 20）。超声在更清晰地定位异物的位置，评估眼内容的状况，寻找不容易通过 CT 检查看到的异物（如木质、玻璃以及塑料）中有着优势。另外，对于巩膜壁附近的异物，超声可以更好地判断异物是在球内还是在球外。

化学和热烧伤常与开放性眼外伤相关，但也可以独立发生。主要的治疗是大量冲洗以及局部使用糖皮质激素和抗生素。尽管如此，在存在开放性眼外伤，修复裂伤是首要的，之后才是化学和热烧伤

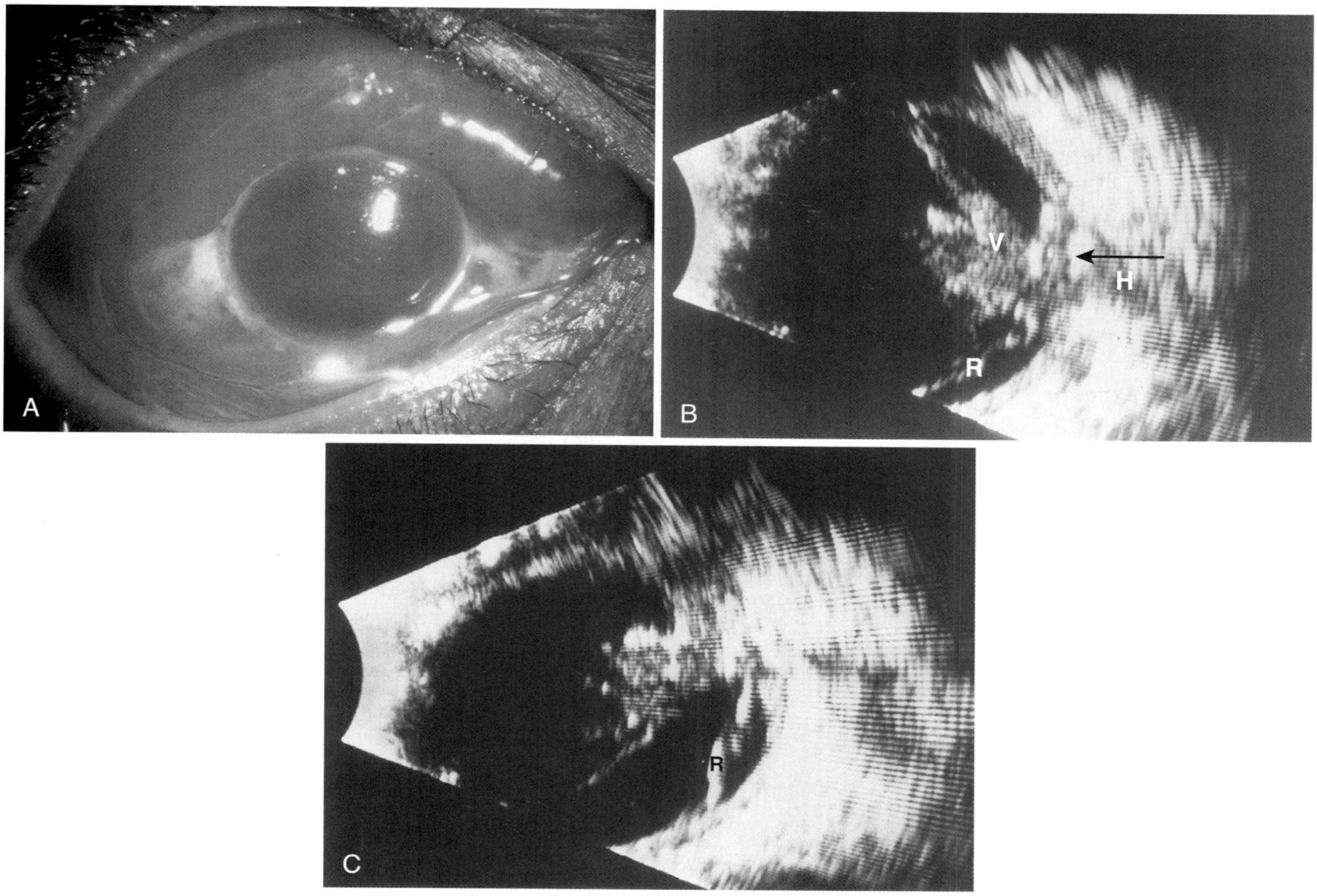

图 18 眼球钝挫伤造成的巩膜裂伤。**A**，前节照相可见前房积血和结膜血肿。**B**，纵向 B 超扫描可见玻璃体积血（V）。可见玻璃体嵌顿于巩膜裂伤处（箭头）以及视网膜脱离（R）。**C**，横向 B 超检查显示玻璃体嵌顿于巩膜裂伤处和视网膜脱离（R）。H，眼眶出血（*From ByrneSF, Green RL: Ultrasound of the eye and orbit, 2nd ed. St. Louis, 2002, Mosby.*）

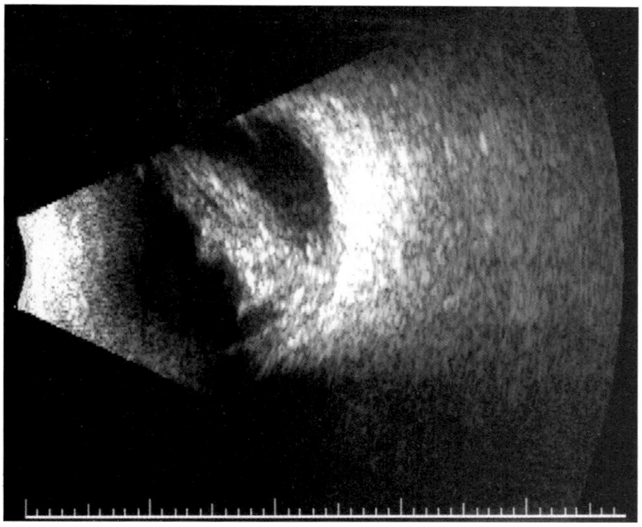

图 19 电击枪探头取出后的血道（见图 11）

的治疗。应使用石蕊试纸测量眼表 pH，并且在最开始就及时地使用 Morgan 镜冲洗眼睛。在每升水冲洗的间隙，应重新测量 pH，然后再冲洗，直至 pH 变为中性。如果 pH 不能恢复中性，应在翻开眼睑的状态下用棉签擦拭上下结膜穹隆去除此处的结晶颗粒。

酸和碱对眼表有着截然不同的影响。酸会造成角巩膜蛋白质的变性和沉积，变性的蛋白屏障会使得酸损伤不会进一步向更深一层发展。酸性物质很少造成穿孔并到达前房而造成进一步的损害。相反，碱会造成角膜表面亲脂层的皂化，使碱性物质更容易穿透到更深的组织中，所以常常会造成眼内结构的损害，从而导致青光眼和白内障。眼部常常异常地平静，以至于烧伤的严重程度被忽视。这时经验性的法则是化学烧伤外表看来越平静，预后越差。这是因为眼表的血管系统被摧毁以至于造成表面不充血、不红的假象。随着时间的流逝，眼表出现炎症和瘢痕（图 21）。这些患者需要大范围的眼表重建。青光眼手术以及角膜移植来恢复视觉功能。伤后数分钟到数小时内积极的冲洗对预后影响最大。在伤后最初的几天局部使用抗生素和糖皮质激素也是无比重要的。这些工作常常在眼部治疗人员诊疗患者之前，急诊和创伤部门就开始进行了。

外伤的解剖定位和损伤分级——眼外伤分类小组

1996 年，眼外伤分类小组为医师和研究人员

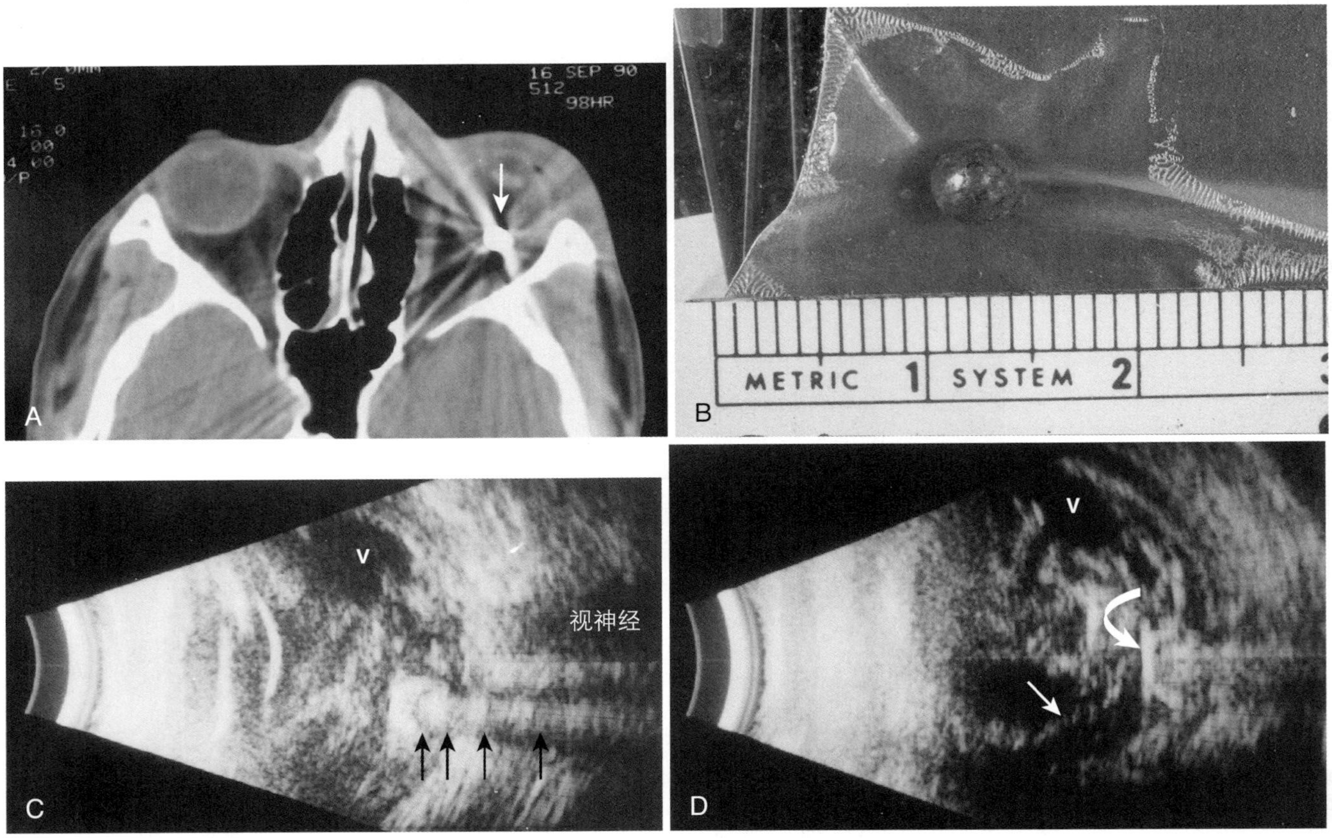

图 20　球内视网膜下 BB 弹（枪击）。**A**，轴位 CT 检查显示球形异物（白色直箭头）位于后部球壁附近。**B**，图 A 中眼内的球形 BB 弹被取出。**C**，轴位 B 超检查可见高反光浓密的玻璃体积血（V）以及 BB 弹的高密度声影，形成 BB 弹造成的特异性的复杂的信号链（彗星尾）（小黑色箭头）。**D**，横向 B 超减少增益后显示视网膜脱离（白色直箭头）和其下的 BB 弹（弯的白色箭头）（*From Byrne SF, Green RL: Ultrasound of the eye and orbit, 2nd ed. St. Louis, 2002, Mosby.*）

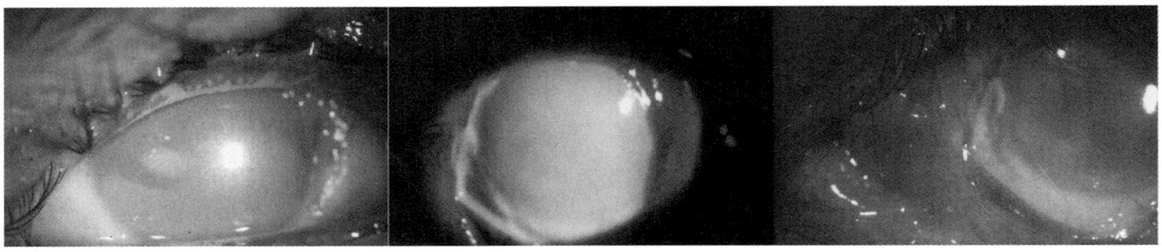

图 21　严重碱烧伤患者。可见白色的平静的眼部表现。钴蓝光下荧光染色后，患者的全角膜上皮缺损。尽管经过非常积极的治疗，患者仍然出现全眼表的烧伤、严重的炎症以及穹窿的消失

可以标准化定义眼外伤而建立了眼外伤的分类。这个过程的一个目标就是可以在描述眼外伤时更好地使用创伤的专业术语。该分类把眼外伤分为开放性以及闭合性的眼外伤（表 5）。Pieramici 等研究了这个针对机械性眼外伤的分类系统的影响预后的因素包括：①受伤的机制。②伤眼最初检查时的视力。③伤眼是否有传入性瞳孔障碍。④眼球壁开放的部位。选择这些变量是因为它们可以很好地提示视力预后，而且可以在最初的检查或最初的外科处理中得到临床评估。眼球壁开放的部位以及是否存在传入性瞳孔障碍对预后是非常强的预测因素。所以对于创伤科医师和急诊科医师而言最重要的就是评估视力以及是否存在传入性瞳孔障碍的状况。即使如此，仍然强烈建议创伤科医师使用 Fox 眼罩将患者的伤眼遮盖，等待专业的眼科医师进行余下的检查。创伤外科和急诊科医师应该能很好地对眼外伤进行分类，并且帮助眼部治疗人员更好地进行有效的药物治疗和手术治疗。

药物治疗和手术治疗

眼眶创伤

眼眶骨折的保守治疗包括口服广谱抗生素和鼻血管收缩剂，特别是在 CT 检查提示鼻窦病变或眶内异物穿通时。如果患者没有复视的主诉并且几乎没有眼球运动的受限，就不考虑外科干预，患者可以每周一次随诊。如果发现临床表现和 CT 上有“白眼”爆裂性骨折（眼部表现正常，眼球运动明显受限）的征象，并且合并无法缓解的心动过缓、房室传导阻滞、恶心、呕吐或昏厥（眼心反射），须要在 24 h 内立即进行修复。对于眶顶骨折，如果出现相关的脑脊液鼻漏和眶骨相关的颅内出血，则须要进行神经外科的评估，常常须要神经外科和眼科医师一起合作进行修复。

当出现眼球突出、眼压升高伴紧绷的眼眶（眼睑非常紧）并且 CT 检查提示球后活动性出血时可以诊断球后出血。如果临床高度怀疑球后出血，可以先行外眦切开，然后再做 CT 检查。做外眦切开时须要在局部麻醉下使用齿镊和直剪来完成。触摸找到外侧眶缘，垂直眶缘从外眦角到眶缘做切开，分离上下眼睑。用镊子夹住下睑，主要的力量用在外眦腱上。可以通过用剪子弹拨的手感来确定肌腱，剪开外眦腱时尽量接近眶缘（图 22）。用同样的方法定位并切开上方的外眦腱。很多医师采用分步的方法，切完下方眦腱后复查眼压。如果眼压正常，上方的眦腱切开就可以暂时不做。降眼压药物包括静脉注射或口服碳酸酐酶抑制剂和 β 受体阻滞剂，应该在最开始就使用高渗透性药物。在完成这些步骤后，通常球后空间的血液被释放，眼可能会变得更突出。尽管如此，最终的结果是眼压的降低和眼血流重新恢复正常。

可治疗的传入性瞳孔障碍的病因包括眶骨筋膜室综合征、机械性视神经压缩伤（被骨折或异物）或创伤性视神经病变。而视网膜中央动脉阻塞、视神经撕脱和视神经管内的神经损伤（骨折或视神经管压缩）则不容易通过药物或手术介入的方法治疗。

表 5　眼部创伤术语的新的标准分类

名称	定义
球壁	巩膜和角膜
闭合性眼外伤	球壁没有全层的外伤
开放性眼外伤	球壁有全层的外伤
破裂	钝性外物导致全层球壁的损害，外力导致暂时性的眼压升高，从而由内向外出现损害
割裂	锐利外物导致的球壁全层伤，损害由外向内形成
穿通伤	锐利外物造成的单纯的眼球壁的割伤
球内异物	造成割伤的外界异物留在眼内
贯通伤	球壁两处割伤（入口和出口），常由锐物或者子弹导致

From Ryan S: Retina, Vol. 3, 4th ed, St. Louis, 2004, Mosby, p 2380, Table 140-1

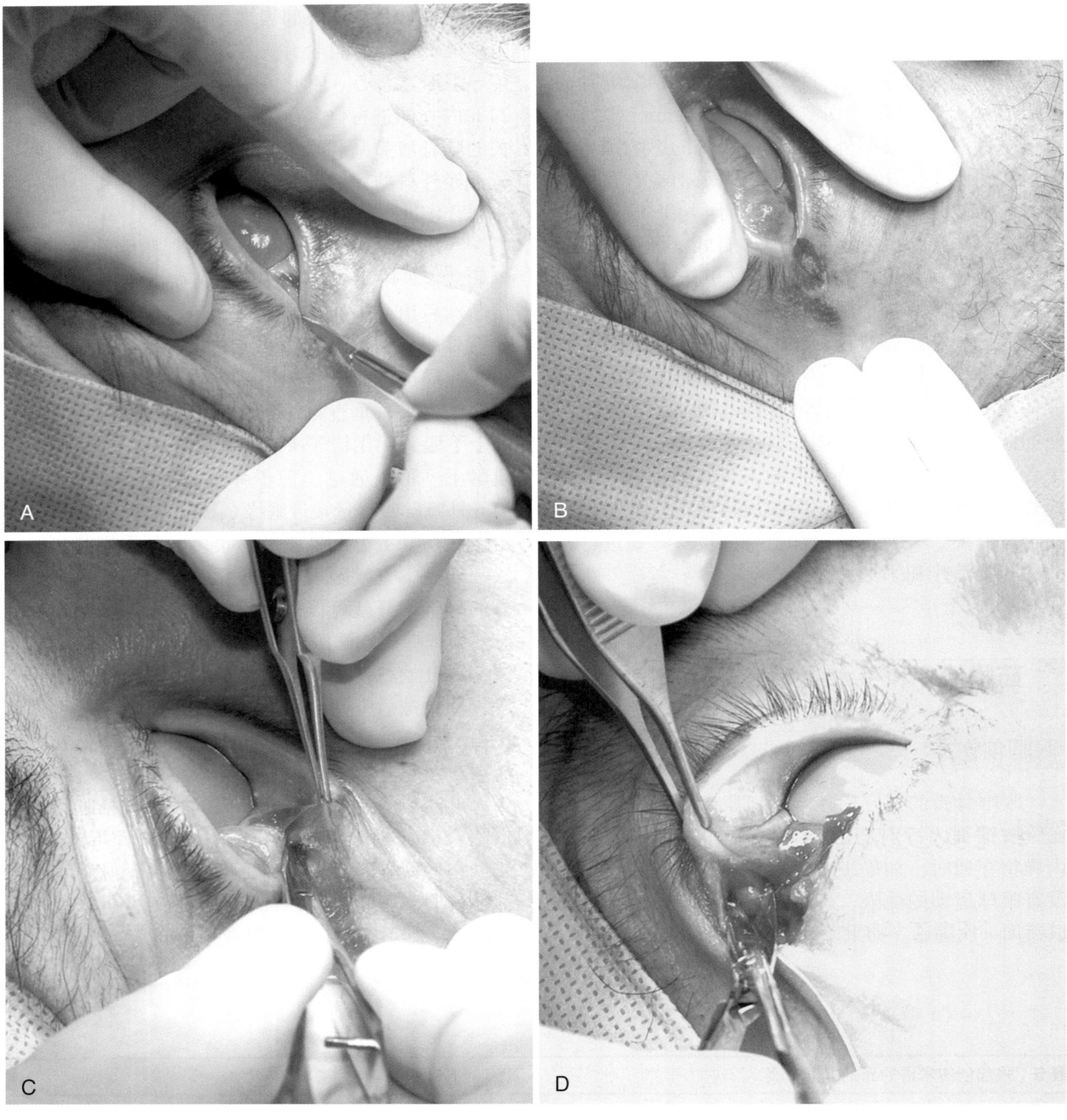

图 22 **A** 和 **B**，外眦角垂直切开。**C**，外眦韧带下方切开。**D**，外眦韧带上方切开

创伤性视神经病变是排除诊断，须要排除其他病因。如果怀疑创伤性视神经病变，建议采用静脉注射甲泼尼龙 5.4 mg/kg Q6 h 连续 3 天治疗。无须再更换成口服激素并逐渐减量。这种治疗是从脊髓治疗的临床试验推测得来的。该试验证实全身使用甾体药物治疗对于长期脊髓损伤患者恢复功能的好处有限。眼科的文献中也没有全身使用甾体药物治疗创伤性视神经病变的确凿证据，但这种治疗方法被广泛接受。所以由于并不明确的治疗效果以及明确的副作用，糖皮质激素在治疗儿童、老人、1 型糖尿病和有感染倾向的患者时要保持最大程度的警惕。

另外一个须要考虑的事情就是眼眶外伤合并有

眼睑和周围软组织裂伤的患者。急诊医师和创伤外科医师是有能力把主要的伤口缝合的，除非眼睑裂伤累及了睑缘和泪液引流系统（泪点和泪小管），或与上睑下垂和眶脂肪外露有关。这类外伤的修复必须在手术室完成，而且常常还合并有眼球的创伤。如果怀疑伤口（例如动物咬伤）有污染，须要考虑预防破伤风以及全身使用抗生素。对深层伤口的缝合须要使用快速吸收的缝线，而浅层伤口的缝合须要使用缓慢吸收的缝线（如 6-0 Vicryl 线），尤其是对那些在 7～10 天时复查有困难的患者（例如儿童，或者复查时有问题的患者）。

针对眼外伤，立即的药物治疗和手术治疗由眼部治疗人员直接进行。急诊科医师和创伤外科医师要通过进行的最初的检查迅速做出决定来获得眼科的紧急会诊以及进行必要的辅助检查。这时对麻醉医师来说，血液和电解质的状况、肺部和神经的状况以及最后一次进食的时间都是重要的资料。在怀疑眼球破裂伤时，麻醉医师避免在手术室使用琥珀酰胆碱也是非常重要的事情。去极化的肌松药会导致眼外肌的收缩，可能会造成眼内容物流出。由眼科医师来完成的眼球壁裂伤的修复包括小心地再次处理球壁以减少术后的散光和眼球变形，并且如果可能，还须为进一步玻璃体手术做准备（图 23）。

结论和处理流程

尽管对眼外伤的进一步处理需要有经验、接受过培训的眼科医师来完成，但对于这些患者而言，急诊科医师和创伤外科医师才常常是做出最重要决定的人。以下是对于本章内容的关键概念的简单总结，以用于快速参考。使用这个逐步式的方法，眼球及眼眶外伤的关键因素可以被记录下来，也可以对下一步的治疗做出快速的选择。

眼球及眼眶外伤的全面检查的关键内容如下：

1. 初始的检查包括视力的评估以及是否存在传入性瞳孔障碍。存在传入性瞳孔障碍（即使视力没有受到严重影响）是视神经损害的表现。潜在的可治疗的病因包括球后出血伴眼压升高（眼眶筋膜室综合征）、眼眶骨折或异物造成的机械性压缩伤和创伤性视神经病变（视神经挫伤）。前两者可以在急诊室由创伤专家诊断，第三者是一个经过影像学检查无法发现问题的排除性诊断。这些情况下须要做 2 mm 的轴位和冠状位的 CT 扫描。如果临床上高度怀疑眼眶筋膜室综合征（明显的上睑下垂和眼压升高），可以在影像学检查结果出来前就进行外眦切开术，而且在病情控制后也可以很容易地进行修复。对于传入性瞳孔障碍，必须排除视网膜动脉阻塞、缺血性视神经病变和视网膜脱离。这些都须要在进行全面的眼部检查后诊断。
2. 下一步的检查是评估开放性眼外伤。如果可见裂伤和穿孔，可以暂时推迟进一步的检查，眼部要先用眼罩遮盖住。要立刻请眼科会诊，并且患者须要全身使用抗生素。须要提醒患者避免咳嗽和 Valsaslva 类型的动作。评估潜在的裂伤的体征：低眼压、前房积血、传入性

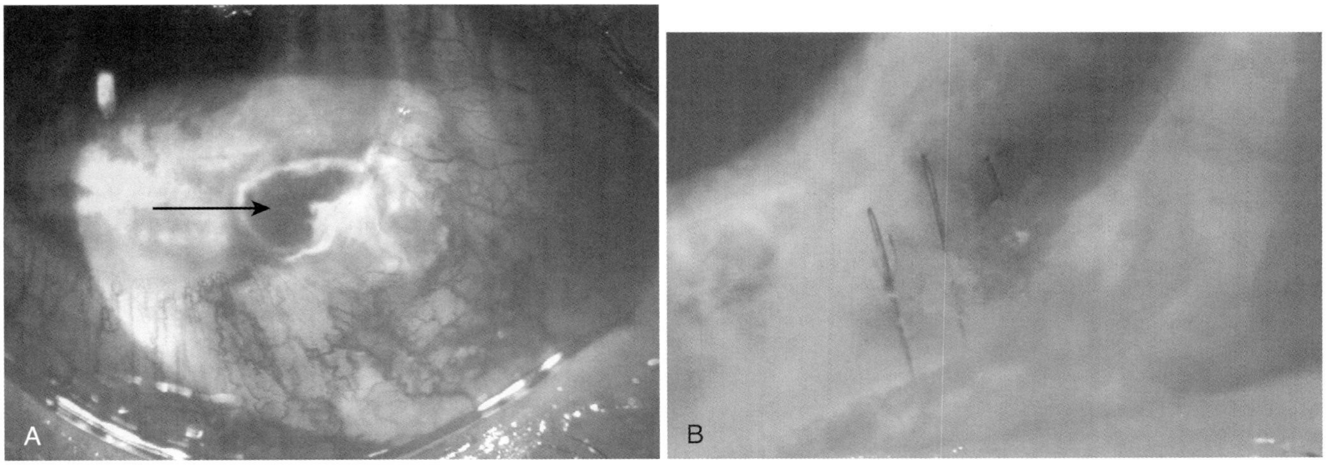

图 23　**A** 和 **B**，患者被空弹击中，怀疑左眼塑料弹壳外伤。荧光素染色后可见房水从角巩膜缘（箭头）延续直达角膜的伤口处渗漏。外科探查发现伤口没有向巩膜方向延续，用 10-0 尼龙线三针轻松地将伤口关闭

瞳孔障碍、玻璃体积血、结膜血肿和尖型瞳孔。如果没有裂伤的证据，而且眼压是正常的，创伤科医师或者眼科医师就可以安全地进行进一步的眼部检查了。对于创伤性的前房积血，使用局部糖皮质激素和局部1%阿托品治疗。创伤性前房积血再出血的最高发时间是在最初的5天，所以这些患者在这段时间内要每天进行检查。对这些患者要密切观测眼压并且局部使用低剂量的糖皮质激素治疗直到积血治愈。

3. 让患者朝主要的四个方向（上、下、左、右）注视来检查眼球运动，并且检查运动是否受限。还要问患者是否有复视，无论是朝正前方还是其他方向上（遮盖一只眼后复视消失）。如果可以见到眼球运动受限，可以在局部麻醉下让患者朝受限的方向看进行牵拉试验，医师用镊子将眼球向相同的方向移动。如果中等程度怀疑眼球运动受限，须要立即进行眶部CT检查来除外眼外肌或眶脂肪嵌顿。预示嵌顿的体征包括心动过缓、恶心、呕吐和昏厥。而且，在儿童如果眼局部表现得很安静，但是出现明显的眼球运动受限（白眼爆裂性骨折）则值得担忧。如果眶部CT检查显示明显的鼻窦疾病（黏膜增厚），推荐使用口服抗生素和鼻血管收缩剂。
4. 如有出现球内异物的病史和表现，须要立即进行眼眶CT扫描，包括2 mm轴位和冠状位扫描。CT检查显示球内异物时须要立即进行眼部超声检查，以更好地定位异物和评估眼球内损伤的程度。木质的、玻璃的和有机异物超声检查显示比眼眶CT检查更好（即使CT扫描不能见到明显的球内异物，也不能除外木质、玻璃和有机异物）。非常有经验的人须要非常小心地进行超声检查，以免对开放眼造成进一步的损害。立即请眼科会诊并开始使用全身抗生素治疗，禁食、水，以为手术进行预先准备。
5. 如果有化学烧伤的证据，要测量眼表的pH。如果pH异常，须要进行眼部冲洗。医生必须警惕化学烧伤后白色、安静的表现是不祥的体征，并且必须立刻治疗。开始并持续使用乳酸林格液或者平衡盐溶液持续的冲洗直到复查pH正常。直接的烧伤可以诊断为热烧伤，并且如果需要的话，可以使用抗生素和润滑液治疗。对于只累及眼睑的烧伤必须要观察直到皮肤修复，因为眼睑可能挛缩，眼球可能暴露。这种情况下润滑是主要的治疗。
6. 眼球后退（眼球向后移位）提示出现较大的眶壁骨折，须要早期的外科修复。对累及范围超过50%的眶底骨折要考虑可能出现眼球后退。这些患者须要在1～2周内预约好外科手术修复外伤。其他眼眶骨折的体征也要进行全面的评估（眼球下方的面部感觉减退、眶缘的骨性错位和眼球运动受限）。
7. 关于儿童的特殊警告　如果眼眶的检查因配合不佳而受阻，与其将有价值的时间浪费在对眼球施加压力的检查中，不如在麻醉下进行检查并且修复可能合并存在的眼球破裂。

本章所叙的观点可以作为急诊室和创伤外科处理中绝大多数眼外伤病例的实用指南。另外，须要关注一些其他创伤，包括非偶然因素的儿童创伤（摇晃婴儿综合征），与颅内和颈部创伤有关的霍纳综合征，动脉瘤压迫脑神经以及偶尔出现的海绵窦动静脉瘘都有可能在与创伤有关的情况下发病。尽管在紧急状态下从严重外伤中挽救患者的视觉似乎是下一步才须要关心的，但对于恢复期的患者和试图恢复正常活动和功能的患者来说，这就是首要的问题了。

第 6 章　颈部损伤

颈部穿通伤：诊断和目前处理

Leonard J. Weireter, Jr. 和 L.D. Britt 著
熊　建　张学民　张立红 译

数百年来，颈部一直是大量创伤外科文献兴趣的源泉。它的解剖紧密度使一些致命的解剖结构彼此非常接近，从而使患者通过一个单一的创伤因素更容易产生一个多系统的损伤。16 世纪 Ambroise Paré 报道一个在打斗中造成颈总动脉和颈内静脉撕裂的患者的治疗以来，关于颈部创伤适当治疗的争论一直延续至今。虽然 Paré 描述的患者存活了，但却遗留了偏瘫和失语。现在，并发症使得对于颈部穿通伤积极外科治疗适当性的讨论依旧很重要。

颈部的解剖

颈部包括大量的致命解剖结构，而且彼此相邻。颈动脉和颈内静脉并列直接走在胸锁乳突肌的深层。咽部以及它和食管的连接处在环咽肌水平直接走行在喉和气管的深层。甲状腺和与之相连的甲状旁腺位于颈前部并叠压在上段气管的表面。胸导管被很好地保护起来，因为它横贯颈部并从颈部左侧胸锁乳突肌的深部进入到颈 - 锁骨下系统。颈椎椎体和脊髓是除了颈长肌外最后面的结构。

颈部以往被分为一系列的三角。最多的外科讨论中心是前三角的解剖，它包含胸锁乳突肌间的区域。功能上，颈部被分为 3 个区（图 1）。Ⅰ区的边界包括环状软骨（上），胸廓入口（下）和胸锁乳突肌（外）。它对于外科的重要性在于这个区域包括重要的颈胸脉管系统，以及呼吸消化道的重要结构。

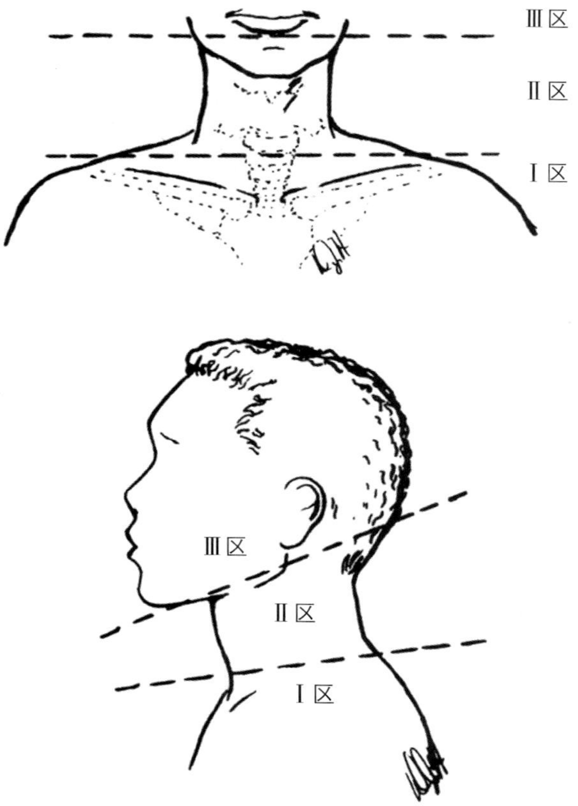

图 1　颈部损伤层次的分区 (*Drawing by Doris Holloman.*)

Ⅲ区是颈部在下颌三角头部的水平区域，它的上边界是颅骨基底。值得注意的是，颈内动脉在这里向头侧进入下颌三角，而且不容易在手术中显露，要被迫使用特殊的方法获得对血管的操作（如手术下颌骨脱位）。但是，Ⅱ区（环状软骨和下颌三角之间的区域）大多数可以通过一个沿胸锁乳突肌前缘的切口较容易地进行手术中的显露（图 2）。

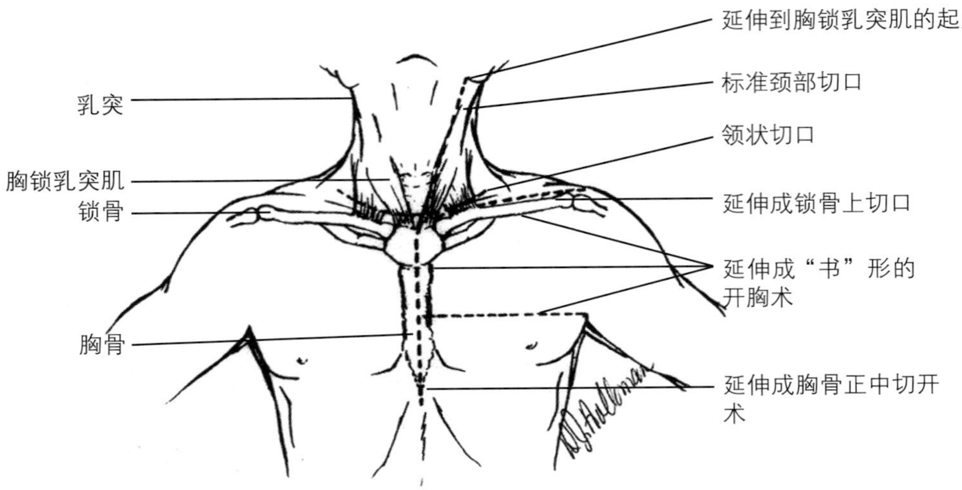

图 2 颈部穿刺伤手术显露的切口 (*Drawing by Doris Holloman*)

初始评价

遭受颈部损伤患者的初始评价应遵循高级创伤生命支持的指南来做。这个指南提供了一个能够快速辨别威胁生命的损伤并适当优化治疗的处理框架。那些需要紧急外科干预的表现通常是指颈部损伤的“硬体征”(表 1)，包括皮下气肿、扩大的或搏动性血肿，或伤口的活动性出血。所有这些发现都提示大血管或呼吸消化道损伤。这些表现的诊断性检查并不重要。最佳的气道管理是最优先及重要的。

没有损伤的“硬体征”即意味着不需要立刻外科干预，就可以进行更多的可选择的或预期的检查、治疗方法。这些可选择的医疗设备包括含或不含血管造影的多排 CT、食管镜、食管造影、喉镜 / 支气管镜或动脉造影。虽然一些细微的发现(软体征)，例如，讲话困难或音调改变能提示这些选择性评估，但主要争论的中心还是在对于Ⅱ区损伤及没有“硬体征”的患者是否应该进行这些选择性处理还是仅仅观察(观察性处理)。

表 1 颈部穿通伤的体征

硬体征	软体征
活动性出血	吞咽困难
扩大或搏动性出血	声音改变
皮下气肿或伤口出现气泡	咯血 纵隔增宽

对于所有的颈部都须进行详细的神经学检查。穿通伤口禁止进行局部探查。这种操作只能作为在手术室正式颈部探查手术的一部分。为了减少患者的咳嗽和恶心，应禁止行鼻胃管插入或鼻气管吸引，如果可能，应在手术室麻醉诱导后进行。

呼吸消化道损伤

由于在颈部气管和食管非常接近，气道和消化道同时损伤十分常见。Asensio 等报道 10% 的穿通伤患者都存在呼吸消化道损伤。如前所强调，理想的气道管理是最重要的。

对于那些需要紧急气道处理的患者，特别是由有经验的医生操作经喉气管插管是最好的选择。当遇到任何可能已经或即将存在困难气道的患者时，应该考虑外科建立气道。气道处理的专家应该努力尝试尽快经喉气管插管。在真正紧急的情况下选择外科建立气道的方法是环甲膜切开术。气管造口术只有在当你怀疑一个成年患者可能存在部分喉气管分离的紧急情况下须建立气道时进行。这种情况下，如果可能，还是应该由气道专家小心尝试经喉气管插管术(图 3)。

如果选择可选择性的处理方法，提供的方法包括可曲式光导纤维喉镜检查、可曲式食管镜检查、可曲式支气管镜检查，以及食道对比造影。使用水溶性造影剂对食管进行多角度的观察，可以安全地排除食管溢出。如果结合食管镜检查，这项研究的灵敏度和特异度可以从 85% 提高到将近 100%。随

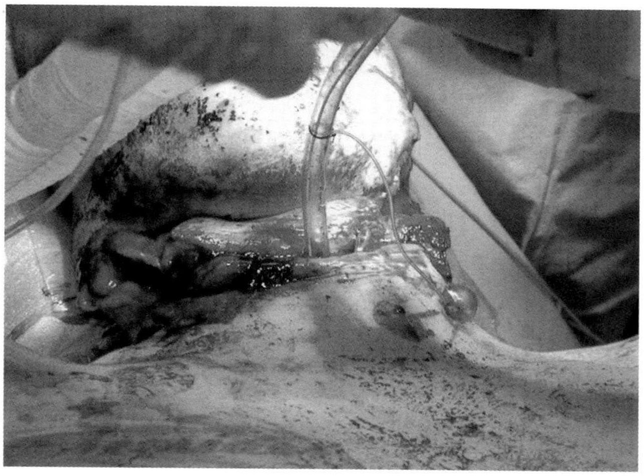

图3 争执中造成的颈部伤口。注意是通过伤口直接插管到受伤的气管中建立气道。使患者保持坐姿直到插管完成，这样可以使气道容易显露，而且减少分泌物窒息的风险

着可曲式纤维内镜检查经验的增加和技术的增强，对于造影检查的依赖越来越小。对于在环咽括约肌下方的颈段食管近端 3～5 cm 的观察比较困难，因为这段区域很容易在内镜插入和拔出的过程中忽略掉。不得不对这个区域进行特殊的检查。

虽然应该直接用喉镜检查是否存在喉损伤，但是一般用纤维支气管镜来检查气管或支气管损伤。此外，颈部 CT 扫描也用来辨别损伤是否需要进一步检查或手术干预。

如果发现气管损伤，应该在适当清除失活组织后用可吸收缝线间断缝合撕裂的气管。如果没有复合伤，一般不须同时行气管造口术。

对于可疑喉损伤的患者，可根据评估团队的推荐以及对更严重损伤的怀疑，选择纤维内镜进行诊断，同时结合外科探查。包括甲状软骨、声带和杓状软骨的喉损伤可能需要特殊的重建。Brent 等提出的分级系统（表 2）回顾并细化了他们对一个 18 年周期内的喉损伤病例的经验。重点是要获得充分安全的气道以及处理所有相关的威胁生命的损伤。对于喉损伤，最好通过气管造口术获得对气道的控制。喉损伤治疗延迟超过 48 h 会导致更不好的结果。但是这种延迟经常反映一个事实，就是患者确实伤得很重，而不能进行确定性处理。黏膜接合和骨折复位应该在最初探查时进行。

颈段食管损伤很难诊断，而且可能会发展成爆发性纵隔炎。Weigelt 等报道的 10 例损伤患者中只有 7 例有食管损伤的症状或体征。作者指出内镜或食管造影都有接近 20% 的假阴性率。当联合这两种方法评估时，假阴性率可以降到 0。Armstrong 等回顾性报道 23 例颈部食管穿通性损伤。食道对比造影只有 62% 的灵敏度，而硬质食管镜有 100% 的灵敏度。随着纤维光学技术的进步和手术经验的提升，可曲式内镜会本质上取代硬质食管镜。

表 2 喉损伤分级

组 1	小的喉内出血或无法发现的骨折的撕裂
组 2	水肿、出血、没有暴露软骨的小的黏膜破裂、CT 扫描上显示无移位骨折
组 3	大面积水肿、黏膜撕裂、软骨外露、声带固定、骨折移位
组 4	与组 3 相同，同时有超过 2 条骨折线或累及喉黏膜的严重创伤
组 5	完全喉气管分离

From Bent JP, Silver JR, Porubsky ES: Acute laryngeal trauma: a review of 77 patients. Otolaryngol Head Neck Surg 109:441–449, 1993.

基本外科原则适用于大多数的食管损伤。应该在两个层面小面积清创后一期闭合伤口。内层用可吸收线、外层用不可吸收线缝合。对于同时有气管和食管损伤的伤口，中间插入有活力的自体组织如肌瓣，是很重要的。如食管狭窄、气管食管瘘和感染等并发症也是很常见的。

经常难以察觉的咽部损伤只需要简单的一期修复和引流。

软组织损伤

对软组织损伤的处理要遵循与对坏死皮肤进行清创相同的原则。虽然可以一期关闭，但为了对软组织有充足的覆盖，须构建皮瓣或游离组织移植物，特别是对于大的开放性伤口。甲状腺的穿通伤最好通过缝合结扎控制，虽然根据出血、血供阻断以及组织破坏的程度可以行甲状腺叶切除术。要辨别颈部主要神经或臂丛神经的损伤，并加以标记，以便于后期的修复。

胸导管损伤

左侧颈部基底的损伤会有胸导管撕裂的风险。

软组织损伤和出血使这种损伤的发现很困难。因此，典型的乳糜样引流液在最初外科探查时显得不那么明显。

颈部血管损伤

在20世纪早期美国的军事战争中，颈部大血管损伤的预后非常差。第一次世界大战后报道用结扎的方法治疗颈动脉损伤有30%的神经损伤率。直到20世纪50年代，随着朝鲜战争中对于血管修复的经验的丰富，颈动脉损伤的修复才变得越来越普遍。好的治疗效果很快被大家接受，关注于血管损伤的诊断和修复的更加积极的处理方法建立了起来。出现在1956年出现了第一个颈动脉损伤的民间报道，当时Fogelman和Stewart总结手术干预是必要的，以及手术时间延后使死亡率增加。这份报告成为接下来的20年对于颈部强制性探查治疗标准的基础。

挑战颈部中央穿通伤强制性探查的报道在20世纪70年代中期大量发表。Sheely等报道632例遵循强制探查原则的颈部穿通伤患者，认为选择合适的患者可以安全地观察，同时可以被有经验的人员治疗。反面观点由Saletta等提出，他们报道了246例颈部穿通伤强制探查的病例。虽然阴性探查率很高，达63%，但致病率低，而且死亡率为0。虽然他们的临床评价为阴性，但13例患者在探查大血管时有所发现。强制性探查被认为是有利有弊的。遵循这个逻辑，Bishara等报道了一组病例，其中53%的患者进行了强制性探查，并有正常的手术发现。然而，23%患者的损伤在术前临床评估时为不可疑。这些患者大多是孤立的静脉损伤或孤立的咽食管损伤。对Ⅱ区损伤的手术探查应该是安全且合适的。然而，高的阴性探查率使许多机构质疑这种方法。Elerding等报道了一组基于强制性探查原则的病例，阴性探查率为56%。所有损伤患者术前都有提示损伤的临床体征。在评估和处理这些患者时选择性探查是非常合理的选择。

Jurkovich等报道结合荧光射线技术及血管造影对血管和呼吸消化道解剖的研究的诊断率为23%。只有9%的患者会从这些检查中受益。使用损伤分区来决定处理的方法，Jurkovich等提出对于Ⅰ区损伤要更积极地使用血管造影术、X线胸片和食管造影术，Ⅲ区损伤要更积极地使用血管造影术。特别强调，如果患者没有症状，Ⅱ区损伤可以安全地进行观察。Obeid等也发表回顾性文章额外支持高选择性方式处理这些损伤，他们提出强制性探查应该被选择性处理原则替代。这背后的理论是基于若干发现而得出的，包括即便对于强制探查患者依然会有没有发现的损伤，以及与阴性探查相关的致病率以及住院天数的延长。Obeid等发现有“硬体征”的损伤患者需要手术干预，而那些体格检查阴性的患者可以观察。那些体格检查发现比较模糊或有变化的患者须进行辅助检查来诊断，以决定是否有任何有临床意义的损伤存在。Belinke等也发表文章对选择性探查原则进行支持。在他们的研究中，44例患者根据体格检查发现而采用选择性探查原则治疗。22例立即探查的患者的阴性探查率为23%。在观察的患者中，没有出现延迟手术或并发症的情况。如果所有患者都立即进行探查的话，那么阴性探查率将会为60%，这促使作者支持对于Ⅱ区损伤进行选择性探查。

Metzdorff等报道83例患者有56%的阴性探查率。当术前有明显的临床体征时，82%的患者会有损伤的发现。而如果术前体格检查是阴性的话，80%的患者没有损伤的发现。

1987年，Meyer等对120例颈部穿通伤患者进行了前瞻性研究。7例患者因为出血进行了急诊探查。其他患者接受动脉造影术、上呼吸消化道内镜术和食管造影结合手术探查治疗。其中5位患者发现了6个大血管损伤，而这些损伤术前并未料到。作者认为，选择性处理会错过太多的大血管损伤，强制性探查是更加谨慎的选择。

Wood等推崇基于体格检查发现的选择性探查方法。模糊的发现需要诊断性检查，以辨别是否需要外科探查。相似的争论中，Narrod和Moore肯定了对这样的患者进行选择性处理的安全性和有效性。Mansour等也支持选择性非手术处理，对119例患者运用此原则时，只有1例患者由于一个极隐匿的损伤而进行了延迟手术。

Beitsch等报道一个对于颈部穿通伤的回顾性研究。阴性的体格检查可以排除99%的血管损伤。在进行了的71次血管造影片中，只有1个患者需要手术修复。体格检查正常时，强制性探查以及血管造影评估的作用被质疑。

Scalfani等报道1项邻近组织血管造影片的研究发现，体格检查有61%的灵敏度和80%的特异度。作者认为，在评估颈部穿通伤时，没有同时对邻近组织进行血管造影术是不成熟的。然而，Menawat

等报道 110 例颈部穿通伤患者，只有 1 例有损伤但没有体格检查的发现。9 个非手术治疗的动脉损伤没有后遗症。Atteberry 等报道了 1 个包括 66 例患者的回顾性研究，没有血管损伤的绝对或“硬体征”的患者可以安全地进行观察治疗。Sekharan 等报道了单独使用体格检查评估有 0.7% 的误诊率。Jarvik 等报道对于临床发现的明显的血管损伤，体格检查有充分的灵敏度和特异度。体格检查有 93.7% 的灵敏度。Azuaje 等的颈部穿通伤病例表明，在发现外科相关明显的血管损伤方面，体格检查有 100% 的灵敏度和阴性预测值。当考虑血管造影发现的损伤时，体格检查有 93% 的灵敏度和 97% 的阴性预测值。这组体格检查阴性的病例中，在不考虑损伤分区的情况下，没有人需要血管修复。

特别提到Ⅲ区损伤，Ferguson 等报道了 72 例穿通伤患者。没有“硬体征”确实排除了外科相关明显的损伤。60% 有“硬体征”的损伤患者进行了探查。这组中只有 1 例患者没有可辨认的损伤。其余有“硬体征”的损伤患者接受了急诊血管造影术，同时接受了血管造影下的血管内治疗。作者推荐有血管损伤“硬体征”的Ⅲ区损伤患者应该接受血管造影术，因为他们可能须进行血管内介入治疗。

很多互补的诊断方法可以用来评估颈部穿通伤。Ginzburg 等强调，在一项对于Ⅰ、Ⅱ或Ⅲ区穿通伤的稳定患者的前瞻性双盲研究中，评价血管造影和双功能扫描，发现双功能扫描有 100% 的灵敏度和 85% 的特异度。

更新的影像设备出现了。Munera 等前瞻性地研究了 60 个患者，报道螺旋 CT 有 90% 的灵敏度、100% 的特异度、100% 的阳性预测值、98% 的阴性预测值。作者总结，螺旋 CT 在评价颈部损伤时是一项非常优秀的诊断方法。Mazolewski 等对Ⅱ区穿通伤的 14 例稳定患者进行了一项前瞻性评价。所有患者都进行了彻底的体格检查、加强 CT 扫描和手术探查。14 例患者中 3 例患者共发现有 5 处损伤。这基于 CT 扫描发现，这几个患者有高的损伤发现概率。虽然只是一个小样本研究，但结果提示，CT 扫描有 100% 的灵敏度和 91% 的特异度，阳性预测值为 75%，阴性预测值为 100%。作者认为 CT 扫描在评估颈部损伤中扮演着关键的作用。Gracias 等用 CT 对 23 例涵盖 3 个区的颈部穿通伤患者进行评估，并进行了回顾性研究。所有患者都没有血管或呼吸消化道损伤的“硬体征”。13 例患者发现了远离重要结构的损伤痕迹，但没有进行进一步的评估。没有不良事件。Gonzalez 等报道了一个没有必须即刻探查的“硬体征”的Ⅱ区穿通伤患者的前瞻性研究。作者认为对于Ⅱ区损伤，CT 能够在体格检查的基础上提供很少的信息。

Hollingsworth 等对 CT 血管造影术（computed tomographic angiography，CTA）探查动脉粥样硬化源性或创伤源性的颈动脉和椎体损伤进行了 meta 分析研究。结果发现没有充足的高质量数据说明 CTA 对创伤灵敏或特异。

Woo 等研究了用 CTA 作为诊断检查方法的Ⅱ区穿通伤患者。他们报告随诊 CTA 使用的增多以及团队经验的加强，与之相关的阴性颈部探查的数量也随之下降了。作者强调用这种成像方法，伤口的轨迹可以被看到。这个发现有助于决定是否需要其他的诊断方式。例如，CT 可以显示损伤的轨迹远离所有重要结构，因此可以排除进一步的检查。另一方面，损伤可以被清楚地显示，也可以据此行外科探查或常规血管造影下的血管内介入治疗。最后，基于有问题的发现，不确定的研究结果可以提示要进行其他的检查。

对于颈部基底的Ⅰ区损伤推荐行血管造影术，因为损伤在胸廓出口，很难诊断和控制。Eddy 等进行了一个多中心超过 10 年的回顾性研究。他们研究 138 例患者，其中有 28 个动脉损伤。然而，这组病例提示，如果体格检查和 X 线胸片均正常，可能不须行血管造影术。

Gasparri 等通过对 100 例患者的回顾也确定了这个发现。所有具有血管损伤“硬体征”的患者迅速行外科探查。81 例没有血管损伤“硬体征”的患者行血管造影术，其中 11 个发现了隐匿的损伤。当结合正常体格检查和 X 线胸片时，它们有 100% 的灵敏度和 80% 的特异度，阳性预测值为 40%，阴性预测值为 100%。这组病例提示只是怀疑损伤，并不推荐行血管造影。

Demetriades 等的一项前瞻性研究分析体格检查在颈部穿通伤中的作用，缺乏血管或呼吸消化道的“硬体征”时有 100% 的阴性预测值，并能可靠地排除所有这类需要手术修复的伤口。这组病例分析时使用的标准特别寻找与血管和呼吸消化道损伤相关的体格检查信息。无症状患者可以安全地观察。

我们自己的处理原则见图 4 的流程图。表现出血管或呼吸消化道损伤“硬体征”的患者应立即去手术室做颈部探查术。如果损伤在Ⅰ或Ⅱ区，食管镜和支气管镜可能成为手术室探查的一部分。手术入路由主治医生慎重考虑。有“软体征”的患者应接受多层螺旋CT（multislice helical CT，MHCT）血管造影。如果伤口轨迹明显远离相关的重要结构，则不用采取特殊治疗。接近意味着伤口轨迹离感兴趣的血管或呼吸消化道结构在5 mm之内。一项研究说明这种邻近可能由于遗留的金属物或其他碎片的伪影而变得模糊，这种情况下应该进一步检查。如何做应由创伤主治医生慎重决定，可能需要食管镜、支气管镜、血管造影或这些检查适当的联合。

根据我们自己的经验，图5显示了颈部软组织里的空气以及残留弹片产生的伪影。患者没有损伤的硬或软体征。这种不确定性以及主要的血管结构可能损伤的情况下应建议行CTA检查。图6是一个类似的没有损伤硬或软体征，但有软组织内气体的患者的侧位像。图7显示的是图6患者颈动脉的正常的CTA表现。图8显示的是Ⅲ区枪伤造成的颈内动脉损伤。这个损伤进行了支架治疗。

对开展MHCT的作用的讨论正逐步进行。事实上，每个身体区域和器官系统已经用这种方法研究，在许多方面MHCT事实上已经成为显像模式的标准了。广泛的使用、图像采集的速度、图像质量、不须依赖特殊团队而只需要随时待命，以及对于特殊研究能够在多层面上进行重建，所有这些都促使这项技术快速进步。对于颈部穿通伤应用这种技术也使不需即刻手术探查成为可能。

Inaba等对于使用MHCT评估不需要即刻手术探查的颈部穿通伤的前瞻性研究发现，CT图像实际上不会错过任何损伤。但这项研究结论的问题在于随访时间短（平均33天）和不完全（评估了84%的患者）。之前的研究以及Inaba的陈述都支持这样的前提，那就是如果不禁用其他检查，MHCT是灵敏度和特异度高的检查。它能够使应用其他诊断方法的需要降到最小。对于那些不需要即刻在手术室探查的颈部穿通伤患者，MHCT看来是非常安全和可信赖的筛查手段。

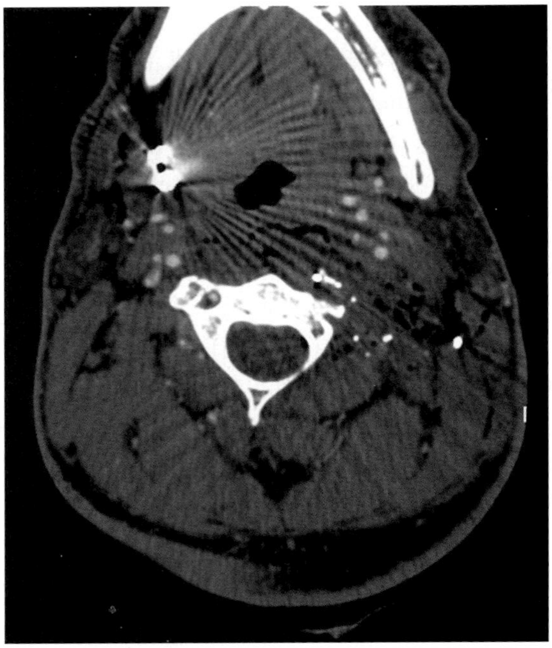
图5 颈部枪伤经CT检查显示软组织窗上的皮下气体

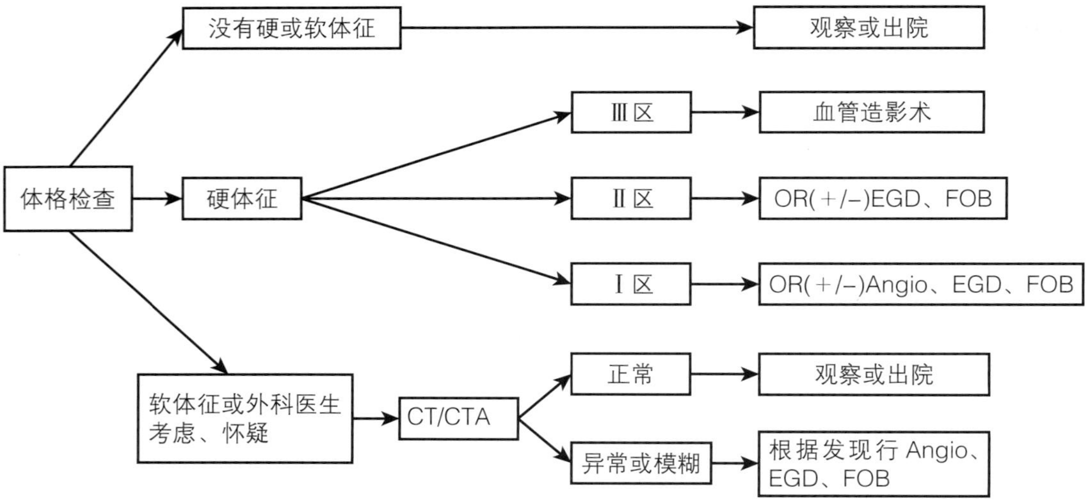

图4 颈部穿通伤的评估流程图。Angio，血管造影术；CT，计算机断层扫描；CTA，CT血管造影；EGD，食管胃十二指肠镜检查；FOB，纤维支气管镜检查；OR，手术室

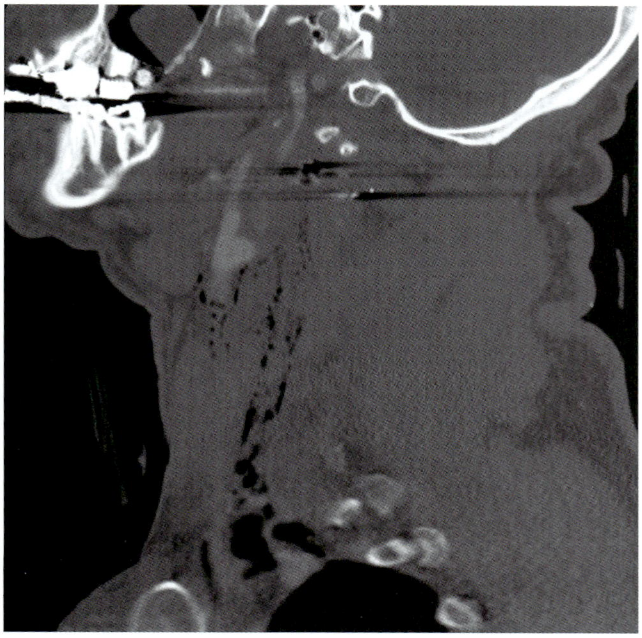

图 6　CT 的侧位像显示软组织内气体

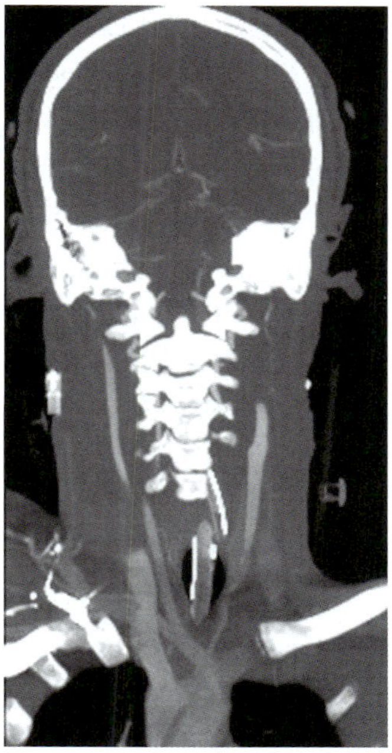

图 8　CT 血管造影显示枪伤后左颈内动脉血流中断

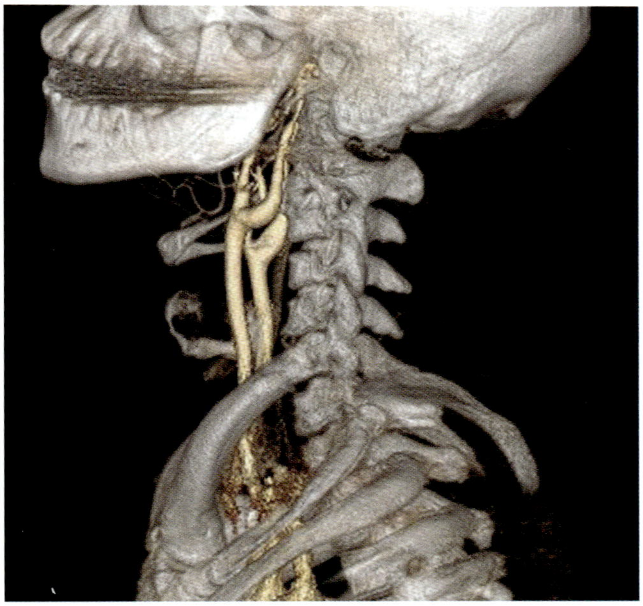

图 7　CT 血管造影术显示正常、没有损伤的颈动脉和椎动脉的解剖

已经很清楚的是，对于颈部Ⅱ区穿通伤的患者应用强制探查原则会导致高的阴性探查率。常规使用辅助诊断手段（选择性方法）将会导致大量时间和精力的消耗，而对有经验性期待治疗。血管或呼吸消化道损伤的“硬体征”的出现需要外科探查。血管或呼吸消化道损伤的不明显的体征可以根据外科团队的考虑分析进行评估。对于血管损伤体征的详细的体格检查能够发现绝大多数需要外科探查和修复的患者。只有在考虑选择影像检查评估是否比体格检查更有计划时，才能够体现 MHCT 的作用。

Steenburg 等写了一个关于颈部穿通伤进行影像学检查选择的优秀的综述。这是从影像学专家的角度写的，但与外科文献观点相同。能够描绘弹片轨迹以及看到邻近感兴趣的血管或呼吸消化道结构，才允许对进一步诊断或治疗的方法进行计划。如果没有这种怀疑，就不需要进一步的干预。

颈动脉损伤的治疗

颈部脉管系统的手术入路是由损伤的区域决定的。Ⅱ区损伤最好的入路是做沿胸锁乳突肌前缘的切口，同时头偏向对侧。在患者的肩下放一个手术巾卷是非常有帮助的。沿这个切口显露，会遇到面总静脉，可以将其结扎，这将可以完全显露颈总动脉、颈动脉球部、颈内动脉近端及颈外动脉、颈内静脉。颈动脉损伤最好用外科修复的方法治疗。使用从邻近的面静脉取下的静脉补片或 Gortex 人工补片修复是直接缝合修复的一种替代方法。这种情况下不常规使用分流术。是修复还是结扎，要在它们带来的并发症——严重缺血和进展性梗死所带来的恶果中做出选择。有固定的神经损伤表现的患者的血供重建能力差。颈内动脉远端的损伤需要特殊的方法才能得到修复。颞下颌关节离断可以使下颌骨向前脱位，从而可接近颈内动脉在下颌角头侧的部分。颅底无法外科显露，可能须介入技术控制。外科探查时，颈动脉有前向血流是好的修复指征。如果没有前向血流，可能会推荐结扎。颈动脉损伤的结扎应该只用于那些完全神经损伤的患者。Liekweg 和 Greenfield 的文献综述发现修复患者比结扎患者有着更低的发病率和死亡率。Unger 等和 Brown 等分别在各自的研究中确认了修复优于结扎的结论。

颈内静脉最好在外侧静脉造影后治疗，虽然有时结扎是合理的选择，尤其是当处理那些静脉几乎完全横断或损伤会导致静脉内腔直径狭窄超过 50% 的病例时。损伤如果向近端延伸进入胸廓出口，可以通过延长胸锁乳突肌前缘切口，同时胸骨正中切开或胸部陷门切口切开显露。如果需要，这样可以一直连续显露到主动脉弓以及颈动脉和锁骨下血管的起始处。同样地，可以将颈前切口向侧方延长以探查锁骨上窝。如果需要，这也可以方便地显露锁骨下血管或椎动脉的起始部。

扩大的颈部领状切口，可以用来进行甲状腺或甲状旁腺手术，也可以用来进行双侧颈部探查。经过颈部的枪伤会有损伤双侧血管的可能。从这个切口进入可以获得更好显露，也更容易从一个体位获得两侧的控制。有时这个切口需要更偏向头侧，以更容易显露。

累及锁骨下血管、颈血管和椎血管的颈部穿通伤的腔内血管治疗正在不断发展。从对于动脉粥样硬化疾病治疗中获得的经验毫无疑问可以用于损伤治疗，但现在并没有充足的经验可以广泛地推广应用。并且，腔内支架的应用也需要对患者终身的随访。

结论

颈部穿通伤在诊断和治疗上还面临着严重的挑战。专注、仔细的体格检查，以发现血管和呼吸消化道损伤的“硬体征”看来是评估颈部穿通伤的最有效的方法。虽然介入治疗在不断发展，但外科治疗通常是最直接有效的。对于没有“硬体征”的损伤，在结合或不结合其他诊断方法的前提下进行小心地观察会是非常成功的策略。对于那些不需要即刻手术探查的患者，MHCT 是可选择的影像学诊断方法。

钝性脑血管损伤

Clay Cothren Burlew 和 Ernest E. Moore 著
张学民 译

在过去的十年中，大量研究证实了钝性脑血管损伤（blunt cerebrovascular injuries，BCVIs）早期筛查和早期治疗的有效性。最初，人们认为 BCVI 会不可避免地造成毁灭性的神经系统损伤。但也有一些报告指出，在缺血性脑血管事件（ischemicneurologic events，INEs）的患者中，抗凝治疗可以改善神经功能。如果不经治疗，颈动脉损伤（carotid artery injuries，CAIs）导致的卒中风险高达 50%，且损伤程度越高卒中风险越大。椎动脉损伤（vertebral artery lnjuries，VAIs）导致的卒中风险为 20%～25%。根据患者的损伤模式和损伤机制建立的筛查方案可以筛查出无临床症状的患者并启动治疗，以免出现神经系统后遗症。目前的研究指出，对 BCVI 患者的早期抗血栓治疗可以减少卒中发生率，并预防神经系统疾病。

体征和症状

BCVI 最早被报道于 30 年前，是 1 例受损伤后发生卒中的患者。患者出现脑缺血症状或者症状的分布往往预示着潜在的脑血管损伤。CAI 导致的卒中往往表现为对侧感觉和运动缺失。当卒中发生在主导大脑半球时会出现失语症，而非主导大脑半球卒中可能会导致半边忽略症。VAIs 的典型症状为模糊的症状，包括共济失调、头晕、呕吐、面部或身体麻木以及视野缺损。颈动脉海绵窦瘘的症状包括眼眶痛、眼球突出、球结膜水肿、结膜充血。

虽然有些患者可能在损伤后 1 h 内出现 BCVI 相关缺血症状，但多数症状具有潜伏期。在有明确损伤而未接受抗血栓治疗的患者中可能会有一段无症状期。这个时间范围可以从数小时至长达 14 年，但大多数患者在 10～72 h 内出现症状。我们的目标是抢在卒中发生前的“沉默期”时诊断出 BCVI。现有的数据证实，如果能在无症状期时诊断出损伤，可以有效地治疗患者，预防卒中发生。在认识到 BCVI 特殊的损伤模式后，20 世纪 90 年代中期首次提出应在无症状期筛查 BCVI。虽然筛选标准仍有待完善，但目前的筛选可以通过他们的损伤方式筛选出高风险患者。

损伤机制与模式

Crissey 和 Bernstein 最早提出了可能导致 BCVI 的 3 种损伤机制。首先是直接击打颈部。这一情况常见于车祸时患者不恰当地佩戴安全带使安全带勒到颈部，也可能发生在休闲运动时颈部受击。第 2 种机制是头部过度向对侧扭转。这是最常见的造成 CAI 的原因，可能造成颈动脉拉伸越过 C1-C3 横突（图 1）。VAI 也可能由于在颈椎横突侧块的椎动脉受到过度牵拉造成。第 3 种机制是由于相邻的蝶骨或岩骨骨折导致的动脉撕裂。这一机制不仅可以导致 CAI 也可能导致 VAI。随着椎孔、横突孔骨折，椎动脉很可能会直接受到损伤。除了以上 3 种损伤机制，还有颈动脉或椎动脉内膜破裂的情况。内膜破裂会导致血小板聚集从而形成血栓或血管阻塞，最终导致随后的卒中。

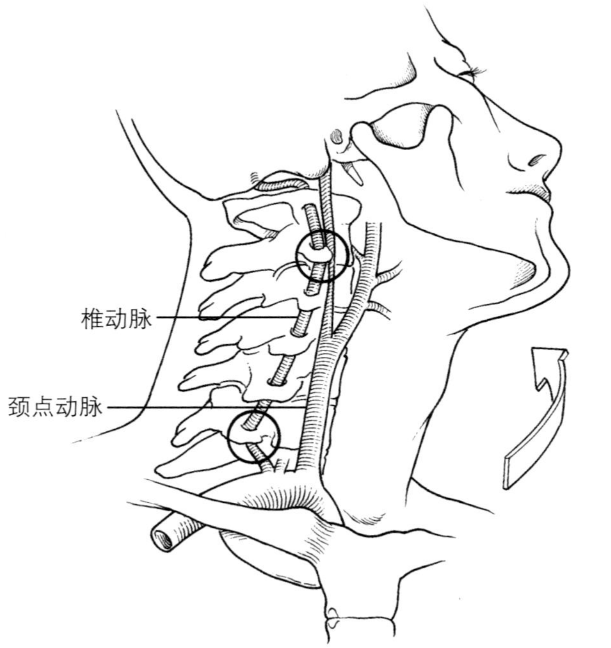

图 1 转动颈部和过度牵拉导致颈和椎脉管牵张损伤 *(Modified from Biffl WL, Moore EE, Elliot JP, et al: Blunt cerebrovascular injuries. Curr Prob Surg 36:505, 1999.)*

虽然损伤机制对于判断 BCVI 高风险患者十分重要，但患者的相关损伤对于判断无症状患者是否需要筛查 BCVI 同样很关键。认识到特定损伤的相关性后对 BCVI 主张积极筛查。目前的筛查因素包括患者的症状或体征，以及高风险的损伤模式（表 1）。随着 CT 血管造影非侵入诊断技术的应用越来越广，且学界认识到既往的诊断方式可能会漏诊约 20% 的 BCVI 患者，目前已提出应拓宽 BCVI 筛查指南范围。以往未包括的损伤模式随着影像学检查的应用也得以丰富，新增的损伤模式包括下颌骨骨折，复杂的颅骨骨折，颅脑损伤伴有胸部损伤，头皮撕脱，胸部血管损伤，绳带类损伤 / 安全带擦伤伴有明显的肿胀、疼痛或精神状态改变。除此之外，所有颈椎骨骨折患者也应进行筛查以排除 BCVI。虽然有观点认

表 1 丹佛钝性脑损伤筛查标准

BCVI 的症状体征	动脉出血
	>50 岁患者颈部杂音
	颈部扩张性血肿
	局灶性神经功能缺损
	神经系统检查与头颅 CT 检查结果不一致
	在二次 CT 扫描中发现卒中
BCVI 的危险因素	与下列有关的高能转化机制：
	面中部骨折移位（LeFort Ⅱ或Ⅲ）
	下颌骨骨折
	复杂颅骨骨折 / 颅底骨折 / 枕骨髁骨折
	GCS<6 的严重 TBI
	颈椎骨折、半脱位或在任何水平的韧带损伤
	接近绞刑的脑缺氧损伤
	绳带伤或安全带擦伤伴有明显肿胀、疼痛或精神状态改变
	TBI 伴胸部损伤
	头皮撕脱伤
	胸部血管损伤
	钝性心脏破裂
	上位肋骨骨折

出自丹佛健康医学中心。

BCVI，钝性脑血管损伤；CT，计算机断层扫描；TBI，创伤性脑损伤

为应对所有脊柱骨折的患者进行筛查，但也有观点认为应该根据机制和骨折模式（颈椎脱位、骨折累及横突孔、C1-C3的上位颈椎骨折）缩小筛查标准。

诊断显像

经过确定的筛查步骤，高风险患者应接受影像学检查来确诊BCVI。过去，四血管造影是诊断BCVI的金标准。但许多临床医生对患者接受血管造影的必要性持谨慎的怀疑态度。血管造影须花费较高的人力物力，且不是全然无风险的。在一些较小的医院，如果没有条件进行血管造影，还须紧急转移患者到有条件的医院进行确定性评估。

CTA是替代以导管为基础的诊断的有效方式。CTA不仅无创，而且大多数需要筛查BCVI的患者往往也有要CT检查其他部位的指征，因此多排CT检查往往对患者"一条线"的CT检查或全身进行从头到脚的多排CT检查。与过去的血管造影相比，CTA随时可用，可以缩短BCVI患者诊断的时间，从而使患者得到更早的治疗。

虽然早先的1至4排CTA在诊断BCVI的准确性上不尽如人意（灵敏度47%~68%，特异度67%），但随着多排螺旋CTA的引入，损伤诊断明显得到了改善。有5项已发表的研究和1篇报告评估对比了16层多排螺旋CTA和血管造影的准确度。Eastman教授等选择了162名做CTA的患者，其中146名同意接受血管造影。在这项研究中，患者检出率为28%，16层多排螺旋CTA对CAI的灵敏度为100%，对VAI的灵敏度为96%，只有一个Ⅰ级损伤未检出。Harborview的研究说明了在运用CTA诊断BCVI时经验的重要性。研究中对82例CTA检测正常的患者进行了血管造影，结果发现CTA漏诊了7例BCVI，阴性预测值达92%。然而，在回顾CTA影像时发现，7例患者中有6例患者有明确的损伤证据，而第7例患者的异常可能是因为没有外伤。此外，所有的漏诊都是发生在研究的前半段。Virginia医学院团队也有相似的发现。该团队筛选了119名患者，其中92名接受了血管造影验证。结果发现CTA的假阳性率为43%，假阴性率为9%，但所有漏诊的BCVI都出现在研究的前半段。研究的后半段CTA检出的灵敏度和阴性预测值均为100%。这些研究都发现，颅底区域的损伤是最难以识别的，对于这个高风险区域的检查应更为仔细、更加重视。最后一项研究在对比CTA和血管造影诊断BCVI时得到了高分辨率CTA最差的结果。16排CTA的灵敏度只有29%，64排CTA的灵敏度只有54%。在缺少质量控制的情况下，我们很难解释这项研究对BCVI筛查方式的影响。与之结论相反的是，在Fakhry等的一项初步报告中指出，CTA诊断BCVI可能过于灵敏。最近Memphis团队的研究中指出，由于CTA可能存在漏诊，血管造影仍然应该继续在BCVI的诊断中应用。

所有符合筛查指征，无抗血栓治疗禁忌证的患者都应尽快接受影像学检查。已发现BCVI的患者应在初次检查的7~10天后复查影像学检查。在Ⅰ级和Ⅱ级损伤的患者中，常规随访进行影像学检查尤为重要。超过一半的Ⅰ级损伤可以痊愈，并停止抗血栓治疗。但是只有不到10%的Ⅱ级、Ⅲ级和Ⅳ级损伤的患者可以痊愈，在已接受治疗的BCVI患者中约12%的损伤会继续进展。在颈动脉或椎动脉闭塞的患者随访中，超过80%的影像学检查没有变化，因此复查影像学检查意义不大。另一方面，一些专家推荐腔内方法治疗假性动脉瘤，因此应对Ⅱ级和Ⅲ级损伤的患者重复进行影像学检查评估。由于重复血管造影的主要风险发生在损伤后的前5天，因此目前认为损伤后的第7~10天是进行复查的最佳时间。

损伤分级量表

BCVI有各种与不规则管腔形态（夹层、闭塞、横断和假性动脉瘤）有关的不同结果，这促使我们建立分级量表从而便于从多方面评估、管理这些潜在的破坏性的损害。损伤分级量表不仅可以准确地描述损伤情况，同时可以根据损伤级别界定卒中风险（图2、3和表2）。在未经治疗的损伤中整体卒中率约20%。CAI中损伤级别越高卒中风险越大，而VAI中不同级别损伤的卒中率都保持在约20%（表3）。

钝性脑血管损伤的发生率

起初，BCVI被认为是一种少见的损伤，目前在所有因钝性创伤住院的患者中诊断率只有1%。在此之前，BCVI相关的卒中往往被归因于患者初期的脑

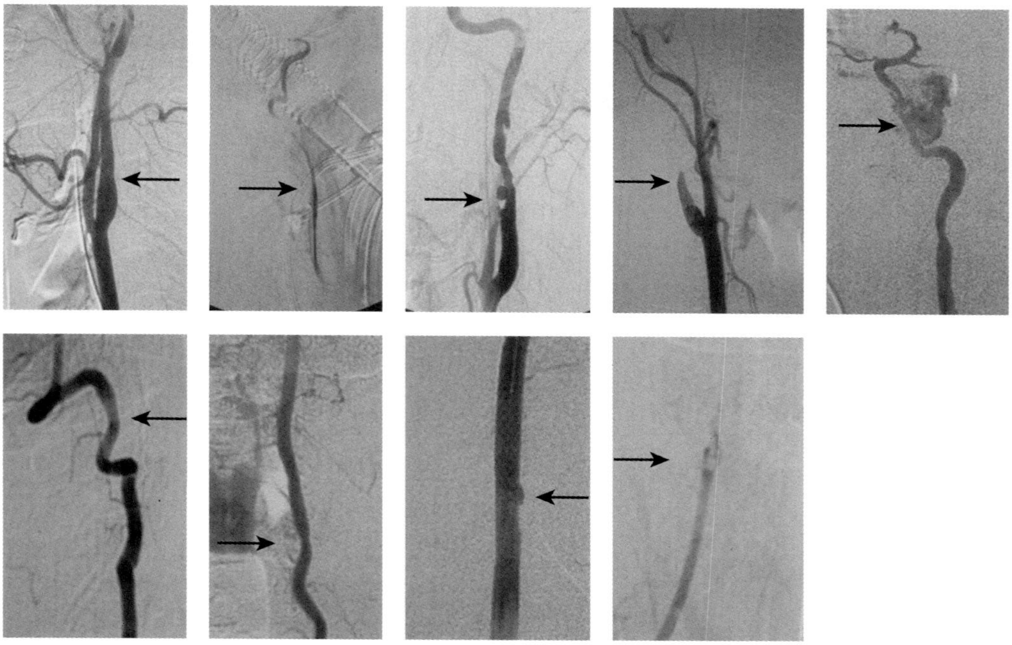

图2　钝性脑血管损伤不同分级的典型血管造影图像。箭头表示受伤区域

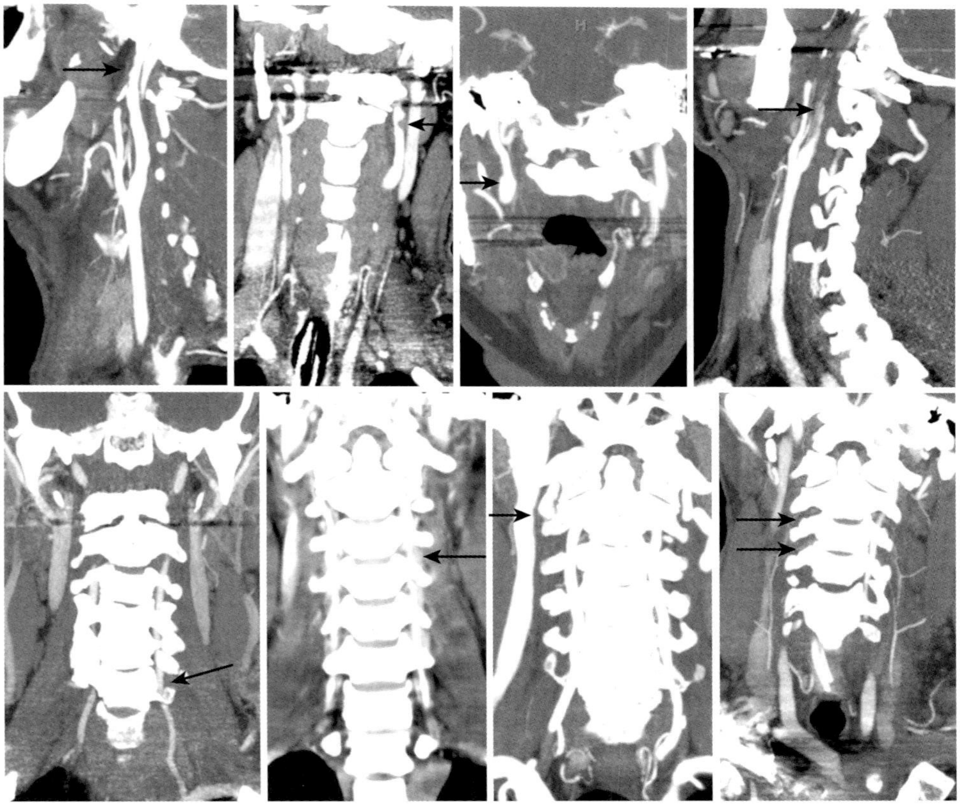

图3　钝性脑血管损伤不同分级的典型 CTA 影像。箭头表示受伤区域

表 2 钝性脑血管损伤丹佛分级量表

Ⅰ级	血管壁不规则或夹层 / 壁间血肿伴管腔狭窄低于 25%
Ⅱ级	管腔内有血栓或可见内膜片抬起，或夹层 / 壁间血肿伴管腔狭窄大于 25%
Ⅲ级	假性动脉瘤
Ⅳ级	血管闭塞
Ⅴ级	血管横断

出自丹佛健康医疗中心

表 3 不同级别钝性脑血管损伤的卒中发生比例

损伤部位	损伤级别	卒中发生比例（%）
颈动脉损伤	Ⅰ	3
	Ⅱ	14
	Ⅲ	26
	Ⅳ	50
	Ⅴ	100
椎动脉损伤	Ⅰ	6
	Ⅱ	38
	Ⅲ	27
	Ⅳ	28
	Ⅴ	100

损伤，而非是颈动脉损伤继发的栓塞性卒中。因此，BCVI 被认为非常罕见，在文献报道的创伤住院患者中发生率不足 0.1%，而钝性 CAI 在外伤性颈动脉损伤中的发生率不足 3%。当学界认识到患者的神经功能改变是源于血管的，并且有了鉴别血管损伤的影像学证据支持时，BCVI 的发病率升高了 2 倍。西部创伤协会主导了第一个多中心的 BCVI 综述，在超过 6 年的时间中，11 个主要创伤中心，只有 49 名 CAI 患者被诊断。BCVI 会显著提高卒中相关的发病率和死亡率，并往往通过一个“沉默期”来识别。具体来说，约一半的患者在受伤后 12 h 后才会出现症状，而这显然是一个宝贵的治疗时机。如果在筛查无症状高风险的患者时发现广泛的损伤，往往意味着明确的 BCVI。目前，在一些有综合筛查能力的中心，高风险患者的筛查量超过 30%。在最近的超过 8.5 年的中心回顾中，0.1% 的钝性损伤患者会出现神经系统症状，且 4% 的患者接受了筛查。其中 34% 诊断为 BCVI，占所有钝性创伤住院患者的 1.5%。

抗血栓治疗

在认识到 BCVI 与患者的神经系统不良事件密切相关后，如何治疗成为一个有争议的问题。如果损伤发生在外科手术可及的颈动脉部位，尤其是颈总动脉，则首选手术治疗（图 4）。然而，绝大多数的 BCVI 发生在手术难度较大的或在无法接近的血管的区域，如靠近颅底的颈动脉管内或横突孔（图 5）。这些部位使得常规血管修复方式（如重建或取栓）变得极富挑战，即使可以实现但也困难重重。肝素可以通过内源性纤溶机制稳定并溶解血块，防止血栓进一步形成，这是最初治疗 BCVI 的主要方式。抗凝治疗被证实可以改善疑似 BCVI 相关的 INE 患者的神经学预后。在包括西部创伤协会的多中心研究等早期的研究中，抗凝治疗组与没有治疗或因禁忌证无法接受抗凝治疗的患者相比，临床结局明显有改善。在这些研究中，高达 45% 的患者神经功能恢复到良好的水平，因此抗凝治疗是改善神经系统结局和提高生存率的独立因素。

随后，静脉注射肝素成为了治疗钝性损伤后无症状患者的治疗选项。起初采用的是标准化肝素治疗方案，但由于多系统创伤的患者有一定的出血风险，肝素治疗方案进行了相应的调整（图 6）。目前，全身肝素抗凝方案采用静脉持续输注肝素 15 U/(kg · h)，无负荷量。肝素滴定至部分促凝血酶原时间达到 40 ~ 50 s。根据我们的经验，调整后的肝素治疗方案中只有不到 1% 的患者会有出血并发症，需要输血。对于肝素禁忌的患者，可以给予抗血小板药物（阿司匹林 325 mg/d）。对于闭合性头部损伤或者脑实质出血的患者，需要神经外科同意才可以开始抗血栓治疗。对于有明确的脏器损伤或复杂骨盆骨折合并腹膜后血肿的患者，必须在生理功能稳定且没有输血需要的 24 h 后才可以开始抗血栓治疗。

目前，对于各种类型动脉疾病的理想抗血栓治疗方案仍有争议，主要集中在抗凝药物与抗血小板药物的比较上。Chimowitz 等的回顾性研究表明，在椎 - 基底动脉闭塞的患者中，华法林具有优势。但同样也是这个研究团队最近发表的，一项前瞻性双盲对比研究中显示，在有症状的脑血管动脉粥样硬化导致动脉狭窄的患者中，阿司匹林是治疗首选。这是因为阿司匹林与华法林相比，预防卒中的疗效相当，且可以减少出血并发症。最新的一项对椎 - 基底动脉疾病的回顾研究表明，抗血小板药物更适

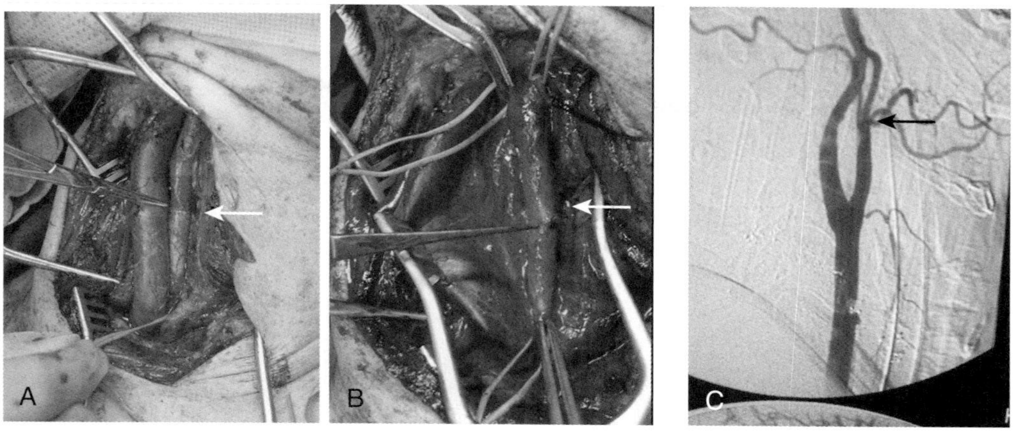

图 4　颈总动脉假性动脉瘤血管造影后手术入路（A）诊断；识别损伤（B）随后一期端端吻合修复（C）

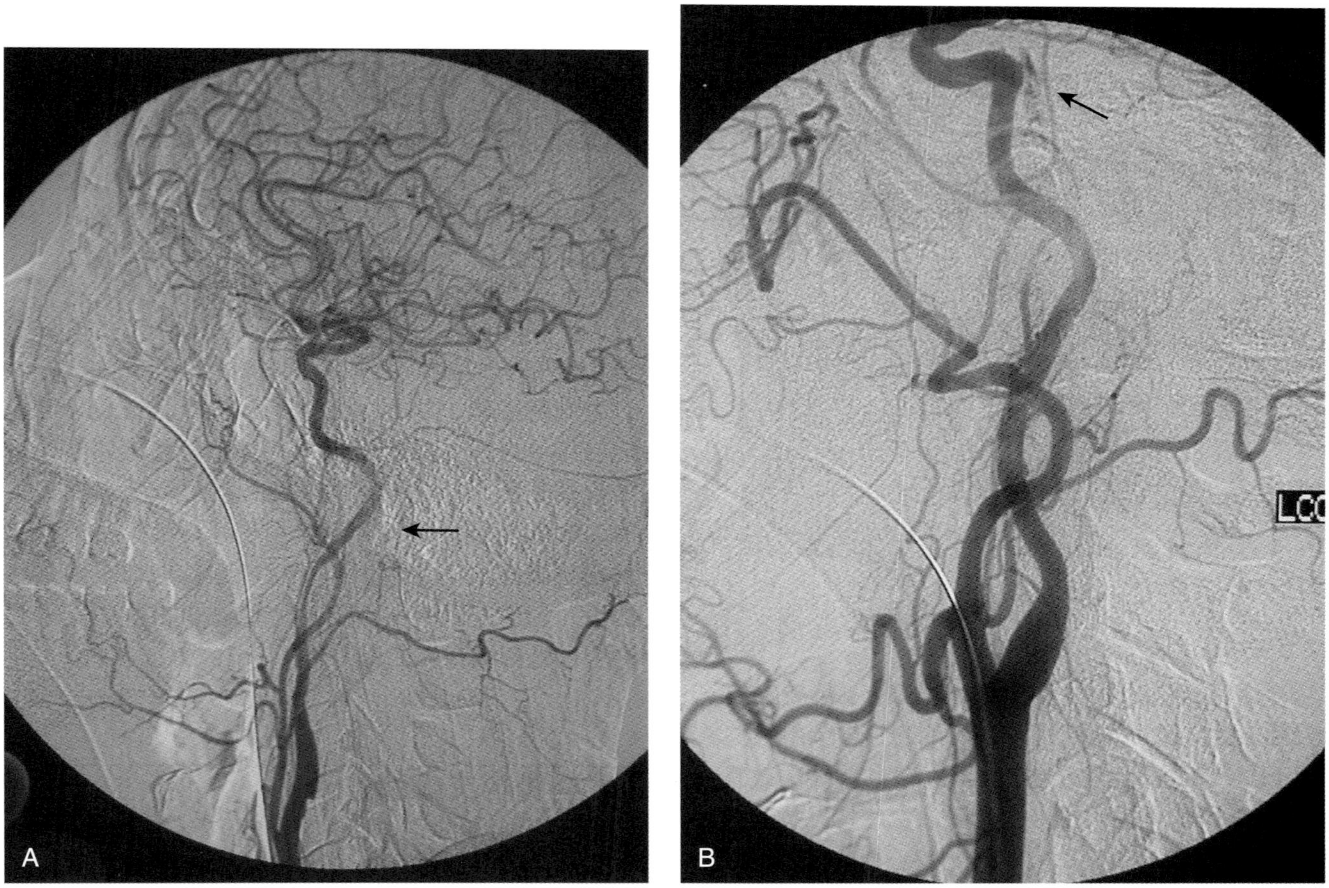

图 5　外科手术操作难度极大或无法到达的损伤，包括颅底的颈动脉损伤（A 和 B）

（续）

合应用于动脉狭窄的患者中，而华法林更适合于严重的、限流性病变或夹层的患者。由于使用简便，抗血小板药物在治疗 BCVI 时更受青睐。虽然最佳抗血栓方案仍有争议，但抗凝治疗和抗血小板治疗对于预防卒中和单个损伤治愈 / 改善率上有着同等的价值。我们的团队主张在急性期的患者中使用静脉注射肝素，且在出院时过渡为抗血小板药物。在出血并发症中，华法林的作用更容易被 FFP 逆转。使用什么样的治疗方式，是否应根据患者的损伤分级来选择抗血栓药物，这些必须在前瞻性研究中

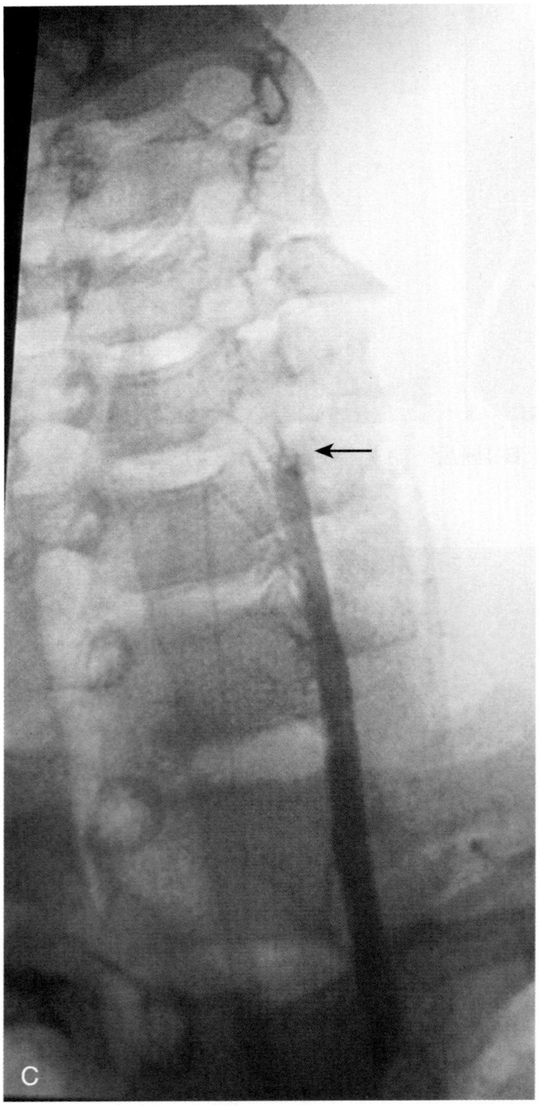

图 5 续 .C. 横突孔内的椎动脉损伤

继续评估。未来血栓弹力图（thromboelastography，TEG）的应用可能将帮助患者制订最佳的治疗方案。由于个体对抗血小板治疗的反应存在差异，改良后的 TEG 和血小板地图将成为评估治疗情况的有效手段。

最重要的是，早期诊断 BCVI 的患者中除 INE 接受抗血栓治疗是普遍的。Memphis 团队的研究表明，未治疗的 CAI 患者卒中风险高达 64%，而在接受抗血栓治疗（抗凝或抗血小板药物）后卒中风险降至 6.8%；同样，VAI 的患者治疗后卒中风险从 54% 降至 2.6%。我们团队最新的研究表明，在 282 名 BCVI 患者中，接受抗血栓治疗的患者卒中发生率为 0.3%，而未治疗患者整体卒中发生率达 21%。虽然最佳抗血栓方案仍有争议，但 2 种治疗（抗凝和抗

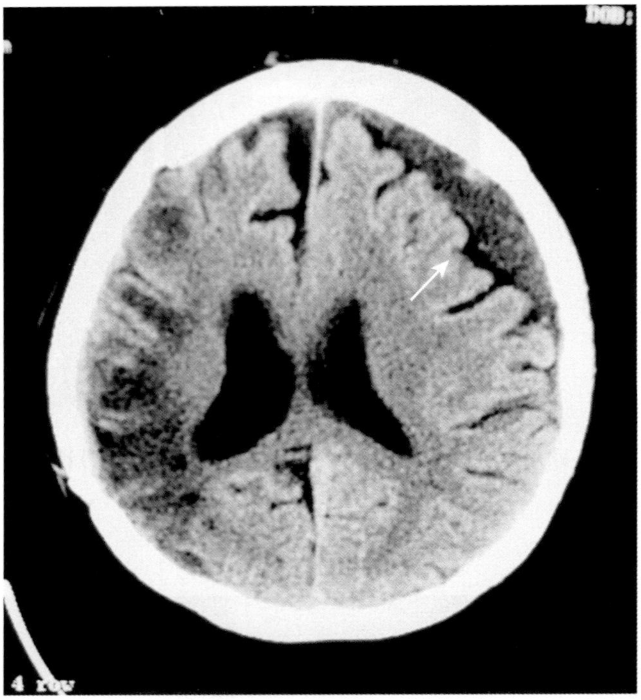

图 6 一例钝性脑血管损伤患者肝素化后出现颅内出血并发症（箭头）

血小板）对于预防卒中有着同等的价值。

根据经验，在再内皮化的假设上，抗血栓治疗应持续 6 个月。虽然根据 7 ~ 10 天复查影像学检查的数据显示，超过一半的 Ⅰ 级损伤可以痊愈，但绝大多数的 Ⅱ 级、Ⅲ 级和Ⅳ级损伤是持续性的。由于目前仍缺乏关于急性期住院患者的长期综合随访数据以及创伤人群调查研究，这些损伤在 3 ~ 6 个月内愈合还是持续存在，尚未可知。

血管内支架的作用

从 21 世纪开始，在外伤性损伤和动脉粥样硬化病变的治疗中，经皮穿刺血管内介入治疗有了巨大的发展。虽然颈动脉支架在治疗动脉粥样硬化疾病中的作用已有随机对照试验研究，但介入治疗外伤性损伤的证据较为不明确。考虑到继发栓塞或者破裂的危险，颈动脉支架已被应用于治疗钝性损伤并发的持久的假性动脉瘤。理论上，颈动脉裸支架可以起到类似过滤器的作用，捕捉假性动脉瘤内的血栓，从而预防栓塞和卒中。支架也可以通过增加颈动脉内支架本身中的层流来减少进入假性动脉瘤内

的血流。减少进入动脉瘤囊内的血流可能会减少囊内血液的排出，从而减少管腔内的湍流。目前有关于颈动脉假性动脉瘤破裂的文献报道，特别是颈动脉管的坚硬部分导致的鼻出血，但是我们没有观察到这一事件。然而，除了个别病例外，文献中还没有其他晚期事件的报道。因此，目前很难证实这些损伤的真实愈合率或者破裂风险或者是否存在迟发的栓塞性卒中。

一些研究主张使用经皮血管成形术和支架术治疗颈动脉损伤。虽然大多数人在随访的放射影像学评估中显示颈动脉支架通畅，但也有一些关于支架植入后颈动脉闭塞的病例报道。在一项对于血管腔内修复的早期评估中表明，急性血管损伤的患者，在常规使用脑保护装置和抗血小板治疗之前，明显的卒中和颈动脉支架内堵塞率与颈内支架放置有关。由于缺乏创伤性假性动脉瘤患者单纯接受抗血栓药物治疗的长期随访数据，很难判断支架和药物处理这两种方案哪个更理想。我们最新的关于血管腔内修复与抗血栓治疗的对比评估显示，抗血栓治疗BCVI可以更有效地预防卒中。常规支架植入术不仅增加经济费用，还有潜在的卒中风险，而且并没有增加获益。在我们的临床实践中，仅建议对有症状的血管狭窄或假性动脉瘤明显扩大的患者使用血管内支架。

长期随访和预后

以目前经验，抗血栓治疗在开始后应持续6个月。6个月内应重复评估患者的损伤并确定抗血栓治疗方案。虽然尚缺乏长期研究数据，目前我们建议使用多排CTA进行长期随访。在复查影像检查时发现有持续性损伤的患者通常须终身服用阿司匹林并长期接受治疗，应使患者充分知晓其中风险。

关于BCVI相关INE的并发症率和死亡率，有较多数据。从既往来看，BCVI患者卒中相关的永久性神经系统并发症发生率大于80%，且相关死亡率为40%。在现代的系列文献报道中，BCVI相关的并发症率有所下降，但死亡率依然很显著。其中CAI患者卒中相关的死亡率为13%～21%，VAI患者卒中相关死亡率为4%～18%。关于神经系统疾病并发症发生率是否会影响急性期患者长期护理需求的研究较缺乏。我们的研究指出BCVI相关的INE患者有更高的院外康复率。这种长期的急性患者照护增加了患者、保险公司乃至整个社会的经济负担。对于多系统创伤的患者而言，计算分析BCVI相关的医疗花费是很困难的，然而，对于患者生活成本的分析更为困难。在我们的一系列研究中发现，在CAI患者中，无神经系统事件的患者死亡率为7%，而发生神经系统事件的患者死亡率为32%。在VAI患者中，无神经系统事件的患者死亡率为7%，而发生神经系统事件的患者死亡率为18%。由于损伤严重度评分中有无INE的患者之间没有显著差异，因此对BCVI相关卒中死亡率的影响似乎和患者的相关损伤无关。

总结

在过去的30年中，学界始终致力于诊断和治疗BCVI的研究，但从20世纪80年代开始才取得了突破性的进展。早期认为BCVI是一个罕见疾病，而如今在钝性创伤入院的患者中诊断率约1%。临床沉默期为损伤筛查提供了可能性，可以根据创伤机制和患者的一系列损伤进行筛查。目前，根据筛查方案，应对高风险损伤的患者进行适当的影像学检查（图7）。患者综合评估有利于在无症状期时早期诊断BCVI，从而及时开始治疗。虽然抗血栓治疗的理想方案仍有争议，但不论是抗凝治疗还是抗血小板治疗都可以降低BCVI相关的卒中风险。BCVI是一种少见的但具有潜在破坏性的损伤。高风险患者应进行适当的筛查并及时治疗，以防止发生INE。

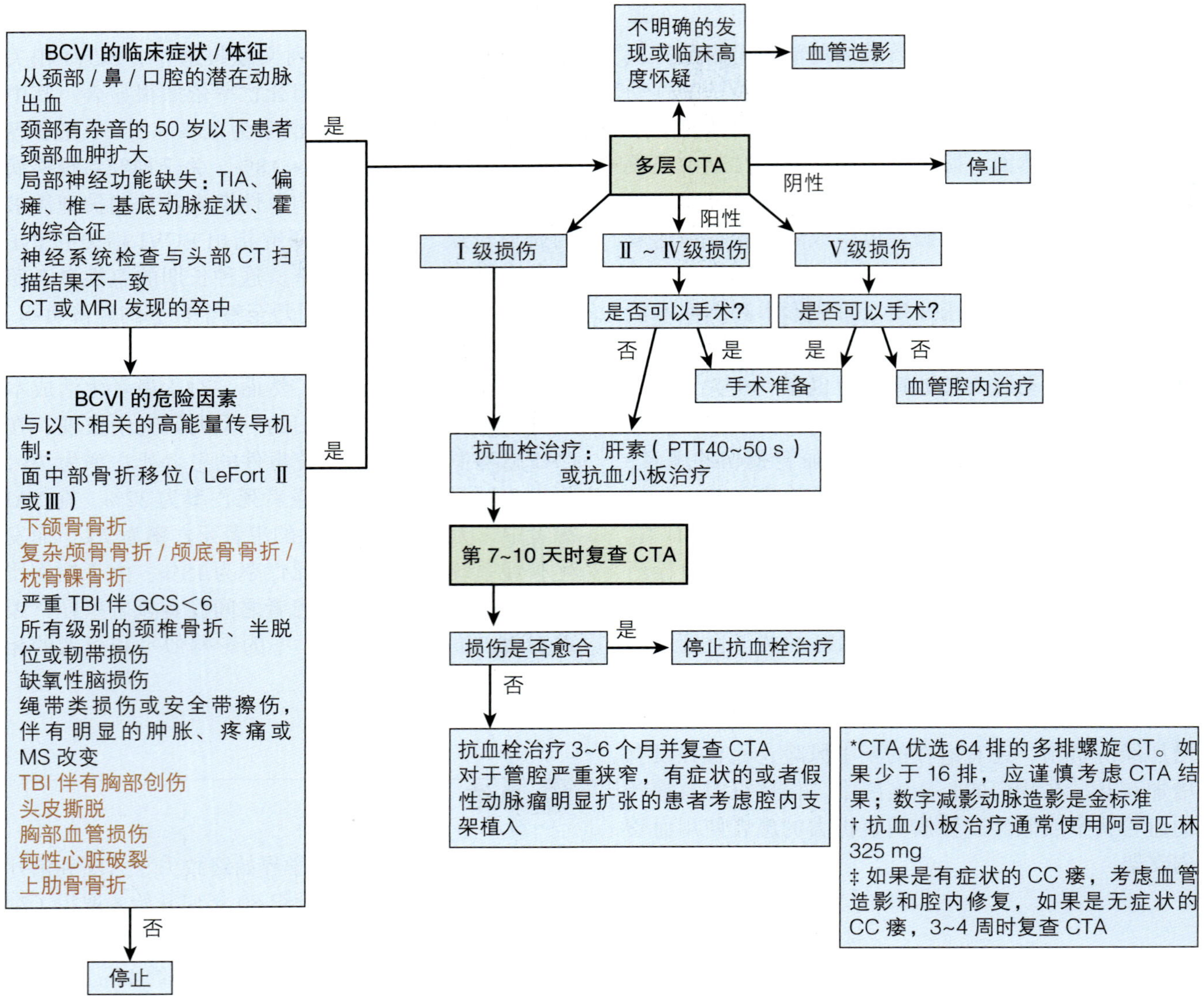

图 7　丹佛健康医学中心的当前 BCVI 筛查流程图。BCVI, 脑血管钝性损伤；CHI 闭合性头部损伤；CT，计算机断层扫描；CTA，计算机断层扫描血管造影；DAI，弥漫性轴突损伤；GCS，格拉斯哥昏迷等级评分；MRI，磁共振成像；MS，精神状态；TBI，创伤性脑损伤，TIA，短暂性脑缺血发作；PTT，部分促凝血酶原时间 *(Courtesy of Denver Health Medical Center.)*

气管、喉和口咽部损伤

Luis G. Fernández, Scott H. Norwood 和 John D. Berne 著

张立红 译 曹　杰　王文伦 校对

上气道具有弹性和可活动性的结构特点，因此其损伤并不多见。前方的下颌骨、胸骨和后方的脊柱的骨性结构也为其提供了保护（图 1）。在大型创伤救治中心的患者中，上气道损伤的患者仅占 0.03%。但这些损伤通常是致命的，这就解释了为何死亡患者的尸检中往往会发现上气道损伤。穿通性损伤往往比钝性损伤更为常见，但二者的发病率目前尚无报道。据统计，21% 的上气道损伤患者在入院后的 2 h 内死亡。非致命性的上气道损伤的诊断常常会有延迟，而这种延迟可能会导致后期的并发症。由于对上气道损伤的手术治疗和非手术治疗的经验往往有限，针对各种不同临床情景的一系列指南也应运而生。对于不稳定的、可立即危及生命的上气道损伤，当机立断地采用任何有效的气道控制措施对于维持患者的生存至关重要。大多数学者认为经

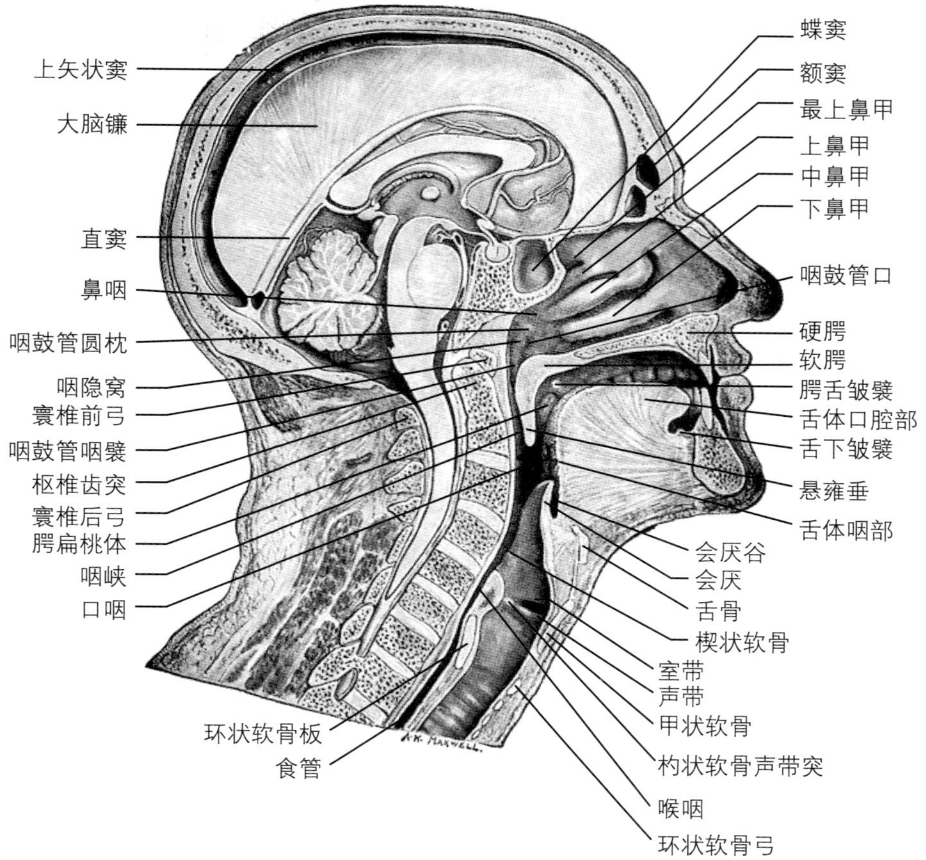

图 1 **A**，头颈部正中矢状位切面

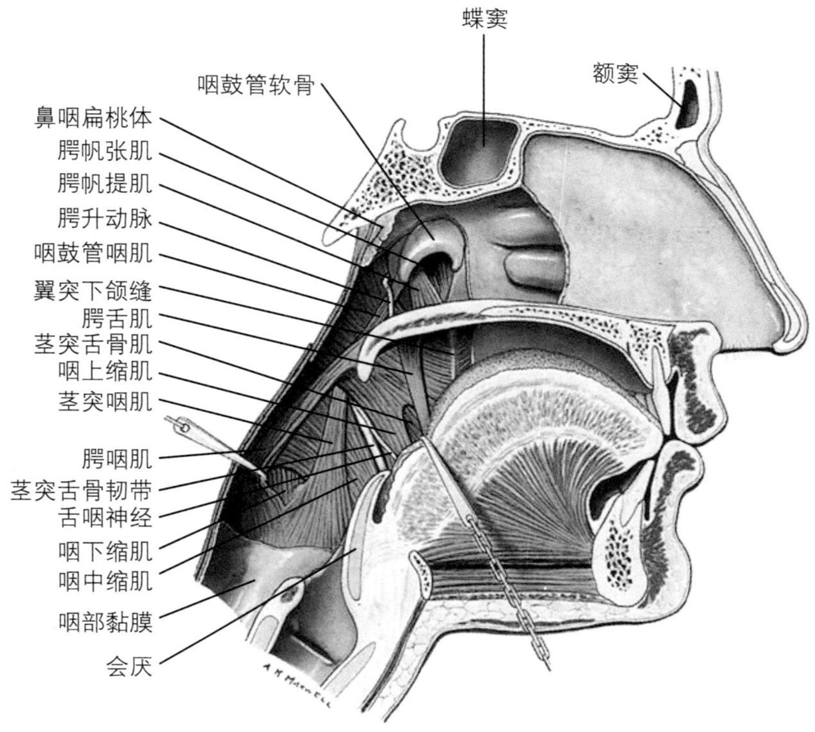

图 1 **B**，头部正中矢状位切面，移去黏膜后显示下咽的解剖（*Gray's anatomy, 39th ed. St. Louis, 2004, Churchill Livingstone, Figs. 35.1 and 35.3.*）

伤口气管插管是一种有效的方法。病情稳定的患者最好在支气管镜的引导下从创伤的远端行气管插管。除非万不得已，尽量不要盲插。上气道损伤即使是对于最有经验的外科医生来说仍然是具有挑战性的，因为此时往往存在着传统气道管理措施的禁忌证。

上气道的解剖

口腔

口腔的主要生理功能是发声和咀嚼，它同时也是上气道系统的一个替代性通道（代替鼻咽）。

边界

前界——口唇
后界——前扁桃体的支柱
顶——硬腭和软腭
底——舌下腺和颌下腺上覆的口底黏膜
侧壁——颊黏膜

内容物

牙槽突和牙齿
舌尖至轮廓乳头的舌体部分
腮腺导管（Stenson 管）开口，正对上颌第二上磨牙的颊黏膜
颌下腺导管（Wharton 管）开口，在口底前部
舌下腺导管开口

咽

外科解剖

咽部包括以下部分：

鼻咽：自后鼻孔至软腭游离缘，后与颅底相连。鼻咽部有腺样体组织和咽鼓管咽口。这一区域无法在直视下观察，须借助鼻咽镜或光学器械才能看到。

口咽：可以经口直接观察。口咽部自软腭至会厌。咽后壁和咽侧壁由咽上缩肌和咽中缩肌构成。

腭扁桃体：淋巴组织在腭咽肌和腭舌肌之间的黏膜皱襞内聚集而成。腭扁桃体被覆复层扁平上皮、上皮延伸至扁桃体隐窝内。腭扁桃体大小不一，可带蒂或者固定。

下咽：会厌上缘以下的咽部。下咽后壁和侧壁由咽中缩肌和咽下缩肌构成。向下延伸至环咽肌，与颈段食管相延续。前方由会厌延伸而来，包含会厌和喉部。喉部两侧的袋状结构是梨状隐窝，其内侧壁由喉的侧壁构成。下咽后壁包括咽后壁和环后区的黏膜（图 2-4）。

咽部损伤

发病率

单发的钝性咽部损伤极其罕见，往往合并有颈部和头面部创伤。穿通性咽部损伤更常见于儿童，系经口吞食异物导致的撕裂。

损伤机制

咽部损伤常由于吞咽异物、钝性损伤或穿通性损伤，以及喉镜或其他内镜操作所致。

诊断

损伤初期的临床表现多种多样。非致命性损伤一般表现为吞咽困难和吞咽疼痛。更严重的损伤可表现为失声、呼吸困难、咯血、严重的急性呼吸衰

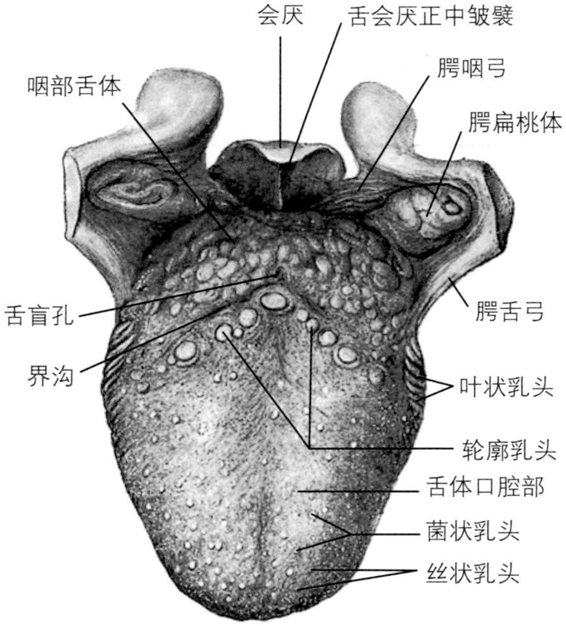

图 2　口咽部结构（*From Gray's anatomy, 39th ed. St. Louis, 2004, Churchill Livingstone, Fig. 33.4.*）

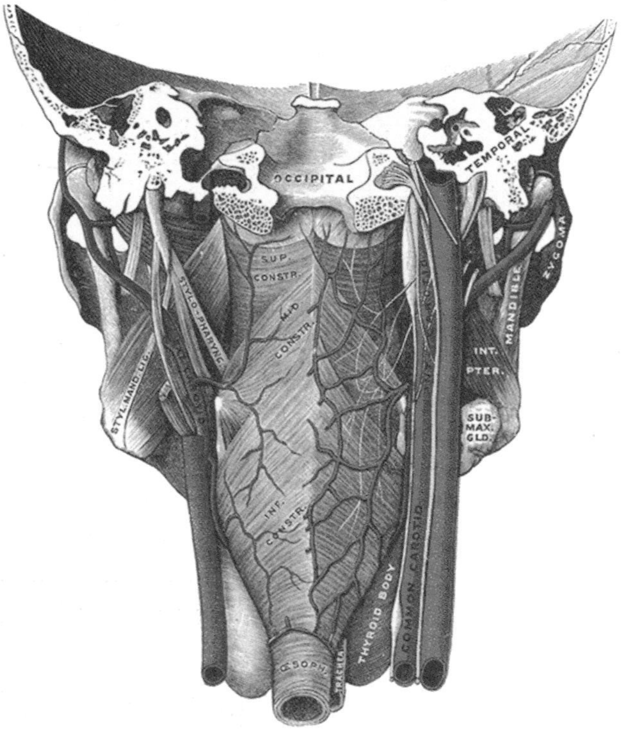

图 3　咽部的肌肉和血供。咽部的肌肉、相关的血管和神经后面观（*Modified from Gray H: Anatomy of the human body. Philadelphia, 1918, Lea & Febiger. Available at www.bartleby.com/107/.*）

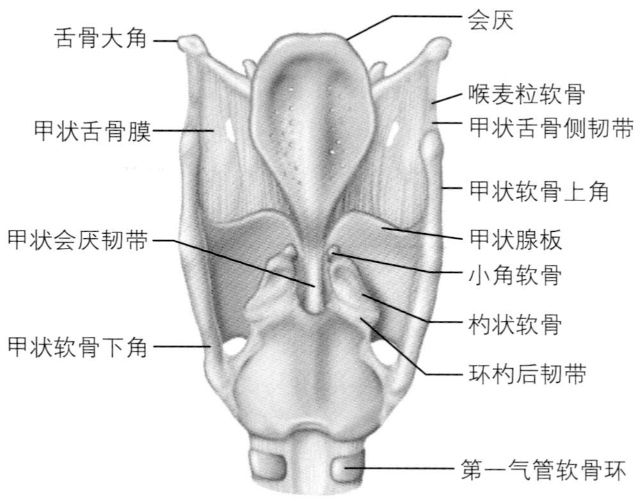

图 4　喉部软骨和韧带后面观（*From Gray's anatomy, 39th ed. St. Louis, 2004, Churchill Livingstone, Fig. 36.3.*）

竭，如果不治疗可迅速引起至窒息。食管和咽部的损伤诊断较为困难，而且常常因为过于关注其他危及生命的损伤而被遗漏。口腔出血、流涎以及皮下气肿都提示着存在上消化道或气道损伤。如果情况允许，应当尽可能在床旁对口咽和下咽进行详尽的检查。

软组织积气可经由颈部侧位平片或 CT 扫描观察到（图 5-6）。如果临床怀疑食管损伤，可以行非离子造影剂食管对比检查或食管镜检查。食管造影的造影剂漏出往往提示着损伤存在（图 5）。

喉

外科解剖

喉是一个将气管与上呼吸消化道分开的功能性“活瓣”。它首先是一个用来言语交流的器官（喉头），其次也有着重要的呼吸调节功能。喉部的存在对于完成有效的咳嗽和 Valsalva 动作（屏气）必不可少。此外，它还能在吞咽时防止误吸。

喉部包括以下组成部分：

骨性成分（图 7）

舌骨：与会厌和带状肌相连。

甲状软骨：前部有声带附着，后部与环状软骨形成关节。

环状软骨：一个完整的环形结构。与甲状软骨和杓状软骨形成关节。

杓状软骨：可以沿环状软骨后面滑动的成对软骨，附于声带的后缘上。

分区

声门上区：覆有含大量黏液腺的呼吸道上皮。

会厌：叶状黏膜附在软骨上，由喉部向上伸出。

杓会厌襞：自会厌侧缘连向杓状软骨。

假声带：真声门上方的黏膜皱襞，与真声带之间有喉室相隔。

喉室：内覆黏膜的囊结构，大小各异，将声门区与声门上区分隔。

声门区：真声带的前联合附着于甲状软骨板交角的面，后联合附着于杓状软骨，可以活动。声带的内收和外展依靠杓状软骨的运动完成。声带的主体由声带肌上覆黏膜构成。声带的游离缘覆有复层鳞状上皮。吸气时声带外展，发声、咳嗽和 Valsalva 动作时声带内收。

声门下区：位于声带下方，下至环状软骨下缘。

神经支配——来自迷走神经的分支

喉上神经：感觉支（内支）支配声门及声门上区的感觉，运动支（外支）支配环甲肌的运动，其收缩

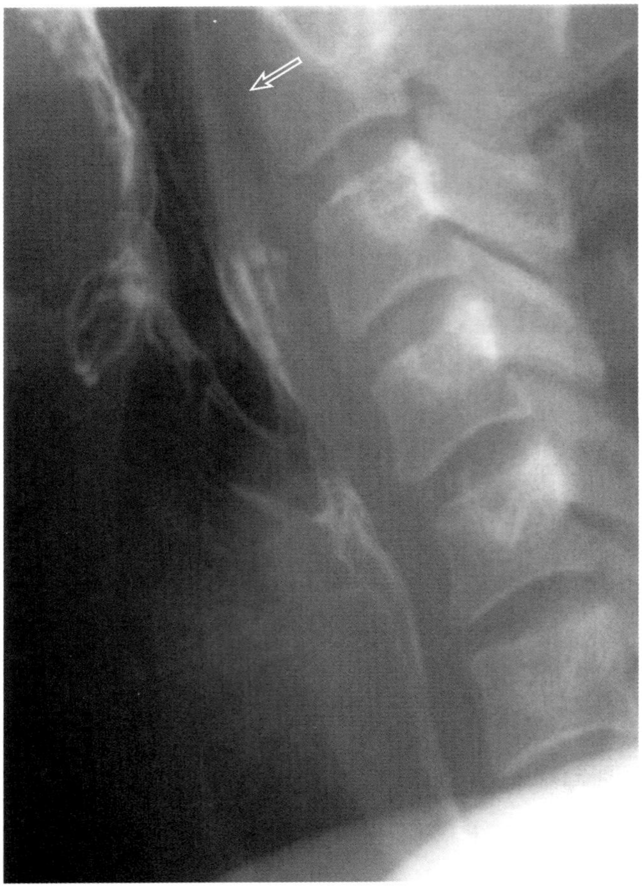

图 5　颈椎侧位片 / 食管成像显示咽后组织积气（箭头所示）

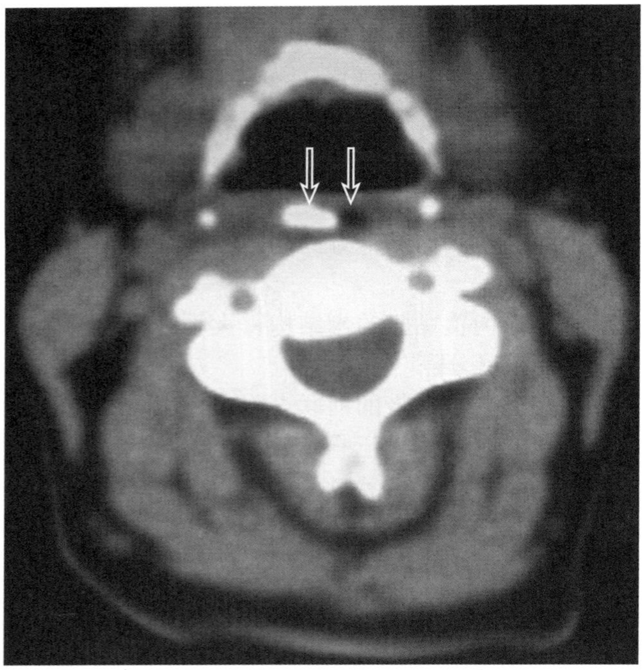

图 6　颈部 CT 扫描示咽后组织积气（箭头所示）

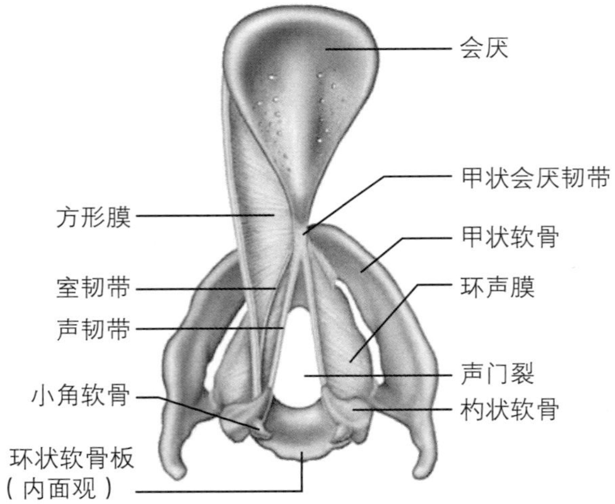

图 7　喉部的环甲软骨方形膜、相关的韧带及膜上面观
（From Gray's anatomy, 39th ed, St. Louis, 2004, Churchill Livingstone, Fig. 36.7.）

时使声带紧张，由迷走神经在颈部高位发出。

喉返神经：感觉支配声门以下的感觉，运动支支配喉内肌的运动。由迷走神经在纵隔内发出，左侧绕行主动脉弓，右侧绕行锁骨下动脉，然后返回颈部。

喉部损伤

发病率

喉部损伤和颈段气管损伤是少见却棘手的疾病，未经合适的诊断和治疗可导致相当高的死亡率和并发症发生率。这类损伤的患者在各主要的创伤中心住院的创伤患者中比例低于 1%，在急诊就诊的患者中仅占 1/30 000。与头颈部的总体损伤相比，这类创伤相对罕见，因此诊疗经验也相对有限。喉部损伤患者相对罕见的原因有很多，一方面由于下颌骨和胸骨的保护作用使喉部不易受到损伤，另一方面全身多处严重创伤的患者常常由于忽视了其喉部的微小损伤造成漏诊，以及由于气道功能丧失或窒息所造成的患者受伤当场死亡等情况的存在，致使目前报道的喉部损伤发病率相对较低。

尽管发病率很低，喉部损伤的初次处理显著影响着患者的生存率和长期的生活质量。喉部是一个保护得很好的结构和功能很复杂的器官。钝性损伤和穿通性损伤都有可能会造成慢性的误吸、发声障碍或呼吸功能不全等问题。

损伤机制

喉部损伤的机制可以分为钝性损伤（包括撞击伤、晾衣绳损伤和勒伤等）和穿通性损伤。喉气管损伤的部位和程度往往是多方面的。Sheely 等发现 88% 的喉部损伤发生在第 4 气管环水平以上。穿通性损伤可以发生在颈部任何水平。

诊断

喉部损伤的患者应当依据 ALTS 进行初步评估。评估患者的 ABCs（气道、呼吸、循环）并采取相应的复苏方法、完善后续的检查对于气道损伤患者的处理至关重要。对损伤机制的质疑和对颈部、胸部细致的体格检查有助于早期识别喉部损伤的患者。相应的临床症状和体征包括喉喘鸣、急性呼吸窘迫、颈部触痛、皮下气肿以及大血管损伤所致的颈部血肿等。咯血通常提示着喉内损伤的可能。这些临床表现常见于穿通性损伤，但也可见于钝性损伤致喉部软骨骨折的情况。如果患者的情况允许，应当尽可能采取合适的检查手段如直接喉镜、纤维支气管镜、颈部多排螺旋 CTA 增强扫描（最低 16 排，64 排以上最佳）等明确诊断。图 8 示一个喉部损伤评估的流程图，可供参考。

治疗

近期的一项对 12 名喉部损伤患者的研究报道，50% 的患者（6 名）接受了非手术治疗。这些患者的喉部骨折均不伴有移位，他们被给予了流食、院内观察、静脉应用地塞米松 10mg Q8h 等治疗。所有患者在治疗后都恢复了正常的发声功能。伴有移位的骨折或粉碎性骨折须行手术治疗，而且一期骨折复位比延迟修复有着更好的功能恢复。喉部损伤的严重程度可以根据 Schaefer-Fuhrman 喉部损伤分级量表[NR1，NR2]来进行分级，这种分级有助于制订后续治疗方案（表 1）。

气管

外科解剖

气管是由软骨和黏膜组成的管状结构。它由喉部向下延续，自第 6 颈椎水平延伸至第 5 胸椎椎体上缘，然后分为左右两个主支气管。气管是一个椭圆形的管状结构，后面相对扁平。成年人气管平均长约 11 cm，直径约 2～2.5 cm。儿童的气管相对较短，位置较深，活动度更高。气管一半位于颈部，一半位于胸腔内。气管的上 2/3 由 18～22 个 U 型的软骨环构成。膜性的气管后壁与食管前壁并列。主气管分叉处在第 4 至第 5 胸椎水平形成气管隆嵴。气管由甲状腺下动脉供血。同名静脉参与构成甲状腺静脉丛。气管的神经起自迷走神经、喉返神经和交感神经链。喉返神经走行气管食管邻近的侧面构成的气管食管沟内，它是由邻近的侧面食管和气管构成的（图 9-11）。

气管损伤

发生率

气管支气管树断裂的情况相当罕见，大多数外科医生对此经验有限。即使是在大型的创伤救治中心，这种病例平均每年也只能见到 1 例。Bertelsen 和 Howitz 等回顾了 1 178 例创伤致死的患者的尸检报告，发现仅有 33 例（2.8%）患者伴有气管或支气管断裂。在这 33 例患者中，有 27 例当场死亡。

颈部气管完全横断的情况更加罕见。颈部横断伤（通常也包括气管支气管损伤）真实的发病率尚不明确。文献可查到有许多相关的个案报道和小型的综述，然而，现有的手术经验相当有限。

掌握气道管理相关的急救知识是必不可少的。在这种临床情景中，气道功能的丧失会迅速导致一系列的严重的并发症甚至患者的死亡。

对于受伤时气道功能仍有部分保存的患者，他们的死亡率取决于其他合并损伤的严重程度。对于能够坚持到进入创伤救治中心接受治疗的单独的气管支气管损伤（包括完全性的气管横断损伤）的患者，一个掌握了困难气道处理方法的创伤外科医生是完全有可能让他存活下来的。

Beskin 于 1957 年报道了第一例成功修复钝性创伤致颈部气管完全横断的病例。1959 年，Hood 和 Sloan 在全世界范围的文献中收集了 18 例气管支气管损伤的病例，发现完全性的气管横断“极其罕见”。近期，Ecker 等报道了一项对 105 例气管支气管的损伤病例的研究，其中 75 例由穿通性创伤所致，30 例由钝性创伤所致。其中仅有 24 例患者转入创伤救治中心时仍然存活。在 30 例遭受钝性创伤的患者中，有 18 例在到达救治中心前就已经死亡。不论何种损伤机制，大多数能够活着到达救治中心的患者，

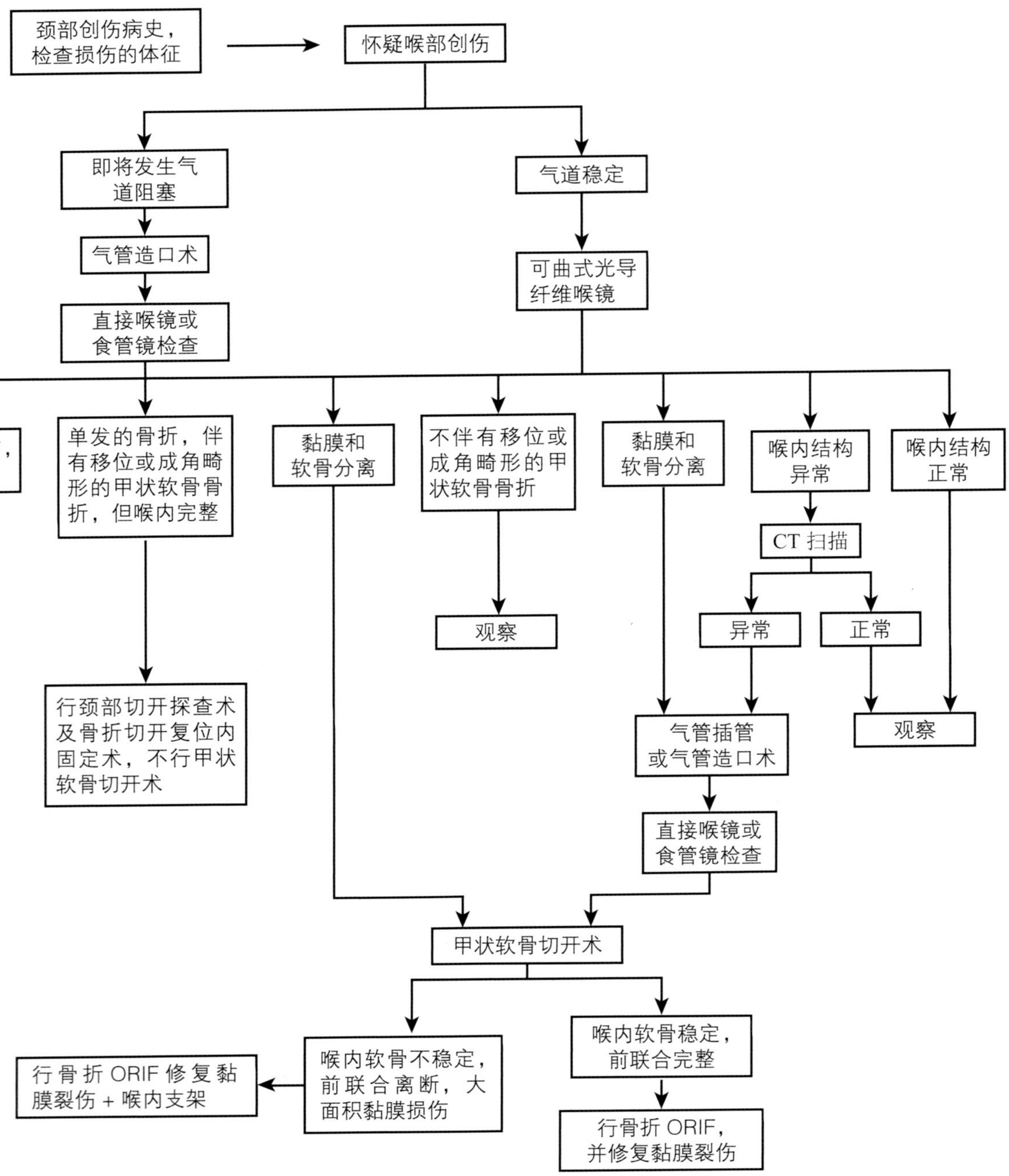

图 8 可疑喉部损伤患者的评估流程。CT：计算机断层扫描；ORIF：切开复位内固定术 *(Modified from Pancholi SS: Fractures, laryngeal. Louisa, KY, Three Rivers Medical Center, Department of Otolaryngology, November 3, 2005. Available at http://www.emedicine.com/ent/topic488.htm.)*

表 1 Schaefer-Fuhrman 喉部损伤分级 [NT1, NT2]

级别	损伤
Ⅰ级	轻微喉内血肿，不伴骨折
Ⅱ级	水肿、血肿、无软骨暴露的微小黏膜破裂，骨折不伴移位
Ⅲ级	广泛水肿、黏膜撕脱、软骨暴露、声带固定、骨折伴有移位
Ⅳ级	在Ⅲ级基础上有多于 2 处的骨折线或者广泛的喉黏膜创伤
Ⅴ级	喉气管完全分离

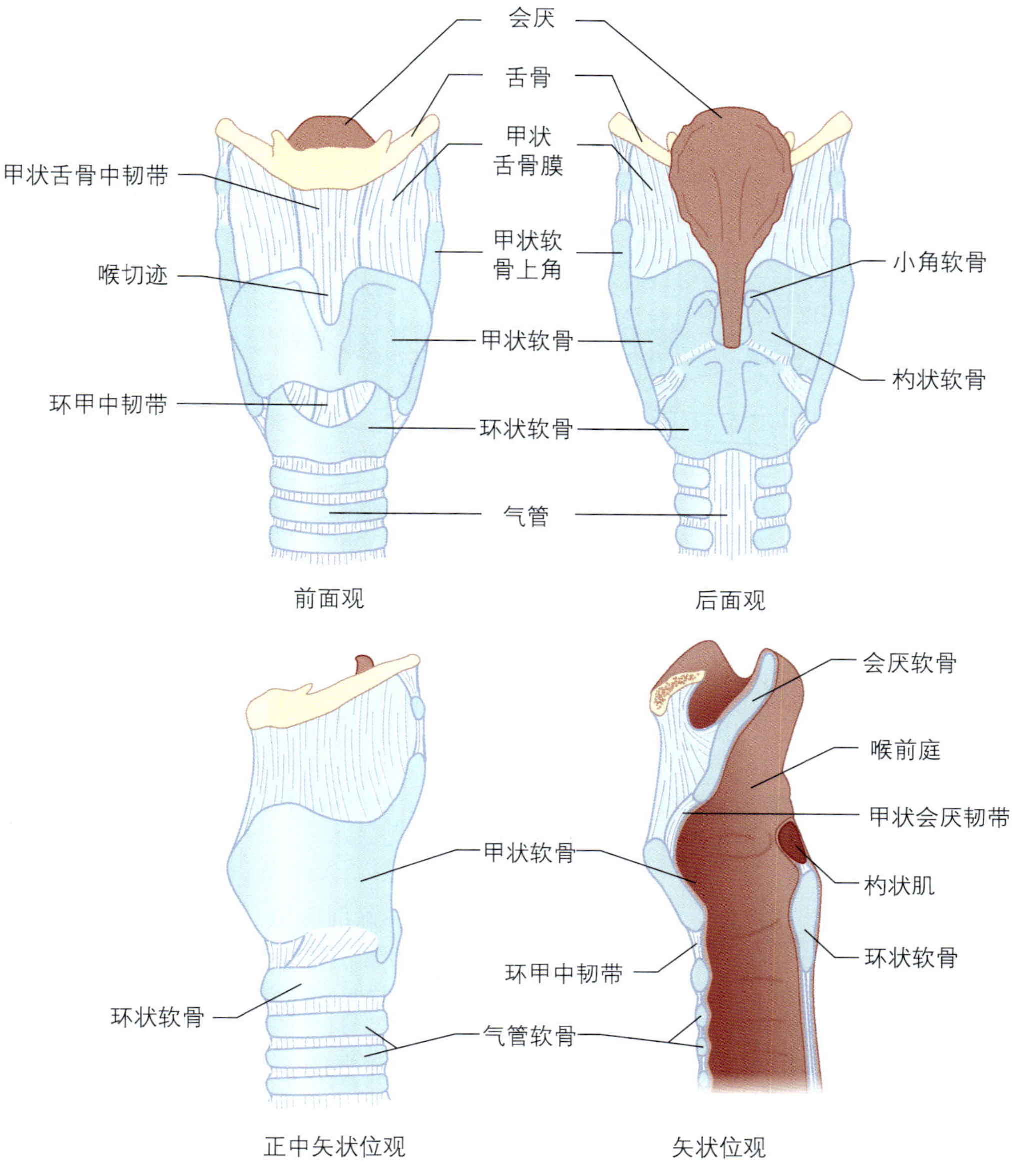

图 9 喉部解剖图示：前面观、后面观、正中矢状位观和矢状位观 *(From Miller RD, et al: Anesthesia for eye, ear, nose, and throat surgery. Miller's Anesthesia, ed 7, chapter 75, Philadelphia, 2010, Churchill Livingstone)*

没有合并其他的损伤 [15/24（63%）]，其余存活的患者也仅合并 1 处其他部位的损伤 [9/24（37%）]，包括食管损伤。这份研究报告同时显示，存活患者中最容易受伤的气管支气管树的节段是颈段气管（37%）。而气管完全横断的患者数量在 Ecker 等的研究中没有明确报道。

Kelly 等回顾了 106 例气管支气管损伤的病例，其中仅有 6 例由钝性损伤所致。他们认为，对于这类患者，外科医生采取迅速的、积极的手术措施才有可能挽救患者的生命。

损伤机制

颈段气管损伤

颈段气管损伤可由钝性损伤或穿通性损伤所致。穿通性损伤相对来说比较直接。除了弹片损伤外，这类损伤往往可以见到利器或子弹所致的组织缺损。刀伤常常位于颈段气管，而枪伤则可发生在气管支气管树的任何部位。

在一项回顾性研究中，颈段气管的钝性损伤在 1 248 名纳入研究的钝性损伤患者中仅占不足 1%。

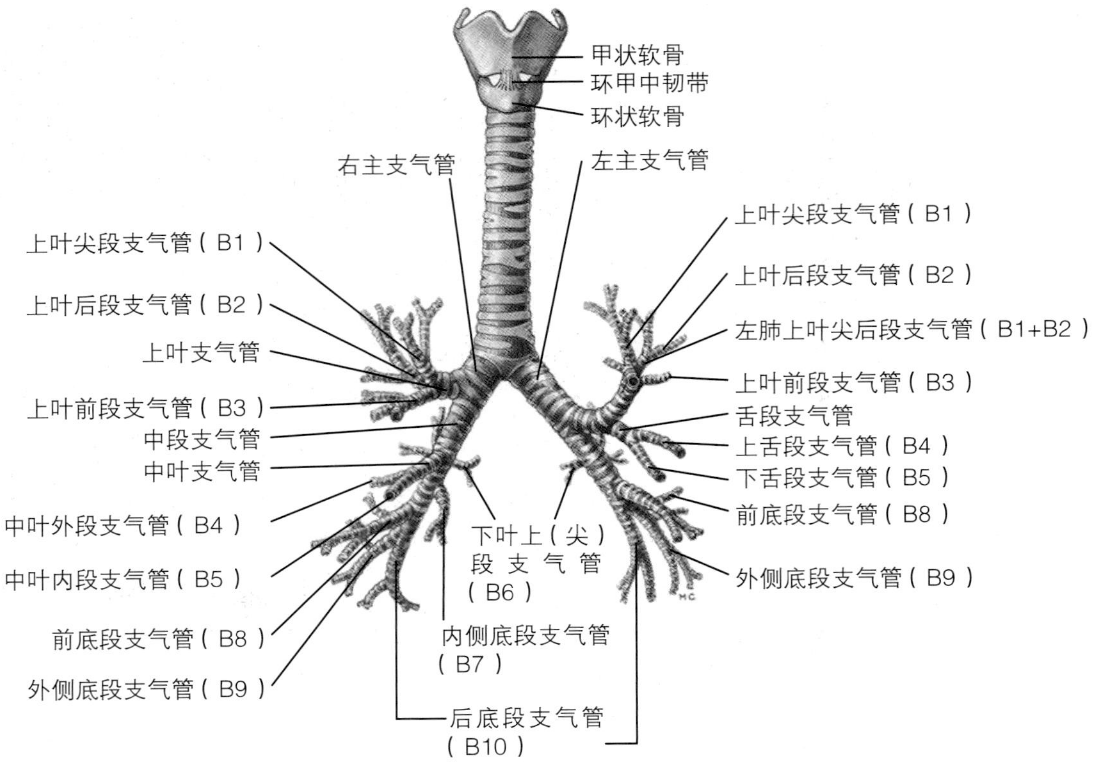

图 10　喉部的软骨，气管和支气管：前面观 *(From Gray's anatomy, 39th ed, St. Louis, 2004, Churchill Livingstone, Fig. 63.12.)*

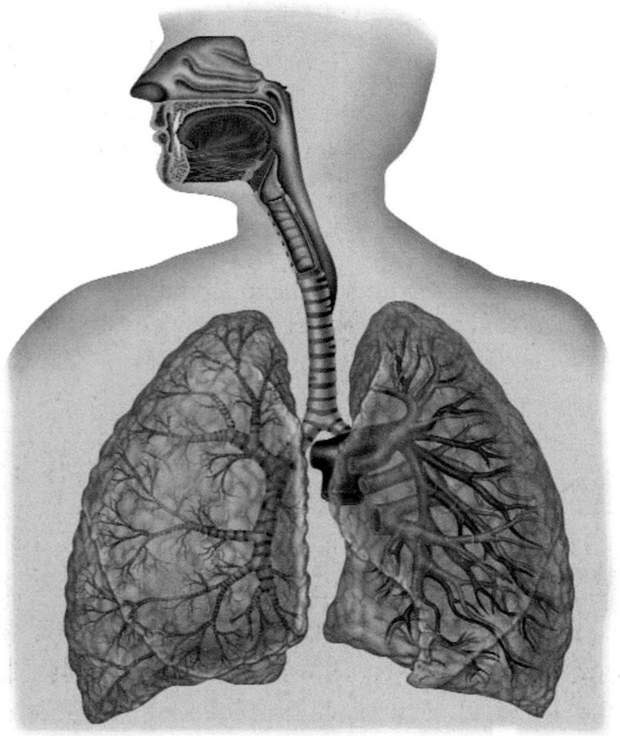

图 11　呼吸道。头部和上段颈部的呼吸道均以矢状位显示，下段颈部转向前方，其余的呼吸道部分均为前面观。右肺显示支气管树，左肺显示肺部血管 *(From Gray's anatomy, 39th ed, St. Louis, 2004, Churchill Livingstone, Fig. 63.1.)*

在这一解剖区域，喉部的钝性损伤往往更为常见。它们通常由机动车事故、运动损伤以及对该区域的直接冲击所致（例如，晾衣绳损伤）。

胸段气管损伤

这一区域的损伤更常见于钝性创伤，但也可见于穿通性损伤。对于前者，具体的损伤机制目前尚不明确，不过目前提出了几项假说。这种损伤往往是由于胸部突然受到强力的压迫所致。假说认为，在声门闭合的情况下，胸腔受到突然的前后方向的压力作用会造成管腔内压力短时间内显著升高。当剪切力作用于相对固定的环状软骨和气管隆嵴之间的气管支气管树时（发生在急剧减速过程中），气管破裂就有可能发生。胸内的气管断裂通常发生在距离气管隆嵴 2 cm 以内的膜性气管与软骨性气管交界处。垂直方向的损伤很罕见，它们通常发生在软骨结构不明显的气管后部。支气管损伤常常发生在距离气管隆嵴 2.5 cm 以内的主支气管。

枪伤是最常见的穿通性损伤。经纵隔的枪伤会显著增加胸腔内气管支气管损伤的概率。这类患者合并心脏、大血管以及食管损伤的情况也相当常见，而且这些合并伤往往是患者出现并发症或死亡的主要原因。

诊断

全面的体格检查和对损伤机制的理解是诊断气管支气管损伤首先和最重要的一步。由于损伤机制不同，各种类型的气道损伤的临床表现也不尽相同。Cicala 等对 9 例刀刺伤的患者进行了研究，其中有 5 例患者的伤口与气道的直接相通，有 3 例患者的查体和颈部侧位片均发现明显的皮下气肿，仅有 1 例患者没有明显的气道损伤的体征和影像学表现。这例患者行支气管镜检查最后在环气管膜上发现了小的穿刺伤口。大多数气管枪击伤的患者会表现出相应体征，或者在颈胸部平片上有气道损伤的阳性发现。在 Cicala 等的研究中，有 2 例颈胸段气管损伤的患者发生了严重的张力性气胸，在心肺复苏时会导致大量气体进入胸膜腔。还有 2 例患者发生了甲状软骨骨折但通气功能却没有受损。有 1 例患者通过触诊直接确诊，其余患者均通过颈部 CT 扫描确诊。咯血症状见于 2 例枪伤的患者。

就诊于创伤救治中心的钝性创伤患者依据颈胸段气管的损伤部位和严重程度会表现出一系列的临床症状和体征。颈段气管的钝性损伤会导致严重的呼吸功能受损，进而导致急性呼吸衰竭和窒息。损伤程度较轻的患者可表现为喉喘鸣、声嘶、咯血和皮下气肿等。

颈部和胸部平片可能具有诊断意义。如果临床怀疑存在主要气道损伤，而且平扫或 CT 扫描发现颈胸部皮下气肿，我们应当考虑行进一步的评估。纤维支气管镜是确诊支气管损伤的首选检查手段。支气管镜的适应证包括大的纵隔气肿，持续性气胸，放置胸腔引流后大量、持续性的漏气，持续性肺不张以及增大的严重皮下气肿。支气管镜在确定损伤部位，判断损伤程度和明确诊断方面是最精确、最可靠的检查手段。目前争论主要集中在硬质支气管镜和可曲式支气管镜孰优孰劣的问题上。硬质镜的缺点是需要全身麻醉，以及不适用于颈椎有问题的患者。可曲式支气管镜不需要全身麻醉，而且可以应用于颈椎损伤的患者。纤维支气管镜不仅可以用来辅助诊断，也可以用来引导气管插管建立人工气道。

对于气管支气管损伤的患者，强烈推荐在术前对声带状况进行评估。直接喉镜对于声带功能的评估恐怕是必不可少的。不论损伤的部位和程度如何，如果存在喉返神经损伤导致的声带麻痹，则提示外科医生可能须行气管造口术。

外科处理

外科治疗包括进行合适的非手术的临床观察（由创伤外科医生完成）和手术干预。初治患者采取何种气道管理措施必须经过慎重考虑。对于能够自主呼吸并保持足够的血氧饱和度和呼吸指数的患者，除非病情恶化，否则不应行气管插管。在到达创伤救治中心前完成气管插管的患者应当尽快行可曲式支气管镜检查。对于因病情进行性恶化、治疗其他致命损伤而要求早期完成气道管理的患者，由有经验的医生进行支气管镜引导下的仔细的气管插管是最佳选择。气管插管操作最好在手术室内进行，这样必要时可以行紧急环甲膜切开术或气管造口术。创伤外科医生必须做好扩大气管造口术的切口行胸骨正中切开术的准备，因为气管断端随时有可能缩入纵隔内。如果损伤位置距离气管造口位置较远，即便使用正压通气，患者的临床情况也可能进一步恶化。对于这种情况，可能须在高频通气或者低潮气量通气的同时行胸廓造口术置管。

非手术处理

对于气管插管造成的小的医源性损伤和微小的钝性损伤通常可以相对安全地进行临床观察。而大多数的高能钝性创伤和所有的穿通性损伤一般不适用保守治疗。

Gomez-Caro 等报道了 17 例在 1993 — 2003 年发生的医源性气管支气管损伤的成功处置病例。其中一些损伤甚至长达 4 cm。研究人员未发现任何由非手术治疗直接导致的并发症和死亡事件。17 例患者中有 14 例在之后的临床随诊和内镜复查中完全恢复。非手术治疗的适应证包括：生命体征稳定、不伴食管损伤、没有须行机械通气或者必要时气管插管的原发损伤、不伴进行性的严重的皮下气肿和纵隔气肿、无脓毒症的征象等。指南公布的非手术治疗的其他要求还包括：单发的较小的气管支气管损伤，其创面长度小于气管周径的 1/3、创缘对合良好、没有明显的组织缺损、不合并其他损伤、不需要正压通气。最好尽量避免行气管插管或气管造口术。Marquette 等提出，必要时还可以将气管插管的气囊置于气管损伤部位的远端。这项技术被作者成功地应用于 3 种临床情景中。非手术治疗的方法包括预防性应用抗生素、应用质子泵抑制剂、密切观察病情变化，以及随时行支气管镜复查等。图 12 提供了一个简明的流程图，可供参考。

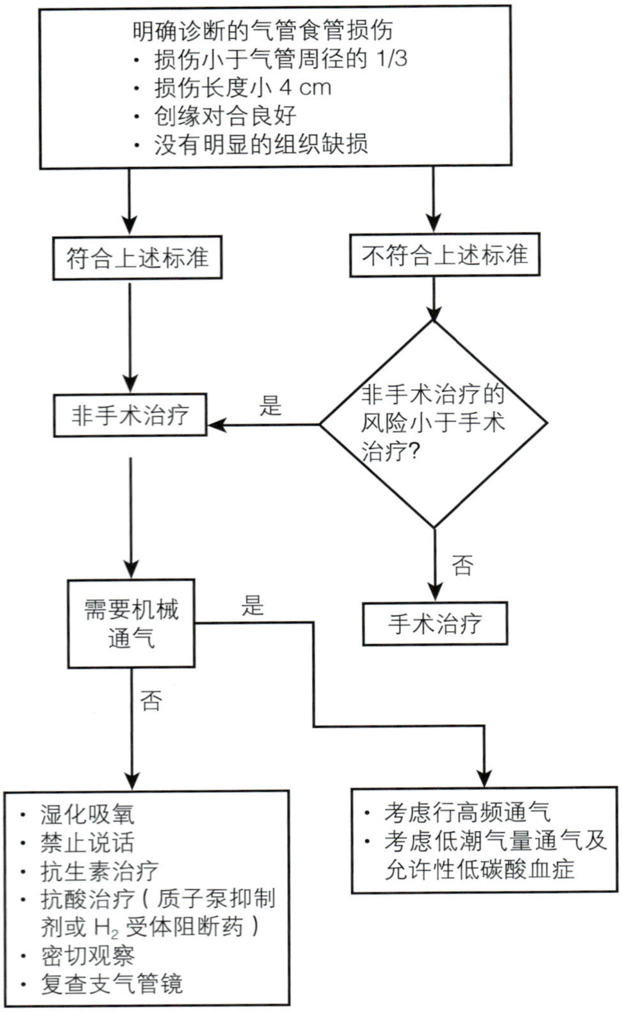

图 12　气管支气管损伤非手术治疗的流程图

非手术治疗的病例报告一例

- 患者女性，43 岁，因交通事故中受到高速撞击致伤。
- 入院时被诊断为严重的钝性胸部损伤，以及由弥漫性肺挫伤和重度低氧血症导致的严重的 ARDS。（图 13-14）
- 由于肺部损伤严重，不能耐受手术，故手术方案未予考虑。

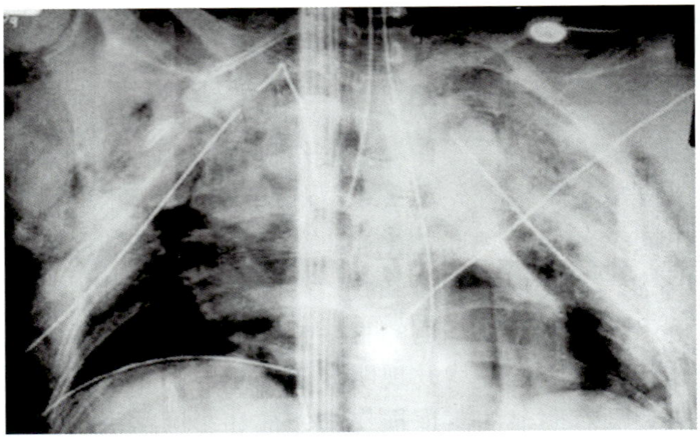

图 13　钝性创伤致远端支气管撕裂伤

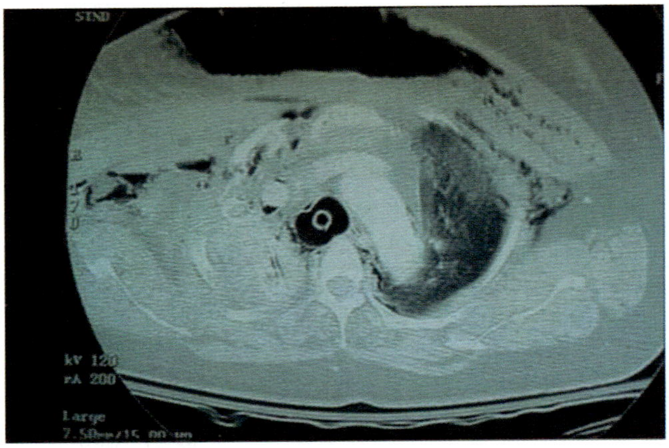

图 14　钝性创伤致远端支气管撕裂伤

- 支气管镜检查可见自右侧后外侧的远端支气管至右侧主支气管的有一处撕裂伤，长约 4 cm（图 15）。
- 予患者低潮气量通气（潮气量 350 ml）及允许性高碳酸血症治疗，调节机械通气的呼气末正压为 15 cmH_2O，并每日复查纤维支气管镜。
- 7 天后裂伤愈合。
- 患者最终得以存活并且恢复了正常功能。

手术处理

确诊为主气管支气管损伤的患者，除非生命体征不稳定或合并有明显手术禁忌的严重损伤，否则均应接受手术治疗。对于这些患者，应当尽一切努力维持患者的生命体征稳定，并保证足够的通气和氧合指数。高频通气可能会对此有所帮助。应用低潮气量通气（小于 5 ml/kg）造成允许性高碳酸血症也有过治疗成功的病例。

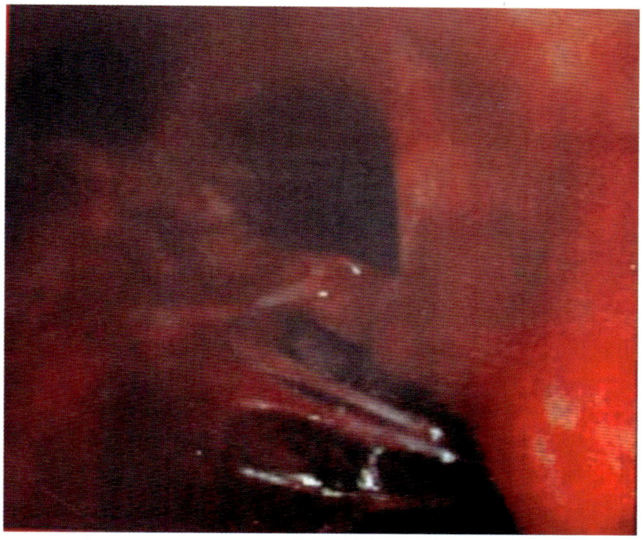

图 15 钝性创伤致一处 4 cm 长的远端支气管撕裂伤

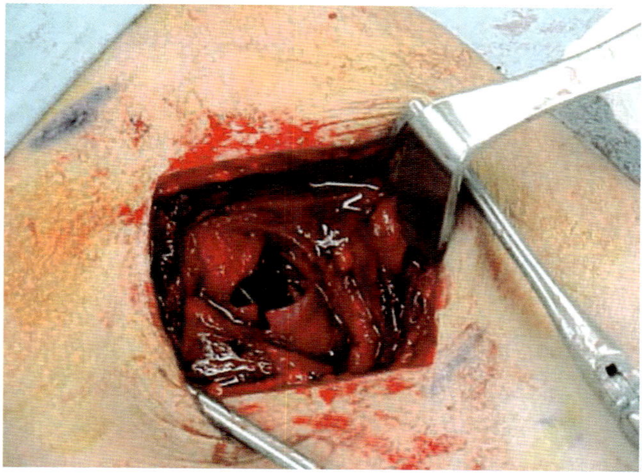

图 16 钝性创伤致颈部气管破裂，通过颈部领状切口暴露

大多数的患者最好早期行手术治疗。损伤的部位决定了手术的入路。这类手术即使对最有经验的医生来说也常常且有挑战性。处理高位颈段损伤时最好咨询一下耳鼻喉科医生的意见，而处理胸廓内的损伤时则应当咨询胸外科医生的意见。

大多数的颈部损伤可以通过颈部横向领状切口进行暴露（图 16）。综合考虑原发损伤以及合并损伤的位置，这种切口在必要时可以沿胸锁乳突肌前缘向头侧延长。对于颈部穿通性损伤，常常行经伤口的切口来直接进行手术暴露。这对于尽快开放气道可能是必需的。

钝性颈部气管损伤也常常通过胸骨上切迹上方 2 cm 处的颈部横行领状切口进行暴露。术前应做好行胸骨正中切开术的准备。如果损伤远端的气管断端缩入胸腔内，应立即行胸骨上段正中切开术。这时往往很难在中线上找到气管。我们曾有过一例患者，开胸后发现其气管断端回缩到胸骨上切迹下方 10 cm、中线左侧 10 cm 的位置。

大多数胸腔内的气管支气管钝性损伤发生在距离气管隆嵴 2～3 cm 以内。经右侧第 4 或第 5 肋间隙的后外侧开胸术可以充分暴露损伤部位，除非损伤位置位于左侧气管隆嵴远端 2～3 cm 以上。而此时应当行经左侧第 5 肋间隙的后外侧开胸术。

术前与麻醉师的沟通也非常重要。各式各样的气管插管、连接管和呼吸机管须在开胸之前就在手术台上备齐。在手术室内行支气管镜引导下气管插管可以将插管置于最佳位置。双腔的气管插管对于单肺通气是有帮助的，但其较大的管径可能会进一步损伤气管或妨碍手术操作。开胸术的体位及术中开放胸腔均有可能导致通气不足和低氧血症，进而导致病情的急剧恶化。必要时可以在迅速地开胸后，经术区直接将气管插管置入主支气管内。外科医生也可以将经口的气管插管从上段气管引导至未受损的支气管，从而实现单肺通气。如果损伤的部位的解剖层次不清，则应在手术室内备 2 台呼吸机，这样必要时可以实现双侧单肺通气。Univent 支气管填塞管可以用于主支气管或段支气管有活动性出血的情况。这种设备由 1 个气管内导管和 1 个可调节的装置组成。这个装置可以在引导下进入并且封闭主支气管、中间干或叶支气管。

气管或支气管修补术要求对所有失活组织彻底清创并一期完成端端吻合。使用可吸收或不可吸收的单股缝线均可。我们更喜欢用可吸收的单股缝线行连续缝合。所有的线结都应打在气管腔的外面，以免形成肉芽肿。表 2 总结了一些处理的“要点”。

表 2 急性喉气管创伤的处理要点

避免探查喉返神经
避免在修补的部位行气管造口术
尽量保留未坏死的气管组织
对合并损伤进行全面的评估
确保有效的气道管理
避免气管缝合处与食管缝合处的位置重合

Modified from Mathisen DJ, Grillo H: Laryngotracheal trauma. Ann Thorac Surg 43:254–262, 1987

并发症发生率

早期并发症

在气管损伤或喉部损伤的初期，气道损伤是最危急的并发症。确定性气道控制的绝对适应证包括各种呼吸功能不全的临床表现，如呼吸困难、呼吸急促、低氧血症以及大量咯血等。当怀疑有喉部损伤时，行气管插管时须格外小心，因为气管插管在通过损伤部位时，有可能会将气管的部分撕裂变成完全撕裂。张力性气胸和广泛的皮下气肿会机械性限制肺的膨胀，进而导致机械通气失败。如果想尝试气管插管，操作时应谨慎。如果存在气管损伤或者怀疑有气管损伤，通过声门时应当格外小心。对于病情稳定的患者，可以考虑在可曲式支气管镜引导下经鼻置入 7 号或更小管径的气管插管。这项操作最好在手术室内或者其他可以立即手术建立人工气道的条件下进行。正确地识别损伤并合适地引导插管，可以将医源性损伤最小化。这项技术对于术前怀疑有完全性或接近完全性气管断裂的患者格外有效。此类操作必须由有经验的支气管镜操作人员完成。即便是气管完全断裂的病例，如果颈部和上纵隔的气管周围的组织仍然完整，仅行遗留气管近端的气管插管也能保证足够的通气和氧合。在这些情况下，手术探查或者尝试手术建立人工气道行颈部切口时须格外小心。如果导管不慎进入此处，使远端气管未与人工气道连接，可引发快速呼吸衰竭和心肺功能衰竭。远端气管一旦回缩至上纵隔内，将难以再从颈部切口探及。为了预防此类情况的发生，对于可疑的完全性气管断裂的患者，可以在进入气管前间隙之前先行胸骨切开术。

张力性气胸如果不能及时发现和治疗，可以迅速导致心肺功能衰竭。尽管张力性气胸的治疗方法有了很大的进步，但胸腔穿刺术仍然是入院前急救和急诊情况下拯救即将发生心肺功能衰竭的气胸患者的有效措施。最理想的治疗方法是迅速地做一处或多处胸廓造口术置管。气管或支气管损伤的患者在该操作后可以引流出大量的气体。此时须采用更高级的机械通气方式，以增加胸膜腔的负压，并改善气体交换功能。低潮气量通气、高频喷射通气和高频振荡通气等机械通气方式都可以有效地降低气道压峰值，提高平均气道压、减少漏气，并促进伤口的愈合。

气管或支气管损伤也可以导致纵隔气肿。尽管有报道表明纵隔内气体的额外压力会引起血流动力学损伤，但这种情况并不常见。治疗方法是积极处理原发损伤。随着损伤的修复，气体会被逐渐吸收，纵隔气肿一般可以完全恢复。

皮下气肿可以很广泛，甚至可以迅速扩展到躯体的所有部位。尽管有学者推荐多数切口或引流的方法，但皮下气肿本身往往不会直接引起后遗症，而且通常可以自愈。

气道内大量的血液往往提示合并有主要血管损伤。治疗的首要目标是明确出血点并控制出血。大量的血液进入气道会直接导致气道阻塞，或因影响气体交换而导致低氧血症。对于这种情况，在确定性气管控制后，应当尽可能地使气管内套囊越过出血部位。支气管灌洗可以清除存留的血液和血凝块，对于改善低氧血症有很大帮助。

其他部位的合并损伤也相当常见，并且导致了很大一部分的早期并发症。初期评估时即应对合并损伤保持高度的警惕。依据 ATLS 指南处理患者可以将此类并发症的发病率最小化。

晚期并发症

气管损伤的晚期并发症通常与损伤部位组织结构的完整性和手术修复的部位相关。

术后气管支气管狭窄的发病率为 3.8%～9.3%。非手术治疗的患者也可能发生气管支气管狭窄。减轻炎症反应的主要措施包括应用类固醇治疗以及应用质子泵抑制剂和 H_2 受体阻断剂来减少酸性胃内容物的误吸。类固醇治疗目前存在争议，因为它在减少瘢痕形成、减轻术后狭窄的同时也有着免疫抑制和使伤口延迟愈合的风险。因此在应用类固醇治疗前必须权衡收益与风险。类固醇在保守治疗的患者可以通过减少肉芽组织增生来减轻狭窄，但是目前还没有大样本量的研究支持或反驳这种治疗观点。气管狭窄的风险与气管损伤的分级和手术修复的时间相关。但手术修复前等待的时间与术后气管狭窄的发病率之间没有相关性。手术修复的时机取决于患者合并损伤的情况以及全身的生理状态。一般应当尽早实施手术以降低潜在并发症的发生率。良好的手术技术可以减轻术后气管狭窄的程度。对失活组织彻底清创。广泛地游离周围组织以充分减少吻合口张力，以及使用可吸收线进行缝合等处理技术都可以减轻炎症反应并促进损伤愈合。将带蒂肌瓣

（通常是胸锁乳突肌或带状肌）缝合到吻合部位作为支撑，可以减少吻合口裂开、漏出以及吻合口瘘发生的概率。气管修补术后出现喉喘鸣、呼吸困难、缺氧等症状时应当高度怀疑气管狭窄。通常这些症状会在几天或几周的时间内逐渐加重，可以同时伴有嗓音的改变。其他表现还包括阻塞性肺不张和肺脓肿等，尤其是在支气管或远端段支气管修补术后。

应用可曲式支气管镜或硬质支气管镜可以在精确诊断的同时进行辅助治疗。目前的多排CT对于诊断气管支气管损伤也有着很高的灵敏度和特异度。CT三维重建可以显示解剖学细节，对于制订手术和介入修复方案有很大的帮助。治疗方案包括：①内镜下扩张配合激素治疗；②置入硅胶、金属或聚四氟乙烯支架；③ Nd-YAG激光消融瘢痕组织；④开放性手术修复。上述治疗方法均有过治疗成功的案例，而且对于特定的患者，必须根据其狭窄的程度、合并症的严重程度、手术医生的经验以及设备技术水平等制订个体化的治疗方案。目前已经发展出许多开放性手术技术，但是它们的基本原则均包括切除气管瘢痕组织，彻底清创、游离气管和使用可吸收线一期端端吻合。

对于气管或食管损伤诊治的延误可能会导致气管食管瘘。无论气管损伤或食管损伤中哪一个被确诊，都应当高度警惕发生另一个的可能性，这时通常须行支气管镜、食管镜和食管造影等检查进行全面的评估。术中应当强制性地进行全面详尽的检查。在游离颈段食管全长后，通过在食管内注入亚甲蓝的方法，可以避免遗漏微小的食管撕裂。一旦确诊迟发的气管食管瘘，则应当在患者生命体征平稳、吸入性肺炎或肺炎得到有效控制、放置胃造瘘管之后延期行修补手术。修补手术包括充分游离气管和食管。彻底清创坏死组织和一期端端吻合。在修复的位置必须移植一块有血管的带蒂肌瓣将气管与食管分隔开，这样可以有效地减少吻合口破裂和瘘管再形成的风险。

喉部损伤愈合后喉部结构的位置关系可能会发生改变，这种情况会导致发音困难和喉狭窄。伴有严重的黏膜破裂、杓状软骨脱位或软骨裸露的喉损伤通常预后不良。有研究表明，损伤时间超过24 h后行手术修复会导致气道狭窄的发病率上升13%～31%。喉内支架置入可以通过保持前联合的正常形态帮助恢复嗓音，尤其适用于一侧或双侧声带仍可运动的病例。由于长期使用会影响黏膜血供，支架应当尽早撤除（通常10～14天）。

气管损伤或喉部损伤后，由于喉返神经受损可能会导致单侧或双侧声带麻痹。喉气管分离合并喉返神经损伤的概率可高达60%，而且通常是双侧喉返神经损伤。神经功能可能会在一年之后部分恢复，有些患者的声带麻痹会因此得到改善。

喉蹼、肉芽肿和肉芽组织增生可能在喉部损伤数月后发生。这些相对较轻的并发症可以通过内镜随访和激光消融术得到有效控制。

其他有潜在致命性并发症

咽部损伤也可以导致严重的并发症，尤其是在诊疗有延误的情况时。咽后脓肿通常比较少见，但如果继发上气道阻塞或纵隔脓肿，这种并发症也足以致命。短期预防性地应用抗生素可以减少此类并发症发生的风险。咽后脓肿通过口咽部和腭扁桃体的查体通常可以明确诊断。咽后组织积气可以通过颈部侧位片发现，如果积气确实存在，则应进一步行颈部CT和胸部CT检查。咽后脓肿的治疗包括手术切开引流和静脉应用广谱抗生素，严重病例则应收入外科重症监护病房进一步治疗，必要时行气管插管。

对于咽后壁刺伤的病例，应该高度警惕颈内动脉损伤。无症状的颈内动脉破裂可能会在数小时至数天内发生动脉闭塞或脑血管栓塞，进而导致严重的神经功能障碍。因此，当临床表现提示有颈内动脉损伤的可能时，应当高度警惕并进行血管造影筛查。随着多排技术的发展，CTA的分辨率近年来有很大的提高。临床经验表明，CTA是筛查颈内动脉损伤的有效检查手段。抗凝治疗可以预防血栓形成和血管闭塞，是颈内动脉损伤患者的标准治疗方案。近年来颈动脉支架的应用也不断增长，这对于某些特定病例也不失为一种有效的治疗方案。由于大多数颈内动脉损伤的位置过深，手术修补通常难以实现。

死亡率

现代气管支气管损伤患者的总体死亡率低于30%。一项大型的文献分析回顾了1873 — 1996年间所有钝性气管支气管损伤的病例，发现到1970年之后，所有到医院就诊时仍然存活的患者，其总体死亡率为9%。左侧损伤、减速伤和挤压伤的患者通常预后不良。尸检表明 80% 的气管支气管损伤患者当场死亡。早期死亡的病例通常死于其他严重的合并损伤或气道损伤。

喉部损伤患者的死亡率可高达 40%，其主要死因是气道损伤造成的窒息。穿通性喉部损伤的死亡率相对较低（20%），其死因多为严重的合并损伤，尤其是食管和主要血管的损伤。

咽部损伤鲜有致命，所以其归因死亡率目前难以评估。患者的直接死因通常为继发的颈内动脉血栓、颈部感染和纵隔炎等并发症。是否可以得到早期的诊断和治疗直接影响着此类并发症的预后。

第 7 章　胸部损伤

胸部及纵隔相关外科解剖学

Leonard J. Weireter, Jr. 和 L.D. Britt 著
王　迅　赵　恒 译

胸部的解剖包括胸壁、纵隔、胸膜腔。胸壁是由胸骨、肋骨、胸椎组成。纵隔是由心包、心脏、食管、气管、大血管、胸导管以及胸腺组成。胸膜腔包含双侧肺。本章节将讨论上述组织结构解剖，它是胸部创伤及外科重症监护的相关基础知识。

胸壁

胸部肌肉、肌腱及骨性结构发挥着重要的功能。胸壁须有足够的强度来保护胸腔脏器，并且为上肢及腹部肌肉提供稳定的附着点，同时足够有弹性，在剧烈呼吸时可以扩展及收缩。

平静呼吸时，胸壁类似于气缸，膈是这个气缸的活塞。吸气时膈收缩，膈顶部变为扁平，像活塞一样，膈降至胸膜腔底部。这种运动形式增加了胸腔的容积，增加了通过气管进入到肺组织中的空气。肺具有很大的顺应性，在没有外力的情况下倾向收缩。呼气时膈舒张，肺的弹性使肺组织回缩、气体排出。最终，肺组织通过外力以及胸壁的固定作用倾向于萎陷。剧烈呼吸过程中，肋间肌、斜角肌以及其他辅助呼吸肌抬高肋骨，以增加比往常更大的胸腔容积。此时，胸壁和膈的运动类似于风箱的活动，增加了胸腔的容积，并在舒张过程中，通过肺组织的顺应性减小胸腔容积。

胸壁的骨性结构包括 12 根肋骨、12 个胸椎骨，以及胸骨。所有的肋骨连接于后方对应的胸椎椎体的横突和上一胸椎椎体。第 1 肋骨到第 7 肋骨通过肋软骨向前连接在胸骨上，被称作真肋。第 8、9、10 肋骨通过上方肋骨的肋软骨连接至胸骨，因此被称为假肋。这样形成了阶梯样的肋软骨结构，最终与胸骨相连，形成肋弓或肋缘的解剖结构。第 11，12 肋骨前方无连接，因此被称为浮肋，浮肋附于腹壁的肌肉组织，主要是腹内斜肌。

因为第 1 肋骨到第 10 肋骨前后固定于胸壁，它们的功能类似于水桶的桶柄（图 1A）。在进行胸廓造口置管术时，前方近胸骨处以及后方近横突处，肋间隙的宽度相对固定、狭窄。离开上述连接点，肋骨相对分离，肋间隙也相对打开。肋间隙最宽的位置位于肋骨的侧面最高点，胸廓造口置管于胸壁侧面较为容易，并且能够减轻患者疼痛（图 1B）。同样，在开胸术过程中，分离肋骨侧面的肋间肌能够提供更加充裕的手术操作空间，并能够避免撕开肋间肌或者肋骨拉钩引起的肋骨骨折。仅仅分开操作部位的皮肤即可，而不须切开整个肋间皮肤。

胸骨由 3 个部分构成，胸骨柄、胸骨体、剑突。胸骨柄宽厚，与锁骨、第 1 肋骨连接，并与胸骨体共同与第 2 肋骨连接。胸锁关节是唯一的胸部与肩部连接的骨性关节。对锁骨角度、胸骨柄以及第 1 肋骨解剖的理解对于放置锁骨下中心静脉导管十分重要。锁骨下动脉、锁骨下静脉通过第 1 肋骨上缘和锁骨下方离开上肢进入胸廓入口。在锁骨下方时，针尖方向平行于锁骨和第 1 肋骨，能够避免在进入锁骨下静脉前进入胸腔造成气胸。进针角度过大，可能导致针尖过快进入和离开锁骨下静脉的三角地带，进而穿透肋间隙刺破肺组织（图 2）。

第 2 肋骨插入胸骨柄连接处，也被称作 Louis 角。胸骨柄和胸骨体在此处形成角度，因此在大多数人中，它是胸骨柄上容易触及的水平方向上的嵴（图 3）。在 Louis 角下方的肋间隙为第 2 肋间隙，

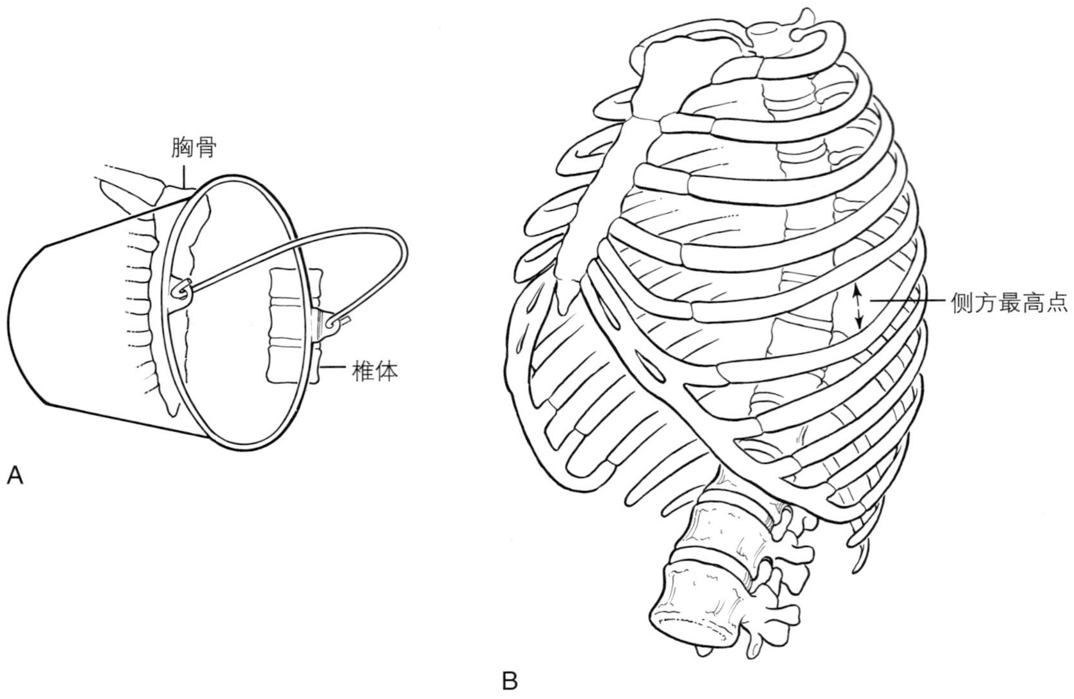

图 1 **A，B** 肋骨形态类似于水桶桶柄，肋骨前端固定于胸骨，后端固定于胸椎。肋骨的活动类似于桶柄。肋间最宽的间隙位于肋骨侧面的最高点（*Modified from Pearson FG, editor: Thoracic surgery, 2nd ed. Philadelphia, Churchill Livingstone, 2002, Fig. 48-3, p1327.*）

Louis 角可作为标志，快速定位第 2 肋骨，并可在此快速放置导管减压张力性气胸。

第 1 肋骨短、宽、平，从前至后角度较大（图 4）。第 2 肋骨与第 1 肋骨相似，但是比第 1 肋骨长（图 5）。前锯肌的第 1 束连接于第二肋骨后 1/3，这一束同样连接于第 1 肋骨下缘。在此附着处后方，前斜角肌也附着于第 2 肋骨。

在开胸术中，计数肋骨能够正确地定位肋间隙。在背阔肌分离、前锯肌后方分离或向前推移的过程中，肩胛骨上移。菲薄的附着物维持着肩胛骨的下表面与胸壁的位置。术者一只手深入至肩胛骨深面，向后靠近脊柱，向顶部能够触诊肋骨。第 1 肋骨依靠其明显宽、扁的轮廓而确定。在此下方，第 2 肋骨可以通过后斜角肌附着点进行定位。这个肌肉可以通过由后向前沿第 2 肋骨轻移手指而触及（图 6）。不确切的是第 3 肋骨的定位，其位于胸顶部和胸部侧面的转角处（图 7）。在侧卧位，肩胛下角位于第 6 肋间隙，男性患者的乳头位于第 4 肋间隙。

胸壁的肌肉

安全的胸腔穿刺术、放置导管的胸膜腔造口术，或开胸术须理解胸壁的结构层次和肋间隙解剖。

前胸壁的大部分被成对的胸大肌覆盖，胸大肌起自锁骨和第 1 肋骨至第 6 肋骨前侧，止于肱骨近端。胸大肌自胸壁起源范围较宽，前开胸术须游离或分离胸大肌纤维。下方的腹直肌插入第 5 肋骨到第 7 肋骨的软骨上以及剑突。在外侧，腹外斜肌插入第 5 肋骨至第 12 肋骨。腹外斜肌与前锯肌交错，前锯肌则附着于第 1 肋骨至第 8 肋骨（图 8）。大部分开胸手术并不穿过腹直肌和腹外斜肌之间的肋间隙。穿过肋缘的胸腹联合切口中会切开这些肌肉。

侧方和后方，两层肌肉筋膜保护肋骨，浅层外侧包含背阔肌。后方，在听诊三角或背阔肌后缘，这层筋膜成为菲薄但坚韧的筋膜层，再向后方包裹斜方肌。第二肌肉筋膜层外侧包含前锯肌，逐渐向后形成一个菲薄但是坚韧的纤维结缔组织，向后方和上方成为大菱形肌以及小菱形肌。胸廓造口术的

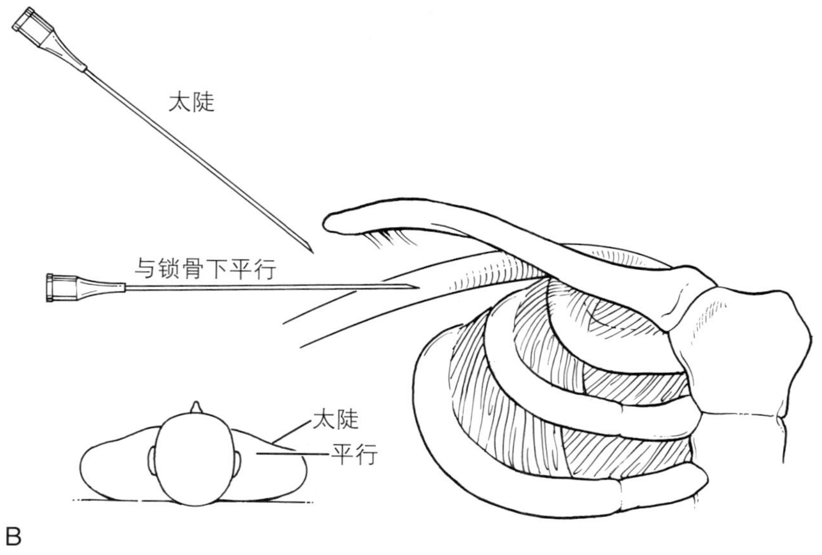

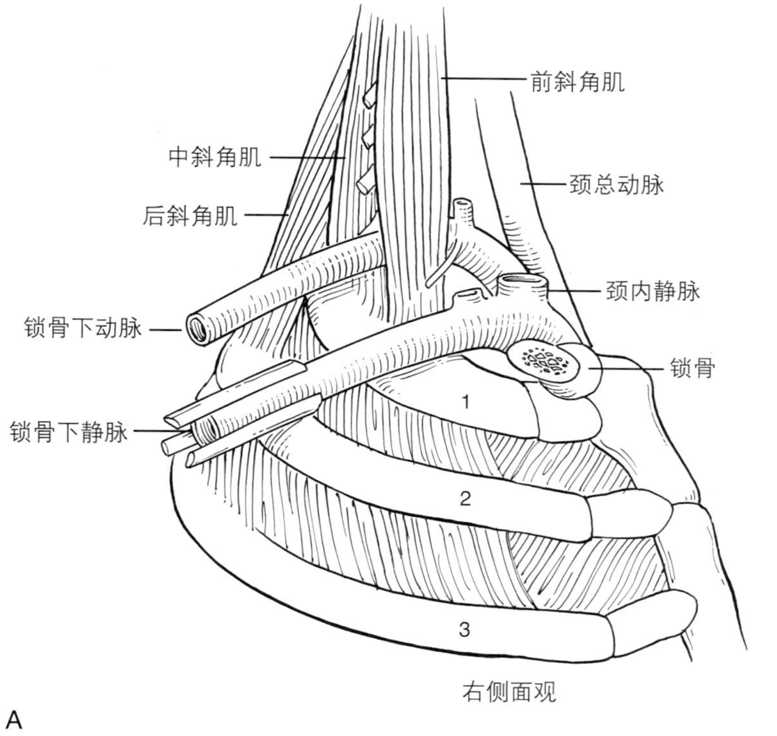

图 2　锁骨下静脉中心静脉置管。**A**，锁骨和胸廓形成了锁骨下静脉通过的三角形。静脉走行大致与锁骨和胸廓平行。**B**，穿刺针一旦到达锁骨下方，方向平行于肋骨廓和锁骨将更有利于找到锁骨下静脉。如果穿刺针的角度太陡，它将会进入三角区后随即离开，穿透肋间隙，然后穿刺到肺（*Modified from Agur AMR, Dalley AF, editors: Grant's atlas of anatomy, 11th ed. Philadelphia, Lippincott Williams & Wilkins, 2004, Figs. 1.8, 6.29, pp 9, 379.*）

导管穿过上述肌肉至肋间时，理解上述解剖层次能够节省穿过它们时间，且可以帮助术者完成手术过程。

通常，胸腔闭式引流放置于腋前线第 5 肋间隙。横穿的胸壁肌肉在此处较薄。从浅层至深层，术者须分离皮肤、皮下脂肪组织、背阔肌 / 斜方肌肌肉筋膜层，前锯肌肌肉筋膜层。在此层，能够清晰地看到肋骨表面的光泽以及肋间外肌的斜形肌纤维。正如之后所讨论的，胸廓造口术在肋骨上缘进行。在未进入肌肉和筋膜层前定位肋骨上缘更为容易。

开胸术须分离或切断上述肌肉层次，全开胸术须从两侧分离背阔肌，并向后分离斜方肌。切口水

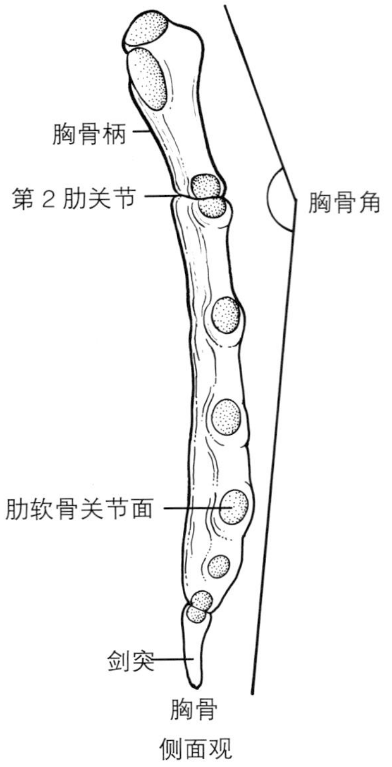

图 3 胸骨，侧面观。Louis 角可在中线处触及，在胸骨柄平面和胸骨体平面的交界处，似一突起的嵴。第 2 肋以关节连接于 Louis 角的外侧（*Modified from Standring S, editor: Gray's anatomy: the anatomical basis of clinical practice, 39th ed. Edinburgh, Churchill Livingstone, 2004, Fig. 57.5, p 954*）

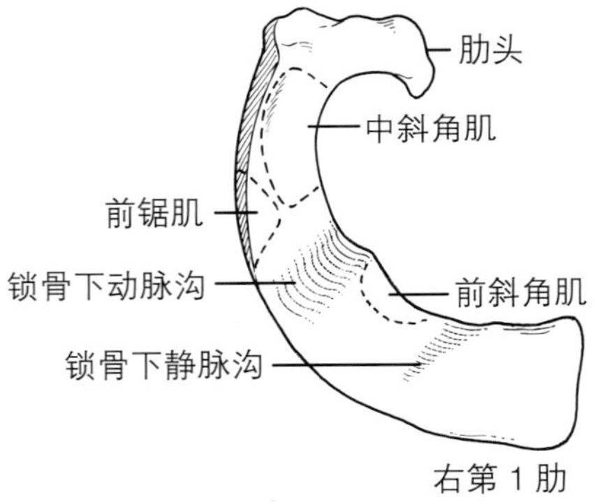

图 4 右 第 1 肋（*Modified from Gray H, editor: Gray's anatomy, 20th ed. Lea & Febiger, 1918, Plate 124.*）

平方向上从侧胸壁延续至脊柱，在后方与脊柱平行。游离至此层的前锯肌可以向前推移或分离。向后，继续分离上的筋膜层和大菱形肌和小菱形肌。斜方肌和菱形肌的神经分布和支配是由内侧到外侧。保留更多内侧肌肉，能够保留更多的肌肉功能。附着

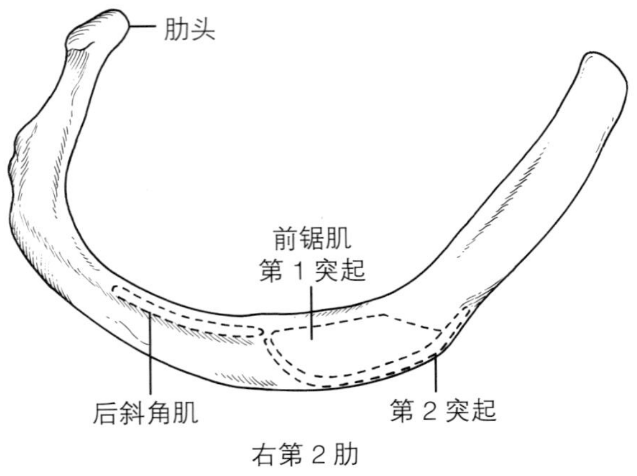

图 5 右第 2 肋（*Modified from Gray H, editor: Gray's anatomy, 20th ed. Lea & Febiger, 1918, Plate 125.*）

于肩胛骨上的肌肉需要更多的保留，以提供更多的缝合部位。肩胛骨附着的肌肉组织不能剔除。沿全开胸切口的后侧及垂直方向（在此位置游离斜方肌和菱形肌）抬高肩胛骨，来接近下方肋间隙。

开胸术可以向前扩展，分离覆盖在肋间隙上的胸大肌。胸骨可以被横向劈开，并且可以继续在对侧进行开胸术。这被称作“蛤壳”开胸术。左侧和右侧的乳动脉位于胸骨两侧旁 1 cm，于肋骨和肋间肌肉的深部、胸膜的浅部。如果为了提高速度这些血管可以烧灼，但是有可能会产生痉挛和迟发性出血。如果可能，尽量找到血管并结扎。当血供恢复时，它们经常会开始出血，此时应当结扎。

肋间隙

由浅到深的每个肋间隙，都有 2 层肌肉和 1 条动脉、1 条静脉和 1 根神经，以及 1 层小的内层肌肉。肋间外肌的肌纤维走行方向和腹部的腹外斜肌一样（方向类似于插在裤兜的手指）。其深部是肋间内肌，走行方向相反。肋间动脉、静脉、神经走行在每条肋骨的下缘，偶尔走行在肋沟的突出部分之下。为了避免损伤这 3 个结构，胸廓造口置管术和开胸术应沿着每条肋骨的上缘或者是肋间隙中间，而不应该在肋骨下缘（图 9）。肋间最内肌位于神经血管束的深处，并且走行和肋间内肌一致。即使在解剖书上提及到，外科手术中，不须考虑分离肋间最内肌与肋间内肌（图 10）。肋间动脉以节段性分支由降主动脉发出。肋间隙，包括潜在的胸膜，可以有后

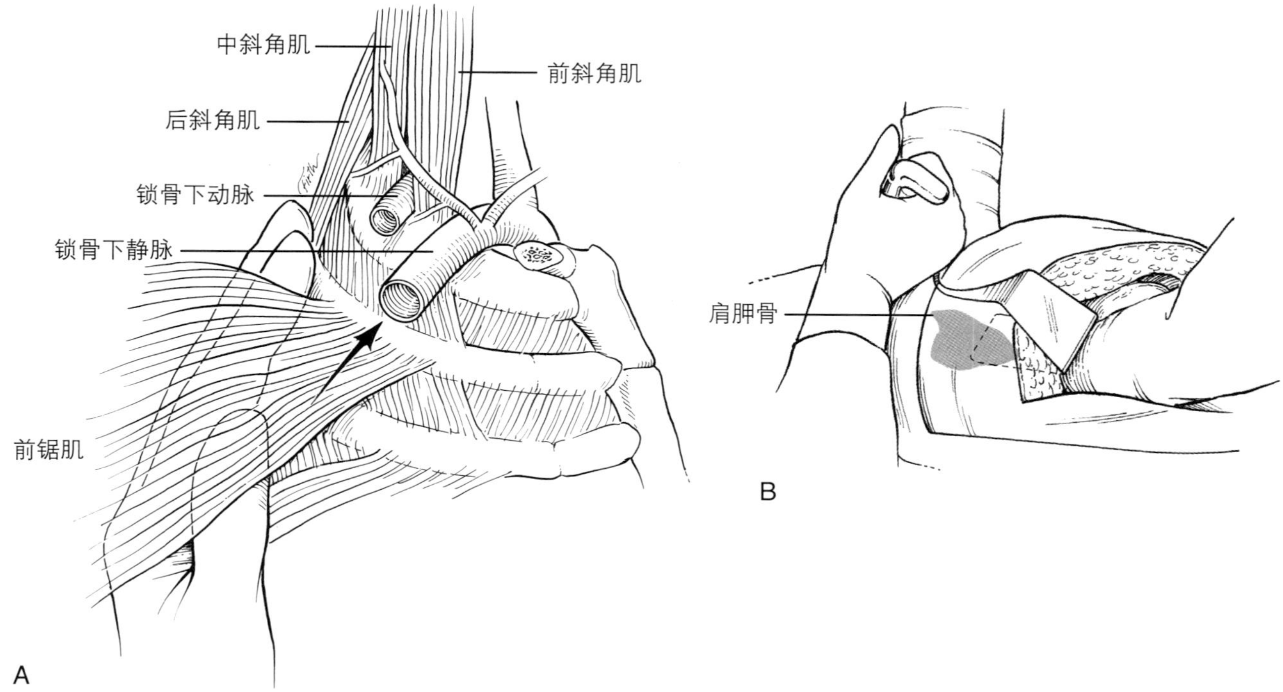

图6　**A**和**B**，计数肋骨。看到胸廓之后，肩胛骨被抬高，可以用手置于其后方和上方来触诊和计数肋骨。注意第1肋较宽、短、平；第2肋有后斜角肌插入；第3肋位于顶端到侧胸壁的“拐弯处”

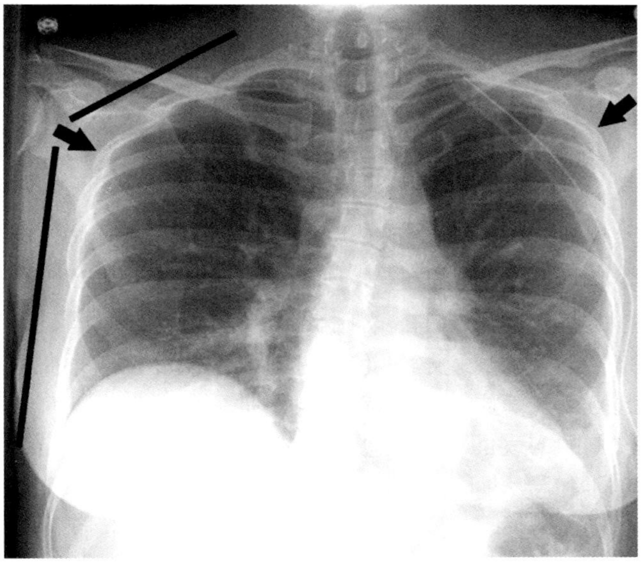

图7　第3肋在“拐弯处”。正位X线胸片显示胸廓形成一个宽松的盒子，第3肋在拐角处。箭头指示第3肋

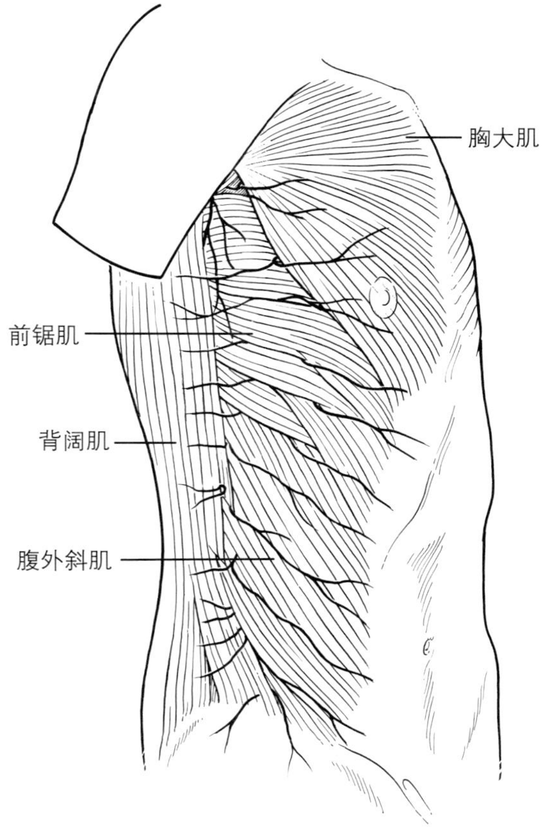

图8　胸部肌肉：左侧面观（*Modified from Gray H, editor: Gray's anatomy, 20th ed. Lea & Febiger, 1918, Plate 392.*）

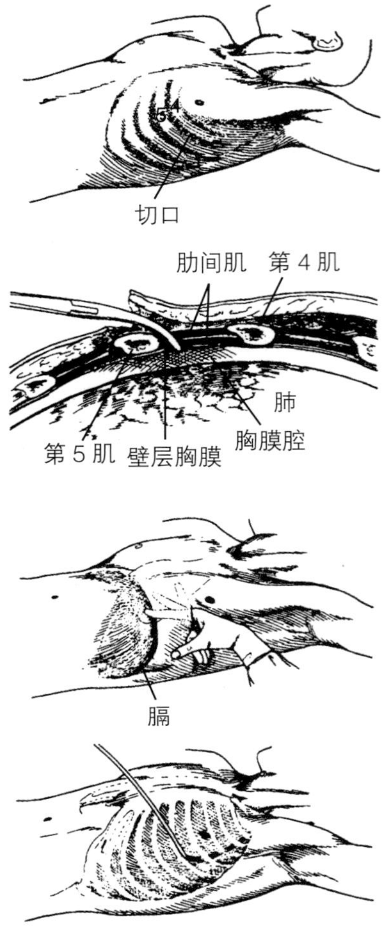

图 9　胸廓造口术置管。创伤后紧急置管被放在腋前线，第 4 或者第 5 肋间。从肋骨上缘进入肋间隙。用手指触摸确认进入胸腔，并避免把管放到肩胛下或者腹腔内或损伤肺（*Modified from Moore FA, Moore EE: Trauma resuscitation. In Wilmore DN, Brennan MF, Harken AH, et al, editors.* Care of the surgical patient. *New York, Scientific American, 1989.*）

方基底的带蒂肌瓣（图 11）。这种肌瓣可以用来加强支气管或者修复食管。

内乳动脉发自锁骨下动脉两侧，并且沿胸壁内下降，大概在胸骨双侧旁 1 cm（图 12）。

胸膜腔

正常来说，肺是通过存在于脏层胸膜与壁层胸膜之间的真空被吸附于胸壁的。如果胸壁穿破，空气从外界进入胸膜腔，或者更常见地，肺穿破而空气从肺内的气腔（肺泡、细支气管、小支气管）进

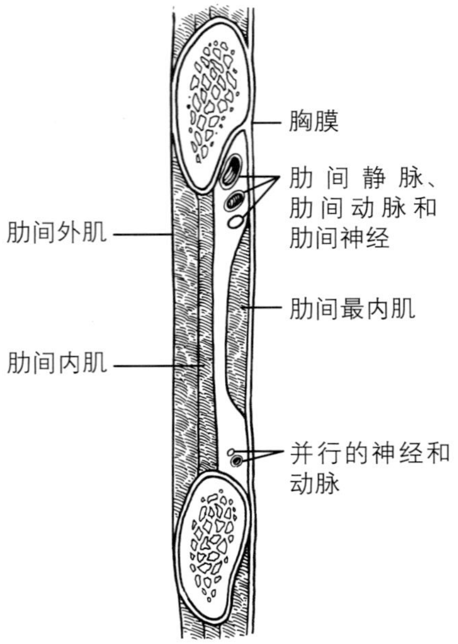

图 10　肋间隙横切面。注意主要肋间血管及神经走行在肋骨下缘。并行的神经和动脉，即使出现也是很微小的（*Modified from Crafts RC:* A textbook of human anatomy, *3rd ed. New York, John Wiley, 1985.*）

入胸膜腔。脏层胸膜和壁层胸膜之间的吸附被破坏，并且潜在间隙即胸膜腔，成为真正的空间。肺的弹性导致它萎陷从而形成气胸。胸膜腔间隙向上扩展至第 1 肋周之上，向下至膈插入肋骨和第 12 肋的位置。在胸膜腔最低处的隐窝，肺可能会或不会出现在膈和肋骨之间。在心包前及胸骨后，两个胸膜腔可以接近但是不会相通。

膈

膈是可动的、圆顶状的肌肉，它分隔胸腔和腹腔。当呼气末时，膈的圆顶可达第 4 肋间隙前部的水平（乳头平面）。吸气末时，膈变平，使胸腔下降到肋骨边缘（前）和第 12 肋（后）水平。膈纤维发自胸骨、肋骨和脊柱。3 组肌纤维汇合形成坚固、纤维性的中心腱。胸骨部分的肌纤维较短，以小肌束起自剑突背面。在剑突两侧，肌纤维起自下 6 个肋软骨的内表面（肋骨边缘）。在后方，肌纤维起自腰方肌和腰大肌上方的一个厚的弓带状结构（外侧弓状韧带、内侧弓状韧带）。成对的外侧弓状韧带从第 12 肋的尖端和下缘以及腰方肌上的弓状结构，延伸到第 1 腰椎的横突。成对的内侧弓状韧带延续之，形成腰大肌上方的弓状结构，从第 1 腰椎的横突尖

图 11　**A**，肋间肌瓣。以肋间动脉和后方的蒂为基础。**B**，瓣的横面观

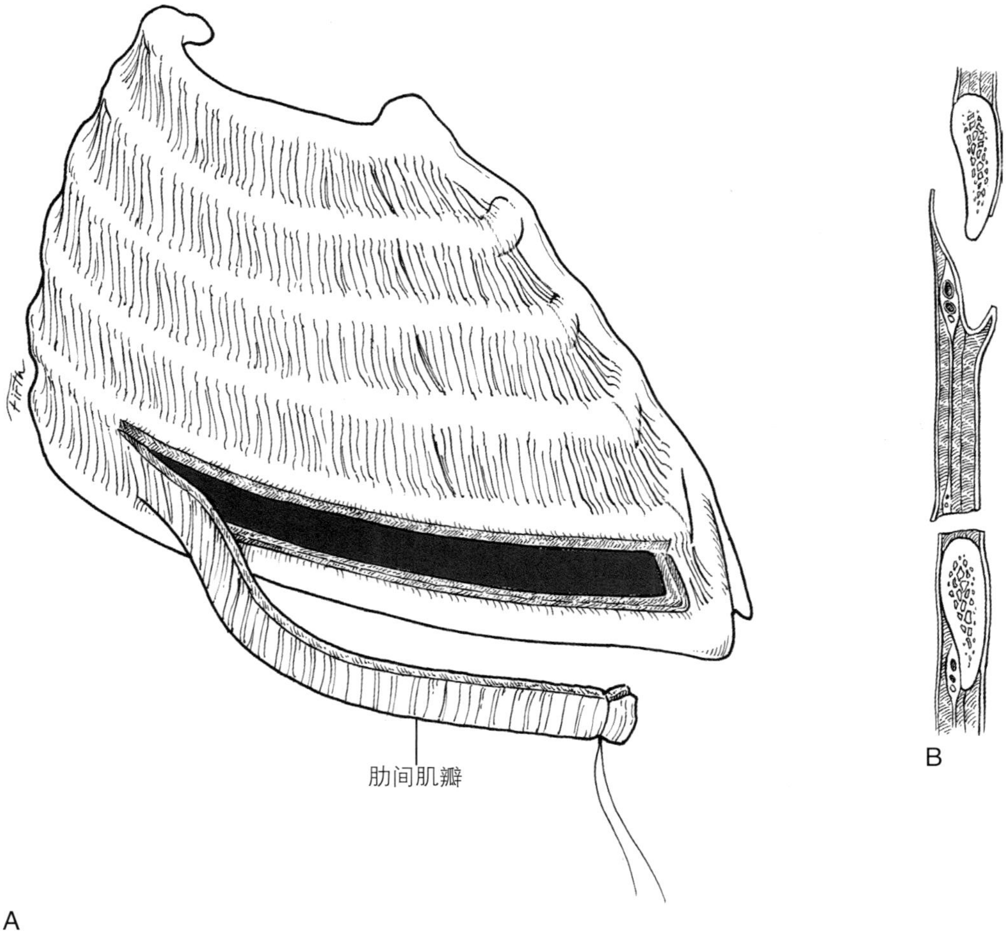

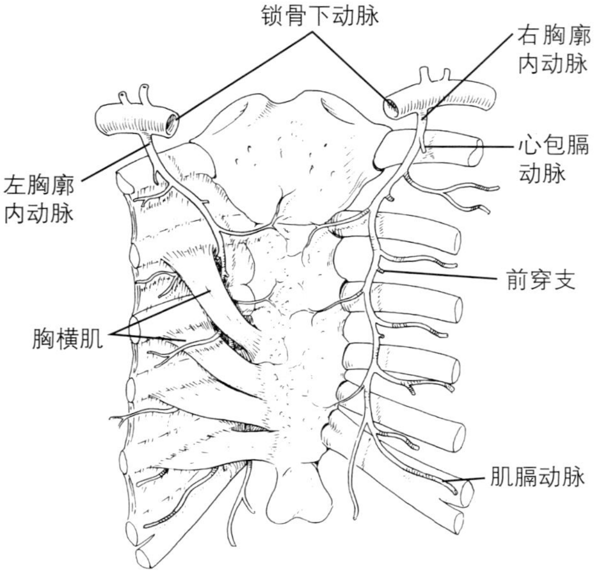

图 12　胸腔内视角观察内乳动脉 (*From Pearson FG, editor: Thoracic surgery, 2nd ed. Philadelphia, Churchill Livingstone, 2002, Fig. 48-8, p 1330.*)

端延伸到每个膈脚（图 13）。

膈的后中部由两个“脚”——一个解剖学上的右脚，起自上 3 个腰椎的椎体；和一个解剖学上的左脚，起自上 2 个腰椎的椎体。在主动脉之前，2 只“脚”的内缘形成一个不完全的拱状结构，称为正中弓状韧带。在这个韧带前方，解剖学上的右脚（64%）或者左脚（2%）或者两者共同（34%）形成了食管裂孔。虽然解剖学家以它们起自椎体的左右来命名脚的左右，但是外科医生以它们与食管的关系来命名脚的左右。在腹腔，看见食管和辨别走行至食管左侧的膈脚可以帮助暴露在腹腔动脉和肾动脉水平之上的远端胸主动脉。在这里可以利用夹钳控制血管，也可以用 Conn 主动脉根压迫器或者用剖腹手术垫包裹的 Richardson 牵开器将动脉压向椎体来阻断主动脉（图 14）。

膈神经和来自下肋间神经的小分支支配膈。膈神经发自 C4 神经根，但也接受来自 C3 和 C5 的神经支配（C3、C4 和 C5 维持人体生命）。在颈部，膈神经发自前斜角肌外侧并在该肌肉表面从外侧下行

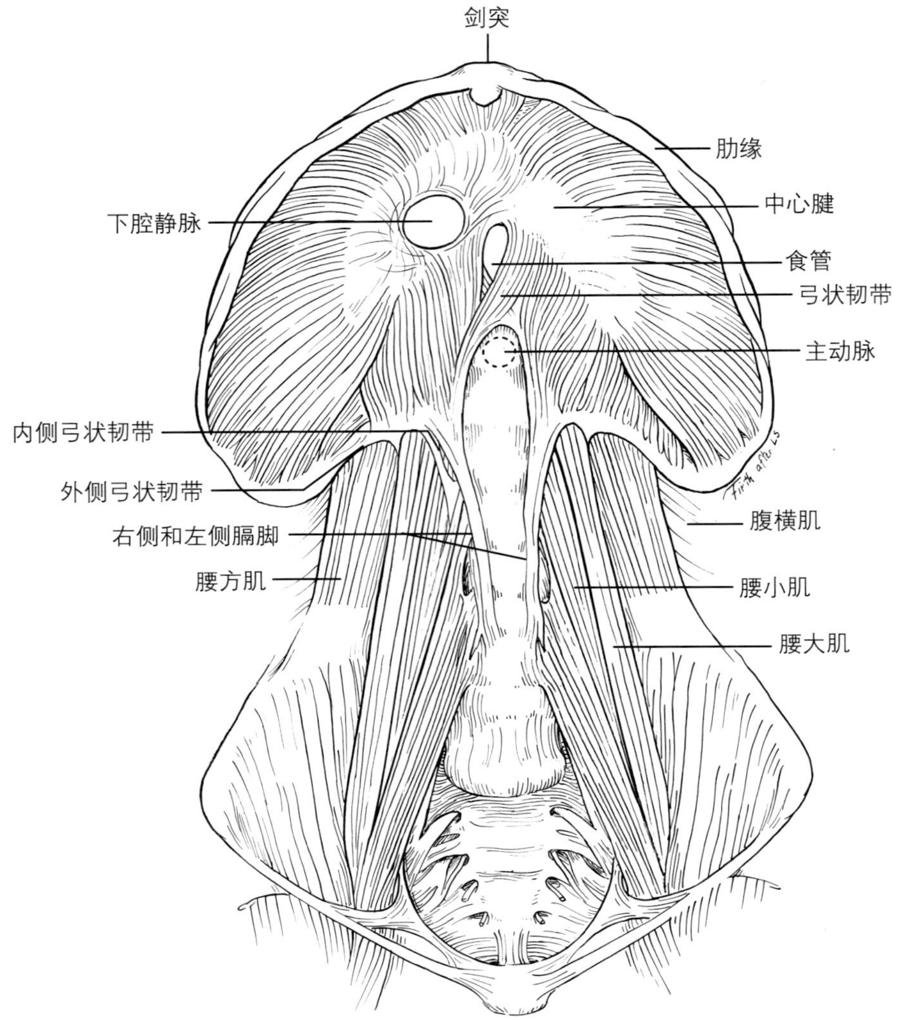

图 13　腹腔内观察膈。膈两侧起自剑突、肋缘、外侧弓状韧带和内侧弓状韧带，汇入中心腱。左右膈脚起自腰椎椎体并汇入中心腱（*Modified from Langley LL, Telford IR, Christensen JB: Dynamic anatomy and physiology, 5th ed. New York, McGraw-Hill, 1980.*）

至内侧，向胸锁乳突肌的深部走行。它进入胸廓入口，并处于纵隔的内侧部分，恰好位于两侧胸膜的深部。在上方，它位于胸腔的前方并且很容易受损，尤其是在胸骨正中切开和分离大血管时，经常不是那么容易看清，但是膈神经非常靠近分离的位置。在左侧，它在心包外下行，位于胸膜深部，经过主动脉弓，并且在肺门及下肺韧带前方。随着靠近膈，它常被心包脂肪遮盖，像窗帘一样悬挂在心包和膈之间。膈神经刚好在心脏左界从侧面分布到膈，其所在的平面要比右侧膈神经更靠前（图 29）。右膈神经沿上腔静脉的右外侧界下降，并经过右肺门前方及下肺韧带前方。当接近膈时它也被心包脂肪遮盖。右侧膈神经在下腔静脉外侧进入膈（图 28）。

左、右侧膈神经进入单侧膈之后都分 3 支进入 3 个肌束。一支向前内侧至胸骨，一支向前外侧，第 3 支向后。后支又分叉一支到第 12 肋，另一只到膈脚。安全切开膈是指避免切断膈神经的主要分支（图 15）。周边弧形切口可以避免除远端细小分支之外的膈神经损伤。亦可行放射状切口，但必须仔细操作以避免损伤膈神经主干。

因为膈的主要神经支配即膈神经，它从中央进入，离心性分布。膈可以被转移到胸廓内更高或者更低的位置，来保护它的神经支配。有时这在修补膈破裂中是需要的。特别是当膈表面部分丢失或者胸壁失去刚性，且不能再保持它的圆柱状功能时。要注意保持膈的圆顶状结构。静息时变平的膈在收缩时会拉着胸壁靠近。收缩时，膈会减小胸腔内容量（而不是增加），并且会成为呼气肌（图 16）。

心包

心包腔比胸膜腔要小得多，并且其内的液体少量增加都会对心脏功能产生相当大的影响。壁层心

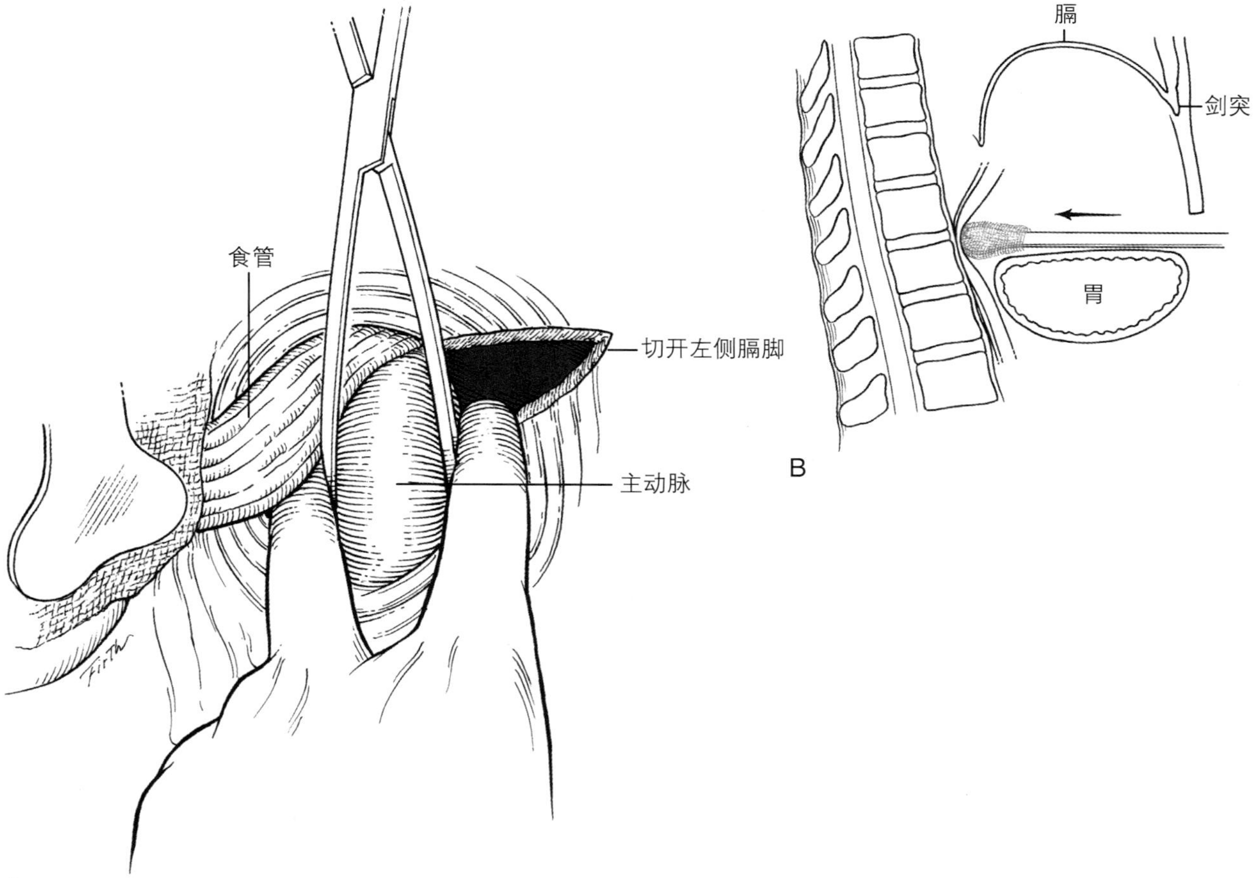

图 14　从腹腔十字钳夹降主动脉胸段远端。**A**，分离膈左脚暴露深部胸主动脉。**B**，侧视图，向椎体压迫阻断主动脉

图 15　膈切口与膈神经分支。此切口能够防止膈大面积地失去神经支配 (*From Meredino KA, Johnson RS, Skinner HH, et al: The intradiaphragmatic distribution of the phrenic nerve with particular reference to the placement of diaphragmatic incisions and controlled segmental paralysis. Surgery 39:189, 1956.*)

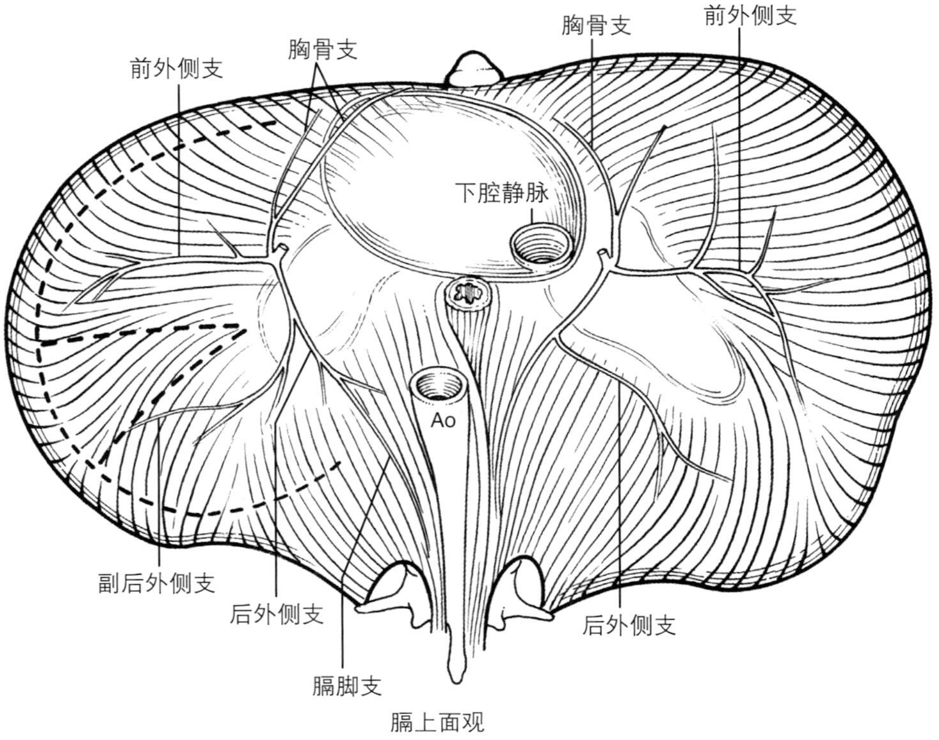

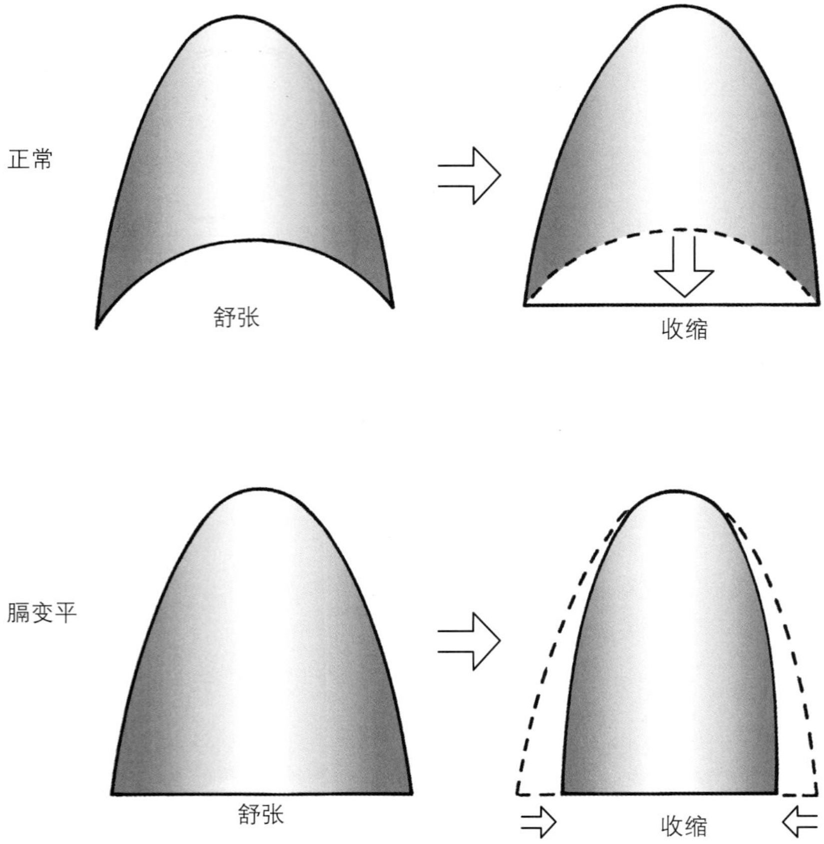

图 16 膈舒张时平坦；收缩时牵拉肋骨，引起呼气，而非吸气

包是一层厚的纤维囊，内层浆膜面包裹心脏、升主动脉近端、上腔静脉远端、下腔静脉远端、肺动脉主干及其分叉、左右主肺动脉近端和所有 4 支肺静脉的远心端的一小部分。从这个描述，可以很直观地想象所有进出心脏的血管都有一小段包含在心包囊内（图 17）。而且，这些血管把心脏固定在心包腔内。如果心脏可以旋转，那么这些血管会扭转和打结，阻碍静脉回流。因为上腔静脉和下腔静脉是压力最低的血管，它们是最容易被扭结和阻碍血流的。随着回心血流减少，心脏输出血量也会减少，体循环血压就会下降。这就是与张力性气胸和心脏疝相关的低血压的生理学机制。

心脏后方有 2 个窦。心包斜窦是心脏后方心包后壁的无效腔，以下腔静脉的附着物和 4 条肺静脉为界。因为心包斜窦的存在，在胸骨正中切开术中，手可以放在心尖周围，并且心尖可以轻轻地向切口上提。这样就可以看清左心室的侧壁和后壁，包括对角支、旋支和钝角缘支冠状动脉的分布。如果没有平行于膈神经垂直打开右心包，这个策略通常是比较难以耐受的。这样心脏右边就可以进入右胸膜腔，并且在被提起时仍保持灌注。而且，极端的Trendelenburg 位和顶部放置的吸引回缩装置可以帮助暴露和改善血流动力学。在实行这个策略前胸内除颤器应该打开并准备好，因为室颤并不少见。

心包横窦可以允许一根手指或钳子从升主动脉右侧放入，在主动脉弓和肺动脉主干后方，经过左侧肺动脉主干和左上肺静脉上方，达到左心耳附近（图 21）。

心包可由胸骨正中切开术、左侧或右侧经剑突下的开胸术或剖腹手术切开。左侧或右侧的开胸术切口应选在平行于膈神经的前方或后方。左侧路进入时，切口后的心包腔为左心室；右侧路进入时，切口后的心包腔为右心房（图 18）。

剖腹手术时，改良的剑突下入路方式可用于进入心包腔。除此之外，膈中央部分参与组成了心包囊纤维层腔壁的下壁，在肺的此位置切开后进入心包囊，可看到心脏的下壁。

剑突下间隙

经剑突下间隙的手术入路方式是诊断和治疗心包积液的常用入路。腹白线和膈都附着于剑突。膈

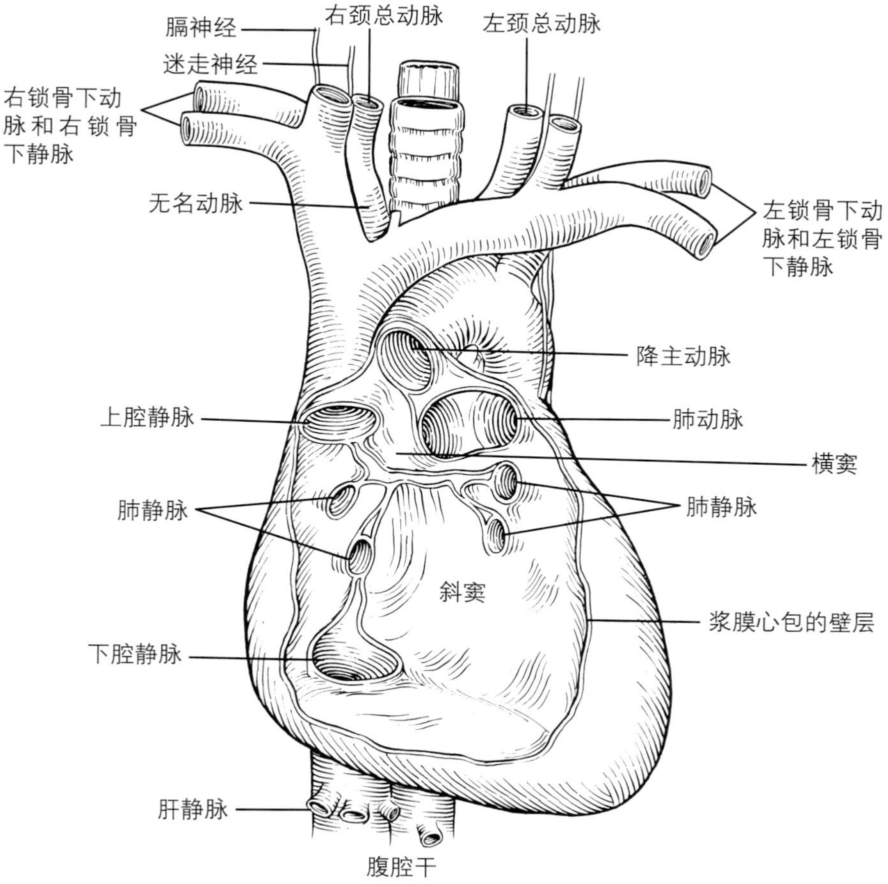

图 17 心包囊，后面及侧面。前面的心包膜已移除。心脏已移除（*Modified from Agur AMR, Dalley AF, editors: Grant's atlas of anatomy, 11th ed. Philadelphia, Lippincott Williams & Wilkins, 2004, Fig. 1.61, p 55.*）

表面的腹膜和前腹壁后方筋膜的深层相连接。从剑突上至剑突下 4 cm 的切口都会经过皮肤、脂肪、腹白线这三层。切开腹白线会暴露剑突的浅面及腹膜的深面。剑突附着的膈可被分为剑突部分和胸骨体 / 肋缘部分。在剑突和肋缘、胸骨体的夹角中常可发现大静脉走行。向后牵拉膈、向上牵拉胸骨可以很好地暴露心包在膈上的反折。这些反折部分经常覆盖有脂肪组织，须用 Kittner 海绵剥离棒钝性分离后才能显露后方的心包。切开心包就能够进入心包腔。透过这个切口可以看见右心室锐利的边缘（图 19）。由于这个切口位于 2 个相互垂直的平面夹角处，因此可以从 2 个不同方向吸出心包积液。首先，从正后方、平行于纵隔，沿着心脏下界吸出液体；其次在上方、平行于胸骨体，在心脏前表面的前面吸出液体（图 20）。

心脏

心脏占据了胸腔的中部及左侧空间，是中纵隔的主要脏器。它四周都被心包围绕。在心包外面，前方是胸骨，后方是食管、椎体和降主动脉。右侧是纵隔胸膜和肺，膈神经走行于肺门的前方。在左侧也是同样的结构，只是膈神经的走行位置更靠前。因此。如果从左侧接触心脏，须更加注意保护膈神经。

心脏的体表标志

心脏的上界体表投影位于第 2 肋间胸骨左侧 2 cm 至第 2 肋间胸骨右缘之间。这标记了主要肺动脉的体表位置。心脏的右侧边界向下延伸至第 6 肋软骨与胸骨体的交界处。这部分主要由右心房构成。心脏下界由第 6 肋软骨向左延续至能触及心脏搏动最强烈的位置，这个位置大多处于左侧第 5 肋间锁骨中线内侧。右心室组成了心脏的下界。心脏的左界向上延伸至左侧第 2 肋间胸骨旁 2 cm 处。左心室构成了心脏的左界（图 21）。

外表特征

心脏由 4 个腔和 3 个沟组成。房室沟中包含了

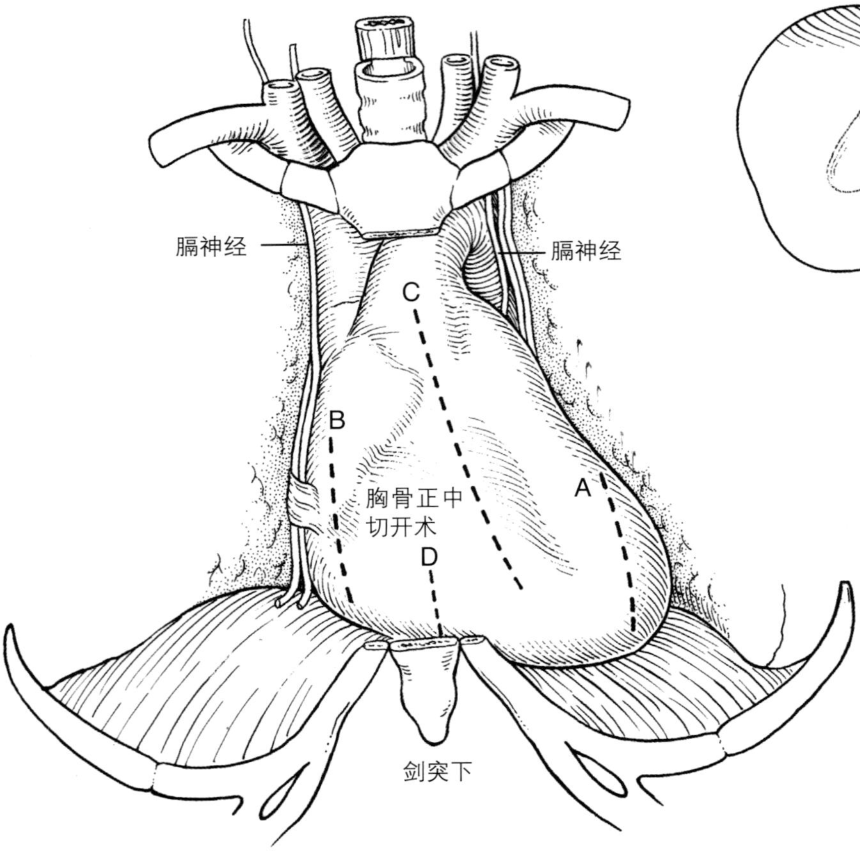

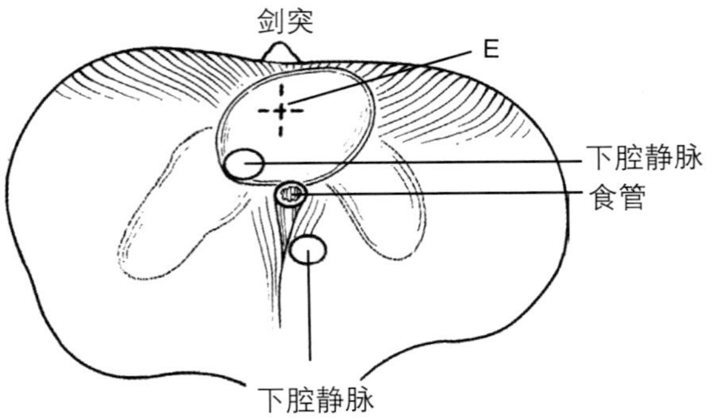

图 18 心包窗的打开方法。心包可以从左胸切口（**A**）、右胸切口（**B**）、胸骨正中切口（**C**）、剑突下切口（**D**）或腹部切口（**E**）打开 (*Modified from Agur AMR, Dalley AF, editors: Grant's atlas of anatomy, 11th ed. Philadelphia, Lippincott Williams & Wilkins, 2004, Fig. 1.49.*)

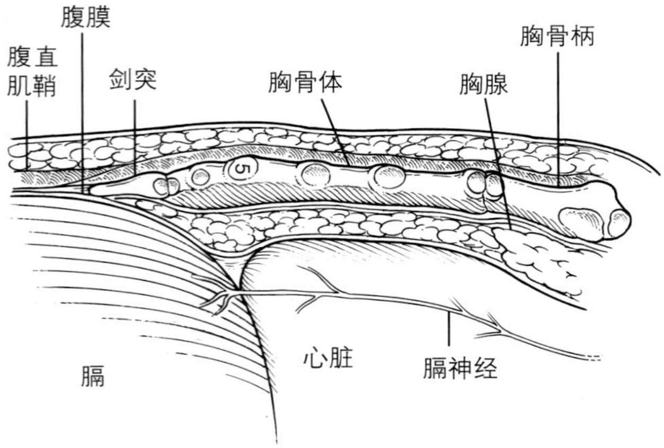

图 19 剑突下空间

冠状窦，这是心脏最大的静脉，从后方开口于右心房。房间沟的前方被升主动脉及肺动脉主干覆盖。房间沟可以在心脏右侧看到，是一条位于上腔静脉及右上肺静脉之间的富含脂肪的线样结构。室间沟在前面走向心间，其中包含了心大静脉。在后方，室间沟于心脏下方继续延续至心脏右侧缘，其中包含了心中静脉。

心脏有 5 个表面：前面、后面、下面、右侧面和左侧面。前面主要由右心室和右心房构成，因此任何来源于前方的外伤会导致这些结构的损伤。2/3 的右心房和右心室朝向前方。心脏的后面和基底面由左右心房组成。两个肺静脉分别从下面和上面两个方向汇入左心房的后壁。上腔静脉和下腔静脉注入右心房。心脏的后面贴附在第 6 至第 9 胸椎，两者之间的结构包括心包、右肺静脉、食管和主动脉（从右到左）。右心室的 1/3 和左心室的 2/3 构成心脏的下面或膈面。心脏的该部分与膈的中心部分接触。右心房和右心室形成心脏的右侧面。它们与心包、右肺和右膈前的右膈神经相邻。左心室和左心房形成左侧面。它们与右侧的相同结构毗邻，但有膈神经穿过表面中央。

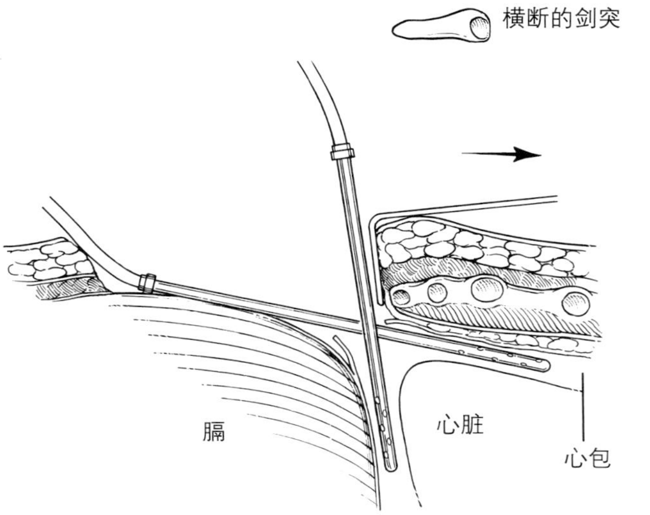

图 20　剑突下心包窗

冠状动脉与静脉

右冠状动脉和左冠状动脉起源于升主动脉。右冠状动脉供应右心房、右心室、室间隔的后 1/3，以及隔膜的下部。左冠状动脉供应左心房，左心室和室间隔的前 2/3。心脏中的侧支循环很少，因此一旦冠状动脉的闭塞会导致特定区域的心肌梗死和功能障碍（图 23）

冠状动脉分布于在心外膜下，心肌的浅面。靠近冠状动脉但侵犯动脉的裂伤可以用 Halsted 的未置入的水平褥式缝合修复，也可以使用置入的水平褥式缝合，置于冠状动脉床下，有效地修复心肌但不阻塞冠状动脉（图 24）。在放置和绑扎缝合线时应注意不要缝入过多的心肌而使冠状动脉扭结。如果左前降支动脉是须避开的血管，则可以用缝线闭塞血管深处的主要房间隔穿支血管。

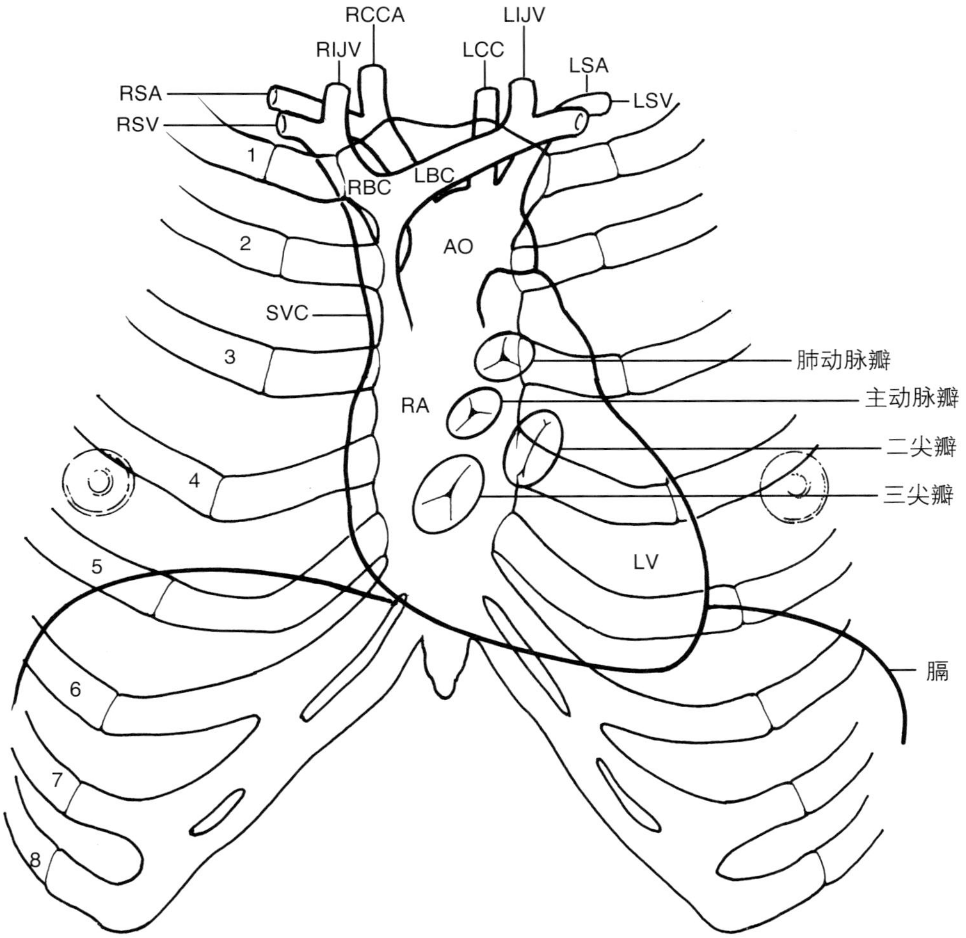

图 21　心脏和肺的体表投影。AO，主动脉；LBC，左头臂静脉；LCC，左颈总动脉；LIJV, 左颈内静脉；LSA，左锁骨下动脉；LSV，左锁骨下静脉；LV, 左心室；RA, 右心室；RBC，右头臂静脉；RCCA，右颈总动脉；RIJV, 右颈内静脉；RSA，右锁骨下动脉；RSV，右锁骨下静脉；SVC，上腔静脉 (*Modified from Gray H, editor: Gray's anatomy, 20th ed. Lea & Febiger, 1918, Plates 1216, 1218.*)

心脏的静脉系统以冠状窦为中心，冠状窦接收来自心脏不同区域的分支，并汇入右心房的后部，汇入部位在三尖瓣上方（图 22B）。

传导系统

窦房结是心脏的起搏器，位于上腔静脉开口处的右上方。脉搏通过心房壁传递到房室结。房室结位于冠状静脉窦开口以上的房间隔隔膜后下部。从

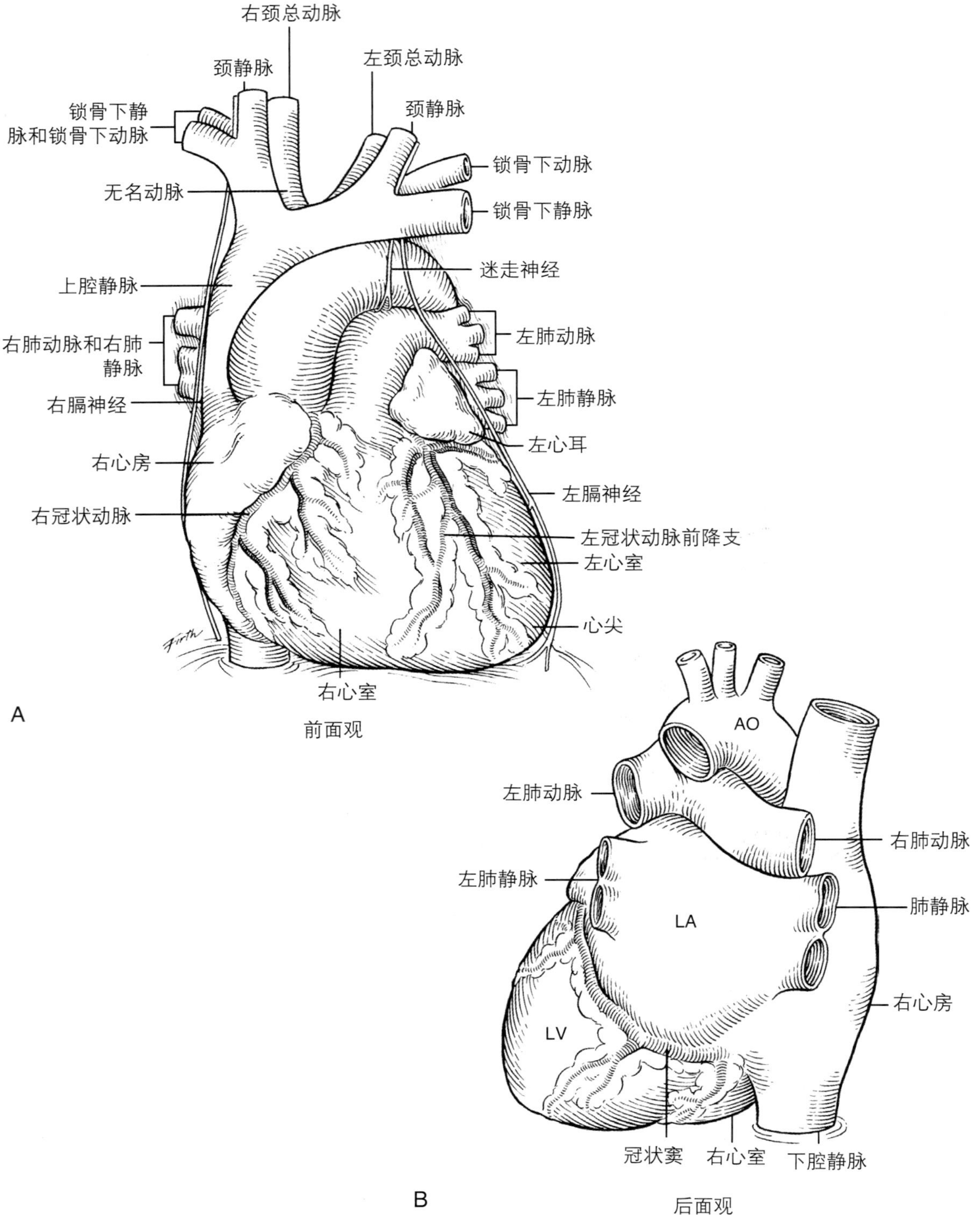

图 22 心脏。**A**，前面。**B**，后面。AO，主动脉；LA，左心房；LV，左心室 (*Modified from Gray's anatomy, 39th ed. Plate 970, and Fig. 60.2.*)

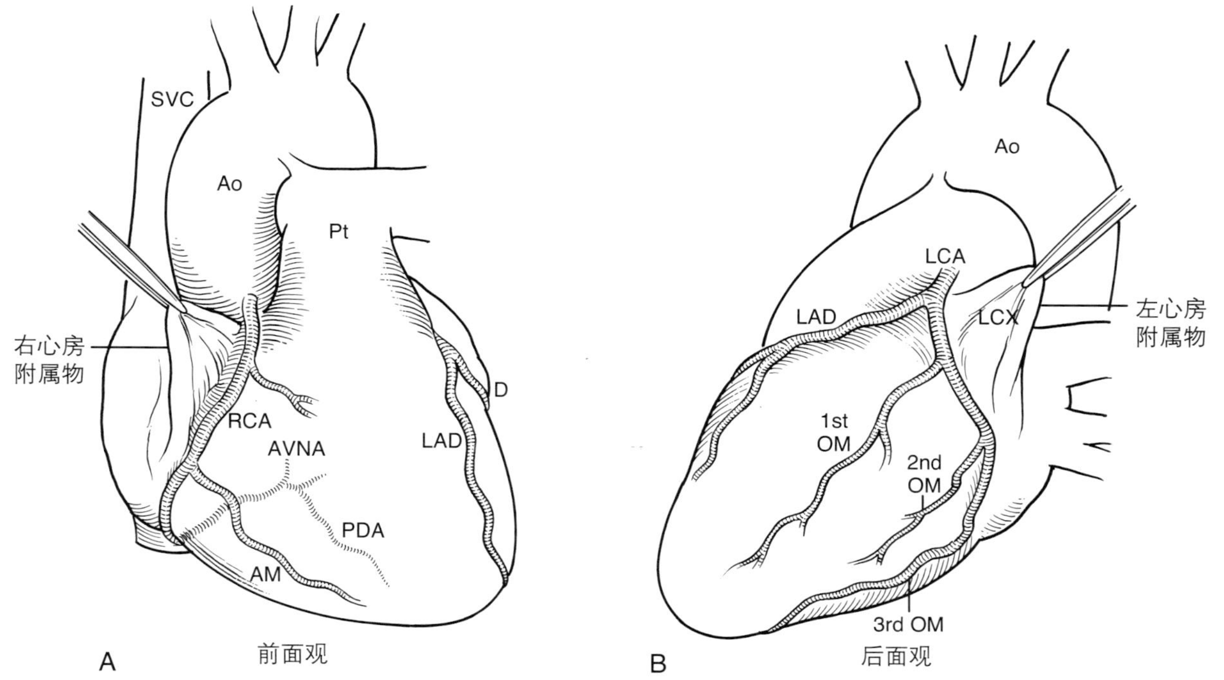

图 23　冠状动脉。**A,** 前面观。**B,** 后面观。AM, 右冠状动脉锐缘支；Ao, 主动脉；AVNA, 房室结动脉；D,LAD 对角支；LAD, 左前降支；LCA, 左冠状动脉；LCX, 左回旋支；OM,LCX 的钝缘支；PDA, 后降支；Pt, 肺动脉主干；RCA, 右冠状动脉；SVC, 上腔静脉

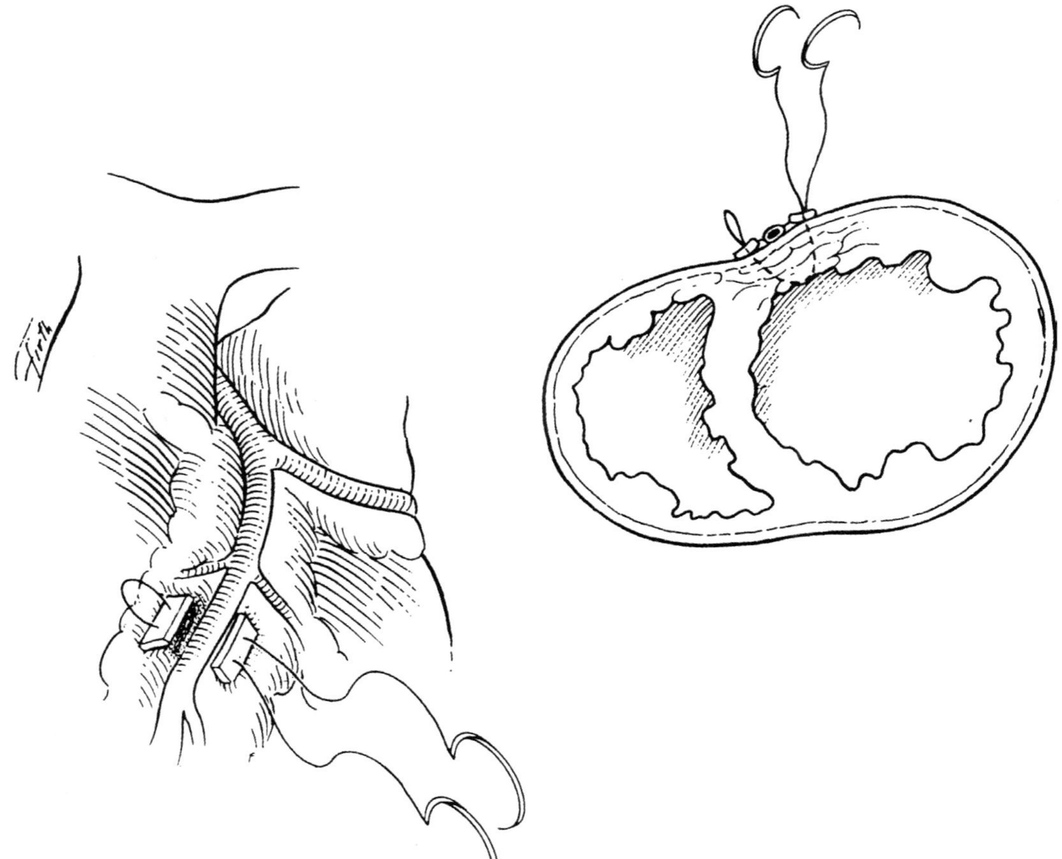

图 24　邻近冠状动脉心脏裂伤的修复

这里，冲动信号沿着希氏束（房室束）传导，从室间隔膜的后上缘传向左、右束支。这些冲动穿过室间隔到左心室和右心室的乳头肌，然后形成心内膜传导网（浦肯野纤维）（图 25）。

心脏腔内的结构

右心房内的后壁表面平滑，是腔静脉和冠状窦的开口。前壁布有小梁的肌肉。中后方是房间隔，其有一凹陷，称为卵圆窝，这标志着以前的卵圆孔或子宫内存在的心房之间的通道。前下方是通往右心室的三尖瓣开口。

右心室是三角形的，布满肌肉，具有来自三尖瓣的流入道和平滑的通向肺动脉瓣的流出道。

心室壁通过三（前、后、中隔）锥形突起支撑起乳头肌。每一个锥形的尖都发出腱索附着到三尖瓣的尖端。瓣膜任何部分的损伤都可能导致瓣膜的失效。中间斜向放置着分离两个心室的室间隔。

左心房呈四边形，壁面光滑。左心耳向左侧突出，是心房可以从前方看到的唯一部分。静脉的开口位于左侧和右侧。房间隔位于右侧和斜后方，使得左心房位于右心房后面。二尖瓣位于心房的前下部（图 30）。

左心室也是肌性结构，并且具有来自二尖瓣的流入道和通向主动脉根部的流出道。心室壁支撑起前后壁的乳头肌，其通过腱索附着于二尖瓣的前、后两个小叶（尖）。前小叶将二尖瓣孔的流入道与主动脉根部的流出道分开。因此主动脉瓣口位于二尖瓣前方。室间隔的位置偏向右前方（图 26）。

肺动脉和 Swan-Ganz 导管放置

肺动脉导管通常通过锁骨下静脉或颈内静脉引入，但也可以使用股静脉。导管通过这些静脉进入上腔静脉或下腔静脉，然后进入右心房。血液流动带动导管尖端通过三尖瓣孔进入右心室，然后通过右心室流出道和肺动脉瓣进入肺动脉。由于肺动脉主干上右肺动脉的方向，导管倾向于优先进入右侧，并暂停置于远端肺动脉中。

偶尔导管可能会穿过右心房而进入下腔静脉或

图 25　心脏传导系统。IVC，下腔静脉；SVC，上腔静脉 (*Modified from Gray H, editor: Gray's anatomy, 20th ed. Lea & Febiger, 1918, Plate 501.*)

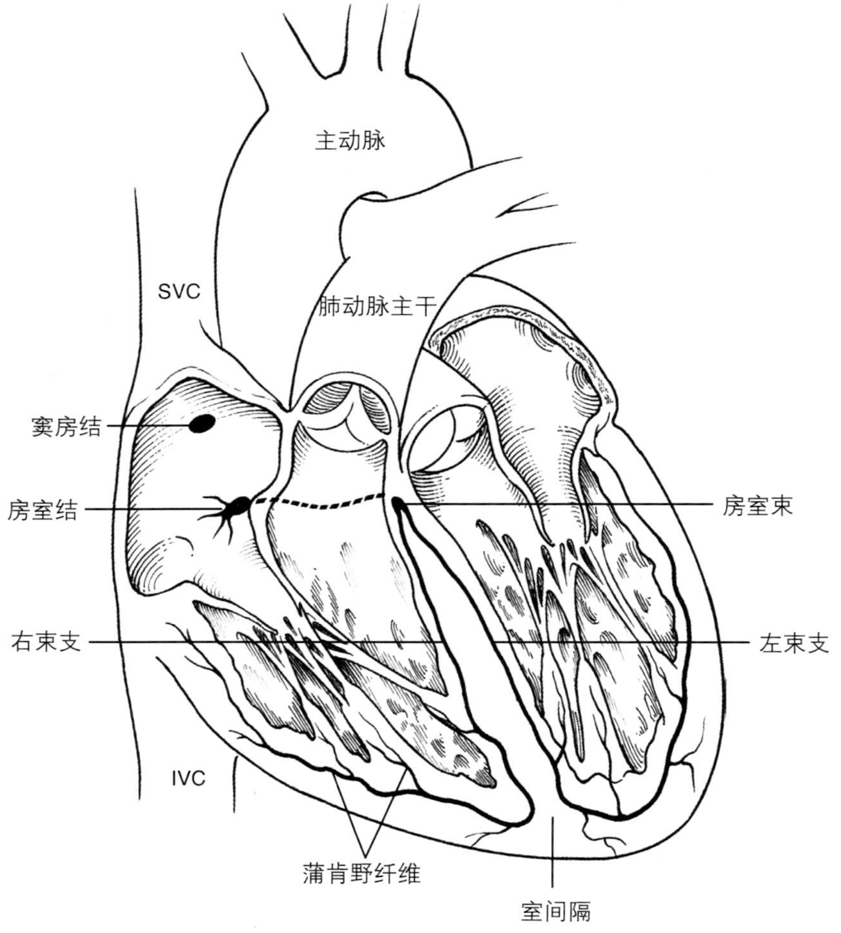

冠状窦。若进入冠状窦，我们可以立刻发现右侧心房踪迹的消失。在导管的长度合适的情况下，若导管在右心房内盘曲或进入下腔静脉，会出现持续的踪迹信号。

传统的肺动脉导管放置的指南包括指导导管的卷曲方向，使得其从上腔静脉进入心房并且被引导通过三尖瓣。导管线圈被盘成冠状面，因为三尖瓣在矢状平面上呈一个孔（图 27A）。然而，真实情况下三尖瓣位于矢状面偏转 40°～50° 的平面（图 27B）。仰卧位的患者，血液从右心房的右后位置经三尖瓣流向左侧。因此，导管的线圈尖端是朝向天花板偏转 40°～50°，而不是直面左壁。 然而，右心室流出道处于矢状面。 一旦压力跟踪表示导管的尖端位于右心室，则应逆时针旋转，使得线圈朝向左侧壁。

肺门

肺门是气道、肺动脉进入肺和肺静脉离开肺的场所。它是相对移动的肺与纵隔相连接的一个固定部位。脏器在胸膜上的移行也发生在肺门，增添了额外的支持。

很多胸外科手术是通过暴露使肺前部或后部回缩或直视肺门前后表面来完成的。两侧膈神经各自走行在两侧肺门的前方。在右侧（图 28），食管、迷走神经、胸导管和奇静脉走行在肺门后方。在左侧（图 29），降主动脉、食管、迷走神经走行在肺门后方。

右肺门

下肺韧带是右肺下叶内侧面脏层胸膜移行而成的结构，连接肺至纵隔。分离此韧带可以显露肺右下叶的视野，以便通过标准的第 5 肋间开胸手术进行检查及修复。分离此韧带时须尽可能地贴近肺组织，并且不损伤肺实质以避免损伤到其下方的胸导管、食管和迷走神经。下肺韧带最上方的结构是下肺静脉。这里可以看到心包膜的反折进入肺部。在下肺韧带顶部常可见一淋巴结位于下肺静脉旁。

在右肺门上方，奇静脉由后向前注入上腔静脉。奇静脉深部即是气管分叉处。走行在奇静脉前下方或内侧的是前方的右主支气管，走行在后下方或后内侧的是食管。右肺动脉主干在上腔静脉下方进入

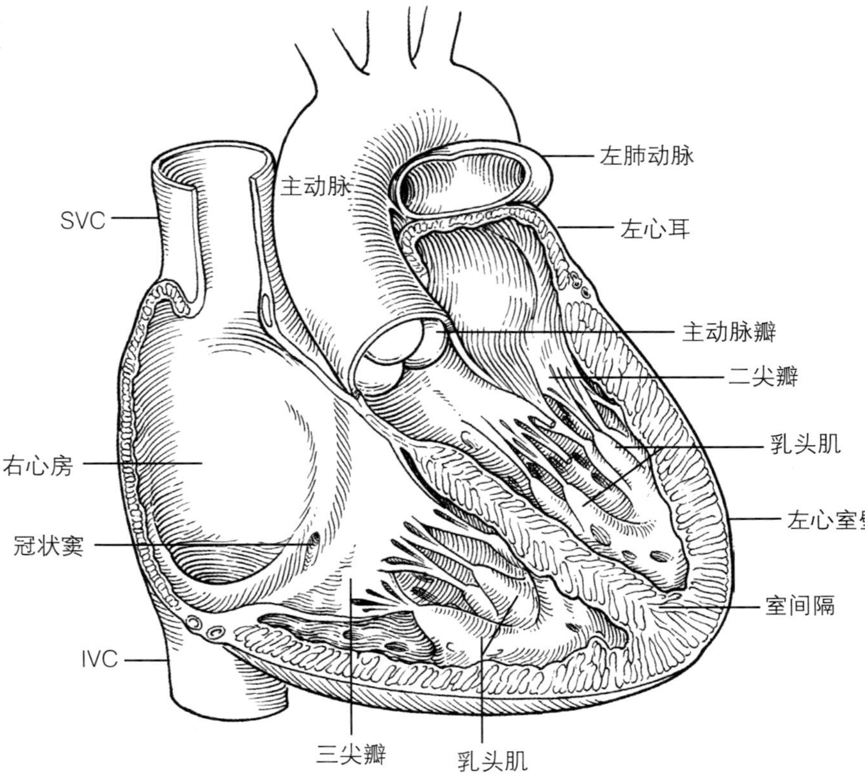

图 26　左心腔和右心腔解剖。IVC，下腔静脉；SVC，上腔静脉（*Modified from Gray H, editor: Gray's anatomy, 20th ed. Lea & Febiger, 1918, Plate 498.*）

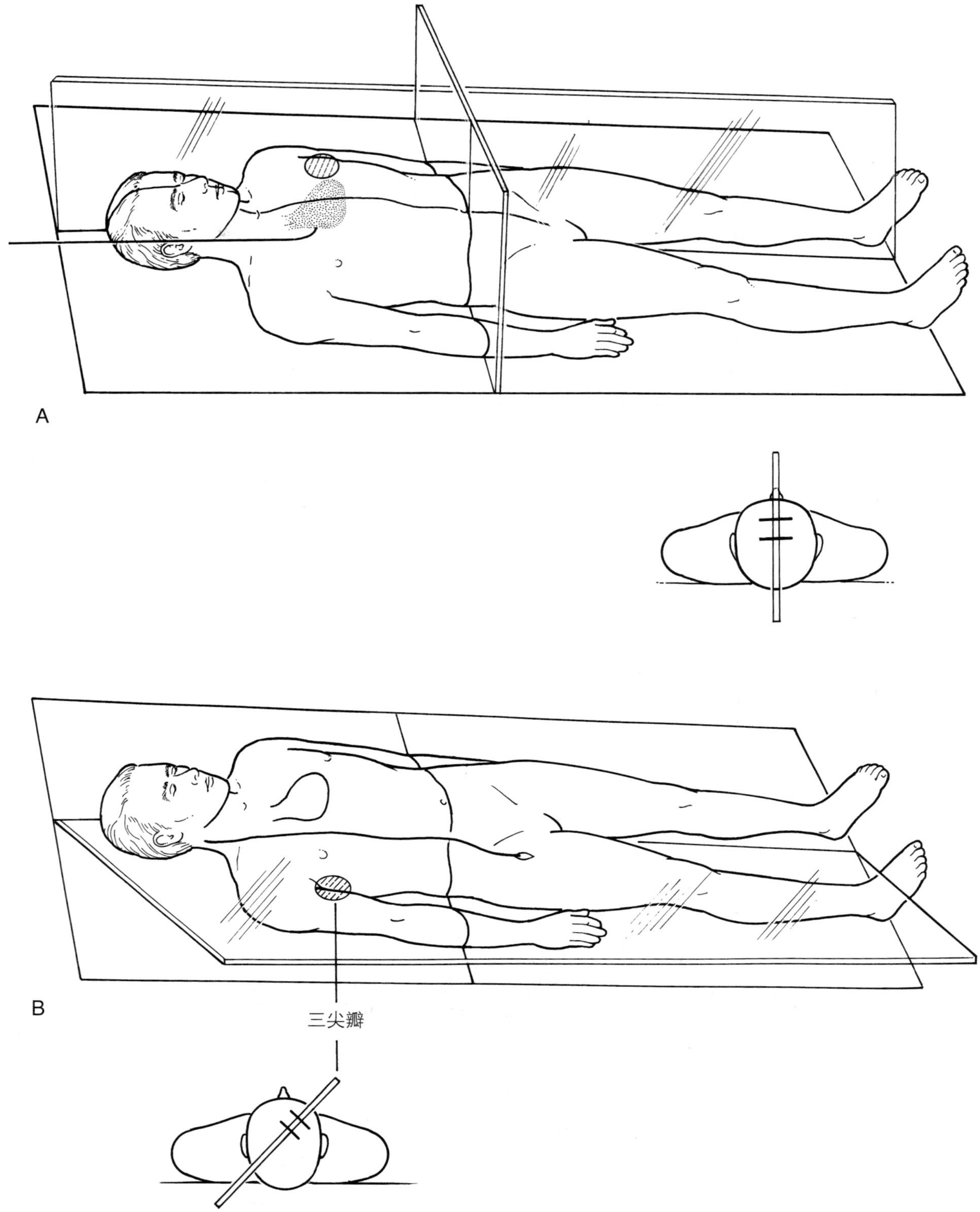

图 27　肺动脉导管的留置。**A,** 传统放置线圈的方法是沿冠状面朝向患者左侧，可认为三尖瓣是位于矢状面上的一个开口。**B,** 实际上三尖瓣是一与矢状面呈 40° ~ 50° 的开口，因此正确的置管方向应朝向天花板偏转 40° ~ 50°

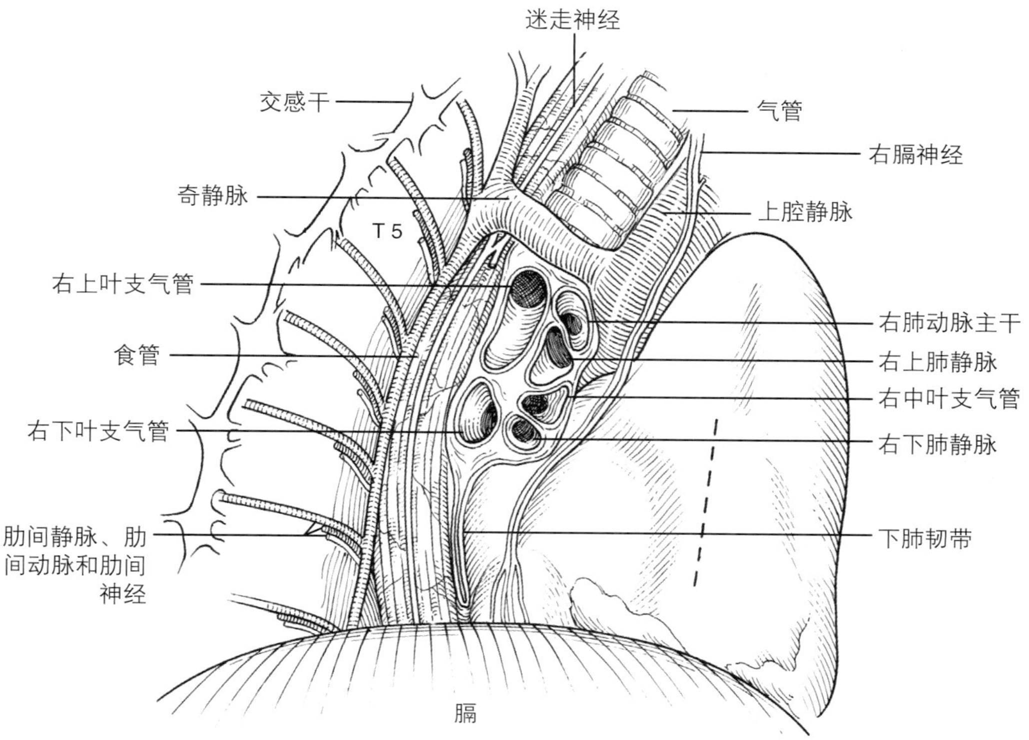

图 28　右肺门。虚线所示经右胸心包开窗切口。PA, 肺动脉；PV, 肺静脉；SVC, 上腔静脉 (*Modified from Agur AMR, Dalley AF, editors: Grant's atlas of anatomy, 11th ed. Philadelphia, Lippincott Williams & Wilkins, 2004, Fig. 1.43, p 40.*)

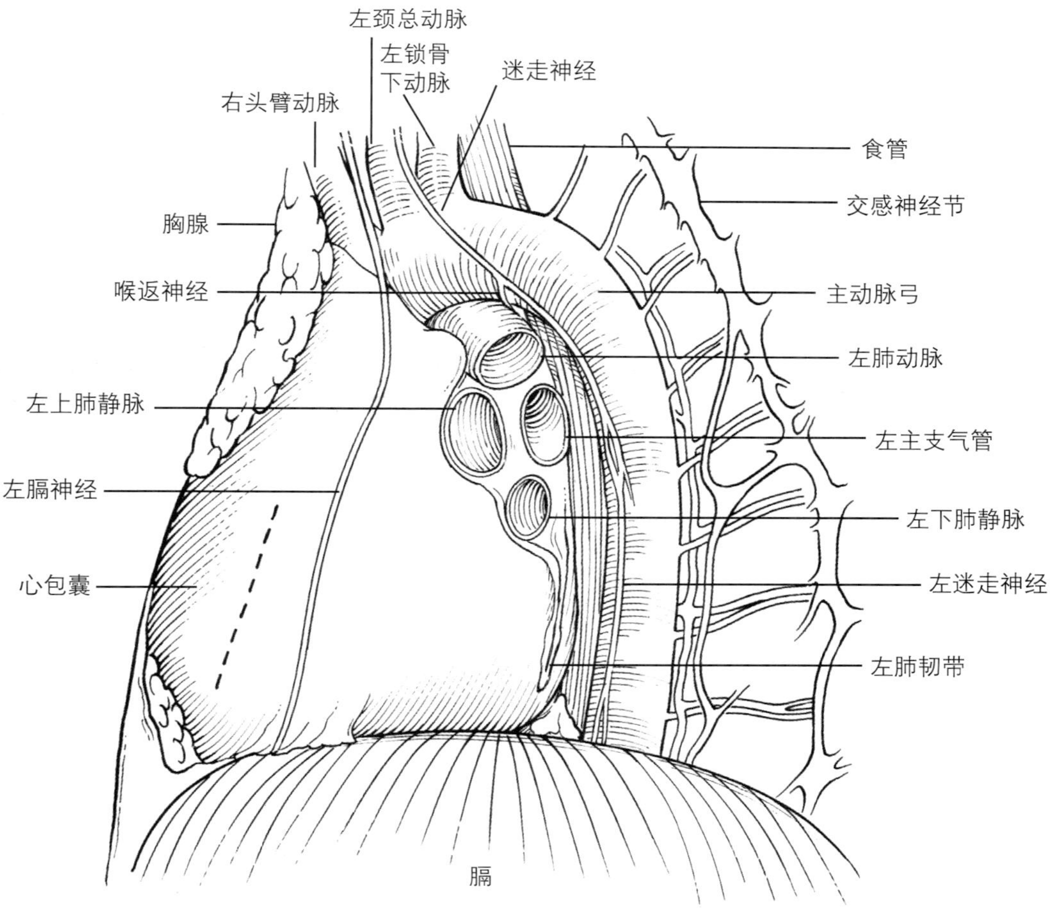

图 29　左肺门。虚线所示为心包开窗切口。PA，肺动脉；PV，肺静脉 (*Modified from Agur AMR, Dalley AF, editors: Grant's atlas of anatomy, 11th ed. Philadelphia, Lippincott Williams & Wilkins, 2004, Fig. 1.44, p 44.*)

胸腔右侧，走行在奇静脉下方、气管和右主支气管的前方。到达胸膜腔之前和在右肺动脉分支前，右肺动脉主干走行的距离长于左肺动脉主干。进入右侧胸腔后，肺动脉突然转折向下到达水平裂和斜裂的最深处，发出分支分别供应右肺上叶、中叶和下叶。须记住的是，肺动脉在肺内的分支就如同阔叶树的分支一样。肺门周围、水平裂和斜裂内可见较大的血管，越接近肺外表面，血管就越来越小（图 30）。右肺动脉主干的第一个分支走行进入右肺上叶。这个分支有可能从肺动脉的近心端分出，并从上腔静脉的下方穿过。此分支经常呈拱形跨过肺门上方，位于右肺上叶支气管的前方和奇静脉的下方。这个位置非常容易造成医源性牵拉损伤，尤其是大力牵拉肺组织下方时。

右肺动脉附近血管的控制可在其经过上腔静脉的下方时，用血管带包绕血管，小心钳夹（图 31）。如有必要，可非选择性钳夹整个肺门（图 32）。一次非选择性钳夹常被指为“流氓”钳夹，因为钳夹是为了及时控制出血的血管，但这种钳夹方法会累及到很多出血血管外的正常结构。

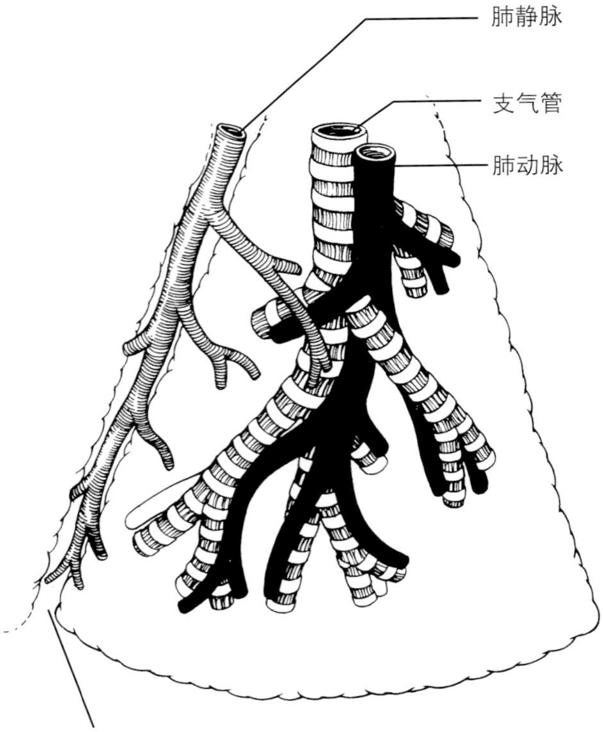

图 30 支气管肺段 (*From Pearson FG, editor: Thoracic surgery, 2nd ed. Philadelphia, Churchill Livingstone, 2002, Fig. 20-1, p 428.*)

在胸腔右侧或胸骨正中切开术中，上腔静脉和下腔静脉可以在心包内钳夹处理。这被称为入路阻断或 Shumacker 法，可造成心搏停顿，耐受时间不超过 3 ~ 5 min。在危急时刻如肺动脉主干或分支大出血时，这种方法为术者创造了时间和视野去控制出血血管。一旦出血被控制住，应在造成不可逆的心脏损害前立即使血液回流至心脏。应提前做好心脏复律的准备，若心脏已有纤维颤动，心脏复律则非常必要。

构成右侧肺门的剩余血管结构是上肺静脉。上肺静脉可在前方被观察到，发出一条向上的分支到达右肺上叶。这条分支在水平裂中走行，在肺动脉前方与之交叉，并向右肺中叶发出多个分支。

在右肺门的后上方可观察到右主支气管。右主支气管是气管隆嵴的分支，走行在奇静脉的下方。从肺门后方观察支气管时，可在任意一侧观察并触及到拱形支气管软骨和气管膜部。

左肺门

与右肺一样，左下肺叶也通过左下肺韧带与纵隔相连。左下肺韧带的最上方是左下肺静脉，韧带中常有一个淋巴结，在此静脉下方。左肺门的上部是从右向左、从前向后交叉走行的主动脉弓。左肺门最上方的结构是左肺动脉，其较右肺动脉主干短。它的第一个分支通向左肺上叶，常常走行在肺实质内侧。此分支在向下牵拉肺时易损伤。左迷走神经在胸腔左侧、左锁骨下动脉前方向下走行，与主动脉弓侧面交叉，跨过降主动脉的前方，并与位置更居中的食管相伴下行。在主动脉弓的下方，左迷走神经发出左喉返神经，其在动脉韧带周围及食管旁下行，在气管食管沟之间向上走行返回颈部支配喉。动脉韧带即为退化的动脉导管，它连接在肺动脉主干分支顶端至主动脉弓之间，为已纤维化或钙化的组织。它在胸腔左侧可见，提示了肺动脉主干分支与左肺门的相邻关系。在此区域内尽量少使用电刀等设备，尽可能靠近肺动脉并远离主动脉和动脉韧带进行解剖分离操作，这样可避免损伤喉返神经。左肺动脉的近端控制可以通过应用血管钳或肺门钳钳夹肺动脉完成。由于左肺动脉非常短，为了不损伤到膈神经，常须在左肺动脉主干前方切开心包。随后，肺动脉主干和在心包内走行的左肺动脉主干就可被观察到、左主肺动脉的钳夹也可完成。如果放置血管钳后血管立即塌陷可能暗示右肺动脉的血

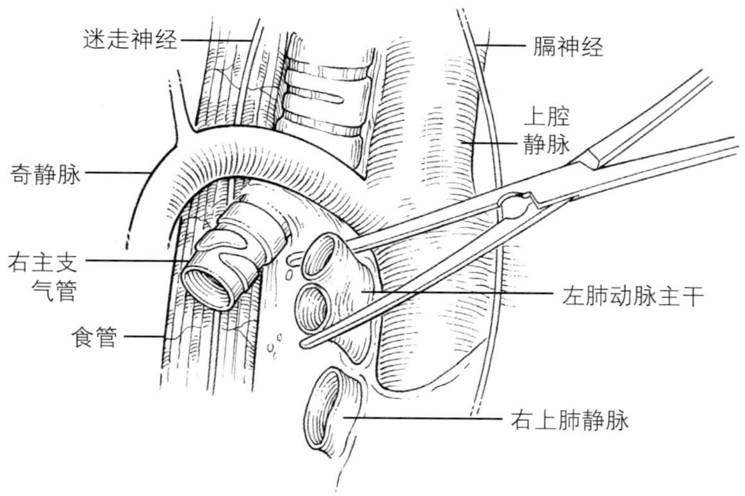

图 31 钳夹上腔静脉下方的右肺动脉主干。PV，肺静脉

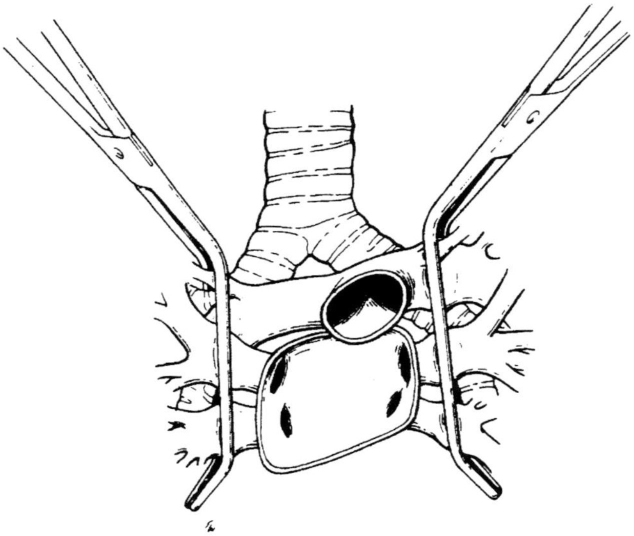

图 32 “流氓”钳夹阻断左侧或右侧肺门 (*From Pearson FG, editor: Thoracic surgery, 2nd ed. Philadelphia, Churchill Livingstone, 2002, Fig. 68-3, p 1837.*)

流也闭塞，此时须重新放置血管钳。左心耳在此位置也可见，它是一个移动的组织，且常对手术操作造成干扰。左心耳在钳夹和回缩等操作中极易发生损伤、出血和空气栓塞，因此应对其谨慎处理。

左肺动脉进入胸腔后立刻转行，并在斜裂的最深处向下走行。像右上肺静脉一样，左上肺静脉仅在前方可见，可以被看作心包进入肺的地方。左主支气管虽然很长，却被主动脉和主肺动脉所遮挡。当没有很好地在后方切开腔壁的反折和脏层胸膜、暴露左主支气管和食管之间的平面，这个结构几乎是完全看不见的。

为达到血管控制的目的，左肺门同样可以被非选择性地钳夹。

肺部解剖

右肺有 3 个肺叶，右肺上叶、右肺中叶和右肺下叶。左肺有 2 个肺叶，左肺上叶和左肺下叶。左肺上叶小舌与右肺中叶类似。肺裂通常存在，但其完整性多变。在右肺，水平裂通常不完整，起自斜裂的后部，将右肺上叶和中叶分开。斜裂将右肺上叶和和右肺下叶的上部分开，并将右肺中叶和右肺下叶分开。右肺下叶位于膈后方，右肺中叶通常位于膈前方，在此位置常被误认为右肺下叶。在左肺，斜裂将左肺分为上、下两叶。左肺下叶位于膈后方。左肺上叶舌段常可向下延伸到膈前方。

图 33 所示为肺段。肺动脉和支气管分别进入相对应的肺段中间，并向外周发出分支。肺静脉在肺段之间的边界区域和沿着水平裂、斜裂的方向走行（图 30）。

主动脉、气管、食管和胸导管

在心脏后方、心包外侧，几个管状结构彼此平行走行，分别是主动脉、气管、食管和胸导管。

主动脉

胸主动脉起自心脏纤维三角的主动脉瓣处。冠状动脉起自主动脉窦，并立即向远离主动脉瓣的方向走行。左冠状动脉通常起自主动脉左窦，位于心脏后方并朝向肺动脉瓣。用 Valsalva 手法发现右冠状动脉起自主动脉右窦，位于心脏前方并向右走行。

可在右冠状动脉自主动脉起始处观察到其从左向右走行穿过右心室前壁。升主动脉很短，结束于主动脉弓处。主动脉大多从前向后弓形弯曲，自中线稍向左运动，恰好沿左侧胸腔内脊柱的左边下行。主动脉弓的顶端由近端到远端、由前向后发出 3 大分支：右头臂动脉、左颈总动脉和左锁骨下动脉。右迷走神经从右头臂动脉前方交叉后下行，并在交叉处向后发出一分支，为右喉返神经，其在右气管食管沟之间向上走行返回颈部。在主动脉弓的下方，动脉韧带连接在主动脉和肺动脉主干之间。上述主动脉弓的三大分支和动脉韧带一同将主动脉弓固定在胸腔内。降主动脉是相对移动的。在左锁骨下动脉远端的主动脉是相对固定和移动的移行区，也是主动脉加速 / 减速损伤的好发部位。降主动脉向胸壁发出多个节段分支，为肋间动脉，同时也向食管、气管、气管隆嵴、近端支气管发出分支。主动脉从 T11 ~ T12 水平的膈主动脉裂孔处下行进入腹腔。T8 至 L2 之间，但通常在 L2 附近处，是脊髓前根动脉（Adamkiewicz 动脉）起源的部位。它是一条大的节段动脉，在左侧最常见，与脊髓前动脉相吻合，并供应脊髓 2/3 的血流量。因此夹闭该血管附近的主动脉可能会引起脊髓缺血。

气管

气管在颈部起自环状软骨，在食管前方，主动脉弓、升主动脉和肺动脉的后方下行进入胸腔。在远端气管隆嵴旁，主动脉弓与气管的左侧相交叉。气管在气管隆嵴处分叉形成右主支气管和左主支气管。气管隆嵴在胸骨角水平，后方是 T4-T5。成年人气管平均长度为 11 cm，并随身高的不同而不同。一个年轻人可以通过颈部向后过伸使 50% 的气管从胸腔进入颈部。相反，一个脊柱后凸的老年人，环状软骨可以在胸骨切迹水平。在颈部，气管位于皮下前方。当其进入胸腔时，它斜向后走行到达后纵隔。一点到一条线的最短距离是过该点与该线相交的垂线。如果把气管看做一条斜向后的直线，那么从皮肤上一点到气管的最短距离是一条稍靠上方的线。了解这种解剖关系有助于选择气管造口术和甲状腺切除术的切口（图 34）。气管前壁由气管软骨构成，其间有很多结缔组织。气管后壁是膜性组织。气管的血供是节段性分布的，气管上部血供主要来自甲状腺下动脉，气管下部血供主要来自支气管动脉。锁骨下动脉、最上肋间动脉、胸廓内动脉和无名动脉也为气管提供血供。上述这些血管同样也供

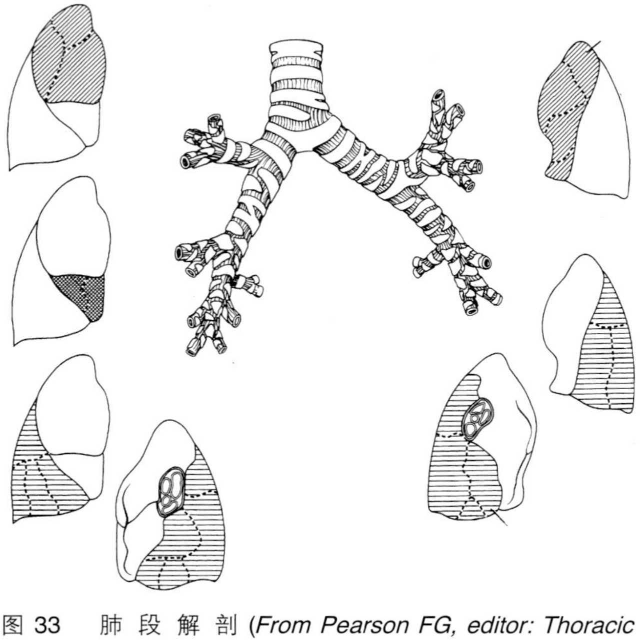

图 33 肺段解剖 (*From Pearson FG, editor: Thoracic surgery, 2nd ed. Philadelphia, Churchill Livingstone, 2002, Fig. 20-2, p428.*)

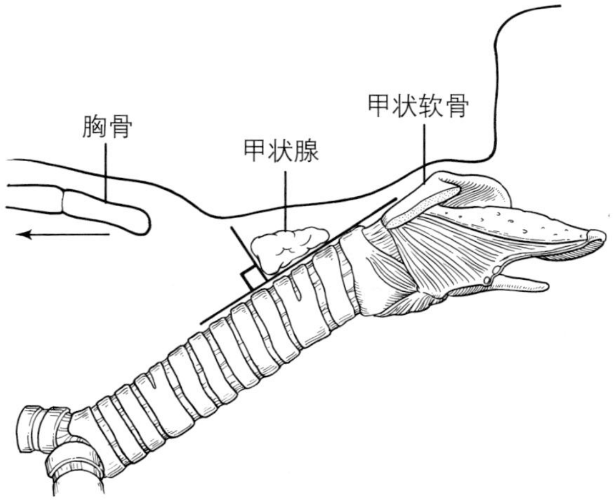

图 34 气管向后方走行离开颈部进入胸部。某点与某线之间最短距离是经过该点与线的垂直距离

应食管的血供。这些血管在 3 点至 9 点方向进入气管外侧。

食管

食管下行穿过后纵隔，走行在椎体前方、降主动脉的右侧和奇静脉的左侧。降主动脉发出节段性的分支供应食管，食管的静脉汇入肋间静脉。在气管隆嵴上方，食管位于并紧贴气管后方。在动脉韧带水平以上，左喉返神经在左侧气管食管沟之间走行。在右头臂动脉水平以上，右喉返神经在右侧气管食管沟之间走行。在气管隆嵴下方，食管紧贴在心包后方。从左到右、从上到下分别有上肺静脉、下肺静脉和下肺韧带。食管在 T10 — T11 水平通过食管裂孔进入膈。在下肺韧带水平和其下方的、进入膈之间的食管的左右区域是一个解剖学的弱点。在此处，食管壁并没有被其他牢固的纵隔结构所支撑，而是暴露于胸膜腔的负压之下。这就是此处最常发生因食管内压增大而导致穿孔（Boerhaave 综合征）的原因。

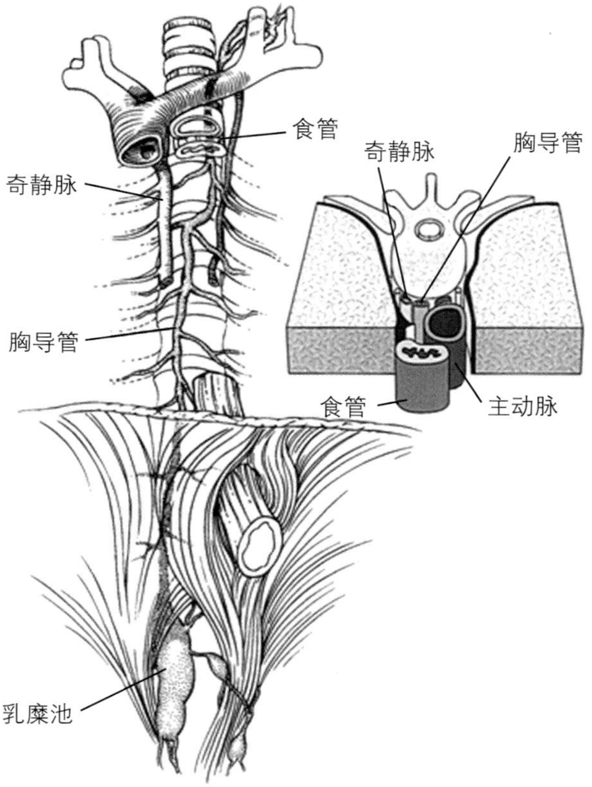

图 35 胸导管 (*From Pearson FG, editor: Thoracic surgery, 2nd ed. Philadelphia, Churchill Livingstone, 2002, Fig. 20-7, p 431.*)

胸导管

胸导管起自乳糜池（图 35）。乳糜池位于腹腔内椎体的前方、主动脉的右侧，在腹腔干水平。胸导管向上走行，在膈处穿过主动脉裂孔进入胸腔。它在后纵隔主动脉和奇静脉之间上行。在主动脉弓上方，胸导管在食管后方走行，在颈内静脉后方形成弓状弯曲，并在颈内静脉和锁骨下静脉交界处注入静脉系统。胸导管管壁很薄，如果没有被淋巴液充盈，肉眼常不可见。胸导管损伤时常可在损伤部位附近观察到淋巴液的漏出。运送至小肠的脂肪在 10 ~ 20 min 内可将淋巴液转变为乳白色，因此变得易于观察。胸导管结扎术要将疑似漏出部位以下所有被 4 个壁包围的脂肪组织和淋巴管全部结扎包括奇静脉、壁层胸膜、食管、主动脉。

胸壁损伤：肋骨、胸骨和肩胛骨骨折；血胸和气胸

David H. Livingston, Carl Hauser, Noelle Salliant, 和 Devashish J. Anjaria 著
刘敢伟 译

尽管许多胸部损伤可能是致命性的，挖掘出的尼安德塔人的骨骼显示了钝伤和穿通伤导致的肋骨骨折被治愈的证据。Edwin Smith 纸莎草在大约公元前 3000 年就详细描述了一些胸部损伤的处理方法，包括软组织损伤和骨损伤。事实上，43 个病例中有 8 个是关于胸部损伤的，表明即使在当时，胸部损伤就占全部创伤的 20 ~ 25%。

胸壁创伤和独立或作为多系统创伤一部分的肺组织损伤仍然很常见，是导致创伤和死亡的常见原因。血胸和气胸虽然理论上没有伤及胸壁，但它们常与上述损伤合并发生，也将被考虑在内。此处仅简要提及连枷胸和其伴随的肺挫伤，在其他章节（肺挫伤和连枷胸）会有详细的介绍。

发病率

胸部损伤仍然很常见，由其导致的死亡直接占全部创伤死亡的20%～25%。胸部损伤通常伴有其他类型损伤，并可使多发伤患者发生器官衰竭。其中肋骨骨折是最常见的损伤形式。一个Ⅰ级创伤中心对7 000名患者的回顾研究所示，肋骨骨折患者占据10%，其中94%合并其他损伤，死亡率为12%。一半肋骨骨折患者需要手术或ICU治疗，1/3患者发生并发症，另有1/3患者最终须在门诊进行简易护理。

气胸和血胸在送往创伤中心的患者中发现率相当，超过20%。使用X线平片可能会低估气胸和血胸的发病率。胸部CT相比于传统仰卧位前后位胸部X线检查气胸和血胸有较大的优势。

锁骨骨折是除了肋骨骨折外最常见的骨折形式，在所有骨折中占5%～10%。胸骨和肩胛骨骨折的发生相对较少（发病率分别为0.5%～4%和0.8%～3%），比锁骨骨折更易合并其他损伤。此外，胸部CT广泛的应用导致更多的肩胛骨和胸骨无移位性骨折被发现。完全的肩胸分离伤比较罕见，但会合并严重的神经血管损伤，属于重型损伤。

损伤机制

胸壁损伤在严重程度上差异很大。常规急诊室处理的胸部创伤多由低能量损伤所致，严重程度相对较轻。相反，在创伤中心治疗的由于机动车碰撞所致的高能量创伤患者常常病情严重且危及生命。成年人胸壁损伤和肋骨骨折最常见的原因是机动车车祸，常由于跌落、胸部直接撞击在钝性物品上导致创伤。须被提及的是，婴幼儿肋骨骨折几乎全部都是由儿童虐待导致。老年人受伤的主要机制是跌倒和被机动车撞伤。

肋骨骨折通常是严重钝性胸部创伤的标志，骨折肋骨数量的增加与发病率和死亡率的增加有关。在成年人X线胸片上发现多于3个肋骨骨折与实质脏器的创伤和高死亡率有关，因此它被作为转运至创伤中心的一个标准。在血流动力学稳定的患者中，存在钝性胸部创伤的患者的发生约为腹部CT检测出腹内损伤患者发生率的2倍。因为儿童骨性胸壁的弹性较好，所以儿童较少发生肋骨骨折。因此，一般情况下儿童可能遭受大的胸腔内损伤却不伴有肋骨骨折，但若发生肋骨骨折通常提示胸部创伤很严重。若儿童发生急性肋骨骨折的原因不明或在不同年龄段发现肋骨骨折，也提示儿童虐待的可能。相反，老年人因骨质较脆，即使发生大范围肋骨骨折，也很少累及胸腔内的损伤。

不同的损伤机制提供了不同的损伤模式。胸部穿通伤导致肺实质撕裂，会造成血胸。胸部伤常为移位的肋骨损伤引起，并可导致血气胸和肺挫伤。胸部钝伤后发生血气胸的机制如下：①胸腔内压突然升高导致肺泡破裂，空气漏出；②因骨折而移位的肋骨使肺组织撕裂；③减速伤导致肺组织的撕裂；④直接对胸部的挤压伤。

诊断

体格检查

快速地对胸部视诊和触诊检查将提供患者受伤的很多信息（图1）。因为创伤急诊科噪音较大，叩诊和听诊检查常常不可靠。低血压、心动过速、面色苍白或发绀提示患者处于休克状态。在已知或可疑有胸部损伤的情况下，必须考虑休克来源于胸腔内。胸部视诊应该包括对提示气道梗阻附属肌肉、胸壁的对称度、伤口的数量和部位、开放性胸部伤口、皮下气肿和连枷胸的评估。颈部气管的偏移常被作为张力性气胸的征兆，但事实上很少见到，即使X线胸片显示有纵隔偏移的患者也是如此。触诊

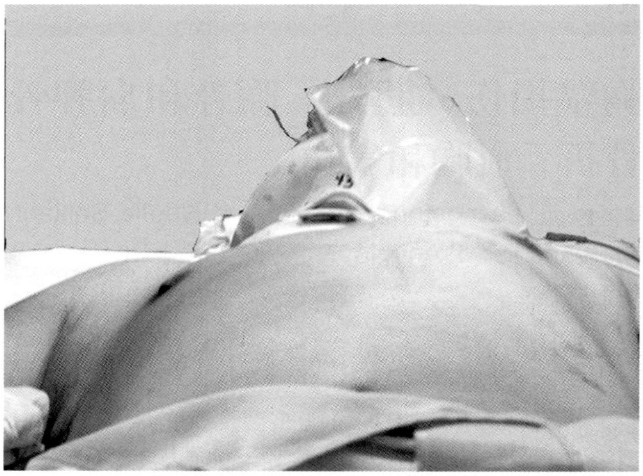

图1 对一机动车驾驶员查体显示左、右两侧胸部不对称.

可以显示胸壁的运动，进一步感受胸壁运动的对称性和捻发感。对创伤患者的听诊特异度很好，但灵敏度差，因此应仅将重点放在能否匀称地吸入空气上。心音（如 Beck 三联征中含混的心音或 Hamman 征中的“纵隔摩擦音”）同样很难在急诊室被清晰地听到。然而，不对称或消失的呼吸音对重大的创伤有着提示意义。在不稳定的患者中，它是临床理论干预的适应证，也是进行影像学检查的禁忌证。胸部叩诊在创伤患者中应用极少，因为它比听诊更难反映患者的伤情。

体格检查经常但不总能显示血气胸的存在。在对血流动力学不稳定的患者进行体格检查时应怀疑是否存在血胸。对伤侧呼吸音极度减弱或消失的患者，应尽快做出临床诊断。呼吸音可从对侧（健侧）肺传导而来，从而掩盖听诊结果。在钝伤或距穿通伤一定距离处发现皮下气肿是需治疗的气胸存在的充分证据。当然，开放性气胸在体格检查中极易发现。一旦确诊血胸或气胸，就应放置胸导管排出血液或空气。

影像学研究

仰卧后 AP X 线胸片检查是最初被应用，有时也是处理胸部创伤最重要的检查。由于患者身体原因、仰卧位、脊柱固定架的存在或便携式 X 线机器的应用，拍摄出的 X 线片经常达不到最佳标准。因此创伤科医生必须很好地辨认并合理解释这些 X 线片。然后便携式 X 线胸片具有很高的阳性预测值（例如 X 线片上的结果通常有很大意义，可以诊断或排除一些危及生命的损伤）。这种 X 线片必须在患者被运送去做其他影像学检查或手术操作前被拍摄并被评估。

胸部 X 线的解读应从肺实质和胸膜的评估开始。肺扩张、肺浸润或挫伤、气管内导管的位置（如果存在）和血胸或气胸的存在应被包括其中。应评估纵隔以查看有无大血管的损伤，纵隔扩大、主动脉结变钝、顶端封闭胸、左主支气管或鼻胃管向内侧移位均提示有大血管损伤。还应注意膈有无升高或损伤。最后，应关注有无骨性胸廓——肋骨、锁骨、肩胛骨的骨折。胸椎是否竖直也可在胸部 X 线片上被评估，但脊柱的全部影像学检查和骨性胸廓结构的特殊位置的 X 线检查应在患者气道、呼吸和心血管状态稳定的情况下完成。

X 线检查对诊断血胸和气胸极为有用。诊断常在第 2 次检查时在便携式 AP 胸部 X 线检查基础上完成。在卧位时的正位胸部 X 线检查仅在胸膜腔积血达到 200 ~ 300 ml 以上时才会显示血胸征象——与健侧对比浑浊或不透明，因为液体向后坠积（图 2）。不过当发生双侧血胸（两侧无差别）或一侧血胸、另一侧同时发生气胸（相对密度减低与对侧相似）时，X 线片会出现假阴性结果。患者发生穿通性胸部创伤时，最好在直立位拍摄 X 线片，以增加血胸和气胸检出的灵敏度。胸部超声可以帮助检出胸腔积液，但灵敏度和特异度尚未明确。

随着躯干（胸部、腹部和盆腔）CT 扫描的应用越来越普遍，许多在 X 线平片检查中先前未显示明显气胸的钝伤患者在 CT 检查中存在气胸。前后位胸部 X 片对气胸的漏诊率约有 20% ~ 35%。尽管患者有呼吸困难和缺氧表现，他的 X 线胸片结果可能仅显示相对较小的气胸。因此这类气胸应行胸部 CT 检查，可以明显地被检出。在稳定的患者中，CT 扫描同样可以显示胸腔积液，并有助于将它们和肺实质损伤如肺挫伤区分开。

对于仅被 CT 检测出气胸的患者，如何正确处理是有争议的（图 3）。据报道，在钝伤的患者中此

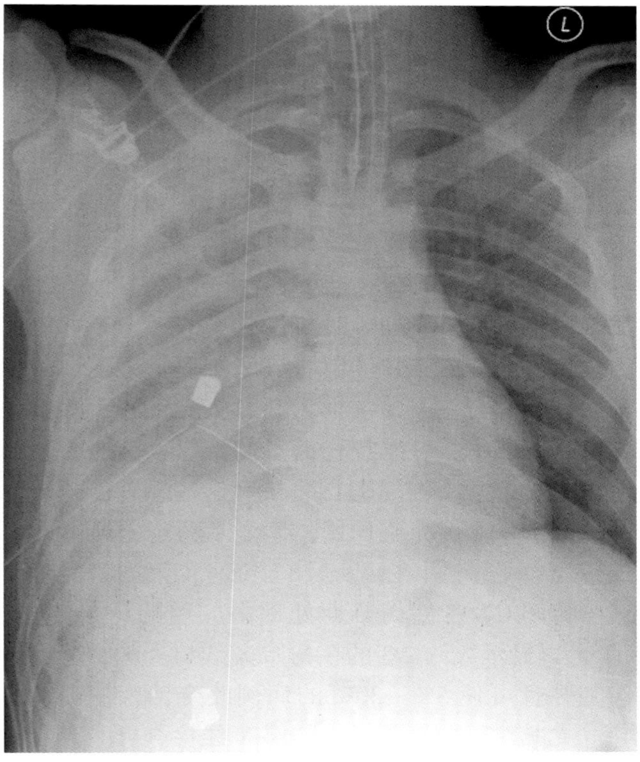

图 2 卧位 X 线胸片显示大片模糊影，诊断为右侧血胸（本病例中胸廓造口术引流不充分）。注意左右两侧的差别

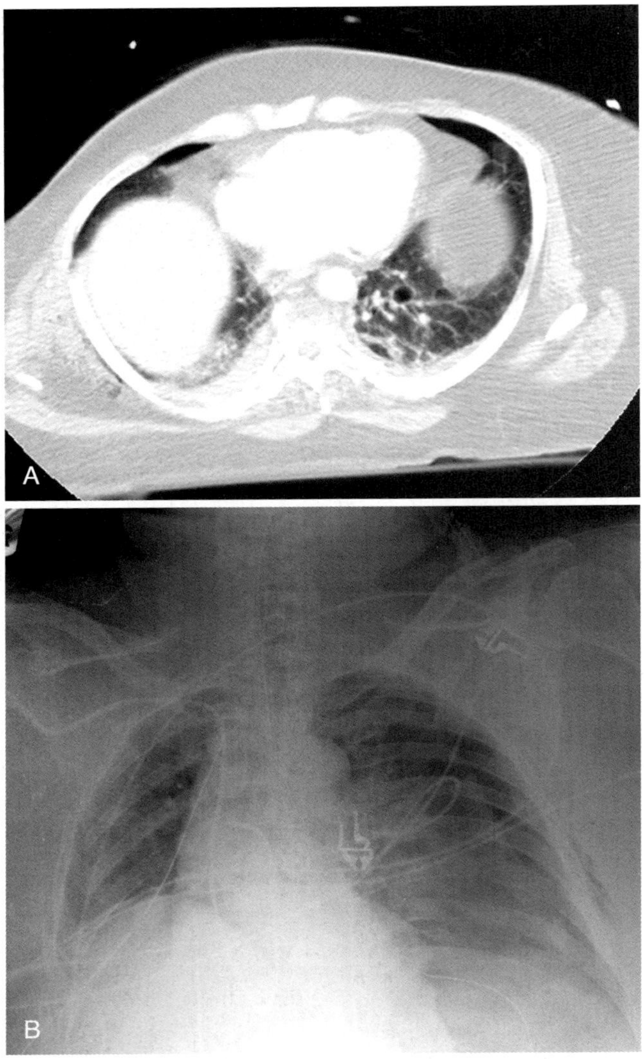

图 3 计算机断层扫描 (CT)(A)，显示两侧“仅 CT”可见的小的气胸 (B)，后续机械通气。左侧大量气胸，显示小的气胸可引起不可预测的结果。该患者右侧始终未发生气胸

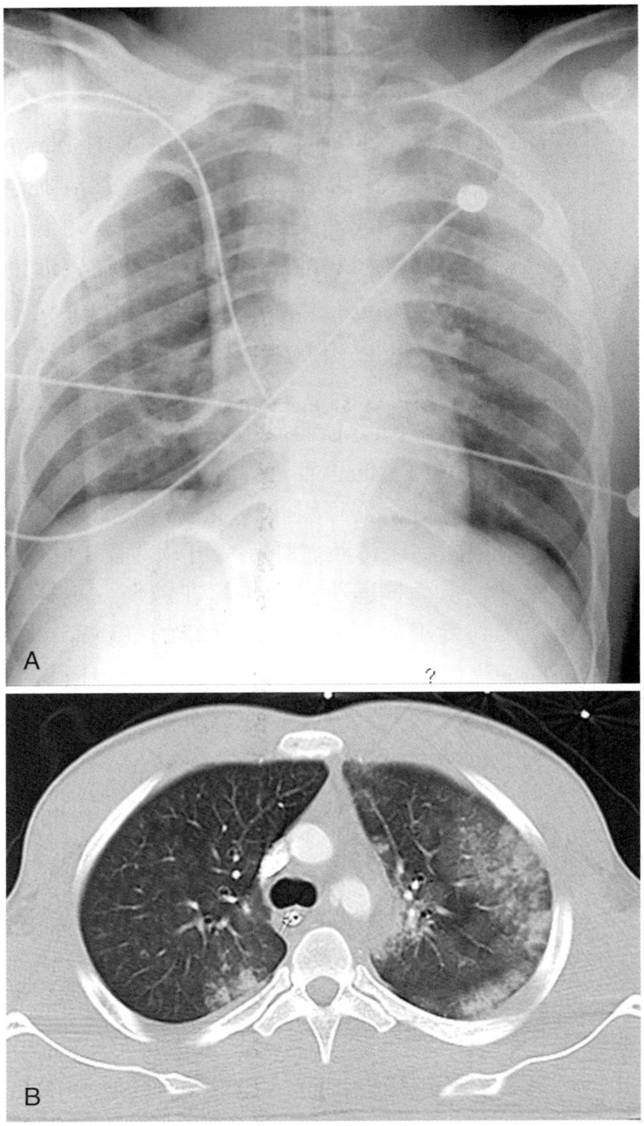

图 4 从高速行驶的汽车中弹出的患者的 X 线胸片 (A)。肺野透亮度基本正常，但是纵隔轮廓不正常。CT 显示 (B) 该患者肺挫伤严重，解释该患者临床上有缺氧表现。此外，可见降主动脉有损伤

类气胸的发生率为 2%～8%。相关文献表明，20% 的患者需要胸廓造口术置管。然而，是否进行胸腔置管应以患者全身情况作为参考。对于处于出血性休克状态或持续性脑损伤的多发伤患者，他们甚至无法耐受一个小的气胸（图 3）。这些患者可获益于胸廓造口术。对于临床影像学显示稳定的患者，应进行持续观察，并在诊断后 6 h 和 24 h 连续摄片检查。

胸部 CT 在创伤早期处理中应用的越来越多。CT 可以显示大约 2/3 的在初始 X 线检查为阴性的损伤，并且可使 5%～30% 的病例改变治疗策略（图 4）。尤其对于肋骨骨折，胸部 X 线检查可能会漏诊大于 50% 的 CT 阳性的肋骨骨折。若初始进行 X 线胸片检查显示肋骨骨折，CT 常会在此基础上额外多发现平均 2 处肋骨骨折。尽管 CT 增加了检出肋骨骨折和肺挫伤的灵敏度，肺部疾病发生率（肺炎、呼吸衰竭）和死亡风险仅受胸部 X 线检查发现的肋骨骨折和肺挫伤的影响，提示 CT 增加的灵敏度不一定有临床意义。

此外，CT 扫描能显示胸部 X 线不明确的额外发现（图 5）。在一些特殊情况下，胸部 CT 对创伤的处理有显著意义。胸椎 CT 是评估椎体和后部骨折的“金标准”，同样也有助于颈胸段连接处的脊柱成像。在 X 线胸片显示纵隔增大的非特异性发现时，

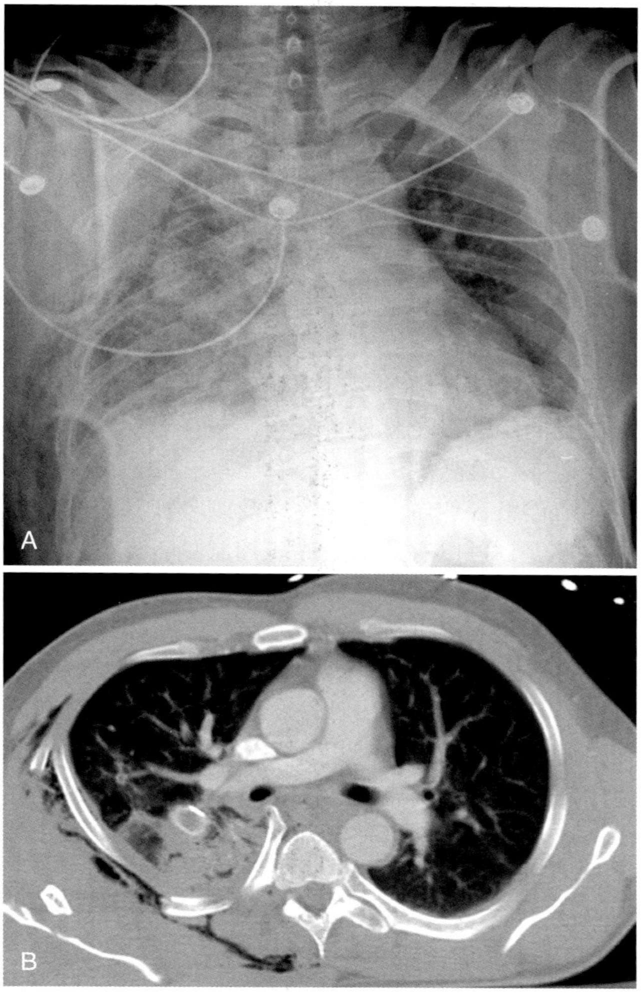

图 5 机动车车祸致胸部严重创伤的 CT 图。右侧上半胸壁体格检查未见明显矛盾运动。A，胸部平片。多根肋骨骨折（7 根），整个右半胸可见斑片影，可见皮下气肿，未见明确气胸征象。B，胸部 CT 可见胸导管影（在体检中发现的皮下气肿处置入），引出少量积血，但无气体引出。证实肺部斑片影是肺挫伤合并少量血胸所致。另外，胸部 CT 扫描发现共有 18 处肋骨骨折，较胸部平片发现更多的肋骨错位。该患者未出现矛盾运动，可能是由于该患者骨折连枷段位置偏后。除此之外，胸部 CT 扫描可发现 1 处肩胛骨无移位性骨折以及 6 处胸椎横突骨折

应用 CT 可以评估主动脉的损伤情况，而不须进行主动脉造影。随着 CT 技术的进步和研究的深入，CT 在胸部创伤中的应用将会越来越明确。

超声检查已在评估腹腔内出血和心包积液等创伤中占有重要地位。近期报道显示超声可能在评估气胸和血胸患者胸膜腔情况时也有用处。探查胸膜腔可以通过将超声探头放置在肋骨之间并寻找气胸的特异性征象来完成。

美国创伤外科协会器官损伤分级

美国创伤外科协会器官损伤分级 (American Association for the Surgery of Trauma-Organ Injury Scale，AAST-OIS) 量表用于评估胸壁以及肺部的损伤是由 Moore 等制订的，详见表 1 和表 2。

表 1 胸壁损伤分级

分级	损伤类型	伤情
Ⅰ	挫伤	任何大小
	裂伤	皮肤及皮下
	骨折	<3 肋，闭合性
		无锁骨移位，闭合性
Ⅱ	裂伤	皮肤、皮下和肌肉
	骨折	≥3条相邻的肋骨，闭合性
		锁骨，移位或开放性
		胸骨，无移位，闭合性
		肩胛骨，开放性或闭合性
Ⅲ	裂伤	全层，包括胸膜的穿通伤
	骨折	胸骨，开放性或闭合性，浮动胸骨
		单侧连枷胸（<3 肋）
Ⅳ	裂伤	胸壁组织撕脱，合并深部肋骨骨折
	骨折	单侧连枷胸（≥3肋）
Ⅴ	骨折	双侧连枷胸（两侧均≥3肋）

Modified from Moore EE, Cogbill TH, Malangoni MA, et al: Organ injury scaling. Surg Clin North Am 75:293–303, 1995

表 2 肺损伤分级

分级	损伤类型	伤情
Ⅰ	挫伤	单侧，<1 叶
Ⅱ	挫伤	单侧，单叶
	裂伤	单纯气胸
Ⅲ	挫伤	单侧，>1叶
	裂伤	远端漏气>72 h
	血肿	实质内，无扩展
Ⅳ	裂伤	大气道（肺段或肺叶支气管）漏气
	血肿	实质内，扩展性
	血管	肺内血管一级分支破裂
Ⅴ	血管	肺门血管破裂
Ⅵ	血管	全肺门横断

Modified from Moore EE, Cogbill TH, Malangoni MA, et al: Organ injury scaling. Surg Clin North Am 75:293–303, 1995

常见的胸壁损伤

胸壁缺损

胸壁缺损常导致开放性气胸，且是潜在的、快速的、致命的。大面积胸壁创伤会导致胸腔内负压消失，胸腔内压和大气压迅速相等，影响肺复张以及肺泡换气，最终因窒息而死亡。实际上，大部分严重胸壁组织缺损的患者常在送至创伤急救室途中因病情恶化而死亡。那些被及时送至医院救治的患者通常为穿通伤，例如近距离枪伤或者穿刺伤。

对于胸壁创伤较小患者，院外急救措施中最重要的是放置三面有遮挡的敷料，控制胸腔内气体只出不进。后续的治疗措施为在皮肤无创清洁区行胸廓造口术置管。置入胸管后，用纱布将创口完全封闭，并及时将患者送入手术室缝合创口。

对于大面积胸壁缺损患者，纱布封堵效果不佳。这部分患者必须及时进行气管插管，予以正压通气。手术中须控制胸壁出血点，探查是否合并其他损伤。胸壁出血有时是致命的，必要时需急诊开胸探查。对于这部分患者，“损伤控制”有时可能是最佳的选择。使用皮肤或者人工材料对胸壁缺损处进行暂时性封堵。这些缺口的确定性关闭可能需要组织移植手术，故手术最好推迟到患者完全复苏和身体能耐受长时间手术时进行。

肋骨骨折和连枷胸

肋骨骨折会导致胸壁疼痛、胸壁出血，少数可出现胸壁不稳定。连枷胸的定义是连续 3 根或者以上的邻近肋骨分段骨折。在有此损伤的患者中，不稳定胸壁及深部的肺挫伤可造成呼吸功能不全。连枷胸的病理生理以及相应的治疗将在另一章节中详细描述（肺挫伤和连枷胸）。

有证据表明胸壁损伤患者如果不进行充分的镇痛，会出现通气不足、分泌物潴留、肺叶萎陷、肺炎和呼吸衰竭等。持续的疼痛可引起持续的应激反应，抑制患者的免疫功能。镇痛不佳时还会影响机械通气患者的拔管的决定。胸部损伤的疼痛管理可使用镇痛药，必要时联合局部麻醉。另外，类似酮咯酸这种非甾体抗炎药对于缓解轻中度的疼痛也是有效的。

麻醉药

麻醉药是创伤患者疼痛管理的基石，它可以口服、肌内注射或者静脉滴注。几十年来，肌内注射一直被认为是标准的给药途径，但是这种方法会增加患者额外的疼痛以及药物吸收的不确定性，因此我们强烈建议不要采取这种方法。对于哌替啶，我们还是建议肌内注射给药。但是，在疼痛管理中，确保有效的药物浓度要远比选择何种药物重要。麻醉药的使用剂量须参照过去和现在的使用标准，根据患者的年龄以及其他可能会影响患者对疼痛感知的因素进行调整。

结合患者疼痛评分量表以及刺激性肺量测定法中的表现，可以有效判断疼痛控制是否充分。现阶段，对于那些清醒的患者，我们的方法是首先使用吗啡或者芬太尼进行镇痛。之后，若出现爆发性疼痛，可改用奥施康定或者美施康定等羟考酮类长效镇痛药。联合使用非甾体药物可抑制炎症反应并增强口服麻醉药的镇痛效果。须注意的是，对于长期使用阿片类药物的患者，应尽量避免他们出现麻醉药诱导性便秘。这可导致剧烈腹痛、恶心、呕吐等症状。

局部麻醉

肋骨骨折的镇痛可以通过肋间神经阻滞的方法。1%～2% 的利多卡因和 0.25% 的丁哌卡因配成的麻醉药注入肋间肌，剂量为 2～3 ml。穿刺点位于肋骨下缘近肋骨骨折处稍后方若干厘米。为了达到最佳的麻醉效果应至少同时阻滞骨折处上下相邻的 2 根肋骨。这项技术的缺点是控制疼痛时间较短，只适用于中部或下部的肋骨骨折。最后，根据我们的经验，该麻醉效果差异较大，也确实存在气胸的风险。

硬膜外镇痛对于中重度胸部创伤患者的呼吸功能影响较大，特别是双侧胸部创伤患者。各种局部麻醉药联合镇痛药的镇痛方法已被广泛使用。在我们中心，最常见的给药方案是芬太尼联合丁哌卡因。联合给药是有益的，其机制主要是以下 2 点：阿片类药物能调节脊髓背角神经元突触前后的递质从而影响它们特定的受体。局部麻醉药通过阻断钠离子通道达到镇痛效果。因此，这 2 种不同类型的药在镇痛中是相互协同作用的。而且，联合给药可降低药物潜在的副作用，原因是联合给药时需要的药物剂量小于单药给药时的药物剂量。

硬膜外镇痛在使用中存在很多风险，包括肠梗阻、皮肤瘙痒、尿潴留和暂时性低血压等。硬膜外镇痛须评估患者脊柱有无损伤，但是对于创伤严重的患者，短时间内可能无法确定其脊柱是否有损伤。另外，通过硬膜外置管，镇痛药联合低分子肝素可能会出现硬膜外血肿导致神经损害。最后，硬膜外置管安全放置时间为7～10天，时间太长可能会继发硬膜外脓肿。因此，强烈建议机械通气患者尽量不要使用硬膜外置管，直到准备脱机拔管时再采用。

很多数据支持硬膜外镇痛这种镇痛方法。Mackersie等证实，使用芬太尼硬膜外麻醉可显著提高患者的肺功能，约85%的患者无须另外使用肠道外的镇痛药。静脉镇痛药会造成血中二氧化碳分压升高、氧分压降低，但是这种现象在硬膜外镇痛中未观察到。在一项前瞻性随机对照试验中，Bulger等报道，硬膜外镇痛组相较于阿片类药物组，患者机械通气时间减少一半。同时，他们也指出硬膜外镇痛的一个局限，即大约有50%的创伤患者因合并相关禁忌证而无法使用这种镇痛方法。尽管硬膜外镇痛存在诸多限制，但是，如果条件合适的话，严重创伤患者可以采用这种方法。它可以明显降低院内感染发生率并缩短机械通气时间。

还有一种局部麻醉替代方法是经胸椎旁导管持续注入丁哌卡因。这种导管可以是硬膜外导管（置于椎旁间隙），或者是On-Q这种便于置入的专用导管系统。前瞻性研究表明，各种硬膜外镇痛方法均能达到相同的镇痛效果，另外，出现肺部并发症的概率也一样，在ICU中治疗的时间也一样。而且，椎旁注射还能降低低血压的发生率。椎旁注射阻滞对于那些有脊柱损伤的患者也有一定的优势：可以和肝素联用，且没有硬膜外出血风险，消除了中枢神经系统感染以及脊椎脓肿的风险。

肋骨手术固定术

在20世纪40年代和50年代，首次报道了可以通过肋骨的内外固定治疗连枷胸。后来因为出现了正压通气以及缺乏有效的修复装置稳定肋骨，故抛弃了肋骨固定术。正压通气不仅能控制疼痛，还能保证足够的氧合和通气。至此，肋骨固定术仅限于胸壁严重畸形的患者或者因某种原因需要开胸术的患者。

有趣的是肋骨固定术在过去15年间又重新得到了发展，起初是在欧洲，而现在是在美国。尽管大家对它的兴趣在增加，但是肋骨固定术的适应证还没有达成共识。有研究表明，对于某些连枷胸患者，在机械通气的同时予以肋骨固定术，可减少机械通气时间并缩短ICU住院时间。尽管肋骨固定术能够改善疼痛的控制，但是对于那些有潜在的肺实质疾病的患者，肋骨固定术后还是可能出现呼吸衰竭，最终依赖呼吸机辅助呼吸。那些支持肋骨固定用于治疗连枷胸的研究，在应何时固定的时间点上并没有达成共识。但是它们都认为固定时间越晚，可能对最终的呼吸机脱机越不利。

虽然相关的文献样本量少，在患者的选择上、时间点上、获益程度上均未达成共识，但是我们依然认为那些胸部开放伤或者胸壁严重畸形的患者是可以通过肋骨固定术获益的。除此之外，当固定作为胸壁关闭的一部分时，也有报道肋骨固定术可在开胸术中进行，用于那些有其他指征（如残留性血胸）的患者关闭胸壁。如急性疼痛综合征和慢性骨折不愈合等情况是能否采用肋骨固定术依然存在争议。

固定肋骨的办法有很多。如果没有商品化内植物的话，可以采用钢丝环扎法固定。这种方法的难点在于固定后有时稳定性较差，以及操作不慎有骨折的风险。如果专用的肋骨固定系统不可用，则可以使用一般的手或面部固定装置的前板、螺钉和线。这两种方法通常在开胸术时使用。多个专用的肋骨固定系统可以使用，可以增强骨的固定，且不用进入胸腔。这些系统包括双皮质螺钉固定前路钢板、骨髓腔内夹板，以及能抓住肋骨上下边界而无须使用螺钉固定的可弯曲Judet支架。U型钢板系统通过连锁螺钉固定前后钢板。除此之外，可吸收的聚乙酸材料也有应用，该技术已被成功用于固定颌面部骨折。对于有感染的胸部开放伤患者，这项技术有其潜在的好处，因为置入之后不用取出，而对于金属物来说不用取出的可能性很小。尽管大家对于手术固定骨折肋骨的兴趣不断增加，肋骨骨折固定装置越来越多，但是目前仍缺乏充足的证据，来证明哪些患者获益最大。

气胸和血胸

肋骨骨折可导致潜在的肺实质损伤，出现血胸和气胸，即使没有肋骨骨折也可能出现上述两种情况。气胸有时是无症状的，但是严重时是致命的。气胸分为3类：单纯性气胸、开放性气胸，以及张力性气胸。单纯性气胸是由于肺实质损伤导致气体进入胸膜腔。开放性气胸是由于大气经开放的胸壁伤口进入胸腔，使得胸腔内外压力相等。张力性气胸是由于形成了“活瓣”，胸膜腔内气体只进不出，最终导致胸膜腔内压力高于大气的压力。其结果是引起心脏和大血管从伤处转移，循环血量进行性减少。

血胸，即胸腔内出现血液。血液既可以来自于胸腔，也可以来自腹腔。来源于胸腔的血胸可能的原因有：肺实质损伤，肋间肌撕裂，或者内乳动脉、心脏、大血管的损伤。来源于腹腔的血胸主要出现于膈合并腹腔脏器的损伤，主要是肝或脾。

气胸的治疗取决于气胸的类型。小的单纯性气胸通常只需观察，严重时可使用胸腔闭式引流。如果患者情况稳定，且考虑是少量气胸，可在干预前行X线胸片检查。此操作有以下几点好处：①确定诊断，避免了不必要地放置胸管；②排除意外的损伤，如膈破裂；③发现一些诸如大的血胸、胸壁血肿之类可能影响置管位置、大小的情况。血流动力学稳定且呼吸正常的轻微气胸患者可通过多次复查X线胸片，动态观察。辅助吸氧可加快气胸的吸收。大的气胸患者应进行标准的胸廓造口术置管，一部分患者也可以使用猪尾管引流。

开放性气胸和张力性气胸需要紧急治疗。开放性气胸首先要暂时性封堵破口，胸廓造口置管术，随后通过确定性手术关闭胸部缺损。张力性气胸应行针刺减压术，并进行胸腔闭式引流。如果怀疑是张力性气胸，且患者表现出任何呼吸窘迫或者血流动力学不稳定的症状，无须等待影像学检查结果立即减压。急诊胸部减压术是在锁骨中线第2或3肋间（大约锁骨下两横指距离）插入14-G IV管。随后置入稍大的胸管（见后续讨论部分）。

和气胸一样，血胸的治疗目标是排空胸膜腔，使肺复张。脏层胸膜和壁层胸膜完全对合说明出血已得到有效控制。只有不到10%的胸部创伤患者需要开胸术。有时候患者可能受伤若干小时后才被送至创伤室，胸管引流了大量引流液。这一般代表出血是缓慢的，而非快速活动性出血，特别是在血流动力学稳定的患者中。如果积血无法通过一根胸管引出，则须置入另一根胸管。闭式引流术后须立即行X线胸片检查，以确认胸管位置是否合适，肺有无复张。如果怀疑胸腔内仍有残留的血，在患者病情稳定的情况下，建议行CT检查。若出血量大，血凝块可能堵塞胸管，积血无法顺利引出，无法评估是否仍有活动性出血，则须手术引流（图6）。在选择的稳定的患者中，手术方式可以是开胸，也可以通过电视辅助胸腔镜手术（video-assisted thoracoscopic surgery，VATS）。

中到重度的大的急性血胸须收集胸管中引出的血液，并自体输血。收集装置应在创伤急救室随时准备着。因为一旦胸管置入便会有大量血液丢失。根据我们的经验，自体输血可减少这部分患者的凝血功能障碍及炎症反应。

对于血气胸患者，若血流动力学稳定、胸管中没有或有很少量的出血、X线胸片见胸膜腔排空、无其他急诊手术指征，患者可先心电监测、持续观察。快速活动性出血或者持续的快速出血说明肺损伤严重。若置入胸管后立即引出超过1 L的血液，须紧急开胸探查。若初始引出量较少，但后续4 h连续每个小时引出量大于200 ml，也应行开胸探查。同时，这部分患者在观察过程中可能会出现胸管的引流液逐渐减少，须复查X线胸片以排除血凝块堵管可能性。

胸腔闭式引流术：技术和处理

一旦决定放置胸管，应把患者摆成合适的体位，暴露第5或第6肋间腋中线。选择这两处的原因是因其在膈之上，胸壁组织最薄，便于操作。首先消毒穿刺点周围皮肤，用1%的利多卡因逐层麻醉胸壁各层直至胸膜。为了延长麻醉时长，保证穿刺过程中患者的舒适性，我们建议使用利多卡因和等体积的0.25%丁哌卡因配比。血流动力学稳定且呼吸功能正常的患者可在清醒情况下给予镇静。沿选择

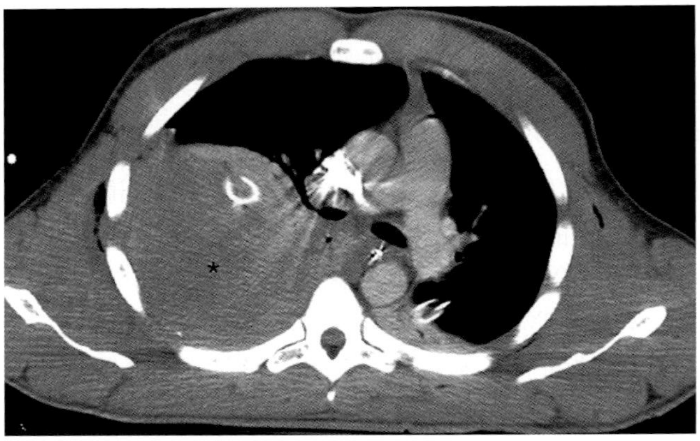

图6 图2所示患者的CT图。右侧大量血胸（星号处），和肺组织界限明显。VATS顺利排出积血

好置入导管的肋间隙的下一肋骨做 2 cm 的切口。锐性分离肋骨，其上缘进入至胸腔内。注意保护上一肋下缘的神经和血管。虽然一般用钳穿透胸腔，但我们建议一直都用手术刀，这样既简单，还能减轻患者的疼痛。一旦进入胸腔，进行手指探查，确认进入的是胸腔而不是肺内或者是腹腔内，以及胸腔内有无粘连。膈可疑损伤、既往有胸部手术史或者肺部感染性疾病患者，手指探查尤其重要。如果没有粘连、没有膈或者肺部损伤，可安全置入胸管。不建议经由套管盲置胸管。

和其他大部分器械一样，胸管也有其特有的标记帮助医生判断置入深度。遗憾的是，根据我们的经验，这些标记很容易被住院医生所忽略，造成胸管放置的位置不佳。一个常见的问题是担心胸管脱出而置入太深，这样容易造成胸管在最后的洞口弯曲导致引流不畅。为了避免这种位置不正，须在皮肤表面找好标记点。如果胸管是从第 5 肋间腋中线置入，则至皮肤表面标记点距离应在 10 ~ 12 cm 之间，若更深，则胸管容易打结。另外，在固定胸管之前要确保胸管能旋转 360°。如果胸管不能旋转 360° 则考虑胸管可疑打结或置入位置不佳。

胸管置入后须连接引流瓶，以 20 cm 水柱的压力水对持续负压吸引。之后须行 X 线胸片检查以判断胸管位置是否合适、胸腔内气体和液体是否排出、肺是否合适地复张。若胸腔内仍有残留气体和液体，根据情况可放置第 2 根引流管。排空胸腔使肺完全复张可减少出血和漏气，同时降低创伤后脓胸风险。胸膜腔持续积血是早期手术干预的一项指征。

每日复查 X 线胸片评估血气胸吸收情况。胸膜腔造口术置管后预防性使用抗生素仍有争议，我们并不采用这种办法。若没有漏气或者引流量 24 h 少于 100 ~ 150 ml，便可拔出胸管。一项前瞻性研究表明，与没有进行水封的胸管相比，6 ~ 8 h 的水封降低复发性气胸的发生率。

若未拔出引流管前再次出现漏气或者肺无法扩张，须考虑各种可能的原因。检查胸管、引流瓶、负压吸引器的连接处。一定要检查管管末端在最后一个洞处是否脱出胸壁。若胸管置入后立即发现脱出，可往胸腔内送入一小段距离。若发现时间较晚，则必须要移除胸管，在不同的地方重新置入。若胸管插入肺裂隙内会使肺的再度膨胀不足，若插入肺实质中则导致肺持续漏气。出现这些情况时，胸管也须移除并重新置入。另外，胸膜腔被分隔成若干小腔以及胸管堵塞的情况并不少见。对于机械通气的患者，即使已置入胸管，也应注意张力性气胸的可能性。

胸骨骨折

胸骨骨折相对来说出现概率较低，大多发生于钝伤后。常见的创伤机制是未系安全带的司机在减速过程中胸骨撞向方向盘。坠落或其他直接作用于胸骨的外力均可造成胸骨骨折。大多数胸骨骨折发生于中、上部。和肩胛骨骨折一样，出现胸骨骨折的患者应格外注意有无其他潜在的合并伤，包括肋骨骨折（40%）、长骨骨折（25%）、头部损伤（18%）等。

胸骨骨折本身无需紧急治疗，超过 95% 的患者可非手术治疗。须常规检查心电图，特别是年龄超过 40 岁的患者，是否需要持续心电监测取决于患者的心功能状态而非有无胸骨骨折。大多数患者可能出现短暂性右心室功能不全。单纯胸骨骨折且急诊评估正常的患者可出院。和肋骨骨折一样，胸骨骨折的处理主要是对症、镇痛及避免活动。若骨折错位严重、疼痛持续剧烈，则需手术复位和内固定（operative reduction and internal fixation，ORIF）以减轻疼痛。目前已有很多技术通过使用钢丝和小钢板等修复胸骨骨折。

肩胛骨骨折

肩胛骨骨折不常见，在钝性伤中约占 1% ~ 3%。由于它的位置和结构特点，肩胛骨骨折多由直接作用力所致。因此，合并伤很常见（80% ~ 98%）。若患者出现肩胛骨骨折应怀疑有严重的胸部创伤。要仔细检查胸腔内的神经、血管以及腹腔内损伤，另须检查是否合并其他骨科的损伤。体格检查可发现局部疼痛、压痛、肿胀、捻发音。虽然大部分肩胛骨骨折在 X 线胸片在很容易辨认，但有时因骨折线模糊而忽略。过去许多的肩胛骨骨折未被发现，但随着现代 CT 技术的广泛使用，更多的非移位性骨折被发现（图 5）。肩关节 CT 用于评估骨折和肩关节的伸展是有必要的。

大部分肩胛骨骨折的最初处理包括镇痛和固定，辅以渐进的物理治疗。很少采用手术方法进行干预，只有那些估计会引起严重畸形的肩胛骨骨折才会考虑手术干预。肩胛骨体部、颈部、喙突、肩峰、肩胛的微小移位性骨折通常无须手术，而且愈合后功能正常或接近正常。关节盂的骨折脱位，不稳定的颈部骨折，喙突、肩峰、肩胛严重的移位性骨折等为了恢复功能则须手术固定。肩胛骨骨折的其他手术适应证包括关节内骨折致关节面缺损大于 5 mm，或关节内骨折造成关节不稳定、肩胛盂颈部骨折成角大于 40°、骨折错位超过 1 ~ 2 cm、肩上方悬吊复合体断裂等。

肩胛胸骨关节脱位

肩胛胸骨关节脱位是由于严重的钝性创伤牵拉肩胛带，导致肩胛骨、肱骨、肩周围肌肉和神经血管结构被拉离身体。虽然这种损伤相对罕见，但可以是广泛性的，不仅涉及肩带的结构，而且与胸部、颅脑和脊髓损伤相关。在包括 58 例患者的综述中，Damschen 报道 81%的患者合并完全臂丛神经损伤，13%合并部分臂丛神经损伤，88%出现锁骨下动脉或腋动脉破裂。因为这些患者受影响的肢体几乎普遍存在严重的神经缺陷，达到较好的功能预后可能性低。故保留须进行大范围重建但基本上无功能的肢体之前，应该牢记这点。

锁骨骨折

锁骨骨折常合并胸部和胸腔外创伤，不像肩胛骨或胸骨骨折等通常为单个骨折。锁骨骨折部位最常见于中 1/3，最常出现于坠落或侧向打击肩部后。临床体征包括局部压痛、捻发音和畸形。若出现骨折错位，可发现肩部向下、向中线移位。大部分这种类型的骨折在前后位 X 线胸片中很容易识别。大部分（85%）锁骨中段骨折无须干预即可自行愈合。初期处理包括使用“8”字形的敷料或者肩部固定器固定肩部。

传统上，手术复位及锁骨骨折固定适用于开放性骨折、移位性骨折和伴有神经血管损伤的骨折。骨折伴有大于 2 cm 的短缩、胸部损伤且有广泛移位的碎片、漂浮肩（锁骨和肩胛骨联合骨折）和骨折不愈合均是手术干预的适应证。手术治疗包括髓内固定或放置固定钢板。

最近，使用非手术悬带固定法受到质疑。据报道，保守治疗骨折不愈合率高达 15%，其功能预后远比手术治疗要差。一项前瞻性随机研究显示，与保守治疗相比，开放复位内固定后 3 个月功能性预后改善，但治疗后 6 个月和 12 个月结果无差异。另一项前瞻性研究显示，手术固定可改善功能性预后，并降低骨折不愈合率。但是，2009 年发表的两篇 Cochrane 综述显示，对于中段骨折的治疗，保守治疗和手术治疗在治疗锁骨骨折上并没有差异。尽管缺乏确凿的证据，在骨科领域通常会选择手术固定锁骨骨折。锁骨试验是一项目前正在英国进行的前瞻性随机试验，该研究旨在招募 300 名成年患者，希望能更好地回答锁骨骨折手术和非手术治疗后不愈合率以及功能预后的问题。

血气胸并发症

脓胸

据报道脓胸的发生率为 0 ~ 18%。至少有一部分细菌培养阴性的钝伤患者的脓液是无菌的，其本质上是炎症介质富集，产生的全身效应在临床上同真正的脓胸很难区分。严重创伤患者的真正脓胸发生率可能接近 5%。但是，随着严重创伤患者的生存率的增加，这种并发症的发生率也随之增加。导致脓胸的危险因素包括胸腔积液引流不充分、损伤的机制、胸管的位置和数量、合并肺挫伤或者肺炎等。

脓胸的临床症状包括不明原因的发热、白细胞计数升高和呼吸衰竭。大多数怀疑患有脓胸的患者都是危重的。对于这部分患者，前后位 X 线胸片可能帮助很少，甚至没有帮助，但是 CT 扫描可以更容易地识别在 X 线胸片上不明显的损伤（图 7）。尽早使用 CT 可以防止延误诊断，进而减少需要更多的手术过程的可能性。

治疗方法包括①通过胸管或 CT 介导置管引流；②胸管引流辅助胸膜内纤维蛋白溶解治疗；③ VATS 和④开胸及纤维板剥除术。随着脓肿从单纯渗出性发展到分隔渗出，又发展到积脓机化，胸膜腔内液体变得越发黏稠，最后须依赖更加具有侵入性的干预措施。因此早期诊断和治疗很重要。

在那些接受纤维板剥除术的患者中，术后第一次 X 线胸片可能看起来更糟而不是更好。然而，患者其实是在逐步好转的，即使 X 线胸片显示没有好转。所有患者都应进行严格的肺部清洁、吸出痰液，并根据细菌培养结果使用特异性抗生素。

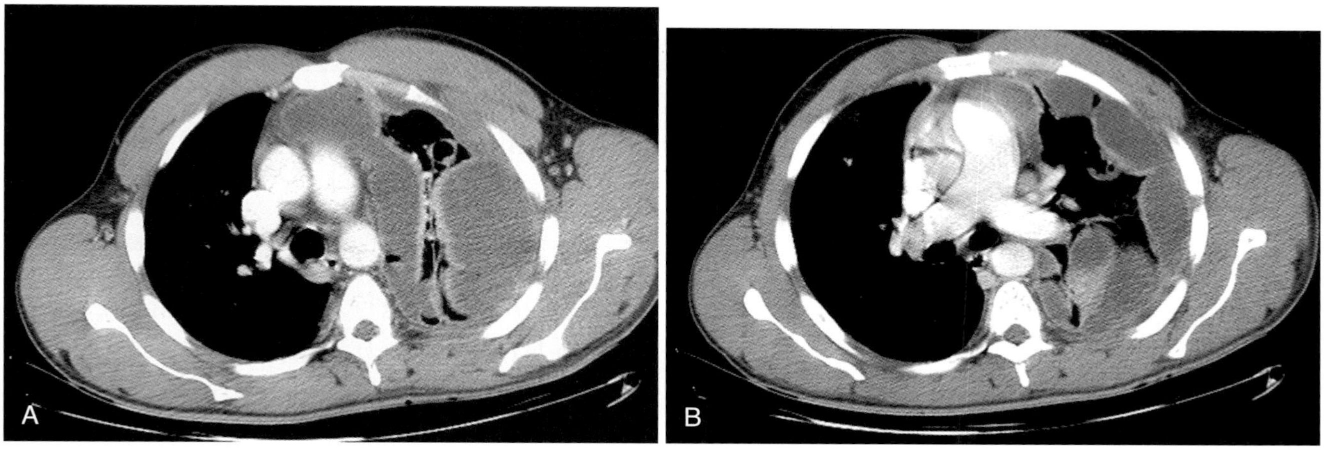

图 7　计算机断层扫描（A 和 B）显示一个胸部枪伤后 2 周的患者产生气胸后出现多分隔脓胸。注意积脓周围的增强区。患者成功地完成了开胸术和纤维板剥除术治疗

肺膨出

创伤后的囊肿或肺气肿可在胸部创伤后出现。这通常是由于气道破裂后肺内的空气聚集，但未与胸膜腔相通。大多数这类损伤不需要特别的治疗，脱离呼吸机后可自动消退。如果病变范围较大，且不断扩大或继发感染，CT 引导下经皮穿刺引流是一种有效的治疗方法。

持续漏气和支气管胸膜瘘

胸部创伤后漏气并不罕见，通常采用胸廓造口术置管进行治疗。然而，出现大量漏气时须检查是否有气管支气管的损伤。如果排除了这种可能性，则完全肺膨胀是治疗的基石。在接受呼气末正压通气（positive end-expiratory pressure，PEEP）的患者中，漏气可持续数天甚至数周，只有脱离呼吸机时漏气处才开始封闭。气管造口术可以通过减少解剖无效腔来帮助降低峰值气道压力，并因此减缓漏气。长时间漏气但血流动力学稳定的患者还可以采用 VATS。

骨损伤并发症

胸部的骨损伤最常见的并发症与疼痛有关。单独或轻度联合损伤的胸骨骨折似乎具有相对较低的损伤后遗症发生率。在一项研究中，在 6 周的随访后，只有 3% 的患者诉求需要进一步干预，包括移位性骨折的手术干预。在同一研究中，21% 的患者在 6 周时报告疼痛，但不需要进一步干预。

肩胛骨骨折很少有不愈合的，但可引起慢性疼痛。如果采用非手术方法治疗骨折，疼痛和功能障碍与关节盂角度和位移的程度有关。

与之相对的是，锁骨骨折确实存在一定比例的不愈合情况，尽管这个数字有些争议。早期研究显示锁骨骨折非手术治疗的不愈合率只有 0.1%。但是最近的研究显示保守治疗锁骨骨折的不愈合率很高，其中中段 1/3 骨折的不愈合率为 15%。即使通过手术固定，也会发生一些不愈合情况。一个对 8 项研究和 14 例病例的中段锁骨骨折的分析显示，总的不愈合率为 4.2%。非手术治疗的不愈合率是 5.9%。当发现移位性骨折时，髓内固定术有 4.8% 的不愈合率，非手术方法治疗移位性骨折的不愈合率为 15.1%。

锁骨骨折的其他长期后遗症包括疼痛、局部畸形和胸部出口压迫。对于这些患者，随后的手术固定可以有效地控制严重的症状。

可以预见的是，肩胛胸骨关节脱位有显著的长期后遗症。一项平均随访时间超过 12 年的回顾性队列研究显示，通过标准的 SF-36 问卷调查，完全臂丛神经撕脱的患者有显著的身体和精神损伤。当出现完全臂丛神经撕脱时，应该考虑进行截肢术来避免无功能的肢体形成，虽然这是一个艰难的决定。

结论

胸壁损伤合并血气胸常常出现在钝性和穿通性

损伤后，是创伤致死率和发病率高的重要原因。由于胸部损伤的种类繁多，它可能为单发的，也可能涉及多系统，故须了解这些损伤的病理生理学以及对患者的影响。虽然大多数胸部创伤可以行非手术治疗，但须警惕那些可能危及生命并需要紧急干预的损伤。更重要的是，这些损伤常常导致呼吸衰竭，从而须呼吸机辅助通气，并增加ICU治疗时间，因此对创伤预后有巨大的影响。

支气管镜和电视辅助胸腔镜技术在胸外伤中诊断以及治疗的作用

Ajai K. Malhotra, Michel B. Aboutanos, and Therese M. Duane 著
刘敢伟　周足力 译

胸部直接创伤以及严重创伤后出现肺部并发症是导致创伤相关并发症和死亡率的重要原因。在过去，胸部内镜检查的作用仅限于借助支气管镜诊断有无气道损伤以及辅助肺部清洁。巨大损伤致气管支气管树损伤、胸腔内严重出血、胸部损伤保守治疗后失败，以及出现严重肺部并发症等无一例外均需要开胸探查，其缺点是其高并发症和死亡率。光导纤维和视频成像技术的进步促进微创手术领域的快速发展。在胸部区域，出现了VATS，拓展了支气管镜检查在诊断和治疗方面的作用。这些微创内镜技术具有显著降低并发症和死亡率的作用。本章重点介绍胸腔内镜（胸腔镜和支气管镜）在胸外伤和创伤后出现严重肺部并发症时的作用。

发生率

在发病率和死亡率方面，胸部创伤占了大部分。20%的创伤相关死亡涉及胸部损伤，胸部创伤的死亡率仅次于头部和脊髓损伤。在紧急情况下胸部创伤所致死亡，与气道损伤、心脏的直接创伤或胸腔内大量出血有关。除了由胸部创伤直接导致的急性死亡外，胸部创伤或任何创伤后出现的肺部并发症均增加胸部创伤的死亡率和发病率。

大多数胸部创伤，包括擦伤、肋骨骨折和通过X线胸片或胸部CT容易判断的气胸等。气胸可以通过简单的措施如肺部清洁、疼痛管理和胸廓造口置管术来治疗。在紧急情况下，开胸探查的适应证包括主气道破裂和胸部或气道中大量出血。大约1%的急诊入院患者须进行开胸术。这种情况下的开胸术具有非常高的并发症发生率和死亡率。对于一部分患者，可以通过支气管镜大大控制出血或置入气道支架以降低开胸术的概率。类似地，在处理胸腔内出血时，VATS是一种风险较低的替代方案。在非紧急情况下，无论是否存在胸部的直接损伤，创伤患者均具有较高的肺部并发症发生率，包括肺炎、血胸、纤维胸、脓肿和急性呼吸窘迫综合征（acute respiratory distress syndrome，ARDS）等，增加了诊疗的难度。在这种情况下，胸腔内镜检查技术在这些并发症的早期诊疗中起着越来越重要的作用，并能改善预后。

电视辅助胸腔镜手术在诊疗中的作用

适应证以及患者的选择

1922年，斯德哥尔摩大学的Hans Christian Jacobaeus首次记录了通过胸腔镜技术诊断与治疗如胸腔积液、脓胸和胸部恶性肿瘤等胸腔内疾病。胸腔镜检查首次用于治疗创伤是在1946年由Branco描述的用于治疗胸部穿通伤所致的血胸。在21世纪，小切口联合电视辅助技术和选择性肺通气技术彻底改变了胸部损伤的诊断和治疗，增加了其应用范围并改善了预后。

VATS应用于胸腹外伤患者时，选择合适的患者非常重要。目前指征包括用于诊断和治疗，以及包括评估结构性损伤（膈、心包、肺实质、胸管等）或引流胸腔积液以及修复任何结构性损伤。除了常见的出血性疾病之外，VATS的主要禁忌证包括状态不稳定或具有潜在肺部和心脏创伤导致无法单肺通气的患者。表1列出了当前VATS使用的适应证和禁忌证。

膈损伤

据报道钝性膈损伤的发生率最低为0.8%，最

表 1　VATS 应用于创伤时的适应证和禁忌证

适应证	禁忌证
持续气胸	血流动力学不稳
胸腔内有内容物	心肺功能差无法耐受单肺通气［慢性阻塞性肺疾病（COPD）、心脏衰竭］
血胸	
乳糜胸	无法侧卧位
双侧	出血倾向史
胸腔积液	大量出血（首次出血大于 1.5 L 或者每小时出血大于 200 ml，持续 3 ~ 4 h）
脓胸	
怀疑胸腔内器官损伤（膈、肺、胸导管、心包）	胸膜腔闭塞（感染、胸膜炎、既往手术史）
胸腔内异物	怀疑心脏损伤
急性出血但状态稳定的患者	剖腹探查的指征

高为 7%。据北美城市创伤中心的数据显示，钝性创伤造成 10% ~ 30% 的创伤性膈破裂（traumatic diaphragmatic ruptures，TDR）。据报道，膈损伤的发生率在胸腹穿通伤中高达 67%。

膈损伤特别难以通过放射性摄影成像技术例如 X 线胸片或常规 CT 来诊断，并且高达 30% 的患者可能被误诊。在大多数城市创伤中心配备了多排螺旋 CT（multidetector row CT，MDCT），可以进行高分辨率的轴向、冠状和矢状重建图像，显著提高诊断膈损伤的准确性。R.Adams Cowley Shock 创伤中心 Stein 等的一项研究报道，使用 4 或 16 层 MDCT 扫描器用于排除由于穿通伤所致的膈损伤，可分别提高灵敏度和特异度至 94% 和 96%。然而，作者同时强调，对于不确定的 CT 结果仍然需要额外的诊断性评估，以明确排除患者有无膈损伤，如膈增厚、继发于弹道碎片的伪影、膈附近的损伤和创伤通道（空气、血液、子弹或者骨碎片勾勒出延伸到膈的轮廓）等。

与其他非手术方法相比，胸腔镜检查联合腹腔镜检查技术，仍然被认为是膈损伤的首选诊断工具。

当腹腔镜检查不是最佳或不可行时，胸腔镜检查特别重要。它有助于评估右侧膈损伤和腋后线到脊柱这部分区域的创伤，同时避免了腹部手术，特别是那些先前有腹部手术史并怀疑存在广泛粘连的患者。

VATS 在治疗膈损伤中的作用已有大量文献记载。在一项包含 24 名接受 VATS 的胸部损伤患者的报告中，10 名患者中有 9 名成功诊断为膈损伤，4 名患者采用了 VATS 膈修复。Martinez 等评估了 52 名来自危地马拉城事故在总医院进行治疗的胸腹穿通伤患者，通过 VATS 成功诊断其中 35 名存在膈损伤。所有 35 例膈损伤均经胸腔镜成功修复。即使相关报道认为通过胸腔镜技术成功修复膈损伤是可行的、安全的和快速的，但目前缺乏长期的随访结果。

怀疑有其他腹部损伤时，应参考外科专家的意见，确定是优先选择腹腔镜手术还是开放手术，也可以使用联合胸腔镜和腹腔镜技术。图 1 示在我们

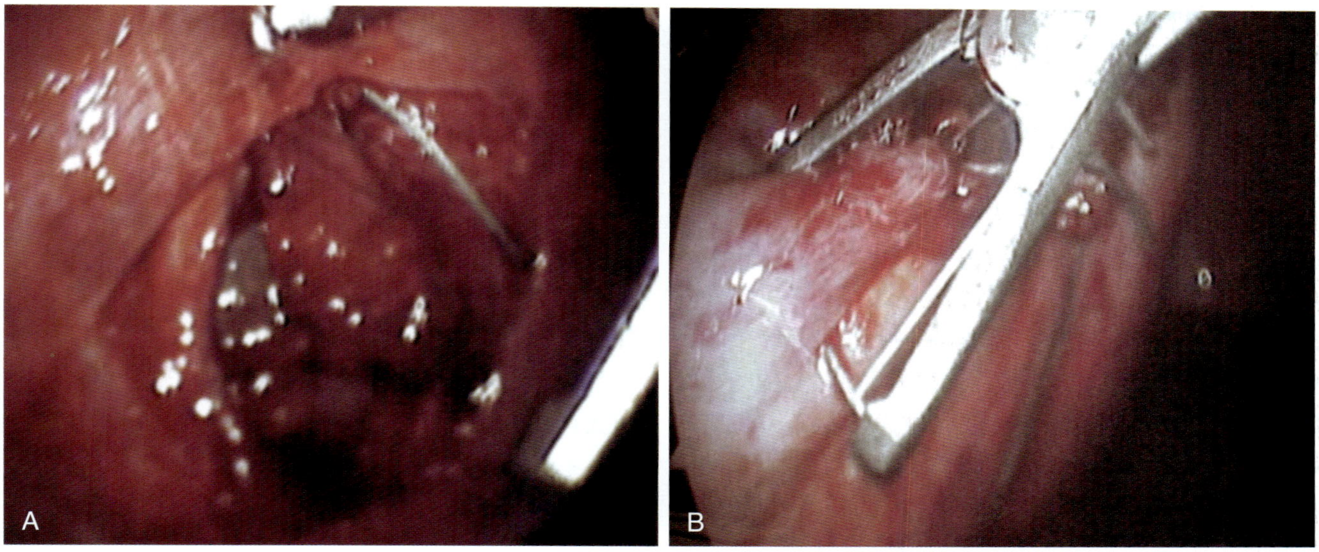

图 1　1 个 48 岁建筑工人被大小约 4 × 4 的木制品扎伤。**A**，超过 5 cm 的膈全层裂伤合并潜在的肝裂伤；**B**，胸腔镜下膈修补

创伤中心，一个胸部穿刺物导致右侧膈损伤的患者，采用胸腔镜进行评估。随后腹腔镜检查确认无出血的肝撕裂或者无相关的腹部损伤后，通过胸腔镜修复膈。所有发现膈损伤的患者，应强烈考虑进行探查性腹腔镜检查或剖腹探查，以排除其他可能的腹腔内损伤。

胸腔内有残留内容物

清除胸腔内积血是 VATS 的手术指征之一。胸膜腔内积血清除不充分或者留置引流管时间过长，会增加患者发展为脓胸和纤维胸的风险，延长住院时间、增加住院成本。胸廓造口术置管后出现残余血胸和脓胸的发生率分别为 4%～20% 和 4%～10%。来自 Parkland Memorial 医院的一项包含 39 例胸部创伤合并血胸的患者的前瞻性随机研究显示，与传统的二次置入胸管的治疗相比，VATS 有更多的优势，如留置引流管时间显著缩短（2.5 天）、住院时间缩短（2.7 天）、住院费用减少（6000 美元）。VATS 的优势主要是因为其可快速并完全清除胸膜腔积血，视频辅助下在合适位置置入胸管，确认出血来源或者其他相关的胸内损伤，并进行处理。

特别要注意的是，这些 VATS 的优点是基于须早期使用 VATS（损伤后 4～7 天）排除胸腔内积血。Morales 等的一项关于采用胸腔镜技术用于排除创伤后出血最佳时机的研究，发现行胸腔镜引流时间越晚，成功的概率越低。创伤后 5 天内行 VATS 可获得最佳疗效（成功率 >80%）。若 5 天后行 VATS 则中转开胸术以及再次手术的相对风险增加 2 倍。来自路易斯维尔大学的多个早期研究报道了类似的成功率（>75%）。VATS 失败与否与从损伤到手术的时间间隔以及积液类型（血胸与脓胸）有关。近期，来自同一机构的一项大型研究证实了早期 VATS 干预（入院 5 天内）的优势，如中转开胸术比例显著降低（8% vs. 29.4%，$P<0.05$）和更短的住院时间（11±6 天 vs. 16±8 天，$P<0.05$）。入院 5 天后行 VATS 出现脓胸的概率显著升高（29.4% vs. 10%，$P<0.0001$）。

VATS 应用于创伤性脓胸时须评估脓胸的病程特点。对于 1～5 天内的急性/渗出性脓胸，VATS 均是有效的。过渡期/纤维性及脓性阶段（6～14 天）VATS 的成功率约为 75%～85%，在机化期/慢性期（>2 周）时，VATS 的成功率急剧下降至约 50%。最近的研究证实，与单纯血胸或持续漏气相比，治疗脓胸时统计学显示存在更高的转换开胸术率和较长的住院时间（lerigth of stay，LOS）。

持续出血

VATS 也可用于缓慢持续出血但血流动力学稳定的患者。疑似胸腔内出血且状态不稳定患者须行开胸探查。Smith 等成功采用 VATS 对 5 个肋间血管持续性出血但血流动力学稳定的患者进行止血。其中 3 个患者使用透热疗法成功控制出血。其他控制出血技术包括止血夹或氩气刀。我们中心成功采用围绕肋骨的体内缝合技术对止血夹无法处理的肋间血管持续出血患者进行止血。胸腔镜控制无血流动力学不稳定患者的出血成功率约为 80%，中转开胸术率为 15%～20%。

持续气胸

持续性漏气并且胸廓造口术置管 72 h 后肺复张的发生率为 4%～23%。持续负压吸引这种保守性处理方法延长胸管留置时间和住院时间，并增加住院费用。VATS 已被证实用于治疗持续性漏气是安全有效的，缩短胸管留置时间和住院时间，并降低住院费用。Smith 等的一项近期报告显示，83 例患者中有 8 例（10%）持续性漏气且超过 72 h 肺仍未复张的患者成功通过 VATS 进行治疗，且无一人中转开胸。须注意的是，只有大约 50% 的患者是可明确漏气来源的。然而，该研究中所有患者均通过 VATS 胸膜固定术成功完成了治疗。在我们创伤中心，内镜下 GIA 吻合器通常用于切断被影响的肺实质。另有一种有弹性的、不透水的、无反应性的外科密封胶（Coseal; Baxter，Freemont，Calif）用于局部封闭的报道。通过化学胸膜固定术或电凝下胸膜瘢痕化术都是可行的办法，尤其适用于 VATS 术后复发患者。Carillo 等报告了 VATS 成功应用于 11 例创伤后持续性气胸损伤患者中的 10 例。第 11 位患者成功地接受了化学胸膜固定术。然而，采用化学胸膜固定术时出现的炎症反应可增加胸部的水肿和引流量，并增加术后的疼痛。在行 VATS 之前，以下几点很重要，积极评估漏气原因、排除胸管故障或位置不佳等可能性、评估是否存在异物或深部穿通的肋骨碎片。通过胸部 CT 和支气管镜检查等对患者进行彻底评估，包括气管支气管树、远端肺实质和胸膜腔。

其他适应证及应用

胸部创伤患者使用 VATS 的其他适应证包括支

气管胸膜瘘的诊断、残留的异物的清除、破损的胸导管的结扎、乳糜胸的引流，以及心脏和纵隔结构的评估。虽然有报道认为，那些可疑存在穿通性心脏损伤但血流动力学稳定的患者可以采用心脏周围检查，这是安全、可行的，但因存在医源性危及生命的风险，目前仍存在争议。对于血流动力学稳定的患者，怀疑心脏损伤时标准的检查方法仍然是先进行超声心动描记术，随后在剑突下心包开窗，有必要时立即行胸骨切开术或左侧开胸术，排出心包积血并修复损伤的心脏。

手术方式

手术须在在双腔气管插管下进行。插管的位置须通过支气管镜确认。患者为侧卧位，并且使髋部弯曲以增加肋间隙。初始打孔约 10 mm，放置位置则可以选择原留置胸管处，或在第 5 肋间腋中线处。该孔的作用是将可以调整 30° 或 45° 视野范围的镜头置入胸膜腔中，并帮助确定另外一个 5 mm 操作孔的位置。操作孔一般最多两个，而直径为 5 mm 的 30° 镜可以充分检查肺和胸膜腔的所有地方。当肺没有完全萎陷时，可以使用吹气法，这可能是有帮助的。在手术结束时，胸腔镜直视下置入胸管并让肺复张。患者自控麻醉联合局部肋间神经阻滞是最佳术后疼痛管理措施。

发病率和并发症管理

据报道，胸腔镜检查术后的并发症发生率小于 10%，漏诊率小于 1%。围术期并发症包括胸腔内出血（胸壁、肋间或肺实质）、复发性气胸和血胸。其他并发症包括肋间神经炎和医源性肺裂伤。据报道，中转开胸术的概率小于 8%，中转开胸术的主要原因有胸腔镜视野不佳、胸膜腔内粘连致密使肺萎陷失败，或出现不可控的出血。这强调了手术时间的重要性，须在创伤后 5 ~ 7 天内进行——及早避免胸膜粘连和纤维化，并确保充分止血。术后持续漏气可能是因为存在潜在的其他肺部疾病，例如肺气肿或肺尖部大疱。晚期并发症少见，包括肺炎、胸腔积液和脓胸。双腔气管插管位置不佳所致的气道并发症以及单肺通气时出现张力性气胸均有类似报道。

支气管镜的诊断和治疗作用

早在希波克拉底时期就有人尝试直接可视化探查气道内部。然而，第一次有记录的支气管镜检查是由德国 Freiburg 的 Gustav Killian 在 1887 年进行。当时唯一可用的仪器是硬质支气管镜。主要适应证是以治疗为目的，最常用于清除吸入气道内的异物。该领域被美国支气管食管系统之父 Chevalier Jackson 改进，因为他设计了现代的硬质支气管镜。1963 年，池田博士介绍了可曲式纤维支气管镜，主要用于诊断。可曲式支气管镜因其更容易使用而被广泛应用。唯一的治疗适应证是从气管支气管树内清除异物。最近由于设备本身的不断改进以及其他治疗工具如支架、电烙术和激光等技术的应用，支气管镜检查在治疗中的作用正逐步建立，并且其诊断作用也在不断扩大。虽然在一些苛刻的环境下，硬质支气管镜有其一定的优势，但因可曲式支气管镜使用的便利性且拥有丰富的操作经验，使得硬质支气管镜已很少应用于创伤的诊治。

可曲式纤维光学支气管镜的基本技术

几乎所有支气管镜检查（无论是否是在急诊环境）只用于气管插管并机械通气的创伤患者，无论是在创伤之后不久还是在肺部并发症之后进行。

准备

患者应预先吸入 100% 纯氧，呼吸机速率设定为每分钟 10 ~ 12 次呼吸。充分镇静对于避免应激很关键，尤其是在头部受伤的患者中更为重要，因为在支气管镜检查期间颅内压（intracranial pressure, ICP）会出现急性升高有详细记录。在我们机构，经常使用苯二氮䓬（氯羟安定或咪达唑仑 2 ~ 4 mg，静脉注射）和麻醉镇痛药（吗啡 4 ~ 8 mg 或相似药物，静脉注射）。虽然支气管镜操作可以在患者没有瘫痪下进行，但是我们发现，使用维库溴铵（10 mg，静脉注射）后，在患者处于临时麻痹的状态下进行支气管镜检查会很顺利。应保证有足够的时间，允许患者预先吸氧并且在药物起效后再开始手术操作。常用的可曲式支气管镜是单平面方向控制的。为了能够在其他平面中操作镜头，须沿纵轴线对整个镜头进行旋转。为了实现这一点，支气管镜的外端要设计成可旋转的。如果支气管镜不是平直的，则旋转运动将不会传递到尖端，因此须调整床的高度以保持支气管镜尽可能平直。

技术

无论是什么适应证，支气管镜检查的基本操作技术是相同的。但是，对于不同的适应证存在一些微小的差异和技术要点。在床的高度调整合适后，患者预先充分吸氧并且达到镇静和麻痹状态，将已润滑的支气管镜插入直角转换头——该适配器允许支气管镜在气管内操作时保持通气，当支气管镜达到气管底部时，可以看到隆嵴。两侧主支气管区分如下①气管环的位置——后方缺如；②支气管的长度——左边更长；③起始的角度——右边更直。要想成功地完成支气管镜检查，术者须掌握两侧肺叶的解剖结构以及各肺叶内肺段的情况。根据患者身体条件，支气管镜可以插入Ⅲ / Ⅳ级细支气管。非常重要的是，虽然在气道内对分泌物的抽吸和清除是支气管镜检查的一个重要部分，但是它确实可引起部分萎陷的肺泡张。因此，像任何其他医疗操作一样，应在开始支气管镜检查前衡量风险和益处，以及决定一次操作须检查多大范围。

监测

在镇静和麻痹下接受支气管镜检查的患者须仔细监测镇静是否充分，以及在手术过程中可能出现的任何心肺并发症。监测最好由另一个人执行，以便连续记录患者生命体征。须监测的重要体征是①心率，②血压，③脉搏血氧仪测定动脉血氧饱和度，以及④ ICP。当患者出现应激时，心率和血压将增加。首先停止操作，达到足够的镇静后再恢复操作。如果脉搏血氧饱和度显示下降到 90%以下，除非在极少数的情况下，应首先移除支气管镜，以便患者能够充分通气和氧合。最后，即使患者保持着足够的氧饱和度，但仍可能出现心律失常，通常是缓慢性心律失常，甚至心搏骤停。这是因为即使通过预吸氧实现高肺泡氧含量、维持氧合，但手术期间的通气被严重干扰，会导致 $Paco_2$ 急剧上升和严重的呼吸性酸中毒。这在头部损伤的患者中变得特别重要，因为它可以导致 ICP 的急剧和严重上升。如果患者出现任何心律失常，应立即退出支气管镜，并确保充分通气。复苏药物应立即用于治疗任何不能自主消退的心律失常。在进行手术前应重新评估支气管镜的风险和益处。

支气管镜并发症

可曲式纤维支气管镜检查后可能出现的并发症已有大量报道（表 2）。操作时间越长、疾病越重，并且以治疗为目的而不是以诊断目的的支气管镜检查，并发症的发生率越高。然而，有经验的医生具备细致的操作也进行了充分的监测，可曲式纤维支气管镜检查是相当安全的。

表 2　支气管镜检查并发症

低氧血症	高碳酸血症
气压伤	低血压
高血压	出血
误吸	颅内高压
感染	喉痉挛
支气管镜损耗	心律失常

可曲式气管镜的诊断价值

急性创伤

气管支气管损伤

创伤后气管支气管损伤是非常罕见的，但损伤后由于漏诊，其后果可能是严重的。虽然一些损伤可以非手术处理，且能够愈合，但如果损伤确实需要修复，修复时间延迟将会显著增加手术失败的概率。纤维支气管镜检查应该在任何可能有气管支气管损伤的患者中尽早进行。在某些情况下，如果患者不是急性缺氧或者怀疑气管支气管损伤，支气管镜检查除了其诊断价值外，还可以对插管和管的放置位置提供帮助。在这些情况下，支气管镜检查应由经验丰富的支气管镜医生操作。硬质支气管镜对颈部气管损伤的患者有作用，其中硬质支气管镜可以辨认远端破裂末端，并使其与近端对准，从而为患者插管创造条件，另外管的球囊也可经过破损位置。一旦诊断气管损伤，支气管镜检查结果可用于制订合适的治疗方案，如选择非手术治疗、开放手术或是支气管镜支架置入术。在 Lin 等的报告中，支气管镜在 1/3 的病例中对于决定治疗策略是有用的。

气管支气管树急性或者迟发性出血

创伤后的气管支气管树内出血通常由肺挫伤引起，且很少由气管树本身的损伤引起。在后期阶段，咯血可能由肺栓塞、感染、气管支气管侵蚀或气管无名静脉瘘造成。纤维支气管镜检查有助于出血原因的诊断和出血部位的定位。它可以辅助暂时性控制出血，隔离出血部位以避免血液进入肺的非出血区，并且在某些情况下，可以提供确切的止血（见后面的讨论）。

吸入性损伤

纤维支气管镜在疑似吸入性损伤患者的诊疗中起着非常重要的作用。任何疑似气管支气管吸入性灼伤的患者应尽早进行诊断性评估。如果存在阻碍气道迹象，并且患者没有气管插管，则支气管镜可用于引导安全插管。在损伤后数小时内可观察到吸入性损伤的支气管镜征象，分为急性、亚急性或慢性。在急性期，最显著的特点是气道水肿、黏膜内烟灰沉积。随着损伤进展到亚急性期，则表现为内层黏膜坏死和出血性气管支气管炎。亚急性期可持续数小时至数天，在该阶段，患者可表现为大量支气管分泌物，可能需要反复行支气管镜检查以维持气道通畅。最后，在慢性期，会出现肉芽组织造成气道狭窄，可见瘢痕形成以及闭塞性细支气管炎。初期支气管镜下所见特征与是否需要机械通气及机械通气的时长无关，与最终预后也不相关。在临床疾病发展过程与支气管镜下所见不相符时，可以考虑反复行支气管镜检查以便更准确地制订治疗计划。

呼吸机相关性肺炎

呼吸机相关性肺炎（ventilator-associated pneumonia，VAP）是现代重症监护室（intensive care unit，ICU）中最常见的院内感染之一。它与高发病率和死亡率相关，每次 VAP 的发生都显著增加护理成本。早期适当的抗菌治疗证实有改善预后的作用。尽管 VAP 有一定的发生率，但是有时候诊断 VAP 是很困难的，特别是创伤患者。造成这一困难的原因主要是肺炎的诊断标准（发热伴咳嗽以及白细胞增多，X 线胸片显示出现新的浸润灶或者原有浸润灶出现变化，痰培养显示一个菌株显著增长）的指标均是非特异性的，且存在假阳性，因为 ICU 内患者气管支气管内常有菌落聚集。下呼吸道标本（灌洗或洗刷）的定量检查已被建议用于准确区分非致病性气管支气管定植和 VAP。来自下呼吸道的支气管肺泡灌洗（bronchoalveolar lavage，BAL）标本可以通过支气管镜容易地获得。这种方法已经被证明是安全的，并且不仅能准确诊断 VAP 还能准确排除 VAP，使得患者免于不必要的抗微生物治疗。图 2 概述了作者的机构中实行的简单诊疗流程。在该方案中，支气管镜检查发挥着最重要的作用，因其显著减少了抗微生物药的使用，并因此降低了 ICU 中

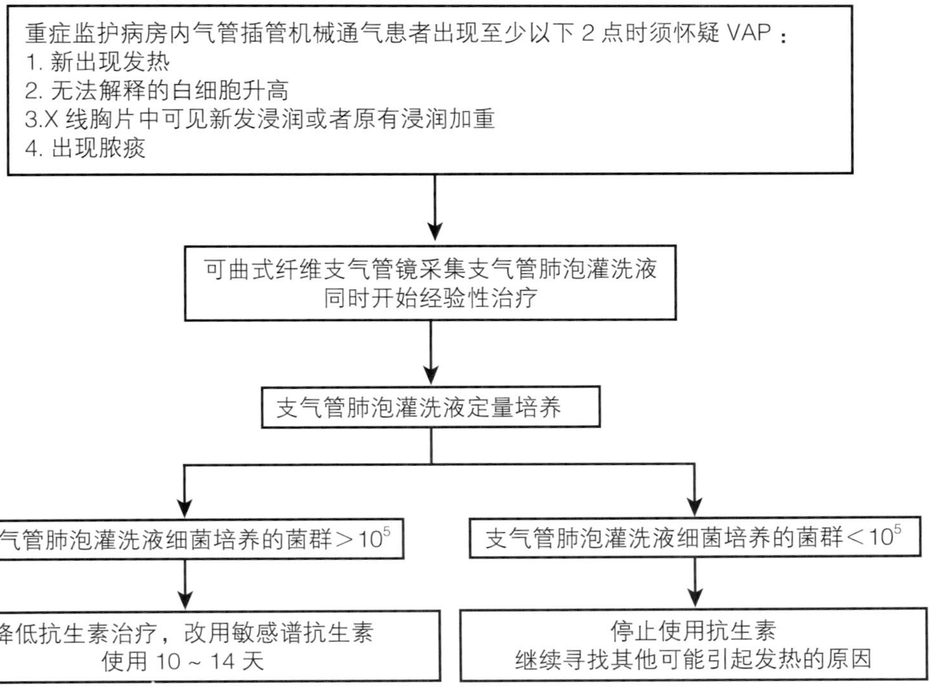

图 2 评估疑似呼吸机相关性肺炎（VAP）引起初始发热患者的简单流程

的微生物耐药性。

通过可曲式支气管镜获得 BAL 标本很简单。支气管镜到达第三级支气管水平后楔入。在支气管镜插入过程中避免抽吸以维持整个支气管镜工作通道的无菌状态。灌洗地点选择依据以下几点：① X 线胸片中新浸润灶；②支气管镜操作过程中发现脓痰最多处；③ VAP 最常见的部位——右下叶。一旦支气管镜楔入选定的细支气管，通过工作口滴入 5 等份的 20 ml 无菌非抑菌盐水并立即吸出。吸出 50% 或更多的滴注盐水并观察吸出物中的浮沫（表面活性剂的证据）提示标本收集良好。然后将该样品送至实验室进行定量培养，并根据 ICU 中的主要菌群开始经验性使用抗微生物药。当最终定量培养结果可用时（通常在 48 ~ 72 h 内）后，须根据药物灵敏度对比曲线和培养结果更改抗微生物疗法。在我们中心的 ICU，超过 10^5 个集落形成单位 / 毫升（CFU/ml）的 BAL 为阈值用于诊断 VAP。其他单位参考的数值更小。一种替代灌洗的方法是使用经保护的标本刷，其内特殊的刷头导管穿过支气管镜后刮擦支气管的内壁。用刷子获得的样本其诊断阈值通常使用 10 CFU/ml。虽然可以通过非支气管镜检查方法获得下呼吸道标本，但是目前还没有比较支气管镜和非支气管镜检查方法的对比性试验。

狭窄

气管支气管树狭窄的原因中大多数与肿瘤有关。在创伤中，狭窄可能是由于长时间插管、先前受伤部位的瘢痕形成或吸入性损伤引起。支气管镜在处理狭窄中具有诊断和治疗作用。最初支气管镜检查可以发现有无狭窄并确定其位置。此外，支气管镜下观察到的狭窄位置、长度和组织特征都可以帮助制订合适的治疗方案。 支气管镜检查可辅助处理狭窄远端的肺段肺不张，并可用于治疗这些肺不张区域的感染。

可曲式气管镜的治疗价值

急性或者迟发性咯血的控制

大咯血的定义是气管支气管中的出血量可导致气道阻塞进而危及生命的情况。支气管镜检查不仅用于诊断出血的来源，还用于清除血液，从而解除气道阻塞。在某些情况下，支气管镜技术可以用于提供临时出血控制，通过手术或支气管动脉栓塞为确定性出血控制做准备。在一些患者中，支气管镜技术甚至可以提供确定性治疗。控制出血方法包括灌洗低温盐水、注射 1 : 200 000 肾上腺素、滴注纤维蛋白胶或其他局部止血剂、球囊填塞、电凝术和激光凝固。尽管关于使用这些技术的大多数报道来自医学文献，但这些技术也正应用于外科 ICU 患者的创伤性出血或迟发性咯血控制。

急性气道创伤支架修复

气管支气管树的巨大破坏是罕见的，但危及生命。过去，唯一可采用的治疗措施是开放手术。最近，已经出现了扩张型金属支架，其可以在支气管镜控制下放置。这种方法为修复那些具有潜在毁灭性的创伤提供了一种低风险的替代方案。疑似气管支气管受伤时，早期通过支气管镜检查进行评估，对诊断或排除损伤以及随后进行计划性治疗均有非常重要的意义。支气管镜可以确定损伤部位，并辅助安全气管插管。一旦患者的气道固定，开始仔细评估损伤的特点，特别要检查气道各分支并确定受伤的范围。虽然开放式修复是传统的治疗方法，但损伤容易修复时，或者患者合并其他损伤不适合手术时应考虑支架修复。如果没有任何支架可用时，可根据具体的损伤的解剖学特点定制合适的支架。

举作者机构的一个例子说明。一名与高速车辆相撞的 18 岁男子，胸部 CT 显示其主动脉横断。除了严重气胸以及胸腔持续存在大量漏气之外，通过支气管镜检查发现其存在远端气道损伤。支气管镜辅助下放置定制的支架，漏气随即停止。几天后，患者通过开胸手术成功地修复了受损的主动脉。后续的支气管镜检查显示气管损伤已经愈合（在支架周围形成肉芽组织）。8 周后，支架被完整移除，移除 2 周后可见黏膜已覆盖于损伤部位。

清除异物

在可利用支气管镜检查从气管支气管树取出异物之前，气道异物堵塞常导致高发病率和死亡率。支气管镜检查的可行性彻底改变了这些患者的治疗方案，因为它提供了一种风险非常低的手术替代方案。虽然起初气道异物清除是通过硬质支气管镜进行的，但目前绝大多数情况都是用可曲式支气管镜进行的。它可以进入更远端的气道，并且具有允许操作器械进入的工作通道。怀疑吸入异物且在急性阻塞中幸存下来的患者，应在进一步干预前先进行仔细规划。这是因为规划不当可能导致患者气道阻塞和死亡。该操作须由经验丰富的内镜医生来执行，须同时准备硬质支气管镜和可曲式支气管镜。虽然该操作可以在患者清醒状态下进行，但更多的是在麻醉下进行。内镜医生与麻醉师之间必须就如何安全管理气道仔细协商。一旦确定了气道管理计划，便可开始支气管镜检查。除了准备2种类型的支气管镜之外，辅助器械对于安全去除各种可能已经嵌入到黏膜中的异物非常有用。这些器械包括气囊导管、特殊抓钳和铁丝筐。此外，已经开发了其他辅助技术用于安全地去除异物。这些技术包括可以使异物黏附到仪器末端的冷冻探针或钕-钇-铝-石榴石（Nd：YAG）激光器（用于分解异物，使周围的肉芽组织汽化而被清除，且钝化异物边缘以便安全清除）。

肺萎陷、大量分泌物及误吸的处理

可曲式支气管镜已经成为管理肺不张和由黏液分泌物造成的完全或部分肺部萎陷的重要工具。在中央气道黏性分泌物堵塞的患者中，观察到使用支气管镜的效果立竿见影。在全肺萎陷或者肺叶不张的患者中，支气管镜抽吸有明显的改善氧合作用。然而，在其他患者中，支气管镜清理气道的作用相较于传统胸部叩击疗法的益处并不明显。在创伤患者中，由于合并其他损伤，有时可能无法接受良好的叩击疗法，支气管镜可能是清除分泌物的唯一有效方法。对于大量吸入胃内容物的患者，早期支气管镜检查和气道灌洗可帮助清理气道，并可能限制化学损伤。尽管出现这类情况时经常使用支气管镜检查，但是没有确凿的研究结果证实其益处。根据已有证据，如果疑似大量误吸的患者已经插管或须在发作后立即进行插管，则采取支气管镜检查和灌洗是有益的。如果患者不需要插管，则须仔细监测，并采取积极的叩击疗法和其他有助于肺部清洁的措施。与所有其他操作一样，有必要平衡潜在的风险和获益。在支气管镜检查期间，呼吸道内大量抽吸会导致肺泡不张，这可能造成氧合不全，气道内的广泛灌洗液会影响弥散，进一步导致氧合恶化（见之前的并发症）。

经皮气管造口术

经皮气管造口术作为开放式气管造口术的替代术已经普及，可以较低的成本在ICU中进行。尽管可以在没有支气管镜检查的情况下进行手术，但是许多人认为，在支气管镜辅助下操作能增加手术的安全性。多年来，在气管造口术前，该操作已从多次扩张改进为一次扩张，使得手术的持续时间更短，且不影响其效果。

该操作包括将针放置在气管内，并在直接可视情况下将导丝穿过针。一旦导丝被放置，则用28 F光滑的导管扩张从皮肤到气管的管道，该导管在末端是逐渐变细的。此步骤之后是将预先装载在24 F扩张器上的8号气管造口术导管通过已建立的通道进入气管。当在支气管镜辅助下进行操作时，可以确保针、导丝和扩张器确实进入气管，而不是在颈部软组织内的假通道中。

经皮气管造口术的适应证与开放性气管造口术相同。皮肤感染、不稳定的颈椎和ICP升高是手术的绝对禁忌证。肥胖、需要高通气、凝血功能障碍以及其他该区域任何解剖学异常都是相对禁忌证。最近一项报告关于在外科ICU中进行的1 000例床边经皮气管造口术的研究表明，该操作几乎可用于所有患者，其并发症发生率仅为1.4%，高危患者并发症发生率升高至1.7%。报道的并发症包括黏膜撕裂、于黏膜下置管、后气管壁穿孔形成气管食管瘘、气管旁置管、气压性损伤，以及对气管内插管和支气管镜的损伤。像开放手术一样，后期可能出现气管无名静脉瘘和声门下狭窄。

支气管胸膜瘘处理

支气管胸膜瘘表现为胸廓造口术中管的持续的漏气。当保守措施，包括持续负压吸引和化学胸膜固定术，不能在1～3周内将瘘关闭，可能须进行手术处理。支气管镜检查可用于明确瘘所在的肺段。将支气管镜置入怀疑存在瘘的各肺段，观察有无新生肉芽组织及是否有气泡从中排出，从而相当准确地确定瘘所在位置。瘘位置确定后，在支气管镜辅助下置入球囊导管，扩张球囊以堵塞瘘。如果发现漏气停止，则瘘的诊断和位置得到进一步确认。一旦诊断明确及位置确认，就可以使用纤维蛋白胶、明胶海绵和铅粒塞子等在手术之前临时封闭瘘。在某些情况下，甚至可以永久性地控制漏气，从而避免了大手术。也可将新鲜的自体血块粘贴到球囊导管的球囊上，从而传递到瘘。当有血块时，滴注抗纤维蛋白溶解剂（如ε-氨基己酸）或四环素或多西环素可以提高成功率。

气管支气管狭窄扩张/激光治疗

创伤患者气管支气管狭窄通常与长时间插管相关。然而，它们也可能由感染后形成的肉芽组织以及手术或支架修复损伤气道造成。虽然手术切除和修复狭窄区域的成功率很高，但是支气管镜下扩张狭窄是一种风险较低的替代方案（无论是否使用激光汽化），可以暂时缓解症状，直到可以进行手术修复，甚至在某些情况下可以永久治愈狭窄。该操作的技术细节超出本文讨论范畴，但强调必须根据每个个体情况设计最佳治疗方案。一些须考虑的重要因素包括狭窄的部位、长度和组织类型，如果选择激光治疗，则可使用 Nd：YAG、CO_2 或磷酸氧钛钾。此外，本专业的知识和经验也是须参考的重要因素。可以与激光汽化配合使用的辅助技术包括球囊扩张、支架放置和丝裂霉素 C 的滴注（降低激光治疗后的复发率）。目前手术切除与激光治疗间疗效的对比缺乏比较试验，通过多学科方法来处理每个患者是获得最佳结果的最佳途径。

肺脓肿的引流

肺脓肿是胸部创伤后或创伤性肺炎后的严重并发症。其发病率高，死亡率高。传统的治疗方法包括适当的早期抗生素治疗和体位引流。如果上述方法均失败，则手术引流是唯一可行的方法，但也具有高发病率和死亡率。通过影像介入技术可以在无需高风险手术的情况下对脓肿进行引流。然而，在肺深处大气道附近放置引流管时，存在发生持续性支气管胸膜瘘的风险。还有一种技术是支气管镜辅助下进行经支气管吸除脓肿，留置引流管允许脓腔灌洗和连续引流。已有报告认为该方法效果良好，但须注意尽量减少脓液溢出进入气道。

结论

内镜技术，包括 VATS 和纤维支气管镜，在任何胸部创伤或创伤后肺部并发症患者的诊断和治疗中的作用越来越明显。在一部分患者中，这些技术可以在急性和非急性环境中作为开放手术的一种风险较低的替代方案。随着技术的进步以及设备的改进，支气管镜检查和 VATS 可能在胸部创伤和任何创伤后肺部并发症的管理中发挥更大的作用。

肺挫伤及连枷胸

Carl Hauser, Noelle Salliant 和 David H. Livingston 著
幸华杰 译

肺挫伤及连枷胸是严重胸部钝性伤后最常见的并发症，二者都能以其独特和具体的方式引起肺部呼吸生理的改变，导致创伤后肺功能不全或者呼吸衰竭。Morgagni 早在 18 世纪就对肺挫伤进行了描述。Laurent 在 1883 年《柳叶刀》杂志上首次提出了胸廓可塑性的概念，认为可以在胸廓骨性结构完整的前提下造成肺部的挫伤，尤其是在年轻人当中。与此相对的是，连枷胸主要发生于老年人，大部分老年患者 60 余岁，而且患者年龄越大，相对预后越差。肺挫伤与连枷胸有时可以并存，但是二者对于呼吸病理生理学的影响截然不同。如果不能准确区分这二者，可能会将一种疾病的研究应用于另一种疾病上，这可能导致治疗上的失误。

发病率

对于肺挫伤及肺出血的最早记录，见于第一次世界大战期间对于战场上死于爆炸创伤的军人的尸体解剖学研究。类似的发现也见于二战期间，当时多使用“肺震荡”这个词，其所表达的意思类似于 Hadfield 描述的在大不列颠之战中受爆炸伤市民的肺部损伤。在现代伊拉克和阿富汗战争中，爆炸引起的肺损伤构成全部创伤的 3%，这一数字也随着爆炸性武器应用的增长而上升。

肺挫伤在非战争情况下的发生率在不同的研究中差异较大。早期的记录见于 20 世纪 60 年代的机动车创伤，当时报道的胸部创伤患者中有 10% 发生肺挫伤。近期的一项由交通创伤研究部和工程网络进行的研究中，分析了 2 187 例受到正面或者侧面撞击的行人，大约一半（52%）的行人伴有胸部钝性创伤。这部分患者当中，大约 32% 伴有肺挫伤［平均损伤严重度评分（Injury Severity Score，ISS）为 17 分］。

诸多因素导致了不同报道之间的肺挫伤的发生

率差异较大。首先，现代影像学技术使得轻度肺挫伤的发现率大大提高。其次，总体研究人群的年龄，对于各个机构数据库在报道发生率的结果有着显著影响。年轻人，尤其是儿童，与老年人相比胸廓的顺应性更好，因此在受到胸部创伤时，更容易把能量传递到肺实质，而不是由肋骨来分担力。胸部创伤患者，年龄低于25岁的，发生肺挫伤的可能性要比年龄偏大者高50%，与此相反，老年人发生肋骨骨折的风险是年轻人的2倍。

类似于肺挫伤，报道的连枷胸发生率也因研究人群不同而有较大差异。儿童受到胸部创伤后，多表现为肺挫伤，连枷胸非常少见（即使是多发伤）。一种少见的情况是，对于患有成骨不全的婴儿来说，可以表现为连枷胸。而在成年人当中，发生连枷胸的概率较高。一项大规模的关于成年人胸部钝伤的观察性研究报道，在有胸壁损伤的患者当中，5%～13%的患者发生连枷胸。在发生明显肺挫伤的患者当中，50%伴有连枷胸。体弱的老年患者胸廓的脆性增加，即使是相对较轻的胸部创伤也会造成连枷胸，而他们很少或没有肺挫伤。

胸部创伤的发生机制

创伤的物理机制

所有的钝伤都是由于能量通过物理方式传递到人体所致。但是由于胸廓坚固的骨性结构，所以除了老年人以外，肺挫伤以及连枷胸基本是由高能量损伤造成的。在普通人群中，多数的胸部钝伤是由机动车相撞或机动车撞击行人引起的，常见的一种情形是没有系安全带的司机撞到方向盘上。高处坠落是引起肺挫伤和连枷胸的另一种常见情况。尽管胸部外压伤没有车祸和坠落普遍，但也能引起肺挫伤。但是因为外压发生的速度较慢，因此这些损伤中的肺挫伤比连枷胸中相对少见。通常这些患者会表现为创伤性窒息。有时候搏斗、钝物打击和踢打过程偶尔会造成肺挫伤。因为这种损伤较少涉及年轻患者，而且生物力学的结果也不太容易造成连续肋骨的多发节段性损伤。婴儿或者儿童的肋骨骨折须特别关注，因为有可能是虐待造成的。在一些罕见的情形中，切线方向的枪击伤也可以在不进入胸膜腔及撕裂肺的情况下造成潜在的肺挫伤。通常这样的损伤是限制性的，仅造成轻微的生理影响。

由于军队作战的重心从传统意义上的参战转向镇压暴乱，简易爆炸装置（improvised explosive devices，IED）已经成为导致美国军人创伤的主要原因。爆炸伤有4种能量传递方式。初始的爆炸伤由冲击波造成，可以单独出现，不伴有弹片造成的明显外伤（二级损伤）、钝挫伤（三级损伤），或者其他爆炸造成的伴随伤（四级损伤）。由于高密度的爆炸物将动能传递至低密度表面，实质组织与含气空腔脏器之间的致密界面倾向于“碎裂”，残余的能量继续传递造成气泡内向破裂。短暂的爆炸损伤（例如由IED造成的）一般引起比较局限的肺部损伤。持续时间较长的爆炸损伤通常是由空投的炸弹或者车载爆炸装置造成的，能够将压缩性的高动量的力传递到肺实质。它是由更大的炸弹引起，如空运炸弹、车载、IED。使用防弹背心以及肢体护具能够有效地提高肺组织抗击爆炸的能力。由于恐怖组织的活动，以上提到的爆炸损伤也可以在普通人群中见到。

病理生理学

能量传递到胸腔能够直接引起肺水肿及出血。由于肺门和肺实质的剪切力惯性不同，可能引起肺裂伤（图1），尽管这种情况并不常见，但是随着常规CT检查的广泛应用，其诊断率也越来越高。另一种创伤后可能造成肺功能不全的机制是冲击导致的细胞变性继发肺血管内皮激活。这种现象在脑血管内皮细胞中有过描述，在肺血管床中可能也存在类似的机制（图1）。

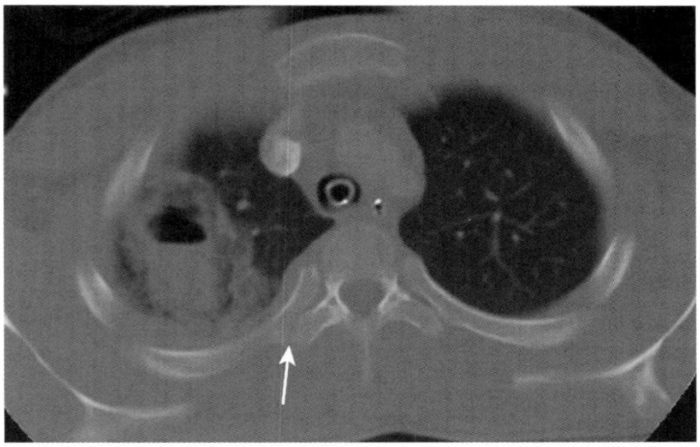

图1 胸部CT图像，来自高速车祸伤的14岁儿童。可以明显看到肺挫伤及肺裂伤，没有明显的气胸或血胸，也没有肋骨骨折，但是可以看到T4-T7椎体右侧横突骨折（箭头所示）。根据我们的经验，CT类似的肋椎关节损伤是比较少见的，其生物力学效应等同于后侧肋骨骨折。CT，计算机断层扫描

第一次世界大战中病例的研究认为爆炸伤主要可以引起肺出血，因此肺衰竭反映了血液填充了肺泡腔。尽管这种理论能够解释伤后肺分流（Qs/Qt）增加的情况，但是还存在其他的一些机制。

最为恰当的做法是把肺部创伤对于肺功能的各种病理生理影响归纳为以下两类：

1. 分流（Qs/Qt）增加引起的低氧血症；

2. 损伤机械性改变呼吸功，继发 CO_2 潴留以及呼吸性酸中毒等呼吸衰竭的表现。

这两种病理生理改变通常会重叠而加重肺损伤。除了上述两方面，损伤对于胸壁机械功能的影响、肺充气的影响，以及由于心脏功能异常导致的肺灌注不足也会影响到肺功能，但是这些方面不在本文中探讨。

分流和低氧血症

损伤后肺出血并不是唯一导致胸部急性损伤 V/Q 比例失调的因素，胸部夹板固定以及治疗不当的疼痛也是进展性的肺不张分流原因之一。系统性休克及缺血 / 再灌注可以催化免疫系统对于肺的攻击，这种情况在肺移植中比较明显，但是在系统性 Z/R 和肠道 Z/R 中也可以看到，它们可以在胸部创伤之后激活固有免疫系统，导致系统性的免疫反应综合征（systemic imflammatory response syndrome，SIRS），最终导致急性肺损伤（acute lung injury，ALI）和肺功能不全。

在有些情况下虽然必须使用呼吸机，但是也会通过许多机制引起呼吸机相关肺损伤。最终，休克、肺炎，不当的机械通气策略或在肋骨骨折固定过程中造成的细胞因子或损伤相关分子模式（damage-associated molecular patterns，DAMP）释放入血，可以造成免疫系统对肺的二次打击。

呼吸功增加和呼吸衰竭

呼吸衰竭、高碳酸血症以及呼吸性酸中毒是损伤后呼吸功增加导致的最为常见的结果。呼吸功增加是多因素的。胸廓的损伤会引起胸壁顺应性下降以及神经肌肉功能的缺陷。与胸壁损伤相关的疼痛和夹板固定可以导致潮气量下降以及解剖无效腔（V_D/V_T）相对增加。因此，胸部创伤的患者须增加每分通气量从而达到正常的肺泡通气量，然而在胸廓神经肌肉功能障碍以及剧烈疼痛的情况下是很难实现的。

在连枷胸的情况下，CO_2 潴留多是由于“摆动呼吸”现象造成的。如果是单侧连枷胸，那么进出向气体都始终在两侧胸腔之间流动。这个概念直观上很好理解，气体不与外界交换的话实际上就造成了病理无效腔。然而实际上并没有这么简单。临床实践中，连枷胸的患者分流分数提高及低氧血症比高碳酸血症更为常见。此外，在急性肺损伤的患者中，摆动呼吸在没有胸壁不稳定的情况下也可以出现。这是由于损伤后非均匀的黏弹性造成的，使得气体可以在顺应性不同的肺段之间交换。明显的连枷胸段导致呼吸过程疼痛且越来越低效。

最后，在继发 ALI 的严重创伤中，在肺实质中同样的免疫攻击可以引起低氧血症、急性肺损伤 - 急性呼吸窘迫综合征（ALI-acute respiratory distress syndrone，ALI-ARDS），也可造成“静止肺”和呼吸功。这种情况导致的肺顺应性下降可以在胸廓外形及生物力学恢复后继续存在。肺外引起肺顺应性下降的情况，常见于腹腔隔室高压。这种情况很难诊断，当膀胱压力超过 20 ~ 25 mm Hg 的情况下尤其需要怀疑。

炎症性的肺损伤

胸部创伤之后肺功能恶化通常都与系统性炎症反应相关。ALI 和 ARDS 就是经常用来反映创伤后肺损伤严重程度的指标。目前认为这种损伤与多形核中性粒细胞（polymorphonuclear neutrophil，PMN）和内皮细胞（endothelial cell，EC）相互作用有关，二者的相互作用激活肺血管内皮细胞，增加内皮的通透性，导致间质及肺泡水肿，最终引起肺泡顺应性及气体弥散功能下降。最近的研究证实，外伤后线粒体中的 DAMP 释放入血是引起 PMN 和 EC 相互作用的动因。ALI/ARDS 通常是一个排除性诊断，在有明确低氧血症的情况下，排除其他可以引起肺衰竭的病因，如肺炎或者充血性心力衰竭，才可以做出诊断。事实上，ALI/ARDS 存在于几乎所有的肺部严重创伤患者。尽管目前对于 ALI 和 ARDS 的处理都是支持性的，但是理解其病理生理机制也非常重要。胸部创伤会使肺有可能受到继发的损伤，而继发的休克、肺炎、脓毒症等情况会使肺有恶化的风险。胸部创伤后，发生肺炎的风险明显升高，而肺炎既能作为肺功能不全的主要因素，也可以作为“二次打击”器官衰竭的诱发因素。一个特殊的问题是胸部创伤有时会伴有长骨骨折，胸部损伤患者在骨折固定后发生肺炎的概率明显升高。

这可能是因为在创伤后早期，骨折部位的骨髓腔被扩大，导致细胞内的DAMP，如线粒体内的多肽片段以及DNA片段大量产生，聚集在骨折部位激活内皮细胞及白细胞。而手术复位的过程会将这些炎症因子释放入血，从而导致ALI/ARDS的发生。目前还需要一些前瞻性的研究来回答，在这类患者中，骨接合的方法是否不利于保护肺功能，或者能否开发出保护骨折相关的肺损伤患者的药物。

肺血管外体液

在肺动脉（pulmonary artery，PA）导管常规应用于临床以前，普遍认为胸部创伤后引起的液体负荷过重以及继发的肺血管外体液过多是造成外伤后肺功能不全的主要原因。目前对此观点有疑议，认为低血容量、低灌注，以及再灌注都是导致炎症性肺损伤的重要原因。此外，右向左分流也会导致通气不佳的肺段灌注增加，因而加重了分流。

胸部创伤有时候会伴有心功能不全，但通常是一过性右心室功能不全，很快就能恢复。休克以及复苏过程会增加血管外的体液量，但是肺淋巴管网的储备可以避免肺间质体液量负荷过重。因此我们主张在胸部创伤患者中保持充足的循环血量。对于肺损伤的患者，建议使用高渗盐水（hypertonic saline，HTS）进行液体复苏，不过目前还缺乏基于人体研究的强有力的证据支持，有限的一些证据仅支持在早期使用HTS。此外，HTS已经被证实能够减少中性粒细胞的激活，导致ALI和休克患者的系统性炎症应答。然而对于伴随基础疾病，如心脏、肾、肝疾病的患者，肺血管外体液增加是一个比较严重的问题。这类患者可能需要强心、利尿，以及渗透压支持。前瞻性的研究证实，使用高张白蛋白（25%）进行血浆容量支持，对于需要利尿治疗的ALI患者有明显的益处。

诊断

体格检查

在有自主呼吸的患者中，连枷胸的诊断可以通过视诊或触诊胸廓的不对称运动来获得。即使X线胸片甚至CT诊断为“连枷胸”或“连枷胸段”（连续3根肋骨存在2处骨折）仍无法解释胸廓黏弹性的特性。肌肉覆盖比较多的区域，可能是由于解剖结构正常或个体更加年轻或健康不容易发生连枷胸。这些区域即使发生了骨折，一般也能够保持胸廓的机械稳定性。对于连枷胸的诊断，矛盾运动不是必须的，只要患侧胸廓有不对称的或者延迟的起伏即可。

胸廓最脆弱的地方，大约在胸骨60°角的地方，因为这个位置肋骨比较平，支撑性较差。肋骨在受到前后向或者侧向的冲击之后，通常会在两个方向上形成骨折。一个是刚才提到的60°旋转角的地方，一个是后方。前后向的压缩可能会导致肋软骨的破坏，引起胸骨连枷。如果骨折线超过腋前线的话，会导致整个前胸壁发生连枷胸，像盾牌一样（图2）。

最后，临床上并不少见的一种情况是被方向盘或者安全气囊撞击，尤其多发生于年龄比较大的人，可以发生胸骨柄前胸壁连接。这可以导致“前胸壁连枷胸”，表现为吸气时剑突下降而胸骨柄上升。伤

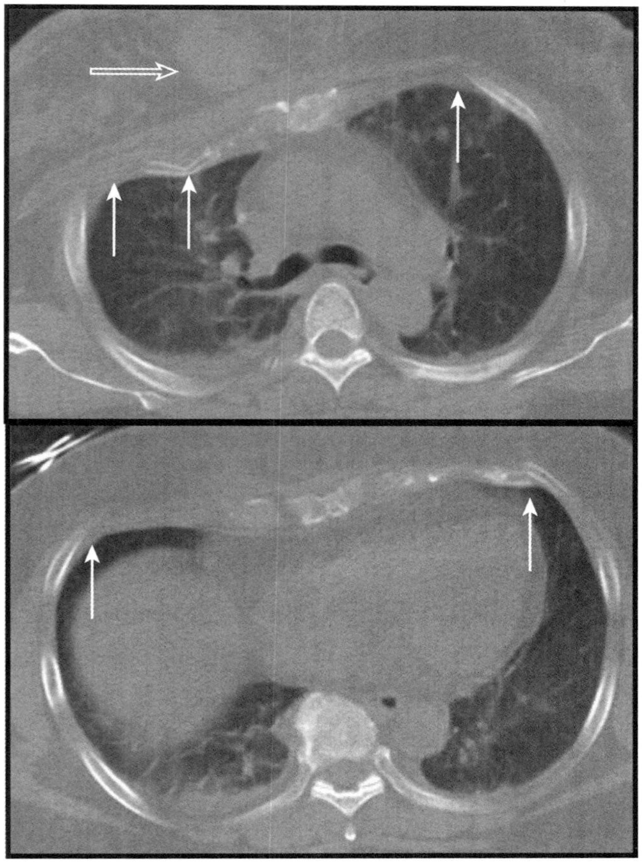

图2 胸部CT图像，来自一位肥胖的老年妇女，车祸时前胸壁撞到方向盘导致连枷胸。可以看到双侧腋中线多发肋骨骨折，累及每一根肋骨（实心箭头所示），伴有肺不张及少量胸腔积液。相对来说肺挫伤程度不重。前胸壁可见动脉血肿（空心箭头所示）。这位患者接受了药物镇痛，没有呼吸功能不全的表现

后早期，肌肉对于胸壁的固定作用可能会掩盖连枷胸段的表现，因此需要细致的体格检查，一般来说触诊的灵敏度会更高。触诊简单、信息量大，但是经常被忽视。对于有自主呼吸的患者，可以把双手分别放在双侧胸腔，感受双侧胸廓运动是否对称。皮下握雪感也比较常见，肋软骨连接处的压痛提示可能存在脱位或者影像学上无法显示的肋软骨骨折。发生连枷胸的患者，预后相对差一些，而且需气管插管的可能性也比仅有肺挫伤大很多。听诊对于诊断肺挫伤或者连枷胸的意义并不大，不过可以在开始进入创伤中心的时候排除气胸及血胸（它们可急性恶化）。

X 线胸片

X 线胸片、CT 等检查对于胸部创伤诊断起着非常重要的作用。严重损伤的患者，初始的前后位 X 线胸片能够发现肺挫伤或者提示连枷胸（图 3）。通过前后位 X 线胸片诊断的胸部损伤通常临床上表现也比较明显。相较于只通过 CT 检查获得诊断的肺挫伤，通过 X 线胸片就能够诊断的患者，须通气支持的比例更高（OR＝2.09, 95%CI 为 1.01～4.14），须进行胸部干预治疗的比例也更高（OR＝4.01, 95%CI 为 1.92～8.37）。X 线胸片的灵敏度比较低，可能会遗漏一些重要的胸廓内损伤。Pape 等的研究表明，仅行 X 线胸片检查的话，在刚入院时仅能发现大约 47% 的肺挫伤。到创伤后 24 h，X 线胸片可以发现 92% 的肺挫伤。尽管 X 线胸片上肋骨骨折也很明显，但是相较于 CT，它能够发现的骨折的部位比较少。

而且 X 线胸片还可能会低估疼痛情况，而且不容易判断肋骨骨折是否会导致机械活动不稳定。因此，尽管创伤早期 X 线胸片对于及时评估是否存在危及生命的损伤非常重要，但是对于肺挫伤、血胸、气胸以及肺裂伤等需要具体干预的并发症的诊断比较有限，在前方的气胸或者后方的液体积聚、共存的情况下尤为明显（图 4）。

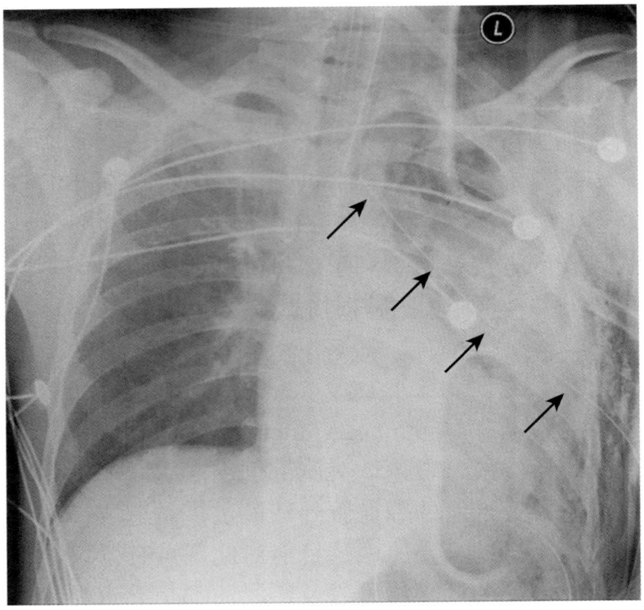

图 3　X 线胸片，来自一位发生皮下气肿、动脉氧合下降后进行胸腔置管引流的患者。可以看到左肺下叶有肺挫伤，胸管位置似乎比较合适（箭头），看不到残留气胸表现。侧位 X 线胸片可见第 4、5、6 肋骨骨折

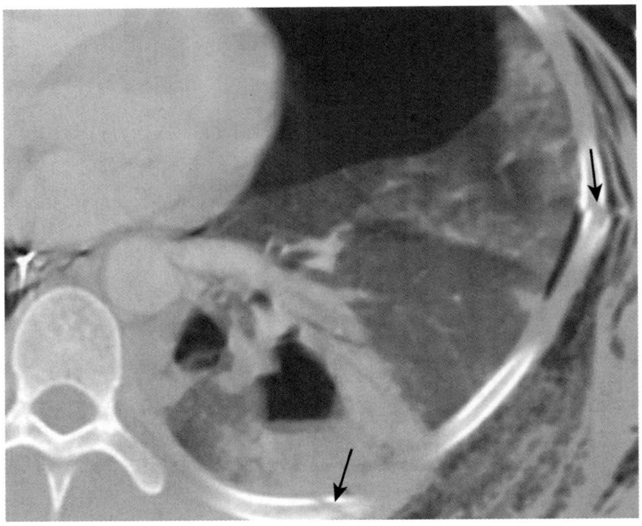

图 4　图 3 中患者的胸部 CT 表现。可见 X 线胸片无法显示的多发肋骨骨折（箭头所示）。尽管 X 线胸片提示胸管在侧方，肺扩张良好，但是 CT 上仍能看到后方的肺挫伤和裂伤，以及前方的气胸。这可能是因为 X 线胸片上气体及液体密度叠加造成的

胸部 CT

胸部 CT 扫描能比 X 线胸片发现更多的肋骨骨折以及肺挫伤（图 5）。Miller 的研究发现，即使只有 18% 的肺实质挫伤，胸部 CT 仍然能够发现，并且作者认为肺受累的范围与严重呼吸功能不全的可能性相关。如果肺挫伤的范围累及肺实质 20% 以上，82% 的患者会发展为 ARDS；如果累及范围小于 20%，仅有 22% 的患者发展为 ARDS。

连枷胸多见于 3 根及 3 根以上连续的肋骨骨折的情况。CT 扫描能够发现连续性的肋骨骨折，并且能提示查体未能发现的胸廓不稳定或功能异常。但

这并不意味着任何位置的CT显示的连续3根肋骨骨折都可以引起连枷胸。

肺挫伤病变区域在胸部CT上显示为浸润灶，其分布与解剖结构没有直接关联。伤后CT上继发出现的浸润影可能提示其他的情况，例如误吸、肺不张以及之后发生的肺炎等。这些情况和肺挫伤不容易鉴别，相反，CT上所显示的非解剖性和非继发性浸润性病灶可能是肺挫伤的特征性表现（图6）。CT上与胸膜相连的“冲击波”样改变是肺挫伤的特有表现（图7）。早期的胸部CT检查有利于评估肺挫伤的程度并预测是否会发生呼吸功能不全。

生理学研究

影像学对于功能评估的作用比较有限，因为很多非解剖性和生理性的导致肺损伤的因素可能会共存。对于肺挫伤以及连枷胸的生理以及功能方面的诊断依赖于对于患者生命体征、动脉血气、血流动力学以及床旁肺功能的评估。

肺挫伤最为显著的生理指标变化是低氧血症，这是由于部分肺通气功能不良引起的。低氧血症定义为在FIO_2稳定的情况下发生动脉血氧饱和度的下降，或者是需要吸入更高浓度的氧气来维持正常的血氧饱和度。低氧血症的情况可以用动脉氧分压与吸入氧浓度的比值（PaO_2/FIO_2）降低来反映。在呼吸机支持的患者当中，PEEP升高、平台压升高，或吸气与呼气比（I/E）逆转都可以提示高的肺血分流率Qs/Qt。此外，肺实质损伤经常导致肺顺应性下降，在自主呼吸或者压力通气模式的患者中可以表现为潮气量下降以及呼吸急促；而在容量控制通气模式下通气的患者中，则表现为气道峰值压的增加。

在单纯的连枷胸患者中，尽管每分通气量和呼吸功（work of breathing，WOB）会增加，但早期很

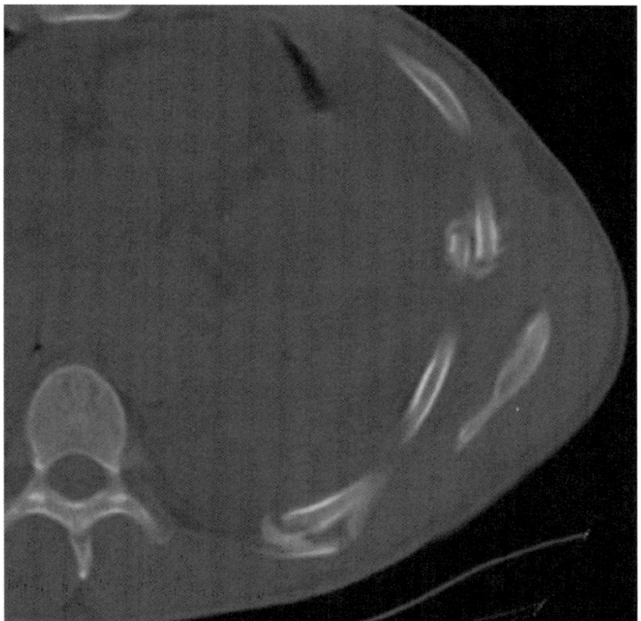

图5　无对比胸部CT图像，显示超过3根连续肋骨骨折。肩胛骨下方的肋骨骨折通过查体很难发现，而且一般也不会导致胸廓不稳定

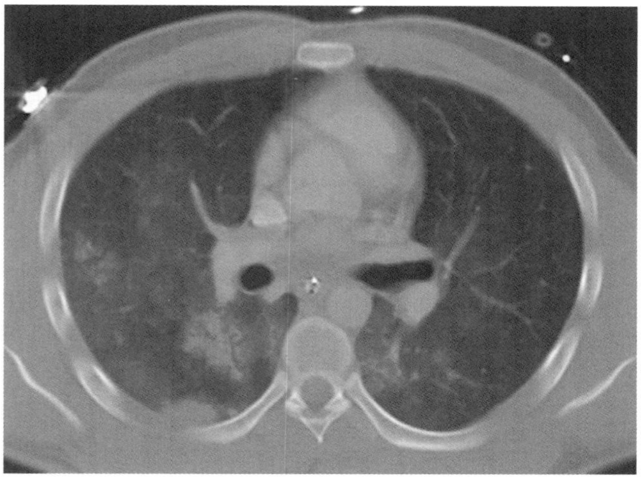

图6　胸部CT图像，来自高速车祸伤后发生严重肺挫伤的19岁患者，但骨性胸廓中仅有锁骨骨折。该患者3天后发展为严重的ALI/ARDS

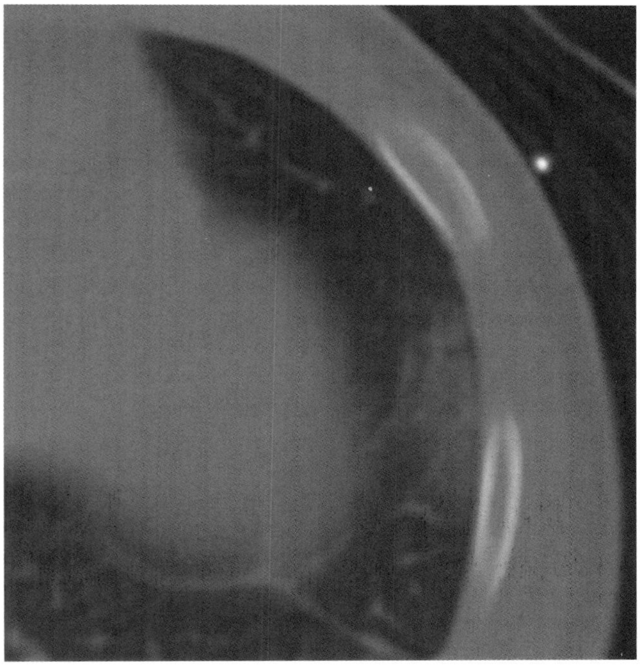

图7　仅能通过胸部CT发现的轻微的肺挫伤

少出现低氧血症，主要表现为浅快呼吸而血氧正常。当通气失败时发展为高碳酸血症和低氧血症。但是部分患者发病初期会伴有一定程度的肺挫伤，因此他们可能会由于肺不张、分泌物清除差或者免疫损伤等因素逐步出现低氧血症。有呼吸机支持的，只要呼吸机的容量压力能够支撑起胸壁和其同步运动，那么一般很少出现呼吸功能不全。

损伤的解剖学位置损伤分级

AAST-OIS 中胸部创伤的部分见 Moore 等总结的表 1、2。须注意的是对于胸廓及肺损伤的评分是分开的，但是二者在创伤中可能有重叠和相互作用。例如，连枷胸伴有肺挫伤的患者，需要气管插管的可能性显著高于仅有肺挫伤的患者，预后也更差一些。而现在 CT 上发现的小的肺挫伤对于预后一般没有明显的影响，或者说其意义仅限于患者须对长骨进行固定的情况。因此，这些量表应该用于 CT 诊断胸腔内损伤时评估（表 1 和 2）。

处理

肺挫伤或者连枷胸可以导致 4 种常见而严重的后遗症：①疼痛；②胸壁机械活动不稳定；③直接性肺损伤；④继发（免疫）性肺损伤。这 4 种后果都能直接或者间接引起肺气体交换功能障碍，因此可能是多系统损伤中影响发病率和死亡率的重要因素。

即时处理

在 20 世纪 80 年代早期，对于肺挫伤 / 连枷胸早期处理的争论点在于是否应积极行气管插管或是否应尝试避免插管。这个争论反映了早期时候插管的患者通常预后要更差。Richardson 等首次证明了，插管与非插管患者预后差异的根本原因在于创伤本身的严重程度，二者并不存在因果关系。后来认可的方法（反映在 ATLS 和其他流程中）为在早期表现为低氧血症的患者中进行气管插管，即选择性气管插管。对于连枷胸患者，如果不能够早期识别出呼吸功明显增加的情况，容易进展为早期通气衰竭而需要急诊插管。这是有争议的，有一些研究支持避免积极的早期插管。分析现有的文献，其实并没有在相同的人群对比早期插管和需求性插管的完全随机前瞻性的研究。现有的研究当中，早期插管的患者病情都相对严重一些。在我们看来，选择性插管导致预后变差是缺乏证据支持的。我们的策略是早期进行快速贯序插管和辅助通气来协助诊断并处理可能存在的严重损伤，如果确认患者能够自主呼吸的话，就及早拔除气管插管。如果在插管情况下呼吸功能仍在持续恶化，那么就需要长期的呼吸机支持并转入重症监护处理。

重症监护处理

肺挫伤会降低肺的顺应性并增加 Qs/Qt，连枷胸会导致胸廓功能下降、疼痛以及通气低效，这些损伤都能够引起通气不足和通气衰竭。减少胸部在连枷段的扩张，减少了功能残气量（functional residual capacity，FRC）相关的系统性损伤、休克以及肺部感染会引起继发的肺实质损伤。这些都可以导致分流和低氧血症。因此，对于连枷胸 / 肺挫伤的治疗是重症监护中创伤救治中很重要也很有挑战性的一方面。

对于连枷胸 / 肺挫伤的处理包括两个方面，一是减少分流比，二是限制畸形的胸腔的机械性问题。针对这两个目标的策略如下：

（1）通过有创或者无创正压通气和呼吸机复位操作来减少肺不张和肺压缩；

（2）通过改变患者的体位促进正常肺优先进行气体交换，或者使用单肺通气法优先正常肺通气；

（3）减少肺炎发展的可能。

对于较轻的损伤，可根据需要采用面罩吸氧。Trunkey 首先提出限制气管插管的应用。他还强调镇痛是临床上治疗肺损伤的有效补充措施。

通气管理的原则

通过紧密贴合的面罩进行持续正压通气（continuous positive airway pressure，CPAP）能够明显改善氧合并维持功能残气量。Antonelli 首先通过随机对照研究证明了在各种原因引起的急性呼吸衰竭的患者中使用无创通气的有效性。Gundez 通过随机对照研究在表现为连枷胸的高选择性、年轻人群（平均年龄 40 岁）中检验了 CPAP 的作用。研究中呼吸窘迫被定义为：呼吸频率大于 25 次 / 分，氧

表 1　胸壁损伤分级

等级	损伤类型	损伤描述	ICD–9	AIS–90
Ⅰ	挫伤	任何大小	911.0/922.1	1
	裂伤	皮肤和皮下	875.0	1
	骨折	<3 根肋骨骨折，闭合性	807.01	1-2
		无移位的锁骨骨折，闭合性	807/02	2
			810.00/810.03	
Ⅱ	裂伤	皮肤、皮下及肌肉	875.1	1
	骨折	>3 根相邻肋骨骨折，闭合性	807.03/807.09	2-3
		开放性或移位性锁骨骨折	810.10/810.13	2
		无移位性胸骨骨折，闭合性	807.2	2
		肩胛骨骨折，开放或闭合性	811.00/811.18	2
Ⅲ	裂伤	全层，包括壁层胸膜	862.29	2
	骨折	开放性或闭合性胸骨骨折	807.2	2
		包含胸骨的连枷胸段	807.3	3-4
		单侧连枷胸段（<3 根肋骨）	807.4	
Ⅳ	裂伤	胸壁组织撕脱，可伴有肋骨骨折	807.10/807.19	4
	骨折	单侧连枷胸（≥3 根肋骨）	807.4	3-4
Ⅴ	骨折	双侧连枷胸（双侧>3 根肋骨）	807.4	5

Modified from Moore EE, Cogbill TH, Malangoni MA, et al: Organ injury scaling. *Surg Clin North Am* 75:293–303, 1995.

AIS，简明损伤分级

这个量表仅限于在胸壁创伤中使用，不适用于合并肺实质损伤或者腹部损伤。因此，上胸部和下胸部或者前胸壁和后胸壁的对比未涉及。Ⅵ级损伤的引入是必要的，胸部挤压并未作为一个描述性词汇。相反，骨折和软组织损伤的分布与程度作为分级的依据

表 2　肺损伤分级

等级 *	损伤类型	损伤描述	ICD–9	AIS–90
Ⅰ	挫伤	单侧，<1 肺叶	861.12 861.31	3
Ⅱ	挫伤	单侧，单一肺叶	861.20 861.30	3
	裂伤	简单气胸	860.0/1	3
Ⅲ	挫伤	单侧，>1 肺叶	861.20 861.30	3
	裂伤	远端气道持续漏气（>72 h）	860.0/1 860.4/5 862.0	3-4
	血肿	位于肺实质，不再扩大	861.30	
Ⅳ	裂伤	严重漏气（涉及肺段或者肺叶）	862.21 861.31	4-5
	血肿	位于肺实质，逐渐扩大		
	血管	肺内主要血管分支损伤	901.40	3-5
Ⅴ	血管	肺门血管损伤	901.41 901.42	4
Ⅵ	血管	肺门血管横断，未受污染	901.41 901.42	4

Modified from Moore EE, Cogbill TH, Malangoni MA, et al: Organ injury scaling. Surg Clin North Am 75:293–303, 1995.

AIS，简明损伤分级

*：对于Ⅰ级和Ⅱ级，如果病变为双侧的话，就在原基础上增加 1 级。血胸归入血管损伤中进行评分

和在吸入 10 L/min 氧气的情况下小于 90%，当 FIO_2 大于 0.5 时 P/F 比例小于 300。结果发现院内感染发生和存活方面 CPAP 组要优于插管组。尽管研究设计是随机化的，但是仍然不可避免地造成创伤相对轻的患者进入非插管组。此外连枷胸 / 肺挫伤导致肺功能不全的自然病程是在创伤发生后的几天内逐渐恶化的。根据我们的经验，胸部创伤的患者如果须使用 CPAP 或者 BiPAP（相关的鼻形式）的话，往往几天后须急诊行气管插管，这也有风险。并且 CPAP 容易引起胃扩张，继而可能发生误吸。因此我们认为在严重胸部创伤的患者中使用 CPAP 来延迟插管可能是不恰当的。严重损伤的气管插管往往是不能避免的，应在病情恶化前插管。正如医学上常讲的，当你觉得该气管插管时，应该已经确实有这个必要了。

通气支持

对于胸部创伤的患者进行呼吸机支持要比其他患者情况复杂一些。插管的患者可能需要一些气体交换的支持，但是只要患者能够进行自主呼吸（不论什么程度），就应该采用自主呼吸模式。压力支持通气（pressare support ventilation，PSV）模式对于存在自主呼吸的患者是首选的，但是对于严重连枷胸的患者须慎重考虑，因为在这种情况下触发呼吸机的负压可能会造成胸壁的不稳定，导致疼痛和延迟愈合，这应该被避免。我们通常在开始阶段使用容量控制通气，如同步间歇指令通气（synchronized mandatory ventilation，SIMV），通过控制每分通气量来保证动脉血 pH 轻度高于 7.4。这样能够在不使用镇静药物的情况下抑制自主呼吸。连枷胸大约可以在一周内稳定，有较厚的胸壁者通常稳定得更快。之后可以换成 PSV，直到后来撤除呼吸机。

最近有研究发现，对于可能发展为 ALI/ARDS 的胸部创伤患者，气道压力释放通气模式（airway pressure release ventilation，APRV）是一种潜在的呼吸机策略。APRV 是一种压力限制的周期性通气模式，通气周期中会从高压迅速转换到低压，从而形成深呼气。呼吸周期中任何时候的自主呼吸都是允许的，来支持 CPAP 呼吸中的患者做功。回顾性的研究结果显示，APRV 能够显著改善氧合情况，并能降低气道压峰值以及呼吸机相关肺炎的风险。

胸部创伤、肺挫伤以及 ARDS 会降低肺顺应性。为了达到与正常肺一样的潮气量，需要更高的气道压力。来自 ARDSNet 的数据显示，应该避免过高的气道压（35 cm H_2O），使用低潮气量（6 ~ 8 ml/g）可以降低气道压峰值。对于有支气管胸膜瘘的患者，限制气道压更为重要。对于镇静的患者，不严格要求正常的 $PaCO_2$，因为适当的高碳酸血症对于胸部创伤后的低氧血症有一定帮助。回顾性的研究显示在 ARDS 和胸部爆炸伤的患者中，适当高碳酸血症是安全的，而且在一些研究发现适当的高碳酸血症明显改善死亡率，但是并没有前瞻性的随机对照研究证实。此外，须注意的是，保持适当的高碳酸血症须注意控制肺泡压，而不能只关注 $PaCO_2$ 的数值。

氧气支持

受到胸部严重创伤的患者都会表现出一定程度的低氧血症。在初期可以通过提高 FIO_2 来改善，但是长时间的高 FIO_2 本身是有害的。因此，低氧血症的长期治疗须包括增加平均气道压的方法来维持和改善氧合。这包括通过不同呼吸机策略实现的 PEEP 或者逆转 I/E 时间。这些措施能促进肺复张，减少肺泡内和间质中的水分。逆转 I/E 时间受到 CO_2 蓄积以及高 I/E 比时自发 PEEP 的限制。传统的高潮气量通气（10 ~ 15 ml/kg）并不能促进肺扩张，在多数情况下也不能改善氧合，而且这种方法会引起通气分布不均衡，导致部分肺泡过度扩张以及 VILI。从 20 世纪 90 年代起，我们开始使用低潮气量通气策略（我们称之为"温和通气呼吸"）。从当时起，低潮气量通气在常规的 ICU 患者中就显示了生存获益，此后我们把这种做法扩展到多数的胸部创伤患者。

在创伤相关的文献中，关于如何使用 PEEP 的资料非常有限。从一份包括 2 299 例 ALI 以及 ARDS 患者的 meta 分析推论得出，使用高 PEEP 以及肺复张呼吸治疗是安全的，而且可能会带来生存获益（>12 cmH_2O）。Schreite 研究了 17 例因为肺挫伤引起 ARDS 的患者的资料，发现肺复张呼吸压在 50 ~ 80 cmH_2O 时能够改善患者的氧合，并且 CT 扫描证实它能够减少肺萎陷，不过对患者的预后并未进行研究。另一种可能改善肺挫伤患者氧合情况的方法是高频振荡通气（high-frequency oscillatory ventilation，HFOV）。使用低潮气量进行高频通气，能够使气道压维持在一定水平，这样最大程度地减少了气压伤，并且能够维持肺泡复张。目前有一些小规模的研究发现 HFOV 能够改善手术后患者的氧合，但还需要更大规模的随机对照研究来得出关于安全和疗效的结论。

在顽固性的低氧血症的患者中，还有一些缺乏循证医学证据支持的方法在广泛使用，包括旋转病床或差别肺通气、吸入一氧化氮、部分液态通气、HTS、输注红细胞，以及使用正性肌力药物提高混合静脉氧饱合度等。这些方法都可能会起到一定效果，某些情况下能延长终末期患者的生存时间，但是都缺乏前瞻性的研究验证。体外膜氧合支持或体外生命支持（extracorporeal membrare oxygenation support or life support，ECMO/ECLS）然而对于创伤后 ARDS 进展的患者来说，也是一种有效的辅助方法，即使是在控制止血时。

对于已经插管的胸部创伤患者，应该优先进行气管支气管清洁，因为患者可能会发生颗粒误吸，或者因为气道分泌物堵塞造成肺叶萎陷。损伤发生时的大量误吸，以及气管插管以后的少量误吸，都会导致气道分泌物增加以及口咽部菌落的定植。气道分泌物增加会继发引起肺萎陷、分流和低氧血症、肺顺应性下降，以及阻塞后气道感染。肺挫伤之后出血会在气道内聚集并形成支气管内血块，插管的患者无法咳痰，这些情况都需要吸引（为了气道清洁）。当分泌物黏稠时，N- 乙酰半胱氨酸类药物可以用于溶解黏液，但是会引起支气管痉挛，因此须同时使用支气管扩张剂。此外长期的 N- 乙酰半胱氨酸类药物治疗会引起支气管黏液溢出。胸部物理疗法对于排痰有帮助，但是叩诊损伤的肋骨会比较疼痛。因此，通常须使用支气管镜去除分泌物和颗粒。颗粒残渣和血块的取出须用到网兜或者将其粉碎后吸出（图 8）

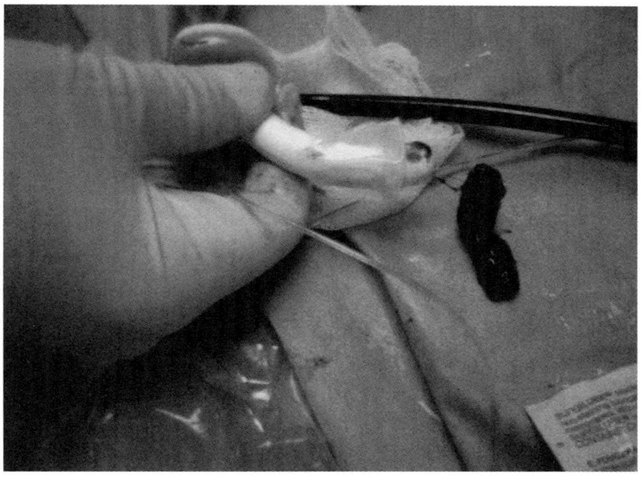

图 8　气管内出血形成的血凝块。这个血凝块体积较大，支气管镜下无法切碎。当用支气管镜取出的时候由于无法通过气管造口管孔道而被迫先撤出，再更换造口管

疼痛管理

对于胸部创伤的处理中，疼痛的控制非常重要。既往认为，合并肋骨骨折的患者，如果通过胸壁夹板固定的方法来减轻疼痛的话，往往会成为肺炎的主要诱发因素，但是这个观点从来没有得到证实。近期的研究提示，创伤的患者发生肺炎，实际上是免疫受到抑制的后果。良好的疼痛控制对于改善患者的一般状况非常重要，并且可能改善患者的肺部清洁情况。胸壁疼痛可以通过系统性的镇痛药物和肋间、胸膜内、胸膜下或者椎旁神经阻滞来实现。条件允许且无禁忌证的情况下，硬膜外阻滞也是镇痛不错的选择。既往采用胸带或包扎固定的方法来止痛是没有科学依据的。

类固醇激素治疗

前文已经提过，所有胸部钝伤都会伴有一定程度的 ALI/ARDS，然而目前还没有公认的对于治疗创伤后 ARDS 有效的药物或者干预。有一些小的研究提示，在 ARDS 后期的纤维增生阶段，系统性地使用类固醇激素可能有效。然而，考虑到类固醇激素使用相关的多种已知并发症，在前瞻性研究得出结果之间，我们不会在晚期 ARDS 患者中常规使用类固醇激素。

气管造口术

和气管插管类似，在严重创伤患者中进行早期气管造口术似乎有些激进，但是，病情恶化后进行气管造口术的风险会明显升高。因此，对于病情较重的患者，有经验的医生会寻找合适的时间窗，将通气途径从气管插管改为气管造口术。早期气管造口术（通常定义为 7 天以内）能够为清洁气道提供更好的途径，也提供了更好的口咽卫生。尽管还存在不同观点，但是这个方法确实可以降低肺炎发病率，缩短脱机拔管时间。正如上文提到的那样，与高通气量和压力相比，低潮气量和低气道压通气会造成较少的肺损伤。而气管造口相较于气管插管，在相同的肺泡通气量时，能够减少解剖无效腔量并降低气道压峰值。这对于顽固性呼吸衰竭、需要更积极的呼吸机设置来维持氧合的患者来说是非常重要的。

手术固定治疗连枷胸

多数的连枷胸通过镇痛、选择性插管及机械通气能获得较为理想的生理学上的控制。手术治疗的指征包括长期的呼吸机支持、严重的胸壁畸形，以及其他需要开胸探查的指征。理论上讲，复原胸壁的三维结构能够帮助纠正连枷胸引起的呼吸功能损伤。

很多方法可以用来实现胸壁稳定，包括钢板、可吸收聚合物板、髓内钉、合成树脂、U 形板等都可以作为可选的固定手段，目前还没有确定最佳干预方法的比较研究。

从解剖学角度来看，由于每根肋骨的骨皮质有限、下方的血管神经束走行接近，且容易形成粉碎性或斜形骨折，因此对肋骨骨折进行手术复位和内固定难度较大。而且，在存在胸管、呼吸道菌群污染，以及创伤本身的环境污染的情况下，在胸壁植入内固定物可能使手术复杂。

EAST 发布的连枷胸的处理指南中，对于需要呼吸机支持和开胸术的严重的单侧胸壁畸形和连枷胸患者，手术内固定是三级推荐，但这个推荐的依据主要是来源于非随机化的、未经过匹配的观察性研究。

然而也有两项随机对照研究值得注意。第一项是由 Tanaka 等进行的前瞻性随机对照研究，入组的 37 例患者通过年龄、ISS 评分、骨折肋骨数量、肺挫伤严重程度、入院时的 P/F 比例进行了匹配。试验组在伤后第 5 天使用合成树脂对 T4 — T10 肋骨进行了固定，对照组给予最佳的呼吸策略（通过 PEEP、SIMV、压力支持保持内部气动稳定）。结果发现试验组明显优于对照组，使用机械通气的时间减少 8 天，ICU 治疗时间减少 10 天，肺炎发生率降低 50%，总的医疗花费也明显降低（\$13 455 vs. \$23 423, $P<0.05$）。但是在 EAST 指南中，这项研究的证据等级被定为 3 级，因为入组的随机化患者数较少，而且对照组中没有使用更为有效的综合治疗策略，例如硬膜外镇痛以及胸部物理疗法等。第二项随机研究是由 Granetzny 等主导的，结果也证明了对于连枷胸患者进行手术固定的优势。共有 40 名患者随机分到试验组及对照组，试验组伤后 24 ~ 36 h 之内进行外科胸壁固定，对照组的连枷胸段使用有弹性的绷带包扎——“捆绑和包扎”。研究结果发现胸壁畸形（胸部萎陷或者肋骨聚拢）的发生率在试验组明显低于对照组（试验组 1/20，对照组 9/20），而且试验组患者伤后 2 个月肺功能（包括用力肺活量、肺总量、75% 用力呼气量）好于对照组，但是研究中使用的解剖学疗效指标以及肺功能的改善程度在临床中是否有意义，这一点还不明确。在有气管插管的患者中（仅有 35% 对照患者和 45% 手术患者，或总病例数 16 人），手术修复组平均机械通气的时间从 12 天减少为 2 天。此外，尽管研究中对于肺炎的定义并不明确，手术组肺炎发生率也明显降低（10% vs. 50%）。这项研究同样存在样本过少的问题，此外，研究中并未对呼吸机策略以及镇痛处理进行控制或者匹配，也未探讨肺挫伤的作用。

Voggenreiter 等在 42 名连枷胸患者中，研究了其是否存在肺挫伤。患者在年龄、损伤严重范围这些方面没有显著差异。他们特别在存在或不存在肺挫伤的患者中检查了胸部固定的效果，结果发现，只有伴有呼吸功能不全的不存在肺挫伤的患者，可以从 ORIF 中获益，这可能是因为这类患者能够早期插管。而伴有肺挫伤的患者，是不能从 ORIF 中获益的。总的来说，对于大多数连枷胸患者来说，手术固定是不推荐的。

目前也慢慢地出现一些证据，认为在一些特定的患者群体中，例如连枷胸胸廓不稳定引起呼吸衰竭的患者和肺实质相对无损伤的患者，早期积极的治疗可能是有效的。此外，因为其他相关的损伤而必须手术治疗的患者可能也会从中获益。目前还需要效能高的多中心随机对照临床试验来证明手术固定对于连枷胸患者中的哪部分患者能够起到作用。目前基于标准的 CT 扫描对连枷胸的评估可能是不准确的，将来需要基于损伤的生物力学作用对连枷胸进行分型，并改进手术的方法。我们认为，非增强的动态 CT 扫描可能会帮助我们明确哪些患者更能从手术中获益。明确骨折的病理解剖学也有助于发现“铰链”和最大机动性的区域。基于这些信息进行手术重建，有利于提高术后的胸廓稳定性，同时减少手术的创伤程度。

死亡率

创伤导致肺挫伤或连枷胸后，多数情况下死亡是由相关合并损伤导致的，例如头颅损伤，但是严重的胸部创伤也是死亡的独立危险因素。在这类情形中，死亡的原因通常包括 ARDS、呼吸衰竭、脓毒症以及多器官功能衰竭（multiple organ failure，MOF）。因此，预后与可能引起这些情况的因素相关，包括患者的 ISS 评分或者急性生理和慢性健康评估（Acute Physiology and Chronic Health Evaluation，APACHE）评分升高、输血次数增多等等。如果连枷胸的患者在胸片上发现有肺挫伤，那么患者需要机械通气的可能性以及死亡率是仅有其中一种情况的两倍以上。Livingston 等研究通过 CT 影像预测，少于 5 根肋骨骨折的死亡率大约是 2%，5 ~ 8 根肋骨骨折的死亡率上升到 9%，多于 9 根的死亡率可以高达 27%。类似的，连枷胸患者的死亡率与年龄及 ISS 评分相关：55 岁以上的患者，年龄每增加 10 岁，死亡率增加 132%；ISS 评分每增加 1 分，死亡率增加 30%。呼吸机相关性肺炎也是胸部创伤患者死亡的独立危险因素，虽然肺炎本身为一个大的系统性创伤的标志。

最后，因为爆炸导致胸部创伤的患者，通常更容易合并高能量引起的全身损伤，因此整体的死亡率要比机动车或行人的创伤要高。一项最近由联合手术室创伤登记发布的报告显示，爆炸伤的患者，在到达医疗机构前的死亡率就高达 66%，早期存活的患者当中 24% 会死于后续的肺部后遗症或相关损伤。

总的来说，肺挫伤以及连枷胸的死亡率很高，尤其是在有多系统损伤或共存疾病的患者当中。不过随着越来越先进的 ICU 管理技术，仅由连枷胸或者肺挫伤引起死亡的情况会越来越少。

结论

- 肺挫伤和连枷胸是胸部钝伤后常见的比较危险的后遗症；
- 肺挫伤和连枷胸通常同时存在；
- 单纯的连枷胸通常见于肋骨质地较脆弱的老年人；
- 单纯的肺挫伤通常见于肋骨质地较柔韧的年轻人；
- 肺挫伤和连枷胸都会因为休克、SIRS 以及炎症性急性肺损伤而引起呼吸功能不全；
- 肺挫伤和连枷胸导致的氧合下降通常是由于 ALI 和挫伤肺内分流引起的（Qs/Qt）；
- 肺挫伤和连枷胸导致的通气功能障碍通常反映了胸壁损伤和机械通气和呼吸功引起的疼痛；
- 严重的肺挫伤和连枷胸患者通常需要 5 ~ 10 天的呼吸机支持；
- 创伤比较轻微的患者可以不需要气管插管；
- 创伤较重的患者须考虑早期插管。

胸壁损伤的手术治疗

R. Stephen Smith，Juan A. Asensio 著
幸华杰 译

胸壁损伤是导致发病和死亡的重要病因，而肋骨骨折是胸廓损伤最常见的表现之一，在很多创伤的患者中都会发生。例如 94% 的系安全带的机动车创伤患者都合并有肋骨骨折，大约 25% 的创伤所致死亡是与胸廓损伤相关的。多数的胸廓创伤仅需要简单的处理，例如辅助供氧气、机械通气、胸廓造口术置管等，不需要手术治疗。胸壁损伤的基本病例生理学改变包括低氧血症、高碳酸血症，以及代谢性和呼吸性酸中毒。连枷胸会涉及上述所有的病理生理学改变。

在创伤中心处理的所有患者中，大约 10% 合并肋骨骨折，这些患者中多数仅需要镇痛、肺部清洁以及其他的对症处理。肋骨骨折的患者当中，大约 10% 为连枷胸。连枷胸是由胸部高能量暴力损伤引起的，传统上定义为有 3 根或 3 根以上连续的肋骨上的至少 2 处骨折。多发连续肋骨骨折的患者呼吸和肺功能受损的表现与连枷胸一致。对于连枷胸的患者，即使有充分的镇痛、肺部清洁以及其他的支持措施，仍有 50% 以上的患者需要气管插管。连枷胸治疗很重要的一点是充分的镇痛。没有通气的患者，如果镇痛不充分的话，会异常疼痛，导致通气不足、分泌物潴留、进行性肺不张、肺叶萎陷、肺炎以及呼吸衰竭。对连枷胸患者最好的镇痛措施为胸廓硬膜外镇痛。镇痛应该及早进行，以免发生进行性呼吸困难。然而这项措施经常被拖延到创伤发生 24 h 以后。如果可以用长效局部麻醉药，也可以采用肋间神经阻滞的方法。经皮置导管向肋骨骨折部位或肋间神经走行区持续给予局部麻醉药也是可行的，但是目前还缺乏证据支持。外用的含有长效局部麻醉药的贴剂和敷料在肋骨骨折和连枷胸的患

者中没有明显作用。发生连枷胸的患者，死亡率可以高达 10%～36%，主要与相关的损伤相关。

手术治疗的指征

大多数的连枷胸患者不需要手术治疗。多数情况下，潜在的肺挫伤是引起低氧血症和需要机械通气的根本原因。肺挫伤引起低氧血症的患者，在氧合没有改善之前，不应该做择期手术。有些患者中多发肋骨骨折和连枷胸的生物力学影响导致无法进行充分的通气，在这种情况下，即使没有肺挫伤，通气不足也会造成呼吸衰竭。

对于肋骨骨折和连枷胸的手术固定的指征在不断变化。伴有急性呼吸衰竭的患者和因为肋骨骨折不愈合引起慢性疼痛及残疾的患者的手术适应证不同。合并其他胸内损伤需要开胸探查的患者，可以同时对骨折肋骨进行手术固定。此外早期没有插管的患者，如果在充分的非手术治疗措施下，肺功能仍持续恶化而需要气管插管，这类患者也可以通过手术对肋骨进行固定。伤后初期就因为肺挫伤需要呼吸机支持的患者，如果在肺挫伤好转后，仍不能脱离呼吸机，可以考虑进行手术固定。广泛移位性骨折，或者前外侧连枷胸伴进展性骨折移位的患者，可以进行手术固定。对于这类患者，手术复位内固定可以避免产生胸廓畸形，更重要的是，能够避免形成假关节以及由此带来的慢性疼痛。对于这类患者，肋间神经阻滞是治疗慢性疼痛的重要方法，这类患者加巴喷丁是治疗肋骨移位和假关节所致慢性疼痛的标准的治疗方案。图 1 所示为制定急性连枷胸手术治疗决策流程图。

解剖和切口

正确显露骨折肋骨进行手术固定须熟悉胸壁的解剖。胸壁的主要肌群包括斜方肌、菱形肌、胸大肌、胸小肌、背阔肌、前锯肌，以及竖脊肌。能够充分显露肋骨骨折端的入路包括经过腋尖的开胸切口、弯曲的腋窝的切口、保留肌肉的水平切口，以及经典的后外侧开胸切口。大约 90% 的固定手术是通过后外侧切口进行的。多数病例都不须进入胸膜腔即可完成肋骨固定，手术可以实现第 3 至第 9 肋的修复，第 1 肋和第 2 肋的显露较为困难。第 10、11、12 肋一般不需要手术来恢复胸廓的机械结构。连枷胸的患者通常会合并胸壁肌肉结构和肋间神经损伤，这些结构的损伤会影响呼吸时胸壁的力学并引起慢性疼痛。

手术技术

在过去的几十年当中，文献中报道了多种对连枷胸进行手术固定的方法，包括人造树脂板、髓内设备（kirschner 线）、垂直桥接假体（如钢板、假体网片以及胸骨钢丝）。目前还没有研究说明哪一种方法更好。近年来也开发出一些新的肋骨骨折手术固定方式能更好地实现肋骨骨折的固定，包括一种 U

图 1　手术治疗急性连枷胸的流程

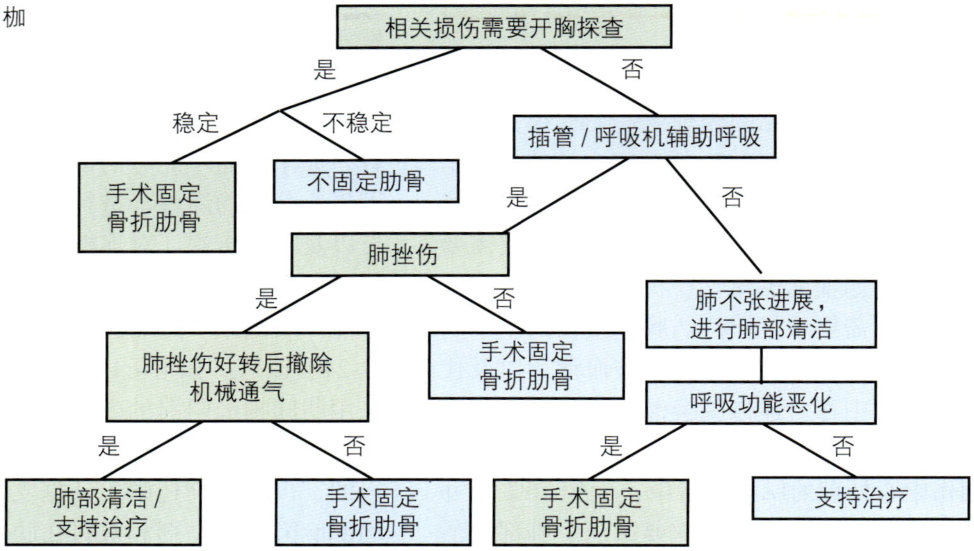

形固定板（Acute Innovations），以及利用弯曲钢板和髓内支架的系统（Synthes）。这两种方法都能够顺利完成肋骨骨折内固定（图2和图3）。假关节的手术治疗相对困难一些，往往需要较大范围的分离及截骨术。

考虑做手术固定的患者，应该在术前进行胸廓的影像学评估。除了常用的X线胸片，胸部CT扫描能够清晰地显示胸壁损伤的程度。三维CT重建能够充分显示胸壁畸形的程度以及骨折端重叠的程度，这对于制订手术计划非常重要。对于肋骨骨折后慢性疼痛的患者，胸部CT对于确定假关节的存在和定位非常有帮助（图4）。

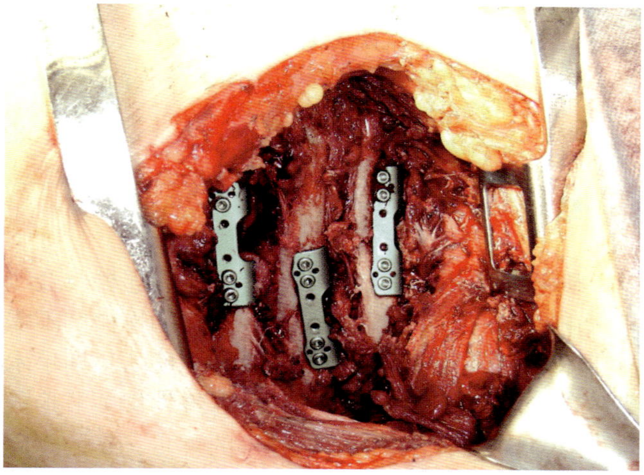

图2 使用特殊设计的U形固定装置对肋骨骨折进行手术治疗

预后

关于连枷胸手术固定的文章有很多，然而多数研究是非随机的回顾性研究，或者是个案报道。多数文献对于手术固定治疗连枷胸的优势都比较认可，包括降低机械通气时间、缩短ICU治疗时间、降低肺炎发生率，以及降低死亡率。手术固定的劣势在于需要全身麻醉、较大的切口，以及植入物造成的术后慢性疼痛。对于发生慢性疼痛的患者，有必要取出植入物。Ahmed和Mohyuddin报告了包括426例胸壁损伤患者的10年回顾性调查，其中64例患者发生连枷胸。连枷胸患者中，26例进行了手术修复。作者把手术患者和38例接受非手术处理的患者进行了对比，手术患者的死亡率更低（8%vs. 29%）、机械通气时间更短、气管造口比例更低、入住ICU时间更短，以及肺部感染率更低。Balci等在9年时间中对64例需要机械通气的连枷胸患者进行了一项前瞻性、非随机研究，其中27例进行了手术治疗。结果发现，手术组机械通气时间、住院时间以及并发症发生率和死亡率都较非手术组降低。Tanaka等也在需要机械通气的连枷胸患者中进行了一项前瞻性试验。手术组和非手术组都首先接受了5天标准的机械通气、镇痛以及肺部清洁治疗。如果5天机械通气后患者还不能拔除气管插管，那么患者被随机分到手术组和继续非手术治疗组。手术组机械通气时间以及ICU治疗时间明显低于非手术组。此外手术组患者术后1个月的肺活量明显高于非手术组，且差异有统计学意义。近期，Solberg等介绍了胸部

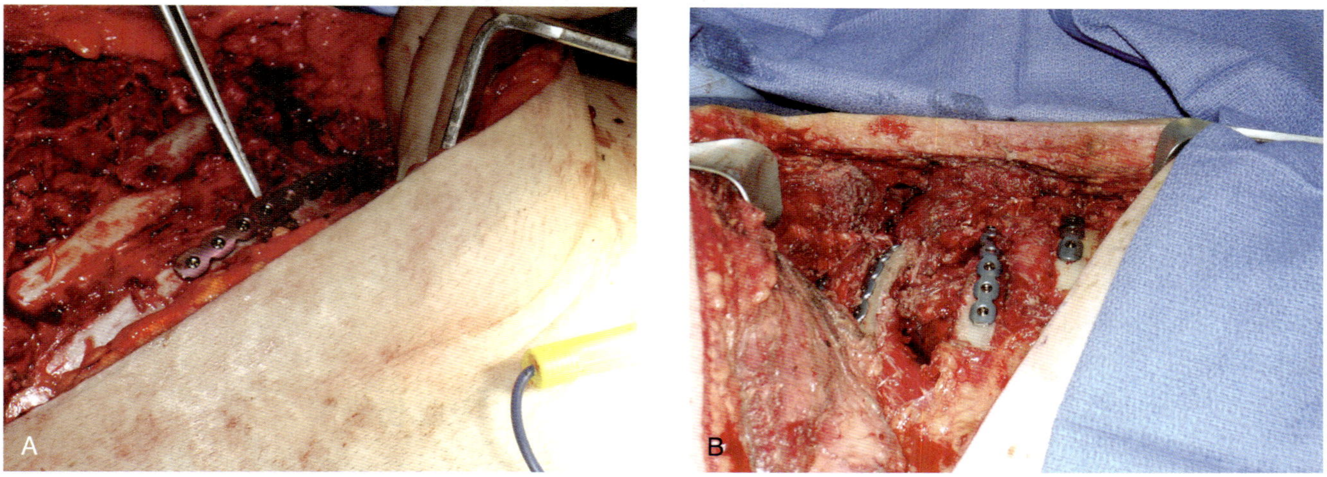

图3 A 连枷胸术中照片，可以看到肋骨骨折断端有明显的重叠。通过可用的与肋骨形状匹配的钢板及锁定螺钉对骨折进行手术固定。B 对连枷段胸段进行手术固定，可以见到肋间肌损伤比较严重

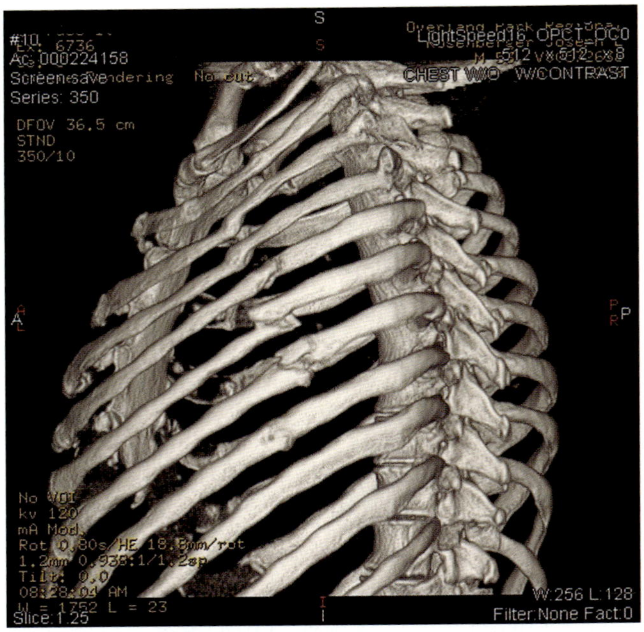

图 4 对肋骨骨折慢性不愈合（假关节）的患者进行胸部 CT 扫描三维重建，可以见到 2 处肋骨有问题。手术切除假关节并对肋骨进行固定可以明显缓解慢性疼痛并改善其伤残

治疗的方法。研究发现，手术治疗的患者，能够较早拔管，ICU 治疗时间也相对较短。Collins 等最近报道了一项长达 60 个月的回顾性对照研究，其中 15 人接受手术治疗，18 人接受非手术治疗。两组患者在年龄、性别、ISS 评分和 GCS 评分这些方面的情况相近。手术组的患者机械通气的时间明显缩短（6.3 vs. 11.8, P=0.036），并且 ICU 治疗时间和总的住院时间也呈缩短趋势。在过去的 5 年半中，我们为 36 例连枷胸患者做了手术，其中 24 例是在连枷胸的急性期，12 例是因为肋骨骨折不愈合，导致严重残疾或者慢性疼痛而做的手术。手术的总体效果良好，但是有 2 例因为植入失效而需要二次手术。

胸骨骨折

胸骨骨折常见于不系安全带的司机遇到减速机动车事故的情况。胸壁钝伤的患者当中，5% 的患者合并胸骨骨折，40% 的胸骨骨折的患者会合并肋骨骨折。既往认为，胸骨骨折相关损伤导致的死亡率可以高达 25%～45%。而近年来文献中报道的死亡率和发病率较前降低。胸骨骨折一般不需要手术处理，骨折不愈合很少见。但是假关节造成的慢性疼痛以及骨折断端重叠畸形需要手术矫正。这种情况下须评估患者有无心、肺、胸段脊髓损伤。

胸骨骨折的患者通常表现为胸骨的局部压痛，多数是横行骨折，发生在胸骨柄和胸骨体的连接处。侧位 X 线胸片或者胸部 CT 扫描可以明确诊断。多数患者仅需要合适的支持治疗就能愈合，包括充分的镇痛以及肺部清洁。如果骨折断端明显重叠的话，早期的手术修复可以使患者疼痛明显减轻、外观改善，并且能够改善肺功能，从而使患者获益。

结论

胸部钝性伤后引起多发肋骨骨折和连枷胸会严重影响患者的生存。多数的肋骨骨折和连枷胸不需要手术处理。经过筛选的部分患者能够从早期手术复位固定中获益。慢性疼痛的患者继发假关节形成也可以考虑手术治疗。随着技术的进步，新的内固定系统的出现提高了外科医生修复连枷胸段的能力。对于胸骨骨折的患者，仅有少部分需要手术修复。胸壁创伤的患者，在决定手术治疗之前，一定要意识到可能有发生并发症和设备故障的风险。

气管和气管支气管树损伤

Preston R. Miller 和 J. Wayne Meredith 著
幸华杰 译

气管支气管损伤可以引起不同程度的后遗症，其中很多都是致命的。如果患者能够被及时送到创伤中心和医疗机构，得到合适的诊治的话，预后一般较好。这需要医生熟悉气管支气管损伤的症状、体征、诊断技术、合适的气道处理方法，以及修复手段。

发病率及损伤机制

气管支气管树损伤比较少见，但是在胸部穿通伤和钝伤中为容易识别的并发症。很多患者因为重要器官的相关损伤，引起出血、张力性气胸、呼吸功能不全等，在到达急诊之前死亡，因此有些诊断是在死亡后才做出的。还有一部分患者表现不典型，只有当气管支气管损伤发展症状严重后才能得到诊断。因此，气管支气管树损伤的准确发病率难以得知。一项对 1 178 例死于胸部钝伤的患者进行尸体解剖的综述发现，有 33 例患者发生了气管支气管树损伤，发病率为 2.8%。其中 27 例在伤后迅速死亡。另一项包括了 15 136 名诊断为胸部钝伤的存活者和非存活者的综述中，49 名（0.3%）发生气管支气管损伤。这个研究显示患者的死亡率高达 67%，但是研究中并没有描述相关损伤的严重程度。Asensio 在一项包括 4 193 例颈部穿通伤的患者的综述中报告其中的 331 例（8%）发生了喉及气管损伤。超过 80% 的气管支气管钝性损伤发生在距离隆嵴 2.5 cm 的范围内，其中 86% 的患者发生主支气管损伤，9.3% 的患者发生远端支气管损伤，8% 的患者为复合型损伤。

穿通伤是一种直接的机制，通常是由刀或者子弹的路径造成的洞。刀伤多见于颈部气管，而子弹伤可以见于气管支气管树走行的任何部位。胸内气管支气管树损伤多见于胸部钝性伤，也可以由子弹伤引起。如果子弹穿透纵隔的话，损伤发生的概率会比较高。合并其他纵隔结构的损伤，包括心脏、大血管、食管等，这些器官的损伤也会使死亡率和发病率升高。

钝性创伤损伤气管和支气管有几种机制，包括直接打击、剪切应力以及爆裂伤。颈部受到直接打击后出现晾衣绳样损伤，会导致颈部气管挤压颈椎椎体，导致气管软骨环或者环状软骨横断。剪切应力导致气管相对固定的部位容易受到损伤，如环状软骨和隆嵴。沿气管支气管树的爆裂伤常见于胸廓受到快速的前后向的挤压，而胸膜内负压导致肺沿胸壁向两侧拉伸，从而在隆嵴处产生牵拉。当这种牵拉超过气管支气管树的弹性范围时，肺被拉向两边，支气管被撕裂。如果声门关闭，外界的冲击会导致气道内压力增高，使气管变硬，造成气管膜部的线性撕裂或爆裂或造成气管支气管的复合型损伤。根据 LaPlaee 准则，通常这种损伤发生在气道内径最大的部位，一般在距离隆嵴 2.5 cm 以内，但也可以发生在气道的任何位置。对于多数气管支气管树损伤来说，一般是上述几种机制共同作用的结果。由于气道一般受到这些结构保护，因此损伤多由大量的高能量转移引起的。

诊断

临床表现

气管支气管树损伤后可以出现多种临床表现，但是多与损伤发生的位置和损伤的严重程度相关。颈部气管损伤的患者，可以表现为喘鸣、严重的呼吸窘迫，或者伴有声音沙哑、咯血、颈部皮下气肿等。胸部气管支气管损伤的表现，取决于损伤是否局限在纵隔区或者是否与胸膜腔交通。局限于纵隔的损伤通常表现为严重的纵隔气肿，有时会出现心包气肿。若损伤穿透胸膜腔，通常会引起单侧气胸，可能有或无张力。如果气胸经过充分的置管引流后仍然有持续漏气的话，提示存在气管支气管损伤以及支气管胸膜瘘。由于肺的总体积会通过引流管丢失，即使留置引流管后呼吸困难症状仍会恶化。其他能够在气管插管时提示气道损伤的影像学证据包括气管插管的尖端发生异常的位移，或者气管插管的球囊过度扩张超出了正常气管的直径范围。

一些回顾性的研究显示，超过 2/3 的气管支气管撕裂不能在伤后 24 h 内被识别出。高达 10% 的病例不会产生任何临床或者影像学表现，直到伤后几个月，产生狭窄症状之后才被发现。伴随多系统损伤的患者，如果即刻进行气管插管，喉段或者高位颈段气管损伤可能会被忽略，这会导致诊断延迟。在气管支气管横断之后，气道周围的结缔组织可以保持完整，远端肺组织仍能通过类似于主动脉横断时维持灌注的方式来持续通气。这种情况如果没有被及时识别出来，损伤处逐渐通过瘢痕和肉芽组织愈合，长时间会导致支气管狭窄及阻塞。在一段潜伏期之后，出现肉芽组织和支气管狭窄。在狭窄的远端，可能会形成肺炎、支气管扩张、脓肿，以及脓胸。支气管完全阻塞且没有感染的话，会导致持续的肺不张及肺功能下降。

即使气管支气管的合并损伤非常多样化，包括大血管、心脏、肺、食管、骨性胸廓，以及神经损伤，这些合并的损伤能够反映创伤发生的部位程度以及损伤机制。医生也可以根据气道损伤发生的情况推断是否合并其他器官的损伤。例如，穿过颈部或者穿过纵隔的穿通性损伤提示可能对穿过的结构造成特定的损伤。这些合并的损伤导致的后果可能会非常严重，在至少一项研究中这些损伤均导致死亡。有研究报道，在有气管支气管树损伤的患者中，超过 30 岁的患者全部合并对应部位肋骨骨折。当然情况也不总是这样，没有胸壁损伤也不能完全除外气道损伤，而存在气道损伤就须进一步检查是否合并其他损伤。高度的警惕性对于及时和适当地诊断和治疗这类创伤非常重要。

评估

首先须根据病史以及前面列出的相关症状和体征做出大致的诊断。对怀疑气管支气管树损伤的患者的评估如图 1 所示。先进的 CT 检查能够提供较为准确的诊断和损伤程度的评估。三维重建能够更为直观地显示出病变的位置及程度。尽管在某些病例中 CT 可以很好地显示气管支气管损伤，诊断性支气管镜检查对于确诊和制订治疗方案还是必要的。除了在 CT 上可见的气管损伤，支气管镜检查的指征包括广泛的纵隔气肿、难治性气胸或者持续漏气。硬质支气管镜或者可曲式支气管镜是目前认为最有效的诊断气道损伤的方法。其中可曲式支气管镜最为常用，可以不实施全身麻醉，且可以在床边进行。若还未插管，它可以避免头颈部活动，在可曲式支气管镜引导下控制性地插入鼻式气管导管。硬质支气管镜无法提供通气能力。检查可能会遗漏或低估存在的损伤，而这些损伤可能会导致更为严重或明显的损伤。也正因为这样，如果病情需要的话，可自由地使用可曲式支气管镜检查。

处理

初期处理

与所有损伤一样，对于支气管气管树损伤患者的救治来说，气道管理是最重要的。如果患者能够维持自主的气道并且通气充分。谨慎地采用非侵入性方式通气可能是个最佳选择，直至其他诊断工作完成或者更为严重损伤状况稳定后。不小心或者错误的插管，如将气管插管经横断或破裂的气管插入软组织中，可能会加重损伤。如果怀疑存在气道损伤的话，最好能在患者清醒的状况下进行详细的评估以便于计划适当的干预。可以通过支气管镜检查对损伤进行评估，如果气道损伤轻微的话，可以在气管镜引导下将气管插管小心地送至损伤的远端。对于可疑喉气管损伤的患者不要尝试经鼻气管盲插管或者使用标准的快速贯序插管（standard rapid sequence intubation，RSI）气管插管。因为这样可能会使导管经过损伤部位导致气管完全横断。

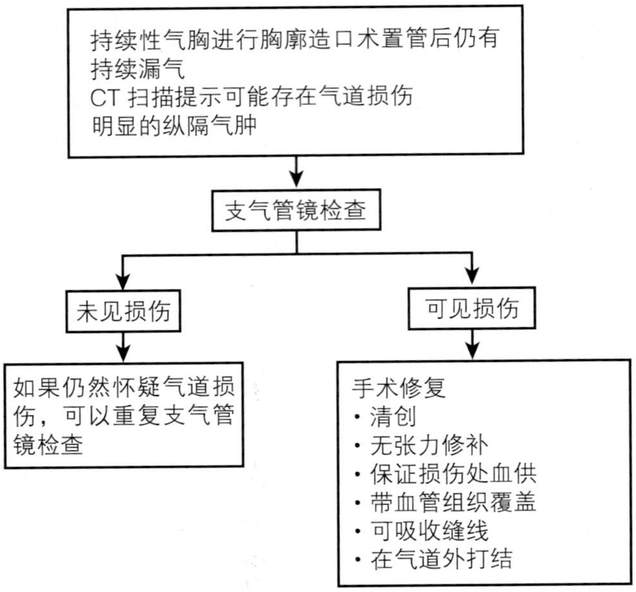

图 1 对可疑的气管支气管损伤进行评估和处理的流程图

在手术室进行气管造口术是最为安全的控制气道的方法，被许多专家推荐使用。为了保证安全，在有足够气道保护的人群中可以在患者清醒状态下造口避免气道损伤。如果气管完全横断，通常远端断端在上纵隔，找到远端后可以插入套囊管。具体的操作方法根据机构选择的器械以及熟练程度的不同而不同。须注意的是，如果损伤位于气管插管远端的话，虽然能够维持通气，但是机械通气的过程会使损伤进一步恶化。这种情况下应该进行胸廓造口置管，并连接抽吸装置。在气道得到有效控制以后，可以进行共存损伤的必要识别，例如使用食管镜、喉镜、血管造影以及剖腹术来诊断存在的合并症，并将患者转至对应的专科进行进一步治疗。图 1 所示为气管支气管损伤处理指南。

手术处理

气道损伤的手术修复需要外科医生与麻醉医生的充分配合。所有的相同的原则都适用。虽然经过初期处理气道已经得到维持，但是手术修复的操作过程中会带来其他的挑战。当气管周围结缔组织被破坏或被修复时，手术台上需要一套无菌的麻醉环路和导管，以便在气管横断部位重新控制患者气道。

若能进行经口气管插管，可以选择单腔气管插管或者双腔气管插管。双腔气管插管能够实现独立通气创伤，但是由于其较粗的口径可能会对气道造成进一步撕裂，因此不令人满意。长的单腔气管插管可以跨过近端或者远端的气管损伤部位进行通气，或者直接插入对侧主支气管进行单肺通气。在可曲式支气管镜辅助下插管可以提高安全性及诊断能力。如果须进行气管造口术，切开位置应选在喉部损伤或者高位气管以下2～3个气管环处，并且应该与气管修复手术的切口保持距离。在修复胸内气管及主要支气管损伤后，在损伤部位近端行气管造口以保护缝线并非必要措施。同样也不推荐在远端气管及支气管损伤中行预防性气管造口术。在极端困难的病例或者进行复杂修复时，气道管理成效往往不尽如人意，则可能须建立心肺旁路。因此须充分考量建立心肺旁路潜在的风险及获益，包括可能须进行系统抗凝，特别是多发创伤患者。

修复完成后，最理想的情况是气道处理也能随手术结束之后的气管拔除一起完成，或者在患者恢复有效自主呼吸后尽快拔除。个别情况下须为患者实施持续气道正压通气，这须借助呼吸机和监护病房的技术来实现，如气管插管须到达损伤部位远端、单肺通气、高频通气甚至体外膜氧合。通过积极治疗肺炎、处理液体及保持肺洁净等方式，来最大限度改善肺的顺应性。

大多数胸腔外气道损伤修复都可以经水平领状切口进入。有时为了充分暴露术野，切口可以向上延伸至颈部以修复颈动脉，或者垂直向下延伸至胸骨，行部分或者完全胸骨正中切开以实现深部暴露。经第4或5肋间右后外侧开胸术因可以避开心脏及主动脉弓，是修复胸内气管、右侧支气管、左主支气管近端损伤的最佳入路。复杂或者双侧气道损伤也因为同样的原因选择右侧开胸入路。修复距离隆嵴超过3 cm的远端左侧支气管损伤，选择第5肋间的左侧开胸入路更加合适。

理想的修复包括充分清创，即清除包括软骨在内的失活的组织和一期气管或者支气管端端吻合。吻合可以通过游离气管支气管前方或者后方组织来减少张力，保留侧方血供。同时可以通过松解颈部气管并将下颌与前胸壁缝合来巩固减张效果。许多研究建议吻合时采用可吸收缝线间断缝合。但是我们发现，用单股可吸收缝线连续缝合是安全的，并且吻合时视野更佳。膜部应该先行无张力缝合，在开始缝合软骨环部时再将缝线收紧。缝合时可以包绕软骨环或者穿透软骨环，但必须尽量做到黏膜与黏膜接近。线结应该打在管腔外侧，以避免日后在线结处形成肉芽肿或产生其他问题。为了防止产生吻合口瘘，在后期修复时通常使用心包补片、来自胸膜的带蒂血管、肋间肌、带状肌、肠系膜及带血管的胸膜，来加固吻合口、帮助支气管愈合。而在早期修复中胸膜由于不够强韧，不适合用来加固吻合口。带血管蒂的肋间肌则既能提供良好的保护，又能促进组织的愈合。因此在开胸时应当保留相应肋间肌的动静脉及神经，而相应的肋骨可以选择保留或切去。切口应该做在肋骨表面正上方，剥下骨膜，然后向上穿过肋骨上缘的骨膜后层进入胸膜腔。相应的肋间肌可从上下肋骨之间剥离，当做肌瓣覆盖并固定在气管上。通过这种办法将有活力的组织置于吻合口周围，可以增加修复部位局部血供，促进愈合（图2）。

颈段气管损伤在修复时或须行气管造口术。简单的气管前壁裂伤在可能的情况下可以进行一期修复而无须行气管造口术，除非是须通过气管造口术来实施短期的气道控制。如果患者近端气管损伤严重，应当即刻修复并在远端气管行保护性气管造口术。喉部损伤应考虑置入支架支撑。有时损伤可能导致气管的进一步失活及污染。在这些少见的情况下，考虑到将来伤口恢复，炎症和瘢痕恢复后需要确定性修复。因此最佳策略是末端气管造口术、缝合近端气管并充分引流。尽管如此，还是应该尽可能地尝试一期修复。

一些气管损伤可以行非手术治疗，但是一些标准和技术因为缺乏足够的数据支持，并没有详细的描述。因此，在此处理中，非手术治疗仅限于熟悉相关操作的专业人员在高度选择的患者身上实施。

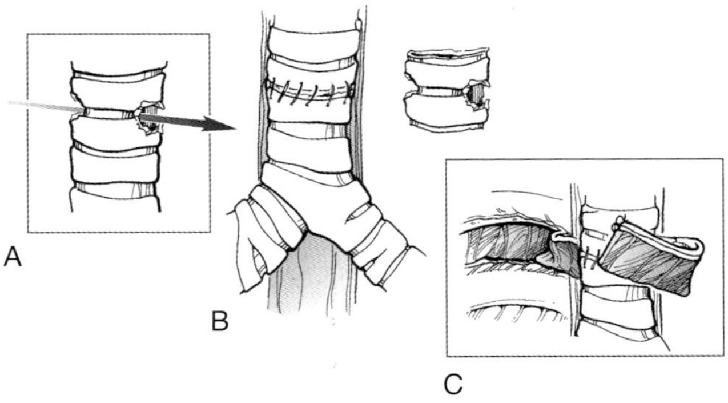

图2　胸段气管损伤（**A**）可以通过清创后可吸收线缝合来修复（**B**）。清创过程如果有需要的话可以去除若干气管软骨环。吻合口可以使用带血管蒂的肋间肌进行包埋（**C**）

预后

良好的预后建立在早发现、早期清创、早期一期修复气管支气管损伤部位的基础上。患者可以恢复正常的解剖及功能，如正常的肺功能及发音等。早期修复同样减少了气管狭窄手术修复的概率。

既往报道的气管损伤死亡率为 3.5%～67% 不等，而最新的系列报道的死亡率小于 30%。大多数早期的死亡多由于缺乏气道管理及存在多发复合伤导致（如血管及食管损伤）。

如果气管损伤未被第一时间诊断，那么在明确气管损伤后应尽快开始处理，或者在处理完其他威胁生命的损伤后尽快开始。不论气管损伤的诊断延迟多久，只要损伤远端没有化脓，都应该尝试进行气管支气管树重建。如果未被发现的完全的支气管断裂导致完全的气道阻塞及无菌性肺不张，也可以稍后再修复。气道阻塞的部分可以切除后按照急性损伤的方式修复，或者按照良性狭窄的方式修复。尽管延迟修复会对肺功能造成一定的损害，但是在修复完成后都可以改善。不完全的支气管阻塞最终会导致化脓和不可逆的肺实质破坏。治疗方法是依据肺实质的损伤程度行肺叶或者全肺切除术。因此，尽管支气管断裂在早期或者在延迟治疗中的效果都较理想，早期诊断可以使感染和其他并发症的风险降低到最小。

尽管并不常见，但是在大型医院依然经常可以看到气管支气管损伤。良好的预后往往取决于成功的早期气道管理以及经验丰富的临床医生对损伤的体征和症状的观察，这些都颇具挑战，例如一些严重的表现如气道断裂、对胸廓造口术置管无反应的气胸和纵隔气肿，或者胸部 CT 难以发现的细微损伤。对于那些预后不佳的、须通过一些过于侵入性操作（如盲法经鼻气管插管或者 RSI）来进行处理的可疑气管损伤患者，其气道管理要谨慎小心。而经过周密气道管理并且接受早期手术干预的患者往往能够获得较良好的预后。

肺部损伤的手术治疗：保留肺组织和标准切除术

Juan A. Asensio, Patrizio Petrone, Alejandro Perez-Alonso, Thomas Templin, Shreya Shetty, Gerd Daniel Pust, Kirby R. Gross, 和 Marcus Balters 著
惠本刚 肖蓉心 译

胸部损伤早在公元前 3000 年的埃德温史密斯外科纸草书就有记载。古希腊书籍同样记载了胸部穿通伤及肺损伤的例子。古希腊人拥有解剖学知识，了解胸部的结构，并且知道肺在一侧胸腔中的位置。在荷马的著作《伊利亚特》中，有普特罗克勒斯杀死萨尔珀冬的清晰描述："他用长矛刺穿他的身体，拔出长矛时带出了他的膈……" 荷马强调了膈的重要性，认为它在解剖上与肺和心脏关系密切。尽管气胸已经众所周知，但是古希腊人知晓了其和胸部穿通伤的关联，并且知道了胸部开放伤的致命性。尽管早期治疗方式的成功率无从知晓，但是似乎在奥林匹克运动会期间，古希腊的医生能够识别出致命的胸部损伤，并且能够尝试进行治疗。

希腊旅行家 Pausanias 描述过一例由 Syracuse 的 Damoxens 对 Epidamnus 的拳击手 Creugas 造成的胸部穿通伤，伤者表现出了明显的肺部损伤症状。Eusebius 在 *Evangelical Preparation* 一书中描述了 Astypalaia 的 Cleomedes 和 Epidamnus 的 Ikkos 比赛："为什么他们崇拜 Cleomedes？因为他打开了对手的肋骨，把手伸进对手的胸腔，扯出了他的肺。"

盖伦（公元 130—200 年），古代最著名的医生之一，记载了角斗士在受到胸部损伤或者可疑肺损伤后的包扎方式。1226 年，Theodoric 的论文中也有肺损伤的记载："我住在 Bolonra 期间，一个 Bologan 仆人被 Hugo 大师救治成功，他的一部分肺被撕掉，并且 Roand 大师目睹了这一切……"

在古代，大多数的胸部外伤及肺部损伤的治疗方法都是随战争发展起来的。1635 年，西班牙探险家 Alvar Nuñez Cabeza de Vaca 从墨西哥北部前往新埃斯帕纳首府时被印第安人俘虏。Vaea 和他的助手 Esteban 切开取出了一个刺入印第安伤者胸部的箭头，并且缝合了伤口。并且他的这一举动使他和他的船员从印第安人手中获得了自由。

16 世纪期间，创伤性肺损伤的救治出现了长足的进展。Ambrorse Pare 通过涂抹油和糖浆的混合

物来覆盖创口以治疗创伤性肺损伤，这是敷料的第一次使用。John Hunter 治疗由滑膛火枪射出的铅弹造成的胸部外伤的经验使他意识到弹丸的射速是决定胸部外伤严重程度的重要因素。Jean-Dominique Larrey 和 Pierre-Joseph Desault 在胸壁裂伤的清创术发展中做出了巨大贡献。不过在这一时期，对胸腔内损伤的治疗并没有特别大的进步。尽管 Larrey 阐述了开放手术修复心脏穿刺伤的技术，但是他在处理肺损伤方面并没有明显建树。

William Beaumont 因为观察胃瘘而成名，他在治疗危重胸部损伤方面也做出过贡献。1822 年，他收治了一位胸部枪伤的患者，并记载了损伤情况："第 6 肋骨前部骨折并缺失，左肺下叶和膈被撕裂，胃被穿透。" 在 18 世纪，争论的焦点是手术治疗胸部外伤及肺损伤能否使患者获益。在德国，Auenbrugger 认为打开胸腔会因为肺压缩导致窒息。1835 年，法国著名外科医生 Dupuytren 罹患脓胸，尽管当时已经准备实施手术干预，但是他基于 Auenbrugger "开胸导致窒息" 的理念拒绝手术，说自己 "宁可死于上帝之手，也不能死于外科医生之手"，并在 12 天后死亡。

在 19 世纪 40 年代，法国医学院依据战争中治疗脓胸的经验制订了治疗指南。在 18 世纪，修森 (Hewson) 发起了胸部钝性创伤导致肺裂伤的机制研究。1886 年，Ashurt 描述了不伴肋骨骨折的脏层胸膜撕裂。1889 年，伦敦圣乔治医院的福尔摩斯（Holmes）医生说："所有的胸部穿通伤，如果较小，都应该迅速闭合并无菌包扎。如果伤口较大并且肺部广泛损伤，最好不要完全关闭外部伤口，并且在胸腔内留置一根粗大的引流管引流积血至抗菌敷料，以预防胸腔积液（血）。" 在 1897 年，Duval 记载了胸骨正中切开术，事实上是胸腹联合切开。1906 年，意大利外科医生 Spangaro 描述了左前外侧开胸术切口。这些切口为处理创伤性肺损伤做出了巨大贡献。

1916 年，门兹（Mentz）报道了肺内异物取出，并且提出开胸手术是相对安全的。第一次世界大战中使用的胸部外伤救治方法中许多都是基于 19 世纪提出的基础理论，特别是血胸的治疗是最令人期待的。血胸不使用抽吸的方法是因为过去认为损伤的肺有压塞。胸部损伤一旦实施手术治疗，只要确保伤口缝合气密性好、异物取出干净，一般都能够有很好的治疗效果。和德国军队相比，美军和盟军军医使用正压麻醉和一氧化氮混合氧气麻醉，实施早期开胸手术，并遵循充分暴露损伤部位、切除受损结构、结扎缝合、胸腔盥洗的原则。术后严密关闭胸腔，不放置引流。这一技术使得死亡率下降了 9%。在此期间，Grey-Turner、Miles、Gask、Duval 和 Bastianelli 提出了治疗肺损伤后持续性血胸的胸膜剥脱术。

在第二次世界大战期间，由于对胸部损伤后血胸并发症高发时认识的提高，军医采用了更加保守的治疗方法。反复胸腔穿刺直到胸腔积血、积液排空、胸腔内不应残留空气。应使肺能够复张并压塞止血，以期肺功能恢复正常。张力性气胸患者须放置水封瓶肋间导管。开胸手术在持续性出血或者明显肺漏气以及其他扩大适应证如胸腹联合伤、纵隔损伤、外伤性开胸、胸部吮吸伤口，以及异物取出时仍须实施。用此方法治疗战时胸部外伤的总体死亡率大约为 8%。

朝鲜战争期间外科医生又面临了新的挑战。陌生的地形和不适的战术条件加上巨大的人员伤亡，使得移动式外科医院（mobile army surgical hospital，MASH 单位）严重超负荷运转。因此创伤性血胸的保守治疗在当时的情形下非常适合。朝鲜战争中，80% 的伤员仅实施了多次胸腔穿刺。然而，使用胸管引流血胸的经验却十分有限。引进更先进的复苏技术有助于解决这些处理所遇到的问题。

在越南战争期间，对肺损伤及血胸的胸管引流被广泛应用。伤员被第一时间从前线转运至医院。组织良好的创伤中心有专业的心胸外科医生按照严格的复苏规范实施手术。由于此情况下胸管引流取得了很大成功，尽管开胸手术的适应证较前没有太大变化，更少的伤员因为血胸而实施开胸手术。胸廓造口术置管成为了治疗创伤性血胸、气胸以及肺创伤性损伤的基石。

近期基于平民和军方经验的认识发现在病情不稳定的患者身上实施（例如解剖性切除及全肺切除等）复杂操作往往耐受性较差，甚至会潜在威胁患者生命。受伤严重的患者往往会发展至低体温、酸中毒、凝血功能障碍及心律失常，导致不可逆的损伤。有效遏制这种损伤同样是外科医生救治胸部损伤患者的一部分。因此治疗严重创伤患者的严重肺损伤的手段更加依赖快捷、简单的保留肺组织的肺切除技术，如楔形切除、非解剖性切除和肺吻合缝合技术和钳夹术。1994 年，Wall 等描述了钳夹神经束切断术能够最大限度地保留肺实质。Asensio 等在 1997 年描述了使用神经束切断。吻合器神经束切断在 40 位患者身上使用，并被充分证明是安全、有价值的保留肺的技术。随后，Cothren 等报道了保留肺技术和肺切除技术相比，显著改善了发病率和死亡率。

包括内镜技术和麻醉术在内的技术飞速进步，使得胸部手术发生了重大变革，宣告了 VATS 时代的来临。VATS 使得创伤科医生能够更加精确、直接地评估肺实质、纵隔及膈损伤，并同时予以治疗。同时 VATS 也被证明可以准确、安全并且可靠地手术处理肺损伤并发症，包括处理创伤后胸腔积液等。

发生率

肺损伤的真实发病率难以通过文献统计得出。胸部构成了人体躯干的一大部分并直接与外界接触，因此易受到损伤。解剖结构复杂的肺、血管及支气管树填满胸腔，在没有外部损伤的情况下胸部穿通伤及挫伤极少发生。既往报道的肺部损伤发病率因作者或研究机构所在地域不同而不尽相同。1979 年，Graham 等报道了 1 年的研究结果，在 373 例肺穿通伤患者中，91 例（24%）接受了开胸手术。其中只有 45 例（12%）开胸是因为肺部本身原因。在这项研究中，仅出现创伤后血胸或气胸就被作者定义为创伤后肺损伤，这个纳入标准是合理的。

1988 年，Robison 等报道了一项在人群中的 13 年的研究结果。它纳入了 1 168 例接受治疗的肺穿通伤患者，然而仅有 68 例须开胸处理肺损伤。在 1988 年，Thompson 等报道了基于 2 608 例胸部创伤患者的 5 年的研究结果，共有 1 663 例患者受到过钝性创伤导致的肺损伤，并且只有 11 例（0.7%）接受了开胸手术。945 例受到穿通伤，15 例（1.6%）接受了开胸手术。Wiencek 和 Wilson 报道了 7 年间的共 161 例因胸部穿通伤须行开胸手术的患者，平均每年 23 例。Wagner 等报道了 4 年间的 104 例严重的胸部钝伤患者，75 例患者共出现 115 处肺裂伤，发生率为 72%。86% 的病例由 CT 诊断，14% 由手术发现。结合手术和影像学发现，作者发表的创伤性肺损伤发病率高于其他研究报道的单纯基于手术发现的肺损伤发病率。

1993 年，Tominaga 等的一项单中心的 7 年研究纳入 2 934 例受到胸部钝伤或穿通伤的患者。其中钝伤占 25%，穿通伤占 75%，损伤发生率为 0.04%，即每年 1.7 例。其中 347 例（12%）须行开胸手术，这一亚组中的 12 例（3.5%）接受了肺切除术。Wagner 等在 1996 年报道了 1 804 例胸部外伤患者的 8 年研究结果。265 例（15%）接受了开胸手术，其中 55 例是因为肺损伤，发生率为 3%，平均每年 6.9 例。

1997 年，Stewart 等报道了一项 10 年的研究结果。研究纳入了 2 455 例胸部外伤患者，包括穿通伤及钝伤。183 例（7.4%）接受了开胸手术，其中 32 例（17.4%）须行肺切除术，即每年发生 3.2 例。Inci 等在 1998 年发表了一项 5 年的研究结果，由 755 例胸部穿通伤患者组成。61 例（8.1%）接受了开胸手术，然而仅仅 3 例（4.9%）因为肺损伤而开胸，平均每年 0.6 例。

1998 年，Wall 等报道了一项 3 年的研究结果，236 例患者因为胸部创伤接受了开胸手术，90 例（38%）须切除或修复裂伤的肺组织，平均每年 30 例。2001 年，Karmy-Jones 等报道了一项来自 5 家Ⅰ级创伤中心的 4 年的多中心回顾性研究，纳入了 43 119 例胸部穿通伤患者。290 例（2.8%）患者接受了开胸手术，这一亚组中有 115 例（40%）患者接受了各种类型的肺切除。Cothren 等的一项纳入 4 087 例患者的研究结果显示，416 例（10%）患者接受了开胸手术，36 例（9%）须行肺的手术干预，发生率为 1%，平均每年 3.3 例。

在最近的报告中，2006 年 Asensio 报道了 101 例须行开胸手术的复杂胸部损伤。在战争地区，Zakharia 等报道 1985 年黎巴嫩冲突造成了 1 992 例伤亡，1 422 例因为胸部穿通伤继发血流动力学不稳定而接受了开胸手术。其中 210 例（15%）存在肺损伤，发生率为 11%。1997 年，Petricevic 等报道了 2 547 例最近的巴尔干地区军事冲突引发的伤亡。在 4 年期间，424 例患者遭受了胸部的穿通伤或钝伤，81 例患者因为肺损伤接受了肺部手术，平均每年 20 例。

病因学

须开胸手术治疗肺损伤的患者大都遭受了肺部穿通伤如枪击伤、刺伤或猎枪伤。须行手术干预的胸部钝性创伤相比之下要少很多。2003 年，Huh 等报道了主要由于车祸伤引起的需要手术干预的胸部钝性损伤的发生率逐年上升，从 1994 年前的 3% 上升至 12%。Tominaga 的研究指出钝性创伤造成的须行开胸手术治疗的肺损伤占 25%。在平民当中，枪击伤是最常见的造成胸部穿通伤并需要手术处理的原因。多位学者报道，枪击伤造成了 33% ~ 80% 的穿通性肺损伤，刺伤造成了 17% ~ 67%。Karmy-Jones 等在一项多中心的创伤性肺损伤研究中指出这一类患者开胸手术的概率在上升。其他受伤机制如穿刺伤和猎枪伤的发生率较低，大约为 1% ~ 5%。

在一项 2006 年开始的研究中，Asensio 等研究了普通人群中 101 例接受了开胸手术的肺穿通伤患者，其中枪击伤占 72%，刀刺伤及其他受伤机制分别占 33% 和 5%。在军事冲突区，Zakharia 等报道，在黎巴嫩，遭受高能枪击伤及炮击伤是最主要的肺部受伤机制。Petricevic 等报道了克罗地亚冲突中造成肺损伤的原因，爆炸伤占大多数（59%），接着是枪击伤（高速和低速兼有，占 37%），刺伤及跌落伤只占 4%。

分类

AAST-OIS 委员会在 1994 年对肺损伤进行了分级。这一分级推动了临床研究的发展，并且提供了一个通用的命名法，这样外科医生就可以描述肺损伤及其严重程度。分级方案基本上是解剖学的描述，按照描述的损伤由轻到重分为 1 级到 5 级。迄今为止，大量研究已经证实损伤等级同死亡率相关联（表 1）。

表 1 肺损伤：OIS，AAST

分级 *	损伤类型	说明 †
I	挫伤	单侧，<1 个肺叶
II	挫伤	单侧，单个肺叶
	裂伤	单纯气胸
III	挫伤	单侧，>1 个肺叶
	裂伤	远端气道持续漏气（>72 h）
	血肿	未延伸至肺实质内
IV	裂伤	严重漏气（肺段或肺叶）
	血肿	延伸至肺实质内
	血管损伤	肺内分支血管破裂
V	血管损伤	肺门血管破裂
VI	血管损伤	完全，肺门血管无限制性横断

* Ⅲ级以上的多发伤上升 1 个级别。血胸根据胸部血管器官损伤分级标准进行评分

† 根据最为准确的尸检、手术或影像学检查

诊断

创伤性肺损伤的诊断由体格检查和辅助检查可以得出。

体格检查

遭受肺损伤的患者临床表现多样，从血流动力学稳定到呼吸心搏骤停均可发生。体格检查可以提供决定患者是否须接受紧急处理的重要诊断信息。

肺损伤的患者可表现出血气胸的症状体征或者有胸壁部分缺损的开放性气胸，也可表现为张力性血胸或者气胸，或更少见的纵隔气肿。这些患者听诊可以闻及 Hamman 征，即收缩期杂音。若出现了心包积气则听诊可以闻及 Brichiteau 风车杂音。肺穿通伤患者很少表现为真正的咯血。偶有患者会合并心脏损伤并表现出相应的症状及体征。

在评估这些患者的伤情时，创伤科医生必须清楚胸腔包括左右两侧，其中还有上纵隔和前、后纵隔。有时致伤物或者弹片会横穿一个或多个腔隙。弹片轨迹通常无法预测，并且当其撞击坚硬的骨性结构（肋骨、胸骨、脊柱）时往往会产生新的碎片，有造成其他严重损伤的可能性。

辅助诊断方法

辅助诊断方法分为有创检查和无创检查的方式。

无创检查方式

这些辅助检查包括超声检查[创伤重点超声评估（focused assessment with sonography for trauma，FAST）]、X 线胸片、CT 扫描和心电图。

创伤超声

创伤超声是二次评估外伤患者时应用的检查方法，是用于检查孤立性肺损伤患者或者多发伤患者是否合并心脏或腹部损伤的有效检查方法。2004 年，Kirkpatrick 等报道了使用超声检查创伤性气胸，并把这一诊断方法称为扩大的创伤重点超声评估。正常的胸部超声表现为彗星尾征，在呼吸过程中在脏层胸膜滑动和重新定位。创伤性气胸的超声表现为彗星尾征消失。这一项研究纳入了 225 例患者，结论是 E-FAST 同 X 线胸片相比有相当的特异

度（99.1% vs. 98.7%）和更高的灵敏度（58.9% vs. 48.8%）。Knudson 等在 2004 年开展的研究纳入了 328 例胸部外伤患者，结论是胸部外伤患者使用胸部超声检查的特异度为 99.7%，阴性预测值为 99.7%，准确性是 99.4%。尽管特异度 (100% vs. 99.7%)、阴性预测值 (100% vs. 99.7%) 和准确性 (100% vs. 99.3%) 相当，相比于钝性创伤，超声在穿通伤的检出上有更高的灵敏度 (100% vs. 88.9%) 和阳性预测值 (100% vs. 88.9%)。基于这些发现，Knudson 认为在损伤患者中超声诊断气胸是可靠的，可以作为伤者完善常规 X 线胸片检查之前的评估手段。

超声也可以用来诊断创伤性血胸，检查方法和上腹部检查方法类似。超声探头可以识别高回声的膈，能够评估双侧膈间隙上方是否存在积液。Sisley 等在 1998 年评估了 360 例有可疑性躯干钝伤或穿通伤的患者。其中 40 例有创伤后积液，39 例（98%）通过超声检查发现，37 例（93%）通过 X 线胸片检查发现。作者得出结论，在发现创伤后积液上，超声比 X 线胸片更敏感（97.5% vs. 92.5%）。然而，两者的特异度均为 97.5%，根据这些数据，作者得出结论，在诊断创伤后积液时，超声同卧位 X 线胸片一样准确，但却明显更快捷。

X 线胸片

标准的卧位前后位胸片是最常用于创伤性肺损伤患者的辅助检查。X 线胸片诊断肺损伤主要基于气胸、胸腔积液、肺内血肿、创伤性肺膨出，以及肺实质挫伤。尽管 X 线胸片诊断创伤后气胸的特异度有 99%，但是灵敏度较低，只有 49%。而它在诊断创伤后胸腔积液的灵敏度为 93%，特异度为 99.7%。

和 CT 相比，传统的 X 线胸片容易漏诊或低估肺实质及胸膜的损伤，判断肺实质损伤及气胸范围的能力欠佳。Wagner 等证实肺实质裂伤通过 X 线胸片诊断容易漏诊。

CT 扫描

CT 扫描诊断创伤性肺损伤比 X 线胸片更加敏感。CT 扫描中最常见的异常分别是肺实质撕裂、创伤后血气胸、创伤后气胸、肺不张、皮下气肿、心包积气、心包积血及胸壁骨折。创伤性肺损伤的补充诊断往往来自于 CT 扫描，例如发现微小或严重的肺挫伤的存在和范围。

Karaaslan 等在 1995 年报道，CT 扫描同样可以发现相关的胸部及纵隔血管损伤、其他胸部大血管损伤、胸腔外损伤、合并的颈椎损伤或腹腔内损伤，这些损伤占 30%。

心电图

创伤患者心电图表现异常并不十分多见。一些变化如窦性心动过速、房性和室性期前收缩多由全身因素引起，例如疼痛、低血容量、缺氧、血清电解质异常浓缩、交感和副交感神经节律改变。但是在某些情况下，创伤也会引起心电图改变，最常见的是心脏穿通伤或者钝伤，心电图会出现新发 Q 波，ST-T 段抬高或压低等类似心肌梗死的表现，或者出现右束支传导阻滞、束支性传导阻滞、房室结传导异常，以及其他心律失常（心房颤动、室性心动过速、心室纤颤、窦性心动过缓和房性心动过速）。

在胸部或肺部创伤患者身上有心电图阳性发现可能提示心包压塞。尽管 PR 段压低及电交替通常也会出现，但 QRS 波低电压与心包压塞程度密切相关（灵敏度为 0 ~ 42%，特异度为 86% ~ 97%）。

有创检查

胸管

放置胸管既是检查手段也是治疗手段。进入胸腔后，创伤科医生插入手指，根据管的位置，触诊确认肺表面是否存在挫伤。膈表面的裂伤部位，以及心包囊来检查是否存在压塞。

胸管中引流液的性状和多少同样十分重要。首次放置胸管引流的血量是决定是否须行开胸手术的指征。胸管持续引流出血液会促使创伤科医生重新评估患者是否需要手术干预。引流液中出现胃内容物说明膈裂伤伴随食管、胃或者小肠损伤，引流管出现气泡说明存在肺裂伤，大量的气泡则指向支气管破裂。

合并损伤

穿通性肺损伤经常伴发合并损伤。肺损伤患者中有 5% ~ 65% 的患者合并有胸部损伤或胸外损伤；文献中报道的合并损伤平均发生率在每例患者有 0.5 ~ 1.9 之间波动。是否伴有合并损伤对预后有明显影响。Gasparri 等报道了合并心脏损伤以及须行开腹探查的腹部损伤对死亡率有显著影响。Asensio 等认为合并心脏损伤是影响预后的独立因素。

Graham 报道了 91 例须接受开胸手术的穿通性肺损伤患者中有 73 例存在合并损伤，平均每例患者合并 0.8 处胸部损伤，最常见的损伤脏器包括心脏（27%）、肋间组织（16%）、锁骨下血管（9%）、上腔静脉（7%）。作者同时也报道了 175 例合并腹部损伤的患者中有 89 例接受了开腹探查，平均每例患者合并 1.9 处腹部损伤，最易伤及的脏器是肝（21%）、脾（19%）、胃（14%）和结肠（10%）。

Robison 等报道在 28 例因创伤性肺损伤接受开胸手术、肺切除术或肺门修补术的患者中，有 11 例患者出现合并损伤，共 14 处。合并损伤的发生率是 39%，平均每例患者合并 1.3 处损伤。11% 的患者出现心脏损伤，剩下的合并损伤包括胸部大血管（7%）、脊髓（7%）、肝（7%）、胰腺（4%）、结肠（4%）、脾（4%）、胃（4%）和周围神经（4%）。

Wiencek 和 Wilson 报道在 25 例中央型肺损伤患者中，19 例患者共出现 35 处主要合并损伤。发生率为 76%，平均每例患者合并 1.4 处损伤。心脏和胸部大血管是最容易受伤的器官，分别占 26% 和 21%。其中 58% 的患者因合并腹部损伤须行开腹探查。Tominaga 等报道了 12 例因创伤性肺损伤接受开胸手术和肺切除术的患者，其中有 10 例患者出现合并损伤，平均每例患者合并 0.8 处损伤。合并损伤包括头部外伤（占 17%）、腹部脏器损伤（须行开腹探查，占 33%）、心脏损伤（占 25%）、大血管损伤（占 8%）。Petricevic 等报道了克罗地亚战争期间遭受胸部外伤的患者的脏器合并损伤的发生率为 4.5%。Stewart 等报道在 32 例因创伤性肺损伤接受开胸手术、肺切除术的患者中，有 21 例（65%）患者出现合并损伤，共 30 处。平均每例患者合并 1.4 处损伤。这些损伤中，腹部损伤占 30%，肌肉骨骼损伤占 30%，神经损伤占 17%，心脏损伤占 7%，其他损伤占 17%。

Gasparri 报道了 70 例因穿通性肺损伤接受开胸手术的患者，41 例（58%）存在合并损伤。最常见的损伤器官中，心脏占 20%，膈占 17%，肝占 11%。Karmy-Jones 等报道在 115 例因穿通性肺损伤接受开胸手术和肺切除的患者中，42 例存在合并胸部损伤，平均每例患者合并 0.36 处损伤。

Cothren 等报道了 36 例因严重肺损伤接受开胸手术的患者，27 例存在合并损伤，平均每例患者合并 0.75 处损伤。合并胸部损伤者占 33%，合并胸外损伤占 66%。Huh 等报道了在须因肺损伤者接受手术干预的患者中，有 28% 的患者合并需要开腹探查的腹部损伤。

Asensio 等在 2006 年报道了一项为期 169 个月、纳入了 101 名需要开胸的肺部穿通伤患者的研究结果。本系列中共出现了 193 处合并损伤，平均每人 1.9 处。其中 39 例（22%）合并胸腔脏器损伤，154 例（79.7%）合并胸外损伤。最常见的损伤的胸腔脏器为心脏（23.7%）、胸部大血管（14.8%）；最常见的损伤的胸外结构为膈（42.5%）、肝（25.7%）和胃（18.8%）。

损伤的解剖学位置

肺损伤的解剖位置在临床和影像学中都描述得不多。Graham 等报道左侧肺损伤率较高，可达 52%，右侧只有 36%，双侧损伤占 12%。Wiencek 和 Wilson 在一系列中心型肺损伤、肺门损伤的研究中发现，在 161 例穿通性肺损伤患者中肺门破裂发生率约为 15%。Robison 等报道的容易因创伤性肺损伤接受肺切除的部位依次是：左肺下叶，28%；右肺中叶，22%；左肺上叶包括舌叶，22%；右肺上叶，17%；右肺下叶，17%。左肺动脉（25%）是最容易受伤的胸部大血管，其次是右肺动脉（14%）、右肺静脉（11%）和左肺静脉（7%）。这些研究结果表明，尽管左侧血管相对右侧更容易损伤，分别是 56% 和 44%，但创伤性损伤更容易发生在右侧肺。

Huh 等报道需要手术干预的创伤性肺损伤更好发于左侧（50%），接下来是右侧（47%），其次是双侧（3%）。Asensio 等在一项纳入了 101 例接受开胸手术的复杂肺穿刺伤患者的研究中发现左侧肺比右侧更容易发生穿通伤（65% vs. 35%）。作者还报道了具体的损伤位置：左肺下叶（40%），左肺上叶（21%），右肺中叶（19%），右肺下叶（11%），舌叶（5%）和右肺上叶（5%）。

处理

尽管近期报道指出军事行动中的胸部外伤提倡早期开胸并积极行肺切除，这与传统的胸廓造口术置管保守治疗方式不同。但是大多数（75%～85%）的胸部外伤患者能够通过放置胸腔引流管和支持治疗成功获得救治。肺复张、血管内压力低及高浓度的组织凝血酶在大多数情况下能够充分止血，但是

9% ~ 15% 的患者仍须手术止血或进行必要的修补。在因为出血而接受开胸的患者中，3% ~ 30% 的患者须通过肺切除术来控制伤情。

肺穿通伤患者的开胸指征如下：

- 心肺骤停
- 阻止心肺骤停并到达急诊科
- 首次放置胸管引流出 1 000 ~ 1 500 ml 血液
- 胸腔引流管引流血量超过 1 000 ml，并持续出血
- 张力性血胸
- 大量胸腔积血
- 胸管明显有气体漏出

手术决策

对于发生心肺骤停的患者，应强制实施急诊开胸手术。须在右侧胸腔放置胸管。这样可能须行双侧前外侧开胸手术。对于收缩压小于 80 mmHg 的患者，应该强制留置双侧胸管，启动每一项高级创伤生命支持流程。如果患者病情仍不稳定，应当立即转入手术室。如果患者病情稳定，则须进行彻底的全身检查。对于存在胸腹联合伤的患者，推荐留置单个或多个胸管。对于需要开腹探查的患者，创伤科医生应该重新评估是否须在手术室中开胸。

手术处理

急诊开胸手术

如果患者来到急诊已经出现心肺骤停，则须立即行急诊开胸手术，目的是：

- 复苏生命垂危的心胸穿通伤患者
- 如果伴随心脏损伤，解除心包压塞
- 如果合并心脏损伤，直接修复心脏裂伤
- 控制胸腔出血
- 防止气体栓塞
- 心肺复苏，可以产生高达正常心脏搏出量 60% 的效果
- 控制肺出血
- 十字钳夹阻断肺门
- 十字钳夹阻断降主动脉

急诊开胸手术只有在患者遭受了穿通性肺损伤并有心肺骤停后由经过专业训练的外科医生按照下列步骤实施：

1. 立刻气管插管，开放静脉通路，同时在复苏时使用快速灌注技术，在右侧胸腔插入胸管。
2. 抬起左臂，快速消毒、进行胸部的术前准备。
3. 进行左侧开胸，向前至左侧胸骨肋骨连接处，从乳头下开始，向侧面到达背阔肌。女性患者乳房被牵向头端。
4. 切口快速穿过皮肤、皮下组织、胸大肌和前锯肌，到达到肋间肌。
5. 三层交叉的肌肉用剪刀锐性分离。打开胸膜。
6. 在一些情况下，第 4、5 肋软骨会被断开以获得充分的暴露。
7. 使用 Finochietto 拉钩分开肋骨。此时外科医生应该评估左侧胸腔内的出血范围。过多的血容量丢失是不良预后的可靠指标。
8. 向中间提升左肺，当降主动脉通过主动脉裂孔进入腹腔时迅速定位它。可以通过触摸主动脉搏动来评估剩余的血容量。
9. 可以暂时朝胸椎椎体方向阻断降主动脉。
10. 在阻断降主动脉之前须钝性、锐性分离结合，以游离主动脉上、下边界，这样才能用示指及拇指环绕主动脉。
11. 经验不足的外科医生往往会将位于主动脉上方的食管误认做主动脉进行阻断。可术前放置鼻胃管作为识别食管和通常为空虚的胸主动脉的引导。
12. 使用 Crafoord-DeBakey 十字钳夹法来阻断主动脉。
13. 如果存在心脏损伤，应该在膈神经上方纵行切开心包，清理心包中的血块和积血，修复心脏损伤。
14. 如果出现肺门血肿或者活动性出血，应使用 Crafoord-DeBakey 十字钳夹法阻断肺门血管。
15. 如果发现肺实质撕裂，应用 Dural 钳钳夹。
16. 如果损伤发生在右侧胸腔，或者先前置入的胸管引流出大量血液，或者损伤伤及对侧胸腔，那么应该横断胸骨，将左侧开胸转为双侧开胸。
17. 如果左侧开胸中转为双侧开胸，应该结扎一侧或双侧内乳动脉。
18. 积极的复苏手段需要压力驱动的快速输液器快速输注温热液体。
19. 须备好除颤仪与除颤电极板，能量在 10 ~ 50 J

之间。

20. 必要时在循环中或左、右心室内注射肾上腺素。
21. 如果怀疑有气体栓塞可能，应当用16号针头行心室内抽吸。
22. 个别情况下可能须使用起搏器，不过这种情况往往预后十分不良。
23. 如果患者复苏成功，应当立刻妥善转运至手术室，进行确定性肺损伤修复。

肺门十字钳夹的效果

优势：①阻断出血，有利于残余血液再分布；②有利于健侧肺的血液灌注；③控制肺门出血；④预防气体栓塞。

劣势：①导致十字钳夹的肺缺血；②增加右心室后负荷；③影响患侧肺的通气和氧合。

不确定因素：影响包括安全的十字钳夹的时间长短和患侧肺与健侧肺的再灌注损伤的发生率。

胸主动脉阻断的效果

优势：①阻断出血，有利于残余血液再分布；②改善冠状动脉 / 颈动脉血流灌注；③减少膈以下血管的血流；④增加左心室的每搏作功指数（left ventricular stroke work index，LVSWI）；⑤增加心肌收缩力。

劣势：①使腹腔脏器的血供大约减少至原来的10%；②肾血供减少至原来的10%；③脊髓血供大约减少至原来的10%；④增加无氧代谢；⑤增加缺氧和增加酸中毒风险；⑥增加巨大的左心室后负荷；⑦极小概率引起截瘫。

不确定因素：影响包括安全的十字钳夹的时间长短和再灌注损伤的发生率。

手术室开胸

器械

在进入胸腔，牵拉，操作及对肺、胸腔内结构行外科干预时须使用特殊的器械（图1）。包括：

- Doyen 肋骨起子（图2)
- Alexander 骨膜刀（图2)
- Cameron-Haight 骨膜起子（图2)
- Bethune 肋骨剪（图3）
- Stille-Horsley 截骨钳（图3）

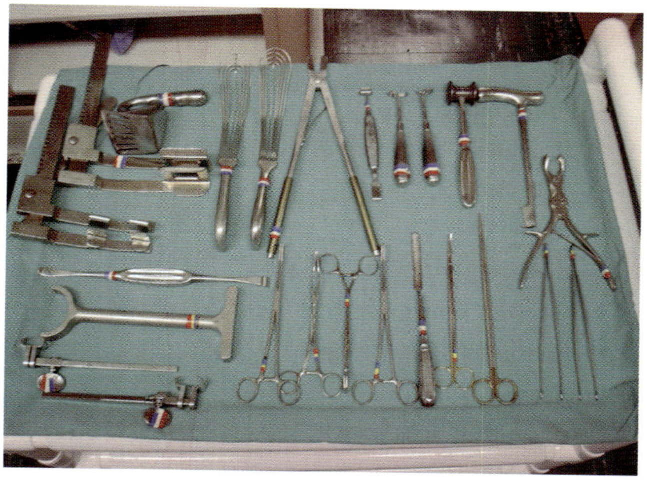

图1　胸部手术工具托盘

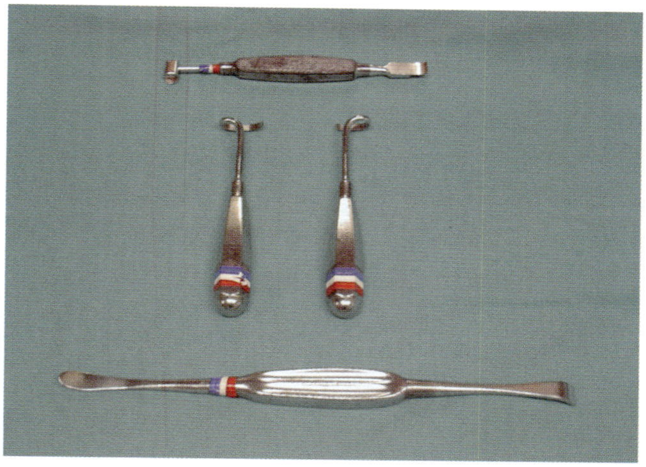

图2　Alexander 骨膜刀、左侧和右侧 Doyen 肋骨起子和 Cameron-Harght 骨膜起子

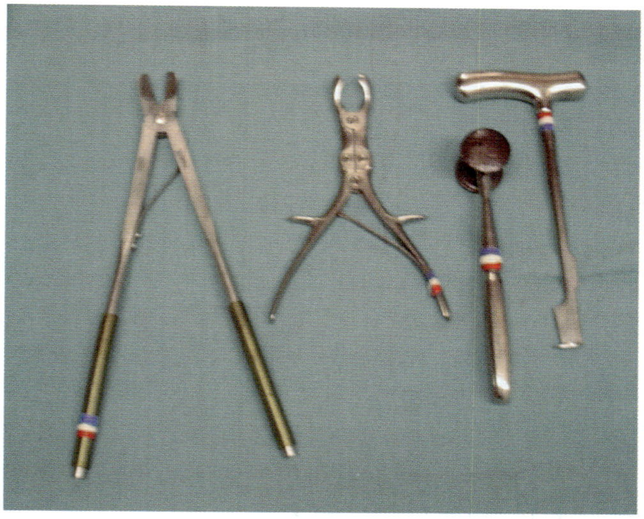

图3　Bethune 肋骨剪、Stille-Horsley 截骨钳和 Lebsche 刀、Lebsche 锤

- Lebsche 刀和 Lebsche 锤
- 肋骨刮匙
- Finochietto 拉钩
- Davidson 肩胛骨拉钩（图 4）
- Allison 肺拉钩（图 4）
- Semb 肺拉钩
- Nelson 肺分离肺叶切除术剪刀（图 5）
- Metzenbaum 长分离剪（图 5）
- Tuttle 胸腔镊子（图 5）
- Duval 肺叶钳（图 6）
- Davidson 肺血管钳
- Sarot 支气管钳
- Bailey 肋骨合拢器（图 7）
- Berry 持针器
- 血管钳

辅助工具

使用双腔气管插管在处理肺部穿通伤患者时非常有用（图 8）。尽管对麻醉医生而言，置入双腔气管插管会比单腔气管插管困难，但是双腔气管插管可以选择性地进行单肺通气。双腔气管插管有两种，一种是插入左主支气管，一种是插入右主支气管。通过扩大球囊来封堵任意一侧主支气管，使肺萎陷并保持静止，方便创伤科医生操作。支气管镜同样作用巨大，可以在肺叶甚至肺段水平确定损伤部位。可以用来吸引气管支气管中的血液，解除支气管痉挛。

通气

手术室使用的呼吸机有两种。传统方式是间歇通气，肺会周期性膨胀和萎陷；高频喷射通气可以

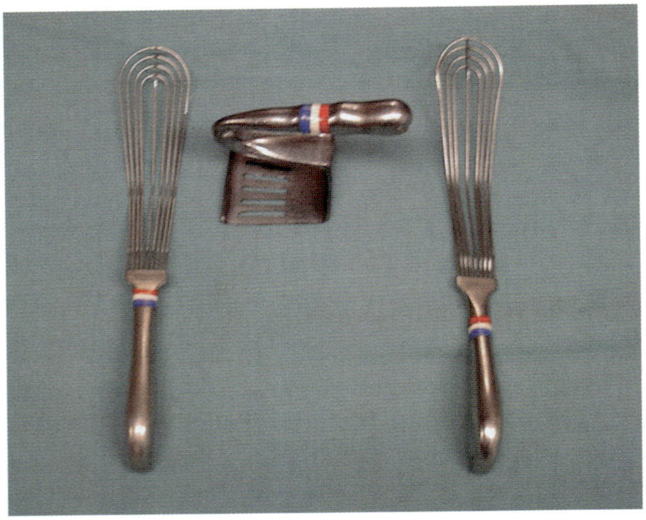

图 4　Allison 肺拉钩和 Davidson 肩胛骨拉钩

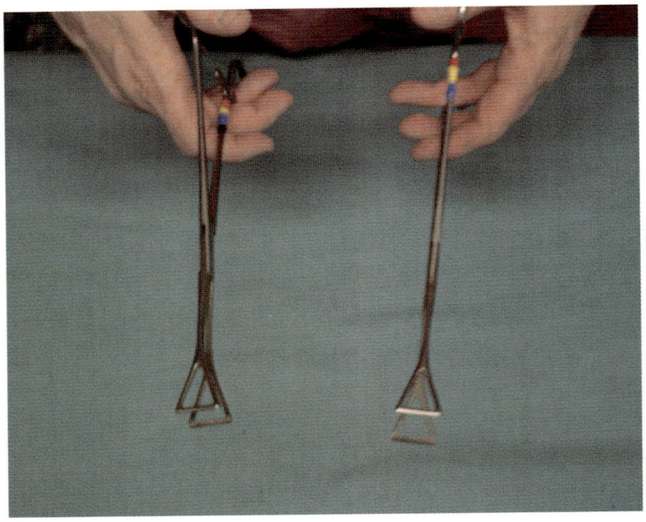

图 6　Duval 肺叶钳

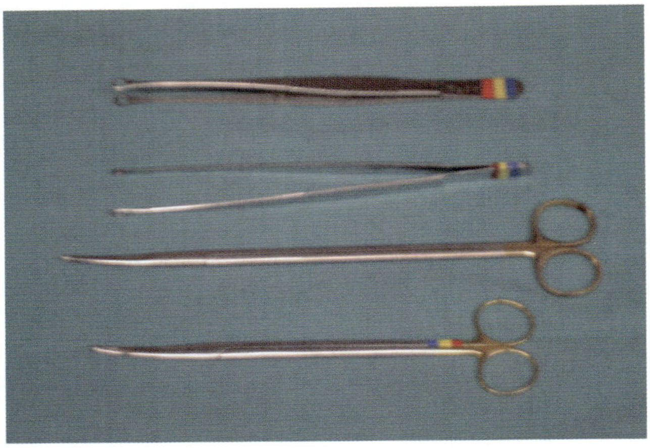

图 5　Nelson 肺分离肺叶切除术剪刀，Metzenbaum 长分离剪和 Tuttle 胸腔镊子

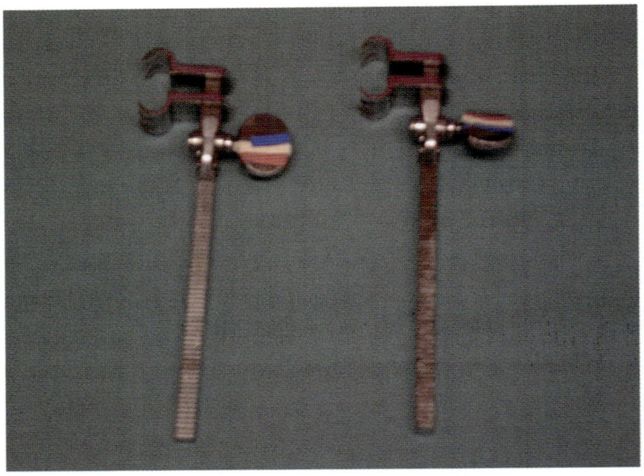

图 7　Bailey 肋骨合拢器

使肺在手术过程中保持静止。如VDR-4型呼吸机（图9）可以提供脉冲气流通气。

手术切口和显露

目前没有任何一个单独切口可以探查到胸腔的所有间隔。处理肺损伤的开胸切口包括前外侧开胸切口（Spangaro切口）、后外侧开胸切口、右后外侧开胸切口、左后外侧开胸切口，以及胸骨正中开胸切口（Dural-Barasty切口）。

前外侧开胸术（Spangaro切口） 这是最常用的开胸切口，用于处理转运到手术室的血流动力学不稳定患者。这个切口提供的术野有限，但可使创伤科医生对左侧或右侧胸腔实施手术。这个切口无法探查到单侧胸腔的后方组织结构。左前外侧开胸可以探查到心脏，在患者出现血流动力学不稳定及心肺骤停时可以通过本切口及时阻断降主动脉。

如果同时发生了腹部相关损伤，可以选择进行前外侧开胸。如果存在双侧胸腔损伤，前外侧开胸切口可以延长为双侧前外侧开胸切口。

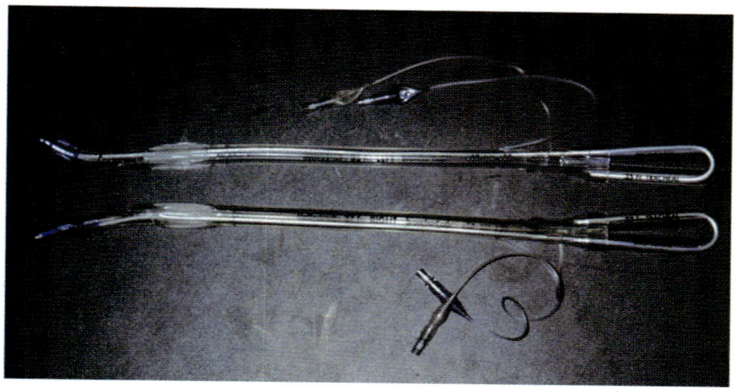

图8 双腔气管插管

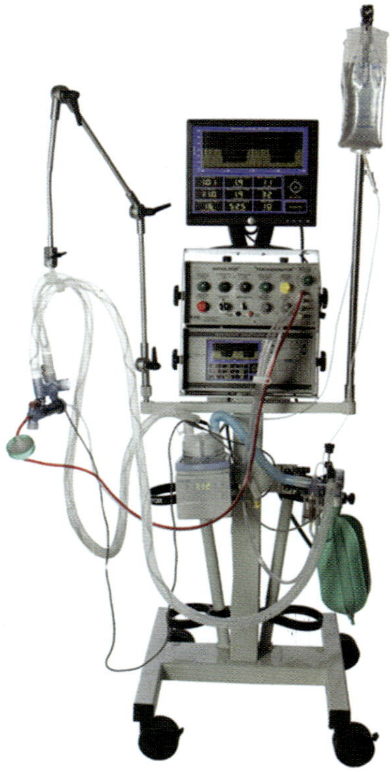

图9 VDR-4呼吸机，可提供脉冲气流通气

后外侧开胸术 本切口可以为手术处理创伤性肺损伤患者提供最好的术中暴露。不足之处在于需要较多的时间，因为患者须被摆成特定的体位。转运到手术室的患者往往血流动力学不稳定，无法耐受这种体位。这一切口也是合并心脏损伤患者的次选方案。

右后外侧开胸术 本切口提供到达右肺和胸段食管跨过胸主动脉前方到达左侧胸腔并且经过胸段降主动脉上方部分的通路。它可以探查到奇静脉和半奇静脉，是处理气管损伤时最常用的切口。

左后外侧开胸术 本切口提供到达左肺、胸段降主动脉和胸段食管最远端的通路，即食管从右侧跨越到左侧胸腔并且经过胸段降主动脉上方的部分。

胸骨正中切开术（Duval-Barasty切口） 本切口适用于处理转运到手术室、合并心脏损伤，并且有生命体征的患者。在锐性横断纵隔胸膜的情况下可以探查到双侧胸腔。它可以探查到双侧肺的前方，但暴露背侧肺的效果欠佳。当肺组织明显向内移动到了手术切口处，应当十分警惕肺门血管是否发生了90°扭转，因其会阻断肺血管的流入和流出，造成严重的血流动力学不稳定。同样的，在处理下肺韧带时应当十分小心，避免发生下肺静脉的医源性损伤。

辅助手段

治疗肺损伤的重要的辅助手段包括：①主动脉十字钳夹；②肺门十字钳夹；③完全的流入血管阻断（shumacker操作）；④肺门血管控制；⑤左、右肺动脉主干控制；⑥控制肺静脉。

主动脉十字钳夹 主动脉只有通过左前外侧开胸才能实现十字钳夹。在钳夹之前要小心地在主动脉通过主动脉裂孔之前钝性和锐性分离它。主动脉必须要小心地环绕，在游离侧壁时一定要仔细，以防对肋间动脉造成医源性损伤。食管位于主动脉前方，一定要在放置Crafoord-DeBaky动脉十字钳之前游离食管。可以通过术前放置的鼻胃管来辨别食管。

肺门十字夹闭 该方法用于存在肺门血肿或者肺门活动性出血时。仔细通过锐性结合钝性的方法分离肺门周围组织，以使手指能环绕肺门所有结构。然后再尽量贴近心包的位置放置 DeBaky 动脉十字钳。

完全血流阻断 当合并右心房侧壁或者腔静脉心房交界处的心脏损伤时须行完全血流阻断，包括在进入心包处钳夹上腔静脉和在 Gibbon 间隙处钳夹下腔静脉。这样可以迅速排空心脏。安全的阻断时间是 1 ~ 3 min，确切的阻断时间不详。

肺门血管控制 肺动脉、肺静脉的出血可以通过这一方式得到控制。游离、结扎或者切断肺动脉及肺静脉的方式不同于体循环血管。肺血管壁薄而且质脆、易撕裂，不能用普通血管钳钳夹，游离过程中要非常小心。血管区的安全快速分离一定要留出足够的血管周空间。在游离动脉或静脉时，要将血管周围 3 个方向完全游离，然后再用 Mxter 直角钳从血管下方通过血管。如果没有这么做，很有可能造成血管穿孔。肺血管不能使用血管钳钳夹因为可能造成撕裂，只有血管外膜可以钳夹。使用 Kittner 剥离器可以安全地牵拉和分离肺血管。

控制左、右肺动脉主干 这项操作可以在胸膜外（肺门处）或胸膜内完成，需要心脏侧壁替代和偶尔的心包横行切开。

控制肺静脉 这项操作可以在胸膜外（肺门处）或胸膜内完成，后者会相对困难。

处理肺损伤的统一流程

处理肺血管损伤的步骤如下：

创伤性肺损伤的统一治疗方法已在前面描述。

1. 清除胸腔内的积血和血块。
2. 暴露受伤的肺组织。
3. 如果血容量严重不足，为恢复血管内容量，选择填塞。
4. 判断是否存在肺门或者中央型血肿和出血。
5. 判断是否须十字钳夹肺门，如果必要，使用 Crafoord-DeBakey 主动脉钳夹闭肺门。
6. 继续寻找肺实质中的出血结构，控制出血，进而解除对肺门的夹闭。
7. 如果肺实质损伤部位远离肺门，则使用 Daval 肺叶钳夹闭损伤部位。
8. 评估纵隔和心包有无损伤；
9. 继续修补损伤；

修复和切除的手术技术

快速切除少量肺组织的切除技术的发展大大降低了创伤性肺损伤患者行肺叶或全肺切除的死亡率。这一技术被称为“肺保留技术”，包括肺缝合技术、选择性血管结扎结合吻合器和钳夹肺神经束切断术。2006 年，Asensio 等报道了 101 例进行开胸手术的创伤性肺损伤患者，其中 80% 使用了肺保留技术。术中的辅助工具包括氩气刀及纤维蛋白胶，成为了创伤科医生手术的有力武器。

下文中介绍的治疗创伤性肺损伤的手术器械可分为 2 大类：组织保留技术和切除手段。

组织保留技术

这些技术包括①肺缝合技术；②使用选择性深血管结扎的肺神经束切断术；③选择性深血管结扎的钳夹的肺神经束切断术；④非解剖性切除。这些技术可以处理大约 85% 的创伤性肺损伤。

这些技术用于控制出血，控制小的漏气和保留肺组织。当肺损伤容易修复重建时也可以使用这些方法。

肺缝合术

使用 Duval 肺叶钳控制出血后，使用 3-0 铬或其他可吸收线缝合伤口的上方、下方及侧面，同时缝线也可用来轻柔地牵引伤口边缘。很好的可塑的丝带拉钩应充分牵开伤口以充分暴露损伤的血管，并用 3-0 铬线或其他类似大小的可吸收缝线选择性结扎。小的支气管使用同样的处理方式。伤口用 3-0 铬线连续锁边缝合。

吻合器肺神经束切断术

1997 年，Asensio 等报道了治疗穿通性肺损伤的方法，使用直线型 Endo GIA 进行选择性结扎血管的神经束切断。1994 年，Wall 等报道了使用动脉血管钳钳夹的神经束切断。使用 Dauvl 肺叶钳稳定肺出血后，找到损伤的入口和出口。必要时可以用剪锐性分离脏层胸膜。使用 55 或者 75 的 3.8 mm 吻合器穿过损伤的入口和出口（图 10-11）。这样可以打开致伤物及弹片造成的隧道，有效暴露受伤血管和支气管，并用 3-0 铬线或类似大小的可吸收线选择性结扎（图 12）。肺实质可用 3-0 铬线或相同大小的

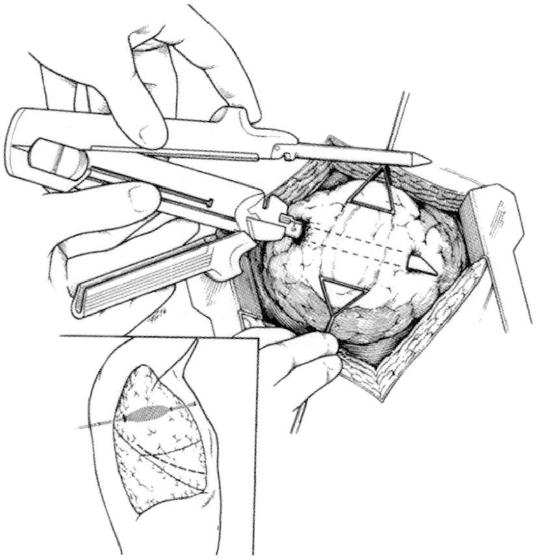

图 10　描述了子弹穿过肺导致的空腔效应。通过通道的入口和出口插入 GIA55

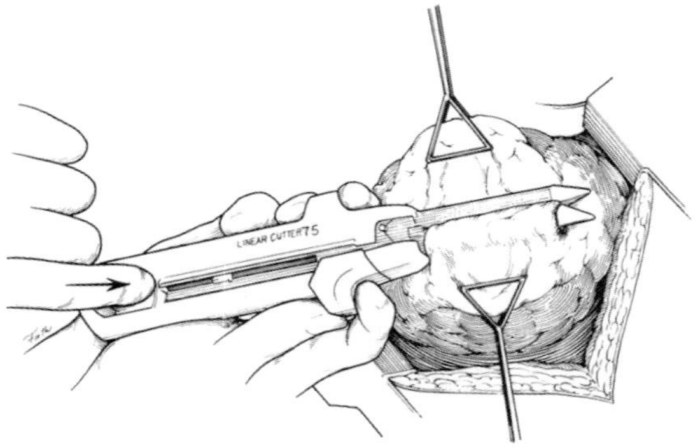

图 11　然后关闭 GIA，并打开弹道

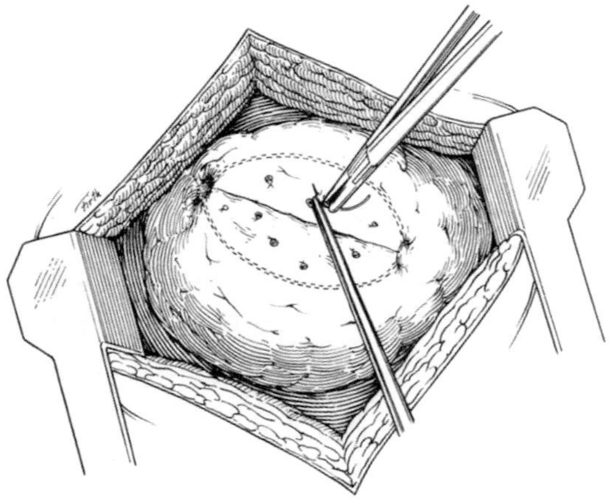

图 12　打开肺部伤道，结扎深部出血的血管（*From Asensio JA, Demetriades D, Berne JD, et al: Stapled pulmonary tractotomy: a rapid way to control hemorrhage in penetrating pulmonary injuries. J Am Coll Surg 185:504–505, 1997*）

可吸收线单纯锁边缝合。隧道的入口和出口保持开放，以引流空气和血流。麻醉医生膨胀肺可以检验缝合的完整性，如果发现漏气，及时修补。

钳夹肺神经束切断术

Wall 等描述的高选择性血管结扎的钳夹肺神经束切断和吻合器神经束切断类似。只是用两把 Crafoord-DeBakey 钳代替吻合器放入损伤隧道的入口和出口，用 Nelson 或 Metzenbaum 剪切断两把钳子之间的肺组织。

非解剖性切除

特别微小的或者外周的肺叶或者肺段损伤可以行非解剖性切除。使用 Duval 肺叶钳固定切除位置，使用 55 或者 75 的 3.8 mm 吻合器直接将损伤处灼烧。可使用 3-0 铬线或相同大小的可吸收线锁边缝合切缘，不过通常没有必要。非解剖性切除也可以非常复杂，须切除主要肺段并行复杂的重建。在损伤的肺叶进行这一操作应当谨慎。

切除技术

切除技术包括正规的肺叶切除和全肺切除。这一操作适用于①控制出血；②切除损毁或失活的肺组织；③控制无法修复的主气管或叶支气管漏气；④控制威胁生命的出血。

标准肺叶切除

标准肺叶切除术适用于肺叶的完全损伤，或者因肺叶的动脉，静脉，叶支气管的大的、破坏性的、不可修复的损伤而出现的无法控制的出血。要实施肺叶切除术，必须要分离叶间裂。在肺门处通过周围血管平面寻找肺的主要血管并在胸膜外进行离断。由叶间裂识别肺叶血管并进行离断。在远端横断下肺韧带可以为双肺下叶提供较好的活动度。所有的肺血管，不论是肺叶还是肺段血管，都可以使用不可吸收缝线连续结扎和缝扎。3.5 mm 的 TA-30、TA-50、TA-90 吻合器或者是血管内吻合器同样可以用来吻合血管。也可以使用 4-0、5-0 或 6-0 的单纤维聚丙烯缝线缝合处理肺血管。

不论是主支气管、叶支气管还是段支气管都应当使用 4.8 mm 的 TA-30、TA-45 或 TA-90 进行吻合和离断，这是处理支气管的最佳方案。也可以使用 Sarot 支气管钳和 4-0 的 Tevdek 缝线结扎支气管。如果决定使用手工缝合的方法，外科医生应当避免使用任何器械来夹持支气管近端切缘。缝合技巧包括钳夹支气管离断部位的远端，横断支气管，近端保留 4～5mm 的残端，并使用 4-0 Tevdek 缝线缝合。缝合不能过紧，以防出现组织切割或阻断支气管血供。缝合 2 针后，延长切缘然后进行进一步缝合。针距为 2～3 mm。对主支气管而言，缝合一般不超过 6 针，叶支气管缝合 3～4 针即可。缝合针数过多会阻断支气管残端血供。缝合结束后应当将支气管残端没入生理盐水中，麻醉医生以 45 cm 水柱的压力膨胀肺，观察残端有无漏气。如果出现漏气，应在漏气部位补充缝合。

在完成肺叶切除后，其余肺叶应当以 2-0 铬线固定在胸壁以防发生扭转，这一点十分重要。可以使用胸膜或者心包外脂肪覆盖支气管残端，这被称为 Brewer 补片。这一技术的实际效果尚未被证实。更好的方法是使用肋间肌的肌瓣，但这会耗费更多的手术时间。

右肺上叶切除术

实施右肺上叶切除术，肺动静脉都须向外周游离以准确定位右肺上叶的供血血管。首先，使用 2-0 丝线结扎肺上叶的前段和尖后段动脉，游离并使用 3-0 丝线缝扎近端血管。在斜裂中可识别出后段动脉，结扎缝扎并使用同样的方法离断。在水平裂中解剖出引流上叶的静脉，小心游离后使用 0 号丝线结扎，2-0 丝线缝扎后切断。此时将肺向前牵引可以暴露后方的支气管通道，可看到右主支气管及隆突，使用 4.8 mm 的 TA-30 或 TA-45 吻合器切断右肺上叶支气管。

右肺中叶切除术

寻找肺动脉的肺中叶分支，使用 0 号丝线结扎，2-0 丝线缝扎后切断。中叶静脉以同样的方式处理。随后仔细分离出中叶支气管并使用 4.8 mm 的 TA-30 或 TA-45 吻合器切断。

右肺下叶切除术

斜裂中有主肺动脉。沿斜裂可解剖出肺动脉的右肺下叶分支。游离肺下叶的上段分支和基底段分支，使用 0 号丝线连续缝合，2-0 丝线缝扎后切断。操作过程中应特别注意避免损伤中叶动脉。随后开始处理下肺静脉，过程中注意保护好引流中叶的静脉。使用 0 号丝线连续结扎，2-0 丝线缝扎后切断下肺静脉。再在斜裂中识别出上段支气管和基底段支气管，分别以 4.8 mm 的 TA-30 或 TA-45 吻合器切断。

左肺上叶切除术

实施左肺上叶切除术时，须结合锐性和钝性分离，仔细分离叶间裂。如果叶间裂分化不良，可使用 3.8 mm TA-30 或 TA-45 切断。在叶间裂中上 1/3 交界处开始游离肺动脉。进入周围血管平面，解剖出上叶动脉各段分支，仔细游离。分别使用 0 号丝线连续结扎，2-0 丝线缝扎后切断。同样方式处理引流左肺上叶的上肺静脉及其下叶的分支。再以 4.8 mm 的 TA-30 或 TA-45 吻合器切断左肺上叶支气管。

左肺下叶切除术

实施左肺下叶切除术的步骤与左肺上叶类似，只是动静脉游离的方向朝向左肺下叶血管。使用 0 号丝线连续结扎、2-0 丝线缝扎舌段动脉。注意部分患者可出现 2 支舌段动脉。随后以 4.8 mm 的 TA-30 或 TA-45 吻合器切断左肺下叶支气管。

肺切除术

右全肺切除术

探查右侧胸腔，定位奇静脉及右肺门。使用锐性分离结合钝性分离结合，识别出右主肺动脉，并用血管环包绕，注意不要过度牵引。锐性离断右上肺韧带。识别上肺静脉和下肺静脉，并用血管环包绕。所有血管均可使用 3.5 mm TA-30、TA-45 吻合器或血管内吻合器结扎或吻合。暴露右主支气管后包绕。注意避免过度牵拉，以防撕裂隆嵴以下的支气管。最后以 4.8 mm 的 TA-30 或 TA-45 吻合器切断右主支气管。

左全肺切除术

仔细探查左侧胸腔，识别膈神经、迷走神经及左侧喉返神经，并注意术中保护。定位左侧肺门，使用锐性分离结合钝性分离分离，识别出左主肺动脉，并用血管环包绕，注意不要过度牵引。锐性离断左下肺韧带。识别上肺静脉、下肺静脉并用血管环包绕。所有血管均可使用 3.5 mm TA-30、TA-45 吻合器或血管内吻合器结扎或吻合。暴露左主支气管后包绕。注意避免过度牵拉，以防撕裂隆嵴以下的支气管。最后以 4.8 mm 的 TA-30 或 TA-45 吻合器切断左主支气管。

全肺切除的其他技巧（左或右）

如果患者出现肺门血管损伤导致的大出血，可使用手指在肺门处压迫止血，使麻醉医生得以及时扩充患者丢失的血容量。随后可使用 Crafoord-DeBakey 主动脉钳在距离纵隔胸膜数厘米处夹闭血管。如果经过处置，威胁生命的大出血得到控制，则须在胸膜外分离肺门血管，并一一结扎。如果无法实施以上操作，或无法控制出血，或血管钳位置需要非常靠近近心端，则须打开心包以控制肺动脉、肺静脉。心包内控制肺静脉较为困难，并且须侧向移动心脏。须在右心耳处钳夹 Satinsky 钳完成该操作。有时甚至须使用 Shumacker 操作完全阻断右心的流入血流。

另一个方法是使用 4.8 mm 的 TA-90 吻合器跨越肺门直接灼烧并离断肺动脉、肺静脉及其分支。在大多数情况下，该方法可控制位于心包外的肺动脉、肺静脉损伤引起的出血。如果该方法无法控制出血，则须心包内控制肺血管。

预后因素及转归

影响肺损伤生存的需要手术干预的因素包括：受伤机制、致伤物类型、院前转运时间、是否当场或即将出现休克、气道是否有缺损、有无合并其他损伤、手术复杂程度，以及损伤位置。

受伤机制及致伤物类型

日常生活中最常见的肺损伤包括钝伤和穿刺伤。最常见的肺部穿刺伤由刀具或者低速发射物造成，而高速发射物致伤的比例也在逐年增高。高速发射物导致的肺部穿刺伤，其死亡率高于低速发射物及刀刺伤。

在一项平民的创伤性肺损伤的多中心研究中，Karmy-Jones 等报道称钝伤倾向于导致更加广泛的肺实质损伤，在需手术的病例中，他们需要较大的手术切除范围。钝伤的死亡风险是穿刺伤的 3 ~ 10 倍。

在战场上，爆炸伤会导致大面积的肺损伤，但是大多数肺损伤是仍是穿刺伤，如炮弹破片、弹片、高速发射物。Zakharia 和 Petricevic 等报道称继发于爆炸装置的肺部损伤和高速飞弹致伤的破坏性损伤的患者的死亡率明显高于刀刺伤和坠落伤。

院前转运时间

躯干损伤患者病情往往随时间推移逐渐恶化，Gervin 和 Fischer 的“伤员迅速转运”理论改善了该类患者的生存情况。Wagner 等报道称对严重肺部穿刺伤患者的快速院前转运可改善预后，因此组建完善的创伤救治流程和组织良好的创伤服务能够提高患者生存率。Petricevic 等也持相同观点，并且指出在战场上救治肺部创伤伤员的关键在于快速、及时将伤员转运至手术中心。

现场或入院前出现休克

众所周知的肺创伤患者预后不良因素包括院前或在急诊出现生命体征及心律消失。同样的，心肺骤停导致的脉搏消失同样伴随高死亡率。Robison 等报道称在抵达急诊室前已经出现心肺骤停的患者中有 85% 最终死亡。Wagner 等报道称遭受肺部穿通伤的低血压患者，若收缩压低于 90 mmHg，其死亡率高达 90%。

Buckman 等对心脏穿通伤患者使用心血管及呼吸道创伤评分（cardiovascular and respiratory components of the trauma score，CVRS）评估后发现，预期的生理评分对预测患者预后有帮助。Asensio 等随后在 2 项处理致命损伤的前瞻性研究中验证了生理因素及 CVRS 是预测患者预后的重要因素。因此有理由推断这些生理因素在遭受创伤性肺损伤的患者身上能够发挥同等重要的预测预后作用。

气道缺损

众所周知，无论在何处抢救重伤患者，包括创伤性肺损伤患者，最首要的复苏措施在于快速、安全保障气道通畅。未经处理的气道缺损通常是致命的。根据 Asensio 等的报道，在有资质的创伤中心的 ED 里，大多数的创伤患者可以通过急诊插管保障气道通畅。对于极少数患者，气管插管无法完成或是其禁忌证，这时就须采用外科方法。在此例中使用环甲膜切开术来开放气道。Inoue 等曾报道过一种保障创伤性肺损伤患者气道通畅的方法，他们用一种带有可移动式支气管阻塞套囊（Univent Fugi Systems Corporation Tokyo）的气管插管选择性停止患侧肺通气，这种方式可以有效防止健侧气道被积血阻塞。

多发伤

多发伤，尤其是合并心脏和胸腔内大血管的创伤，会增加患者的死亡率。相似地，合并复杂腹部创伤的患者死亡率也会升高。

外科治疗的复杂程度

一些作者指出，外科治疗的复杂程度与创伤患者的死亡率密切相关。Wall 等、Velmahos 等，以及 Cothren 等指出，接受保留肺手术的患者比接受扩大肺切除手术的患者死亡率低。文献中报道的肺缝合术、吻合器肺神经束切断、钳夹肺神经切断束，以及楔形 / 非解剖性肺切除术的死亡率是有差异的。与此相对地，解剖性肺叶切除术的死亡率是 40% ~ 50%，全肺切除术的死亡率是 60% ~ 100%。

Wagner 等曾报道，行全肺切除术的创伤患者的死亡率为 50%。Thompson 等报道行肺叶切除术的患者的死亡率为 54.5%，而行全肺切除患者的死亡率是 100%。这一系列事件的总死亡率是 28%。行肺缝合术和神经束切断术的患者死亡率分别为 3% 和 17%。在 1993 年，Tominaga 等曾报道肺手术患者的总死亡率为 33%。作者研究了死亡率与手术复杂程度的相关性，结果发现非解剖性肺切除术、肺叶切除术、全肺切除术患者的死亡率分别为 20%、33% 和 50%。在 1991 年，Velmahos 等曾报道，须开胸手术治疗的肺穿通伤患者的死亡率为 5%。在这个研究中，作者的关注点在于处理这些创伤的方法。须行保肺手术的患者死亡率为 3%，相比之下，须行肺切除术的患者的死亡率为 20%。Stewart 等报道，须行肺切除术的肺损伤患者的总死亡率为 12.5%，并指出采用吻合器切除是此系列低死亡率的因素。Karmy-Jones 等曾报道，肺损伤患者的死亡率随外科技术的复杂程度增加而升高：接受肺缝合术、吻合器神经束切断术、楔形切除术、肺叶切除术，以及全肺切除术的患者的死亡率分别为 9%、13%、30%、43%、50%。在 2002 年，Cothren 等曾报道，36 位须接受开胸手术的严重肺损伤患者的总死亡率为 30%，相比之下，须行解剖性肺切除术的患者的死亡率为 77%，而行非解剖性肺切除术的患者的死亡率仅为 4%。作者还报道，接受吻合器神经束切断术的患者死亡率会明显下降。Huh 等也把关注点放在肺手术的复杂程度上，他们总结的肺缝合术、神经束切断术、楔形切除术、肺叶切除术，以及全肺切除术的死亡率分别为 24%、9.1%、20%、35% 和 69.7%。

损伤的位置

Wagner 等指出，有肺门脉管束损伤的患者的死亡率高于 70%。Wieneck 和 Wilson 曾报道，枪伤所致的持续性的中心型 / 肺门型肺损伤患者的死亡率为 63%，刺伤所致的肺门损伤患者的死亡率为 44%。这些创伤患者的死因主要是失血和可能存在的空气栓塞。这些作者也报道了中心型肺穿通伤的总死亡率为 56%。Petricevic 等指出，肺损伤合并 1 个或多个肺外损伤的患者会有更高的死亡率（6% ~ 14% 至高达 55%）。

死亡率

根据 Asensio 等的报道，创伤性肺损伤或其外科处理的并发症可分为 3 类：术中并发症、术后短期并发症，以及术后长期并发症。

术中并发症

这些并发症可分为单心室衰竭（多为右室）以及双心室衰竭两类。

术后短期并发症

从技术层面分类，短期并发症可分为以下几类：

- 肺疝
- 肺扭转
- 支气管胸膜瘘
- 动静脉瘘
- 支气管残端瘘
- 支气管残端破裂

从生理学层面短期并发症可分为以下几类：

- 右心室衰竭
- 肺动脉高压
- 难治性肺动脉高压
- 双心室衰竭

术后长期并发症

这些并发症可被分为以下几类：

- 持续性支气管胸膜瘘
- 支气管狭窄
- 气胸
- 肺脓肿
- 支气管扩张
- 动静脉瘘

1979 年，Graham 等研究了 373 例持续性肺穿通伤患者，其中 108 例出现了术后并发症，死亡率为 29%，平均每个患者会遭遇 1.43 个并发症。最常见的并发症包括：术后出血，发生率为 32%；肺不张，发生率为 13%；复发性气胸，发生率为 10%；持续性漏气，发生率为 9%；伤口感染，发生率为 8%；肺炎，发生率为 6%。术后出血和漏气是外科再干预后的主要并发症。Robison 曾报道过，须行开胸肺切除术的肺损伤患者的死亡率为 70%。最常见的术后并发症包括咯血、支气管胸膜瘘、空气栓塞、脓毒症和呼吸功能不全。

死亡率

据文献报道，创伤性肺损伤患者的总死亡率为 1.7%～37%。有许多因素与死亡率密切相关，其中反复被提到的预后决定因素包括患者的生理状况、肺手术的复杂程度、多发伤的数目（尤其是合并的心脏损伤）和是否有额外手术干预的需求。

1979 年，Graham 等报道了持续性肺穿通伤患者的总死亡率为 8%。仅须行胸廓造口术置管与须行开胸手术患者的死亡率分别为 3% 和 6%。这些患者的死因主要包括呼吸功能不全、休克 / 失血、脓毒症、中枢神经系统损伤、空气栓塞和气管食管瘘，这些并发症的发生率分别为 36%、32%、11%、11%、7% 和 4%。1988 年，Robison 报道持续性肺穿通伤患者的总死亡率为 2.4%，主要的死因为脓毒症、多发伤、空气栓塞和失血（众所周知，这在中心型肺损伤中很常见）。

1988 年，Wiencek 和 Wilson 报道持续性中心型 / 肺门血管损伤患者的死亡率为 56%，并总结出他们最主要的死亡原因是失血和空气栓塞。1993 年，Tominaga 等曾报道上述患者的总死亡率是 33%，他们还注意到，肺手术的复杂程度与死亡率密切相关，非解剖性肺切除术、肺叶切除术、全肺切除术的死亡率分别为 20%、33% 和 50%。1999 年，Velmahos 等曾报道，行开胸手术治疗的肺穿通伤患者的死亡率为 5%。作者还注意到救治措施与创伤患者死亡率之间的关系，并报道需要保肺手术和需要肺切除术的患者的死亡率分别为 3% 和 20%。

1997 年，Petricevic 等报道，在克罗地亚战争中，持续性肺穿通伤患者的总死亡率为 1.7%。死因主要为两种，30% 是由于出血和难治性休克，70% 是由于感染性并发症。Stewart 等曾报道，须行肺切除术的肺损伤患者的总死亡率为 12.5%，并总结出采用吻合器行肺切除术与患者低死亡率相关。

2001 年，Karmay-Jones 等报道，在一项为期 4 年的回顾性多中心研究中，451 名须行开胸手术治疗肺损伤的创伤患者的总死亡率为 9%。根据创伤机制分层分析后，研究人员发现这些患者中，68% 的人有钝性损伤，19% 的人有穿通伤。这些患者的死亡率随所需手术的复杂程度的增加而升高：肺缝合术、吻合器肺神经束切断术、楔形切除术、肺叶切除术和全肺切除术的死亡率分别为 9%、13%、30%、43% 和 50%。同穿通伤相比，钝性损伤的死亡率高 10 倍。通过多变量分析得出的致死因素包括损伤机制（钝性损伤 vs. 穿通伤）、高头 / 颈损伤 AIS 评分、需要开腹手术处理、入手术室时收缩压下降。结合外科对肺损伤修复 / 切除的方式——缝合、吻合器肺神经束切断术、楔形切除术、肺叶切除术和全肺切除术等——把这些因素逐步通过一个回归分析模型分析后，明显影响预后的因素包括损伤机制、入急诊室时收缩压下降和肺切除量的增加。

2001 年，Gasparri 等报道，需要肺实质损伤干预患者的总死亡率为 16%，那些收缩压较低、体温低、ISS 评分高、失血量大、合并心血管损伤和需要腔镜手术治疗的患者死亡率普遍较高。然而，作者发现手术干预的复杂程度与患者预后无关。Cothren 等的一项关于 36 位须接受开胸手术处理的严重肺损伤患者的研究报道，接受解剖性肺切除术和非解剖性肺切除术的患者的死亡率分别为 77% 和 4%。作者报道，接受吻合器肺神经束切断术的患者死亡率会显著下降。Huh 等曾报道，须行开胸手术处理的创伤性肺损伤患者的总死亡率为 28%，而且，如果患者同时须接受腹腔镜手术，死亡率会增加到 33%。作者还注意到干预复杂程度与患者死亡率的相关性，肺缝合术、吻合器肺神经束切断术、楔形切除术、肺叶切除术和全肺切除术的死亡率分别为 23.9%、9.1%、20%、35% 和 69.7%。2006 年，Asensio 等在研究了 101 名须行开胸手术的肺穿通伤患者后报道，这些患者的总死亡率为 37%，其中 7 名（19%）患者由于须行 EDT 而未入手术室。

结论

须行开胸手术处理的肺损伤患者在忙碌的城市创伤中心十分常见，为了减少术后并发症，外科医生须有精湛的技艺来处理创伤。通常外科医生会采用相对简单的肺缝合术和肺楔形切除术来救治这些患者。吻合器肺神经束切断术是最常用的保肺手术，可以有效处理 85% 的需要外科干预的肺损伤。虽然现在创伤外科的手术技术和外科监护水平飞速发展，创伤性肺损伤，尤其是需要手术切除的创伤患者，仍然有很高的概率出现术后并发症，甚至死亡。

肺及胸膜损伤的并发症

Thomas K. Varghese, Jr., Riyad Karmy-Jones 和 Gregory J. Jurkovich 著
肖蓉心 译

在创伤患者的死因中，胸部损伤被视为一个主要元凶，它占创伤患者死因的 25%，虽然实际上只有 5% ~ 15% 的胸部损伤患者需要急诊手术干预。基于这一理论，人们普遍认为，虽然胸部创伤发生率很高，但是须行急诊手术处理的概率很小。同时，虽然没有确切的统计数据，但是这些手术中还有一部分是为了处理迟发的并发症。不同中心报道的这些事件的发生率均不同，钝伤与穿通伤的比例、总的损伤程度会导致差异。创伤患者的肺部并发症既可以由直接肺损伤所引起，也可以继发于对胸外创伤的反应。如果创伤患者的肺功能严重受损，就可能对肺通气和肺灌注造成负面影响。因此，处理的措施应该包括急性复苏、对肺损伤的高度警惕、积极处理和预防并发症。

肺部并发症

肺挫伤

据报道，有 75% 的胸部钝性损伤患者会罹患肺挫伤，文献中这部分患者的死亡率可以高达 40%。损伤导致肺实质内出血，引发下游一系列级联式的病理生理学改变。通常，这种病变在创伤后的 48 h 内最严重，7 天内消退。在救治这些患者时，由于影像学检查也会有滞后的表现，所以要在早期就提高警惕。CT 检查比 X 线胸片更能灵敏地显示病变。影像损伤的因素包括以下几方面：机械力，如肋骨骨折或胸壁压缩撕裂肺组织；直接受影响的肺区域出血流入周围肺段内，导致支气管痉挛；挫伤肺周围肺不张；肺泡组织损伤，导致黏液分泌增加，肺表面活性物质分泌减少，诱发呼吸衰竭。挫伤肺组织的肺泡通气功能也会下降，肺泡通气 - 灌注失衡会导致肺内分流增加（由于局域血管收缩），进而导致肺的顺应性下降。在细胞水平，黏膜纤毛、肺巨噬细胞和淋巴细胞的功能不全会导致患者更易感染肺炎。

对于肺挫伤的处理措施主要在于支持治疗，目的是提高呼吸功能、清理支气管肺的分泌物和减少挫伤肺周围的肺不张。及时补液、控制胸壁损伤相关的疼痛和维持血流动力学稳定在疗程的前几天至关重要。肺挫伤的范围越大，患者需要机械通气的可能性就越大。处理重症单侧肺挫伤患者时可能会须双腔气管插管行独立机械通气，来避免健侧肺的气压伤和伤侧肺治疗不足。在使用机械通气时，应该根据肺内分流（Qs/Qt）的评估结果来调整潮气量和 PEEP。虽然在治疗非创伤性的急性低氧性呼吸衰竭的患者时可以使用无创正压通气（noninvasive positive pressure ventilation，NPPV），但在澳洲进行的一项针对 75 名患者的研究中，经过反复的测试，研究者认为将此项技术应用于急性创伤患者时须提高警惕。间歇正压通气呼吸模式会将一定体积的气体打入气道，直到达到预设气道压。然而，这种治疗措施可能引发一系列并发症，包括增加有潜在肺疾病患者的气胸发生率、加重肺实质损伤

导致的漏气和气体进入消化道后导致的腹胀等。因此，在急性创伤环境中分清哪部分创伤患者可以从 NPPV 中获益是救治过程中的一大难题。现行的 ATLS 措施中推荐，有明显低氧血症（不吸氧时 Pao_2＜70 mmHg，Sao_2＜90%）、低通气量（$Paco_2$＞45 mmHg）或精神状态改变的患者须立刻插管抢救。

持续性的漏气

胸部创伤患者肺持续性的漏气分为 3 种情况：肺实质损伤后、解剖性肺切除术后和接受机械通气后。

肺实质损伤后的持续性漏气

肺实质的损伤的病因可以是肺穿通伤、有胸壁软化或肋骨贯穿的钝性损伤、患者已有的基础肺实质疾病（如大疱性肺气肿）等，此时可以按照自发性气胸的处理原则来治疗。在超过 80% 的病例中，单纯行胸腔闭式引流术就足以复张因创伤而萎陷的肺。一项前瞻性的研究表明，在 48 h 后，胸腔闭式引流接水封瓶可以加速漏气的愈合，因为这样可以减小跨胸膜的压力梯度。排除技术因素的影响（如引流管移位或脱落），对于超过 3 天的漏气或合并复发的气胸患者，使用胸腔镜比持续胸腔闭式引流更有效。Schermer 等回顾了 39 位创伤患者的病程，这些患者若非漏气已经可以出院（漏气多于 3 天）。其中的 25 位同意接受 VATS，这缩短了他们的带管时间（带管时间，分别为 8 天和 12 天；住院时间，分别为 10 天和 17 天）。

CT 扫描可以确定肺损伤的位置，从而有助于肺楔形切除术或应用生物黏合剂的术中定位，也有助于病程早期进行 VATS。Carrillo 等曾报道了一项纳入 11 位遭遇胸部创伤后持续漏气的患者（平均 6 天）的研究。这些患者中有 10 位遭受钝性损伤，有 10 位患者漏气的破损处可以定位，可行肺段吻合切除，最后一位患者由于无法定位漏气点因而接受了化学胸膜固定术。术后所有患者都在 48 h 内拔除了胸管，9 位患者在 72 h 内出院。在很多病例中，只要单纯在胸腔镜直视下分解软组织小腔并置入胸管就足以使患者受益。在胸膜固定环节，我们尽可能采用胸膜摩擦术而非使用化学胸膜固定术，从而避免肺实质的粘连和化学物质对于年轻患者的远期影响。合并基础肺部疾病的患者须同时维持未受伤的治疗。对于有手术禁忌和有少量漏气、无手术指征的患者，可予 Heimlich 瓣膜然后离院观察，80% 的患者可以在 3 周内愈合。

行肺切除术后的持续性漏气

由于在处理创伤患者时很少采用肺叶切除术和全肺切除术，因此在术后发生漏气（支气管胸膜瘘或 BPF）的概率很小。然而，急诊肺切除术本身就比选择性切除术有更高的概率发生此类并发症。危险因素包括残端过长、血供阻断和感染性血胸。在理想状态下，行肺叶切除术 / 全肺切除术后应该第一时间将残端在切除部位加固，或者随后用胸膜、肋间组织或其他肌瓣加固。一旦发生漏气，处理措施由病程的不同时间段（术后 7 天以前或以后）、严重程度（是否有足够的代偿性通气、缺损是否能在内镜下可见）、患者的一般生理状况和患者是否接受通气决定。对于状况较稳定的患者，BPF 可表现为新发的排痰性咳嗽、胸腔积液的液平面下降 1～2 个肋间隙（全肺切除术后）、新发的液气平。接受通气的患者主要会出现脓胸和潮气量的损失，抢救的首要目标是避免误吸。非插管患者最好取直立位或患侧卧位。引流位置不当时一定要及时调整，若患处没有引流，则须在原胸廓造口的瘢痕上方重置胸管，因为膈会上升至瘢痕处并产生粘连。如果漏气的破口较小，或破口无法在直视下准确定位，就可以采用支气管镜下胶黏合。

在病程的前 7 天内，仍有机会进行二次手术闭合残端，但是可能伴发的脓胸会增加手术的失败率。初次手术与二次手术之间间隔的时间越长，难度就越大。在全肺切除术后，纵隔会产生炎性反应，此时肺门的脉管束残端会很难显露且不能移动。因此，在全肺切除术后，最好的选择可能就是用网膜封堵残端、胸腔填充，并且定期灌洗直到缺口闭合。另一种选择，尤其是对于右侧全肺切除术后的患者，就是行隆嵴下右主支气管切除术。残端已被固定，无法移动，但是其黏膜可用烧灼法处理，同时可以用其他活体组织加固新的残端。外科医生可以自己选择脓胸腔的治疗方式。对于行肺叶切除术的患者，可以采取与上述措施相似的处理方式，但是可能须扩大切除范围（例如，右肺下叶切除术后的漏气患者须补充切除右肺中叶）。对于残留空间，可采取开放引流，或用各种残留空间填补方式填充，具体措施会在脓胸处理的章节阐述。

机械通气患者的持续性漏气

机械通气患者若出现持续性漏气却没有明确的

破损病变，通常是由于肺泡胸膜瘘导致的，而非BPF。很显然，患者的基础肺疾患与预后密切相关，发生支气管胸膜瘘的急性呼吸困难综合征（acute respiratory distress syndrome，ARDS）患者的死亡率高达80%。无论解剖学基础如何，出现漏气的机械通气患者死亡率会明显升高。Pierson等曾研究过39名（从1 700名机械通气患者中选出）出现漏气且持续时间超过24 h的接受机械通气患者。其中27名是创伤患者，并总结出致命的危险因素，包括入院早期未发生而在后期发生的漏气（早发与晚发的死亡率分别为45%和94%）、每次呼吸有超过500 ml的漏气（少于与超过的死亡率分别为57%和100%），还有合并胸部创伤（合并和不合并的死亡率分别为56%和92%）。

这些研究结果都表明，虽然创伤患者的漏气是一个良性的病程，但是仍是一个须慎重处理的并发症。另一方面，漏气本身很少致死，漏出的气体可以引发持续性气胸，甚至是张力性气胸，进而影响通气，这时就须放置胸管（有时须放置多根）。在某些更少见的情况下，漏气可能会影响氧合。救治措施中最主要的就是减小肺泡压，呼气末平台压是公认的反映指标。理想的呼气末平台压应该不超过30 cmH_2O，最常用的实现这一模式的方法就是结合低潮气量和允许性的高碳酸血症。Marchenkov等曾报道过一项纳入74名机械通气后持续漏气的胸部钝伤患者的研究。他们每天接受3～5次双相气道正压通气（bilevel positive airway pressure，BiPAP）或同步间歇指令通气（synchronized intermittent mandatory ventilation，SIMV）模式通气，峰值压力为33.4 ± 0.2 cm H_2O。PEEP为16.1 ± 0.2 cm H_2O。研究者强调，病程早期更积极的肺复张措施可以加速漏气愈合。如果这一治疗失败，备选方案包括高频喷射通气或独立肺通气。须强调的是，虽然高频通气可以成功治疗中心型气道损伤的患者，但是它既不能在术中持续降低患者的平均气道压，也不能减少漏气或改善氧合。因此，不应常规应用于肺泡胸膜瘘患者。

还有一种暂时性的方法，是用支气管镜技术分离出主要漏气源的肺叶，用Swan-Ganz管或球囊导管按顺序封堵对应支气管。如果此操作后可以消除或明显减少漏气，再注射封堵材料（明胶海绵、纤维蛋白胶、加入四环素的血液等等）。近期有人推荐使用一种侵入性更小、更好的控制方法，那就是经灵活的支气管镜置入可回收的单向活瓣。在多数情况下，当气道压力降低时漏气会减少。如前所述，处理这类并发症时外科手术也是一种干预方式，但是对于有弥漫性肺实质损伤、肺部炎症、重症肺气肿或使用类固醇类药物的患者来说，吻合失败的风险会升高，甚至可能漏气加重。如果医生认为患者确实有接受手术的必要，则可以考虑使用加固吻合线（用牛垫片）、肺尖填塞（将肺尖的胸膜游离并覆盖在切除区域）或解剖性肺叶切除术（如果主要为一叶漏气）来缓解症状。

肺膨出或肺内血肿

当肺实质被破坏，气体或血逸出进入肺实质内而非向肺外渗漏，则会形成肺膨出。这种并发症在肺钝性损伤时较常见，有时也会发生在深刺伤或小口径枪弹伤患者中。因此，这些损伤最好被描述为肺裂伤或继发于肺裂伤。肺膨出常常是单发的，有时可呈多叶状，偶尔为多发。肺膨出在病程初始时很难在X线胸片中被发现，原因可能是因为直径太小或叠加的肺挫伤或出血遮挡。随着病程的进展，逸出的气体和液体向薄壁的空腔内弥散。肺膨出的位置和尺寸由机械力因素决定，压缩会导致破裂，因此最常见的机制为中心型损伤。肺受压后，产生剪切力，纵隔旁腔隙沿着从肺门到膈的方向被拉伸，有时它会与包裹性气胸混淆。肋骨断端穿通也会导致肺膨出，这时病变通常靠近外周且直径较小。粘连组织裂伤是最少见的病因。大多数的肺膨出都是良性疾病，在个别病例中，肺膨出可能导致持续性漏气或感染，这时可以按照脓肿的治疗原则来处理。

血肿的产生机制与上述肺膨出相同。血肿可为实性的，或部分排空形成液气平，甚至可以被纤维壁包裹在肺表面形成真菌球样的新月形气腔。通常，血肿会在3～6个月内消退，这也是血肿与恶性肿瘤在影像学上的鉴别点之一。

肺炎

肺炎可能是胸部创伤患者中最常见的并发症，其危险因素包括误吸、机械通气、直接损伤、肺挫伤和由于疼痛导致的持续性肺不张。肺炎的发病率在无插管患者中为6%，在机械通气患者中为44%。但即便有如此高的发病率，仍然没有数据可以支持对创伤患者预防性使用抗生素。所有诊断肺挫伤的患者中有半数会并发肺炎、气压伤或大面积肺不张，1/4 的患者会进展至 ARDS。VAP 是指患者在机械通气超过 48 h 后发生的肺炎，这种肺炎在界定和诊断上比较困难。在 Harborview 医疗中心，我们发现 VAP 在机械通气超过 7 天的患者中的发病率约为 20%，同时，住院前的气管插管并不是创伤患者发生 VAP 的危险因素。通常，新发炎性浸润、反复发作的发热、白细胞升高或气道内分泌物的改变在临床上提示 VAP 发生的可能性。然而，鉴别微生物定植与感染还需要一些特殊检查，支气管分泌物的定量培养可以提高诊断的特异度（虽然可能会降低灵敏度）。每个检测机构都要基于患者是否已经使用抗生素界定出须临床应用抗生素的阈值（表 1）。

表 1　呼吸机相关性肺炎的诊断性检查

样本	域值	灵敏度 (%)	特异度（%）
气管内吸出物	任何致病原	20 ~ 95	<50
气管内吸出物	≥10^6CFU/m	25 ~ 70	70 ~ 85
支气管镜			
PSB 培养	≥10^3CFU/m	30 ~ 100	80 ~ 100
BAL 培养	≥10^4CFU/m	55 ~ 95	70 ~ 100
BAL 细胞学标本	2 ~ 7%CAB	30 ~ 85	65 ~ 100
非气管镜			
PSB	10^3CFU/m	60 ~ 100	75 ~ 100
BAL	10^4CFU/m	70 ~ 100	65 ~ 95

From Skerrett SJ: The diagnosis of ventilator-associated pneumonia. In Karmy-Jones R, Nathens A, Stern E, editors. Thoracic trauma and critical care. Boston, Kluwer Medical Publishers, 2002, pp397–402.
BAL，支气管肺泡灌洗；CAB，细胞相关细菌；CFU/m，每毫升菌落形成单位；PSB，受保护的样本毛刷

肺感染性坏死

肺感染性坏死的病程在临床上表现为“三部曲”：肺脓肿、坏死性肺炎和肺坏疽。这 3 个部分有时可有重叠或同时发生，3 个环节都是由于肺灌注不足导致组织血供阻断。简而言之，肺脓肿可以解释为一个被周围肺实质包裹的肺叶内的坏死区域；而肺坏疽则是肺叶或全肺的坏死，通常仅在边缘留有少量组织。典型的肺坏死表现为斑块状，通常于解剖结构无关，由于灌注不足致使肺实质破坏，在影像学上常表现为多个小脓腔。虽然这三部曲可以分开来讨论，但在大多数病例中均为两部分或三部分共存，因此其处理原则也可重叠。

在 ICU 中的患者产生肺脓肿的原因包括误吸、肺炎的并发症、异物残留、感染性栓子和创伤感染。在创伤患者中更加特殊的病因包括误吸（伴有或不伴气道阻塞）、感染性肺膨出、肺切除术后切口感染（尤其是急诊神经束切断）和晚期的 VAP 并发症。总体来说，在创伤患者中这些更加少见。7 年来，因肺脓肿、坏死性肺炎和肺坏疽而在 Harborview 医疗中心行急诊肺切除术的 45 名患者中，仅有 4 名是伤后就进行手术的。

肺脓肿的诊断可能相对容易一些。当患者有发热、咳脓痰或咯血的表现时，及时行 X 线胸片检查，可以看到有代表性的液气平。在另一极端情况下，ICU 里持续发热的患者可能须在脓腔形成之前就行 CT 扫描来协助诊断。

在 20 世纪 50 — 70 年代的超过 30 年的时间里，医学界的一些进步将肺感染性坏死患者的死亡率从 50% 降低到 10%，这些进步包括认识到抗生素的重要性、防止误吸、清洁气道的高需求（包括支气管镜的使用）、影像引导下导管引流和手术干预。经皮导管引流术可以在多数患者（甚至是机械通气患者）中使用，它可以减少开胸手术的数量。虽然人们会担心并发脓胸和 BPF，但是前者通过胸腔闭式引流很容易处理，后者很少严重到影响氧合。有些患者，无法放置经皮导管而导致引流不出的液体蓄积，诱发持续性脓毒症或引流不充分或持续性 BPF 等，就需要外科手术干预。在这些情况下可选择的术式通常有 2 种，对于大的中心型脓腔可行肺叶切除术，对于小的周围型脓腔可行清创术（有 / 无肌瓣关闭腔）。这些手术是对外科技术的挑战，一些技巧的应用有助于减少并发症，例如在侧卧位之前隔离患侧肺以避免误吸、在手术早期即暴露主肺动脉以便于控制出血、放置鼻胃管或食管镜防止食管解剖结构难以辨认、尽量避免切除小于 2 cm 的小脓肿来尽量保留有活性的肺实质。术后不常发生漏气、术后应持续灌洗残余空间，这部分内容会在脓胸部分详细讨论。

肺坏疽的特征性鉴别点在于中央血管血栓形成和支气管阻塞，从而导致严重的空穴现象和肺叶 / 全肺液化。与肺脓肿相比，肺坏疽没有坚硬的、边界清晰的包膜。这些特点可以通过增强 CT 鉴别，任何一项都能证明肺脓肿保守治疗的失败。因为保守治疗的成功需要两方面因素的支持，一是有丰富的血供以使抗生素达到有效的血药浓度，二是有开放的气道来排出脓性引流物。在一个历史研究中，Schamaun 等随访了 14 位单侧全肺坏疽的患者。其

中 4 位接受药物治疗后死亡，但 10 位接受肺切除术的患者均存活下来，生存率为 100%，有些患者有弥漫性的双侧肺疾患。当面对持续感染的迹象时，如果存在原发灶，并且仍有手术可能，即使患者不能耐受独立肺通气也应该实施肺切除术。有趣的是，此时肺裂和血管的分离会变得更容易，因为坏死组织更易被剥除。但若患者正在使用升压药物，则不应予以外科切除术，此时采用胸腔镜治疗相关的脓胸和经皮引流大的脓腔才是更好的选择。

坏死性肺炎的特征性表现是病变区域实变、斑片状血流灌注，常伴有小的空洞形成。在这种情况下经皮引流术无效，通常也不推荐行肺实质切除术。然而，CT 扫描有助于定位病变发展的分界线，当出现持续性的肺源性脓毒症时，可以行外科切除术。

支气管狭窄

在气管远端或细支气管钝伤的患者中，有 10%～20% 的患者最终会被诊断为气道狭窄。这一诊断通常不能在创伤发生时立刻做出，而是须滞后一段时间。这些患者中约有 2/3 者会在受伤后的 1～2 周出现化脓、持续性的肺不张和咯血。剩下的人群中，后遗症可能会在受伤后的几年后出现，临床表现为哮喘、劳力性呼吸困难或迟发性的肺实质坏死。任何年轻患者，若在遭遇胸部创伤后的 1～2 年新发哮喘，都应该进行气道评估，即使患者曾经做过影像学和支气管镜检查，并且当时结果无异常。根据具体情况，行支气管镜、CT 扫描、CT 支气管造影和流速 - 容量环等检查有助于作出诊断。如果患者出现了阻塞后的肺实质破坏，则须行阻塞远端肺切除术。若狭窄远端的肺实质未被破坏，则狭窄气道的切除和重建就足以重新复张狭窄远端的肺组织。部分患者会演变为慢性病程，这可能提示患侧肺血流灌注不足。当没有证据支持有败血症或肺坏死时，处理的主要目标是重建气道，因为此时的灌注不足是由于低氧造成的血管收缩。一旦通气被纠正，这个过程仍是可逆的。对于病情极不稳定的患者，可以暂时用气管支架维持气道通畅。对于几年后出现气道慢性纤维性狭窄的患者，除手术干预外，还可以选择球囊扩张或反复植入支架来治疗。

肺扭转

肺叶扭转在创伤后极少发生，较常见的是出现在右肺上叶切除后，中叶由于可以在残余空间内自由摆动因此容易发生扭转。为了降低这种情况发生的可能性，外科医生在术中会用吻合器或缝线将中叶固定在下叶上。有时，在行开胸手术中将肺牵拉至前方以暴露后纵隔会导致肺扭转，尤其是在下肺韧带已被断开的情况下。预防这一并发症的关键在于关胸前确认肺已扩张。原发性的肺扭转虽然极其罕见，但是并非从未发生。Schamaun 回顾了包括 26 例肺扭转患者的文献报道，发现有 5 例是在创伤后。发生的机制可能是由于损伤局限于肺叶内而肺裂完整，从而导致病灶处肺实质迅速扭转，或是由肺出血、水肿诱发的延迟性扭转。在临床上，当出现肺叶实变、发热、咯血，最终演变为症状明显的肺脓毒症时，就要怀疑肺扭转的发生。支气管镜检查可以确诊，在镜下可以看到病变支气管呈“鱼唇”样改变，通常还间断有血性或间歇引流的脓性分泌物。一旦确诊，就需要立刻手术。若肺叶还未发展至坏疽程度，则须将其扭转回来避免坏死；若肺叶已坏死，则须行肺叶切除术。有时还须将肺叶吻合至邻近肺叶上以防止其再次扭转，或者用可吸收缝线行肺叶固定术，将其缝合至邻近肺叶。

肺内残留弹片

肺实质内残留的异物，尤其是形状不规则的异物（比光滑物体常见），可能会诱发并发症，因此须被及时移除。来自 Heidelberg 大学的学者回顾总结了 55 例肺内子弹残留的患者，其中的 34 例有反复发作的咯血（8 例咯血为单发）。芬兰学者进行的一项持续数年的、纳入 502 位患者的研究，结果表明，20% 的创伤患者出现了需要手术处理的并发症，包括慢性支气管炎（39 位）、肺脓肿（31 位）、支气管扩张（5 位）、脓胸（24 位）和 BPF（10 位）。目前实行的许多指南都源于第二次世界大战及其后 20 年内的数据支持，包括上述几项研究。在第二次世界大战中，在受伤后早期和晚期移除异物的患者的死亡率分别为 0.9% 和 7.3%。然而，研究者也注意到，等待 2～6 周再取出异物，由于受损肺实质附近的炎症反应已消退，既可以使操作更简便，又能减少患者如大出血、漏气和脓胸等并发症。取出弹片的方式跟病变的位置以及异物的性质相关，周围型的异物可通过肺楔形切除术移除；更深部的异物可采用神经束切断术治疗；当肺叶受损严重、坏死或感染时，可直接行肺叶切除术。在一些比较罕见的情况下，随着时间推移，中心型的异物可侵蚀支气管，诱发阻塞性肺炎和肺脓肿，这时可以借助支气管镜取出异物。若肺实质破坏严重，可行肺叶切除术治疗。有时，中央型的异物会向外周迁移，导致脓胸，这时可以通过 VATS 或开胸手术来治疗。

胸膜并发症

残留血胸

在大约 5% 的病例中，胸管无法彻底排出胸腔积血。这可能会产生包括脓胸和纤维胸的并发症，这种并发症在长时间机械通气、肺炎、积血穿破胸膜（胸廓造口术置管后），以及合并其他部位感染的患者中更易出现。另一方面，病情稳定、无机械通气的少量血胸（血胸量 < 25%）的胸部钝伤患者，若无胸膜破损，常常不会有残留血胸这一后遗症。这些患者的治疗重点为观察。

许多综述报道，在放置胸管时就使用抗生素，尤其是抗革兰氏阳性菌的抗生素可以有效降低许多、并非全部患者出现脓胸的风险。然而，即使在支持预防性使用抗生素的文献中，也没有人提出抗生素多次使用、持续使用超过 24 h 或使用至拔管的好处。

有证据表明，血胸的早期排空可以降低并发症（尤其是脓胸）的发生率。最好是在病程的前 7 天内，这时脓腔还未形成分隔，清创相对容易。然而，血胸的严重程度仍然是一个很难判定的问题，X 线胸片的检查不但可能低估肺实变的程度，还可能低估残留积血的量，尤其是在机械通气的患者中。胸 CT 对血胸的评估会更为精确，但胸 CT 结果的解读须结合患者的实际情况个体化判断（图 1）。有中量积液的机械通气患者或合并其他危险因素的患者在做 CT 时要积极放置引流引出积血。

残留血胸一经诊断，最简便迅速的方法就是再放置一根胸管引流。若在 1 ~ 2 天后诊断，引流可能不但没有治疗效果，反而加重患者的疼痛、制动的可能性以及发生肺炎的风险（有微生物在胸膜腔内播散）。而采用胸膜内注射链激酶、尿激酶或最近出现的重组组织型纤维蛋白酶原激活物治疗的有效率高达 65% ~ 90%。并发症包括发热和疼痛，但再出血的风险微不足道。这种治疗的不足之处是恢复时间会比直接手术引流长许多天，而且无法降解血胸中的小腔。除此之外，溶栓失败的费用高昂。因此，

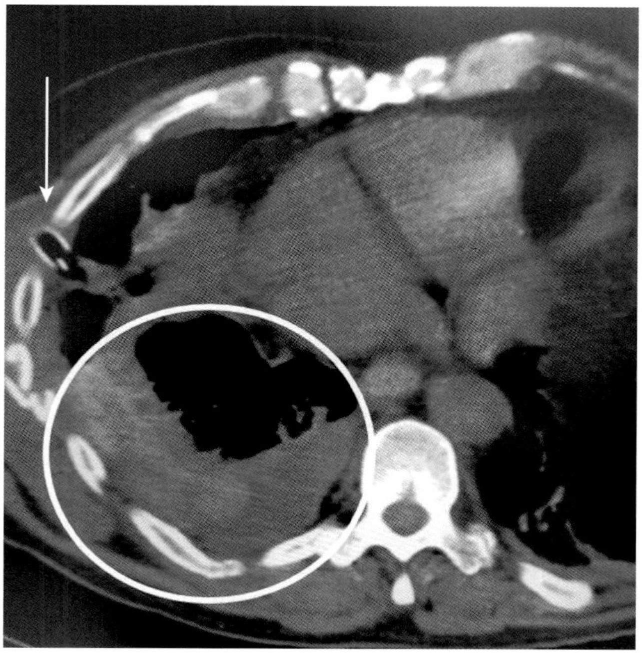

图 1　CT 显示残留血胸。该患者钝伤后出现骨折和血胸。X 线胸片提示右下肺突变。CT 显示胸管在原位（箭头）、右下肺突变和密度不均匀的积液（圆圈）入院 6 天后，患者出现低热和白细胞计数轻度升高

这种治疗最好用于清创术后，并且在血栓较软的患者中应用。

胸腔镜手术在完全移除残留血块时有着明显的优势，它也不会像传统开胸手术一样有许多并发症。Meyer 等将二次放置胸管与胸腔镜手术进行了对比，结果表明胸腔镜组的患者带管时间较短、住院时间短（2.7 天）、住院费用也低（$6000），而且术中并没有出现胸腔镜手术失败、手术并发症或中转开胸等情况。相比之下，二次置管组中有超过 40% 的患者都未能成功引流出残余血胸，须手术治疗。

在高选择性病例中，小切口开胸手术就足以取出柔软的胶状的脏层胸膜硬壳，从而使肺扩张（图 2-3）。用温盐水灌洗有助于血栓移除。血栓粘连越紧越需要充分暴露，如果前一次手术预期已经剥除了脏层的粘连，就须采取标准方法处理，可以通过骨膜下切除一段肋骨来安全地辨认胸膜。

总而言之，对于有残留血胸，并且有脓胸风险的患者，应该采取更积极的治疗措施救治，最好是尽早行胸腔镜手术引流积血。有时，有患者在受钝伤的几天后出现迟发性的渗出病变，可能是起初处理时遗漏了一些小的血胸灶，或是反应性地继发于胸水蓄积。对于充分疼痛控制、渗出病灶小（少于一侧胸腔的 25%）和无明显感染征象的患者，并不

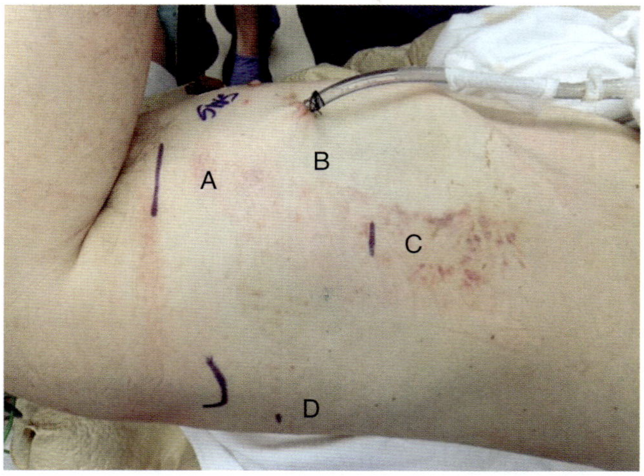

图 2 电视辅助胸腔镜（VATS）手术入路。有许多可行的入路。图中所示内图 1 中患者。第一个切口应一直保持，因为肺可能与胸壁粘连，对于许多病例，早期 VATS1～2 个切口就够了，而对于慢性病例，切口就越需要大一些。

A，不辅助牵开肋骨的小切口，可充分清创及操作，类似于进行 VATS 肺叶切除术，背阔肌保留。

B，前方切口通常为首先做的切口。因为肋间隙较宽，可通过小切口获得空间以避免损伤心脏、膈和肺。该病例中首先插入胸管，然后用手指分离内部空间操作

C，腋中线切口。在经切口 B 的直视下建立，通常放置摄像头，根据术中发现可做 5 mm 小切口

D，根据需要建立后侧切口。常为 5 mm。如果胸腔内器械＞5 mm，不使用切口以免损伤肋间神经

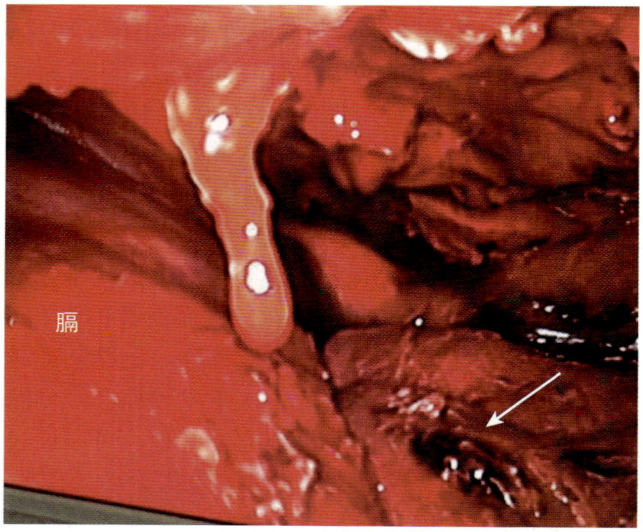

图 3 图 1 和图 2 中患者 VATS 术中所见。右肺下叶突变并且有一裂缝（箭头），胸膜腔内的游离液体排空后仍有很多碎片，通过钳夹和灌洗清除。肺的裂缝已不漏气。胸腔经清理后正压通气可使右肺下叶复张。患者恢复迅速，术后 2 天拔除胸廓造口术置管，肺功能和清洁功能恢复后康复迅速

须常规放置胸管，因为出现纤维胸的可能性很小。对于出现纤维胸的慢性（创伤后 3 个月以上）血胸患者，因为他们大多会有重构和适应的过程，须先行非手术治疗 6～9 个月，此时再实施手术治疗就不会增加操作难度。

脓胸

胸廓造口术置管的创伤患者中有 2%～7% 患者会出现脓胸。发病的危险因素包括 X 线胸片可见残余血胸、合并肺炎、影响咳嗽的疼痛和胸外感染，可能还包括机械通气和放置胸管。创伤患者易形成革兰氏阳性菌脓胸，其特征是早期就形成的脓腔和由血胸导致的紧密粘连。这些影响和纤维组织为细菌定植提供了有利条件。这些因素也导致单纯的引流术对于创伤所致脓胸患者的疗效比常见肺周围脓胸患者差。

脓胸的诊断依据是渗出性胸腔积液，其特点为胸腔积液 / 血浆 LDH 比值升高（>0.6）。在约 25%～30% 的病例中，由于使用了抑菌但非杀菌剂量的抗生素，培养可能是阴性的。无反应的过程也较常见，常发生在无法脱机的机械通气患者中，这些患者即使持续有胸管引流也会一直有 CT 或 X 线胸片可见的胸腔积液。增强 CT 常可见“环状征”，这提示有进行性的炎症。在许多情况下，一旦将这些“受污染的胸腔积液”引流出来，临床状况会立刻改善。

脓胸的病程常被描述为 3 个阶段，第一阶段是发病后 1～7 天，即所谓的“急性期”或“浆液渗出期”。这一阶段的鉴别十分重要，因为渗出液较稀薄，是单纯胸腔引流治疗的最佳时期。通常，严重的炎症反应（pH＜7.0）预示着这一措施的失败。对于有复杂性渗出的患者，无论有无小腔的形成，除非有其他可能的感染灶，开放引流也是恰当的治疗手段。无论用何种引流方式，必须要保证的就是充分引流。若无法实现，则须在进展性胸膜腔闭塞发生、病程进展到第二阶段或亚急性期甚至终末期或慢性期前尽早手术引流。行胸廓造口术时触及小腔或 CT 上显示有小腔存在，则提示外科医生单纯的引流术可能会失败。

若想施行微创手术治疗，则越早进行成功率越高。因为随着时间的推移，胸膜腔闭塞和与纤维板形成会使肺实质粘连。既增加了中转开胸的风险，也增加了腔镜手术的失败率。正如前面提到的，与

非创伤性的脓胸患者相比，创伤患者的脓胸需要外科手术干预的概率更高。

治疗脓胸的基本原则是充分引流胸腔积液和促进肺扩张，有一些个体化的因素可能会影响手术方式和预后（表2）。其中最主要的两个因素是否有小腔和限制性脏层纤维板的形成。在急性期，尤其是临床迹象提示有活动性感染时，治疗的首要措施就是引流。若有证据表明已有小腔形成时，单纯置管引流治疗会失败，这时可以选择的治疗方法包括影像学引导下的导管置入引流、胸腔镜引流和小切口或全切口开胸术治疗。溶栓治疗也是一种被提倡的可以代替手术的干预措施。但现有的数据表明，与胸腔镜手术相比，溶栓治疗有着更高的失败率、更长的住院时间和更高昂的开销。它对于手术风险极高和小腔为薄壁的患者来说不失为一种选择。在极罕见的情况下，患者若有临床感染并且极其虚弱，但还未行气管插管，上述原则就不再适用。因为一旦患者开始机械通气，手术的原发并发症（呼吸衰竭）就已经出现了。对于行手术剥除术后早期的患者，若仍有小腔内液体残留，溶栓治疗也有重要的地位，此时若纤维粘连较软，则可能被溶解。

已有许多研究来比较开胸手术与腔镜手术，包括VATS和胸腔镜（使用纵隔镜手术）在内。结果显示，VATS可以降低术后并发症的发生率、减少住院时间，但VATS常在住院早期小腔未形成时实施，此时患者的病情也较稳定。对于除外孤立肺和致密胸膜联合的高机械通气需求的患者来说，VATS的实施可能在技术上不可行。此时，硬质胸腔镜或称纵隔镜技术就是另一个选择，这些患者可以接受纵隔镜手术。以其CT图像作为参考，切口越大，清创术和积液吸引术就越容易完成。这种术式也可以用于剥除脏层纤维板，除非是高度纤维化的病例。

在某些病例中，术后灌洗是一项有效的辅助治疗，其目的可能是冲洗术中的出血，从而避免新的、强力的粘连形成。此外，局部应用抗生素可以加强对耐药菌的局部治疗（如念珠菌或耐甲氧西林微生物）。灌洗系统可以根据环境来修改（如通过三通管将Jackson-Pratt引流管连接至静脉输液管）。灌洗液的量是不定的，虽然通常我们设定为100 ml/h。为了避免引流液从切口或引流口溢出，需要紧密封闭，灌洗须一直持续至胸部引流物清亮、培养阴性为止。术后灌洗的一个可能的缺陷就是阻止了胸膜粘连，这会导致残余空间的形成。另一方面，如果医生判定已有残余空间形成，那灌洗就是一项尤为有效的措施。实际上，在某些病例中，当拔出胸管后，如果条件允许，尽量在原有单纯引流通道置入Jackson-Pratt引流管，这样可以提高患者的耐受性。

治疗后的胸膜残余空间仍是一个需要灵活处理的问题，主要取决于肺是否能够扩张（表3）。在创伤性脓胸患者中，肺复张失败的主要原因就是脏层纤维板的形成，但对肺创伤患者来说，脏层纤维板、肺实变和肺切除术在残余空间成因中所占比例相同。

若想对脓胸患者实施开胸手术，我们建议不要从肩胛骨下开始计数肋骨。这可以减少污染和肩胛下脓肿形成的可能。如果医生怀疑已有致密胸膜顶和重要的胸膜联合形成，则骨膜下肋骨切除术可以提供更安全的胸腔入路。当患侧肺通气时脏层剥除术会更易实施，因为此时纤维板-肺实质的界线会更明显。当估计肺可以充分扩张并填充胸腔时，明显的外周肺漏气是可以接受的。若肺实变过于严重以至肺无法扩张，或是脏层胸膜切除术无法进展（技术难题、大量漏气、出血），可能就要放弃胸膜切除术，转而处理残余空间，如引流、灌洗、组织瓣覆盖或开放引流等。

无论脓胸的引流如何，需要再评估潜在的肺的状况的都是很重要的。一旦肺开始扩张，需要进一

表2 治疗脓胸所涉及因素

残余空间
肺实质的质量
肺压缩程度
小腔密度
患者是否机械通气
目前漏气和预期漏气
肺脓肿

表3 残余空间的处理

冲洗＋抗生素
正压通气以使突变的肺复张
支气管镜检查排除和治疗气道梗阻
脏层胸膜纤维板剥除
慢性病程行开放引流，尤其对虚弱的患者
组织瓣
联合方案：Clagett术式

步干预的肺脓肿和其他坏死过程就会变得更加明显。此外，在影像学上胸膜腔会比术前看起来更明显，这有助于临床上评估胸膜脓毒症是否存在更困难。还有一种方法就是监测胸管引流物的LDH水平，水平降低表明炎症的消退和治疗的成功，升高则相反。

总而言之，脓胸的治疗原则如下：胸腔引流、胸膜清创、促进肺复张。若肺无法扩大则考虑组织瓣覆盖（如果小）或慢性开放引流和关闭严重的BPF。越早干预，阻止病程进展的成功率越高。当不是VATS手术适应证时仍然可考虑坚持硬质胸腔镜下操作，但不要延误开胸手术。

乳糜胸

原发性的创伤性乳糜胸极其少见，它可以发生在胸廓入口的穿通伤、跨纵隔的损伤或钝伤中。有趣的是，只有20%的脊柱骨折患者会出现乳糜胸。乳糜胸可以为迟发型复发性积液，可表现为胸膜腔内持续反复渗出牛奶样液体，或仅仅是张力性乳糜胸。乳糜胸常出现在修复主动脉损伤或食管切除的患者中，诊断的标准是渗出液的三酰甘油浓度超过110 mg/dl，并且主要为淋巴细胞浸润。如果为急性乳糜胸，一定要立刻考虑是否伴发胸导管周围组织的损伤，尤其是食管或主动脉。乳糜胸最主要的并发症是损害营养和免疫。最开始的处理原则是引流、确保完全肺扩张（机械通气患者要加大PEEP）和肠外营养支持。虽然低脂饮食可以减少乳糜液的量，但是饮水都可以增加乳糜液。疗程的长短不定，取决于患者的生理状况，但多短于4周。术后即刻发生的乳糜胸最好再次手术处理，操作如下述。

淋巴管造影（CT、核医学、常规淋巴管造影片等）可能有助于定位破损处、确定有无侧支和乳糜漏的量，这可以预测干预是否成功。如果没有明确的渗漏，并且有侧支引流至静脉系统，保守治疗就有较高的成功率。配合肠外营养和严格NPO（禁食）后，乳糜液立刻终止是保守治疗成功的预示，生长抑素也被用于辅助治疗。如果可以定位胸导管，经腹栓塞术就可以成功治疗。持续的残余空间（尤其是胸膜剥除术后）、大范围的破坏（如食管切除术后）或内科干预后，引流量仍然较高的患者常常内科治疗无效，须尽早外科干预。最终，若乳糜漏在持续超过2周就要考虑外科手术，超过4周，患者的免疫和营养状况恶化或其他手术指征则考虑手术。延迟性出现的乳糜胸患者其处理原则相似。我们建议，若患者保守治疗1周后引流量持续在1500 ml/24 h以上，并且营养状况明显恶化，那么对于这些患者中的大多数我们会尝试弹簧圈栓塞，若栓塞难以实施或失败，可以考虑开放式结扎。

手术既可以用开胸的方式也可以用胸腔镜辅助的方式，有时破损处可以直视，这就可以直接结扎（脱脂棉缝合线）或用胶粘连破损处。通过让患者术前口服奶油有助于定位破损处。在右侧膈上结扎胸导管可以缓解双侧的渗漏。准确辨认胸管至关重要，其周围组织可能较脆，因此结扎时可能会造成新的渗漏。此外，结扎点附近可能有侧支，因此我们发现，确保纤维板完全剥除（促进肺复张）、胸膜摩擦或在情况不定的情况下持续机械通气24 h以促进肺充分复张在治疗过程中地位十分关键。我们还要求患者在术后7天内禁食。

纤维胸

在讨论残留血胸的部分我们曾提到，有症状的纤维胸会造成过度的恐慌。在医院中，感染性血胸患者出现纤维胸的概率最高，也最快。纤维胸是否须行手术治疗的问题与慢性呼吸道疾病的关系包括：在许多情况下，要根据CT是否有胸膜增厚的情况决定是否手术，术后的影像总是与术前相同。有持续性胸部多发伤的患者有时出现慢性痛是因为创伤本身而非纤维胸，这时开胸手术会加重疼痛而非缓解症状。

外科治疗要点

- 对于持续漏气或血胸的患者，早期行胸腔镜手术干预可以缩短住院时间。
- VAP的诊断较困难，是基于临床判断和不同灵敏度和特异度的诊断试验确诊的，对于接受抗生素治疗的患者阈值要降低。
- 肺膨出和血肿是主要的不需要干预的影像学表现。
- 肺感染性坏死的处理须个体化，然而，灌注不足常会导致药物治疗失败和外科手术干预。若患者由于感染性休克正在使用血管活性药物，则须延迟肺切除术，先行胸腔引流术或胸腔镜检查。
- 创伤患者发生脓胸的危险因素是置管后X线

胸片示脓液残留，为避免粘连加重，须尽早行胸腔镜下引流术。

- 对胸部损伤后新发哮喘的患者，须评估是否存在气道狭窄。若无肺坏死发生，无论采用气管支架或直接气道重建都能取得好的疗效。
- 气道内异物残留，尤其是不规则形状的异物，可能会导致远期并发症的出现。大的、中央型不规则异物须在损伤后 2～3 周取出，以待周围组织炎症的缓解。
- 乳糜胸可以通过保守治疗或其他方法缓解。持续的乳糜漏或患者营养状况恶化是积极手术的指征。手术的目的不仅仅是结扎胸导管，也是确保肺充分复张。

心脏损伤

Juan A. Asensio, Patrizio Petrone, Alejandro Perez-Alonso, Zachary Torgersen, Brian Biggerstaff, Brittney J. Maloley-Lewis, Pulkesh Bhatia, Jeffery A. Bailey, Juan A. Sanchez 和 Elias Degiannis 著
陈　彧 译

穿通性心脏损伤

历史回顾

关于心脏损伤的描述最早可以追溯到公元前 3000 年荷马所著的《伊利亚特》以及《艾德温 · 史密斯纸草文稿》中。希波克拉底认为，所有心脏的创伤均为致命的。安布罗斯 · 帕雷，著名的法国创伤外科医生，曾基于解剖学研究描述了 2 例穿通性心脏损伤。1642 年，Wolf 最早对 1 例已愈合的心脏创伤进行了描述。Senac 在 1749 年总结为，尽管全部的心脏损伤均很严重，但仍有一部分创伤是非致命的，并可以愈合。Larrey 首先报道了到达心包、解除心包积液的外科手段，他被认为是心包开窗技术的开拓者。Billroth 于 1875 年及 1883 年曾先后指出，其对于修复心脏损伤的任何尝试均持强烈的反对态度。此后于 1882 年，Block 用兔子建立了心脏损伤的动物模型，并成功实现修复，这提示相同的技术也许可以应用在人类身上。同样，Del Vecchio 在狗的模型上证实了，心脏的创伤可以通过缝合技术实现愈合。

尽管如此，将修复心脏损伤的尝试应用在人类身上仍需要很大的勇气：来自挪威的 Cappelen 在 1895 年尝试修复 1 例左心室 2 cm 的裂伤，其中包括对冠状动脉左前降支远段的一个较大分支进行结扎。其后，意大利的 Farina 在 1896 年同样尝试修复左心室的损伤。然而 2 例尝试均以患者死亡而告终。1896 年，德国的 Rehn 成功修复了 1 例位于右心室的创伤；1902 年，Hill 成为美国首位成功修复左心室损伤的医生。

Duval 医生曾对胸骨正中切开术的切口进行描述，而 Spangaro 在 1906 年则描述了左前外侧的开胸术切口。1909 年，Peck 首先报道了对右心房刺伤进行成功修补的病例，共 11 例患者。针对心脏损伤，Smith 则最先建立了一套完善的管理计划，并首次指出心律失常在心脏手术中的危害。他同样提出，在缝合心脏的过程中，可以使用组织钳夹住近心尖的部位来拿住心脏，并使心脏保持稳定。

1942 年，Beck 介绍了冠状动脉血管床下的心脏褥式缝合技术。同年，Griswold 进一步完善了心脏损伤处理的相关技术，并建议所有大型的综合医院均应该配套有无菌的设备以及可供 24 h 使用的手术室。Elkin 在 1944 年建议手术前进行静脉输液，以扩充血容量及增加心排血量。Beall 等则首次引入了急诊开胸术的概念。同时，Mattox 等再次完善并规范了急诊开胸术与心脏缝合术，包括急诊心肺旁路术的使用。正是这些具有标志性意义的贡献使得如今那些遭受穿通性心脏损伤的患者能够存活。

发生率

Feliciano 等在 1983 年报道了他们在休斯顿 Ben Taub 医院 1 年内诊治的 48 例心脏损伤患者的经验。Mattox 团队则于 1989 年介绍了他们的 539 例心脏损伤患者的诊治经验（平均每年 18 例）。Asensio 等报道了洛杉矶市南加州大学医疗中心的 2 个连续的前瞻性研究，总共囊括了 3 年内的 165 例心脏损伤患者（平均每年 55 例）。在 2006 年的一份综述中，Asensio 等通过美国外科医师学会（American College of Surgeons，ACS）的国家创伤数据库（National Trauma Databank，NTDB），确定了 2 016 名遭受穿通性心脏损伤的患者，并计算出其全国发生率为 0.16%。因此，穿通性心脏损伤是一类罕见的创伤性疾病，并通常仅在较大城市的创伤中心中可见。

病因

对城市市民来说，穿通性心脏损伤的常见病因是枪伤和刺伤，偶见于猎枪伤和碎冰锥刺伤。根据近期的综述报道，在美国，63% 的心脏损伤为枪伤，36% 为刺伤，猎枪弹伤及穿刺伤占 1%。在军队，Rich 和 Spencer 回顾了 96 例越战中的心脏损伤病例，其中大多数创伤由枪弹碎片所致，另有一部分患者则被镖弹所刺伤。

临床表现

典型的心包压塞表现为 Beck 三联征，即心音遥远、颈静脉扩张、低血压。Kussmaul 体征是心包压塞的另一个经典体征，表现为吸气时颈静脉扩张。然而这些体征却不常在实际的临床病例中见到。据估计，仅约 10% 的心脏损伤患者会出现经典的 Beck 三联征。

穿通性心脏损伤的患者，会出现完全的血流动力学不稳定和心搏停止。实际上，有些甚至具有欺骗性。穿通性心脏损伤的临床表现也可能与其他因素相关，包括受伤的机制、受伤到接受救治的间隔时长，以及受伤的严重程度——严重的心肌受损总是会导致左侧胸腔内的过多出血。另外，失血是临床表现的另一个相关因素，当血容量丢失 40% ~ 50% 时，患者会出现心搏停止。左心室的肌肉组织较为丰富，比右心室肌肉组织更多的丰富的心肌也许能够在一定程度上对该部位的穿通性损伤起到封闭的作用，阻止大出血，使患者到达创伤中心时还有一些生命体征。

心包压塞是穿通性心脏损伤的典型表现。心包由坚硬的纤维组织构成，弹性较差，顺应性低，当心包内压力急剧升高时，右心室薄壁受压严重，使其接受回心血量的能力下降，左心室的充盈及射血分数明显降低。这将导致心排血量和每搏输出量的骤降。而左、右心室射血分数的下降则会加重心脏负荷与心肌的张力，心肌耗氧量上升，却难以维持，最终导致心肌的低氧血症和乳酸性酸中毒。

众所周知，在出血速度缓慢的情况下，心包腔可以容纳一定程度的血量，使出血不会立即导致心包腔内压力的急剧升高，而影响心室充盈能力。因此，心包压塞在损害心脏功能的同时也具有保护性作用。它一方面会导致心包腔内压力快速上升和心肺骤停，另一方面它也限制了左侧胸腔内的心包外出血，而起到保护作用。在一项纳入 100 例穿通性心脏损伤患者的回顾性研究中，Moreno 等发现其中 77 例具有心包压塞的表现，并且其生存率（73%）远高于没有心包压塞的患者（11%）。这说明其是保护因素，这一结果具有显著的统计学意义，且心包压塞是患者生存的独立因素。

Asensio 等在另一项纳入 105 例患者的为期 2 年的前瞻性研究中却并未发现心包压塞与生存率之间存在统计学关联，也无法确定其为患者生存的独立因素。目前尚无法判断，心包压塞的保护性作用究竟在持续多久后会失去，何时这种转变发生转而为对心功能的不良影响。

诊断

体格检查

心脏穿通伤的患者的临床表现轻则血流动力学尚能维持稳定，重则出现心搏停止。血气胸及同侧胸腔的呼吸音减弱是常见的征象。有时，心前区损伤的患者会表现为躁动及拒绝平躺，这往往是心包积血或早期心包压塞的提示。穿通性心脏损伤患者最为致命的表现则为心肺骤停，需要急诊开胸手术进行干预，以挽救生命。需要指出的是，心包穿刺术目前对于建立诊断的意义不大。

剑突下心包开窗术

心包开窗的技术最早由 Larrey 在 19 世纪提出，发展至今其技术改变甚少。然而近年来随着二维超声心动图显像的出现以及 FAST 评估法的应用，心包开窗术的使用显著减少。然而在一些缺少超声设备的国家，这项技术仍然被广泛采用。

心包开窗术须在手术室内全身麻醉的情况下进行。在剑突的表面做一 10 cm 的正中切口，触及心脏搏动后通过钝性及锐性分离显露心包位置，将其游离后使用两把 Allis 钳夹住心包并将其轻轻向下牵拉。在心包上做一个 1 ~ 2 cm 的纵行切口，注意保护心包下的心肌组织，避免医源性损伤。纵行切开心包后，其内的液体会流出，若液体性质为血性，则为阳性诊断，提示潜在的心脏损伤可能，此时应进一步行胸骨正中切开术继续进行心包开窗术。另外，若心包内的积血已形成血凝块，则不会流向术野内。

这项技术的优点是它能够安全有效地对穿通性心脏损伤做出诊断，操作相对简单，所有创伤外科的医生在设备齐全的条件下均可进行。缺点则在于患者必须接受全身麻醉以及外科操作。

二维超声心动图显像

作为FAST的一部分，超声心动图显像已成为评估穿通性心脏损伤患者的金标准。它的优点在于其能够无创、快速、准确地评估病情，具有可重复性，最重要的是，它不为患者带来额外痛苦。基于2个中心的研究数据均显示，超声心动图评估创伤具有较高的准确性，且易于操作，应成为评估穿通性心脏损伤的首选方式。其他技术加TEE显像却因其无法实现即刻评估而未能广泛应用。

微创方式

胸腔镜

Morales等报道了采用胸腔镜心包开窗术用于诊断心脏损伤的研究，他们认为这项技术的准确性高、并发症少、患者易耐受，并推荐用于排空保留的血胸。然而我们认为，胸腔镜心包开窗术不适用于穿通性心脏损伤患者的紧急评估。

腹腔镜

与胸腔镜相似，腹腔镜曾被用于进行腹部穿通性损伤中的腹膜侵犯的诊断。在胸腹联合伤中，它可用于评估实质脏器以及膈的损伤，同时也可评估心包的情况。尽管如此，我们同样认为腹腔镜技术不适用于穿通性心脏损伤患者的紧急评估。

处理

院前处理

大城市的急诊医疗系统能够对穿通性心脏损伤的患者进行快速转运至创伤中心，从而为挽救生命争取机会。对于心搏停止患者，现场急救应包括气管插管与闭式心肺复苏。多项研究表明并强烈提倡将创伤性胸部损伤患者即刻转运至创伤中心。通过气管插管的方式实现气道的开放是唯一能够预测预后的因素。气管插管已被证实能够增加使用时间短于5 min的心肺复苏的持续时间和耐受性，为患者的存活提供了最佳机会。

急诊室处理

所有穿通性心脏损伤的患者均应按照ATLS进行快速地评估与复苏。在评估阶段，患者根据自身状况分为3层：第一层为血流动力学稳定，并能够进行诊断性研究的患者；第二层为血流动力学不稳定，但能够通过液体复苏维持相对平稳，并快速转运至手术室的患者；第三层为出现心搏停止，需要通过急诊开胸术等外科干预挽救生命的患者。首选快速评估病情的手段为FAST以及X线胸片，心电图检查则作为备选手段。对于复苏，乳酸盐林格液以及O型血或相同血型的血应作为液体复苏手段。动脉血气分析可协助了解初始酸碱度、碱缺乏以及乳酸水平。然而大部分患者仍会进展至临终状态，需要进一步干预去挽救生命。

急诊室开胸手术

急诊室开胸手术对于符合指征的患者来说意义重大。对于城市创伤中心接收到的临终患者，这项手术应常规进行。当进行紧急手术时，急诊开胸术、主动脉十字钳夹术，以及心肌缝合术能够挽救约10%的穿通性心脏损伤患者。在确定性心脏修补完成后，开胸心脏按压有助于提高心脏射血分数。相似地，胸腔内大血管的撕裂同样可以通过血管钳的钳闭予以控制。

提示预后较差的院前因素包括无生命体征、瞳孔固定和散大、心脏节律消失、四肢运动消失、脉搏消失以及心肺骤停。

通常手术指征包括因穿通伤导致的心搏停止、收缩压低于60 mmHg的重度失血性休克或心包压塞。钝性损伤导致的心肺骤停通常是手术的禁忌证。

手术的目的是使具有穿通性心胸损伤的老年患者得以复苏，解除心包压塞，控制胸腔内的大量出血、预防空气栓塞，以及通过开胸心脏按压使心脏恢复功能。其他目的包括对穿通性心脏损伤进行确定性的修补，以及控制胸腔内血管损伤导致的大量出血。另外，术中还可以通过短时间十字钳夹降主动脉重新分配剩余的血量，以灌注颈动脉和冠状动脉。

应在进行急诊开胸手术的同时进行对患者的评估与复苏。这一过程必须由受过训练的外科医生在ATLS的指导下实行。同时，应快速开放静脉通路，进行快速液体复苏。左前外侧切口可在左侧胸肋交界处的侧缘，位于乳头下方，向侧方延伸至背阔肌。女性的乳房可适当向头侧牵拉。切口应通过皮肤快速到达至肋间肌，并予以锐性切断。放置 Finochietto 拉钩打开肋骨，将肺叶向内上侧牵拉，暴露胸主动脉，可见其向下走行，并通过主动脉裂孔进入腹腔。通过触诊主动脉来判断剩余血容量的情况，也可通过手指将胸主动脉向低位胸椎体挤压从而暂时性地阻断血流。通过钝性及锐性分离主动脉上下缘的结缔组织，使得拇指与示指能够环形握住主动脉，可以为充分阻断主动脉提供可操作的空间。接下来，创伤外科医生应探查心包并寻找损伤部位。此时心包往往由于压塞而具有较高的张力并且变色。在膈神经的前方纵行切开心包囊，并上下延长切口。通常要抓住心包，用 Metzenbanm 剪打开心包，做一个小切口

打开心包后，应取出其内的血凝块，医生应迅速判断是否有心跳及节律，以及穿通性损伤的部位。若心脏没有活力，缺乏有效的正向泵运动，则高度提示预后较差。其他预后较差的提示因素包括冠状动脉内无血流，提示在冠状动脉存在空气栓子。

在缝合心室损伤部位的同时，用手指去压迫裂口控制出血，能够预防进一步的失血。我们建议使用单丝缝线进行缝合，如 2-0 聚丙烯线。如果心脏裂口很大，也可采用 Foley 导管插入伤口，膨胀球囊压迫止血，为心肌缝合术或快速转运到手术室进行其他抢救措施争取时间。我们不建议使用如聚四氟乙烯补片等生物材料进行修补，因为这是一项耗时的操作，更应该在手术室进行而不是急诊室。

尽管目前已有医生将吻合器应用于心脏损伤的修复，但根据我们的经验，吻合器不仅无法有效控制出血，还有可能进一步使裂口扩大，并难以取出。

窦性心律的恢复通常需要严格的药物调控以及电复律的辅助。当心脏节律恢复，但仍无有效泵血机制时，可以观察到患者进行急诊开胸术的心肌的进一步坏死，表现为右心室与左心室的依次扩张以及收缩运动停止。

穿通性心脏损伤预后

目前关于穿通性心脏损伤的研究中，生存率的差异较大，0～72% 均有报道。这些研究大部分为回顾性研究，并且患者以刺伤居多。Asensio、Wall 和其他美国外科医师学会创伤委员会工作组的成员通过对相关文献的广泛研究（表 1），制订了急诊室开胸手术的实践管理指南。

心脏创伤修复技术

切口

穿通性心脏损伤的手术切口主要分为 2 种：胸骨正中切口及左前外侧切口。胸骨正中切口由 Duval 报道，适用于心前区的穿通性损伤，且患者存在一定程度的血流动力学不稳定，需要术前评估。左前外侧切口由 Spangaro 报道，适用于已进展为临终状态的患者。急诊室使用这种切口的主要目的是进行复苏。此切口可进一步延长至跨过胸骨，形成双侧前外侧开胸术。跨中线的双侧剖胸切口同样适用于因纵隔贯通伤导致血流动力学不稳定的患者（图 1）。须指出的是，这种横断胸骨的切口亦会导致双侧内乳动脉的横断，因此必须在恢复灌注压后予以结扎。当胸腹联合伤的患者在接受剖腹术的过程中情况进一步恶化时，同样可以选择左前外侧切口作为手术入路。

辅助操作

创伤外科医生必须能够掌握多种处理穿通性心胸损伤的辅助操作。全心脏流入血流阻断术须在心包内同时对上腔静脉及下降静脉实施十字钳夹，从而阻断进入心脏的全部血流（图 2）。这项技术适用于右心房最外侧或交界处的心脏损伤。尽管文献中经常提到血流阻断时间不能超过 1～3 min，但目前对于安全时长仍不清楚。

对于联合肺损伤，尤其是肺门存在中央血肿或活动性出血的患者，肺门的十字钳夹术是另一个行之有效的操作（图 3）。它能够阻止肺的进一步出血，并防止空气栓子进入循环系统。然而当存在酸中毒、低体温，以及缺血时，右心室可能无法耐受这种操作，进而引发纤颤甚至停搏。

有时，外科医生须将心脏搬至心包外来进行损伤修复。如果出血能够通过手指压迫进行控制，则可以逐渐放置多个填充物将心脏垫高，这样能够使心脏更容易耐受操作，从而降低发生心律失常的概率。

心房损伤的修复

心房损伤通常可以通过放置 Satinsky 钳来部分钳夹予以控制，从而为创伤外科医生实施心肌缝合术创造机会。我们建议采用单丝 2-0 聚丙烯线进行连续缝合或间断缝合。充分显露心房损伤的两个面

表 1 心脏损伤的急诊室开胸手术

作者与年份	研究类型	生存人数/总例数（穿通性损伤）	生存人数/总例数（急诊室开胸手术）
Boyd, 1965	R	0/0	17/25
Beall, 1966	R	3/16	42/197
Sauer, 1967	R	12/0	12/13
Sugg, 1968	R	0/0	63/459
Yao, 1968	R	0/0	61/80
Steichen, 1971	R	7/21	35/58
Beall, 1971	R	29/52	42/66
Borja, 1971	R	0/0	24/145
Carrasquilla, 1972	R	8/30	20/245
Beall, 1972	R	0/0	67/269
Bolanowski, 1973	R	0/0	33/44
Trinkle, 1974	R	0/0	38/45
Mattox, 1974	R	25/37	31/62
Harvey, 1975	R	0/0	22/28
Symbas, 1976	R	0/0	50/98
Beach, 1976	R	0/4	26/34
Asfaw, 1977	R	0/0	277/323
Sherman, 1978	R	32/41	31/92
Trinkle, 1979	R	0/0	89/100
Evans, 1979	R	0/4	29/46
Breaux, 1979	R	39/44	78/197
Mandal, 1979	R	0/38	26/55
Gervin, 1982	R	4/21	4/21
Demetriades, 1983	R	2/16	40/125
Demetriades, 1984	R	1/11	0/45
Tavares, 1984	R	21/37	64
Feliciano, 1984	R	5/15	2/3
Mattox, 1985	R	50/119	204
Demetriades, 1986	R	1/18	70
Moreno, 1984	R	4/69	100
Ivatury, 1987	R	28/91	-
Jebara, 1989	R	4/17	-
Attar, 1991	R	21/55	-
Knott-Craig, 1992	R	5/13	-
Buchman, 1992	R	1/2	23
Benyan, 1992	R	1/13	-
Macho, 1993	R	12/24	-
Mitchell, 1993	R	7/47	-
Kaplan, 1993	R	2/23	
Henderson, 1994	R	6/122	215
Coimbra, 1995	R	0/20	
Arreola-Risa, 1995	R	11/40	
Karmy-Jones, 1997	R	3/6	16
Rhee, 1998	R	15/58	41/96
Asensio, 1998c	P	6/37	6/37
Asensio, 1998a	P	10/71	10/71
Tyburski, 2000	R	12/152	12/152
Asensio, 2006	R	47/830	47/830

EDTs，急诊室开胸术；P，前瞻性研究；R，回顾性研究

注意：不包括钝性创伤生存者

很重要，尤其对于子弹所致的损伤，因为这类损伤所导致的组织破坏较严重，在关闭前常须进行全面而仔细的清创。对于这类创伤，诸如聚四氟乙烯补片等生物材料并不推荐使用。

心室损伤的修复

心室损伤通常会导致明显出血，须通过手指压迫止血的同时进行间断缝合或 Halsted 的平行褥式的连续缝合。对心室刺伤的心肌缝合术，难度往往要小于枪弹伤。子弹所导致的损伤常会因爆破效应使心肌纤维缩短，因而需要多次缝合才能控制大出血。这种情况下，常常须使用生物材料（如聚四氟乙烯带和脱脂棉）对缝线进行进一步加固（图 4）。我们仍然推荐使用针和 2-0 单丝聚丙烯线进行缝合。

冠状动脉损伤

邻近冠状动脉的心室修补较为困难。为了避免对冠状动脉或其分支造成损伤使其狭窄或闭塞，缝合的操作推荐在冠状动脉血管床以下进行。冠状动脉通常分为 3 个节段：近段、中段及远段。近段的冠脉损伤须在心肺旁路的辅助下进行修补，中段的损伤须接受主动脉球囊反搏技术的辅助，并进一步

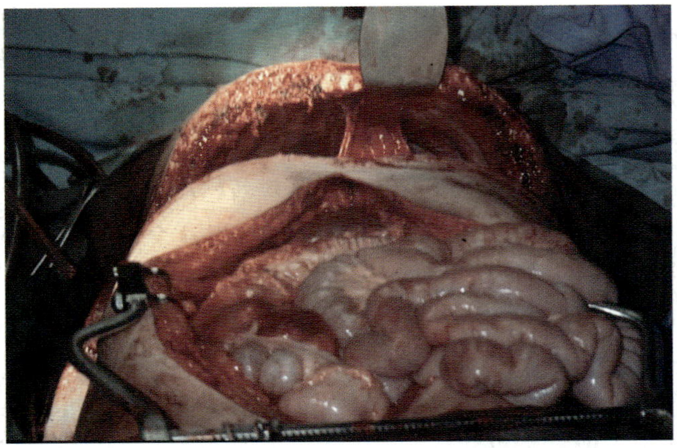

图 1　危急的胸腹联合伤患者的双侧开胸术与剖腹术

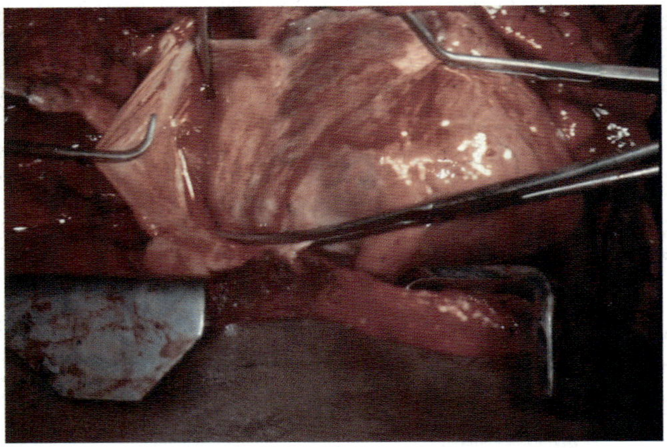

图 2　上下腔静脉均被钳夹。下腔静脉在 Gibbon 空间内被钳夹。钳夹并牵拉右心耳有助于更好的显露

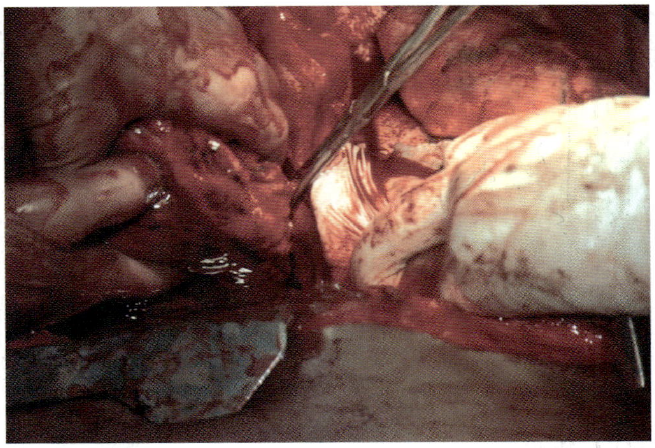

图 3　钳夹肺门的血管。这种方法有助于控制穿通性肺损伤的出血及肺门处的血肿

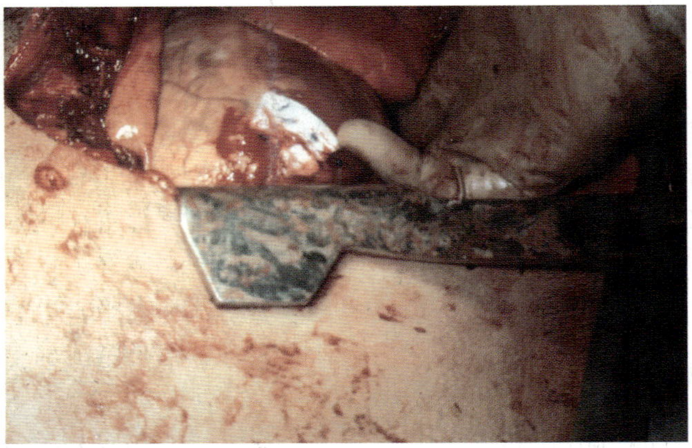

图 4　应用聚四氟乙烯补片对左心室枪伤进行修补

实施主动脉冠状动脉旁路术。远段的，尤其是最远的第三节段的冠脉损伤则可予以结扎。

复杂性和联合损伤

相当一部分的穿通性心脏损伤的患者同时存在其他部位的损伤。复杂性损伤即为心脏损伤联合颈部、胸部、胸部血管、腹部、腹部血管，以及周围血管的损伤（图 5-6）。这类损伤的处理相当棘手，其原则为首先处理导致失血最严重的或威胁生命的损伤。

损伤的解剖学位置

既往文献中关于心脏的心腔损伤的报道存在较大差异（表 2）。心室损伤的发生率占全部心脏损伤的 37%～67%，其中左心室损伤的发生概率在 19%～40% 波动。对于心房而言，右心房损伤的发生率为 5%～20%，而最深处的左心房的发生率为 2%～12%。

相关损伤

刺伤的位置基本位于心前区，其所致的穿通性心脏损伤通常仅累及单个心腔。然而枪伤的部位则更为广泛，从心前区至心前区外，因此枪伤更有可能导致多心腔的联合损伤。

预后因素

为了对心脏损伤进行统一的描述，AAST-OIS

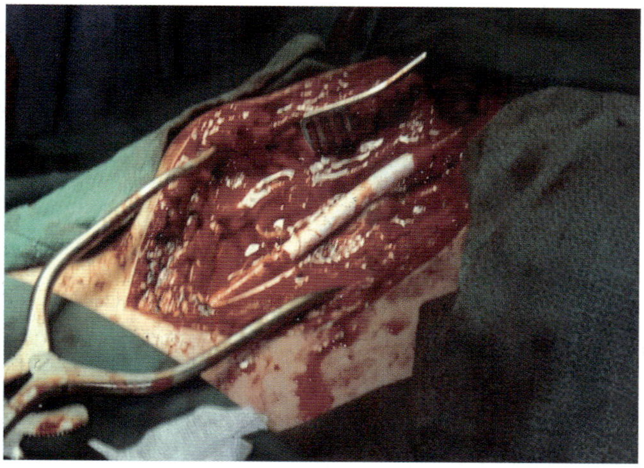

图 5 用聚四氟乙烯实行股 - 股动脉旁路术以及股静脉的结扎。该患者因枪弹伤致左心室、左肺、左侧股骨以及右手的损伤

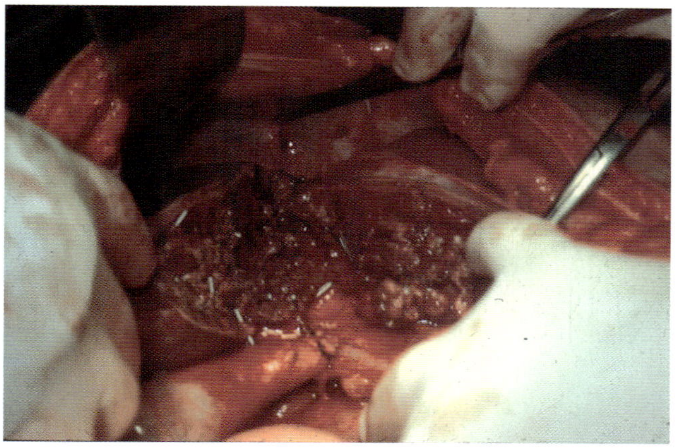

图 6 AAST 器官损伤Ⅳ级肝损伤合并心脏损伤。图为复杂肝切开术与缝合术，注意多个夹子用于控制出血

委员会对器官损伤制订了一套评分系统（表 3）。这套评分系统对损伤进行了系统性描述，并于 1994 年投入使用，尽管如此，几乎没有研究将心脏损伤的分级与死亡率建立起联系。

Asensio 等在一项纳入 105 例患者的为期 2 年的前瞻性研究中，将心脏损伤的 AAST-OIS 评分与死亡率进行关联。研究中 99 例（94%）患者为Ⅳ ~ Ⅵ级损伤，且死亡率随着分级的上升而增加：Ⅳ级损伤的死亡率为 56%，Ⅴ级损伤为 76%，Ⅵ级损伤为 91%。学者们认为，这些研究可以发现死亡率与器官损伤级别之间的关系，损伤程度分级与死亡率的相关性仍有待进一步的研究去证实。此外，作者相信所有心脏损伤均应该通过这项评分进行分级。

多种预后因素包括损伤机制，受伤、转运和救治时的生理学状态，如术后有瞳孔的反应、自主呼吸、颈动脉搏动、可测血压、窦性心律、肢体活动，以及是否需要气管插管及心肺复苏，和救治前等待时间超过 10 min。上述因素均已通过多项前瞻性研究得以证实。另外，心搏停止作为预后不良的预测因素也已经得到证实。同样，Buckman 等的研究也确认了一些由创伤评分（tranma score，TS）的 CVRS 测得的生理学参数同样是影响预后的相关因素。

钝性心脏损伤

发展历史

第一例明确的心肌挫伤是由 Akenside 在 1764 年报道的，而第一例钝性心腔破裂则由 Borch 在 1679 年记录的。据 Warburg 所述，在 1676 — 1868 的近 200 年间，仅有 27 例钝性心脏损伤被记录在文献中。

1958 年，Parmley 等回顾了部队病理研究所的 207 548 例尸检报告，并描述了其中的 546 例非穿通性心脏损伤病例，其发生率为 0.1%。在这一项标志性的研究中，他们发现了 353 例心脏破裂的患者，其中 273 例为孤立的心脏破裂，另 80 例合并有主动脉的破裂。66 例心脏破裂的位置位于右心室，59 例位于左心室，41 例位于右心房，26 例位于左心房。另外，总共有 106 例患者存在多个心腔的损伤。

机制、病理生理学与发生率

对于钝性心脏损伤（blunt cardiac injury，BCI）的准确定义一直以来存在不同的理解，它曾一度被理解为心脏挫伤，并多被称为“心脏震荡”。这是因为，钝性心脏损伤的概念实际上并不单指一种情况，而是包含了几种不同的情况。

钝性心脏损伤可以是轻微的心肌挫伤，也可以是明显的心腔破裂，同时也包括心脏震荡的少见情况，例如由于心脏撞击胸骨致使突发的心搏停止，进而导致心源性休克的情况。钝性心脏损伤可以继发于挤压、减速、爆破，以及直接作用于胸部的外力。高速运动的车辆相撞导致使胸腔受到挤压，或高处坠落的物体砸向胸骨，均会直接使心脏被压于胸骨和脊椎之间，而从造成损伤。同样，高处坠落伤或爆炸伤也是引起 BCI 的原因。BCI 的真

表 2　损伤的解剖学位置

作者	年份	跨　度（年）	例数	心腔				多腔联合	合并冠脉损伤
				右心室	左心室	右心房	左心房		
Ivantury	1987	20	228	90(39.4%)	44(19.2%)	15(6.5%)	6(2.6%)	38(16.6%)，位置未报道 20(8.8%)	11(4.8%)
Buckman	1993	2.25	66	单腔	42(63.6%)			24(36.3%)	NR
Henderson	1994	6	251	96(38.2%)	98(39.8%)	57(22.7%)	31(12.3%)	101(40.2%)	NR
Arreola-Risa	1995	7	55	29(52%)	17(30%)	7(12%)	2(3%)	11(20%)	1(1.5%)
Wall	1997	20	711	284(40%)	284(40%)	171(24%)	21(3%)	14(1.9%)	39(5,4%)
Asensio	1998c	1	60	40(66.6%)	15(25%)	11(18.3%)	3(5%)	NR	5(8.3%)
Asensio	1998a	2	105	39(37.1%)	26(24.7%)	8(7.6%)	5(4.7%)	23(21.9%)	9(8.5%)
Tyburski	2000	17	302	121(40%)	75(24.8%)	17(5.6%)	6(1.9%)	83(27.4%)	NR
Totals			1778	699	559	328	74	314	65

LA，左心房；LV，左心室；NR，未报道；RA，右心房；RV，右心室

表 3　AAST-OIS：心脏损伤

级别 *	损伤描述
Ⅰ	钝性心脏损伤伴有轻微心电图异常（非特异性 ST 段或 T 波改变，房性或室性期前收缩，或持续性心动过速） 钝性或穿通性心包损伤不伴有心脏损伤、心包积液或心脏疝
Ⅱ	钝性心脏损伤伴有传导阻滞（右或左束支传导阻滞、左前分支传导阻滞或房室传导阻滞）或缺血性改变（ST 段压低或 T 波倒置），不伴有心功能衰竭 穿通性心肌切割伤，伤口未扩张，且不伴有心脏压塞
Ⅲ	钝性心脏损伤伴有持续性（≥6 次 / 分钟）或多源性室性期前收缩 钝性或穿通性心脏损伤伴有隔膜破裂、肺动脉瓣或三尖瓣关闭不全、乳头肌功能不全或冠状动脉远段闭塞，但不伴有心功能衰竭 钝性心包裂伤伴有心脏疝 钝性心脏损伤伴有心功能衰竭
Ⅳ	不累及心包的穿通性心肌切割伤，伴有心脏压塞 钝性或穿通性心脏损伤伴有室间隔破裂、肺动脉瓣或三尖瓣关闭不全、乳头肌功能不全或冠状动脉远段闭塞，导致心功能不全 钝性或穿通性心脏损伤伴有主动脉瓣或二尖瓣关闭不全 位于右心室、右心房或左心房的钝性或穿通性心脏损伤
Ⅴ	钝性或穿通性心脏损伤伴有冠状动脉近段闭塞 钝性或穿通性心脏损伤导致左心室穿孔 右心室、右心房、左心房损伤导致＜ 50% 的心腔组织损失
Ⅵ	钝性心脏撕脱，穿通性损伤导致＞ 50% 的心腔组织损失

* 单腔的多处穿通性损伤或多腔受累，则严重程度上调 1 级。

实发病率仍然很难从文献中估计。

临床表现

钝性心脏损伤包括多种损伤情况，因此其临床表现并不唯一，可表现为血流动力学不稳定，也可以表现为心肺骤停。典型的心包压塞体征也可能会出现。一些患者表现为胸痛，并难以与心肌梗死的胸痛区分。其他可能出现的症状与体征包括前胸壁的疼痛与肌紧张、挫伤、瘀斑、肋骨骨折，以及连枷胸。

诊断

协助诊断的手段包括 X 线胸片、心电图、动态心电图、心肌酶、经胸超声心动图、经食管超声心动图、放射性核素血管显像术（radionuclide angiography，RNA）铊 201、单光子发射计算机断层摄影术（single-photon emission computed tomography，SPECT）和多门控影像采集扫描（mul-liple-gated image acquisition scans，MUGAs）。所有创伤患者均应常规接受 X 线胸片的检查，以了解是否存在肋骨骨折、连枷胸甚至球形心脏轮廓（罕见）等。心电图则用于排查心脏传导系统的异常和筛查患者。然而，目前还没有可以可靠诊断 BCI 的发现。

过去，人们认为当血清的肌酸磷酸激酶（creatine phosphokinase，CPK）或肌酸激酶（creatine kinase，CK）升高至一定程度时，BLI 的诊断则能够建立。之后有研究发现，肌钙蛋白 T 与肌钙蛋白 I 具有更好的心肌特异性。Fulda 等使用心电图、血清肌钙蛋白 T 浓度及 CPK-MB 和标准心电图对 71 例胸壁损伤的患者进行评估，研究显示肌钙蛋白 T 预测临床异常的灵敏度与特异度分别是 27% 和 91%。这次研究认为，对于进展中的有意义的心电图改变，最好的预测因素是首次心电图提示的异常以及升高的肌钙蛋白 T 水平，因此心电图与血清肌钙蛋白 T 的检测均应是诊断钝性心脏损伤的手段。

Salim 等研究了肌钙蛋白 T 与心电图如何提示钝性心脏损伤患者进一步产生并发症的风险。在这项纳入 115 例患者的前瞻性研究中，他们将出现心源性休克、需要治疗的心律失常，以及出现心脏结构异常的患者定义为明显 BCI 风险。所有患者在诊治过程中，每 8 h 接受一次心电图检查，并于入院的第 0、4、8 h 检测肌钙蛋白 T 的水平。在这些患者中，19 例（16.5%）为明显损伤，其中绝大部分患者在伤后 24 h 以内均出现症状。在 115 例患者中，58 例提示心电图异常，27 例则存在肌钙蛋白 T 水平的上升。这项研究认为，心电图联合肌钙蛋白 T 的检测有助于判断患者是否存在明显的钝性心脏损伤。

对于可疑钝性心脏损伤的患者，二维经胸超声心动图检查被广泛应用在评估与诊断上。当患者心电图、心肌酶和肌钙蛋白出现异常时，应接受这项检查。超声心动图能够对阶段性室壁运动异常以及瓣膜功能异常进行评估，然而它评估并发症以及预测疾病预后作用有限。同时，当胸壁存在水肿或结构异常如肋骨骨折或连枷胸时，超声心动图的应用也受到限制。最重要的是，它无法对心电活动的不稳定性进行评估，而这恰是钝性心脏损伤的重要标志。

经食管超声心动图同样是评估心脏损伤的重要辅助手段，它在检测 BCI 的能力上比较多样。但其创伤较大，操作复杂，且使用有时间的限制。

过去，一些基于核医学的检查被用于诊断 BCI，但均尚不足以提供可靠的灵敏度和特异度来识别 BCI，现多已不再使用。

钝性心脏损伤的范围

临床上，钝性心脏损伤可分为两类：急性与亚急性。急性损伤包括心脏破裂合并急性心包压塞、心脏与心包联合破裂导致胸腔出血，以及急性心肌损伤与心源性休克。急性损伤通常为灾难性损伤，在无外科干预的情况下患者会即刻或快速死亡。亚急性损伤包括心肌挫伤、亚急性心包压塞、心肌梗死、瓣膜损伤、心内分流、附壁血栓，以及心律失常。这类损伤可能不会导致患者即刻死亡，但会影响血流动力学，使患者存在发展为心律失常及各类并发症的风险。

心包损伤

心包的钝性破裂可由直接高能量冲击或腹内急性压力突然增高所致。心包破裂可发生于膈面和胸膜面，常与左侧膈神经的走行相平行，心脏可能会突入腹腔，甚至引起大血管的急性扭转。心包破裂的患者可表现为血流动力学的不稳定，也可以严重至发生心肺骤停，大血管的继发扭转以及合并心腔破裂同样可见。通过 X 线胸片可发现心脏轮廓移位、心包积气。若患者血流动力学稳定，应接受 FAST 的评估和心电图的检查。剑突下心包开窗术可以确认诊断，可能会提示血性心包积血。若如此，则须进一步行胸骨正中切开术。

瓣膜、乳头肌 / 腱索、间隔损伤

钝性心脏损伤很少导致瓣膜的损伤。其中主动脉瓣损伤最常见，其次是二尖瓣。重要的临床表现包括新出现的心脏杂音、震颤、响亮的音乐性杂音。相似地，急性左心功能障碍、心源性休克、相关的肺水肿也是重要的临床体征。

胸腔受到冲击和挤压时，心室舒张期心腔内的血流可能会发生快速的异常流动，使得瓣膜、乳头肌、腱索发生撕裂，从而导致瓣膜功能不全。正是因为这个原因，主动脉瓣最容易受到损伤。同样，任何原因导致的主动脉内压力突然升高均会导致瓣叶的破裂，以及乳头肌的拉伸和血肿形成。乳头肌结构的突然改变会导致其功能异常，进而影响瓣膜活动。

间隔损伤同样并不常见。Hewett 在 1847 年首先报道了钝性创伤导致的室间隔破裂。之后，Bright 和 Beck 在 1935 年报道了，在 152 例发生致命性心脏损伤的患者中，有 11 例发生了间隔破裂。

冠状动脉损伤

钝性冠状动脉损伤极为罕见。胸部直接的钝性冲击伤可能会导致冠状动脉的急性血栓形成，并进一步引发内膜破裂。冠状动脉的损伤常常与严重的心肌挫伤有关，累及左前降支分布的部位。这类患者的临床表现无法与急性心肌梗死区分。此损伤的远期后遗症可能进展为室壁瘤形成，以及相关并发症，如心脏破裂、心室功能不全、血栓形成及恶性心律失常。

心腔破裂

钝性损伤导致的心脏破裂并不常见。这类患者中，仅少数能够存活至医院。车祸造成的心腔破裂常会导致患者即刻死亡，往往通过尸检才得以诊断。关于钝性心脏破裂的发生机制有如下假说：心前区直接受到冲击，压力由腹腔逆向传导至心脏导致破裂，心脏受挤压，加速或减速导致心脏与大血管连接处发生撕裂，爆炸效应，恶性心律失常继发致命性的心脏震荡。

钝性心腔破裂的临床表现多为持续性低血压以及心包压塞。大量出血可进一步诱发心肺骤停。这类患者应立即接受 FAST 的评估。对于血流动力学稳定的患者，剑突下心包开窗术可作为明确 FAST 诊断的方式之一。然而，对于心肺骤停的患者，急诊开胸术可能是挽救其生命的唯一机会，尽管其预后很差。

Türk 和 Tsokos 报道，钝性心房损伤较心室损伤更为常见。最常见的心腔损伤部位为右心房，其次是右心室，左侧心腔损伤相对更为少见。过去有一些多心腔破裂的报道，但这些患者中尚未有存活者。

心肌挫伤

心脏挫伤是所有钝性心脏损伤中最容易被忽视的，也是最难被定义的。心肌挫伤的定义曾在创伤外科医生的讨论下经历数次更改。Mattox 等曾建议删除心肌挫伤的概念，并以钝性心脏损伤伴随心功能不全、复杂性心律失常，以及心电图或心肌酶的微小异常来代替。在此基础上，他们不推荐把无症状的创伤患者留置在外科重症监护室，也不建议对其进行心电图和心肌酶的监测，以及进一步心脏影像学的检查。

Civetta 等认为，对于年轻的胸部创伤患者，严重的心脏事件并不常见，并且他们指出心电图的异常能够较好提示临床损伤的患者有心脏并发症。

经过全面的文献回顾，Pasquale 等总结了一些高质量的相关研究和综述。基于此，EAST 制订了如下推荐：

Ⅰ级

对于怀疑钝性心脏损伤的患者，心电图检查应常规进行。

Ⅱ级

1. 如果心电图异常，患者应接受连续 24 ~ 48 h 的心电图监测。如果心电图正常，则无需进一步诊断。
2. 如果患者血流动力学不稳定，应接受影像学检查。若经胸超声心动图检查无法实施，则患者须接受经食管超声心动图检查。
3. 与超声心动图相比，核医学检查无法提供更多信息。因此在超声心动图能够实施的情况下，没必要采用核医学检查。

Ⅲ级

1. 既往有心脏病的老年患者、病情不稳定的患

者，以及心电图异常的患者，可在严密监测下进行手术治疗。对于这类患者，放置肺动脉导管应予考虑。

2. 胸骨骨折不是钝性心脏损伤的预测因素，且也不意味着这类患者须进行监测。
3. CPK 与循环肌钙蛋白 T 均无法对钝性心脏损伤患者是否已发生或将要发生 BCI 相关并发症进行有效预测。

结论

心脏损伤仍为一类极具挑战性且有吸引力的疾病。对这类致命性创伤的处理方式（图 7），仍有待于进一步科学严谨的前瞻性研究。

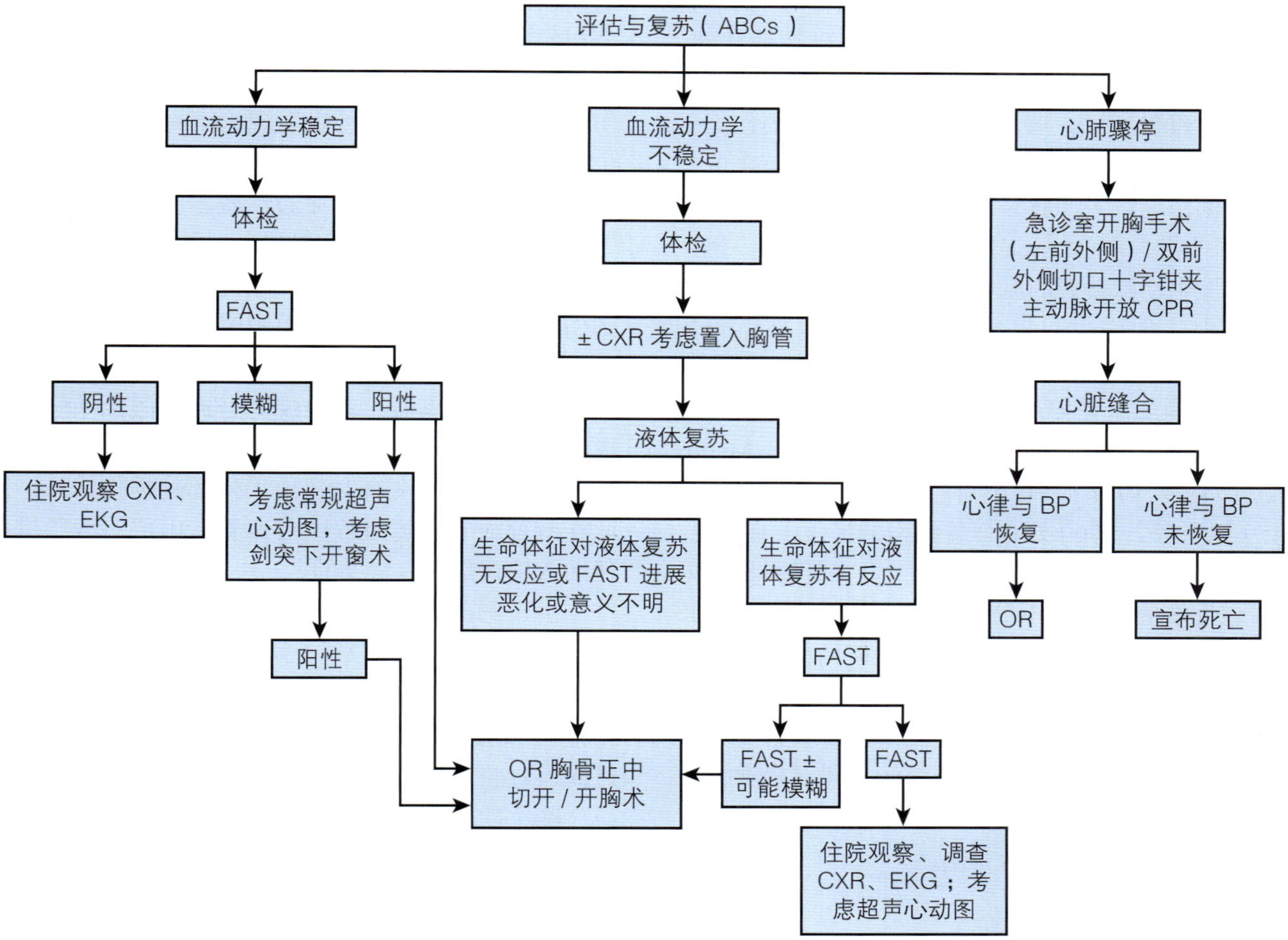

图 7　穿通性心脏损伤的管理流程。ABC，气道，呼吸，循环；BP，血压；CPR，心肺复苏；CXR，X 线胸片；ED，急诊室；ECHO，超声心动图；EKG，心电图；FAST，创伤重点超声评估；OR，手术室

胸部血管损伤

Peter I. Tsai, Ramyar Gilani, Kenneth L. Mattox 和 Matthew J. Wall, Jr. 著
张学民 译

心脏、主动脉及其大血管是胸腔内的主要部分，被椎体、肋骨、锁骨、胸骨柄和胸骨保护。大血管穿通伤可以导致类似钝性创伤的完全破坏的状态，引起立即出血、横断和假性动脉瘤、内膜下血肿和内膜瓣上继发血栓。最早的一篇胸部血管损伤报告是 1557 年由 Vesalius 描述的一个从马上摔下来的男性钝性创伤导致主动脉破裂。直到 1959 年，Passaro 和 Pace 才报告由 Klassen 在 1958 年完成的第一例一期创伤性主动脉破裂的成功修补。

在现代创伤中心发展前，大多数胸部血管损伤个体在到达医院前死亡。随着快速反应创伤系统的到来，胸部血管损伤患者活着到达医院的数量增多，损伤的复杂程度更有挑战性。这一点从 Mattox 等的 1958 — 1987 的 30 年间德克萨斯州的休斯顿的 4 459 例患者、5 760 处心血管损伤的报告中有体现。

胸部血管损伤是个特别的挑战，创伤科医生对近端、远端的暴露是不简单的。未仔细规划的切口会导致灾难性后果。鉴于胸部血管损伤到达创伤中心所增加的损伤的复杂性，外科医生制订系统的方式和行动计划以避免这种损伤相关的并发症和死亡是重要的。另外，技术的进步继续提供了越来越高的诊断和治疗能力，但我们必须不断客观地评估之前公布的患者治疗流程的变化。

发生率

胸部创伤占所有创伤死亡的 50%。在大系列的胸部创伤患者中，主动脉和大血管损伤占 4%。超过 90% 的胸部大血管损伤由穿通伤造成。在存在穿通伤的情况下，所有胸部血管都可能受伤。升主动脉的解剖学位置使其成为刺伤最常损伤的胸部大血管，而枪伤常导致胸降主动脉损伤。钝伤可以导致全部胸主动脉和静脉的潜在损伤，尤其是无名动脉起始部、肺静脉、腔静脉和最常见的胸降主动脉。

损伤机制

大量胸部大血管损伤由穿刺伤或医源性创伤引起。穿刺性胸部血管创伤的损伤机制通常是直接裂伤或血管穿通伤。损伤类型可以表现为外出血或内出血。内膜瓣引起的血栓形成或假性动脉瘤。由于穿通性血管损伤涉及各种类型的枪弹，所有胸部血管结构都有风险。有趣的是，骨结构也可以有独特的损伤表现，如导致子弹 / 碎片弹跳或改变穿刺伤最初的方向。胸廓出口血管损伤时从皮肤破口有大量外出血，而内出血通常发生在主动脉和腔静脉损伤。胸内大血管损伤可以表现为至纵隔、胸腔或心包腔的内出血。重要的是远侧脉搏正常可触及不能排除近心端血管损伤。穿通性血管损伤可完全被血管外膜包裹而保持远端血流。

没有明显大量的出血不能排除穿通性血管损伤。刺伤的血管损伤经常导致内膜瓣或夹层形成，进而最终导致受损血管部分或完全血栓。小血管破坏最初可能不表现出血，而表现为延迟的假性动脉瘤形成。枪弹冲击导致的血管损伤往往被低估，因为内膜破裂的严重程度有时超出了外部的损伤体征。因此在胸部血管重建过程中对血管从内部对内膜进行仔细的检查是很有帮助的。

由于胸部血管直径大，子弹可以直接进入血管并向远侧迁移（图 1）。子弹栓塞的诊断经常延误，因为子弹的弹道可能不明显。子弹栓塞经常发生在髂血管和股血管。入路可能因为出血首先被控制，进而通过腔内介入或另做动脉切开去除子弹栓塞。

胸主动脉和大血管钝性损伤有两种可能的机制。在胸部前后位冲击时，主动脉及其分支可能被“夹”在胸骨和脊柱之间导致血管破裂。无论前面或侧面的机动车事故导致的胸部快速 - 减速伤，肺静脉和腔静脉附着点和降主动脉在动脉韧带和膈水平相对的固定增加了破裂的易感性。与主动脉内膜病变的患者相比，他们的外膜是限制屏障，完整的胸膜壁层会包裹血肿，避免了大量的血胸。

诊断

胸部血管穿通伤患者经常因大量失血死于现场。随着急救医疗体系（emergency medical system，

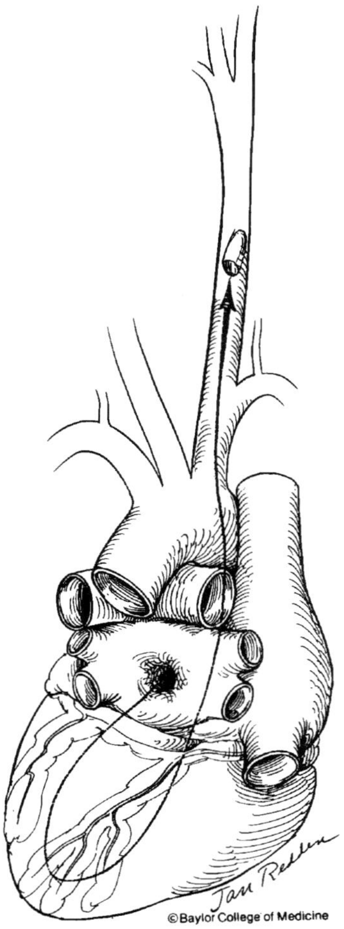

图 1 从左房到左颈动脉子弹栓塞 (*Courtesy of Jan Redden, Baylor College of Medicine, 1980.*)

EMS）转运的进步，越来越多的患者活着转运到急诊室。这些患者可以表现因未控制的出血流入纵隔、胸腔、心包囊而血流动力学不稳定，须紧急转运到手术室行外科治疗。这些损伤能典型地在开胸急救术中诊断。相比之下，胸部钝伤患者最初血流动力学稳定，多数的其他损伤可能掩盖他们明显的血管损伤。

在创伤室重点询问病史和体格检查有助于特定血管损伤的诊断。在穿通伤中，凶器的类型、刀的长度、枪的口径和患者与枪手的距离有助于诊断。虽然这些信息经常不可信，但可以帮助外科医生重建子弹损伤的弹道和形成外科治疗方案。在胸部钝伤中，损伤机制特别重要，外科医生可以据此估计动能转化的数量，和与之相关的患者躯体在受伤时的形态。急诊医疗病案也可以提供关于现场失血量和转运过程中血流动力学稳定性的信息。

可能的胸部血管损伤的指征列于表 1。单独的、最重要的胸部血管损伤的筛选工具是正位 X 线胸片。表 2 列出了许多 X 线胸片发现提示胸部血管损伤。一个最可靠的影像学发现提示胸部血管钝伤是 X 线胸片上主动脉结轮廓突出。

动脉造影仍是评估可能的胸部血管损伤的影像学“金标准”。对可疑胸部血管损伤血流动力学不稳定的患者，术前造影从不作为依据指标。在可疑无名动脉、颈动脉或锁骨下动脉穿通损伤的血流动力学稳定的患者中，术前应做造影以提供这些主动脉分支近端控制的切口类型的信息（图 2）。进而，接

表 1　胸部血管损伤可能的指征

损伤机制
坠落、机动车事故和行人与机动车碰撞导致的严重减速伤
挤压伤
有轨迹提示胸部穿通伤，包括纵隔横贯枪伤
暗示性体征
胸廓出口血肿
不均匀的周围脉搏或血压
前胸部方向盘挫伤
触及胸骨骨折
局部神经功能不全
胸片发现
纵隔异常或增宽
主动脉结轮廓消失
气管或鼻胃管侧向偏移

表 2　影像学发现提示大血管损伤

上纵隔增宽 >8 cm
左主支气管受压 >140°
主动脉结消失
鼻胃管或气管插管或气管向右偏移
第 1 或第 2 肋骨、锁骨或胸骨骨折
左胸膜顶帽
在侧位 X 线胸片上主肺动脉窗闭塞
侧位 X 线胸片上气管前移
胸椎骨折脱位
主动脉结钙化影
主动脉明显双重轮廓
多发左侧肋骨骨折
大量血胸

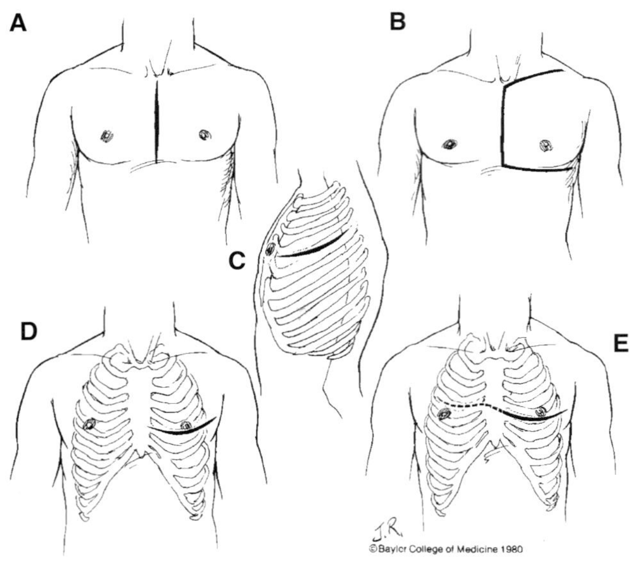

图2 可以用于治疗胸部血管损伤的各种胸部切口。**A**，胸骨正中切开术。**B**，前外侧开胸术联合锁骨上切口（不常用胸骨切开形成“门扇”切口开胸）。**C**，后外侧开胸术。**D**，前外侧开胸术（极端情况的患者的通用切口）。**E**，左前外侧开胸，从翻盖切口扩展到右侧（*Courtesy of Jan Redden, Baylor College of Medicine, 1980.*）

近弹道的头臂动脉血管造影是除外损伤的指标。在胸部钝伤中，动脉造影须取决于体格检查、X线胸片筛查和损伤机制的高度怀疑。50%的胸部血管钝伤患者没有表现出外部损伤的征象。7%的主动脉及其分支血管钝伤的患者X线胸片筛查中的纵隔看似正常。而基于损伤机制被怀疑的患者需要进一步的影像检查。

胸部增强螺旋CT血管造影（CT angiography，CTA）应更加频繁地使用以评估胸部创伤。CTA对胸部血管损伤的灵敏度为54%～80%。胸部CTA对胸部血管损伤评估的阴性预测值接近100%。而对损伤机制明确、入院X线胸片看似正常、体检无特殊发现的稳定患者，用胸部CTA作为排除潜在胸部血管损伤的筛查工具也是合理的。然而，有阳性或模糊的CTA结果的患者应当进一步检查，大多数患者采用血管造影术在术前明确胸部血管损伤。CTA也用于术前血管内修复的规划。它可以得到关于侧支血管和锚定区的详细信息。有了这些信息就可以决定腔内修复的可行性和选择恰当器械。此外可以评估覆盖范围和是否需要如颈-锁骨下动脉旁路的辅助过程。

然而，CTA用于胸部血管不是没有限制的，主动脉根部和升主动脉损伤由于心跳影响经常在标准CTA上看不清。心脏门控CTA是个应对移动物体的急诊技术，正广泛用于近心端主动脉的成像并潜在性地用于创伤。除CTA异常发现外有许多正常变异，如动脉导管隆起、漏斗状的上位肋间动脉或Kommerell憩室，像主动脉损伤却无须治疗。最后，血流动力学不稳定的患者可能有一过性的血管直径缩小，这可以理论上导致支架偏小和器械失败。腔内血管超声（intravascular ultrasound，IVUS）提供了360° 实时影像，提供血管壁和管腔异常的信息。此图像对运动不敏感，可以用于近端主动脉成像的应用。内膜血肿在血管造影无法看到或内膜损伤被造影剂掩盖时，用实时IVUS可以看到。进而，当评估CTA模糊的患者时，IVUS诊断钝性主动脉损伤（blunt aortic injury，BAI）表现好于传统血管造影。

磁共振血管成像（magnetic resonance angiography，MRA）既不是理想的、也不是经验丰富的评价急性损伤的方法。因为患者在磁共振线圈里难以监测和治疗，因此不推荐用MRA来评估损伤患者。

经食管超声心动图（transesophageal echocardiography，TEE）提供了一些和动脉造影相比评估胸部血管损伤的潜在的优点。它避免了静脉内注射造影剂，可以得到相应的心功能信息，其便携性与动脉造影相比也有潜在的优势。发表的文章报告，诊断动脉损伤时TEE的灵敏度和特异度分别为85.7%和92.0%，而动脉造影分别为89.0%和100%。TEE也是高度依赖操作者的技术。而且升主动脉、近端主动脉弓和主动脉血管分支用TEE很难看到，合并胸部损伤/血肿的时候情况更糟。因此，不将其作为评估胸部血管损伤的常规推荐。

美国创伤外科协会，器官损伤分级

表3列出基于创伤大小和严重程度，AAST设计的胸部血管损伤器官损伤分级，从Ⅰ到Ⅵ级。

Ⅰ级损伤通常包括胸部小血管，Ⅱ级损伤累及有名字的上腔静脉分支静脉，如无名静脉、颈内静脉、锁骨下静脉和奇静脉；主动脉血管分支如无名动脉、颈动脉和锁骨下动脉构成Ⅲ级损伤；Ⅳ级损伤包括心包外大血管结构损伤；Ⅴ级损伤包括心包内大血管结构损伤；Ⅵ级损伤时是未控制的，完全的胸主动脉或肺门横断伤。

外科处理

胸部血管损伤急诊外科干预的指征列于表 4。切口选择依损伤位置而不同（图 2）。对不稳定的可疑而未确诊的胸部血管损伤患者，最恰当的切口是仰卧位的左前外侧开胸切口。该切口提供了良好的心脏和主动脉急救显露，而且可以通过扩大切口到对侧很容易地转为翻盖式切口，以提供右侧肺门、升主动脉和右侧锁骨下血管的良好显露。胸骨正中切口是无名动脉、右侧锁骨下动脉、右侧颈总动脉和近端左颈总动脉损伤的切口。可以附加颈部斜切口或锁骨上延长横切口以提供进一步显露。在侧卧位的左后外侧开胸术提供对已知胸降主动脉和左肺门的最佳显露。

升主动脉 / 横主动脉损伤患者很少生存到足以转运到创伤中心。大多数这些钝性损伤须使用心肺旁路术或循环停止下间置移植物。在特定的小的升主动脉前侧壁或外侧壁穿通裂伤可以一期修补而无需心肺旁路术。包含升主动脉后方和肺动脉的复合伤也需要心肺旁路术。延长胸骨正中切口分离无名静脉到颈部可以使横弓显露得更好。

就恰当的治疗而言，最近的重点在于 BAI。有证据表明在血流动力学稳定的患者中，有目的地推迟手术结合使用 β- 受体阻断药药物抗脉冲（dP/dT）治疗和严密监测可能是急诊修补手术的安全的替代方法。此外，诸如小的内膜瓣或壁间血肿的“小”的 BAI 可能倾向于非手术治疗。

治疗胸降主动脉损伤的手术原则是近 / 远端控制、处理损伤节段、重建血流连续性。大多数钝性损伤在胸降主动脉，起源于动脉韧带水平的内侧。近端控制的迅速有效的方法是追寻左锁骨下动脉向近端到主动脉弓的部分，并在左颈总动脉和左锁骨下动脉之间环绕主动脉弓放置套带。大多数胸降主动脉的钝性损伤起源于动脉韧带水平的内侧。套带也缠绕左锁骨下动脉。要注意避免损伤走行在主动脉弓周围的靠近动脉韧带后方的左侧喉返神经。下一步控制损伤远端血管。检查胸降主动脉全长非常重要，以分辨任何其他裂伤，特别是在膈水平。有几个方法可以实现胸降主动脉基本的血管修复。第一是钳夹和缝合技术，不用左心转流。一些外科医生推荐使用积极的部分左心转流修复胸降主动脉损伤（图 3）。这种手术最常用于一直有冠脉疾病、射血分数尚可的老年人。所有这些附加技术应当是治疗此型损伤的外科医生所熟悉的。在近端和远端控制完成后，进入血肿。肋间动脉不常规缝扎。从主动脉外面和里面检查损伤范围。简单的主动脉部分裂伤可以用 4-0 聚丙烯线一期连续缝合关闭。复杂的损伤经常要用人工血管。

文献上对是否积极行远端灌注以减少可怕的截

表 3　胸部血管损伤分级

级 *	损伤表现
Ⅰ	肋间血管 内乳血管 支气管血管 食管血管 半奇静脉 无名血管
Ⅱ	奇静脉 颈内静脉 锁骨下静脉 无名静脉
Ⅲ	颈动脉 无名动脉 锁骨下动脉
Ⅳ	胸降主动脉 胸腔内下腔静脉 肺动脉 / 肺静脉，实质内分支
Ⅴ	升主动脉 主动脉弓 上腔静脉 肺动脉主干 肺静脉主干
Ⅵ	未控制的胸主动脉或肺门血管的完全横断伤

美国创伤外科协会 (AAST) 修订。

* 多发的Ⅲ级损伤或Ⅳ级损伤中血管受累 >50% 周径时，损伤分级增加 1 级。Ⅳ级损伤如果血管受累 <25% 周径时，损伤分级降低 1 级

表 4　胸部大血管损伤手术修复的指征

从胸导管最初失血 1500 ml
从胸廓造口术置管中继续出血＞ 200 ml/h
创伤后心包积血
心包压塞
胸廓出口扩张性血肿
锁骨上穿通伤口的活动性出血
急性胸部大血管损伤的影像证据
慢性胸部大血管损伤并发症的影像学或其他影像证据

瘫发病率有持续的热烈讨论。而多数研究表明术后截瘫发生率是多因素的，不能归咎于单一原因。所有的远端灌注技术都有潜在的并发症，包括由插管部位和全身肝素使用引起的。不考虑使用的技术，在各种研究中，术后截瘫的发生率平均为 8%。

在过去十年，胸降主动脉 BAI 治疗有重大进步。Demetriades 等在 2008 年及其后的两篇关于 AAST 多中心研究随访报告中将最初的诊断方法改为 CTA。胸主动脉腔内修复（thoracic endovascular aortic repair，TEVAR）近年来也得到普遍应用，成为大多数中心修复的方法。没有 TEVAR 和开放性修复的随机对照研究，而 TEVAR 和开放手术相比表现出更低的死亡率，更少的失血、截瘫率和更低的脑卒中率。还有一些对 TEVAR 的担忧，如有报告称器械并发症率达到 20%，且长期随访研究还很有限。结果尽管已上市，器械经历了几代改进，对年轻患者使用仍不理想。这种趋势体现在我们自己医学院过去 3 年的实践中。

对 BAI 做 TEVAR 就像对动脉瘤一样。已知 BAI 的最常见位置，经常须覆盖左锁骨下动脉以获得良好的近端锚定。基于已发表的指南，如果需要覆盖，要评估患者是否需要血管再生。在多发伤患者中，全身肝素化是禁忌，不能进行。术后随访指南还没有，但似乎可以用动脉瘤的相似的指南。

无名动脉和近端左颈总动脉损伤最好用胸骨正中切口，如有必要可以做颈部延长。分离无名静脉可以提供良好的弓部显露以达到近端控制。在小的部分撕裂的远端无名动脉患者中用 4-0 聚丙烯线一期修补经常是可行的。在大多数病例中，旁路旷置技术是无名动脉损伤最好的治疗措施（图 4）。这个方法可以不用全身肝素化、心肺旁路或低温循环停止。一个 10 mm 编织的管状移植物用于从近端升主动脉到远端无名动脉旁路术。完成旁路术后，对动脉起始部的损伤进行缝合。近端左颈总动脉的损伤也可以用类似方法处理。

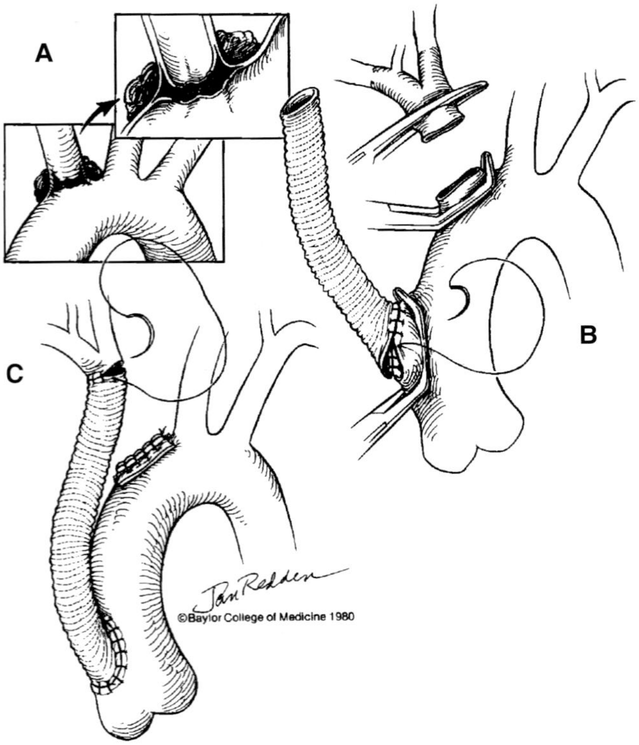

图 3　治疗无名动脉损伤的旁路旷置技术。**A**，严重的内膜破损可能和小的外膜血肿有关。**B**，选择一个部位沿升主动脉切开，用人工血管端侧吻合。部分钳夹的血管钳置于无名动脉起始处，另一把血管钳钳夹远端无名动脉，在两个钳之间切断动脉。**C**，通过人工血管和远端无名动脉的端端吻合和缝合无名动脉在主动脉的起始处完成修补。(*Courtesy of Jan Redden, Baylor College of Medicine, 1980.*)

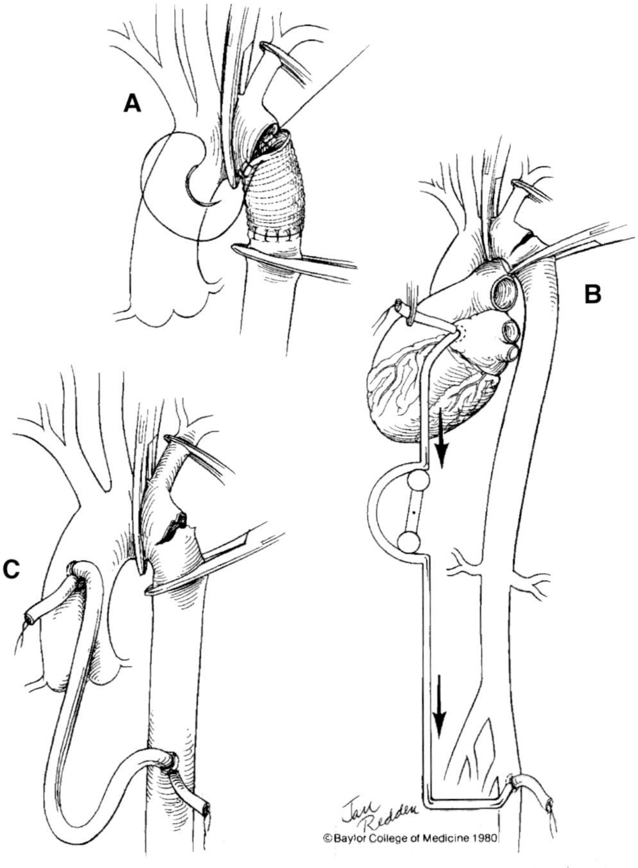

图 4　胸降主动脉损伤治疗的辅助。**A**，用血管钳的近端和远端控制的简单钳夹和缝合技术。**B**，主动的左房股旁路和左侧心脏旁路。**C**，被动的胸升主动脉到胸降主动脉分流 (*Courtesy of Jan Redden, Baylor College of Medicine, 1980.*)

胸骨正中开胸术伴右颈部延长切口是右锁骨下动脉损伤的切口选择。近端左锁骨下动脉损伤最好是通过左第4肋间后外侧开胸术修补。远侧锁骨下动脉显露可以通过左侧锁骨上切口，近端控制通过第3肋间前外侧切口。虽然少见，左锁骨下动脉多阶段损伤可以用通过结合这两个切口形成“门扇”切口治疗。应当避免在显露锁骨下动脉时损伤在前斜角肌前方的膈神经。如有必要可以切开或切除左侧锁骨，以提供更好的显露。在近端和远端控制后，一期修补或间置缝合或使用聚四氟乙烯人工血管取决于损伤范围。因为锁骨下动脉的柔软性质，移动它做端端吻合通常很困难。锁骨下动脉损伤经常合并臂丛神经损伤，而术前神经学检查有帮助。锁骨下静脉损伤显露和锁骨下动脉相似。静脉损伤修补用一期静脉缝合或结扎。

腔内技术当然可用于治疗大血管损伤，以减少显露的困难和暴露相关并发症。无论具体的方法是什么，对于此类损伤的血管内手术，必须坚持与开放手术类似的血管创伤原则。适当选择患者的早期系列研究中已确立血管内修复的可行性。尽管在早期研究中是成功的，开放手术仍推荐用于低血压、完全横断伤或血栓形成的患者。然而，最近的报告描述了血管内技术跨越了这些障碍，并达到可与开放手术媲美的可接受的临床结果。在特定状况下，在进行开放手术修复前，通过血管腔内方法达到近端和远端球囊控制是有好处的。混合的过程证明了熟练掌握开放手术和血管内技术对最佳处置这些复杂损伤的重要性。

心包内肺动脉损伤最佳路径是胸骨正中切口。打开心包就能看到主肺动脉和近端左肺动脉。近端分离上腔静脉和升主动脉显露右肺动脉。小的前部损伤用部分阻断血管钳、4-0聚丙烯线连续缝合。更复杂的和后壁损伤须使用心肺旁路术。远侧心包外肺动脉损伤由开胸切口显露。在特定患者中，肺切除可能是大的肺门损伤的救命的选择。

由于解剖学位置的原因，胸部腔静脉损伤特别难以手术。胸骨正中切开术提供了最佳显露。单纯前壁裂伤可以用部分阻断的血管钳一期修补。后壁损伤需要完全心肺旁路或循环停止。随后的修复是从右心房内完成的，偶尔腔静脉内转流可能是个有用的辅助方法。

心包内肺静脉损伤罕见，在经验性急诊开胸手术中诊断。最佳切口是左前外侧开胸，可以到达心脏后部。心包外肺静脉损伤在稳定的患者中可以经后外侧开胸显露。单纯裂伤可以一期缝合。可以用临时肺门阻断控制大出血。如果为救命，不须结扎肺静脉，接着要做适当的肺叶切除。

由于奇静脉引流直接进入上腔静脉，奇静脉损伤可能潜在致命。这种类型的损伤术前甚少诊断或怀疑。当在手术室发现奇静脉损伤最好用一期修补或切断两端缝扎。类似的，内乳动脉和内乳静脉损伤可以导致大出血，经常在术中诊断。最佳治疗方式是单纯结扎并在手术记录中恰当记录，排除使用内乳动脉作为之后潜在的冠状动脉旁路术的导管的可能性。

在一个垂死的胸部血管损伤的患者，损伤控制开胸是一种治疗选择。左前外侧开胸切口提供最好的初步显露。开胸损伤控制的原则包括用尽可能简单的技术达到一次迅速控制出血或临时措施控制出血，待患者生理状态恢复到更适合生存的水平后，有计划地进行二期手术确定性修补。肺门血管损伤可以通过使用吻合器肺切除或肺叶切除迅速控制。对超过5 mm的血管，人造血管可用于减少获取自体静脉的时间。临时结扎和放置血管内转流管可以控制出血，直到患者的生理状态恢复到恰当水平做确定性修补。左锁骨下动脉结扎经常耐受性好，可用于控制损伤。开胸切口可以用巾钳快速关闭。而使用大的针把全部肌肉层一次整体关闭可以更好地止血。对心功能不全的患者为了避免压迫心脏也可以用 Bogota 袋或补片临时关闭。

年轻患者通常胸腔有非常柔软的中型或大的有名字的动脉，没有粥样硬化疾病。在手术修补胸部血管时任何缝合针轻微的横向偏离自然曲线可转化为增加针孔出血。在某些情况下，可能会导致进一步的动脉撕裂和致命的结果。当使用人工血管时，低血压患者的血管可能明显痉挛也须考虑。轻柔、精细的技术能提供最好的修补。

并发症率和治疗并发症

神经功能缺损经常作为附加相关的损伤或术后并发症伴随胸部血管结构损伤。因此，术前恰当记录患者神经状态非常重要。如前所述，降主动脉修复术后截瘫的平均发生率为8%。血管内修复显著降低截瘫率到1%。上臂丛和锁骨下血管解剖上邻近是锁骨下血管损伤相关的臂神经丛病高发的原因。建议和患者及其家庭成员详细探讨相关的神经并发症。一些患者表现为持续的开胸术后疼痛，这可能使其社会和情感功能恶化。因此，早期活动和康复是护理这些患者的重要辅助。在特定的患者，肋间神经阻滞有其益处。

大多数胸部血管损伤患者有相关的多器官损伤。因此，这些患者中的大部分在ICU中病情也很重。各种肺并发症，如肺不张、肺炎、急性呼吸窘迫综合征成为术后早期最常见的并发症。合并肺挫伤的患者发展为急性呼吸窘迫综合征的风险增加。积极的肺灌洗、适当的疼痛控制、详细的重症护理是预防这些并发症的基本要素。

死亡率

由于合并其他体腔内损伤的高发生率，胸部血管损伤有任何器官系统损伤的最高死亡率，升主动脉损伤患者极少能活着到医院。升主动脉损伤到达创伤中心时生命体征平稳的患者死亡率仍高达50%。中心肺动脉和静脉损伤是高致命性的，死亡率超过70%。类似的胸部腔静脉损伤不常见但极难控制，死亡率超过60%。不考虑使用的手术技术，胸降主动脉损伤死亡率为5%～25%。无名动脉损伤的总死亡率在1960－1992年报告为25%。锁骨下动脉损伤预后最好，Graham等报告其总死亡率低于5%。

结论

胸部血管损伤患者的治疗需要擅长的技术和出色的外科判断。基于此，关注此类损伤患者既有挑战性又有回报。

与腹部损伤不同，中线垂直切口是标准的探查切口，稳定的胸部血管损伤患者需要仔细的术前规划。因为硬质的胸壁，错误定位的切口和不正确的肋间进入会明显干扰胸部血管损伤出血的近/远端控制的显露。腔内修复需要股血管或肱血管入路，可以避免不同的胸部切口，但需要熟练的技术。虽然胸部血管损伤有所有损伤中最高的死亡率，高超的手术判断与手术精度将转化为患者护理和预后的改善。

胸主动脉损伤的开放和血管内治疗

K. Shad Pharaon 和 Donald D. Trunkey 著
张学民 译

1557年，Vesalius首次描述了钝性创伤主动脉破裂，报告了他在一个从马上摔下后死亡的男性中的发现。1946年，DeBakey和Simeone报告了第二次世界大战期间的胸部血管损伤。1959年，Passaro和Pace报告首次成功一期修复主动脉创伤性破裂，1994年Dake等首次报告一例胸降主动脉瘤血管内修复。

主动脉损伤代表对创伤外科医生的特殊挑战，因为部分主动脉可以通过胸骨正中切开、左侧开胸和正中剖腹手术显露，哪个切口最好并不总是明确的。正常解剖、解剖变异和走行的知识对任何外科医生都很重要，无论选择开放或导管治疗。胸主动脉损伤（thoracic aortic injury，TAI）开放手术和明显的并发症和死亡风险有关。虽然证据质量很低，胸主动脉血管内修复（thoracic endovascular aortic repair，TEVAR）现在作为自选手术技术。因其与开放性修复相比，改善了预后，特别是其有更低的死亡率和脊髓缺血的发生率（图1-4）。

发病率

TAI的发生率不为人所知。一些估计基于尸体解剖学研究。机动车碰撞（motor vehicle crash，MVC）是最常见的导致TAI的损伤机制，其次是行人被机动车和摩托车碰撞。大多数死者是男性（71%），酒精或非法药物的使用和39%的病例有关。胸主动脉破裂见于34%的死者，最常见的损伤位点是狭部/胸降主动脉（66%）。TAI患者被发现也和心脏损伤、血胸、肋骨骨折、腹内损伤和盆腔骨折有关。尽管机动车安全性和我们的院前急救系统有改善，据估计仍有大约80%的这些损伤患者在现场因出血死亡。

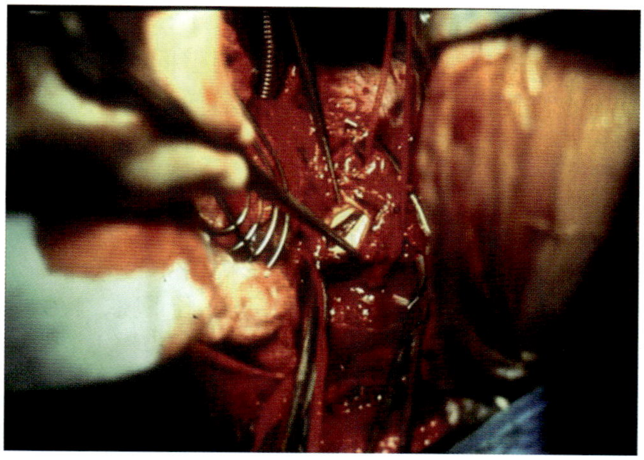

图 1　胸主动脉用涤纶移植片修补 (*Courtesy of J.A. Asensio, MD.*)

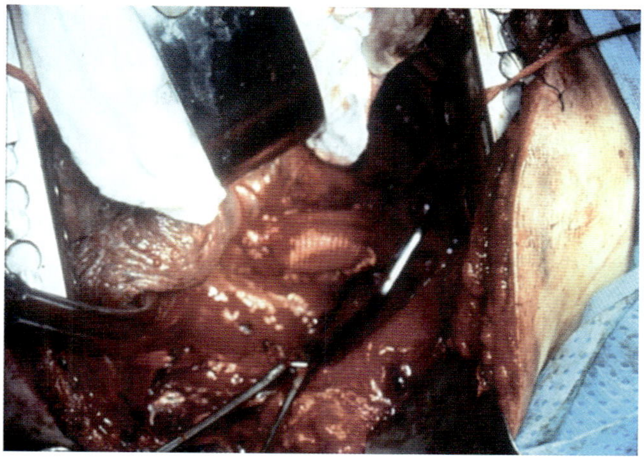

图 2　左后外侧开胸显露破裂处 (*Courtesy of J.A. Asensio, MD.*)

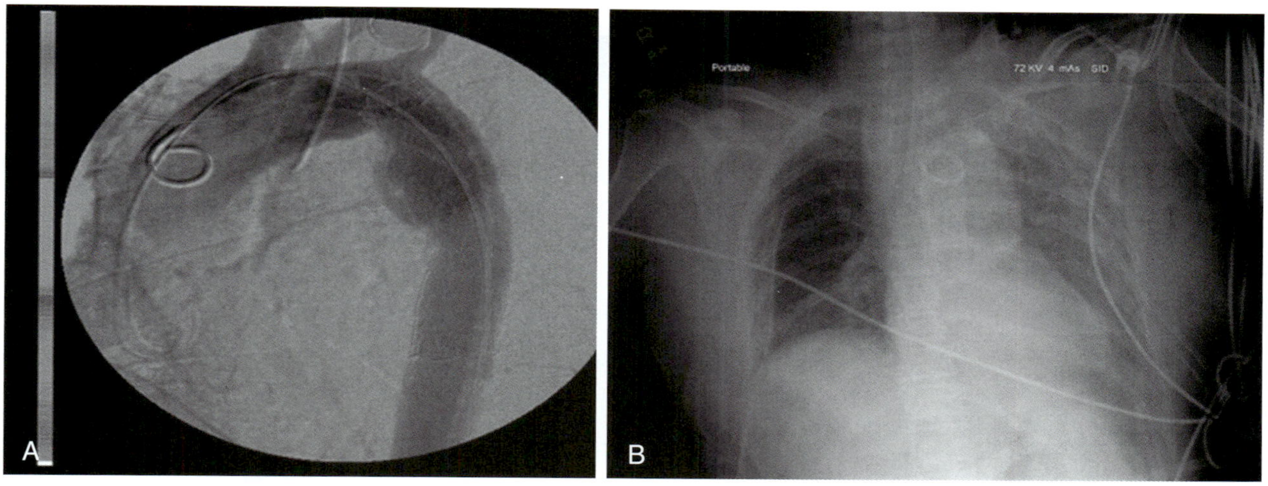

图 3　A 和 B，破裂的胸主动脉瘤用导丝支持下血管内胸主动脉修复 (*Courtesy of J.A. Asensio, MD.*)

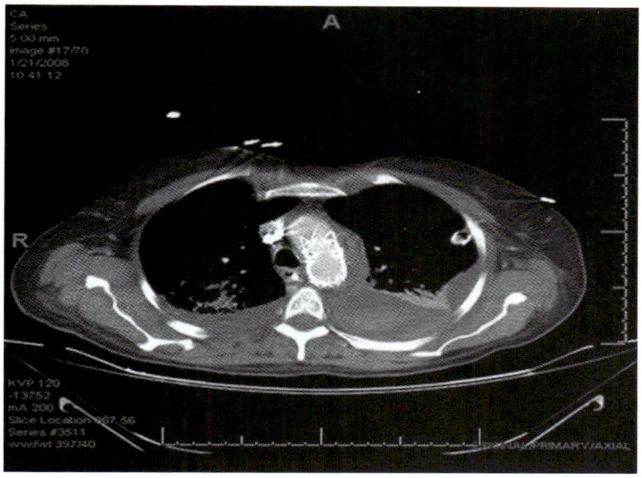

图 4　胸主动脉血管内修复完成后，CT 扫描显示胸主内支架 (*Courtesy of J.A. Asensio, MD.*)

损伤机制

由于它们的位置靠前，主动脉弓、无名动脉和颈动脉在如刺伤的穿通伤的情况下受损。胸降主动脉位置靠后，易于在如机动车碰撞、坠机和坠落的钝性损伤中受损。胸降主动脉在动脉韧带和膈处固定，是近端降主动脉最易损伤的部位。

诊断

作为可疑躯干钝伤、穿通伤患者的完整的检查的一部分，应该在急诊室做仰卧位 X 线胸片，任何减速伤患者都应考虑创伤性主动脉损伤。对于胸部穿通伤，在伤道的进口和出口放置放射学标记有助于影像的理解。而且，X线胸片可以提供气胸、血胸、子弹和弹片等异物的证据。放射学发现提示可能的创伤性主动脉损伤发现，包括纵隔增宽、主动脉弓异常、左顶帽、左主支气管受压、食管内鼻胃管偏移和气管侧向移位。

纵隔包含心脏、大血管、食管、器官、膈神经、胸导管、胸腺和淋巴结。主动脉钝伤的最敏感的指征是异常或增宽的纵隔，定义为前后位胸片上主动脉弓水平纵隔宽度超过8 cm。正常情况下，可以看到从弓到膈的清楚的主动脉轮廓。如果这个清晰的轮廓缺失，是另一个潜在的提示TAI的放射学发现。左侧顶帽（血液积聚在肺上胸膜外间隙）、左主支气管受压或器官侧移是提示胸部大血管损伤的其他线索。

分类

TAI最好用CTA诊断，为了治疗的目的分成1至4级（Ⅰ－Ⅳ级）。Ⅰ级损伤表现为只有内膜损伤，治疗为血压控制。大约6周复查CTA，随访损伤。Ⅱ级损伤表现为中膜损伤，表现有壁间血肿。一旦血肿在中膜内发展，经常改变血管轮廓。Ⅱ级损伤可以考虑做血管腔内移植物修复。Ⅲ级损伤扩展到外膜，导致假性动脉瘤形成。Ⅱ级和Ⅲ级损伤应视为紧急而非急诊手术修复。而Ⅳ级损伤是急诊手术。由于主动脉破裂，TAI有很高的死亡风险（图5）。

TAI可以同时合并脾、肝、肠、肠系膜、胰腺或胆囊损伤，这些损伤一旦出现，经常剖腹探查。一旦患者在腹内损伤修复中生存下来，就可以用血管内修复治疗主动脉损伤。传统上，主动脉修复经由胸骨正中切开术或开胸术（取决于位置），用“钳夹缝合”技术完成。

初始评估和治疗

大多数TAI患者因大量失血死于现场。在最初的主动脉损伤中幸存下来的患者可能有其他的损害，这对他们的生命造成了更为直接的威胁。一旦发现

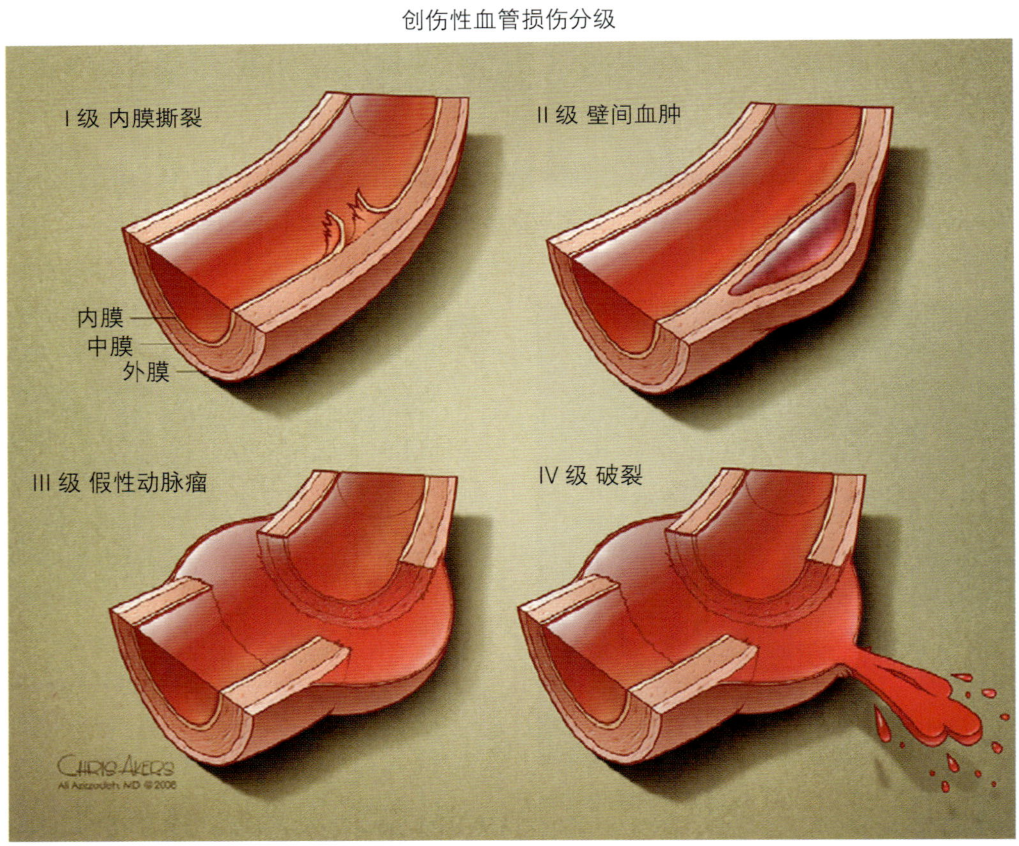

图5 主动脉损伤创伤分级，Ⅰ至Ⅳ级 (*From Dua A, Desai SS, Holcomb JB, et al, editors:* Clinical review of vascular trauma. *New York, Springer, 2014, p 160.*)

TAI，我们倾向于重点关注主动脉，忽略其他危及生命的伤害。因此，如果患者存活至急诊室，最初的管理应该从 ATLS 指南开始，稳定是最优先的。应对患者的气道、呼吸、循环、残疾和暴露进行评估。在可容忍的低血压和维持满意的脑灌注压之间应该有适当的平衡。80 mmHg 的平均动脉压是目标。血流动力学稳定的患者通常接受初始和随后的随访，胸部和盆腔平片，以及胸、腹、盆腔 CT。近期证据提示某些 TAI 根本不需要修复。

非手术处理

Ⅰ级 TAI 患者可以药物治疗，用尼卡地平和艾司洛尔静脉滴注降压。理想的心率在每分钟 100 次以下，舒张压低于 100 mmHg。随后可以将静脉滴注（Ⅳ）改为口服药物。Ⅰ级患者应当在 6 周内复查影像。

血管内修复

TEVAR 术通常在安装有常备影像设备的手术室内进行，有时称之为“混合”手术室。特定损伤级别的 TAI 患者的 TEVAR 和非手术治疗相比，预后有明显改善，大多数患者选择这种方式，而不是开放手术修复。CTA 对诊断和治疗的方案是个可选择的方法。磁共振成像不能在紧急情况下广泛使用。传统血管造影术不再作为常规诊断程序推荐。一旦得到 CTA，则测量血管、选择支架，将患者送入混合手术室，植入支架。胸、腹、双侧腹股沟和双腿到膝盖都要备皮。经股动脉路径做诊断性主动脉造影（图 6）。患者静脉注射肝素抗凝，根据主动脉横断片测量选择支架。有 4 种类型的支架可供选择：Valiant (Medtronic), TX2 (Cook), TAG(W.L. Gore) 和 Relay (Bolton)。目前最小的支架是 21 mm，可用于 16 mm 直径的主动脉。当植入支架后，如有必要获取近端锚定区，可以覆盖左锁骨下动脉。对完全横断的主动脉和纵隔内出血患者应立即行血管内治疗，尽管仍有人声称这是开放手术的最后的指征（图 7）。

开放性修复

传统上对降主动脉 TAI 患者，最合适的切口是仰卧位左前外侧开胸。虽然许多外科医生用“钳夹缝合”技术，避免转流或旁路的需要，主动脉弓以远的灌注可以通过心肺转流实现（图 8）。流出通道

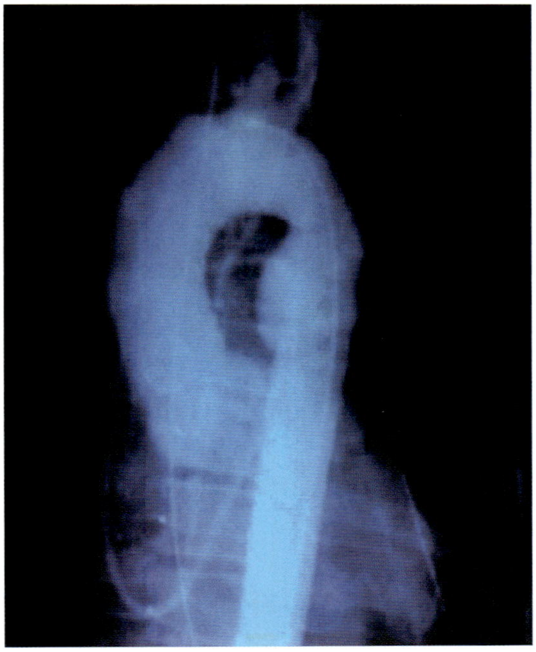

图 6　胸主动脉造影显示胸主动脉内膜破裂 (*Courtesy of J.A. Asensio, MD.*)

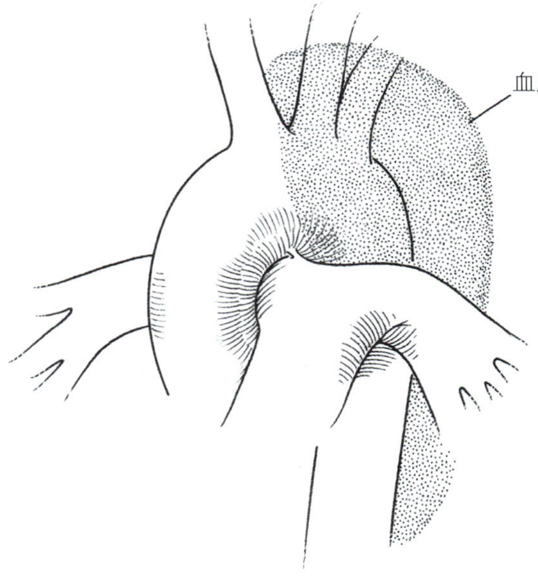

图 7　活着到达创伤中心的钝性胸主动脉损伤患者通常是有外膜包裹大的血肿。现在绝大多数患者通过 TEVAR 治疗，而很少需要开放技术、心肺旁路术或部分旁路术。因为其他技术很少采用，作者尝试描述开放技术

从心脏或升主动脉到降主动脉远侧或左股总动脉。处理胸降主动脉损伤的原则是近端 / 远端控制、处理损伤部分和重建血流连续性。患者治疗性肝素化。近端控制通过在主动脉弓左颈总和左锁骨下动脉开口之间缠绕胶布带（图 9）。胶布带也缠绕左锁骨下动脉。在动脉韧带附近通过主动脉弓后方时要避免左侧喉返神经损伤。接着控制胸降主动脉远侧（图 10-11）。简单的主动脉侧壁裂伤可以用 4-0 Ethicon 线一期缝合。复杂损伤经常须间置 Dacron 血管移植物（图 12）。不考虑所选择的技术，术后截瘫发生率平均为 8%。

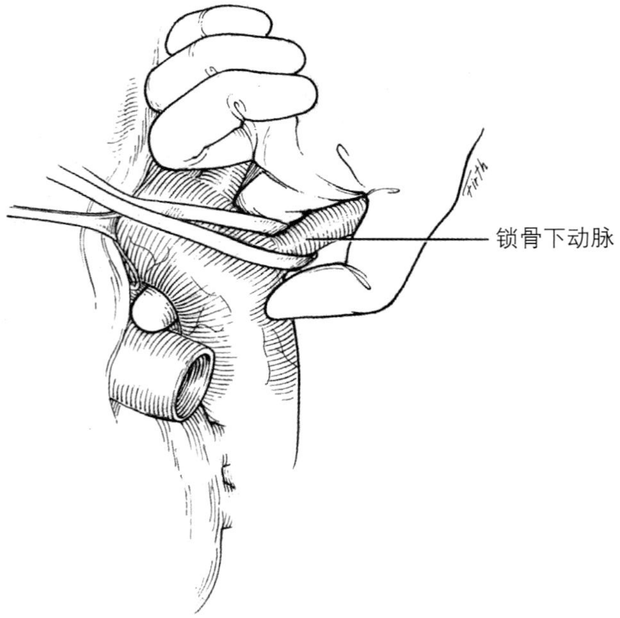

图 8　在部分或完全心肺旁路后，主动脉通过左后外侧开胸显露。主动脉弓被精细分离。图示左锁骨下动脉起始部环绕。血肿经常很大，向上和外侧延伸。钳夹缝合技术因有大量的并发症，尤其是截瘫，而放弃

胸骨正中切开术提供了上纵隔的入路。分开左无名静脉改善显露，并供外科医生显露主动脉弓及其分支。修复主动脉弓通常需要心肺旁路术。偶尔，无名动脉小的损伤可以一期修复。更多情况下，无名动脉的损伤需要旁路旷置技术。升主动脉到远侧无名动脉用一段人工血管间置缝合。近端无名动脉缝合。左颈总动脉横断伤，用聚四氟乙烯人工血管端端吻合建立主动脉旁路术更好。股腘浅静脉也用于无名动脉和颈总动脉重建。

右侧和左侧锁骨下动脉，根据损伤部位与椎动脉的位置显露不同。右侧锁骨下动脉可以经过右侧锁骨上切口显露，如果须在更近端显露切口，可以向胸骨正中延伸。左锁骨下动脉可以用锁骨上切口与锁骨切除显露，左前外侧开胸术和胸锁皮瓣（翻转门）作为最后的方法。

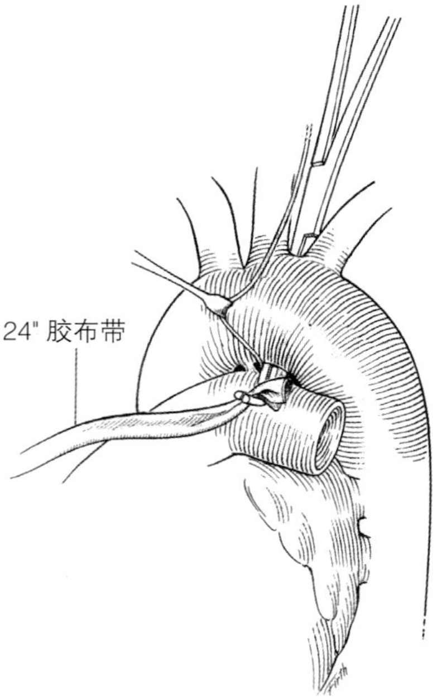

图 9　胸主动脉在颈动脉远侧和左锁骨下动脉之间环绕，在使用血管钳之前，执行此操作以确保近端控制。左喉返神经于此绕过主动脉弓和向上走行，注意保护

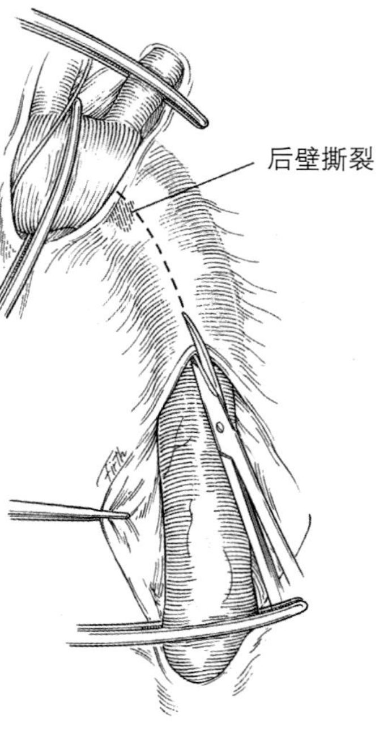

图 10　分离降主动脉，在近端控制前切开主动脉上的胸膜进入血肿，获得近端和远端控制

并发症发生率和并发症的处理

最可怕的开放手术的并发症是截瘫。肠缺血和肾衰竭是长时间阻断的结果。TEVAR 几乎不存在截瘫问题，因此很有吸引力。接受 TEVAR 的患者需要长期随访。在 1 个月、6 个月、1 年和之后的每年通过 CT 影像监控。TEVAR 特殊的并发症是内漏、支架移位、支架移植物不通畅、器械不完整。TEVAR 和开放手术相比，有低位脊髓缺血、终末期肾病和全身及支架感染等并发症。TEVAR 患者支架相关并发症与二次介入有关，而 TEVAR 的花销和开放手术没有明显不同。

死亡率

TAI 有很高的死亡率，部分原因是合并了身体其他筋膜室的损伤的高发生率。升主动脉损伤患者很少存活。高级别损伤的非手术治疗与开放手术和 TEVAR 相比有更高的死亡率。生命体征平稳到达创伤中心的升主动脉损伤患者，死亡率仍高达 50%。

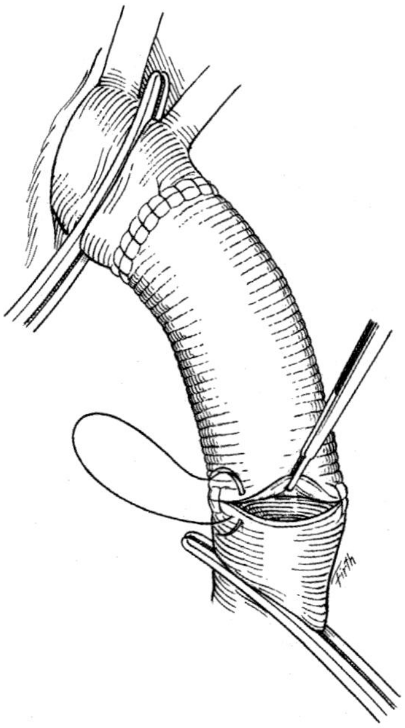

图 12　损伤的胸降主动脉用编织的 Dacron 移植物重建。人工血管直径在测量主动脉后选择。大多数成年人主动脉在 18～29 mm 之间。2-0 或 3-0 聚丙烯单股编织线用于端端吻合。肋间动脉的出血必须控制

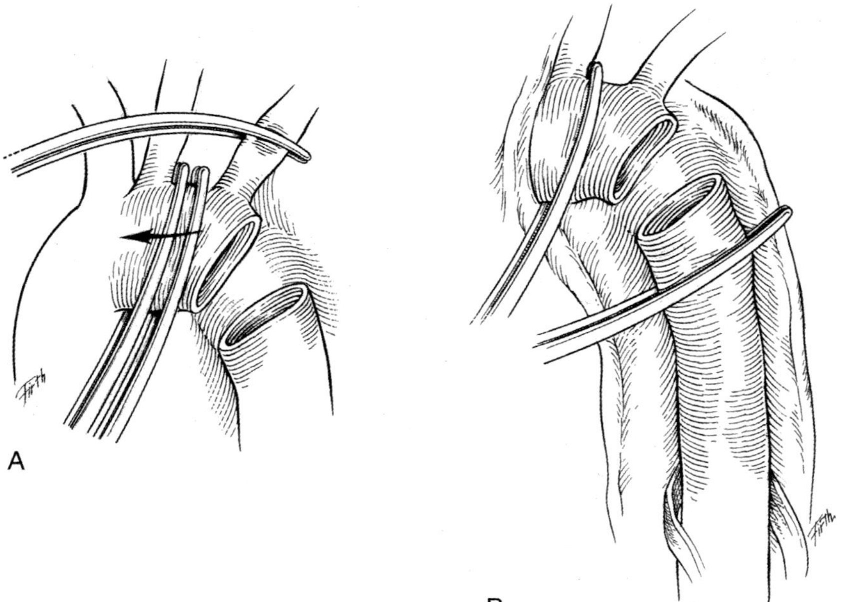

A

B

图 11　**A**，精确近端控制是最重要的。左颈总动脉和左锁骨下动脉之间的空隙通常是小的，须对主动脉和左锁骨下动脉双重钳夹，直到损伤更好显露。**B**，在切开损伤的降主动脉节段前可以重置钳子

结论

TAI发生在近1/3的钝性损伤死亡病例中，大部分死亡发生在现场。TAI幸存者，要做ATLS评估。患者应当完整地评估其他合并的致命损伤，因为许多TAI患者有其他腹内损伤，在治疗主动脉损伤前需要剖腹探查。Ⅰ级TAI可以通过单纯血压控制治疗。对于大多数需要治疗的主动脉损伤患者，即便是一个濒死的胸部血管损伤患者，TEVAR仍是一个治疗选择。开放手术有更高的死亡率、更高的截瘫率、更高的肠缺血发生率和更多的急性肾损伤。

食管损伤的治疗

A. Britton Christmas 和 J. David Richardson 著
赵　辉　周足力 著

发病率

食管损伤发病率不高，多伴发于穿通伤。直到第二次世界大战时食管创伤才被人们注意，在第二次世界大战、朝鲜战争以及越南战争的记载中一共仅有18例报道。在多数报道中，创伤性食管损伤的发病率不足1%，在穿通伤中其发生率远高于钝性损伤。在食管的创伤机制中，发生率最高的是枪伤（70%～80%），其次是刺伤（15%～20%）和猎枪伤（3%～5%），由钝伤导致的食管损伤在所有食管损伤中所占比例不足1%，极其罕见。从损伤部位上来看，最常见的是颈部食管处于过伸位时从前方的打击致伤。胃处于过伸位时从前方快速打击腹部也可能导致食管远端裂伤，最常见的损伤原因仍是刺伤和枪伤。

颈段食管损伤发生率最高，胸段和腹段食管损伤的发生率次之。实际上，所有遭受食管伤的创伤患者都伴有其他的呼吸、消化和血管系统损伤。因此，创伤外科医生必须提高警惕，以免延误诊断。虽然这些创伤的发生率极低，但是其死亡率却高达20%～30%。

诊断

根据文献报道，食管损伤的诊治若被延误，创伤患者并发症和死亡率会增高。导致延误的原因有很多，其中就包括此损害不常见的原因。由于食管损伤常伴多系统创伤，因此在开始评估食管前，诊断延误就可能发生了。而且，对于食管的损伤，即使是“单纯”的穿孔也可能诱发严重的炎症反应与纵隔组织破坏，使完整性的修复更加复杂。

在处理穿透颈阔肌的颈部穿通伤、跨纵隔的枪伤和合并支气管损伤的重症胸部创伤患者时，必须要警惕食管的损伤。食管损伤的患者最常见的临床表现包括颈痛和吞咽困难，还可能出现触诊时的肌紧张、被动运动和声音嘶哑。在没有明显的口咽部创伤时，如患者出现明显的呕血、咯血或血性鼻胃管引流液，则提示可能有食管损伤。颈部血肿的扩散当然也可能导致发热、咳嗽和喘鸣，外科医生须提高警惕。在皮下触诊时有捻发者或气肿，或是在影像学上看到椎旁积气可能提示患者存在食管损伤，胸部CT检查可能会显示皮下气肿或上纵隔积气。

胸段食管损伤早期在临床的表现上可能是非特异性的或是隐匿的，可能表现为腹部压痛或肌紧张、由于纵隔气肿导致的颈部捻发音或Hamman征（纵隔听诊时有摩擦音）。胸部穿通伤患者若出现纵隔气肿及胸腔积液时，医生须对食管损伤提高警惕。

膈下食管损伤在临床上常常表现为腹部压痛或肌紧张，患者常常以腹痛为主诉，可能进展为腹膜炎表现。直立位X线胸片或CT扫描可能会有气腹的表现。

虽然对于血流动力学不稳定的颈部或胸部穿通伤患者来说，常常须立刻寻找是否合并其他部位的创伤。但是对于血流动力学稳定的患者来说，多发伤的诊断是一个挑战。在过去，所有颈阔肌受损的颈部创伤患者都须常规探查食管是否受损。而现在许多创伤中心仅对患者进行选择性地处理，这些处理措施需要一些研究来排除食管损伤。对于病情稳定的患者，我们推荐先使用水溶性造影剂行食管造影，若未见损伤，可再用安全的稀释后的钡剂造影予以排除。因为食管造影的假阴性率高达25%，若高度怀疑患者有食管损伤，可行食管镜检查以确诊或排除。食管造影和食管镜检查的串联试验在排除食管损伤的诊断试验中特异度为 100%。即使是血流动力学稳定的颈部患者，我们也建议行食管镜探查，因为积血或血肿可以进一步定位损伤部位。由于积血污染组织，可能会影响食管损伤部位的辨别。由于诊断时间的延误与并发症发生率和死亡率密切相关，所有的诊断试验都必须尽快完成，一旦确诊食管损伤，在手术前应立刻予禁食、胃肠减压、静脉注射液体复苏和广谱抗生素治疗。

外科治疗

虽然多数颈部穿通伤可以保守治疗，但是所有的被确诊的食管损伤都应该急诊手术，外科干预的具体方式应视损伤部位、患者病情稳定程度、诊断的时间，以及联合损伤的情况而定。

在我们看来，无论哪一节段的食管损伤，都应按照统一的原则处理，这些原则包括：①尽可能用某些方法关闭所有缺损；②利用附近的组织瓣覆盖以加强或直接修补缺损，最好是肌瓣；③在修补部位附近放置引流管。根据有无浆膜层的缺损，不同食管损伤的愈合过程会有所不同。因此，支撑物的使用有助于减少愈合过程中食管漏的发生，破损处附近的肌瓣是覆盖创面和修补破损的很好选择。

颈段食管入路损伤的手术可以取领状切口或前面的胸锁乳突肌前切口；颈部单侧单发损伤患者可以取单侧前入路；颈部中线、多发或双侧颈部损伤可以取颈前切口入路。由于食管位于气管深处，因此放置胃管时经常须依靠触诊引导。在术中分离食管时，一定要避免伤及位于气管食管沟内的喉返神经；若须扩大暴露，则须离断肩胛舌骨肌。在充分游离后，可以用 Penrose 引流条环绕牵引食管，以辅助进一步的游离。

胸段食管损伤的手术最好根据损伤的程度经开胸切口处理。除了上述因素外，选择切口位置时还须考虑造影时是否有胸腔积液或食管漏。上 2/3 的胸段食管损伤最好行第 5 肋间右侧开胸切口，下 1/3 的胸段食管损伤最好行第 6 肋间左侧开胸切口。

最远段的食管损伤须行腹部切口处理，但要预留左侧开胸切口的术野以备需要。要想进一步暴露则可以取 Trendelenburg 位或移开肝左叶，正中切口可以根据暴露须向上或向剑突以左延伸 1 ~ 2 cm。分离胃食管交界部时须辅以 Penrose 引流条牵引，并手动钝性分离，如有需要，可以扩大食管裂孔，以暴露胃食管交界部的损伤。

如果能及时诊断，多数的食管损伤都可以一期修复，小的食管损伤可以横向缝合，2 ~ 3 cm 的损伤须纵向缝合以避免张力过大。不幸的是，食管损伤常被延误诊治，导致严重的纵隔炎症甚至脓毒症。此外，缺乏浆膜层会导致在此环境下非常易碎的食管组织更难一期近接处理。食管损伤可通过胸腔引流等非手术方式、食管切除和转流与旷置等方法处理，胸膜和心包补片也已被广泛用于一期修补。近些年，医生们使用了各种肌瓣来一期修补食管的缺损。然而，食管损伤手术成功的关键依然在于充分的清创、无张力修补和有效的引流。

颈段食管

当出现颈段食管损伤时，须对颈部进行探查，须仔细探查食管，以定位损伤部位，并探查有无气管和血管的损伤。探查中一旦发现有无用或坏死的组织，须彻底清创刮除，直至暴露正常组织的边界。破损处要尽可能双层闭合，用可吸收线缝合黏膜层，用不可吸收线缝合肌层。当有严重的炎症反应时，可能只能行单层闭合。所有食管破损都须用胸锁乳突肌肌瓣一期闭合，可以游离该肌肉的胸骨附着点，再将肌肉覆盖在修补后的创面上。用肌肉修补破口时也可以用可吸收线缝合。修补食管时均须用 Penrose 引流条或 Silastic 管牵引。当患者合并心血管损伤时，须从损伤对侧行颈部漏液引流，以避免造成远期的血管并发症。

有时，食管损伤的诊断延迟会导致颈部严重的炎症反应，如果损伤部位不明显、难以确定，可以在术中将食管浸入无菌水中并通气以辅助定位，也可以通过管腔内灌入亚甲蓝来定位损伤部位。若无法定位损伤处，直接采用引流以及广谱抗生素治疗也常常可以取得满意的疗效。

若食管损伤的诊断已被延迟，此时就须对患者进行充分清创、冲洗和引流。对于这些患者，一期修补是不够的。因此，可以将胸锁乳突肌瓣覆盖在吻合口上。同时，须仔细探查、冲洗以及引流食管旁及颈前组织，以防感染。在我们治疗过的患者中，一部分人的破口较大，无法用肌瓣一期关闭；还有一部分人的食管损伤由于未能及时诊断，可以用胸锁乳突肌覆盖在破口上修补。

胸段食管

如前所述，患者一旦被诊断有胸段食管损伤，就须即刻行开胸手术探查，这些患者常常会伴发急性凝固性坏死、弥漫性组织出血和严重的炎症反应，因此在处理时须打开纵隔并彻底冲洗。有时，炎症反应过重以至于破损处难以定位，这时，可以从远离破损的部位环绕，再向破损的方向游离。为了直视创口，须精细探查，破损处的黏膜层和肌层都须探查。通常伤口黏膜层的缺损会大于肌层，因此，常常须同时向近端和远端扩大肌层的切口以充分显露黏膜层的缺损。若无法完全暴露黏膜层缺损，可能会导致关闭不完全和随后的修补处的漏。若条件允许，尽量行黏膜层和肌层近接双层关闭，而且要用附近的组织覆盖在修补处上加固。

在很多病例中，胸段食管损伤的一期修补会失败。下段食管血供不丰富，且缺乏浆膜层，吻合时组织较糟脆，因此医生们经常会用周围组织支撑或一期修复损伤处。胸膜瓣被广泛应用，但它的强度有限，且有时无法完整覆盖创面。当炎症反应导致胸膜增厚时，胸膜瓣的效果可能更好。用心包做组织瓣可能听起来不够明智，因为那样会将破损处的心包腔直暴露于污染环境中。根据我们的经验，在覆盖破口或直接修补食管缺损处时，使用肌瓣的效果更好。

对于气管附近的食管损伤，用足够的组织覆盖就更为重要了，因为这样可以有效减少术后气管食管漏的发生率。若同时发生气管和食管的损伤，我们会尝试在两部分损伤的缝线之间放置肌瓣，它有更高的强度和更大的覆盖面积。常常有人建议使用肋间束用作肌瓣来支撑提供，但我们在临床中常常发现它并不能提供足够的组织，尤其在一期修补时。

在前文中我们提到，即使损伤范围达到食管直径的2/3，用肌瓣充分完全关闭破口也不会增加术后食管狭窄的发生率。上、中段食管的损伤可以用菱形肌来修补（图 1），这条肌肉可以通过肩胛骨旁切口与肩胛骨上的附着点分离，再将带蒂肌瓣置入开胸切口。对于无法用胃底支撑的远段食管，我们建议用膈肌瓣来修补（图 2）。从膈的中间部位游离一块带蒂肌瓣，并用它支持缺损或加固修补处。这块肌瓣的基底部在后方，并且注意避免损伤膈神经。膈带蒂肌瓣可以达到奇静脉水平，膈的边缘用粗的不可吸收缝线缝合。最好能双层关闭，这样还有助于折叠膈。

若胸段食管损伤未被及时诊断，后续的手术将面临重大挑战。长时间的食管穿孔会引发纵隔炎症和继发性的脓肿，使缺损处的定位复杂化。要想成功处理非包裹性的食管漏，须注意以下几点：坏死组织的清创、充分灌洗和彻底的纵隔和胸腔引流。虽然食管缺损的修复也很重要，但是我们发现这一措施在胸段食管损伤诊断延误的患者中并无意义。

所有的胸段食管损伤患者都须行广泛引流，广泛切除纵隔胸膜，并且在修补处附近放置大直径胸管。对于那些食管有大面积创伤、诊断延误或手术失败风险很大的患者，我们建议常规放置鼻胃管行胃肠减压。为了保证充足的营养支持，也可以考虑放置空肠营养管。

腹段食管

腹段食管损伤常伴发腹腔内或胸腔内的创伤，若想处理这些部位的损伤，最好通过左侧剖腹探查术，并准备开胸手术的术野。远端食管穿孔或损伤应该先用不可吸收缝线紧密分层关闭，再用 50 或 60 F 探条的 Nissen 胃底折叠术、Thal 补片或膈肌瓣来修补加强。无法直接吻合的损伤应该用膈肌瓣修补，修补区域周围应该用 Silastic 管充分引流。同时，应该放置鼻胃管以行胃肠减压，并放置空肠管以行肠内营养。

无法修补的食管损伤

有时，创伤患者会遭遇毁灭性的食管损伤。此时无法修复食管，只能采取相对姑息的技术，如食管切除、T 导管放置和伴 / 不伴食管旷置的颈段食管切除术。

在一些特殊的病例中，可以采取食管切除术，但是本团队的高年资医生在行医 35 年来从未遇到过必须行食管切除术的病例。很显然，那些无法修补的或腐蚀性损伤的食管损伤患者须急诊行食管切除术，此时，可以使用胃或结肠旁路的延期重建术。

有时，医生会遇到无法修补的食管大缺损，虽然我们会尝试用肌瓣修补破损处，但是也有报道可以采用 T 导管控制瘘。T 导管的短臂应放置在破损处，长臂穿过胸腔。根据我们的经验，如果食管的

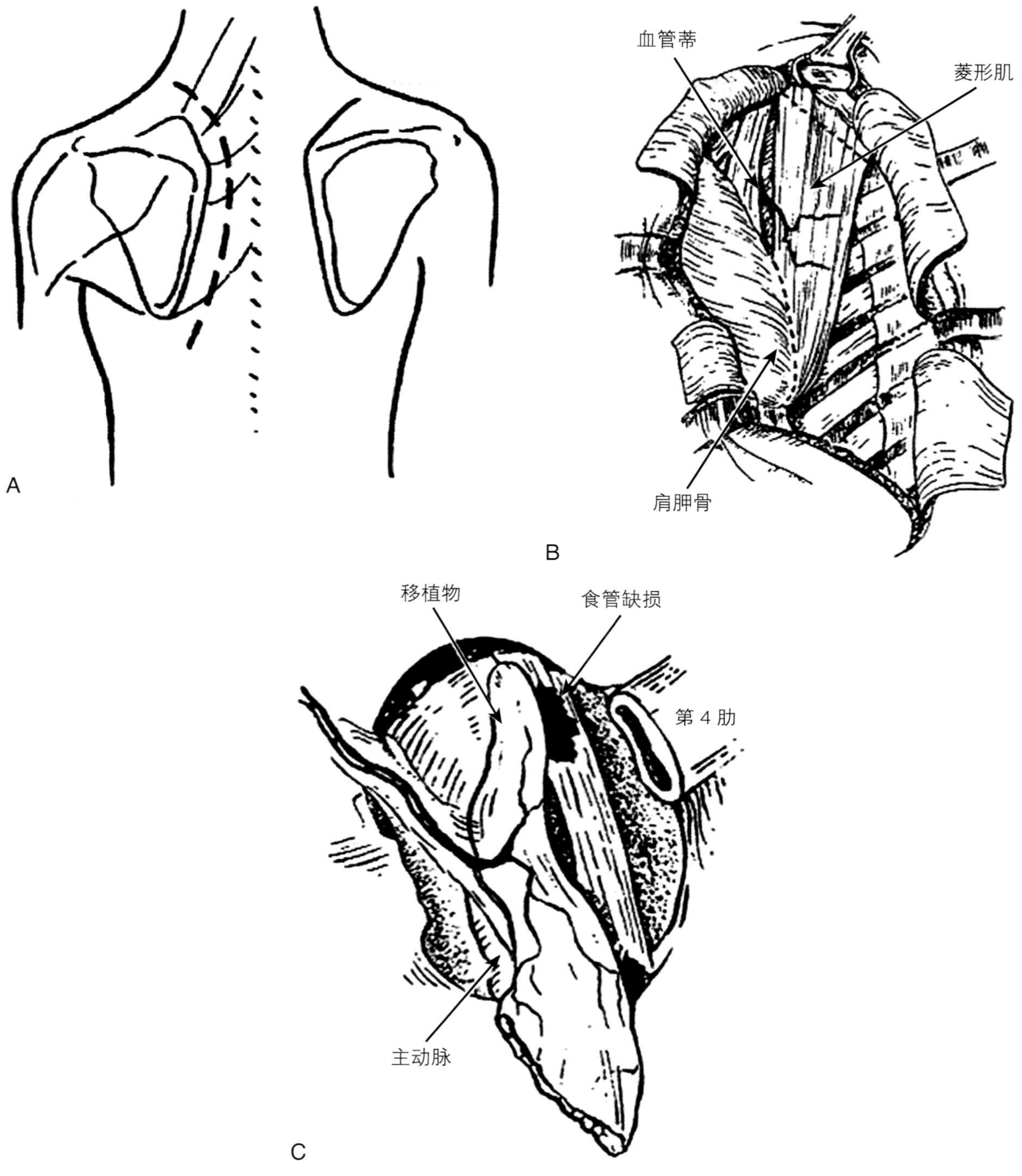

图 1　**A**，虚线所示为显露菱形肌所做的肩胛旁切口。**B**，仔细分离菱形保护其后肌血管蒂。**C**，切除肋骨以使肌瓣转入胸腔，并覆盖于食管缺损之上 (*From Richardson JD, Tobin GR: Closure of esophageal defects with muscle flaps. Arch Surg 129:541–548, 1994.*)

穿孔过大无法通过导管封堵，可以用组织瓣覆盖封闭。这种方法在诊断延误的患者中也可以使用。

不应对食管损伤的患者常规行颈段食管切除术，因为术后重建极难。根据我们的经验，术后须对患者行食管旁路分流，以避免无法控制的食管漏引发脓毒症或其他致命的并发症。如果可能的话，可以行环状食管造口术，这样就为食管损伤愈合后一期闭合食管造口创造了条件。末端食管造口术需要复杂的重建。

若已行食管分流术，在远端食管结扎时，我们

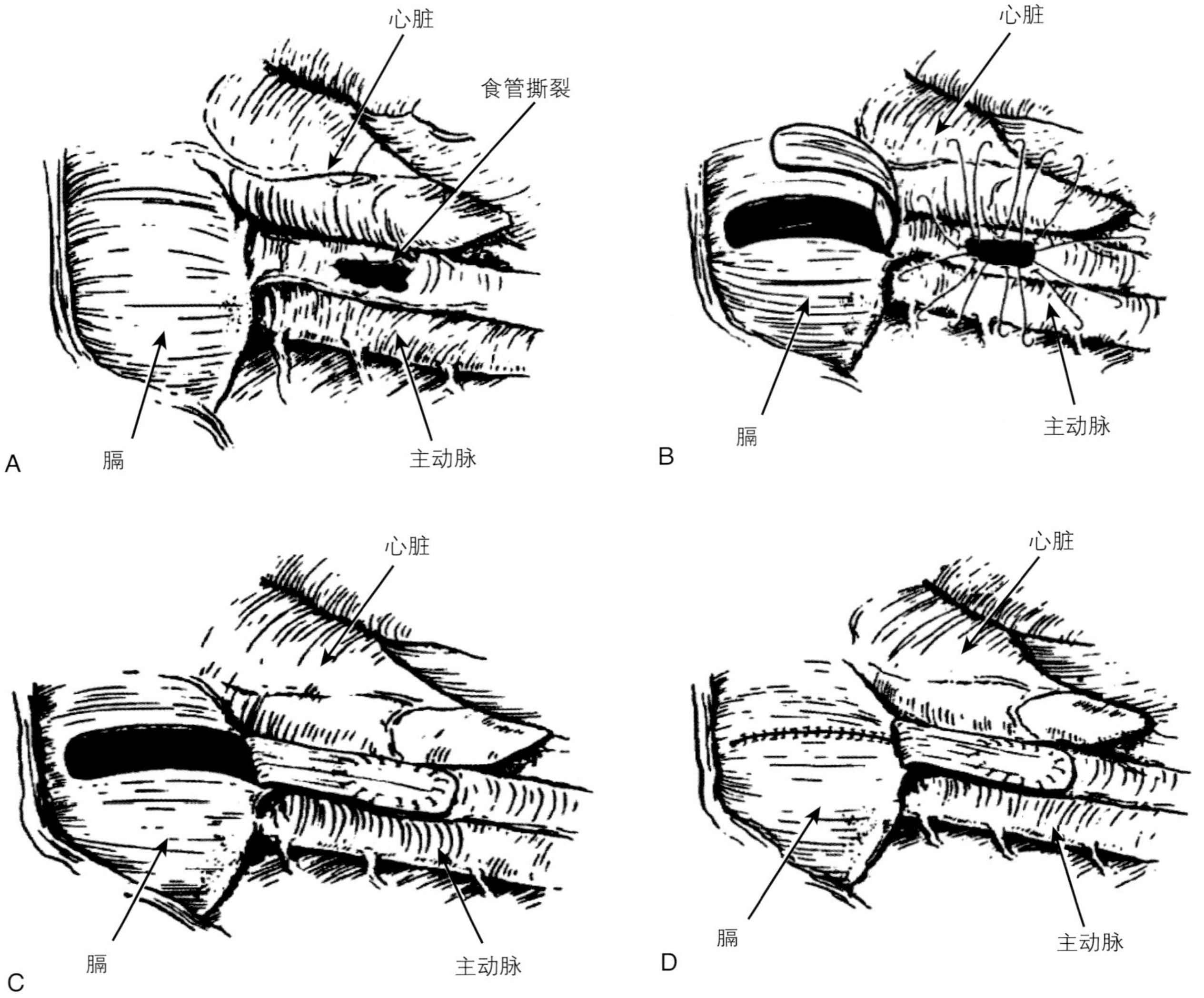

图 2 **A**，食管远端 1/3 的缺损通常邻近膈。膈可以用来修复胸中部的缺损。**B**，食管缺损的边缘经过清创并游离出一个膈肌瓣。经过食管缺损用双重缝线将膈肌瓣完整覆盖于缺损之上。**C**，膈肌瓣缝合到位。**D**，双层缝合关闭膈缺损（*From Richardson JD, Tobin GR: Closure of esophageal defects with muscle flaps. Arch Surg 129:541–548, 1994.*）

就很少再旷置食管，因为结扎会导致食管远端梗阻，并且此时的食管唯一出口就是破口，很容易滋生细菌。因此，即使近端已经分流，我们也不愿意结扎旷置远端食管。若损伤极重，必须旷置食管，那此时应行食管切除术。对于一些创伤复杂的患者，我们可以用肌瓣重建食管的功能。

食管支架的应用

在过去的 10 年中，共发表了超过 300 篇关于食管支架的报道。食管支架可以用于处理多种导致食管穿孔的情况，包括医源性损伤、吻合口漏、肥胖症治疗术的并发症，以及食管的自发性穿孔等，在复杂的慢性食管漏中，食管支架也已被证明是一种有效的治疗措施。虽然这些的大部分均为个案报道，但是也有许多为系列性的研究，可其中没有一例研究是针对创伤患者的。迄今为止，用食管支架治疗食管创伤的报道不足 5 例。由于发病率低且须紧急处理合并损伤，也不可能有更大样本量的研究报道。可能性更大的应用场合就是手术失败后处理持续的吻合口漏。

目前还没有循证医学的研究推荐在创伤性食管损伤的患者中采用覆膜食管支架治疗。对于一般状况稳定，且临床怀疑为单纯食管损伤的患者，采取此种措施是恰当的。但是如前所述，创伤患者的病情常常很复杂，会合并其他损伤。

并发症的处理

颈段食管损伤的患者出现并发症的概率高达16%，多数并发症都是由于诊断的延误和继发于食管内容物污染的感染产生的。由于组织破坏更严重，枪伤比刺伤发生并发症的概率更高。

有研究证明，诊断和治疗的延误会增加并发症的发生率。然而，几乎没有文献报道创伤性食管损伤的患者的长期预后和食管功能。当然，食管损伤最严重的并发症就是大血管和气道的损伤导致的严重出血或急性呼吸功能失代偿。继发于吻合口漏的纵隔炎、脓毒症和呼吸衰竭也为治疗带来挑战。休克、剧烈移动、清创不彻底和张力过大也是缝线开裂的危险因素。约有50%的食管漏是无症状的，只有在术后行食管造影时才能发现。一旦确定漏存在，应该立刻充分引流、应用广谱抗生素、行肠外营养或放置空肠营养管行肠内营养支持，以及禁食。这些治疗对于患者来说至关重要。介入影像学的发展技术与经皮穿刺引流的出现，对于复杂损伤的处理也有很大帮助。多数的漏可以通过保守治疗自愈。腔内支架也越来越多地被用于处理食管漏。虽然我们从未在一期治疗中使用过支架，但曾经在2个病例中，我们用食管支架来治疗创伤后迟发性漏的患者。

结论

虽然食管损伤并不常见，但是对于颈部或胸部穿通伤的患者，需要格外警惕。这些患者多合并有血管、气道或腹腔内的损伤，因此常常需要急诊手术处理。对于血流动力学稳定的患者，须立刻完善检查，排除食管损伤，以避免延误诊治。先行水溶性造影剂的食管造影，若未发现漏再行钡餐造影。因为前者的假阴性率高达25%，还可行食管镜检查以确诊。食管镜检查联合食管造影检查诊断食管损伤的特异度接近100%。若患者有颈部血肿，我们建议术中在探查前先行食管镜检查。当患者有出血、气道阻塞或血流动力学异常时，也要在术中行食管镜检查。一经确诊，须立刻应用广谱抗生素、严密的外科手术修补、术中充分清创，以及术后引流来保证治疗的成功。

第 8 章　腹部损伤

膈损伤

Charles E. Lucas 和 Anna M. Ledgerwood 著
刘敏伟　翁文翰 译

解剖和生理

膈起于腹膜与脏胸膜交汇的平面，是由胸骨后缘、下方 6 个肋软骨和后部腰肋角构成的环，向中心延伸。肌肉群由左、右和中央 3 叶构成，向中央汇聚于中心腱（图 1-2）。膈的中后部边缘大部分由膈脚构成，中央的肌瓣还参与心包的构成。左、右后外侧的肌瓣若闭合不全会导致胸腹膜裂孔疝。部分闭合可能导致胸膜和腹膜不连，影响中心腱的完整性，导致所谓的膈膨升（图 3-4）。

膈会随着呼吸收缩。充分呼气时膈顶会上升至胸腔内，深吸气时膈会下沉呈盘状。上下的幅度可达 3 个肋间。膈后部下沉到最低位置时可达第 2、3 腰椎，后沟可以向下延伸至肾中部。上腹部枪伤或刺伤的患者常常伴发后沟处的易忽略的穿孔，此部位穿孔导致的血胸须行开腹探查术来诊断治疗。

膈上有 3 个大的裂孔，分别有主动脉、食管和下腔静脉穿行（图 1）。前部较小的裂孔为 Morgagni 裂孔，位于剑突后方，内乳动脉从中穿行。膈的正中部分从 Morgagni 裂孔延伸至食管裂孔，称为正中缝。这部分膈由于缺乏血管，因此可以一分离用于暴露下纵隔（图 2）。膈静脉可能在食管裂孔上 1 cm 的位置穿行于中部平面，因此，这一部位的无意中的损伤可以导致大出血。膈神经起于 C3–C5，并在

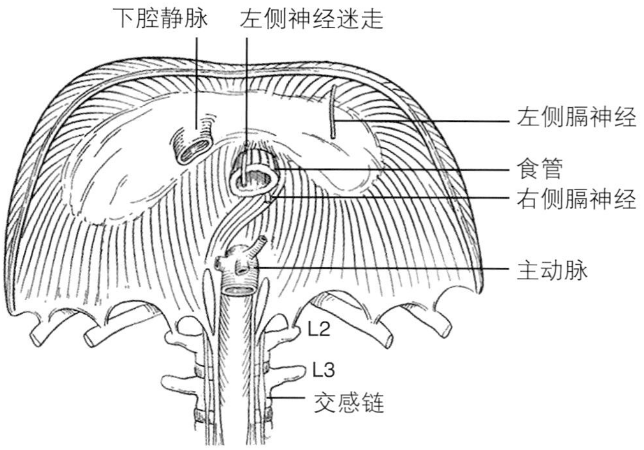

图 1　膈的下面观。突出位于后方的孔和中心腱。IVC，下腔静脉 (*From Asensio AA, Petrone P, Demetriades D: Diaphragmatic injuries: operative techniques in general surgery, Philadelphia, 2000, Saunders.*)

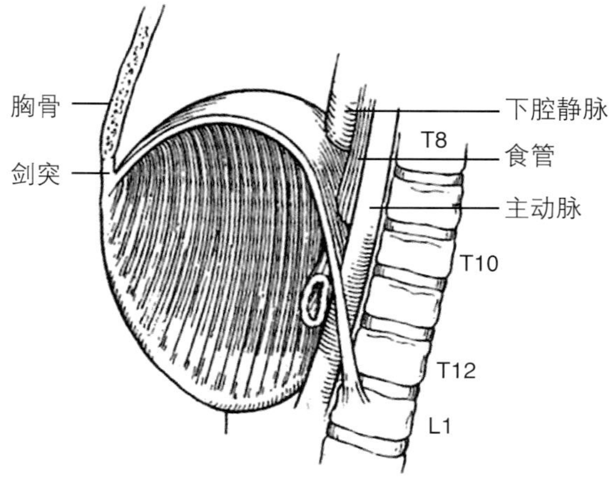

图 2　膈的侧面观。注意剑突和前方的胸骨附着物，以及膈脚向后方的延伸。IVC，下腔静脉 (From Asensio AA, Petrone P, Demetriades D: Diaphragmatic injuries: operative techniques in general surgery, Philadelphia, 2000, Saunders.)

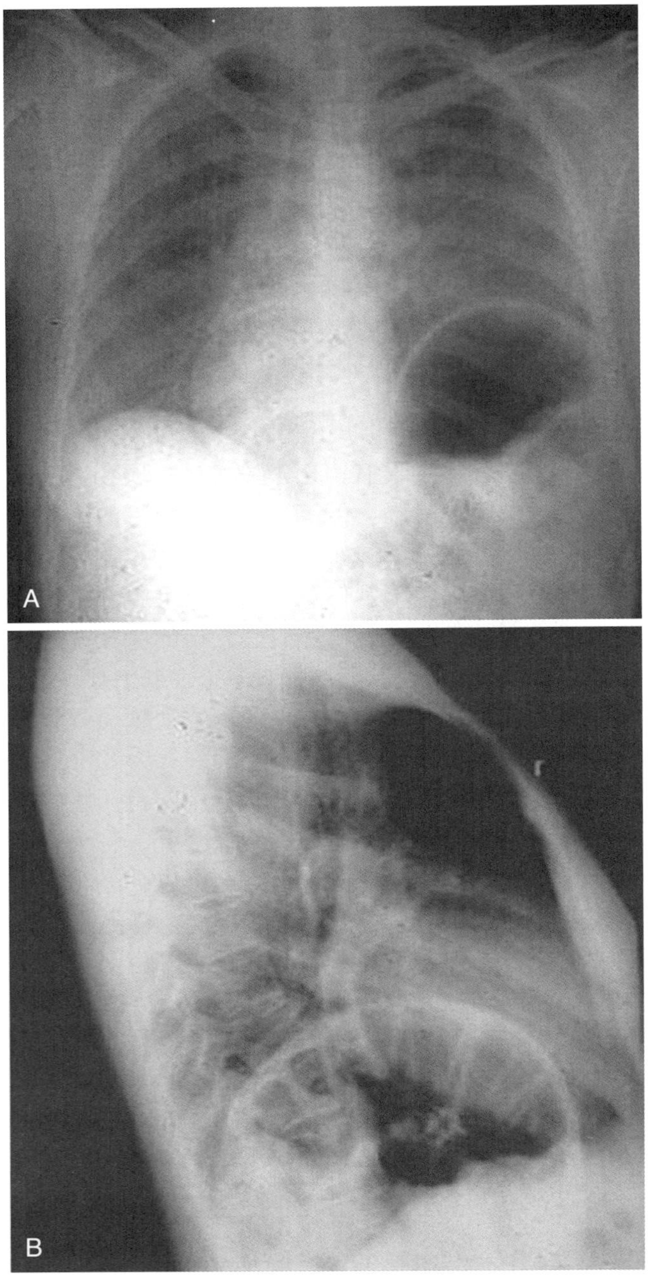

图 3　术前正侧位胸片显示膈膨升误诊为车祸伤后膈破裂

纵隔内向下穿行至膈，并向前、侧、后方发出分支（图 1）。

发病率

Asensio 等在一个多中心的研究中曾报道，在所有经历躯体创伤的患者中，膈损伤的发病率为

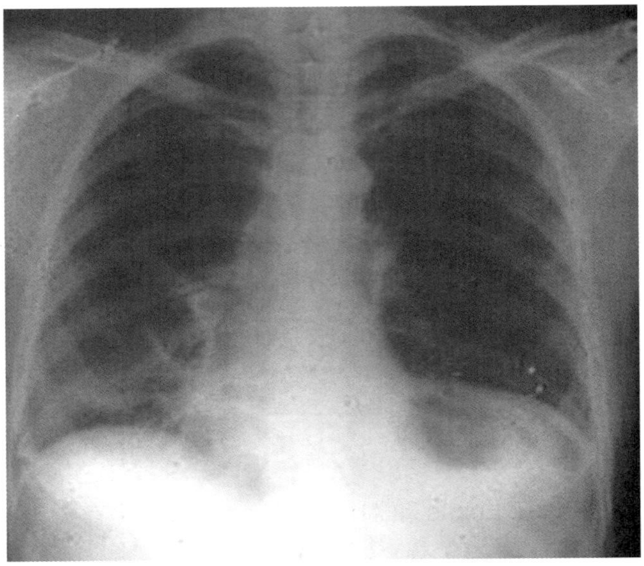

图 4　膈膨升折叠术后误诊为膈破裂

0.8%～5.8%，平均为 3%；各中心报道的发病率差别很大，反映了各中心处理的损伤种类的差别，以及不同中心确认膈穿孔时的谨慎程度。在乡村地区的创伤中心里钝伤较多见，而城市内部的创伤中心则主要收治穿通伤患者。膈破裂的发生率在不同中心报道也不同，这同样反映了穿通伤患者在不同中心的治疗策略的差异。目前，多数穿通性锐器刺伤腹腔的患者，若无腹膜炎或腹腔积血的征象时都行非手术治疗（nonoperative management，NOM），这类创伤还包括造成血胸的下胸部刺伤。过去人们推测，在剖腹术探查时可以发现合并的膈穿孔，若仅行导管胸廓造口术则可能会漏诊膈穿孔（图 5）。最后，合并右侧血气胸的右上象限枪伤患者，即使伴发不少于 2 处的膈穿孔和肝的穿通伤，也单纯行导管胸廓造口术。这些未被诊断的膈穿孔也没能在创伤注册系统中编码。对下胸部穿通伤的患者，须常规行诊断性腹腔灌洗（diagnostic peritoneal lavage，DPL），当灌洗液呈粉红色且红细胞计数低于 100 000 细胞 / 平方厘米时，就可以预测患者有膈穿孔，这一推测可通过后续的剖腹术来证实并治疗。超声（ultrasonography，US）可以替代 DPL，且对于检测少量出血灵敏度较低。上腹部穿通伤导致的膈穿孔即使经剖腹术探查也可能会漏诊，因为弹片可能只穿透了腹横肌部分。术后的血胸可以证实有漏诊的膈损伤，此时可以行导管胸廓造口术治疗。在 20 世纪 70 年代，医生会常规对多数腹部穿通伤的患者行开腹探查术，那时的枪

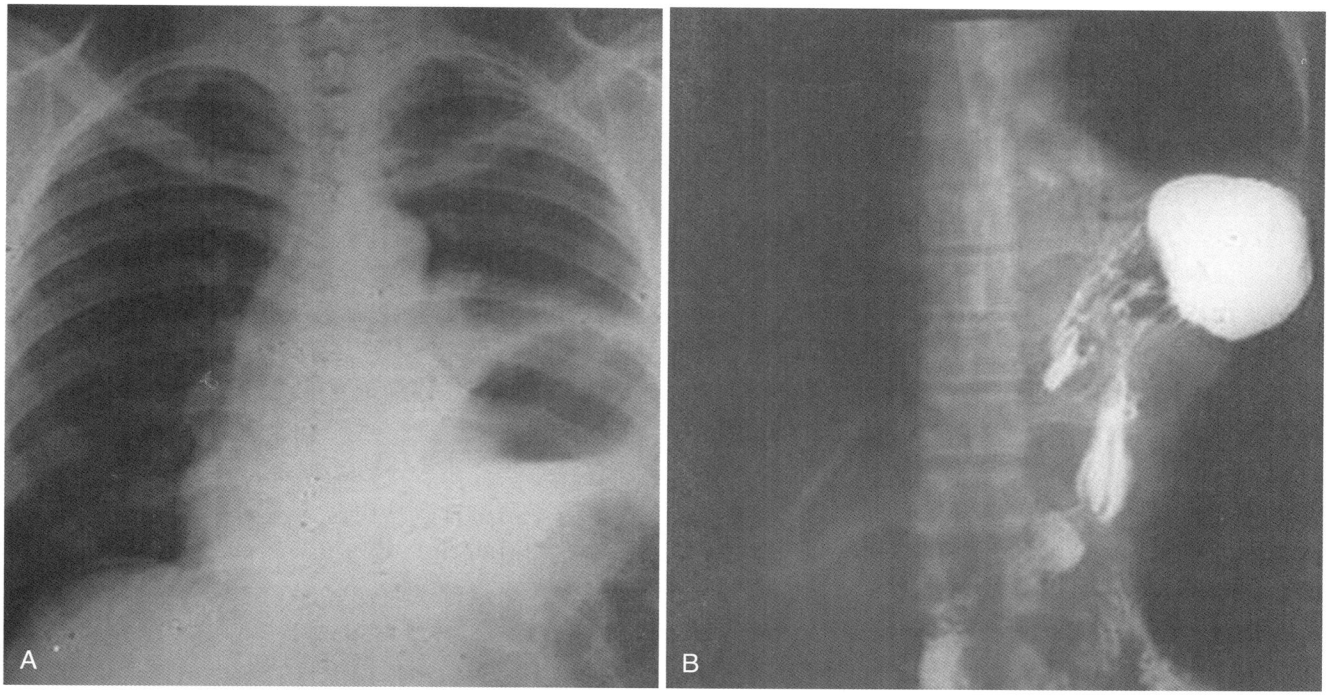

图 5　**A**，胸部前后位 X 线片，显示 18 个月前曾通过导管胸廓造口术治疗左侧胸部刺伤的患者出现膈疝。**B**，泛影葡胺确认左侧胸部存在胃

伤和刺伤所致的膈穿孔发病率分别为 19% 和 11%；自非手术治疗时代起，这两种损伤的发病率分别为 8% 和 2%。在同样的住院治疗中，钝伤患者的膈损伤被漏诊得更少。然而，在经历严重的躯体钝性创伤的患者中，有很大一部分患者会在伤后数年出现膈疝，而这类损伤在当初就诊时常会被漏诊。相似地，现今报道的躯体钝性创伤导致膈损伤的发病率不到 1%，行剖腹术的钝伤患者发生膈破裂的发病率约为 3%。

损伤机制和部位

根据损伤机制的不同，膈穿孔的部位也不同。Lopez 等注意到，那些无症状的腹部穿通伤且行 NOM 的患者，膈钝性破裂的发生率为其他患者的 4 倍（从 13% 升高至 66%）。钝伤经典的发生机制是机动车迎面撞击（motor vehicle collision，MVC），或侧面碰撞（T 骨）导致腹内压明显升高，进而导致膈过度伸展破裂。破裂常发生在中心腱的左后外侧部，破损经常延伸到肌部。膈的钝性破裂还可以继发于攻击、冲压、高处坠落和爆炸伤。破裂最常发生在后外侧，也可发生在食管裂孔附近、右肝上方裸区附近，以及伴发的包内疝时的双侧剑突下的部位。在一篇包括 1 589 名患者、32 篇出版的文献综述中，Asensio 等发现左侧膈破裂的患者有 1 187 人（75%），右侧破裂的有 363 人（23%），双侧破裂的有 39 人（2%）。既往，人们将右侧膈破裂的低发病率归功为肝的缓冲性保护作用；人们也提出了左侧膈相对薄弱的理论，但却从未证实。穿通性穿孔的位置可以在膈的任何部位。双侧穿孔多发生于流弹伤。刺伤所致穿孔常位于膈周围。

损伤的严重度分级

膈破裂严重程度的判断主要依据美国创伤外科学会提出的 5 级器官损伤量表。Ⅰ级损伤是挫伤或未破裂的血肿。Ⅱ级是直径小于 2 cm 的裂伤。Ⅲ级是 2～9 cm 的裂伤。Ⅳ级是 10～25 cm 的裂伤。Ⅴ级损伤则是大于 25 cm 的裂伤。穿刺伤和低速枪伤的患者最有可能受轻伤（Ⅰ级和Ⅱ级）。钝伤患者的膈更有可能出现Ⅲ级或Ⅳ级裂伤。大面积膈损伤（Ⅴ级）通常见于近距离射击枪开枪后、高速步枪穿过身体或爆炸之后。

诊断

钝伤后膈破裂的诊断常常基于X线胸片检查，显示左侧胸腔内出现胃泡（图6）。通过鼻胃管注射的造影剂流入胸腔，填充疝入胸腔内的胃。膈破裂的其他征象包括肋膈角模糊。单侧膈明显升高及左侧胸腔内出现结肠（图6）。存在胸部和骨盆等的多系统损伤合并低血压患者更容易发生膈损伤。当初始X线胸片检查不能明确诊断时，后续可对躯干进行CT扫描，以发现膈的损伤；然而，CT并不那么灵敏。

当钝伤发生于右侧胸部时，肝可能会阻止腹内脏器进入右侧胸腔。然而，钝伤合并右侧气胸伴严重出血的患者应怀疑肝裸区附近的右侧膈撕裂，并且这是出血的来源（图7）。双侧膈破裂出现的概率要低得多，但是，当出现双侧膈破裂时，由于两侧膈均可抬高，故可能造成诊断延迟。另外，双侧肋膈角均显示不清有助于双侧膈破裂的诊断（图8）。对于这部分患者，重复进行胸部检查后常会发现单侧或双侧膈的进一步抬高（图8）。当X线胸片检查显示左侧膈破裂范围似乎很大，但患者症状轻微时，应再次询问病史，排除之前左膈就存在解剖学变化的情况，如有可能，最好拿到既往的X线胸片资料（图3）。

当X线胸片未能明确有无膈破裂时，可能要借助其他检查。胸腹部CT扫描可能有用，但灵敏度不高；腹腔镜检查在识别膈损伤方面已经变得越来越流行，尤其是伤口为穿通伤时。另外，锝扫描已被采用，但价值有限。DPL可能有助于发现下侧胸部穿通伤患者的膈损伤，但用于躯干钝性伤患者则不太可靠。胸腔镜检查已被用于先前被漏诊的膈损伤患者。最后，我们也尝试使用磁共振成像，但其价值有限。

膈穿通伤的诊断通常在剖腹术中治疗其他器官损伤时发现。因此，由于在大多数躯干刺伤和一些枪伤之后医生使用NOM较多，许多膈穿孔未被诊断。当下侧胸部刺伤引起无症状的患者血胸时，少量腹腔积血的DPL强烈提示膈穿孔。腹腔镜检查可对小穿孔进行确认并修复。对这部分患者的漏诊可能导致其后期出现膈疝（图5）。周围粘连的存在，可能增加修复这类损伤的复杂性，但通常可通过经腹的手术方式顺利完成。当穿孔出现在膈中间部分近食管时，疝入的脏器可能延伸到心包周围，使得诊断更为困难。

膈中间部分的破裂增加了用剖腹术进行其他损伤修复时漏诊膈破裂的可能性（图9）。完成相关的腹内损伤治疗后，外科医生应仔细检查膈的所有表面，包括三角韧带后方的膈后部。

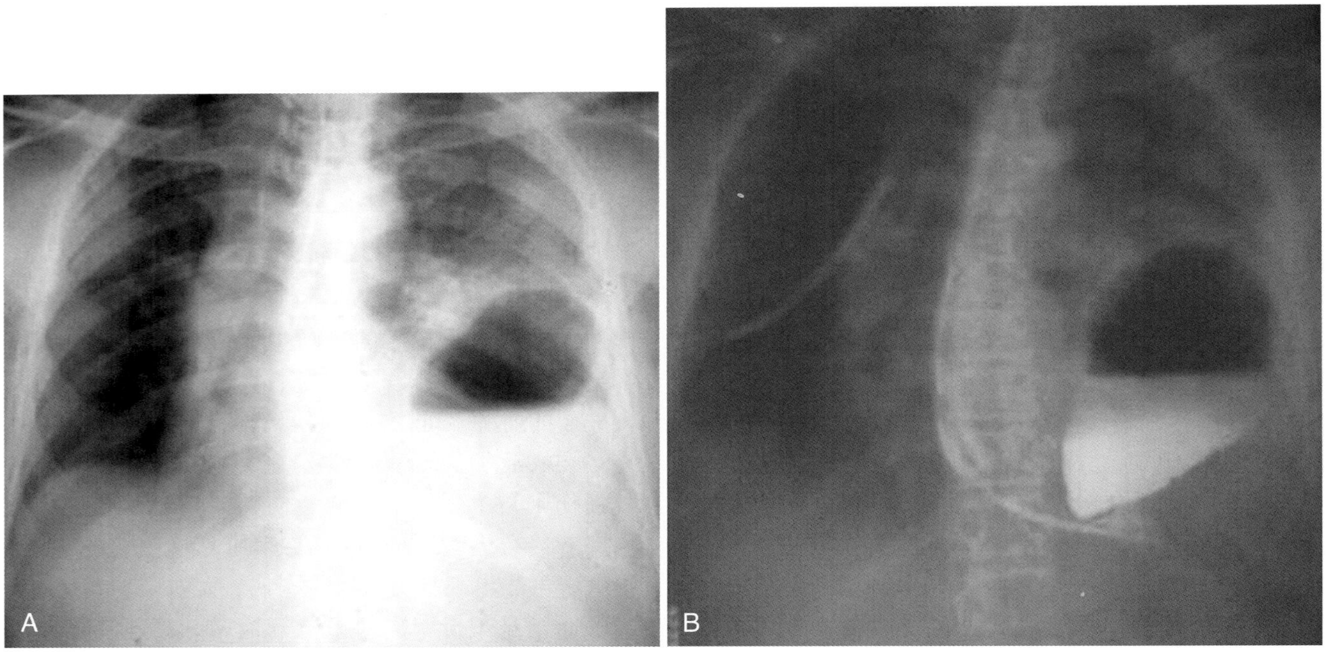

图6 **A**，前后位X线胸片显示钝性创伤后左侧胸腔内出现明显的胃泡。**B**，通过鼻胃管注射造影剂证实存在胃填充

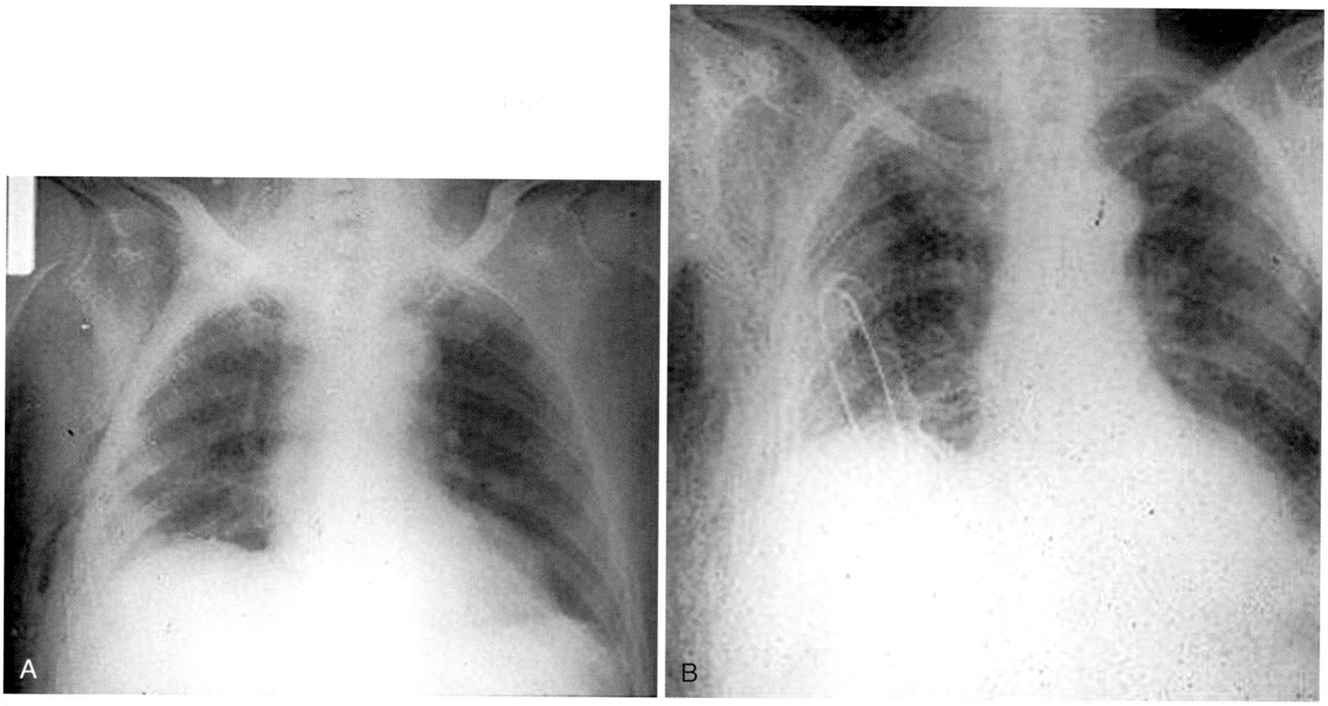

图 7　**A**，这名 86 岁的男子被一辆公共汽车撞伤，存在右肋骨折、皮下气肿和血胸。注意肋膈角模糊。**B**，右侧胸管引出 500 ml 血液，在接下来的一小时内继续出血 300 ml。剖腹术探查发现膈顶部有一巨大裂口、肝损伤Ⅳ级，均已修复

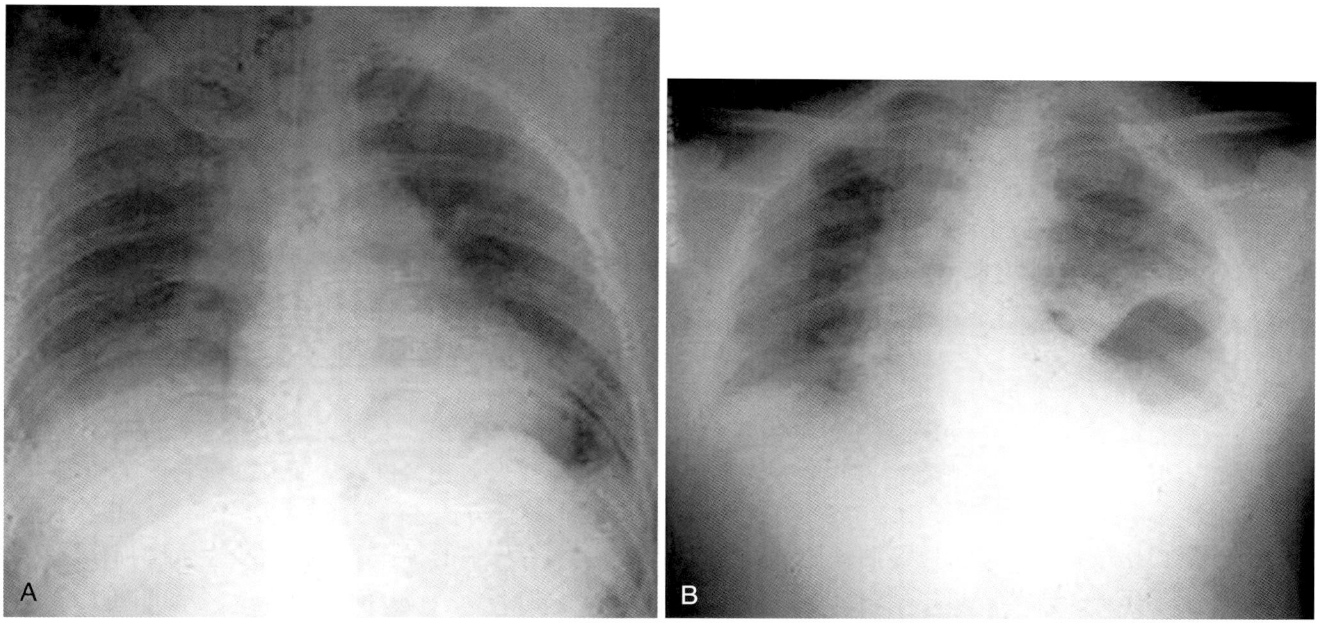

图 8　**A**，老年患者与方向盘撞击后，**X** 线胸片显示，左侧与右侧相比没有膈抬高，但左肋膈角模糊。**B**，**2 h** 后，双侧膈均升高，双侧肋膈角均模糊。剖腹术探查发现双侧 膈破裂

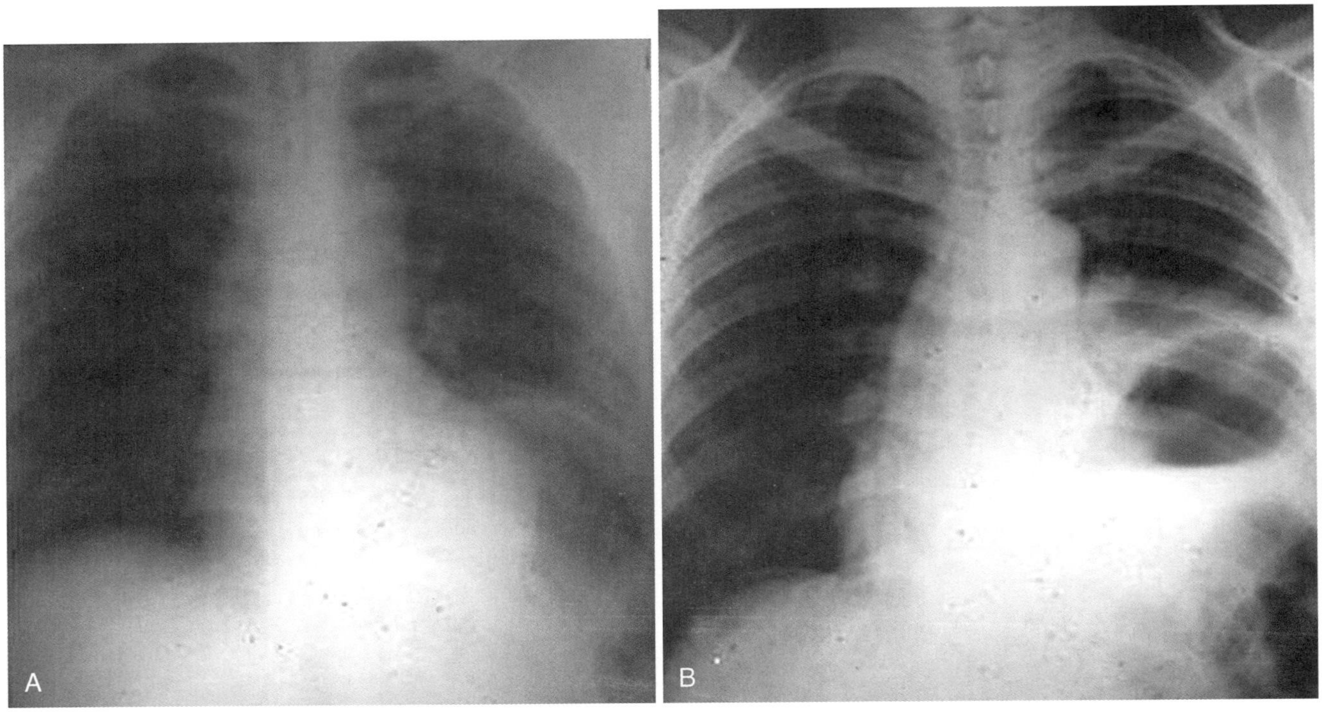

图 9 **A**，术后 **X** 线胸片，剖腹术后 1 天，Ⅲ级肝钝性损伤修复后，显示左侧胸部有气泡，认为是膈膨升。**B**，这个气泡 1 天后变大，再次手术，发现左侧三角韧带后方与食管裂孔相邻处的膈存在 4 cm 的纵向撕裂

处理

膈损伤的严重度以及相关损伤的程度决定了手术治疗的最为合适的策略。关于休克患者的复苏以及特定器官损伤处理的顺序在本书中的其他部分讨论。应使用抗生素。多数Ⅰ级损伤（挫伤或者血肿）是在因为其他原因做剖腹术或者开胸术探查时发现的，这类损伤不需要手术干预，但是术者必须进行全面探查以免遗漏更为严重的损伤。如果发现有较小的膈全层穿孔，推荐进行简单关闭（图 10）。如果是在做腹腔镜手术过程中发现的，较小的损伤可以在腹腔镜下进行缝合。使用缝线的类型根据术者本人的习惯而定，作者倾向于使用 2-0 或 1-0 可吸收缝线。如果损伤位置靠后，可以使用长的直角钳通过穿孔钩住膈来放置缝线，可以暴露穿孔。第一个缝线可以作为后续缝合暴露膈的把手（图 11）。

较大的Ⅲ级损伤，长度为 2 ~ 10 cm。如果损伤裂口是线性的话，例如大的刀刺伤和部分患者钝伤，也可以通过上面描述的方法进行缝合（图 11）。然而由高速弹片或者钝伤引起的Ⅲ级裂伤，通常裂口是不规则的。术中在显露裂口后，可以先进行几针“策略性缝合”以对合不规则的裂口，从而有利于后续缝合。对于不规则的组织碎片，小范围的清创也有利于保留更多的组织，以利于对合。作者习惯于先使用 1-0 可吸收线间断缝合，以对合不规则的裂口，然后用 1-0 可吸收线连续缝合，来进行确定性关闭。

对于撕裂超过 10 cm，并伴有中度组织缺损的Ⅳ级裂伤来说，手术重建的难度较大。这类创伤有时会伴有腹腔脏器疝入左侧胸腔，常见的包括胃、脾、结肠，也会有小肠及网膜进入胸腔。术中在显露裂口后，须将这些器官在腹部重新定位。首先可以尝试轻柔的牵拉，如果内脏抵抗牵拉，可以将手通过裂口伸入胸腔，托起脾，将其从胸腔推回到腹腔。如果膈裂口太紧，卡住疝入内脏的话，以依据内脏的半径适当切开裂口，从而方便术者的手伸到疝内容物上方，方便还纳入腹腔。这个措施可以保护脾，经过术者仔细的操作，一般很少发生脾损伤。多数的Ⅳ级损伤，不使用补片或者改变膈的附着位置即可完成修复。膈在放松状态伸缩度很高，因此对合后一般不会产生明显的张力。尽管一期关闭后膈修补的一侧可能突出会减少，但是这对远期的影响非常小。如果裂口边缘难以对合的话，可以尝试改良的 Z 形成形术。理论上讲，Z 形成形术所做的切口须从膈中心放射状延伸到外周，有利于保护膈神经。

但是实际上，即使切断了部分膈神经分支，膈修复的远期效果都不错。对较大的缺损进行修复时，首先应该对合缺损的中间部分，侧部分则可以精确地重新分布从而避免形成“狗耳形”的闭合口。

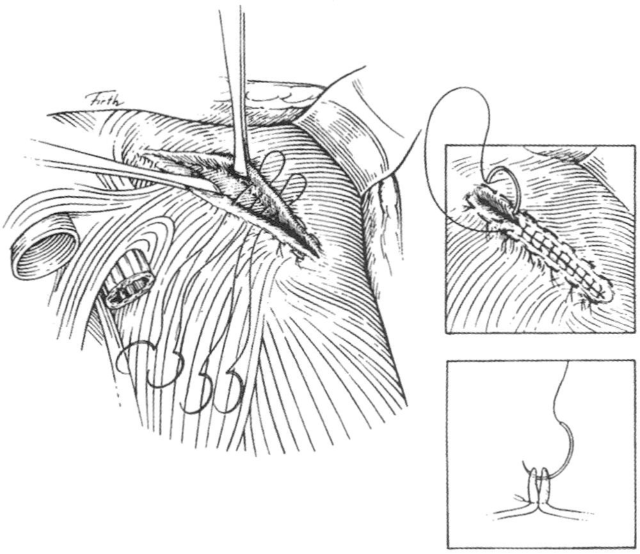

图 10　多数的轻度膈损伤可以通过间断缝合或者连续缝合进行修复。作者习惯于使用 0 号可吸收聚羟基乙酸线进行连续缝合。如果损伤相对较重的话，可以补充几针间断缝合进行加强（*From Asensio AA，Petrone P，Demetriades D*: Diaphragmaticinjuries: operative techniques in general surgery，*Philadelphia，Saunders，2000.*）

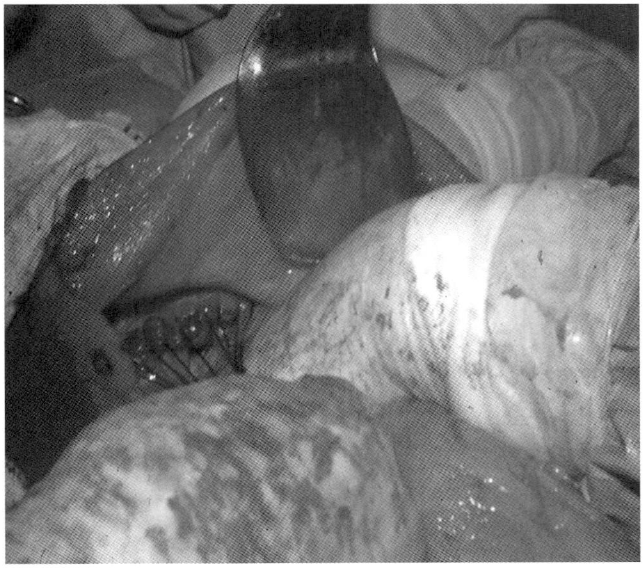

图 11　Ⅲ级钝伤后膈穿孔，用 0 号不可吸收线连续缝合进行修复

Ⅴ级膈创伤通常伴有超过 25 cm 的组织缺损，手术难度非常大。一般来讲，如果邻近的胸腔及腹壁是完整的话，较大的伴主要组织丢失的缺损可以一期关闭。如果在肌松状态下都不能完成无张力对合的话，可以先切断膈外周的附着点，将膈边缘上移 2 ~ 3 个肋间的距离后再附着。这样能够松解出较多的正常组织，从而有利于无张力缺损修复。手术的远期效果不错。

死亡率

由于损伤原因、损伤严重度及累及器官的范围不同，目前已有报道的膈损伤发病率及死亡率差异很大。大部分严重的并发症及死亡病例都是由于合并损伤造成的。Lopez 等表示目前膈破裂后死亡率的显著升高主要是因为膈钝性破裂的比例较高。大部分躯干锐性伤都通过非手术治疗，因此膈轻微锐性损伤被忽略了。钝性膈损伤的患者常常合并肝、脾甚至更严重的肺的损伤。同时合并的多根肋骨骨折及肺挫伤常导致呼吸功能受损，需要长时间的通气支持，它最终导致死亡的情况并不少见。

Asensio 等的综述提出膈损伤总死亡率为 4.3% ~ 41%，平均死亡率为 13.7%。较低的死亡率的情况主要发生在膈穿通伤患者中。较高的死亡率情况由 Boulanger 等报道，主要囊括了合并肋骨、肺及脑部损伤的患者。他们在同一时期报道的穿通性膈损伤患者的死亡率低于 4%。对于合并低血压及腹膜炎的躯干伤患者仍然需要手术治疗。在这种其他器官致死性损伤发生率显著高于膈，膈穿孔会仅被当作轻微损伤。因此，膈穿通伤死亡率可能超过 30%，主要是因为合并其他损伤而失血造成的死亡。

损伤机制还会影响治疗方法的选择以及钝性创伤后出现危及生命的相关损伤的可能性。高速车祸伤的患者更容易出现涉及肺、脑和盆腔等脏器的危及生命的合并损伤。气囊保护减少了市区内车祸中的膈损伤。相比之下，无力偿还毒品债务而导致的坠落伤及冲击伤患者更可能仅存在孤立的损伤。这个现象反映在市区内膈钝性破裂患者死亡率相对较低。我们在 2004 年治疗的 11 例膈钝性破裂患者中无死亡病例发生，但是 2010 年有 6 例已无生命体征的创伤患者，在尸检中被发现有包括膈钝性破裂在内的多发损伤。

发病率

与死亡率类似，能见到的膈损伤主要来源于其他器官的损伤。肺功能不全主要是由于多发肋骨骨折后的肺不张、肺炎及肺挫伤导致的。枪伤后更容易出现肺内血肿感染，发展为肺脓肿。在Ⅳ级或Ⅴ级损伤中为了达到一期关闭，偶尔会在膈修补过程中由于广泛游离而导致膈在手术中破坏。然而膈修补失败并不常见。其他膈损伤并发症包括膈神经麻痹、膈上脓胸和膈下脓肿等。RoDriguez-Morales 等报道肺不张的发生率为 65%，脓胸发生率为 5%。

胸部创伤中的复杂膈修补

对于合并有胸壁或腹壁损伤的Ⅴ级膈损伤，手术难度较大。这些巨大损伤常常由于近距离枪击或高速步枪导致。关于这类罕见损伤的手术技巧描述很少，很可能是因为这类损伤死亡率极高。这类巨大损伤须同时重建膈与躯干壁才可能成功修复。重建手术分几步完成。

这些患者典型表现为休克，因为经常合并大血管、肺或腹腔内脏器（尤其是肝）的损伤。在快速复苏过程中，术者必须谨记躯干壁与大的膈破裂的复杂修复需要有双侧主支气管的独立气道控制。双腔导管气管插管可以保证在胸腹壁的重建及膈修补过程中患侧肺的萎陷。同时双腔导管气管插管还能避免患侧的积血通过重力从隆嵴流向对侧，这会导致术后严重的呼吸衰竭。术中首要目标是快速控制出血，可能须对受损严重的肺进行肺叶切除术（图 12）。术者首先须对胸壁及膈上失去活力的组织进行清创（图 13）。巨大损伤后的缺损经常会影响一期修补的成功。如果损伤仅限于腹部，就可以使用腹壁填充技术来处理。然而，如果损伤累及胸腔，那么开放性填充胸腔是无法做到的，因此，须使用一些充满想象力的修补方法。某些情况下可以将膈移动，固定到胸腔更靠上的位置（图 14）。这个方法须将膈前侧、后侧及外侧的附着游离，然后将其重新固定到受损胸壁的上方内侧（图 15）。这个方法保证了胸腔的密闭性，而胸壁的缺损在肋骨中。仅暴露了腹腔，这个缺损就可以使用腹腔填充技术来处理了。持续的换药可以让肉芽组织在腹腔脏器上充分生长，然后将游离厚皮瓣覆盖在肉芽组织上（图

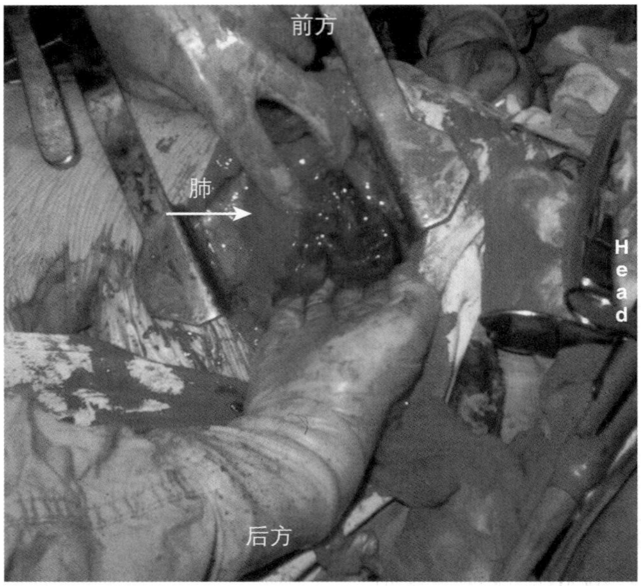

图 12　该患者遭受近距离枪击，左侧胸壁及左下肺巨大损伤

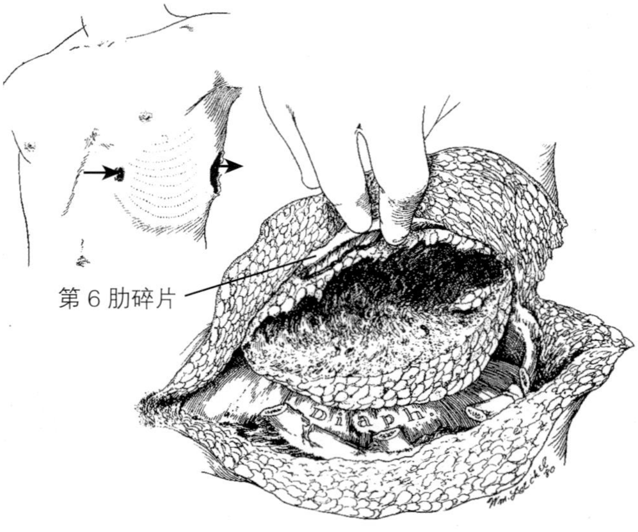

图 13　经过广泛胸壁组织清创和左肺叶切除止血后，该患者出现胸壁全层缺损

16）。晚期缺损的重建可以等患者创伤康复后，通过旋转筋膜移植物来完成。

膈是一个中心性供血的巨大肌性器官，因此分离与重新缝合相对较容易。由于膈是天然组织，感染风险较低。即便部分膈在爆炸中损坏，剩下的部分一般仍然足够重建。这个方法对于低位全层胸壁缺损非常有效。枪伤后高位胸壁缺损可以通过上叶切除合并胸廓成形术的伤口覆盖以及旋转背阔肌瓣

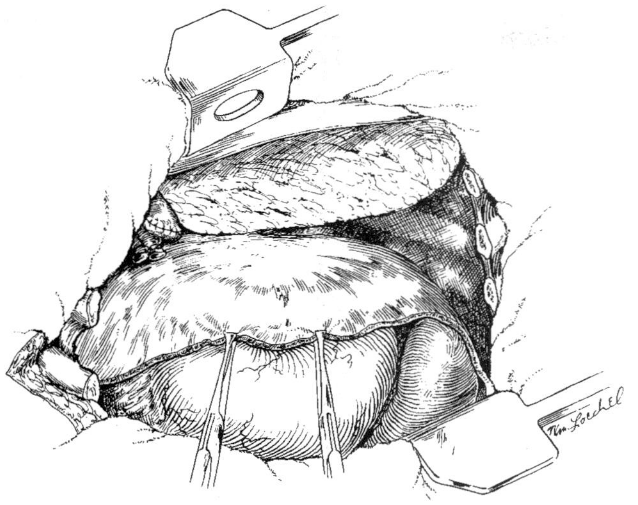

图 14 如图 13 显示的广泛清创后，游离膈前侧、后侧及外侧后，将其重新固定到更高位置的 3 个内部空间，以便将胸壁缺损转变为腹部缺损

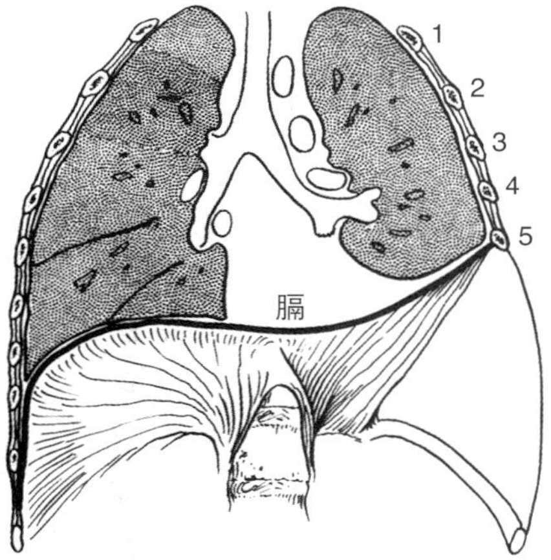

图 15 将膈重新安置在胸壁全层缺损上方的内部空间中，将胸壁缺损转变为腹壁缺损，然后再填充修补

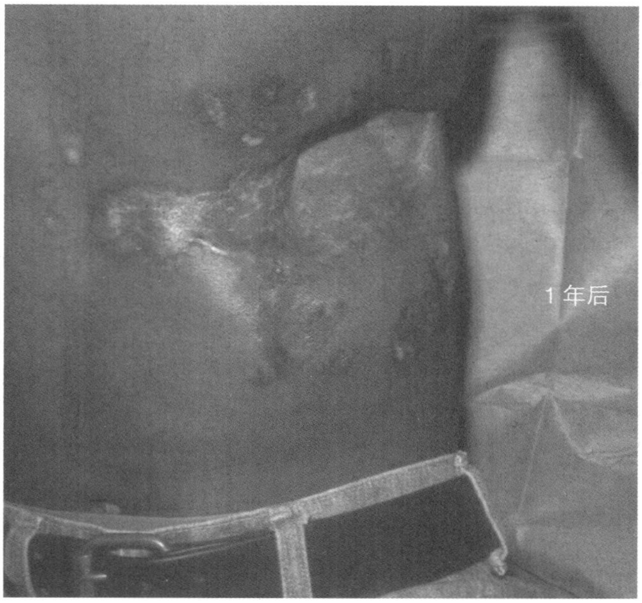

图 16 原来的胸壁缺损经过皮肤移植后现在覆盖腹腔脏器；在患者恢复后进行重建，是否恢复可以通过恢复正常活动和增加体重判断

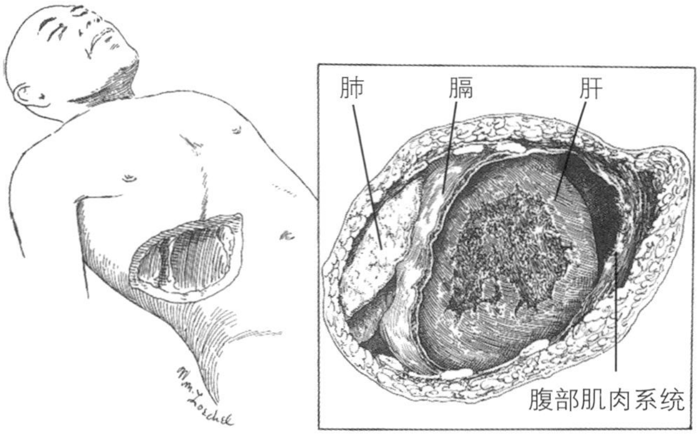

图 17 该年轻男性患者的右上腹及胸壁的右下部分遭受了近距离枪击。将坏死的肝、膈、右肺下叶及胸壁清创后，联合缺损面积为 25 × 18 cm

覆盖的办法来处理。位于胸壁前方的创伤缺损损伤了同侧乳房和下方的胸壁后，可以使用未损伤的对侧乳房或同侧胸大肌重新定位来处理。

合并胸腹壁损伤的膈破裂

膈撕裂伤同时合并胸腹壁损伤的手术修复难度更大。此损伤技术难点最好通过 1 例成功治疗的近距离枪击创伤的男性年轻患者来阐述。该患者在被枪击数分钟后右下和外侧胸壁及上侧、外侧腹壁损伤后幸存，并于数分钟内送医（图 17）。在快速复苏过程中，双腔气管插管保证了出血不会误吸到左侧肺。巨大腹壁、胸壁及半侧膈损伤不会影响术者为获得一期关闭对坏死组织小范围的清创。可能的后果包括组织缺血、感染和肺组织暴露，这些后果都是致命的。完成合理的清创后，须使用一些特殊技术来完成无张力修补。不同种类的补片都应该尝试，但如果存在结肠膨出则修补失败。这类合并缺损的成功修复需要伴有多处肋骨碎片的胸壁和腹壁肌肉组织的肌瓣旋转（图 18-20）。首要目标是完整

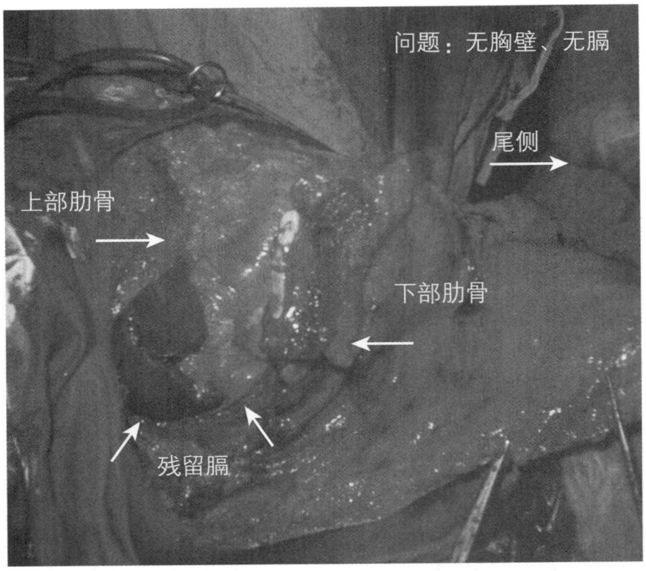

图 18 部分胸壁缺损通过游离第 7 - 10 肋前方与胸骨的连接部，并将其向外上方旋转充当膈来修补。膈后保留的部分向缺损上方移位来封闭膈。剩余的胸壁和腹腔缺损通过向外上方旋转腹壁全层肌瓣来修补，右侧腹部缺损使用皮肤及皮下组织来覆盖

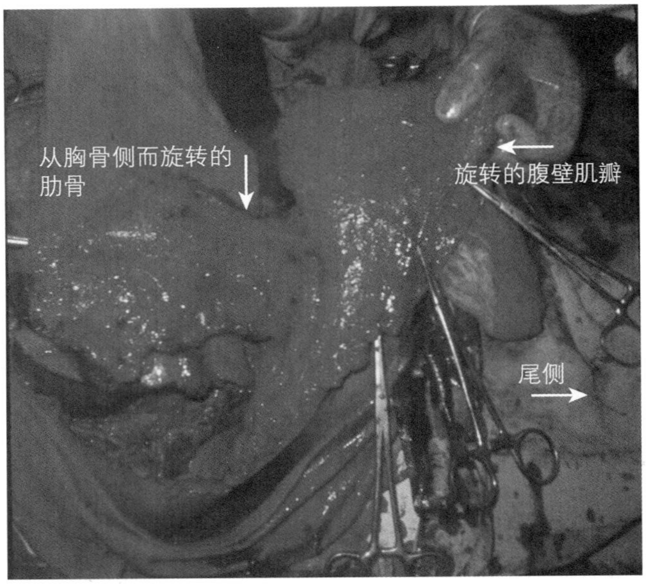

图 20 旋转的腹壁肌瓣保证了暴露的下胸部及上腹部的无张力闭合

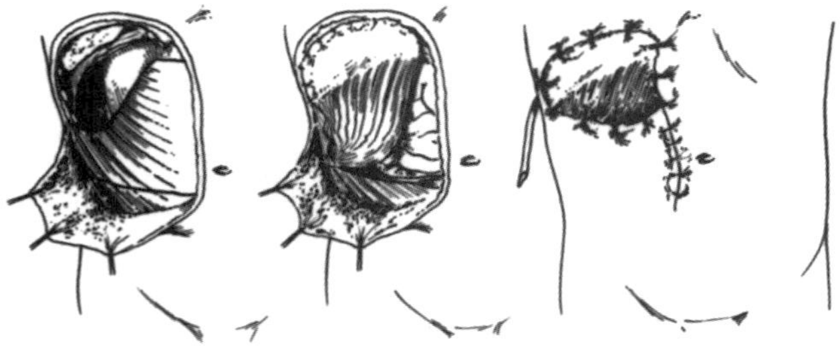

图 19 保留侧方血供的右侧全层腹壁肌瓣向上方旋转，来覆盖腹腔脏器并形成新的肋弓

覆盖，疝可以等患者康复后后期修补。暴露的无皮肤的组织可以通过频繁换药和后期皮肤移植来治疗（图 21）。在去除皮肤移植物和一期关闭后这名选中的患者描述腹壁全层缺损没有修补（图 22）。

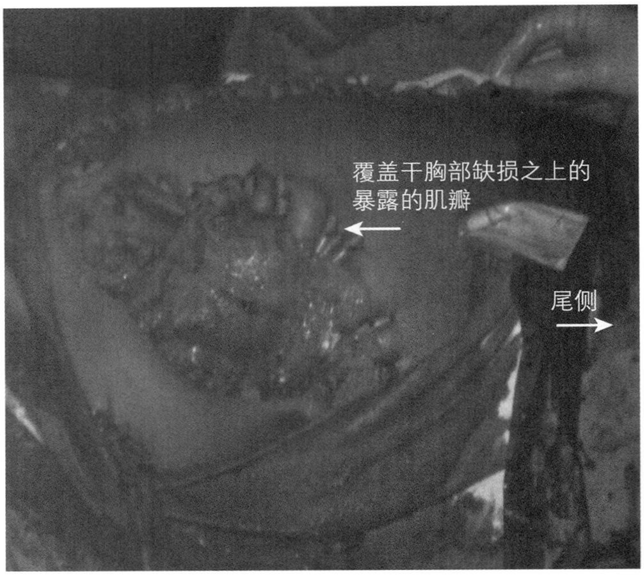

图 21 图 16 中显示的暴露的旋转肌瓣通过频繁换药及后期皮肤移植来治疗

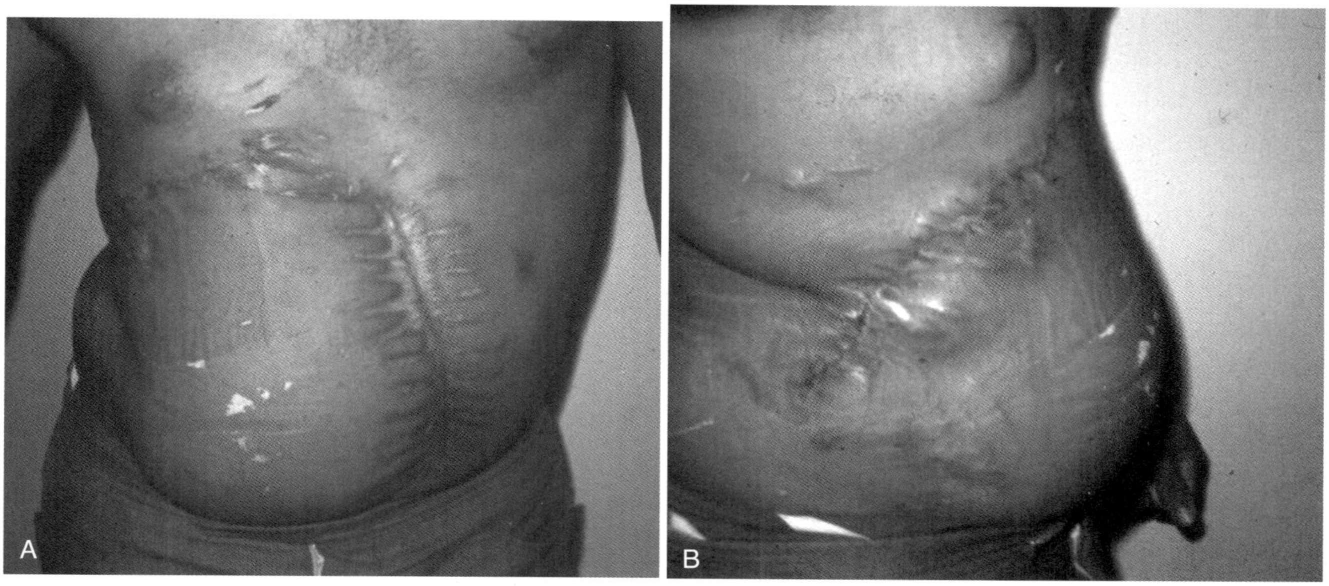

图 22 图 A 与图 B，1 年后，分离移植物去除后皮肤基本闭合。患者拒绝了腹壁全层缺损的修补而选择了腹部束带

腹腔和腹膜后腔的外科解剖

Joe DuBose 和 Thomas M. Scalea 著
沈 凯 译

腹腔和腹膜后彼此紧靠并以腹膜相隔。某些器官诸如小肠和结肠，都各有一部分区域位于腹腔和腹膜后。某些器官，例如肠系膜上动静脉也穿过这两个间隔。透彻地掌握腹腔和腹膜后解剖对寻找躯体外伤正确的手术入路至关重要。

大多数腹腔和腹膜后创伤手术都采用相同的手术入路，正中剖腹术。某些特殊区域的外伤，例如腹腔干上方主动脉或盆腔脉管系统，可能须将正中切口结合对侧切口或者分离切口，例如胸廓入路、腹股沟入路，或者直接从腹膜后入路来确诊和修复特定的损伤。在本章节内，我们会综述腹腔和腹膜后的解剖关系，尤其强调创伤外科治疗过程中的功能解剖学概念。

做切口

腹腔和腹膜后显露一般都采用腹部正中切口，通常为了充分显露采用从剑突到耻骨的长切口。只有在术前即有一个较为明确的诊断时才能使用稍小的切口。长度充分的正中切口可以最大限度地探查所有腹腔和腹膜后结构。为增大某些特定区域的显露也可采用额外的切口。

胸腹联合切口有利于显露上腹部的特定结构。该入路一般采取第 7 或第 8 肋间前外侧切口剖胸并延至胸骨。将肋骨充分与胸骨分离。从胸壁上将膈以放射状切开。靠近胸壁保留 1 ~ 2 in（1 in = 2.54 cm）膈以便后期重建。左侧膈应一直游离至主动脉，右侧应一直游离至腔静脉。左侧胸腹联合切口可能是腹腔干上方主动脉的最佳显露入路。而右侧胸腹联合切口可以更好地显露肝右的后部叶和肝后腔静脉。

正中切口也可延长至可以进行胸骨正中切开术。这样可以为进入前纵隔结构做好准备。如果为了救治肝后腔静脉损伤，需经右心耳行心房腔静脉分流术。胸骨切开术是完成操作最快的入路。如果为了完整游离肝血管而要在心包内控制下腔静脉（inferior vena cava，IVC），胸骨切开术或右侧胸腹联合切口将为外科医生提供良好的入路来完成操作。

经标准剖腹术探查切口显露盆腔深部血管也比较困难，可能需要增加显露的操作。有许多操作可经腹股沟切口可以在腹股沟韧带水平控制股总动脉、股总静脉。全长剖腹术加腹股沟切口有助于快速修复腹股沟韧带附近的血管损伤。

腹股沟韧带可以被牵拉或离断以便探查远端髂外血管。另一种选择是采取在肾移植中使用的腹膜后切口。这种可探查腹膜后腔的“曲棍球棒”形切口能够显露远端髂外动静脉，但只能应用于病情稳定的患者。患者的末端盆腔血管修补可在随后完成。尽管发生率极低，但是采取移植切口加正中切口时应注意，切口间皮肤、皮下组织和筋膜有可能发生缺血或梗死。

探查腹腔

在剖腹探查时切开筋膜后，仔细观察腹膜表面很有用。如果腹膜膨出且发蓝，一般提示张力性腹腔积血，张力在切开腹膜时会被释放。此时应准备好血液收集以应对可能使用细胞循环设备的自体血液回输。钝性损伤最常受伤的脏器是肝和脾。这两个脏器的损伤可以通过术中对右上腹或左上腹的触诊来进行检查。术者随后将小肠和结肠向中线牵拉，然后探查是否存有较大的腹膜后出血。之后探查小肠系膜来寻找系膜损伤。

为使术者彻底探查脾的各个面，完全游离脾非常重要。这有助于明智地选择脾切除术还是脾修补术（图 1）。务必游离脾的所有韧带才能将脾向前、向靠近腹壁中线牵拉，这样有助于术者做出正确决定。

游离肝的原则与脾类似。镰状韧带应一直向下游离到腔静脉水平。两侧的三角韧带应完全切开。这两步操作完成后，与肝相连的结构将仅剩肝静脉和肝门结构。此时，术者就可以旋转并把肝从右上

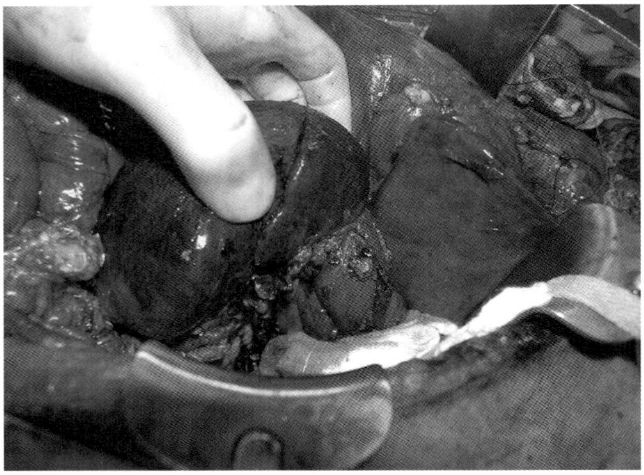

图 1　完全游离脾，能探查脾各个面

腹深部向外取出。这个操作对于探查肝右后叶损伤特别重要。此时应当考虑是否须行胸骨切开术或右侧开胸术游离膈来加强显露。

尽管现在的大部分肝钝伤都可经过保守治疗处理，但是严重的肝损伤出血常常是持续且大量的。在这些出血的病例中，用手直接压迫或填充可以暂时控制出血。Pringle 手法经常具有诊断和治疗双重作用，因为这个操作可以暂时控制出血。Pringle 手法动作须在肝十二指肠韧带处横向放置血管钳，因此可以暂时阻断门静脉和肝动脉血流。使用这种操作可以让术者在有活动性出血，且损伤较小的环境中探查和修补肝。如果在肝门处压迫也不能止血，术者必须怀疑患者是否存在肝后下腔静脉损伤、肝静脉损伤或者肝动脉血管变异，该变异存在于 10%～25% 的患者中。有 10%～20% 的患者其肝总动脉或肝右动脉是从肠系膜上动脉（superior mesenteric artery，SMA）上发出的，在大约 5% 的患者中存在从 SMA 上发出的副肝右动脉。另外，接近 5% 的患者中存在变异的肝左动脉（自胃左动脉上发出）。

Pringle 手法虽然经常是有效的，但是也会造成肝全面缺血，有造成术后肝功能损害的可能。虽然有证据表明，在择期肝切除的患者中，肝可以耐受长达数小时的热缺血，此时肝有时间形成侧支循环，但在休克患者或急性肝外伤的患者中，肝叶间不能形成侧支循环。此时 Pringle 手法可能会使情况变得更糟。主刀和助手夹持血管钳的手会影响显露。而且，严重的肝损伤病例几乎总是伴随有肝静脉损伤，这也限制了 Pringle 手法的作用。

对更加严重的肝外伤病例，也可以考虑使用 Heaney 手法，该操作须全面游离肝血管。使用该技术时，须在肝上方和下方分别钳夹阻断腔静脉。联合使用 Pringle 手法或腹腔干上方主动脉阻断，可以阻断肝血流，提供相对干燥的操作面使得术者能够修补肝或者处理肝静脉损伤。肝后腔静脉的侧支可能会继续出血，但这种出血一般都是可控的。尽管这种血管阻断技术是有效的，但是，除非经胸骨切开术或开胸术打开心包或切开膈，否则想要钳夹肝上腔静脉非常困难。肝下腔静脉阻断须在肾静脉汇入点近端完成，如果阻断钳放置过低，肾静脉汇入下腔静脉的血管会持续出血给显露制造困难。

为了完全阻断肝血流而阻断腔静脉会使得心脏前负荷明显降低。低血容量患者可能无法耐受这种

状况从而导致明显的心力衰竭甚至呼吸、心搏骤停。

所有静脉输液通路都应在锁骨下或颈内静脉放置。可以通过压迫或钳夹腹腔干上方的主动脉来代偿增加后负荷，这种方式可能提高耐受性和降低心血管破坏的风险。由于同样的原因，彻底游离血管时也可同时行静脉旁路循环，使得静脉血流回心（图2）。但是在大部分中心都没有能力立刻完成这种操作，这也限制了它的应用。

一种临时处理含有血管成分损伤的肝外伤的方法是在伤处中心手工压迫。压迫可以阻断受伤处的一切血流，然后可以对受损的肝清创。撤去压力时可以分辨并结扎肝血管。更大的肝动脉和门静脉分支也可以采用同样的手压暂时放松法来结扎（图3）。

十二指肠和胰头的前方位于腹膜内。十二指肠和胰头的后部位于腹膜后腔。完整的Kocher手法（切开侧方腹膜返折并完整游离十二指肠和胰腺）是探查这两个部位损伤的必要手段。胰体位于小网膜囊内。为探查胃后壁必须切开小网膜囊，也能同时探查胰体前方。要完成这个操作最好切开大网膜。

沿着胃大弯侧可将大网膜一直游离到胃食管（gastroesophageal，GE）结合部。这步操作须结扎靠近脾的胃短血管。一旦胃结肠网膜分离完成，术者可以更好地进入小网膜囊并探查胃后壁。探查胃壁

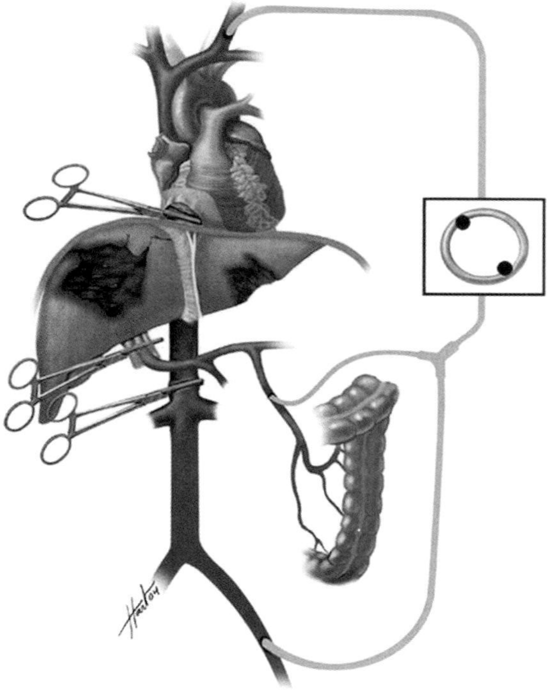

图2　肝静脉阻断结合静脉静脉旁路术（*Courtesy ATOM, Dr. L. Jacobs, Cine-Med, 2004.*）

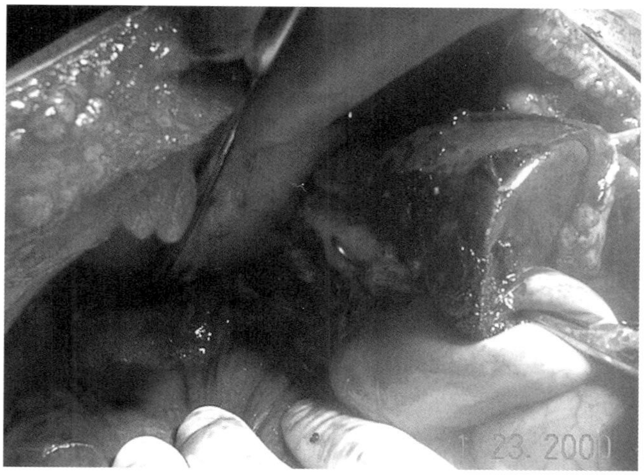

图3　右肝清创切除术后。注意放置在创面上的止血钳

很有必要，特别是GE结合部附近的区域，这样可以避免漏诊小的损伤。如果有必要的话，可以利用Penrose引流管向下牵拉增加显露来游离腹段食管。在GE附近使用海绵棒使胃变成三角形，使此处胃前后壁变平也有助于游离。这些方法使探查更彻底，降低漏诊高位胃壁微损伤的风险。

肝门区域包括肝动脉、门静脉和胆总管。肝门结构均被腹膜覆盖。当切开腹膜时，首先探查到的结构是胆总管。通过内部存在的可触及的搏动和震颤可以确认肝动脉。肝动脉常常位于胆总管的内侧，但这里也存在解剖变异。门静脉位于胆总管后方。上述每种结构都可单独游离和探查，并进行必要的修补。

一旦大血管和实质脏器损伤得到控制，应当进一步探查小肠。有必要彻底探查小肠，以避免漏诊肠道损伤。完整地评估小肠须用手逐段触诊。探查的每一步都须翻动肠袢，以确定肠袢两面都被探查到。将肠袢牵开可以探查对应的系膜。所有靠近肠袢的系膜出血必须被探查到。在关腹前应再次探查小肠以避免漏诊。

探查腹膜后腔

腹膜后一般分为3个区（图4）。1区是腹膜后中心区域，含有的结构包括主动脉、腔静脉和其大血管分支，也包括肠系膜上静脉（superior mesenteric vein，SMV）和脾静脉。任何来自1区的腹膜后出血通常都能被探查到。2区是两侧盆腔上

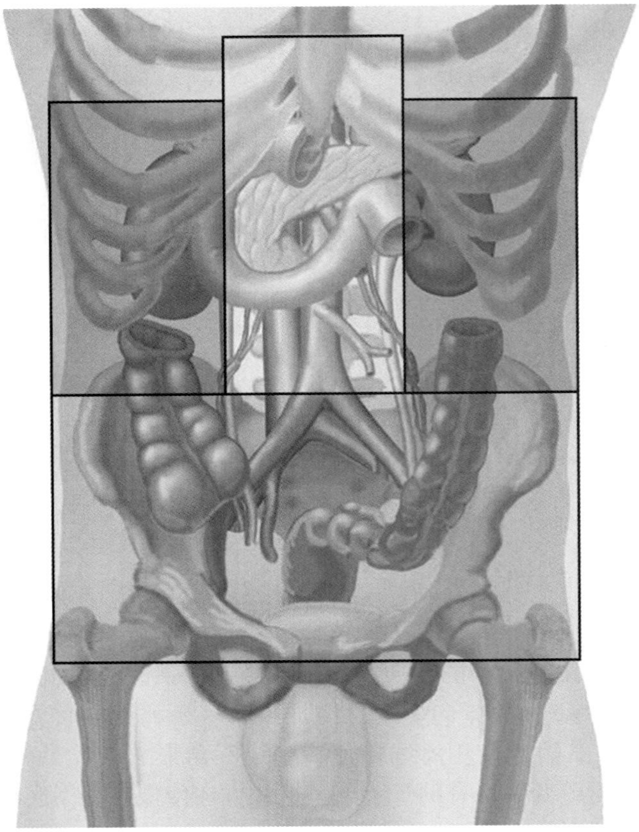

图 4　腹膜后血肿。1 区（中央的方框）：强制探查。2 区（两侧的部分）：在所有穿通性损伤和有增大或搏动性血肿的钝伤时探查。3 区（底部方框）：只在穿通性损伤时探查（*Courtesy ATOM, Dr. L. Jacobs, Cine-Med, 2004.*）

方的外侧肾周区域。2 区容纳肾、输尿管、肾动静脉。一般来说，在探查完所有的穿通性损伤后应探查 2 区是否出血。在某些行术前影像学检查的病例中可观察到肾周损伤和完整的肾周血肿。2 区的钝伤可行保守治疗，除非已知该处伤情须行手术处理，例如输尿管破裂或血肿持续增大或成搏动性。3 区包括所有的盆腔器官，包括髂总动脉和髂外动脉以及髂内动脉。乙状结肠下端和远端输尿管也位于 3 区。

只在穿通性损伤的探查 3 区的血肿。一般来说，不建议外科探查钝性损伤引起的盆腔腹膜后血肿。髂内动脉较短，且分支成众多的小血管。去掉盆腔血肿的顶部有无法填塞止血的风险。钝伤后的 3 区出血使用外加压或者血管内栓塞治疗可能更明智。腹膜外盆腔加压填塞是近年来治疗钝伤出血的方法。这项技术应采用后方切口进入腹膜后空间，而不是经腹腔进入。

有几种外科手段探查腹膜后腔。无论左侧或右侧脏器都须翻向内侧。从 Toldt 白线切开可将脏器翻向内侧。先在白线上做一小切口，然后以电灼术或剪刀将白线切开，将一指伸入腹膜后腔来保护深部组织。切口应一直延伸到结肠肝曲或脾曲。我们一般是用一手将结肠提起，再用探查海绵、海绵棒或手将腹膜后结构向下牵拉。这样可以保护结肠系膜，并且可以快速进入腹膜后腔。

左侧脏器内翻的技术最早是由 Creech 和 DeBakey，在 1956 年经胸腹联合切口处理肾动脉上方主动脉瘤时，首次描述。这些操作包括将左侧结肠沿 Toldt 白线一直切开到脾曲，并向内部翻起脾、胰尾和胃至主动脉、腹腔干、肠系膜上动脉。

所谓的“Mattox 手法”包括将左侧脏器翻起到内侧（图 5）。游离左结肠的方法如前所述。这种方法可以让术者进入将腹膜后腔。在肠系膜基底部可看到主动脉。因为无分支，主动脉也可在 3 点钟方向的侧边继续快速游离，直到分出左侧肾动静脉。

Mattox 手法与 Creech 和 DeBakey 的操作相似，只是还要翻起肾（图 5）。我们一般把肾留在原位，

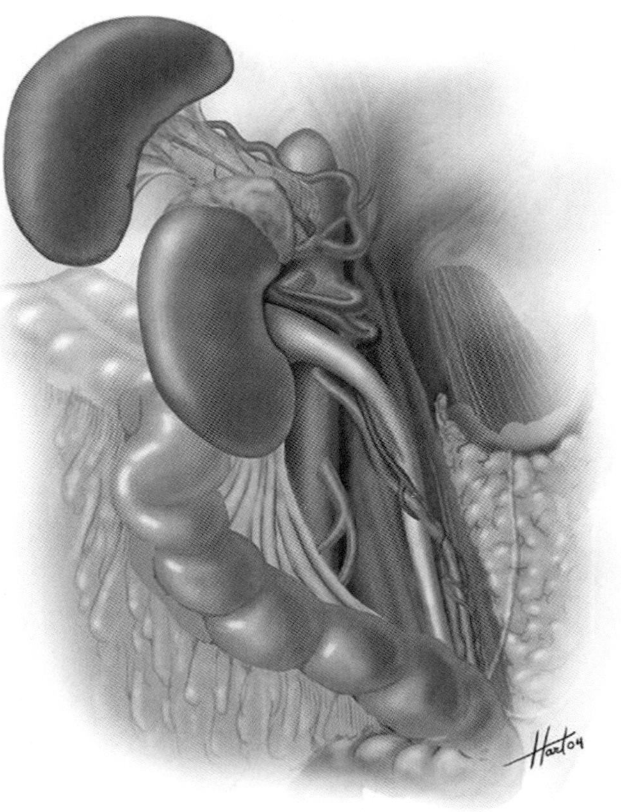

图 5　主动脉显露：Mattox 手法（*Courtesy ATOM, Dr. L. Jacobs, Cine-Med, 2004.*）

如果有需要再最后游离。脾曲必须完整游离到小网膜囊。脾和胰尾游离后可以将主动脉一直显露到主动脉裂孔处。我们认为这是在膈水平控制主动脉的最佳方法。膈脚比外科医生通常认为的位置要低。通常有必要松解一些膈脚纤维才能控制腹腔干上方主动脉。将左侧脏器向内翻起也有助于获得左肾动静脉的良好通路。如果要探查患者的盆腔穿通伤，左侧脏器内翻有助于在血管分叉上方控制主动脉。这也是在根部控制 SMA 的合理显露方法。如果患者须显露较长的 SMA 血管，我们一般联合使用小网膜囊切开和左侧脏器内翻的方法。

我们坚信髂上主动脉血管阻断必须将主动脉完全游离。无论从前方还是侧方，盲目地钳夹阻断主动脉几乎肯定会导致钳夹松脱。我们将食管从主动脉前方游离，再从左侧伸一根手指环绕至右侧，然后可以在脊柱前方将包绕主动脉的纤维钝性分离。当手指可以环绕主动脉时，术者可在主动脉周围轻柔地放置阻断钳，阻断主动脉血流。

腹腔干上主动脉阻断可以通过小网膜囊进入的方式（图 6）。可以通过分开胃结肠韧带或小网膜的方式大范围切开小网膜囊，术者可以将小网膜囊一直游离到胰腺前方。再将胰腺游离，并将食管和胃钝性分离。此时术者可以向下探查主动脉。为了更好地进入主动脉可能须游离膈脚。显露主动脉以后可以横向钳闭主动脉，或者使用 Conn 动脉压缩机在腹腔干上方临时阻断主动脉血流。

我们愿意选择左侧脏器内翻有几个理由。有一定数量的食管支发自主动脉前方。如果从小网膜囊入路进入，由于游离带有一定程度的盲目性，因此有损伤食管支的风险。另外，我们发现从小网膜囊入路进入很难将主动脉环周游离。若选择经此入路，使用阻断钳控制动脉一般都有一些盲区，因此经常脱落。

右侧脏器内翻法，即所谓的 Cattell-Braasch 手法，可以显露右侧腹膜后结构（图 7）。游离右侧结肠的方法同所描述的左侧方法。类似地，游离应直到肝曲，然后进入小网膜囊。十二指肠和胰头应使用 Kocher 手法完整地游离。这个操作的要点还包括小肠系膜向对侧牵拉，以及横结肠向头端牵拉。这个操作可以使术者可以一直向下游离到 IVC。术者也可控制 IVC，并一直探查它到左、右肾静脉汇入点。腔静脉有一段较短的肾上腺节段，后转移到肝后。

Cattell-Braasch 手法是显露腔静脉和右肾及其脉管系统的理想方法。配合 Kocher 手法，还可以完整探查十二指肠和胰头。另外，右侧盆腔脏器也可以通过这种方法显露。盆腔血管通过 Cattell-Braasch 手法显露比左侧入路效果好。左结肠系膜限制了

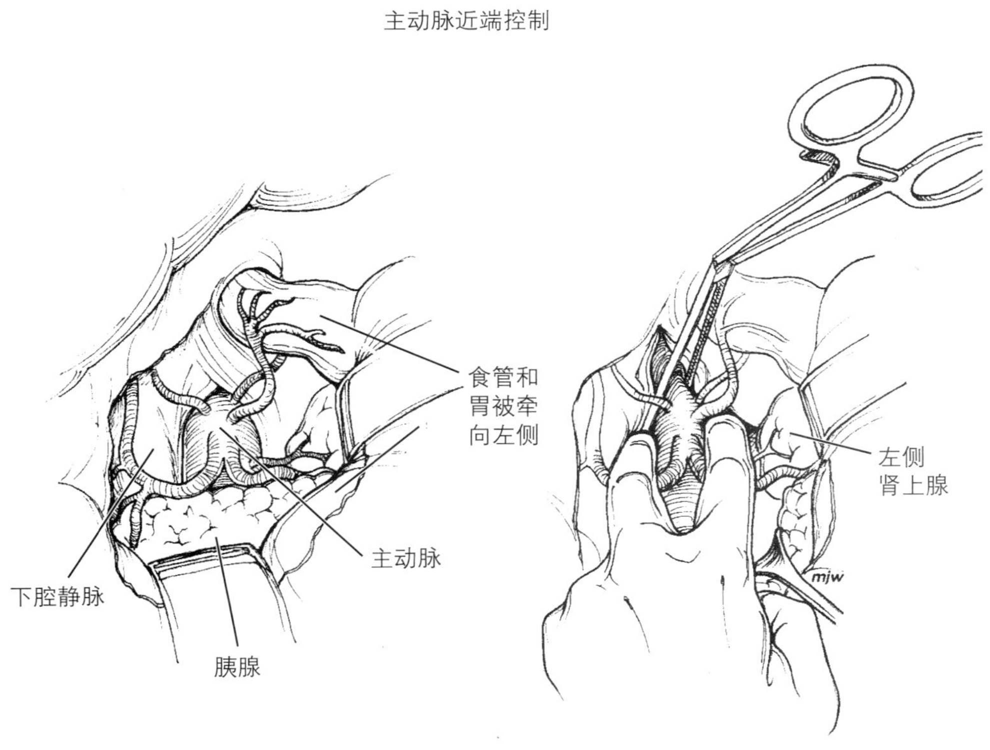

图 6　主动脉近端控制

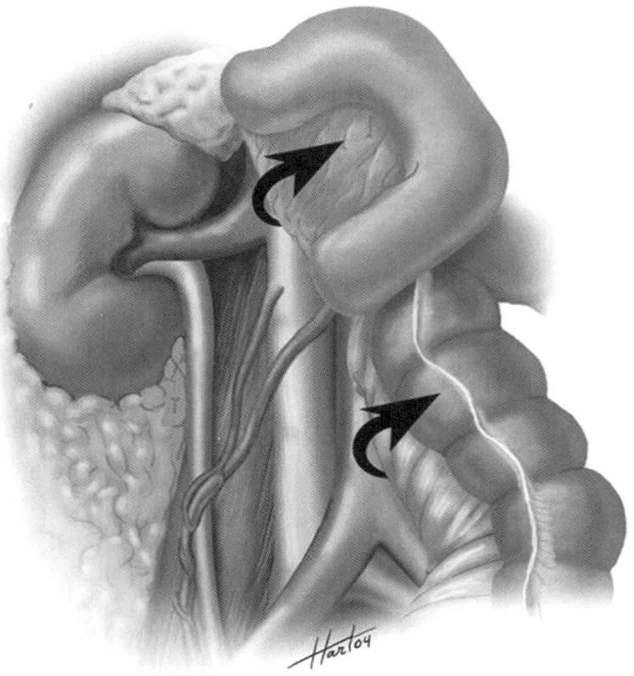

图 7 Cattell-Braasch 手法或右侧脏器内翻。Kocher 手法。将右侧结肠沿着 Toldt 白线游离（*Courtesy ATOM，Dr. L. Jacobs，Cine-Med，2004.*）

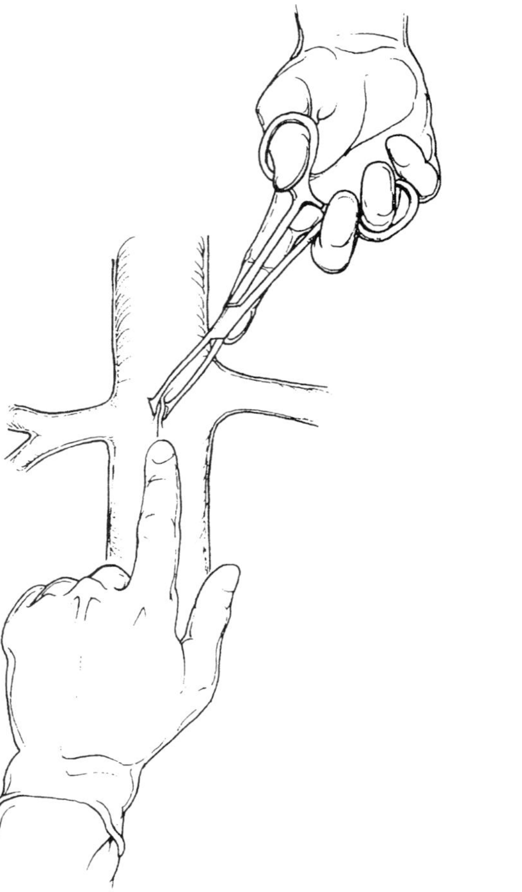

图 8 用指压法临时控制静脉出血，使用肠 Allis 钳夹闭出血点，在钳下方连续缝合修补静脉（*From Henry SM，Duncan AO，Scalea TM: Intestinal Allis clamps as temporary vascular control for major retroperitoneal venous injury. J Trauma 51:170–172，2001.*）

Mattox 手法的显露效果。而右侧没有系膜阻挡视野，因此 Cattell-Braasch 手法显露范围更大。

小肠系膜也可切开，以提升主动脉和腔静脉，这种手法类似于血管外科医生在主动脉手术过程中使用的操作方法。配合 Cattell-Braasch 手法，可以更好地显露主动脉后的腹膜后脉管系统、盆腔中的腔静脉。

腹膜后血管损伤采用标准技术处理。必须采取近端和远端血管阻断，再采取直接修补、旁路移植或者分流。髂总动脉和髂外动脉连接处的损伤和髂内动脉损伤可以使用近端胃下动脉作为导管来处理。将髂内动脉游离出盆腔并结扎。再在髂内动脉和髂外动脉之间进行端端吻合。

腹膜外静脉损伤是最难处理的，特别是腔静脉和髂外静脉汇合处的损伤和近肾下腔静脉损伤。已描述过许多技术来临时性控制出血，包括使用海绵棒、止血钳和指压法。我们喜欢使用小肠 Allis 钳（图 8-10）。血管出血首先在远端用指压控制出血，然后用 Allis 钳在出血点处钳夹，之后可以提起 Allis 钳。这样有利于恢复静脉血回流入心。此时可决定行修补或结扎，在钳下连续缝合即可修补出血点。

在小网膜囊内显露 SMV 的方法问题很多。SMV 在胰腺后方走行，并汇入脾静脉形成短小的门静脉。SMV 损伤常常合并严重的失血。偶然的情况下，可以将胰腺越过 SMV 向上游离，把损伤显露出来。但是 SMV 有许多细小的分支，游离的过程中这些分支都必须独立地结扎。如果这些分支被撕裂了，仅仅是它们造成的出血都很难控制。

有些情况下，术中辨认 SMV 的损伤位置比较困难，特别是损伤点位于胰腺后方或者与脾静脉汇合的位置。在这些病例中，我们一般采取在 SMV 的水平分离胰腺。操作的方式是在胰腺后方。SMA 和 SMV 的上方（在这个位置 SMA 和 SMV 有两个前支）伸进一根手指将胰腺从 SMV 上游离开。用 Penrose 引流管指引 GIA（胃肠吻合用）闭合器来切开胰腺。这种方法显露 SMV 和 SMV 与脾静脉和门静脉汇合处的效果极佳。此处几乎所有的损伤都可被探查到

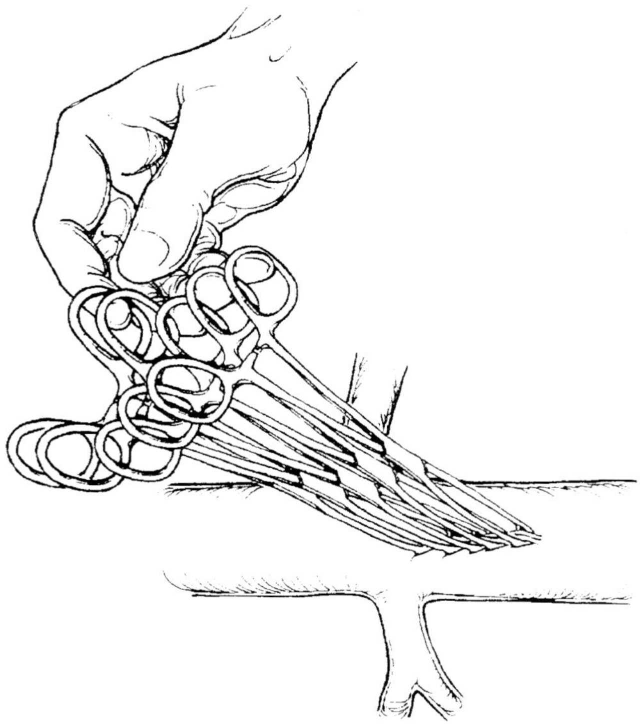

图 9 用指压法临时控制静脉出血，使用肠 Allis 钳夹闭出血点，在钳下方连续缝合修补静脉（*From Henry SM, Duncan AO, Scalea TM: Intestinal Allis clamps as temporary vascular control for major retroperitoneal venous injury. J Trauma 51:170–172, 2001.*）

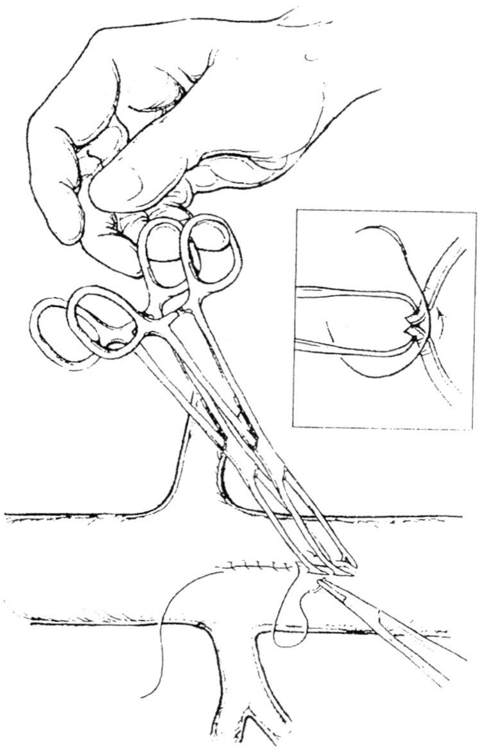

图 10 用指压法临时控制静脉出血，使用肠 Allis 钳夹闭出血点，在钳下方连续缝合修补静脉（*From Henry SM, Duncan AO, Scalea TM: Intestinal Allis clamps as temporary vascular control for major retroperitoneal venous injury. J Trauma 51:170–172, 2001.*）

并加以修复。随后可以把切断的远端胰腺切除或插入回肠环中，采用哪种方式取决于术者。

显露盆腔脉管系统特别具有挑战性（图 11）。操作的要领是要寻找到近端主动脉，并且确认它。严重的失血性休克可导致年轻的患者产生严重的血管痉挛。此时髂总动脉可能会被误认为是髂外动脉，甚至是主动脉。只有明确地找到并控制主动脉和下腔静脉，术者才能进一步显露髂总动脉、髂外动脉和腹下动脉。这几支动脉都必须单独控制。输尿管经过腹膜后跨过髂动脉进入盆腔，这是一个稳定无变异的解剖关系。在盆腔暴露过程中，应当辨认并保护输尿管。

盆腔内静脉粗大且易碎。一般位于动脉后方，静脉的医源性损伤可以是极其严重的。即使患者已处于深度休克状态，术者也应慎重操作避免加重创伤。暂时控制出血可以采用填塞或者分别识别各支静脉并系环的方法。由于髂内动脉的存在，显露近端髂内静脉是受限的。一旦静脉损伤得到修复或结扎，动脉一般都能顺利结扎。

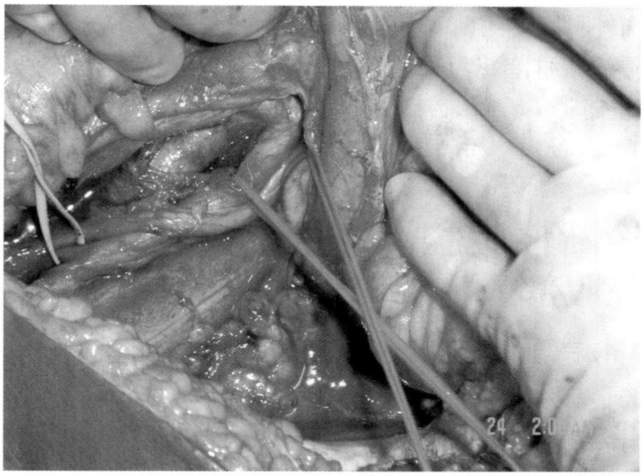

图 11 盆腔血管解剖。注意输尿管跨过髂血管分叉

未来的挑战

需要手术治疗的创伤病例在减少。NOM 成为了大多数实质脏器钝伤的救治常规。甚至手术治疗穿通伤的病例数也在下降，并且集中在少数中心。那

么未来我们如何训练外科医生认识这些复杂的解剖结构和手术技术？

大部分普外科医生几乎不会在腹膜后腔、小网膜囊或者GE结合部附近做手术。曾经需要开腹手术的外科情况现在由于有了更好的药物、微创手术或者内镜技术得以免于开刀。普外科的手术越来越多地采用腹腔镜的方式进行。其结果是，普外科住院医生结束住院医师培训时参与的手术量不足700例，这个数量远少于过去的住院医生实施的数量。而对于社区外科医生来说，他们可能选择将适宜的外伤患者转送到上级医院救治，但是如果患者循环已不稳定，这几乎无法实现。

显然我们必须设计一套不同于现在的外科培训计划，来让将来的外科医生做好手术治疗创伤的准备。现在已经有一些解决方案。模拟器有一定的用处，尽管现在的技术还不能够替代实际操作。尸体解剖也有助于外科医生理解解剖关系。不幸的是，在尸体组织上操作和在正在出血的患者身上操作的感觉非常不同。尸体处于稳定的状态，完全体现不出在一个鲜活的生命体上做手术的紧迫感。

我们已经引进了来自美国康涅狄格州Hartford的高级创伤外科治疗课程（Advanced Trauma Operative Management，ATOM），该课程由Lentworth Jacob和一群其他的知名和受人尊敬的创伤外科医生团队开发。参与课程的学生必须在50 kg重的猪身上练习修复损伤。这些损伤包含了腹部所有的器官系统和胸部的部分器官系统。例如，学生必须成功修复膀胱、输尿管、胰腺损伤，还有更常见的肝、脾、肠道损伤。最后的2项课程包括IVC的严重损伤和右心室刀刺伤。培训课程在一个完整的手术室环境中进行，使用真实的器械、消毒技术和铺单。学生没过多久就会忘记这是一个动物实验，而完全沉浸在创伤救治的节奏中。

另一项新近开发的培训以尸体解剖为基础，叫做创伤治疗高级外科显露技巧培训，课程从解剖的角度显露腹膜后血管。在这个过程中学生关于此区域内血管结构显露的经验也有了潜在的提高。我们强烈推荐在接收急救的单位工作的高年资住院医生和主治级别的外科医生参与这两项培训。

总结

全面了解腹腔和腹膜后结构的解剖关系对快速有效地控制出血和修复损伤是绝对必要的。在接诊严重躯体外伤患者前，理解并完全掌握这些解剖关系对外科医生至关重要。需要手术治疗的创伤患者在减少。因此，外科住院医生接触的创伤手术越来越少。我们强烈敦促将已有的创伤救治训练纳入到住院医生和专科医生的培训体系中，这样才能保证将来的外科医生面对创伤治疗手术的挑战时能做好充分的准备。

诊断性腹腔灌洗术和腹腔镜探查在腹部外伤中的评估

Amy Rushing 和 David T. Efron 著
沈　凯 译

现代科学技术为创伤外科医生提供了多种诊断方式，如何选择适当的方式来快速准确地确认损伤成为目前的一个挑战。大约50年前，Root等介绍了DPL用于评估隐匿性腹腔出血。这种方法很快成为腹部内脏损伤检查的标准诊断方法之一，目前仍然是美国外科医师协会的高级创伤生命支持（Advanced Trauma Life Support，ATLS）学院的学习课程内容。随着先进的CT和超声技术的发展，许多外科医生认为，DPL在腹部损伤患者的评估中已不再起重要作用。尽管其应用有所减少，DPL仍然有一定的临床应用价值，因此仍值得我们对该技术进行回顾。

诊断性腹腔镜探查也允许创伤外科医生评估患者潜在的腹腔和膈损伤，同时避免了非治疗性剖腹术的相关并发症。这一章，我们将回顾诊断性腹腔镜检查在穿通性腹部创伤中的应用发展及其对目前临床实践的影响。

诊断性腹腔灌洗术

1965年，Root等首次描述了DPL这一方法，它被用于诊断那些由于精神状态改变或合并脊髓损伤的而难以评估的腹腔内血管或内脏损伤的患者。其优势在于可快速实施，不须转移患者至特殊地点，并且具有较高的灵敏度。其缺点是特异度较低，不能再重复，而且冲洗液可能会影响后续的CT扫描。对于以下血流动力学不稳定的腹部钝性损伤的患者，美国外科医师学院建议把诊断性腹腔灌洗作为创伤重点超声评估（Focused Assessment with Sonography in Trauma，FAST）的替代：

- ■继发于颅脑损伤、酒精中毒或非法用药的精神状态改变；
- ■脊髓损伤导致的感觉减退；
- ■合并肋骨下部、骨盆和腰椎损伤；
- ■可疑的体检结果；
- ■由于腹腔外损伤或血管造影而进行全身麻醉，从而影响体格检查；
- ■"安全带征"阳性并有可疑肠管损伤

表1显示了DPL、FAST及CT检查在诊断腹部创伤中的相对优缺点。

表1 DPL、FAST及CT检查在诊断腹部创伤中的优点及缺点

检查方式	优点	缺点
DPL	可快速获取 不需移动 对空腔脏器的损伤特异度较高	有创操作 不可重复 漏诊腹膜后损伤或膈损伤
FAST	可快速获取 不需移动 可重复	漏诊腹膜后损伤或膈损伤 非常依赖操作者水平
CT扫描	最灵敏 可获得最佳解剖学信息（包括腹膜后腔）	须移动患者到特定检查区域 昂贵 需要硬件设施

CT：计算机断层扫描；DPL：诊断性腹腔灌洗术；FAST：创伤重点超声评估

诊断性腹腔灌洗术可分为开放法、半开放法和经皮法。Root认为开放法是最安全的。操作前胃和膀胱用鼻胃管和Foley导管减压。取脐上或脐下做2 cm切口显露白线。对于骨盆骨折的患者，切口应取脐上。找到筋膜后切开并游离、分开腹膜。将腹膜透析管插入腹腔并向下植入盆腔。类似大小的导管很重要，另外也有几种商业化的工具包可供选择。荷包缝合筋膜层，然后抽出腹腔内液体，获得超过10 ml的血液、胆汁、肠液或蔬菜样物质，即可认为试验阳性。若抽吸的血液少于10 ml，将1 L盐水灌入后，把空的盐水袋放在地板上进行虹吸。恢复不少于300 ml的液体随后进行检测，出现下列结果之一即可认为检测阳性：每毫升液体中红细胞个数超过100 000个，每毫升液体中白细胞个数超过500个，发现革兰氏染色细菌。若操作规范，DPL灵敏度可达83%～96%，特异度可达87%～99%（表2）。

表2 诊断性腹腔灌洗术阳性的定义

迅速抽出至少10 ml如下液体：	实验室检查至少出现下列结果之一：
血液	红细胞＞100 000个/毫升
胆汁	白细胞＞500个/毫升
肠液	存在革兰氏阳性细菌
未消化的微粒物质	

RBCs，红细胞；WBCs，白细胞

尽管20世纪自60年代以来，DPL彻底改变了腹腔内损伤的诊断方式，但多层螺旋CT与超声的发展使DPL成为很少用到的诊断方法。批评者认为DPL缺乏特异性，导致非治疗性开腹探查率达36%。假阳性结果可能来自于骨盆骨折或者肝、脾的裂伤，而这些情况多采取非手术治疗。扩大的腹膜后血肿和膈裂伤往往导致DPL阴性，而这两种情况多需手术干预。另外，操作DPL的并发症发生率为0.8%～1.7%，这些数据来自于2 500例DPL操作的报道，不良事件包括以下几项：肠道或膀胱损伤、最少液体恢复、腹壁渗液、伤口愈合问题。与现代影像诊断相比，DPL有一个较长的禁忌列表，如既往腹部手术史、已知的凝血功能障碍、肝硬化和病态肥胖。骨盆骨折和怀孕也会影响DPL的安全操作。

问题是DPL在现代创伤护理中是否仍有作用。Wang等最近研究了64例腹部钝伤行DPL的患者。这些患者行CT检查后考虑行保守治疗，并行DPL评估可能存在的空腔脏器损伤。其中19例患者DPL阳性，4例患者存在小肠损伤。总体灵敏度和特异度分别为100%和75%，无空腔脏器损伤患者被漏诊。相比之下，CT成像对于腹部钝伤后空腔脏器损伤诊断的灵敏度为64%～95%，4例小肠损伤的患者的CT扫描均未能确诊，而这些患者依照先前的CT结果，治疗选择是不同的。Wang的研究规定应用细胞计数率来定义DPL阳性。细胞计数率是由Fang

等提出的用于提高 DPL 的特异度和降低非治疗性剖腹术的使用率。其定义如下：

（冲洗液白细胞计数 / 冲洗液红细胞计数）:（外周血白细胞计数 / 外周血红细胞计数）

如果细胞计数率大于 1，则 DPL 为阳性。Fang 等报告应用细胞计数率的阳性预测值为 89%。原始研究对于标本收集有一定的要求，DPL 得到细胞计数率>1 需 3 h。这种延迟测试是不实用的，导致患者不能及时接受手术治疗。尽管如此，当射线照片的评估不可靠时，这种 DPL 的新方法可以作为 CT 成像的辅助诊断方法。

Cha 等最近报道了在Ⅰ级创伤中心 10 年的 DPL 实践历史。研究显示即使 PDL 预测患者治疗性剖腹术的总体准确率为 77%，在血流动力学不稳定的患者中，其准确率为 100%。对于血流动力学不稳定的需开腹手术的患者，创伤重点超声评估的阳性率仅为 46%。另外，Cha 等报道 7% 的患者 PDL 为阴性，但最终须行治疗性剖腹术。这说明 DPL 技术在评估超声检查失败的创伤患者时，仍有一定作用。基于这些数据，作者推荐对于血流动力学不稳定的患者，若创伤重点超声评估为阴性，而患者的前腹壁穿刺伤伴有可疑腹膜破损时，应立即行 DPL。

许多医生认为 DPL 已无必要，最著名的例子为 Jansen 和 Logie 写的“诊断性腹腔灌洗 - 讣告”一文。此文作者认为 DPL 可被 CT 扫描和超声取代。CT 和超声确实是无创的，并具有较高的特异度，文献报道其特异度可达 98%。但是 CT 检查须移动患者至特殊的放射检查室，而超声则依赖操作者的技术水平。对于不稳定的昏迷患者，若无 24 h 急诊超声可用，DPL 可用于这类患者的诊断。

诊断性腹腔镜探查

很少有技术进步能像腹腔镜一样带来外科手术的革命。1976 年，Gazzaniga 等报道了应用腹腔镜探查来评估腹部创伤的经验，研究认为在诊断脾及小肠损伤时，腹腔镜检查具有很高的灵敏度和特异度。从那以后，腹腔镜探查也被用于钝伤或穿通伤导致的膈裂伤。该技术大大降低了非治疗性剖腹术的使用及相关并发症的发生。

诊断性腹腔镜探查的适应证包括穿通性腹部外伤或胸腹联合伤且血流动力学稳定的患者。这些患者无剖腹探查的典型征象，如腹膜炎或膈膨升。对于那些有胸腹联合伤的患者，特别是穿通伤，诊断性腹腔镜可用来评估膈损伤。由于继发性膈疝导致腹腔内脏嵌顿的病死率高达 36%，所以腹腔镜探查是非常重要的。超过 20% 的胸腹区域穿通伤会出现膈裂伤，所以进一步的评估是毋庸置疑的。

创伤后的腹腔镜探查与外科的微创手术技术层面本质上无明显不同。前腹壁经脐部置入气腹针或 Aasson 套管针，并进入腹腔的选择何种方式进腹依据医生的选择及患者的既往手术史。进腹后，充入二氧化碳建立气腹。由于持续的下腔静脉外的压力会加剧原有的低血压，故这种方式适应于血流动力学稳定的患者。通过套管接入 30° 腹腔镜进入腹腔，仔细评估腹腔，尤其是枪伤或穿刺伤进腹的区域。必要时使用另外套管针以便于牵拉肠道。为全面探查膈，须行反 Trendelenburg 位，使内脏下移。若明确损伤须进一步干预，则可中转为剖腹术，进行确定性修补。

既往研究显示，对于血流动力学稳定的腹部穿通性损伤患者，高达 60% 的患者行腔镜探查后未见明确腹膜异常，从而避免了非治疗性剖腹术。这种情况尤其适用于前腹壁穿刺伤的患者。尽管腹腔镜探查诊断腹膜穿通伤的灵敏度达 100%，但对空腔脏器损伤的诊断成功率不高。既往研究显示，腹腔镜探查诊断小肠损伤的灵敏度仅为 18%。这个结论可能与医生对腹腔镜技术的适应度相关。现在微创手术已经成为现代外科训练的基础，对于血流动力学稳定的患者，我们相信未来的外科医生会很容易地发现空腔脏器损伤，并行腹腔镜下修补（图 1）。

DPL 和腹腔镜探查联合应用已成为一种新的诊断手段。Vinces 和 Madlinger 最近报道联合应用腹腔镜探查和灌洗（laparoscopy exploration and lavage，LELA）来排除空腔脏器损伤。28 例前腹壁穿刺伤患者行腹腔镜检查来评估腹膜受损情况。17 例患者被证实存在腹膜穿通伤，8 例患者发现脏器损伤，紧急中转为剖腹术，剩余 9 例患者行 LELA。阳性的定义为红细胞计数>5000/ml 或白细胞计数>150/ml，或发现胆汁、血液、肠液、蔬菜样物质。4 例患者灌洗液阳性，行剖腹手术证实结肠或小肠受损。剩余 5 例患者灌洗液阴性，避免了剖腹术。这个研究显示联合应用两项技术避免了其各自的缺点，使腹部穿通性损伤的诊断更确切。

对于膈损伤的评估，腹腔镜可提供足够的视野来发现隐匿性裂伤。在最大呼气量时，膈顶位于第 5 肋间水平，在胸腹区域外伤时有损伤风险。其解剖定位的体表投影位于胸骨缘前内侧，上方平乳头下缘连线，并在后外侧向两侧肩胛骨顶端展开，在后内侧向棘旁肌展开。下方由肋骨缘的前、侧及后方构成。这个梯形区域的穿通伤容易发生膈裂伤。

对于左侧胸腹联合伤可能导致的潜在膈损伤，大部分创伤外科医生认为腹腔镜探查还是很有必要的。腹腔镜探查可以用来早期识别和修复膈的损伤，从而避免腹腔内容物形成膈疝的风险。而如果发生右侧胸腹联合伤，因为肝作为天然屏障的存在，可以避免右侧膈疝的形成。理想情况下，应在探查之前观察一部分时间，以便空腔脏器的体征潜在性的演变。如果患者的病情没有进一步进展，外科医生就更加确信可以在腹腔镜下修复膈损伤，从而避免中转为剖腹术（图 2）。但是，对于那些患者的一般状况并不稳定（包括精神状态不稳定），或者临床资源有限，或者患者高度怀疑损伤（枪伤、CT 发现有问题）等这些情况，观察并不是很适合。

Friese 等做了一个样本量为 34 人的前瞻性研究，这些人都是胸腹穿通伤，但是早期都没有临床症状。研究中所有患者均行诊断性腹腔镜探查，之后再用剖腹术或者电视辅助胸腔镜来证实创伤是否存在。研究证实腹腔镜探查术的灵敏度和特异度分别是 87.5% 和 100%。基于更多样本的数据，Powell 等在 3 年间评估了 108 位胸腹穿通伤患者。这些患者都进行了诊断性腹腔镜探查，其中 22（20%）名患者有膈的断裂伤。有趣的是在这 22 人中，有 15 人（68%）X 线胸片未发现损伤。在 X 线胸片上，

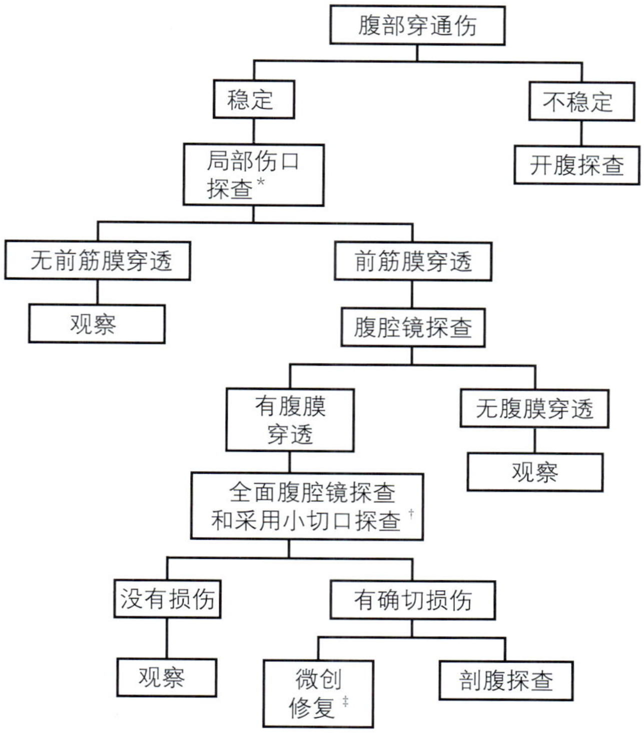

图 1　空腔脏器损伤的诊治流程。*局部伤口探查在急诊室进行。†通过腹腔镜完成主要探查；对于小肠，可以通过一个 4 cm 的小开腹切口完成小肠探查。‡如果创伤不大，对于外科能力精湛的医生，可以实施腹腔镜下创伤修复

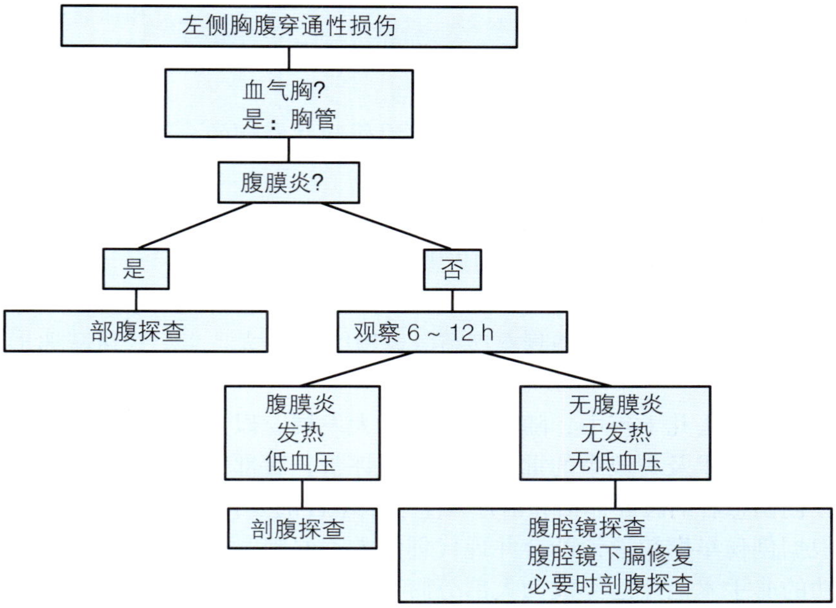

图 2　左侧胸腹穿通伤诊治流程

也没有患者出现腹腔脏器疝的证据。这些研究都表明，腹腔镜探查不仅仅在微创技术领域，在创伤手术领域内都有很高的价值。

总而言之，对于腹部创伤的患者，DPL 和诊断性腹腔镜探查有着各自的优势。对于腹腔内脏器损伤，DPL 是最敏感的技术之一，而且可以直接在床旁实行；而诊断性腹腔镜探查可以早期识别腹膜损伤。这些可以帮助外科医生排除需手术干预的严重的腹腔内损伤，避免对患者实施不必要的剖腹探查，同时可以缩短患者的平均住院日。此外，腹腔镜探查也被用来诊断隐匿性的膈损伤，这些损伤经常是胸部影像学无法发现的。这些诊断方式揭示了过去 50 年创伤评估方法的进步，同时也为创伤医学提供了评估危重患者的选择。

腹部钝性创伤和穿通性损伤的非手术治疗

Matthew J. Martin 和 Peter Rhee 著
沈　凯 译

腹部钝性损伤

外科治疗要点

1. 腹部 CT 联合使用静脉造影剂是评估全腹腔脏器最可靠、最准确的方法。
2. 然而，初始 CT 扫描并不全面，可能会遗漏某些重要损伤，特别是胰腺损伤。
3. 大部分腹腔实质脏器损伤可以无须剖腹探查而成功处理。
4. 决定进行非手术治疗的主要依据是患者生理状况和现有治疗条件，而不是损伤分级和影像学表现。
5. 应由经验丰富的创伤外科医生做出非手术治疗的初始决策，并不断进行再评估。
6. 介入和微创方法应是处理某些损伤和并发症的辅助手段。
7. 适时转入手术治疗应该被认为是救治成功的措施，而不是非手术处理的失败。

介绍

在过去几十年中，随着科技的巨大发展，以及对处理技术及其成束的批判性的重新评价，腹部钝性创伤患者的腹腔评估和治疗发生了根本性的变化。根据创伤早期快速诊断合并现代创伤救治原则，成功的非手术治疗已经成为大部分腹部钝性伤的治疗方法而不是另外的选择。尽管有些患者可能需要立即手术或者延期手术，但是无论患者的年龄大小，损伤是否合并伤，非手术治疗可以安全地应用于大部分腹部钝性伤患者。然而，不恰当的非手术治疗，以及没有严格遵守治疗原则和流程将会导致严重不良后果，包括延误治疗、增加并发症发生率和可预防的死亡。

发病率

腹部钝性损伤的发病率因人群、受伤机制和各中心纳入的研究不同而差异较大。经过 CT 检查，在所有腹部钝性创伤患者中，大约 12% 的患者有 1 处及以上的腹腔内损伤，其中，46% 的患者为严重损伤，30% 的患者需要手术或者血管介入治疗。实质脏器损伤最为多见，如脾和肝，然后是肾、肠系膜、小肠、结肠、胰腺。腹部损伤可分为实质脏器（肝、脾、肾）、空腔脏器（胃、十二指肠、小肠、结肠、输尿管、膀胱）、内分泌器官（胰腺、肾上腺）和血管损伤。总之，超过 80% 的实质脏器钝性损伤可以通过非手术治疗处理，其并发症发生率与手术治疗相比相似，甚至更低。

损伤机制

钝性创伤可以通过多种机制导致腹部损伤，包括能量直接传导引起腹部组织破裂或空腔脏器爆裂，快速减速形成的剪切伤，腹腔脏器直接压迫至脊柱造成的损伤，肋骨、脊柱骨折或异物相关的穿刺伤或者撕裂伤。尽管外力严重程度和腹部损伤数量没有线性相关关系，但是速度越快、外力越大，腹部脏器的损伤越广泛、越多。外力的直接传导主要被大的实质脏器吸收，如肝、脾和肾，引起其实质的断裂。快速减速力主要影响固定脏器或者系膜结构，如肾、十二指肠、肠系膜，导致组织撕裂或者根部撕脱。尽管安全带的使用降低了创伤性脑损伤的发生率及死亡率，但是空腔脏器的损伤却增加了2倍。毗邻或者固定在脊柱上的器官也可受到外力直接挤压，包括远端十二指肠、胰腺和大血管。低位肋骨骨折可直接撕裂上腹部器官，包括膈、肝、脾、肾。

诊断

腹腔钝性损伤的诊断首先在进行基本病史询问和重点的体格检查。出现低血压应考虑是否由腹腔损伤引起，除非证实是其他情况引起。腹部体格检查可能受到全身其他损伤和沮丧的神智状态的限制，但应该重点关注患者有无腹膜刺激征、局部压痛、外部杂音、“安全带”征和腹部膨胀。实质脏器损伤不会引起腹膜炎，单纯的腹腔积血也不会导致弥漫性腹膜刺激。目前，创伤重点超声评估（FAST）常是初始检查方式之一。即使检查发现腹腔游离液体，即FAST检查阳性能够准确提示腹腔损伤，但是阴性结果并不能排除严重腹腔损伤。不能认为它是确定性检查。尽管超声检查常用于特定器官损伤的确认和分级（如肝、脾），但其可靠性和可重复性并不高。

目前，创伤超声的应用已经超过FAST标准四个区域，而且受到越来越多的关注，特别是躯干钝性创伤。与标准的创伤重点超声评估相比，扩大的创伤重点超声评估（extended FAST，E-FAST）还包括短时间内进行胸腔的检查以诊断气胸和血胸。E-FAST的诊断技术易于传授给主治医生和住院医生，并且已经证实较X线胸片更加准确。在急性创伤的情况下，超声还用于有效评价容量状态和液体反应性（使用腔静脉的直径和呼吸变量），也可以用于引导过程，如超声引导下进行经皮血管穿刺。在大多数情况下，经DPL已经被FAST检查和CT扫描所代替，并不常使用，而在体格检查和CT检查结果不一致的情况下，可用于某些可疑空腔脏器穿孔的患者。然而，诊断性腹腔穿刺（diagnostic peirtoneal aspirate，DPA）可发现明显的腹腔内出血，特别适用于低血压而FAST检查阴性的患者。所有患者均应进行尿液分析，一旦发现明显血尿，应该全面评估泌尿系统（肾、输尿管、膀胱）。

CT已经成为大多数确定腹部钝性损伤诊断的标准检查，应该积极使用。没有发现的腹腔内损伤，特别由于缺乏完善检查造成的漏诊是创伤后可预防的死亡的最常见原因。现代新型螺旋CT扫描能够提供腹腔器官的详细图像，包括腹膜后结构和大血管。其诊断实质脏器损伤的灵敏度和特异度接近100%，并且为损伤分级提供可靠的解剖学细节。其中CT对胰腺损伤诊断和分级方面尚有限制，特别是在创伤之后立即进行CT检查，可能会低估创伤程度。最近，美国创伤外科协会（American Association for the Surgery of Trauma，AAST）开展的一项多中心研究发现多层螺旋CT检查检出胰腺损伤的灵敏度只有60%。强调需要更准确的辅助诊断方法。在损伤初期48～72 h之间，连续测定淀粉酶和脂肪酶的水平可有效诊断胰腺重大损伤。但是对于大约30%的胰腺轻微损伤，这些指标可能正常。

“造影剂填充”可以为活动性出血和动静脉瘘提供证据。因此，在条件允许的情况下，腹部CT检查都应该使用静脉造影剂。虽然既往有些系列研究认为CT检查对空腔脏器穿孔以及十二指肠和胰腺损伤不可靠，但是越来越多的证据表明高质量的CT扫描能正确地识别大多数损伤。然而，在少数情况下，如果高度怀疑有未发现的损伤或者初始CT检查诊断不清，应该考虑复查CT（如无剖腹探查的指征）或者进行DPL。在进行腹部CT检查时，我们仅使用静脉造影剂。口服造影剂在创伤时应用获益不大，并且存在过度延时和误吸的风险。在后期进行CT检查评价空腔脏器穿孔或者更好地显示已知或可疑的胰腺和十二指肠损伤时，口服造影剂或许有效。

损伤的解剖学位置和美国创伤外科协会器官损伤分级

腹腔分为腹膜腔和腹膜后腔两大区域。钝性创伤所致的大部分损伤主要为腹膜腔内结构，如肝、脾、小肠、肠系膜，常引起腹痛、压痛和腹部膨胀等临床症状和体征。与创伤外科相关的腹膜后损伤的主要结构有肾、十二指肠、胰腺、大血管和部分结肠。即使在严重损伤的情况下，腹膜后脏器损伤常不表现出相应的临床症状和体征，或者会延迟一段时间才出现。所幸腹膜后空腔脏器损伤相对少见。

根据美国创伤外科协会器官损伤分级（AAST Trauma organ Injury，AAST-OIS系统，表1），腹部损伤分级依据CT进行。这一分级为讨论和研究腹部损伤提供了统一、可参考的标准，并且可用于指导非手术处理的级别和监测时长。最近，通过国家创伤数据库的损伤和预后分析，已经验证了脾、肝、肾的AAST-OIS分级的有效性。虽然损伤程度越重，发病率和非手术处理的失败率越高，但是损伤分级并不是决定是否进行非手术治疗的主要因素。在适宜的临床环境中，任何程度的损伤均可成功地实施非手术治疗。后续治疗决策还应关注和考虑到其他因素，包括血胸的量、患者年龄、合并症状况、并存损伤是否存在（特别是创伤性脑损伤）和造影剂是否填充存在。

表 1 腹腔部分器官 AAST–OIS

分级	描述
脾 *	
Ⅰ	裂伤深度 <1 cm 被膜下血肿 <10% 表面积
Ⅱ	裂伤深度 1 ~ 3 cm 被膜下血肿为 10% ~ 15% 表面积 实质内血肿直径 <5 cm
Ⅲ	裂伤深入皮质 >3 cm 或累及小血管 被膜下血肿 >50% 表面积或呈扩展性 / 破裂 实质内血肿直径 >5 cm 或呈扩展性 / 破裂
Ⅳ	裂伤累及脾段或脾门血管，导致 >25% 脾无血供
Ⅴ	脾破碎 脾门血管损伤致全脾无血供
肝 *	
Ⅰ	裂伤深度 <1 cm 被膜下血肿 <10% 表面积
Ⅱ	裂伤深度 1 ~ 3 cm，长度 10 cm 被膜下血肿 10% ~ 50% 表面积 实质内血肿直径 <10 cm
Ⅲ	裂伤实质深度 >3 cm 被膜下血肿 >50% 表面积或呈扩展性 / 破裂 实质内血肿直径 >10 cm 或呈扩展性 / 破裂
Ⅳ	实质破裂累及一叶的 25% ~ 75% 或局限于一叶内的 1 ~ 3 个肝段
Ⅴ	实质破裂 >75% 或一叶内多于 3 个肝段 肝后下腔静脉或肝静脉主干损伤
Ⅵ	肝撕脱
肾 *	
Ⅰ	血尿影像检查正常 被膜下血肿
Ⅱ	裂伤深度 <1 cm，无尿外渗 无扩展的肾周血肿
Ⅲ	裂伤深度 >1 cm，无集合管系统破裂或尿外渗
Ⅳ	裂伤累及皮质、髓质和集合管系统 主要肾动静脉损伤伴局限性血肿
Ⅴ	肾完全破碎 肾门断裂致全肾无血供
胰腺 *	
Ⅰ	浅表裂伤，不伴胰管裂伤 轻度挫伤，不伴胰管损伤
Ⅱ	重度裂伤，不伴胰管损伤 重度挫伤，不伴胰管损伤
Ⅲ	远端胰腺横断或有胰管损伤的实质损伤
Ⅳ	近端胰腺横断或累及壶腹的实质损伤
Ⅴ	胰头广泛破坏
腹部血管	
Ⅰ	无名分支、膈动 / 静脉、腰动 / 静脉、生殖腺动 / 静脉、卵巢动 / 静脉
Ⅱ	肝动 / 静脉、脾动 / 静脉、胃动 / 静脉、胃十二指肠动 / 静脉、肠系膜下动 / 静脉， 及其他有名称的主要的动 / 静脉（需结扎或修补）
Ⅲ	肠系膜上静脉主干、肾下腔静脉、肾动 / 静脉、髂动 / 静脉、髂内动 / 静脉
Ⅳ	肠系膜上动脉主干、腹腔干、肾上腔静脉、肾下主动脉
Ⅴ	门静脉、实质外肝外肝静脉、肝后或肝上腔静脉、肾上膈下主动脉
十二指肠 *	
Ⅰ	血肿限于一段 部分裂伤
Ⅱ	血肿多于一段 裂伤 <50% 周径
Ⅲ	裂伤为 50% ~ 70% 周径（第 2 段）或 50% ~ 100% 周径（第 1、3、4 段）
Ⅳ	裂伤 >75% 周径（第 2 段） 累及壶腹部或胆总管远端
Ⅴ	十二指肠复合的广泛破坏 十二指肠完全无血供

Modified from Moore EE, Cogbill TH, Jurkovich GJ, et al: Organ injury scaling: spleen and liver (1994 revision). J Trauma 38:323 – 324, 1994; Moore EE, Cogbill TH, Jurkovich GJ, et al: Organ injury scaling III: chest wall, abdominal vascular, ureters, bladder, and urethra. J Trauma 33:337 – 339, 1992; Moore EE, Cogbill TH, Malangoni MA, et al: Organ injury scaling, II: pancreas, duodenum, small bowel, colon, and rectum. J Trauma 30:1427–1429, 1990; and Moore EE, Shackford SR, Pachter HL, et al: Organ injury scaling: spleen, liver, and kidney. J Trauma 29:1664–1666, 1989.

AAST-OIS，美国创伤外科协会器官损伤分级

* 同一器官多处损伤增加 1 级，到Ⅲ级截止

处理

对于已知或者可疑的腹腔内脏器损伤患者，其初始治疗的选择取决于临床检查和患者的血流动力学状态。对于经过充分的液体复苏，腹膜炎仍无好转或者血流动力学仍不稳定的患者，应该立即进行剖腹探查。在创伤评估早期阶段，液体复苏应该谨慎且仅在必须的情况下进行。过于积极的液体复苏，导致平均动脉压升高，从而加重损伤器官的出血，或者引起血液稀释，可能导致医源性血红蛋白的降低。我们建议给予少量容量负荷，然后由经验丰富的创伤外科医生快速评估患者反应。有些证据认为与标准晶体或胶体补液方法相比，高渗晶体液有利于复苏和免疫调节，但是此方法仍有争议。使用少量高渗液体（100 ~ 250 ml，3% ~ 7.5% 盐水）能够降低组织水肿、改善气体交换、降低全身和器官特异性炎症反应，其安全性较高。对于相关创伤性脑损伤患者，高渗盐水还能够降低液体复苏时的颅内压。对于重大外伤须大量使用血液制品的患者，使用 1∶1 比例的浓缩红细胞和血浆似乎能够改善预后。然而，如果需要大量液体或者输血进行液体复苏，应该果断放弃尝试非手术治疗，而转入手术室治疗。

适宜的监测和频繁的重新评估患者的临床检查和实验室检查是安全处理这些损伤的前提。患者护理级别（重症监护室还是普通病房）和监测的频率应该由患者的临床状态、相关的损伤和器官损伤的严重度决定。所有医护人员应该警惕患者腹部损伤的存在和类型，对任何变化的监测和预警，创伤救治小组应该有明确的计划。非手术治疗失败一般出现在损伤发生的 48 h 内，因此这段时间应该严密监测。

患者年龄、合并症情况、相关损伤也是指导创伤救治的其他重要因素。既往认为，老年患者以及多发伤患者，特别是重度创伤性脑损伤患者是腹腔实质脏器损伤非手术治疗的禁忌证。然而，随着医学影像技术的发展和监测手段的提高，很多医学中心都有这种比较复杂患者进行非手术治疗成功的报道。有研究称在多发伤患者中，非手术治疗成功率超过 90%，而并发症发生率与单个脏器损伤相似。这种损伤应该在具有治疗复杂的多系统创伤经验和专长的中心进行，同时需要相关外科科室间的协调与合作，如神经外科和骨科。虽然大多数合并症并不显著影响非手术治疗的成功率，但是对发生于肝硬化患者的腹部钝伤应该提高警惕。进展期肝硬化的患者存在门静脉高压和脾静脉高压、器官硬度增加、肝脾大以及全身凝血功能障碍，严重影响钝伤所致的肝或脾裂伤的止血。此外，肝硬化患者的生理储备往往极差，在这种情况下，非手术治疗和手术治疗的死亡率和并发症发生率均较高。据报道，在肝硬化患者中，脾损伤的非手术治疗的失败率高达 92%，与迅速剖腹术相比，死亡率明显较高。

脾和肝

明确有肝或脾损伤的患者应当送往医院进行至少 24 ~ 48 h 的住院观察。对于较严重的损伤（Ⅲ至Ⅳ级损伤，图 1-2），建议在外科监护病房或稍低一级的病房进行监测。观察的首要目的是监测有无其他腹腔脏器损伤，以及监测有无持续的或反复的肝、脾出血。此类患者中出现漏诊的概率较低，大约为 2%，但并不影响其非手术治疗的策略。对患者的体

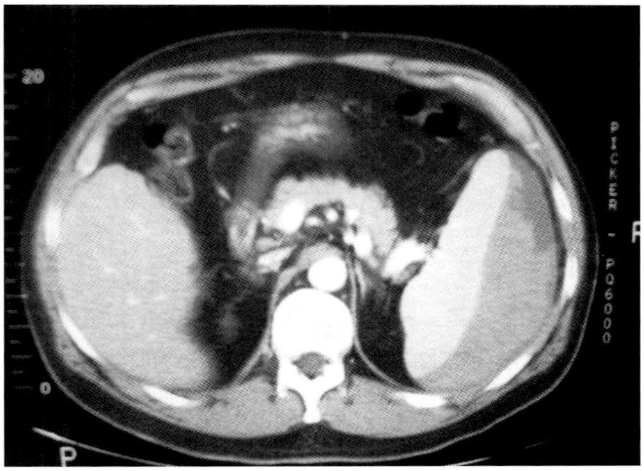

图 1　腹部 CT 显示脾被膜下血肿（Ⅲ级），未见造影剂外渗

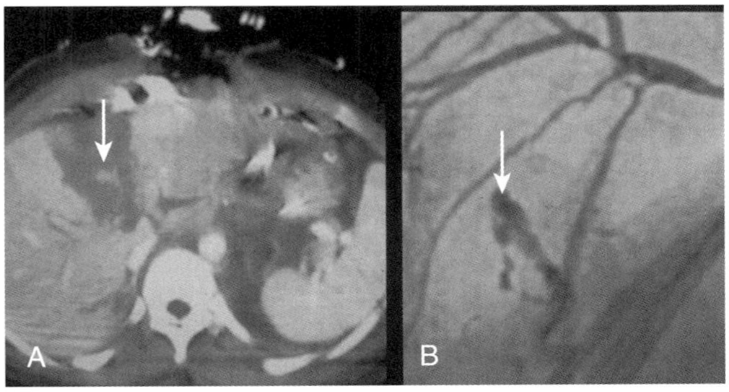

图 2　**A**，腹部 CT 显示肝实质裂伤（Ⅲ级），可见造影剂外渗或者浓聚（白色箭头）；**B**，同一损伤行肝血管造影显示造影剂从右肝动脉渗出（白色箭头）

格检查应当注重以下几个方面，如患者的血流动力学状态，有无加重的腹部压痛、腹胀和腹膜炎。系列实验室检查至少要有全血细胞分析。应当有一些监测患者灌注状态和酸中毒的指标，如乳酸或碱缺失，有助于此类患者的治疗决策。如何适时地进行输血治疗目前仍存在争议。即便原来认为需要输血就是手术指征，但现在已经大有不同。例如脾损伤的患者需要输血的量超过1～2个单位，我们会最大限度地选择进行手术或血管介入治疗。但对于肝损伤的患者，如果需要输血大于4～6个单位，我们才会采取手术治疗。理想情况是既不输血也不手术，但对于实质脏器损伤的患者，何时输血以及何时手术实际上是一门艺术，而非科学。这须经验丰富的创伤外科医生在患者血流动力学状况崩塌的瞬间作出精准的判断，避免差错而延误手术。

既往要求腹部损伤患者卧床休息和限制活动，但没有临床数据或科学证据来支持这种做法。应该避免长时间制动，并且允许患者早期活动。尽管对所有损伤患者应进行常规复查超声或CT，似乎并不能获益，也不能取得良好成本效益比，但对某些患者如重度损伤者或者平常活动量大者，如运动员、消防队员和警察，我们建议进行复查。对所有Ⅳ至Ⅴ级脾损伤患者，因为脾可能失去功能，应考虑进行适龄免疫接种预防。为保证依从性，免疫接种应在出院前进行。

肾

大部分肾钝性损伤可以经非手术治疗治愈，据报道非手术治疗成功率超过90%，即使Ⅴ级损伤也可达50%。这对保护肾功能尤为重要，可避免大部分肾钝性损伤手术探查时行肾切除术。肾位于腹膜后，周围有坚韧的纤维囊（Gerota's筋膜）包裹，因此肾实质出血可因此压迫止血。住院原则、监测和系列评估方案同肝脾损伤。除了监测血红蛋白评估出血量之外，入院时还应检测肾功能指标[血尿素氮（blood ureanitrogen，BUN）、肌酐、肌酐清除率]，并且在住院期间定期复查。肾损伤初期观察应留置尿管监测尿量和血尿程度（如果存在）。对于III至Ⅴ级肾损伤，我们建议可以复查影像学检查，包括肾功能，以评价损伤严重程度和残余肾实质功能。

肾的钝性损伤中，必须将肾实质损伤和肾血管损伤严格区分对待。肾血管损伤常常是由于牵拉或撕裂的机制造成血管的栓塞或破损，可能累及肾动脉、静脉或二者皆有。血尿突然消失需要立即剖腹探查，此类损伤造成肾缺血坏死常推迟或突然出现在CT检查时（图3）。通过开放手术或血管内修复的方法恢复肾灌注，可能导致不良后果，包括修复失败、需要肾切除、感染、肾血管性高血压和死亡。西部创伤协会的一项多中心研究证实了血管修复的不良结果，而伤后立即或者延迟肾切除能够带来更好的预后。初始评估以及其他紧急损伤处理完毕之后，大多数患者应该经非手术治疗观察或延迟行肾切除手术。血管再通通常仅用于早期即获得诊断（2～4 h内）且肾功能开始恶化、双侧肾损伤或孤立性功能肾的患者。

十二指肠和胰腺

腹部钝伤较少引起十二指肠和胰腺损伤，儿童较成年人常见。十二指肠和胰腺位于腹膜后，少有异常临床体征，而CT扫描常显示较差，因此诊断较为困难。与其他腹腔器官不同，一旦确诊十二指肠和胰腺损伤，大部分需要手术探查修复和引流。然而，某些轻微损伤可以经过非手术治疗治愈。大部分Ⅰ级十二指肠损伤（血肿或者非全层裂伤）无须剖腹探查，可以自行恢复。患者如有较大的壁内血肿，特别是儿童，可能会有肠梗阻表现，需要住院营养支持治疗直至血肿消退以及梗阻症状消失。复查口服造影剂的影像学检查有利于评价患者梗阻缓解程度或者病情进展程度。

胰腺损伤是否需要手术治疗取决于胰腺实质破裂的程度和是否有胰管的损伤。在患者血流动力学

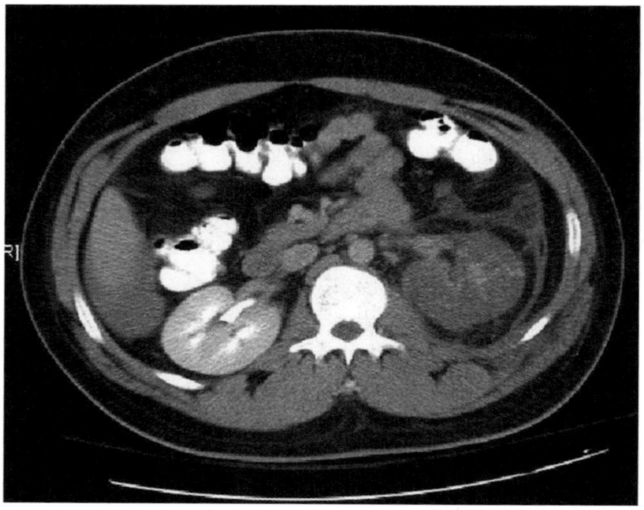

图3 腹部CT扫描显示左肾动脉钝性损伤导致的缺血性改变，右肾造影剂显示正常强化

稳定、临床症状轻微的情况下，CT 评估的Ⅰ级和Ⅱ级损伤（无胰管损伤的挫伤或裂伤）可以经观察处理。行体检和胰腺酶学测量（淀粉酶和脂肪酶）以监测胰腺损伤和炎症进展还是缓解。在病情恶化或者有实验室化验证据显示损伤加重时应复查胰腺增强 CT。如果局部积液或者胰腺脓肿形成，应尝试进行经皮引流，而不是手术引流。如果怀疑胰管损伤，应行经内镜逆行胰胆管造影术（endoscopic retrograde cholangiopancrentography，ERCP）诊断，同时也能介入性治疗（支架或者括约肌切开）。然而，如果有证据显示胰管严重破裂，强烈建议行剖腹探查。同样，胰腺钝伤非手术治疗的经验有限。

血管造影术干预的作用

随着介入放射学的技术发展和疗效的提高，目前已经广泛应用于腹部创伤治疗，其在某些损伤的非手术治疗中具有重要作用。腹部损伤中最常见的应用是通过栓塞出血血管（选择性）或近端主要供血血管（非选择性）从而控制肝、脾的活动性出血。尽管最初血管栓塞技术被积极推广，用于高级别实质脏器损伤，尤其是脾损伤，但经验积累之后发现它应该慎重采用。多个系列研究概述了这些损伤血管栓塞的局限性，包括末端组织坏死导致脾脓肿、囊肿以及很高的再出血率。西部创伤协会的多中心研究发现脾血管栓塞后严重并发症发生率达 20%，强调在脾活动性出血时应谨慎思考和进行患者选择。

CT 扫描显示造影剂渗出或者有证据支持活动性出血时，如果患者无容量依赖并且血流动力学稳定足以坚持介入操作，应该考虑进行血管栓塞。虽然没有预防性血管栓塞的明确标准，但对于复杂的肝损伤（Ⅳ和Ⅴ级）患者，其再出血率和非手术治疗失败率较高，我们建议采用血管栓塞。目前治疗血管栓塞多放置弹簧圈，这可以使血管永久性栓塞，还可以使用可吸收性明胶海绵。明胶海绵通常仅提供暂时性栓塞，在 8～96 h 内血管可以再通，在这段时间内应严密监测再出血的发生。

类似导管介导的溶栓和血管支架的血管介入治疗，如果在血管损伤发生的数小时内进行，可以选择性地对某些血管损伤有作用，特别是对于肾血管损伤。虽然血管造影术越发普及成为非手术治疗的一部分，但是一种侵入性操作，在治疗选择或权衡时也应考虑其明确的并发症。因为这是一个新兴领域，需要进一步的研究和经验积累，以明确其适应证和治疗相关预后。

并发症发生率和并发症处理

腹部钝伤非手术治疗并发症发生率与特定器官损伤、是否有相关损伤及程度、患者年龄、合并症等患者因素有关。避免剖腹术并不等同于避免了任何疾病，在某些情况下，其并发症发生率与手术治疗类似甚至更高。实质器官损伤导致出血的漏诊通常是创伤患者可预防的并发症和死亡发生的最常见原因，但在现代专业的创伤中心中极少见。大约 25% 的腹腔脏器损伤的患者经过非手术治疗后会发生严重并发症，从而需要进一步治疗，而这其中超过 80% 的患者无需手术治疗即可治愈。

腹部损伤患者最常见的并发症也见于其他任何损伤和住院患者。其中包括局部和全身性感染、单个和多个器官功能衰竭、静脉血栓栓塞、住院时间延长和功能障碍。其他与损伤相关的并发症包括延迟性出血、器官坏死或者脓肿形成、假性动脉瘤或者动静脉瘘、胆漏或胰漏、胆道出血、尿外渗和动静脉血栓造成的终末器官组织缺血。

对于腹部钝性损伤的患者，使其预后最佳的关键点是预料其可能出现的常见并发症，以及形成多学科协作的团队来进行诊断和处理。任何患者的临床状况的变化或主诉（如疼痛、发热、呕吐、肠梗阻、出血、黄疸）均应立即再次评估。可以选择 CT 来检查这些器官相关的并发症，并且可以看到器官的坏死或缺血。液体聚集（脓肿、胆汁瘤、尿性囊肿、假性囊肿）、胆管扩张，以及评判已有的器官损伤是继续恶化还是好转。应用静脉造影剂可以显示绝大多数的血管相关并发症，如假性动脉瘤、动静脉（或门体静脉）瘘、内膜夹层和血栓形成。如果 CT 检查不能确认，可采用血管介入造影协助诊断和治疗。腹部透视造影技术，如静脉肾盂造影或逆行尿道造影术可以用来检查有无尿道损伤和尿漏。怀疑胆道和胰腺损伤（漏、瘘）的患者须进一步行 MRCP、ERCP 或经皮肝穿刺胰胆管造影（percutaneous transhepatic cholangiography，PTC）进行检查和治疗。

对于器官并发症的治疗要参照并发症的程度、患者的临床状态，以及可用医疗资源和设备。然而绝大多数的并发症可以采用非手术治疗或微创技术治疗来治愈。目前没有关于腹部损伤预防性使用抗生素的指南。但是，如果出现或怀疑感染，应当使用适当的抗生素治疗。如果腹腔有液体积聚，应当在 CT 或超声引导下进行经皮穿刺引流，吸出物应当进行革兰氏染色，同时进行细菌培养。其他检验如总胆红素、尿素氮、肌酐、淀粉酶和脂肪酶检查会有助于诊断可能出现的胆汁瘤，尿囊肿和胰漏，并指导下一步治疗。严重肝损伤患者如果有持续的胆漏，应当行 ERCP 或 PTC 来进行胆道支架治疗。支架通过十二指肠壶腹还可以治疗或减轻胰胆漏。与此类似，持续的尿外渗可以用经皮穿刺引流及输尿管支架治疗。随后可以通过影像学复查来观察治疗效果，以及判断何时拔除引流管或支架。

任何腹腔脏器的实质损伤都会不同程度地造成组织坏死，随后会出现组织的再生、塑形或瘢痕形成。大量的坏死组织或被继发感染的坏死组织会造成局部或全身的并发症。尤其常见于那些通过血管栓塞止血而造成器官灌注减少的患者。大多数患者通过输液和抗生素治疗可好转，如果发现有大量的液性坏死物质积聚应考虑经皮穿刺引流术。但仍有一部分患者须进行剖腹探查来清理坏死和感染的组织（图 4）。最终，腹部钝伤造成的血管相关并发症会在受伤后任何时间出现，甚至数年以后。轻微而无症状的血管瘤和动静脉瘘可以采取观察并定期成像的治疗策略（图 5）。严重的有症状的病变最好采用血管造影栓塞术治疗。肝钝性损伤的患者出现上消化道出血、右上腹痛和黄疸（Sandblom's 三联征），应当考虑到上消化道出血的可能，可以采用血管造影栓塞术治疗。

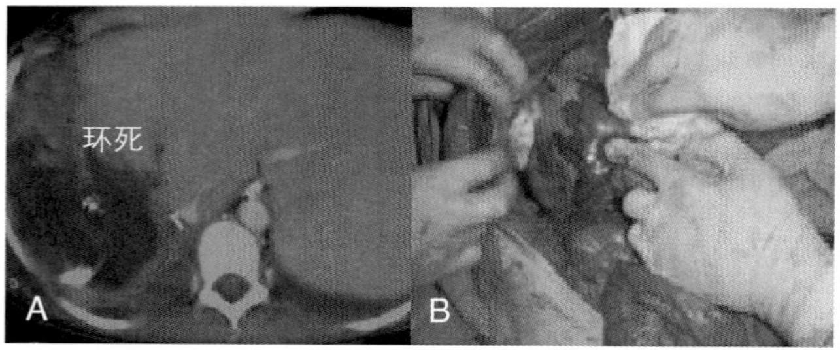

图 4 **A**，腹部 CT 扫描显示肝右叶侧方大量坏死组织需要手术清创。**B**，术中发现显示肝右叶部分坏死区域

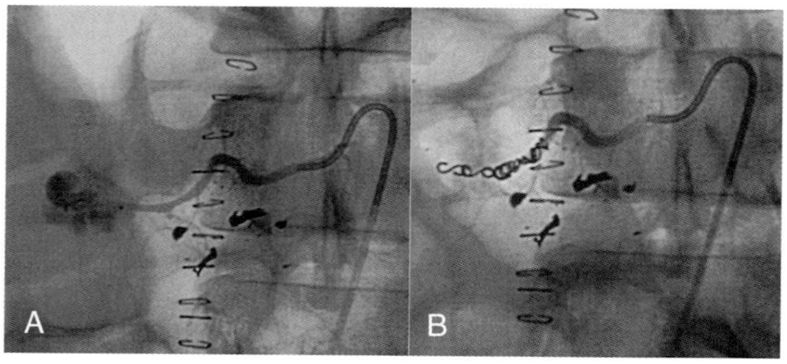

图 5 **A**，肝损伤后 10 天行动脉造影显示肝动脉假性动脉瘤。**B**，血管栓塞术后复查动脉造影，显示弹簧圈位置良好，假性动脉瘤消失

死亡率

腹部钝性损伤的患者死亡率与患者的调查分布、涉及器官的特异性和其严重程度有关。患者死亡的主要原因并非腹部脏器本身，而是其他损伤或患者本身合并疾病。超过一半的患者死亡是因为其他合并损伤，常见的是闭合性头部和胸部外伤，仅有 10% 的患者是因为腹腔脏器出血死亡。近期的数据表明，脾损伤的患者进行非手术治疗，总体死亡率约 6%，如果患者年龄超过 55 岁，死亡率加倍。非手术治疗失败会明显增加 12% ~ 30% 的死亡率。肝损伤的患者有更高的非手术治疗失败率、持续出血率及合并损伤率，因此其死亡率明显高于脾损伤。肝损伤非手术治疗的总体死亡率约为 12%，但如果肝损伤严重（Ⅳ或Ⅴ级损伤），其死亡率最高达 80%。如果患者合并其他脏器损伤（脾和肾），非手术治疗失败率、器官持续出血率和患者总死亡率会加倍。在其他的器官损伤的非手术治疗研究中也得到类似的结果，但须强调的是死亡率与患者的自身因素和受伤机制相关。

总结

现代化文明社会里的损伤大多是钝性高速外伤，经常会导致腹腔内脏器损伤。所有的创伤外科医生必须熟知其流行病学、诊断方法和现代治疗策略，以对此类复杂的患者达到最佳治疗效果和预后。对此类损伤患者采取非手术治疗绝不是单一的流程化模式，须考虑到很多其他因素和决策点，更要有经验的医生凭借经验并随时警醒地护理治疗。血流动力学稳定的情况下，可以对绝大多数腹部钝性损伤的患者采取非手术处理。其失败率较低，不良预后较少。最有效提高此类患者治疗效果和预后的关键点是相关创伤团队和专家的专注治疗。

腹部穿通性损伤

手术要点

1. 对于所有腹部穿通性损伤患者须立即进行全面

检查以排除腹腔内脏器损伤的可能性。

2. 对于有腹膜炎或者生命体征不稳定的患者须立即进行剖腹探查。
3. 清醒有知觉的患者的体检才可用来排除腹腔内的严重损伤，对这些患者可以选择非手术治疗。
4. 对于准备进行非手术治疗的腹部枪伤患者须进行 CT 弹道重建。
5. 膈损伤患者的临床症状不明显，所以对于所有上腹部或下胸部受伤的患者须排除膈损伤的可能性。
6. 对于非手术治疗的腹部穿通性损伤患者须进行严密监测和观察，至少为 24 ~ 48 h
7. 实质脏器穿通性损伤的患者须进行重复的腹部 CT 检查。
8. 大部分感染和器官特异性并发症可以用非手术治疗的多学科手段治愈，如介入性放射学和内镜治疗。
9. 对患者中转手术治疗的评估需要严格的标准和低阈值。

介绍

很少有手术能像腹部穿通性损伤患者的“紧急剖腹探查术”一样能让外科医生精神振奋而肾上腺素激增。虽然在电影和电视节目中经常出现，平民生活和战争中的腹部穿通性损伤的发生率近年来正逐步降低。因此除了有些大城市的创伤中心之外，外科医生和住院医生对于腹部穿通性损伤的治疗缺乏经验。相对于对腹部钝性损伤患者的革新性治疗理念，腹部穿通性损伤的诊疗在过去 50 年没有显著的变化。传统认为对于疑似腹部穿通性损伤或者腹膜炎的患者必须进行剖腹探查手术，目前也有些非手术治疗的经验表明可以将其选择性地应用在不严重的腹部穿通性损伤的平民患者。即使非手术治疗已经被很好进描述，是通常被应用在被锐器刺伤的患者。然而对枪伤患者的非手术治疗一直是一个广泛争论的领域，大部分创伤外科医生和创伤中心还没有广泛接受这种观念。

发病率

总体来说，由于各种因素的影响，腹部穿通性损伤的发病率近年来有显著降低。在所有外伤患者中，即使是在最专业、外伤发病率最高的美国创伤治疗中心，腹部穿通伤患者仅占 10%。有些大城市的创伤治疗中心可以见到约 40% ~ 50% 的腹部穿通性损伤患者。2013 年国际外伤数据库的研究表明，在 850 000 平民外伤患者当中，由枪伤引起的腹部穿通性损伤仅占 4.34%，而锐器伤引起的占 4.51%。大部分腹部穿通性损伤患者集中在 15 ~ 35 岁之间的群体。一项最近对于伊拉克和阿富汗军队的医疗研究发现，外伤的原因由单纯的枪伤引起改变为简易爆炸装置（improvised explosive device，IEDs）爆炸。其引起的外伤占外伤总数的 81%。虽然防弹衣被广泛应用，与先前相比，腹部和胸腔的伤害被大大减弱，美国军队外科医生仍可能面对较多的腹部穿通性损伤。

在讨论非手术治疗对腹部穿通伤的有效性时，最重要的一点就是腹腔内脏器损伤发生率及其类型。大量文献研究表明，腹部刺伤的非手术治疗一直都比枪伤更可行。粗略估计，有一半的前腹部刀刺伤患者和 30% 的腹膜异常的患者并没有明显的腹腔内损伤。腰部和背部刀刺伤的患者发生腹腔内脏器损伤和腹膜后损伤的概率比较低。所以对患者刺伤部位的检查变得尤为重要。正确地对所有刺伤（甚至仅有腹膜异常的患者）检查可以使非治疗性的剖腹术率降低至 30% ~ 50%。

虽然有人声称 90% ~ 95% 的腹部枪伤的患者会出现腹腔脏器损伤，从而须接受剖腹手术。然而这个数据大多应用于由城市内中、大口径手枪引起的枪伤或者在军队对抗中遭受的高速度的伤害，在这一章中我们不进行讨论。一项单因素研究表明，30% ~ 40% 的前腹部枪伤患者和高达 70% 的后腹部枪伤患者没有明显的腹腔脏器损伤，从而不须进行外科治疗。成功的非手术治疗可以帮助减少不必要的剖腹术引起的并发症，但是对非手术治疗的运用须要加倍小心，以减少腹腔内脏器损伤的漏诊或延误治疗。一项单中心研究表明，约 20% ~ 40% 的腹部枪伤和至少 50% 的腹部锐器刺伤，不需要剖腹术也可以被有效地治疗。然而，这些研究还没有被广泛接受。

损伤机制

武器类型不同，腹部穿通性损伤引起的组织和器官损伤可以有很多种损伤机制。刺伤的通过速度很慢，会在接触时造成通过区原始组织的破坏和血行阻断。组织损伤的程度和临床症状主要取决于伤口的确切位置和深度。锐器刺伤会产生较为规整的伤口（针眼，裂口），会对周围的组织造成极小的损伤或者没有损伤。尽管大部分刺伤随刀片刺入、拔出造成直接、线性的损伤。有一点须注意，在某些情况下刺伤会产生轴向旋转或扭转的损伤。中心点位于皮肤，这个“壶样”的致伤机制会造成皮肤很小的损伤，但却在腹腔里造成大规模撕裂伤（图 6）。

相反的，枪伤由于不同的损伤机制和受累组织数量的多少而大不相同。子弹穿透组织时，通过机械撕裂、破坏会造成一个特殊的通道或腔。没有配弹头壳的子弹会造成更大的创伤，其原因在于这种子弹撞击人体之后（或再次击中骨骼时）的碎片产生大量小的碎片，会增大腔的大小和组织损伤的范围。子弹在受到阻力时变形或旋转同样会明显增加主要创面腔的范围。除了固有组织损伤外，子弹撞击周围组织的能量产生一个撞击波或临时残腔，会造成更大范围的组织损伤和失活。

尽管目前已有很多关于平民和军队枪伤的研究，但其中有很多众所周知的弹道学方面的观念是错误的。尽管高速武器会对组织产生更大的撞击力，但组织损伤的数量及空腔形成绝大多数决定于子弹（子弹的包壳、变形、旋转和偏航的多少以及轨道）的作用而不是速度。例如，一枚高速配弹头壳子弹会干净快速地穿过组织而产生很小的损伤，但一枚低速无弹头壳子弹则非常容易粉碎、变形、且会产生明显更大的损伤和组织坏死（图 7）。除此之外，临时残腔的大小及临床意义被过度夸大，大大小于有研究提到的为子弹直径的 20 ~ 30 倍。某些研究所指出的所有高速子弹伤均须对临时腔做广泛的清创术，并没有被动物实验和临床数据所支持，其引申出的低速子弹伤不需要清创同样不被支持。

诊断

如何对血流动力学稳定的腹部穿通性损伤患者进行诊断目前有很大争议，须根据损伤机制、创伤部位和患者的临床状态的不同而区分对待。诊断的规范由确定腹膜是否有异常逐步向损伤是否需要外科干预决定转变。评估应着重于快速明确这些患者的损伤，是否存在像空脏器穿孔或持续出血等需要急诊剖腹术的情况，同时须评估腹部以外有无严重损伤。

腹部枪伤的术前检查一般来说比较少，因为大多数损伤都是在剖腹探查手术过程中诊断的。在急诊抢救过程中，应彻底探查体表并明确标记伤口位置。影像学检查（胸、腹、盆腔）可以快速明确残余的弹片和碎片的数量和位置。血流动力学稳定、清醒、意识清楚的患者，体格检查可靠（没有醉酒、

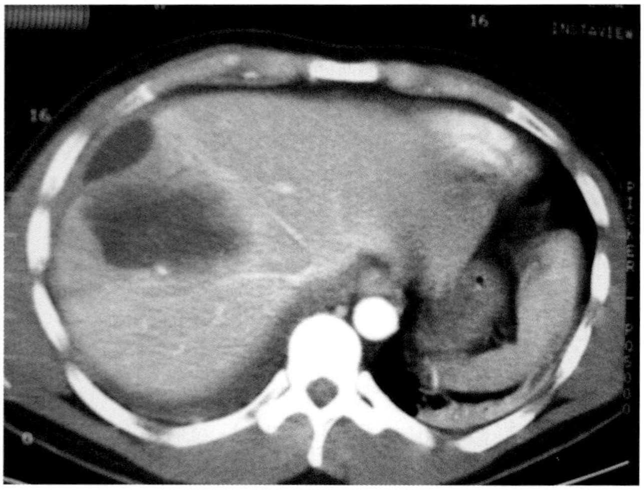

图 6　前腹部刺伤，腹部 CT 显示肝右叶Ⅲ级实质损伤

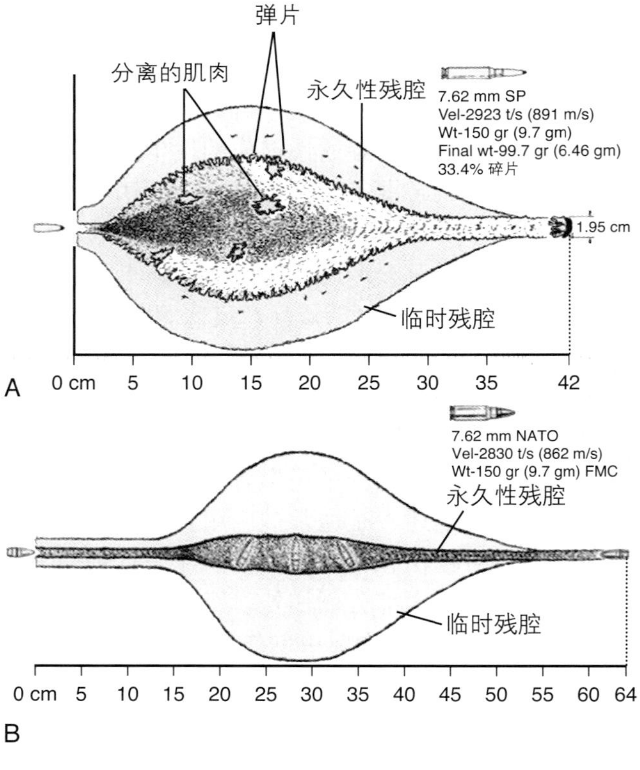

图 7　**A** 图为 7.62 mm 北约组织的制式步枪配软头（SP）狩猎子弹造成的创伤的组织破碎及播散，**B** 图为 7.62 mm 北约制式步枪标准弹。应注意到尽管有相似的通过速度和弥散区域，**A** 图中 SP 子弹比 **B** 图中的标准弹有明显更大的主要残腔

滥用药物及重大的其他损伤），没有其他外科手术或全身麻醉的指征情况下，可以考虑非手术处理。大多数创伤患者并不能符合这种临床表现。这些患者须进一步行急诊腹部CT检查扫描创伤区域或创伤腔道的平面。除了明确有无实质脏器损伤或其他损伤之外，CT还可以重建弹道以明确可能损伤的毗邻结构。在整个影像学评估过程中，有经验的外科医生密切的监测病情是非常重要的，以时刻评价任何临床状态的变化是否需要急诊手术。但须注意的是CT检查明确损伤情况并不是决定性的标准。

上腹部刺伤应当检查胸片，一旦有任何胸部受累的证据（气胸、血胸）应当考虑膈损伤。侧腹部及背部的锐器刺伤应当行腹、盆腔增强CT检查，除非伤口极其浅表。尽管有一些文献推荐应用三重对比（静脉、经口、经直肠）CT，但也有其他研究质疑三重对比CT的必要性。我们并没有发现三重对比CT是必需的，我们更倾向于仅行腹、盆腔静脉增强CT检查。前腹部锐器刺伤不须必须行CT检查，但在高度怀疑创伤位置可能造成实质脏器损伤、创伤重点超声评估阳性（腹腔存在积液）或有血尿时，应当考虑施行。大多数患者的血流动力学稳定。神志清醒、感觉正常且没有腹膜炎的患者并不需要进一步的影像学检查。这些患者会安全地持续接受临床监测，在出现临床状况恶化或腹膜炎进展时行外科手术探查。传统认为，前腹部锐器刺伤的局部伤口探查术（local wound exploration，LWE）是决定性的诊疗措施，如果没有腹膜穿透可继续观察或出院；如果探查阳性即腹膜穿透，则须行剖腹探查。两项西部创伤协会的多中心研究表明，局部伤口探查阴性能可靠排除腹腔脏器损伤可能，但探查阳性并不能准确指示剖腹探查的必要。因此，局部伤口探查可用于排除损伤，但探查阳性的患者并不一定需要强制性剖腹探查，而须通过密切观察腹部体征和临床评估来分类，决定是否需要手术探查。

损伤的解剖学位置及AAST-OIS分级

创伤部位的解剖主要由创伤机制及创伤的伤道决定。锐器刺伤往往局限于一个腹部分区或腹部象限中，通常只损伤一个器官或结构。枪伤可能累及腹部多个分区，经常贯穿其他体腔（胸部、盆腔），而且还可能是经轴的（跨越中线）。损伤或伤道累及上腹部或下胸部，即肋骨下缘到乳头连线圆形区域则须怀疑有膈损伤，直至排除。器官损伤分级应按照我们之前提到的表1中的腹部钝性创伤的AAST-OIS分级表来评价打分。尽管CT所示的弹道解剖并不是决定治疗方式的主要因素，但可以帮助评判是否施行剖腹探查。

处理

对腹部穿通性损伤安全、成功地实施非手术处理，最重要的因素就是合理地选择患者及有经验外科医生的监管。如果按先前所述的流程完成诊断性评估，患者应当送至可以密切观察、监测至少24 h的区域。腹部钝性损伤的患者的治疗，须进行一系列的实验室检查以及监测评估。推荐体格检查由同一位医生（主治医生或高年资住院医生）施行以便能及早发现病情微小的变化。一旦出现临床症状的恶化或腹膜炎体征的进展则立即行剖腹探查。持续性心动过速、发热、白细胞数升高、代谢性酸中毒加重（碱缺失或乳酸）等其他因素也应考虑立刻行剖腹探查。尽管外科医生一直以来通常被教导体格检查并不可靠，有可能遗漏损伤，但我们发现体格检查在评估是否需要外科干预时是准确、可靠的。

可以药物治疗疼痛，但必须慎重决定，并且患者腹痛加剧须立即行再评估。住院后不久即可以饮清水，没必要因为可能需要手术探查而让患者长期禁食。没有发现长期制动有明显的益处（和明显的损害），因此鼓励早期下床活动。密切监测的时间因腹部损伤性质和相关的条件而异。出血、腹膜炎进展等明显的问题常发生在伤后24～48 h内。出院的标准应当与先前所述的腹部钝性损伤一样。在出院前应安排好门诊随访以及急救护理措施。

血管造影术以及其他一些微创技术能否应用于腹部穿通性损伤，目前尚未深入研究。血管栓塞治疗实质脏器损伤出血等介入技术的实用性以及适应证实际上和之前所说的腹部钝性损伤类似（图8-9）。除此之外，对于高级别的肝损伤（Ⅳ或Ⅴ级），或者因其他原因已经行血管造影检查，应当考虑施行预防性血管栓塞术。即使在成功施行非手术治疗之后，对于某些高风险致伤位置（同前所述）或穿通性损伤累及肝、脾、肾上极的患者，须行腹腔镜或胸腔镜探查以明确有无膈损伤。但是，这应当是一项可选择性措施，应在患者观察至确保临床症状稳定，且没有其他进展的剖腹探查指征时实施。

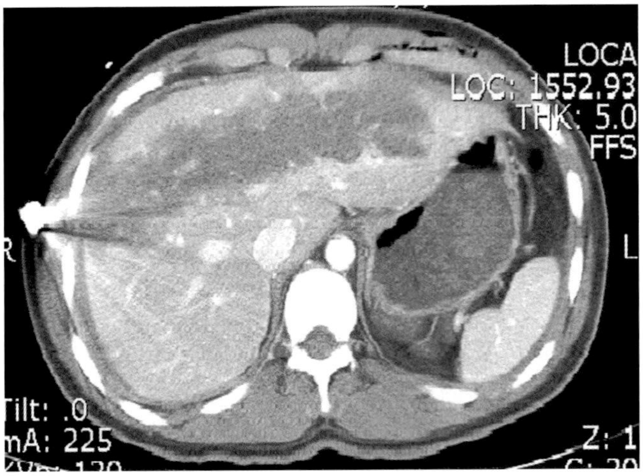

图 8　腹部 CT 所示枪伤造成肝损伤（Ⅳ级），成功接受非手术治疗

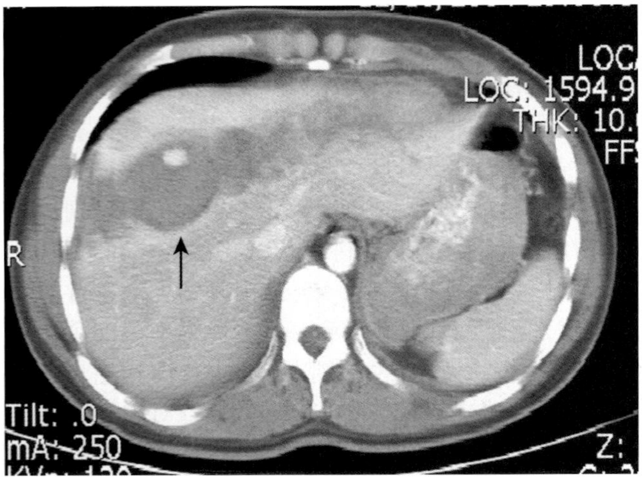

图 9　损伤 1 周后再次对图 8 中创伤情况行常规 CT 复查，可见巨大假性动脉瘤（中央有造影剂填充），随后用血管栓塞术成功治愈（黑箭头所指）

发病率及并发症处理

对于这些患者最主要的忧虑就是非手术治疗失败。尽管总体上大多数腹部穿通性损伤患者需要手术探查，但在这些损伤中有极少一部分像前面所提到的患者可接受选择性非手术治疗。无论是腹部刺伤还是枪伤，接近 4% 最初接受非手术治疗的患者在逐渐出现广泛的腹膜炎体征时最终须接受剖腹探查。延迟剖腹探查的并发症发生率和死亡率很低，与伤后立即行剖腹探查的发生率基本相同。但是，选择性非手术治疗可显著地将非治疗性剖腹探查的概率由 30% ~ 50% 降低到 5% ~ 10%。剖腹术的减少会明显合理利用资源，降低患者并发症发生率，减少医疗卫生系统花费。

患者出现感染或特定器官并发症，非手术治疗跟之前提到的腹部钝性损伤的治疗基本相仿，这里就不做过多赘述了。是否须进行影像学的复查，以明确有无遗漏或判断不清的无症状临床的腹部穿通性实质脏器损伤并发症，目前仍无定论，应当由主管医生决定。严重的实质脏器损伤后期的影像学检查（伤后 7 ~ 10 天）可以明确 50% 以上患者有无脏器相关性并发症，且这其中有一半的患者都没有临床症状。由目前相关的研究和数据，我们推荐出院前和创伤几个月后复查腹部 CT。明确有无腹腔积液、血管损伤等并发症（假性动脉瘤、动静脉瘘），主要可采取微创或介入的非手术方法治疗（图 9）。尽管外科医生不倾向于非手术治疗，但在大多数病例中非手术治疗会改善患者的预后。

死亡率

根据 2013 全国创伤数据库，腹部锐器刺伤的总死亡率为 1.8%，明显低于枪伤总死亡率 16%。死亡率主要由创伤的严重程度、患者的基本情况（年龄、合并症），以及创伤后治疗的合理性决定。很多大型研究表明，几乎没有腹部刺伤的患者接受非手术治疗出现死亡，即使是那些非手术治疗失败再行剖腹探查术的患者。同样地，枪伤非手术治疗患者的死亡率＜1%，明显低于手术患者的 10% ~ 20%。防止非手术治疗死亡最重要的因素是合理选择患者、密切监测病情变化、适时中转为手术治疗。

尽管遗漏腹腔内创伤以致死亡是质疑非手术处理的最大忧虑，迄今为止的数据显示适当选择非手术治疗是安全有效的。实际上，降低腹部穿通性损伤患者较高的非治疗性剖腹探查比例可明显减少总体发病率和死亡率。然而，腹部的枪伤患者存在很严重的穿通性损伤，选择性非手术治疗必须由经验丰富的创伤外科医生决策，且需要密切观察，严格遵从临床评估。一旦出现化验检查和临床症状的恶化或可疑情况，立即行剖腹探查术。应当注意的是，腹部枪伤患者的非手术治疗，并未得到大多数创伤外科医生或创伤中心的认可，目前仅有很少几篇研究支持这一临床实践。这些研究的发现和结果仍需要其他中心以及更大样本量的后期研究来验证。

结论和诊疗流程

尽管大多数腹部钝性器官损伤的非手术治疗在现代创伤中心非常常见，但由于经验不足目前并不愿意将这种治疗手段推广应用于腹部穿通性损伤患者。选择性非手术治疗在适合的患者中可以安全实施，但必须在充足的医疗条件和有经验的监护下进行。特别是腹部枪伤患者的非手术治疗，其安全性评估必须严格遵从先前提到的评价原则。我们相信随着经验的不断积累，选择性非手术治疗的应用会更多地被接受。减少非治疗性剖腹探查术，可以节省医疗花费及降低并发症发生率，从而使患者个体和整个医疗系统都获益。

图 10 列举了我们现在应用的没有腹膜炎的腹部穿通性损伤患者的诊疗流程。

图 10　腹部穿通性损伤患者选择性非手术治疗诊疗流程。CT，电子计算机断层扫描；OR，手术室。非手术治疗由创伤外科医生评估决策。监测环境中，在观察期间至少每 24 h 评估一次临床体征及实验室检查

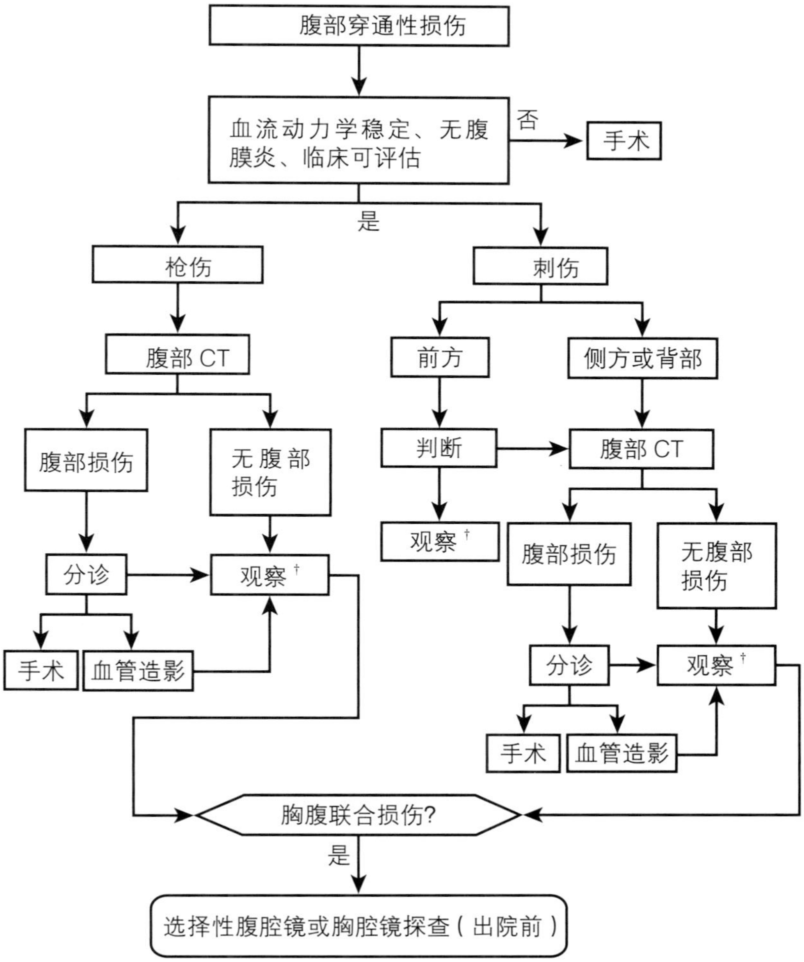

胃损伤

Lawrence N. Diebel 著
沈 凯 译

胃是一种相对壁厚、血供良好的脏器，其在腹膜腔内的位置可以发生变化。尽管下段肋骨可以起到一定保护胃的作用，但是由于胃的容积并且其位置关系，使得胃有被损伤的可能，特别是来自腹部或下胸部的穿通性损伤。

胃的大量血供主要包括胃左动脉——腹腔干的分支，胃右动脉——肝总动脉的分支，胃网膜右动脉——胃十二指肠动脉的分支，胃网膜左动脉——脾动脉的分支，以及胃短动脉，常来源于脾动脉。由于其血供丰富，故胃损伤常出现严重的出血，须在修复中精确止血。但是好的血供同时也有益于大部分胃损伤外科修补术后的康复，即使是在最差的临床情况下。

胃周围包含了许多重要的解剖学脏器，如膈、肝、脾、胰腺，以及横结肠和结肠系膜。如果伴随邻近结构的复合损伤，通常也意味着须着重关注胃钝性和穿通性损伤带来的后果。

发病率

胃损伤常因穿通性损伤导致，大约发生于 20% 的枪击伤和 10% 的刺伤中。钝性胃损伤通常不常见。美国东部创伤外科学会对于空腔脏器损伤的多机构研究显示 0.06% 的进行评估的腹部钝性损伤患者会出现钝性胃裂伤，而在有空腔脏器损伤的患者中，其发生率为 2.1%。

损伤机制

左侧胸腹区域的刺伤有损伤胃的风险。超过 50% 的此类患者会发生单发的胃穿孔。但通常会合并周围邻近脏器的损伤。90% 的枪伤患者会出现 2 处以上的胃伤口。尽管枪伤伤口常合并周围结构的损伤，但这种损伤常常仅发生在高速子弹射伤情况下。近距离（ <15 ft，1 ft = 0.31 m ）枪伤常造成腹壁、胃及腹腔内脏器的大面积创伤。

胃的钝性损伤常见于车祸或者机动车碰撞行人创伤。其他相对少见的原因还包括坠落伤、被袭击，以及不恰当的心肺复苏。钝性胃损伤包括线性撕裂伤和完全胃破裂。钝性胃损伤的可能机制包括胃力压突然升高导致“气球爆破”样损伤、后方脊柱压迫性损伤（座椅 - 安全带损伤），或剪切应力的减速损伤导致胃前壁撕裂。

诊断

钝性损伤导致的胃穿孔常破损较大，并且腹腔内污染通常明显。腹膜刺激征常明显，须尽早外科干预。钝性胃裂伤患者常常由于其他脏器损伤如脾和肝的破损导致休克。

刺伤的患者出现低血压、腹膜炎或者两者均有时，应及时接受剖腹术。对于无症状的患者如不合并中枢神经系统损伤（脑损伤或脊髓损伤）、不涉及药物或饮酒等情况，可以考虑反复体格检查观察。对于其他患者，局部伤口探查、DPL 或者腹腔镜探查可以作为选择。腹腔镜探查对于诊断胸腹刺伤是否合并膈损伤非常重要。FAST 对于空腔脏器损伤造成的少量积液可能无法确诊，因此复杂情况可能被误认为是单纯的胃损伤。

对于有症状的腹部枪伤应尽早外科干预。极少情况下对于病情稳定的患者可以发现切线性枪伤，或者在经过 DPL 或腹腔镜探查后发现类似的伤口。腹部 CT 对于诊断这种状况亦有所帮助。对于怀疑有钝性和穿通性胃损伤的患者，放置鼻胃肠管有所帮助。正确放置鼻胃肠管可以减少误吸的风险，并且一旦发现血性引流液应高度怀疑胃损伤可能。对于钝性胃损伤没有明显腹膜刺激体征的患者，卧位腹部平片只能发现不到 50% 的患者出现游离气体。同样情况下，腹部 CT 诊断游离气体的灵敏度更高。

外科处理

通过正中切口进行腹腔探查。鼻胃肠管减压有助于胃的显示。控制出血是首要治疗目标，其次是控制肠漏。胃的伤口开始可以通过可吸收缝线连续锁边缝合快速控制。随后在术中可以应用不可吸收缝线加固浆肌层缝合。这不仅是为了止血，也是为了控制胃内容进一步渗漏造成腹腔污染。此外也可以选择 TA（胸腹）吻合器、Allis 钳或者 Babcock 钳进行暂时性控制。

在关注其他更可能导致生命危险的损伤之后，就该处理胃可能出现的损伤了。首先应当仔细检查胃小弯或胃大弯有无瘀斑或血肿。探查以下区域可能有一定困难，如胃食管结合部、胃底高位、胃小弯、胃后壁。在剑突旁延长正中切口、应用自动牵引拉钩、对血流动力学稳定的患者采用反 Trendelenburg 体位，这些可能有助于显露上述探查困难的部位。另外切开左侧三角韧带并游离肝左外叶可以更好显露胃食管结合部。沿胃大弯的侧胃网膜血管弓外打开胃结肠韧带可以显露胃后壁。分离胃短血管对于显露胃底近端可能是必要的。少数情况下，通过将胃浸入生理盐水后经鼻胃管注气，可能会发现一些隐匿的伤口。切线伤口和胃单发穿孔确实会发生，但这须排除其他情况才能获得诊断。

胃损伤一旦确诊，应按照其严重程度进行治疗（表 1，图 1）。大多数胃壁内血肿（Ⅰ级和Ⅱ级）可以通过仔细排空、止血和非可吸收缝线浆肌层缝合关闭来治疗。小的Ⅰ级和Ⅱ级穿孔可以通过单层或者双层缝合关闭。由于胃血供丰富，因此作者更喜欢止血后双层缝合关闭伤口。

表 1 AAST 的胃损伤分级量表

AAST 分级	损伤特点
Ⅰ	胃壁内血肿 <3 cm，胃壁部分全层撕裂伤
Ⅱ	胃壁内血肿 >3 cm，小（<3 cm）的胃壁撕裂伤
Ⅲ	大（>3 cm）的胃壁撕裂伤
Ⅳ	大的胃壁撕裂伤并损伤胃大弯侧或胃小弯侧血管弓
Ⅴ	广泛（>50%）破裂，胃血供阻断

美国创伤外科学会（AAST）修订

靠近胃大弯侧大的（Ⅲ级）损伤也可以使用相同的技术关闭或者应用 GIA（胃肠吻合）吻合器关闭。这种缺损同样也可以应用 TA 吻合器关闭。吻合器钉合线可以通过不可吸收缝线缝合浆肌层加固。须注意的是要避免食管和幽门的狭窄。幽门的伤口可以进行幽门成形术以避免这一区域可能的狭窄。广泛的伤口（Ⅳ级）由于破损严重，常须行近端或远端胃大部切除术。重建手术可采取毕Ⅰ或毕Ⅱ式吻合，具体选择由是否合并十二指肠损伤来决定。极少数病例，如发生Ⅴ级损伤，往往须行全胃切除术和 Roux-en-Y 食管空肠吻合术。

如果胃穿孔合并膈损伤，胃内容物污染胸膜腔可能造成麻烦。大多数情况下，关闭胃穿孔后通过

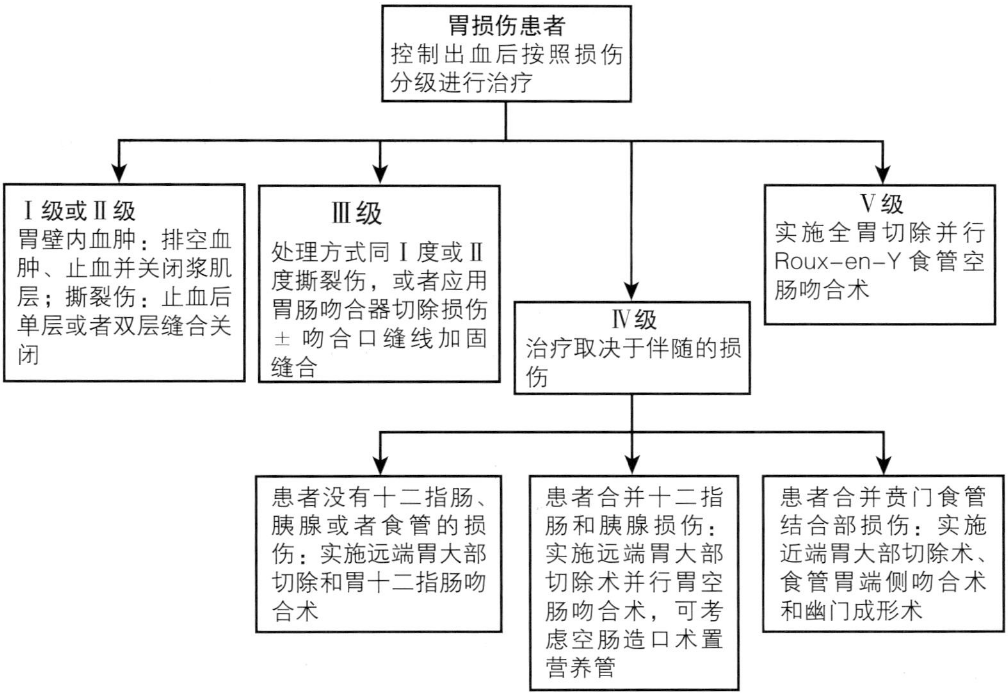

图 1 胃损伤处理流程

膈伤口就可以充分清理胸膜腔。扩大膈伤口有助于彻底清理胸膜腔的污染。外科修补胃后，须关闭膈伤口并放置胸管。少数情况下，胸腔污染可能非常严重，特别是手术干预较晚的病例，可能需要单独的开胸手术，以达到充分引流胸膜腔的目的。用胸腔镜清理胸膜腔胃内容物污染，随后置入胸管也可以作为一种选择。

死亡率

胃损伤的死亡率与损伤机制、是否合并休克和输血需求，以及合并其他损伤的数量相关。有报道表明，钝性胃破裂的死亡率为 0～66% 不等，平均约 30%。同时合并腹腔内和腹腔外损伤也比较常见。常见的腹腔内合并损伤包括脾、肝、小肠和胰腺。最常见的腹腔外损伤如胸腔、四肢和头部。绝大多数的死亡是因为其他合并损伤造成的失血性休克和相关并发症。

胃穿通性损伤的总体死亡率为 14%～20%。早期死亡通常与其他损伤造成的不可逆的失血性休克相关。损伤的脏器数量增多，死亡率会明显升高。最常见的合并损伤包括肝、膈、结肠、肺和小肠。脾、胰腺和腹腔大血管损伤也十分常见。穿通性或钝性胃损伤造成死亡的可能性较低。这种情况造成死亡，往往是由于吻合口裂开、脓肿或瘘形成，以及后续造成的器官衰竭。

并发症发生率

胃损伤主要的并发症包括腹腔内脓肿形成、出血、吻合口破裂、脓胸形成等。胃损伤的严重程度和腹腔污染的程度主要影响腹腔内脓肿的形成。胃钝性损伤造成的腹腔内污染通常更加明显。

穿通性损伤造成的孤立性胃损伤和结肠损伤，两者腹腔内脓肿形成和外科手术刀口感染的风险类似，均较低。但如果合并肝、肾、胰腺或者十二指肠损伤，由胃损伤和结肠损伤造成的腹腔脓肿形成的概率会明显升高。如果同时合并胃和结肠损伤，其协同效应会造成腹腔内脓肿形成概率升高。如果穿通性胃损伤合并膈损伤，则脓胸的可能性会明显升高。手术区域或胃吻合口的术后出血可能造成二次手术。少数情况下吻合口出血可以通过内镜技术治疗。胃损伤极少数情况下会需要吻合口和胃切除，吻合口狭窄可能须进一步手术来纠正。

结论

大多数胃损伤需要清创和缝合。少数情况下，须进行更复杂的操作，如胃切除和吻合。休克和合并其他损伤会影响总体预后。

小肠损伤

Kimball Maull 著
沈　凯 译

小肠损伤

自古以来就有肠损伤的描述。亚里士多德曾描述“没有皮肤损伤的轻微的击打可造成肠破裂”，希波克拉底首次描述了穿通性损伤造成的肠损伤。1275 年，De Salicet 首次报道了横向缝合修复肠损伤的方式。1686 年，Bonet 描述了被鹿撞后猛烈撞击树干引起的钝性肠损伤。Autopsy 描述了回肠末段和盲肠的破裂。1761 年，Morgagni 报道了几例直接撞击腹部造成小肠钝性损伤的病例。他强调腹部体征的迟发性和隐匿性，这项发现和现在的临床观察非常贴近。首次修复完全断裂的小肠是在 1889 年由 Croft 报道的。20 世纪初，俄日战争期间 Gedroitz 的经验证实了对于腹部损伤早期手术干预的优势。她将手术室设在前线，选择 4 h 内的急诊创伤进行治疗，结果显示可以改善预后。20 世纪末，认识到早期修复的优势，并伴随着诊断技术的提高，预后明显改善。然而，考虑到有风险的患者的诊断和治疗方法，上述结果仍然有争议，还未达成一致。因此，外科医生须对于肠损伤的诊断和治疗的误判提高警惕。

发生率

小肠损伤应根据其受伤机制不同进行分类。由于小肠占据了腹腔绝大多数空间，因此在穿通性损伤后小肠常常受累。大多数情况下枪伤累及小肠或小肠系膜的发生率为 90% 或更高，刺伤的小肠损伤发生率为 25% ~ 30%。钝性损伤中，虽然小肠是第三位最容易受伤的器官，仅次于肝和脾，但近年来的观点认为其发生率比以往认为的要低（表 1）。钝性创伤后小肠损伤发生率为 1%，而腹部钝性创伤后小肠损伤的发生率增加到 3%，钝性腹部损伤中小肠穿孔率仍然小于 1%。这些特点可能令人误解。Nance 等运用宾夕法尼亚损伤系统数据库，显示了实质脏器损伤数量和空腔脏器损伤有显著相关的可能性。总的发生率为 9.6%，但是随着实质脏器损伤数量的增加，比如 3 个或以上实质脏器损伤，空腔脏器损伤发生率可上升至 34%。单独的胰腺损伤后空腔脏器损伤发生率为 33%。只有空腔脏器的简明损伤分级（Abbreviated Injury Scale，AIS）评分≥3，才能被包含在数据库内，但这个数据库还包含胆囊和膀胱的损伤。

表 1　钝性小肠损伤的发生率

	钝伤入院（n=227 972）		腹部钝性伤（n=85 643）	
	任何损伤	穿孔	任何损伤	穿孔
小肠	1.1%	0.3%	2.9%	0.8%
空肠 / 回肠	0.9%	0.3%	2.5%	0.7%

Modified from Fakhry SM, Brownstein M, Watts DD, et al: Relatively short diagnostic delays (<8 hours) produce morbidity and mortality in blunt small bowel injury: an analysis of time of operative intervention in 198 patients from a multicenter experience. J Trauma 48:408–415, 2000

损伤机制

没有几个解剖学位置像空腔脏器一样，损伤机制在决定诊断的难易或者治疗的确定性上发挥重要作用。穿通性力量会引起的小肠损伤，包括火器伤、猎枪伤和刺伤。虽然最近有研究报道证明火器伤保守治疗有效，但大多数外科医生坚信对于腹部的火器伤，或者伴有下胸部开放伤、臀部伤等导致腹部处于危险状态的损伤时，手术还是很有必要。因为在有腹部火器伤的情况下，外科意义上的损伤可能性超过 80%，因此适用剖腹探查。即使没有穿透进入腹腔，但产生近端创伤的冲击波效应可能导致脏器穿孔，尤其是当冲击的火器处于高速状态时（>2 000 ft/s）。火器伤的损伤性质与子弹的大小和射击距离有关，大口径枪弹、距离近则损伤大。刺伤极少致命，但由于多数是选择性治疗，所以那些被忽视的损伤相对于需要手术的损伤风险性较高。

小肠可能因为非穿通力造成损伤。高速交通方式和安全带的普遍使用增加了小肠钝性损伤的风险。过去交通事故常常造成现场死亡或快速致命的中枢神经系统损伤，对交通安全的努力改善减少了死亡事故，然而却增加了不同类型的损伤。安全带综合征就是其中一种类型，包括小肠损伤。事实上，Fakhry 等的 2003 例多机构的报告指出，安全带的使用增加了小肠穿孔的风险。在许多损伤病例中，主要导致综合征的原因是安全带的不正确使用，比如太松、太高或者身体大小不符合，如小孩用成年人的安全带。

钝性外力造成小肠破裂的发病机制仍待确认，但不同程度地归因于挤压、剪切或爆炸力。当暴力直接作用于腹部，可挤压位于外力和脊柱之间的肠管。这种机制常伴随其他器官的损伤。由突然减速造成的典型的损伤常发生于相对固定位置，如 Treitz 韧带和末端回肠或者有附着束的部位。有些研究者总结上述为损伤机制，在某些书中引用的某些研究发现小肠损伤分布相对均匀。肠管末端暂时关闭造成部分肠管膨胀，若此时外力作用于此段肠管可使小肠破裂。这就解释了小肠在相对小的外力情况下可能破裂的原因，而且已经在犬模型中得到证明。总之，小肠多处破裂伴随肠系膜毁损伤和广泛小肠挫伤是挤压伤的发病机制（图 1）。小肠损伤且伴有孤立的明确定义的破裂位置，可能代表着爆炸伤和撕裂伤，尤其是在 Treitz 韧带、盲肠或者其他固定点附近，这样的损伤很可能是由剪切力造成的（图 2-图 3）。

诊断

由于新技术和微创外科技术的应用，腹部穿通伤的诊断方法逐渐发展起来。1960 年，Shaftan 提出异议并提出外科判断对于穿通伤的患者是更好的方法，而不是强制性剖腹探查。他提出的锐器刺伤评

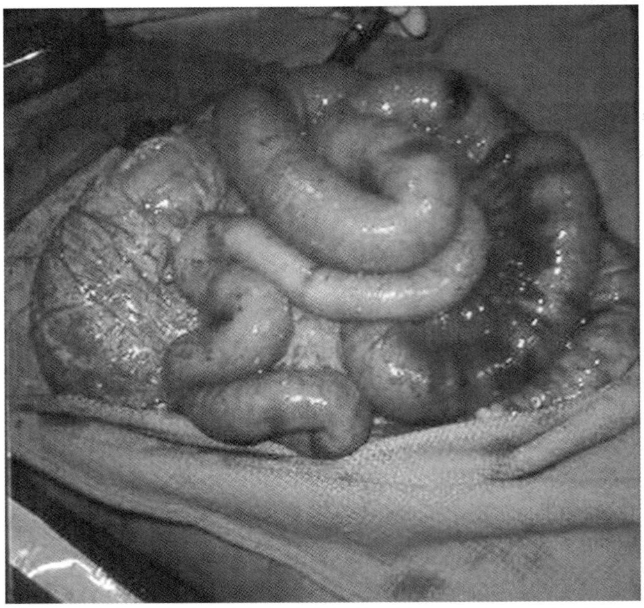

图 1 由挤压力造成的小肠损伤。注意广泛的无活力的肠管

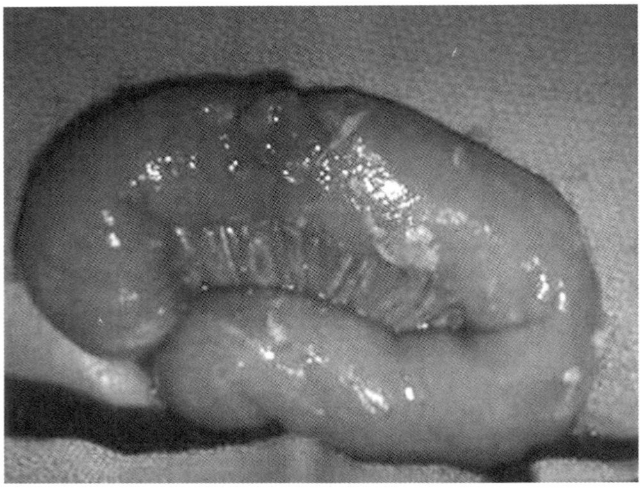

图 2 部分小肠爆炸伤

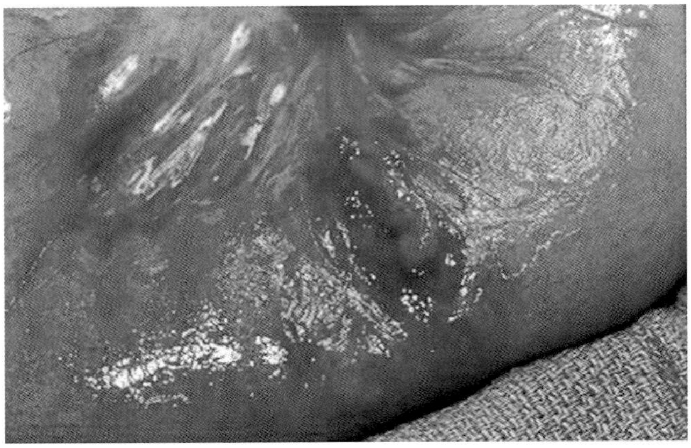

图 3 小肠线性穿孔，由剪切损伤机制引起

估逐渐得到了支持。刺伤分为 3 类：一类是没有进入腹膜腔，一类是进入腹膜腔但是没有造成脏器损伤，还有一类是造成损伤，并须手术修复。须认识到强制性剖腹探查可能造成 2/3 的患者接受阴性或非治疗性剖腹术。选择性的治疗是现代普遍的做法。2001 年，Chiu 等报道一项前瞻性研究，对血流动力学稳定的穿通伤患者进行三重对照 CT 的应用研究。这项试验包括了连续选择的 75 名患者，60% 有火器伤或者猎枪伤。CT 检查阴性的患者中，96% 的患者经过非手术处理成功治愈。尽管有这些令人印象深刻的系列试验，绝大多数外科医生仍然用剖腹探查手段治疗火器伤，这会导致 15% 的阴性或非治疗性的剖腹探查。在一些研究机构，手术和选择性非手术处理共存，当怀疑腹腔内有穿通性损伤或者损伤位置低时，也就是说，有侧腹部伤和肝区的损伤，这些情况应该考虑外科干预。

手术适应证遵循以下通用的流程图（图 4-5）。当符合标准时，大多数外科医生进行手术治疗。随着有经验的微创外科医生的出现，穿通伤后剖腹手术的适应证开始被修改，尤其是可能损伤半侧膈或

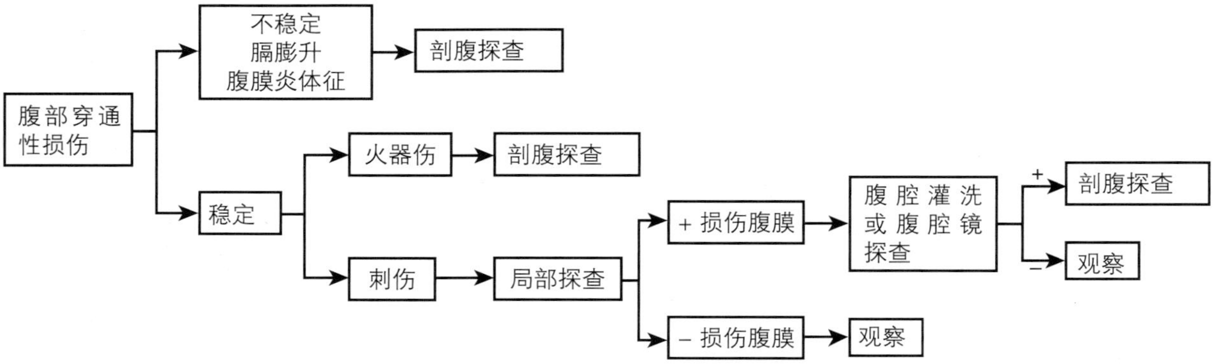

图 4 小肠穿通性损伤的处置流程图

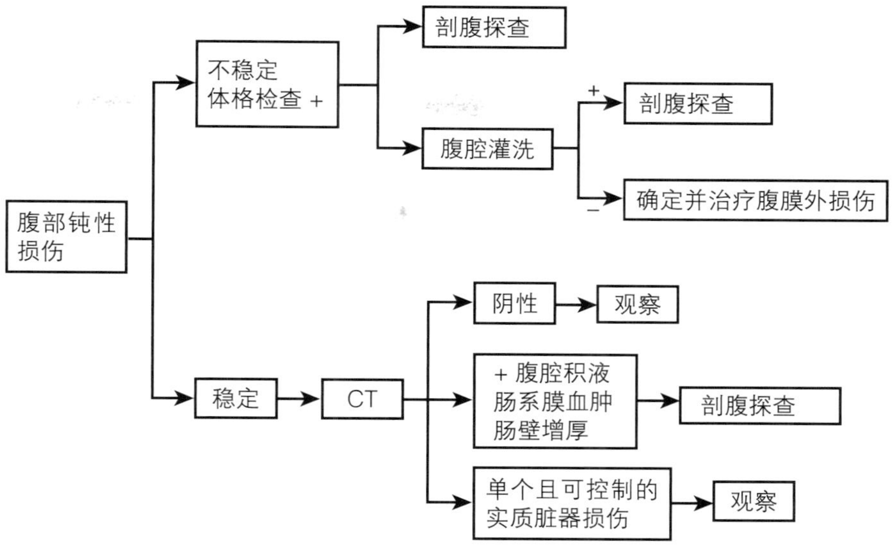

图 5　小肠钝性损伤的处置流程图。
CT，计算机断层扫描

可疑的腹部穿通伤。这些增强的技能支持腹腔镜由最初的诊断手段逐渐演变成集诊断和治疗为一体的工具。膈损伤能够被看到并修复。其他器官系统的损伤在很多情况下可以探查到，进行损伤严重程度分类，在部分情况下，进行修复或控制出血治疗。小肠损伤仍然存在问题。明显的损伤可能会被腹腔镜外科医生用其余的简单或者更小侵入性的操作检测到，如体格检查、CT 和 DPL。不管用何种诊断方法，隐匿性的损伤在最初可能会被忽略，但是用局部伤口探查或腹腔镜直视损伤而排除腹膜穿通都是有用的。

小肠钝性损伤的诊断并不是那么明显。小肠钝性损伤根据程度可包括钝性小肠伤伴或不伴浆膜撕裂、肠壁内血肿、肠壁完整性缺失。后一种情况常在直接损伤后立即发生，但仍有很多延迟穿孔的病例，可能是外伤后缺血导致肠壁坏死引起。肠系膜的损伤可引起类似的结果，或者仅仅引起创伤后狭窄和肠梗阻的延迟症状。受伤的患者伴有穿孔，其症状常表现为腹痛和腹膜刺激征，包括腹部叩痛，深触压痛和直接、间接反跳痛。这种情况没有额外的诊断也具有手术适应证。在多处损伤的患者中，以下情况可能出现体格检查阴性，如合并头外伤、醉酒或服用其他药物，或有其他损伤转移了患者的注意力。在这些情况下，CT、超声、DPL 或腹腔镜探查等诊断方法可能会有效。小肠损伤的诊断须注意以下几点：

1. 清醒患者的体格检查才可信；
2. 没有单个的诊断方法能确诊小肠损伤，除了剖腹探查；
3. 没有出现穿孔的小肠和肠系膜损伤也需要手术处理。

小肠损伤时 CT 扫描的可靠性仍有较大争议。如 CT 检查时口服造影剂是否增加准确性也有争议。对于腹腔有游离积液但没有实质脏器损伤的患者如何处理亦有争议。DPL 能否作为 CT 的补充诊断方法有争议。没有争议的是，即使 CT 检查正常，仍可能发生小肠损伤，包括小肠穿孔。某些研究中，CT 检查诊断小肠损伤的概率小于 50%（图 6）。腹部 CT 已经成为腹部损伤最常用的检查方法。这样，在 CT 检查阴性的患者中，很大可能遗漏了小肠损伤的诊断，以及推迟了恰当的手术治疗。2000 年，Malhotra 等评价了不同代 CT 扫描仪对确诊钝性小肠损伤的能力。与早期的 CT 仪器相比，新一代螺旋 CT 更加灵敏。然而，在他的研究中，有 7/47（15%）的 CT 诊断阴性的小肠或肠系膜损伤的患者

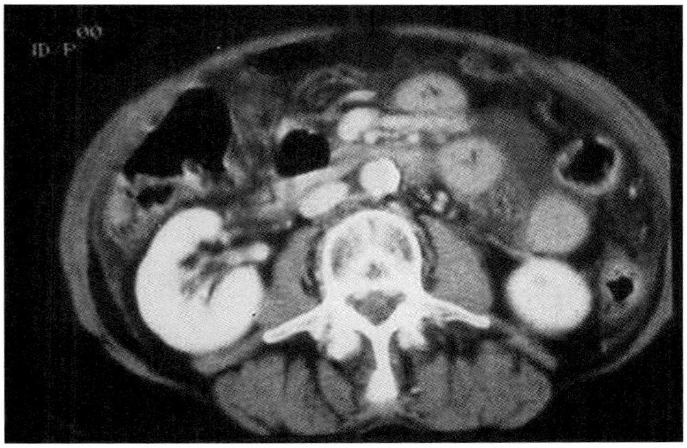

图 6　小肠破裂患者 CT 阳性表现：肠壁增厚伴附近游离腹腔积液

须行手术治疗。Malhotra 的研究结果与东部创伤外科学会多机构临床试验的研究结果相似，后者证明了 CT 诊断小肠损伤有 13% 的错误阴性率。2004 年，Allen 等的回顾性研究表明，腹部增强 CT 在诊断钝性小肠损伤和肠系膜损伤中的灵敏度和特异度分别为 95% 和 99%。然而，他们实际损伤的病例数少。2001 年，Gonzalez 等报道了 CT 检查前运用 DPL 的方法，他们将患者随机分成 DPL+CT 组和仅用 CT 检查组。如果红细胞数大于 20 000 个 / 微升，便可用 CT 检查。主要研究那些仅行 CT 检查并发现腹腔有游离液，且不伴有实质脏器损伤的患者。运用 DPL 筛查法，他们发现非治疗性剖腹术使用率较低，提高了成本效益。CT 扫描联合腹腔镜探查可提高诊断的准确性。2005 年，Mitsuhide 等报道了选择性腹腔镜探查应用于体格检查或 CT 检查怀疑小肠损伤的患者。腹腔镜探查发现肠穿孔或缺血则须中转为剖腹术。他们得出结论，CT 联合腹腔镜探查能避免非治疗性剖腹探查和减少诊断延迟。2000 年，来自于 AAST 的报告称关于小肠损伤诊断和治疗，他们对任何可实施的诊断方法均没有绝对的信心。在如何处理 CT 报告显示有腹腔游离液体而没有实质脏器损害，且有神经系统受损的患者方面存在很大差异（表 2）。可以选择观察、手术，在怀疑时可以使用 DPL 等方法。对于儿童，当出现腹部压痛和腹腔游离液体时，则高度怀疑小肠穿孔。

表 2　患者处理：无实质脏器损伤、游离液体、不可靠的检查

治疗选择	头部损伤（%）	中毒（%）
观察	28	51
重复 CT	12	11
诊断性腹腔灌洗	42	26
手术	16	10

Modrhied from Brownstein MR, Bunting T, Meyer AA, Fakhry SM: Diagnosis and management of blunt small bowel injury: a survey of the membership of the American Association for the Surgery of Trauma. J Trauma48:402–407, 2000

损伤分级

小肠损伤程度的分级较简单，但损伤结果复杂。理由很简单——小肠损伤发生时，有些病例非初次诊断。许多病例从损伤到愈合没有症状，有些发生坏死，则表现为腹腔内严重的疾病症状，有些症状延迟，常须后期手术治疗。AAST 的器官损伤分级见表 3。注意Ⅱ级至Ⅳ级损伤，相当于穿孔且很可能损伤后立即出现症状。Ⅴ级损伤，即肠管横断伴有节段性组织缺失或血供阻断，症状可以明显也可能隐匿，但都会引起肠管完整性丧失并需要小肠切除。在某些无法分类的缺血事件，即有部分血供阻断不伴有肠壁全层坏死，愈合后会出现狭窄而引发延迟性肠梗阻症状。出现上述问题多数需要手术干预。

外科处理

大多数情况下，外科治疗即指手术治疗。然而，外科评价在决定是否行肠切除、切除范围以及修复和切除方法上有确切的作用。小肠损伤常是单纯的损伤，但在腹部穿通伤或钝伤机制下也常常合并其他腹腔内损伤。外科决策对于相关损伤的治疗和是否应用损伤控制外科理念极为重要。2000 年，Hackam 等将小肠损伤患者与伴有和不伴有其他腹腔内损伤的患者做了比较。虽然伴有其他损伤的患者能够更早得到诊断和实施剖腹探查，但合并其他损伤的患者死亡率高，住院时间长（length of hospital stay，LOS），腹部并发症多。

小肠损伤需要手术处理的情况包括小肠穿孔、肠壁内血肿、挤压伤使肠管丧失活力、肠管撕裂、肠系膜创伤致肠系膜撕裂、出血、血肿增大和小肠缺血。小肠损伤是行修补、切除，还是损伤控制要基于患者的临床条件、损伤的解剖学情况、损伤是累及单个区域还是节段小肠、多处损伤分布于小肠

表 3　小肠损伤分级

分级*	损伤类型	损伤描述	AIS 评分
Ⅰ	血肿	挫伤或血肿，没有血供阻断	2
	裂伤	局部增厚，无穿孔	2
Ⅱ	裂伤	裂伤 <50% 环周	3
Ⅲ	裂伤	裂伤达 50% 环周，没有横断	3
Ⅳ	裂伤	小肠横断	4
Ⅴ	裂伤	小肠横断伴节段组织缺失	4
	血管	小肠节段性血供阻断	4

AIS，简明损伤分级

* 多发伤分级为Ⅲ级

多个节段。外科医生应注意单个穿孔或损伤的数量。虽然这可以用切线伤或找到肠内子弹解释，但系膜内小肠壁穿孔更容易被忽视。所有的小肠系膜血肿都应打开探查确认肠壁完整性。

修补最好是直接缝合。如果有肠切除的指征，吻合器和手工吻合具有相同的效果。然而，2 种形式的切除吻合与单纯修补相比有更高的并发症发生率。因此，能修补的损伤尽量修补，除非有多处的近端损伤，从技术上说节段切除比逐个修补更容易。在损伤控制模式下，可用吻合器快速闭合伤口以防止肠内容物持续溢出。没有确定性的吻合方法。

创伤的剖腹探查包括开始探查时即要积极止血，然后全面探查确定所有损伤部位。剖腹探查遗漏的损伤往往是最致命的损伤。因此，要尽全力确认所有腹腔内损伤，尤其是在损伤控制方法的情况下，持续的污染可导致预后不良。空腔脏器的损伤导致的渗漏应用非损伤肠钳或助手用拇指和示指控制，或者可以用 Babcock 钳控制。探查从胃食管结合部到直肠的消化道，计数损伤，并记录或用缝线标记确认。血肿的部位应该仔细检查。大多数损伤是局限于浆膜的损伤，最好将浆肌层边缘内翻缝合加强。真性肠壁内血肿需要外科评价。如果面积局限、没有增大，血肿很可能自行吸收，不需要特殊处理。面积大的或逐渐增大的肠壁血肿，或者累及的一段肠管活力无法确认，则需要处理。推荐血肿清除和受累肠管切除。本文作者倾向于后者。穿孔损伤应仔细切除以能见到活力组织，展开边角处牵拉的缝线，横向双层关闭肠壁（图 7–9）。两个相对紧邻的穿孔，应转换成单个缺损，并以同样的方法缝合（图 10）。位于较短距离内的多处穿孔最好使用肠切除和吻合（图 11）。肠系膜缺损应连续关闭（图 12）。

肠系膜损伤程度不同，可能是小血肿，也有可能是广泛的危及生命的撕裂伤。大范围的或逐渐增大的肠系膜血肿以及紧邻的肠壁血肿须探查和缝扎血管（图 13）。必要时应修补保证肠壁完整性。肠系膜撕裂可能造成累及的肠段缺血，这时行肠切除很有必要（图 14）。所有的撕裂需缝合（图 15）。

微创技术在小肠损伤包括钝伤和穿通伤的诊断和治疗中应用得越来越频繁。微创技术的成功使用很大程度上依赖于外科医生的熟练程度和患者的稳定性。由于存在潜在的漏诊损伤的可能性，因此小肠损伤的微创方法只能选择性使用，而且只有那些腹腔镜技巧高超的医生能使用、其安全性有待进一步证明。

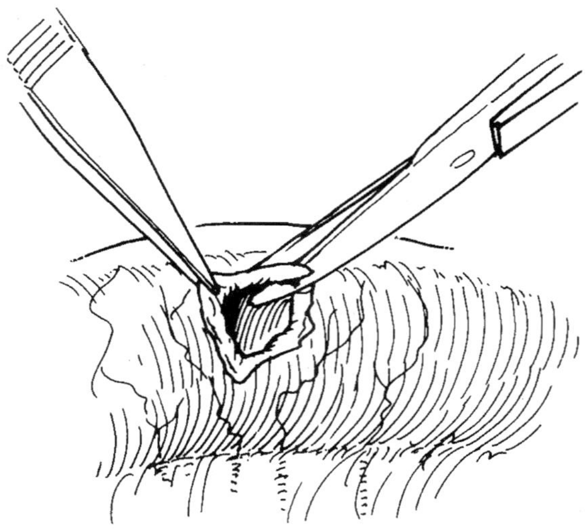

图 7　穿孔损伤应仔细清创以显露有活力组织（*From Maull KI: Stomach, small bowel and mesentery injury. In Champion HR, Robbs JV, Trunkey DD, editors:* Rob and Smith's operative surgery: trauma surgery, *4th ed, London, 1989, Butterworth-Heinemann, pp 401–413.*）

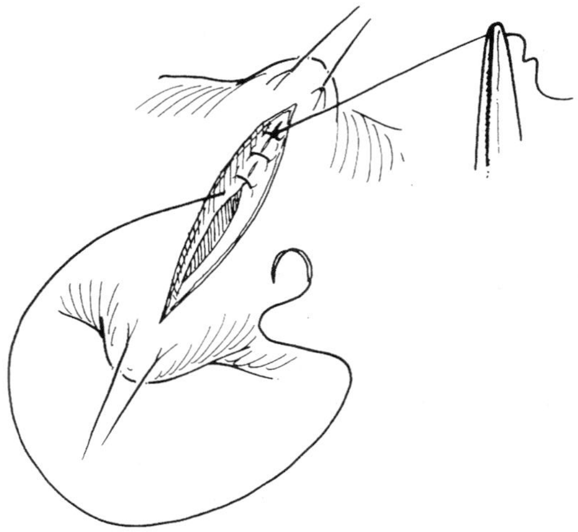

图 8　穿孔处用边角缝线牵拉展开（*From Maull KI: Stomach, small bowel and mesentery injury. In Champion HR, Robbs JV, Trunkey DD, editors:* Rob and Smith's operative surgery: trauma surgery, *4th ed, London, 1989, Butterworth-Heinemann, pp 401–413.*）

并发症

小肠损伤的并发症由于损伤机制不同而异。对于钝性损伤，首要关心的是诊断的延迟。2000 年，Fakhry 等通过 8 个创伤中心的研究报道，损伤后 24 h 内手术与 8 h 手术相比，单纯的小肠穿孔患者合并伤

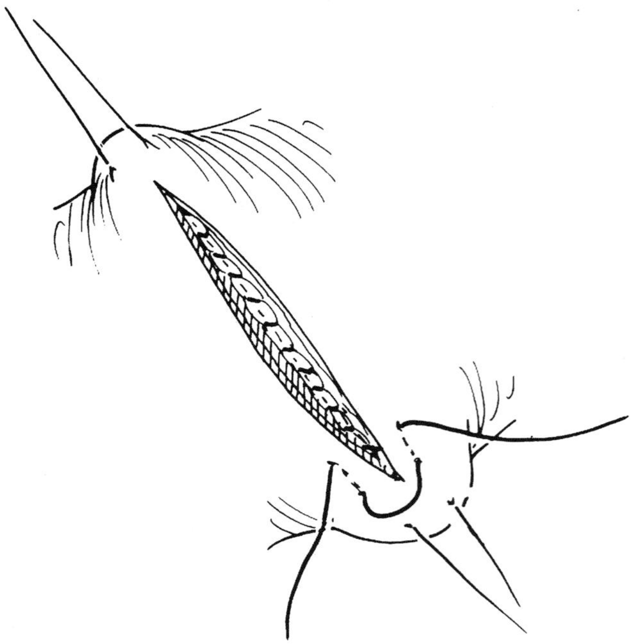

图 9 穿孔处横向双层关闭肠壁（*From Maull KI: Stomach, small bowel and mesentery injury. In Champion HR, Robbs JV, Trunkey DD, editors:* Rob and Smith's operative surgery: trauma surgery, *4th ed, London, 1989, Butterworth-Heinemann, pp 401–413.*）

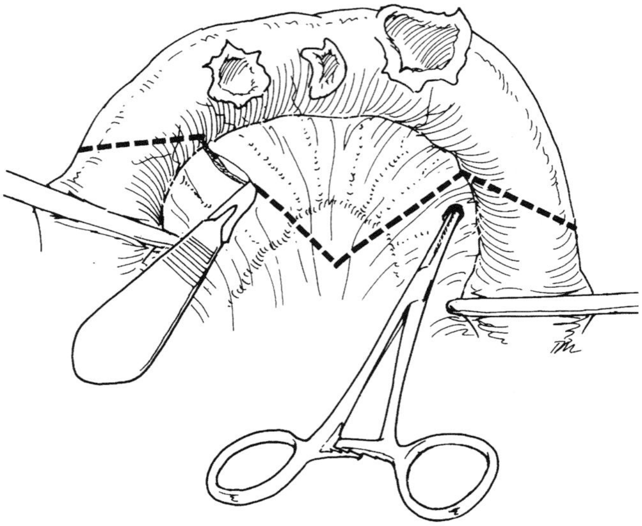

图 11 位于某一短肠段内的多处穿孔最好使用肠切除和吻合（*From Maull KI: Stomach, small bowel and mesentery injury. In Champion HR, Robbs JV, Trunkey DD, editors:* Rob and Smith's operative surgery: trauma surgery, *4th ed, London, 1989, Butterworth-Heinemann, pp 401–413.*）

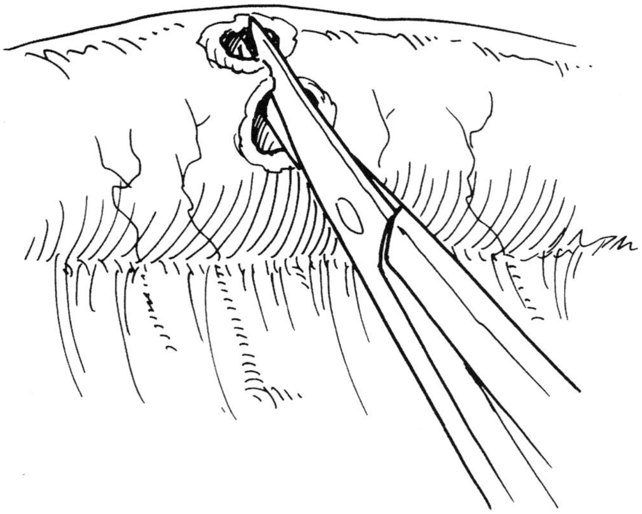

图 10 2 个紧邻的穿孔，应转换成单个缺损，并以同样的方法缝合（*From Maull KI: Stomach, small bowel and mesentery injury. In Champion HR, Robbs JV, Trunkey DD, editors:* Rob and Smith's operative surgery: trauma surgery, *4th ed, London, 1989, Butterworth-Heinemann, pp 401–413.*）

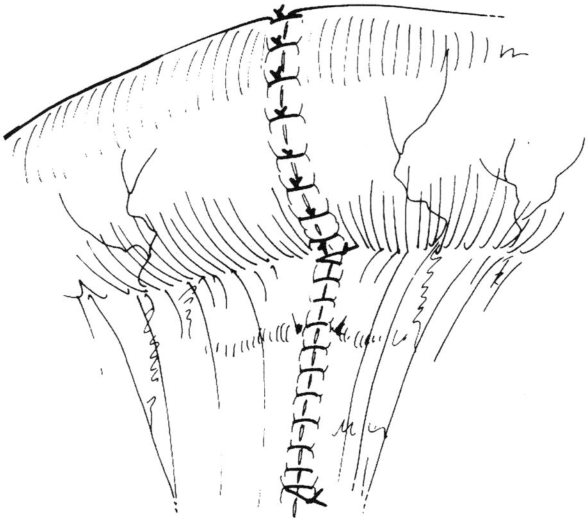

图 12 肠系膜缺损应连续缝合关闭（*From Maull KI: Stomach, small bowel and mesentery injury. In Champion HR, Robbs JV, Trunkey DD, editors:* Rob and Smith's operative surgery: trauma surgery, *4th ed, London, 1989, Butterworth-Heinemann, pp 401–413.*）

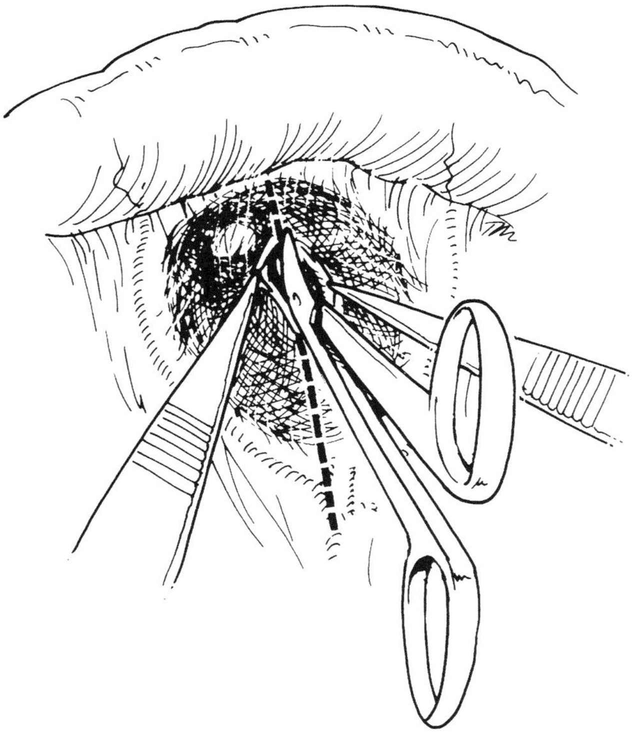

图 13　大范围的或逐渐增大的肠系膜血肿以及紧邻肠壁的血肿须探查和通过缝扎直接控制血管（*From Maull KI: Stomach, small bowel and mesentery injury. In Champion HR, Robbs JV, Trunkey DD, editors:* Rob and Smith's operative surgery: trauma surgery, *4th ed, London, 1989, Butterworth-Heinemann, pp 401–413.*）

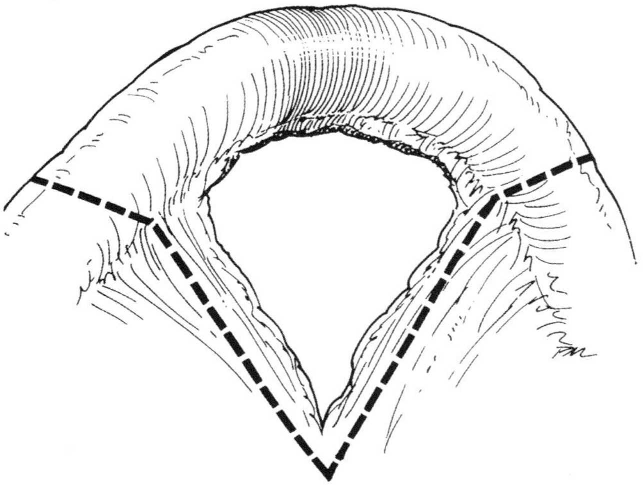

图 14　肠系膜撕裂引起受累肠段缺血，有必要行肠切除术（*From Maull KI: Stomach, small bowel and mesentery injury. In Champion HR, Robbs JV, Trunkey DD, editors:* Rob and Smith's operative surgery: trauma surgery, *4th ed, London, 1989, Butterworth-Heinemann, pp 401–413.*）

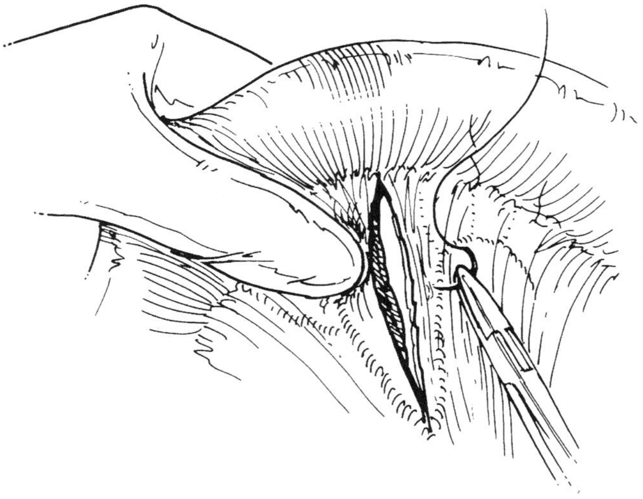

图 15　缝合关闭所有撕裂的肠系膜（*From Maull KI: Stomach, small bowel and mesentery injury. In Champion HR, Robbs JV, Trunkey DD, editors:* Rob and Smith's operative surgery: trauma surgery, *4th ed, London, 1989, Butterworth-Heinemann, pp 401–413.*）

口感染、伤口裂开、腹腔内脓肿、急性呼吸窘迫综合征（acute respiratory distress syndrome，ARDS）、脓毒症的风险增高。Fang 等研究显示损伤 24 h 后手术并发症发生率急剧升高。Bensard 等称对于儿童，钝伤致小肠破裂，诊断延迟超过 24 h 不增加并发症发生率和死亡率。

并发症与联合损伤以及小肠损伤是否需要修补或切除肠管有关。钝性损伤后发生多系统损伤的概率高达 70%。且它不仅与并发症发生有关，还与最终预后相关（图 16）。吻合口相关并发症包括吻合口漏、吻合口瘘和腹腔内脓肿。这些并发症不常发生但单纯修补后发生率高。损伤控制处置后吻合口相关并发症发生的可能性增加。

肠梗阻属于晚期并发症，与未识别的小肠或肠系膜损伤后肠粘连和缺血性狭窄有关。对于后一种情况，患者症状常出现在损伤后 6 周中，症状包括轻度腹痛、梗阻症状。此时有必要手术切除肠段，缓解梗阻。

死亡率

虽然有报道称小肠钝伤后的死亡率高达 25% 或更高，但通常认为死亡率接近 10%。2000 年 Fakhry 等的多中心研究称单独的小肠损伤和小肠

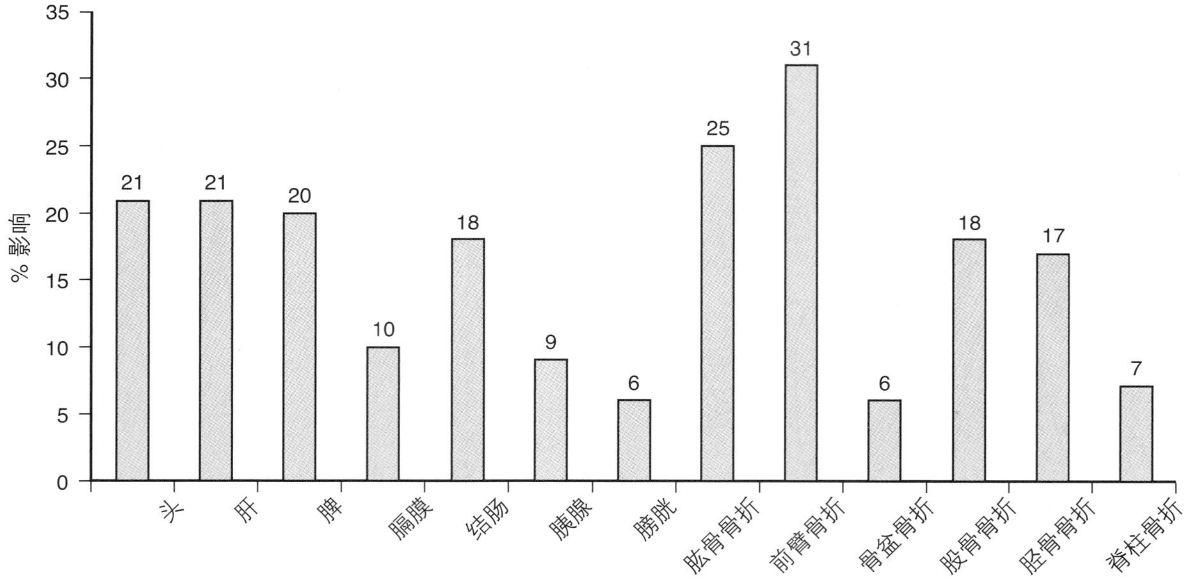

图 16 伴有小肠钝性伤的典型损伤。(*Modified from Neugebauer H, Wallenboeck E, Hungerford M: Seventy cases of injury of the small intestine caused by blunt abdominal trauma: a retrospective study from 1970 to 1994.* J Trauma *46:116–121, 1999.*)

损伤合并其他多处损伤的死亡风险没有差异。而延迟诊断则与近一半的死亡发生直接相关。事实上，诊断延迟超过 8 h 并发症发生率和死亡率增高。穿通伤后死亡与腹腔内其他损伤和腹膜后损伤相关。

结论

小肠损伤分为钝伤和穿通伤。小肠钝性损伤的主要问题是如何辨识损伤的存在。有联合损伤需要手术的患者或有火器伤的患者，应能迅速甄别有无小肠损伤。基于 CT 的非手术处理和早期损伤后 CT 的不准确性倾向使单纯的小肠钝性损伤有诊断延迟的风险，并发症发生率和死亡率也会增加。损伤机制和体格检查的重要性常常被忽视。感觉正常的患者常有腹部压痛，许多患者就诊时还有腹膜发现。安全带造成的损伤需要提高警惕。损伤在横向肠修补术后很少引起术后并发症，这与钝伤和穿通伤后是否联合其他相关损伤密切相关。需要外科评价确保早期诊断和适宜的手术处理。

十二指肠损伤

Gregory J. Jurkovich 著
沈 凯 译

十二指肠损伤并不常见，但也并不罕见，因此外科医生和急诊科医生须掌握常规的诊断及治疗策略。来自美国宾夕法尼亚州 6 年来的回顾记录中，仅有 0.2%（206/103 864）的钝伤患者存在十二指肠损伤，其中仅有 30 名患者存在十二指肠全层损伤。钝性十二指肠损伤来自上腹部的直接冲击受力，如成年人常发生于超速驾驶时方向盘撞击损伤，儿童常来自于自行车手把、拳头或其他类似机制的冲击损伤。穿通性损伤是更常见的病因，十二指肠损伤治疗研究报道中约有 75% 的患者发生穿通性损伤。这一数字大概反映了大城市学术性创伤中心对穿通伤的机制及处置更具有经验。穿通性十二指肠损伤应通过剖腹探查，须系统性探查伤道进行诊断。钝性十二指肠损伤表现更为隐匿，初诊困难。尽管具备常规检查条件，十二指肠损伤的诊断延误仍困扰着创伤外科医生并严重影响患者救治。

预后的决定性因素

以十二指肠损伤为直接原因的死亡率为2%～5%，这是由于伤后出现常见并发症，如伤口裂开、脓毒症和多器官功能衰竭。十二指肠患者死亡风险的相关原因可从20世纪后期的大量研究报道中获得。这些报告显示十二指肠损伤患者的平均死亡率为18%，但报告变化性较大，波动于6%～29%。十二指肠损伤后的并发症发生率为30%～63%，虽然仅有约1/3与十二指肠损伤本身直接相关。并发症发生率和死亡率数据变异性原因包括损伤机制、其他合并损伤和初诊时间。例如，Ivatury等连续回顾了100例穿通性十二指肠损伤病例，记录得到25%的死亡率，与钝性损伤患者的12%～14%的死亡率相比具有明显差异。

十二指肠损伤导致的早期死亡，特别是穿通性损伤，是由于相关的血管、肝或脾损伤引起的。十二指肠与其他重要组织结构的密切关系导致孤立的损伤不常见，但并不是不存在。虽然大量出血和其他相关的损伤是早期死亡的原因，但感染和多系统器官衰竭是大多数晚期死亡的原因。在最初48 h内存活的患者中，有高达1/3的患者发生与十二指肠损伤相关的并发症。吻合口破裂、瘘、腹腔内脓肿、肺炎、脓毒症和器官衰竭是常见的并发症。十二指肠损伤患者的晚期死亡通常在损伤后1～2周或更长的时间后发生，约1/3的晚期死亡归因于损伤本身。

从损伤到接受治疗的时间也是晚期并发症发展和随后的死亡的重要因素。Roman等发现了10例十二指肠损伤的诊断延迟超过24 h的患者。10例中有4例死亡，有3例患有十二指肠瘘。在经典的创伤学读物中，Lucas和Ledgerwood证明了十二指肠损伤诊断延迟的显著重要性（和周期性）。在他们的报告中，53%的患者发生了超过12 h的诊断延迟，28%的患者延迟超过24 h。在诊断延迟超过24 h的患者中，死亡率为40%，而在24 h内接受手术的患者死亡率为11%。Snyder等证实了这些观察结果，报告显示有钝性十二指肠创伤并诊断延迟的4例患者中，2例死亡，另外2例发展出现十二指肠瘘。Cuddington等也指出，100%的十二指肠损伤的死亡病例都有诊断延迟。

这些研究结果发现，治疗十二指肠创伤的优先措施应是控制出血。下一个优先事项是限制来自结肠或其他肠道损伤导致的细菌污染发生，以防止晚期感染。明确十二指肠损伤的程度应作为下一个优先事项，重点是确认胰腺的状态，因为这影响治疗计划制订。遗漏十二指肠损伤的诊断是致命的，因此对相关损伤机制、早期临床表现和影像学特点的警觉意识是创伤外科医生和急诊医生的关键职责。

解剖学和生理学

十二指肠是小肠的第一部分，起始于脊柱右侧的第1腰椎的水平位置，从幽门环延伸到十二指肠空肠曲，通常被称为“Treitz”韧带。十二指肠命名来自拉丁语duodeni，名为“每十二个”，因为它总长度25～30 cm，约为12个手指长。为了便于描述，十二指肠被分为4个部分，通过方向的改变来区分。十二指肠上部或第一部分（D1）向后和向上朝向胆囊颈部，该部分大部位于腹膜内。降（垂直）部或第二部分（D2）与第一部分形成锐角并下降7～8 cm。这部分包含胆管和胰管开口。该部分（和十二指肠的其余部分）完全位于腹膜后，通过Kocher手法分离。十二指肠的水平部或第三部分（D3）横向延伸，跨越输尿管、下腔静脉、腰椎和主动脉，终止于第3腰椎的左侧边缘，长度为12 cm。肠系膜上动脉在十二指肠的第三部分的前向表面向下延伸。十二指肠升部或第四部分(D4）向上并略向左延伸2～3 cm，沿着脊柱到达悬吊十二指肠的Treitz韧带。

十二指肠的动脉血供源自胰十二指肠动脉。胰十二指肠上分支发自肝动脉，胰十二指肠下分支发自肠系膜上动脉。这两条动脉在十二指肠的降部、水平部和胰头部之间的沟槽中走行。连续的边缘动脉使其具有良好的侧支循环。静脉回流与动脉血供平行，后上方汇入门静脉，而前下弓汇入胃结肠干。

十二指肠黏膜类似于其他的小肠节段，与黏膜下层的Brunner腺具有最相近的组织学特征。这些腺体分泌的黏性、黏液状、碱性液体可中和胃酸，保护十二指肠。胰腺和胆汁与胃流出物的混合通常也发生在十二指肠。十二指肠平均每天通过2 500 ml胃液、1 000 ml胆汁、800～1 000 ml胰腺分泌物和800 ml唾液，总共约5 L液体。每日有如此大量的液体流量，因此明确十二指肠的完整性是至关重要的，有助于解释十二指肠瘘是十二指肠损伤的严重并发症。

诊断辅助检查

在最初的腹部平片或胸部X线片上的十二指肠损伤的放射学特征通常是十分细微的，轻度脊柱侧凸或右侧腰肌的缺失有时会提示腹膜后十二指肠损伤。腹膜后气体的存在是十二指肠损伤的明确征象，但这通常难以与其背覆的横结肠区分。CT仍然是早期诊断十二指肠损伤的最佳方法，但并非绝对可靠。超声在紧急情况下几乎无用。准确诊断的关键是口服和静脉碘剂双重对比造影显像的联合应用。因为口服造影剂显像不是大多数创伤性腹部CT扫描的标准路径，所以是否采取该检查的权利在临床医生身上，面对可疑的十二指肠损伤患者须采取该检查（图1）。1997年的报告，回顾了全州6年的十二指肠损伤的经验，Ballard等报告说，在记录的30例钝性十二指肠损伤中，初始CT扫描漏诊率为27%。检查必须对可疑的伤害进行解释，影像描述的不确定性是手术探查的充分理由，而不是进一步进行延迟和重复检查。假阴性检查结果时常发生。在某个CT诊断十二指肠和其他小肠损伤准确性的研究中，只有59%（10/17）的术前扫描提示小肠损伤，而经过手术探查评估后，再回顾性观察术前的CT可以发现小肠损伤的概率增加到88%（15/17）。这些研究者强调，使用CT诊断钝性小肠破裂须谨慎地通过检查和技术来发现细微的征象。

相较CT更为复杂的替代方案是上消化道造影（upper gastrointestiual，UGI）检查。先使用水溶性造影剂，如为阴性，再考虑用钡剂。部分专家认为如果初始CT检查结果难以解释，则应推崇以上检查。但作者认为CT影像中的细微发现是进行手术探查的充分理由。在96例CT提示有可疑十二指肠损伤的患者中，随后进行的十二指肠造影检查的灵敏度为54%，特异度为98%。对于需要手术修复的损伤，CT的灵敏度仅为25%，且具有25%的假阴性率。Allen等证明，83%的钝性十二指肠损伤延迟诊断的患者具有细微的CT影像学发现，包括气腹、不明原因的腹腔内液体和异常肠形态学表现。这些研究强调，十二指肠损伤后腹部CT的细微发现指示了剖腹术的必要性。

DPL在检测单纯的十二指肠和其他腹膜后损伤是不可靠的。然而，DPL有助于诊断，因为约40%的十二指肠损伤患者具有相关腹内损伤，这将导致腹腔内灌洗结果阳性。灌洗液中发现淀粉酶或胆汁是提示可能发生十二指肠损伤的特异性指标。血清淀粉酶水平也是非诊断性的，但若淀粉酶水平升高，则须对是否存在胰腺或十二指肠损伤进行补充检查评估（CT或剖腹探查）。在剖腹探查中，上腹部腹膜后发现血肿、胆汁染色或气体提示须完全显露并检查十二指肠。1997年，Asensio等介绍了十二指肠和胰腺的术中暴露方法。

治疗

治疗原则由十二指肠损伤的严重程度和修补后

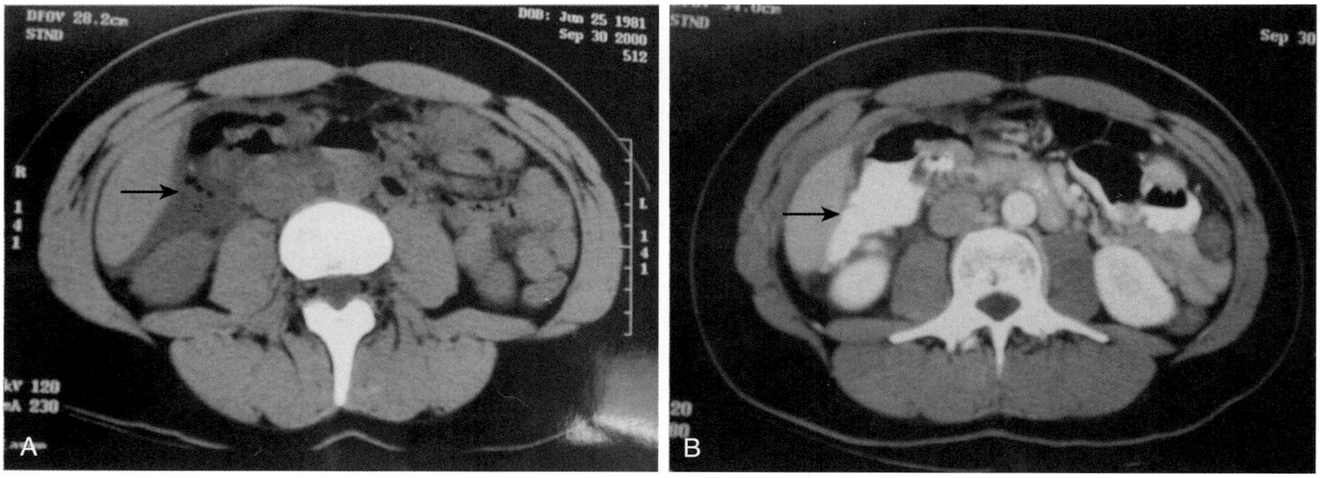

图1 **A和B**，十二指肠穿孔。A，一名19岁的女性，腹部被一个185（83.25 kg）的杠铃坠落砸伤，4 h后就诊于急诊科，伴有轻微的腹痛和恶心，无发热，血流动力学稳定，有持续的上腹部压痛，无腹膜的刺激征。白细胞计数为16 000/ml，淀粉酶114U/L。箭头指向腹膜后的非肠腔内气体和造影剂的外渗

可能出现的并发症来决定。约 70% 的十二指肠损伤可一期修复，其余 30% 为“严重”的损伤，需要更复杂的术式操作，虽然研究趋势主张几乎所有的十二指肠损伤都可行一期修复（Asensio，Rickard 等，2005；Talving 等，2006；Velmahos 等，2008）。Snyder 等对十二指肠损伤是否可行一期修复进行因素分析。他们对 247 例十二指肠损伤接受治疗的患者行回顾研究，报告存活超过 72 h 的 228 名患者中总的十二指肠瘘率为 7%，死亡率为 10.5%。研究者认为表 1 中列出的前 5 个因素与十二指肠损伤的严重程度和随后的发病率和死亡率风险最显著相关。如表中所指出的，因素列表中最近增加的因素是存在胰腺损伤，是提示晚期发病率和死亡率风险的重要指标。这些因素，单独或组合，已被用于开发各类十二指肠损伤分类系统。Snyder 等表明，轻度十二指肠损伤的患者的死亡率为 0，十二指肠瘘发生率为 2%，而严重十二指肠损伤的患者的死亡率为 6%，瘘发生率为 10%。通常，具有轻度十二指肠损伤和无胰腺损伤的患者可以行一期修复。

更严重的十二指肠损伤患者需要更为复杂的治疗策略。图 2 提供了用于控制十二指肠损伤的有效流程。AAST 已开发了用于所有器官损伤的分类系统，并称之为器官损伤分级（Organ Injury Scale，OIS）。十二指肠损伤的分级详见表 2，十二指肠损伤分为 Ⅰ 级至 Ⅴ 级，从轻到重。对 8 个创伤中心的 164 名十二指肠创伤患者进行 AAST-OIS 分类方案评估，其中有 38 名 Ⅰ 级患者，70 名 Ⅱ 级患者，48 名 Ⅲ 级患者，4 名 Ⅳ 级患者和 4 名 Ⅴ 级患者。117 名患者接受单纯一期修复手术（占总病例数的 71%）。其中 108 名 Ⅰ 级或 Ⅱ 级损伤患者中，有 90 名患者行一期修复。56 例（46%）Ⅲ 至 Ⅴ 级损伤患者中有 26 例（占总病例数的 29%）进行更复杂的十二指肠治疗策

表 1　十二指肠损伤严重程度的决定因素

参数	轻度	严重
损伤严重程度的决定因素		
损伤机制	锐器	钝性或枪弹
大小	<75% 肠壁	≥75% 肠壁
十二指肠部位	3，4	1，2
损伤 - 修复间隔时间（小时）	<24	≥24
相关损伤	无胆总管损伤	有胆总管损伤
	无胰腺损伤	有胰腺损伤
预后		
死亡率	6%	16%
十二指肠并发症发生率	6%	14%

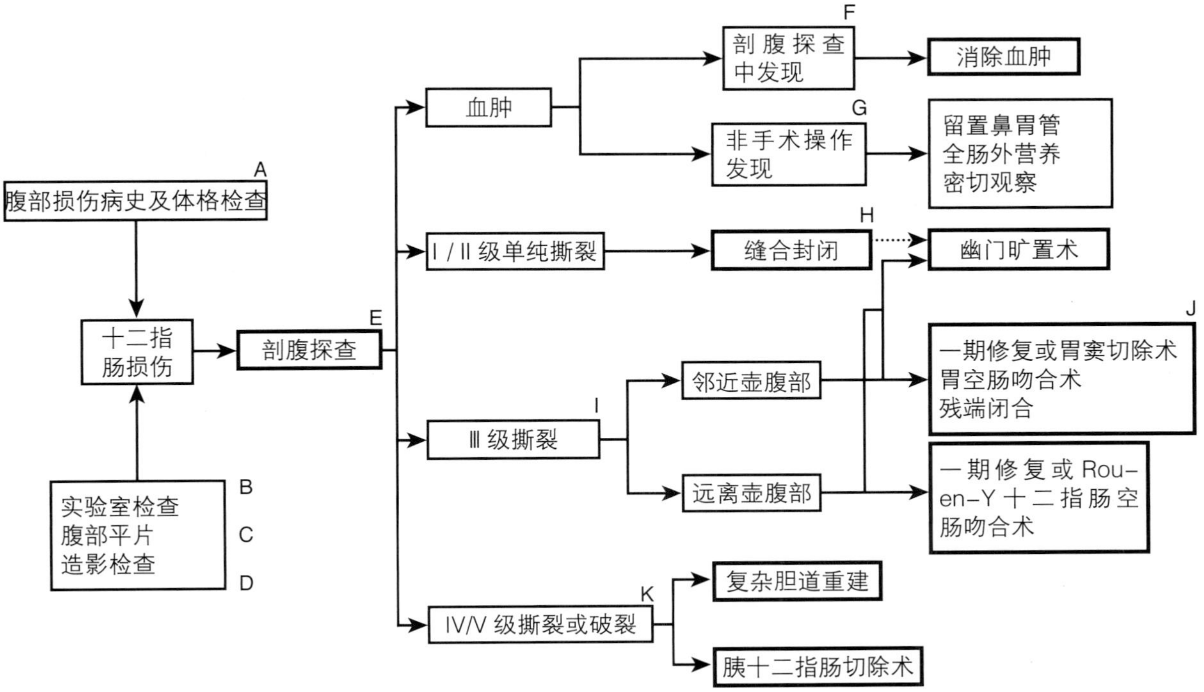

图 2　十二指肠损伤的处理流程图（*From Jurkovich G: Duodenal injury.In McIntyre R, Van Stiegmann G, Eiseman B, editors: Surgical decision making, 5th ed, Philadelphia, 2004, Elsevier, pp 512-513*）

表 2　十二指肠损伤严重性 AAST-OIS 分级

分级 *	类型	描述
Ⅰ	血肿 裂伤	十二指肠单一位置 非全层肠壁
Ⅱ	血肿 裂伤	超过一个位置 <50% 环周
Ⅲ	裂伤	50% ~ 75% D2 50% ~ 100% D1、D3、D4
Ⅳ	裂伤 累及壶腹或远端胆总管	≥75% D2
Ⅴ	裂伤	胰 - 十二指肠复合物大范围损毁 / 血供阻断

Modified from American Association for the Surgery of Trauma（AAST）。AAST-OIS，美国创伤外科协会器官损伤分级；D1，十二指肠的第一位；D2，十二指肠的第二部分；D3，十二指肠的第三部分；D4，十二指肠的第四部分。＊将同一器官多发性损伤一级

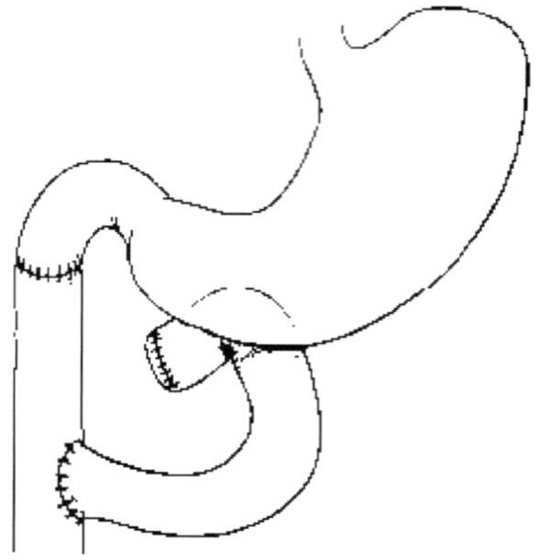

图 3　十二指肠大面积破裂可通过用端端 Roux-en-Y 十二指肠空肠吻合术治疗（*From Asensio J, Feliciano D, Britt L, Kerstein M: Management of duodenal injuries.* Curr Probl Surg *11: 1064, 1993, Fig.9*）

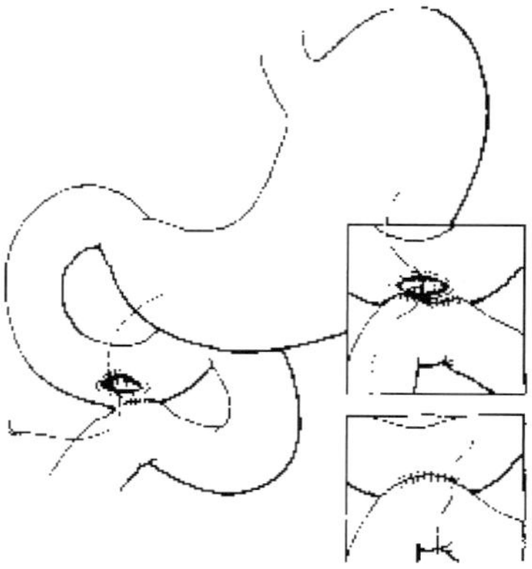

图 4　浆膜补片技术。应用指征较少，这种修复方法选择性用于十二指肠壁缺损，且无法一期修复或切除修复的情况。将空肠袢的浆膜缝合到十二指肠缺损的边缘（*From Asensio J, Feliciano D, Britt L, Kerstein M: Management of duodenal injuries.* Curr Probl Surg *11: 1060, 1993, Fig.6*）

略，包括幽门旷置术、十二指肠十二指肠吻合术、十二指肠空肠吻合术或胰十二指肠切除术。

一期修补通常是治疗十二指肠损伤的最简单、最快、最理想的治疗方法。如果几乎没有组织损失、不涉及壶腹，且黏膜边缘可以清创和无张力地闭合，则一期修补适合于十二指肠的部分或完全横断损伤。十二指肠修复类似于其他小肠修复。双层封闭，或者可密封液体的、浆肌层单层连续缝合修补同样可以接受。然而，如果无法进行无张力修复，或损伤非常接近壶腹有损伤胆管可能，那么通过 Roux-en-Y 术式将空肠与近端十二指肠吻合，同时修补远端十二指肠损伤是最合理的选择（图 3）。不太理想的选择是通过空肠补片修复，其中小肠浆膜缝合作为十二指肠缺损表面的补丁（图 4）。虽然一些试验证据表明十二指肠周边带的黏膜可能在浆膜补片上迅速重铺，但该技术应用于临床时面临各类并发症的困扰。在近期的严重多发性十二指肠损伤的多中心试验中，它从未被使用过。其中有 5 名患者（3%）进行十二指肠十二指肠吻合术或十二指肠空肠吻合术修复。Ivatury 等在 1985 年的报告比较了一期修补与修补加肠造口减压或浆膜补片的十二指肠损伤患者的预后，证明了不推荐这种重建方法的原因。在本报告中，60 例穿通性十二指肠损伤患者中，11 例十二指肠枪伤患者的腹部严重感染发生率为 64%，死亡率为 27%。相比之下，30 例一期修复或类似损伤的 Roux-en-Y 吻合修复的患者中，有 7% 发生腹腔脓毒症，死亡率为 0。在同一系列中，发生十二指肠刺伤的 17 名患者中，十二指肠伤口一旦使用“吸盘补片”修复，并发症发生率也升高。“吸盘补片”为改良补片修补术，即小肠的 Roux-en-Y 环的开放端被缝合到十二指肠缺损处。鉴于以上报道，完整修复伤口、分离边缘，并且进行直接端端十二指肠十二指肠吻合是推荐的处理方法。如果十二指肠末端不能充分游离，则应该进行 Roux-en-Y 端端吻合术。几种术式可以帮助保护十二指肠修补伤口。使用大网膜（作者偏好）或空肠带的一个“浆膜补片”对修复处进行支持是合乎逻辑的，但这种方法的益处并未得到证实。胃内容物的改道是另一种选择，

最常见的是通过 Vaughan/Jordan 幽门旷置术完成。该技术在 1904 年被首次记录，Summers 用其进行十二指肠伤口的辅助治疗。相比 Berne 和 Donovan 等倡导的十二指肠“憩室形成手术”，幽门旷置术的破坏性更小（图 5）。

十二指肠憩室形成手术通过十二指肠伤口的一期封闭、胃窦切除术、迷走神经切断、端侧胃空肠吻合术、T 形管胆总管引流和侧管十二指肠切除术完成。该术式的观念是完全转移胃和胆汁内容物远离十二指肠损伤，肠内营养通过胃空肠吻合实现，并将潜在的不受控制的十二指肠瘘转换成可控制的瘘。一个操作性强并较少破坏性的术式选择是“幽门旷置术”，它无需切除术、胆道转流或迷走神经切断术（图 6）。该过程通过胃切开术进行，用

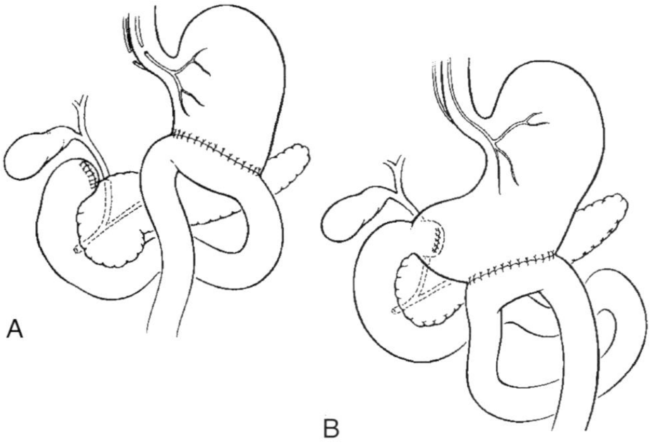

图 5　**A**，Berne 十二指肠憩室化手术 和 **B** 幽门旷置术（*From Jurkovich GJ: Duodenum and pancreas. In Moore EE, Feliciano DV, Mattox K, editors: Trauma, 5th ed, New York, 2004，McGraw-Hill, p717*）

Babcock 夹钳抓住幽门，用可吸收 0 号的聚乙醇酸或聚乳酸、Maxon（聚葡糖酸盐）或 PDS（聚二氧杂环已酮）缝线缝合闭合幽门，并建立胃空肠吻合。吻合器法或使用不可吸收的缝合线（例如，Prolene）关闭幽门都是不推荐的。虽然曾经被认为同样有效，但大多数这类关闭术不能再通，经常导致严重并发症。十二指肠旷置数周后，等待十二指肠和胰腺损伤愈合，幽门会自行再通（2 周至 2 个月），胃空肠吻合口会功能性关闭。1993 年，Asensio 等制作了一本经典专著，详细描述了十二指肠损伤治疗中的所有外科技术。台湾长庚医院的 Fang 等描述了控制开放幽门旷置环的技术方法，从而定时控制幽门闭塞的再通。据报道，在 5%～33% 的患者中，在胃空肠吻合部位存在边缘溃疡，这促使一些学者在该手术基础上增加迷走神经切断术。然而，大多数外科医生没有在幽门旷置术式中增加迷走神经切断术，因为几乎所有幽门旷置都在几周内开放。边缘溃疡可以在临床上进行内科药物治疗。某些文献数据支持在“严重”十二指肠损伤或延迟诊断的情况下使用幽门旷置和胃空肠吻合术，尽管没有前瞻性随机试验证明胃转流手术的真正益处。此外，增加的操作时间和额外的吻合应建议明确用于其适应证。

幽门旷置现在被广泛用于十二指肠修复的辅助治疗中，最近的研究对其效用提出了质疑。Nassoura 和 Ivatury 等报道了 1986–1992 期间治疗的 66 例穿通性十二指肠损伤患者，7 例患者在 48 h 内死亡。在 59 例幸存者中，56 例进行了一期修补，只有 3 例（5%）采取幽门旷置术作为十二指肠和胰腺复合损伤的辅助治疗。其中 4 例患者死亡，1 例为十二指肠相关死亡（1.7%）。这些研究人员建议使用幽门旷置术作为穿通性腹部创伤指数大于 40 或

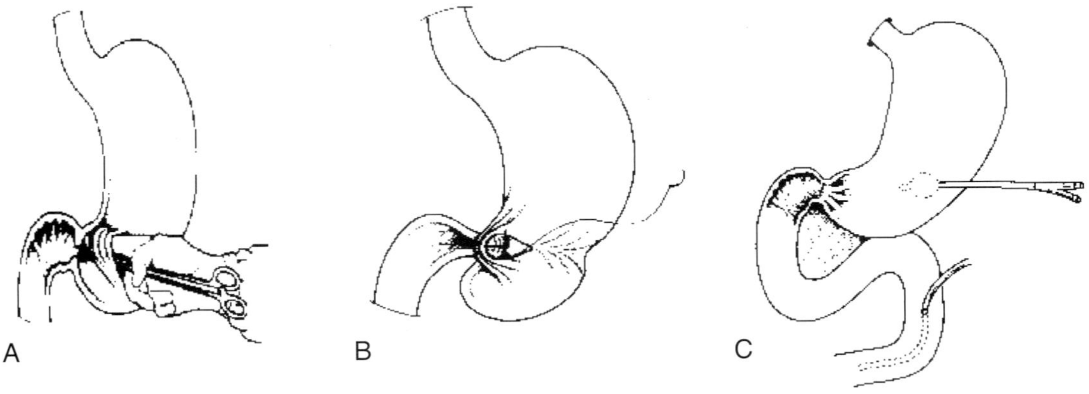

图 6　**A** 至 **C** 幽门旷置技术

复合胰腺损伤的患者的辅助治疗，而不是使用表 1 中的 Snyder 标准。复合胰腺损伤存在于另外 3 名死亡患者（2 名仅进行一期修补术），术后均发生十二指肠吻合口瘘，证实了复合胰腺损伤导致并发症高风险情况。类似的幽门旷置术适应证建议来自国家创伤数据库研究（Dubose 等，2008）。Dubose 等访问了 NTDB 5 年间的滚动记录，它记录了超过 950 000 名患者，发现了 147 名严重十二指肠损伤患者（AAST 级≥3）。28 名患者（19%）接受幽门旷置术治疗，与另外 119 名仅行一期修补术患者的进行对比分析。虽然差异并未达到统计学意义，但相比之下 28 名幽门旷置术患者的平均损伤严重度评分（Injury Severity Score，ISS）（26 vs. 23）更高，及 ISS>20 的比例更高（75% vs. 56%）。多变量分析显示各组之间死亡率或腹部感染性并发症的发生率差异无统计学意义。最后，Velmahos 等连续回顾了 1992–2004 年期间洛杉矶医疗中心治疗的 193 例十二指肠损伤患者。总共 50 例患者发生严重的十二指肠损伤（AAST Ⅲ、Ⅳ或Ⅴ级）。68% 的患者行一期修补治疗，幽门旷置术作为辅助治疗用于 32%的患者，使用幽门旷置术组具有更严重的十二指肠损伤情况、更多相关胰腺损伤，以及更多十二指肠第一部分或第二部分的损伤。他们报告 2 组之间的死亡率或并发症发生率没有差异。以上最近的研究显示，一期修补中幽门旷置术等辅助治疗在很大程度上是不必要的。或者，这些报告可以提示术者对严重十二指肠损伤患者是否选择幽门旷置术进行仔细的判断，且没有更糟糕。准确地定义哪些患者受益于幽门旷置已经因为缺乏前瞻性随机试验而受到阻碍。严重十二指肠损伤的相对罕见导致前瞻性随机试验难以开展。然而，作者的实践在持续进行中，即在伴随胰腺损伤和严重的十二指肠损伤的患者中（修复困难）进行幽门旷置术。

与十二指肠损伤直接相关的致死性因素是十二指肠破裂，以及随后出现的难以控制的脓毒症和多系统器官衰竭。对于十二指肠破裂和十二指肠瘘致死性的认知诱使外科医生采取幽门旷置、吻合加固和十二指肠切除术以修复Ⅲ或Ⅳ级十二指肠损伤。如前述，伴发的胰腺损伤作为高危因素也应包括在十二指肠修复是否附加幽门旷置术的考虑范围内。在一篇 40 例穿通性十二指肠损伤的患者报告中，有 14 例患者合并十二指肠和胰腺联合损伤。5 例伴有这种损伤的患者单独行一期十二指肠修复，2 例发生十二指肠瘘，3 例患有联合损伤的患者采取幽门旷置术作为辅助治疗，未发生十二指肠瘘。

胃转流术的替代或补充治疗是通过逆行空肠造口术置入导管引流对十二指肠减压。Stone 和 Fabian 报道，在各种通过逆行空肠造口术置管引流治疗的十二指肠损伤中，十二指肠瘘发生率小于 0.5%（1/237）。未使用减压的十二指肠损伤患者并发症发生率为 19.3%。逆行十二指肠引流优于侧向十二指肠造口术。直接在缝合处行导管引流导致 23% 的胃高位破裂或瘘发生率。Hasson 等回顾了截至 1984 年的关于穿通性十二指肠创伤和十二指肠切除置管术的相关文献，评估了 8 个回顾性研究和超过 550 个患者。研究表明无减压处理下患者总死亡率为 19.4%，十二指肠瘘发生率为 11.8%，而减压处理的患者死亡率为 9%，十二指肠瘘发生率为 2.3%。同时得出结论，置管引流应通过胃造口术或逆行空肠造口术进行，因为此类方法的瘘发生率较低，总死亡率低于侧向置管十二指肠造口术。尽管如此，如同用于胃转流的幽门旷置术，由于缺乏对于十二指肠置管引流术效果的前瞻性随机分析，当前并非所有外科医生都支持使用肠减压技术。

在十二指肠近端和胰头部的大范围损伤中，壶腹和近端胰管或远端胆总管的结构破坏可能导致重建困难。此外，因为十二指肠和胰头部具有相同的动脉供应，所以不可能完全切除其中一个，而不出现另一个缺血的情况。因此发生以上损伤情况，须进行胰十二指肠切除术，相当于损伤后创面的完全清创处理。1961–1994 年期间，共报告了 184 例因创伤行 Whipple 手术治疗的患者，其中 26 例死亡（14%），39 例延迟死亡，总生存率为 64%。明确适应证标准，用于治疗创伤的胰十二指肠切除术可以达到和肿瘤患者类似的并发症发生率和死亡率。最近，Asensio 等进行了最大样本量的胰腺十二指肠切除术或 Whipple 术式报道，包括 18 名患者，报告的死亡率为 33%，文献综述包括了共计 247 名患者。作者验证了 Facey 和 Fry 方法对于创伤后 Whipple 手术的效果。

十二指肠血肿

十二指肠血肿常见于儿童嬉闹或儿童虐待发生的损伤，但也可发生在成年人。在一份报告中，50% 的儿童十二指肠血肿病例来自儿童虐待。值得注意的是，十二指肠在最常见的腹部钝性损伤的腹内器官的排名是第四。十二指肠损伤发生在2%～10%的儿童中。几乎1/3的患者在损伤48 h后表现出不明显的梗阻症状，可能是液体转移至高渗十二指肠血肿的结果。十二指肠血肿通常代表非手术治疗的损伤，在保守治疗或非手术处理中可获得最好的结果。它可以通过增强CT扫描或UGI检查来诊断（图7）。最初可采用水溶性造影剂造影检查（使用泛影葡胺），也可以用钡剂以获取更细节的影像学特征表现，被称为螺旋弹簧或堆叠硬币征。虽然十二指肠壁内血肿的特点特异，但这一特点仅存在于大约1/4的血肿患者中。

虽然初始治疗是非手术治疗，仍须排除其他相关的损伤，特别是胰腺损伤。Desai等报道了42%的十二指肠损伤（穿孔或血肿）的儿科患者伴有胰腺损伤，Jewett等发现十二指肠血肿患者的胰腺损伤发生率为20%。应该使用鼻胃管置入，持续减压，并开始全肠外营养。如果梗阻的迹象没有自行解除，应每隔5～7天用UGI对比检查评估患者。超声也已可用于十二指肠血肿缓解情况的随诊。相关研究指出，无法缓解的十二指肠血肿可通过经皮穿刺引流，通常在保守治疗2周后推荐进行手术探查和解除血肿，以排除狭窄、十二指肠穿孔和胰头部的损伤等其他导致梗阻的因素。对6例因钝性创伤导致十二指肠和空肠血肿的患者进行的综述研究显示，6例患者中有5例患者采取了非手术治疗，平均住院时间为16天（范围为10～23天），平均总肠外营养时间为9天（范围为4～16天）。第6例患者有UGI检查完全肠梗阻的影像证据，在保守治疗18天后未能解决。剖腹探查显示该患者空肠和结肠狭窄与纤维化，通过手术切除治疗。另一项研究包括19例十二指肠血肿的儿童，17例（89%）采取非手术治疗，2例患者在发病24 h内采取手术或引流治疗，且在手术治疗前未尝试非手术治疗。鼻胃管减压和全肠外营养平均使用9.3（±7.7）天（范围为2～29天），平均住院时间为16.4（±17.8）天（范围为2～37天）。

如果在剖腹探查术中偶然发现十二指肠血肿，则必须全面检查以排除穿孔。这须通过扩大的Kocher手法以有效引流浆膜下层血肿。目前尚不明确是否应当将十二指肠浆膜大范围切开以“排除”血

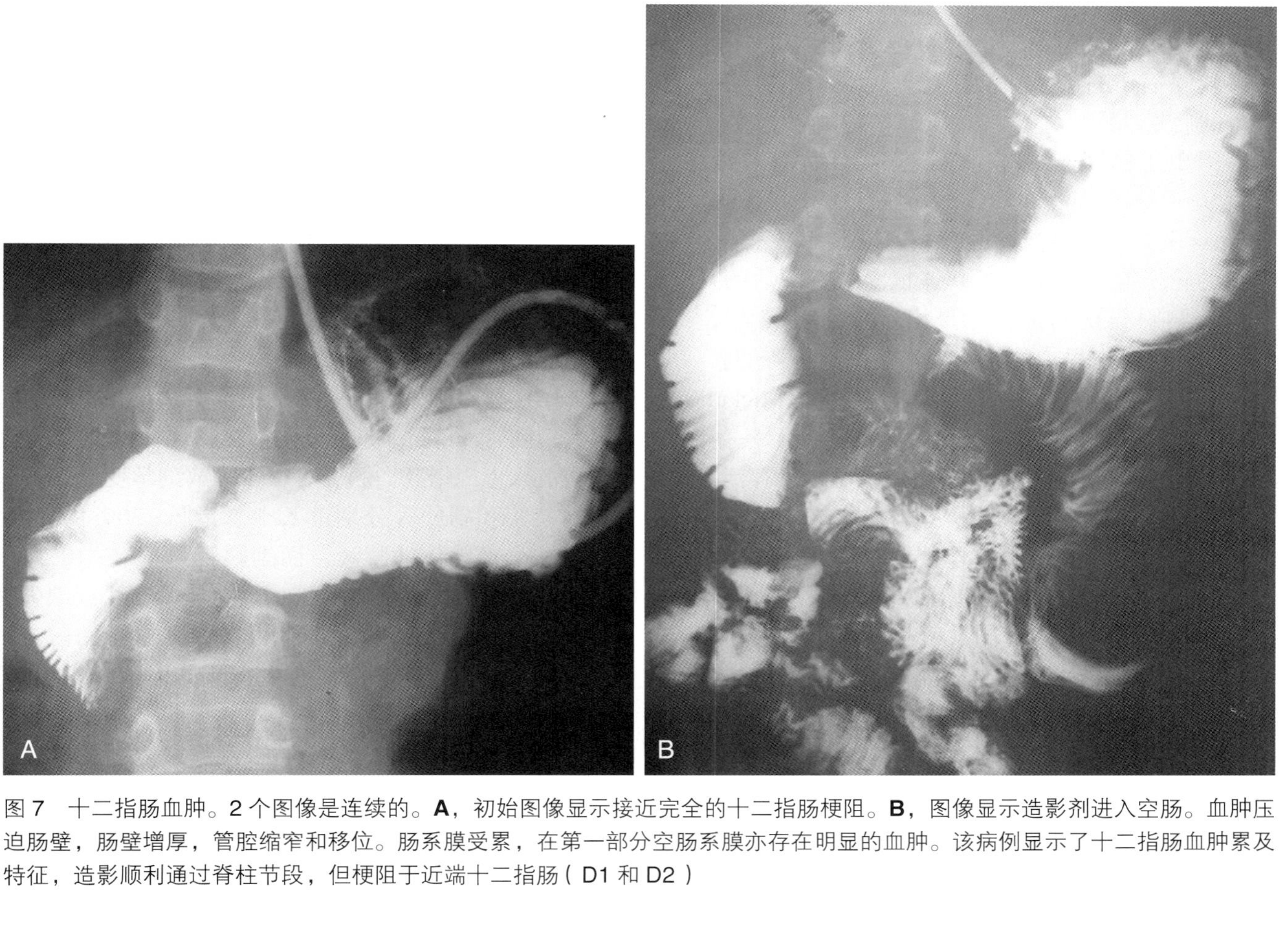

图7　十二指肠血肿。2个图像是连续的。**A**，初始图像显示接近完全的十二指肠梗阻。**B**，图像显示造影剂进入空肠。血肿压迫肠壁，肠壁增厚，管腔缩窄和移位。肠系膜受累，在第一部分空肠系膜亦存在明显的血肿。该病例显示了十二指肠血肿累及特征，造影顺利通过脊柱节段，但梗阻于近端十二指肠（D1和D2）

肿，或它是否实际上增加了将部分十二指肠壁撕裂转化为完全穿孔的可能性。作者的经验是除非高度怀疑十二指肠肠壁全层损伤，通常不打开十二指肠血肿，而是全面仔细地检查。应该进行空肠造口术置营养管，因为可能需要更长时间的胃肠减压。

胰腺损伤和胰十二指肠切除术

Louis J. Magnotti 和 Martin A. Croce 著
张大方 译

胰腺是一个位置比较深的腹膜后器官，相对受到较好的保护。正因如此，胰腺损伤虽不常见，但也并非罕见，诊断常充满困难。尽管现代化的创伤治疗不断进展，如损伤控制性手术以及影像学技术的进步，但胰腺损伤对于创伤外科医生来说仍然是一大挑战。实际上，过去的 25 年间，胰腺损伤相关的死亡率和并发症发生率并没有很大的改善，其死亡率仍然徘徊在 9% ~ 34%。胰腺损伤后的并发症依旧频繁发生发生率高达 30% ~ 60%。并发症发生率如此之高可能与诊断延误和漏诊有关。如果能早期诊断，大多数胰腺损伤的治疗方案很明确。相反，如果胰腺损伤的诊断和治疗受到延误，则可能造成严重的后果。

历史上有关胰腺损伤处理的详细记录很少。首次关于胰腺损伤的记录来自于 1827 年伦敦 St. Thomas 医院的一份尸解报告，一位患者被一辆公共马车的轮子撞到，造成了胰体横断。在随后的几十年里，胰腺损伤的报告零星出现。到 1903 年，经过确认的文献上报道的胰腺损伤病例只有 45 例，其中 21 例为腹部穿通伤，另 24 例为钝伤。Mickulicz-Radecki 指出其中 20 例保守治疗的患者无一存活，而 25 例接受手术的患者则有 18 例（72%）存活。通过上述发现，他建议对于胰腺损伤应该采用正中切口进行全面手术探查、缝合止血以及充分引流，这与现代的治疗方式非常相似。

胰腺损伤的并发症同样很早就被指出并在相当长的时间里成为一个主要问题。1905 年，Korte 首次报道了一例胰腺断裂后胰瘘的病例。该患者的胰瘘自行闭合，患者也得以存活。Whipple 在 1935 年首次描述了胰十二指肠切除术，随后又报道了相关的并发症，如继发性出血、瘘形成、十二指肠漏，以及腹膜炎。

本章试图说明胰腺损伤相关的解剖和生理学基础，同时阐明胰腺损伤的具体诊断和治疗方式。

解剖

全面掌握胰腺相关解剖对于选择适当的治疗方式并理解损伤相关并发症的发生是非常必要的。胰腺长 15 ~ 20 cm，宽 3.1 cm，厚 1 ~ 1.5 cm。平均重量 90 g（范围为 40 ~ 180 g）。下腔静脉、主动脉、左肾、双侧肾静脉和右肾动脉位于胰腺的后方。胰头被十二指肠包绕，胰体横跨脊柱，胰尾在脾门中。脾动静脉沿胰腺上缘走行。肠系膜上动静脉位于胰颈部后方，钩突在其后方环绕。钩突可以小到几近缺失，也可以大到将肠系膜上动静脉几近完全包绕。

胰头被肝十二指肠韧带悬吊在肝下，被十二指肠的第二部分和第三部分紧密固定。门静脉及其向下延续的肠系膜上静脉是胰头和胰颈的分界线。胰颈部长约 1.5 ~ 2 cm，位于第 1 腰椎水平。胰颈被其下方的肠系膜上血管和其上方的腹腔干所固定。肠系膜上血管左侧的胰腺组织在技术上被定义为胰体。胰体和胰尾并没有真正的解剖学分界线，同样，胰头和胰颈也没有真正意义上的分界线。

主胰管（Wirsung 管）起源于胰尾，通常穿越胰腺全长，与胆总管汇合后进入十二指肠。主胰管在胰体尾走行过程中位于胰腺的中部（上下）偏后的位置。副胰管（Santorini 管）通常在胰颈发自于胰管并独立汇入十二指肠。胰管有很多种解剖学变异：60% 的主胰管和副胰管分别进入十二指肠；30% 的主胰管收纳全部腺体的胰液，而副胰管为盲端；10% 的副胰管收纳全部腺体的胰液，而主胰管很小或缺失。但无论哪种情况，胰管都走行在胰腺血管的前方。不论如何，外科医生在处理胰腺损伤时应非常了解这些解剖变异。

胰腺的动静脉血供相对恒定。胰腺的动脉血供来源于腹腔干和肠系膜上动脉。胰头的血供最丰富，胰体尾其次，而胰颈最少。胰腺的静脉同动脉一样，走行在胰管的后方，静脉位于动脉的表面，并与动脉平行走行。胰腺的静脉回流至门静脉、脾静脉和肠系膜上静脉。

生理学

胰腺由腺泡和导管构成，兼具内分泌功能（胰岛素、胰高血糖素、生长抑素）和外分泌功能（消化酶原、碳酸氢盐）。内分泌细胞在组织学上独立形成细胞巢，被称为 Langerhans 胰岛。最主要的 3 种胰岛细胞分别为 α 细胞（产生胰高血糖素）、β 细胞（产生胰岛素）和 δ 细胞（产生生长抑素）。虽然这些细胞遍布胰腺的任何部位，但大部分位于胰尾。正因如此，远端胰腺切除患者术后胰腺内分泌功能会受到较大影响。然而，如果剩余的胰腺是正常的，那么只有切除超过 90% 的胰腺才会造成胰腺内分泌功能不足。事实上，胰腺部分切除会促使剩余胰岛细胞肥大，并且活性增加。在动物实验中，Dragstedt 首先证实，如果剩余胰腺是正常的，并且胰液仍能通过胰管进入上消化道，则切除 80% 的胰腺既不会显著影响碳水化合物和脂肪的代谢，也不会影响食物的消化和吸收。

诊断

任何时候诊断胰腺损伤时，一定要特别注意是否存在主胰管损伤，因为这是影响胰腺损伤预后最重要的独立危险因素。这一观念最早可追溯到 1962 年。此后，学者们已经证实并反复强调检查胰管是否损伤的重要性。Heitsch 等发现，与单纯引流相比，远端胰腺切除术治疗胰管损伤可以显著降低患者的术后死亡率和并发症发生率。这一发现在 10 年之后被再次证实，在胰管损伤部位的近端切除胰腺可以使死亡率从 19% 下降至 3%。尽管影像学技术不断发展，CT 在评价多发伤患者的胰管状态时并没有足够高的灵敏度。而 MRI 对于急性创伤患者通常很不方便。因此，早期、准确的判断主胰管状态是非常具有挑战性的。

胰腺损伤的成功诊断需要对可疑损伤的高度警惕，以及尽量缩短损伤到确定性治疗之间的时间。损伤的机制、是否需要剖腹探查，以及距最初腹部检查的间隔时间，这些将引导创伤医生进行最适当的检查。如果患者须立即行剖腹探查，则术前检查可能很少甚至没有，胰腺损伤的诊断只能在手术中完成。相反，患者不需要手术探查则可能需要更多的检查，以证实是否有胰腺损伤。因此，早期诊断隐匿的胰腺损伤须对可疑损伤高度警惕，同时也需要一套完整的诊断和观察流程。

胰腺损伤通常是由于上腹部受到高能损伤而造成的。对于成年人来说，机动车事故是胰腺损伤的首要原因，通常继发于方向盘的撞击。对于儿童来说，最典型的损伤原因是上腹部撞到把手。无论是哪种情况，外伤时的能量直接作用于腹部上方（上腹部或季肋部）导致腹膜后结构的挤压。腹膜后损伤的典型表现包括上腹部受到撞击（包括挫伤）与体检有与上腹疼痛不成比例的发现。

血清淀粉酶升高并不是胰腺创伤的可靠指标。在一项研究中，钝伤后血淀粉酶升高的患者只有 8% 是胰腺损伤。事实上，淀粉酶作为腹部钝性创伤的监测手段的阴性预测值为 95%。检测血清胰淀粉酶含量并不能提高诊断胰腺损伤的灵敏度或特异度。但是，血清淀粉酶升高确实应该引起是否存在胰腺损伤的高度怀疑。

无症状的患者如果血清胰淀粉酶升高须继续观察并复查淀粉酶。淀粉酶持续升高或出现腹部症状则需要进一步的检查，可能包括 CT、ERCP 或手术探查。尽管很大程度上取决于检查者的经验、扫描的质量以及距受伤的时间，但腹部 CT 扫描诊断胰腺损伤的灵敏度和特异度都在 80% 以上。Patton 等曾报道，在 26 名钝性胰腺损伤的患者中，15 名早期 CT 扫描怀疑存在胰腺损伤；4 名（21%）CT 未显示损伤，导致手术时间延迟（平均 3.8 天）。其他患者则因为其他指征进行手术探查。

胰腺损伤的 CT 表现包括胰腺实质的断裂、胰腺内部血肿、小网膜囊积液或积液导致脾静脉与胰体部分离、胰周水肿、左侧肾前筋膜增厚，以及腹膜后血肿或积液。显然，有些表现比其他表现更有可靠性，上述表现全部出现在 1 名患者的情况也很少发生。有些胰腺损伤的 CT 表现并不是在损伤后立即出现，而是需要一定时间才会出现。这一点很重要，尤其是在评估患者腹部症状恶化，而最初 CT 扫描有没有明显异常时。

ERCP 在诊断胰管破裂时很有价值。此外，它可以帮助诊断遗漏胰腺损伤所造成的并发症，有时甚至还可以帮助治疗。Louisville 大学的一篇报道显示，对于淀粉酶升高、持续性腹痛、CT 异常或可疑异常的血流动力学稳定患者，在其损伤后早期阶段进行 ERCP 是一项非常有用的胰管评估检查手段。对于那些初始评估胰腺损伤诊断的患者，ERCP 也是一项非常重要的评估方法。对于这些患者，ERCP 可以帮助评估胰腺损伤、制订手术方案、胰腺内支架置入、胰腺脓肿的经胰管引流。但是，ERCP 并不是任何时候都能实施，患者临床表现恶化时不应因 ERCP 而延迟手术。对于血流动力学不稳定的患者也不应采用 ERCP 进行评估。

磁共振成像，特别是磁共振胰胆管造影术（magnetic resonance cholangiopancretography，MRCP），已经成为了另一种可以评价胰管的检查方法。在一些特定的环境下，MRCP 已经成为了一种切实可行的评价胰腺损伤患者胰管情况的方法。然而，MRCP 对于创伤患者来说经常不太实用。

为了成功诊断胰腺损伤是否存在以及其损伤程度，外科医生必须了解与胰腺损伤相关的各种表现，并充分观察整个胰腺。此外，还必须确定胰腺实质的完整性和主胰管的状态。胰腺损伤根据胰管的状况和胰腺损伤的解剖学位置进行分类。其他相关的损伤往往使胰腺评估复杂化。若存在中央腹膜后血肿或覆盖胰腺的血肿、腹膜后皂化或胆汁染色，则需要完整的胰腺探查。

再一次必须强调的是，如有可能，在手术探查时一定要确认胰管的情况。大多数胰管损伤可以通过胰腺的局部探查来诊断。胰管损伤在胰腺创伤时的发生率约为 15%，通常是穿通性损伤的结果。钝伤也可导致主胰管断裂，可以合并或不合并胰腺完全横断。胰腺实质的轻微挫伤和裂伤通常不须进一步探查胰管。然而，胰腺被膜完整不能消除胰管完全横断的可能性。

直视胰管破裂、胰腺腺体完全横断、胰液渗漏、涉及胰腺直径一半以上的裂伤、胰腺中央穿孔，以及严重裂伤合并或不合并大块组织破裂，这些术中所发现的征象预测主胰管损伤的准确率很高。然而，在胰管情况不确定的情况下，术中胰管造影已被用作主胰管的可视化技术。虽然术中胰管造影可能听起来很吸引人，但通常是不切实际的。

胰管造影有 2 种方法，可以通过切开十二指肠直接在 Vater 壶腹插管，也可以通过切断胰尾找到主胰管进行插管。插管可以使用 5 F 儿童饲管，使用 2 ~ 5 ml 造影剂。Vater 壶腹插管须切开十二指肠，除非有相关的十二指肠损伤。须注意的是，识别壶腹可能是困难的，胰尾切除也不一定能确保看到胰管。

最简单的技术是胆囊胆管造影。该技术首先在靠近胆囊管的胆囊处荷包缝合。然后将 18-G 血管导管插入胆囊。胆囊的剩余部分可以用肠钳夹闭。然后直接注入水溶性造影剂进行透视。造影结束后并不必须切除胆囊。该方法可能显示，也可能不能显示胰管。

胰腺损伤的分级

尽管目前有一系列不同的胰腺损伤分类方法，AAST 器官损伤标准制定委员会解决了胰腺实质破裂和主胰管损伤的问题，同时结合损伤的解剖学部位对胰腺损伤进行了分级（表 1）。近端胰管损伤的治疗方法不同于远端胰管和胰腺实质损伤。胰腺实质破裂和主胰管损伤的患者在治疗上困难更大。该分型方案通过胰管和胰腺实质损伤的解剖学位置（近端与远端）来提供有用的治疗指南。

表 1 AAST 胰腺损伤分级

分级	损伤类型	损伤描述
Ⅰ	血肿	轻微挫伤，没有胰管损伤
	裂伤	表浅裂伤，没有胰管损伤
Ⅱ	血肿	严重挫伤，没有胰管损伤或组织缺失
	裂伤	严重裂伤，没有胰管损伤或组织缺失
Ⅲ	裂伤	远端胰腺断裂或胰腺实质损伤，合并胰管损伤
Ⅳ	裂伤	近端胰腺（肠系膜上静脉右侧）横断或胰腺实质损伤
Ⅴ	裂伤	胰头大范围破坏

AAST，美国创伤外科协会

胰腺损伤的外科治疗

和其他任何腹部损伤一样，手术的首要目标是控制活动性出血和胃肠道污染。在这些目标完成后，应对腹腔进行全面的探查，以辨认和评估胰腺损伤的可能性。

对胰腺适当的评估须完整显露胰腺。打开小网膜囊以充分显露胰腺。该步骤是在胃网膜血管下方打开胃结肠韧带，这样胰体尾的前面和上下缘就获得显露。将横结肠向下牵拉，将胃向上牵拉（图 1）。胃后壁和胰头前面常有粘连，须切开。鼻胃管可能被放置于胃大弯侧，可以有助于牵拉胃。充分的 Kocher 手法可以完整显露胰头和钩突。该步骤是切开十二指肠外侧腹膜，钝性和锐性分开结合部位，将十二指肠的第二和第三部分翻向中线（图 2）。如果存在较大的腹膜后血肿，应该将鼻胃管进一步向下放置通过幽门，同时用手触摸引导，以防止出现医源性损伤十二指肠壁。Kocher 手法应该充分，直至左肾静脉可以轻易显露。有时须松解结肠肝曲以充分评估胰头。如果胰尾损伤，则要显露脾门。切开脾结肠韧带有助于显露。这样就在脾、结肠、胰腺后方和肾前方制造了一个平面。该手法可以用于检查胰腺后缘（图 3）。

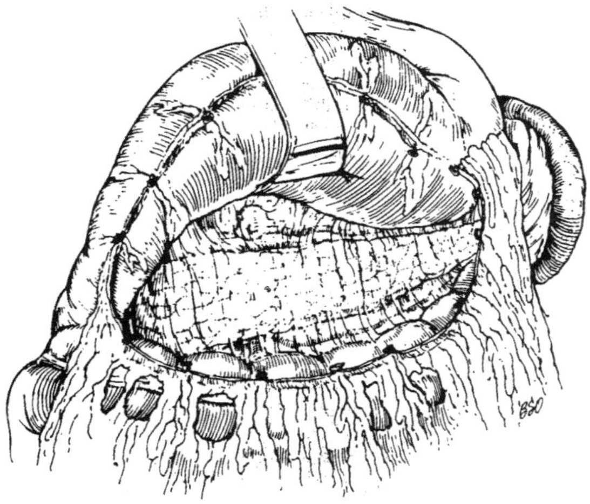

图 1　打开小网膜囊以显露胰腺。切断胃结肠韧带，将胃向上牵拉，将横结肠向下牵拉，充分显露胰体尾 (*From Asensio JA, Demetriades D, Berne JD, et al: A unified approach to the surgical exposure of pancreatic and duodenal injuries.* Am J Surg *174:54–60, 1997.*)

大约 60% 的胰腺损伤为轻微挫伤、血肿和被膜撕裂（图 4）。胰腺实质裂伤不伴主胰管破裂或胰腺组织缺失占胰腺损伤的 20%（图 5）。这些损伤只需要止血和适当的外引流。不要试图修复被膜撕裂，这容易造成假性囊肿形成，而受控的瘘通常是自限性的。任何胰腺损伤的引流都应使用闭式负压引流。这些引流的耐受性好，能够减少腹腔内脓肿形成，引流物收集更可靠，皮肤剥脱发生更少。通常，这些引流至少留置 10 天以上，因为如果发生胰瘘，在术后 10 天时应该比较明显。

营养支持可以经口或经胃管，几乎可以立即开始提供。然而，如果是更严重的损伤，胃肠梗阻时间更长和潜在的胰腺并发症可能会影响标准的进食方式。此外，大多数管饲营养制剂会增加对胰腺的刺激，反过来会增加胰液量和淀粉酶浓度。要素饮食（低脂肪、高 pH）对胰腺刺激较少，更适合这些情况。对于所有Ⅲ至Ⅴ级损伤患者，应考虑初次探查时进行空肠造口术置营养管。这保证了术后早期

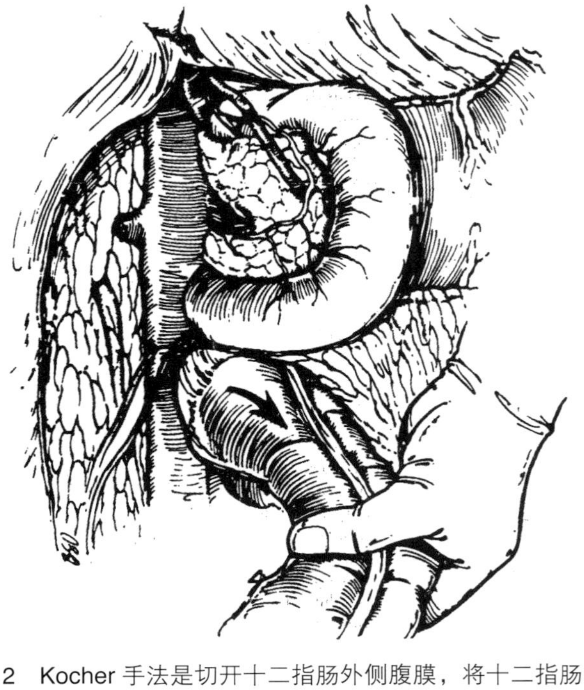

图 2　Kocher 手法是切开十二指肠外侧腹膜，将十二指肠的第二和第三部分翻向中线 (*From Asensio JA, Demetriades D,Berne JD, et al: A unified approach to the surgical exposure of pancreatic and duodenal injuries.* Am J Surg *174:54–60, 1997.*)

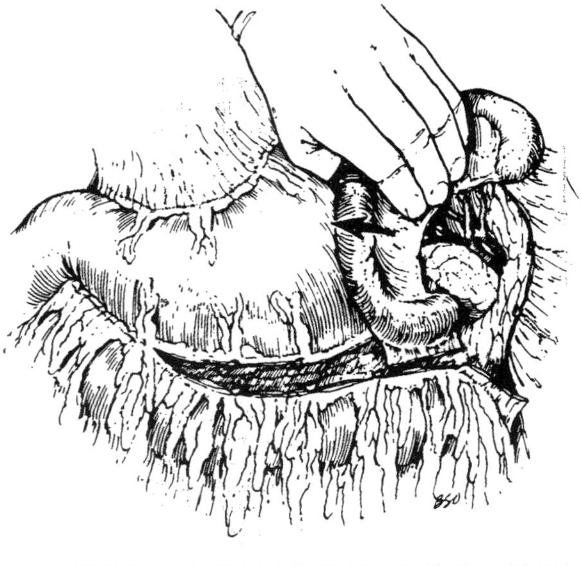

图 3　显露脾门以直视损伤的胰尾。将脾从左侧翻向中线，这样可以直视脾和胰尾的后面 (*From Asensio JA, Demetriades D, Berne JD, et al: A unified approach to the surgical exposure of pancreatic and duodenal injuries.* Am J Surg *174:54–60, 1997.*)

就可以进行肠内营养，并避免对那些不能耐受口服或经胃管管饲的患者进行全肠外营养。

远端胰腺实质横断，特别是主胰管破裂（图 6），最好采用远端胰腺切除术。一般来说，近端和远端胰腺之间的解剖学分界标志是在胰头和胰体交界处的通过胰腺后面的肠系膜上血管。如果近端胰管正常，则应使用"U"型缝合或"8"字缝合封闭胰管断端。尽管胰腺切除术后 90% 的患者内分泌和外分泌功能仍正常，但应努力保留至少 20% 的胰腺组织以尽量减少术后并发症。

胰腺断面的处理方式取决于个人偏好。使用非吸收缝合线从前到后贯穿整个腺体的"U"型缝合有助于减少胰腺断面的潜在渗漏。还有人喜欢使用吻合器关闭胰腺实质。无论使用何种技术对胰腺进行切除和闭合，胰管（如果可见）应被找出并单独结扎。如果可行，可以胰腺断面出用小网膜加以覆盖，但这不是必需的。在靠近切断线处应留置闭式负压引流，与其他损伤外引流类似。

远端胰腺切除术可以联合或不联合脾切除术。保留脾的远端胰腺切除术须将脾动脉的分支血管单独结扎，并且避免损伤脾门（图 7）。这可能会导致手术时间增加和潜在的失血。因此，如果决定保留脾，需要患者血流动力学完全稳定且体温正常。脾切除术后脓毒症的风险尽管很小，但也应注意。即使是尝试保留脾，也必须首先将全部胰腺和脾进行充分游离。将损伤处的胰腺远端胰体游离抬高，仔细结扎沿胰腺上缘走行的动脉和静脉分支，最后在靠近损伤处的近端切断胰腺。

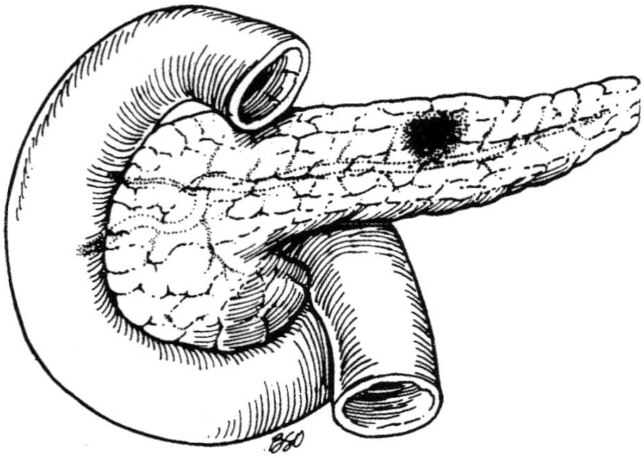

图 4 胰腺挫伤或轻微血肿没有损坏胰腺被膜 *(From Asensio JA, Demetriades D, Berne TV:* Atlas and textbook of techniques in complex trauma surgery, *Philadelphia, 2005, Saunders.)*

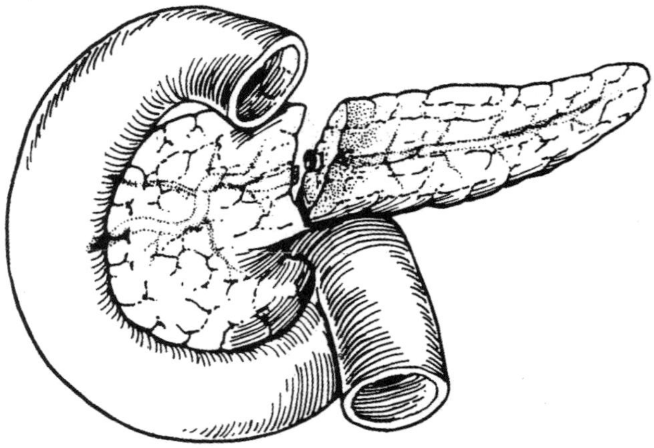

图 6 胰腺实质破坏伴胰管损伤 *(From Asensio JA, Demetriades D, Berne TV:* Atlas and textbook of techniques in complex trauma surgery, *Philadelphia, 2005, Saunders.)*

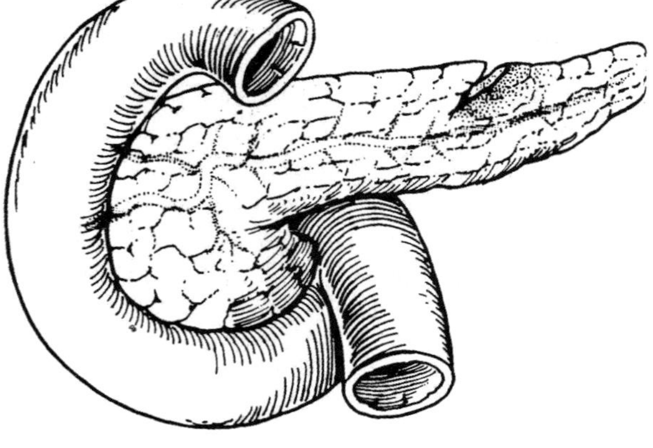

图 5 胰腺实质损伤不伴胰管损伤 *(From Asensio JA, Demetriades D, Berne TV:* Atlas and textbook of techniques in complex trauma surgery, *Philadelphia, 2005, Saunders.)*

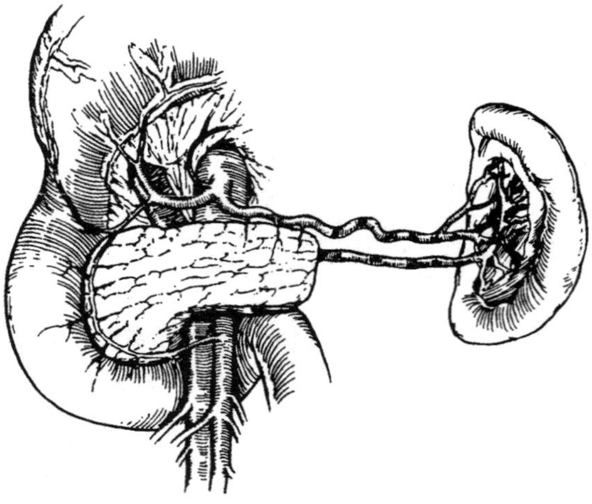

图 7 保留脾的远端胰腺切除术 *(From Asensio JA, Demetriades D, Berne TV:* Atlas and textbook of techniques in complex trauma surgery, *Philadelphia, 2005, Saunders.)*

胰头损伤的处理最为棘手。虽然对所有胰腺损伤都很重要，但是对于所有近端胰腺损伤，必须明确胰管解剖。如果对损伤的局部检查和探查不能排除胰管损伤，术中胰管造影术又无法实施，那么应实施广泛的外引流和术后ERCP。事实上，由于近端胰管损伤相关的并发症发生率相当高，所以几乎所有近端胰腺损伤都应使用闭式负压引流。

充分的外引流非常重要。受损伤的胰腺永远是一个不能被遗忘的器官。胰液的消化能力很强，不受控制的胰腺分泌液（特别是胰酶）渗漏可能会消化腹膜后组织和用于修复肠管和血管的缝线，从而对患者造成严重伤害。

在没有主胰管损伤的情况下，充分的外引流对胰头和胰颈的损伤是有效的。类似地，如果患者血流动力学不稳定，并且近端胰管情况不确定，则推荐采用广泛外引流联合术后ERCP。Patton等报道了单纯引流对近端胰腺损伤的疗效。在接受腹腔闭式负压引流治疗的37例近端胰腺损伤患者中，只有13.5%发生瘘或脓肿。因此，胰腺损伤的治疗变得相对直接。对于远端胰腺损伤，如果可能涉及胰管损伤则进行远端胰腺切除，如果不涉及胰管则单纯引流。对于近端损伤，无论是否涉及胰管，都采用引流。这种简化的方案不需要术中胰管造影。

在不完全胰腺实质断裂的情况下，有些外科医生采用空肠对胰腺的端侧吻合。这种方法仅仅是为了历史的意义而被提及，但并不推荐。因为它难以确保吻合的完整性，而且损伤的后面发生高流量胰瘘的可能性很大。Stone已经证实了这种过时技术的并发症发生率相当高。在238例患者中，7例患者使用了该技术，5例（71%）发生瘘，3例（43%）死亡。

幸运的是，严重的胰头十二指肠复合伤很少见。这些损伤最常见的原因是穿通伤，常合并腹腔多发脏器损伤。由于可能的损伤类型多种多样，没有哪种单一的治疗方式对所有患者都有效。最佳治疗方案取决于远端胆总管和壶腹的完整性，以及十二指肠损伤的严重程度。因此，对于任何胰腺和十二指肠复合伤的患者，在决定具体的治疗方式之前都至少应进行术中胆管造影，除非明显没有胆管损伤。

胰腺十二指肠复合伤患者死亡的首要原因是大血管损伤。一旦血管获得控制，对于十二指肠和胰头严重破坏的患者，Whipple切除仍然是首选治疗方案。基本上，在这些患者中，胰十二指肠切除术是对失活组织的彻底手术清除。对于那些血流动力学不稳定、低体温、凝血功能障碍和酸中毒的患者来说，分阶段的手术方法往往是最佳的治疗方法。对于合并胆总管明显损伤的患者，在出血得到控制后，应原位保留胆囊（假设胆囊无损伤），并在纠正低体温、凝血功能障碍和酸中毒后（通常在24～48 h内）进行Whipple切除。通过保留未受伤的胆囊，可以进行胆囊空肠吻合术，这比在胆总管正常的患者中实施胆管空肠吻合更容易。

西雅图Harborview医疗中心6年中的117名胰腺损伤患者中，有10名由于无法重建的壶腹部损伤或严重的胰十二指肠复合伤而进行了Whipple切除。术后并发症包括4例腹腔脓肿，2例胰腺炎和1例胰瘘。更重要的是，所有患者都得以存活。在一篇有129例胰十二指肠复合伤的综述中，24%的患者接受了简单的修补和引流，50%的患者进行了修补和幽门旷置术，只有10%的患者需要Whipple手术。由于这个原因，每位胰腺十二指肠复合伤患者都需要胆管造影，同时评估壶腹和胰管。当胆总管和壶腹完好无损时，应该对十二指肠进行修补，并应根据损伤位置和主胰管状态处理胰腺损伤。

儿童胰腺损伤

幸运的是，大多数儿童胰腺损伤是Ⅰ级或Ⅱ级，没有主胰管损伤。事实上，儿童钝性腹部创伤后主胰管损伤的发生率仅为0.12%。因此，一些作者建议所有儿童钝性胰腺损伤都可以采用非手术治疗。然而，40%～100%的主胰管损伤儿童会出现假性囊肿形成以及远端剩余胰腺萎缩，需要进一步住院和介入治疗（如ERCP支架置入、经皮穿刺引流）。

并发症发生率和并发症处理

虽然大多数与胰腺损伤相关的并发症都是自限性或可治愈的，但继发脓毒症和多器官功能衰竭导致死亡的情况还是真实存在的，可以占全部胰腺损伤死亡数的30%。

胰瘘是胰腺损伤后最常见的并发症，发生率为7%～20%。通常，胰瘘定义为任何可测量的引流液中淀粉酶水平大于血清水平的3倍。大多数的胰瘘是低流量瘘（引流量小于200 ml/d），通过充分的外引流可以自愈。然而，引流量大于700 ml/d（高流量瘘）的患者通常需要较长时间的外引流，并可能需要手术干预。ERCP 已被证实有助于治疗持续性高流量瘘。ERCP 既可以帮助确定瘘的原因，又可以通过留置胰管支架管起治疗作用（减少瘘流量）。在此期间，营养支持至关重要。低脂肪、较高 pH 值的要素饮食会减少胰腺刺激，应在全肠外营养之前进行尝试。在初次或再次手术探查时，空肠造口术留置营养管方便提供肠内营养，对于长期胰瘘患者来说非常有帮助。

有文献报道使用长效生长抑素类似物醋酸奥曲肽治疗选择性胰腺切除术后的并发症。这种合成类似物的使用已经扩展到创伤后胰瘘的治疗，但在文献中支持其有效的数据很少。事实上，文献报告的结论是矛盾的。

胰腺损伤后脓肿形成取决于损伤的数量和类型，发生率为 10% ~ 25%。腹腔脓肿通常位于筋膜下和胰腺周围。真正的胰腺脓肿很罕见，通常是由于坏死组织清除或初始引流不足造成的，通常需要开放式的清创和引流。无论如何，这些患者的死亡率仍然保持在 25% 左右，再次强调及时引流（经皮或开放）的重要性。

胰腺损伤术后的另一个常见并发症是胰腺炎，发生率为 8% ~ 18%。这种类型的胰腺炎，其特征是短暂的腹痛和血清淀粉酶的升高，胃肠道休息，伴或不伴鼻胃管减压和营养支持，有助于缓解。这类胰腺炎通常是自限性的，可以自愈。出血性胰腺炎很少见，发生率不到 2%。

胰腺损伤术后继发出血的发生率为 5% ~ 10%。该并发症尤其常见于胰腺坏死组织清除引流不足以及术后出现腹腔脓肿的患者。这些患者通常须再次手术探查和止血，但血管栓塞也是一种可行的选择。

未被发现的胰腺损伤患者经非手术治疗后出现假性囊肿并不罕见。如上文所述，重要的是要记住，胰腺损伤后最主要的预后指标和首要治疗决定指标是胰管的状态。事实上，如果胰管完好无损，观察性等待或经皮引流通常就解决假性囊肿。相反，如果胰管损伤，经皮引流不能完全治愈，而是会形成胰瘘。显然，如果对胰管状态有任何疑问，应在经皮引流之前进行内镜逆行胰管造影。

胰腺损伤后内分泌功能和外分泌功能不足都不常见。无论是动物实验还是人体试验都已证实，10% ~ 20% 的正常胰腺就可以维持正常的胰腺功能。因此，远端胰腺切除的耐受性很好，即便存在术后生理后遗症也是很轻微的。一项多中心的研究已经证实了该结论，在该研究中只有 1 例出现了内分泌功能不足，没有患者出现外分泌功能异常。

结论

创伤后胰腺损伤相对不常见。因此，即使经验丰富的外科医生也容易漏诊。这是胰腺损伤的并发症发生率和死亡率相对于其总发病率显得很突出的重要原因。而这与诊断的及时准确性、手术过程的全面性，以及术后须细致关注的各种细节（以确定和治疗与胰腺损伤相关的潜在并发症）都有很大的关系。及时的诊断须对各种可疑表现的高度敏感（术前和术中），并且及时进行适当的检测。随后的手术治疗要根据损伤的类型和严重程度决定。事实上，只要能早期诊断，大多数胰腺损伤的手术治疗是直接的，具有可接受的低并发症发生率和死亡率。然而，一旦最初诊断延迟或错过，会导致病情持续而复杂，而且往往具有毁灭性的后果。

肝损伤

Manish S. Parikh, Susan I. Brundage 和 H. Leon Pachter 著
张大方 译

肝损伤是最常见的腹部器官损伤，约占 30% ~ 40%。绝大多数肝损伤是轻微的，出血几乎总是可以自行停止，很少需要手术干预。另一方面，复杂肝损伤即便对于最有经验的创伤外科医生仍然是很大的挑战。自 1908 年格拉斯哥皇家医院 J. Hogarth Pringle 编写的《创伤引起的肝出血的注意事项》出版以来，肝损伤一直是一个吸引人的话题。作者们首次发表了严重肝创伤处理的科学的尝试，描述了迄今为止仍然是肝出血控制的主要手术操作之一。

也许在过去二十年来肝损伤治疗方面取得的最大进展就是非手术治疗钝性肝损伤获得了显著进展和巨

大成功。其他进展包括肝门阻断、指捏法（肝切除）和网膜填塞复杂肝损伤的联合应用，以及对已表现出“死亡三联征”体征（酸中毒、凝血功能障碍和低体温）计划再次探查的患者进行肝周填塞，同时强化浓缩红细胞、新鲜冰冻血浆和血小板的 1∶1∶1 比例的输血策略，目的是预防术中凝血功能障碍。

在新千年之后，“多学科联合”概念已经演变为治疗复杂肝创伤的标准模式。除了及时的手术干预外，当有指征时，辅助介入技术如肝血管造影、ERCP、胆道支架置入和经皮 CT 引导引流已成为创伤外科医生全部治疗手段中的一部分。

发生率

大约 5% 的住院创伤患者存在肝损伤。在全美国范围内，穿通性肝损伤的发生率稳步下降。但是，钝性损伤似乎在上升，主要是因为在钝性创伤的患者中常规使用 CT 扫描更容易发现其存在。然而，复杂肝损伤的发生率在过去 25 年中保持相对稳定，为 12%～15% 不等。MVC 继续占据肝损伤原因的榜首（约 80%），其次是行人和汽车碰撞、跌倒、袭击和摩托车事故。

大多数钝性肝损伤患者都合并其他损伤，可以是腹腔内损伤，也可以是腹腔外部损伤。伴随的胸部创伤是钝性肝损伤最常见的合并伤，发生在超过 50% 的患者身上。右下肋骨折的患者，特别是第 9 至第 11 肋骨折，至少有 20% 的可能性存在肝损伤。尽管上述胸部相关创伤的发生率高，但脑损伤仍然是影响总生存期最重要的单个决定因素。在钝性创伤的非手术治疗时代，遗漏损伤的风险，尤其是膈或小肠，应受到主要重视。经验丰富的人员通过对影像学研究的细致解读，应将漏诊限制在 1%～2%。

穿通性胸腹部创伤患者中有 30%～40% 存在肝损伤。损伤的程度与所用武器的类型直接相关。相关的腹腔内损伤（例如胃、十二指肠、结肠和胰腺）很常见，但术前难以发现。

损伤机制

钝性肝损伤

在 MVC 中，最容易受到肝损伤的人是未系安全带的前排乘客。这些乘客特别容易受到压缩伤害，特别是在快速减速期间。虽然前腹壁已经停止，后腹壁继续向前移动，腹内器官被“困住”并压缩，导致肝在其血管和结构附着物上的拉伸 / 撕裂。由于肝仅有部分被肋骨保护，因此方向盘撞击引起的肝损伤是驾驶员受伤最重要的因素之一。

在侧向（侧面或“T 骨”）碰撞中，目标车辆在其侧面被撞击并且在其之前行进方向 90° 方向快速加速。未系安全带的乘客同时受到压缩和剪切伤害，导致拉伸和撕裂，有时会导致肝的撕裂。此外，在侧向撞击损伤中，由于脊柱和后腹壁不在冲击线上，与正面撞击伤害相反，腹内器官的相对运动更多，导致受伤的可能性更大。

穿通性肝损伤

由穿通伤引起的伤害取决于投射物的动能以及组织的密度和弹性。低能量武器如刀只能切割而不能产生临时空腔。中等能量和高能量火器不仅直接损伤投射物路径中的组织，还会损坏投射物路径两侧的组织。当投射物穿过相对无弹性的肝实质时，会产生一个临时空腔（投射物前表面积的大小的 3～6 倍，持续几分之一秒）和一个永久性空腔（对于检查者来说是可见的）。更高能量的火器产生更大的临时和永久性空腔，导致更广泛的组织损伤。这个较大的空腔所产生的真空会将衣物、细菌和其他碎屑从周围区域吸入伤口。

诊断

血流动力学不稳定患者

有血流动力学不稳定（收缩压 <90 mmHg）和对适当液体复苏不能迅速做出反应的患者，无论其受伤机制如何，均应毫不犹豫地立即迅速送至手术室。不要在此时做进一步的诊断性评估，因为这些不必要的延误可能会造成患者接下来的死亡。

在血流动力学不稳定的钝性骨盆骨折创伤的患者中，DPL，这种目前已经成为快速诊断性腹腔穿刺（diagnostic peritoneal aspirate，DPA）筛查的方法被广泛使用。或者仅由 DPL 初始吸入部分进行 DPA，联合 FAST 是目前用于检测腹腔内血液存在的诊断方式。对 DPA 强阳性（肉眼血液 >10 ml）应立即进行手术干预。在大多数创伤中心，FAST已经取代DPL/DPA作为确定不稳定钝性上患者腹腔出血的首选诊断方式。虽然FAST对于大于1 L的腹腔积血灵敏度为97%，但具体的损伤部位无法可靠地识别。当腹腔液量小于400 ml时，FAST的灵敏度急剧下降。Kuncir和Velmahos的前瞻性研究显示，DPA对于血流动力学不稳定的钝性创伤患者的灵敏度和特异度分别为89%和100%，而FAST为50%和95%。如果在血流动力学不稳定的创伤患者中FAST检查结果模糊，则应进行快速DPA。

血流动力学稳定患者

另一方面，血流动力学稳定的创伤患者可以进行进一步的诊断研究。然而，血流动力学稳定性不应该将创伤外科医生延伸到虚假的安全感中，生命体征和腹部检查正常的患者也可能存在严重的腹腔内损伤。对于钝性创伤患者，单独体格检查评估是否存在严重的腹腔内损伤的准确性很差。腹腔或体格检查正常的患者中高达20%~30%的患者随后在影像学检查或剖腹术时会发现存在严重的腹腔内损伤。

CT扫描是血流动力学稳定的腹部或下胸部钝性损伤患者的首选诊断方法。静脉注射造影剂后，采用螺旋扫描仪进行高速扫描。在大多数创伤中心，腹部盆腔CT扫描筛查腹部钝性创伤时不再常规使用口服造影剂。口服造影剂通常用于对特定的空腔脏器损伤的评估，例如识别十二指肠撕裂或血肿。以2 ml/s的速率注射120 ml非离子化碘造影（碘海醇）后，获得层厚5 mm的CT影像。注射后50 s的扫描即为相应的肝扫描的门静脉期延迟显像。

扫描后应立即由CT放射科上级医生根据美国创伤外科协会肝损伤分级（表1）进行判断和分级，创伤科住院总医师和上级医生应通常在场共同完成判断。由于创伤科上级医生通常比值班的放射科医生更有经验，因此外科上级医生参与完成CT扫描的初步诊断至关重要。在场的创伤科上级医生对是否实施非手术治疗做出最终决定。应该注意的是，CT上的损伤分级或腹腔积血严重程度不能成为是否需要手术干预的唯一依据。患者血流动力学稳定，且如果患者同时伴有空腔脏器损伤，但没有腹膜炎表现不需要剖腹探查，才能做出非手术治疗的决定。相反，CT扫描的作用仅仅是为外科医生提供损伤的大体解剖学表现，识别需要手术干预的相关腹部损伤，并且可以为治疗后的肝损伤和腹腔积血吸收情况提供信息。CT还可以识别涉及肝裸区的损伤，其通常表现为很小量腹腔出血腹部体征少，且DPL/DPA往往为阴性。

FAST作为血流动力学稳定患者筛查手段的作用正逐步受到重视。目前，许多创伤中心在初始FAST检查阴性的稳定患者中不再进行CT扫描，仅在6 h后重复行FAST。然而，只针对游离液体进行扫描有其诊断限制，因为并非所有的钝性肝损伤都会导致腹腔积血。Richards等在最近的一项针对钝性肝损伤超声检测的灵敏度的研究中显示，基于单独检测腹腔游离液体，FAST对于钝性肝损伤（所有等级）的总灵敏度为67%。另一方面，很明显，大多数FAST显示无腹腔游离液体的实质脏器官损伤通常临床意义很小。目前，大多数创伤外科医生都认为，对于血流动力学稳定的患者，如果初次FAST检查存在腹腔积血或下胸部和上腹部查体阳性，应进行CT扫描，以特异性识别可以非手术治疗的肝损伤或脾损伤。一旦确定为肝损伤，必要时可以复查超声。

诊断性腹腔镜探查（diagnostic laparoscopy，DL）是一种安全的手术，对于可能没有穿透腹膜的刺伤或枪伤患者，可以避免不必要的剖腹探查，有着重要的作用。钝性肝损伤患者DL的作用不太明显。DL可以准确评估大多数肝损伤，并且随着腹腔镜设备的进展，也可以用于修复一些肝损伤。然而，DL漏诊肠系膜损伤和其他腹腔内损伤的报道很多，这明显限制了DL的应用。

损伤的解剖学定位和损伤分级

综合的肝解剖学知识对创伤性肝损伤的合理治疗至关重要。Couinaud基于肝静脉回流描述了肝的功能性解剖学信息（图1）。肝的韧带附着物如图2所示。

AAST创建了器官损伤分级委员会，对各个器官的损伤严重程度进行标准化评分，以促进临床观察和结果研究。AAST肝损伤分级见表1。

处理

钝性肝创伤的非手术治疗

目前，非手术治疗是成年人钝性肝损伤的标准治疗方法。大约 85%～90% 的成年人和儿童肝损伤可以成功地进行非手术治疗。最近的文献报道了提交给国家创伤数据库的 14 919 例肝损伤数据，结果显示所有肝损伤病例中，只有 13.6% 的患者接受了手术治疗。不同级别肝损伤进行手术治疗的比例分别为：Ⅰ级和Ⅱ级 8.5%（n=10 178），Ⅲ级 21%（n=2793），Ⅳ级 27.2%（n=1462），Ⅴ级 37.4%（n=439），Ⅵ级 42.6%（n=47）。初始血流动力学稳定或在中度液体复苏后血流动力学达到并维持稳定是肝损伤患者非手术治疗最关键的条件。一旦确定了血流动力学稳定性，还必须满足以下标准：

1. 没有腹膜刺激征
2. 精确的 CT 扫描描述和 AAST 分级（见表 1）
3. CT 扫描上没有看到需要手术干预的相关的腹腔内或腹膜后损伤
4. 避免过度的肝相关输血

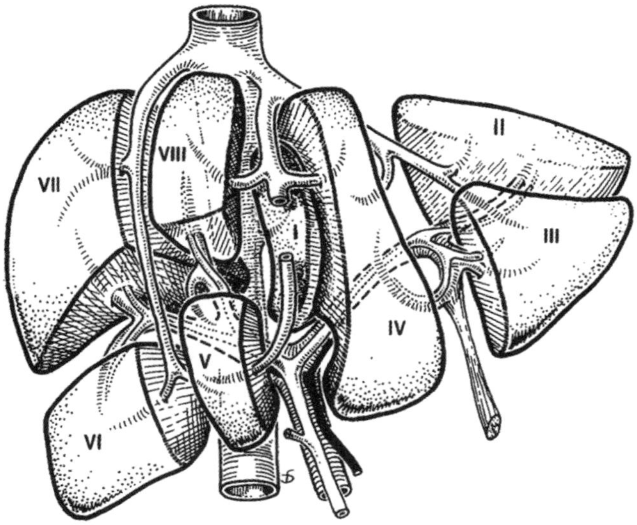

图 1 Couinaud 法将肝功能性分段 *(From Mattox KL, Feliciano DV, Moore EE, editors: Trauma, 4th ed, New York, 1999, McGraw-Hill, Fig. 30-1. Originally appeared in Blumgart LH, editor:* Surgery of the liver and biliary tract, *New York, 1988, Churchill Livingstone.)*

以往列举的纳入标准如神经完整性不再有效，因为神经功能障碍患者可以在监测的环境中非手术地进行安全地处理。此外，重复 CT 扫描以证明损伤得到改善或稳定是不必要的，并且对患者的预后几乎没有贡献。总之，患者的临床过程决定是否须进行额外的评估。

有趣的是，Pringle 在 1908 年的代表作中描述了肝门阻断控制肝出血的方法，他还提到了用腹壁进行生理性填塞和非手术处理损伤不严重的患者潜在优势：“这些情况下，仅仅打开腹部，不管以哪种方式打开腹部，我觉得都会增加患者出血及输血量。门静脉压力并不高，由于局部损伤和血液外渗，导致腹部肌肉稳定收缩的状态。腹壁变得非常坚硬，呈板状，引起腹腔内张力升高，必须达到至少防止血液的快速外溢的水平，并可能导致其完全停止。

今天，大多数钝性肝创伤患者可以成功非手术治疗。虽然非手术治疗最初仅限于 AAST Ⅰ至Ⅲ级

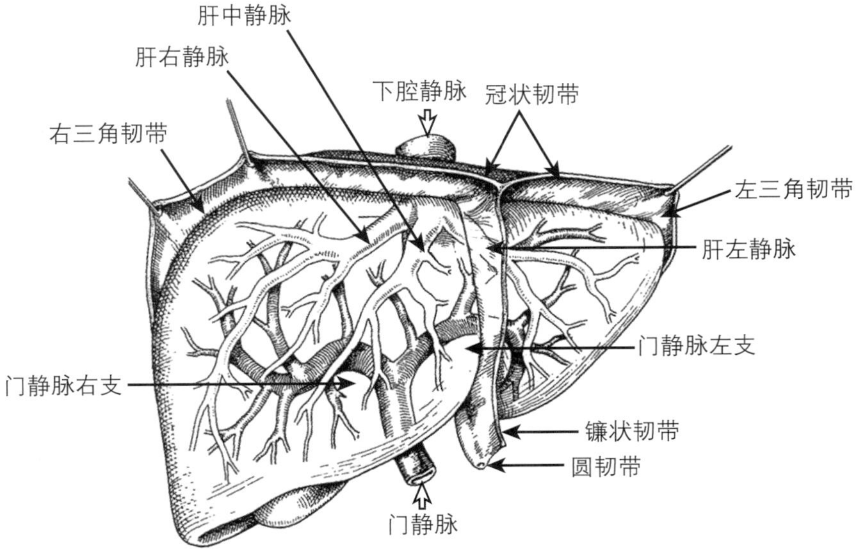

图 2 肝手术解剖 *(From Mattox KL, Feliciano DV, Moore EE, editors:* Trauma, *5th ed, New York, 2004, McGraw-Hill, Fig. 30-2.)*

表 1　美国创伤外科协会肝损伤分级表

分级 *		损伤描述	ICD-9	AIS-90
Ⅰ	血肿	位于被膜下，<10% 肝表面积	864.01–864.11	2
	裂伤	被膜撕裂，实质裂伤深度 <1 cm	864.02–864.12	2
Ⅱ	血肿	位于被膜下，10% ~ 50% 肝表面积；实质内血肿直径 <10 cm	864.01–864.11	2
	裂伤	实质裂伤深度为 1 ~ 3 cm，长度 <10 cm	864.03–864.13	2
Ⅲ	血肿	位于被膜下，>50% 肝表面积或仍在继续扩大；被膜下或实质内血肿破裂；实质内血肿直径 >10 cm 或仍在继续扩大		3
	裂伤	实质裂伤深度 >3 cm	864.04–864.14	3
Ⅳ	裂伤	实质破裂累及 25% ~ 75% 的肝叶或在单一肝叶内有 1 ~ 3 个 Couinaud 肝段受累	864.04–864.14	4
Ⅴ	裂伤	实质破裂累及超过 75% 的肝叶或在单一肝叶内有超过 3 个 Couinaud 肝段受累		5
	血管	近肝静脉损伤，如肝后腔静脉 / 肝静脉主支		5
VI	血管	肝撕脱		6

From Moore E，Cogbill T，Jurkovich G，et al: Organ injury scaling: spleen and liver（1994 revision）. J Trauma 38:323–324，1995.

* 如为多发性肝损伤，则损伤程度增加 1 级，最高至Ⅲ级

损伤，但清楚的是，患者的血流动力学状态，而不是 AAST 分级，是确定是否需要手术干预的最重要因素。部分Ⅳ级和Ⅴ级损伤患者也可以非手术治疗。然而，多数Ⅳ和Ⅴ级损伤患者通常会存在血流动力学不稳定或合并其他损伤，因而需要手术，从而排除了非手术治疗方法。在一项多中心研究中，Ⅳ级和Ⅴ级患者占全部非手术治疗失败随后需要手术的患者的 67%。因此，虽然血流动力学稳定性决定了哪些患者可以非手术治疗，但复杂肝损伤（Ⅳ级和Ⅴ级）的亚组患者治疗失败的风险更高，因此应在重症监护病房中给予密切关注。

相反，这些基本标准适用于 AAST 分级较低的患者（即Ⅰ至Ⅲ级）。在这些情况下，初始损伤可能“不明显”，在血流动力学不稳定或血细胞比容下降时也会尝试避免手术干预，这须依赖进一步的补液和输血。这一行为充满缺点，应避免这样的治疗，以尽量降低并发症发生率和死亡风险。总而言之，在各种指标中，血流动力学稳定性似乎是最关键的，被认为是非手术或手术的分水岭。

造影剂“浓聚”的 CT 表现

初次 CT 扫描在使用静脉造影剂之后，出现造影剂“外渗”“浓聚”或肝实质造影剂“聚集”的征象时应特别引起重视。这种征象提示活动性出血。即使患者血流动力学稳定，无论为何种 AAST 损伤等级，都应做好手术准备，因为患者可能突然出现不可预测的病情恶化。如果患者血流动力学保持稳定，则应尝试用血管造影术对撕裂的血管进行栓塞（手术室随时可用）。经验丰富的介入放射科医生在选择性导管插入和栓塞受损血管方面几乎没有困难。为实现可靠和永久的栓塞，最常用的栓塞材料是不锈钢弹簧圈，而不是吸收性明胶海绵。栓塞成功后可以允许继续非手术治疗。由于肝内血管外渗的自然史是未知的，因此对于这种情况应立即处理，以避免可能出现的突发性出血、假性动脉瘤形成和迟发性胆道出血。

应该避免长时间反复尝试血管造影控制出血血管。如果血管栓塞失败，采用血管造影作为解剖学标志进行手术止血，可以更快速地达到肝内止血的效果，应该迅速被采用。

手术处理

基本原则

肝创伤手术治疗的 4 个基本原则是止血、充分暴露、预防凝血功能障碍和损伤控制。清除坏死组织和引流也是重要的考虑因素。在处理肝损伤时，可以通过使用指捏法切割肝实质来切除肝实质，通常联合 Pringle 法暂时阻断肝门止血。随后可以对受损伤的肝组织进行广泛的清创，然后用有活力的有蒂网膜填塞和闭式负压引流。

在切口切开之前，患者应接受一剂能够覆盖需氧和厌氧微生物的抗生素，并使用加热毯。外科医生必须牢记，体温过低是严重肝损伤患者复苏和手术的常见并发症。减少低体温发生的适当措施如表2所示。采用这些措施常可以预防术中凝血功能障碍的发生、出血过多，以及继发于低体温的致命性心律失常。

表2 预防/减少严重肝损伤患者低体温发生的方法

温晶体液（37°~40℃）进行复苏
用高流量血液加热器进行复苏
塑料袋包裹患者头部
将患者置于加热毯上
下肢使用Bair Hugger动力充气型升温仪，如开胸则胸部也使用
开放体腔用温盐水冲洗
麻醉机使用加温装置

Modified from Pachter H, Liang H, Hofstetter S: Liver and biliary tract trauma. In Feliciano DV, Moore EE, Mattox KL, editors: Trauma, 4th ed, Stamford, 2000, Appleton & Lange, p 637

皮肤准备从下颌到膝部，并行标准的正中切口。正中切口不仅能很好地显露整个肝，而且可以广泛地进入所有腹腔和腹膜后结构。延长正中切口并使用大的“上部”牵开器在大多数情况下可以避免开胸和进一步暴露腹部的必要。应该记住，将正中切口延伸到胸骨上切迹（例如胸骨正中切开术）会开放暴露患者的2个体腔，增加患者低体温和凝血功能障碍的风险。

活动性出血仍是肝创伤患者术中最主要的直接死因。一旦失去了压塞效果，大量血液可能从腹腔的切口处流出。此时，所有的工作都应针对术中复苏，可以采用各种损伤控制技术、临时肝填塞、在ICU纠正凝血功能障碍和低体温与延迟手术探查。在没有适当的术中复苏的情况下，手术止血的尝试常导致全身低体温和严重的凝血功能障碍，并导致严重后果。应该不惜一切代价避免这种根本性的错误。

无论肝损伤的严重程度如何，几乎所有的肝损伤都可以通过手工用纱垫压迫暂时控制（图3），从而争取时间让麻醉团队恢复患者的血流动力学和代谢稳定性。在低血容量和酸中毒未纠正之前就试图手术处理肝损伤可能导致患者心搏骤停继而死亡。一旦实现了术中复苏，则可以缓慢释放对肝的压迫，

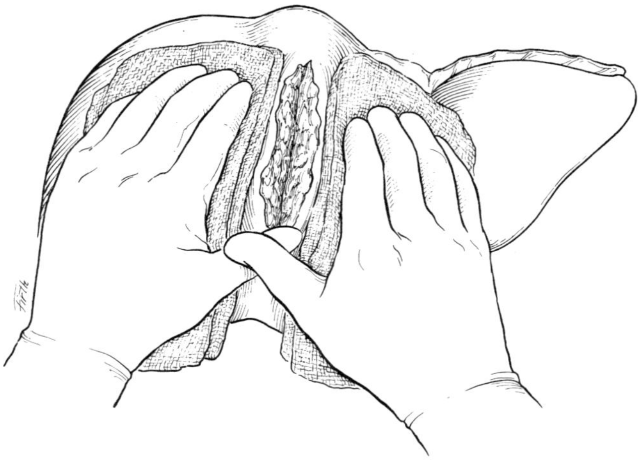

图3 严重肝损伤手工纱垫压迫

从而对损伤进行更准确的评估。

切开镰状韧带以利于在切口中放置“上部”自持牵开器。为了更好地显示肝叶的上部或外侧的损伤，通常须将肝搬动至正中线处。然后再小心牵引肝可以帮助显露肝顶部和肝上腔静脉、肝下腔静脉。可以将纱垫放置在肝后以获得进一步的显露。切开左右三角韧带可以移动左右肝叶（图4）。如果三角韧带肝叶内有血肿，最有可能发生肝静脉或下腔静脉损伤。如果血肿无扩张，不须立即控制活动性出血，不建议进入稳定的肝后血肿。甚至在牵引时也要非常小心，以免破坏稳定的血肿，造成大出血。

轻微损伤（Ⅰ级和Ⅱ级）

控制出血的简单方法包括5~10 min的压迫、局部止血材料（如纤维蛋白胶）、电凝/氩气集束电凝，以及缝合止血（图5）。在许多肝被膜撕裂的患者中，5~10 min的压迫经常可以控制任何出血。如果没有肉眼可见的胆漏，则不需进一步治疗。局部止血材料，如纤维蛋白胶、Surgicel和Avitene，在Glisson鞘撕脱时是有用的。将止血材料施加到出血表面之后再用纱垫压迫5 min。解除压迫后，可以用电凝处理任何剩余的出血点。纤维蛋白胶或其他止血材料可以覆盖大的吸收性明胶海绵，以形成一个非黏合的表面，有利于再用纱布剖腹术垫压迫。如果没有明显的胆漏，引流不是必需的。

肝缝合历来是Ⅱ级和部分Ⅲ级肝损伤止血的主要方法。首先进入肝的伤口创面，并选择性结扎任何开放或撕开的胆管或血管。通常采用2-0或3-0 Prolene线“8”字缝合。或者，也可以使用2-0或3-0线习惯性缝合或血管夹。肝实质的小缺损可以用

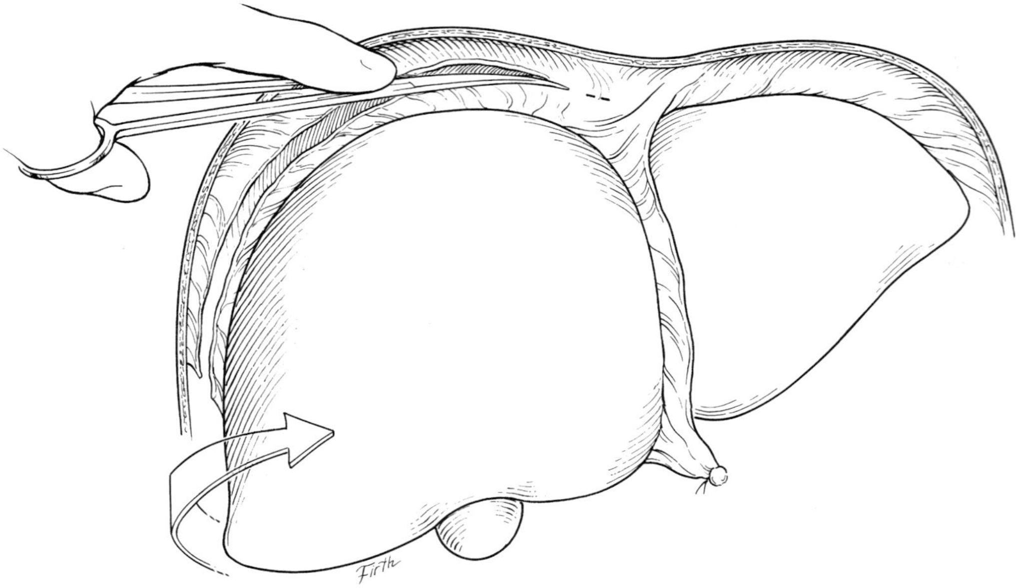

图 4 切开右三角韧带以搬动右肝

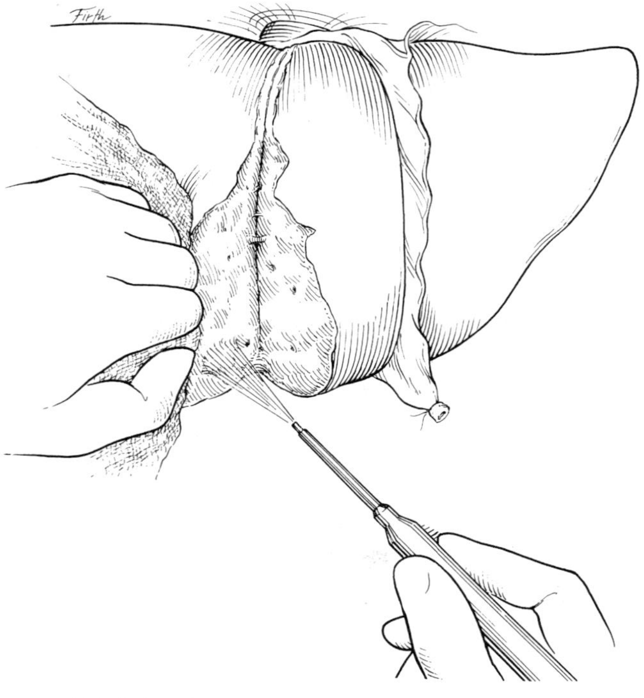

图 5 使用氩气刀控制出血

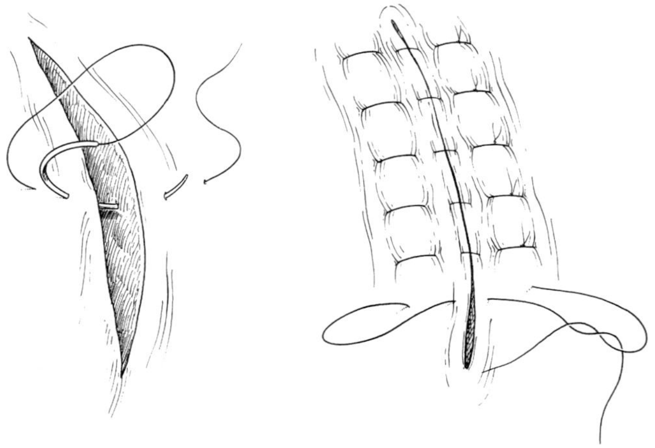

图 6 肝缝合

0- 铬或 2-0 铬常规或钝头肝针进行单纯间断缝合（图 6）。对于较深的裂伤，不应尝试关闭肝缺损。相反，应将带蒂的网膜置于肝实质缺损内，然后用肝针间断缝合将其保持在适当的位置（图 7）。重要的是缝合边缘不要太紧，如果缝合太紧，则缝线下的一部分肝可能在术后发生坏死。

复杂损伤（Ⅲ级和Ⅳ级）

如果在手工压迫肝放松后存在明显的活动性出血，应使用无创血管钳进行肝门阻断（Pringle 法，图 8）。在超过 85% 的复杂肝损伤患者中，肝门阻断可以暂时止血。这种方法联合指捏法以暴露撕裂的血管，进行直接修复，是死亡显著减少的主要原因。

复杂肝损伤（Ⅲ级和Ⅳ级）可以通过遵循以下几个连续的关键步骤得到最佳治疗：

1. 肝门阻断（Pringle 法）
2. 指捏法切开肝实质，显露出撕裂的血管和胆管，直接结扎 / 修复
3. 可以暂时采用纱垫压迫，使患者得到适当的术中复苏

图 7 网膜填塞

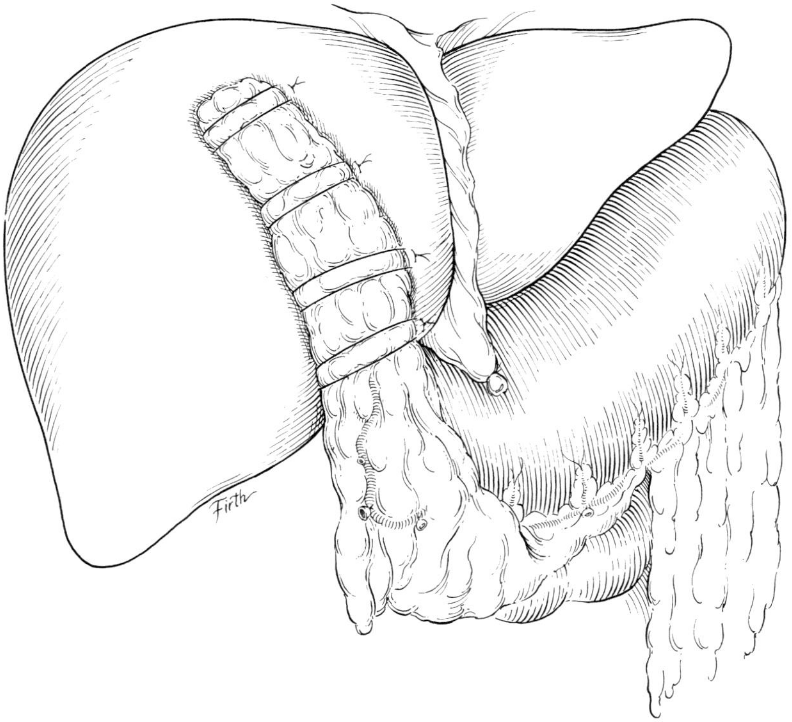

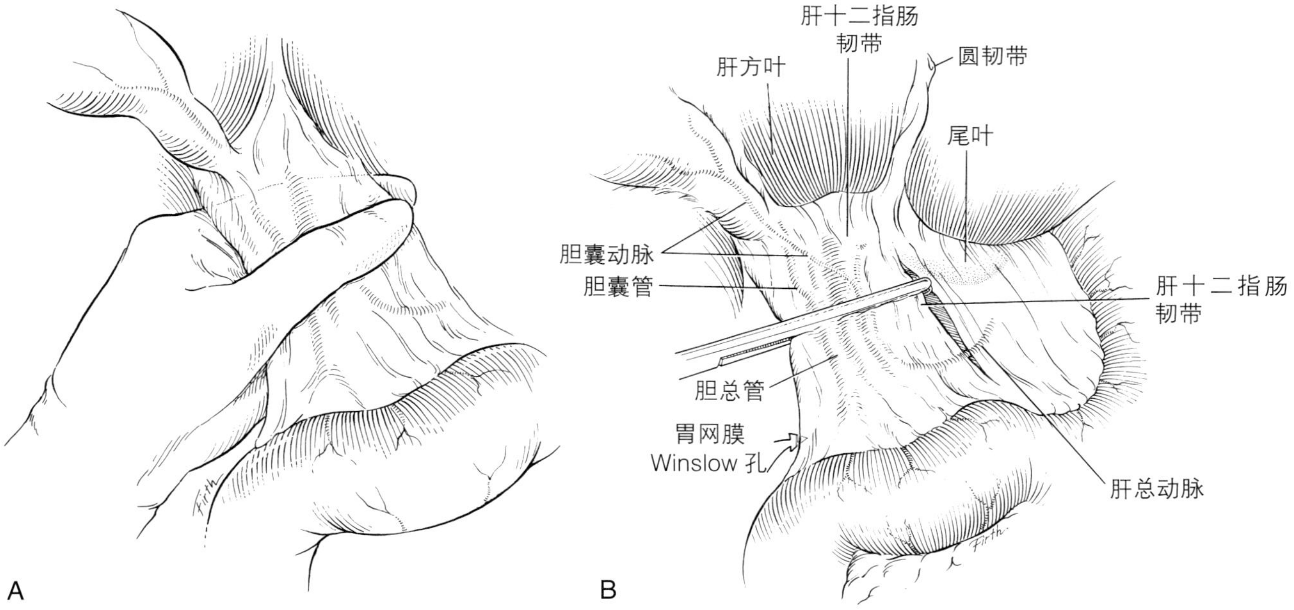

图 8 **A** 和 **B**，Pringle 法阻断肝门

4. 可以使用止血材料（如 Nu-Knit 等）暂时进行肝内填充
5. 清除没有活力的肝组织
6. 将带完整血供的网膜置于损伤部位内
7. 闭合负压引流

由 Pringle 法产生的正常体温缺血时间存在着很多争议。数据显示，复杂肝损伤手术过程中可以连续钳夹阻断肝门长达 75 min，而无不良后遗症。通过防损伤的血管钳阻断肝门，外科医生可以沿损伤方向打开肝实质（图 9）。虽然最初看起来很粗糙，但指捏法可以获得快速而充分的显露，已经成为了标准方法。具体来说，使用电刀将 Glisson 鞘向受损

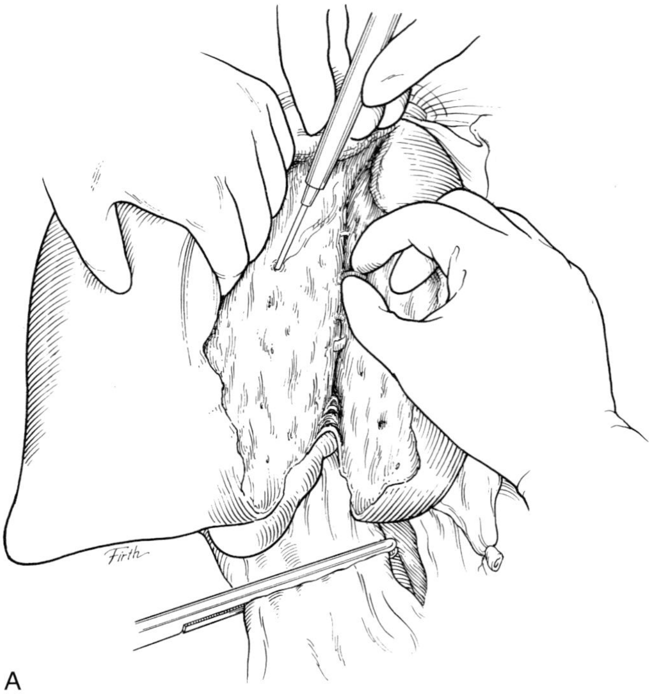

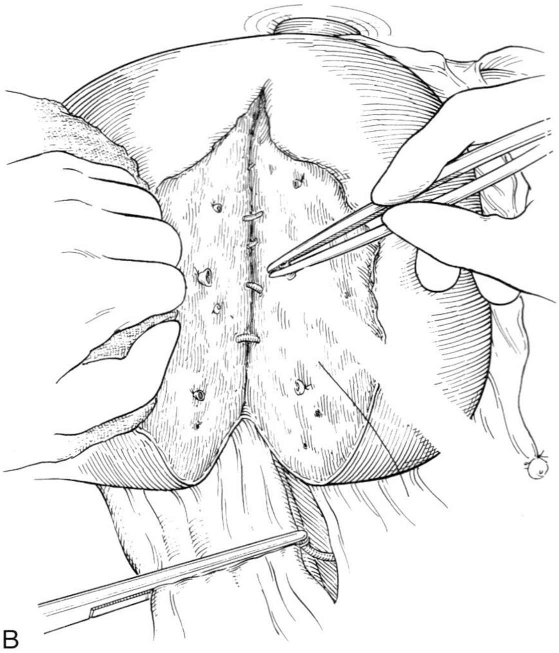

图 9 **A** 和 **B**，指捏法技术

伤的方向切开。然后外科医生用拇指和示指（或神经外科手术吸引器）将正常的肝实质挤压，从而迅速显露出受损血管和胆管，然后在直视下修复或结扎。窄拉钩或可伸缩拉钩可以插入肝切开处，以获得更好的肝内显露（图 10）。肝叶内的门静脉或肝静脉大分支的裂伤可以使用 5-0 Prolene 缝线以横向方式修复（图 11）。

肝内止血成功后，血管阻断的肝组织的彻底清除对于避免术后脓毒性并发症至关重要。网膜的使用在复杂肝损伤的治疗中是非常有益的，因为它提供了可行的组织来填补无效腔、填塞压迫小静脉渗血，并且提供了可以帮助抵抗感染的丰富的巨噬细胞来源。

肝损伤引流的选择是有争议的。如果术中发现存在胆漏，引流不仅没有争议，而且是必需的。推荐的引流方法是在损伤部位的前方和后方留置闭合负压 Jackson-Pratt（JP）引流。关于择期肝切除术中不必要的引流的数据并不能应用于复杂肝创伤，失血、低血压和须频繁终止手术是复杂肝创伤手术当天的常见情况。此外，损伤“区域”可能会延伸数厘米至似乎正常的肝实质内，导致最终的肝坏死和脓肿形成。虽然择期肝切除术后常规引流可能是多余的，但在创伤手术中可能存在的变数太多，复杂肝损伤手术使用闭式负压引流是值得考虑的。

McSwain 等在一篇值得注意的文章中回顾了 Charity 医院的 164 例肝创伤，其中 12 例随后出现了腹腔脓肿，作者分析了各种引流类型相关的感染

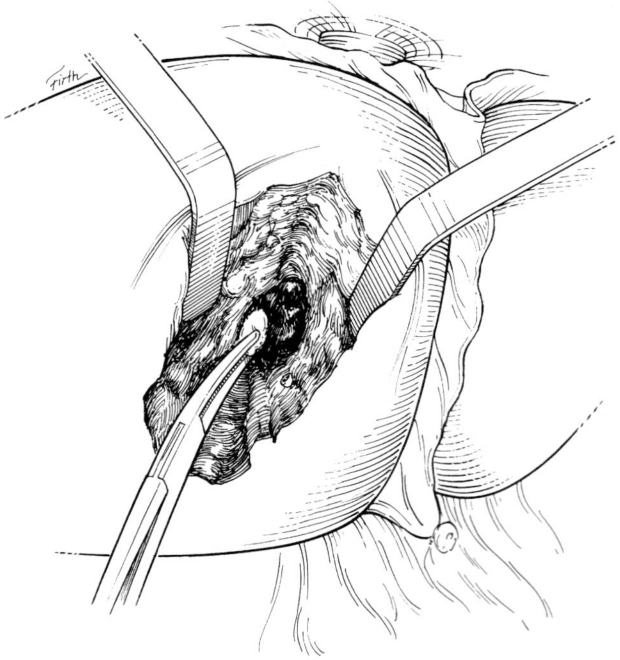

图 10 放置窄拉钩能够更好地显露

图 11 用 Prolene 线或血管夹结扎大的血管分支

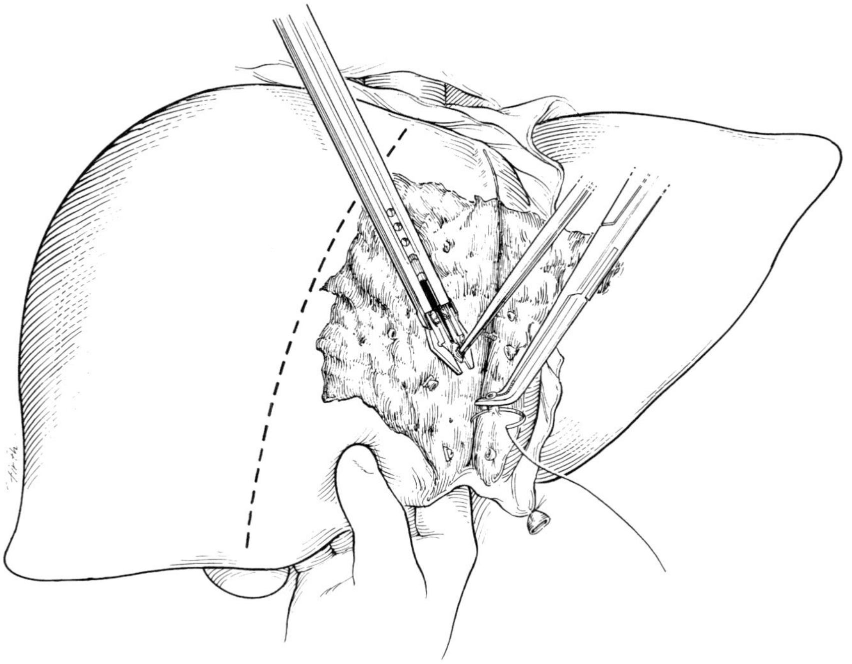

率。34% 的患者没有进行腹腔引流，脓肿发生率为 1.8%。JP 类型的闭式负压引流的相关感染率最低，有 18% 的患者使用，脓肿率为 0。14% 的患者为开放式 Penrose 引流，感染并发症发生率为 8.7%。19% 的患者使用 Penrose 引流联合储水式引流，并发症发生率最高，达 22.5%。封闭的 JP 引流是肝创伤的首选。由于脓肿形成率过高，故应避免使用开放式引流，如 Penrose 引流或储水式引流。

损伤控制：肝周压迫和计划性再探查

复杂损伤的肝患者由于常存在活动性出血、低体温（低于 34℃）、酸中毒（pH <7.2）和大量输血（超过 10 单位 PRBCs）造成的凝血功能障碍，导致常规治疗方法可能难以对其起效，肝周填塞已经成为这种情况下的基本救命方法。肝周填塞的有效性与肝损伤处受到了压塞有着直接关系。具体来说，填塞会增加腹内压（intrabdominal pressure，IAP），引起低压静脉和非机械性毛细血管出血被压塞。肝周填塞成功的关键是在手术过程中出现反复发作的低血压之前尽早插入填充物。

肝周填塞的主要适应证如下：

1. 术中出现凝血功能障碍
2. 双侧肝大范围损伤，出血无法控制
3. 逐渐扩大的大血肿或已破裂的血肿
4. 严重低体温，可能会导致血流动力学不稳定，可能会造成手术中止
5. 其他方法无法控制出血
6. 患者须转至 I 级创伤中心
7. 近肝静脉的损伤

一般情况下，在填塞之前应该搬动肝，以帮助建立压塞的效果。然而，如果在三角韧带内存在明显的血肿（提示下腔静脉或肝静脉损伤），则忌进一步搬动，因为可能造成不可控的大出血。大多数情况下，将干的多层纱垫放置在受损伤肝的顶部，直到达到同侧膈（图 12）。为了减少纱垫撤出时肝表面的出血，可以在肝表面上常规放置 Steri-Drape（3M，St.Paul，Minn.），在受损伤的肝和纱垫之间形成一个隔离面。另一种方案是在肝表面放置大的不可压缩的吸收性明胶海绵为止血辅助材料，当撤除纱垫时，可以提供防止出血的保护层。

填塞压迫止血通常是一种有排战性的情况。在这种情况下，可以用巾钳快速关腹。用几个聚乙烯酮碘浸泡过的大 Steri-Drape 覆盖整个切口，包括所有巾钳。巾钳关腹在几分钟内就可以完成，有助于将患者快速转运到监护病房，在那里改善患者的代谢状态，也可以使用消毒的静脉输液袋（通常称为 Bogata 袋）关腹。经过商业设计的创伤 VAC（真空辅助闭合）系统也可用于这种情况，伤口 VAC 和该系统目前得到广泛的应用的新版本 -ABThera 开放式腹部负压治疗系统装置（KCI，San Antonio，Tex.）是非常有用的。

由于肝周填塞会升高 IAP，监测围术期的 IAP

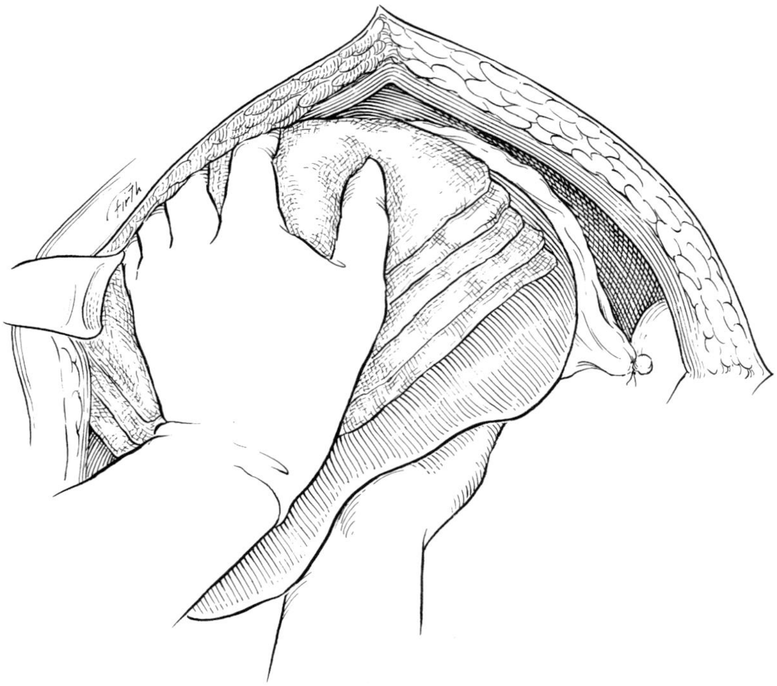

图 12 肝周填塞压迫

对于避免腹腔隔室综合征（abdominal compartment syndrome，ACS）的发展至关重要。直到患者的低体温、酸中毒和凝血功能障碍得到纠正后才能去除填塞物。这一目标通常可以在 36～48 h 之内完成。肝周填塞后肝周脓毒症的发生率为 20%～30%。早期移除填塞物、清除腹膜内血凝块和彻底清除坏死肝组织可以减少该并发症的发生率。

近肝静脉损伤（Ⅴ级）

近肝静脉损伤，尤其是钝性伤，往往是致命的，死亡率高达 50%。Pringle 法阻断肝门后，深处裂伤、弹道或刺伤的出血仍不能得到控制时，强烈提示存在近肝静脉损伤。无论采用哪种方法处理这些严重损伤，早期识别并及时修改手术方法才是至关重要的。

以往，创伤外科医生插入心房下腔静脉分流管抢救这些患者，但死亡率极高（60%～100%）。目前，心房下腔静脉分流术已经被废弃了，这种困难的损伤有时可以通过一系列措施得以救治。

目前，创伤外科医生的普遍共识是，如果肝后腔静脉或肝静脉损伤（Ⅴ级）可以通过肝周填塞得到控制，则在初次手术中不应开始进一步的修复。当充分的复苏已经完成，在去除填塞物之前可以考虑损伤的血管内支架置入。即使没有血管内支架，当进行计划内再次探查手术时，经常发现出血已经停止。如果填塞物移除后发生出血，由于患者的血流动力学状态已得到改善，而且有足够的医护人员可以进行血管分流。因此这时可以进行确定性的治疗。

另一种方法是沿肝正中裂直接切开肝，达到受伤的肝后腔静脉或肝静脉。在手工压迫、强力复苏和长时间肝门阻断后，可以将肝向正中线旋转、移动，从而提供显露肝后腔静脉和肝静脉的途径。向损伤部位行快速和广泛的指捏法，直至显露出撕裂的肝后腔静脉或肝静脉，并在直视下修复。手术医生必须准备通过正常平面或频繁地在非解剖性平面用指捏法切开肝实质。由于这些患者通常也有肝实质损伤，肝门阻断有 2 个目的：首先，它有助于控制肝动脉和门静脉的肝内分支出血；其次，它可以减少入肝血流，从而有助于指捏法并减少失血。

第三种方法则包括静脉静脉旁路术、血管阻断和一期修复。通过静脉静脉旁路术（联合 Pringle 法肝门阻断并在钳夹肾上腔静脉和肝上腔静脉）进行全肝血流阻断，这样就可以直接缝合、修复静脉损伤。这种方法的优点是通过静脉静脉旁路术进行血管阻断避免了心内分流。静脉静脉可以通过大隐静脉和腋静脉切开，在外周插管进行。静脉静脉转流已经用于一小部分严重肝后肝损伤的治疗，总生存率为 88%。

最后是全肝切除和延期肝移植。全肝切除和二期肝移植术可能是所有常规治疗失败的严重肝损伤的最后的可能挽救生命的治疗方法。肝周填塞、全肝切除并门腔分流可以在初治医院完成，然后将无肝患者转运到移植中心进行最终的肝移植。虽然这种激进的治疗方法的并发症发生率和死亡率很高，但如果在出现难治性多器官功能衰竭之前有此计划，并进行全肝切除和门腔分流，则预后会更好。

肝门损伤

肝门损伤是死亡率很高的复杂损伤，大出血是其最常见（85%）的死亡原因，因此肝门损伤手术的首要任务是控制出血，特别是 Pringle 法阻断肝门手工压迫止血。广泛的 Kocher 切口和结肠肝曲的游离可以将升结肠向中线旋转，从而更好地显露门静脉结构。胰后部分门静脉损伤的显露可能须横断胰腺，在血管修复完成后可能需要远端胰腺切除。虽然门静脉结扎可以迅速处理门静脉损伤，但更理想的治疗方法是门静脉缝合修补，大多数文献报告生存率为 51%～60%。

肝动脉损伤一般可以通过结扎进行处理。但是，在结扎后必须评估肝实质是否缺血，特别是存在门静脉损伤或休克的情况下。此外，如果行肝动脉结扎，应该切除胆囊。肝外胆管部分损伤（＜50% 的周长）可以一期修复，联合或不联合支架置入。完全性或复杂胆管损伤最好采用 Roux-en-Y 胆肠吻合术治疗。对于不稳定的患者，结扎与胆管外引流和二期重建是一个合理的方法。

手术辅助治疗

Asensio 等描述了一种多学科团队治疗复杂肝损伤的方法，其中包括立即外科手术，充分采用外科方式中各种最复杂的技术，包括广泛的肝切开、肝造影和选择性深部血管结扎、非解剖性切除和清创，甚至肝切除术以及填塞后临时关腹，随后 ICU 团队在场进行复苏的情况下在血管造影室进行血管造影和血管栓塞结扎。之后，患者在生理异常纠正后返回手术室去除填塞物，进一步清创、非解剖性或解剖性肝切除、引流并关闭腹壁。术后如出现并发症则采用 CT 引导下经皮穿刺肝内容物引流，如出现严重胆漏则采用 ERCP 和支架置入治疗。

随后，Asensio 等发表了 103 例 AAST-OIS Ⅳ级和Ⅴ级损伤患者的治疗结果，他们主张对所有Ⅳ级和Ⅴ级损伤患者行早期肝血管造影和血管栓塞。结果显示，即刻手术以控制危及生命的出血、必要时早期肝填塞，以及随后患者直接从手术室转移到血管造影室进行肝血管栓塞，这些可以提高患者生存率。显然，血管栓塞对复杂肝损伤的治疗至关重要，无论是由钝伤还是穿通伤引起的。

在唯一的前瞻性研究文献中，Asensio 等采用他们的多学科方法治疗 75 例 AAST-OIS Ⅳ级和Ⅴ级复杂肝损伤，证实了该方法的价值以及血管造影和血管栓塞的价值，并报告了这些损伤的生存率得到显著提高：Ⅳ级损伤生存率为 81%，Ⅴ级为 43%。

早期血管栓塞也可用于可以非手术治疗但血细胞比容持续性下降的多发伤患者。在这种情况下，患者应立即进行重复 CT 扫描，而不是随意增加输血量。如果重复 CT 扫描证实肝损伤恶化，但患者保持血流动力学稳定，则应尝试血管栓塞。在任何时间，如果血管栓塞不能阻止活动性出血或血流动力学不稳定，应立即进行剖腹探查。

如果出现胆道出血、术后腹腔引流出血，以及随访 CT 扫描时发现血管异常，则应进行晚期血管造影。

西部创伤协会最近发表的一篇有趣的研究报告，概述了钝性肝损伤手术治疗中的关键决策点和推荐的治疗流程图。这些推荐是基于可获得的已发表的前瞻性、观察性和回顾性研究数据以及西部创伤协会专家意见制订完成的，希望能够传播这些资深创伤外科医生的专业共识。有趣的是，由于近几十年来肝创伤非手术治疗的成功，外科住院医生在手术室治疗肝损伤方面几乎没有任何经验。Lucas 和 Ledgerwood 在最近出版的《医学院在教授学生实质器官损伤止血技术时所面临的挑战》一书中指出，平均来说，毕业生在整个住院医生培训过程中只能执行手术止血技术 1.2 次。由于肝损伤的手术越来越少见，如本章所提供的这样的详细说明在提供培训和教育方面变得更加重要，如 ATOM 课程的手术和互动课程。

穿通性肝创伤的非手术治疗

至少根据 AAST 标准，大多数平民穿通性肝损伤的肝实质损伤程度比钝性创伤更轻。因此，对于没有腹膜炎证据、血流动力学稳定的孤立性穿通性肝损伤患者，非手术治疗是可行的。

Renz 和 Feliciano 对 13 例穿透性右胸腹部枪伤的患者进行了非手术处理。作者强调连续腹部查体和对比增强 CT 扫描在成功的非手术处理中的重要性。Demetriades 等通过成功地处理了单纯性肝枪伤患者证实了这一观点。这些作者得出结论，无腹膜炎证据、血流动力学稳定的Ⅰ级和Ⅱ级肝损伤患者，非手术治疗是可行的。然而，应该指出，近 1/3（5/16）的“观察组”患者最终需要延期剖腹探查。

Omoshoro-Jones 等对 33 名肝枪伤患者进行了非手术处理，其中 31 例治疗成功，其中包括Ⅲ至Ⅴ级损伤。虽然较高级别的损伤会出现更多的并发症（大多数非手术治疗），但非手术治疗的总体成功率并不取决于肝损伤的 AAST 等级。最近，USC / LAC 的同一团队描述了他们 2005 — 2007 年 178 例穿通性肝损伤的患者的治疗经验。总体而言，142 例患者（79.8%）合并其他腹腔内损伤，膈为最常见的受伤器官（39.3%），其次为胃（30.9%）和结肠 / 直肠（29.2%）。178 例患者中有 55 例（30.9%）血流动力学稳定，入院时 CT 扫描无腹膜炎。根据这些 CT 发现，30 例（54.5%）被认为是孤立性肝损伤，并接受了非手术处理（2 例患者行血管栓塞），另外 25 例（45.5%）接受了剖腹探查。非手术处理的 30 例患者中，1 例（3.3%）Ⅱ级肝损伤患者由于枪伤后的结肠损伤被漏诊（CT 假阴性发现），而导致非手术处理失败。患者入院后 9 h 进行一期修复手术，随后出院，无术后并发症。总体而言，所有穿通性肝损伤的 16.2%(29/178)，包括 6 例Ⅲ至Ⅴ级损伤，换句话说，80.6%（29/36）的单纯性肝损伤患者，用非手术方法成功处理。3 例高级别损伤患者非手术治疗成功治愈。

作者得出结论，2/3 的穿通性肝损伤患者由于血流动力学不稳定、腹膜炎或无法评估腹部而须进行急诊剖腹探查手术，因而无法进行 CT 评估。1/3 的穿通性肝损伤患者可以进行 CT 评估，这可以预测非手术处理能否成功。然而，作者警告说，空腔脏器损伤可能不易发现，建议无论最初的临床检查和 CT 扫描结果如何，都要保持高度警惕，并对所有非手术处理的患者定期复查白细胞。

显然，非手术治疗穿通性肝创伤最困难的方面是患者选择，因为只有 30% 的肝枪伤患者才适合非手术处理。此外，鉴于大部分非手术治疗经验是从单个大容量中心发布的，所以在这个患者群体中其他脏器损伤漏诊的风险必须与非治疗性剖腹探查肝损伤的风险相权衡。至少，血流动力学稳定、神志清楚允许反复腹部查体、无腹膜炎体征并且 CT 上没有活动性出血证据，是成功的非手术处理所需要的。

并发症发生率及治疗

非手术处理失败

成年人钝性肝损伤非手术处理的生存率将近 100%。总体并发症发生率为 0 ~ 13%。由于非手术治疗的死亡率将近 0，研究的重点转变为相关并发症的处理和描述上。原发性肝疾病情况包括出血、胆道并发症、ACS 和感染并发症等。

Kozar 等在最近的一项大型多中心研究中提出了非手术治疗早期并发症的危险因素。在 699 例患者中，453 例（65%）采用非手术治疗，13% 出现并发症。常见的并发症包括出血（总共 38 例出血患者中共有 35 例发生在非手术治疗组，8%）、胆道并发症（总共 29 例胆道并发症患者中共有 17 例出现在非手术治疗组，6.5%）、ACS（5 例，1%）和感染（15 例，3%）。出血和 ACS 通常出现在受伤早期（3 天内），但是胆道并发症和感染通常发生较晚（3 天后）。在Ⅲ级损伤的患者中，肝并发症的发生率为 5%（13/264）；在Ⅳ级损伤的患者中，肝并发症的发生率为 22%（36/166）；在Ⅴ级损伤的患者中，肝并发症的发生率为 52%（12/23）。单因素分析提示并发症的危险因素如下：24 h 内晶体液量、总的和首个 24 h 内的 PRBCs、FFP、血小板、冷凝蛋白质的需要量和肝损伤分级。多因素分析显示肝损伤分级（Ⅳ级 OR = 4.439，Ⅴ级 OR = 12.001）和 24 h 内输血需要量（OR = 6.446）是非手术治疗发生并发症的独立危险因素。

早期并发症：出血和腹腔隔室综合征

出血

血流动力学稳定的钝性肝损伤患者出血的比例是 5% ~ 10%。除非螺旋增强 CT 上能看到浓聚区，否则肝损伤出血的可能性较低。CT 扫描可见浓聚区的患者提示不良事件可能性增加，即便患者未出现失代偿期休克的表现，仍因警惕血流动力学是否稳定。因为出血导致的非手术治疗失败通常发生在伤后首个 24 h 之内。需要剖腹探查的迟发性出血的发生率大概为 2% ~ 3%。

肝损伤的术后出血通常较为凶险，可以快速地从术野沿着引流管流出。然而，更加不典型的是，血流动力学稳定的患者的表现较为轻微，可有局部腹胀且伴有血细胞比容下降。过去，肝损伤术后再次手术止血的指征是酸中毒、低体温和凝血功能损伤。目前，如果没有血流动力学的异常，主张先对症处理。

血流动力学不稳定的患者需要再次手术探查。有可能用到手工肝压迫伴术中液体复苏、Pringle 法和指压法等。如果担心扩大肝切开时会累及重要血管、胆管等结构，可以通过外侧叶肝动脉结扎或用Penrose球囊填塞和红色橡胶导管。如果仔细寻找后仍未发现出血点，首先应考虑有无输血相关的凝血功能障碍。在这种情况下，应快速对肝进行填塞压迫，具体根据前面的填塞压迫指南所述。

最近的军方数据发现使输血方法产生变革，且增加了预防凝血功能障碍的可能性，从而停止和防止出血。现代的输血方法是以1：1的方法输注PRBCs和FFP，这样可以更好地减少凝血功能障碍，对于降低死亡率有很大作用。过去以4：1的方法输注PRBCs和FFP，总体死亡率为大于65%，当仅改变比例为1：1.8后，总体死亡率降至19%。现在PRBCs和FFP的目标比例为1：1，理想范围为1：1至1：1.8。更频繁地输注血小板同样是可接受的，虽然具体比例尚无定论，这些在输血上的改进对肝损伤患者减少凝血功能障碍和处理出血有重要影响。但是，此方法的输血方案对于高级别肝损伤的预后的影响尚无定论。

腹腔隔室综合征

ACS是肝损伤非手术处理后的一种少见并发症，发生率大概为1%，多见于受伤后的1～3天。患者通常因为持续性出血进入腹膜腔导致的血流动力学不稳定，而非ACS而进行手术治疗。ACS最常见的原因是肝损伤后出血通过动脉栓塞得到控制，但是此患者在复苏过程中输注了大量的血液制品。进行复苏的肝损伤患者应该进行常规流程的膀胱压力监测，正如进行肝填塞的患者容易导致IAP增高和ACS的发生，非手术处理的患者同样也有ACS的风险，应该高度怀疑并严密检测腹腔内压力。治疗ACS最合适的方法是剖腹减压术。

晚期并发症：胆道并发症和感染

回顾相关研究发现，胆道并发症和感染多接连出现，二者的发生率皆为3%～6%。有趣的是，最近关于肝损伤非手术治疗并发症的多中心研究发现，2种并发症都可能晚期才发生。胆道并发症的平均发生时间为损伤后12天，范围为2～38天。感染并发症的平均发生时间为损伤后15天，范围为1～90天。

胆汁积聚／胆瘘

非手术处理肝钝伤可能导致胆汁积聚（胆汁瘤）或胆瘘形成。虽然肝损伤多合并胆管撕裂导致的胆漏，临床上明显胆漏的报告发生率较低（2%～3%）。经核成像（HIDA扫描）证实的胆汁外溢通常不需要外科干预，因为经皮引流通常亦能有效。治疗胆漏最关键的方法就是充分引流，即便是严重胆漏（大于50 ml/d，大于14天）也可以通过充分引流好转。如果充分引流无效，建议行ERCP支架置入加括约肌切开术。Anand等最近的一项研究纳入了26例严重肝创伤后胆瘘行ERCP治疗的患者，结果示治疗胆瘘的有效率为100%。54%的肝损伤继发于腹部钝性创伤，其余是腹部开放伤。可以联合ERCP下Oddi括约肌切开术和CT或超声引导下胆汁或肝的其他液体引流术治疗胆瘘。ERCP可以在2天内平均降低72%的胆汁引流。没有患者发生ERCP相关并发症。此研究是最大型的关于ERCP和括约肌切开术成功治疗胆瘘的文章。

胆汁胸膜瘘是一种罕见的并发症，见于胸腹联合穿通性创伤的患者。受伤的机制可能是遗漏难以修复的小范围膈损伤。经皮引流胸腔积液和内镜下括约肌切开术能有效治愈该并发症。须对该并发症进行早期诊断，以避免胆汁对肺和胸膜腔的侵蚀。

胆道出血

胆道出血是肝损伤少见的并发症，发生率最多为1%。胆道出血可能由于腹部钝伤和穿通伤，或者深部肝缝合时造成的医源性损伤引起。胆道出血通常会出现胃肠道出血、右上腹疼痛和黄疸（Sandblom三联征），通常发生于损伤后4天至1个月。反复的内镜检查通常无发现，通常须结合创伤病史和腹腔干血管造影。如果胆道出血是出血的原因，血管造影可发现肝动脉假性动脉瘤，可以进行弹簧圈、吸收性明胶海绵、丙烯酸酯胶栓塞治疗。弹簧圈可以达到最永久的栓塞，其他材料可能会产生血管再通，有再出血的风险。通常不需要手术干预，即便手术干预，也难以到达出血血管，因为出血血管通常位置在肝实质深部，除非胆道出血处为大的肝内空腔或者不能血管造影检查。如果要进行手术治疗，最佳方案是肝切除手术，切除范围包括受损肝和假性动脉瘤。在切除和清创大的肝内空腔和假性动脉瘤之前，进行血管控制（术中Pringle手法或直接肝动脉结扎）是非常重要的。

肝内胆管损伤和晚期狭窄

肝内胆管损伤是罕见的并发症。正常和断裂的肝内胆管周围的肝实质损伤自然愈合后的长期后遗症仍不清楚。尽管肝内二、三级胆管常发生断裂，但是晚期肝内胆管狭窄形成非常罕见。

肝周脓毒症 / 脓肿

肝周脓毒症 / 脓肿是肝损伤后的复杂后期并发症，发生率通常为 3% ~ 6%。肝周脓毒症，特别是在多发伤的患者中，容易导致休克、全身炎症反应综合征和多器官功能衰竭，导致患者处于晚期死亡风险中，属于 Baker 和 Trunkey 描述的创伤患者死亡三峰分布中的最后一峰。非感染的因素同样可能引起严重的全身炎症反应综合征，使患者多器官功能衰竭和死亡。

肝创伤的术后肝脓肿的危险因素，包括合并肠道损伤、实质损伤程度、输血需要、在初始手术中清创和引流不足。多数时候，以下方法可以避免手术治疗肝创伤引起的肝脓肿：仔细止血、充分清除肝实质坏死组织和避免开放引流。

多数脓肿可以通过经皮引流治疗。如果脓毒症的患者经皮引流 24 ~ 36 h 后失败，应该考虑再次 CT 扫描明确引流管位置是否需要再调整或是否需要外科干预。若需要手术，应该对脓肿进行开窗引流、清理失活组织和闭式引流。少数情况下，须进行坏死肝组织切除，甚至需要肝叶切除手术，以根除脓肿腔或感染的胆汁瘤。

观察后 CT 扫描

肝损伤后肝的生理功能以可预测的方式修复，可以使肝在 3 个月的时间内完全恢复。通常认为，对于Ⅰ、Ⅱ级无症状的肝损伤患者观察后的 CT 扫描对临床处理意义不大。对于Ⅲ、Ⅳ级且无需严密护理监测的患者，定期复查 CT 或超声，可作为识别此患者的宝贵方法。对于此类患者，最佳的复查 CT 时间是受伤后 7 ~ 10 天。

恢复正常体力活动

Dulchavsky 等的实验模型表明，肝损伤 3 周后伤口的强度可以与正常肝相似，甚至超过正常肝实质。此外，3 ~ 6 周后二次干预的肝损伤的伤口愈合的强度等于或超过肝缝合或肝缝合加网膜填塞术。切口强度增加的机制包括纤维细胞和肝实质的增生和 Glisson 鞘的增生。肝组织的恢复可以在 6 ~ 8 周左右完成。对于大多数损伤，可以让Ⅱ级或以上的肝损伤患者在 CT 扫描正常 3 个月后恢复正常活动。

死亡率

在多数人数众多的研究中，肝损伤非手术治疗的肝相关死亡率是 0.5%。当按照损伤严重程度进行分层时，显然，排除Ⅳ、Ⅴ级损伤以外的肝损伤患者，影响死亡率的因素是合并其他脏器损伤，特别是脑和心脏损伤。在大多数的研究中，合并脑损伤的死亡率为 60% ~ 70%。

大多数肝相关的致命损伤是复杂肝损伤（Ⅳ、Ⅴ级），特别是近肝静脉损伤和肝门损伤，这些损伤的死亡率较高。最近 20 年来，复杂肝损伤的死亡率较前下降，主要是因为肝出血的死亡率下降。主要的原因包括入肝血流阻断的时间延长、切开肝的选择性血管结扎、早期填塞和再次探查，还有辅助的介入手段，特别是肝动脉血管栓塞术。

结论和处理流程

非手术治疗对大多数肝钝伤和部分肝穿通伤的患者有效。非手术治疗的基础是血流动力学稳定。无论损伤的 CT 分级如何，增强 CT 显示造影剂的“浓聚”提示须立即血管造影。成功的血管栓塞治疗提示可以继续进行非手术治疗。如果患者血流动力学不稳定或有腹膜炎体征，无疑须马上进行手术干预。

如果肝损伤须进行手术治疗，须谨记 4 点：①损伤部位的压迫止血；②复苏；③评价损伤；④ Pringle 手法阻断入肝血流。即便是经验不足的新手，这 4 点基本可以保证患者生命安全。复杂的肝损伤（Ⅳ、Ⅴ级）是对手术医生和医疗中心的一个考验。大多数患者血流动力学不稳定、合并其他损伤、需要大量输血和有一定的死亡率。为了手术成功，外科医生须谨记以下 5 点：

- 肝切开和肝缝合
- 填塞和计划性再次探查

- 非解剖性和解剖性肝切除
- 血管栓塞
- 内镜逆行胆管造影术、乳头切开手术和内镜下支架置入术

肝损伤处理流程图见图 13-14。

图 13　钝性肝损伤的处理流程

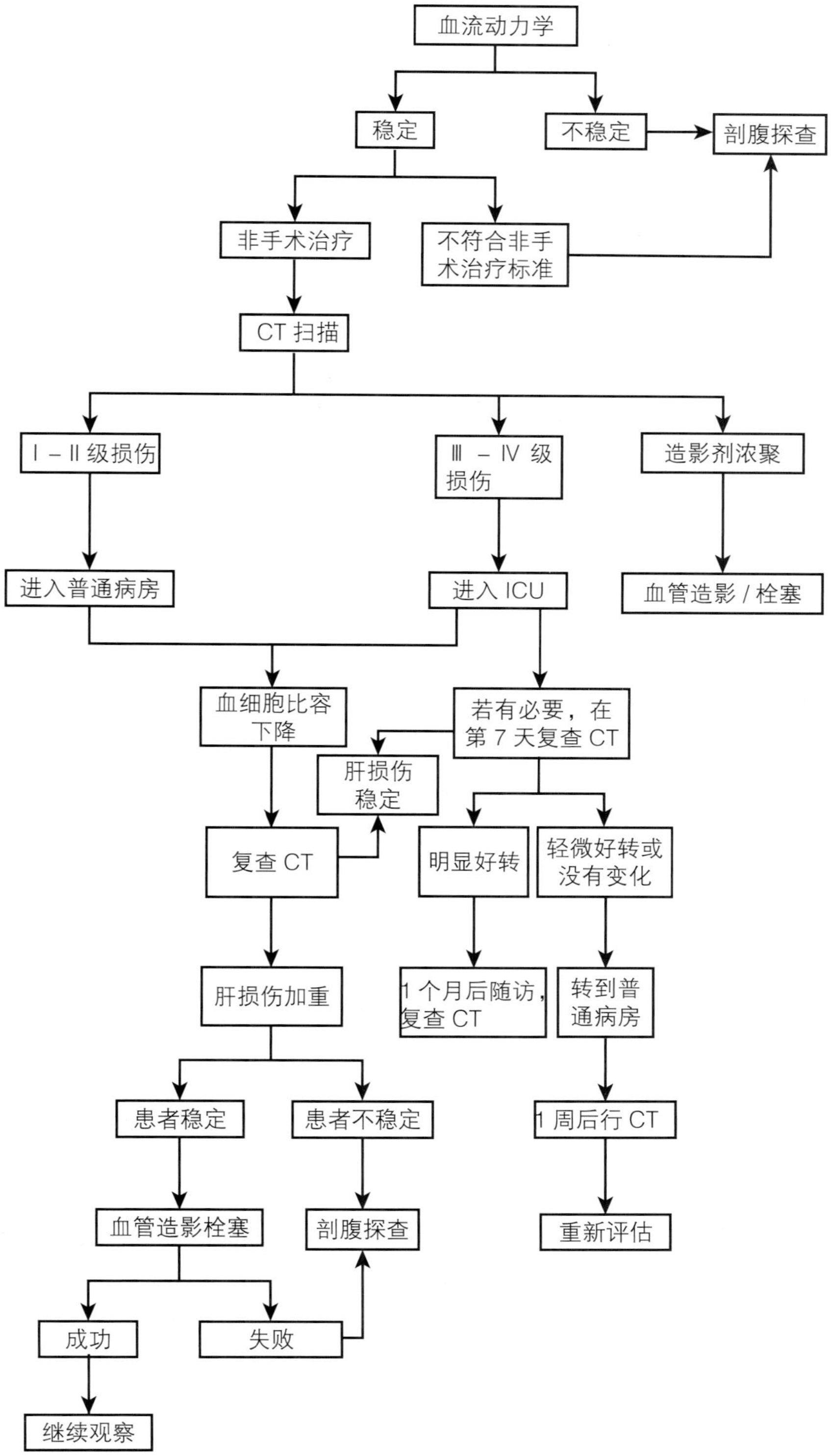

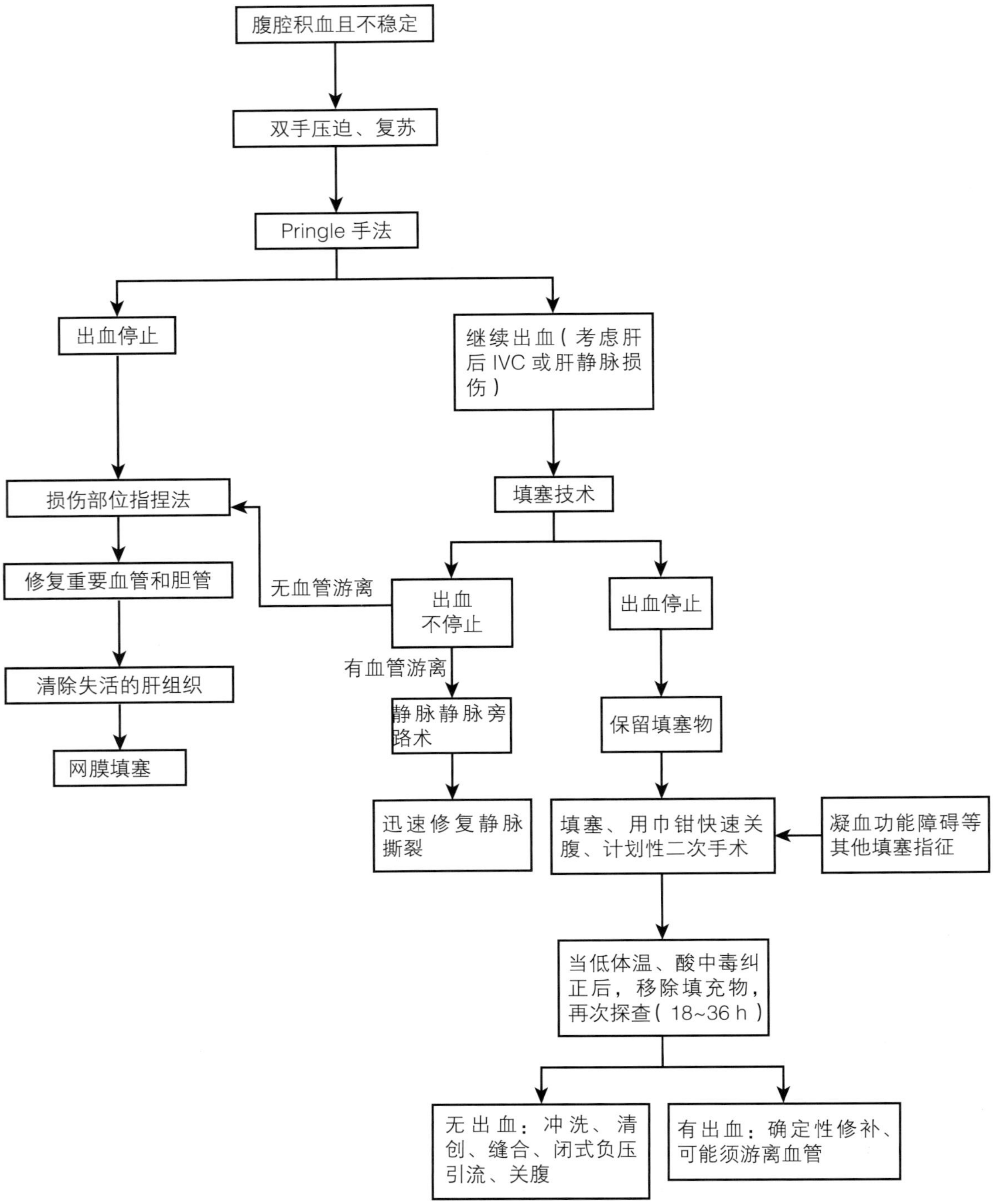

图 14　复杂肝损伤的术中处理流程图。IVC，下腔静脉

脾损伤

Joseph M. Galante 和 David H. Wisner 著
张大方　刘以俊 译

脾在医学历史的医疗主题和经验中有着举足轻重的地位。古希腊和罗马人认为脾可以滤过人的不良情绪，这和一些现代观念有异曲同工之处。上个千年时期的中叶，印度破坏女神凯莉的崇拜者们（Thuggee 组织）是职业的暗杀组织，他们把暗杀当做是对神灵的崇敬。他们除了以绳索扬名，还经常攻击左上腹脾区，当时的人们的脾通常因疟疾而脆弱和肿胀。如果没有输血和现代手术支撑，斗殴中的脾损伤很可能是致命的。

随着我们对脾损伤认识的增加，处理方法也随之增加。因此，我们逐渐从传统的积极手术治疗转向现在的非手术治疗。随着现代医学的进展，我们仍须保持警惕：脾损伤是可能致命的，脾破裂的患者可能死于失血性休克，正如在 Thuggee 组织时一样。

脾损伤的发生率和机制

腹部钝伤后，脾是最容易或第二容易受损的腹内实质脏器。在增强 CT 出现之前，脾被认为是最容易损伤的实质脏器。显然，肝也同样容易受损，因此有研究认为肝才是最容易受损的腹内脏器。无论如何，我们仍须时刻警惕脾损伤的发生。一项大型、多中心研究提示，脾损伤的发生率为 2.6%（6308/227 656 例），脾损伤是经过 CT 或剖腹术确诊的。

脾损伤的发生机制有 3 种：穿通伤、钝伤、间接损伤。一项回顾性研究纳入 Grady 纪念医院和 Ben Taub 总医院的穿通伤患者，腹部枪伤的脾损伤发生率为 7%～9%，远远少于空腔脏器和肝。刺伤所致的脾损伤同样发生率较少。

脾钝伤可能导致即刻出血或延迟性出血，延迟期是保守治疗中的一个重要时期。迟发性出血可能导致保守治疗的失败，其发生率根据损伤分级的不同而不同。延迟性出血的假说之一是，被膜下血肿在伤后数天的破裂，破裂后进入腹腔隔室，损伤区域的渗透性活动性微粒增加，导致更多体液向该处聚集。这导致损伤区域体积增大，直至超过被膜张力，导致被膜破裂和新的出血。即便是没有被膜下出血，血肿周围的炎症及纤维蛋白分解可能减弱血栓强度，从而导致重新出血。

第三种损伤机制是直接损伤，特别是结肠镜镜检过程中。脾损伤是结肠镜的一个常见、难以发现的、被低估的并发症。对脾结肠韧带的牵拉可能导致脾被膜的撕裂。虽然此并发症罕见，但其死亡率可达 5%，并且需要与其他原因所导致的脾损伤一样的处理。

诊断

正如其他创伤的患者一样，脾损伤须根据 ABCs（气道、呼吸、循环）的方式进行复苏。复苏过程中非常重要的一点是，应及早发现难治性休克，在适当时机予以手术治疗。

在病史采集过程中，须重点记录手术史，特别是脾切除史。如患者有左侧胸部、左上腹部的击打并伴有疼痛，都应警惕脾损伤。其他可能导致脾大或异常的原因也应考虑。应该询问患者或疑似患者有无肝或门脉疾病的病史、是否正在进行抗凝治疗、是否有出血倾向和近期服用阿司匹林或非甾体消炎药物的用药史。

体格检查中，须着重检查患者是否存在左侧季肋区疼痛或肌紧张。因为脾位于左侧季肋区，因此此处，特别是后部尤为重要。在儿童中，由于胸廓具有良好的弹性，在存在潜在脾损伤的情况下，上方的肋骨可能无骨折。稍年长的患者可能无明显的季肋区疼痛和其他阳性体征，除非存在严重的胸廓损伤和潜在的脾损伤。腹部查体可发现局部腹肌紧张或全腹腹肌紧张，但是并不是所有的脾损伤都会有腹膜炎的表现或其他阳性体征。没有血栓形成的出血可能不会产生容易被引出的腹膜炎表现。在神智改变的患者中，体格检查的可靠性下降。因此，对于血流动力学稳定的患者，影像学检查是诊断和处理的重要组成成分。

过去，DPL 是腹部损伤的重要诊断方式，但现在使用已经越来越少了。它在初步诊断、决定下一步试验和手术干预中的作用已经被腹部 CT 和超声所取代。在超声不可行或不可靠时，腹腔灌洗仍有一定作用，其可明确血流动力学不稳定的患者是否仍然有腹腔内的活动性出血。

超声检查腹腔内的游离液体，FAST 广泛用于钝伤后腹腔内出血的诊断。和 DPL 一样，其适用于血流动力学不稳定的患者，但是其对明确出血部位的作用有限。对于用超声明确特定脏器损伤的尝试大多尚未成功。通常使用 FAST 以探查有无腹腔游离液体，决定是需要更进一步的影像学检查还是急诊手术（图 1）。

腹部 CT 是脾损伤的一个主要的非手术性诊断方法（图 2-4）。患者可能在初步复苏后直接行 CT 检测，或者在腹部超声检查后再决定是否须行进一步 CT 检查。增强 CT 对诊断更有帮助。口服造影剂对脾损伤的诊断帮助小，且几乎无法增加其灵敏度。

CT 中提示脾损伤的引起众多关注表现为脾组织可见“断裂”的实质或高密度区域（其中有造影剂浓聚）。当出现时，浓聚代表活动性出血，从而导致造影剂溢出。其他研究也指出浓聚提示持续性或迟发

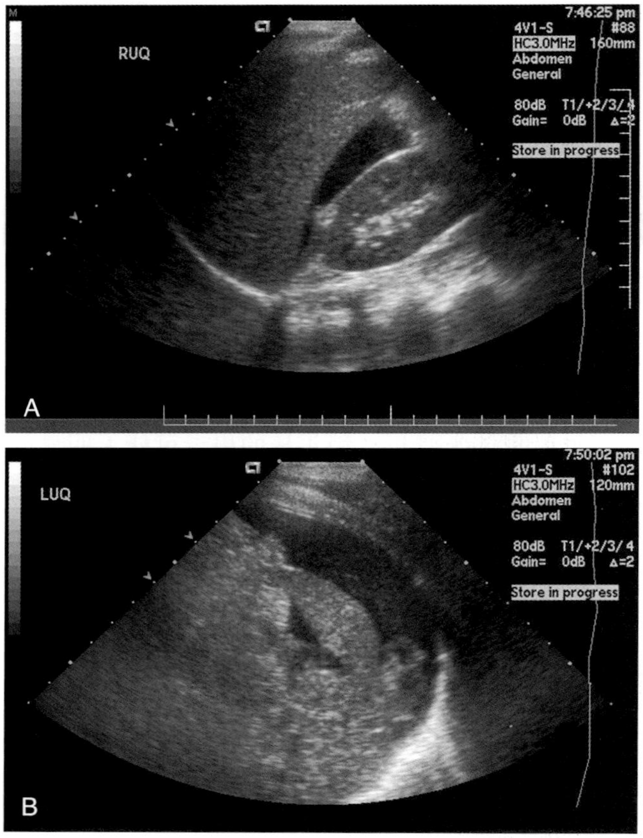

图 1 FAST。肝肾隐窝的积液。积液是黑色区域，后界是肾，前界是肝（A）。积液在左上腹围绕脾。积液是侧方的黑色区域（B）

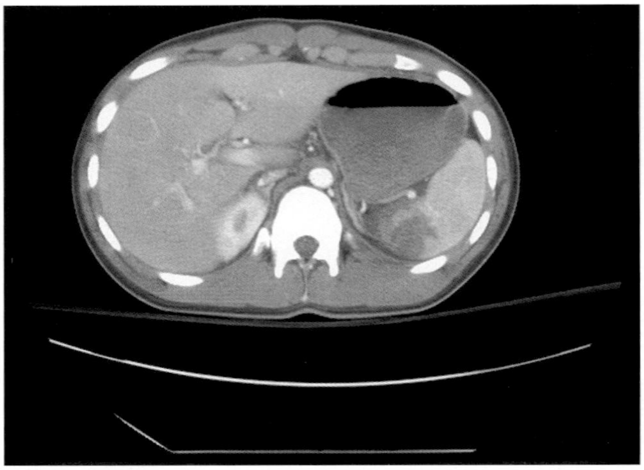

图 2 脾钝伤 CT 扫描，Ⅲ度。脾实质的前界和后界中断，形成被膜下血肿

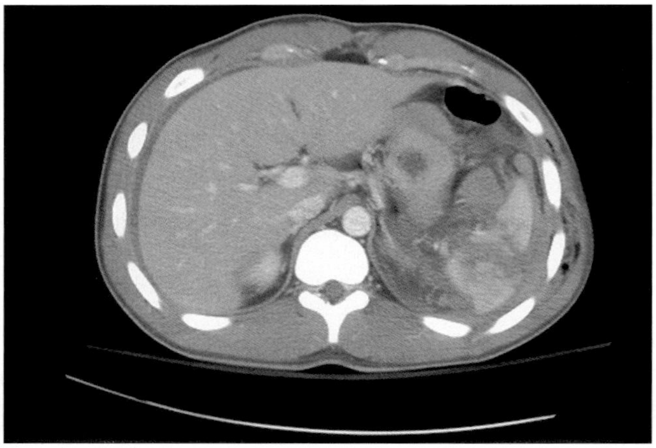

图 3 脾钝伤 CT 扫描，Ⅳ度，可见脾实质的裂伤及被膜的断裂

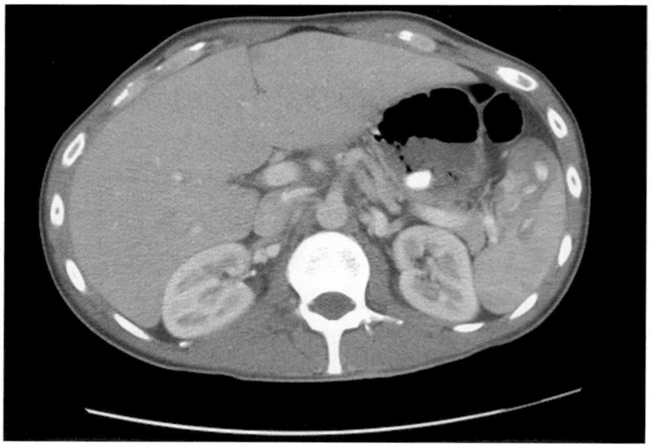

图 4 脾钝伤 CT 扫描，Ⅲ度。可见脾前部的裂伤，脾实质可见“浓聚”

性出血可能，以及保守治疗失败的风险增加。然而，这样的发现并不要求改变血流动力学稳定患者的初始处理，尤其在儿童患者中，更应警惕非手术治疗失败的可能（图 5）。

损伤的解剖学部位及损伤分级，美国创伤外科协会器官损伤分级

组织学上，脾被分为皮质和髓质。皮质含有许多通道，以过滤衰老红细胞及捕获细菌。滤过红髓质空隙中的细菌使细菌壁的抗原呈递给位于白髓质的淋巴细胞。白髓质中充满了淋巴细胞，它们可以暴露于微生物或在循环中的抗原。淋巴细胞接受抗原刺激后可以产生抗体，最常见的是 IgM。

脾起源于左侧、背侧胃系膜处，逐渐向左部迁移至左上腹。在成熟过程中，相对大小不断变化。当儿童的骨髓成熟后，脾的作用的重要性下降，相对身体其他器官的大小减小。在脾被膜和实质的连续性上，儿童和成年人有一定区别。儿童的脾被膜比成年人要厚，并且脾实质的连续性要比成年人更加稳定。这两点区别将影响非手术治疗的成功。儿

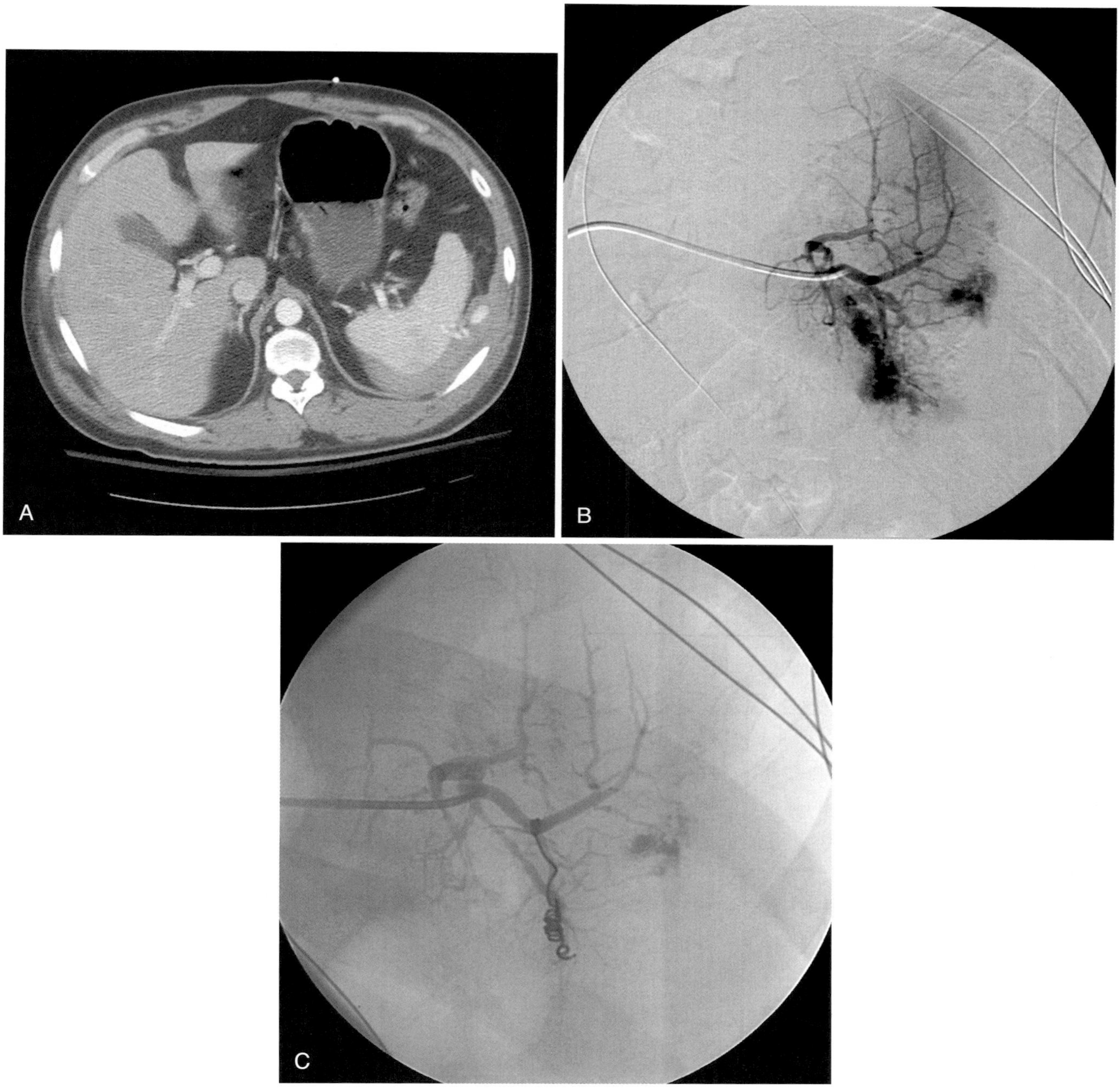

图 5 通过基于导管的方式治疗脾损伤。CT 提示 II 级脾损伤（**A**）。动脉造影提示持续性出血（**B**）。栓塞治疗损伤区域（**C**）

童的脾损伤保守治疗成功率更高。

解剖学教材上的前后视角可能不够直观。但是脾通常位于上腹部的后侧。除了脾门外，其余脾都有腹膜覆盖。脾的后面和侧面与左侧膈、左后侧和外后侧的肋骨相连，脾的侧面和腹壁的后外侧和左侧膈相连。腹壁的外侧（脾膈韧带）之间有许多连接组织，这些在游离脾时都须分离。脾的后方与左侧髂腰肌和左侧肾上腺相邻。脾的中后部与胰体尾相邻。将脾从左上腹提起时，游离胰体尾将有所帮助。脾的前中部和胃大弯相邻。脾的后下部与左侧肾相邻。游离脾时，须分离脾与左肾相连的韧带（脾肾韧带）。最后，脾的前面和横结肠远端与结肠脾曲相邻。脾的下极和结肠相连（脾结肠韧带），脾游离时此韧带须分离。脾的主要动脉血供来自于脾动脉，脾动脉由腹腔干分出，在走行于胰体、尾上方时走行可能有所变异。脾门处与脾动脉的分支数量变异较多。脾的其他血供有胃短动脉，在胃大弯处连接胃网膜左动脉和脾循环，因此，脾的动脉与胃大弯有相同的血液循环。脾静脉回流主要通过脾静脉和胃短静脉。

对脾损伤的程度的分级设计了不同的评分系统。这些评分主要根据 CT 发现的脾撕裂和术中所见。最常用的是 AAST 提出的评分体系（表 1）。AAST 评分也许是较明显的判别方法。分数在脾实质损伤的长度和深度增加、存在累及脾门、有脾的多处损伤时增加。

脾损伤的 CT 表现和术中所见有较大的个体差异，部分是由于检查和手术的时间之间损伤进展造成的。但是，CT 扫描对描述脾撕裂的病理学解剖可能存在较大缺陷。基于 CT 表现的脾损伤评分可能高估或低估的术中所见的损伤的严重性。可能 CT 提示的脾轻微损伤，在术中发现其实是严重的脾破裂。同理，CT 表现看起来像严重脾破裂，术中可能发现其实程度并不如报告所言严重。通常，CT 扫描和相关评分会低估术中所见的脾损伤的严重程度。

重要的是，临床预后可能与基于 CT 的损伤程度并不紧密相关。尽管 CT 为基础的评分与手术干预的频率及非手术处理的失败率有一定程度相关，但是也存在不少例外。脾损伤评分，特别是 AAST 的评分主要作用在于术语的客观标准化和确保用他人可理解的确切词语描述个体化损伤。标准化器官损伤分级其对描述脾损伤患者群体和制订治疗标准有一定作用。

表 1　AAST 脾损伤评分

分级	损伤类型	损伤描述
Ⅰ	血肿	被膜下血肿，<10% 表面积
	撕裂	被膜撕裂深入实质<1 cm，无腹腔出血
Ⅱ	血肿	被膜下血肿，10%~50% 表面积
	撕裂	被膜撕裂深入实质 1~3 cm，不涉及小梁血管
Ⅲ	血肿	被膜下血肿，>50% 表面积或扩大，或者被膜下破裂和实质血肿；实质内血肿 5 cm 或扩大
	撕裂	被膜撕裂深入实质 >3 cm，或累及小梁血管
Ⅳ	撕裂	实质内血肿破裂有活动性出血，累及脾门或段的血管撕裂，导致血供阻断的脾>25% 表面积
Ⅴ	撕裂	完全粉碎
	血管	脾门血管损伤，脾血供阻断

Modified from Moore EE, Cogbill TH, Jurkovich GJ, et al: Organ injury scaling: spleen and liver. J Trauma 38:323, 1995.

AAST-OIS, American Association for the Surgery of Trauma Organ Injury Scaling.

* 多发损伤增加Ⅰ级，最高至Ⅲ级

处理

非手术处理

虽然大部分患者可以进行非手术处理，但是恰当的患者选择仍然是非常重要的一环节，主要根据血流动力学状态决定患者进行非手术处理的合适性。血流动力学稳定并没有明确的定义，是一个虚幻的概念，但是低血压（成年人收缩压<90 mmHg，老年人的水平更高）须引起足够的重视。院外的或急诊时的低血压是格外危险的，须高度怀疑持续性出血，在存在时须立即处理。在大多数情况下，血流动力学不稳定的患者不建议进行腹部 CT 检查。除了复苏外，此类患者须直接进行手术治疗，或用腹部超声或 DPL 明确有无腹腔积液，从而指导下一步治疗。

假设血流动力学稳定，保守治疗的方案考虑主要取决于腹部检查。如果患者为清醒的，且对体检有反应，应该明确患者有无弥漫性、持续性的腹膜炎。虽然脾损伤常会有继发于腹腔内出血的左上腹的局限性疼痛和压痛，但是明显的弥漫性腹膜炎体征可提示小肠损伤，且需要腹部探查。

如果患者进行了CT检查，并选择了随后的非手术处理，重要的是连续地对患者进行查体。如果腹部体征恶化，可能存在小肠钝伤。小肠损伤的常见CT表现为腹腔游离液体。在存在脾损伤的患者中，可能把腹腔游离液体仅归结为脾损伤，从而漏诊了小肠损伤的存在。在此情况下，腹部体格检查就尤为重要。

儿童脾损伤非手术处理的成功率为95%或更高，成年人为80%或更高。如此高的成功率可能存在误导。研究选择的患者群体为选择非手术处理的患者，而非脾损伤的全部患者。当把需要立即脾切除的患者纳入研究，非手术处理的成功率仅为50%～60%。应注意的是，计划行保守治疗，却在行CT检查时或在急诊时就情况恶化改行手术治疗的患者并未纳入研究。发表的论文中的非手术处理的脾损伤仅纳入了足够稳定、可行CT检查，并扫描发现脾破裂的患者。

除了血流动力学稳定和腹部查体发现外，选择合适的非手术处理时的其他重要考虑有医疗环境以及一些患者特点。仅在患者可以密切观察的情况下，可以进行非手术处理。如果密切观察患者不可行，应该选择剖腹探查。相似地，在迟发性出血或持续性出血时难以快速转运至手术室和快速手术干预，应进行初始手术干预。

如果在持续保持稳定的患者可以行CT检测，并且发现脾撕裂，那么非手术处理是合理的。除了生命体征，我们还须观察患者的血细胞比容。我们须制订一个血细胞比容的下限，如果血细胞比容低于该下限，就应该进行手术治疗。当患者无相关损伤以及未进行栓塞时，此方法可行性最好。如果存在其他损伤，将很难判断血细胞比容的下降是由于脾出血还是其他脏器出血。如果对脾损伤的患者进行输血治疗，应该牢记有证据显示输血治疗会导致有害的免疫反应，这是创伤患者预后的独立危险因素。研究提示，年龄大于55岁的患者的非手术处理预后较年轻人更差，但也有研究认为年轻和年老者预后相同。虽然此部分研究的结果不一致，但最近一项大型的多中心研究发现，年老患者非手术处理更容易失败。这是由于年轻患者脾的密度更高，是血栓形成的更好的平台。

合并严重的相关损伤，特别是脑损伤，是脾损伤的非手术处理的另一个相对禁忌证。之前的经验认为，观察多脏器严重损伤的患者血细胞比容有很多问题。其次，对于头部损伤的患者，如果脾出现迟发性出血将严重影响严重头部损伤的预后。虽然并不建议对此类患者都强制进行手术治疗，但是在个体基础上，此类患者或持续性出血手术治疗的阈值应该更低。

尚无科学的证据指出该如何对脾损伤的患者进行非手术处理，多数的推荐仅是共识和建议。大部分的患者包括Ⅱ级及以上脾损伤患者和有多发相关损伤的患者应于ICU接受治疗，因为后续的查体和血细胞比容难以判断他们的病情。

一开始患者应禁食、水以免保守治疗失败，它通常发生于受伤的早期。如无特殊原因，可以不插入鼻胃管。大多数非手术处理的指南中均要求卧床休息，但是也有研究提出早期活动并不会增加非手术处理失败的风险，而创伤患者会得益于早期活动。应该严密监测患者的血流动力学和尿量。连续进行血细胞比容检测，并多次对比，并与入院数据对比。

应给予嗜血杆菌、脑膜炎球菌和链球菌的疫苗。虽然脾切除的患者在围术期须预防性使用抗生素已成为共识，但是抗生素的使用时间仍无定论。择期脾切除手术应该在术前接种疫苗。此作法推荐立即接种，即便是非手术处理的患者。有许多理论上的原因表示在脾切除术前接种疫苗将更有效果，也有研究提出术后接种肺炎链球菌疫苗更加有效。

ICU的住院时间尚无定论。大部分中心会让患者在ICU中停留24～72 h，如果病情平稳且其他损伤允许，即可转入普通病房。转入普通病房后，如果没有需要禁食的其他损伤，患者就可以经口进食了。仍须持续监测血细胞计数，但是频率可以有所减小。

最佳的住院时间尚无定论，这方面不同中心差异较大。大的多机构的研究显示，保守治疗的失败通常发生于受伤后的6～8天。留院观察的主要原因是以防出现潜在的致死性的脾撕裂影响，特别是在急救手术医疗不发达的偏远地区。本机构的方法是保证住院时间是7天，涵盖了可能发生迟发性出血的主要时间段。

对非手术处理的脾损伤患者随访的CT扫描的时间同样存在争议，大多数中心不复查CT或者复查CT的频率较低。复查CT会增加患者射线暴露的危险，特别对于儿童是个大问题。我们仅对1周后仍有腹部阳性体征和症状的患者进行研究，偶尔此类患者复查CT可发现脾假性动脉瘤，可能在初始CT上未有浓聚显示。我们不知道如果不治疗此类假性动脉瘤，患者的自然转归如何，他们可能在外观上很明显，可用动脉栓塞治疗。

应该建议患者出院后避免对抗性的体育运动，持续的时间尚不明确，但是一般会建议患者持续2~6个月。有经验证实，脾需要6~8周方可恢复正常的完整性强度，因此建议避免接触运动2~6个月似乎是合理的。

经导管栓塞治疗

对撕裂的脾的出血区域的动脉栓塞是非手术处理的重要的辅助手段。仍无指南建议动脉造影术和栓塞的时机，目前经导管动脉栓塞主要用于高级别的脾损伤和CT提示有造影剂浓聚的证据（无论损伤分级）的患者的干预。动脉栓塞的理论基础是自明的，但是尚无数据证实其有效性，而且关于栓塞治疗的报告结果差异较大。

手术处理

脾切除或其他腹部创伤手术的最佳入路是前正中入路。此入路作用多样，方便向上或向下延续。而且在干预的速度很重要时，此入路最快。对于脾损伤的手术，此入路能方便地向上延续或向左侧绕过剑突，这可方便对左上腹的暴露，特别是对于体型较大的患者和肋角较窄的患者。

正如所有的创伤性剖腹术，须快速探查、填塞腹部的4个象限，特别是一般情况不稳定的患者。初步的检查应该是非确定性地、快速地检查4个象限，并且填塞。当所有象限都被填塞后，有充足的时间寻找凝血块。凝血块通常聚集于损伤处，脱纤维的血液可能弥散于腹腔中。

一旦把重点放在左上腹，应该对左上腹所有的结构都仔细检查一遍。须对胃大弯和左侧膈进行检查。完成脾游离后，应该再一次检查左侧膈。肝左叶、左侧肾、胰尾同样需要检查。未游离脾时胰尾的检查比游离脾后更简单。

脾的游离应该是分步骤的，分步有助于提供更好的游离和更大程度地减小医源性的脾或胰腺的损伤。在保脾和脾修补的患者中，脾游离的顺序同样重要，直到脾门结扎。若患者血流动力学不稳，或合并其他危及生命的损伤，可由有经验的外科医生快速切除脾。

游离脾的第一步是切除脾的脾膈韧带、脾肾韧带和侧方连接物。此步骤应从锐性分离开始，然后是钝性分离结合锐性分离。侧方和上方的连接物须一直切除至食管处的平面上。在分离腹膜之前，用手指或血管钳预先达到潜在平面之下，然后钝性分离至潜在的平面可能有助于侧方连接的游离。在体型较大或者脾位置很靠后的患者，可能须凭感觉进行锐性分离。

完成侧方连接物的分离后，应该将脾和胰尾作为一体从侧面游离至中间。此操作更简单的方法是，将右手手指甲背部置于脾和胰腺的下面，以让他们靠近左侧肾，肾可被轻易地触及。因为，左肾很坚固，且可以指引术者正确地分离平面。此时常犯的2个错误是：其一，想单独游离脾，并没有与胰腺一起游离；其二，进入了Gerota筋膜，同时游离了左肾。这两种错误都会减少脾的活动度，并且使避免脾、胰尾、肾胰源性损伤更困难。在将脾从侧方游离至中间的时候有可能对脾门产生医源性损伤。这些问题可以靠最佳的游离程度和可见度来减少。

当脾和胰腺作为一个整体被游离至中线时，下一步是离断胃短血管。因为脾有双重供血系统，也通过胃短血管供血，分离胃短血管后并不损伤脾的活力。分离胃短血管的最佳方法是，让助手将脾和胰腺抬至术野中央，然后安全地结扎血管，从胃大弯近端开始。在胃大弯上的位置的鼻胃管，可以作为回拉胃时的把持处，从而提高胃短血管的可见度。胃短血管正如其名，长度较短，因此在钳夹胃短血管的过程中容易钳夹到少量胃壁组织。胃短血管和胃的小部分的结扎会导致部分胃组织的坏死，增加延迟性胃瘘的风险。可以通过对胃行缝合来处理这个问题。

完全游离脾的最后一步是游离脾结肠韧带连接物，它连接脾的下极和远端横结肠、结肠脾曲（图6）。在分离胃短血管和脾结肠韧带的过程中，可以通过手指压迫脾门来控制脾出血。如果患者虚弱且出血较多，可以在游离脾的最后钳夹脾门止血。大范围的钳夹仅可用于极端情况，因为可能伤及胰尾。

当脾完全游离后，可以进行仔细的检查，同时可以检查脾的后方和胰尾。在游离后填塞脾窝可控制小出血，同时有助于暴露脾和胰尾。在填塞的过程中，可以再检查左侧肾上腺和左侧膈。

如果损伤和出血皆较小，可以置入止血剂后将脾移回正常的位置。电凝难以起到良好作用。在动物模型上，氩电刀有一定作用。如果患者损伤小，一般情况不太严重，可以进行脾修补术，虽然随着

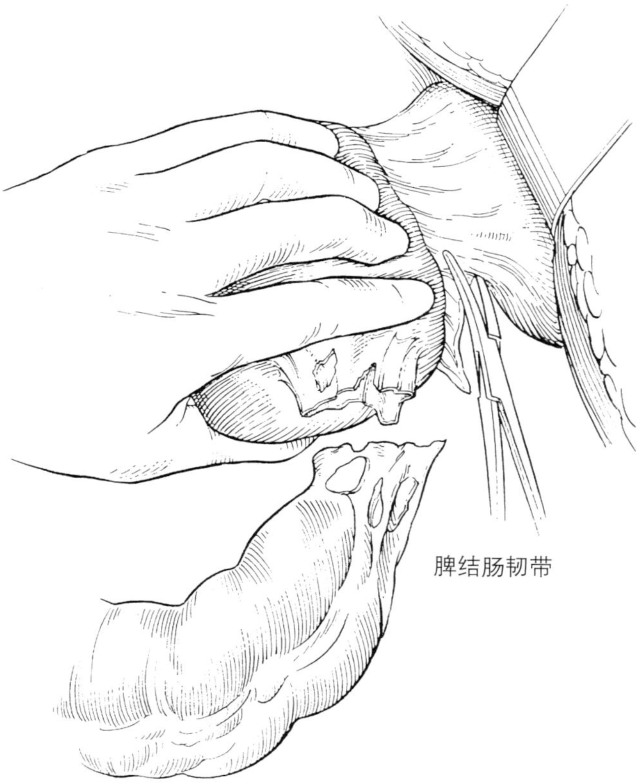

图 6 抓住脾，分离侧腹膜韧带。分离脾结肠韧带可松解脾曲（*From Khatri V, Asensio JA: Operative surgery manual, Philadelphia, 2002, Saunders, p189.*）

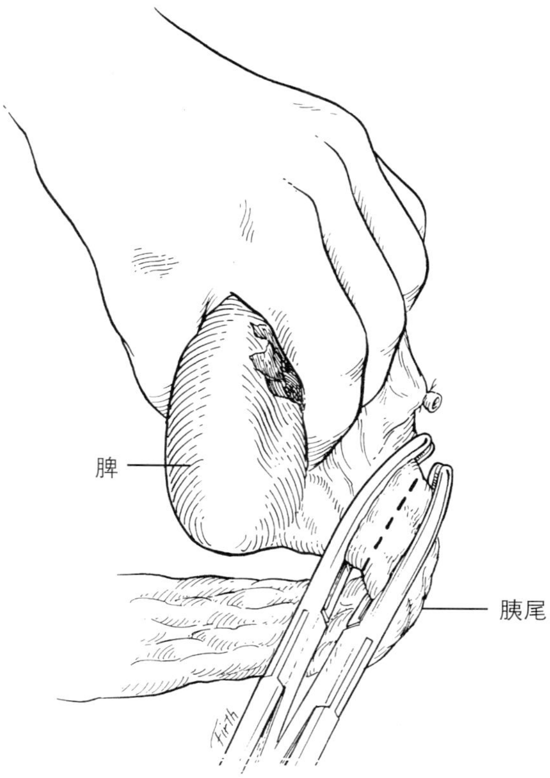

图 7 完全游离脾后，钳夹脾门血管并分离，避免损伤胰尾（*From Khatri V, Asensio JA: Operative surgery manual, Philadelphia, 2002, Saunders, p189.*）

非手术处理的发展，术中发现需要修补的脾损伤的数量在下降。其他须考虑的问题是，脾内部的损伤可能比手术观察到的更加严重。

如果决定行脾修补手术，可以缝合脾损伤，特别是在被膜完整的情况下。但是，脾不能提供很好的缝合张力，因此建议使用纱布。用可吸收的补片包裹整个或部分脾是可行的，但是此技术耗时较多。脾部分切除术同样可以，因为脾根据血供而分段，通过结扎受损区域的血管，可以在脾上看到缺血线。在切除无活力的脾的同时，可以通过对暴露脾实质缝合及包裹补片的方法止血。脾修补术的并发症发生率高于脾切除术，术中进行决定的时候应该仔细考虑这一点。此外，由于大部分脾损伤的患者都进行非手术处理，因此需要手术的患者可能更倾向于行脾切除手术。

不稳定或相关损伤严重的患者应该行脾切除手术。脾损伤分级最高（Ⅳ、Ⅴ）时，如果选择手术处理，建议行脾切除手术。脾门结构须连续分离，大血管须缝扎。

当切除脾后，须对脾床进行仔细检查。剖腹探查中，此步须分 3 步进行：从侧面到中间。在腹膜后腔时从后面到前面和脾窝。虽然此法可以探查手术视野的全部，最重要的是探查胃短血管，发现在游离过程中尚未结扎或结扎不稳的胃短血管。胃短血管的出血是术后最常见的出血原因。

脾切除和脾修补手术术后常规不放引流管，因为留置引流管可能增加并发症的发生率。只有在担心胰腺或肾损伤（术后尿瘘）时才留置引流管。

并发症发生率及其处理

保守治疗最主要的并发症是持续性出血。保守治疗失败会增加损伤程度，另外的风险是延误对其他需要手术的腹腔内脏器损伤的诊断，最常见的是肠道损伤和胰腺损伤。适合非手术治疗的患者，合并严重的相关损伤的发生率很低，只有 5%～10%，但对一位脾损伤患者做出非手术决定时一定要警惕合并小肠或胰腺损伤的可能性。在一开始漏诊的损伤初期，腹部查体尤为重要。

即便对保守治疗的患者进行了动脉导管栓塞手术，仍然有失败和并发症的风险。栓塞与并发症相关的几项研究报道，动脉栓塞的主要并发症发生率高达 20%。并发症包括脾脓肿、脾梗死、损伤漏诊。行导管栓塞后，应该警惕该患者可能有更大的可能需要手术治疗。

无论是何种干预方法，在脾切除或脾修补术后，都有出血的风险。出血的来源可能是修补后的脾实质、胃短血管、脾窝和脾门。凝血功能障碍应该被处理，如果患者一般情况不佳，尤其是脾未被切除时，术后出血通常存在。脾切除后可发生胃排空障碍，通过鼻胃管胃肠减压可能能起到良好效果。胰损伤可能是因为术中分离所致，也可能是原发性损伤。

静脉血栓栓塞并发症是创伤后通常发生的状况，脾损伤时情况更差。保守治疗或脾修补手术可能影响患者抗凝治疗和早期活动。本中心会对血细胞比容稳定 24 h 以上的患者进行抗凝治疗。脾切除可能导致血小板增多，但是并没有证据表明脾切除引起的血小板增多会增加深静脉血栓的发生率。

虽然经常提到，脾切除后凶险性脓毒症的发生很罕见。脾切除术后患者的脓毒症发生率的具体值尚无报道，但有文献估计成年人一生中的发生率是 0.026%，儿童一生中的发生率是 0.052%。肺炎链球菌和脑膜炎链球菌是最常见的病原体，预防流感嗜血杆菌同样重要。由于脾切除术后脓毒血症的发生率较低，疫苗的有效性将难以证明。然而，疫苗注射已成为脾切除的常规步骤。

死亡率

单纯的脾损伤的死亡率非常低，原因可能是患者经过仔细选择和非手术处理，以及脾切除的确切疗效好。根据包括将近 15 000 名脾损伤患者的国家数据库所示，死亡率大约是 1% ~ 3%。脾损伤的死亡损伤的风险主要在于合并其他损伤，特别是脑损伤。

结论和流程

腹部损伤并且可能合并脾损伤的患者应该按照 ABCs 的方法进行初始创伤复苏（图 8）。如果血流动力学不稳定，并且超声和 DPL 提示有腹腔内出血，须进行急诊手术探查。如果发现脾损伤，须进行脾切除手术，特别是当患者有血流动力学不稳定和合并其他损伤的时候（图 9）。

如果患者血流动力学稳定，须进行腹部 CT 扫描检查。如果有没有显示浓聚的损伤和血流动力学稳定，应该予以保守治疗。如果患者出现弥漫性腹膜炎或腹膜炎加重，或存在进行性出血现象（血细胞比容下降和血流动力学不稳定），须进行剖腹探查，并且手术治疗脾损伤（图 10）。

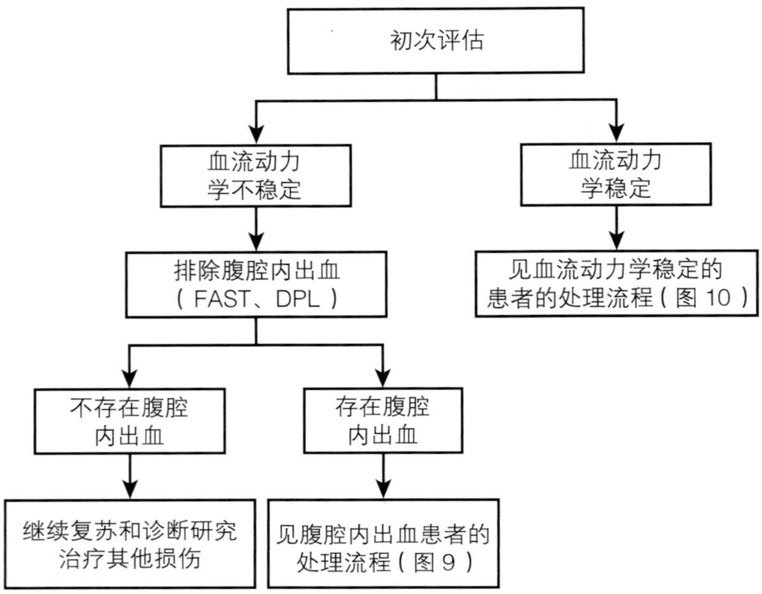

图 8 腹部损伤、怀疑脾损伤患者的首次评估流程。DPL，诊断性腹腔灌洗；FAST，创伤重点超声评估

在脾损伤患者的整个处理过程中，从急诊室的初始复苏到随后的手术或非手术处理，始终应牢记，脾损伤可大出血，如果处理不当，可以导致严重的并发症甚至死亡。

致谢

感谢 Glenn Tse 医生对本书上一版的贡献。

图 9　血流动力学不稳定的腹腔内出血患者的处理流程

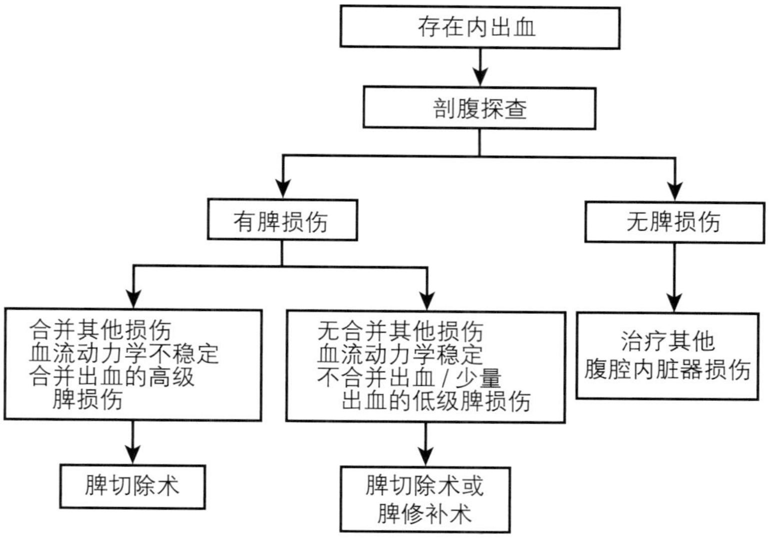

图 10　血流动力学稳定的患者的处理流程

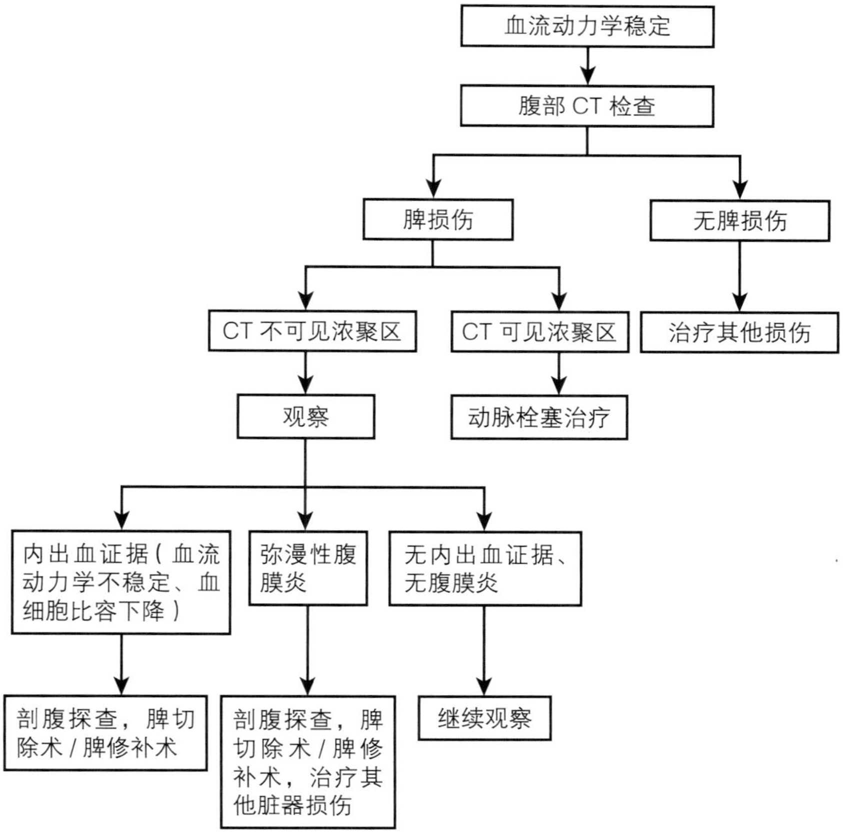

腹部血管损伤

Christopher J. Dente 和 David V. Feliciano 著
张学民 译

主要腹部血管结构的损伤称为腹部血管损伤（abdominal vascular injury，AVI）和钝性或穿通伤后明显的并发症发生率和死亡率有关。损伤可能迅速致命，涉及的血管很大，所以很重要的是要对快速显露的手术操作有全面的了解。

虽然在军事冲突中很罕见，AVI 在城市中心更多见。在 20 世纪 70 — 80 年代，AVI 在几个研究中占全部心血管损伤的 18.5%～33.8%。在当代，Feliciano、Mattox 和 Asensio 各自在 20 世纪 90 年代报告治疗了超过 300 个患者，尽管穿通性损伤减少，AVI 仍是明显的问题。AVI 在平民经验中与军队相比显著高的数量似乎反映手枪的损伤能力更弱，以及在美国大多数城市地区院前转运时间更短。而且，军用防弹衣的优点使损伤转向肢体而不是躯干，尽管在最近的文献复习中无法压迫的（躯干）出血仍是出血致死的主要原因。

病理生理学

钝性创伤

机动车事故中快速的减速或导致从大血管分出的小分支撕脱进而出血或内膜撕裂并继发血栓形成。腹部挤压伤，如被安全带勒住或从后面击打脊柱也可能导致附在其上的血管继发血栓形成。直接击打可以导致暴露血管的完全破坏，如肠系膜上动脉或系膜根部的静脉，导致腹腔内大出血，甚至肾下腹主动脉部分破裂，导致假性动脉瘤形成。

穿通伤

相比之下，穿通伤产生和肢体血管损伤同样类型的腹部血管损伤。它们包括爆炸反应与内膜瓣和继发血栓形成，侧壁缺损伴出血或搏动性血肿和完全横断伤出血或血栓。罕见地，穿通伤产生动静脉瘘，大多累及门静脉和肝动脉、肾血管或髂血管。另外，医源性损伤在许多中心还是一个老问题。

诊断

病史和体检

如前所述，AVI 可以表现为游离腹腔内出血，血肿或血管内血栓形成。因此，症状、体征表现基于涉及的血管和有无活动出血，而有所不同。来自腹主动脉大血管的活动性腹腔内出血通常导致严重失血性休克，在高级创伤生命支持过程里称为“无应答”。相反，有稳定血肿的患者，尤其是有静脉损伤的患者，可能是非常稳定的或表现为瞬时响应，或仅在手术室中血肿时失代偿。最后，主要血管结构的血栓患者会表现为血流动力学正常，但会经常有严重疼痛或下肢有脉短绌。

影像

在稳定和不稳定的患者中，快速的由外科医生做的超声着重于 FAST，对确定腹腔、胸腔或心包腔出血的存在是有用的。在稳定的腹部枪伤患者中，常规腹部平片有诊断价值，因此子弹的轨迹可以从放置在伤口上的标记或残留子弹的位置来预测。

在穿通性损伤后术前腹腔内血管造影不在证实腹腔内血管损伤时常规使用。事实上，大多数患者的这种伤口不够稳定，不能在血管造影室中做大血管的研究。在钝性伤患者中，主动脉成像用于诊断和治疗与骨折相关的深部盆腔动脉出血，用于诊断不常见的损伤，如前述的肾下主动脉、髂动脉或肾动脉内膜撕裂和血栓形成。偶尔有患者适合腔内治疗，这将在后面讨论。

随着 CT 扫描技术的进步，更多外科医生和放射学家赞成基于多排扫描和正式的 CT 血管成像得到的数据决定治疗方案。大量文献关注用 CT 诊断创伤性主动脉破裂，至少 1 个小的前瞻性研究表明 CT 血管造影对肢体创伤的诊断准确性可以接受。相反，关于使用 CT 血管造影作为诊断 AVI 的方法的数据仍然是初步的。的确，在最近的一项研究中，增强 CT 和血管造影相比，在诊断活动性出血方面有 94% 的灵敏度和 89% 的特异度。

初始治疗和复苏

在可疑腹部血管钝伤或穿通伤患者现场复苏应当仅限于基础气道，插入静脉导管用于注入晶体液成为转运到医院期间最好的措施。和腹部血管穿通损伤患者不灌注晶体液相比，没有一致的证据支持在城市环境下短暂的院前时间须积极灌注晶体液。当前损伤控制复苏的做法，支持限制晶体复苏，成为许多创伤中心的护理标准，将在后面讨论。

在急诊科，复苏的程度明显取决于患者到达时的情况。在枪伤后有板状腹的濒死患者，急诊室开胸十字钳夹降主动脉可能对维持脑和冠状动脉有帮助。创伤手术室和急诊室相距很远是该项操作的指征。不幸的是，重度的 AVI 患者在急诊室开胸后生存者很少。事实上，在 Feliciano 等的大研究序列中，59 例患者仅 1 例有孤立的腹部穿通伤者在急诊室初步开胸术后生存下来。

腹部钝伤患者，若有低血压和一个外科医生做 FAST 结果为阳性 / 腹部穿通伤和低血压 / 腹膜炎，急诊室时限少于 5 min 是强制性的。现在已经认识到，控制出血是最有效的第一步复苏，只能在手术室获得对这些潜在的致命伤害的控制。

损伤控制复苏和大量输血

最近 7 年，主要基于伊拉克的军事行动经验，许多中心的危重患者的复苏理念发生了戏剧性的变化。“损伤控制复苏”的军事复苏理念被看作 20 世纪 90 年代初由 Rotondo 等提出的“损伤控制手术”一词的概念扩展。在大多数民用中心，新鲜全血不足，损伤控制复苏的中心原则是以高频或固定频率早期、积极使用成分血（新鲜冰冻血浆和血小板）维持红细胞。在多数中心，这种做法需要血库的支持和高度组织化的大量输血协议（massive transfusion protocol，MTP）。事实上，有多个发表的研究用了机构特有的 MTP，一般伴有患者预后的明显改善。很多 AVI 患者将需要大量输血，手术医生应当熟悉他们机构存在的所有 MTP 的设计和实施。

手术

手术准备

在手术室，从颏部到膝盖的整个躯干须术前皮准备和常规铺单。防止体温过低的操作应当包括手术室加温、覆盖患者头部、用加温毯覆盖上下肢，以及在麻醉机上使用加热叶栅。

总原则

当患者到达时血压低于 70 mmHg，一些中心会进行手术室开胸十字钳夹胸降主动脉。如果心脏仍在跳动，这可能会维持脑和冠状动脉血流，并可在腹腔填塞放松时防止心搏骤停。不幸的是，它对腹腔内血管损伤的影响不大，因为腹腔内血管可以通过反流持续出血。

做腹部正中切口，用吸引器清除或移除所有血凝块和血液。快速探查是否有血肿或出血区域。如果有来自大的腹内动脉的活动性出血，可能需要从简单的手指压迫到正式的近端和远端控制的各种技术来暂时停止出血。一般说来，若要进行血管修复，则须进一步分离来充分暴露和控制受损的血管近端和远端。相反地，静脉损伤可以用一系列 Judd-Allis 钳用于穿孔边缘的有效控制，不需要常规的近端和远端控制。一旦穿通伤患者血管损伤的出血暂时控制，在血管修复期间，尽可能迅速地隔离多的胃肠道穿孔，以避免腹部的进一步污染。一旦完成了腹部的冲洗和血管修复，则须软组织覆盖修复。

相反，如果患者开腹时有腹膜后血肿，医生有时首先要在游离腹腔进行必要的胃肠修复。医生要换手套，在打开后腹膜暴露潜在 AVI 前冲洗腹腔。

与腹部血管损伤有关的血肿或出血通常发生在如前所述的 Ⅰ 区，后腹膜中线；Ⅱ 区，上外侧后腹膜；Ⅲ 区，盆腔后腹膜；右上象限肝门 - 肝后区。使用美国创伤外科协会器官损伤分级记述损伤量级，见表 1。

腹部血管按区显露

血管的大小及其位于后侧的位置使得 AVI 的手

术治疗成为创伤外科医生最困难的任务。相反，如果血管年轻或在没有动脉粥样硬化的健康人，虽然很可能血管收缩或血管相对小较细，但在血管显露后，可直接修复血管。因此创伤外科医生会对所说的每种技术非常熟悉，并在各种情况下，选择正确的手术思路。

如前所述，腹膜后分成几个区，每个区可以通过一个或多个手术步骤显露。这些适当的手法总结在表 2 和本章后面的流程图里（图 3）。

I 区，结肠系膜上区域

如果血肿或出血在这个区域，有几项技术可以在膈裂孔处控制主动脉近端。当存在一个包裹性血

表 1 腹部血管损伤评分

级 *	损伤描述	ICD-9 编码	AIS-90 评分
I	无名字的肠系膜上动脉或静脉分支	902.20/.39	无评分
	无名字的肠系膜下动脉或静脉分支	902.27/.32	无评分
	膈动脉或膈静脉	902.89	无评分
	腰动脉或腰静脉	902.89	无评分
	生殖动脉或生殖静脉	902.89	无评分
	卵巢动脉或卵巢静脉	902.81/.82	无评分
	其他须结扎的无名字的小动脉或静脉结构	902.90	无评分
Ⅱ	肝右动脉、肝左动脉或肝总动脉	902.22	3
	脾动脉或脾静脉	902.23/.34	3
	胃右动脉或胃左动脉	902.21	3
	胃十二指肠动脉	902.24	3
	肠系膜下动脉或肠系膜下静脉、肠系膜干	902.27/.32	3
	有名字的肠系膜动脉分支（如髂结肠动脉）或肠系膜静脉	902.26/.31	3
	其他须结扎或修复的有名字的腹部血管	902.89	3
Ⅲ	肠系膜上静脉、肠系膜干	902.31	3
	肾动脉或肾静脉	902.41/.42	3
	髂动脉或髂静脉	902.53/.54	3
	下腹动脉或静脉	902.51/.52	3
	腔静脉、肾下腔静脉	902.10	3
Ⅳ	肠系膜上动脉、肠系膜干	902.25	3
	腹腔干	902.24	3
	腔静脉、肾上腔静脉和肝下腔静脉	902.10	3
	主动脉、肾下主动脉	902.00	4
Ⅴ	门静脉	902.33	3
	实质外肝静脉	902.11	3（肝静脉） 5（肝 + 静脉）
	腔静脉、肝后腔静脉或肝上腔静脉	902.19	5
	肾上主动脉、膈下主动脉	902.00	4

From Moore EE, 等 : Organ injury scaling. III: chest wall, abdominal vascular, ureter, bladder, and urethra. J Trauma 33:337–339, 1992.

AIS，简明损伤分级；ICD，疾病国际分类；NS，没有评分

* 该分类体系用于实质外血管损伤。如果血管损伤在器官实质 2 cm 以内，参照特定器官损伤分级。累及超过 50% 血管周长的多个Ⅲ级或Ⅳ级损伤增加 1 级，在Ⅳ或Ⅴ级损伤时，损伤小于 25% 血管周长降 1 级

肿的时候，外科医生通常有时间翻起全部左侧腹腔内脏器，包括结肠、肾、脾、胰尾和胃底到中线（左侧内脏内侧翻转，图 1）。由于有致密的腹腔神经丛和丰富的淋巴结包绕腹腔上主动脉，通常在两点位置横断膈主动脉裂孔左脚，有助于显露裂孔上方的远侧降主动脉。可以获得额外的几厘米显露，在这一致密、有限的解剖区域内做复杂的血管修复非常重要。虽然这个操作需要几分钟，并可能对脾、肾和左侧结肠造成损害，但它允许广泛显露腹主动脉的全长。

相反，如果活动性出血来自这个区域，外科医生可能试图手工控制或用主动脉压迫设备。如果失败，替代的方法是手工分离小网膜，将胃和食管牵拉向左侧，并将主动脉裂孔的肌纤维用手指分离，以获得更快、更相似的显露。如果显露区域有限，用前述方法暴露。

这个区域的主动脉的远侧控制由于腹腔干和肠系膜上动脉的出现显得尴尬。在一些患者中，腹腔干必须分离结扎，以获得更大的空间来进行远侧主动脉钳夹，进而修补血管。胆囊坏死是可能的后遗症，通常推荐胆囊切除，尽管也可以在必要时再次剖腹手术。

表 2　腹膜后区域的手术手法

区域	手术手法
Ⅰ（结肠系膜上）	内脏左侧中线翻转 中线肾上主动脉显露
Ⅰ（结肠系膜下）	内脏右侧中线翻转 中线肾下主动脉显露
Ⅱ	肾门中线显露 肾门侧方显露
Ⅲ	中线肾下主动脉显露 右髂总静脉 / 腔静脉汇入处显露 全部盆腔游离
肝门	肝门显露 门静脉胰后显露

Ⅰ区，结肠系膜下区域

结肠系膜下区域主动脉损伤的显露通过和择期切除腹主动脉瘤时获得近端主动脉控制一样的手法实现。横结肠系膜向患者头端提起，小肠向手术台

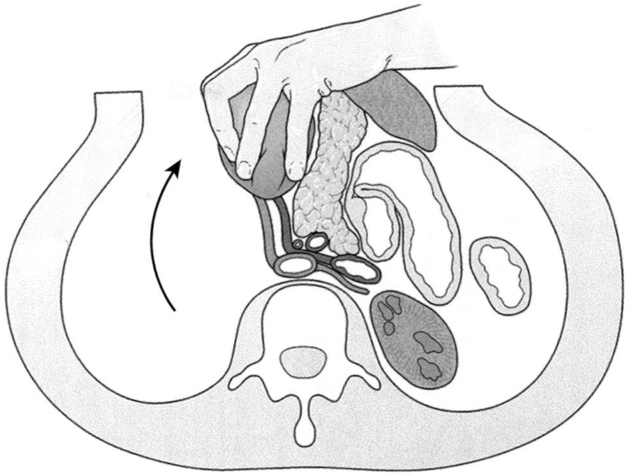

图 1　钝性和锐性结合分离提起左侧结肠、左肾、脾、胰尾和胃底，实现左侧内脏中线翻转。(*From Feliciano DV: Injuries to the great vessels of the abdomen. In Ashley SW, Cance WG, editors: ACS surgery: principles and practice, 7th ed, Canada, 2014, BC Decker, Inc, Fig.3, p.3.*)

右侧取出。打开后腹膜中线直到左肾静脉显露，可以在其下放置近端主动脉阻断钳。分离后腹膜中线到主动脉分叉，将视野显露到足以在血管下放置远侧血管阻断钳，避免损伤左侧起源的肠系膜下动脉（当显露需要时可以牺牲）。

如果主动脉是完整的或如果有活动性出血来自升结肠或结肠肝区肠系膜，可能是肾下下腔静脉或近肾下腔静脉损伤。尽管可能通过之前描述的后腹膜中线切口看到下腔静脉，更广泛地显露下腔静脉可以通过游离右侧结肠和十二指肠 C 袢、保留右肾在原位（右侧内脏向中线翻转，图 2）来实现。如此可以使全部下腔系统从髂静脉汇合部到肝下肾上腔静脉显露清楚。很难精确定义腹部大静脉哪里有破损，直到大多数疏松腹膜后脂肪组织从血管壁剥离。一旦完成剥离，出血位置可以确定，通常很容易控制。

肝下的下腔静脉有 2 个区域的近端、远端控制特别困难，一个在髂总静脉汇入部，一个在下腔静脉和肾静脉交界处。虽然海绵棒压迫髂总静脉和腔静脉可以很好地控制汇入部出血，这一区域穿通伤的显露受横向穿过其上的主动脉分叉的干扰。在显露困难的病例中，一项技术是分离并结扎右侧髂内动脉，可以向外侧和头端牵拉右侧髂总动脉以显露静脉损伤。一个替代和有意思的，但很少采用的方法是暂时分离其上的右髂总动脉，将主动脉分叉推向左侧。这个技术提供了髂总静脉汇入部和远侧腔

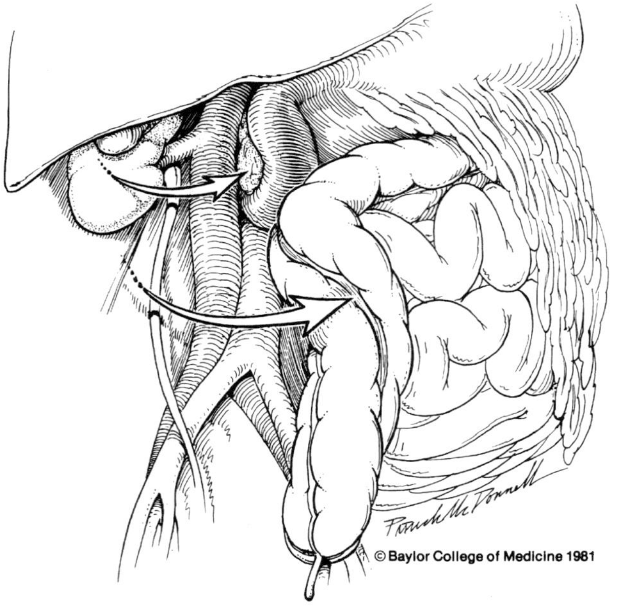

图 2 右侧脏器向中线翻转。右侧腹部脏器（除肾外）向中线翻转可以看到全部肝下下腔静脉 (*From Feliciano DV: Abdominal vascular injury. In Moore EE, Feliciano DV, Mattox KL, editors: Trauma, 5th ed, New York, 2004, McGraw-Hill, Fig.36-5, p765. Copyright 1981 Baylor College of Medicine.*)

静脉更广泛的显露。右侧髂总动脉之后再通过端端吻合重建。当穿通伤发生在肾静脉和下腔静脉结合部时，可以用海绵棒或手指直接压迫。随后一个助手钳夹或压迫肾下腔静脉和肝下腔静脉并用血管阻断带分别环绕肾静脉，再使用角度血管钳直接阻断。

Ⅱ区

如果血肿或出血在外上后腹膜，有可能使肾动脉、肾静脉和肾损伤。患者腹部穿通伤探查伤道时发现肾周血肿。如果血肿不迅速扩大，没有腹腔内游离出血，一些外科医生会在结肠系膜根部中线用血管阻断带环绕同侧肾动脉。左肾静脉也可以在此处套带；而近端右肾静脉须移开十二指肠 C 形袢、剥离肾静脉汇入处的下腔静脉才能控制。应该指出的是，肾周血肿探查前获得近端血管控制是有争议的。事实上，在一项研究中，肾门的初步血管控制对肾切除术率、输血需求或失血量没有影响。许多外科医生采用直接的方法打开损伤肾外侧的后腹膜，在伤口处用手抬起肾。用大血管钳在左中线或下腔静脉右外侧阻断肾门近端，控制远侧出血。

钝性伤患者可能表现既有肾血管损伤也有肾实质损伤。在前者，通常表现肾血管阻塞，将在后面章节讨论。若腹部钝伤患者影像学证实肾有血流，也没有其他原因急诊剖腹探查的话，就没有理由探查肾周血肿。

Ⅲ区

第 4 个主要的血肿或出血区域是盆腔后腹膜。如果穿通伤后表现为血肿或出血，可以用剖腹垫或手指或用手简单地抓住出血血管作为近端或远端血管控制。近端髂总动脉显露通过解剖游离小肠到右侧和将后腹膜中线分离到主动脉分叉处来完成。如果创伤患者年轻，通常在此处髂总动脉和静脉没有粘连，可以迅速通过血管阻断带环绕近端动脉。远侧血管控制在髂外动脉腹股沟韧带近端的出骨盆处。此区域的主要问题是髂内动脉血液回流。动脉显露可以通过进一步打开同侧盆腔后腹膜、提起近端髂总和远侧髂外动脉血管阻断带、十字钳夹或结扎分离大的下行入盆腔的髂动脉分支来实现。当双侧髂血管损伤时，整个盆腔分离技术，包括在分叉部位十字钳夹阻断主动脉和下腔静脉以及在远端十字钳夹阻断髂外血管，可以减少来自髂内血管的血液回流。

髂静脉损伤可以通过前述髂动脉损伤类似技术显露。不常须在这些血管周围穿过阻断带，因为对它们进行可以压迫。如前所述，右侧髂总静脉显露有些困难，不好到达，由此有建议暂时横断右侧髂总动脉或结扎同侧髂内动脉，以改善此处显露。

肝门

肝门血管损伤可能合并胆总管损伤，必须注意显露此区域。当有血肿出现时，切开血肿之前，近端肝十二指肠韧带须用血管阻断带或非挤压血管钳控制（Pringle 手法）。如果有出血，手指压迫出血血管就够了，直到在此处放置血管钳。Pringle 手法控制远侧胆总管和出血血管，但德克萨斯州的休斯顿的 Ben Taub 总医院的一项旧的肝损伤研究中患者只有 1 例出现胆总管狭窄。因为多数患者肝门段很短，很难在远侧放置血管钳钳夹右侧肝缘，且手压已经足够。

肝十二指肠韧带的门静脉损伤与肝动脉的损伤几乎完全隔离。静脉后方，显露这些损伤更困难。

将胆总管移向左侧，伴随扩大的 Kocher 手法，可以得到胰腺上损伤的视野良好的显露。近端伤口在肠系膜上动脉或肠系膜静脉，在罕见情况下，用非挤压肠钳或用闭合器分离胰腺颈部，显露胰腺后门静脉部。在此处显露门静脉须分离胃十二指肠动脉，做选择性胰十二指肠切除术。暴露和处理肝后和膈上下腔静脉将在本书其他阶段探讨。

根据区域的手术治疗（图 3）

如前所述，血管损伤的治疗，一旦恰当显露，就相对比较直接。作为最初修补的标准技术，端端吻合和间置移植物，外科医生应当牢记损伤控制原则——许多血管可以结扎。就像我们下面要讨论的，许多重要的有名字的腹部血管可以结扎。偶尔也须结扎主要的血管结构，在仔细考虑前不要这么做，因为这样的决定会严重使患者术后病程复杂化。

Ⅰ区，结肠系膜上区域

肾上主动脉

主动脉在此平面的小的穿通伤，最好用 3-0 或 4-0 聚丙烯线侧壁缝合。如果缝合穿孔导致严重狭窄，或如果有一部分动脉壁缺失，就要用聚四氟乙烯主动脉补片成形。另一种方法是切除损伤主动脉的一小段，尝试端端吻合。不幸的是，这经常是不可能的，因为两端主动脉在这个平面上活动度有限。许多患者同时合并肠损伤，关于在腹主动脉置入人工血管的问题已经得到了广泛的关注，而美国文献中描述这些损伤的数据并不支持对人工移植物潜在感染的关注。

肾上腹主动脉穿通性损伤的生存率报告在 1970 年代和 1980 年代平均为 35%。更近期的文献综述表明腹主动脉损伤（肾上和肾下）生存率有明显下降，至 21.1%～50%，即便排除了修复前出血和仅仅单纯

基于损伤区域的手术手法的选择

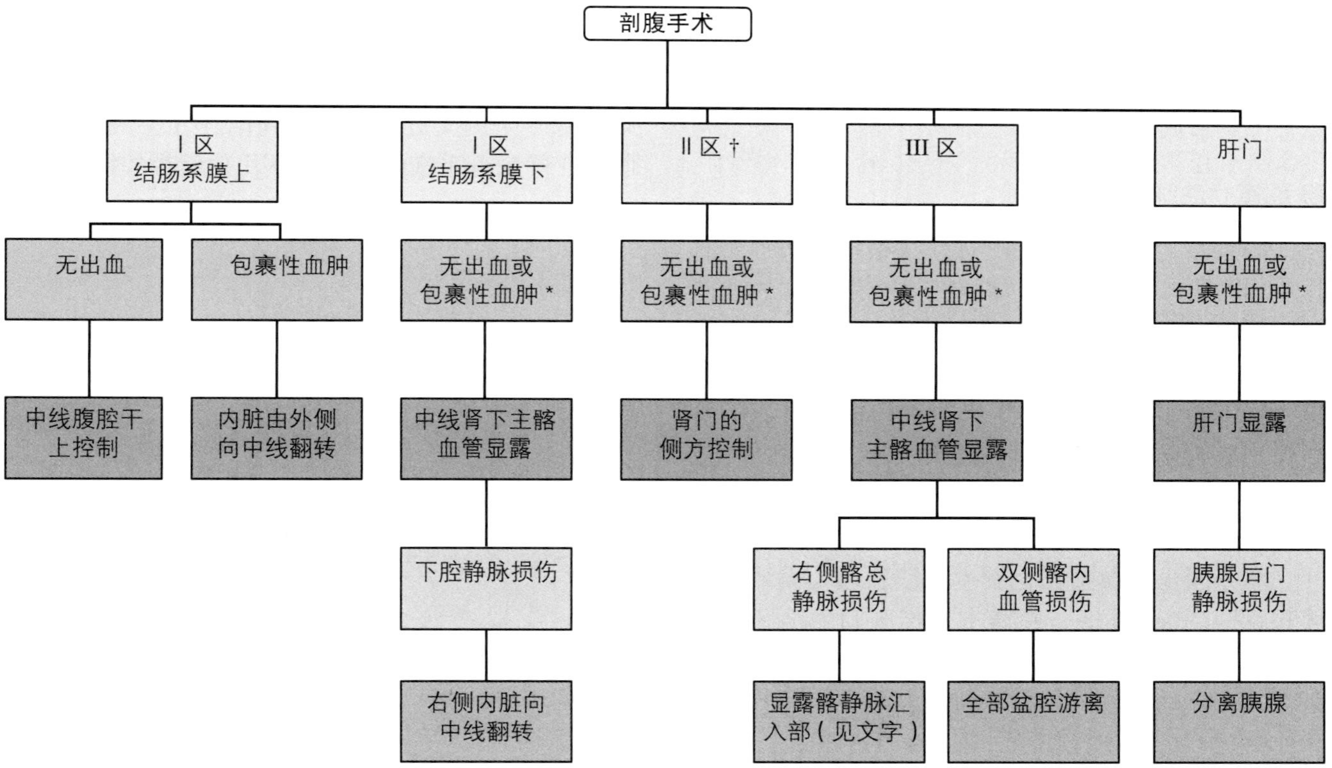

* 如果血肿是包裹性的，控制肠道污染要优于血肿探查。
† Ⅱ区：如果有包裹性血肿，要考虑肾门中线控制，但没有患者生存改善或保肾率改善（见文字）

图 3 流程图：基于损伤区域的手术方法选择

结扎的患者。文献综述中所述生存率下降的原因还不清楚，虽然可能的原因是出血患者在深度或不可逆昏迷的心肺骤停期前到达中心，这表明急诊医学服务的进步。

肾上主动脉钝伤极其罕见。尽管胸降主动脉的钝伤在创伤文献中已有详细描述，直到 1997 年 Roth 等的文献综述只有 62 个腹主动脉钝性伤病例。其中只有 1 例记录是肾上主动脉。这些损伤通常表现为主动脉血栓的症状和体征，而不是出血，治疗讨论得更广泛的是肾下主动脉损伤节段。

腹腔干

腹腔干损伤罕见。最大宗的报告来自 Asensio，记录了 13 例这种少见损伤的治疗。12 例是穿通伤，总死亡率是 62%。11 例患者结扎治疗，1 例一期修复，1 例治疗前失血而亡。更广泛的文献复习可以查到 33 例先前报告的病例，均是穿通性损伤。而且，没有幸存者是用其他复杂修复治疗的。Schreiber 等报告 1 例伤及腹腔动脉的钝性伤，而且患者之前就有正中弓状韧带综合征。鉴于这些结果，对于那些伤及腹腔干且无法进行简单动脉缝合的患者应该进行结扎，这样可以减少短期内的并发症，但不包括之前所述的胆囊坏死风险。根据前肠和中肠的侧支循环情况，腹腔干主要分支近端结扎的后遗症也可以被降到最低。

肠系膜上动脉

肠系膜上动脉的损伤处理应该根据损伤平面而定。1972 年，Fullen 医生等将肠系膜上动脉的损伤进行了解剖学分类，该分类被后来的文献作者间断使用。如果肠系膜上动脉损伤在胰腺下方（Fullen Ⅰ区），胰腺可能要在无挤压肠钳之间横断来显露出血点。因为肠系膜上动脉在此区域分支很少，一旦覆盖的胰腺被分离，近端和远端血管控制相对易于实现。

肠系膜上动脉损伤也发生在胰腺远处横结肠系膜根部（Fullen Ⅱ区，在胰十二指肠和中结肠动脉分支之间）。虽然这里有更多空间可以操作，胰腺近端和接近动脉修补部位的胰瘘风险使该区域的损伤比更近端的损伤操作更加困难。不幸的是，尽管近端肠系膜上动脉结扎在理论上可行，但血流动力学不稳定的患者的侧支循环通常不足以防止肠坏死。所以，与其在损伤控制过程中结扎，不如外科医生在肠系膜上动脉的清创端插入临时腔内转流管。如果有必要置换稳定患者的近端肠系膜上动脉，最安全的方法是在远端肾下主动脉用大隐静脉起始段或人工血管搭桥，远离胰腺和其他上腹部损伤（图 4）。这个位置的移植物应量身裁剪，以便它通过小肠系膜的后方。然后以没有显著张力的方式端侧缝合到肠系膜上动脉。要求用后腹膜脂肪或可用的带蒂大网膜覆盖动脉缝线，以避免后期主动脉十二指肠瘘或主动脉肠瘘。

更远的肠系膜上动脉损伤（Fullen Ⅲ区，在中结肠动脉分支前）和在肠道分支平面（Ⅳ区）上的损伤应当修补，因为结扎此区域是在前肠和后场侧支吻合以远。若因血管太小而无法修补结扎可能导致广泛回肠和右侧结肠切除。

无论是在 Feliciano 和 Asensio 的以前的或更新的研究中，肠系膜上动脉穿通伤患者的生存率在 55%～60% 之间。

肠系膜上静脉

另一个腹部大血管，近端肠系膜上静脉在肠系膜上动脉右侧，可能在结肠系膜根部受损。最近端的损伤接近和脾静脉的汇合部，很难显露，如前所述，胰腺颈部可能必须横断才能显露。通常，静脉可以压迫或外科医生用手指挤压同时助手用 5-0 聚丙烯缝线在穿孔边缘连续缝合。如果有后壁穿孔，此处有多条侧支进入静脉，须结扎才能翻转显露。偶尔，静脉近乎横断，两端须用血管钳控制。一个

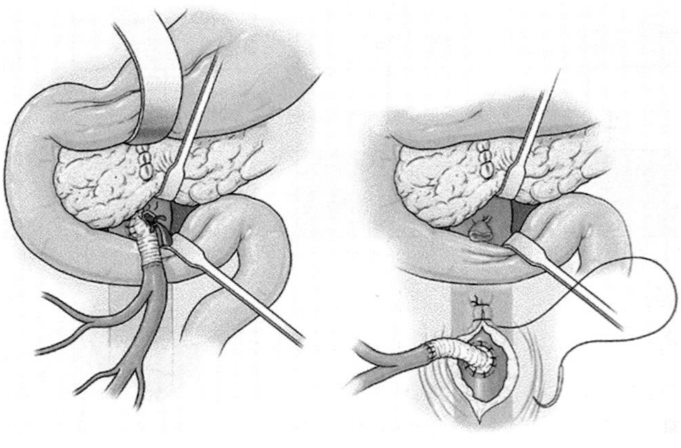

图 4 肠系膜上动脉（SMA）重建。**A**，当需要 SMA 移植手术时，近端缝合线接近胰腺损伤是危险的。**B**，近端吻合口应当在低位主动脉，远离上腹部损伤，并用后腹膜组织覆盖（*From Feliciano DV: Injuries to the great vessels of the abdomen. In Ashley SW, Cance WG, editors:* ACS surgery: principles and practice, *7th ed, Canada, 2014, BC Decker, Inc, Fig.3, p.3.*）

助手将小肠及其系膜向胰腺推，外科医生可以无张力使静脉两端接近。

当上腹部多个血管和脏器损伤和肠系膜上静脉严重损伤时，年轻创伤患者可以结扎。Stone 等强调这些患者需要积极的术后液体复苏，因为结扎肠系膜上静脉后至少 3 天后脾血容量过多，这会导致周围血管低血容量。在以往的研究中肠系膜上静脉损伤患者的生存率约为 70%，最近的研究中生存率降到 60% 以下。

Ⅰ区，结肠系膜下区域

肾下主动脉

肾上主动脉损伤、肾下腹主动脉穿通伤或钝性伤用 3-0 或 4-0 聚丙烯缝线缝合或补片成形。端端吻合或间置人工血管的方法。因为年轻患者后腹膜组织经常很薄，在关闭后腹膜前要用带蒂网膜覆盖广泛的主动脉修补处或吻合口缝线。

绝大多数的肾下主动脉损伤是穿通性质的，一小部分是钝性损伤。在前述综述的 62 例研究中中，Roth 报告在 1997 年前机动车碰撞占 57%，其中 47% 由安全带造成。患者通常表现为前述的急性动脉供血不足症状，尽管有一小部分表现为延迟的间歇性跛行、阳痿或罕见的延迟破裂。

肾下腹主动脉损伤患者的生存率在旧的研究中平均约为 45%，更近期的研究提示肾下主动脉损伤患者的生存率为 34.2%。

肝下下腔静脉

下腔静脉前壁穿孔最好用 4-0 或 5-0 聚丙烯缝线横行连续缝合。如果血管控制满意，后壁穿孔可以通过延长前壁穿孔显露，后壁穿孔可以在腔静脉内修补，第一针打结在腔外。广泛修补可以导致静脉“小时玻璃”效应，在不稳定患者会出现凝血功能障碍，不要试图进一步修补。而在稳定患者，要有理由才用肠系膜下静脉、卵巢静脉或薄壁 PTFE 补片做静脉补片。

年轻患者中的出血有必要广泛修补肾下下腔静脉，结扎该血管通常稍加注意的话耐受性好。首先，要注意的是测定大腿前隔室的压力，在第一次手术时如果压力是 30 ~ 35 mmHg，行双侧膝下四筋膜室切开。在 48 h 内双侧大腿筋膜切开可能也是必要的。患者需要大量液体复苏和调高下肢，术后早期用弹力绷带包扎。另外，当开始下床行走时，患者须穿戴医用弹力带。如果在出院时弹力带包扎下有残余水肿，患者应配全长定制弹力袜。在最近的 100 例下腔静脉损伤患者的综述中，25 例结扎，其中有 22 例损伤在肾下下腔静脉。出院生存率为 41%。9 例幸存者中对 7 例进行了 1 年随访，没人有明显的下肢水肿。虽然大多数患者似乎没有或有很轻的长期水肿，偶尔报道术后严重水肿须后期间置移植物。

下腔静脉损伤患者的生存率明显依赖于损伤位置。从 1970 年代和 1980 年代已发表文献中如果除外膈上和肝后腔静脉损伤，平均生存率大约为 75%。最近的两项研究根据部位分层，表明总生存率较低（40% ~ 60%）。最后，对下腔静脉修补后短期通畅率做了研究。28 例患者先前进行了下腔静脉侧壁缝合，记载的通畅率为 86%。

Ⅱ区

肾血管损伤：肾动脉

肾动脉是特别小的血管深埋在腹膜后。偶尔，小的穿孔可以通过侧壁动脉缝合或切除端端吻合修补。对广泛损伤，只有当有希望保留肾时，才有间置大隐静脉或 PTFE 移植物的指征。多发腹内损伤患者或术前长期缺血、术中触摸确认有正常侧支循环者，肾切除可能是个相对好的选择。在 2 个旧的研究中，肾动脉穿刺性损伤患者的生存率约为 87%，保肾者只有 30% ~ 40%。在 3 个最近的研究中，保肾者生存率为 65.1%。

肾动脉钝性损伤患者的诊断更困难。各种机制可以导致肾动脉内膜撕裂、继发血管的血栓形成，患者主诉上腹部和腰部疼痛。如果 CT 扫描显示肾动脉闭塞，外科医生必须决定是否需要外科手术或腔内介入。损伤发生的时间间隔似乎是最重要的保留受累肾的因素。其中一个研究发现在 12 h 内保留某些肾功能有 80% 的概率，到 18 h 就降到 57%。如果做手术，若受累肾动脉活动度大，则允许在腹主动脉起始处的 2 ~ 3 cm 的内膜撕裂处做有限的切除，以及端端吻合重建血管。更常见的情况，腔内技术用于肾动脉损伤后肾血管重建，将在后面讨论。

肾血管损伤：肾静脉

肾静脉比动脉大，既可以用手指直接压迫，也可以直接用血管钳钳夹控制出血。静脉侧壁缝合是最好的修补技术。如果有必要对右肾静脉进行结扎、控制出血，肾切除可以在最初手术或有必要进行损伤控制、进行再次手术时进行。然而只要肾上腺和生殖静脉完整，左肾静脉中部就可以结扎。但外科医生更倾向于修补，因为在以往的研究中结扎后有更高的概率出现术后肾并发症。既往的文献中，肾静脉穿通伤患者生存率为42%～88%，差异可能是由于相关的内脏和血管损伤数量较大。在最近的3个综述中，肾静脉穿通伤患者生存率为44.2%～70%，平均为60.4%。

肾实质损伤另外讨论。

Ⅲ区

髂总动脉、髂外动脉和髂内动脉

髂总动脉或髂外动脉损伤需要修补或临时转流，因为在低血压患者中任何一个血管结扎会导致进行性下肢缺血，需要高位截肢。相反，一侧或双侧髂内动脉可以安全结扎。

对稳定患者的髂总动脉或髂外动脉损伤的治疗方法包括动脉侧壁缝合，部分横断和端端吻合，损伤区域切除和大隐静脉插入或PTFE移植，同侧髂内动脉转移作为髂外动脉替代，如果伤在分叉处，伤口一侧的髂动脉转位到对侧髂动脉。

须注意的是当盆腔有明显的肠道或粪便污染时，复杂的髂总动脉或髂外动脉重建还是一个严重问题。在此区域内端端修补或间置移植物会发展为术后假性动脉瘤，或因初始污染导致盆腔感染继发破裂。因此，外科医生在这些区域应当考虑解剖外转流如股股血管交叉。这就须用4-0或5-0聚丙烯缝线行髂动脉残端双重结扎，然后用无损伤的后腹膜或有血管的带蒂网膜覆盖。如果外科医生直到患者在外科ICU情况稳定，才选择股股血管交叉手术，应当做同侧膝下四筋膜室切开，因为膝下缺血、水肿经常导致筋膜室综合征。

髂动脉的钝伤较少见，因其被骨性骨盆保护，位于后腹膜深部。有报告部分横断、撕脱或内膜损伤与继发血栓同骨盆骨折有关。1997年的文献，报告了10例患者有钝性血栓，少数使用一期修补，大多数用人工血管移植。只有1例需要截肢。如前述，最近研究国家创伤数据库的患者，报告骨盆骨折和髂动脉相关损伤的截肢率为7.7%。

髂动脉损伤患者的生存率依据相关的髂静脉、主动脉和下腔静脉损伤程度的不同而不同，旧文献中为45%～81%，近期文献报告45%～55%。

髂总静脉、髂外静脉和髂内静脉

髂总静脉或髂外静脉损伤用4-0或5-0聚丙烯线侧壁缝合或结扎。如果采用结扎下腔静脉后使用同样的预防措施，年轻患者中结扎的耐受性通常较好。一些中心强烈推荐修补而非结扎损伤血管。当侧壁缝合导致髂总静脉或髂外静脉明显狭窄时，为减少血栓和（或）肺栓塞风险，要进行术后抗凝。

髂静脉损伤的生存率不同，但大多数旧的文献报告超过70%，最近的文献报告的生存率大约为65%。

肝门

肝动脉

由于较短，肝动脉任何部位的损伤罕见。很少用血管插管替代受损的肝总动脉，因为大多数肝门血肿或出血的患者有显著的相关损伤如肝、右肾或下腔静脉。的确，适当的或肝总动脉的结扎似乎在年轻创伤患者耐受性好。由于有广泛的侧支循环，甚至可以在胃十二指肠起始点前结扎。由于右肝动脉或左肝动脉直径小，侧壁修复通常是困难的，后叶血管会阻塞，要经常随访。

1995年，Jurkovich发表了较大的多中心经验，记录了99例肝门损伤病例。该组中，28例患者有29个肝动脉损伤，19例随后结扎，8例存活。1例肝坏死，须清创，患者有同一肝叶的相关的广泛损伤。7例试图修补，仅1例存活，2例在治疗前出血。明显地，选择性结扎右肝动脉确保了胆囊切除术的可行性。

门静脉

如前所述，任何部位的门静脉损伤比肝动脉损伤更难处理，由于静脉的位置靠后、管壁脆、血流量大。静脉修补技术不同，但用4-0或5-0聚丙烯线静脉壁缝合是首选。偶尔成功使用的、更广泛的手法包括切除加端端吻合、间置移植物、脾静脉向下转位到肠系膜上静脉代替近端门静脉、门腔端侧分流，或从肠系膜上静脉转流到远侧门静脉或下腔静脉的静脉静脉。如此积极地尝试恢复血流是因为考虑到如果结扎门静脉，中肠的活力。然而，静脉结扎 Pachter 和 Stone 所强调的，生存率尚可。Pachter 在 1979 年的文献综述中报告，6 例门静脉结扎导致门静脉高压的患者中只有 1 例生存。1982 年 Stone 的研究中包含了 18 例门静脉结扎患者，其中有 9 例幸存。本质上，如果有广泛的损伤存在，患者需要损伤控制手术，门静脉可以结扎。外科医生要准备大量输液，以扭转继发于脾高容量的瞬间周围血管低血容量。

最近，Ivatury 等报告 14 例门静脉损伤患者，其中 3 例出血，10 例行静脉缝合（其中 6 例存活），结扎 1 例（生存）。最后，Jurkovich 报告了 56 例门静脉损伤，33 例行一期修补（死亡率 42%），1 例行复杂修补（死亡），10 例行结扎（死亡率 90%），另外 11 例患者在治疗前死亡。

肝后和膈上下腔静脉损伤在本书另外的地方讨论。

血管内介入治疗

虽然表现有活动性出血的 AVI 患者通常须立即开腹探查，一小部分表现有出血或血栓的患者可以用血管内治疗。虽然血管内移植物现在已作为破裂胸主动脉和血管栓塞的治疗被广泛接受，成为一个特别成功的非手术治疗实质器官损伤的辅助物，这些类型的介入的作用在真性 AVI 中尚不明确。事实上，描述这些灾难性损伤情况中使用血管内血管技术的文献主要由病例报告和小病例组构成，已经在其他地方做了综述。

血管内治疗在治疗肾血管损伤和骨盆骨折出血方面有着长期而确定的作用。如前所述，肾血管损伤难以手术治疗，特别当涉及肾动脉的时候。由于诊断经常某种程度的延误，肾开放手术的血管再通的功能较差，开放修补的热情已经减弱。多数作者描述了肾血管损伤的腔内处理。回到 20 世纪 80 年代，在良好肾保护的情况下进行肾动脉及其主要分支栓塞。如 Sclafani 报告 8 例肾损伤患者血管造影栓塞治疗。有趣的是，8 例中有 7 例手术成功，所有 7 例都保留了肾，1 例因持续性血尿而进行肾切除。最近的研究报告了 8 例患者的治疗，其中 7 例成功血管造影栓塞，避免了开放手术。出院时，所有幸存者肾功能正常，所有患者血压正常。这样，在血流动力学正常的患者中，经导管栓塞成功用于处理各种肾血管损伤并提供器官保护。最近几年，随着技术的改进，使用自膨式支架而非导管栓塞的方法，保留流向肾实质的血流的方法得到越来越多的关注。至少 3 例报告记录了各种支架的成功使用，避免了肾动脉损伤患者使用内膜皮瓣，保留他们的肾功能并且没有短期并发症。

2006 年发表了最大的一组非胸部血管损伤用覆膜支架治疗的文献。在这个多中心试验中，6 年用 Wallgraft 腔内覆膜支架治疗了 62 例患者。这包括 33 例髂血管损伤患者，4 例动静脉瘘患者，1 例假性动脉瘤患者和 1 例夹层患者。技术成功定义为术后完全隔绝，除 1 例外全部髂动脉损伤外技术成功，这些患者的 1 年一期通畅率为 76%。早期不良事件出现于 14% 的患者，大多是穿刺位点的并发症。后期不良事件发生在另外 6.5% 的患者中，1 例患者为全身感染，1 例患者为闭塞，3 例患者为修补处狭窄。全部患者术后早期死亡率为 6.5%，后期随诊率为 17.7%。没有支架导致的死亡。

预后

腹部血管修补后并发症和肢体一样多见，包括如血栓形成、缝线开裂和感染等问题。当血管细小、压缩时，闭塞并不少见（如肾动脉或肠系膜上动脉、侧壁动脉缝合的动脉）。这些患者，在体温、凝血功能异常和血压恢复正常后，术后 12 ~ 24 h 的二次探查是有价值的。做完这些，纠正血管血栓形成才可能成功。

腹部血管缝线开裂在 2 个部位时有发生，前面都已经讨论过。第一，如果在术后发生小的胰漏，可在胰腺损伤邻近的肠系膜上动脉内插入替代血管导管。第二，髂动脉端端吻合和导管缝线的开裂，在有明确盆腔肠或粪便污染和考虑早期解剖外旁路的患者，如果肢体有存活风险，可以通过限制修补的程度避免。

最后，腹部特有的血管并发症是术后血管、肠瘘。这个并发症最常发生于主动脉前壁修补、主动脉移植或从主动脉向肠系膜上动脉移植的患者。同样，这个问题可以通过用后腹膜组织或有活力的带蒂大网膜适当覆盖和用系膜血管做受体血管来避免。

总结

腹部血管损伤常见于腹部穿通伤患者。他们表现为腹膜后、肠系膜或门静脉血肿或活动性出血。当出现压塞的时候，在打开导致填塞的血肿之前的近端和远端血管控制是重要的。如果有活动性出血，用手指、手、压肠板或海绵条在损伤部位直接压迫出血血管是必要的，直到近端和远端血管控制住。血管修复通常用聚丙烯线缝合，可以做单纯动脉或静脉侧壁缝合和插入替代转流管，修补方法同肢体血管损伤一样多。偶尔有患者表现血流动力学正常、血栓形成后遗症或 AVI 后延迟状态，血管腔内技术能在治疗上起作用。总体而言，如果出血可以迅速控制，恢复远侧灌注，许多腹部大血管损伤患者可以挽救。

结肠和直肠损伤

David J. Ciesla 著
沈　凯 译

结肠和直肠损伤的外科处理在第二次世界大战以后经历了飞速的发展。基于战时的伤亡救护经验，当时广为接受的治疗原则是手术切除病变肠管并行末端结肠造口术。尽管认识到平民和军队的创伤治疗有所不同，平民的创伤外科医生通常会参照军队同行的治疗方式。在朝鲜战争和越南战争后的几十年里，一期修补术逐步取代了“仅行结肠造口”作为非战时的治疗理念。很多平民医学中心设立的前瞻性随机对照研究已经证实，一期修补术适合作为大多数结肠和直肠损伤患者的首选治疗。

损伤的机制和发生率

结肠和直肠损伤的机制可以分为以下几种：刺伤或枪伤等异物对结直肠管壁的直接穿通伤，钝性损伤时对肠壁造成的高压力挤压伤，由于系膜撕裂造成的肠管继发血供阻断。绝大多数的结肠损伤是由穿通伤造成的，其中火器伤约占结肠穿通伤的 75%～90%。在腹部穿通伤中，结肠的易受损程度仅次于小肠。腹部穿通伤时结肠更容易受到损伤的原因正是由于其在腹腔内的体积和分布决定的。相反，钝性结肠损伤十分少见，在腹部损伤中发生率低于 5%。常见于高速车祸时对结肠壁的爆炸性损伤或系膜撕裂。约 80% 的直肠损伤由火器伤引起，10% 由钝性损伤引起，6% 由经肛门损伤或异物插入引起，3% 由腹部刺伤引起。

诊断

结肠损伤通常可以在剖腹探查中被发现。尽管难以在术前做出特定器官的损伤诊断，但在术前的胸部平片、腹部平片或腹部 CT 检查时常出现的腹腔游离气体，也可以表现为术前肛门指诊有血迹或潜血阳性。对于任何有发热、心动过速、腹膜炎和白细胞升高的外伤患者都应怀疑肠道损伤。术前 CT 检查发现腹腔积液而没有实质脏器损伤时，通常提示应当进一步检查，例如采取诊断性腹腔灌洗检查。侧腹部穿通伤的患者没有明确的腹腔内损伤的证据时，三重对比 CT 扫描可能更有应用价值。

钝性结肠损伤通常在外伤附近的结肠壁大面积爆炸性损伤或邻近结肠的系膜的剥脱撕裂伤中分布较均匀。尽管多数的结肠穿通伤比较明显，漏诊通常由于小口径枪伤或刺伤部位难以检查，如结肠脾曲和直肠乙状结肠交界处。穿孔不明显、粪臭气味、血肿或系膜沾染都提示需进一步检查。应当充分游离可疑损伤的部位。通常须分离 1～2 支的末端系膜血管来充分评估可能潜在的系膜边缘损伤。最终诊断的手法是挤压受损肠管的近端和远端，来形成关闭的环，慢慢将肠内容物向可疑损伤处挤出。如果有粪样肠内容物或气体被挤出通常具有诊断意义，反之则可以排除结肠损伤。

所有躯干的刺伤或枪伤的患者，下腹部、臀部、会阴或大腿上部穿刺伤的患者，以及任何在肛门操作后有下腹部和盆腔疼痛的患者都应怀疑有直肠损伤。评估应当从直肠指诊开始，如果发现血迹或潜血阳性应当进行进一步检查。但是须强调的是，直肠指诊阴性不能完全排除直肠损伤。任何怀疑直肠损伤的患者都应接受硬直肠镜检查。已经通过剖腹手术控制出血的患者如果仍有血流动力学不稳定，应当临时关腹并变换体位进行直肠镜检查。触诊或直视下发现穿孔会直接证实直肠损伤。但直肠损伤常常仅表现为腔内出血或黏膜下血肿。对于这类直肠远端损伤患者，经腹腔探查并充分游离直肠并不能提高直肠损伤的确诊概率，反而可能增加血管损伤、泌尿系统损伤和神经损伤的概率。因此，这类患者应当按确诊直肠损伤的患者对待。

损伤的解剖学定位和损伤分级

结肠从回盲瓣开始一直延续到直肠乙状结肠交界处。血液通过肠系膜上动脉所属的回结肠动脉、右结肠动脉和中结肠动脉，以及肠系膜下动脉所属的左结肠动脉和乙状结肠分支动脉来供应。静脉回流通过肠系膜上静脉的静脉网和肠系膜下静脉回流至门静脉系统。直肠开始于直肠乙状结肠交界处，止于肛管的齿状线。直肠的血液由肠系膜下动脉的分支直肠上动脉和髂内动脉或阴部内动脉的直肠中动脉、直肠下动脉分支来供应。直肠的静脉与动脉连接，通过直肠上静脉回流到门静脉系统，通过直肠中静脉、直肠下静脉回流到髂内静脉。

美国创伤外科协会的器官损伤分级委员会已经制定了结直肠损伤的评分系统，可以有效地将患者按创伤程度分级，同时可以识别出哪些是容易出现术后并发症的高危患者（表 1 和表 2）。直肠损伤进一步分为腹膜内区和腹膜外区有助于外科方案的制订（图 1）。

表 1　AAST 结肠损伤分级

分级 *	类型	损伤描述
Ⅰ	血肿	挫伤或血肿，没有血供阻断
	裂伤	局部增厚，没有穿孔
Ⅱ	裂伤	裂伤＜肠周的 50%
Ⅲ	裂伤	裂伤＞肠周的 50%
Ⅳ	裂伤	结肠横断
Ⅴ	裂伤	结肠横断并部分缺失

Modified from Organ Injury Scaling Committee of the American Association of the Surgery of Trauma, Moore EE, Cogbill TH, Malangoni MA, et al: Organ injury scaling II: pancreas, doudenum, small bowel, colon and rectum. *J Trauma* 30:1427, 1990.

AAST，美国创伤外科协会

* Ⅲ级以上的多发生应上升 1 个级别

表 2　AAST 直肠损伤分级

分级 *	类型	损伤描述
Ⅰ	血肿	挫伤或血肿，没有系膜血管损伤
	裂伤	局部增厚，没有穿孔
Ⅱ	裂伤	裂伤＜肠周的 50%
Ⅲ	裂伤	裂伤＞肠周的 50%
Ⅳ	裂伤	全层裂伤延伸至腹腔
Ⅴ	系膜血管损伤	部分肠段血供阻断

Modified from Organ Injury Scaling Committee of the American Association of the Surgery of Trauma, Moore EE, Cogbill TH, Malangoni MA, et al: Organ injury scaling II: pancreas, doudenum, small bowel, colon and rectum. *J Trauma* 30:1427, 1990.

AAST，美国创伤外科协会

* Ⅲ级以上的多发伤应上升 1 个级别

外科处理

目前，结直肠损伤的处理策略是由近几十年来平民创伤中心科学地建立的，因为患者可以接受及时的急救复苏和抗生素治疗，且在损伤后很快接受了手术治疗。对于结肠损伤治疗，现在普遍认同的外科处理原则包括：一期修补和结肠造口。一期修补术即对肠管破损部位直接关闭或将病变肠管切除、一期吻合，指初始进行确定性手术，而不需要再次手术干预。结肠造口术包括近端末端结肠或回肠造

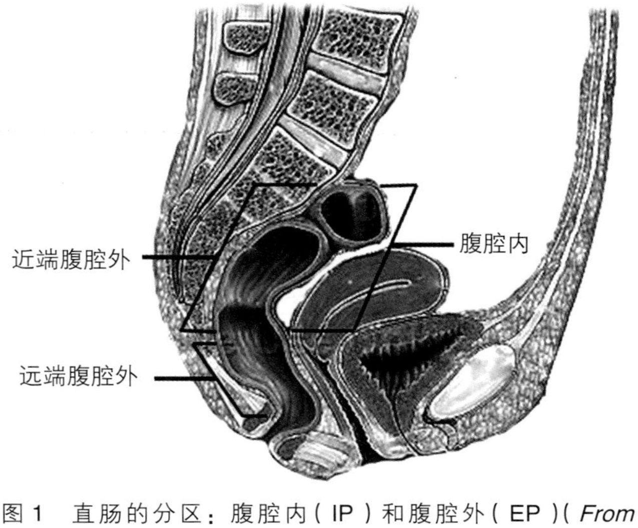

图 1　直肠的分区：腹腔内（IP）和腹腔外（EP）（*From Weinberg JA, Fabian TC, Magnotti LJ, et al: Penetrating rectal trauma: management by anatomic distinction improves outcome. J Trauma 60:508–514, 2006.*）

口伴远端黏膜瘘或远端关闭（Hartmann 手术）、直接将损伤部位肠管拖出（不进行修补）而形成的结肠袢式造口，或损伤部位缝合修补后的近端结肠转流性造口。

对于结肠损伤，大多数作者同意现在的一期修补或结肠造口的治疗策略。虽然结肠损伤的一期修补术在非军事环境中是非常理想化的治疗方案，但常常事与愿违。治疗成功的关键是根据损伤部位和程度以及患者的生理状态来选择合适的患者进行修补。例如非损毁性外伤而不需要肠段切除（AAST-OIS 分级Ⅰ至Ⅲ级），选择的治疗为一期缝合修补。清创术的目的是尽量去除污染物和缺血组织。我们通常采用单股可吸收线在结肠两端几毫米的地方开始进行横向缝合。缝合采用 Lembert 法对合浆肌层连续缝合（图 2）。或者，有些外科医生会采用双层缝合，即可吸收线缝合全层然后用不可吸收缝线 Lembert 法缝合外浆肌层。

对于损毁性结肠损伤，到底采用一期缝合修补还是结肠造口术是非常复杂的。首先须考虑的是患者的生理状态。有明显的新陈代谢损伤的患者应当首先考虑损伤控制手术。严重损伤的患者如果出现酸中毒、凝血功能障碍或低体温，常常提示很高的死亡风险。损伤控制性手术是基于患者的状态不稳定、没有充足的时间对所有的创伤进行修复的原则上。紧急状况下应优先控制出血和腹腔污染、临时关闭腹腔、送患者到外科监护病房积极复苏、纠正凝血功能障碍和复温。最便捷的控制粪便污染的方法是用胃肠道吻合器（GIA）切除病变肠管，然后用有黏性的塑料布临时关闭腹腔。然后等患者充分复苏之后，通常 24 h 之内，再行确定性手术来处理创伤。

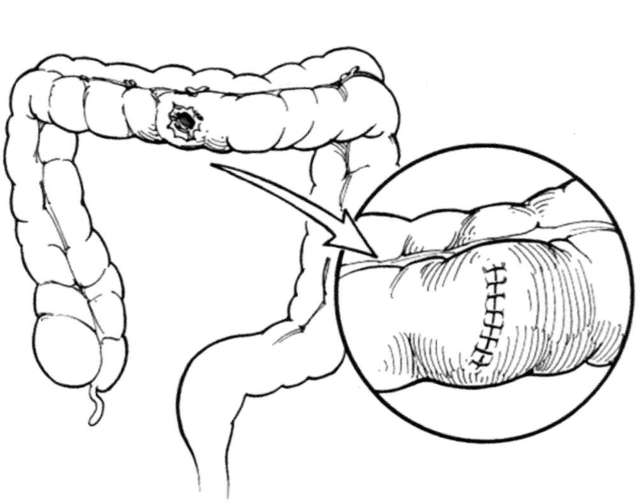

图 2 非损毁性结肠损伤通过单层连续缝合行一期修补（*Courtesy of Baylor College of Medicine.*）

一期修补手术是损毁性结肠损伤的最理想治疗方案。如果损伤部位是在结肠中动脉的近端可以行右半结肠切除并回肠结肠吻合术。紧急状况下，回肠结肠吻合术是一个可行的技术，吻合口漏的发生率很低，因此可以作为结肠中动脉近端所有结肠损伤的治疗。对于结肠中动脉远端结肠的损毁性损伤，可以采用横向的单纯缝合修补、肠段切除和结肠结肠吻合术来治疗。一些近期的回顾性研究和前瞻性随机对照研究都表明，一期修补在术后并发症方面等同或优于传统的结肠造口术。研究中指出有一些危险因素会导致缝合失败，如失血、合并实质脏器损伤、粪便污染、损伤的机制、修补时间较晚和患者年龄。另外须考量的客观评价指标是修补时肠管水肿的程度。由于大容量复苏造成的内脏水肿会使缝合的安置及张力变得不确定，进而使其愈合难以预料。因此，如果损伤发生在结肠中动脉的远端而且存在明显的肠壁水肿时，应当考虑结肠造口术。

尽管有很多种方法来进行回肠结肠吻合和结肠结肠吻合，我们更倾向于使用单股可吸收线进行端端单层缝合（图 3）。缝合开始于系膜边缘，使用两头的单股 3-0 PDS 缝线，然后在距离肠管断端 3～4 mm 的地方进针缝合肠壁近全层（不包含黏膜层）。然后两端缝线向沿肠管缝合直至在对系膜缘打结形成吻合。肠管的直径差异可以通过给小肠系膜游离部的边缘来扩大较小边缘的肠切除术。再用可吸收线连续缝合关闭系膜裂口。也可以用双层缝合技术来进行修补。

对于结肠中动脉远端的损毁性结肠损伤，如果有多种危险因素可能导致修补失败，应当进行结肠造口术。可以用线性切割吻合器（GIA）将病变肠管切除，然后在近侧断端行结肠造口。结肠造口时关键的技巧是保证造口结肠断端可以毫无张力地提到皮肤水平，以维持造口结肠断端的血供良好，保证黏膜和皮肤间的造口可以无张力地快速形成。无功能的远端结肠旷置，断端用吻合器闭合。远端结肠应用黏膜皮肤瘘管的治疗应当避免，因为其耗时、没有更多的益处、可能形成第二造口，并且增加随后结肠造口关闭的手术难度。

直肠损伤的层面决定其治疗。如前所述，直肠损伤可能仅表现为肛门镜检查时的腔内出血和黏膜下血肿。如果损伤发生在腹腔内和近端腹腔外区直肠时，如果术中评估的 AAST-OIS 分级为Ⅰ至Ⅲ时，一般不需要肠切除，一期单纯修补就可以。这类损伤通常是肠管周围组织损伤不重的撕裂伤，通过近端直肠游离容易被暴露并缝合修补。修补方法类似于前面介绍的结肠损伤修补方法，一般用 3-0 聚二恶烷酮缝线连续单层缝合。放置盆腔引流并非必须，可能增加瘘管形成的风险。如果有大片的直肠壁缺失或缺血（AAST-OIS Ⅳ和Ⅴ级），最佳治疗方案是切除受损肠管然后近端结肠末端造口。在游离远端直肠后，用 TA 吻合器在距离肛缘几厘米处来切断直肠。另外可以使随后使用圆形端端吻合器进行择期结肠造口关闭。事实证明，对于损毁性直肠损伤，这种治疗比一期修补术更加安全。

如果损伤发生在直肠远端腹膜外区域，应当行结肠造口术。应当避免进行过度的游离来明确损伤部位，因为这样会有可能损伤血管、神经、泌尿系统，甚至造成医源性直肠损伤。对于怀疑直肠损伤的患者，应当按直肠损伤来对待，而行近端粪便转流性造口术（图 4）。尽管有很多种方法来进行近端转流，关键的事项是要选择合适的手术技术来将粪便从损伤的直肠处转流。我们习惯将乙状结肠在患者的左下腹部行袢式造口，应当纵向打开肠壁、保证造口两端的肠袢的共用肠壁和运输完全高出皮面，促进造口与皮肤迅速愈合，以此来保证粪便的完全转流。这样的袢式结肠造口术就可以完全转流粪便。

骶前引流术一直被认为是直肠远端损伤治疗必不可少的部分，但有些报道对此提出了质疑。毋庸置疑的是，一些学者支持进行骶前引流术，以减少盆腔脓肿的感染性并发症，如盆腔脓毒症。在肛门后方行弧形切口，钝性游离骶前间隙直至骶骨水平。将引流管放置到接近损伤的部位而与损伤部位不相连。将引流管与皮肤用丝线缝合固定，然后通常在损伤后 4～7 天的时候拔除。

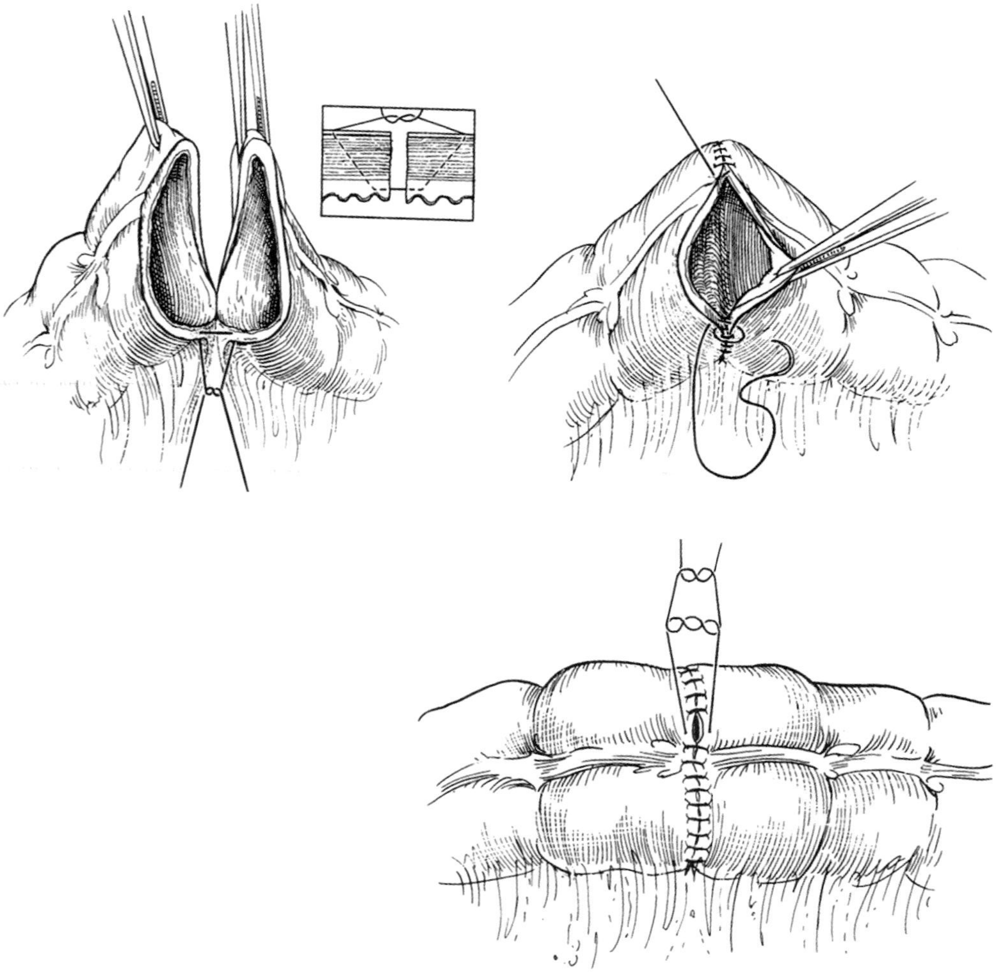

图3　损毁性结肠损伤行肠切除和一期修补术，采用单层连续缝合完成端端吻合（*Courtesy of Baylor College of Medicine.*）

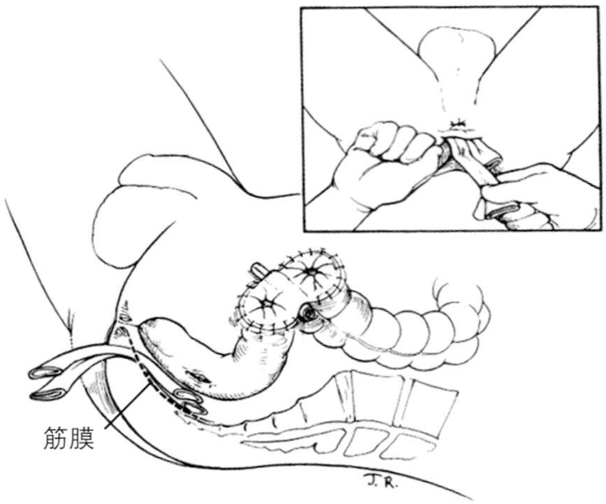

图 4　近端结肠袢式造口加骶前引流治疗直肠下段损伤（隐匿性或无法修补的损伤）(*Courtesy of Baylor College of Medicine.*)

并发症发生率和治疗

腹腔内脓肿是结肠修补术后最常见的感染性的相关并发症，发生率约 5%～15%。小于 2 cm 的小脓肿通常通过静脉内抗生素治疗而不需要引流。多数的腹腔内脓肿可以通过影像介导下的经皮穿刺进行引流。有时经皮穿刺引流会形成潜在的瘘。对于这类患者，如果患者没有明显的脓毒症，可以持续保留引流管，直至证实没有脓肿残腔后再拔除。这种情况下应当缓慢逐步地拔除引流管。对于无法通过经皮穿刺进行引流的大的腹腔内脓肿，如果患者有脓毒症的症状，应当进行手术引流。

无论采取哪种治疗方法，都可能发生缝合修补失败和粪瘘，发生率约为 1%～8%。延伸至切口的瘘经常合并有腹腔内脓肿，并且患者会有脓毒症的表现。瘘管造影可以帮助判断有无腹腔内的广泛肠漏，而腹部 CT 可以观察有无腹腔内脓肿。控制良好的瘘管可以经过非手术治疗愈合，但必须仔细检查伤口是否合并坏死性筋膜炎。已控制的瘘常需要外科干预，通常治疗方法是切除瘘管和渗漏的一段结肠，然后行末端结肠造口和近端转流。

造口相关并发症包括肠管缺血坏死、梗阻、造口周围膈膨升和皮下脓肿，发生率约为 3%～14%。多数的造口相关并发症需要手术治疗。

结直肠损伤的患者伤口感染发生率最高达 50%，但并不将其作为修补术的并发症。实际上，如果在关腹时将伤口开放可以避免伤口的感染。初次手术时也可以直接关闭伤口，仅限于损伤轻微、皮下脂肪少、污染轻，且没有经历过长时间休克的患者。

穿刺伤和枪弹损伤感染率非常高，并且当患者有全身性脓毒症时要考虑到这个可能。应当尽力取出穿过结肠并残留在软组织内的子弹以及其他异物，避免软组织感染和坏死性筋膜炎的可能。

死亡率

合并结直肠损伤的复合伤患者，早期死亡常常是由于其他损伤的严重出血所致。结肠损伤相关的晚期并发症发生率约为 1%～4%，最常见的是脓毒症和多器官功能衰竭。进行结肠造口的患者死亡率更高，但实际上结肠造口术反映了损伤的严重性，而不是治疗方法。

总结和治疗流程

尽管近些年来对于结直肠损伤的治疗有很大的变化和发展，但其治疗的核心原则并未改变。尽早发现、控制出血、控制肠内容物的播散污染是紧急抢救的重要环节，随后再进行肠道重建或粪便转流。尽管应当根据患者的损伤情况、复合伤的评估和患者的生理状态来进行个体化治疗，但仍应当总结出一套普通的方法来评估治疗预后。

基于以上考虑，我们制订了图 5 所示的流程图来指导结直肠损伤的治疗。对于结肠损伤的患者，至关重要的决策判断因素包括：生理代谢状态、是否需要肠段切除、损伤部位和修补时肠管的状态。参照这样的流程进行治疗，可以对 70%～90% 的患者进行一期修补。对于直肠损伤的患者，最重要的是能否发现损伤并进行修补。在初次手术中，直肠上段的非损毁性损伤可以进行一期修补术，但如果需要肠段切除的患者最好进行结肠造口而不是一期吻合。直肠下段的损伤由于解剖学位置的原因不容易被充分暴露和修补，因此应当进行其近端结肠转流，同时考虑是否在骶骨前方留置引流。

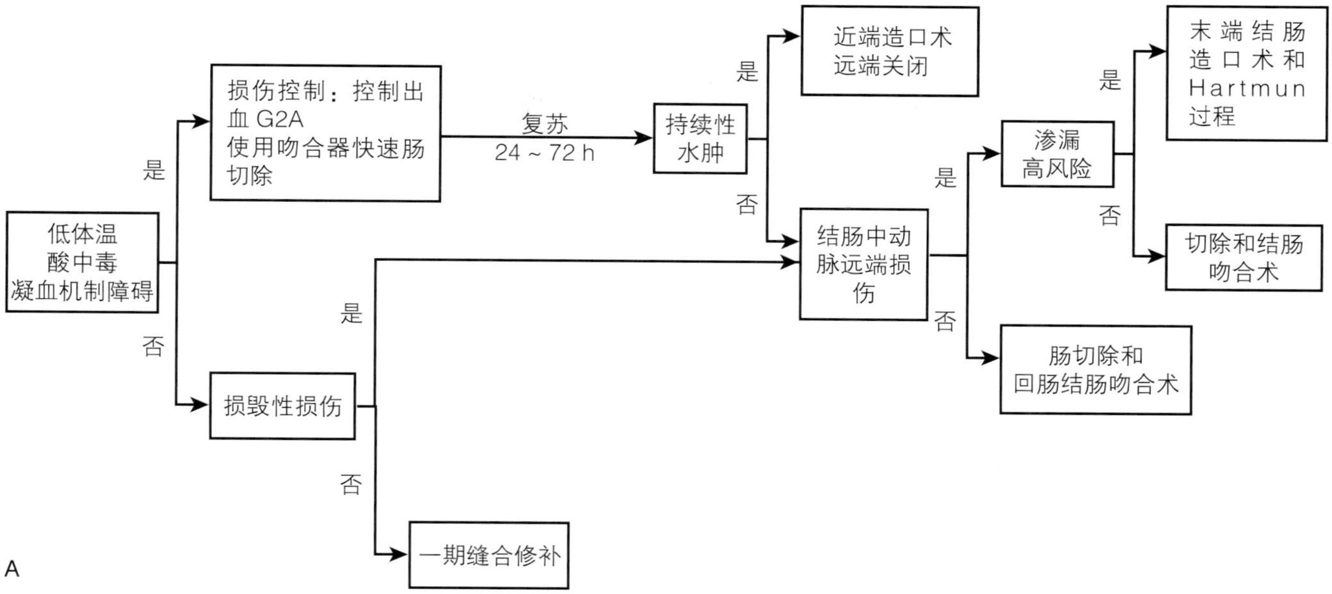

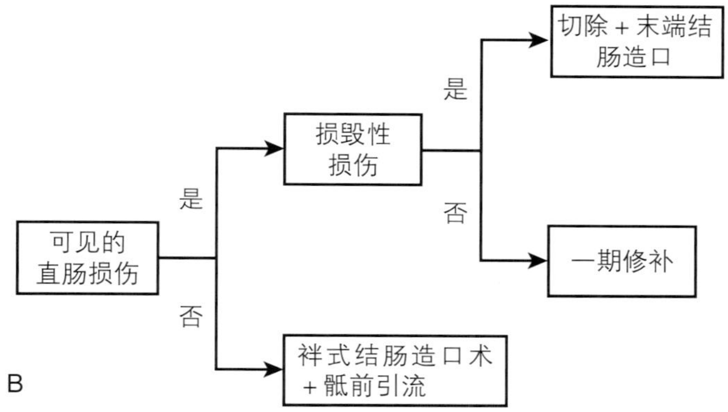

图 5　结肠损伤（**A**）和直肠损伤（**B**）的治疗流程图。ICU，重症监护病房

泌尿生殖系统损伤

Lucas R. Wiegand 和 Steven B. Brandes 著
刘士军 译

肾创伤

发病率及损伤机制

在大多数城市创伤中心，肾损伤主要为钝伤（80%～90%），少部分为穿通性损伤（10%～20%）。在所有创伤病例中，肾损伤约占 5%。由于儿童肾相对体积较大、肾周脂肪薄弱、肋骨骨化不完全等原因，更易遭受钝伤。大多数肾损伤较轻微，可自愈。仅有 4% 的钝伤和 70% 的穿通性肾损伤较为严重。

诊断

症状与体征

血尿是肾损伤的特征性表现。但血尿程度与肾损害的严重程度并不相关。约 40% 的肾蒂损伤不会出现血尿。通过病史采集，可以定量患者遭受肾损伤的暴力程度。高处坠落伤和高速机动车车祸伤预示减速损伤的可能，须对肾蒂及肾盂输尿管连接处（ureteropelvic junction，UPJ）进行评估和检查。胁部、腹部、下胸部损伤的患者，以及出现胁部瘀斑、压痛或下后肋骨骨折，或腰椎横突骨折时，应考虑是否存在肾损伤，并应行影像学检查。此外，若肾本身存在先天性畸形（如 UPJ 梗阻），可能在肾区遭受轻微创伤时即出现严重肾损伤。

对于枪伤（gunshot wounds，GSW）所致的肾损伤，鉴别损伤是由高速子弹还是低速子弹导致十分重要。高速子弹可导致广泛性肾损伤和延迟性肾坏死。子弹的入口和出口应使用不透 X 射线的标志物标记。如果刺伤（stab wound，SW）的入口在腋前线之后、乳头平面以上，则发生腹膜内器官损伤的可能性较小，一般无须行开腹探查。

影像学检查

对于可疑的肾损伤，行影像学检查的指证包括：

1. 钝伤合并肉眼血尿
2. 钝伤合并镜下血尿（每高倍镜视野下多于 5 个红细胞）及休克（收缩压 <90 mmHg）
3. 巨大加速性或减速性损伤
4. 胁部、背部、腹部穿通伤后出现镜下或肉眼血尿，或子弹路径经过肾区
5. 儿童创伤患者出现任何程度的血尿
6. 有其他部位的损伤，体征提示可能有潜在肾损伤

对于一般状况较稳定的创伤患者，静脉尿路造影（intravenous urography，IVU）可替代腹部 CT 作为肾损伤的检查手段。对于一般情况较差，需要开腹探查的患者，泌尿科医生主张在术前，特别是腹膜后（肾周）血肿探查前，行单次注射 IVU 检查。一般按每千克体重 2 ml 注射静脉造影剂，10 min 后行单次腹部摄像。单次注射 IVU 主要用于对侧肾功能的评价，以避免在手术中将孤立肾切除。临床实践中，单次注射 IVU 的图像总是“很模糊”，难以评价解读。大多数创伤外科医生则不采用单次注射 IVU 方法，而是通过触诊对侧肾是否存在或采用静脉注射甲基蓝或靛胭脂染料，并临时闭塞同侧输尿管的方法进行评价。如果 Foley 袋中出现蓝色尿液，则提示对侧肾功能尚可。

CT 一般用于评价肾实质损伤、肾周或腹膜后血肿、尿外渗、肾门及大血管损伤和其他相关腹腔内脏器损伤情况。肾动脉阻塞、肾梗死呈肾实质强化不充分表现或呈“肾皮质边缘征”表现。动脉期影像（用于评价大血管损伤）和延迟肾实质期影像（用于评价造影剂外渗）对肾损伤的准确分级十分重要。

超声检查（ulrasonography，US）评价肾损伤情况主要在欧洲使用，但价值有限。超声检查对肾周积液显像较好，但难以对新鲜血液和外渗尿液进行区分。动脉造影和超选择性栓塞是评价和治疗 CT 中造影剂“毛玻璃样”改变影像或延迟性肾出血（假性动脉瘤）的重要手段。在一些病例中，血管造影和腔内支架植入能有效控制闭合性肾损伤所致的肾动脉内膜撕裂和栓塞形成。

损伤分级

详细的泌尿生殖创伤评分请至 http://www.aast.org/library/traumatools/injuryscoringscales.aspx. 查看

处理

肾损伤的治疗流程图如图 1 所示。钝性肾损伤多采用保守治疗。只有在肾碎裂和肾蒂撕脱伤，须对积血进行清创引流时，才有手术探查指证。在 UPJ 没有完全破裂的情况下，从肾外渗的尿液多可自行恢复。选择保守治疗前，须进行影像学检查和准确分级。肾损伤的保守治疗包括严格卧床休息直至尿液变清澈、规律复查血细胞比容，对于有显著尿液外渗（表现为造影剂外渗）的患者应在 2 ~ 3 天后复查影像学检查。若患者持续出血，须重复影像学检查，行血管造影，甚至应行手术探查。恶化或有伴有临床症状的漏尿患者须放置输尿管支架。大多数穿通性肾损伤需要手术探查，因为这类损伤级别较高并常伴有重要器官损伤。大约 75% 的肾枪伤和 50% 的肾刺伤须进行手术探查。3 级和 4 级穿通性肾损伤可以观察治疗，但其中仍有 25% 须进行后续血管栓塞治疗。

手术治疗

手术探查的绝对适应证为持续性、可能危及生命的肾出血。这类出血常发生于肾碎裂伤或肾蒂撕脱伤。持续性肾出血的主要体征是出现有搏动的、持续增大的、界限不清的腹膜后血肿。手术探查的相对指证为：

1. 失活的肾实质大于 50%。
2. 尿液外渗本身并非手术指证。在多数病例中，外渗尿液通常在 72 h 内自行恢复。如果出现 UPJ 撕脱，则须快速手术修复。
3. 如果不能对损伤进行确切分级，则须做进一步影像学检查或行肾的手术探查。
4. 对于双侧肾正常的患者，对于与大出血或尿液外渗无关的肾动脉血栓，宜采用保守治疗。因为即使行血管再通也不能挽救大部分肾功能。一般在双侧肾动脉都发生闭塞或孤立肾单侧血管闭塞时考虑血管再通。
5. 当存在其他腹腔内脏器损伤须行手术探查时，可一并探查高级别肾损伤。对于高级别闭合性肾损伤，是否应手术探查尚存争议，一般应由有经验的泌尿外科医生实施手术。
6. 高级别穿通性肾损伤由于有很高的延迟出血概率，一般需要手术探查。

手术探查一般取正中经腹膜切口，以便充分暴露肾。对于 1 区血肿，应在探查肾前，先控制近端血管。否则，贸然探查肾会使肾筋膜内压塞的血液迅速流出，造成大出血，难以控制的出血增加肾切除术的风险。对于 2 区血肿，是否应持续控制肾蒂内的近端血管目前尚存争议，因为可以通过钳夹肾门或手工压迫的方法有效控制出血。控制血管后应迅速充分暴露肾和损伤区域，暂时阻塞肾血管以防大量出血，锐性切除所有失活肾组织，小心止血并缝合集合系统以防尿液渗漏，最后用丝线加强缝合缺损的肾实质。

并发症

肾损伤的并发症通常包括长期尿液外渗、延迟性出血、肾动脉假性动脉瘤、脓肿、尿瘘及肾积水。肾损伤后的肾血管性高血压通常是一过性的。在十

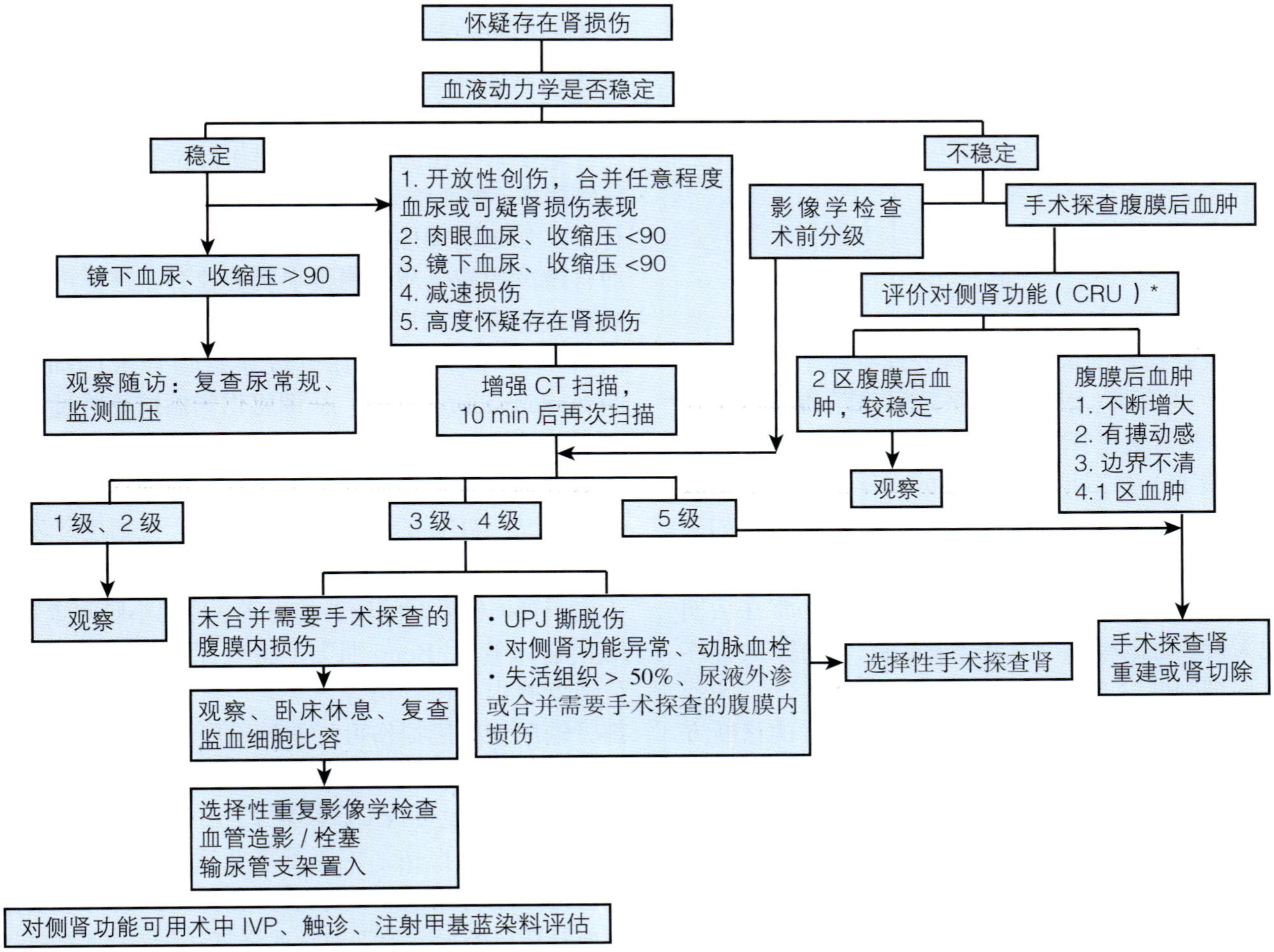

图 1 肾损伤治疗流程图。UPJ：肾盂输尿管连接处；CT：计算机断层扫描

分罕见的情况下，会出现由于包膜外血肿压迫肾实质（肾实质变薄，“纸肾”）而产生的持续性高血压。

输尿管损伤

发病率及损伤机制

外源性损伤

外源性输尿管损伤十分罕见。95% 为穿通性损伤，5% 为钝伤。输尿管邻近部位的枪伤可产生爆震效应及对输尿管造成严重钝挫伤。减速创伤使肾异位，会导致 UPJ 固定点及肾门血管撕脱。另一种损伤机制是背部过伸，由于腰椎和下胸椎的拉扯而导致输尿管撕脱。这种机制的损伤经常发生于身体柔软的儿童，他们被机动车碰撞后会出现上述的背部过伸。

医源性损伤

医源性输尿管损伤常见于复杂或出血较多的盆腔手术。盆腔手术中发生输尿管损伤的概率大约是 0.5% ~ 1%，最常发生于经腹子宫切除术，也可见于泌尿系统、结直肠（经腹会阴切除或低位前部切除）、血管手术。

诊断

症状与体征

输尿管损伤的成功的外科处理有赖于对损伤的早怀疑、早诊断（因此泌尿系统影像学检查的指征应放宽）和对输尿管解剖和血供的熟悉。血尿（包括肉眼和镜下）并不是十分可靠的指征，45% 的开放性损伤和 67% 的闭合性损伤都不会出现血尿。如果能在术中及时发现并修复，后期输尿管损伤的发生率将会大大降低。未能发现的输尿管损伤常在后期表现为持续性肠梗阻、发热 / 脓毒症、腹痛 / 胁部疼痛、白细胞减少或瘘管。

直接手术探查是对输尿管损伤最准确的诊断方法。经静脉或逆行性注射靛胭脂或甲基蓝染料，观察蓝色染料从损伤部位外渗，也有助于发现输尿管损伤。

影像学检查

单次注射 IVU 并不是诊断输尿管损伤的可靠方法，它一致性差，不推荐。逆行肾盂造影（retrograde pyelography，RPG）是判断有无输尿管损伤的准确方法，它能通过造影剂外渗观察到具体损伤部位，但操作繁琐、用时较长。RPG 不能用于紧急创伤的诊断，仅能用于一般状况较为稳定且其他影像学检查未能明确诊断的患者。一般也不单独进行，而是在输尿管支架置入的同时实施。随着尿路造影中延迟显像技术的进步，CT 能够获得造影剂在输尿管全程走行的准确图像，因此 CT 在诊断输尿管损伤中的应用越来越普遍。造影剂在肾周向内侧渗漏常提示 UPJ 集合系统损伤。

处理原则

输尿管损伤的治疗流程图如图 2 所示。治疗应考虑到患者的一般状况、是否存在其他损伤、损伤与诊断的时间间隔，以及输尿管损伤的位置和程度。对于损伤后很快就被发现并诊断的损伤，应积极行手术探查及重建。邻近部位枪伤爆震导致的输尿管钝挫伤、擦伤应尽快进行输尿管支架植入和引流。如果挫伤较为严重，应行输尿管节段性切除，应在切缘出血部位进行清创，行支架无张力再植，并与相关损伤部位分离，外接 Jackson-Pratot 引流管。

输尿管损伤的治疗也与损伤部位有关，远端输尿管损伤（髂血管分支以下）一般采用输尿管膀胱吻合术。如果远端输尿管缺损较大，可行腰肌栓系，即将游离的膀胱与同侧腰小肌腱缝合。这样可以建立远端输尿管的联系，以便下一步行输尿管再植。同时，还可以行经输尿管输尿管吻合术（transureteroureterostomy，TUU），即将伤侧输尿管跨过中线缝合至健侧输尿管的侧面。这种术式多用于合并其他损伤（直肠、盆腔、血管）或膀胱较小、顺应性差的情况。TUU 的相对禁忌证很多，包括反复发生的肾结石、上尿路移行细胞癌、对侧肾异常等。对于输尿管损伤后时间较长的患者，可用小肠间置（小肠代输尿管）、Boari 肌瓣（膀胱尿道肌瓣）、肾移位或盆腔内自体移植等方法采用进行复杂重建。大部分输尿管中段损伤可行初始输尿管输尿管吻合术（ureteroureterostomy，UU，端端吻合）。对于输尿管上 1/3 损伤，也可行 UU 修复。UPJ 撕脱伤是最常见的钝性输尿管损伤，主要见于儿童患者。UPJ 撕裂伤可采用期待疗法，但 UPJ 撕脱伤须积极行手术修复或肾造口术置入导管和延迟修复。

如果患者一般状况不稳定，不能接受长时间的输尿管重建。可暂时行“损伤控制”，即经皮输尿管造口术或在结扎输尿管后做经皮肾造口术。待患者一般状况改善后再行确定性重建。

并发症

输尿管损伤后识别时间较长是常见的。然而，即使是及时发现并修复的输尿管损伤，也会有出现严重并发症的风险。并发症包括脓毒症、脓肿、肾积水、肾功能丢失、输尿管狭窄、瘘管，以及尿性囊肿。

膀胱创伤

发病率及损伤机制

大部分膀胱损伤的原因是腹部钝性创伤，如机动车事故伤或挤压伤。90% 的外源性膀胱损伤会合并骨盆骨折，10%～15% 的骨盆骨折会合并膀胱破

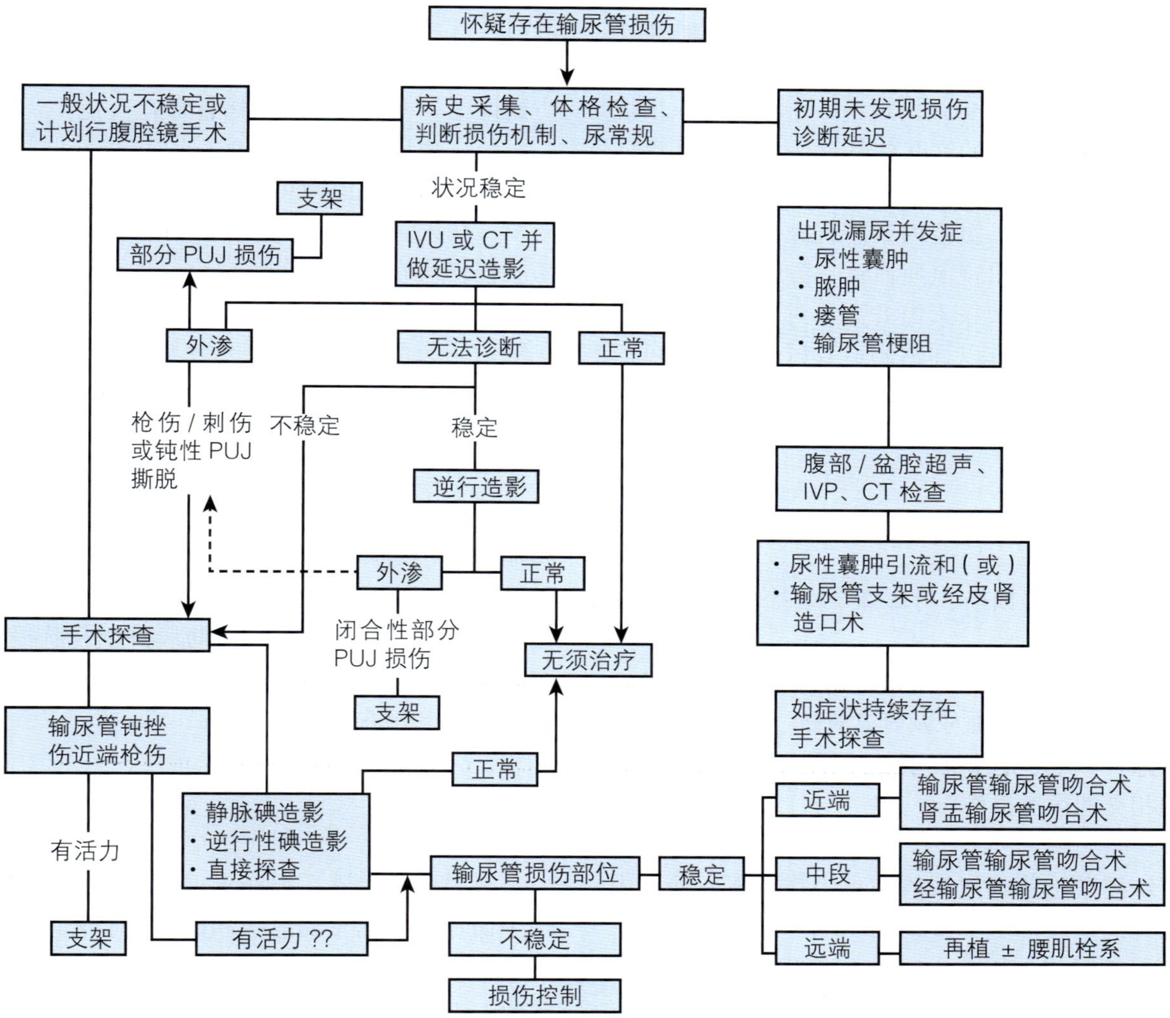

图 2　输尿管损伤治疗流程图

Algorithm for ureteral trauma. Abd, 腹部；CT, 计算机断层扫描；Extrav, 外渗；GSW, 枪伤；Inj, 损伤；IVP, 静脉肾盂造影；IVU, 静脉尿路造影；PCN, 经皮肾造口术；PE, 体格检查；PUJ, 肾盂输尿管连接处；SW, 刺伤；Sx, 体征和症状；TUU, 经输尿管输尿管吻合术；Tx, 治疗；UA, 尿液分析；UP, 肾盂输尿管吻合术；US, 超声；UU, 输尿管输尿管吻合术 (*Modified from Brandes SB, Coburn M, Armenakas N, et al: Consensus on genitourinary trauma, diagnosis and management of ureteric injury: an evidence-based approach.* BJU Int *94:277–289, 2004*.)

裂。60% 的膀胱破裂为腹膜外型，30% 为腹膜内型，10% 为混合型。医源性膀胱损伤常见于盆腔手术，如经腹子宫切除术。

腹膜内型膀胱破裂多为严重的钝性下腹部或盆腔创伤导致膀胱扩张或充盈。破裂多发生在膀胱顶部。空虚的膀胱很少发生损伤。因为存在相关损伤，所以该病的死亡率很高。腹膜外型膀胱损伤几乎与骨盆骨折共同存在。损伤主要由剪切力所致，但在极少数情况下也会出现破裂的骨质刺破膀胱。

诊断

症状与体征

几乎所有的闭合性膀胱破裂都会出现肉眼血尿（95%～100%），余下的 5% 也会出现镜下血尿。穿通性膀胱损伤大约有 50% 出现镜下血尿，50% 出现肉眼血尿。膀胱损伤的症状包括盆腔或下腹部疼痛与排尿无力。膀胱破裂的体征包括耻骨上压痛、尿量减少和肉眼血尿。腹膜内型膀胱破裂如未能及时诊断，可能在后期出现氮质血症、酸中毒、高钠血症、高钾血症和血清尿素氮升高。对女性患者，还应做详细的盆腔检查以评估阴道及尿道撕裂的可能性。如果术中怀疑膀胱损伤，可通过尿管逆向注入甲基蓝染料染色的生理盐水，观察是否有蓝色染料漏入腹部。

影像学检查

对于可疑的肾损伤，行影像学检查的指征包括：

1. FAST 提示存在盆腔游离液
2. 钝性损伤：肉眼血尿及骨盆骨折
3. 穿通性损伤：任何程度的血尿或出现任何与膀胱相交的通道损伤

传统膀胱造影通过尿管在重力作用下向膀胱内灌注稀释的造影剂至少 300 ml 或直至在荧光透视下可见造影剂外渗。因为此方法可能漏诊 10%～15% 的病例，因此须再灌注后引流时拍摄平片。膀胱造影中膀胱损伤可分为膀胱挫伤、间质破裂、腹膜内型破裂（造影剂能显示出肠管轮廓或能够充盈盲管）、腹膜外型破裂（造影剂以火焰或星爆炸状外渗）和盆腔血肿（造影剂呈泪滴状）。CT 膀胱造影也是一种可选的当前经常在医院使用的影像学检查形式。可在 CT 中看到向膀胱逆行灌注至少 300 ml 造影剂及造影剂外渗的全过程。这种检查方式具有与传统膀胱造影相同的准确性，同时具有不用在后续引流过程总再次拍摄平片的优势。

处理

膀胱损伤的治疗流程图如图 3 所示。对于钝性腹膜内型损伤，膀胱多在顶部发生损伤，损伤可达数厘米之长。这种损伤难以仅靠尿管持续引流尿液自愈，须用可吸收线进行开放缝合修复。一般推荐两层缝合。对于穿通性膀胱损伤，也须进行手术探查，因为可能存在其他腹部脏器损伤或输尿管、膀胱三角区损伤。子弹所致的膀胱损伤必须进行探查，并对碎片或失活组织进行清创，用可吸收线进行缝合。膀胱修复后，应长期留置尿管引流尿液。在极少数情况下可于耻骨上置管引流。

与之相反的是，大多数钝性腹膜外型膀胱损伤仅靠留置尿管引流即可处理，无须进行探查和缝合修复。在尿管充分引流尿液的情况下，接近 90% 的膀胱损伤可在 2 周内自行愈合。如果探查是否存在其他腹部脏器损伤，应同时修复腹膜外型膀胱损伤。一般使用腹部正中切口以充分暴露膀胱，一般在膀胱顶部打开以避开盆腔血肿。如果开放了盆腔血肿，可能会造成细菌感染，还会造成填塞的血液释放引发大出血。探查中应注意检查膀胱颈及输尿管开口是否存在损伤，如果发生输尿管开口处损伤可能需要输尿管再植。膀胱颈损伤须进行手术修复，如果未修复可能在日后发生压力性尿失禁。由骨折碎片或相关直肠、阴道损伤导致腹膜外型膀胱损伤由于存在严重出血 / 血凝块，仅靠尿管引流膀胱尿液无法自愈，也须进行修复。

并发症

腹膜内型膀胱后损伤延迟诊断可能导致患者出现生命危险。迟发的症状和诊断会显著增加本病的死亡率。本病的并发症包括代谢性酸中毒、肠梗阻、腹痛 / 盆腔痛、脓毒症，也可能出现腹膜炎。

尿道创伤

尿道损伤相对而言并不常见。通常分为前尿道损伤和后尿道损伤。后尿道损伤多由骨盆骨折造成，前尿道损伤多由骑跨伤所致。穿通性尿道损伤多为枪伤所致的前尿道损伤。尿道损伤的治疗目标是减少尿失禁、阳痿、尿道狭窄等使人虚弱的并发症的出现。

后尿道损伤

发病率及损伤机制

约 3.5% ~ 15% 骨盆骨折会合并后尿道损伤，完全性尿道损伤约占 73%，部分性尿道损伤约占 27%。固定的前列腺和游离的膀胱间的剪切力导致了膀胱颈损伤，固定的尿道膜部和游离的尿道球部间的剪切力导致了尿道膜部的损伤。与男性不同，女性尿道和膀胱颈的损伤主要是由碎裂的骨片所致。

诊断

症状与体征

后尿道断裂的症状包括排尿无力、下腹部肿胀和血尿。男性尿道损伤的体征包括尿道口渗血（灵敏度 98%）、肉眼血尿、会阴部瘀斑 / 血肿、阴囊或阴茎血肿、插入尿管困难、膀胱扩张和排尿无力、前列腺高浮。当骨盆骨折的女性患者出现阴道流血和撕裂、血尿、阴唇肿胀或排尿无力等表现时应高度怀疑尿道损伤。

影像学检查

在骨盆平片中，如果出现骨盆环断裂、双侧耻骨支骨折或垂直剪切骨折，则提示可能存在尿道损伤。逆行尿道造影（retrograde urethrographyRUG）可用于评估尿道损伤。经尿道灌注少量（20 ~ 30 ml）造影剂并在荧光透视下检查。RUG 也可用来对尿道损伤进行分级。尿道生殖隔将盆腔和会阴分隔，是重要的标志。

处理

尿道损伤的治疗目标是保存排尿功能和勃起功能，避免出现盆腔血肿。尽管之前存在争议，但一般认为阳痿、尿失禁等并发症仅与损伤本身相关，与处理方法无关。最传统的治疗方法为耻骨上置管尿道转流，二期手术处理尿道闭塞。重建中断尿道的主要方法是放置尿道膀胱导管，为一期重新排列。当患者一般情况稳定后即可进行此项操作，或待骨科修复骨盆骨折几天后再行操作。如果能在膀胱镜及荧光透视配合下置入尿管，后续手术修复将会十分简单，须行开放手术重建尿道的比例将降到 50%。

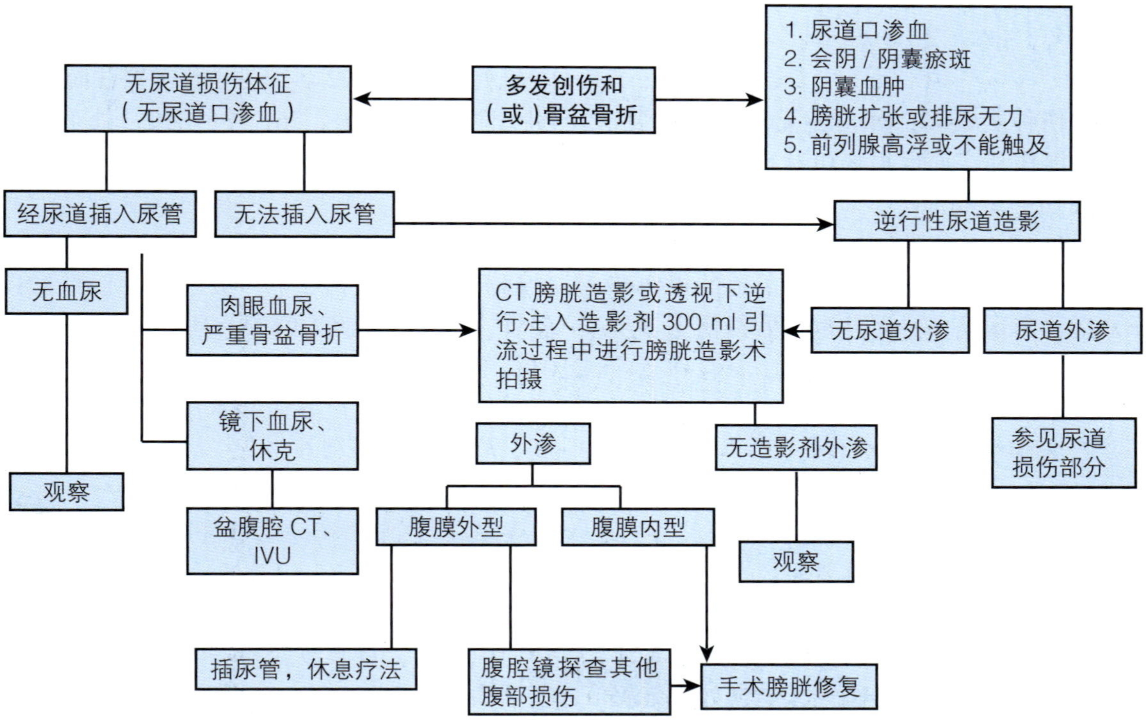

图 3 膀胱损伤治疗流程图 *(Modified from Brandes SB: Trauma to the genitourinary tract. In Rakel RE, Bope ET, editors:* Conn's current therapy, *57th ed. Philadelphia, 2005, Saunders.)*

对于尿道不完全撕裂者，仅靠尿管留置引流尿液即可自愈。

前尿道损伤

发病率及损伤机制

钝性前尿道损伤多是因为阴茎和尿道直接遭受损伤，合并其他损伤少，死亡率相对较低。穿通性尿道损伤中，18% ~ 57% 是阴茎枪伤，50% 是会阴部枪伤。

诊断

症状与体征

前尿道损伤的症状包括血尿、排尿无力。当患者报告直接会阴部创伤或骑跨伤病史，穿通性阴茎、会阴部创伤（如枪伤）病史，出现尿道口出血（最重要的预测因素）、阴囊或阴茎肿胀 / 瘀斑或压痛（即"蝴蝶样"血肿）、阴茎袖样血肿、排尿无力等体征时，有可能为前尿道损伤。

处理

不完全的钝性损伤一般行尿道转流 2 ~ 3 周即可成功处理。完全钝性挤压伤应行耻骨上置管，不宜做一期重新排列和立即修复。随后尿道狭窄发生率较高，须在延期开放性手术时进行修复。对于刺伤和低速枪伤所致的尿道损伤，主要采用一期吻合尿道成形术进行修复。如果尿道缺损广泛，需先行造袋及尿液转移，后期再做重建。

并发症

诊断和治疗的延迟会导致生殖器脓肿形成、脓毒症和筋膜炎。长期并发症包括尿道狭窄、阴茎弯曲、阴茎缩短、勃起功能障碍和尿失禁。

妇产科损伤：妊娠期及非妊娠期子宫和女性生殖器损伤

Patrizio Petrone 和 Areti Tillou 著
候弘毅　王志启 译

妇产科损伤种类繁多，相对少见且有挑战性，主要包括钝性损伤和穿通性损伤机制。机动车事故是导致孕妇损伤的主要原因，而几乎所有输卵管、卵巢、非妊娠期子宫损伤都是由于穿通性损伤所致。骨盆骨折和骑跨伤往往会导致会阴、阴道的损伤和一小部分子宫、宫颈损伤。而外生殖器损伤更多与人为暴力有关，因此在此情况下应治疗。

妊娠期损伤

创伤是孕妇妊娠期死亡的首要原因，同时也是导致胎儿死亡的最主要原因。女性在 10 ~ 50 岁之间均具有生育能力，因此女性患者受到创伤后一定要考虑其是否处于妊娠期。所有医务人员在处理妊娠期创伤患者时，一定要认识到并理解妊娠所带来的女性生理和解剖学上的变化（表 1）。

发生率

有研究发现，近 50% 的孕妇死亡与创伤有关。6% ~ 7% 孕妇孕期受到过创伤，0.4% 的患者需要住院治疗。1995 年，Weiss 报道了为期一年的流行病学研究，在 16 722 名因为创伤需要住院治疗的育龄期女性中筛查妊娠，761 名（4.6%）处于妊娠期。孕期受创伤的数量是被低估的，尤其是因家庭暴力所导致的创伤。

2011 年，Petrone 等进行了一项为期 155 个月的研究，研究包括 2 个一级创伤中心的 321 名孕期患者，其中 291 例（91%）是由于钝性损伤，30 例（9%）是穿通伤。这项研究的结论之一是由于腹部穿通伤，胎儿死亡率和母体并发症发生率依旧非常高，分别是 73% 和 66%。

损伤机制

交通事故是孕期发生创伤的最常见原因。随着孕期的进展，重心改变和身体灵活度下降可能导致跌倒和意外损伤的发生。其他常见原因有机动车行人碰撞和火器伤。22 ~ 25 岁的年轻孕妇妊娠期发生创伤的风险更高。

表 1　妊娠期母体生理变化

生理改变	结果
心排血量和血容量增加	失血量 >40% 后休克
血液稀释	生理性贫血
动脉压和静脉压下降	生命体征不反应血流动力学状态
脉搏增加	解剖
乳房增大	胸部手术（如胸廓造口术置管）中应注意解剖学标志的改变
膈升高	
胸骨下角增大	
功能残气量减少	呼吸暂停或气道阻塞时 Po_2 迅速下降
耗氧量增加	
仰卧位时气道关闭	
潮气量和每分通气量增加	Pco_2 和碳酸氢盐下降
麻醉剂需求减少	须调整镇静剂量
胃动力下降	误吸风险
胃食管括约肌松弛	

年轻孕妇遭受殴打的风险也更高。据报道10% ~ 30% 女性在孕期遭受过虐待，5% 因此造成胎儿死亡。在受伤的怀孕患者中，17% 受到过故意创伤，其中 60% 长期遭受家庭暴力。躯体遭受虐待时损伤部位往往是身体近端和中线部位，如颈部、胸部、面部、上肢和大腿侧部，而非远端，也有一些少见的损伤如香烟烧伤和咬伤。

诊断

要注意监护母亲和胎儿。子宫血供与母体血压直接相关，同时缺乏自我调节机制，因此，与非妊娠期创伤患者的救治重点相同，对胎儿的最佳治疗就是对母体进行有效复苏。全面的查体和影像学检查对发现孕妇的特殊情况十分重要，例如子宫钝性损伤和穿通性损伤、胎盘早剥、羊水栓塞、同种免疫反应、胎膜早破。

院前抢救

由于母体的生理变化，应及时给予吸氧，以防在运输和抢救中发生母体和胎儿缺氧。即使没有低血容量和休克体征，也要进行补液治疗。为了避免子宫压迫下腔静脉所造成的仰卧位低血压，在转运妊娠第二、三期孕妇时应使其左侧倾斜，同时要注意颈椎的固定。如果孕妇处于仰卧位，应使右侧髋关节抬高 4 ~ 6 in（10.16 ~ 15.24 cm），同时向左侧手推子宫。这种方法可以使心排血量增加 30%，从而恢复循环血量。虽然只有 10% 的孕妇在仰卧位时会出现休克症状，但是当母体血压正常时也有可能出现胎儿窘迫，因此包括在手术过程中，均应持续抬高右髋。

院内抢救

首先应评估气道、呼吸和循环情况，包括补充血容量和控制出血。然后询问产科病史、体格检查、评估和监测胎儿宫内情况。病史询问应包括末次月经、预产期、此次妊娠和既往妊娠的异常情况，例如早产、胎盘早剥。妊娠期高血压、妊娠期糖尿病等共存情况也应记录。

腹部检查十分重要，子宫的大小（图 1）可以帮助我们判断妊娠周数和胎儿成熟度。妊娠周数与子宫大小不符提示子宫出血或子宫破裂。当出现腹膜刺激征、由于子宫外的位置导致的腹部触及胎体、触及不到宫底时应怀疑子宫破裂。同时，由于妊娠期增大的子宫使肠管向上及两侧移位，使腹膜伸展，使腹部体检不可靠。

胎龄的测定非常重要，将指导对早产的处理。大多数医疗机构可以接受 24 ~ 26 周的早产，胎儿生存率为 20% ~ 70%。影像学评估胎龄的误差在 1 ~ 2 周。除非受孕日期十分确切，胎龄并不容易确定。可根据手测宫底高度判断胎龄。母婴状况评估流程见图 2。

对孕妇的身体评估必须针对孕妇的以下 6 个妊娠相关急性情况检测：

- 阴道出血：提示宫颈过早扩张、早产、胎盘早剥和前置胎盘的先兆。轻微创伤后胎盘早剥的发生率在 2% ~ 4%，重大创伤后发生率上升至 50%。发生胎盘早剥后母亲死亡率不足 1%，但胎儿死亡率为 20% ~ 35%。
- 胎膜破裂：除了使感染风险增加，还可导致脐带脱垂，造成脐动脉、脐静脉受压。
- 会阴肿胀：这通常是受胎儿先露压迫所致。
- 存在子宫收缩和其类型：对子宫肌层直接和间接损伤会导致花生四烯酸的释放，引起子宫收缩。虽然大部分宫缩会自行消失，但仍要做好

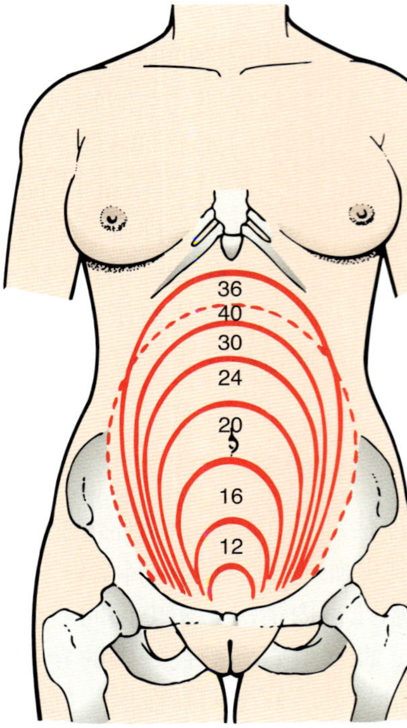

图 1 不同孕周子宫的位置和大小（*Modified from Wilson SF, editor: Assessment of the pregnant client, Health assessment for nursing practice, ed 4, Mosby, 2009; Original credit Seidel et al, 2006.*）

早产的准备。

- 胎心率和心率异常：是胎儿出现平衡主要异常的最早征象。在创伤复苏期，应听胎心或行持续的胎心外电子监护（electronic fetal heart rate monitoring，EFM）来进行胎儿评估。妊娠 24 周及以上的存活胎儿在创伤后须行监护。在抢救室就应开始行至少 4 h 胎心监护。当出现宫缩过频（每小时大于 6 次）、腹部或子宫压痛、胎膜破裂、阴道出血或低血压时，应胎心监护至少持续 24 h。
- 胎母输血综合征：8%～30% 的孕妇受到创伤后会出现胎母输血综合征，即胎儿血液通过胎盘进入相对分开的母体血循环中。创伤程度和胎龄与胎儿出血的速度和量无关。KB 试验可用于检测创伤后母体血循环中的胎儿红细胞，通过计数胎儿红细胞与母体红细胞的比例，可以计算出胎儿进入母体循环的血量。胎母输血综合征的并发症有母体 RH 血型致敏作用、胎儿贫血、胎儿阵发性房性心动过速、因失血导致死胎。当胎儿失血量小于 5 ml 时，低于典型的实验室 KB 试验的灵敏度水平，但却能使 Rh 阴性血型母体致敏。因此所有有腹部外伤史的 Rh 阴性血型孕妇应在创伤后 72 h 内预防性给予 300-μg Rh 免疫球蛋白（抗 D 免疫球蛋白，RhoGAM）。母体血循环中每发现 30 ml 胎儿血须给予 300-μg Rh 免疫球蛋白。只有 3.1% 的重大创伤病例须多次给予 300-μg Rh 免疫球蛋白治疗。妊娠 16 周前不须做 KB 试验，因为胎儿血容量小于 30 ml。

影像学检查

妊娠期胎儿受到辐射损伤分为 3 个时期。在妊娠 3 周以前射线暴露，无论是在胚胎植入前或在早期植入时，都会导致流产。妊娠 3～16 周是器官形成期，射线可能造成胎儿神经管形成的损伤，导致中枢神经系统发育异常。妊娠 16 周以后，神经功能缺失是射线暴露最常见的并发症。产前射线暴露也可能与某些幼年时期的恶性肿瘤有关。

尽管妊娠期射线暴露的危害得到普遍关注，但在大多数情况下妊娠期行射线检查是利大于弊的。一般认为，胎儿暴露的射线剂量小于 5～10 rad 并不会明显增加胎儿先天畸形、宫内发育迟缓和流产的风险。常用的影像学检查的辐射剂量见表 2。对于非妊娠期妇女，也要实施必要的 X 线检查（图 3），同时也应避免不必要的重复检查。

表 2 X 线平片和 CT 的辐射剂量

前后胸部 X 线平片	<0.005 rad
盆腔 X 线片	<0.4 rad
头颅 CT 扫描（1 cm 断层）	0.05 rad
上腹部 CT 扫描（20 1 cm 断层）	3.0 rad
下腹部 CT 扫描（10 1 cm 断层）	3.0~9.0 rad.

CT：计算机断层扫描

腹部评估

妊娠期患者的腹部检查是具有一定难度的。受到扩大的子宫的影响，腹腔内脏器上移，使得腹腔内器官的解剖学结构发生改变（图 4）。尤其要注意患者因药物、酒精或脑损伤引起的肋骨骨盆骨折、不明原因低血压、血液丢失、血尿或感觉中枢改变等症状。

针对创伤患者的 FAST 对于腹部情况判断具有

图 2　母婴状况早期评估流程。ABC，气道、呼吸、循环；C-section，剖宫产；DPL，诊断性腹腔灌洗；OB，产科；US，超声（*Modified from Knudson MM, Rozycki GS, Paquin MM: Reproductive system trauma. In Moore EE, Feliciano DV, Mattox KL, editors:* Trauma, *5th ed, New York, 2004, McGraw-Hill, pp 851–875.*）

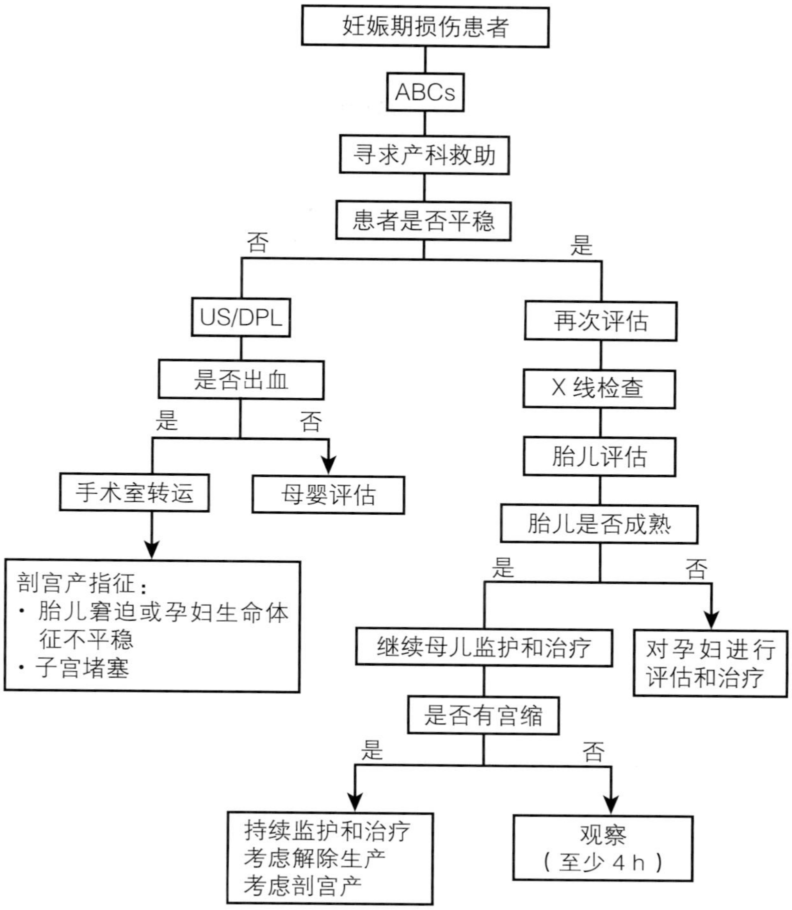

重要意义，因为它能快速检查母体腹腔、心包情况和胎儿状况。在血流动力学正常的患者中，CT 对母体和胎儿的评估是安全的。行 CT 检查时，应按需给予口服或静脉注射造影剂。诊断性腹腔灌洗的不足是其为有创操作，穿刺部位应使用位于脐上的开放技术。

AAST 对妊娠子宫的损伤分级如表 3 所示。

手术治疗

钝性损伤

血流动力学稳定的孕妇实质脏器损伤时可采取非手术治疗，相反，血流动力学不稳定或者存在肠损伤的孕妇要尽快手术治疗，因为低血压或者感染对胎儿是有害的甚至是致死性的。

对于孕妇来说骨盆骨折是最为严重的一种钝性创伤。因腹膜后静脉扩张，会造成大量出血和致死

表 3　AAST 对妊娠期子宫的器官损伤分级

分级	损伤情况	AIS–90 评分
Ⅰ	无胎盘早剥的血肿或挫伤	2
Ⅱ	浅表性撕裂深度 <1 cm 或部分胎盘剥离 <25%	3
Ⅲ	孕中期撕裂深度 1 cm 或胎盘剥离面积为 25%~50%；孕期第二期深度撕裂	3~4
Ⅳ	撕裂延展至子宫动脉、撕裂深度达 1 cm，合并胎盘剥离面积 50%	4
Ⅴ	孕期第二和第三期子宫破裂、完全性胎盘剥离	4~5

Modified from Moore EE, Jurkovich GJ, Knudson MM, et al: Organ injury scaling VI: extrahepatic biliary, esophagus, stomach, vulva, vagina, uterus (non-pregnant), uterus (pregnant), fallopian tube, and ovary. J Trauma 39:1069–1070, 1995.

AAST-OIS，美国创伤外科协会器官损伤分级；AIS，简明损伤分级

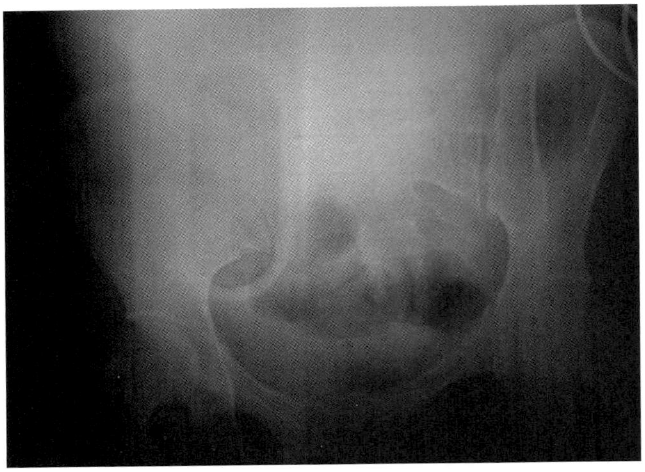

图 3 一位妊娠期钝性损伤患者骨盆 X 线片：可见胎儿脊柱及其他部分

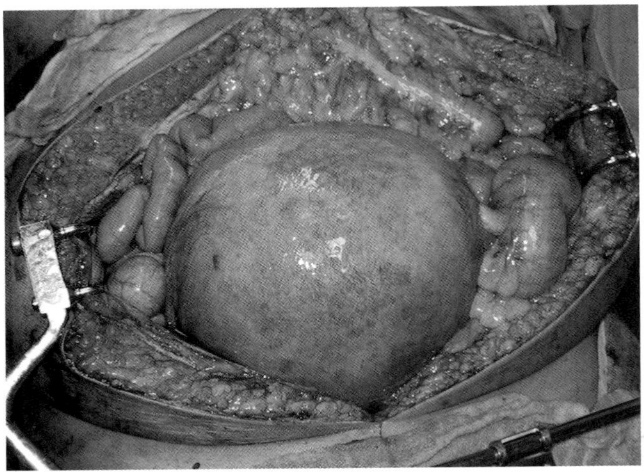

图 4 孕妇遭机动车碰撞后剖腹探查可见：妊娠子宫取代内脏

性的出血性休克。孕妇骨盆骨折时胎儿死亡率接近 25%，是引起胎儿死亡的最常见原因。对于非妊娠期患者，血管栓塞是治疗骨盆出血的常规方法，但是治疗过程中的放射剂量对于孕妇来说却是过量的。

腹壁、子宫肌层和羊水可在受到钝性创伤时起到缓冲作用。胎盘早剥可引起胎儿缺氧、早产、出血，是引起胎儿死亡的最常见原因，临床表现有腹痛、阴道出血、子宫压痛和宫缩。胎盘早剥最严重的并发症是弥散性血管内凝血，主要是由胎盘促凝血酶原激酶进入母体血液循环引起的。

穿通性创伤

子宫在盆腔内逐渐增大，更容易受到穿通性损伤。子宫肌层可以吸收速度较慢的穿通性损伤的能量，但是当上腹部受到损伤时往往会引起孕妇较严重的创伤，这可能引起孕妇死亡。枪伤引起的胎儿损伤占穿通性创伤的 60% ~ 70%，其中胎儿死亡率为 40% ~ 65%。如果子弹穿透子宫而胎儿尚且存活，应行剖宫产（表 4）。

若母亲死亡，胎儿尚且存活（24 ~ 26 周），应行围死亡期剖宫产。时间是至关重要的，因为在产妇死亡的 5 min 或更短的时间内完成分娩，胎儿存活的概率相对较高。随着时间的增加，胎儿存活的可能性逐渐减小。在极少情况下，孕妇脑死亡但生命体征仍平稳，可在至胎儿成熟后终止妊娠（图 5）。

表 4 穿通性创伤的剖宫产指征

孕产妇休克
任何原因的威胁生命的大量出血
孕产妇损伤无法修复
子宫严重损伤
存活的胎儿产生胎儿窘迫
胸腰椎不稳定损伤
妊娠近足月
孕产妇死亡

对创伤患者行急诊剖宫产手术时，相较常用的横切口，贯穿全层、直达子宫的纵切口更为安全、迅速。纵切口从两侧进入子宫可以避免对子宫血管造成损伤。

妊娠 24 ~ 32 周，在进行紧急剖宫产前，无主动脉十字钳夹的开胸心肺复苏是十分重要的。如果开胸心肺复苏成功，则分娩就有可能后延，那么胎儿出生后成活率就会得到提高。创伤后实施紧急剖宫产抢救流程见图 6。

发病和死亡率

在美国创伤已经成为引起孕妇死亡的最常见原因。旧的报道将 80% 的孕妇死亡的主要原因归结于羊水栓塞所导致肺的血栓栓塞。感染、出血、高血压和血栓栓塞造成的孕妇死亡率逐渐下降，而创伤导致的孕妇意外死亡率逐渐升高。虽然因腹部枪伤所造成的孕妇死亡率在 7% 左右，但是由此造成的胎儿死亡率高达 73%，孕妇总体并发症发生率为 66%。与胎儿不良结局相关的危险因素见表 5。

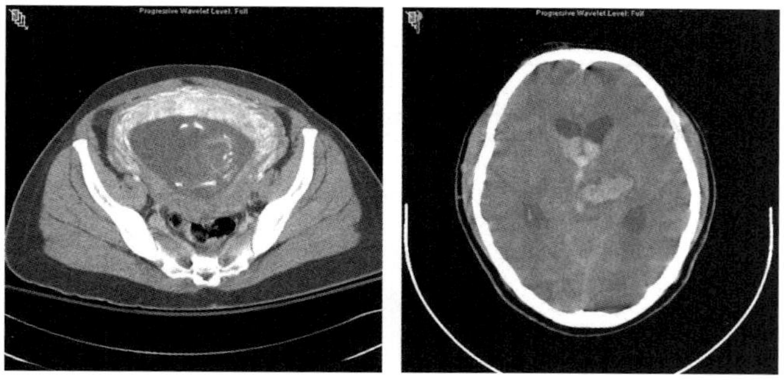

图 5 一个妊娠 18 周的孕妇颅内出血脑死亡（右图）。胎儿已经死亡，患者家属同意器官捐献

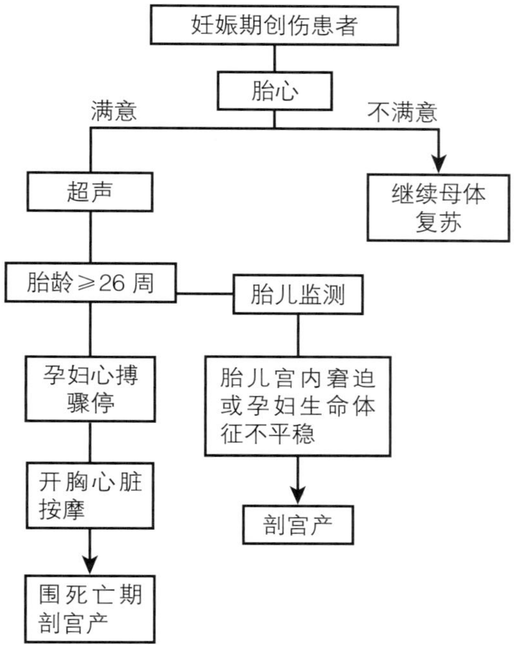

图 6 创伤后紧急剖宫产处理流程（*Modified from Morris JA Jr, Rosenbower TJ, Jurkovich GJ, et al: Infant survival after cesarean section for trauma.* Ann Surg *223:481–488, 1996.*）

表 5 胎儿结局预测

孕妇死亡
孕妇低血压
孕妇创伤性脑损伤
损伤严重度评分（ISS）高
骨盆骨折
交通事故中孕妇从车辆内甩出
孕妇严重腹部损伤

结论

创伤已经成为年龄在 34 岁以下的女性和孕妇死亡的主要原因。育龄期女性创伤患者的评估一定要考虑其是否处于妊娠期。妊娠期特有的病理生理改变影响创伤性损伤，其需要更为仔细和谨慎的处理。

非妊娠期女性生殖器损伤

在非妊娠期女性患者中生殖器损伤并不常见，更多见于内生殖器的病理性增大和产后早期的损伤。错过治疗时机或者治疗不恰当会导致出血、脓毒症、内分泌紊乱和生育能力受损。

发病率

关于女性生殖器损伤只有一些个案报道或数量少的样本，其发病率尚不可得知。骨盆骨折所导致的阴道裂伤发生率大约 3.5%。尿道和膀胱损伤也相对常见。

损伤机制

与骨盆骨折相关的女性生殖器钝性损伤最为常见。骑跨伤和意外的穿通性损伤会导致外生殖器损伤。滑水、体操、骑自行车意外被报道过会引起外生殖器的钝性损伤。尽管有报道过子宫和卵巢钝性创伤，但一般情况下内生殖器的损伤均是穿通性创伤。

妊娠期和非妊娠期女性的外生殖器损伤大多是由暴力损伤引起的，尤其当损伤原因不明时，暴力损伤可能要考虑在内。如果发生性侵犯，进行病情评估时一定要得到患者的知情同意。

在两性关系中，家庭暴力的绝大多数受害者是女性，跨越种族、年龄、国籍、性取向、宗教和社会经济地位。通常，家庭暴力是经常性发生的而非一次性事件。医务人员在治疗创伤患者时应识别出是否存在家庭暴力的可能，将患者转至合适的机构，并提供一定的社会支持。

诊断

首先应对创伤患者进行初步的评估和复苏。其次应对患者进行仔细的会阴部体格检查。对于有严重疼痛或活动性出血的患者，可能须在麻醉下进行体检。一个完整的检查应包括双合诊、阴道窥镜检查和肛门直肠检查。有人建议麻醉下进行会阴部创伤检查评估损伤程度。

盆腔内生殖器损伤通常需要剖腹探查。在非妊娠期患者中，钝性损伤更常见于内生殖器的病理性增大，腹部 CT 和 DPL 可以帮助诊断，但后者不常用。妇科损伤的详细分级见表 6-10。

表 6 AAST 对妇科损伤的器官损伤分级：阴道

分级	损伤情况	AIS-90 评分
Ⅰ	钝挫伤或血肿	1
Ⅱ	累及黏膜的浅表裂伤	1
Ⅲ	累及黏膜下脂肪或肌层的深度裂伤	2
Ⅲ	累及宫颈或会阴的复杂裂伤	3
Ⅴ	损伤邻近器官	3

Modified from Moore EE, Jurkovich GJ, Knudson MM, et al: Organ injury scaling VI: extrahepatic biliary, esophagus, stomach, vulva, vagina, uterus (non-pregnant), uterus (pregnant), fallopian tube, and ovary. J Trauma 39:1069–1070, 1995.
AAST-OIS，美国创伤外科协会器官损伤分级；
AIS，简明损伤分级

表 7 AAST 对妇科损伤的器官损伤分级：外阴

分级	损伤情况	AIS-90 评分
Ⅰ	血肿或钝挫伤	1
Ⅱ	仅累及皮肤的浅表裂伤	1
Ⅲ	累及皮下脂肪或肌层的深度裂伤	2
Ⅲ	皮肤、脂肪或肌肉撕脱伤	3
Ⅴ	损伤邻近器官	3

Modified from Moore EE, Jurkovich GJ, Knudson MM, et al: Organ injury scaling VI: extrahepatic biliary, esophagus, stomach, vulva, vagina, uterus (non-pregnant), uterus (pregnant), fallopian tube, and ovary. J Trauma 39:1069–1070, 1995.
AAST-OIS，美国创伤外科协会器官损伤分级；
AIS，简明损伤分级

表 8 AAST 对妇科损伤的器官损伤分级：非妊娠期子宫

分级	损伤情况	AIS-90 评分
Ⅰ	血肿或钝挫伤	2
Ⅱ	浅表裂伤深度 <1 cm	2
Ⅲ	裂伤深度达 1 cm	3
Ⅲ	裂伤延展至子宫动脉	3
Ⅴ	子宫血供阻断或撕脱	3

Modified from Moore EE, Jurkovich GJ, Knudson MM, et al: Organ injury scaling VI: extrahepatic biliary, esophagus, stomach, vulva, vagina, uterus (non-pregnant), uterus (pregnant), fallopian tube, and ovary. J Trauma 39:1069–1070, 1995.
AAST-OIS，美国创伤外科协会器官损伤分级；
AIS，简明损伤分级

表 9 AAST 对妇科损伤的器官损伤分级：输卵管

分级	损伤情况	AIS-90 评分
Ⅰ	血肿或钝挫伤	2
Ⅱ	裂伤 <50% 周长	2
Ⅲ	裂伤达 50% 周长	2
Ⅲ	完全横断	2
Ⅴ	有血供阻断的节段	2

Modified from Moore EE, Jurkovich GJ, Knudson MM, et al: Organ injury scaling VI: extrahepatic biliary, esophagus, stomach, vulva, vagina, uterus (non-pregnant), uterus (pregnant), fallopian tube, and ovary. J Trauma 39:1069–1070, 1995.
AAST-OIS，美国创伤外科协会器官损伤分级；
AIS，简明损伤分级

表 10 AAST 对妇科损伤的器官损伤分级：卵巢

分级	损伤情况	AIS-90 评分
Ⅰ	钝挫伤或血肿	1
Ⅱ	浅表裂伤深度 <0.5 cm	2
Ⅲ	裂伤深度达 0.5 cm	3
Ⅲ	部分无血液供应	3
Ⅴ	完全性实质破裂或撕脱	3

Modified from Moore EE, Jurkovich GJ, Knudson MM, et al: Organ injury scaling VI: extrahepatic biliary, esophagus, stomach, vulva, vagina, uterus (non-pregnant), uterus (pregnant), fallopian tube, and ovary. J Trauma 39:1069–1070, 1995.
AAST-OIS，美国创伤外科协会器官损伤分级；
AIS，简明损伤分级

手术处理

单纯的会阴裂伤在修补前应行有效的冲洗和清创，可引流或不引流。对于较大的会阴血肿应行切开引流，以防止感染和脓毒症发生的高风险。外阴裂伤应用可吸收线缝合。

由于血供丰富，阴道和宫颈裂伤的处理相对较困难。可吸收线常用于黏膜层和黏膜下层的缝合。对于骨盆骨折患者，应快速诊断出这些损伤，任何处理的延误都有可能导致脓毒症甚至死亡。

子宫损伤缝合用缓慢吸收线行双层连续或间断“8”字缝合。因创伤行子宫切除术是十分罕见的，仅用于损伤极其严重或有活动性出血的情况下。输卵管和卵巢损伤根据严重程度行修复或切除手术。常常使用阴道填塞抗生素 24 h。

并发症发生率和死亡率

并发症发病率与相关损伤有关。会阴、阴道、宫颈和子宫的大量出血可导致失血性休克，这些出血往往难以控制。忽略与骨盆骨折同时发生的会阴损伤可能是致命的。远期并发症有性功能障碍和不孕不育。

结论

非妊娠期女性子宫等生殖器官损伤比较少见，常见于暴力行为受害者和直接会阴创伤、骨盆骨折、盆腔穿通伤患者。在手术室进行全面查体、迅速的外科治疗可以改善某些潜在的致命性损伤结局。

骨盆骨折的多学科治疗：手术和非手术处理

Thomas M. Scalea 和 Deborah M. Stein 著
周　靖 译

很少有损伤能够像多发伤和骨盆骨折那样复杂。骨盆是一个复杂的解剖区域。骨性骨盆对所容纳的结构起着很重要的保护作用。骨盆中容纳着胃肠道、泌尿生殖道、血管和神经结构。使骨盆骨折的外力是非常大的。因此，每个骨盆骨折都应该被认为是一种高能量损伤。骨盆因邻接腹部，所以出现复合伤较为常见。骨盆骨折患者通常也伴有其他合并伤。超过 50% 的患者合并创伤性脑损伤或相关的长骨骨折。

伴有骨盆骨折的多发伤患者的最佳治疗方案也许是真正的多学科治疗的最佳实例。这一点对于血流动力学不稳定患者尤其适用。在处理这些患者的过程中，急诊内科医生、创伤外科医生、骨科医生、泌尿科医生和介入放射科医生都起着关键作用。治疗选择的多样性依然存在。每一个患者的正确选择取决于骨性损伤的解剖学功能、患者的血流动力学状态、是否合并其他损伤、每个治疗机构的专业技能。

对于一个治疗机构来说，在患者就诊之前预先制订一个严重骨盆骨折患者治疗管理策略至关重要。每个治疗机构都应该具备一个与该机构实力相匹配的切实可行的处理流程。专业技能和治疗机构的资源能够一天 24 h 不间断、一周 7 天不间断地用于治疗这些复杂患者。在这一章节，我们将试图描述所有可行的治疗选择及各自优缺点。我们希望读者能够理解这一复杂疾病，希望我们的工作能够成为治疗机构建立其指南的基础。

发生率

钝性伤所导致的骨盆骨折占所有骨性损伤的 2%～8%。多发伤患者中，高达 20% 的患者存在骨盆骨折。在一项系列研究中，报道骨盆骨折发生率为每年每 100 000 人群中有 37 人，而另一项研究报道为每年每 100 000 人群中有 24 人。骨盆骨折的发生有两个高峰，高能量不稳定骨折发生在青少年和年轻成年人群，低能量骨折最常发生在老年人群。

损伤机制

骨性骨盆由机体最坚强的韧带维系在一起。因此，导致骨盆发生骨折并产生骨盆韧带不稳定的外力是很强大的。骨性骨盆环由两个髋骨和一个骶骨组成，但骨盆的骨性结构没有内在稳定性。髋骨和骶骨主要是由骨盆韧带维系成一个结构性整体。这些韧带复合体提供骨盆关节连接的稳定性。

鉴于骨盆的解剖结构，相较其他某些损伤机制来说，更可能导致骨盆骨折。在大多数环境中，车辆事故是骨盆损伤最常见的原因。按发生频率来说，依次是汽车行人相撞、高处坠落、摩托车事故和挤压伤。由于骨盆会出现许多年龄相关的变化，低能量损伤机制如轻微的机动车事故和机械性摔倒，通常成为老年患者骨盆骨折的原因。尽管这种骨折在特性上与高能量骨折模式中看到的骨性不稳定程度并不相关，但它们可能与明显出血和血流动力学不稳定是相关的。

诊断

患者出血流入的部位有 5 个：胸腔、腹腔、腹膜后、肌肉间隔和体外。对于多发伤患者，识别出血来源是最重要的。骨盆骨折患者中高达 20% 的患者同时伴有胸部损伤。胸腔内出血可以结合体格检查和 X 线胸片或超声检查来作出诊断。应该迅速识别张力性气胸和大量血胸，并进行胸廓造口术置管治疗。肌肉隔室出血应该通过体格检查逐步鉴别，而外向性失血一般是通过院前急救者提供的病史和体格检查来诊断。救治者应该牢记对于低血压患者，一旦得到复苏并血压回升后，其外向性失血可能会更加明显。腹腔内出血和腹膜后出血之间的鉴别可能是最难的。腹部和骨盆的复合伤是非常常见的。体格检查发现例如腹痛、腹胀或压痛，并不能区分腹腔内出血和腹膜后出血。此外，体格检查的发现可能是非常没有特异性的。患者可以表现为大量出血流入腹腔和腹膜后，而体格检查发现很轻微。过去，对于血流动力学不稳定的患者，腹腔内损伤的诊断一般是通过 DPL 来作出的。然而，FAST 的出现，对于腹腔内损伤的早期诊断起到了革命性的作用。FAST 是一种可以在数分钟内做出腹腔内损伤诊断的快速床旁技术。FAST 很方便，并且在结果可疑时易于重复操作。尽管 FAST 快速，且可以在复苏过程中稳步实施，但它并没有特异性。它能够识别出血但并不是一个有器官特异性的检查。CT 能够对腹腔内以及腹膜后结构的出血进行成像。它能够对这两个隔室的失血都进行识别。尽管 FAST 结果确实是阴性的，但仍有 25% 的骨盆骨折患者存在腹腔内损伤。因此，对于所有骨盆骨折患者，在评估过程的某个时间，都应该进行 CT 扫描，但是 CT 扫描须患者由急诊室转运、相对耗时。因此，对于血流动力学不稳定的患者，它的使用还是受限的。

任何一个骨盆骨折患者都应该怀疑是否存在腹膜后出血。骨盆 X 线片检查是一种快速扫描检查，能够提醒医生存在骨盆出血的可能性。作为一种扫描 X 线片检查，它通常是和 X 线胸片检查一起作为最初评估的一部分来进行。尽管骨盆 X 线片检查是一种很好的扫描检查，但它仅能在二维方向描述骨盆解剖学结构，会大大低估后方骨盆骨性损伤的程度。在骨盆 X 线片上证实的影像学损伤模式，例如增宽的耻骨联合分离、骶髂关节增宽，以及所有 4 个耻骨支都骨折的“蝴蝶型骨折”，提示这是一种严重的损伤模式，并且通常须进行骨盆血管造影。因为这些骨折通常合并有严重骨盆出血。

初期对于骨盆的体格检查在评估骨性稳定性上是有用的，甚至是在进行 X 线片检查之前。尽管有些人提倡用力摇晃骨盆，但我们相信这是一种存在潜在风险的操作。对于骨性不稳定的骨盆骨折患者，这将产生极度的疼痛，并且，骨折块的移位将会加重之前本已减弱的出血。代之，我们鼓励医生在髂骨翼水平向内侧轻柔挤压骨盆。如果骨盆的骨性结构稳定，则不会发现存在活动。如果骨盆存在“弹性”，患者几乎确定都存在骨性不稳定的骨盆骨折。

区分骨性结构不稳定的骨盆骨折患者和血流动力学不稳定的患者是很重要的。骨性结构的稳定性显示了骨盆骨折的骨性架构。血流动力学稳定性显示了患者的生理反应。并不是所有骨性结构不稳定的骨盆骨折患者都存在血流动力学不稳定。此外，骨性结构稳定的骨折患者仍然可能存在大量血液流入腹膜后的情况。

骨盆骨折患者、FAST 结果阳性，以及血流动力学不稳定，几乎可以确定最好要立刻实施剖腹探查手术。在许多患者当中，当腹腔中积液达到 400 ml 时，FAST 能够检测出腹腔积血的存在（图 1）。尽管游离液体肯定是来源于相对较小的腹腔内损伤或空腔脏器破裂，如膀胱。对于血流动力学不稳定的患者，诊断性剖腹探查术可能是最快，以及最确定的检查手段。如果发现损伤较小并且识别出出血是来源于骨盆，应该缩小剖腹探查的范围，并且采取其他措施控制骨盆出血。

损伤的解剖学位置和损伤分级

大量分类系统可以用于描述骨盆骨折的骨性结构。可能最常使用的是 1986 年 Young 等根据外力的矢量阐述的分类系统（表 1）。每一个类型进行细分来描述骨盆稳定性的程度，这在描述骨折解剖学特点和指导初期止血方面是很有用的。然而，关于

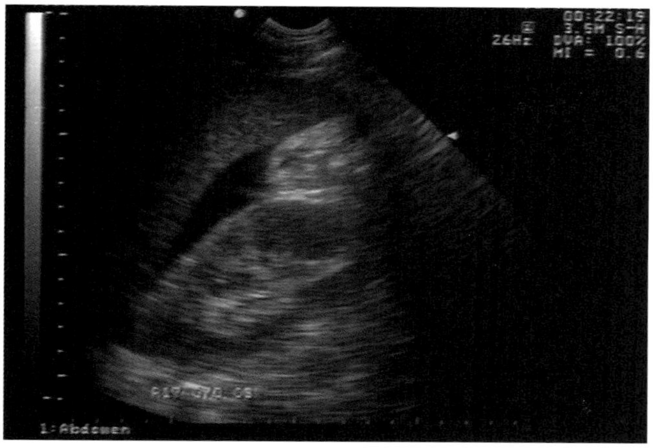

图 1　腹腔积液可能提示创伤重点超声评估结果（FAST）阳性、骨盆骨折和血流动力学不稳定。这样的患者几乎可以确定最好要立即实施剖腹探查手术

骨折解剖学特点能够预测出血的观点是存在争论的。一项来自 Wake Forest 的研究报道了使用血管造影和栓塞来进行骨盆止血，并且在这项系列研究中，低程度的前后压缩型骨折最常需血管造影。来自于我们机构的一项研究表明，Young 等分类系统能够预测输血的需求。

表 1　骨盆骨折分型

骨折类型	描述
前后压缩型	
Ⅰ型	耻骨联合断裂，分离小于 2.5 cm；没有明显的后方骨盆损伤
Ⅱ型	耻骨联合断裂大于 2.5 cm，伴有骶髂前韧带、骶棘韧带，以及骶结节韧带撕裂
III 型	耻骨联合和后方韧带复合体完全断裂，伴有半侧骨盆移位
侧方压缩型	
Ⅰ型	不伴有韧带断裂的骶髂关节后方压缩；斜行的耻骨支骨折
Ⅱ型	骶髂后韧带破裂；半侧骨盆相对前方骶髂关节轴向内旋并骶骨挤压性损伤，以及耻骨支斜行骨折
III 型	Ⅱ型损伤合并对侧半骨盆前后压缩型损伤

Data from Young JWR, Burgess AR, Brumback RJ, et al: Pelvic fractures: value of plain radiography in early assessment and management. Radiology 160:445

侧面碰撞导致的侧方压缩型（lateral compression，LC）骨盆骨折通常发生在侧方车辆事故或汽车行人相撞（图 2）。侧方压缩型骨折会导致骨盆直径急剧缩小。骨盆环不会打开而是“关闭”。骨盆韧带一般保持完整。因此，这种骨折通常不会出血。侧方压缩型骨折后出现的血流动力学不稳定更可能来源于躯干损伤，例如腹腔内出血或胸腔内出血。例外的情况发生于老年人，看起来相对温和的骨折模式，对于他们来说，却存在很高的出血风险。我们发现侧方压缩型骨折更常发生于年龄大于 55 岁的患者，并且他们需要输血的概率是年轻人的 2 倍，而且须输注更多的血（7.5 单位 vs. 5 单位）。这些侧方压缩型骨折较轻，但仍大量出血。很容易理解为何老年患者的总体死亡率更高。

前后向压缩型骨折通常是发生在前方机动车事故时或可能是在骨盆遭受前后方向外力挤压伤时（图 3）。在这种机制下，骨盆直径增宽，并且打开。如果骶髂关节破裂，那么这种损伤可以是单纯的韧带损伤，甚至没有明显的骨性损伤。骨盆血管损伤非常常见。前后向压缩型骨折存在最大的出血风险，这种骨折的患者，输血需求是最大的。

垂直剪切型（vertical shear，VS）损伤发生于患者足部呈过度伸展位着地，这通常发生在高处坠落或摩托车事故时，尤其是患者骑行时腿部处于过度伸展位（图 4）。在垂直剪切型骨折中，应力会向上传导至中轴骨，并通过后骨盆。后方的骨折和韧带破裂是很常见的。如果前侧和后侧部分都出现完全

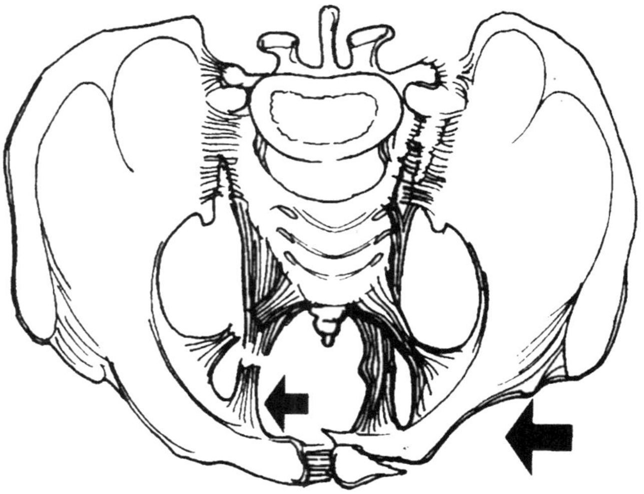

侧方压缩 III 型

图 2　侧方压缩型骨盆骨折 *(From Moore EE, Feliciano DV, Mattox KL:* Trauma*, 5th ed, New York, 2003, McGraw-Hill.)*

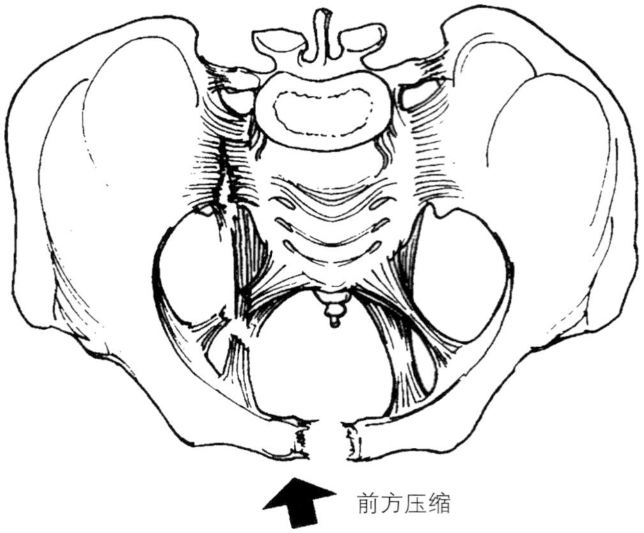

图 3 前后压缩型骨折 *(From Moore EE, Feliciano DV, Mattox KL:* Trauma, *5th ed, New York, 2003, McGraw-Hill.)*

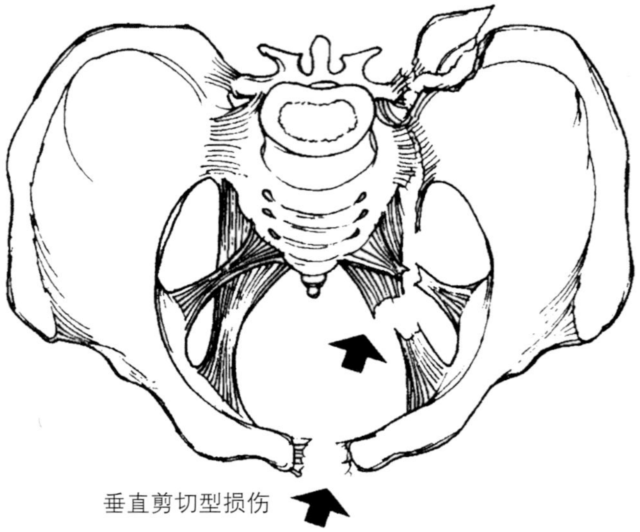

图 4 垂直剪切型骨折 *(From Moore EE, Feliciano DV, Mattox KL:* Trauma, *5th ed, New York, 2003, McGraw-Hill.)*

破裂（马尔盖涅骨盆骨折），腰肌会毫无阻力地向头侧牵拉半骨盆。这一点可以在骨盆 X 片上显示出来。在骨盆骨折的 Young 和 Burgess 分类系统中，垂直剪切型损伤存在中度的出血风险。

骨盆骨折并不总是表现为单一形式，例如当行人被斜向撞击。因此，一个清晰的分类系统可能并不容易。出血部位通常和骨盆骨折的解剖学特点相关联。前后压缩型骨折的出血通常是来自于阴部动脉或闭孔动脉。垂直剪切型骨折的出血最常见是来自于臀上动脉。而如果是侧方压缩型骨折出血，则实际上出血可以来自于任何血管结构。

尽管骨折的解剖学特点可以预测出血的可能性和位置，但显然它还远不完美。机敏的医生会意识到任何骨盆骨折的患者都可能出血。存在进行性失血证据的患者很明显应该探查其他体腔失血。如果没有发现，就应该假定患者的出血可能是来自于骨盆。不管骨盆骨折的解剖特点如何，都应该采取措施进行止血。

处理

许多技术可以用于骨性骨盆的止血。骨盆出血可以通过一些途径来遏止。出血绝大部分是静脉来源的，虽然可以出血量很大，但出血倾向是相对自限性的，因为骨盆血肿会填塞这一低压力的血管损伤。患者出血也可以来自骨折块本身，也可以来自小的骨盆动脉损伤。大动脉，如下腹部区域的主要分支（阴部、闭孔或臀上动脉），通常是大量骨盆出血的来源。主要血管结构，例如近侧腹下动脉或髂外动脉或髂总动脉，很少是典型骨盆骨折的主要出血来源，但是当这些血管损伤时，通常出血很多，并且患者几乎总是血流动力学不稳定。

骨盆骨折出血的止血技术包括外加压装置、骨折固定、血管造影栓塞和术中控制。外加压装置装置可以减少骨盆容积，帮助减少静脉出血。外加压装置能够帮助“稳定已经形成的血凝块”。此外，复位骨折块可以控制直接的骨性出血。稳定骨折块也可以限制骨折的再移动，并且应该有利于预防再出血。许多装置可以帮助达到外加压的效果。

也许最简单的方法是使用床单。理想的情况是，床单放在担架上，甚至是在患者到达之前。或者是，轻柔地抬起患者并且将床单放在患者下面。然后床单在骨盆前方交叉，并且系住（图 5）。这种技术含量比较低的操作被证实十分有用。在那些资源有限并且不可能拥有复杂技术的小型社区急诊室（emergency department，EDs）可能尤其有利。通常我们建议急诊医生紧贴伤者的身体系住床单而不要过紧。然后患者可以在医院中进行转运或者进行更高级别的救护。

军用抗休克服（military antishock garment，MAST）最初是被用在入院前阶段的一种复苏技术。

MAST开创性地通过下肢容量血管进行自体输血。目前清楚的是血压的上升是由全身血管阻力增加而引起的，并不是心脏前负荷增加所导致的。MAST是一种有效的骨盆和下肢的夹板，并且能够维持骨盆骨折复位，就像床单那样。如果腹部和骨盆部分都充气了，那么下肢部分必须充气。如果MAST的压力设定过高，腹腔内压力就会增加，将会导致ACS。必须小心仔细监测患者的这一并发症。MAST的应用大部分已经被放弃，因为它被证实在院前场所治疗低血压时是没有价值的。

对于骨盆外加压来说后方骨盆C型钳是另一种选择。C型钳从后方插入来复位后方的骨折块。在许多欧洲创伤中心，这种方法是在急诊室通过经皮操作进行的。在大多数美国创伤中心，它则是在手术室荧光透视引导下进行，这限制了它作为一种急诊复苏工具的有效性。C型钳的前方部分可以被旋开，以利于进行血管造影或剖腹探查。显然，如果针置入的位置不好，可能会发生包括胃肠穿孔或医源性神经损伤的并发症。

过去，外固定架是一种经常用于骨盆止血的加压装置。外固定架在外固定装置中最坚硬，并且能够确切地闭合骨盆（图6）。在具备专业技能的中心，外固定架可以在急诊室快速应用。在其他中心，它通常是像C型钳那样放置于手术室。在某些病例中，外固定架可以提供确切的骨折固定。外固定架的前部可以像C型钳那样旋转，这样有利于进行血管造影或剖腹探查。在复苏阶段使用外固定架要求这些器械立即可以使用。外固定架可能会降低CT影像质量，并且可能在进入CT工作台时干扰患者的活动。外固定针置入髂骨翼，然后在前方连接框架。对于那些后侧部分严重移位的骨盆骨折患者，收紧外固定架所引起的向内移动，可能会导致后方骨折块的进一步移位，并且增加失血。

事实上许多美国的创伤中心放弃了所有其他的外加压装置，并且专门使用方便购得的骨盆带。骨盆带是一种可以对骨盆施加均匀、直接压力的尼龙搭扣装置。压力是由尼龙搭扣和系带系统在骨盆带的前方部分施加的。这种骨盆带可以快速使用，并且只需要最低限度的专业技能。这种方便购得的骨盆带可以减少前后位骨折中的耻骨分离（图7）。骨盆带应该跨过股骨大转子来使用，而不是跨过下腹部。然而，正确放置骨盆带会使在腹股沟区进行血管造影受到限制。如果须进行血管造影，可以在骨盆带上剪一个孔或者把它轻柔地跨过大腿上段，从而将其放得更高或更低。判断外加压是否有益决定于骨盆骨折的解剖学特点。广泛开放的、前后向Ⅲ型骨盆骨折理论上须通过外加压来治疗。向心性内聚（而不是外向性爆发的侧方压缩型骨盆骨折）不太可能通过外加压而获益。垂直剪切型损伤则可能是以一种间接的方式来表现。在使用外固定架的时代，这种讨论是非常恰当的。骨盆带的出现消除了这其中许多的讨论。尽管骨盆带不太可能使侧方压缩型

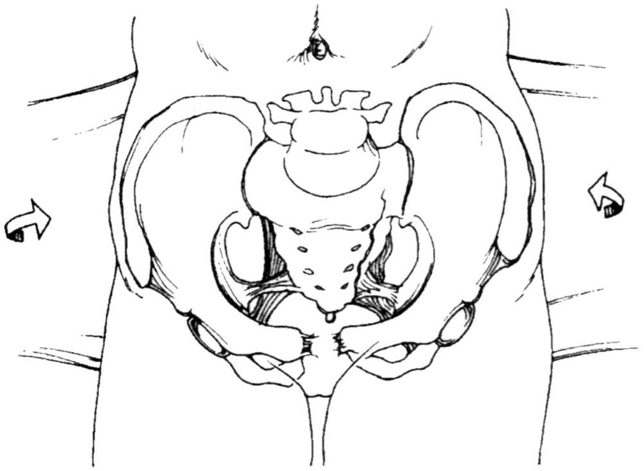

图5 通过围绕患者包裹床单，跨过骨盆在前方交叉，来获得外加压 *(From Moore EE, Feliciano DV, Mattox KL:* Trauma*, 5th ed, New York, 2003, McGraw-Hill.)*

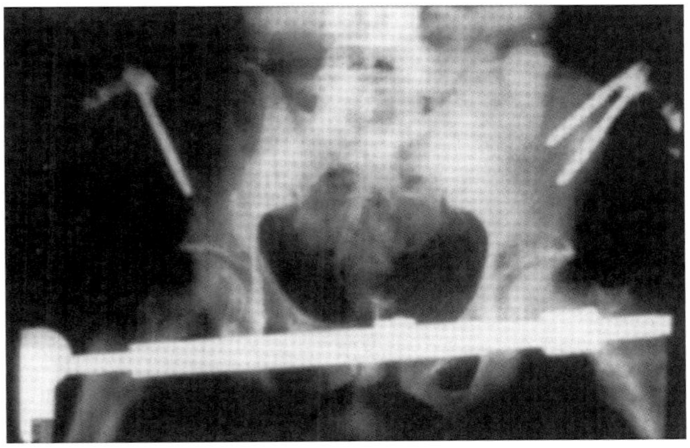

图6 外固定架，过去通常作为骨盆止血的一种加压装置。外固定架在外固定装置中最坚硬，并且能够确切地闭合骨盆 *(From Moore EE, Feliciano DV, Mattox KL:* Trauma*, 5th ed, New York, 2003, McGraw-Hill.)*

骨盆骨折获益，但它能够快速应用，并且一定不会加重出血。骨盆带可以作为一种骨盆夹板，并且在患者转运到CT扫描仪、手术室或血管造影室的过程中，限制骨折块的活动。因此，我们在使用骨盆带时非常灵活，并且事实上任何一个血流动力学不稳定的骨盆骨折患者都会应用它。

骨盆出血的血管栓塞已经应用超过30年。诊断性的骨盆血管造影应该能够识别出所有部位的骨盆动脉损伤。骨盆骨折患者进行血管造影的适应证包括血流动力学不稳定、大的骨盆或腹膜后血肿，以及假性动脉瘤或CT时造影剂外渗。输血触发，例如24 h大于4 U或48 h大于6 U也是被提倡的（表2）。吸收性明胶海绵栓塞、不锈钢线卷，或者两者并用，在获得骨盆止血方面都是非常有效的。有许多血管造影技术可以使用。医生应该尽可能慎重地选择骨盆栓塞，以限制潜在的并发症，如阳痿或远端缺血导致的骨盆或臀肌坏死。然而，选择性更高的技术，使用它需要更多时间和专业技能。代替选择性栓塞的是，使用不锈钢线卷的近侧腹下血管盲栓塞。这种方法是想降低下腹部区域的灌注压进而产生自发性止血。这种方式产生的止血不是最满意的，因为在骨盆血管网中有丰富的侧支循环。伴随腹下动脉近端栓塞，如果出血复发，获得止血的血管造影窗被关闭。使用吸收性明胶海绵微粒的腹下动脉盲栓塞可以达到像线卷栓塞一样的目的。

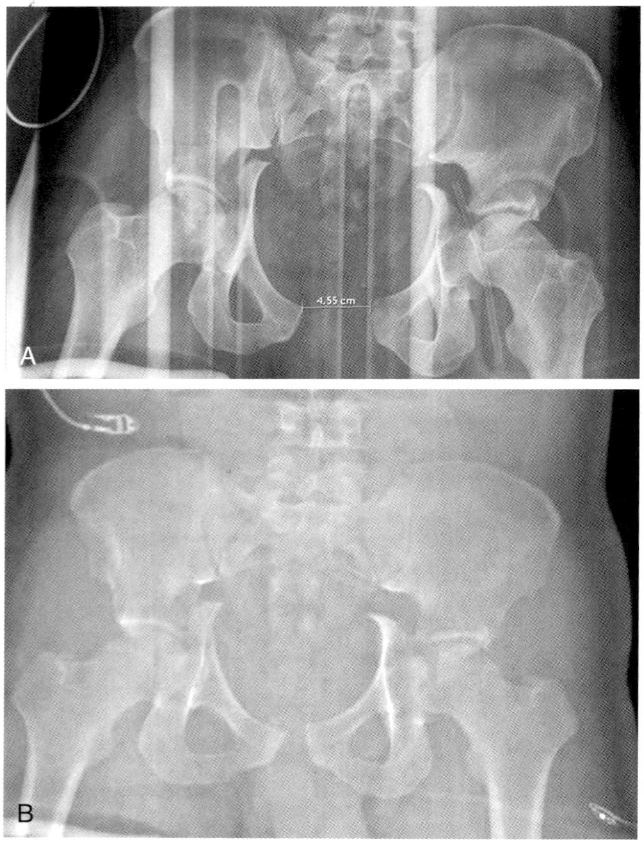

图7 对前后向骨盆骨折应用骨盆带，一种可以对骨盆施加均匀，直接压力的尼龙搭扣装置，应用前X线片（**A**），应用后X线片（**B**）

表2 血管造影的适应证

24 h 4 单位血量
48 h 6 单位血量
创伤重点超声评估（FAST）/诊断性腹腔灌洗结果阴性的低血压
计算机断层扫描（CT）或术中发现大的骨盆血肿
CT 显示假性动脉瘤

Data from Moore EE, Feliciano DV, Mattox KL: Trauma, 5th ed, New York, 2003, McGraw-Hill

手术止血总的来说是令人失望的。剖腹探查并不能够使外科医生直接看到受损的血管。打开腹膜后放松压塞可能使已经减弱的出血再次出现，尤其是静脉出血。腹下动脉主干是一个非常短的结构。在大多数患者中，它仅仅几英寸长，然后很快分支成大量更小的血管，深入到骨盆中。识别出损伤血管极其困难，并且试图去做这一点通常会使情况更糟。经验性的腹下动脉结扎是一种选择，类似于腹下动脉近端栓塞。它确实冒着暴露骨盆血肿的风险，也存在侧支血流出血的风险。在许多创伤中心，腹下动脉栓塞能够在和腹下动脉结扎在大约同样的时间内完成。然而，如果血管造影栓塞不能马上使用，并且患者还在出血，腹下动脉结扎仍不失为一种选择。对于处于紧急关头的患者，术中腹下动脉栓塞是另一种选择。近端腹下动脉是独立于血管环路的。外科医生混合止血物质，包括新鲜冰冻血浆和小微粒吸收性明胶海绵。腹下动脉经血管导管介入并且进行盲栓塞。文献中关于腹下动脉栓塞的经验很有限。除非没有其他选择，否则这种情况应该尽量避免。

某些患者几乎肯定可以从直接手术止血的尝试中获益。表现为失血性休克和单侧股动脉搏动消失的患者可能存在髂总动脉或髂外动脉的损伤。通常来说，这些患者需要创伤性半侧骨盆切除术（图8）。产生这种损伤需要极大的外力，并且这些患者通常都是处于难治性休克的状态。使用内侧内脏翻转的直接手术入路，结合直接显露髂动脉，对于这些患者来说可能是救命的。这些损伤可以通过结扎或单纯修复来治疗。简单的技术不能控制的那些损伤通常应该以损伤控制的模式进行分流。

近期，腹膜外填塞的观点再次获得了明显的欢迎。患者手术入路为下腹正中切口或 Pfannenstiel 切口。在中线劈开下腹部肌肉然后直接显露骨盆血肿。清除骨盆血肿然后将骨盆进行填塞（图 9）。保持在腹膜外很重要。当填塞应用于对抗腹膜时，会增加腹膜的压塞效应。腹膜后筋膜能够闭合来加强填塞或患者通过真空敷料延缓病情。有时，骨盆填塞和剖腹探查协同进行。在这种情况下，我们通常使用横切口，以避免腹部切口和腹膜后切口相交。以同样地方式劈开肌肉和填塞骨盆。当与某种骨性骨盆稳定技术协同使用时，腹膜后填塞是最成功的。在骨盆填塞的时候可以放置外固定架或 C 型钳。或者，可以简单地代替骨盆带。这种技术也可以和更正式的骨盆骨折固定方式结合使用，例如骨盆接骨板或

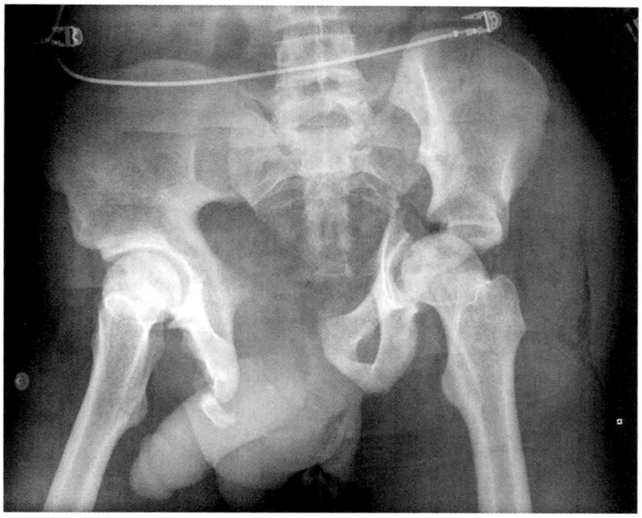

图 8　创伤性内侧半骨盆切除术

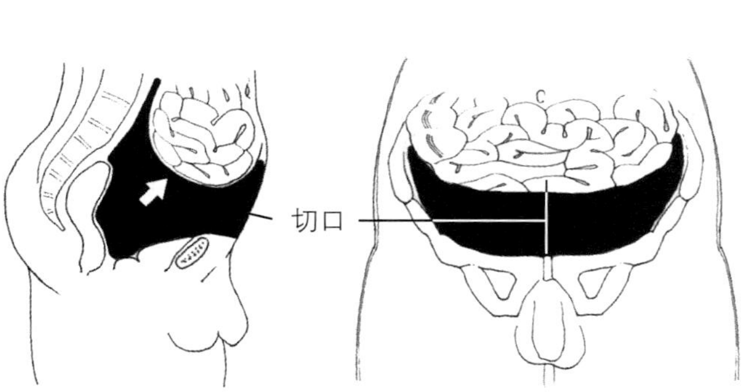

图 9　下腹正中切口显露骨盆血肿 (*From Moore EE, Feliciano DV, Mattox KL: Trauma, 5th ed, New York, 2003, McGraw-Hill.*)

经皮放置骶髂螺钉，这取决于患者的临床情况。

严重骨盆骨折患者早期进行稳定固定是最好的。骨折块的确切复位对于获得止血是非常有用的。然而，早期切开复位内固定增加了大量失血的风险。经皮骶髂螺钉固定能够以最少的失血来复位后骨盆。这些经皮螺钉在透视引导下穿入，并且牢固地复位骨盆（图 10）。我们通常将这种技术应用于前后 Ⅱ 型或 Ⅲ 型骨折。患者必须血流动力学足够稳定以确保能够经受手术操作。然而，这种技术在严重休克的患者并不推荐。经皮骶髂螺钉可以达到骨盆骨折的良好复位，恢复骨盆容积，以及保持血块的稳定。一旦骨折以这种方式确切地固定，患者可以离床活动，将肺部并发症的风险降到最低。

在血流动力学稳定的患者，前方骨盆的固定也可以在进行创伤剖腹探查术时同步完成。在这种情况下，患者接受剖腹探查术以及腹腔内损伤的治疗。当腹部部分完成，可以延长切口或再做一个独立的 Pfannenstiel 切口。前方骨折块通过手法复位，然后放置前方骨盆接骨板。此外，这种方法提供了确切的前方骨折固定，避免使用其他技术，例如外固定架或骨盆带。

开放性骨盆骨折则面临不同的问题。它可能是严重的体外失血的根源。由于在这种情况下失血是流向体外，所以通常没有明显的腹膜后出血。诊断应该基于体格检查来建立。由于患者通常是仰卧位，检查会阴很重要。进行阴道或直肠检查来鉴别撕裂可能是必要的。然后腹部应该通过应用 FAST 来评估。FAST 阳性的患者应该进行剖腹探查，而 FAST 阴性的患者应该进行进一步的诊断性评估。

开放性骨盆骨折的出血最初可以通过填塞来控制。如果与外界相通的出口较小，那么有必要加宽这个出口，以使得填塞物能够深入至骨盆中。描述骨盆骨折的解剖学特征很重要。这一点通常可以结合体格检查和骨盆 X 线片来完成。骨盆骨折应该使用之前讨论过的加压装置中的任何一种来复位。应该对整个多学科团队进行预警，包括手术室、骨科和血管造影室。尽管出血看似是静脉出血，并且可以通过填塞来控制，我们还是提倡对这些患者进行血管造影。患者应该到手术室进行局部探查、重新填塞，并且通过局部控制来获得所有的止血。这一点可以在血管造影团队准备血管造影室时进行。当患者在去除填塞和探查时出现迅猛出血，重新填塞是最明智的方法。一旦获得止血，患者应该手术清除没有活力的软组织和肌肉。对于直肠周围受累的

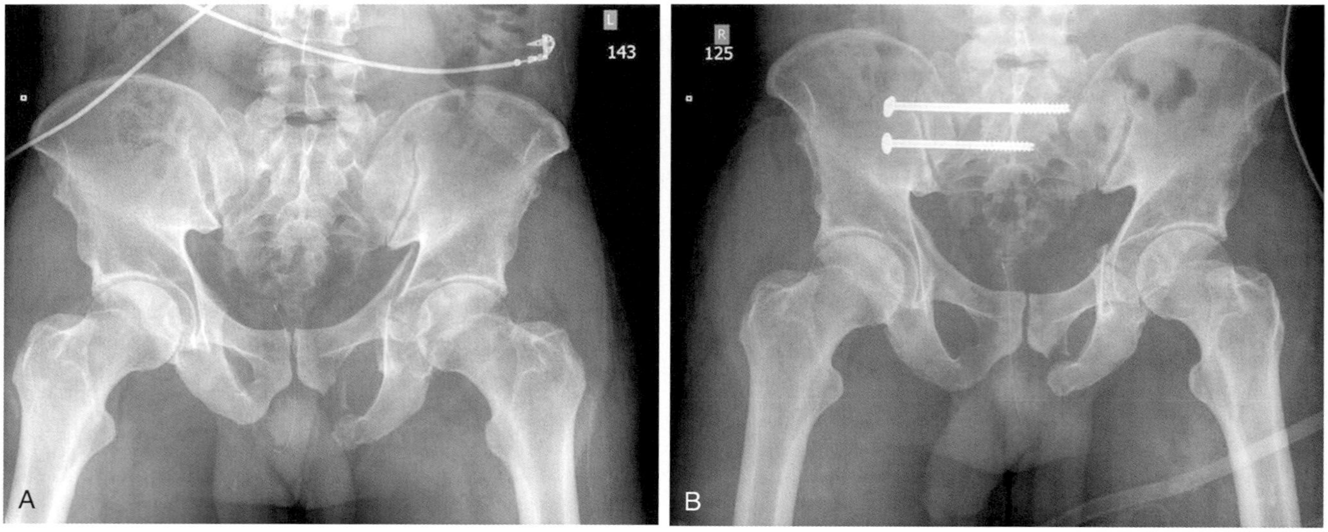

图 10 伴有骶髂关节分离的骨盆骨折经皮骶髂螺钉放置前（**A**）后（**B**）

患者进行粪便转流通常是需要的，但不应是急诊手术，而可以推迟到患者血流动力学稳定和出血被控制后。

并发症发生率和处理

在混合系列研究中报道的骨盆骨折患者的死亡率大约为 6%。传统上来说，大多数死亡是由于骨盆出血，但是最近越来越多的死亡是由合并损伤导致的出血所引起的。据推测，更早识别骨盆是失血的潜在来源，将会减少死于骨盆出血的患者数量。致残和致死的其他主要常见原因包括创伤性脑损伤、脓毒症和多器官衰竭。

短期来说，骨盆骨折患者存在发生与骨盆骨折本身直接相关的众多并发症的高风险。软组织损伤可因止血措施而加重进而导致皮肤、皮下组织和肌肉缺血。伴有软组织坏死的患者须接受手术清创。骨盆深部感染也会发生，尤其是对于开放性骨折患者，并且可能会导致多器官功能障碍以及衰竭和死亡。这些感染应该通过细菌培养及针对性的抗生素和外科引流来积极治疗。拆除外固定可能也是需要的，否则会导致患者长时间的制动。

骨盆骨折患者也面临着发生同多发伤和制动患者一样的众多常见并发症的异常高的风险。骨盆骨折增加了深静脉血栓（deep vein thrombosis，DVT）的风险。骨盆骨折患者面临着血栓栓塞的特殊风险，因为他们都有一定程度的骨盆静脉损伤，并且要制动一段时间。最好的治疗策略是通过早期骨折固定和活动来进行预防，这也可能是预防深静脉血栓的最好方式。发生呼吸衰竭通常是由高风险的肺不张、肺炎、脂肪栓塞、肺栓塞和误吸所引起。院内感染，例如泌尿系统感染和呼吸机相关性肺炎，应该给予积极的诊断和治疗，来预防发生脓毒症和多器官衰竭。

不幸的是，严重骨盆骨折存活的患者通常出现明显的长期残疾。从以往经验来看，将近 50% 的患者可能有严重的疼痛和功能障碍。骨盆的充分复位和残端移位的程度可能起到重要的作用。新型联合手术方法的功能结果可能比传统报道的要好，较新的研究报道，严重骨盆环损伤的患者中有超过 2/3 者有总体良好的功能状态。特别要说，开放性骨折和不良的功能预后相关。骨盆骨折患者其他的长期并发症包括性功能问题、阳痿和性交困难。

结论和流程图（图 11）

伴有骨盆骨折的多发伤患者是创伤治疗面临的最大挑战之一。出血的诊断方法和高效实施的复苏以及恰当的治疗都是至关重要的。众多技术可用于评估患者并且帮助止血。制订一个与救治机构的专业技能和资源相适应的处理流程是非常重要的，这样能够为那些严重创伤患者提供高效、快速、协调和有效的救治。

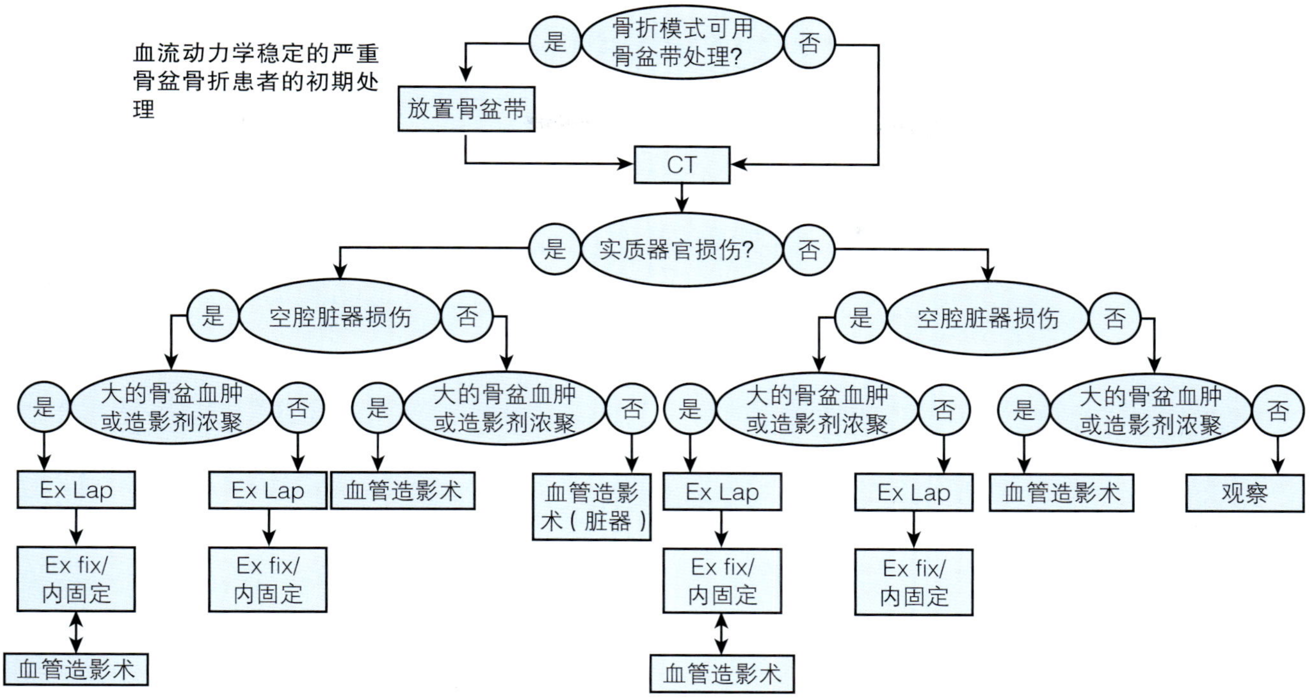

A

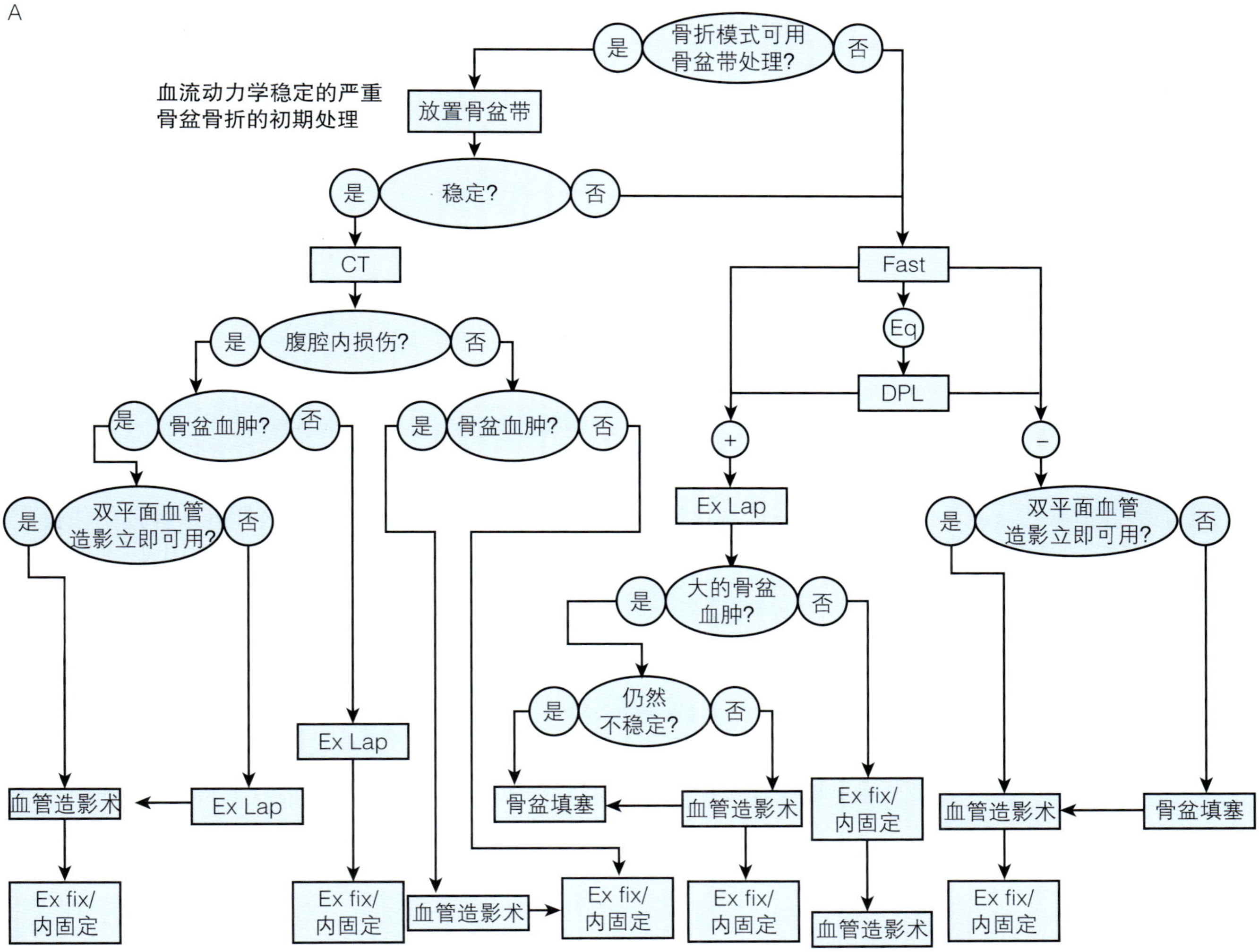

B

图 11 **A**，血流动力学稳定的严重骨盆骨折患者的初期处理流程图。**B**，血流动力学不稳定的严重骨盆骨折患者的初期处理流程图。Angio，双平面血管造影；CT，计算机断层扫描；DPL，诊断性腹腔灌洗；Ex fix，外固定架；Ex lap，剖腹探查术；Eq，不明确；FAST，创伤重点超声评估

第 9 章　主要躯体损伤中的特殊问题

失血性休克诊断与治疗的新概念

Juan Carlos Puyana, Samuel Tisherman 和 Andrew B. Peitzman 著
朱凤雪　李　纾 译

失血性休克的单一普遍诱因是严重的急性出血，但其临床综合征却各不相同。这种情况的诊断和处理起初看起来很简单。然而，休克是如何发生的以及个体代偿机制如何应对损伤本身和疾病的干预可转化为一个复杂的疾病谱。这种疾病谱包括从快速的循环衰竭到伴随着复杂的炎症的全身缺血再灌注损伤与在许多情况下会演变成多器官功能障碍的抗炎反应。本章的目的是对当前存在的问题进行回顾以及从临床角度来看休克的诊断和治疗。

重症失血性休克的流行病学

创伤是全球第二大死因，也是美国人丧生的主要原因之一。创伤引起的严重出血是导致可预防性死亡的主要原因。总的来说，创伤大约每年导致 150 000 人死亡，创伤性出血引起的严重低血容量是其中近半数人死亡的一个主要因素。死亡的主要原因仍然是头部损伤和出血。这些研究结果已经出现在民用期刊和军事发现中，包括越南冲突和最近的伊拉克和阿富汗战争。大约 1/3 的创伤性死亡发生在医院外；失血过多是创伤后 4 h 内发生死亡的主要原因。在越南战争中战场损伤的分布显示，25% 的死亡的发生是由于大量失血导致无法挽救。另外 19% 的死亡被视为可挽救的，这些死亡是由躯干失血（10%）和周围血管失血（19%）导致的。最近在平民创伤早期进行输血的数据表明，58% 的死亡是由于出血导致的。大多数患者（66%）在入院 3 h 内发生死亡，而入院 24 h 后的脑损伤和多器官功能衰竭成为死亡的主要原因。

临床观点：复苏观念的转变

重度失血性休克的特点是冰凉、湿冷、苍白或青紫的皮肤。患者会出现心动过速和低血压，这些临床表现的严重程度可能会有所不同，这与患者的年龄、潜在的心血管疾病、服用的药物或如毒品和酒精等的有毒化合物有关。低血压是休克的标志，它很容易被检测到，它的存在一直是预后不良的预测因素。然而休克的严重程度只能部分根据低血压的存在来判定。显然，快速大量的血液流失会使患者创伤后短暂地出现明显低血压。复杂的设备或监测技术没必要应用在快要死亡的患者身上。及时和有效的干预措施必须立即制定，目的是控制出血和改变血容量。不幸的是，创伤后未出现低血压也不能排除休克的存在。事实上，它可能误导缺乏经验的临床医生认为患者处于安全状态，不须进行积极的复苏。

受伤患者到达创伤中心后处于低血压状态或有短暂性低血压病史的仅占创伤患者总数的 6%～9%。从实用的角度来看，失血性休克患者可分为 3 组。1 组患者是活动性出血。他们通常有导致心脏或大血管损伤的明显的胸部创伤、大量破坏性腹腔内脏损伤或明显的腹膜后出血（如骨盆骨折）。这组代表了低血压患者的 1/3 或创伤患者总人数的 2%。他们能活着到达我们的创伤中心是由于有序的院前创伤处理系统。这组患者的输液反应是最小的，甚至完全不存在，这些患者被称为无反应者。

剩余 1/3 的低血压患者（2% 的总创伤患者）构成第 2 组，该组患者是中度至重度出血，比第 1 组出血速率慢。第 2 组患者如果没有接受恰当及时的治疗和出血控制，可在 6～12 h 内死亡。他们对最初的复苏有反应但时间很短暂，即使处理得当他们也可能会发展为器官衰竭或感染。

第 3 组占创伤患者总人数的 2%，包含出现短暂低血压的患者，他们的代偿性反应可以充分实现其生命体征的自发稳定。这些患者的最终预后较好，但是由于处于未恢复状态或者说是未识别的低灌注或代偿性休克的时间会引起一些并发症或器官衰竭。

随着对创伤后死亡原因的理解的加深，我们认为躯干出血是潜在的可预防性死亡的主要原因。患者在胸腹部有严重的穿通伤，且大量胸腹部血管受损，他人到达创伤中心后须进行积极的干预措施包括急救手术和大量输血（massive transfusion，MT）。中东过去 10 年的战争经验使我们更好地理解了晶体、血液制品的使用，以及创伤诱发的凝血病的治疗。最新的研究结果表明过度使用晶体会产生毒害作用，失血性休克患者会不断地出现创伤诱发的凝血病，这将使我们重新思考创伤高级生命支持（Advanced Trauma Life Support，ATLS）课程教授的传统复苏策略。这些患者送入急诊时有严重凝血功能障碍，死亡率大大增加。

最新的知识挑战了关于液体复苏的传统观念，它可以追溯到 20 世纪 70 年代开始将捐献的全血根据成分不同将其分成多个部分时。需要大量输血的患者现在通过输入更高比例的血浆和血小板来进行不同的处理。然而在提供给平民创伤患者的最佳血液制品的比例上并没有达成广泛的共识。显然，经典的复苏方法须进行改变，尤其是对于那些正处于休克状态、可能需要大量输血的患者。

MT 患者通常需要针对损伤的控制干预措施，并且在出血得到控制之后依然会出现严重的低体温和凝血功能障碍以及循环衰竭。由于低灌注、缺血，对全身进行再灌注在不同的临床方案中有明显的差异性，所以今后的治疗干预将更加复杂并须具有明确地靶向性。液体复苏、明确的血液产品替代率和凝血功能障碍的积极治疗措施将会进一步发展。并且随着人们对这一复杂的病理生理过程的理解不断提高，其他特定的干预性措施也亟待被发现。

对于进展性或较难治疗性休克的认知增强和在出血患者早期治疗中减少循环衰竭的发生可以让我们重新定义“黄金 1 小时”（即有效复苏的机会之窗）。

休克的临床症状和用于研究的动物模型之间的差异

在设计失血性休克模型时，2 个有时相互矛盾的目标让这一领域的研究者受到了挑战。首先，研究者希望减少实验动物间的差异性。其次，研究人员试图造一个具有临床意义的模型。在临床环境中，出血通常是不受控制的。随着持续出血和动脉压降低，出血速率趋于缓慢。当血压足够低时，止血机制开始发挥作用，以使出血能够完全停止。实际上，复苏时可通过升高血压移除新生的血块，从而激发复发性出血。许多失控性出血的动物模型已被报道。这些模型通常用于研究新的止血方法，确定最佳的复苏时机，或确定最佳的复苏参数 / 终点。失控性出血模型虽然因其临床实用性而对研究者具有一定的吸引力，但是也有实验动物之间的变异。因此，在使用这些模型进行新药的临床前药效学研究时，要求比较大的样本量，以获得具有统计学意义的数据。

另一方面，控制性低血压最早是由 Wiggers 提出，可以对损伤做一个更规范的分级。当使用 Wiggers 模型诱导失血性休克时，最初须定期地抽出额外的等分的血液以维持目标血压，因为机体自身对急性血容量降低有代偿性反应。然而，当休克状态持续了一段时间后，就不太可能用抽血来维持目标血压。相反，这时须再输注等分的血维持目标血压。这个阶段与临床实践中的表现没什么相似之处，但是在实验室中它用于描绘“失代偿的终点”，也就是从抽血到输血的转变点。这种转变点通常发生在休克 90～120 min 后，具体时间取决于物种间的差异。这个模型也并不是十分理想，因为不同动物之间失代偿终点出现的时间具有差异性。显然，Wiggers 模型可以模拟一个更具有可重复性的损伤。虽然与临床实际病例的相似性却很低，但是它仍然促进了对于机制或原因 / 结果的研究，并且被广泛应用于的出血后许多细胞和分子作用过程的描绘，这超出了本章范围。

现在已经在小鼠身上开发出了新的出血模型，该模型可以对许多在失血引起的死亡中起到一定作用的有害信号的级联反应做出复杂的分析。在评估生物系统（即系统生物学）中取得的进展，使科学界进一步了解复杂的生理网络和强调休克病理基础的细胞通讯模式。

休克的诊断

测量血压不一定总是可行的，在初次检查时不须开始治疗。事实上，可以通过检测脉搏的特性对灌注的充分性做一个快速的整体评估。休克的明显体征足以诊断和确定血容量损失的严重程度。一些额外的信息，例如血压、心电图、脉搏血氧计和二氧化碳图都可能起到一定的作用。其次在引起严重低血压和休克的其他原因被排除的情况下，如张力性气胸、心包压塞或神经源性休克，在静脉（intravenous，IV）通路中输入常温液体。

理想状况下，任何液体治疗都必须伴随出血控制。可通过在床旁评估特定伤害的血液流失来估计创伤后的血容量不足。单侧胸腔积血可能含有 3 000 ml 血液，腹部可容纳 2 000 ~ 5 000 ml 的血液，并且腹部膨胀不明显。其他沉积大量出血的损伤包括骨盆骨折伴有腹膜后腔 1 500 ~ 2 000 ml 的血液流失，且无任何创伤的外部体征。股骨骨折可出血 800 ~ 1 200 ml，胫骨骨折可出血 350 ~ 650 ml。

创伤引起的凝血功能障碍的早期诊断和凝血功能障碍的严重程度的量化可通过使用治疗性血栓弹力图（thromboelastography，TEG），这是治疗严重休克的一种很有前景的新方法。创伤后使用 TEG 的实用技术取得了更多的进展，这将有助于在出血早期针对各种特定的凝血疾病更加合理地使用血液制品、凝血因子，以及抗纤维蛋白溶解治疗。

缺血和再灌注现象已被广泛地研究。休克和复苏在功能上是一种全身缺血再灌注损伤。SIRS 和 MODS 是缺血、再灌注相关事件的一种集合表达。不幸的是，我们依靠非特异性的整体方法提供的有关组织灌注的间接信息。目前我们面对的挑战是要确定一种创新的方法来量化休克的分级。指导这个领域未来研究方向的问题包括患者的生理储备、机体代偿性反应和个体器官对缺血的耐受 / 反应间的相互影响是如何最终体现的，以及确定最好的方法来精确测量每一个组分。目前，我们对这些问题知之甚少并且使用着最原始的方法来进行测定。术语“组织灌注”多指不容易量化的一个实体。实际上，我们用碱缺失（base deficit，BD）和乳酸作为整体参数来评估组织灌注。在 ICU，我们通过血流动力学参数来解释相关的标准，这些参数通常要通过有创监测技术才能够得到，例如热稀释法测定心排血量、连续性中心静脉以及混合静脉循环的血氧饱和度。

组织灌注评估

BD 和乳酸可以提供无氧代谢程度的信息。乳酸是对缺氧的一种间接的测量。BD 是指使体液 pH 回到 7.40 并且 CO_2 分压为 40 mmHg，使用的缓冲液的量。Davis 等用 BD 对患者进行分级，轻度为 2 ~ 5，中度为 6 ~ 14，重度为 >15。最初的 BD 大小与低血压和液体复苏的进一步需要直接相关。另外，65% 的 BD 持续恶化的患者尽管已经进行了复苏，仍然持续出血。BD 是休克和多种创伤患者需要输液的可靠指标。Davis 等还发现尽管在动物失血性模型中平均动脉压、心排血量、混合静脉血氧饱和度、氧摄取等已经有所改善，BD 仍可以处于异常水平。Rutherford 等发现，BD、年龄和头部损伤对病死率均有额外作用。BD 是一种适宜而灵敏的检测灌注不足的程度和持续时间的方法。作为一种有效的临床工具，它促进了其他创伤评分的预测能力。

乳酸是无氧糖酵解的最终产物。作为一种更直接的测评缺氧引起的组织酸中毒的指标，它已被证明可以很好地判断患者的预后情况。血清乳酸正常值在第 1 个 24 h 内低于 2 mmol/L 与 100% 的生存率密切相关。若休克后 24 h 至 48 h 乳酸含量持续上升，只有 78% 的患者可以存活。休克后 48 h 乳酸值持续上升，则死亡率大于 85%。Sauaia 等证明早期（12 h）乳酸值升高至 2.5 mmol/L 以上与多器官衰竭相关。Manikis 等进一步发现乳酸水平的初始值和峰值以及高乳酸血症持续时间均与创伤后 MODS 的进展相关。大范围损伤的炎症和宿主反应的合作课题（Glue Grant）中的最新研究数据证实，BD 和乳酸在一个严重的闭合性创伤患者的队列的预测价值。早期乳酸水平的升高和损伤后 12 ~ 24 h BD 的升高和持续出现的休克证据，被认为是多器官功能衰竭的独立预测因素。

总之，初始乳酸水平和恢复乳酸正常值的时间与 MODS 的风险和死亡相关。然而，使用乳酸或 BD 作为改善生存率的复苏终点的观点还并未被证实。

休克的处理

创伤性出血患者的处理重点在于呼吸道控制、通气和氧合。复苏的目标是阻止出血和扩充血管内血容量使其最大化地向组织输送氧。心排血量、血压和向重要器官氧合血的供应是决定预后的重要因素。

休克在ICU中从损伤开始到病情稳定过程的持续护理中给予处理，我们可以通过不同的策略进行处理。入院前的干预措施可以挽救生命，但是也会受限于地点中的特定环境，例如城中的内部城市、偏远的农村、战争区域或是刚刚经历一场大规模伤亡事件的地方。入院阶段，可以在护理条件下实施更多明确的治疗手段，同时这也取决于接收医院的能力。当情况更严重时，须将患者转移到Ⅰ级或Ⅱ级创伤中心。因此，具有类似损伤程度的患者可能会受到差别很大的护理，这取决于之前提到的各种变量、创伤系统区域化的情况，以及创伤中心的成熟度。

治疗危及生命的出血患者时快速的外科手术控制出血是成功的关键。熟练的操作和对血管解剖结构的全面了解，是后续继续进行抢救生命的治疗措施的奠基石。然而，介入放射科医生和在血管造影室的血管外科医生现在正处理着越来越多种类的创伤性血管损伤。然而在这一章中，我们将根据生理机会或治疗窗来重点描述可能有效的临床治疗策略。这些措施可能从控制出血的辅助措施、增强代偿性反应、替代血容量的减少和支持固有低灌注时的器官到一个特定的临床情景。及时的气道控制和出血的应急控制显然是最基本的原则。

严重出血患者的血管通路

血管通路是迅速恢复循环容量的关键。在考虑获得血管通路的过程时，解剖学位置、损伤大小、技术水平和护理人员专业知识是最重要的因素。应避免在受伤肢体获得静脉通路。在出现膈下损伤的患者，至少应在上腔静脉的分支上放置一个支流，因为下腔静脉可能出现血管中断。为了快速处理大量的液体，应该使用短的大直径导管。2倍的静脉导管内径使流经导管的液体增加至16倍。一个14 G、5 cm的周围静脉导管注入液体的速度是16 G、20 cm的导管的2倍。当使用8.5 F的肺动脉导管导引器时，侧端口应该被移除，因为这增加了约4倍的阻力。

ATLS指南推荐快速放置2个直径（16 G或更大）静脉导管在严重损伤和失血性休克患者体内。静脉输液的首选应该是肢体周围静脉。最适合的位置在手腕、手背、手臂肘窝，以及腿部大隐静脉。之后依次为颈外静脉和股静脉。正确放置静脉导管并发症发生率低。血管内放置大直径静脉导管应检查血液是否回流。不应在静脉注射部位施加额外的压力。压力作用于渗透的输注静脉时，静脉输注液体会渗到软组织，会出现隔室综合征。紧急情况下一个患者在创伤后无脉搏时，须切开股静脉。

锁骨下动脉和颈内静脉（internal jugular，IJ）置管不应常用于低血容量性创伤患者。静脉塌陷导致并发症发生率高，成功率低。快速的周围皮下静脉注射在下述情况下很难达成：患者血容量低和静脉塌陷、水肿、肥胖、有瘢痕、有静脉吸毒史或烧伤。在这样的情况下，大直径导管的中央通路可以通过皮肤和股动脉穿刺或切开完成。锁骨下静脉穿刺置管为有经验的医生提供了快速的静脉通路。锁骨下静脉穿刺最常见的并发症是气胸。气胸更可能发生在身体左侧，因为左侧胸膜顶的解剖学位置更高。锁骨下动脉和IJ导管应插入患者损伤侧胸部，减少健侧肺萎陷的可能性，特别是在一个胸廓造口术置管已经到位的情况下。一个简单的气胸可能导致肺挫伤或对侧胸部气胸的患者呼吸功能损伤。静脉空气栓塞是中央静脉插管的另一并发症。

虽然IJ皮下导管放置是获得快速大直径导管通路的一个很好的手段，但这并不是创伤患者常用的静脉插入位点，因为它可能导致颈椎外伤并需要颈环固定。

股静脉插管是另一种可选择的通路，它的急性并发症较少。有可能会发生肠穿孔，特别是对于有股疝的患者。髋关节的渗透可能导致脓毒性关节炎。血栓性动脉炎相较于IJ和锁骨下静脉插管更易发生于股静脉插管。然而，血栓性静脉炎的发生最有可能与长期使用导管有关。

静脉切开时，进行快速、安全、大直径静脉插管是可取的，而经周围或中央通路是不当或不可实现的。应采用严格的无菌技术并戴好外科口罩和帽子。静脉切开处由于解剖学损伤而具有低电位。皮神经损伤是最常见的问题。急性期感染率相对较低，但随着时间的推移，感染率有所增加。因此，一旦通过标准的经皮静脉导管或中央静脉导管完成静脉通路，则建议静脉切开导管可以移除。此外，患者的情况允许的话，在没有严格的无菌技术时，创伤患者的复苏过程中放置的任何线都应尽快被移除。

控制出血的辅助措施

局部出血的控制

许多药剂被用于实现局部止血。此类药物可用于局部或全身止血。局部止血剂包括血管收缩剂，例如肾上腺素和促凝血药，促凝血药包括凝血酶、“止血纤维蛋白”、明胶和纤维素物质。

止血粉是一种新型药物，被设计成诱导与血管病变相关的大伤口的局部止血。它是一种沸石矿物颗粒粉，能增加伤口中凝血因子的浓度。应用于四肢动脉损伤和肝撕裂模型，效果良好。止血粉已经被应用到美国的军事部署中。在最近的研究中，Rhee 等报道了 103 例止血粉使用病例：69 例应用于在伊拉克的美国军队，20 例为平民创伤外科医生使用，14 例为平民最初急救者使用。有 83 例应用于外伤，20 例由军队和平民外科医生应用于体内。总的有效率为 92%。失败出现于严重损伤的患者，在不可能将药物直接送至出血源的情况下作为最后的手段使用。由于止血粉使用时的放热反应，患者会出现轻度至重度疼痛和不适。

全身出血的控制

氨甲环酸

氨甲环酸抑制纤溶酶的生成，它分布于机体所有的组织，它在血浆中的半衰期为 120 min。推荐在其抗纤维蛋白溶解作用的基础上进行使用，可以减少出血和输血的需要。最近出版的 CRASH-2 试验提出氨甲环酸的使用改善了创伤患者的预后。这项研究包括超过 20 000 的大出血或有大出血风险的创伤患者，他们随即分为氨甲环酸治疗组和安慰剂组。氨甲环酸为 1g 的药丸，间隔 8 h 给药。

氨甲环酸治疗组死亡率为 14.5%，相对于安慰剂组的 16%，相对危险度为 0.91（95% 置信区间为 0.85 ~ 0.97；$P=0.0035$）。氨甲环酸组出血相关的死亡率为 4.95%，而安慰剂组为 5.7%。致命或非致命性血管血栓的数目并没有增加。建议有痉挛高风险的患者应该在入院时注射 1 g 氨甲环酸，随后控制超过 8 h 后，连续输入 1 g。对于有纤维蛋白溶解亢进实验室证据的患者，氨甲环酸持续输注应增加至 20 mg/(kg · h)。一旦出血已充分控制，则氨甲环酸治疗应持续。

凝血因子 VIIa

凝血因子Ⅶ a（F Ⅶ a）是在 1999 由美国 FDA 批准用于治疗血友病患者和带有凝血因子Ⅷ和Ⅸ抑制剂患者的出血。然而，与血友病患者不同的是创伤患者的所有凝血因子，以及血红蛋白和血小板整体缺乏。而当对患者进行损伤控制时，使用无标签的 F Ⅶ a 仍然显示出有希望的结果。2005 年的一个包括闭合性和穿通性创伤患者的随机临床研究暗示，虽然重组凝血因子Ⅶ Ia（rF Ⅶ a）显著降低Ⅶ a 患者输血的需求和 ARDS 的发生率，它对总体死亡率没有影响。后续的Ⅲ期随机试验因无效，提前终止（1 502 例患者中的 573 例）。

可能除试验外 F Ⅶ a 最大规模的使用是美国军队在中东冲突时的大量使用。尽管有成功的病例，但给予 rF Ⅶ a 治疗的 506 例患者与对照组相比，进行分析（n = 266 例，每组），发现药物与提升生存率或降低 MT 的需要并没有明显的相关性。其他发现也报道了使用无标签的 rF Ⅶ a 会增加血栓性并发症的风险。

凝血酶原复合物

给使用华法林的创伤患者使用凝血酶原复合物（prothrombin complex concentrates，PCCs）的结果暗示 PCCS 可能是扭转维生素 K 依赖性凝血因子相关的凝血病的一种重要的辅助治疗，特别是对于创伤性脑损伤（traumatic brain injury，TBI）的老年患者。当 PCCS 与标准处理方法［新鲜冰冻血浆（fresh frozen plasma，FFP）或维生素 K］进行比较时，RCT 也在需要外科手术或 TBI 纠正凝血功能障碍的患者中不断进行。

液体复苏的时间和体积

出血无法控制时，给患者静脉注射液体的最佳体积是能达到组织氧输送的改善和由于提高血压所增加的血液流失之间的平衡。通过尝试积极的液体复苏来达到正常的血压应该优先于止血，控制出血有可能加剧血液流失，从而增加死亡风险。对于给失血性休克患者输液的最佳时机的相关知识要追溯到大约 1 个世纪之前，然而研究强调的大量复苏的作用和入院前最佳的液体管理战略存在矛盾。然而，这项工作表明在出血得到控制之前不进行液体复苏并不会增加死亡风险。Cochrane 系统评价数据库也关注出血患者液体复苏时机和体积的问题。他们发现只有 6 个 RCT 未发现任何证据支持（或反对）对未控制出血的患者进行早期或大量静脉补液。基于这些信息，我们有理由建议对没有 TBI 的穿通性损伤患者复苏至一个可容许的较低的血压（低血压复苏），以防止“出现血凝块”，直到手术或局部控制住出血。这一战略和相关器官低灌注对脑损伤的影响表明，应为中枢神经系统（central nervous system，CNS）损伤的患者提供较高的血压终点。

流体类型

类晶体

Shires 最初对晶体体积置换的研究发现，相比于单独使用血液或血浆，晶体体积置换在生存率方面有着令人印象深刻的改善，以至于这些研究数据被飞速地应用于临床实践。然而值得注意的是，在使用乳酸林格氏液扩容和复苏长达半个世纪之后，最近才有研究者提出晶体复苏具有有害作用。这些效应包括免疫功能损伤以及中性粒细胞和其他参与宿主防御机制的细胞的促炎作用的增加。此外，过去 30 年的证据表明过度使用晶体与 ARDS 的出现有关，增加肠道和心脏间质液以及腹部和四肢隔室综合征。最近的一篇综述指出不仅这些积极复苏的有害的临床作用会出现，在此基础上还会出现细胞、代谢和免疫功能的紊乱。晶体的使用正在被重新审视，像任何其他药物一样，液体也须规定出适当的适应证、正确的使用剂量以及可能出现的副作用和并发症。目前的趋势是更具选择性和限制性地使用晶体液，通过血液和血液制品的早期置换限制总体积。测量复苏终点的一种简化的方法是基于适当的脉搏和心理状态而不是一个目标血压，这对限制液体总体积也有一定的作用。在出血得到控制之前限制液体复苏的速度和补液量应该成为大型创伤中心的标准规范。有趣的是，并不是所有的晶体都是一样的，在一个随机对照试验中对比乳酸林格氏液和生理盐水，Waters 等发现生理盐水和出血增加相关。生理盐水治疗组的患者需要更大量的血小板输入（生理盐水组 478 ± 302 ml；乳酸林格氏液组 223 ± 24 ml）。值得注意的是生理盐水治疗组被给予了更多的血液制品（$P = 0.02$）。

胶体

白蛋白

白蛋白在危重症患者中的使用已在 Cochrane 报告中进行了分析。作者对低血容量、烧伤或低白蛋白的危重患者的随机对照试验进行了系统性回顾。这些试验对比了用白蛋白或血浆蛋白治疗患者和用晶体溶液治疗的结果。总共有 1 419 例患者参与 30 个不同的试验进行研究。对于不同的患者组别，白蛋白治疗组的死亡风险均高于对照组。对于低血容量患者，白蛋白处理后相对死亡风险为 1.46（95% 置信区间为 0.97 ~ 2.22），烧伤患者的相对风险为 2.40（1.11 ~ 5.19），低白蛋白血症的相对风险为 1.69（1.07 ~ 2.67）。然而，这篇综述是基于相对较小的样本，只有少数死亡病例。因此，这些结果需要谨慎的解释。最后，生理盐水和白蛋白溶液的安全性评估的试验在澳大利亚和新西兰进行（安全性评估是由澳大利亚和新西兰的重症监护协会临床试验小组合作完成），结果表明 7 000 例患者在双盲随机试验中，生理盐水组和白蛋白组的死亡率和器官衰竭发生率没有区别。治疗低白蛋白血症的患者时，必须努力纠正潜在疾病，而不是主要尝试纠正低白蛋白血症。严重低血容量的创伤患者，使用人血白蛋白快速纠正是不现实的。对比于其他血浆替代品，白蛋白纠正低血容量的创伤患者并未显示出更高的生存率。相反，根据安全性评估试验数据的后续分析，发现相比于非白蛋白治疗组，白蛋白治疗组死亡率明显升高。

人造血浆

人造血浆（Abbott 实验室，北芝加哥，Ill.）是一种改良的，生理性“平衡”的第一代大分子羟乙基淀粉（hydroxyethyl starch，HES）制剂（平均分子量约 670 kDa；MW，550 kDa）。它包含平衡电解质（Na，143 mmol/L；Cl，124 mmol/L；乳酸，28 mmol/L；Ca^{2+}，2.5 mmol/L；K，3 mmol/L；Mg^{2+}，0.45 mmol/L；葡萄糖 5 mmol/L）。人造血浆是目前战场伤亡复苏时选择使用的液体，由于其相较于乳酸林格氏液能更大地影响血管容量。不像以前使用的淀粉制剂，如右旋糖苷或羟乙基淀粉制剂，人造血浆对凝血功能的影响较小，但即使是这个观察结果也是有争议的。动物研究表明，人造血浆在出血或头部损伤合并出血模型中有充足的扩容作用。此外，人造血浆比小淀粉有更有效的扩容作用。临床研究表明，人造血浆以其新颖的缓冲方式平衡电解质配方，与含6%羟乙基淀粉的生理盐水对治疗低血容量，具有同等的疗效。在严重创伤的液体，复苏研究中，在南非一个创伤中心的115例严重闭合性或穿通性创伤患者中，比较了在复苏中使用HES和0.9%生理盐水的区别。两组闭合性创伤患者无明显差异。在穿通性创伤中，HES 130 / 0.4显著降低了机体对液体的需求，但比预期值要小，且没有影响正常胃肠功能。FIRST研究员报告称穿通性创伤患者接受HES治疗后，肾功能和乳酸清除率明显改善。然而有趣的是，他们观察到钝性创伤患者受到HES治疗后，血液制品的输入增加。经HES治疗的钝性创伤患者平均须输入的浓缩红细胞（packed red blood cells，PRBCs）为0.9%生理盐水组的2倍，FFP为3倍，血小板为5倍。遗憾的是，这项研究被发现预设与实际评估终点之间存在差异。此外，研究组的基准匹配较差，样本量小，未能报告关键数据，且在统计分析出现一些不足，使我们难以得出在创伤中使用HES的有效性和安全性的坚定结论。

高渗盐水

高渗盐水的特点是它的渗透性能可以吸引液体进入血管腔内，而额外的右旋糖酐或羟乙基淀粉可以通过结合入体的水分延长它的作用。使用高渗溶液复苏，须按体重快速输入的剂量为4 ml/kg 7.2%～7.5%的氯化钠（NaCl），这相当于一个成年患者须摄入250 ml的制剂。它与胶体溶液结合使用。这种治疗方式已被证明在循环中有快速的疗效。研究表明，高渗盐水似乎优于常规容量治疗，可更快地恢复休克期间的正常微血管灌注和早期的器官功能恢复。头部创伤联合全身性低血压患者尤其受益。

复苏预后联盟，在美国和加拿大9个主要地区形成临床研究中心网络，进行了2次独立试验，研究休克患者和TBI患者的高渗盐水治疗效果。2009年2月停止了对闭合性创伤或穿通性创伤的低血容量休克患者的研究。这项休克的研究是为了确定高渗复苏对低血容量休克的创伤患者生存率的影响。该试验停止是因为相比于生理盐水治疗，受到浓缩盐溶液治疗的患者更没有可能存活，尽管死亡率没有升高，但是浓缩盐溶液治疗组更早地出现死亡。使用相同干预措施研究TBI的平行试验也在2009年5月被停止。本研究旨在确定高渗复苏对长期（6个月）神经系统预后和生存的影响。这项研究被停止是因为已确定高渗盐水的解决方案不优于生理盐水标准治疗，并且继续招收新患者不太可能改变研究结果。

红细胞输血

复苏中决定输血应基于临床评估，可以通过估计损伤机制、失血速度和失血量、心肺储备程度和患者整体的氧气消耗情况来辅助评估。血库以外的任何血液制品的储存是困难的，在许多机构都不太可能实现。因此，根据医生的判断来订购血液制品是存在医生低估输血需求的内在风险的。

在过去40年中，大量出血性创伤患者的输血治疗进展显著。Shires和Carrico于1976年发表了关于休克处理的相关的文献，这也是他们对这一领域作出的最后的贡献。当时他们建议在全血可以获得的情况下适度使用晶体（不超过2 L）。同时，血液成分疗法开始被推广，血库开始从血液中分离所有成分。没有进行任何研究，也基本没有循证医学的依据的情况下，美国大多数急救部门开始使用PRBCs代替全血。多年来只有共计不超过80例患者的3个关于创伤患者治疗中血液制品所扮演的角色的临床研究被发表了。ATLS建议对创伤患者血浆的使用应参考1985年Lucas等提出的FFP和PRBCs 1 ∶ 3的比例。该研究阐述了PRBCs的局限性和不足，描述了存放24 h后PRBCs氧气输送效率的降低，每输入1单位的PRBCs，在老化细胞中钾和白细胞介素-8的浓度升高、凝血因子消失MODS发生的概率增加。

回顾之前的发现，无意的血液稀释、晶体的过度使用，以及过度复苏导致的ARDS和腹腔隔室综合征都可能与输血治疗的时间相关，可能全血已经不再有效。

对真实的创伤引发的凝血功能障碍的发病率的了解以及“损伤控制复苏”概念的介绍已经彻底改变了现在对创伤患者以及其他情况下严重急性出血患者的治疗。伊拉克和阿富汗战争后，公布了以下基本原则：①避免晶体复苏；②尽可能在情况允许下维持低血压；③通过血液制品的早期使用防止凝血功能障碍；④积极打破酸中毒、凝血功能障碍和低温的恶性循环。

根据战场经验，美国军队现在为战争中使

用超过10单位PRBCs（MT）的患者制定了PRBC：FFP：血小板应用比例为1：1：1的策略。然而并没有设计较好的随机对照试验可以明确血液成分的最佳配比。

2006年，一篇国际性输血指南证实只有10个出版物描述了如何进行大量输血。自那以后，许多证实大量输血具有治疗功效的研究开始出现。一项历史对照研究由Cotton公布，它对比了在输血后94例患者在18个月期间的死亡率和相似患者在之前18个月的匹配队列的死亡率。研究发现，按照指南操作可以减少30天死亡率（51% vs. 66%，$P<0.03$），减少术中晶体使用（4.9 L vs. 6.7 L，P＝0.002），并且可以降低术后血液制品的使用（2.8U PRBCs vs. 8.7U RBCs；1.7U FFP vs. 7.9U FFP；0.9U 血小板 vs. 5.7U 血小板）。

虽然需要进一步的前瞻性研究才能确定精确的比例，但已有令人信服的证据表明，血液成分输入的标准操作规程的执行有助于改善治疗过程，减少整体血液成分的使用，并可以改善预后。

血液替代品

只有通过管理PRBCs才能恢复携氧能力，但它们的供应是有限的，并且它们的使用会带来广泛的不利影响，包括免疫调节。19世纪30年代开始，人们尝试发展人工携氧载体。最大的障碍是其基质污染的毒性作用。基于血红蛋白的人工氧载体的血红蛋白分子须更具稳定性，以防止α2β2-血红蛋白四聚体解离。这样可以使其在血管内滞留时间延长，消除其肾毒性。

早期的血液替代品的制剂被发现只有有限的价值。严重的不良反应包括高血压、心肌损伤和血管并发症。几种产品开始产生，包括琥珀酰水杨酸交联血红蛋白（HemAssist）、重组人血红蛋白（rhb1.1和rhb2.0）、聚合牛血红蛋白携氧载体（HBOC-201）、人多聚血红蛋白（PolyHeme）、血红蛋白类携氧剂（Hemolink），以及马来酰亚胺活化的聚乙二醇修饰的血红蛋白（MP4）。

PolyHeme的最近的研究表明在PolyHeme治疗组中，心肌梗死的发病率有所升高。一个盲法的析因分析召募患者，来客观地确定是否在每个真正遭受心肌梗死的患者中，都能发现PolyHeme与心肌梗死无关联。然而，因为有出现更严重的不良反应的趋势，本试验公布后，PolyHeme没有获得FDA的批准。Northfield实验室随后宣布破产，停止生产和检测PolyHeme。

血液替代品的发展旨在克服这些限制。MP4的研究在欧洲完成选择性关节成形术的患者中完成，MP4研究组与对照组相比，具有类似的不良反应发生率。然而，最近没有在严重出血的创伤患者中使用MP4的研究。

药物疗法

抗利尿激素

抗利尿激素的出现是各种休克情况治疗的一个潜在的重大进展。抗利尿激素在临床上的使用日渐增多，这是由于人们对它在休克内源性反应中的重要性和它的作用机制有了认识。相比于血管扩张性休克时肾上腺素的使用，抗利尿激素可以产生更多的血液分流，使血液从非重要性器官流向重要器官。正常情况下，抗利尿激素没有或有很少的升压作用，并且由于其他不受监管的激素释放的影响使血浆中抗利尿激素明显升高（即抗利尿激素分泌不当综合征）也不会导致高血压。

抗利尿激素在休克中的可能作用可能与其对血管平滑肌的作用有关。抗利尿激素可以抑制三磷酸腺苷－敏感性钾（K^+ATP）通道和一氧化氮诱导的环鸟苷酸的累积。Landry等已经表明激活的K^+ATP通道促进多种类型休克中的低血压，包括失血性休克。此外，NO合成的激活也促进这种情况下的低血压。因此，抗利尿激素抑制在失血性休克后期促进低血压和血管低反应性形成的血管舒张作用。低动脉压是抗利尿激素分泌的主要刺激，刺激主要通过主动脉和颈动脉窦的动脉压力感受器起作用。如果中心静脉压降低，那么这些受体首先刺激促尿钠排泄因子分泌、交感神经系统和肾素分泌。当动脉血压降低到一定程度不再能通过血管压力感受器的主导作用进行代偿时，抗利尿激素开始分泌。抗利尿激素增强儿茶酚胺的血管加压功效。然而，在冠状动脉和脑血管区域它具有的更大的优势是可使血管收缩不明显。它可使肾功能改善，尽管这些数据还有待证实。它对人体内其他区域的循环的作用还有待进一步明确。

新的治疗可能：低温和失血性休克

失血性休克时出现的低温状态是一把双刃剑。实验室研究不断发现轻度（33℃ ~36℃）至中度（28℃ ~32℃）低温可提高失血性休克的生存率。相反，回顾以往的临床试验表明，低温的创伤患者相较于正常体温的患者会出现更严重的损伤和更高的死亡率。

实验室研究已经证明了失血性休克过程中低温对个体器官以及整个机体的有益作用。例如，Mizushima 等发现相较于维持正常体温或长时间低温，大鼠失血性休克过程中维持轻度低温状态，并在复苏后复温，可以使左室功能和心排血量最佳。Meyer 和 Horton 同样发现在狗的失血性休克过程中，低温较常温可以保持更好的心脏性能。它们也表现出生存率的升高。Wu 等在大鼠模型研究中发现在失血性休克过程中模拟暴露在低温环境中的患者，相较于复苏过程中积极地复温的患者，冷却后维持低温状态更加有益。轻度低温在长时间的失血性休克中也有益处。

临床上回顾以往的研究，Luna 等和 Jurkovich 等表示低温的创伤患者较正常体温的创伤患者死亡风险增加。因为越严重的创伤患者更可能出现低温，很难将低温的作用与其他混杂因素分离开，例如休克的程度、损伤的严重程度、液体和血液制品输入的体积，以及手术的需要。最近 Wang 等进行了一个全亚洲的大型数据回顾性分析，得出入院后体温在 35℃或以下与死亡风险的增加独立相关（OR = 3）。

唯一关于创伤患者体温管理的前瞻性试验由 Gentilello 等完成。低温创伤患者被随机分为在 ICU 进行标准复温措施的一组和使用逆流换热器（Ⅰ级技术，罗克兰，马萨诸塞）通过经动静脉持续性血液复温法（continuous arteriovenous rewarming，CAVR）进行更积极复温的一组。CAVR 组复温速度更快，并且所需的液体量更少，但两者的院内死亡率却相似。

想要了解失血性休克的实验室研究和创伤患者的临床发现之间的区别，我们须考虑到在创伤患者中十分常见的不受控的暴露性低温，与寒战和交感神经反应阻断的受控的治疗性低温在生理上的区别。另一个问题是低温时潜在的凝血功能障碍，除非体温低于 34℃，否则临床上不会出现明显变化。

总结

失血性休克是一种复杂的综合征，其临床表现可能与损伤程度和复苏类型或缺乏复苏相关。从损伤至明确的复苏中针对许多治疗窗口的创新性干预措施是有效的，且已经被讨论。在这方面的积极研究将带来新的突破，并让人们更好地了解这个复杂的疾病。

失血过多综合征：控制损伤的可靠模型

Juan A. Asensio, Robert Bertelotti, Federico N. Mazzini, José Ceballos Esparragon, Chris Okwuosa, Steven Cheung, Riaan Pretorius, Luis Manuel García-Núñez 和 Alicia M. Mohr 著
朱凤雪　李　纾 译

失血过多已被定义为一种极端的持续出血形式，如果不通过手术控制，会导致死亡。失血过多是仅次于神经损伤的引起创伤患者死亡的原因。因此，失血过多的创伤患者从入院前、急诊、手术室到 ICU 的移动速度对生存率至关重要。失血过多的症状由 Asensio 进行描述。损伤的特定情况和复杂性需要损伤控制，以避免失血过多。本章将主要介绍可用于术前和术中，以改善预后效果的敏感指标。本章还将概括当前创伤患者损伤控制相关规定的指南。本章的重点是介绍当前重要研究定义的损伤控制指标。对这些准则的认识可以改善主要脏器损伤和出血的预后，并且有助于防治广为人知的损伤控制的后遗症的—创伤后开腹。

发展史

20 世纪 80 年代初，创伤后救助 / 损伤控制外科

手术已成为外科实践中的一大进展。损伤控制外科手术未遵循传统手术教学中的明确的手术治疗流程，并慢慢地开始被人们采用。目前，损伤控制技术被创伤外科医生们改良已成功应用于胸腹部外伤、下肢外伤，以及周围血管损伤。此外，损伤控制手术已经被外推至应用于全身、血管、心脏、泌尿科，以及骨科手术。

1983 年，Stone 等首次提出了对严重损伤患者实施分期手术的“紧急救援”办法。这种方法的出现是由于他们观察到早期的创伤引起的死亡与机体代谢和生理紊乱伴随大量失血的损伤有关。在创伤和急诊手术中，大量输血超过 2 单位血容量后，严重的机体生理功能紊乱随之出现，并且死亡率大于 60%。严重的休克伴随大量血液丢失导致了低温、酸中毒和凝血功能障碍的恶性循环。正是此时，低温、酸中毒和凝血功能障碍被称为“创伤死亡三角”或“血腥的恶性循环。”Asensio 后来补充的第 4 个要素是心律失常，这通常预示着患者的死亡。凝血功能障碍、酸中毒和低温使创伤患者长时间的确定性的手术治疗危险性增加。这种新的方法，现在被称为“损伤控制，”它描述了多个手术阶段，在纠正机体生理异常后继续手术。

代谢障碍

体温过低是严重的失血性损伤和随后复苏的后果。严重的出血导致组织低灌注和氧输送不足，从而减少热量的产生。如果体温降至低于 36℃超过 4 h，此为临床上具有重要意义的低温。低温可导致心律失常、心排血量减少、全身血管阻力增加以及血红蛋白氧解离曲线左移。低温对心肌具有负性肌力作用，可使左室收缩功能减弱。低温时，最初看到的心电图的改变是窦性心动过速，但随着核心温度的降低，开始出现渐进性心动过缓。低温时心脏对儿茶酚胺的反应也会减弱，并且低温下心脏组织几乎不耐受高血容量或低血容量。低温还会导致凝血功能障碍，抑制凝血级联反应、血小板激活和血小板功能。低温还会损伤宿主免疫功能。由于环境因素或手术干预导致的热量损失会使低温加剧。治疗创伤患者的多学科团队必须尽力减少热量丢失，以及帮助纠正低温。

超过 25% 的创伤患者在入院时表现出明显的凝血功能障碍，它使患者死亡的风险增加了 3 倍。严重创伤患者的凝血功能障碍的病因是多因素的，包括血小板和凝血因子的消耗与稀释，以及血小板和凝血系统功能障碍。临床凝血功能障碍的发生是由于低温，低温时血小板和凝血因子功能异常、纤维溶解系统激活、大量复苏后血液稀释。血小板功能障碍继发于血栓素和前列环素在低温状态下的失衡。低温和血液稀释对凝血功能障碍产生叠加效应。置换 1 单位血容量（5 000 ml 或 15 单位浓缩红细胞）后只有 30% ~ 40% 的血小板保留在循环中。因此凝血酶原时间（prothrombin time，PT）、部分促凝血酶原时间（partial thromboplastin time，PTT）、纤维蛋白原水平和乳酸水平不能预测严重凝血功能障碍。

低灌注的重复性及持续性发作导致的主要生理缺陷是代谢性酸中毒。当休克期间持续灌注不足时，无氧代谢开始，导致乳酸的产生。酸中毒降低心肌收缩力、心排血量、功能性血栓的风险，以及栓子强度。酸中毒也会由于多次输血、使用血管加压药、十字钳夹主动脉和心肌功能受损而恶化。很显然，在酸中毒、低温、凝血功能障碍和各因素相互的作用之间存在复杂的关系，一旦恶性循环发生并且没有中断的话，则会导致死亡率明显升高。

损伤控制模型

Stone 等在 1983 年的原始论著中只提及将术中观察到凝血功能障碍作为紧急救治的指征。在这项研究中，17 例患者接受紧急救治程序，包括一个初始的剖腹手术。之后是观察患者的临床凝血功能障碍的情况，一旦凝血功能障碍得到改善就继续进行手术操作。这使得最终有 11 名幸存者，死亡率为 35%。随后，Rotondo 等描述了对腹部损伤且失血过多的患者进行治疗的多阶段方法，但在术中损伤控制过程中没有定义任何客观的参数。作者报告了一个非常小的亚组其中患者的生存率为 77%。这组患者主要是血管损伤和 2 个或 2 个以上的身体损伤。Burch 等提出了一种核心温度为 32℃或更低、pH 值为 7.09 或更小，以及 PRBCs 输血超过 22 单位的模型，预测患者可以存活 48 h。作者还描述了“致死三联征”。一个包括 39 例患者的研究中，Sharp 定义了一个温度 33℃或更低，pH 值为 7.18 或更小，PT 为 16 s 或更长，PTT 为 50 s 或更长，以及输血超过 10 单位 PRBCs 的目标参数，以表明早期填塞的需要。

Morris 等描述了 107 例患者，他们进行了剖腹探查和腹部填塞。他们提出在患者体温小于 35℃，BD 大于 14 mEq/L，并存在凝血功能障碍性出血的基础上，在手术过程中进行早期损伤控制。同样，Moore 描述了渐进性凝血功能障碍是剖腹手术最具说服力的理由。严重的凝血功能障碍的状态被描述为 PT 和 PTT 大于正常值的 2 倍、4 h 内大量快速输血超过 10 单位。持续性休克被定义为氧消耗小于 110 ml/min · m^2、乳酸水平大于 5 mmol/L、pH 值小于 7.2、BD 大于 14 mEq/L，以及核心低体温低于 34℃。推测凝血功能障碍发病的能力对建立损伤控制具有重要意义。另一个危及生命的凝血功能障碍预测模型包括收缩压低于 70 mmHg，温度高于 34℃，pH 值小于 7.10，以及 ISS 大于等于 25。

没有一个单一的模型能够准确地预测损伤控制应该建立的时间。pH 值小于 7.1 或核心温度低于 33℃可以表明“出血的恶性循环”已经到晚期，不能中断。同样地，在所有医院我们都很难在术中获得 PT、PTT、纤维蛋白原，以及乳酸水平，或在手术室放置 Swan-Ganz 导管。

定义失血过多和死亡风险最高的患者时，必须确定 pH、温度阈值水平，以及评估的最大失血量。因此，为了制订“损伤控制 / 救治”的术中指南，Asensio 首次回顾性评估了 6 年内 548 例由于诊断失血过多而收入大型城市创伤中心的患者。入选标准为术中失血大于 2 000 ml，在最初复苏过程中最低输血需求量大于 1 500 ml PRBCs，并诊断为失血过多。须收集的数据包括人口统计数据、院前急救及入院时的生命体征和预后的生理预测因子、修正创伤评分（Revised Trauma Score，RTS）、格拉斯哥昏迷等级评分（Glasgow Coma Scale，GCS）评分、ISS、复苏液体的体积、EDT 的需要、手术室的补液量、在手术室行开胸术（thoracotomy in the operating room，ORT）的需要以及术中并发症。在这些患者人群中，RTS 为 4.38，平均 ISS 为 32，表示患者具有生理缺陷并且受到严重损伤。其中 180 例患者在 EDT 进行了主动脉钳夹十字和开放式心肺复苏术（cardiopulmonary resuscitation，CPR），99（55%）例患者在急救中死亡。除了 81 例患者行 EDT 后幸存，117 例患者须行 ORT。共计 198 例患者要行 EDT 和 ORT，其中 56 例患者（28%）存活，离开了手术室和医院。在这一系列流程中，记录的 pH 平均值为 7.15，在手术室的平均体温为 34.3℃，这些患者平均接收了 14 165 ml 的晶体、血液以及血液制品。总体来看，449 例患者存活至到达手术室并有生命体征，281 例患者死亡。其中 37% 的患者在损伤控制后存活。表 1 记录了客观的术中参数以预测预后情况，并基于现有的发现为何时建立损伤控制提供指导方针。这一系列试验也提供了影响生存率的独立风险因子，其中包括 ISS 小于 20、急诊室自主通风、未进行 EDT 或 ORT，以及未出现腹部血管损伤。本文全面介绍了失血过多的综合征以及损伤的指标。这些观点后来也得到了其他人的证实。

损伤控制后存活的患者的后遗症之一为腹部的伤口。这些指导意见前瞻性地在 139 例经历了损伤控制和创伤后开腹的患者身上得到了验证。本研究包括 2 组患者：86 例患者在制订指南之前进行回顾性研究，53 例患者在制订指南之后进行前瞻性研究。两组之间就所有相关参数进行比较。尽管两组之间死亡率并没有明显差别（每组为 24%），术中输血次数差异有统计学意义。预期组患者低温和肠水肿更少，术后感染和胃肠道并发症更少，ICU 和医院治疗时间更短。这项研究中的另一个重要发现是 93% 的患者能够在住院期间接受确定性腹部闭合手术，而之前的数据统计只有 22% 的患者可以。

进行损伤控制之前了解潜在触发因素的伤害是至关重要的。对 68 例经历损伤控制性手术的患者的研究发现无法将 pH 值纠正至大于 7.21 以及 PTT 大于 78.7 s 者，预测死亡率为 100%。此外，体温小于 32℃和年龄增长可以在损伤控制后独立预测死亡率。为了在损伤控制后尝试预测预后情况，Karirinos 提出了以下损伤控制的方程：

$$x=(0.012)\mathrm{Age}-(0.707)\mathrm{pH}-(0.032)\mathrm{Temperature}+6.002.$$

如果 x 大于 0.5，那么更可能发生死亡。同样，Ordonez 发明了死亡率的临床预测模型预测死亡率，

表 1　评估损伤控制需求的生理指标

低温 34℃
酸中毒 pH 7.2
血清碳酸氢盐 15 mEq/L
输血 4 000 ml PRBCs
输入 5 000 ml 血和血液制品
术中容量置换 12 000 ml
术中凝血功能障碍的临床证据

结合使用ICU记录的pH值、低温、24 h内PRBC的输注量，以及年龄。推迟承认对伤害控制的需要以及与麻醉和护理团队沟通不畅，对护理多发伤患者来说都是十分不利的。

患者选择

并非所有的创伤患者都需要损伤控制措施。除了损伤控制机制的生理指证（表2），在术前和术中对某些条件和复杂性的损伤进行评估，决定是否须进行伤害控制（表2）。多个大规模伤残和EDT须评估是否需要损伤控制。在持续腹部损伤的多发伤患者中，须及时地评估其他腹外伤害，这也表明须进行损伤控制。失血过多的患者相较于幸存者，术前低血压（收缩压<90 mmHg）持续时间有显著差别（45 min vs.85 min）。因此，除去其他因素，例如术前对低温和凝血功能障碍的评估，持续性低血压超过60 min表明须进行损伤控制。术中，某些复杂的损伤也预示着需要这项技术。这些损伤包括腹部大血管听见伤、复杂的肝损伤、胸部大血管损伤以及术中胸部切口。

表2 提示须进行损伤控制的术前和术中状态

术前	术中
多个大规模伤残	需要术中开胸术
多系统创伤伴大的腹部损伤	腹部血管损伤
骨盆开放性骨折伴腹部损伤	胸部血管损伤
腹部损伤并须进行腹外损伤评估	严重的复杂肝损伤
创伤性截肢伴腹部损伤	持续性低血压
需要 EDT	凝血功能障碍
持续性低血压	低温
凝血功能障碍	
低温	
血管栓塞的辅助使用	

失血过多的患者也许是接受损伤控制的最佳人选。Asensio提出了关于失血过多的防治流程，涉及3个阶段（图1）。第一，将患者归类为失血过多；第二，根据ATLS的指南开始进行复苏（图1）。须手术控制出血的患者开始进行损伤控制复苏和进行大量输血。这是一个分为3部分的损伤控制复苏，结合高血浆和血小板的比例、允许性低血压，以及

1期
- 根据失血过多将患者分类
- 血流动力学不稳定
- 初始失血量 >40%
- 大规模的持续失血
- 损伤易出现失血过多

2期
- 根据 ATLS 指南进行复苏
- 晶体 2～3 L（乳酸林格氏液）
- 血液（无交叉反应、特定类型或交叉反应）
- 湿热液体的快速输入
- 确定 EDT 和胸主动脉交叉钳夹的必要性

3期
- 更便捷的方法
- 确定 ORT 和主动脉交叉钳夹的必要性
- 控制出血源
- 使用辅助技术
  - 快速输液器
  - 自身输血
  - 填塞
  - 分流
  - 损伤控制
- 防止低温和凝血功能障碍
- 适当补充血液和血液制品

图1 失血过多的防治流程。ATLS, 高级创伤生命支持；ED，急诊；OR，手术室

有限的晶体后，发现选择的创伤患者生率出现上升。第三个阶段须快速将患者转运至手术室（穿通性损伤导致的失血过多是一种引人关注的疾病，它的防治要医务人员具有领导能力、敏捷的思维、积极的手术干预能力和深思熟虑的计划）。快速的损伤控制手术和损伤控制复苏可以有效地处理失血过多，提高患者生存率。

损伤控制技术

早期进行损伤控制的首要目标是患者的生存率。Johnson等最近在一个含有24例患者的研究中定义了一个四阶段的损伤控制方法，这些患者经历了损伤控制并与经历了十年前由Rotondo等提出的损伤控制方法的患者进行比较研究（图2）。“零级”阶段包括入院前阶段和急诊室的早期复苏。零级阶段包括医护人员在现场的短暂时间和在急诊室中根据损伤模式鉴别是否须进行损伤控制和在创伤中心进行损伤控制复苏和复温治疗。

损伤控制意味着快速控制危及生命的出血、通过快速的切除或闭合控制胃肠道的感染、使用腔内分流器、通过临时腹腔关闭进行谨慎的腹部填塞。特别是

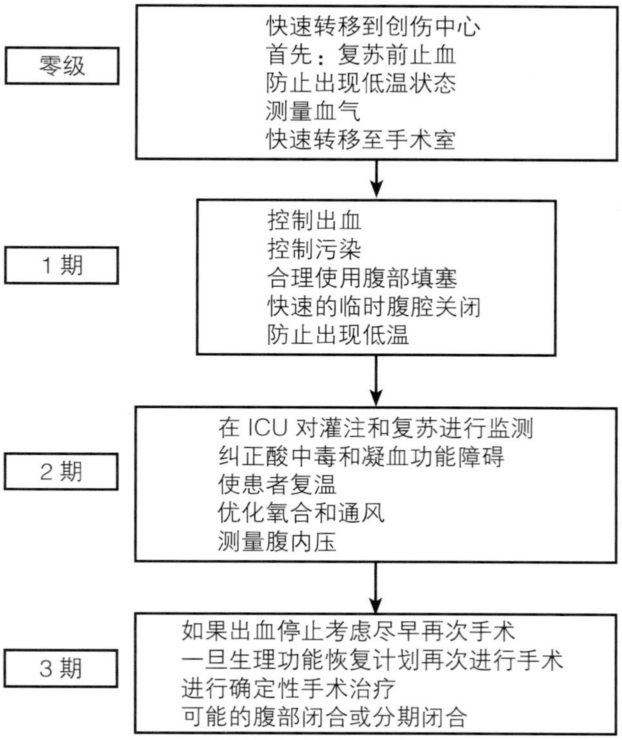

图 2　损伤控制的 4 个阶段。ICU, 重症监护病房；OR，手术室

胸部损伤时，应进行心血管损伤的修复，如 Asensio 所描述的进行使用吻合器的肺神经束切断术。如果需要的话可以进行填塞，放置胸管并缝合皮肤。针对腹部损伤，损伤控制涉及控制大出血、肝的填塞、胰管引流、快速的吻合切除、脾切除术、肾切除术、血管蒂原位夹持，以及使用腹腔内血管分流器。通常，这些患者患有腹腔隔室综合征。因此，创伤后开腹后临时腹腔关闭被用作损伤控制的延伸。在手术室的最短时间是非常重要的，并进行分期手术。

第二阶段始于 ICU，在这里患者的代谢紊乱得到纠正。复温的患者优先进行损伤控制，因为只有当体温恢复正常，凝血功能障碍和酸中毒才能被纠正或维持。损伤控制性复苏持续进行，晶体被慎重地使用。然后进一步检查，以确定在初步筛查中没有被检测到的损伤。24 ~ 72 h 内须纠正代谢紊乱。

损伤控制的最后一个阶段涉及当关键的步骤被执行后再次手术的时机。如果大出血持续的话，须考虑早期再手术，通常在代谢紊乱的纠正和全身炎症反应综合征或多器官功能衰竭发生之间有一个窗口期，是初始损伤后 36 ~ 48 h。在这个时期，关键的步骤被执行。全面的再次探查是为了检测一些额外的损伤并进行胃肠道连续性恢复与血管恢复。可以放置临时进食通道，其次是腹腔冲洗并试图确定性关闭腹腔。患者再返回 ICU 作进一步护理。

结论

失血过多的防治需要领导力、敏捷的思维、积极的手术干预和周密的计划。需要 MT 的创伤性失血过多的患者有遭受酸中毒、低温和凝血功能障碍的多因素相互作用的极大的风险。最终的目标是及时和有效地控制出血源。推迟进行损伤控制会导致更高的发病率和死亡率。因此，损伤控制是多发伤患者进行治疗的重要部分，应该在代谢衰竭之前进行。

损伤控制复苏：一项基于证据的报道

Juan C. Duchesne, Chrissy Guidry, Louis A. Aliperti, Lance E. Stuke 和 Norman E. McSwain, Jr. 著
张　茂 译

在过去的几年，损伤控制复苏（damage control resuscitation，DCR）成为越来越热门的话题。40% 的创伤患者的死因是创伤导致的继发性出血，它同时也是可避免死亡的创伤患者死亡的首要原因。目前 DCR 在军事和民用方面的研究很多，研究的主要方向集中于提高严重出血患者的生存率。应该强调的是，大多数创伤患者并不需要 DCR，它大多数时候是用在损伤最严重的患者身上。对于这些患者，快速和有效地控制出血和纠正急性创伤性休克凝血功能障碍是非常关键的。

大量输血方案（massive transfusion protocol，MTP）的目标是使用新鲜冰冻血浆（fresh frozen plasma，FFP）、血小板（Plts）和浓缩红细胞（packed red blood cells，PRBCs）以接近 1 : 1 : 1 的输注比例进行复苏。早期和持续使用 FFP 的过程中还须补充纤维蛋白原和凝血因子。在一系列数学研究中，Hirshberg 等指出，在复苏过程中使用超过 5 单位的

PRBCs 将会导致稀释性凝血功能障碍，并且校正该凝血功能障碍的理想方式是以 2∶3 的比例补充 FFP 和 PRBCs。Ho 等的另一项研究表明，当凝血因子缺乏时，每单位的 PRBCs 输注必须给予 1 ~ 1.5 单位的 FFP。

应该强调的是，仅仅补充 FFP 不能纠正创伤患者因严重出血而引起的凝血功能障碍。数量上和质量上的血小板功能障碍在凝血机制中也占有至关重要的地位。虽然不像 FFP 一样被广泛研究，但是作为输血方案的一部分，补充血小板也被用来研究，以确定 Plt 与 PRBCs 的最有效输注比例。Hirshberg 等提出，当 Plt ∶ PRBCs 的比例为 8 ∶ 10 时，能有效地防止血小板被稀释到止血阈值以下。须注意的是上述两个研究都是理论模型，没有考虑到诸如低体温、酸中毒、血小板减少症和急性创伤休克性凝血功能障碍等因素的影响。Hirschberg 等和 Hoetal 提出的关于补充 FFP 和血小板的这些量化方案已经被全世界的大量输血方案所参考和采纳。

历史上，很早之前就有对小样本患者的研究来确定输血方案。更多的原始数据是从战争中获得的，尤其是美军在“伊拉克自由行动和持久自由行动”中获得了很多数据。此外，许多民间机构也已开始在大量输血方案中应用 DCR。然而，不同的民间机构的大量输血方案存在差异，产生差异的原因可能最终来源于患者群体的变异，尤其是损伤机制的复杂性。

创伤患者的大量输血已被确定为预测多器官功能衰竭（multiple organ failure，MOF）和全身性炎症反应综合征发生、损伤后感染率增加和死亡率升高的独立因素。然而，在这些患者中，大量晶体液复苏相关的并发症不能被忽视，包括心脏和肺的并发症、腹腔隔室综合征、凝血功能障碍，以及免疫和炎症介质功能障碍。我们在此提供一些有循证医学证据的关于血液制品输注的相关文献，并总结了最新的观察性试验，包括并发症、死亡率、复苏中血液制品的特殊输注比例、输血时间和总体输血的影响。

证据分类

本文采纳了 57 篇文献，这些文献时间跨度从 1985 年到 2011 年，根据脑与创伤基金会的质量评估方法和美国东部创伤外科协会（www.east.org）接受的情况，将它们以科学证据的强度分为 Ⅰ 到 Ⅲ 类。文章概述在本章的附录中，可以在网上找到。评估的依据包括输注血液制品的比例、输血量、输血时间、与输血相关的并发症发生率和死亡率、大量输血方案和生存偏倚等。分析后，根据脑与创伤基金改进、东部创伤外科协会应用的质量评估工具被分为 3 个级别。

Ⅰ 类：前瞻性随机对照试验，这是临床试验的金标准。然而，一些前瞻性随机对照试验因为设计不良、数量不足或方法学上的不足并不具有临床意义，只有 1 项 Ⅰ 类研究被采纳。

Ⅱ 类：基于明显可靠数据的前瞻性和回顾性分析。这些类型的研究包括观察性研究、队列研究、现患调查和病例对照研究。在这一类别中有 17 项研究，其中 10 项涉及前瞻性收集数据的回顾性综述，7 项前瞻性研究。

Ⅲ 类：大多数回顾性收集数据试验。这一类使用的证据包括临床系列、数据库或注册表、病例综述、病例报告和专家意见。在这一类别中采纳了 41 个研究。

证据报告

新鲜冰冻血浆与浓缩红细胞的比例

最佳的 FFP∶PRBCs 的比值在大量输血和损伤控制复苏领域尚未有定论。而数学模型确定最佳的 FFP ∶ PRBCs 比例在 1∶1 至 2∶3 之间。这些数学模型被归为 Ⅲ 类证据，以指导临床应用。

人们确定 FFP∶PRBCs 最佳比例的研究方法有所不同。Sperry 等将患者分为两组（2 组均须输注 >8 单位的 PRBCs），第一组接受超过 1∶1.5 的 FFP∶PRBCs 输注，第二组则小于 1∶1.5 的 FFP∶PRBCs。FFP∶PRBCs 比例为 1∶1.5 或更高的患者死亡的风险显著降低，特别是受伤后 48 h 内死亡率显著下降。Gunter 等进行了一项包含 259 名患者的回顾性观察性研究，通过比较接受高比例和低比例 FFP∶PRBCs 的患者，发现其比例为 2∶3 或更高的患者可以明显地改善死亡率（30 天死亡率分别为 41% 和 62%，P=0.008，）。Shaz 等证实了高 FFP∶PRBCs 输注比例的患者 30 天生存率为 59%，而低 FFP∶PRBCs 输注比例的患者为 44%（P=0.03）。

有 18 个 Ⅲ 类研究来解决 FFP∶PRBCs 比的问题。Kashuk 等比较了输注不同比例的 FFP∶PRBCs（1∶1、1∶2、1∶3、1∶4 和 >1∶5）的患者的死亡率，发现输血比范围为1∶2至1∶3之间的死亡率最低。其他针对平民的研究将患者分为接受低比例和高比例两组，发现接受高FFP∶PRBCs比例的患者表现出较低的死亡风险和较高的生存率。Holcomb等将接受高比例FFP∶PRBC和Plt∶PRBCs的患者和低比例者进行比较，发现接受高比例者的30天生存率显著提高了59.6%，而低比例只有40.4%（$P<0.01$）。Duchesne等的纵向研究调查了止血复苏在创伤诱发凝血功能障碍中的作用。接受超过10单位PRBCs且FFP∶PRBCs比例为1∶1的患者与比例为1∶4者比较时，死亡率存在显著差异（28.2% vs. 51.1%，$P = 0.03$）。此外，接受FFP∶PRBCs比例为1∶1比1∶4的住院患者的重症监护病房住院时间（length of stay，LOS）更短（10天vs. 23天，$P<0.01$）。总共有6个其他Ⅲ类研究比较了输注3种或更多种FFP∶PRBCs比例的影响。这些研究表明，高比例FFP∶PRBCs输注患者的死亡率有所改善。只有一项Teixeira等的研究表明，任何FFP∶PRBCs比例高于1∶3的血液制品输注似乎对提高生存率没有优势。

血小板与浓缩红细胞的比例

创伤患者中Plt和PRBCs的使用也有所不同。Hirshberg等的在前述的数学模型中指出最佳的Plt∶PRBCs的比例为8∶10。Gunter等将患者分成2组，接受Plt∶PRBCs的比例大于1∶5或小于1∶5，发现那些接受1∶5或更高比例的患者，30天死亡率更低。由此证明输注高比例Plt∶PRBCs可以作为生存率的独立预测因子。

4个Ⅲ类研究讨论了有关Plt∶PRBCs的比例问题。Shaz等将患者分为2组：①接受Plt∶PRBCs比例高于1∶2；②接受其比例低于1∶2的。接受高比例者与低比例者相比，30天生存率明显改善（63% vs. 33%，$P<0.01$）。第二个Ⅲ类研究，Perkins等将患者分为3类：①Plt∶PRBCs比例高于1∶8的；②1∶16和1∶8之间的；③低于1∶16的。3组患者的24 h生存率分别为95%、87%和64%（$P<0.001$），显然接受高比例血小板输注的患者24生存率更高。另外，接受高或中等比例组的患者比低比例组者，30天生存率更高（为75%和60% vs. 43%，$P<0.001$）。在Holcomb等的一项包含16个一级创伤中心和466名大量输血患者的FFP∶PRBCs和Plt∶PRBCs比例的更大范围的研究中，他们发现接受高Plt∶PRBC比例组治疗的患者比低比例组具有更高的30天生存率（59.9% vs. 40.1%，$P<0.01$）。然后，他们观察了由以下患者组成的4组：①高FFP和高血小板比例；②高FFP和低血小板比例；③低FFP和高血小板比例；④低FFP和低血小板比例。他们注意到高FFP和高血小板组与其他组相比，6 h、24 h和30天生存率显著增加。有趣的是，他们发现高FFP和高血小板比例组与低FFP和高血小板比例组之间，30天生存率没有差异。Inabaet发现随着Plt∶PRBCs比例的增加，生存率逐步改善。高Plt∶PRBCs比例与24 h生存率独立相关。

输血单位的量

几项研究表明，每增加1单位输注的PRBCs也预示着并发症风险的增加。增加FFP∶PRBCs和Plt∶PRBCs比例可以减少PRBCs的总量，同时可以降低院内并发症的发生率。57项研究中的4项表明，在大量输血过程中，输注较高比例的FFP∶PRBCs患者可以减少输血的总量。Cotton等证实，根据创伤输血方案（包括6单位的PRBCs，4单位的解冻血浆和2单位同一供体血小板）治疗的患者的24 h血液制品使用量，比未按照方案进行输血的患者使用的血液制品明显减少（31.8 ± 19vs. 39 ± 29，$P<0.017$）。Sperry等在他们的Ⅱ类研究中表明，接受FFP∶PRBCs比例大于和小于1∶1.5的两组患者中，比例较大组在24 h内输血液制品的需求明显下降（16 ± 9单位vs. 22 ± 17单位，P=0.001）。先前描述的Zink等的Ⅲ类研究表明，在前6 h中接受比例小于1∶1FFP∶PRBCs的血液创伤输注的患者在前24 h内需要PRBCs单位的中位数为18，而接受比例大于1∶1者只需要13单位的PRBCs（$P<0.001$）。Arulselvi等观察研究了3个方面：①需要输血的患者占创伤患者的94%；②输注血液制品的比例为3 PRBCs∶2FFP∶1Plt；③计算交叉配型量和输血量的比值（C∶T比例）。关于PRBCs的C∶T比例，在206例钝伤患者中，交叉配型953单位的PRBCs，仅输血450单位（C∶T比例为2∶1）。对于146例穿通性创伤患者，交叉配型612单位的PRBCs，输血248单位，C∶T比值为2∶4。因此，在这项研究中，无论钝伤患者还是穿通性创伤患者，交叉配型2单位的红细胞，仅有1单位被实际应用。

血小板、纤维蛋白原和抗纤维蛋白溶解剂的应用

在57篇论文中，有一项Ⅲ类研究，对象为大量输血的战伤患者，该研究是回顾性观察性研究，研究使用的纤维蛋白原：PRBCs的比例。Stinger等发现高纤维蛋白原：PRBCs（0.48g/U±0.2 vs. 0.1g/U±0.06）与低死亡率相关，主要是通过减少出血而降低了死亡率。Schoechl等公开了2个研究，表明用纤维蛋白原浓缩物或凝血酶原复合物治疗的创伤患者的死亡率明显下降。他们的研究并没有局限于大量输血患者，收集的是接受5单位的PRBCs或更大剂量PRBCs的创伤患者。在其中的一篇论文中，Schoechl等研究人员结合创伤损伤严重度评分（Trauma Injury Severity Score，TRISS），将对照组的死亡率与治疗组进行比较，发现两者的死亡率差异为24.4% vs. 33.7%（P= 0.032），排除TBI患者之后，两者的死亡率为14% vs. 27.8%（P=0.0018）。在他的另一项研究中，Schoechl发现用纤维蛋白原或FFP治疗的凝血功能障碍患者具有更好的预后，使用纤维蛋白原组比未使用组有更低的住院天数（23天 vs. 32天，P=0.005）。

有几项发表的Ⅲ类研究是关于血小板使用和死亡率之间的关系的。在一项Ⅲ类研究中，Inaba等发现随着输注Plt：PRBCs的比例上升，生存率会得到提升。死亡的相对危险度（relative risk，RR）随着血小板所占比值的下降而上升，从1.67（高比值）增加到2.28（中比值）再到5.51（低比值）。Perkins等的回顾性研究发现，高Plt：PRBCs比例与生存率的改善独立相关。研究组分为接受高、中或低Plt：PRBCs比例组。他们发现24 h的生存率分别为95 %、87 %和64 %（P<0.001）。Holcomb等证实了高血浆：PRBCs比例（≥1：2）相对于低血浆：PRBCs比例（<1：2）治疗的患者的30天生存率明显升高（59.6% vs. 40.4%，P<0.01）。他还观察到输注高Plt：PRBCs比例（≥1：2）血液制品的患者相对于低Plt：PRBCs比例（<1：2）的患者，30天生存率增加（59.9% vs. 40.1%，P＜0.01）。

最近的一段时间里，抗纤维蛋白溶解剂成为讨论的焦点。一项多中心Ⅰ类CRASH-2研究表明使用抗纤维蛋白溶解剂组比安慰剂组有更高的生存率，它是唯一一个已知的对比试验。CRASH-2试验涉及40个国家的20 000名患者，10 115名患者接受安慰剂，10 096名患者接受氨甲环酸（一种抗纤维蛋白溶解药）。氨甲环酸组的全死因死亡率为14.5%，而安慰剂组为16.0%（RR＝0.91，95%置信区间为0.85～0.97；P=0.0035）。大量出血引起的死亡风险在治疗组中为4.9%，而在安慰剂组中为5.7%（RR=0.85，95%置信区间为0.76～0.96；P=0.0077）。这项试验表明，当出血性创伤需要大量输血治疗时，可以使用抗纤维蛋白溶解药。

有3个Ⅲ类研究关注在凝血功能障碍性创伤患者的治疗过程中使用纤维蛋白原。Stinger等的战伤相关凝血功能障碍病理研究证明，使用高纤维蛋白原：PRBCs比值与死亡率的下降独立相关，与低比率相比，高纤维蛋白原：PRBCs比例组死亡率较低（24% vs. 85%，P<0.001）。Schoechel等比较了创伤性凝血功能障碍患者中纤维蛋白原-凝血酶原复合物和FFP的使用。他们证明使用纤维蛋白原可以避免使用大量的PRBCs，并且在减少PRBCs输注量的方面可能比FFP更有效。通过使用纤维蛋白原和凝血酶原复合物，29%的患者避免了PRBCs输注，而使用FFP的患者只有3%。此外，当使用纤维蛋白原-凝血酶原复合物时，91%的病例中避免了血小板输注，而使用FFP的患者仅有56%。同时两组的死亡率差异无统计学意义。在Schoechl等的另一项研究中，使用纤维蛋白原浓缩物、凝血酶原浓缩物、FFP或所有3种治疗的患者中，使用纤维蛋白原可以改善死亡率。定向回顾性治疗是基于血栓弹力图进行的。

输血时间

没有一个试验直接研究输注FFP与PRBCs的时机的疗效。然而，在许多情况下血浆治疗的早期启动经常由于创伤中心不能立即获得血液制品而有所延迟。实际上，有证据表明凝血功能障碍的病理学变化在复苏过程中比先前想象的要早得多。一项Ⅲ类研究显示，进入ICU时（包括急诊室的复苏），患者的凝血功能障碍仍然未纠正与持续的输血需求和不断发展的凝血功能障碍相关。Zink等研究表明，FFP和血小板的早期输注非常关键，它可以造成入院早期6 h内死亡率的巨大差异。Magnotti等证明6 h死亡率与是否早期高FFP：PRBCs比例输注相关。Moore等研究了在复苏早期死亡的患者，发现这些患者存在凝血功能障碍（平均INR为2.4），尽管他们已经输注了平均26.4单位的PRBCs和平均6.5单位

的 FFP，其中 12%的患者没有输注 FFP。由此，研究人员认为早期死亡患者的凝血功能障碍没有得到很好的纠正。

大量输血方案的建立和有效性

大量输血方案（massive transfusion protocol，MTP）的概念在迅速地被接受，在过去十年中实施频率有所增加。Malone 等 2006 年的文章发现，在美国和其他国家，MTP 的实施只是少数的。在过去几年中，MTP 的实施急剧增加。Hoyt 等 2008 年的一项调查显示，全世界只有 45%的受访者严格遵循 MTP，19%承认并没有严格遵循 MTP，34%的受访者表示没有制订 MTP。Schuster 等 2010 年发表的一篇关于美国创伤中心和其管理者的文章（186 名外科医生和 59 名中心主任回复了调查）发现，85%的受访者有 MTP，65%的 MTP 是在过去 5 年建立的。作者注意到，不同中心的方案在启动、输血组分比例和时间方面存在着很大差异。Núñez 等建议在大型 Ⅰ 级创伤中心设定一个方案，它涉及一种团队方法，目的是最终改善临床生存情况和减少整体血液使用，减少浪费。他们描述了一种通过观察 ABLS（气道、呼吸和循环）的识别方法，以及基于 4 个参数的评分方法：①穿通伤；②创伤重点超声评估阳性；③在到达医院时，收缩压≤90 mmHg；④在到达时心率≥120 次 / 分钟。用这种评分方法，评分大于或等于 2 分对于预测是否需要大量输血的灵敏度为 75%，特异度为 86%。

MTP 试图解决输血实践过程中不同实施者所造成的结果差异性。一些试验已经验证了这些方案的有效性。Parkland 医院的一个回顾性研究显示，在实施 MTP 后血液成分的使用明显减少，此外还带来更快的周转时间和单个患者的治疗成本的减少。通过血液制品使用总量的减少，MTP 使患者患输血相关性并发症的概率减少。Cotton 等证明，严格遵循机构的 MTP 与生存率的升高独立相关（86.7% vs. 45.0%，P<0.001）。不遵循既定的 MTP 是浪费血液制品的独立预测因子。作者指出，他们机构的遵循率是 27%。Cotton 等的另一项研究表明，遵循 MTP 的患者的严重脓毒症 / 感染性休克和多器官功能衰竭的发生率较低。Gunter 等证实，根据 MTP 接受血液制品输注的患者与在方案制订之前患者相比，30 天死亡率显著降低（41% vs. 62%，P<0.008）。Dente 等证明，根据 MTP 输血的患者除了 30 天死亡率得到显著改善（34% vs. 55%，P<0.04）之外，总体死亡率也明显下降（36% vs. 17%，P<0.008）。重要的是，Riskin 等证明，尽管在 MTP 之前和 MTP 之后，血液制品使用的比例不变，MTP 的实施降低了死亡率。他们的数据强调了一旦 MTP 启动，血液制品快速输注的重要性。一些相互矛盾的证据表明 MTP 可能不会对严重出血的死亡率产生影响。Simmons 等调查了在伊拉克自由 / 持久自由行动期间建立 MTP 之前和之后的死亡率，并没有发现明显的变化。

输血并发症

死亡率

57 项研究中有 24 项专门论述了输注 FFP 对死亡率的影响。使用高比例的 FFP：PRBCs 的 Ⅱ 类证据非常充足。然而，这项结论缺乏前瞻性随机对照研究的支持。在 8 个 Ⅱ 类研究中，大多数结果显示随着 FFP：PRBCs 比例的增加，死亡率会下降。Cotton 等发现，在 MTP 治疗过程中，补充 10 单位 PRBCs，4 单位解冻血浆和 2 单位血小板，患者的调整风险后死亡率降低 74%（P<0.001）。Dente 等的结果显示，FFP：PRBCs 比为 1：1 的大量输血患者 30 天和总体死亡率下降。24 h 死亡率从 36%降低到 17%（P=0.008），30 天死亡率从 55%下降到 34%（P=0.04）。Sperry 等比较了输入 FFP：PRBCs 比例大于 1：1.5 的患者和接受 FFP：PRBCs 比例小于 1：1.5 的患者的死亡率，发现早期（24 小时）死亡率有显著差异（3.9% vs. 12.8%，P<0.012），但在最终粗死亡率方面的差异没有显著统计学意义。Gunter 等证明，FFP ：PRBCs 比为 2：3 或更高的接受 MTP 的患者 30 天死亡率下降（41% vs. 62%，P=0.008）。此外，接受 Plt：PRBCs 比例为 1：5 或更高的血液制品的患者组，30 天死亡率较低（38% vs. 61 %，P=0.001，不使用 DCR）。Bochicchio 等证明了血液制品使用比例的增加和不良预后之间线性相关。该研究比较了输注血液制品治疗的创伤患者与未输血组患者，发现输注血液制品组有更多的不良事件产生，特别是感染的增加有显著统计学意义（34% vs.9.4%，P<0.001）。死亡率在输血组中也有所增加（21.4% vs. 6.5%）。然而，作者承认，用血液制品输血治疗的患者 ISS 显著增加（27 ± 13 vs. 19 ± 11，P<0.001），INR（1.8 ± 1 vs. 1.1 ± 0.09，P<0.001）也明显升高。因此，他们更有可能因为创

伤和凝血功能障碍而死亡。Simmons 等比较了实施临床实践指南（Clinical Practice Guideline，CPG）的军队队列。他们发现，实施 CPG 后群组确实获得了较高的 FFP：PRBCs 比例血液制品的输注，并且患者呈现了高血红蛋白水平和正常的体温。然而，总体死亡率（没有一个特定的结果变量）在 2 组之间没有统计学差异（24% vs. 19%，P=0.115）。Scalea 等也未能发现死亡率的显著差异，原因可能是研究没有把 FFP：PRBCs 比例作为连续变量［比值比（odds ratio，OR）为 1.49，P=0.37］或将 FFP：PRBCs 的比例为 1：1 作为二元变量（OR=0.60，P=0.35）进行分析。然而，该研究入选的 806 例患者中的 250 例，在 24 h 内接受了超过 1 单位的 RBC 和 FFP，研究突出了采用的各种复苏措施，而不是仅仅只关注 DCR。Magnotti 等试图质疑 DCR 的原则，包括在创伤性出血的救治中使用高比例的 FFP ：RBC。结果显示早期使用高比例的 FFP ：PRBCs 的血液制品可改善患者的生存率。然而，这项研究缺乏生存偏倚方面的支持。因此创伤患者的生存偏倚可能影响该研究的结论。他们指出，输注高比例 FFP：PRBCs 血液制品的患者的休克严重程度较低。此外，他们的结果显示，高比例组 6 h 死亡率较低（10% vs. 48%，P<0.002）。

大多数Ⅲ类研究能够证明输注更高比例的 FFP：PRBCs 复苏的患者死亡率显著改善。6 项研究，包括一项多中心临床分析，发现当 FFP：PRBCs 的比例高于以前使用的较低比例时，能够改善死亡率。5 项研究能够独立地证明输注高 FFP：PRBCs 比例血液制品能够改善死亡率。Mitra 等的 1 项研究得出结论，较高的 FFP：PRBCs 比例与提高早期生存率相关，但是当排除前 24 h 的死亡时，FFP：PRBCs 比与死亡率无关。因此，Mitra 等认为需要进一步的试验来确定最佳比例。在大量输血的 TBI 患者的研究中，Peiniger 等发现高比例组的死亡率在统计学上比低比例组低（独立于时间，无论存在或者不存在 TBI）。在一项军事研究中，复苏时接受比例为 1：1.4 与 1：1.7 的 FFP：PRBCs 的患者在死亡率方面没有显著差异，在两组中均无死亡病例。

Inaba 等在急性复苏期间使用不匹配的血液作为影响预后的变量，显示接受不匹配血液的患者比接受匹配血液的患者具有更高的死亡率（39.6% vs. 11.9%，P<0.001）。因此，使用非交叉配型的血液是死亡率的独立预测因素。有趣的是，在一项不同的军事研究中，通过比较全血输注与成分输血治疗的效果。结果显示，与成分输血相比，全血输注的患者的 24 h 和 30 天生存率升高。

并发症发生率

大量研究已经证明，医院内并发症发生和血液制品输血之间有剂量效应关系。Silver Board 等在一项Ⅱ类研究中证明，输入更大量 PRBCs 的患者中 ARDS 的发病率增加。在本研究中，患者分为 3 组，分别为需要 0～5 单位的 PRBCs 组、6～10 单位的 PRBCs 组和大于 10 单位的 PRBCs 组，其 ARDS 发病率依次为 21%、31% 和 57%。在 Bochicchio 等的一项前瞻性Ⅱ类研究中，通过风险调整，多变量分析发现每补充 1 单位的 PRBCs 会增加 5% 的感染风险，住院时间长度、ICU 住院天数和呼吸机使用天数增加 0.64、0.42 和 0.47 天。Sadjadi 等的Ⅱ类研究显示，输血患者与未输血患者相比，观察到的感染率升高（61% vs.20%，P<0.01）。两组患者 ISS 相似，然而输血组比未输血组的感染风险要高 8 倍（OR＝7.97；95% CI 为 2.3～27.5；P<0.001）。Dunne 等根据军事数据进行的另一项Ⅱ类研究显示，接受大于 4 单位的血液的患者伤口愈合率会下降（54% vs.9%，P<0.05）、ICU 入住率升高（78% vs. 9%，P<0.01）、围术期感染率增加（89% vs.27%，P<0.01）、住院时间延长、血清炎症标记物增加。

几项研究已经表明了与输注 FFP：PRBCs 比例相关的并发症。Sperry 等在Ⅱ类研究中显示，输入较高 FFP：PRBCs 比例血液制品的患者须补充较少的血液，拥有较低的死亡率，在脏器功能衰竭或院内感染中没有显示出差异，但是发展为 ARDS 的风险为两倍。这些结论由 Chaiwat 等的另一个回顾性研究所证实，其表明接受至少 5 单位的 PRBCs 的患者发展为 ARDS 的风险高 2.5 倍。每个额外单位的 PRBCs 输注会带来 ARDS 的患病风险高 6%（OR＝1.06，95% CI 为 1.03～1.10）。Watson 等得出结论，输注 1 单位 FFP，死亡风险降低 2.9%，但 MOF 风险增加 2.1%［风险比（hazard ratio，HR）1.021，P=0.029，95% CI 为 1.002～1.04），ARDS 的风险增加 2.5%（HR＝1.025，P=0.038，95% CI 为 1.001～1.049）。Cotton 等比较了实施早期、预先制订的输血方案的效果，包括 FFP：PRBCs 比例为 3：2 的血液制品，显示在肾衰竭或全身性炎症反应综合征方面没有差异。但是，实施方案组肺炎、肺衰竭、剖腹术和腹腔隔室综合征的发生率更低。他们发现实施早期输血方案组的严重脓毒症/感染性休克（9% vs. 20%，P=0.011）和多器官衰竭（16% vs. 37%，P<0.001）的发生率较低。

许多关于FFP输注和并发症的Ⅲ类研究结果是相互矛盾的。Peiniger等的研究表明输入较高FFP：PRBCs比例的血液制品患者脓毒症和MOF的发生率并没有升高。Zink等表明，接受包括较高比例的FFP：PRBCs的MTP的患者与接受低比例的患者相比，机械通气天数相近。Holcomb等表明，高血小板比例和高FFP比例可以改善30天生存率，但是ICU住院天数和呼吸机使用天数更长，而多器官衰竭导致的死亡没有差别。Fox等证实了输注较高FFP：PRBCs比例的血液制品军队患者有较低的截肢率和较好的生理恢复。Mahambrey等证实了补充大量RBC的患者的48 h的器官功能不全增加，但住院患者的死亡率没有增加。Khan等证明了，危重患者接受FFP输注（不论是否有其他成分输注）发生ALI和ARDS的风险增加2.48倍（95% CI为1.29～4.74），而接受任意单位红细胞输注的（不论是否有其他成分输注）风险只增加1.39倍（95% CI为0.79～2.43）。Sarani等的研究提示每输入1单位FFP，感染的风险上升，OR为1.039（1.013～1.067）。作者还证明了在FFP输注中，所有类型感染的RR为2.99（95 % CI为2.28～3.93）。Maegele等的一项大型Ⅲ类欧洲研究显示，在接受高FFP比例的患者中，30天死亡率有所改善，但呼吸机使用天数和ICU住院时间延长。

尽管输注血小板被认为具有比输注FFP更少的并发症，但不代表它没有过敏反应、输血相关的急性肺损伤（transfusion associated acute lung injury，TRALI）、ARDS和细菌感染的风险。在一项Ⅲ类研究中，Khan等在他们的回顾性队列研究中证明，在接受任何比例的血小板的患者中，急性肺部感染和ARDS的风险增加3.89倍（95% CI为1.36～11.52），而输注PRBCs的患者（无论是否有其他成分输注）风险增加1.39（95 % CI为0.79-2.43）。然而，Watson等的一项多中心前瞻性Ⅱ类研究证明，在初始创伤事件中存活下来的有出血性休克的钝性创伤患者中，FFP与MOF和ARDS发生的高风险独立相关，而冷凝蛋白物与MOF的低发生率相关。

生存偏倚

57项Ⅲ类研究中有3项经过生存偏倚调整后研究FFP：PRBCs的最佳比例。Snyder等发现在24 h内较高的FFP：PRBCs比例和生存率提高相关。然而，在分析中调整生存偏倚后，关联不再具有统计学意义。Rajasekhar等在11个不同的研究中观察了输注FFP：PRBCs比例为1：1的血液制品者的生存优势。他们得出结论，生存偏倚和研究之间的异质性妨碍了关于FFP：PRBCs比例的统计学比较，并且没有足够的证据支持高FFP：PRBCs比例患者存在生存优势。Magnotti等的第3项研究结论，在第1个24 h内接受较高血浆比例的患者的生存率得到改善。他们指出，患者不会直接因为FFP：PRBCs比例低而死亡，低比例只是其死亡的原因之一。

建议

定义与分级

Ⅰ级建议

这是基于现有的科学数据而得出的非常可靠的建议。它通常基于Ⅰ类证据；另外，充分的Ⅱ类证据也可以作为Ⅰ级建议形成的基础，尤其是当该问题不适合以随机对照的形式进行试验。相反，较弱的或自相矛盾的Ⅰ类证据不能形成Ⅰ级建议。

1. 补充FFP：PRBCs比例为1：1与更少的输血相关。足够的证据显示输FFP将减少所需输血的次数。这里须指出的是，没有随机前瞻性的Ⅰ类试验来验证。将来进行这方面的试验对于更好地理解创伤救治输血的理想方案是至关重要的。

2. Ⅰ类证据支持在大量输血中使用抗纤维蛋白溶解剂。最近完成的CRASH-2试验表明，使用抗纤维蛋白溶解剂可以降低各种原因引起的死亡率以及出血引起的死亡率。应进行进一步的Ⅰ、Ⅱ和Ⅲ类研究，来支持这些发现。

Ⅱ级建议

这项建议的得出是基于现有科学证据，同时得到了来自重症监护领域专家的强烈支持。它通常由Ⅱ类证据或较强的Ⅲ类证据来支持。

1. MTP能改善创伤复苏的结果。这项治疗策略在具体实施过程中面临很多挑战。许多民间机构，甚至Ⅰ级创伤中心，尚未能实施MTP。然而，简单的如1：1的FFP：PRBCs输血是有益处的，而且相对较高的血浆占比似乎能改善预后。这项方案可以促进更多中心来研究复苏和出血的控制。

2. 高 FFP：PRBCs 比例由Ⅱ类和Ⅲ类证据支持，在需要大量输血的创伤性凝血功能障碍患者的治疗中应该考虑采用。Ⅱ类和Ⅲ类数据表明，尽管存在以下负面效果：ARDS/ALI、住院天数和 ICU 治疗时间增加、呼吸机的使用时间增加，大多数研究仍旧呈现出较低的死亡率。因此，这些治疗的实施使得总体治疗效果得到改善。

Ⅲ级建议

这些建议得到现有数据的支持，但缺乏足够的科学证据。它们通常由Ⅲ类数据支持。此类推荐是有指导意义的，并且对于指导未来的研究是有用的。

1. FFP：PRBCs 比例增加会改善大量输血患者的预后，但是也带来了严重并发症的可能性。通过改善 MTP 的实施和依从性，可以降低死亡率和并发症发生率。

2. 高 Plt：PRBCs 比例的使用由一些Ⅱ类研究和几个Ⅲ类研究支持。高 Plt：PRBCs 比例近年来已成为 DCR 的一个组成部分。

3. 几项Ⅲ类研究证明，使用纤维蛋白原可以改善死亡率。在创伤诱导的凝血功能障碍和 DCR 中使用纤维蛋白原应在Ⅰ类和Ⅱ类试验中进一步研究。

4. 早期给予较高 FFP：PRBCs 比例血液制品输注能改善大量出血的预后。因为输血需求降低，输血继发的并发症风险也随之降低，并且能更好地纠正创伤性凝血功能障碍，高 FFP：PRBCs 比例血液制品输注的患者可以得到益处。虽然关于高 FFP：PRBCs 比例降低死亡率尚未达成共识，但似乎存在死亡率降低的趋势。从当前的实践中来看，优化后的方案将有助于对变量的标准化。

结论

在创伤救治中优化输血成分比例的作用仍然需要进一步验证。有足够的证据证明当输注 FFP：PRBCs 比例为 1：1 的时候，所需的输血量更少。此外，迄今为止能收集到的证据表明，将这些原则纳入 MTP 将通过使输血实践的变异性最小化，而有助于减少总的输血量。更少输血总量将有助于减少输血相关的并发症。在临床上考虑到以下几个方面，在各种不同的损伤机制中较高比例 FFP：PRBCs 输注、不同的输血时间和实际输血的单位量的差异，以上得出的这些结论还须进行验证。

DCR 的目的主要是在复苏的初始阶段延长生命。关于高比例 FFP：PRBCs 和 Plt：PRBCs 与改善预后（包括死亡率的改善）之间的关联仍然存在不确定性。几项Ⅲ类试验表明死亡率降低，但并发症增加。此外，许多Ⅱ类研究试图对创伤患者的广泛差异性（由于损伤机制、患者的人口统计学情况和损伤严重程度不同引起）进行说明。尽管这为找到 FFP、血小板和 PRBCs 的理想比例提供了一定程度的证据，但是最终的结论只有在将来的前瞻性随机试验中才能得出。

胸部、腹部、骨盆和肢体损伤控制的外科技术

Greta L. Piper, Kimberly A. Davis 和 Fred A. Luchette 著
都定元 译

介绍

不断演变的损伤严重程度及创伤谱，给现代创伤外科医生提出了不同于以往的巨大挑战。日益先进的武器拥有更加强大的破坏力，同样地，能引起多器官损伤的高能量钝性创伤也能导致更严重的损伤。在实际生活中，尽管这些类型的损伤多会导致患者的直接死亡，但随着这种紧急情况下院前转运和创伤复苏的不断改进，使得越来越多的濒死患者能够活着到达医院。基于这一目的，损伤控制外科得到了重视和发展，即优先处理危及生命的损伤，推迟确定性修复，直到代谢和生理紊乱得以纠正。

损伤控制有 3 个独立且截然不同的管理阶段。第一个阶段包括快速扩容、迅速控制出血以及空腔脏器损伤污染最小化。在临时的伤口管理策略中，填塞物经常留置于原处，用来压塞止血。第二个阶段，主要是发生在重症监护病房，涉及对低体温患者的积极复温，纠正凝血功能障碍，以及使用晶体液和血

液制品的持续复苏。一旦正常的生理功能得到恢复，第三阶段就是损伤患者的确定性的手术处理。

损伤控制手术的目标是在面对严重失血性休克的灾难性损伤中保住生命。Moore 等的研究指出，损伤控制策略的适应证包括：①持续的凝血功能障碍导致无法确切的止血；②技术上的困难或无法显露的主要静脉损伤；③在面对无法得到复苏的休克的情况下，消耗时间去完成一个操作；④须解决的其他危及生命的损伤。这些适应证已经延伸到包括因高能量钝性躯干损伤或多发性穿通伤所致的血流动力学不稳定的患者，或任何出现休克伴低体温和凝血功能障碍的创伤患者（框 1）。除了最常应用于腹部损伤以外，损伤控制的方法同样也成功地被用于致命的胸部损伤和骨损伤。

框 1 损伤控制手术适应证

因出血性休克所致的血流动力学不稳定
存在凝血功能障碍或低体温
主要的腹部血管损伤伴或不伴相应的内脏损伤
复杂的肝损伤伴或不伴相应的内脏损伤
多空腔脏器损伤伴出血性休克
多系统创伤，处理的优后顺序不明确
代谢性酸中毒 pH＜7.3
大量输血的必要性

Modified from Rotondo MF, Zonies DH: The damage control sequence and underlying logic. *Surg Clin North Am* 77:761–777, 1997

致死三联征

损伤控制手术试图在发展到不可逆的生理紊乱之前缩短外科干预的时间。非控制性出血会导致全脑的缺血性损伤，但复苏患者在再灌注期间有可能导致更进一步的损伤。这就不可避免地发展为致死三联征，即低体温、凝血功能障碍及酸中毒。这些并发症单独存在时即可造成对生命的潜在威胁。由于这 3 个并发症同时发生的发生率呈指数级增长，如果不能及时纠正而导致恶性循环的话，最终将造成患者的死亡。损伤控制手术，通过缩短外科手术时间、将患者送回 ICU 纠正致死三联症，从而提高生存率。

低体温被定义为中心温度低于 35℃。在初、中期研究中，中心温度通过热辐射的方式丢失的过程，从院前处置开始时一直持续至到达急诊室后。未复温的复苏液的使用和在手术室中暴露的腹膜和胸膜表面的蒸发作用都会使体温持续丢失。临床上创伤剖腹探查术后的低体温发生率为 57%。低体温将明显增加死亡的风险，特别是在中心温度低于 34℃的患者中。而低于 32℃的中心温度对创伤患者来说是致命的。

低体温具有全身性的影响，包括对血流动力学（降低心率和心排血量、增加全身血管阻力）、肾功能（减少肾小球滤过率）和中枢神经系统（抑制精神状态）的负性作用。体温的降低是影响凝血级联反应的独立因素，因为血凝块的形成依赖于一系列温度依赖性的酶促反应。研究表明低温会延长 PT、凝血酶时间、PTT。低体温也会影响血小板功能，导致门静脉循环阻断以及出血时间延长。

失血性休克后的代谢性酸中毒主要是因为低灌注期间发生了从有氧代谢到无氧代谢转变。酸中毒的不利影响包括心肌收缩乏力以及对正性肌力药物反应的减少，导致室性心律失常的发生，使颅内压进一步增高。最终，酸中毒通过延长 PTT 以及减少因子Ⅴ活性，加重凝血功能障碍，从而导致 DIC 的发生。

即使没有低体温和酸中毒，凝血功能障碍也会继发于包含大量晶体液和无凝血因子的 PRBCs 复苏后。组织损伤后继发的组织因子暴露通过激活凝血级联反应，引起凝血因子的消耗，最终导致凝血功能障碍。

初始复苏的关注

美国创伤外科委员会的 ATLS 课程已经颁布了对创伤患者初步处理的系统办法。在该课程提及的初、中期研究中，要求能够快速识别危及生命的损伤，让外科医生可以优先对不稳定的创伤患者进行后续的手术治疗。一个存在过多出血的患者应该迅速被转运到手术室，并根据患者的生理参数、体温以及血管内容量状态，在手术早期制定出损伤控制的策略（框 1）。对明显须持续进行复苏的患者，应放置中心静脉导管进行积极的容量复苏。考虑到多种因素可导致患者发生凝血功能障碍，在启动损伤控制复苏时就应该事先考虑到这一问题，具体的内容将在后面的章节（现代战场上的躯干创伤）中提及，主要是在标准的晶体液和 PRBCs 复苏以外，对凝血因子（FFP 和冷凝蛋白质）和血小板的早期应用。最近的文献指出在复苏时，PRBCs、FFP、血小板按照 1∶1∶1 的比例搭配使用，同时试图减少晶体复苏的使用。

第一阶段：损伤控制手术

损伤控制性剖腹术

大多数的损伤控制程序在腹部完成。最早的损伤控制手术的类型主要涉及严重肝损伤的患者，针对这类患者实施纱布填塞和分期手术处理，使其并发症发生率和死亡率均得到降低。启动损伤控制程序最常见的损伤是严重的肝损伤和主要的血管损伤。

控制肝出血的主要方法是填塞，填塞的技巧尤其重要，同时取决于肝损伤的解剖学类型。肝的大裂伤须完全游离肝，在肝门处进行阻断能减少出血。直接结扎深部裂伤的出血血管是必要的，从而达到外科止血的目的。一旦大血管出血被控制，就可以在肝的前方和后方分别进行填塞，从而形成类似于双手压迫受损肝产生挤压作用。在第三阶段中，对于肝动脉分支出血的患者，应优先考虑进行介入栓塞止血，而不是选择去除填塞后的再探查术。在穿通伤患者中，行肝周填塞的同时行腔道的球囊填塞可以救命。

有几种可供选择的方法来处理主要的血管损伤。填塞对一些静脉损伤有作用。但是持续的出血仍需要手术干预。许多腹部血管的损伤可以通过结扎出血的血管来处理（表 1）。但是，在大动脉和靠近肠系膜上动脉的损伤中，患者无法耐受结扎，结扎在肝后腔静脉的损伤中也是不可行的。这些损伤在最初通常是尝试尽量修复，或是安置临时的血管腔内分流管后通过二期手术修复（3 期）。通常，Argyle 颈动脉分流和 Javid 分流被用于此手术。当需要较大的导管进行分流时，可以选择胸管。分流应使用脐带、血管环或是缝合加以固定，并且不需要抗凝，以保持通畅。处理血管损伤的另一种方法是将导管插入损伤血管内，使球囊充气来控制近端和远端的出血。这种技术可以修复相对充盈欠佳的血管损伤。最后，在某些罕见的情况下，肝后腔静脉的出血可以使用填塞来控制出血，同时腔内静脉造影术也是一个选择。

对于这些需要损伤控制手术的患者往往都涉及空腔脏器的损伤。处理这些损伤的目的是控制污染。小肠裂伤可以通过手工缝合、线性钉合或吻合器闭合的方式处理。如果肠切除术是必需的，那么腹腔内胃肠道将是不连续的。并且后期是进行吻合还是造口，要等到患者稳定后能够返回到手术室行确定性处理时再决定（3 期）。相关的胆或胰腺损伤通常是选择放置闭式引流管，计划二次手术来修复损伤。

导致血流动力学不稳定的脾裂伤须立即行脾切除术。同样，因为广泛的肾裂伤（Ⅳ级）或肾蒂Ⅳ损伤（Ⅴ级）而导致的失血性休克应该行肾切除术，尤其在尝试肾周填塞后失败的患者。在损伤控制过程中，一经诊断输尿管损伤，应立即置入支架、结扎或是行经皮尿道造口术。腹膜后膀胱损伤应迅速缝合，直到二次手术行确定性的处理。

在损伤控制手术后，由于要通过容量复苏来恢复组织的灌注，以及前期缺血组织再灌注导致的水肿，一期手术缝合关闭腹壁将增加 ACS、ARDS 和 MOF 发生的风险。临时腹腔关闭有很多种选择。临时腹腔关闭的目标是保持腹腔脏器容量、控制腹水、确定填塞到位，并且保存筋膜的完整性以便用于后期缝合。

临时腹腔关闭所涉及的简单技术是用缝线或巾钳关闭皮肤。当凝血功能障碍、酸中毒及低体温得到纠正后，使用这种技术可以帮助填塞止血。然而，这样处理后并不能明显地扩大腹腔容积，并且可能为后期再发 ACS 创造条件。在 ICU 中，当发生 ACS 时，应用下面这些临时腹腔关闭的患者可以很容易地通过重新开放腹腔来进行减压。扩大腹腔容积的技术包括使用 Bogota 包覆盖脏器、3 L 尿袋缝合皮肤。Bogota 包相对于后面将提及的真空辅助技术的优势在于其内脏的可视性和脏器活力评估的可行性，这对重要血管损伤进行分流或结扎后的观察处理是非常重要的。

临时腹腔关闭的负压辅助技术得到了很好的效果。创面覆盖后负压的建立须先在内脏表面放置非贴壁洞巾，然后覆盖无菌手术巾。安置 2 个密闭的负压引流后，使用有黏性的塑料布密封伤口，并固定在皮肤上。这种技术的好处包括维持腹壁筋膜的张力，以减少其缺失的风险，便于后期筋膜的延迟修复。市面上有几个可以购买到的设备能够提供类似的功能。临时关闭腹腔的另一个潜在技术就是 Velcro 魔术贴，将其缝合在筋膜上并依次收紧，来到达关腹的目的。在急性期，临时腹腔关闭的假体

表 1 腹部血管结扎和可能的并发症

血管	并发症	建议
腹腔干	无	
脾动脉	如果胃短动脉完整则无	
肝总动脉	如果门静脉完整则无，可能胆囊缺血	胆囊切除术（可二次探查手术时进行）
肠系膜上动脉	肠缺血	二次探查手术
肠系膜上静脉	肠缺血	二次探查手术
门静脉	肠缺血	二次探查手术
肾上下腔静脉	可能肾衰竭	包裹并抬高大腿，评估筋膜室综合征
肾下下腔静脉	下肢水肿	包裹并抬高大腿，评估筋膜室综合征
左肾静脉（近端）	无	
右肾静脉	肾缺血	肾切除术
髂总动脉和髂外动脉	下肢缺血	同侧小腿筋膜切开术或解剖外旁路术
髂总动脉和髂外静脉	下肢水肿	包裹并抬高大腿
髂内动脉	无	
髂内静脉	无	

Modified from Shapiro MB, Jenkins DH, Schwab CW, Rotondo MF: Damage control: collective review. J Trauma 49:969–978, 2000

材料几乎没有作用。由于没有前瞻性的试验来比较各种临时腹腔关闭的优劣，目前主要由创伤科医生自行决定采用何种方式，而且通常是各个医疗机构各异。然而，回顾性资料表明采用负压辅助闭合比起其他选择，在早期探查术中更易于筋膜缝合。

损伤控制性开胸术

穿通性胸部损伤的患者在紧急情况下应接受 ED 开胸术。ED 开胸术在钝性损伤或胸部以外的穿通伤患者中很少成功，因此在这些情况下应避免急诊室开胸术。

ED 开胸术的经典位置是在第 4 或第 5 肋间水平的左前外侧。这种探查方法可以快速暴露胸腔，并排查心包压塞的可能性。进入胸腔以后，首先应排空胸腔积血，然后探查心包。如果心包压塞是存在的，那应施行从头至尾的纵向心包切开术，在此过程中避免膈神经的损伤。在某些紧急情况下，可以游离下肺韧带，进入后纵隔，十字钳夹主动脉。

心脏裂伤的临时处理方法有很多种。直接用手指按压裂伤或穿孔处往往是非常有效的，但是要注意手指不能插入裂伤或穿孔处，避免扩大损伤范围。Foley 导管可以轻柔地穿过损伤到达心室，然后通过扩张球囊来控制出血，并能提供一定的牵引力。最后，在急诊室中，简单的心肌损伤可以使用皮肤吻合器来修复裂伤的心肌。

同样，肺损伤导致的出血也可以通过多种方法来进行控制，包括直接按压、填塞、肺门十字钳夹以及在肺轴处的肺扭转。在手术室，穿通性肺损伤可以通过 Asensio 提出的肺神经束切断术来控制。使用线性吻合器敞开伤道，可以达到很好的止血作用。通过连续的吻合后，伤道的基底部被充分暴露，这时就可以直接结扎出血部位。漏气的部位可以选择性地进行缝合。使用肺神经束切断术控制出血的患者，其死亡率较肺叶切除术明显降低。

损伤控制性开胸术后，关闭胸腔而不增加胸腔内压力通常是不可能的。而增加胸腔内压力将增加肺泡压和气道压，从而导致呼吸机不能提供足够的潮气量。若填塞对出血的控制是必要的，那暂时的胸腔关闭可以完成。留置胸腔引流管后，只有通过关闭皮肤才能提供足够的填塞。常规的切口关闭可以延迟到 48 ~ 72 h 完成（3 期）。

骨科损伤控制

骨科的损伤控制特点是快速、暂时稳定骨折。

这种观念特别适用于股骨干骨折、骨盆骨折，这类患者严重的软组织损伤和失血可能增加不良预后的风险。骨科的损伤控制之所以能够得到发展，是因为我们观察到有严重头、胸、腹部损伤的患者，在合并有持续的低体温、凝血功能障碍、酸中毒等并发症时，进行确定性的骨折固定将导致预后不良。

下肢骨折后最常见的技术是应用外固定装备来临时固定骨折部位。无论是在手术室还是在重症监护病房的病床旁，外固定都能迅速并且安全地实施。外科医生分别在骨折的上下端各置两颗钢针，注意避开神经、血管。用荧光透视法调整骨折力学对线。外固定支架固定在钢针上，跨越骨折线以保持其稳定性。尽管已经提出针孔脓毒症所导致的深部感染会有所增加，但明显增加的局部感染尚未有报道。

创伤导致的骨盆环破坏有一定的发病率和死亡率。骨盆骨折在所有的骨折中占 3%～8%，多是由于机动车碰撞所致的高能量损伤所致。在急性期，治疗的目标应是控制出血。完整的后腹膜可以容纳多达 4 L 的血液，出血将一直持续至达到生理性填塞。如果腹膜后间隙或皮肤（开放性骨折）被破坏，就不能形成生理性填塞，出血就得不到控制，除非使用无菌纱布对创面进行填塞，以重建封闭的腹膜后间隙及盆腔。

在骨盆骨折导致出血的损伤控制管理中，第一步仍然是通过恢复正常的骨盆解剖来减少盆腔内容积。这可以通过多种方法来完成，包括在骨盆周围系一张床单或一些市售的骨盆悬带和腰带。外固定器和骨盆 C 夹也可用于此目的，是骨盆环中断的理想选择。外固定支架须在每个髂嵴上安置两个经皮的钢针。钢针与铁杆连接，然后手动调节使耻骨联合的边缘靠近。外固定架能够减少对骨折联合的干扰并且降低骨盆容积。C 夹包括两颗钢针，分别固定在骶髂关节区后方的髂骨上。这个装置在髂骨骨折和经髂骨骨折脱位的患者的应用中是相对禁忌的。

对于骨盆骨折应用外固定装置后仍然有血流动力学不稳定的情况的患者，那么必须考虑来自髂内动脉分支的出血。不稳定的骨盆骨折患者中，只有 10% 的患者发生动脉出血。在这种患者人群中，髂内动脉造影行血管栓塞是最佳的选择方法。在不能进行介入栓塞的情况下，剖腹探查术对同侧髂内动脉结扎和盆腔填塞是一个可行的替代方法，尽管有报告指出，更改治疗方法的死亡率为 25%。鉴于腹膜内盆腔填塞的高死亡率，Cothren 描述了剖腹探查术中行腹膜外盆腔填塞时成年人的 6 个填塞部位以及儿童的 4 个填塞部位（图 1）。在最近的一项关于血流动力学不稳定的骨盆环损伤的研究中，Papakostidis 通过早期稳定骨盆环、腹膜外填塞止血，以及必要时选择性血管栓塞的方法，有可能达到最佳的生存优势的结果。

第二阶段：ICU 复苏

损伤控制手术后，患者将返回 ICU 纠正生理紊乱，包括低体温、酸中毒和凝血功能障碍。积极的低体温纠正是至关重要的。外部复温技术包括室内升温、呼吸机回路以及加温器的应用。所有的液体和血液制品应通过一级液体加热器供给。对于体温

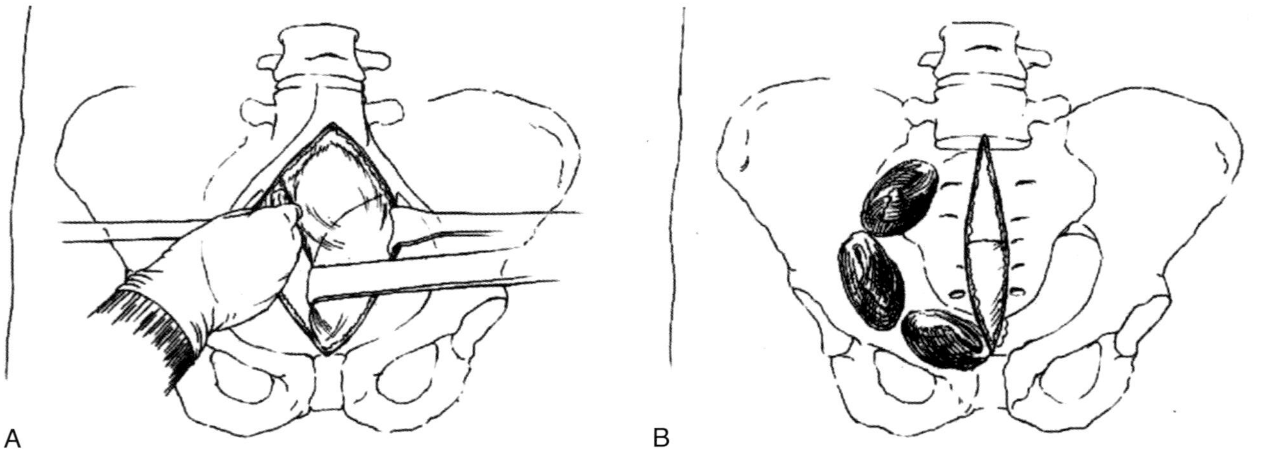

图 1 **A** 和 **B** 显示腹膜外骨盆填塞 *(From Cothren CC, Osborn PM, Moore EE, et al: Preperitoneal pelvic packing for hemodynamically unstable pelvic fractures: a paradigm shift. J Trauma 62:834–839, discussion 839–842, 2007.)*

低于 32℃的严重的低体温患者，应考虑给予经鼻胃管、胸管、腹腔灌洗或 Foley 导管行体腔灌洗治疗。最近，除了留置导管以外，几种外置装置已经开发用来促进系统复温。体外循环是侵入性很强但有效的复温技术，同时也能够为因深度暴露易于出现心律失常和心搏骤停的低体温患者提供循环支持。

损伤控制手术后酸中毒的患者最有可能被复苏，并且须优化氧气输送以进行矫正。侵入性的监测，包括监测中心静脉压或 Swan-Ganz 监测，可能有必要在术后进行，以早期指导复苏。另外，心排血量的无创监测可能用于指导复苏。患者充分复苏后持续的酸中毒可能是使用生理盐水进行积极复苏后所致的高氯性酸中毒。阴离子间隙可以用来区分乳酸酸中毒和高氯性酸中毒。高氯性酸中毒可以导致一个狭窄的阴离子间隙，乳酸酸中毒可以导致一个宽泛的阴离子间隙。

虽然纠正酸中毒和低体温将有助于纠正损伤控制术后出现的凝血功能障碍，但这些患者须持续输注 FFP、冷凝蛋白质和血小板，或进行持续的损伤控制复苏。所有血液制品都应通过液体加热器输入，以缩短复温时间。重组人凝血因子Ⅶ被发现在这些人群中是有用的，因为它能快速纠正凝血功能障碍，即使它的使用并没有被证明能降低死亡风险。

第三阶段：确定性手术处理

随着生理参数的正常化，特别是在酸中毒、低体温及凝血功能障碍等致死三联征得到纠正后，患者就应回到手术室完成先前被延期的修复。再手术的时机尚未形成统一标准，但大多数创伤外科医生会在 48 ~ 72 h 内进行再手术，因为 72 h 之前的再探查术可以降低并发症发生率和死亡率。

在再探查术中，进行常规的探查以确定在损伤控制手术当中可能错过的任何损伤。出血控制后移除填塞物，重建肠道的连续性。小肠损伤可以安全地直接吻合，结肠损伤可以吻合或旷置，这依赖于损伤的程度和外科医生观察的能力。应考虑延期缝合腹膜，虽然如果水肿持续存在，这不太可行。大多数患者（80%）可在伤后 5 ~ 7 天内缝合关闭腹膜。Velcro 魔术贴也可以应用，它可以延迟关闭筋膜至伤后 21 天。不适用分层厚皮片移植物的开放性腹部损伤，可以使用横跨的人工合成的可吸收材料或生物网片关闭腹腔筋膜。腹壁疝的修复可以延迟至 6 ~ 12 个月。

损伤控制开胸手术后，患者可以在所有的生理紊乱得到纠正后回到手术室。在取出填塞、控制出血或漏气之后，才可能进行胸腔引流（胸廓造口术置管）和确定性的胸腔闭合。

有大量的文献表明确定性的骨科固定时机应推迟到 72 h 以后。这表明在初始损伤控制手术后的第 2 ~ 4 天并不是确定性稳定骨折损伤的最佳时期，因为这个时期存在持续的全身炎症反应和广泛的水肿。据报道，在第 2 ~ 4 天稳定骨折的患者比在第 6 ~ 8 天实施手术的患者，其多系统器官功能障碍的发生率在统计学上明显增加。

损伤控制手术后并发症

早期并发症

损伤控制性剖腹术后最常见的并发症是 ACS。尽管 TAC 的应用很广泛，但由于内脏肿胀的加重、持续的出血以及腹腔内填塞的机械性压迫，都可能导致腹腔内压力的增高。ACS 的症状包括腹胀、气道压峰值的持续升高、酸中毒的不断加重、进行性少尿到无尿，以及心排血量减少导致的全身低血压。腹腔隔室综合征的发生、发展既可以很急，也可以很隐匿。通过 Foley 导管测量的膀胱内压可以替代腹内压。当压力大于 25 mmHg 时，就要进行腹腔减压。另外，腹腔灌注压是可以测定的（平均动脉压减去腹内压），腹腔灌注压小于 60 mmHg 时须进行减压。减压要么是重新打开先前的剖腹手术切口，要么是调整 TAC。原发性 ACS 须沿正中线行剖腹手术，这可以在对 ICU 的清醒患者充分镇静后进行。当腹腔减压后，内脏灌注、肾灌注、心功能以及呼吸机制将立即得到改善。

尽管进行了积极的复苏和对致死三联征的纠正，对于术后持续出血的患者，非计划性再手术仍有可能是必要的。在表 2 中列出了损伤控制手术后第一个 24 h 内重返手术室的适应证。

迟发并发症

损伤控制手术后的患者发生 ARDS、MOF 及死亡的风险都比较高。脓毒症的存在、预计输血大于 15 U 浓 PRBCs、肺损伤和长骨骨折已被证明是发生

表 2 早期返回手术室的适应证

持续的出血和凝血功能障碍（在 12 h 内输入大于 6 ~ 10 单位的红细胞）
腹腔隔室综合征
缺血组织引起的代谢紊乱
腹部胃肠修复失败、未发现损伤或钉线破坏导致的胃肠道污染

Modified with from Martin RR, Byrne M: Postoperative care and complications of damage control surgery. *Surg Clin North Am* 77:929–942, 1997

创伤后 ARDS 的独立危险因素。休克、感染、多次输血和重度损伤都与 MOF 的发生相关。损伤控制手术后的死亡率大概为 20% ~ 67%。在损伤后第 1 周，当腹部伤口未正常关闭时，开放的腹腔增加了瘘形成的风险。当切除瘘管时，这些患者往往需要腹壁重建。

总结

损伤控制手术对于多发伤的患者来说是救命的。损伤控制要求迅速解决威胁生命的问题，并缩短手术时间，然后在 ICU 恢复正常的生理功能。要等到致死三联征（低体温、凝血功能障碍、酸中毒）得以纠正后，才能进行后期确定性手术，从而提高患者的生存率。而这一部分患者在以前可能会死于他们的损伤。

腹腔隔室综合征、损伤控制和开放式腹腔

Oliver L. Gunter, Jr., Nathan J. Powell 和 Richard S. Miller 著
张大方 译

目前的关键生命支持措施使得严重受伤和生理损伤的患者能够生存，否则这些损伤可能是致死性疾病。广泛的复苏的主要手术影响之一是腹壁的状况。尽管目标一直是在剖腹术后关闭腹部，但由于情况复杂，一期闭合在技术上可能是无效或有害的。在本章中，我们将讨论创伤后腹部的治疗，首先讨论腹腔隔室综合征（abdominal compartment syndrome，ACS）。接下来是对损伤控制原则和临时腹腔关闭（temporary abdominal closure，TAC）的回顾。本章将总结开放式腹部的特殊考虑的讨论，包括腹壁重建、营养支持和预后。

腹腔隔室综合征

腹腔内高压（intraabdominal hypertension，IAH）的作用首先在 19 世纪被 Marey 和 Burt 描述，他们确定了胸内压力与 IAP 升高之间的关系。Kron 等和 Richards 等报告说，尽管患者在正常的平均动脉血压和心脏功能，但不同的系列中的患者术后都发展为腹部膨隆，肺动脉和 IAP 升高。所有这些患者腹部减压改善。尽管原发性 ACS 可能是腹腔内损伤的直接结果，但 ACS 也被证明可以在没有腹部损伤的情况下由于复苏而发展。因此，ACS 应被认为是潜在可预防的（图 1）。

由于提出的定义种类繁多，世界腹腔隔室综合征大会成立了，并批准了一个明确的分类系统。IAH 定义为 IAP 高于 12 mmHg，并进一步分为Ⅰ级至Ⅳ级（框 1）。

一般而言，隔室综合征是一种条件，其中在限制空间中增加的压力对循环产生不利影响，并威胁该空间内组织的功能和活力。隔室综合征可能发生

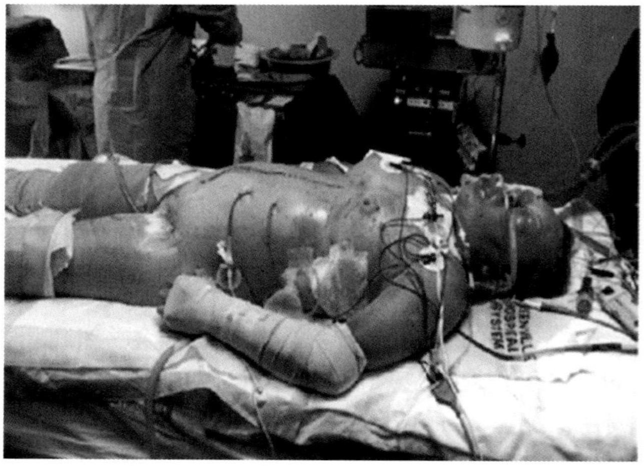

图 1 腹腔隔室综合征高风险的术后创伤患者

框 1　腹腔内高压在 WCACS 上的分级

Ⅰ级：IAP 为 12 ~ 15 mmHg
Ⅱ级：IAP 为 16 ~ 20 mmHg
Ⅲ级：IAP 为 21 ~ 25 mmHg
Ⅳ级：IAP>25 mmHg
IAP，腹腔内压力；WCACS，世界腹腔隔室综合征大会

在四肢、眼球、颅骨和腹腔。ACS 指临床上的整体，其中 IAH 减少腹部器官的血液流动并损害肺、心血管、肾和胃肠功能。ACS 的发展取决于 IAH 的程度以及压力增加的速度。根据世界腹腔隔室综合征大会，ACS 定义为 IAP 高于 20 mmHg 和新发多器官衰竭（图 2）。

ACS 可进一步表征如下：

1. 原发性 / 急性：腹腔内直接和近端损伤导致的隔室综合征。

2. 继发性：无明显的腹内损伤，但腹部受伤会导致液体积聚。（原发性和继发性 ACS 之间的差异可能是重要的，因为继发性 ACS 已经显示出更糟糕的结果。）

3. 慢性：ACS 发生在肝硬化和腹水存在的情况下，通常在疾病的后期阶段。

恶化的隔室综合征导致暴发性多器官功能障碍，如果不治疗，通常是致命的。严重受伤的有 ACS 发展危险的患者的重症监护管理应以预防以及早期识别 IAH 的体征和症状为重点。

尽管我们对 ACS 的病因了解甚少，但病因代表了炎症高反应和对休克的反应（图 3）。ACS 的解剖学作用机制开始于腹膜内和腹膜后结构的直接压迫。

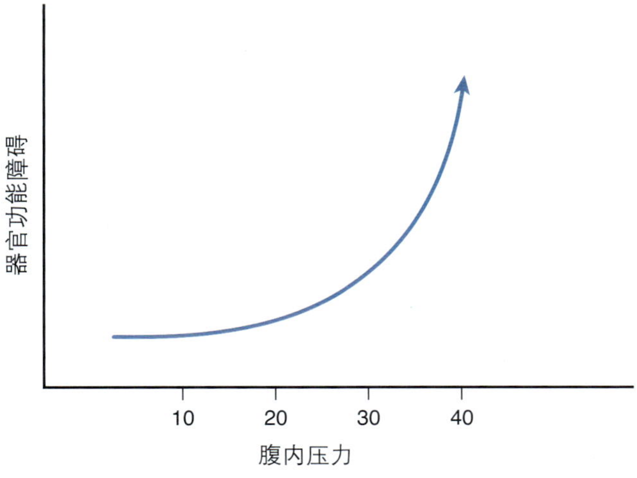

图 2　进行性器官功能障碍与腹内压力恶化

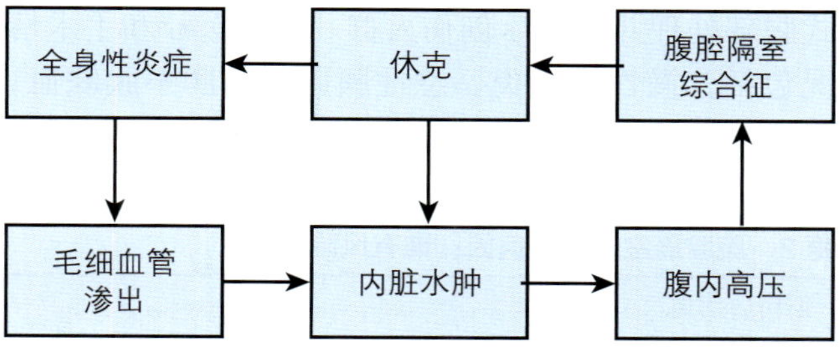

图 3　产生腹内高压和腹腔隔室综合征的缺血循环

受到严重影响的是肠道和静脉系统等低压系统甚至它们甚至有可能崩溃。

直接影响如血栓形成或肠壁水肿可伴随细菌产生物质的易位，导致额外的液体积聚，进一步增加 IAP（表 1）。在细胞水平，氧输送受损，导致缺血和无氧代谢。血管活性物质，如组胺和 5- 羟色胺，增加内皮通透性。进一步的毛细血管渗透会损害红细胞运输，使缺血情况恶化。虽然目前的实践管理指南是由于在创伤环境中 ACS 发展的经验而产生的，但重要的是要认识到损伤控制性剖腹术和开放

表 1　腹腔内高压对器官系统的影响

器官或组织	结果
头	颅内压↑
	脑灌注压↑
心	心排血量↓
	静脉回流↓
	肺动脉阻力和中心静脉压↑
	全身血管阻力↑
肺	吸气压峰值↑
	肺动脉楔压↑
	动态顺应性↓
	动脉氧分压↑
	动脉二氧化碳分压↑
	肺内分流↑
	部分无效腔的分数达到潮气总量（V_D/V_T）↑
肝	门静脉血流↓
	线粒体↓
	乳酸↑
肾	尿量↓
	肾血流量↓
	肾小球滤过率↓
肠	腹腔血流↓
	肠系膜上动脉血流↓
	黏膜血流↓
腹壁	腹壁顺应性↓
	腹直肌血流↓

式腹部处理并不排斥创伤人群。各种医疗和手术情况包括弥漫性腹膜炎、急性胰腺炎和肠系膜缺血，可能使患者发生 IAH 和 ACS 的风险增加（框 2）。

框 2 腹腔隔室综合征病因：谁有风险？
创伤后出血
腹膜内出血
腹膜后出血
腹膜外出血
任何需要积极液体复苏的患者
休克后内脏水肿
“致命三联征”——低温、酸中毒、凝血功能障碍
频繁的腹腔隔室综合征前兆

ACS 的发展的其他危险因素包括腹水或腹内液体积聚、腹膜内或腹膜后出血 / 血肿、肾替代治疗、怀孕、腹部烧伤、大容量复苏，用于控制出血的腹部填塞、肠缺血后再灌注损伤、肠梗阻、腹内肿块、在张力过大的情况下关闭腹部。

测量 IAP 的最实用可靠的方法是通过膀胱作为被动导管。膀胱传导 IAP，而其自身的肌肉组织不会施加任何额外的压力。将盐水注射到完全排水的膀胱中。再将一个 Foley 导管吸入口和一个 16-G 针插入该端口，然后连接到换能器系统，髂嵴被用作零参考点。商业工具包也可用于测量膀胱压力。

预防 ACS 须识别有风险的患者，及时对主要问题进行外科干预（例如出血）和明智的液体管理。医疗管理仅限于镇静 / 化学麻痹、胃和膀胱减压、减少潮气量呼吸机策略、液体限制和利尿。然而，更严重的隔室综合征形式需要外科手术，包括早期减压性剖腹术。尽管在 ICU 中可以安全地进行减压作为床旁手术，但在手术室中最好处理 ACS 的出血源（图 4）。一旦完成，减压性剖腹术通常会迅速逆转 ACS 的不良反应，并改善氧合和肺顺应性，使吸气压峰值恢复正常，并迅速逆转少尿与轻度利尿。在减压之前，尝试纠正酸碱和电解质紊乱（包括钾、镁和钙不平衡）可以减轻减压后的心律失常。减压后维持开放式腹部须用 TAC 维持开腹或腹腔镜造影（图 5）。

未经治疗的 ACS 被认为是致命的，尽管使用腹部减压，但生存率可能低至 50%。虽然 IAH 是进展为 ACS 的一部分，但单独的 IAH 可能不会对多器官衰竭和死亡等结局产生不利影响。在预防 ACS 方面，IAH 的鉴定至关重要，因此可采取医疗或外科手段来制止综合征的进展。

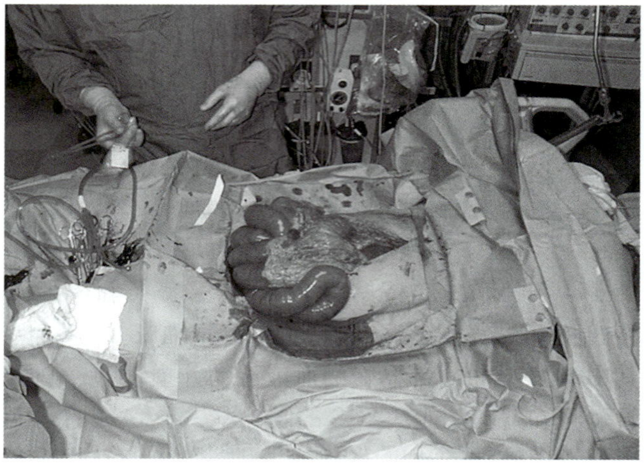

图 4 腹腔隔室综合征的床边减压性剖腹术。注意大量小肠水肿

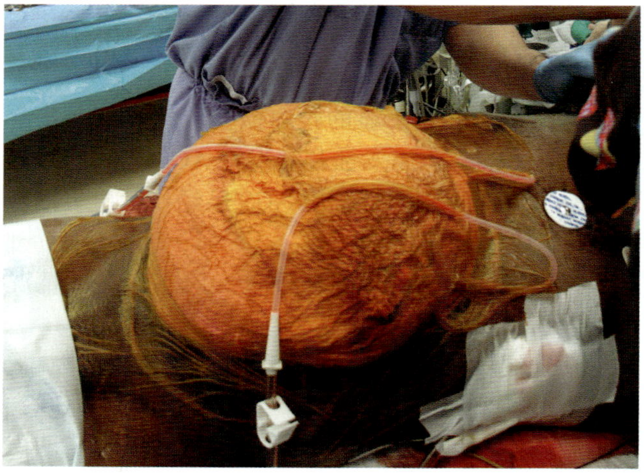

图 5 使用负压吸引设备临时腹腔关闭

损伤控制

损伤控制手术是过去 20 年来极端患者手术治疗的主要进展之一。传统上，损伤控制定义如下：

1. 快速控制出血和污染
2. TAC
3. 代谢紊乱的生理复苏
4. 延迟确定性手术

由于多损伤创伤患者的手术管理的范式发生变化，我们认识到危重患者更可能死于其术中代谢功能紊乱，而不是完全的手术修复失败。部分有凝血功能障碍、低温和代谢性酸中毒的“致命三联征”特征的代谢功能障碍患者常常死亡。这推动手术外科医生认识到这种生理学，并预判它须进行基于快速初始损伤程度的损伤控制，因为不这样做可能会增加死亡风险。

然而，为了解决一个问题，又创造了另一个问题：创伤后开放式腹部，被定义为大的术后腹疝，腹部内脏被临时用敷料或闭合覆盖。在管理与这些危重患者有关的并发症方面，我们已经吸取了许多经验教训。通过这些经验教训，开放式腹部管理的4项基本原则已经演变为：

1. 肠道保护
2. 保护筋膜，以防止腹内容物丢失
3. 如果可能，一期关闭腹部
4. 减少计划性腹疝和延迟重建

损伤控制技术的最早描述之一是1908年的Pringle，他描述了在肝创伤的情况下使用纱布填塞来进行出血控制。虽然这些技术后来基于战时的经验而不被鼓励，但对于严重创伤的缩略腹部手术的兴趣在20世纪后半叶重燃。Harlan Stone的有价值的文章首先描述了“救援”技术，开创了缩略剖腹术和损伤控制的时代。当“损伤控制”技术应用于严重腹部血管损伤的患者时，Rotondo等对它改善生存率的描述，有助于将外伤手术的范例从创伤患者的第一次手术必须是确定性手术的范例改变。目前的损伤管理方案已经包括4个阶段（图6）。

在急诊部，大量出血患者的初步术前评估和复苏可以视为损伤控制连续期（DC0）的序章。DC0期间的最高优先事项是：①鉴定失血患者；②启动血液和凝血因子治疗；同时③准备确定性出血控制。必须明确提供复苏，因为血液制品的大容量复苏、凝血因子和晶体的解决方案可能与ACS的发展有关。不鼓励大容量的基于晶体的复苏，因为这不仅会增加IAH，而且还会导致出血和凝血功能障碍的恶化。早期止血复苏优于全血或血液成分治疗以逆转创伤诱发的凝血功能障碍和休克。越来越多的证据支持低血压复苏，其重点是维持循环和止血，而不考虑血流动力学参数的正常化，特别是在血管损伤的条件下。尽管在文献中有一些争议，但许多报告显示，大量输注血浆和血小板：红细胞比例高的血液制品可以改善患者的生存，并可能降低总体输血需求。

在初始创伤性剖腹术（DC1）期间，重要的是估计每个患者的生理储备，以做适当的操作决定。

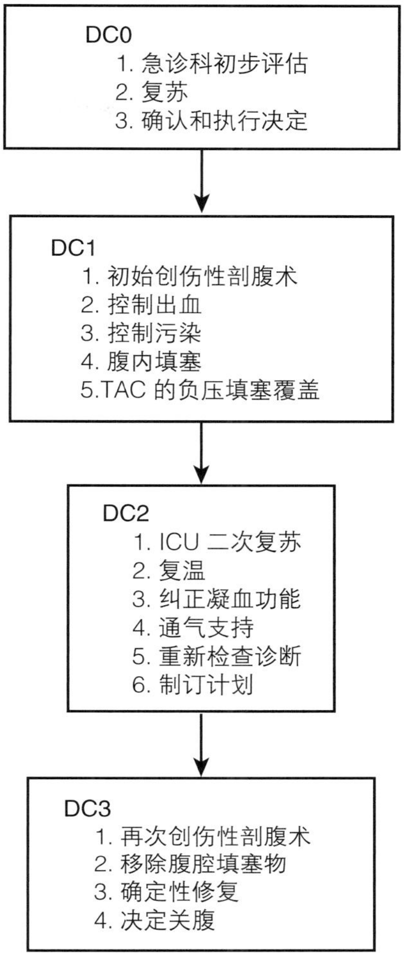

图6　损伤控制方式。DC: 损伤控制；Dx: 诊断；ED: 急诊科；ICU: 重症监护病房；TAC: 临时腹腔关闭

生理储备被定义为个体容忍受损伤的独特能力，是几个主要因素（包括年龄、性别、之前存在的疾病、遗传和免疫能力）的功能决定的。在每个患者的生理学和估计储备的背景下，可以最好地评估损伤程度。因此，损伤严重程度决定了导致生理性耗竭的斜率（图7）。由于生理储备在出血性休克期间耗尽，发生局部和全身性的灌注不良，导致生理性耗竭和随后的死亡。

与麻醉队进行围术期沟通可改善患者的生存，并减少并发症。该沟通包括维持手术室尽可能温暖。建议麻醉人员预期失血量，并避免在出血手术前过度复苏。

在初始创伤性剖腹术期间，外科医生必须认识到须立即控制主要出血和污染，最大限度地替换凝血因子，包括血小板、FFP和冷凝蛋白质，以及某些情况下因子Ⅶa用于微血管出血。术中监测温度、动脉血气和复苏容量对于确定患者是否生理曲线下

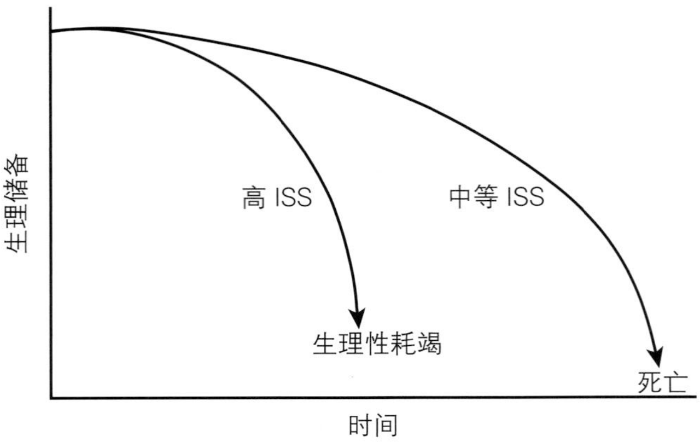

图 7 由于伤害严重度而导致的生理储备的消耗。ISS，损伤严重度得分

降到生理性耗竭是重要的。此外，对于有空腔脏器损伤的患者，用线性吻合器控制污染物，以横断肠道末端，并使其不连续，直到患者能够承受重建。

若已经确定了临床参数，应该敦促手术组开始损伤控制操作、中止手术，并返回 ICU 进行复苏和恢复储备（DC2）（表 2）。在达到生理性耗竭的上限之前，应尽早着手损伤控制。使用这些损伤控制需要的术中预测因子，Asensio 等在随访研究中证实，创伤后腹部开放的患者的体温降低较少，术后并发症较少，包括腹内脓肿和瘘管形成。早期损伤控制的患者也被发现有较少的肠水肿，并且在其初次住院期间更可能进行确定性的腹壁关闭。

表 2 中止初步创伤性剖腹术和启动损伤控制操作的临床指南

问题	描述
低体温	＜35℃
酸中毒	pH＜7.2 碱缺失≥8 mEq/L 乳酸≥4
凝血功能障碍	活化部分促凝血酶原时间＞60 s INR＞1.6
持续复苏	顽固性休克伴收缩压＜90 mmHg ＞10 L 的晶体 ＞10 单位的浓缩红细胞
操作时间	腹腔开放时间＞60 ~ 90 min

Asensio 等在一项涉及 548 例失血和需要损伤控制的患者的标志性研究中，描述并统计验证了能够早日建立损伤控制的标准。这些标准包括 pH 低于 7.2，HCO_3^- 在 15 mEq/L 以下，温度为 34℃或更低，替换大于 12 的 XXX 体积，以及高达 4 000 ml（10~12 单位）的 PRBCs。

一旦患者满足损伤控制的要求或因 ACS 的体征和症状进行减压，外科医生必须使患者接受创伤后腹部开放和 TAC（框 3）。

临时腹腔关闭

TAC 定义为在急性期护理期间含有腹部内脏的任何技术。历史上，在急性期护理期间，已经使用了多种 TAC 技术来容纳腹部内脏（框 4）。尽管 TAC 有多种选择，但我们认为，“真空填塞”技术最符合创伤后开放式腹部管理的前两项原则：①保护肠道，②保留筋膜。Barker 等描述的这种方法通过将穿孔的非黏附塑料材料放置在筋膜下位置的腹部内容物上，来保护肠和腹部内脏。然后放置通过伤口上部引出的两个大引流管和外科手术巾（图 8）。整个腹部缺损被一个大的黏合性敷料覆盖，并且引流管连接到壁来吸引以产生连续的负压。这种技术还抵消了筋膜边缘的侧向收缩，并保留了腹直肌肌筋膜复合体，以供随后关闭（框 5）。

开放式腹部管理的最终目标是实现延迟的一期筋膜闭合。然而，某些临床情况使筋膜无法一期闭合或对此提出技术挑战，并且继续开放式腹部处理可能是必要的。这些患者可能表现出持续的污染和生理损伤、延长的炎症反应、严重扩张的内脏，预期须在 12 ~ 96 h 内再次手术，或失去腹部区域。这些患者，指出了延迟性一期闭合与腹壁重建的策略。

确定性重建与闭合（DC3）

TAC 有 3 个潜在的阶段：

框 3 临时腹腔关闭的适应证

生理储备消耗
不是由肠水肿导致的腹壁过度紧张而无法关闭筋膜
避免大容量复苏后腹腔隔室综合征发展
计划返回手术室
不填塞
重建肠道连续性
肠内通道
彻底探索来重新评估已知的伤害，并识别遗漏的伤害
处理异常威胁生命的伤害（例如主要盆腔骨折、严重闭合性头部损伤）的相关需求

框 4 临时腹腔关闭选择

Bogota 袋
巾钳
拉链
Wittman 补片
仅皮肤的闭合
Barker 负压填塞
负压伤口系统
人造网片
纱布填塞

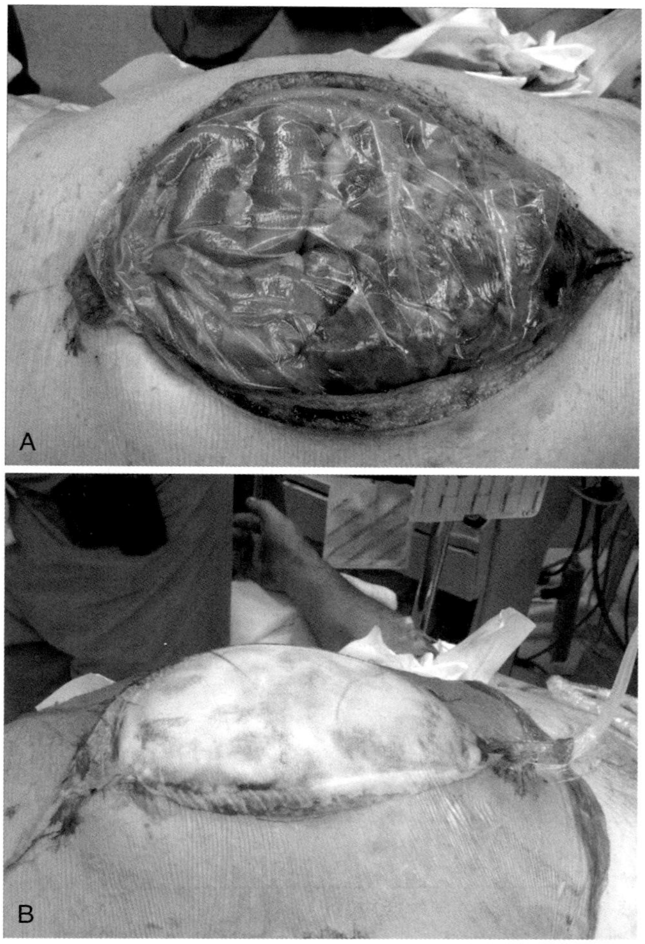

图 8 负压填塞临时腹腔关闭。**A**，肠隔离袋。**B**，具有大引流管和黏合性屏障的无菌手术巾

1. 在 ICU 内复苏至生理终点为止
2. 恢复或再手术和早期筋膜闭合的尝试（数天至数周）
3. 重建或计划性腹疝和延期筋膜关闭

复苏

ACS 的损伤控制或减压性剖腹术后 ICU 复苏的目标是偿还持续的氧债、恢复足够的灌注以满足代谢需要，以及逆转出血性休克。这包括凝血功能障碍的纠正、乳酸性酸中毒的纠正、电解质紊乱的纠正和温度的恢复（框 6）。应该考虑腹部压力的连续监测，因为这些患者发展为 ACS 的风险很高。对于温度正常，酸碱状态和凝血功能障碍的患者仍然表现出持续的输血需求，应该考虑到及时进行手术再次探查，因为这表明出血控制不足。

框 5 真空填充技术的优点

保护肠道，并将它保持在筋膜下方
保留筋膜，防止失去腹部区域
易于使用、快速应用、轻松拆卸
保持患者的干燥和洁净
量化液体损失
预防腹内高压 / 腹腔隔室综合征
简单、无创、经济

ICU 管理中的额外的复苏措施还包括使用动脉造影和栓塞，特别是对于严重的盆腔动脉出血和广泛的肝血管损伤患者。肢体和骨盆骨折也可以使用外固定器暂时重新对齐、推迟复杂的骨科重建，直到炎症反应消失、患者进入病程的后期阶段。

恢复

在 ICU 复苏和纠正在初始创伤性剖腹术或 ACS 减压术后发生的生理和血流动力学紊乱后，TAC 患者返回手术室进行进一步评估。在再次探查期间，外科医生必须再次作出重要的临床和技术决定。仔细去除所有保留的肝周和腹内圈垫，防止血块超过肝损伤，并避免黏附于肠的圈垫的浆膜撕裂。重新评估已知的伤害，并进行彻底的探索，以识别遗漏的伤害。如果在初始损伤控制性剖腹术期间需要肠切除术，则建立 GI 连续性并建立肠内通路。重要的是保护缝合线或钉线，并将其放置在腹腔内，并尝试用未受影响的肠襻或网膜覆盖吻合口。如果造口术是必要的，放置处应该保留随后的恢复手术和可能的腹壁重建的可能性。损伤控制性剖腹术后，患者尽管在 ICU 得到生理恢复，吻合口破坏的风险增加。在这种情况下，应仔细考虑肠道分流。

在重建阶段应插入鼻饲管或手术放置肠内通道。放置在经过胃肠减压的 Treitz 韧带或打开的胃空肠吻合口的鼻饲管是长期肠内通路和营养补充的选择。

进行任何进一步血肿的清洗和移除，并制订关

框 6 重症监护病房复苏清单

复温 / 纠正低体温

心脏导引器中心线

快速输液器（Ⅰ级），热交换器设置在 40℃

静脉注射（IV）液体、血液、血液制品

通风口上的加湿器设定在 40℃

对流暖气机（Bair Hugger）

放在整个躯干上

盖住手、脚、头

防止无知觉者的热损失

保持环境温度 >85°F

纠正凝血功能障碍、酸中毒、电解质不平衡

测量血红蛋白和血细胞比容、凝血酶原时间、部分促凝血酶原时间、国际标准化比率、血小板计数、纤维蛋白原

替换为浓缩红细胞、新鲜冰冻血浆、血小板、冷凝蛋白质、因子Ⅶa

纠正动脉乳酸、碱缺失、纠正 K^+、Mg^+、Ca^+ 缺乏

监测

插入血氧计肺动脉导管，以维持氧气输送并获得复苏终点

Do_2I（氧气输送指数）500 ml/min

心脏指数（CI）>3 L/min

舒张末期容积指数（EDVI）120~140 ml

动脉血氧饱和度（Sao_2）>95%

静脉血氧饱和度（Svo_2）>65%

温度 >36.5°

血细胞比容 >21%

如果对复苏没有反应，检查是否为肾上腺功能不全

随机皮质醇水平

促肾上腺皮质激素（ACTH）刺激试验

药物

预防消化性溃疡

H_2 阻断剂或质子泵抑制剂

深静脉血栓形成预防

低分子肝素

序贯压缩装置

胰岛素滴注

维持血糖 80~110 mg/dl

静脉镇痛及镇静

连续输液

广谱抗生素应用 24 h 或直到腹腔内包扎

覆盖革兰氏阴性微生物和厌氧菌

护理

抬高床头 30°

清洁胸部、腰部和骶骨

频繁的气管吸引和口腔卫生

使用鼻胃管

负压填塞的引流管的抽吸

Foley 导管

检查每小时尿量

检查膀胱压力

压力点垫垫圈减少褥疮（枕部、颏部、肩胛骨、骶骨、脚踝）

于确定性关闭的计划。如果肠水肿很小或完全解决，并且筋膜边缘可以很容易地接近而没有过度的张力，则可以进行一期筋膜闭合。在闭合期间与麻醉小组的沟通至关重要，特别是在通气压力方面。如果吸气压峰值在筋膜接近期间从基线上升到高于 10 mmHg，则应放弃对一期筋膜闭合的尝试。在过度紧张的情况下闭合可导致腹壁坏死、复发性 ACS、严重感染性并发症和呼吸功能不全。如果在此阶段成功关闭筋膜，必须对所有患者的腹腔进行常规术后放射学评估，以确保没有计划外的异物残留。

如果在第一周结束时腹腔不能关闭，则肉芽组织可能开始发育，第二周结束时“腹部冰冻”明显。这为早期筋膜闭合创造了一个敌对的环境，因此需要计划性腹疝和延迟性重建。由于担心在确定性关闭被大大延误时增加并发症发生率，所以我们主张在术后第 8 天尝试确定性关闭。在有可吸收网片和肉芽组织发展的背景下，分层厚皮肤移植物（split-thickness skin graft，STSG）可以应用在肉芽组织床上。然后患者需要 6~12 个月的蛋白质和热量储存的恢复期，才可以进行成功的腹壁重建（图 9）。这项决定虽然可以挽救生命，但是是非常昂贵的，可能导致生产性生活方式的丧失和无法返回劳动的后果。

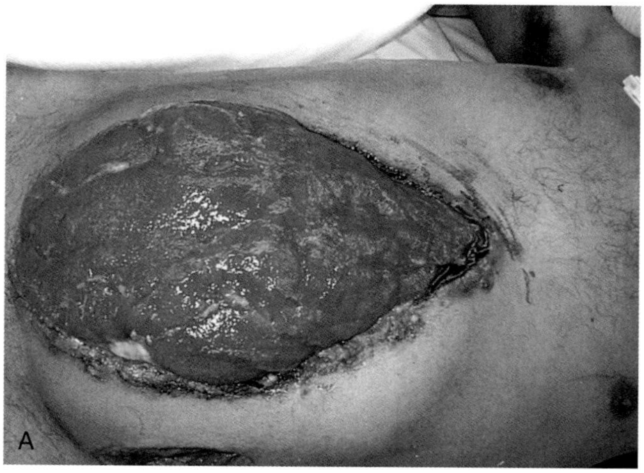

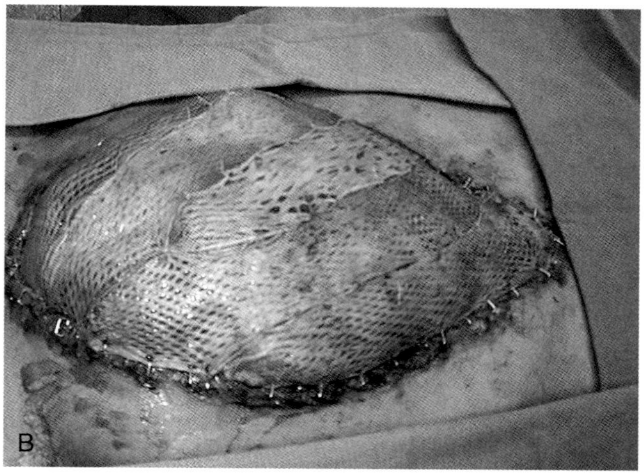

图 9　**A** 和 **B**，开放式腹部的成熟的肉芽组织，然后用分层厚皮肤移植物覆盖

虽然可吸收网片植入是许多中心的常规做法，但与创面中“大气压内”瘘的发展相关的复杂性促使了对替代技术的研究。聚乳糖网片已被广泛使用，因为即使在受污染的区域使用时，其有吸收性，也能促进肉芽组织的发育。尽管有这些优点，肠瘘的发生出现于高达 21% ~25% 的用聚乳糖网状物关闭腹膜的患者中。由于在这些情况下并发症发生率高，文献已经描述了在创伤后开放式腹部中采用生物材料获得闭合或筋膜一期闭合的积极方法。替代方法使用负压填塞、负压伤口装置和生物假体材料的组合来补充腹部筋膜中的间隙，甚至在初始损伤控制生程或减压性剖腹术后 3 周进行。

类似于负压填塞，在市场上有多个负压伤口真空系统，其使用封闭在黏合屏障内的海绵状材料（图 10）。这些装置用于保护肠道并保留筋膜，同时重新恢复腹部损失的区域（框 7）。

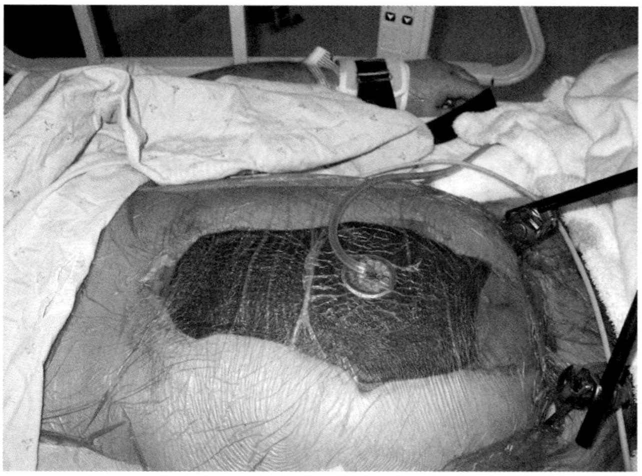

图 10　负压辅助伤口装置。注意损伤控制骨科手术的外部固定器

与身体认为是外来物质并导致被包裹的合成假体材料不同，生物假体材料支持细胞生长和整合、快速血供重建和向患者自身组织转变。这些材料用作天然自体组织的生物支架（图 11）。用于这些植入物的组织可以在化学处理后从牛、猪或人中获得，使其具有生物相容性，并使免疫原性最小化。生物假体材料容易受到污染，并且在禁止使用合成材料的情况下可用于关闭腹腔（图 12）。在细胞水平上，当化学交联时，生物网片植入物可具有较高的初始强度。然而，天然组织向内生长受损，导致类似于非生物假体植入物的被包裹的现象。

尽管关于复发率和腹壁松弛发展的长期结果尚不知道，但是这种方法与计划性腹疝处理方法相比，肯定具有如上所述的固有的高风险伤口并发症的优势。负压伤口敷料和辅助使用生物假体网片的组合实现了创伤后开放腹部的最终基本原则：早期腹壁关闭。

重建

一旦早期一期筋膜闭合的机会窗已经错过，发

框 7　负压：伤口系统的优点

- 减少频繁更换敷料的需求
- 除去多余的间质液
- 增加伤口血管
- 减少活菌数
- 改善伤口收缩
- 延迟“冰冻腹部”的发作——防止肉芽组织粘连筋膜
- 扩大筋膜闭合的机会窗

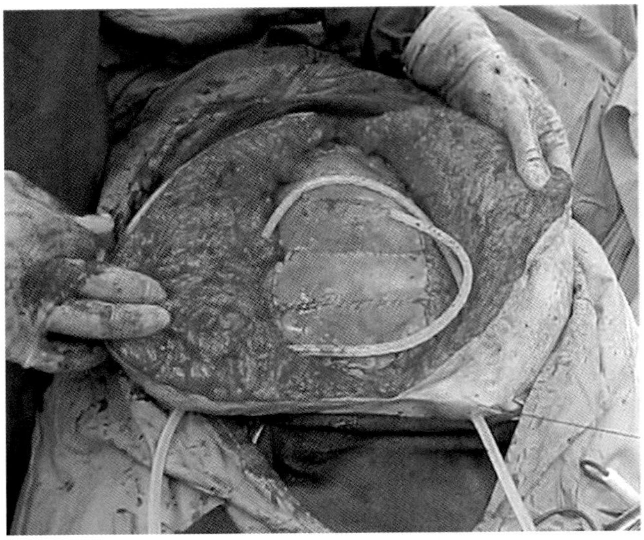

图 11 具有上覆皮瓣的生物假体植入物的腹壁重建

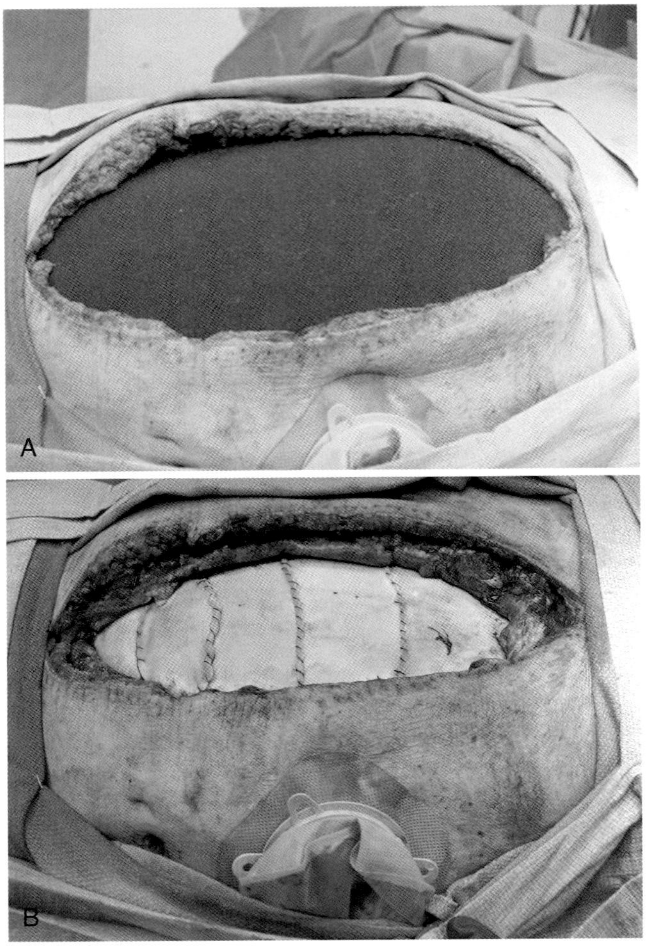

图 12 **A** 和 **B**，在有负压伤口系统的被污染的腹部开放性伤口上，用于桥接筋膜间隙的生物假体放置在生物性筋膜替代物上

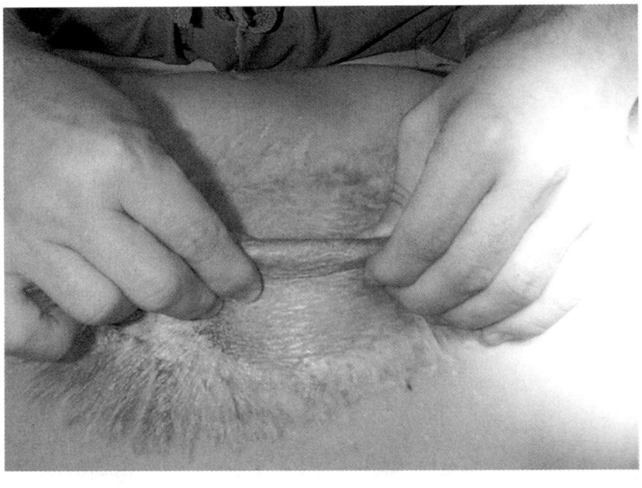

图 13 夹紧试验

生了继发的炎症反应和肠水肿，需要延迟、分期关闭腹壁。因为开放式腹部仍然具有传染性并发症的高风险，使用合成假体材料进行重建不推荐用于确定性重建，虽然有最终使用假体材料的分期重建的描述。一旦 STSG 可以从下面的肠道升高，就可以假定炎症反应已经解决，下面的内脏通常是可移动的（图 13）。这种组织分离通常需要 6~12 个月才能发生，并且是重建期间防止肠损伤的关键。移除 STSG，并且从周围组织移动筋膜。然后将皮肤和皮下组织沿外周提起，作为侧向皮瓣（图 14）。此时桥接筋膜间隙的选项包括成分分离技术和生物假体材料的关闭。

成分分离技术重建筋膜缺损是通过将外斜肌插入直肌鞘，并将其外侧部分肌横切，且从内斜肌分离。直肌可以沿中线前进，并在中线缝合以闭合缺损（图 15）。这种技术可以拉近 10 cm 的缺损，而没有产生过高的张力。使用改良的成分分离技术，可以通过将直肌与后直肌鞘分开来获得几厘米的移动。无增强的成分分离操作的复发率为 22% ~32%。因此，我们目前的做法是通过使用生物假体植入来补充。

损伤控制技术和预防措施，以避免 ACS 的发展现在是处理创伤性休克的护理标准。在复苏的早期阶段使用 TAC 的负压填塞，保护肠道并保留筋膜。可以通过在恢复阶段期间使用 KCI VAC 时，不在高度张力下关闭筋膜，并维持腹部区域来避免并发症。然后可以一期或者通过使用生物材料来安全地进行筋膜闭合的多次尝试，以便在初次住院期间桥接筋膜间隙。

在创伤后进行开腹是不再需要的，它会造成大的腹疝和重建延期，除非有长时间的炎症反应阻止早期筋膜接近的异常情况。

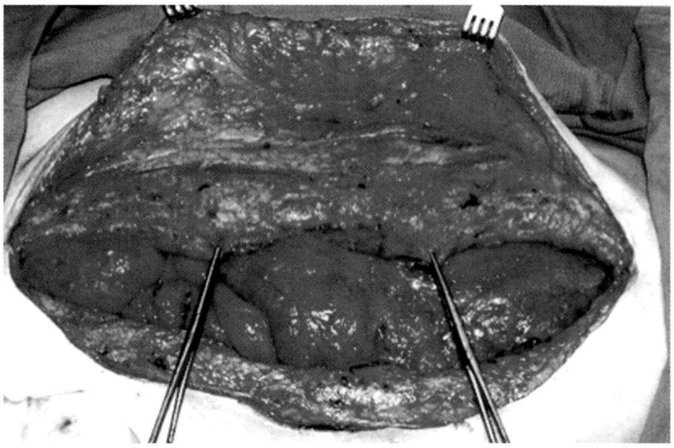

图 14 从周围组织释放出的筋膜边缘和从直肌的侧边缘提起的皮瓣

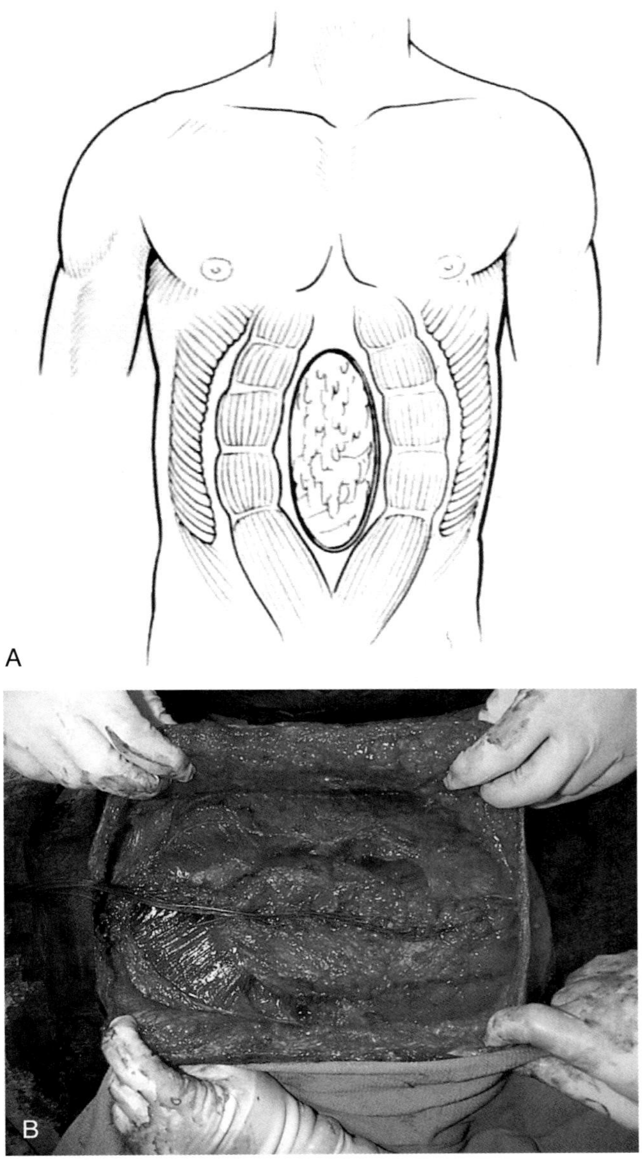

图 15 **A** 和 **B**，成分分离技术

特别考虑：营养支持

在损伤控制手术后，在最大的生理压力期间产生大的腹部伤口缺陷，有持续的代谢需求和分解代谢。所以密切注意营养支持和热量需求对减少早期和晚期并发症这两者至关重要。开放式腹部的理想的营养支持应从恢复阶段开始，腹内填塞被去除，GI 连续性重新建立，并进行凝血功能障碍、酸中毒和低体温的纠正。

在过去 10 年，非开放式腹部的肠内营养优于肠外营养已经被文献反复验证，肠内营养路径的益处包括减少感染风险。

血流减少与微生物易位、肠黏膜血流减少和最终的多器官失败相关。可通过防止萎缩和异常渗透性肠内营养已显示改善肠黏膜的完整性。一些研究表明从“早期”开始的肠内营养（24~48 h 内）有益处。尽管有这些发现，对于它的使用、安全性和危重患者安排腹腔造影的时间上还有不情愿和不确定的使用。开放式腹部患者不给予肠内营养的原因包括不耐受的恐惧、肠梗阻和肠水肿的发展，潜在的抽吸可能性、小肠坏死和在血管加压剂使用时吸收不良的风险、对葡萄糖控制困难的担心，损伤控制手术后，肠道不连续以及无法给予肠内营养（框 8）。肠外营养与肠内营养相比，制造和使用相当昂贵，还须频繁监测电解质，并还可能存在与之相关的严重并发症，如中枢系统并发症、中枢相关血流感染、伴可能的细菌易位的肠绒毛萎缩、代谢紊乱和胆汁淤滞。

Tsuei 展示了肠内营养在开放式腹部患者中的可行性，绝大多数患者（75%）进食后达到 77% 的热量需求。早期肠内营养（36 h 内）也不会实质性地减少呼吸机相关性肺炎的发生率，对损伤控制后腹

框 8 拒绝肠内营养的理由

关注是否有不耐受
麻痹性肠梗阻
肠水肿
误吸风险
关注使用加压药后的小肠坏死
吸收不良
胰岛素和葡萄糖处理困难
损伤控制后肠道连续性中断
临床偏好 / 不适

部闭合率也无不良作用。最近的研究表明，早期肠内营养可能早期筋膜闭合相关，它还降低了肠外皮肤瘘形成率。

我们目前的建议是在早期复苏后的护理阶段开始肠内营养，无论腹壁的状况如何，都可以提供肠道的连续性。获得肠内通路应被视为损伤控制患者的高度优先事项，特别是对于预测可能延长疗程的患者。在这种情况下，早期肠内营养应和肠外营养联合使用以达到可接受的蛋白质及热量的目标。此外，在其他腹外的操作和手术中，肠内营养可以安全地持续。

表 3　开放式腹部相关的并发症

腹部	腹外
伤口感染	呼吸机相关性肺炎
伤口开裂	吸入性肺炎
腹壁筋膜炎 / 坏死	血液感染
腹腔内脓肿 / 脓毒症	泌尿系统感染
肠吻合口瘘	深静脉血栓形成 / 肺栓塞
	压疮（枕骨、肩胛骨、骶骨、跟骨）
	多器官功能障碍综合征 / 多器官系统衰竭

开放式腹部的预后和并发症

多项研究验证了在 DCC 和 ACS 患者中使用开放式腹部后，其并发症发生率降低、生存率下降、长期预后改善。虽然维持开放式腹部是 ACS 患者或需要损伤控制性剖腹术的创伤患者的潜在救命措施，但该处理策略使患者面临潜在的破坏性并发症的风险。创伤后患者与损伤控制相关的死亡率估计高达 31%，这通常归因于多器官系统衰竭的后果。

其他并发症包括输血需求增加、ICU 使用和医院费用增加、瘘形成、腹疝，以及暴露的内脏中有明显的液体、电解质和蛋白质丢失。在持续性开放式腹部的患者中，医疗相关感染，如手术部位感染、血液感染和呼吸机相关性肺炎也增加了（表 3）。

2005 年，Miller 等出版了 344 例开放式腹部患者的经验：与开放式腹部相关的并发症发生率为 25%，一期关闭达 65%。初次剖腹术后第 1 周的一期筋膜闭合与并发症发生率非常低（9%）有关。然而，并发症发生率明显升高有 3 种情况：

1. 在张力太大的情况下一期闭合筋膜
2. 在使用 STSG 之前等待肉芽组织的形成
3. 使用非生物假体材料进行关闭

腹腔关闭延迟的并发症包括伤口感染、脓肿和伤口裂开，从初次干预 8 天后发病率显著上升（图 16）。还应注意的是，尽管我们主张在可行的情况下进行一期腹壁关闭，但是在损伤控制 / 开放式腹部的情况下一期关闭的长期结果仍然未知。Vogel 等通过将持续性开放式腹部与手术部位感染、血液感染和呼吸机相关性肺炎的较高发生率相关联，来证实了这些结论。

与损伤控制相关的死亡率估计高达 31%，这通常归因于多器官系统衰竭的后果。

可疑的是，持续性开放式腹部最具破坏性的并发症之一是瘘管形成，昂贵的劳动密集型和不健康的并发症。瘘形成的原因是多因素的，包括腹部感染、肠缺血和梗阻的存在、不小心的肠切开、肠道长时间暴露于大气中（引起干燥），以及使用的填充

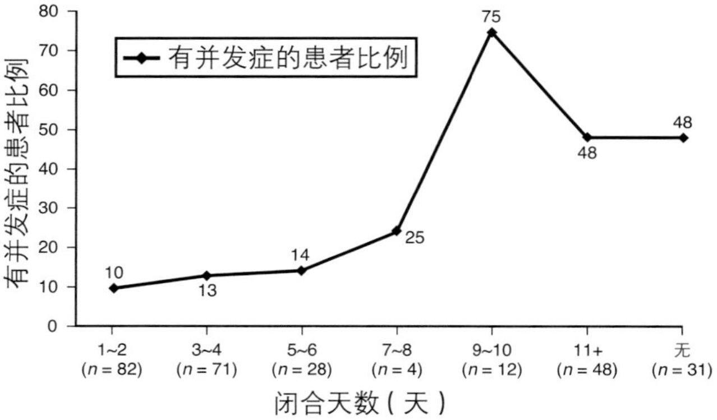

图 16　有伤口并发症患者的比例与筋膜闭合天数之比

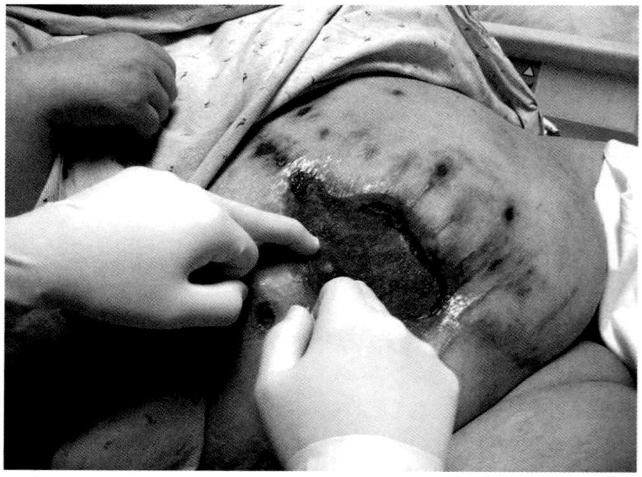

图 17　肠吻合口瘘

物、敷料或假体材料黏附于肠浆膜（图 17）。使用负压填塞的肠道损伤和干燥、适当的营养支持和腹壁早期无张力关闭都是很好的预防措施。然而，一旦形成瘘管，相邻内脏必须被保护，并且来自瘘管

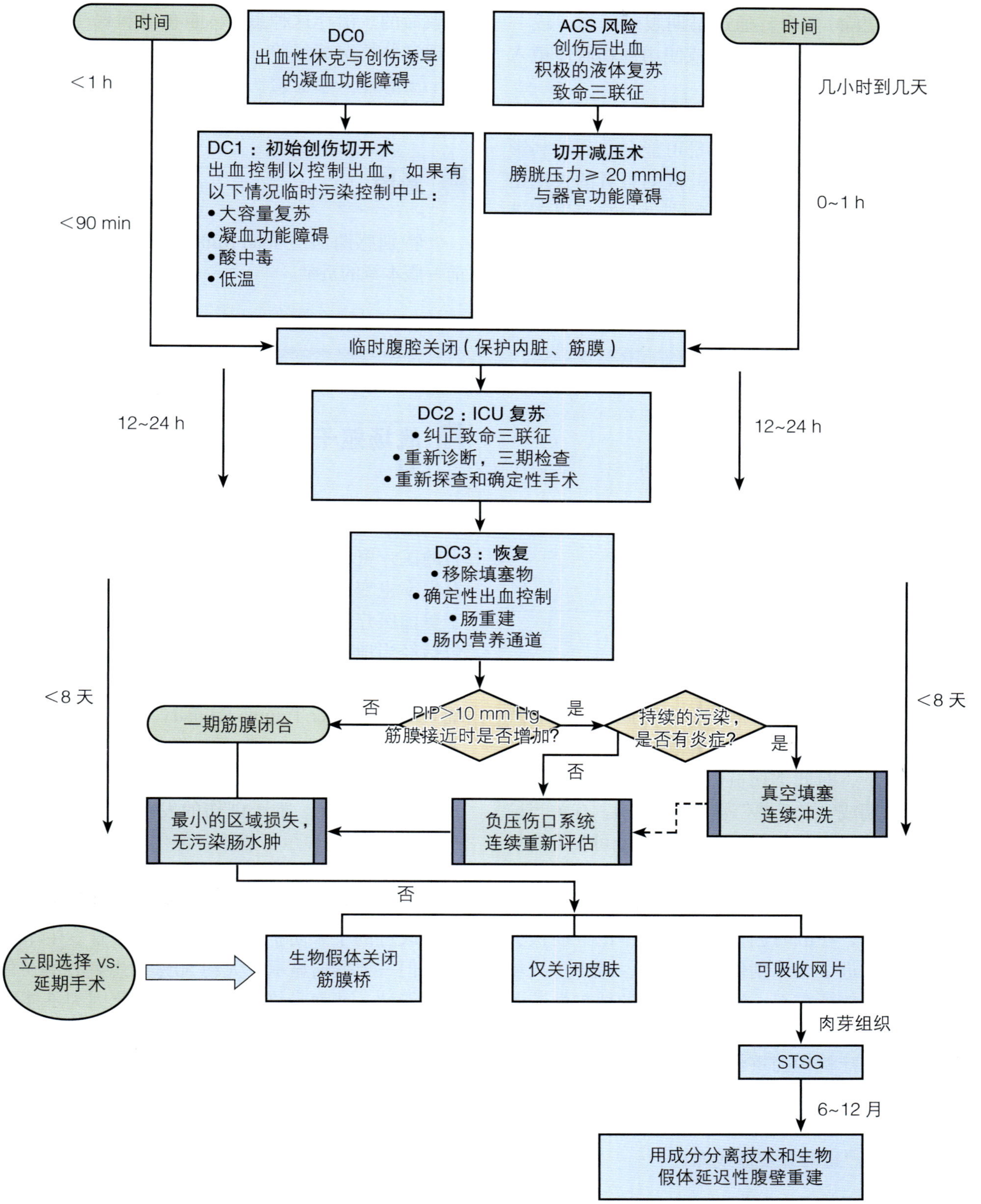

图 18 开腹手术治疗流程。ACS，腹腔筋膜综合征；DC，损伤控制；ICU，重症监护病房；PIP，吸气压峰值；STSG，分层厚皮肤移植物

的流出物必须被控制。由于炎症改变和解剖学障碍，早期修复瘘管通常是不可行的。需要复杂的伤口管理系统来控制瘘出口，并允许肠道肉芽组织形成。伤口愈合有时需要 STSG 覆盖，同时等待延迟的腹壁重建和瘘切除 / 闭合。通过早期腹壁闭合，或一期修复直肠缺损、仅皮肤关闭或使用生物假体植入物都可以使瘘的流速最小化。

开放式腹部对每位患者的社会心理影响很重要，患者甚至在几年后，生活质量都可能会受到不利影响。有数据表明，计划性腹疝开放的患者的长期结果接近能够一期关闭的患者，特别是当腹疝患者进行重建时。

总结

对受伤和危重患者的损伤控制技术的应用可能是救命的。治疗这种患者人群的外科医生必须具备处理这些情况的经验，这需要广泛的潜在手术和生理干预措施。参见损伤控制方法（图 18）。

致谢

特别感谢医生 John Miller 和 John Morris 为本书前一版本章的贡献。

现代战场躯干创伤

Colonel Matthew J. Martin 和 Colonel Brian Eastridge 著
黎檀实　孙荣距 译

战场躯干创伤介绍

在当今时代，战场创伤救治中经常可见之前冲突中出现的快速致命的腹部损伤，除此之外还有严重创伤和生理学的改变。要求军医在有限的人力和设备的情况下，对此类伤员可能要进行手术，尤其是在战斗早期或“未成熟”阶段（图 1）。有关当前军事医学系统早期部署的详尽概述随处可见（战场检伤分类）。本章的重点是战场环境下躯干创伤（胸部、腹部或胸腹联合伤）伤员的特殊问题和管理策略。纵观历史，在战时创伤救治过程中的经验极大地帮助我们改进了全球创伤救治技术，减少了战场躯干创伤伤员的死亡率。然而，改进的保护性装备和院前救治措施以及缩短的转运时间，使得被成功转运至前线医疗机构的重伤员数量上升了。现代战场的军医必须掌握快速且有条不紊的方法，对躯干创伤患者进行评估和早期管理，因为任何的拖延和失误都将导致严重的并发症或死亡。

战场躯干创伤的发生率和流行病学特点

由于在复杂的实际操作过程中收集完整的且有力的医疗资料的困难性，因此统计准确的战时创伤发生率也变得很困难。这些有限的数据基本都来源于美国医疗机构和军队人员的数据分析，而且还不包括经当地或军地联合医疗机构进行救治的大量非军队人员的伤员。一项来源于联合战场创伤登记系统（Joint Theater Trauma Registry，JTTR）包含 3102 名伤员的数据显示，胸部损伤的发生率为 6%，腹部损伤为 11%。在 JTTR 的一项后续的分析中显示，2001 — 2009 年，躯干创伤的发生率为 15%（未公布数据）。表 1 显示了躯体各部位创伤与以前数次战争中的发生率的对比。

现今战场中严重的胸部创伤的显著减少主要归功于改进的个人防护装备和车辆。尽管发生率降低了，但一项数据显示，大约 50% 的患者有潜在存活的可能性，然而最终死亡的伤员的死因为不能压迫止血的躯干创伤大出血。因此，对于此类伤员的早期救治仍然需要高度重视。还有须我们警惕的是尽管在受伤的战士中，躯干创伤发生率降低了，但在那些没有武装和保护性装备保护的平民中，躯干创伤的发生率仍然居高不下。战伤，尤其是躯干创伤，以其独有的严重性和本质，推动了当前一种军事专用评分系统的广泛应用——损伤严重度评分（Injury Severity Score，ISS）。

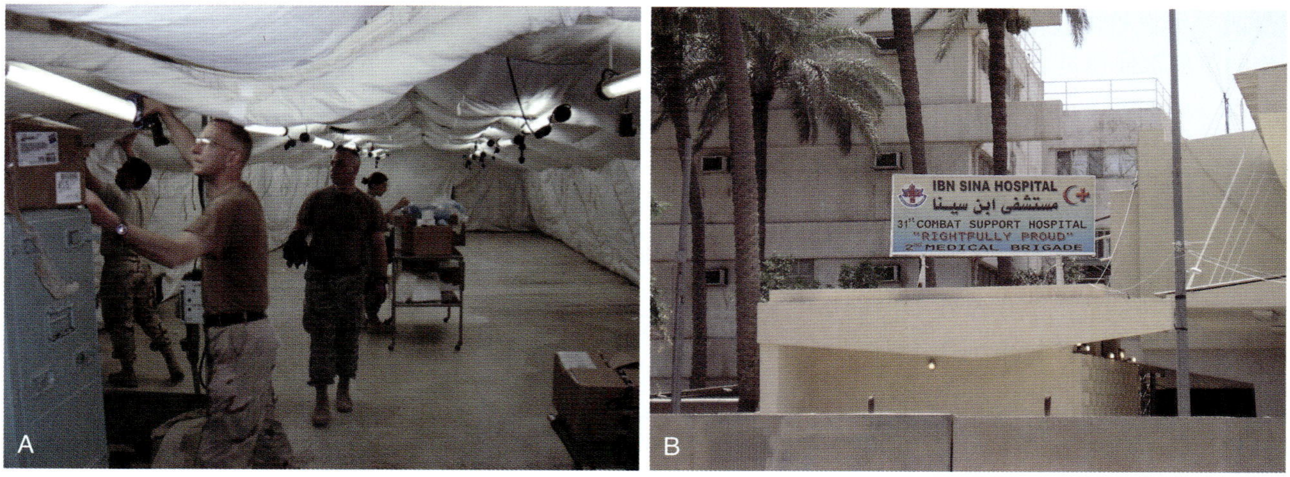

图 1　先期部署设施根据条件和能力灵活多变。**A**，伊拉克提克里克的创伤手术室开设于一顶帐篷中。**B**，位于伊拉克巴格达的装备齐全、现代化的 Ibn Sina 医院

表 1　自第二次世界大战以来躯体各部位战伤分布比例

部位	第二次世界大战	越南	OIF 和 OEF
头颈	21%	16%	30%
胸	14%	13%	6%
腹	8%	9%	9%
四肢	58%	61%	55%

From Owens BD, Kragh JF Jr, Wenke JC, et al: Combat wounds in operation Iraqi Freedom and operation Enduring Freedom. *J Trauma* 64:295–299, 2008

OEF：恒久自由行动；OIF：伊拉克自由行动

表 2　不可压迫的躯干出血的诊断标准和流行病学

部位	生理	相对发生率	死亡 OR 值
胸腔	收缩压 <90 mmHg 或需要紧急手术	32%	1.9
实质器官损伤 >3 级		20%	1.0
重要的躯干纵行大血管		20%	3.4
骨盆环断裂		15%	0.80

Modified from Morrison JJ, Rasmussen TE: Noncompressible torso hemorrhage: a review with contemporary definitions and management strategies. *Surg Clin North Am* 92:843–858, 2012

SBP, 收缩压

不可压迫的躯干出血：定义问题

腹部或胸部的活动性出血与创伤死亡率密切相关，约占平时环境下潜在可预防死亡中的 60%~70%，战时环境下的 80%。尽管长期以来，我们已经认识到战时环境下的“不可压迫”大出血的存在，但对其认识程度一直都受限于缺少可被广泛接受的定义或分类（评分）系统。然而，近期公布的一项关于大出血和战时躯干创伤的分析阐述了一系列有关不可压迫的躯干出血（noncompressible torso hemorrhage，NCTH）的诊断和分类标准问题的进展（表 2）。通过这样的定义，13% 的战地伤员归类于躯体损伤标准，2% 的伤员属于 NCTH。其中最致命的是躯干大血管的损伤（OR = 3.4），占 NCTH 伤员的 20%。在平民创伤中，NCTH 有相似的发病率，为 2%，但是相当大的比例为钝伤。类似于战时数据统计，在平民创伤中心，NCTH 也在因出血所致潜在可预防死亡中占据相当大的比例（45%~85%）。不同于周围血管或连接部位血管创伤，在院前或 ED 阶段，此类创伤不能通过直接压迫或简单的血液阻断（止血带）等方式实施止血。因此，对其进行止血的方法引起了人们极大的兴趣，并对其不断进行创新。对于此类危重 NCTH 伤员的处置措施是：①最大程度缩短从急救机构至 OR 的转运时间（或直接转运至手术室进行复苏）；②尽可能保持低血压，直到出血血管得到控制；③在早期应用血浆的情况下，达到平衡或进行“止血”复苏；④应用氨甲环酸（tranexamic acid，TXA）等止血剂；⑤当有指征时进行损伤控制手术或血管内分流术。当前能够直接影响 NCTH 伤员生存率的创新性手段已经得到应用，包括用于临时血管控制的主动脉内

球囊闭塞等血管内技术，同时在药理学上或激素类药物的革新都使伤员更加能够耐受严重的大出血。

战时躯干创伤机制

现代战争的特点是日渐复杂多变且致死性的武器，使得其所造成的创伤是在平民创伤中心未曾出现过的。尽管在很多城市创伤中心，子弹穿通伤也很常见，但是却都是由一些低速武器所造成的，和战场高速武器所造成的组织毁损性损伤相比就是小巫见大巫了。在面临战时爆炸伤时能发现两者的最显著的差别。通常爆炸伤、贯穿性碎片伤、钝器伤（如翻车）和热损伤的结合，常导致包括多部位截肢、四肢损毁伤、头颈联合伤、主要躯干损伤等严重的多系统损伤（图 2）。在先前的战争中，这些类型的损伤多见于迫击炮、火箭弹、地雷等军事爆炸装置所引起。在当今以对抗叛乱者为特征的伊拉克和阿富汗战争中，损伤多由于作为敌对势力武器之一的简易爆炸装置（improvised explosire device，IED）所引起。躯体各部位主要战伤机制见图 3。这与早先的以枪伤为主要致伤原因的战争形成明显的对比。然而致伤的高速军事武器仍然占据主导地位，而且能产生毁损性且富有挑战性的战伤（图 4）。

美国军方认为抵抗 IED 产生威胁的原因中，最重要的 2 点是：①越坚硬的车辆外壳对于爆炸的抵抗能力越强；②包括躯干装甲、头盔、手套和护眼

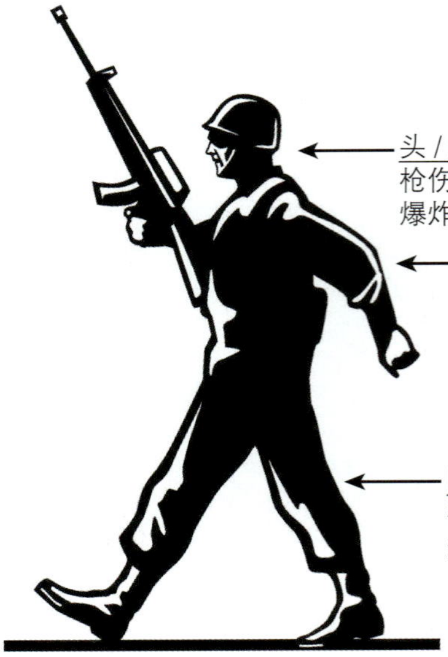

图 3　躯体各部位主要战伤机制

GSW，枪伤 *(Dnta from Owens BD, Kragh JF Jr, Wenke JC, et al: Combat wounds in Operation Iraqi Freedom and Operation Enduring Freedom. J Trauma 64:295–299, 2008.)*

等个人防护装置的改进和普及。这些进步和发展，其最显著的作用就是使得在躯干创伤的发生率中，相比于先前的战争，胸部创伤的发生率降低了 50%。以作者在伊拉克和阿富汗战争中的经验来看，这些保护性装置已使得致死性战伤以及包括胸壁挫伤、肋骨骨折等无生命威胁的损伤的发生率降到了相当低的程度（图 5）。

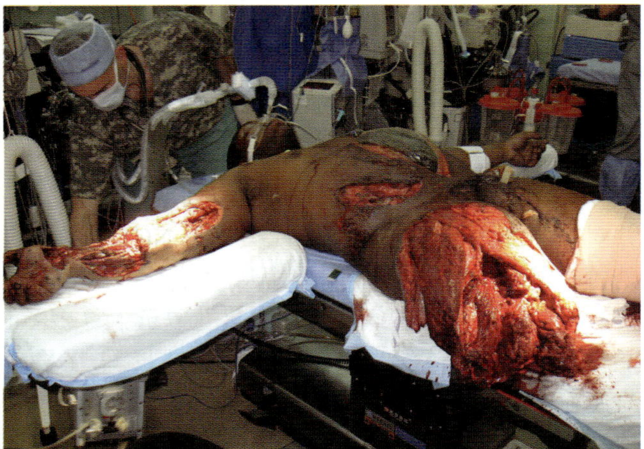

图 2　图中为 1 名在由简易爆炸装置所导致的军用车辆撞击事件中出现的行人伤员，包括肢体毁损 / 截肢伤，空腔脏器穿通伤、骨盆骨折，肱动脉撕裂伤以及肺挫伤

初始评估

对于存在躯干创伤伤员的初始评估必须快速、有序，然而却通常由于环境混乱、创伤严重而变得很难。面对伤员极端的伤情（但是没有生命危险），救护员通常容易产生慌乱的情绪，但只要止血成功，这些情绪就会消失。所有伤员都应优先评估气胸和不可压迫的内出血，直到排除。一些物理检查，包括 X 线胸片、超声可以在数分钟内完成，而且应该用来识别任何来源的大出血。图 6 显示的是躯干评估方法。在初始评估中最重要的方面之一就是避免任何拖延，以及避免对不稳定的伤员或有明显手术干预指征的伤员实施不必要的影像检查。此外，在战场环境下，手术探查的指征应该放宽，这是由于缺少高分辨率的影像设备、有极大可能性存在腔内

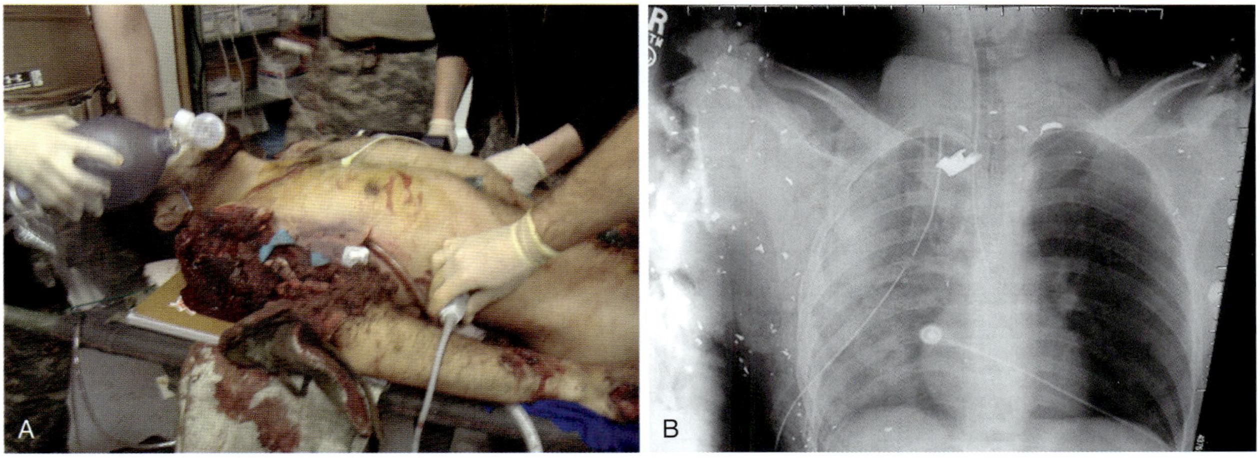

图 4　单纯右肩部的高速枪伤导致了近乎截肢的软组织毁损性损伤（**A**），相应部位的 X 线片显示骨损伤和破碎弹片（**B**）

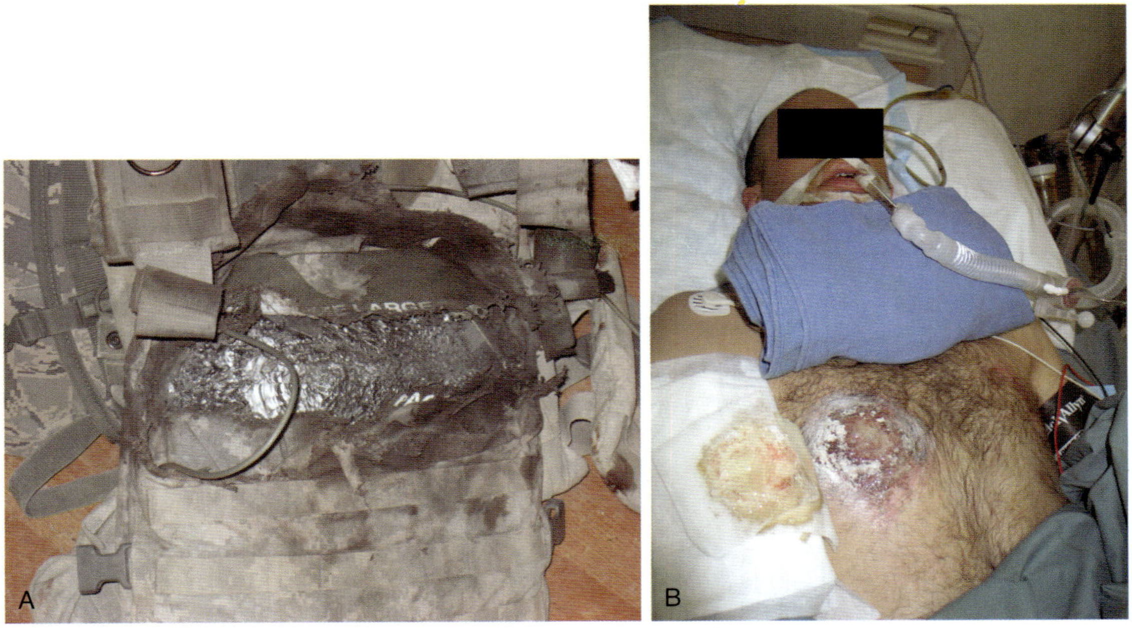

图 5　**A**，士兵胸甲遭到火箭弹打击至胸部受到撞击，但这名士兵的躯干没有受到严重创伤。**B**，这名士兵因导弹撞击胸甲导致胸壁挫伤

损伤，缺乏对大批量伤员进行一系列检查和监测的能力，以及须快速后送至其他医疗机构。尽管很多设置机构在前沿的医疗单元没有行 CT 扫描的能力，但高质量的便携式超声设备可及性很强，因此应广泛使用。即使没经过额外训练，一名医生也能快速且可靠地评估气胸、血胸、心脏压塞，以及心肌收缩力和容量状态（静脉腔大小和呼吸变化）。这一技术甚至已经被延伸到战场环境下的院前救治阶段，而且可以加快识别和救治潜在致命性创伤，尤其是气胸。

手术干预

对于战场环境下多种躯干创伤手术的干预措施已经在本章节前面部分进行过描述，而且目前还有一些涵盖了这一方面细节问题的优秀战创伤指南可供参考。本书中包含的大多数有关躯干损伤的手术技术方面的论述也和平民创伤手术技术并没有什么区别。然而，要想取得最佳的手术效果，就须了解和平民创伤所不同的重要方面的问题，以及遵循一

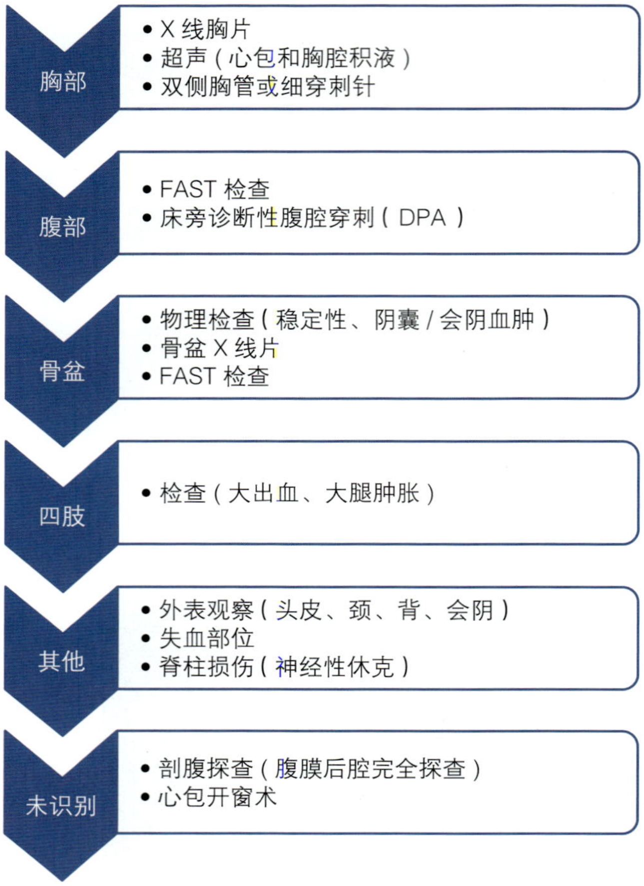

图 6　快速评估和探查战创伤患者大出血部位方法。FAST，创伤重点超声评估 *(From Martin M, Beekley A, editors: Front line surgery: a practical approach. New York, 2010, Springer.)*

系列战伤手术的基本原则。第一，也是最重要的就是严重创伤合并低血压的躯干创伤伤员应迅速转运至手术室，并给予血液制品复苏，同时准备手术干预。

伤员全身的所有损伤部位（包括四肢伤）都应做好手术准备，并且处于同一手术野。只要有条件，头/颈部或四肢损伤应该由一个专门手术团队同时进行处置。只要资源上允许，所有的紧急手术，尤其是胸部和腹部手术，都应该由至少 2 名外科医生协作完成，以便最大程度地彻底暴露术区，同时最大程度缩短手术时间。急诊开胸术（emergency department thoracomy，EDT）应该有选择性地为那些存在躯干或主要肢体损伤且等极危重的伤员实施，生存率为 11%。然而，对于批量伤员，EDT 就不应该实施。而且，应该经常充分考虑对于血液制品等有限资源预期的消耗量。接下来的部分内容主要概括了一些详细原则和一些常规战场躯干创伤的处置方案。

切口的选择

没有经验的手术医生选择“随机的”手术入路，旨在最大程度简化术式和暴露术野，代价是丧失了灵活性和选择性。一个好的手术医生通常宁可损失一部分术野（但总是足够的）来换取最大程度的灵活性和选择性。一个典型的例子就是使伤员侧卧位以便暴露存在出血或其他损伤的一侧胸部。但是如果出血部位是在腹部、纵隔或者对侧胸部，这种情况将是灾难性的。对于躯干部位的探查手术，大多数情况下伤员都应该取仰卧位，以便保留对颈部、双侧胸部、纵隔、腹部和腹股沟区进行手术的可能。如果存在暴露上的困难，应该避免小切口和随意扩大切口。对于前外侧开胸术，最好的、最充分的扩大术野的方式是延长皮肤切口 5~10 cm 到达对侧胸壁并分离胸骨。对于所有短期致命性的胸部创伤，若要获得最完全合适的暴露的方式，要么选择前外侧胸壁入路，要么选择胸骨正中切开术，而不是后外侧胸部入路，这种方法对于择期手术更合适。

胸部损伤控制

胸部损伤控制手术遵循和腹部损伤控制手术一样的原则，但在实践上却迥然相异，因为解剖结构上的不同和术者经常不断升级的不舒适感。在腹部创伤中唯一随时可能威胁生命的危险因素是出血，但在胸部创伤中却有多种因素，包括生理上的紧张、心脏压塞、难治性低氧血症/高碳酸血症、心律失常和空气栓塞等。单肺通气通常不能快速实现，而且暴露的肺很容易因为手术过程中的压迫和肺内气体呼出而出现不张。对于处置出血，最先应该做的是人工移除血凝块，然后进行直接控制出血或填塞止血。在一些胸腹联合交通伤伴有进行性出血的病例中，辨别活动性出血是来自腹部还是胸部是很困难的。快速临时封闭所有大的隔膜缺损来重建体腔的结构能极大地帮助辨别出血来源和控制出血。大多数的隔膜在修复后都会出现相关的术后渗出，因此应该总是于修复的表面留置胸腔引流管。要想避免严重的低氧血症和呼吸性酸中毒，最关键的就是与麻醉师进行密切交流并严密观察各项通气指数变化，而且在手术过程中应该在一系列关键点进行血气分析。最后，虽然选择临时胸腔关闭和临时腹腔关闭没什么差别，但是关胸后要保证患者有一定程度上的正常呼吸和胸壁的力学，避免未充分排空渗出物的关胸造成的张力性气胸或心脏压塞。作者更倾向于放置 2 根大口径胸腔引流管达到充分引流的目的，同时放置一根中号引流管以引流肌肉、筋膜和皮肤之间的渗液。

肺损伤手术

相比于民间，战创伤中的胸部穿通伤更倾向于需要手术干预。来自克罗地亚战争中的数据显示，63% 的战争相关的胸部创伤需要手术，而且 34% 需要肺修复或切除。标准的肺损伤手术技术应用于简单且通常由民用低速手枪造成的穿通性损伤的情况少之又少。战中肺损伤所累及的肺组织通常被广泛浸润而且有出血，适用于民间穿通性肺损伤的用吻合器的肺神经束切断束通常并不适用（图 7）。是实施吻合肺楔形切除还是常规肺叶切除主要取决于所累及的需要处理的肺实质范围。随时可能出现的空气栓塞须时刻警惕，预防方法是快速控制损伤，在损伤部位得到控制前夹住肺门，或用盐水没过损伤部位。最后，对于不稳定或情况恶化的伤员，应避免尝试长时间的肺部血管修复或广泛的组织切除。肺门夹闭、临时关胸或吻合肺切除术等损伤控制可以在数分钟内完成，但是必须做好处置术中或术后瞬时心肺功能不全的准备（图 8）。

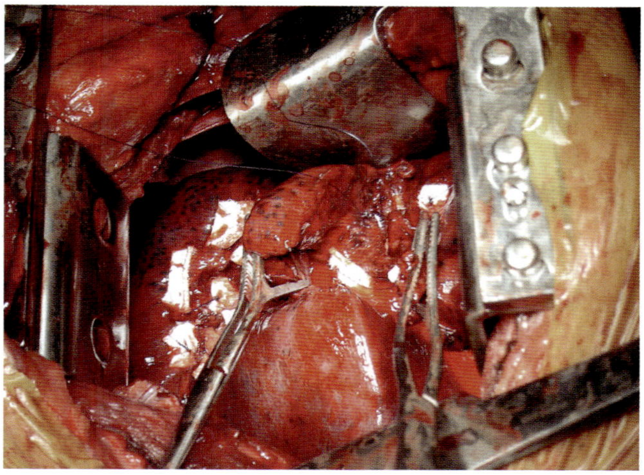

图 7　高速致伤武器造成的肺损伤需要肺楔形切除，修复破损的肺实质来控制出血和气体泄漏

大量血胸

尽管立即行胸廓造口术置管是大量血胸的标准治疗方案，然而在战场中常常还须对活动性出血行立即或延期的介入治疗。将患者送进手术室（如果情况允许），并完成以下程序，更有利于救治：让患者处于仰卧位，轻度抬高患侧，无菌巾覆盖胸部。使用胸廓造口术置入 2 cm 的导管，插入 Poole 吸引管引流管穿刺引流血液，灌洗以清除血凝块，之后于切口放置大直径胸管。如前期失血量较多或有活动性出血，则采用前外侧开胸术或胸骨正中切开术，根据笔者的经验，这种方法不会延误后续的手术或

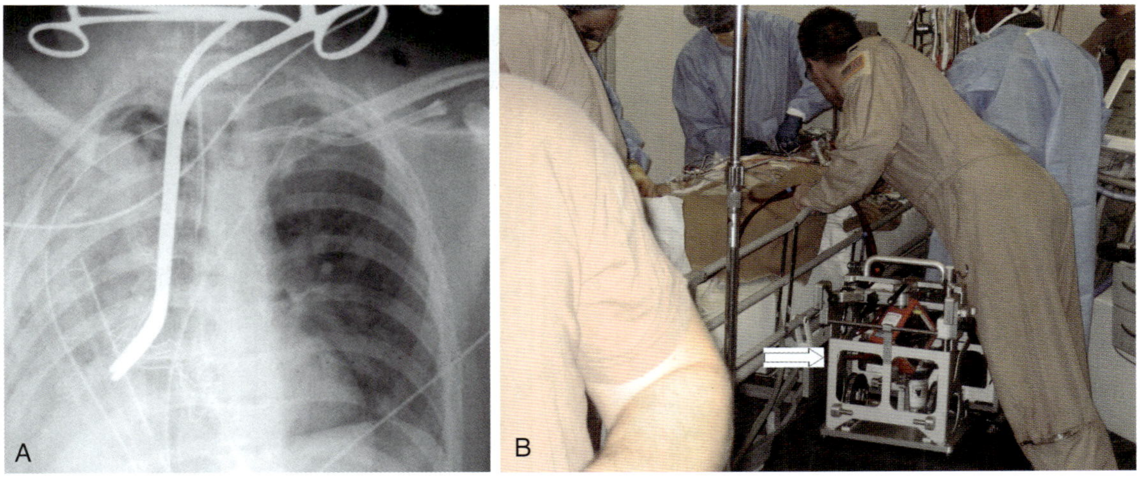

图 8　**A**，一名遭受破坏性肺损伤的士兵在经过损伤控制性胸部手术后的 X 线胸片，在其右肺门部可见止血夹；**B**，这名士兵在便携式体外循环氧化膜的支持下从阿富汗转往德国 *(Courtesy of CDR Rodd Benfield and CDR Eric Elster, U.S. Navy.)*

介入治疗时间，并且降低残余血胸的发生率，也有利于后续的开胸术或胸腔镜（前外侧切口或胸骨正中切口）治疗。

躯干多处碎片伤

爆炸装置造成的伤员中，小的躯干碎片伤并不少见，其中有些类似于平民猎枪伤，但损伤面积更大一些（图 9）。从外观上，很难区分它们仅仅是表面的损伤还是同时有重要脏器的损伤。我们往往借助侧位 X 线片辅助正位片来确定碎片的深度和位置。这些碎片可能在血管上造成小洞，但同时止住出血，也对判断血管损伤造成一定困难。这样的血管损伤如果没有持续的出血或未造成严重缺血，就没有立即处理的指征，但仍然需要一个标准的或 CT 血管造影检查来确定是否有碎片的位置接近主要血管结构。这种情况下仅依靠 CT 或荧光透视难以准确定位损伤，故常与手术探查相结合。在少数病例中，碎片进入周围动脉或静脉，形成栓子，这就须结合 X 线胸片和周围血管成像等检查加以排除。如果心脏超声怀疑有心脏损伤、X 线胸片上可以看到碎片、患者出现不明原因的血流动力学不稳定，这时，有必要施行剑突下或经膈的心包开窗术。

血流动力学不稳定且体检高度怀疑腔内损伤的患者须立即送至手术室开始探查手术。即使开始的 X 线胸片未见明显损伤，仍有很大可能对患者行胸廓造口术置管，特别是将要行正压通气或要立即被后送的患者。躯干的碎片伤的非手术治疗将取决于现场情况和所用的资源。在Ⅱ级救治场所，若没有 CT 设备或无法完成检查，除非能够认定伤口只存在于表浅部位，否则应进行手术探查。在条件更好的Ⅲ级救治场所，体格检查结合 CT 扫描、选择性非手术治疗躯干碎片伤是安全、有效的（灵敏度 98%）。

腹部实质脏器损伤

虽然孤立的腹部实质脏器损伤（solid organ injuries，SOI）是典型平民钝伤，它们在战斗中也时有发生，包括弹片或碎片伤、爆炸伤、车辆事故等。战场中的实质脏器损伤，无论钝伤或穿通性 SOI 造成，与非战场情况下的处理非常不同，认定的 SOI 更倾向于手术治疗。因此，在战时，除非有足够的时间与资源对伤员进行非手术管理，大多数的腹部外伤患者应进行手术探查。战时的 SOI 损伤严重程度更大，常伴有其他伤情，且密切观察监测患者的时间、能力极其受限。因此，腹部创伤和 FAST 检查阴性的多数患者，或 CT 显示的明显 SOI 患者（2 级以上），应行手术探查，除非有足够的资源和人力进行适当的非手术处理。SOI 的另一个特点是，以

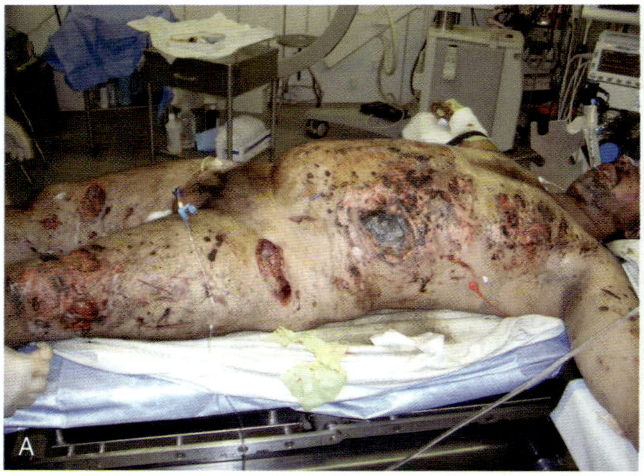

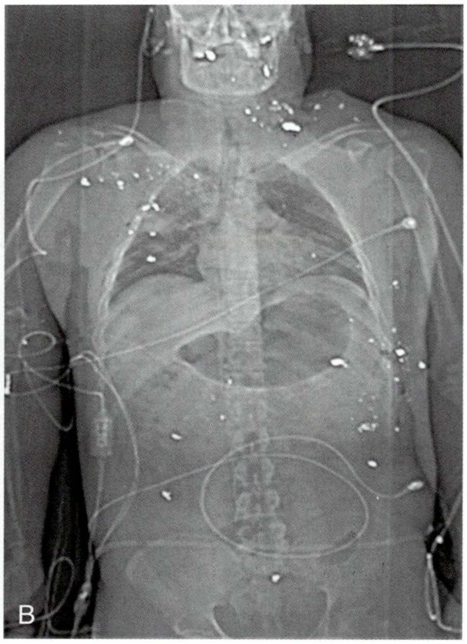

图 9　在简易爆炸装置爆炸中受伤的患者。**A**，由爆炸碎片伤造成的从头到脚的不同深度、范围的损伤。**B**，X 线片显示散布于躯干的爆炸碎片

爆炸伤或高速弹道伤为首，组织破损的范围和程度极大。战场肝损伤可能更具挑战性，须及时探查、清创或切除等（图 10）。解决个体 SOI 问题的同时，必须要考虑到复合伤的严重程度、复苏要求，继发的凝血功能障碍和严重出血。这些可能是第一次探查未发现的小的 SOI 引起的。

肠损伤

肠损伤的最佳处理方案一直是一个充满争议的热点，从第二次世界大战时期强制性结肠造口术或结肠旷置术到现今的选择性政策。初次手术并无太多争议，大部分的损伤使用损伤控制方法，而之后的修复之路上，则是重建和造口术的对决。大肠、小肠战伤行一期修补的失败率较非战伤高，所以最好由吻合器切除。高速弹片对小肠造成破坏性损伤（图 11A），碎片伤造成较小的洞，因此必须进行细致的检查以防遗漏。伤后有独特的发现，弹片伤周围肠管有显著的热损伤，这在平民创伤中是罕见的（图 11B）。虽然造成的缺损很小，但整个烧伤面积必须完全切除。肠系膜有大的破损，肠壁却是完整的，此时应根据血管离断的程度和随后预计发生肠坏死的风险及时切除受累部分（图 12）。选择近端分流与一期修复的方式，不仅要考虑标准患者因素，也要考虑战场现实因素，如是否有多位急需手术的伤员和是否需要立即后送而被限制的密切观察术后吻合口的能力。虽然结肠造口术对于绝大多数结肠伤口肯定不是强制性的，但在战场上应相对平民损

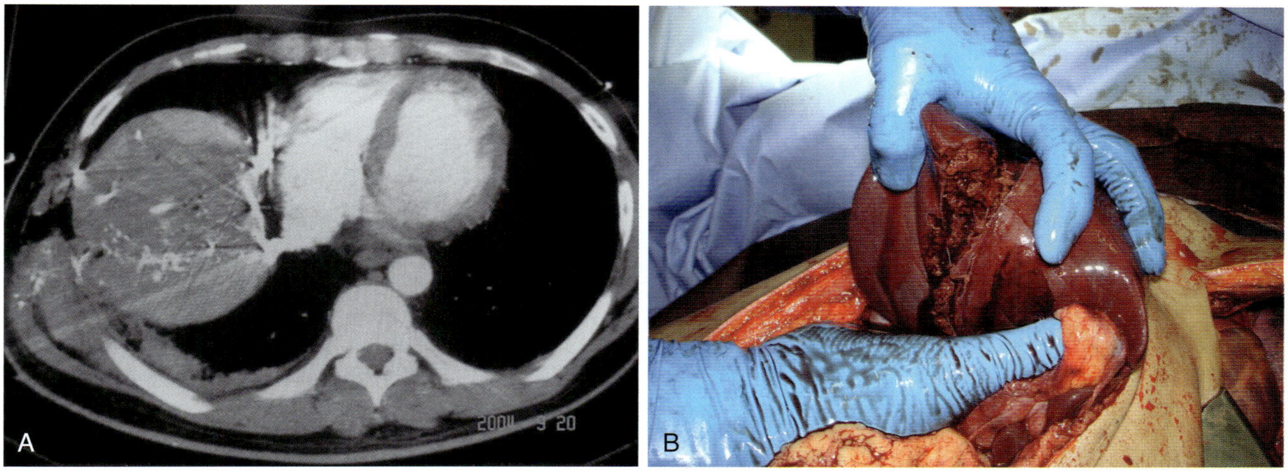

图 10　**A**，计算机断层扫描提示肝右叶爆炸 / 碎片伤。**B**，术中发现肝实质损伤，行切除性清创

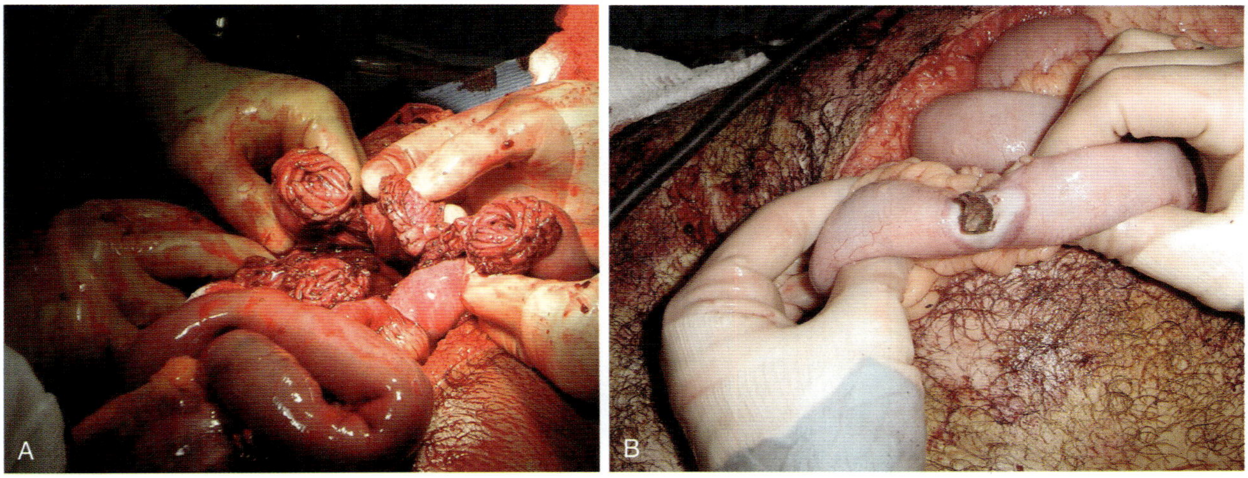

图 11　**A**，单口径 50 的机枪导致的多发性肠破损。**B**，小肠碎片伤，伤口周围见热损伤（*From Martin M, Beekley A, editors: Front line surgery: a practical approach. New York, 2010, Springer.*））

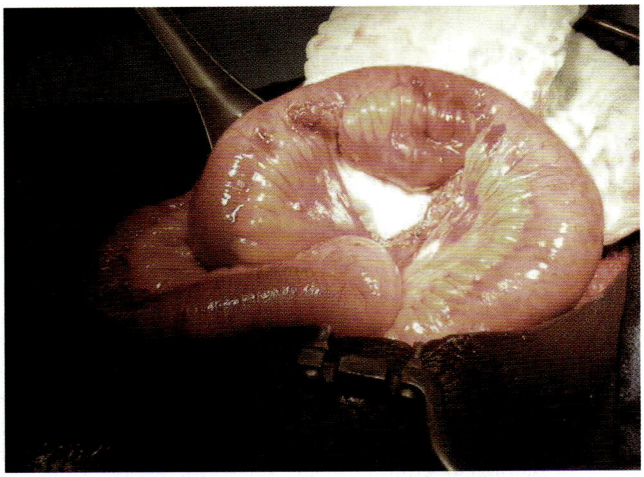

图 12　小肠肠系膜撕裂。虽然无肠壁破裂，仍应切除受累的缺血部分

伤放宽应用指征，尤其是与相关的高危腹部损伤，如胰腺或十二指肠损伤。如须进行造口术，首选环或“闭环”造口，它不仅提供了粪便转流，且更容易修复（通常不需全腹剖腹探查术）。

腹壁和会阴 / 骨盆伤

当前战争中爆炸事件增加，导致了腹壁或骨盆 / 会阴伤发生率的增加，这些通常伴有明显的皮肤和皮下组织的丧失，使一期修复不可能。在腹壁全层丢失伤后，相关脏器脱出的可能性大，须立即剖腹探查（图 13）。大块腹壁缺损的处理非常具有挑战性，可能需要复杂皮瓣覆盖，但初步处理时，负压辅助关闭设备的广泛使用，步骤已大大简化（图 14）。IED 爆炸中最具挑战性和也是最不幸的常见伤口是广泛会阴 / 骨盆伤口，通常伴随下肢损毁伤或截肢，这会使损伤的复杂度和并发症发生率增加。因为有严重出血、污染及相关损伤（大血管、骨盆、大肠、膀胱、直肠）等情况，处理上更加复杂棘手（图 15）。这些患者须进行复苏，应尽快送至手术室。可以完全绕过急诊室就诊阶段。最初的手术干预通常包括 2 个阶段：①处于仰卧位控制出血和处理胃肠膀胱损伤；②进行随后的清创术及进一步止血手术。无论有无肛门直肠受累，均建议行结肠转流造口术，但并不适用于初次手术中。

广泛是会阴 / 骨盆创伤和大腿近端截肢的治疗难点之一控制活动性出血。虽然骨折和软组织损伤看似更为严重，但达到适当的血管控制才是一开始关注的重点。一些病例中，可在直视下快速控制伤口处的股血管出血，但在有替代方案的情况下，应该放弃在活动性出血和混乱场合直接暴露的尝试。高位髂腹股沟血管损伤导致的严重动脉和静脉联合出血，通过剖腹术或腹膜外腹部血管暴露达到近端主髂血管控制，或暴露腹部血管直接控制出血（图 16A）。控制住近端出血后，我们开始直接暴露大腿 / 腹股沟血管，尽快修复大动脉损伤（而不仅是结扎）。临时分流可以迅速替换来恢复血流及延迟确定性修复，直到患者更加稳定或进行复苏后（图 16B）。即使患者可能仍需要近端截肢，修复股骨血管可显著改善截肢水平面保留尽可能多的肌肉功能。整个躯干和损伤的肢体都应准备好进入手术区域，以使腹部或胸部暴露、近端血管控制和多学科团队对躯干和肢体同时进行手术。一旦于血管近端控制住大出血，就可以创造手术探查的条件。大腿和腹股沟部位的损伤，根据组织的受损严重度与动静脉血供情况，决定是否需要髋关节离断术。

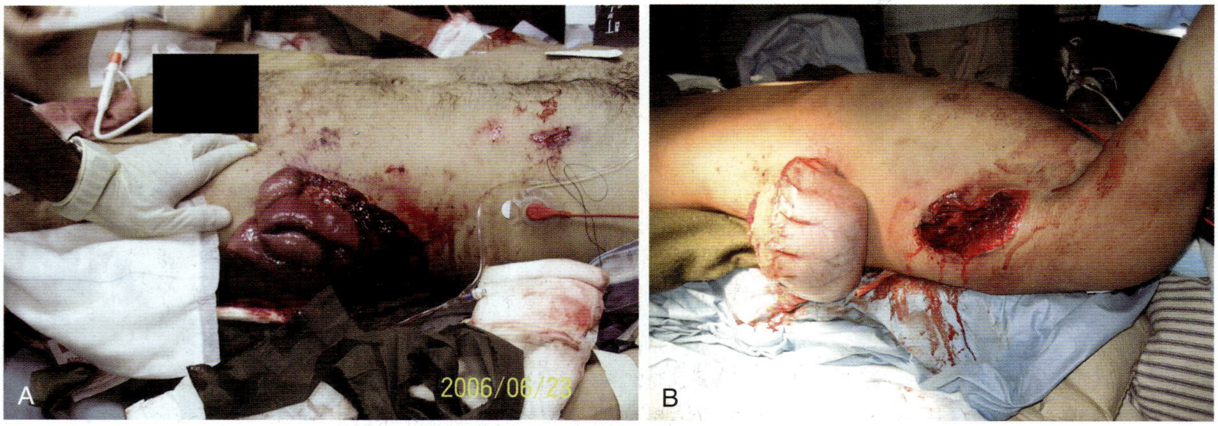

图 13　涉及腹壁及筋膜损伤的爆炸伤。**A**，小肠部分切除手术。**B**，侧面躯干外伤致胃膨出

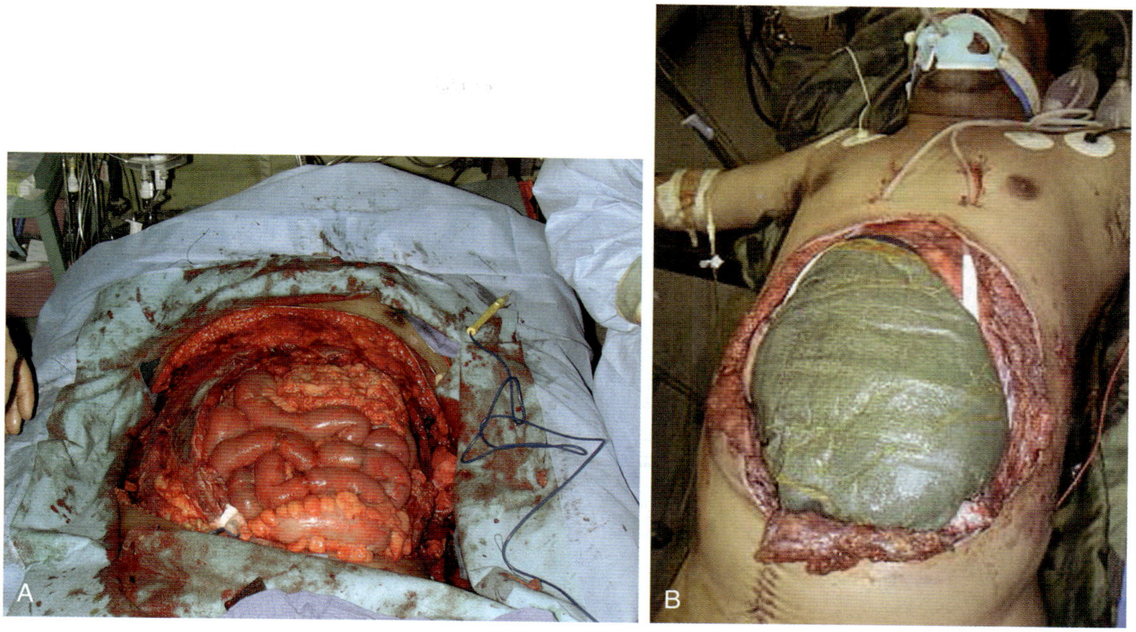

图 14　**A**，爆炸伤引起的整个前腹壁近乎完全丧失。**B**，早期处理这种复杂伤口时，我们简化地应用负压辅助临时关闭装置来保护伤口

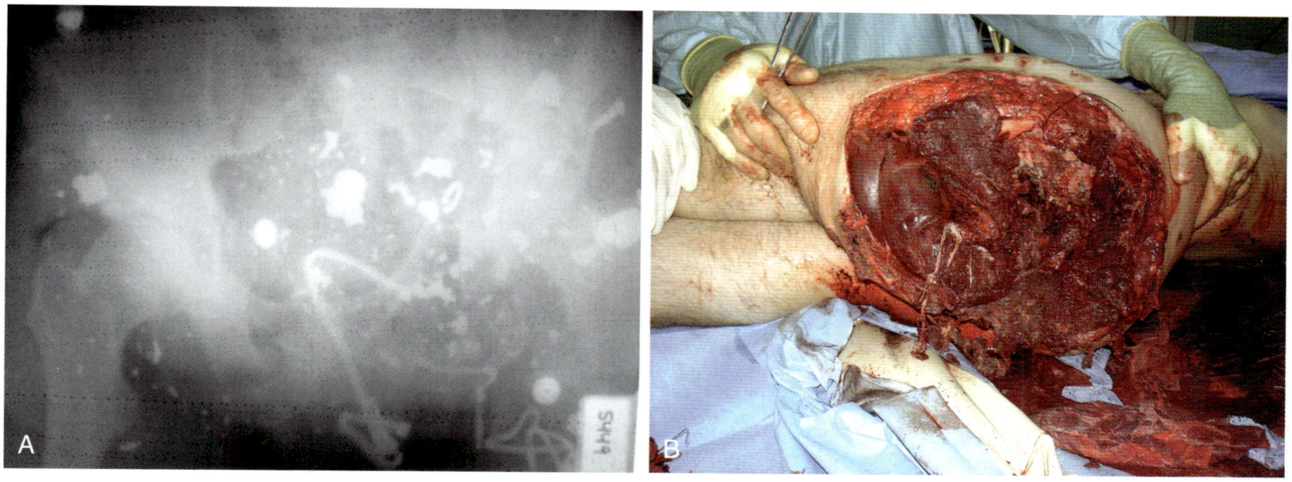

图 15　**A**，骨盆 X 线片显示了 IED 损伤的多处碎片和异物。**B**，广泛的会阴伤口包括肛肠复杂损伤，需要广泛清创、结肠转流造口术等治疗

展望

虽然我们在处置躯干伤的认识和管理上取得了巨大的进步，但是仍有多处领域有待改进和创新。可以说其中最重要的就是提高有不可压迫的出血的患者的生存，改善其预后。典型的病例就是胸腹部伤。这就要求我们不仅要关注液体扩容和复苏的策略的新改进，还要关注那些有潜力能够诱发细胞忍受休克状态能力的新干预措施。这种“需求方”的出血方式尚处于起步阶段并被寄予厚望，它将实现创伤梦寐以求的目标——严重创伤后临时假死状态的诱导。许多有前景的化合物，如丙戊酸、硫化氢、雌二醇等，在动物失血性休克模型中已经表现出了它们的优势，并可能最终进化为可供创伤外科医生甚至前线的医务人员实施的治疗方案。

其他有前途的研究方向包括推行在战场和后送过程中更先进的诊断和治疗能力。通过关于诊断危

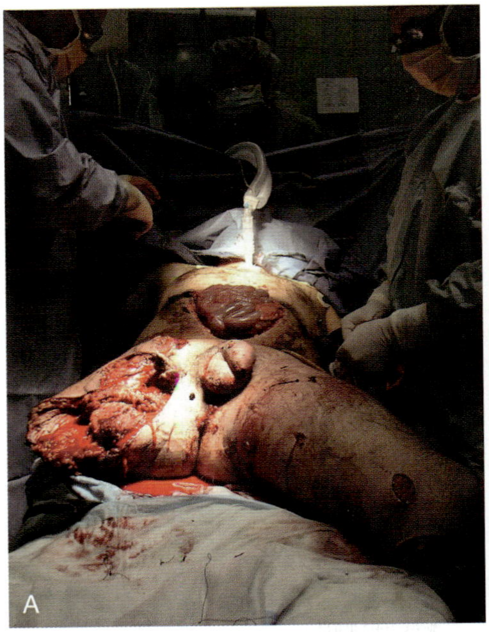

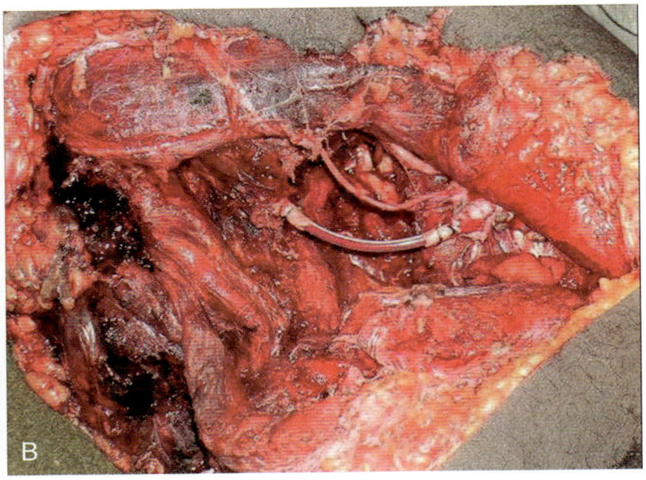

图 16 **A**，高位髂腹股沟血管损伤的严重动脉和静脉联合出血。**B**，暂时性的大腿血管分流术

及生命的躯干伤和引导干预措施的初步试验，便携式超声在前线医务人员和飞行机组人员中的使用有一定的前景。目前战场的院前复苏只依靠有限的冷晶体或胶体溶液，但随着冰冻或冻干血液产品技术的研发，血浆和其他血液制品在固定的医院设施外有很大的潜在使用空间。最后，加强院前MEDEVAC（医疗后送）的能力，在队伍中加入如重症监护护士或创伤医生等专业人才。一些国家，如英国医疗急救反应小组，已经实际应用了这种模式，允许在创伤的发生现场、直升机、地面运输途中进行介入治疗及使用血液制品复苏。最近一项关于阿富汗地区战斗经验分析的文章指出，由英国医疗急救反应小组最新转运模式运送的重伤患者死亡率，较传统转运方式有所降低（12% vs. 18%，P=035）。我们还将后续研究院前转运团队的最佳组成结构、最佳的患者人群构成、分捡标准，以能够充分利用资源达到最好的救治效果。军事医学专家不懈的付出和资源的共享，为战伤研究的开创性发展提供了强有力的支持。此外，过去十年在伊拉克和阿富汗的作战行动促成了国家外科团体和专业组织的合作发展，也很大程度上促进了学术交流、战场经验的共享、最新进展的迅速传播、前沿科技的应用转化。有这样一种说法“每一场战争都会成就医学”，我们须谨记，有些教训的代价太高，以至于我们没有浪费的机会。

第 10 章　周围血管损伤

肢体血管解剖

Norman M. Rich 和 David R. Welling 著
张学民 译

早在多个世纪前的埃及、希腊、罗马，肢体血管损伤就已经得到了认识和治疗。随后，从现代军事冲突中我们又得到关于血管损伤治疗的知识。拿破仑的外科医生 Larrey 是个快速截肢的能手，他记录了在 1812 年的博罗迪诺战役期间，在 24 h 进行了 200 例截肢。在美国内战期间，截肢是公认的肢体创伤的治疗方法，包括血管损伤。历史学家至今仍在争论截肢是否被过度使用，但在过去，“生命优于肢体”。尽管 20 世纪的前半个世纪已经有损伤动脉和静脉修复的经验和临床观念，截肢仍然是救命的方法。DeBakey 和 Simeone 报告二战期间血管损伤有 49% 的截肢率。在朝鲜战争中（1950 — 1953）Hughes、Spencer 和其他人报告了修复受损的动脉和静脉是可以成功的，哪怕环境不理想。在 20 世纪的后半个世纪，在朝鲜战争和越南战争中，外科的进步使截肢率降低到大约 13%。在 21 世纪早期，在阿富汗战争和伊拉克战争中，美国伤亡管理有了进一步的提高。过去 50 年来，血管创伤的平民管理比战场上的管理取得的效果更好。战伤经常有比低速平民伤更广泛的损伤。

搏动性的鲜红出血、远侧无脉、远侧肢体发凉、苍白、神经缺损和扩大的或搏动性血肿都和动脉损伤有关。受伤部位的震颤或杂音会警示动静脉瘘的出现。静脉出血会导致广泛出血，因为含氧量低，血是暗红的。接近穿通伤口、先前的出血已经停止、骨损伤、血肿和神经功能不全都提示血管损伤。进一步诊断检查是有帮助的。血管创伤的基本护理理应当遵循 ATLS。透彻的解剖知识非常重要。今天，全面的解剖教学并没有达到大多数医学院所希望的程度。血肿引起的组织层次破坏、变形挑战着血管外科医生。在大的创伤中神经周围出血看上去像血栓形成的动脉，更容易混淆，增加了治疗的困难。

上肢血管解剖

腋动脉和静脉

腋动脉作为锁骨下动脉的直接延续起源于第 1 肋外侧边缘，从顶部进入腋窝，穿过第 1 肋间沿着腋窝外侧壁走行。随之动脉出现在肋锁区下部，它和臂丛关系紧密。神经包绕腋动脉最终在腋动脉远侧形成正中神经、桡神经、尺神经。神经血管束包绕在腋鞘内，和腋静脉分开。腋静脉在腋动脉下方。动脉和静脉的邻近关系常导致创伤性动静脉瘘。

腋动脉在大圆肌外侧边缘延续为肱动脉。腋动脉走行在胸小肌后方，后者起于胸壁，插入喙突。肌肉将动脉分为 3 部分。第一部分在胸锁筋膜后方和几大重要肌肉的锁骨头处，从第 1 肋外侧边缘向胸小肌上缘走行。胸大动脉是此平面的唯一分支。第二部分位于胸小肌的后方，作为最短的部分，它有 2 条临床上比较重要的分支：胸肩峰动脉和胸外侧动脉。臂丛神经包绕此部分的腋动脉。第三部分起于胸小肌外侧边缘，止于大圆肌外侧缘。这部分腋动脉有 3 条分支：肩胛下动脉、旋肱前动脉和旋肱后动脉。

肱动脉和静脉

在大圆肌下 1/4 处腋动脉延续为肱动脉。肱动脉位于正中神经旁，在肘窝桡骨颈对面分成尺动脉和桡动脉。肘关节处有丰富的侧支网络，当肱动脉受阻时，对保留前臂和手的灌注非常重要。

桡静脉和尺动脉、尺静脉

桡动脉通常是肱动脉较小的分支。桡动脉分出2个主要分支：邻近起源的桡侧返动脉和掌浅支，后者参与形成掌浅弓。桡动脉主干前行形成腕部的掌深弓。尺动脉是肱动脉2分支中较大的一条。在尺动脉起源附近可以见到前和后尺侧返动脉起自骨间总动脉。远侧尺动脉移行为掌浅弓。伴随静脉较小且无关紧要。

下肢血管解剖

股动脉和股静脉

股总动脉是髂外动脉的直接延续，在腹股沟韧带后方进入股三角，位于髂前上棘和耻骨结节连线中点。在股三角内，股总动脉位于股神经内侧，股静脉在股动脉内侧。在后面，可以见到腰大肌和耻骨肌。在股总动脉起源附近，它分出腹壁浅动脉、旋髂浅动脉、阴部外浅动脉和阴部外深动脉。走行4～6 cm后，它在股三角深部分为股浅动脉和股深动脉。

股浅动脉一般是2条分支中粗的一条，通过大腿下行在缝匠肌内侧、股内侧肌前外侧、长收肌和大收肌后侧。隐神经在动脉前方。动脉在内收肌裂孔穿过大收肌成为腘动脉，分出膝上内侧动脉和膝上外侧动脉分支。股浅静脉紧密伴随股浅动脉。股浅静脉经常有多支和重叠。

股深动脉提供大腿的大部分血液供应。它起自股总动脉的后外侧壁，向下行于股浅动脉后外侧，接着，行于大腿长收肌深部。股深动脉起源后，股动脉外侧旋股动脉和旋股内侧动脉很快分出，这些重要的分支作为侧支环绕臀部。3条穿动脉在股深动脉分出供应大腿肌肉，它们通过丰富的吻合相连，静脉伴随动脉。

腘动脉和腘静脉

腘动脉起自内收肌裂孔，是股浅动脉的直接延续。它略向外侧走行，在股骨远侧后方下行进入腘窝。这是个重要的解剖区域，因为所有从大腿到小腿的神经血管结构均从这个区域通过。腘窝在膝后方呈钻石形。腘动脉在股骨髁间的腘窝底部直至到达腘肌远侧边缘，终于胫前动脉和胫腓干。3对分支形成重要的膝关节周围侧支。腘静脉可能是两支，并与腘动脉伴行。

胫动脉和胫静脉

胫前动脉是腘动脉较小的终末分支，起自腘肌下缘。它穿过骨间膜进入小腿的前间隔，在踝部延续为足背动脉。全长被两支交错、并行的静脉和腓深神经包绕。胫腓动脉是腘动脉大的终末支。它在比目鱼肌弓正后方起源和下行。复杂和薄壁的静脉血管网络包绕动脉。胫神经伴行动脉。胫腓动脉有各种长度，在分为胫后动脉和腓动脉前可以长达5 cm。在一小部分患者中，起自腘动脉的可以形成三分叉远端3支胫骨血管动脉。胫后动脉是胫腓干的直接延续。在后间隔下行，在远侧1/3更浅些。其末段走行在内踝与跟骨内侧结节的连线中点。一对深静脉作为动脉的伴行静脉。胫神经沿动脉全程伴行。腓动脉从胫腓干分出后在腓骨外侧下行。在踝部动脉发出分支穿过骨间膜，与腓动脉的外侧和后侧踝分支形成踝周吻合网络。一对深静脉伴行动脉，却没有大的神经伴行动脉。

隐静脉

下肢的隐静脉没有相关动脉。大隐静脉是人体最长的静脉，起自足背内侧缘静脉，与隐神经相伴行。经过腿的全长，进入股三角，加入其他侧支静脉后进入股总静脉。小隐静脉作为足外缘静脉延续，起自外踝后方，上行在腓肠肌两头间，终于腘静脉。在小腿下1/3，小隐静脉与腓肠神经关系密切，在上2/3，它与腓肠内侧皮神经关系密切。

血管创伤的诊断

John T. Anderson 和 F. William Blaisdell 著
张学民 译

血管创伤的诊断通常不是问题，大多数损伤表现为明显失血、休克或脉搏减弱或消失。而在特定条件下，损伤可能无法在最初识别，仅表现为外伤后期伴随突然的继发性出血或严重器官或肢体缺血。

大多数会立即引起临床医生注意的血管损伤与动脉有关。因为静脉出血一般容易被周围软组织控制，大量侧支循环可以代偿阻塞性病灶。后期血栓形成和肺栓塞是静脉损伤相关的并发症。

诊断

应当首先识别和处理威胁生命的损伤和治疗休克。除了头部损伤，几乎所有迅速致命的损伤都和心血管系统有关。

在评价与治疗同步进行时，应遵守 ATLS 指南。源自内出血的休克可以通过心脏按压或颈静脉快速观察识别出来。如果颈静脉充盈，推断心脏受压源于心包压塞、张力性气胸或心力衰竭。颈静脉塌陷意味着低血容量，对液体治疗无反应决定了迅速手术干预的最可能的体腔。这通常决定了急诊 X 线胸片的必要性。外出血通常是明显的，有必要立即控制。一般直接压迫作为暂时控制措施是有效的。

休克的出现可以导致肢体脉搏微弱与混淆血管损伤的位置。相关骨折和脱位会影响血管通畅性，应当在做任何有关血管损伤的决定之前去除。

我们的目的是及时的复苏和血管损伤的识别和处理，以尽量减少死亡率的风险，并防止永久性肢体缺血性损伤。

病史

应当询问院前急救人员现场出血情况和患者是否伴有休克。须考虑复苏和液体容量补充。要决定是否使用和使用止血带的时长，要确定事故现场的失血量和性质。鲜红的搏动性出血史提示动脉损伤，暗红色出血提示静脉来源。在许多情况下，当患者到达急诊室时，出血可能已经停止，这会导致一种错误的安全感。这种类型的患者，尤其是动脉损伤的患者，随时可能发生继发性出血。

应询问患者和院前急救人员患者的损伤机制。大多数城市穿通伤是来自低速机械伤，如刀或手枪。在这些病例中动脉损伤是典型的直接损伤的结果，也就是刀或子弹直接损伤。应收集信息，以帮助确定损伤的轨迹和潜在的结构损伤。这可能包括刀的类型和长度、子弹的数量和方向，以及在受伤时的身体位置。钝性血管损伤的机制通常是由相关骨折或脱位引起的拉伸或压缩的结果。四肢骨折、脱位或灌注改变的证据应描述。此外，特定的机制，如“汽车保险杠”损伤或膝关节后脱位往往与血管损伤有关，应做适当调查。

神经系统症状的信息应包括感觉和运动缺失的信息。潜在的混杂因素如患有周围血管疾病、糖尿病或神经病变应记录。

查体

患者应该脱掉衣服，彻底检查。腋下或会阴和臀部的皮肤褶皱不要忽略，在这些地方的穿通性创伤造成的伤口可能会漏查。应识别骨折或脱位造成的畸形。在穿通性创伤的情况下，应注意伤口的位置和数量，以确定致伤物的轨迹（特别指大动脉）。

应查找活动性出血或血肿形成的证据。出血的特点、搏动性血鲜红或稳定的暗红色渗血应注意。有张力的或扩大的血肿表示存在动脉损伤，出血被周围软组织所包裹。对侧健肢应评估作为比较。慢性周围血管疾病一般对称。非损伤腿无脉支持原有周围血管病的诊断。

检查应包括损伤近端和远端的脉搏。损伤远侧的皮温和毛细血管充盈情况和运动功能测定可以进一步评估灌注和组织活力。这些参数的任何改变需要进一步评估。相反，明显的“正常”脉冲不能排除血管损伤的可能性。在高达 30%～33% 的后来证实的血管损伤患者中，脉搏可触及，且评估为正常。同样，应用对侧无损伤肢体作为一个有用的比较。

偶尔会通过受累动脉段杂音听诊确定动静脉（arteriovenous，AV）瘘。通常动静脉瘘会随时间进展——经常在损伤早期杂音不明显。当有开放性损伤时，手套应放在听诊器外，以确保听诊器不沾到血。

全面的神经学检查应该记录在案。解剖学上的血管和神经的位置都靠近彼此。神经缺损可能提示存在相关的血管损伤。而且这种检查在评估预后中很重要，功能预后依赖于完整的感觉和运动功能。“休克手套”缺失经常暗示缺血导致的神经功能障碍——周围神经易受缺血损伤，因为代谢率高和糖原储备低。血流应当及时重建，以防止肌肉死亡和坏疽发生。

血管损伤的硬和软体征

根据病史和体格检查，血管损伤的表现可分为两大类：硬体征和软体征（表 1）。

表 1　血管损伤的硬、软体征

硬体征	软体征
活动性动脉出血	邻近血管的神经损伤
无脉 / 缺血证据	小到中等大小的血肿
搏动性血肿扩大	无法解释的低血压
杂音和震颤	现场失血量大
动脉压指数 < 0.90，短绌脉搏	损伤（有穿通性机械伤、骨折或脱位）邻近大血管

From Anderson JT, Blaisdell FW: Diagnosis of vascular trauma. In Rich N, Mattox KL, Hirshberg A, editors: Vascular trauma, 2nd ed, Philadelphia, Saunders, 2004

硬体征是存在动脉损伤和需要急诊手术干预的强预测指标。明显的体征包括鲜红的搏动性出血或迅速扩张的血肿。肢体缺血的证据（表现为 6P——无脉、苍白、疼痛、瘫痪、感觉异常和变温）和杂音或震颤是附加的体征。对于肢体创伤，我们把动脉压力指数（arterial pressure index，API），也称为踝肱指数，小于 0.90 作为一个硬体征。API 由损伤肢体收缩压除以非损伤肢体收缩压得出。Johansen 等证实 API 小于 0.90 鉴别隐匿性动脉损伤的灵敏度为 95%，特异度为 97%。超过 0.90 的 API 的动脉损伤的存在有 99% 的阴性预测值。API 易于在床边获得，应被视为体格检查的延伸。一个重要的提示是无分支血管如股深动脉的 API 可能是正常的。

软体征是动脉损伤的暗示，尽管比硬体征的强度要小得多（表 1）。这些由中度脉短绌、轻微杂音、非扩张性血肿、靠近大血管的骨折或伤口构成。有这些发现的动脉损伤的实际发病率变动很大。例如，临近大血管的损伤作为唯一发现的患者，血管损伤发病率小于 10%，而且，许多这样的伤害不需要除单纯观察以外的额外治疗。大多数血管损伤评估的争议围绕着有软体征患者的评估。

额外的辅助测试

辅助成像包括平片、双功能超声扫描，CT 血管成像和常规血管造影。推荐基本上全部患者需要 X 线胸片和可疑血管损伤部位平片。当动脉损伤部位不明显的，或各式各样的损伤（如胸主动脉）时，或已获得信息可能强烈暗示需要后续治疗时，在这些时候对有软体征的患者使用这些方法是最有利的。在许多患者中，动脉损伤的存在是显而易见的，需要手术干预，这些患者通常最好及时手术，无需额外的测试。

X 线胸片和平片在急救室容易获得，应该是对伤员的初步筛选的一部分。不透 X 线的标志物应放在所有怀疑穿透性机制导致的开放性伤口上。射线照片应涵盖全部损伤区域。通常这需要对重叠区域的躯干成像，以确保足够的覆盖范围。X 线胸片应仔细观察异物、骨折和脱位。尽可能评估损伤的轨迹，确定的子弹数和伤口数目相加应为偶数。否则，应评估患者的额外不明伤口和拍片定位额外的子弹。值得注意的是先前的损伤留下异物的可能性。有时，子弹作为可以移动的栓子在血管系统移动到进入点远侧的地方。偶尔，荧光透视（或 CT 扫描探测）可以协助定位额外子弹。如果异物的出现较模糊，应注意，因为这意味着异物移动、异物与血管结构紧密接触或异物在血管内。

应使用双功超声扫描结合二维成像评价解剖学细节，多普勒超声评估流动特性。一些研究人员已经证明了其在不同解剖学部位的血管损伤的检测中的高灵敏度和特异度。存在血管损伤的情况下双功超声检查比 API 更敏感，重要的是，双功超声检查可以确定非主干血管如股深动脉损伤（API 可能还是正常的）。然而，双功超声检查是有局限性的，因为它依赖于技术人员，大多数中心在下班后不能进行。

近年来，大家认可 CT 血管造影作为对多个解剖学部位的血管损伤的诊断方法。它的主要优点包括极强的可用性和三维的细节。与常规血管造影相比，介入放射学家不须在检查时在场。总的来说，该检查比常规血管造影能更迅速地完成，特别是在发病几个小时后。成像分辨率和软件已有明显的技术进步。3D 可以很轻易地重建动脉解剖的细节，而该方法只能用于诊断。随后的血管造影可用于治疗性栓塞。值得注意的是，CT 血管造影和随后的血管造影的造影剂总负荷很大。另一个技术局限是 CT 血管造影的金属碎片比常规血管造影中更易于混淆。CT 血管造影在怀疑胸部血管损伤时具有一定的价值，已被证明是一种高度敏感的筛选试验。而单独的纵隔血肿，若无破裂证据，需要动脉造影来证实是否有大血管损伤。

动脉造影长久以来被认为是判定动脉损伤的金标准。它的耐受性好，并发症发生率低。在大多数创伤中心，典型的年轻人群中，大的并发症如医源性假性动脉瘤或动静脉瘘并不常见。动脉造影的主要优点是可以提供治疗选择（如栓塞）。此外，与 CT 血管造影相比，常规动脉造影不易分辨金属碎片。甚至在那些依靠 CT 影像作为主要诊断方法的中心，常规动脉造影仍然作为确认或进一步确认模糊的 CT 发现的诊断方式。后一点对评估颈动脉损伤特别有用，在颈动脉中，即便是轻微的损伤可能也是重要的。偶尔有患者须在动脉造影或 CT 血管造影之前进行紧急手术。对这些患者，同样，外科医生可以在手术室内做动脉造影。例如，可以经股动脉插管注射造影剂，从而得到平片或荧光透视影像。O'Gorman 等证实腋动脉可以通过在肱动脉注射造影剂同时用血压套袖膨胀阻断远侧流出道（压力超过动脉收缩压）可视。最近流行的腔内技术的好处已经提升了手术室中使用动脉造影的可行性。事实上，一些中心有在手术室做盆腔或脏器血管栓塞的能力，从而排除了须转运不稳定患者到一个影像学装置可能不在手术室的地方的可能性。

损伤的特定区域

一些主要的解剖学区域表现出一些独特的症状或需要诊断筛选的血管损伤。这些部位包括颈部、胸部、腹部和四肢。

颈部血管损伤可以表现为最初的外部出血、扩大的血肿，或同侧半球缺血症状，如半身麻木、轻偏瘫或单眼失明。后者的神经系统症状必须假设由颈动脉中断或血栓形成引起，除非证明为其他原因。颅神经 IX、X、XI 和 XII 功能不全表明血管损伤的可能性，因为它们靠近颈动脉和颈静脉。穿通伤与出血或假性动脉瘤有关，而钝性损伤总是通过血栓产生症状，可以即刻或延迟出现。在大的颈部损伤中，双功能超声大大促进了对内膜中断或夹层的筛查，被一些机构广泛使用。CT 血管造影最近被确定为一种可行的替代血管造影的方法，以筛选钝性颈动脉损伤，也可用于评估穿通性颈部损伤。在可疑的病例和偶尔一些需要栓塞的椎动脉破坏的患者中，常规血管造影仍然被视为金标准。

胸大血管损伤是指颈根部和胸主动脉的损伤。正如所有穿通性损伤一样，大出血是这些一个或多个血管损伤的常见表现。在这种情况下，根据假定弹道路径的损伤部位、刺伤的位置和 X 线胸可能提示应积极手术。由于延误诊断的重要性，许多稳定的患者和有颈根部穿通伤的患者应该进行动脉造影。CT 血管造影在有新一代多排 / 高分辨率 CT 扫描仪和影像学专家的中心是一个恰当的选择。钝性创伤，特别是减速伤，与创伤性破裂有关。不同于小血管，即便有内膜中断，锁骨下动脉、无名动脉、主动脉损伤很少有血栓症状。临床上完全的血管破裂是罕见的，死亡通常是瞬时的。幸存的患者表现有假性动脉瘤存在的血管损伤、纵隔或颈部血肿、顶端覆盖。对这些损伤，CT 扫描是个非常好的筛选工具。然而，除非证实了脏器破裂，否则应做动脉造影证实血肿，因为许多这种情况和小血管破裂有关，不需要外科手术。

穿通伤后的腹部血管损伤总是和出血有关。有失血的大多数下胸部和腹部枪伤和刀刺伤有剖腹术的指征，通常在术中确诊动脉或静脉损伤。由于腹部大血管受到保护，钝性损伤相当罕见，可出现股动脉搏动减弱或消失。由于前述原因，在处理腹部血管损伤时很少需要特殊的诊断方法。CT 扫描经常用于评估持续性出血来源，但更重要的是确定具体的器官损伤，而不是大血管损伤。值得注意的例外是持续不稳定的骨盆骨折，可能需要造影与出血的证据。动脉造影可以用于评估髂内动脉和栓塞性治疗出血。CT 血管造影对钝性创伤造成的不稳定骨盆骨折有作用，以确定可能区域为后续栓塞的目标。通常 CT 扫描可以在等待血管造影的时候做。此外，附带的腹内和盆腔的损伤可以明确并获得关于骨盆骨折的类型的 3D 信息。

前文已经描述了肢体血管损伤的诊断和筛选策略。这些患者分为三大类：①有无脉 / 缺血、活动性出血或搏动性血肿的证据的患者；②有硬体征和可触及的脉搏的患者；③软体征或与血管损伤相关的损伤的患者。首先，所有患者应该充分复苏、复位和稳定相关的脱位和骨折。初步治疗后要重新评估血液灌注。在某些情况下，灌注的正常化可以使后续工作更审慎地进行。如图 1 所示，对疑似肢体血管损伤的患者进行评估将在下面讨论。

在第一类患者中，有无脉 / 缺血证据、活动性出血或搏动性血肿的患者，迫切须注意防止出血或组织缺血坏死。一般这些患者应当尽快进手术室。如果是完全缺血，如用止血带，4 h 会导致肌肉坏死。幸运的是，通常有一些侧支血流延长了这个关键的时间段。在大多数情况下，受伤的位置是显而易见的，由病史、体格检查和初步的平片获得，手术干预可以据此进行。在其他情况下，受伤的确切位置和程度不明显（表 2）。为减少热缺血时间，应即刻血管造影。在一些中心，血管造影可以在手术室进行。

第二类患者表现为硬体征，但没有活动性出血或无灌注的证据。这些患者可以进行更深思熟虑的、可能是权宜之计的评估。通常情况下损伤的位置和程度通过血管造影确定。最近，CT 血管造影受到热捧，血管造影的优点是可以实施血管内干预治疗，如肌肉出血或假性动脉瘤或动静脉瘘的栓塞。如上所述，在某些受伤相关的情况下，在紧急手术干预前可以行血管造影。在这种情况下，在手术室进行血管造影或血管造影是可行的选择。

表 2 动脉造影指征：肢体损伤

血管损伤部位或范围不清
广泛软组织损伤
骨折或脱位
弹道与动脉平行于动脉
多发伤
枪伤
周围血管疾病

From Anderson JT, Blaisdell FW: Diagnosis of vascular trauma. In Rich N, Mattox KL, Hirshberg A, editors: Vascular trauma, 2nd ed, Philadelphia, Saunders, 2004

最后一类涉及疑似肢体血管损伤、只有软体征的患者。许多关于血管损伤的争论涉及这一类，在创伤邻近大动脉处的患者（虽然没有硬体征）中，影像学异常可能出现在 10% 的造影患者中。然而，需要手术干预的患者比例更小——几个系列研究表明此范围为 0.6% ~ 4.4%。Dennis 等提出有说服力的争

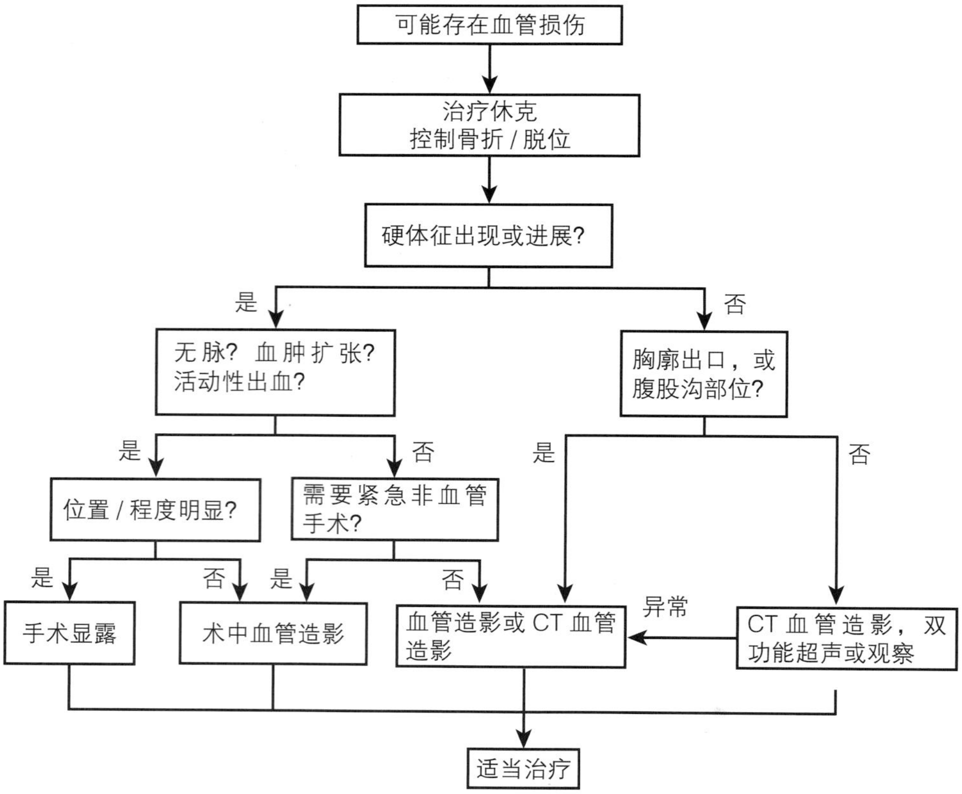

图 1 流程图：肢体损伤的评估。CT，计算机断层扫描 *(Modified from Anderson JT, Blaisdell FW: Diagnosis of vascular trauma. In Rich N, Mattox KL, Hirshberg A, editors: Vascular trauma, 2nd ed, Philadelphia, Saunders, 2004.)*

论支持对这个患者群单独体检，他们提出将需要手术干预的患者从硬体征后续发展的患者中识别出来的必要性。典型的患者需要短期观察。考虑到患者对随访依从性差和应尽快识别严重损伤（理想的是到达急诊室后尽快恰当引导安置）使许多人使用替代方案，包括超声或CT成像。最终，选择往往取决于成本、可用性、创伤中心的体量/资源和当地的专业人士。

虽然任何2条前臂血管或3条下肢血管的损伤可能会导致出血，需要治疗。在大多数情况下，除非临床症状倾向于干预，否则手术很少用于损伤筛查。这些血管有丰富的侧支循环，因此损伤导致的任何一条血管闭塞很少会出现症状，血管破裂的出血通常可自行停止。

须提及的2种情况是膝关节后脱位患者和腹股沟或胸廓出口损伤。由于膝关节周围侧支循环差，未能识别的腘动脉损伤可导致迟发性血栓和严重的远端缺血。由此，膝关节脱位与髁上和胫骨近端大的骨折须做血管筛查。至少要进行双功能超声评估或严密观察/检查，最好用血管造影。另一个重要区域涉及走行在大腿深部的股深动脉，它可能和需要干预的深部出血血肿有关。当对损伤有任何疑问的时候，股动脉造影是最好的筛查方法，而且这个方法同时可以对远端出血（近端损伤最好显露和修复）进行栓塞。在没有血管损伤硬体征的情况下，患者在腹股沟区、胸廓出口或颈部的损伤一般应用常规血管造影或CT血管造影进行评估。双功能超声对锁骨下和髂血管损伤的作用有限。及时评估是强制性的，因为错过了这些部位的血管损伤可能会导致过多失血进入胸腔或腹膜后间隙。

颈动脉穿通伤：少见复杂且致命的损伤

Juan A. Asensio, Patrizio Petrone, Alejandro Perez-Alonso,Joe DuBose, Irony C. Sade, Erin Hale, Peter Collister, Thomas P. Brush 和 Frank Plani 著
张学民 译

颈动脉损伤是最难处理和最能迅速致命的穿通性损伤。其活动性出血和潜在气道阻塞使手术非常具有挑战性。其潜在的神经上的致命后果要求创伤急救医生在确定性处理过程中具有出色的判断力（图1）。通常，这些创伤出血的快速性导致颈部筋膜内的广泛出血，从而引起气道阻塞，往往需要气管插管或通过外科环甲膜切开开放气道。由于出血导致解剖学标记扭曲使建立外科气道成为一个困难的操作。手术过程充满危险，由于切口的血肿减压导致大出血，可能会使手术部位显露不清，患者有误吸风险。这些损伤有高并发症发生率和致死率。神经并发症也是灾难性的，好在并不常见。

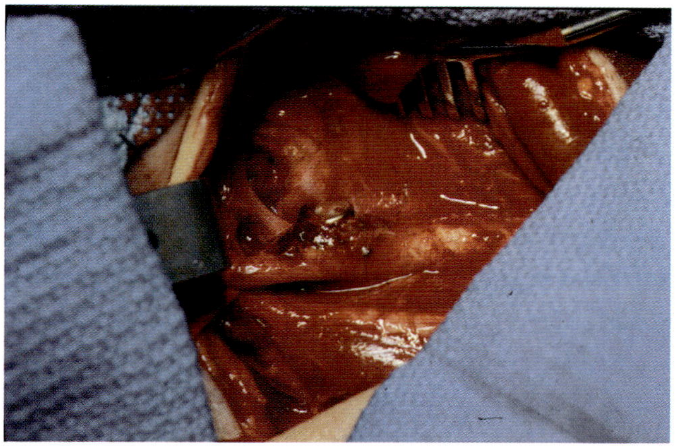

图1 高速枪伤伤及颈总动脉分叉以下

历史回顾

颈部血管损伤最早的文字记载是法国外科医生Ambroise Paré（1510－1590）提供的，他结扎了一个受伤士兵的破裂的颈动脉和颈静脉。患者生存下来，并伴有永久的神经功能不全，包括失语和左侧偏瘫。1803年，Fleming结扎了一个海员的破裂的颈总动脉，患者成功生存。1811年，Abernathy结扎了一个被公牛顶伤的患者的裂伤的左侧颈总和颈内动脉。患者留下了永久的偏瘫继而死于这次损伤。在第一次世界大战期间，Makiins报告了128例颈动脉结扎患者中，30%的患者遗留神经功能不全。这些并发症促使医生对急性颈动脉损伤采取保守的方法，对有并发症的损伤采取手术干预。第二次世界大战期间，Lawrence报告了2例颈动脉损伤修复，朝鲜战争期间Hughes报告了4例颈动脉损伤修复尝试。Both Cohen 和 Rich报告越南战争中有50例颈

动脉损伤，发生率为 5%，其中 38 例为颈总动脉损伤，12 例为颈内动脉损伤。直到 20 世纪 70 年代，大量的平民报告出现在文献中，与军事经验相结合（表 1）。

发生率和损伤机制

颈动脉损伤估计在所有颈部穿通伤中占 6%～13%。Asensio 报告颈动脉损伤占全部颈部穿通伤的 11%～13%。Demetriades 报告颈动脉损伤占全部颈部穿通伤的 6% 和全部颈血管损伤的 22%。Weaver 估计颈血管受累占头颈部穿通性损伤的 25%，颈动脉损伤占全部动脉损伤的 5%～10%。1970 年，Rich 报告在他的来自越南的标志性 1 000 例动脉损伤系列中颈动脉损伤的发病率为 5%。损伤的穿通机制是颈动脉损伤的主要原因。枪伤、罕见猎枪伤与偶尔由锯齿和锐器（如玻璃）导致的裂伤产生了这些伤害。

解剖

颈部解剖是独特的，身体没有哪部分像这样，有那么多重要结构位于如此狭小的范围内，也没有任何躯体其他区域包含如此多不同系统的代表性结构——心血管、呼吸、消化、内分泌和中枢神经系统。所有颈部结构由 2 个筋膜包绕：浅层筋膜包裹颈阔肌，颈深筋膜包裹胸锁乳突肌。气管前筋膜附在甲状软骨和环状软骨上，并和胸腔内的心包融合。椎前筋膜包绕椎前肌，与包有锁骨下血管的腋鞘融合。颈动脉鞘由颈深筋膜的 3 部分构成。如此致密的颈部筋膜室结构限制了血管损伤的出血，由此减少了失血的机会。

颈部是分为 3 个解剖区：Ⅰ区从锁骨到环状软骨，Ⅱ区从环状软骨延伸至下颌角，和Ⅲ区从下颌角延伸至颅底。这些区域被用来描述颈部损伤的位置。双侧颈总动脉的起源不同，左侧颈总动脉起源于主动脉弓，而右侧颈总动脉起源于头臂动脉。而在颈部，解剖是相同的。

颈总动脉起源于胸锁关节后面的颈部，动脉从此关节后方向上斜行至甲状软骨上缘水平，在此分为颈外动脉和颈内动脉。颈动脉是颈部最粗大的动脉。它有一个扩大的部分叫颈动脉窦及其分叉，由舌咽神经的一个分支——Hering 神经支配。颈动脉窦包含一个特化的感觉器官，称为颈动脉体，是一个血管化学感受器，位于分叉后内侧。颈总动脉、颈内静脉和迷走神经包于颈动脉鞘内。在分叉前，颈总动脉没有分支。颈外动脉是颈总动脉的 2 条分支中较小的一个，从甲状腺软骨的上部延伸到下颌

表 1　颈动脉损伤的解剖部位

作者（年）	患者数	损伤数	颈总动脉	颈内动脉	颈外动脉
Cohen 等 (1970)	85	85	66	19	0
Bradley (1973)	24	26	17	7	2
Rubio 等 (1974)	72	81	61	10	10
Thal 等 (1974)	60	60	48	12	0
Liekweg 等 (1978)	18	19	17	2	0
Ledgerwood 等 (1980)	33	33	23	10	0
Unger 等 (1980)	564	564	415	49	0
Brown 等 (1982)	129	143	103	20	20
Demetriades 等 (1989)	124	124	104	10	10
Ditmars 等 (1997)	13	15	0	11	4
Mittal 等 (2000)	18	18	9	7	2
Navasaria 等 (2002)	32	34	24	4	6
Ferguson 等 (2005)	6	6	0	3	3
总计	1160	1189	870 (73%)	262(22%)	57 (5%)

角。颈内动脉起自甲状软骨上缘，上行入颅，经破裂孔穿行入颅通过颞骨的颈动脉管，终于颅内，分成大脑前动脉和大脑中动脉。

在Ⅱ区的上缘外科医生会见到面总静脉，在显露颈动脉损伤时经常结扎或回缩。在颈部Ⅱ区上缘，舌下神经在前方跨越颈内动脉。面神经下颌缘支直接位于下颌骨下缘。

诊断

体检发现存在颈部血管结构损伤的表现包括搏动性血肿或扩大的血肿、无脉、杂音和活动性出血，作为可靠的指征。与失语或偏瘫有关的大的神经学功能不全同样标志着潜在的血管损伤。然而，全面的神经学检查不能经常进行，因为许多患者入院时休克，无法配合这样的检查。确立血管损伤的诊断，极大地促进了可用的诊断工具的可靠性。一些外科医生认为，体检是一种非常安全和可靠的方式，用于检测需要治疗的重大血管损伤。Demetriades 在一个包含 335 例颈部穿通伤患者回顾性研究中，在详细的书面文件的基础上评估血管结构损伤，减少了血管造影的次数。Demetriades 和 Asensio 报道的另一项前瞻性研究包括 223 例患者根据书面报告的临床检查。47 例未接受血管造影评价，因为存在危及生命需要急救操作的问题（19 例）或因为他们拒绝造影（28 例）。其余 176 例患者行四血管造影。176 例患者中有 34 例（19.3%）有异常的血管造影发现，但只有 14 例（8.0%）患者须治疗血管病变。其余 20 例患者成功接受非手术治疗。共 160 例（71.7%）患者无临床症状提示血管损伤，均无需手术或任何其他形式的治疗（特异度和阴性预测值均为 100%）。127 例患者进行了血管造影，另外 5 例因为其他相关的损伤进行了手术。5 例颈部探查患者均未出现血管损伤。血管造影显示有 11 例血管损伤患者（8.3%），均不需要任何类型的治疗。该项研究支持用体格检查排除需要四血管造影的患者。

虽然血管造影仍然是颈部血管损伤评价和诊断的金标准，但应保留经彩色血流多普勒（color flow doppler，CFD）作为发现Ⅰ区和Ⅲ区的血管损伤的方法，也作为探查Ⅱ区损伤的技术选择。一些作者的许多研究报告 CFD 对颈动脉损伤的诊断确立有一致的高达 95% 的灵敏度、特异度和准确性。

目前，我们建议对所有疑似颈动脉损伤的患者进行全面细致的体格检查。那些出现与颈部血管损伤或血流动力学不稳定有关的临床症状者应立即运至手术室。血流动力学稳定的患者可临床观察或用 CFD 或血管造影检查。Nemzek 等在 1996 年提出 CT 血管造影（CT angiography，CTA）可以作为一个创伤筛查手段替代常规血管造影。Munera 等在一个对比 CTA 和血管造影的研究中证实 CTA 有非常好的结果，它有 90% 灵敏度和 100% 的特异度、100% 的阳性预测值和 98% 的阴性预测值。任何需要进一步确定的损伤可以用血管造影证实。应保留血管造影作为评价血流动力学稳定患者和隐匿的Ⅰ区和Ⅲ区的血管结构损伤的评估方法。

损伤的解剖学位置

大多数颈动脉损伤仅限于颈总动脉。我们回顾了 1 160 例患者中的 1189 例颈动脉损伤。这些患者中有 870 例（73%）有颈总动脉损伤，262 例（22%）有颈内动脉损伤，57 例（5%）有颈外动脉损伤（表 1）。

外科治疗

在手术室中，患者仰卧在手术台上，头部伸展并旋转到被显露区域对侧。肩下垫毛巾卷有助于显露。面部、颈部、锁骨上、胸部包括在手术野里，如果有必要，将切口向上延长到下颌角或通过开胸切口显露和治疗Ⅰ区和Ⅲ区损伤的近端和远侧颈动脉。如果需要一段大隐静脉作为自体移植物修复颈动脉损伤的话，要准备和覆盖对侧腹股沟。

颈部探查通过从下颌角到胸锁关节的、在胸锁乳突肌前缘的标准切口（图 2），可以向胸锁乳突肌起点延长。对于位于Ⅲ区的损伤，可以通过切开到二腹肌，以便更多地显露。进一步显露二腹肌以上的颈内动脉可以通过使下颌骨向前半脱位实现。下颌关节半脱位的固定可采用弓形杆或更简单地通过经鼻金属线缝合下牙床完成。这将Ⅱ和Ⅲ区域的交界处的狭窄的三角域转换为一个更宽的矩形开口，从而允许进一步暴露颈内动脉到颅底。进一步暴露可通过延长耳垂周围的皮肤切口和向上牵拉腮下叶实现。这种显露方法由 Fisher 和 Dossa 描述（图 3）。

在Ⅰ和Ⅱ区交界处下部，常切断肩胛舌骨肌以获得更多显露。如果有必要，显露Ⅰ区的颈动脉起

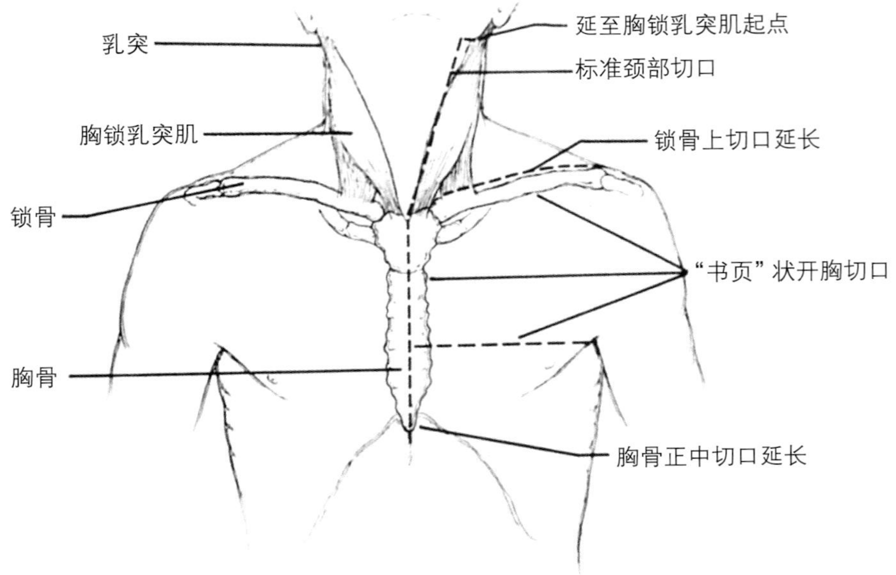

图 2　Ⅰ区和Ⅱ区损伤的显露

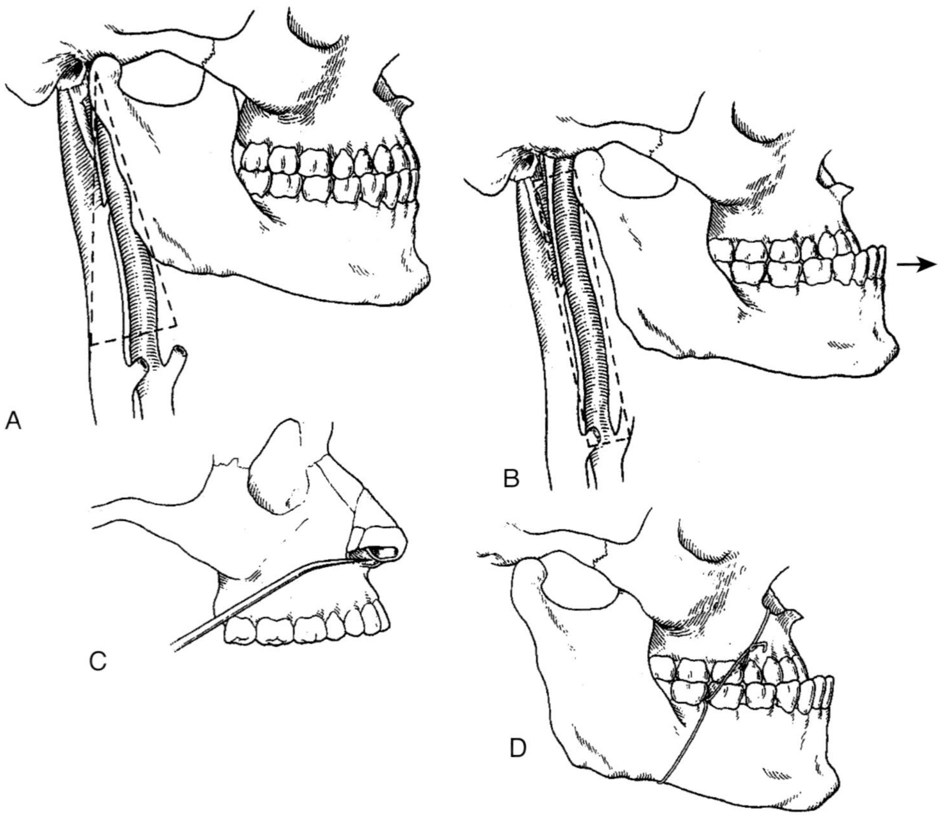

图 3　Ⅲ区损伤的显露

始部，可以选择胸骨正中切口。可以允许将颈动脉的起始处从主动脉弓分离，将右颈总动脉从头臂干上分离。极少情况下，在有锁骨下血管损伤时，做锁骨切口控制和显露这些血管。当有必要行双侧颈部探查时，胸锁乳突肌前缘切口可以通过横切口连接，如此可以使创伤外科医生向头端提起皮瓣从而显露全部颈部中线结构。

一旦显露，第一要务是立即控制危及生命的出血。在解剖学控制颈动脉近、远端及其分支的同时用手指控制出血位置。最重要的是迅速而精细地解剖颈动脉鞘，并仔细观察保护其内的结构。颈根部的颈总动脉比较容易定位。切开甲状舌骨肌更容易显露。这一手法可以快速控制近端血管。可以用 45° 的 DeBakey 血管钳控制近端，也可以用

60° DeBakey 或 Castaneda 钳（图 4）。同样的钳子可以用来控制颈内动脉近端和颈外动脉。对这些血管的完全控制是非常重要的。右或左 Kitzmiller 钳对颈内动脉近端的控制最好（图 5）。

血管外科修复的常规技术可以用于颈动脉损伤。损伤动脉侧壁缝合作为基本修复方法得以采用。而造成颈血管壁严重破坏的损伤应当切开，并用 Potts 剪小心清理。如果内膜边缘呈锯齿状应当用 Penfield 或 Freer 起子小心掀起，羽状的边缘用 6-0、7-0 或 8-0 聚丙烯线固定。应能看到近端颈动脉回血。良好的回血意味着足够的经过 Willis 环的跨脑灌注。创伤外科医生必须认识到 Willis 环完整者只占人群中的 20%。一些医生会选择测量残端压力作为何时使用转流的客观依据。如果残端压力为 40 ~ 50 mm Hg 是一个安全的压力，表明没有必要用转流。而我们的团队提倡对复杂颈内动脉或颈总动脉损伤，如果患者有任何低血压经历，或需要自体或人造移植物广泛重建，则使用颈动脉转流（图 6-8）。

将 Fogarty 球囊导管送入损伤颈内动脉近端开通血流通道是创伤外科主治医生在有充分经验的情况下作出的决定。这是一个特殊的区域，如果造成导管相关的医源性损伤可能是毁灭性的。尽管一些作者不喜欢对颈动脉损伤患者进行全身肝素化，创伤医生必须认真考虑使用肝素作为一个有效的辅助以完成这些修复。对所以颈动脉损伤，我们倾向于全身使用 5 000 U 肝素。

颈总动脉如果是切线伤可以直接修复。偶尔，在血管没有张力的情况下可以行端端吻合。有张力

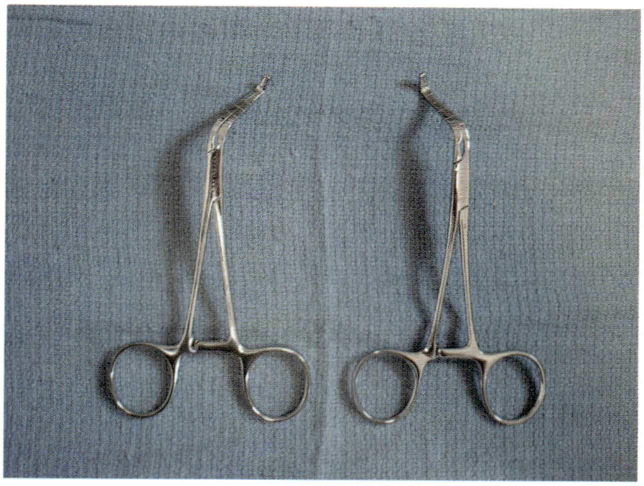

图 4　右 Kitzmiller 钳和左 Kitzmiller 钳

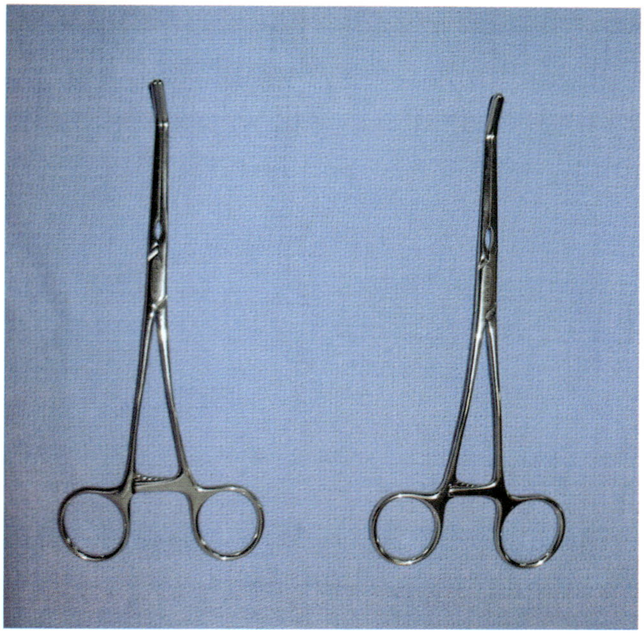

图 5　Castaneda 钳

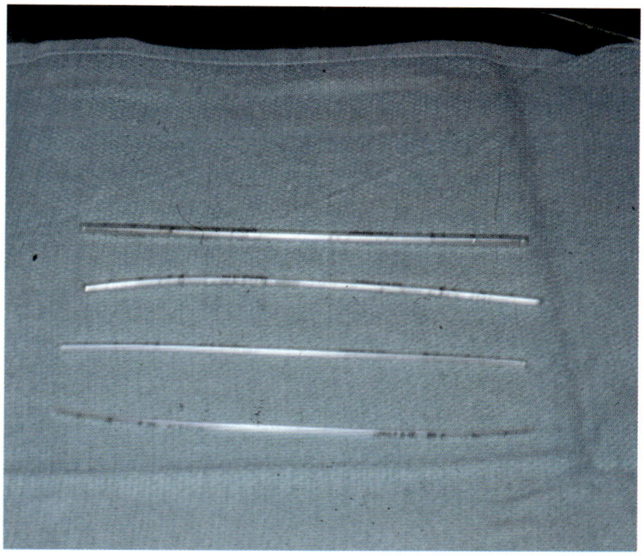

图 6　Argyle 转流管

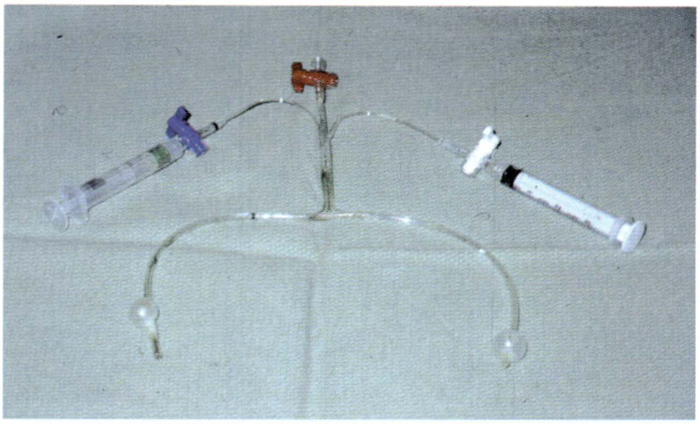

图 7　Pruitt-Inahara 转流管

的情况下最好间置移植物。修复颈动脉损伤最好用自体大隐静脉。而对没有这样的管道的颈总动脉损伤，可以用聚四氟乙烯人工血管。对颈内动脉损伤要尽可能使用自体大隐静脉（图 9-14）。完成颈动脉损伤修复后，在完成吻合前，最先松开近端钳，让近端碎片或血栓冲出来。然后再替换远端钳前，松开近端冲出碎屑或血栓。然后颈外动脉释放，再次松开近端阻断钳，使可能的碎屑或血栓冲入颈外动脉。在完成这些后，如果有转流管就移除，缝合最后几针完成吻合。使用转流的时候全身肝素化非常重要。我们通常用 6-0 聚丙烯线吻合。

Asensio 最近对几个颈动脉损伤处理的系列进行综述。一共包括 433 例患者的 456 例损伤。392（86%）例患者一期修复 64（14%）例结扎。为修复颈动脉损伤做了各种尝试，结果是一期修复更好。如果有致命性出血或其他方法不能控制的出血，损伤颈动脉的结扎也是个选择。对探查前已有确定的有固定且严重神经功能不全患者，远端血栓形成或无法重建的颈内动脉损伤可以结扎（表 2）。

结果和死亡率

Liekweg 和 Greenfield Fry、Ledgerwood，以及 Weaver 的大量报道证实如果施行一期颈动脉修补，预后将得到很大的改善。Unger 分析了 722 例颈动脉损伤的患者。其中 186 例患者有严重的神经功能缺损，如果接受了一期手术修补，34% 的患者将得到恢复，而与之对比的是接受结扎或没有接受手术治疗的患者，仅有 14% 得到恢复。我们回顾了 1 647 例颈动脉损伤的患者，死亡率为 0%～30%。颈动脉损伤患者的平均死亡率为 15%（表 3）。

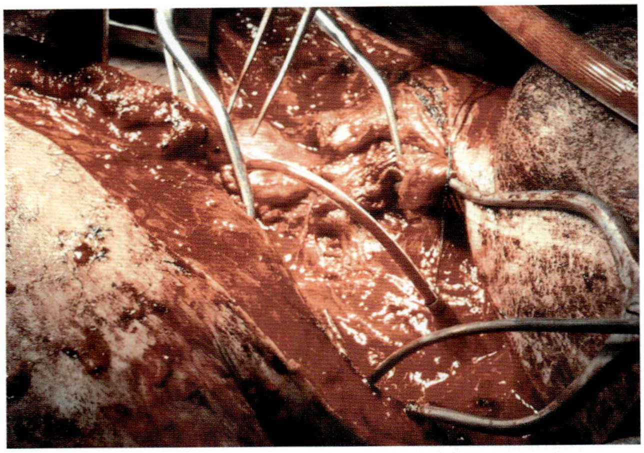

图 8　在顺行自体大隐静脉旁路术前在左颈总动脉植入 Argyle 转流管

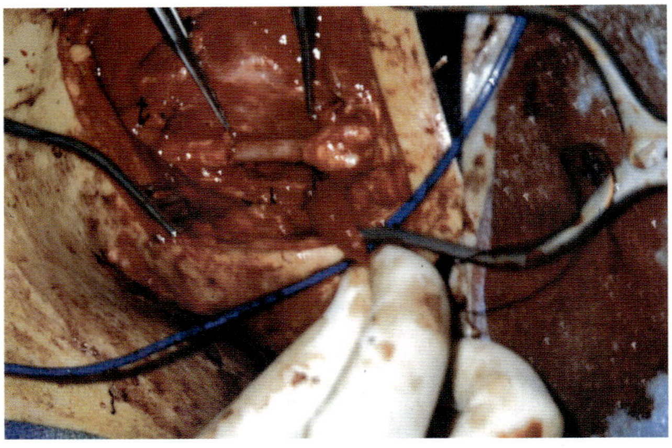

图 9　顺行自体大隐静脉旁路术修复颈总动脉分叉以下损伤

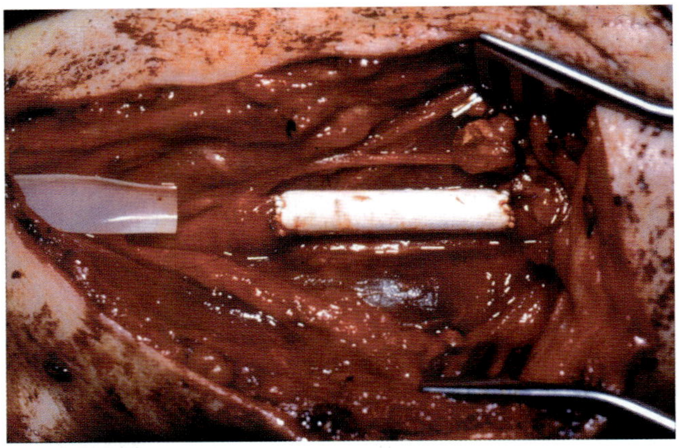

图 10　聚四氟乙烯人造血管用于颈总动脉修复

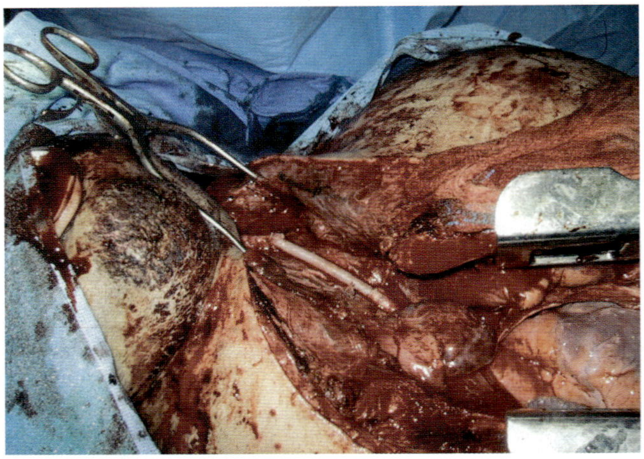

图 11　顺行自体大隐静脉旁路术用于修复从主动脉弓发出的 3 cm 的颈总动脉起始段。由于患者损伤在胸内，需要胸骨正中切开术

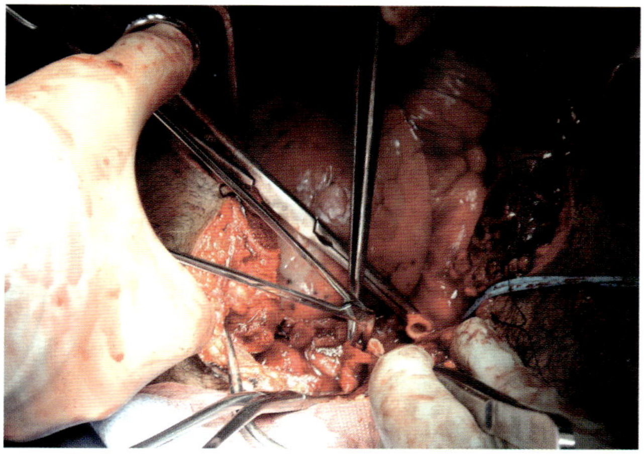

图 12 胸内左颈总动脉枪伤。注意近端和远端控制，动脉正在用 Potts 剪修剪

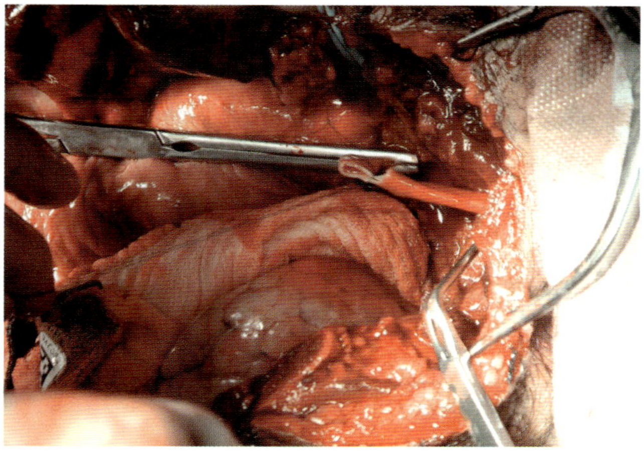

图 13 游离后使用端端吻合修复

表 2 颈动脉损伤的手术治疗

作者（年）	手术修复例数	损伤例数	修复	结扎
Cohen, 1970	85	85	78	7
Bradley, 1973	22	22	20	2
Rubio, 1974	72	81	69	12
Liekweg, 1978	18	19	15	4
Ledgerwood, 1980	36	36	31	5
Fry, 1980	54	54	42	12
Brown, 1982	125	139	115	24
Richardson, 1988	39	39	37	2
Ditmars, 1997	3	5	2	3
Mittal, 2000	18	18	16	2
Navsaria, 2002	32	34	28	6
Ferguson, 2005	6	6	3	3
总计	492	519	441 (85%)	78 (15%)

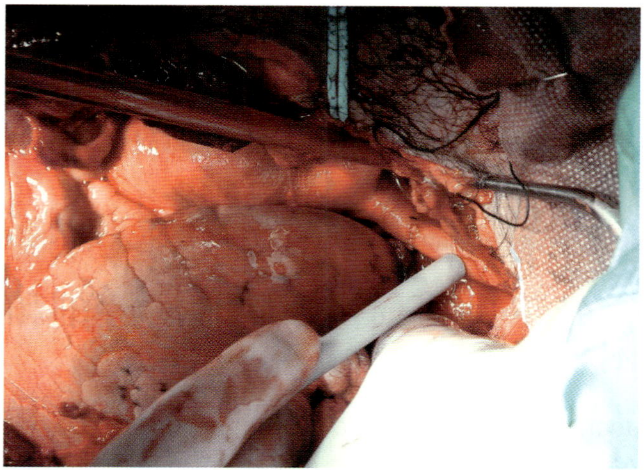

图 14 主动脉弓上大约 2 cm，修复完成。用多普勒探头检测三相血流信号

表 3 颈动脉损伤的死亡率

作者（年）	例数 *	死亡率（%）†
Cohen 等（1970）	85	15.0
Bradley（1973）	24	33.0
Rubio 等（1974）	72	23.4
Thal 等 (1974)）	60	8.3
Liekweg 和 Greenfield（1978）	233	10.0
Ledgerwood 等（1980）	36	16.0
Fry 和 Fry（1980）	54	10.0
Unger 等（1980）	722	21.0‡
Brown 等（1982）	129	20.9
Richardson 等（1988）	45	6.6
Demetriades 等（1989）	124	22.0
Ditmars 等（1997）	133	0
Mittal 等（2000）	18	16.6
Navsaria 等（2002）	32	6.3

* 总计 1 647 例。
† 平均计算死亡率 =15%。
‡ 确切纳入的只有 513 例

发病率

颈动脉修补术的短期并发症包括急性血栓形成、远端栓塞、脑梗塞范围扩大，出血伤口发生血肿、伤口感染，以及舌下神经或下颌神经损伤。最严重的并发症是大范围的脑梗塞扩散导致的脑死亡或永久的植物状态。

总结

颈动脉损伤是一种不常见但极有挑战性的疾病。颈动脉损伤的修补需要精细的手术技术来避免严重的后果。它将导致高死亡率和并发症发生率。必须尝试所有可能的方法来修复颈动脉损伤，因为相对于结扎，一期手术会有更好的效果。

锁骨下血管损伤：困难的解剖和困难的领域

Juan A. Asensio, Patrizio Petrone, Alejandro Perez-Alonso,Mamoun Nabri, Gerald Gracia, Michael Ksycki, Paul W. White 和 Robert F. Wilson 著
张学民 译

胸部和胸部相关的血管损伤对创伤科医生的复杂挑战有代表性。特别是锁骨下血管损伤不常见，但高致命性。无论机制如何，这样的伤害可能会导致显著的高的并发病发生率和死亡率。锁骨下血管损伤经常和致命性多发伤有关。多年来，随着复苏、急救医学转运系统和创伤识别系统的进步，总体死亡率有持续的改善。

历史回顾

Halsted 1892 年成功实施首例锁骨下动脉瘤结扎。由于锁骨下血管损伤罕见，医生在战前处理经验少。一般的做法是单纯结扎。第一次世界大战期间，美国和英国医生估计总的血管损伤率为 0.4%～1.3%。1919 年，Makins 报告英国在第一次世界大战中的死亡案例中有 45 例锁骨下动脉损伤。DeBakey 和 Simeone 1946 年里程碑式的研究报告了第二次世界大战中美国士兵的 2 471 例动脉损伤中有 21 例锁骨下动脉损伤，发生率低于 1%。朝鲜战争中，Hughes 的研究报告 304 例大动脉血管损伤，只有 3 例为锁骨下动脉损伤。在战争史中可能因为战场失血死亡的病例相对较少。越南战争期间穿通性锁骨下血管损伤在全部血管损伤中少于 1%。在此期间，48 个不同的医生治疗这种创伤，只有 2 个处理这类创伤超过 1 次，总共报道了 68 例。Rich 在越南战争期间急性动脉血管患者损伤的越南血管注册原始报告中一共报告了 63 例锁骨下动脉损伤。

在近期的伊拉克和阿富汗战争中，总的血管损伤发生率比之前的战争中报告得略多。这种增加可能是与出血控制改进、疏散时间缩短有关，生存得以改善。爆炸或枪伤的高速损伤占这些损伤的大部分。有趣的是，在伊拉克，血管损伤的发病率较阿富汗高，分别是 12.5% 和 9%。White 等确定了 1 570 名美军，在伊拉克和阿富汗与战争有相关的血管损伤。其中，12% 为躯干血管损伤，锁骨下血管损伤占 2.3%。在 24 个月内，Clouse 等发现 301 个动脉血管损伤，其中 3.7% 是由于锁骨下腋血管损伤。然而，管理和治疗策略都已经从各种战争和战场的时间经历进化（表 1）。

表 1　锁骨下血管损伤的军事经验

冲突	作者（年）	总动脉数	锁骨下动脉	百分比
第一次世界大战	Makins (1919)	1191	45	3.8
第二次世界大战	DeBakey 和 Simeone (1946)	2471	21	0.9
朝鲜战争	Hughes (1958)	304	3	1
越南战争	Rich (1970)	1 000	8	0.8
阿富汗战争	Sherif (1992)	224	锁骨下动脉 / 腋动脉结合	N/A

解剖

左锁骨下动脉和右锁骨下动脉有不同的起源。右锁骨下动脉在右侧胸锁关节后方起自无名动脉；左锁骨下直接起自主动脉弓。锁骨下动脉分成 3 部分。第一部分起自前斜角肌内侧缘。第二部分位于该肌肉后方。第三部分起自前斜角肌外侧缘，上行到第 1 肋骨外侧缘（图 1）。

右锁骨下动脉的第一部分起自右胸锁关节后上方，并向上外侧走行到前斜角肌的内侧缘。它上升到略高于锁骨的水平，在不同的情况下，它的程度有所不同。颈内静脉和椎静脉、迷走神经和迷走神经心脏支、交感神经锁骨袢（走行在血管周围形成一个圈）会跨过它。颈前静脉在动脉的前外侧走行，在胸骨舌骨肌和胸骨甲状舌骨肌旁分开。

左锁骨下动脉的第一部分在第4胸椎水平，起自左颈总动脉后方，在上纵隔内上行到颈根部，然后弓向外侧到前斜角肌内侧缘。其解剖学关系如下：前方，与其平行的迷走神经、心脏、膈神经；左颈总动脉；左颈内和椎静脉；无名静脉起始部。它被胸骨甲状肌、胸骨舌骨肌、胸锁乳突肌覆盖。左锁骨下动脉第二部分在前斜角肌后方。它很短，构成血管弓的最高部分。

在右侧颈部，膈神经在前斜角肌旁和动脉第二部分分开，在左侧其靠近肌肉内侧缘跨越动脉第一部分。血管后面是胸膜和中斜角肌，上面是臂丛神经，下面是胸膜。锁骨下静脉在动脉前下方，被前斜角肌分开。

左锁骨下动脉的第三部分从前斜角肌侧缘向下、向外到第1肋骨外侧缘，在此成为腋动脉。颈外静脉穿过其内侧部分并接受肩胛横静脉、颈横静脉和颈前静脉，在动脉前形成丛。在静脉后方，支配锁骨下肌的神经在动脉前下行。动脉的终末部分在锁骨后方和锁骨肌处被肩胛横血管跨越。锁骨下静脉在动脉前面，且比动脉稍低。在后面，介于它和中斜角肌之间有最低的臂丛神经干，上面及其外侧是臂丛上干和肩胛舌骨肌。

锁骨下动脉的分支是椎动脉、内乳动脉、甲状颈干和肋颈干。在左侧，所有4个分支一般来自血管的第一部分；但右侧肋颈干通常起源于血管的第二部分。在颈部两侧，前3条分支在前斜角肌内侧边缘一起上行。大多数情况下动脉开端和最近的分支开端存在一个1.25～2.5 cm的距离。

发病率

锁骨下血管损伤占全部血管损伤的大约5%。繁忙的城市创伤中心报告每年接收2～4例锁骨下血管损伤患者，而一些国际创伤中心报告每月接收多达4例锁骨下血管损伤。锁骨下动脉损伤占全部急性血管损伤的1%～2%。虽然大多数这些损伤是穿通性的，但超过25%的损伤和钝性机械损伤有关。锁骨下动脉损伤的低发病率主要是因为解剖学位置和锁骨和胸廓提供的保护屏障。Demetriades等结合了前瞻性和回顾性文献综述，报道孤立的锁骨下动脉

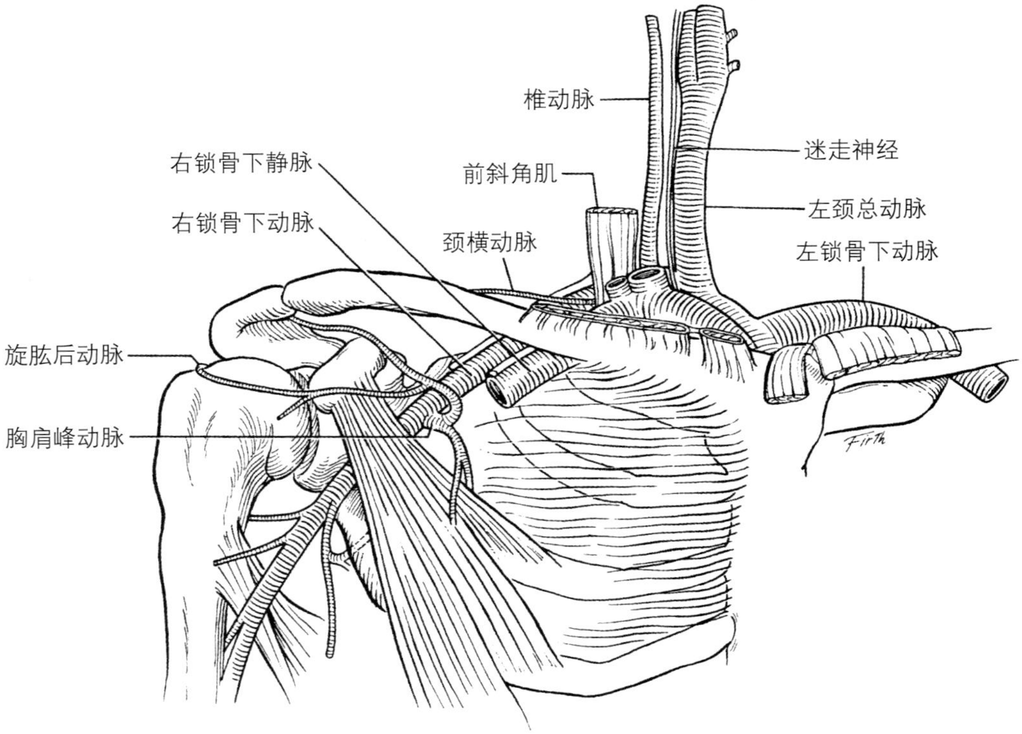

图1　锁骨下血管解剖

损伤占 39%，复合损伤大约占 17%。另一方面 Lin 等报告 54 例患者中的 24 例有锁骨下动脉和相关的静脉的可能损伤。

锁骨下血管受到其上方的锁骨和第 1 肋骨的相对比较好的保护。它们和其他邻近骨结构骨折可能导致严重的致命性损伤。在已发表的文章中的最大一个系列，Natali 报告了 10 例有锁骨骨折相关损伤的患者。锁骨骨折和相关的锁骨下血管损伤估计发病率低于 1%。Richardson 等发现第 1 肋骨骨折是严重上胸部创伤的有用的指标。在这项研究中，对 55 例第 1 肋骨骨折患者进行了评估，其中 5.5% 提示有相关的锁骨下动脉钝性损伤。在一个比较性综述中 Phillips 提出当第 1 肋骨移位时有相似的发现，9% 的患者有相关的锁骨下动脉损伤。

大部分城市居民的锁骨下血管损伤是穿通性损伤。在过去的几十年里，由于民用武器使用的增加，美国枪支相关的伤害稳步上升。几个发表的系列研究观察到美国相对于全球各地的发病率，有低的钝伤发病率与高的穿通伤发病率。Graham 的超过 24 年的最大的居民系列研究，报告了 93 例有锁骨下动脉损伤患者，其中只有两例是非穿通性损伤。Lin 回顾分析了超过 10 年的 54 例锁骨下动脉穿通性损伤患者，其中 85% 是枪伤。相反，McKinley 报道，82% 的锁骨下动脉损伤源于刀刺伤，10% 源自低速枪伤，趋势和美国区域创伤中心不同（表 2）。

另一方面，锁骨下动脉钝性损伤很少发生。城市创伤中心报告将近 1%～3% 的源自钝伤的锁骨下动脉创伤。钝性血管创伤的相对低发生率是由于锁骨下血管解剖学位置受到保护。快速减速伤和骨折是此动脉钝性损伤的原因。然而，不寻常的是，正常体检结果后损伤仍然无法识别。在其他情况下，患者在最初损伤后症状延迟出现，而导致治疗延误。

临床表现

可能有胸廓出口穿通性损伤的患者并表现为血流动力学不稳定者应当尽早插管，明智的液体复苏和迅速治疗有表现的危及生命的损伤。对有锁骨下血管损伤的血肿扩张导致的颈部或纵隔肿胀者应当立即行对侧上肢或下肢的完全静脉通道建立和气管插管。

DeGiannis 等在一个锁骨下血管损伤的回顾性研究中，报道 50% 的患者最初的收缩压低于 100 mmHg。

表 2　锁骨下血管损伤：平民报告

城市	年	作者	损伤
Louisville	1962	Cook	3
Memphis	1964	Pate 和 Wilson	12
Rochester	1968	Matloff 和 Morton	3
Chicago	1969	Amato	14
Houston	1970	Bricker	14
Baltimore	1970	Brawley	11
Durban	1978	Robbs	24
Johannesburg	1987	Demetriades	127
Johannesburg	1994	Degiannis	56
Houston	1999	Cox	56
Los Angeles	1999	Demetriades 和 Asensio	79
Durban	2000	McKinley	260
Atlanta	2000	Kalakuntla	25
Chicago	2003	Lin	54
Istanbul	2004	Aksoy	12
Houston	2008	Carrick	15

一些发表的研究证实了类似的血流动力学发现符合低血容量休克表现。在 Agarwal 的经验中，更重的休克见于 80% 的锁骨下动脉和静脉均损伤的患者。不稳定的低血容量休克患者，对复苏反应不好者应当立即转移到手术室。

任何锁骨下动脉穿通性损伤伴搏动性出血者应当立即直接外部压迫控制。如果可能，手法压迫应持续到在手术室控制血管。在锁骨后穿通伤病例中，直接压迫可能无效，而球囊压塞是可以救命的选项。在一个结合了回顾性和前瞻性研究中，Demetriades 等报告患者首诊后有伤口活动性出血者占 65%，有休克发现者占 72%。超过 20% 的锁骨下血管或腋血管损伤患者由于失血，到达医院时没有生命体征或立即心搏骤停。特别要注意的是这些患者中 28% 有相关的胸腔内损伤。一旦开放气道，患者应当立即在损伤侧行 EDT，如果必需，切口可以延长到对侧。

在 McKinley 等对 260 例患者的前瞻性研究中，将近 25% 的锁骨下动脉损伤有轻微症状和延迟的并发症，这会促使患者就医。在 Lim 等报告的研究中，只有 24% 的患者有短绌脉。在颈根部和上胸部明显的软组织瘀斑和血肿可对体检提供诊断线索。其他特征性发现包括臂丛神经麻痹、上肢肿胀、搏动性血肿或可能提示创伤性动静脉瘘的杂音。

诊断

锁骨下血管损伤的早期诊断非常重要。在有穿通伤的患者，体格检查发现锁骨下动脉损伤比见到明显搏动性出血更敏感。其他靠近锁骨下血管的合并伤是高度可疑为神经血管损伤。上肢神经功能不全，表面可闻及杂音，肱动脉、桡动脉或尺动脉脉搏减弱或消失和同侧锁骨或肋骨骨折是诊断线索。通过全面的血管检查发现冰冷、无脉、苍白的上肢，可以明确临床诊断。锁骨下动脉损伤的特异性标志还包括在锁骨上窝或腋下扩大或搏动性血肿，而血肿沿神经鞘走行。臂丛神经损伤也可以是一个潜在的锁骨下动脉损伤的可靠的预测。

放射学检查只能用于血流动力学稳定的患者。在这些患者中要立即行 X 线胸片检查。Graham 等报告 93 例锁骨下穿通伤患者中 16% 的患者有纵隔增宽。锁骨下血管近端部分损伤在 X 线胸片上可以表现为血胸和纵隔增宽。其他诊断检查包括测量血流动力学稳定患者的简单的踝肱指数（ankle brachial index，ABI）。ABI 小于 0.9 为异常，可视为潜在动脉损伤的表现。而由于侧支循环丰富，即便存在锁骨下动脉损伤也可以表现为正常 ABI。

彩色血流多普勒（color flow doppler，CFD）检查是另一个用以评估锁骨下血管损伤的非侵入性技术。不幸的是，CFD 在体型大的患者中观察主动脉弓、无名血管和左锁骨下动脉不是最理想的。使用静脉注射造影剂的快速螺旋 CT 扫描已经成为鉴别血管损伤的最佳选择。CT 血管造影是个潜在替代选项，可以替代 85% 的病例的血管造影。

急诊血管造影的价值有限，仅限于经过恰当复苏后血流动力学稳定的患者使用。理想状态下，医生应陪同患者到血管造影室。如果发生急性呼吸困难症状就放弃血管造影，将患者转运手术室。在内膜夹层、假性动脉瘤和包含物断裂的病例中，实验室检查阳性而无临床发现者推荐对受伤部位手术探查。许多人推荐对锁骨下动脉损伤常规使用血管造影。这些观点有利用精确手术计划的制订和额外动脉损伤的识别。

在 Graham 的研究中，20% 合并动脉损伤的患者通过血管造影明确。然而，现在，比传统的血管造影，更频繁地使用 CFD 和 CT 血管造影。血管造影却仍是“金标准”，用于没有任何血流动力学损害证据的患者。

手术处理

锁骨下血管损伤的手术方法须非常熟悉局部解剖。对近端和远端控制血管外科手术的基本原则是必须要执行。历史上各种经典手术显露对处理锁骨下动脉损伤已有描述。手术方式取决于临床表现和损伤部位。患者最初为仰卧位同侧上肢外展 30°、头偏向对侧。若计划切开锁骨，最初的切口在胸锁关节区域向锁骨内侧延伸，如有必要扩展到胸三角肌间沟（图 2-5）。邻近的肌肉附着点从锁骨上剥离，以方便向上牵拉。锁骨切除和胸锁关节离断是可以提供近端损伤的额外显露的手术技术。Henly 锁骨下钳是实现近端和远端控制的好用的工具（图 6）。

胸骨正中切开术向锁骨延伸可以提供右锁骨下损伤的良好的近端控制。已详细描述了既不推荐、现在也不经常使用的“活板门”切口，它可以显露左

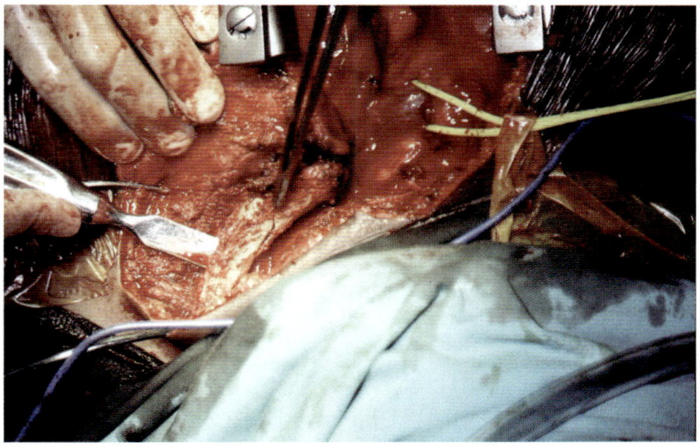

图 2　枪伤。锁骨下切口切除锁骨，暴露锁骨下血管

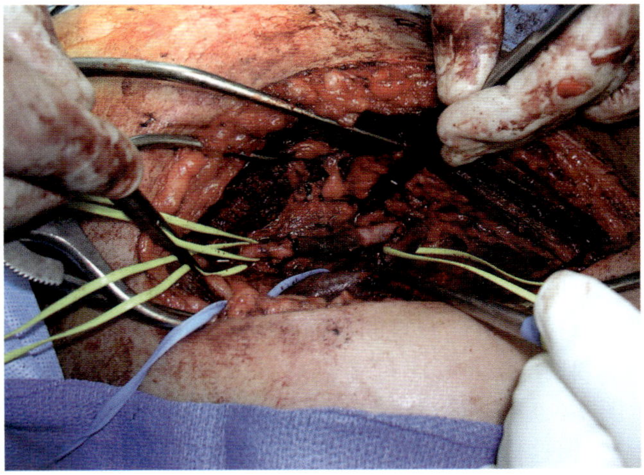

图 3　枪伤后血栓形成的右锁骨下动脉

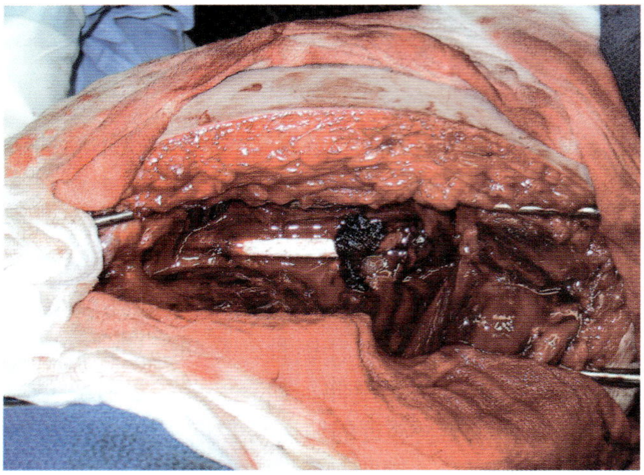

图 4 8 mm 直径的聚四氟乙烯人工血管

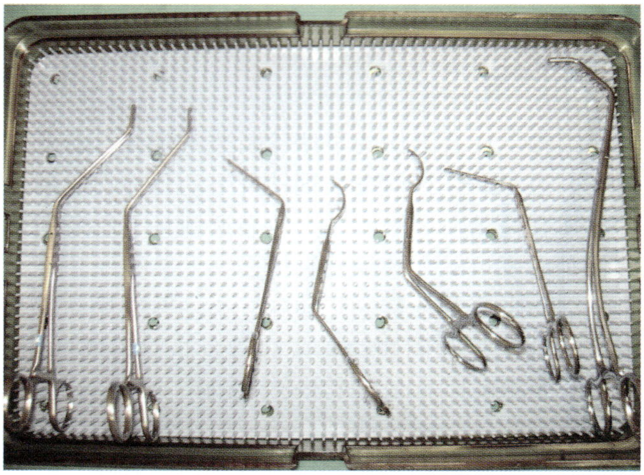

图 6 Henly 锁骨下钳

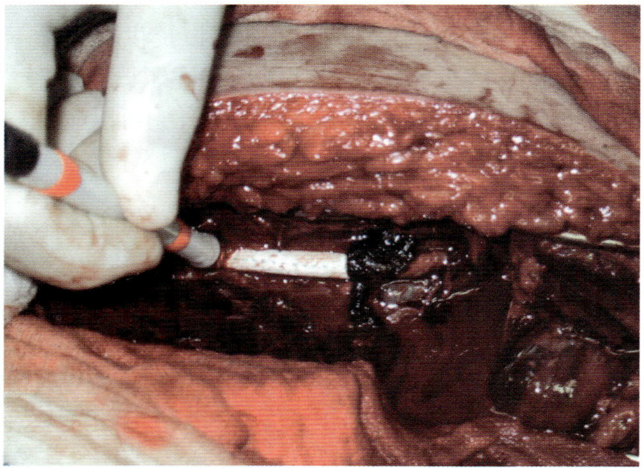

图 5 多普勒探头用于确认修复后血管的血流和流速

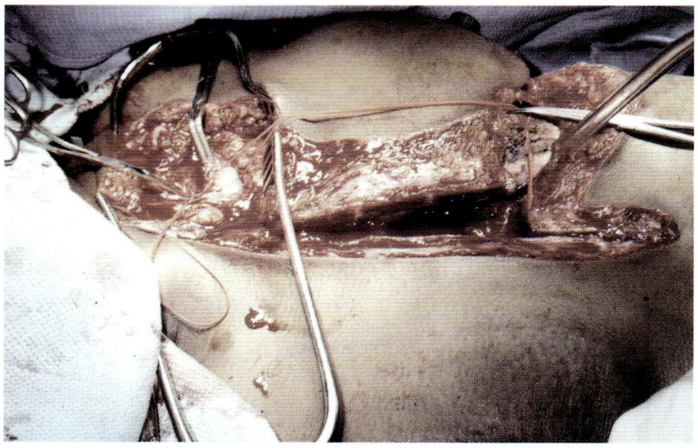

图 7 年轻女性左胸廓入口刺伤，入院时心肺骤停。她需要左前侧开胸术和开放性心肺复苏。在手术室需要胸骨正中切开术和锁骨上切口控制左锁骨下动脉损伤，钳夹控制血管近端和远端

锁骨下动脉第一和第二部分。这种入路的组成包括锁骨切口、限制性胸骨正中切开术和前外侧开胸术。这种暴露只对左锁骨下损伤有优势，而不是右侧，因为右侧血管位置偏后。这些手术入路要根据个体和外科医生的经验逐个病例选择手术对象。

传统上，锁骨下动脉损伤的手术治疗包括结扎、一期修复或间置移植物。血管修复的选择受损伤程度和水平的影响。结扎可用于那些多种致命损伤、广泛肩损伤、感染或动脉瘤的破裂病例。解剖上，有经过甲状颈干的广泛的侧支，允许安全地结扎锁骨下动脉。任何时候只要有可能就要重建动脉。偶尔，对需要后期修复的动脉可以用暂时转流。

刺伤有时可通过清创和修复进行适当的处理（图 7-8）。单纯动脉侧壁缝合在恰当病例是首选技术，但这个方法只能用于 20% 的情况下（图 9-11）。结扎多个动脉分支在一期修复时可以提供额外的长

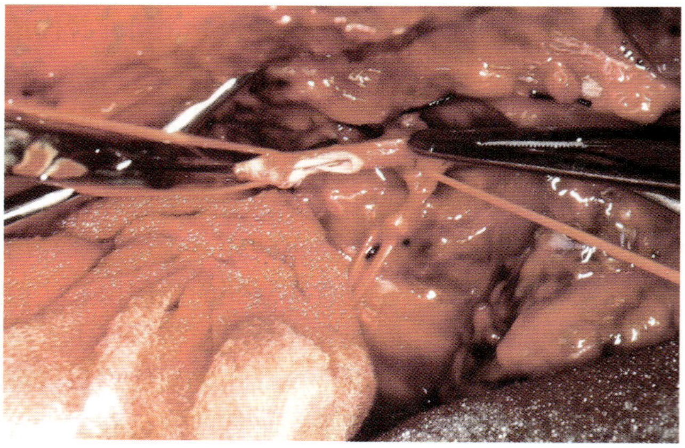

图 8 上述患者左锁骨下动脉部分横断。须切除横断部分和自体大隐静脉移植物间置

度，但明显的牵拉应当慎重，因为这些分支为上肢提供了广泛的侧支网络。另一方面，枪伤通常导致线明显的爆裂伤，经常须间置移植物（图 12-13）。

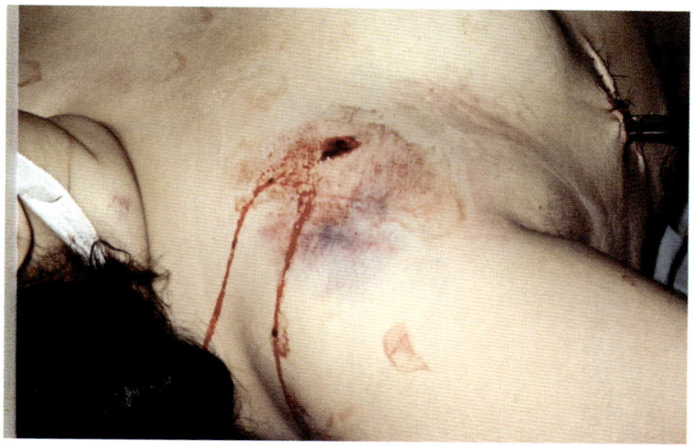

图 9　右锁骨下区域枪伤

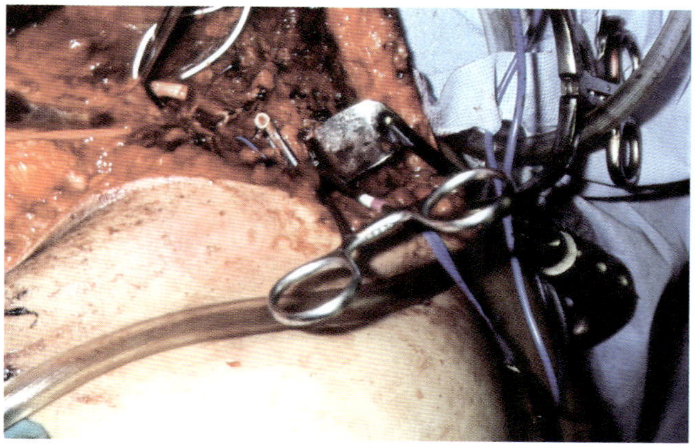

图 10　损伤的右锁骨下动脉节段性切除

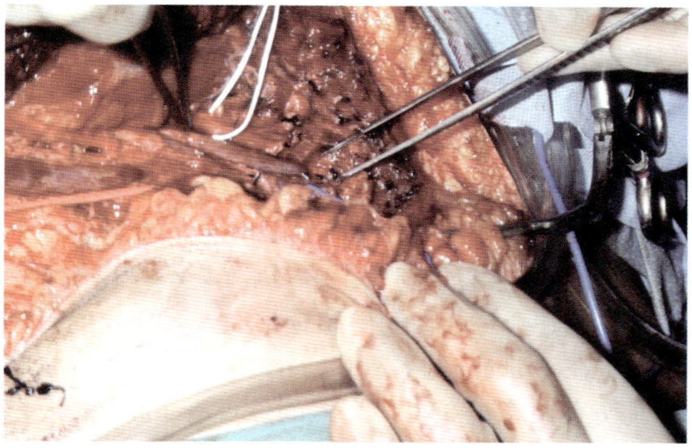

图 11　用自体大隐静脉修复

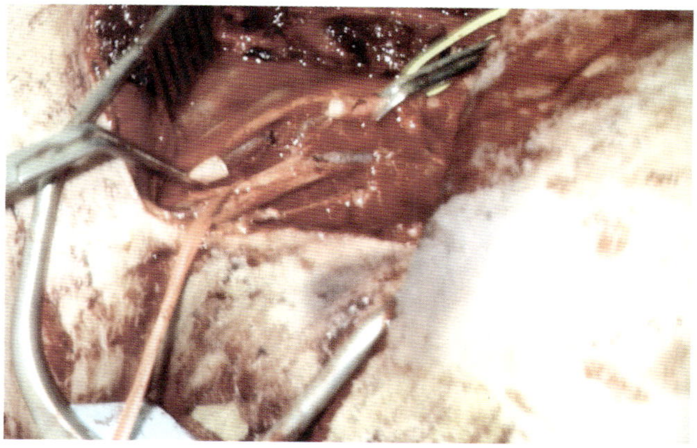

图 12　右锁骨下动脉枪伤。血管清创和切除

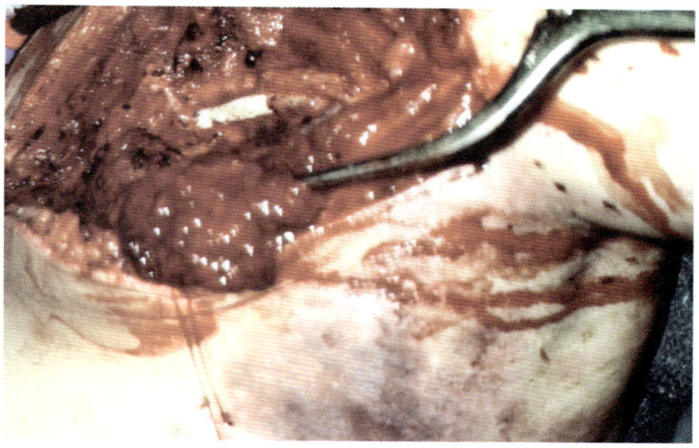

图 13　间置 6 mm 聚四氟乙烯移植物

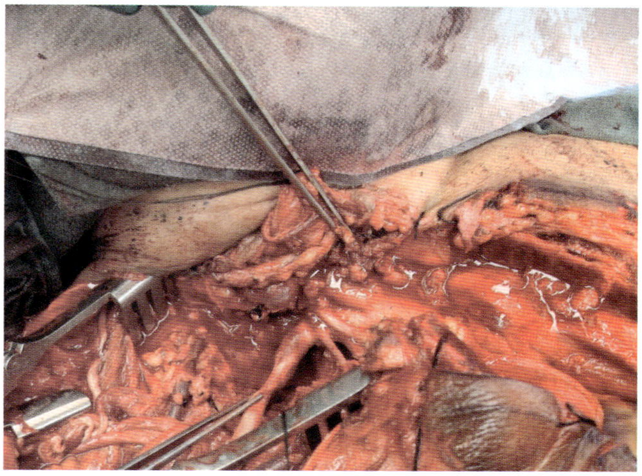

图 14　右锁骨下动脉在头臂干起始处钝伤。右颈总动脉起始处

清创后进行自体大隐静脉或人造移植物端端吻合是应对动脉损伤的常规方法。人造移植物可以安全使用，报道中移植物感染率低（图 14-16）。同时，相比取自体静脉延误时间，人造移植物提供更好的应急措施。锁骨下静脉损伤如果不导致明显的管腔狭窄，可以静脉侧壁缝合（图 17）。如果不可行，简单结扎也可以接受，它的并发症很少。

近期腔内技术的进步提供了另一种可靠的方法

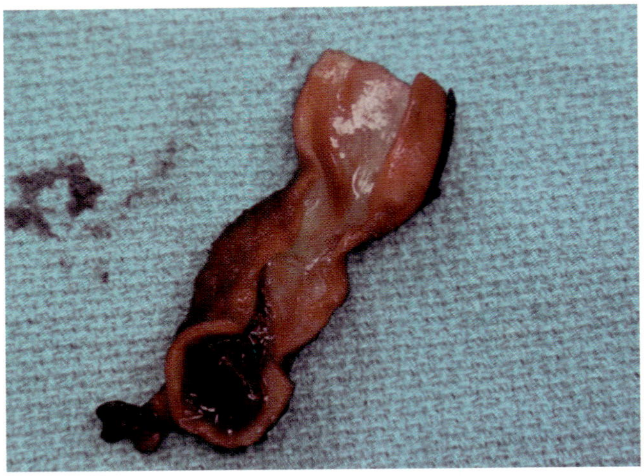

图 15　锁骨下动脉切除段，可见内膜瓣

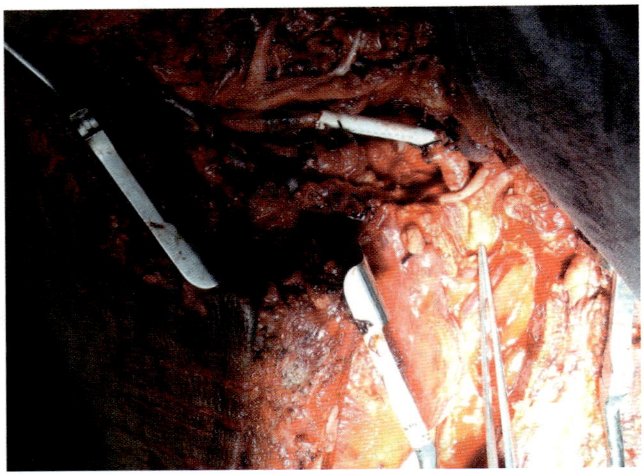

图 16　从右锁骨下动脉起始处开始的 8 mm 聚四氟乙烯移植物间置，头臂干

治疗那些不适合外科手术的患者和那些有苛刻标准的患者。微创方法治疗锁骨下动脉损伤有希望作为这些损伤的替代治疗方法，且已经被记录。仔细选择的患者，如那些有动脉狭窄、假性动脉瘤或动静脉瘘的患者可以通过介入手术植入基于导管的支架处理。不幸的是基于导管的覆膜支架技术并非没有不良反应。然而就目前而言，血管内修复似乎并不优于传统的手术治疗，但对特别仔细选择的患者不失为一个替代治疗方案。同样，也没有可用的数据报告他们的长期预后（表 3）。

并发症发生率

诊断延误、复杂的手术显露和相关损伤都是影响患者入院时的总的并发症发生率的因素。Kalakuntla 报告锁骨下动脉损伤治疗的 6 年回顾性综述指出，到达医院时血流动力学代偿也对应较高的并发症发生率和较长的住院时间。锁骨下动脉损伤并发症发生率和死亡风险受合并损伤数量的影响。在穿通伤中，损伤严重性和位置、枪伤患者的子弹速度有关。附近结构，特别是锁骨下静脉、臂丛神经、肺、锁骨、第 1 肋骨最可能损伤。

总的来说锁骨下动脉损伤的长期并发症发生率和臂丛损伤的出现密切相关。因挫伤或挤压伤（直接创伤）和牵拉伤使同侧感觉神经衰弱，导致臂丛症状。在 Graham 的系列中，65 例患者中研究与臂丛损伤有关者占 35%。类似的发现有 Johnson 报告的 43%。在这个研究中他们在随访期间发现了 83% 的患者有部分臂丛损伤，证实了某些功能有所改善，说明了神经失用症是初始的神经功能不全。不幸的是，在完全臂丛神经切断和二次神经修复的情况下，患者只能恢复最小的功能改善，这代表患者有永久性功能障碍。

已知的血管并发症如血栓形成、移植物感染和动脉瘤形成是常见的术后缺陷。同时，对有上肢神经麻痹症状的损伤的关注的延迟可能由大的假性

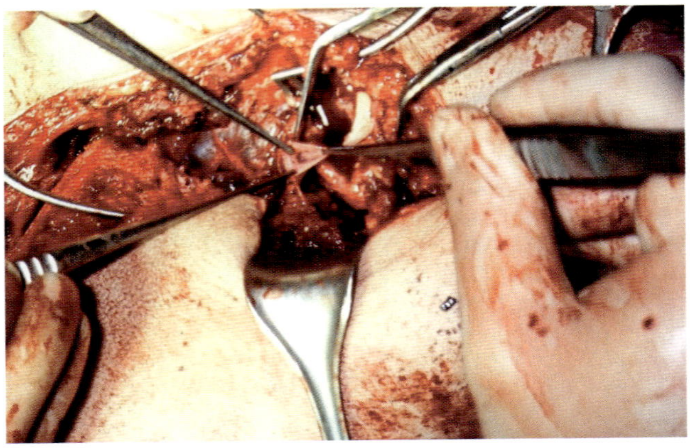

图 17　左锁骨下静脉裂伤

表 3　锁骨下动脉修复结果

作者	年份	损伤数	修复数	并发症	截肢	死亡
Amato	1969	14	13	0	0	0
Bricker	1970	14	11	0	0	3
Rich	1970	8	7	1	0	0
Drapanas	1970	16	0	0	1	4
Perry	1971	23	0	0	0	1

动脉瘤压迫臂丛导致。这些患者，即使进行介入，预后仍不好。在静脉结扎病例中，Demetriades 和 Asensio 观察到一过性上肢肿胀，而没有明显静脉相关并发症。经过几天抬高患肢，症状可以有明显改善。锁骨分离也有潜在不良后果如骨畸形愈合、假关节和骨髓炎。

治疗锁骨下血管损伤后的其他并发症有患者局部手术伤口感染、凝血功能障碍、大量输血、胸管损伤、空气栓塞。人造血管感染的风险也存在，但仍然不高，而人造血管的长期通畅率为 94%。肩胸关节分离虽然罕见，但无疑是源于高能创伤的灾难性损伤。一系列损伤包括锁骨骨折或脱位、肩部肌肉撕裂和神经血管破坏。在臂丛无功能的病例中，不须尝试血管重建，应直接肩下截肢。

预后和死亡率

锁骨下血管穿通性创伤和偶尔的钝伤在院前都导致明显的失血和失血性休克。特定的患者转运时间内出血被血肿压迫或血栓控制，表现为血流动力学状态在到院前改善，有较好的生存率。穿通伤住院死亡率为 5%～35%，钝伤的死亡率更高。文献报告总的死亡率为 39%～80%，大多数患者死于院前。这些糟糕的统计学数据和出血和头部钝伤有关。McKinley 等的研究证实这些发现，并对超过 4 年的暴力致死患者进行详细的最终评估，他记录 135 例死亡是由于孤立的锁骨下动脉损伤和出血导致的。

已发表的城市系列研究报告手术死亡率为 4.7%～30%，锁骨下动静脉合并损伤时死亡率更高。在一个包含 228 例锁骨下血管穿通伤的大病例组中，61% 的患者到院时死亡。在这些系列研究中，静脉损伤比动脉损伤有更高的死亡率，分别是 82% 和 60%。类似的发现也见于其他已发表的包含 20 例病例的系列研究，其中单独锁骨下静脉损伤死亡率为 50%。这些高死亡率可能是由于静脉栓子或静脉损伤持续出血导致的，静脉损伤不像动脉损伤会发生血管收缩效应。

锁骨下动脉损伤的并发症发生率和死亡率受相关损伤数量的影响很大。Lin 报告有 3 处或更多相关损伤的患者死亡率为 83% 而孤立锁骨下动脉损伤患者的死亡率为 17%。同时，表现低血压的患者与没有低血压的患者相比，死亡率更高，分别是 57% 和 18%。

结论

锁骨下血管损伤的罕见性时使许多创伤外科医生或创伤中心缺乏治疗的相关经验。这些创伤和明显的并发症和死亡有关。转运中幸存的患者可能有潜在的损伤，甚至可能死亡。这些损伤的治疗根据血流动力学稳定性、损伤机制和相关损伤的不同而不同。除非有显著进步，锁骨下血管损伤的死亡率还会维持高水平。

手术显露和腋血管损伤的处理

Juan A. Asensio, Patrizio Petrone, Alejandro Perez-Alonso,Angela Osmolak, Jason Loden, Gerald Gracia,Michael Ksycki, D' Andrea Joseph, Takashi Fujita 和 Yasuhiro Otomo 著
张学民 译

腋血管损伤是创伤外科医生遭遇的不常见，但有挑战的损伤。该血管和其他静脉相邻，包括腋静脉、臂丛。肩和上肢的骨性结构与大多数相关损伤有关。腋血管，特别是腋动脉出血，如果不控制，会导致汹涌的出血，也可能导致失血。这些血管经常难以显露和控制，特别是在穿通伤时。腋血管损伤可以导致严重的残疾、肢体缺失甚至死亡。

历史

1920 年，Makins 阐述了第一次世界大战英国穿通性血管损伤的经验。他回顾了全部 1 191 例动脉损伤，其中有 108 例腋动脉损伤，发生率为 9.0%，但它们都没有被修复。1946 年，DeBakey 和 Simeone 发表了第二次世界大战的美国经验。他们报告了 2 471 例血管损伤，其中有 74 例腋动脉损伤，发生

率为 2.9%，肢体缺失率高达 43.2%。在朝鲜战争中，Hughes 报告了总共 304 例动脉损伤，其中 20 例为腋动脉损伤，发生率为 6.5%。Rich 1970 年报告了 1 000 例越南战争血管损伤，其中有 59 例腋损伤，发生率为 2.6%（表 1）。

发病率和损伤机制

大的冲突的军事经验报告揭示了腋损伤发生率占战伤引起的全部动脉损伤的 2.9% ~ 9%。其发生率和平民经验报告非常相似，后者为 1.5% ~ 8.6%。近期的平民研究系列表明腋动脉损伤占全部上肢血管损伤的 4.7% ~ 42.9%（表 2）。

表 1　军事经验中腋动脉损伤的发生率

冲突	作者	总动脉数	腋动脉	发生率
第一次世界大战	Makins	1 191	108	0.9%
第二次世界大战	DeBakey和Simeone	2 471	74	2.9%
朝鲜战争	Hughes	304	20	6.6%
越南战争	Rich	1 000	59	5.9%
伊拉克战争	Clouse	163	10	6.1%

表 2　平民上肢血管损伤中腋动脉损伤的发生率

作者（年份）	总上肢动脉数	腋动脉	百分比
Orcutt, 1986	150	20	13.3%
Oller, 1992	361	17	4.7%
Andreev, 1992	50	6	12.0%
Pillai, 1997	21	5	23.8%
Sriussadaporn, 1997	28	12	42.9%
Prichayudh, 2009	52	3	5.8%
Franz, 2009	30	3	10.0%

穿通机制占腋血管损伤的绝大多数。Graham 最近报告在 65 例腋血管损伤患者中，95% 的损伤源于穿通伤，只有 5% 源于钝伤。类似地，越南战争中的经验发现，98% 的腋动脉损伤源自枪伤和碎片伤（如手榴弹或弹片），只有 2% 源自钝伤。

解剖

腋动脉大约 15 cm 长，是锁骨下动脉的直接延续。腋动脉起自第 1 肋骨外侧缘，终止于大圆肌下缘，在此移行为肱动脉。

胸大肌将腋动脉分成 3 部分。第一部分在肌肉近端，分出一条分支——胸上动脉，靠内侧走行，供应前 2 个肋间的肌肉。第二部分在肌肉下行走分出 2 条分支——胸肩峰动脉和胸外动脉。胸肩峰动脉是非常重要的分支，形成丰富的侧支循环。其起始呈一短干，分出 4 条分支供应三角肌和胸肌，也供应肩锁关节区。胸外侧动脉沿胸大肌下缘走行供应胸壁。

第三部分位于肌肉外侧，分出 3 条分支：肩胛下动脉和旋肱前动脉、旋肱后动脉。肩胛下动脉是最大的分支。起自关节窝水平的腋动脉沿肩胛下缘下行到腋后壁肌肉，与肱深动脉降支在肱三头肌下方吻合，构成这一区域的侧支血供。旋肱前动脉和后动脉在肱骨颈周围形成环形。旋肱后动脉和肱深动脉的升支吻合提供另一个重要的侧支循环。

腋静脉是由肱动脉的两并行静脉连接形成，肱静脉与贵要静脉。它进入腋窝，一旦行至锁骨下就成为锁骨下静脉，穿过 Halsted 韧带进入胸腔。手臂外展时腋静脉覆盖腋动脉。这种解剖学关系导致穿通性损伤后动静脉瘘的形成。

臂丛也邻近腋动脉。事实上，它们经常在一个共同的筋膜鞘里。臂丛的 3 个大束（内、外和后）包绕腋动脉的近端部分。上肢主要的周围神经从这些束发出。内侧束在前方，尺神经居中，桡神经在腋动脉后方。

诊断

所有锁骨周围或腋损伤的患者应对血管创伤的存在进行评估。诊断血管损伤的硬体征包括明显的出血、大的扩张的血肿、周围脉搏减弱或消失和听诊杂音。软体征提示血管损伤，包括稳定的血肿、慢性而持续的出血、相关的神经损伤和近端损伤。远处脉搏存在不能确切地排除有丰富侧支循环的重要的近端动脉损伤。

臂丛要进行评估，臂丛相关损伤见于 33% 的腋血管损伤的患者中。要注意识别相关的胸部损伤，如继发于胸部损伤的气胸或血胸，见于 28% ~ 30% 的患者。

当出现严重低血压、活动性大出血或危及肢体的时候，患者应当立即转运到手术室。如果患者血流动力学条件允许可以拍 X 线胸片，可能发现需要处理的血胸、弹头或纵隔血肿。

踝肱指数和肱肱指数（如患侧肢体收缩压和对侧的比例）是个有用的检查，可以对所有稳定患者测量。异常的指数（小于 0.9）是诊断或高度可疑诊断动脉损伤的条件。然而，由于该血管有丰富的侧支循环，明显的腋动脉损伤指标可能是正常的。

血管造影可以用于稳定的有血管损伤软体征表现的患者，很少用于有硬体征而损伤部位不明确的稳定患者，如那些多发枪伤、猎枪伤或多发骨折（图 1-3）。腋动脉近端损伤、没有完全确切的手术探查指征的患者可以做血管造影，因为血管造影可以呈现明确的损伤，由此可以识别无症状的患者。假性动脉瘤、动静脉瘘和腋动脉内膜损伤可以通过血管内支架成功处理，但这部分的经验仍十分有限。

CTA 是另一个有用的诊断方法，可能最终替代或成为血管造影的补充。多排螺旋 CT 的使用（64 排）和三维重建提高了分辨率，减少了扫描时间。研究发现 CTA 在上肢和下肢损伤的灵敏度和特异度分别为 95% ~ 100% 和 87%。CTA 的局限性包括难以区分痉挛和闭塞，若人造物体和高衰减结构，

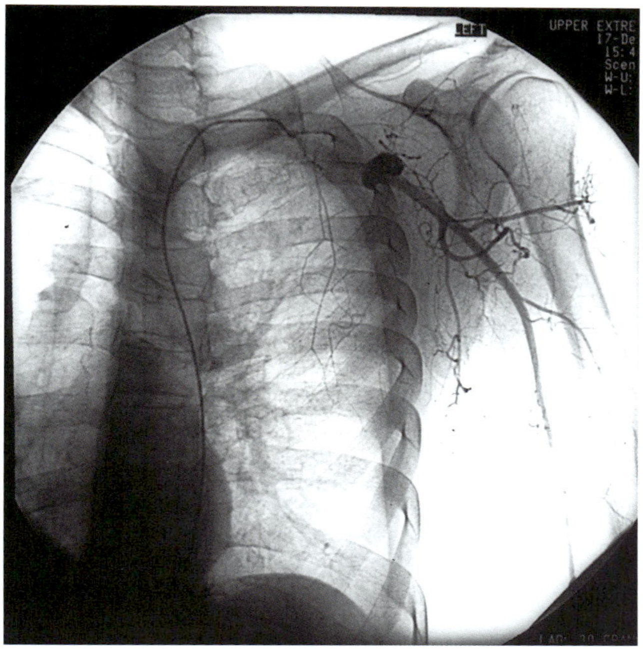

图 1　左腋动脉枪伤。血管造影发现腋动脉第二部分损伤

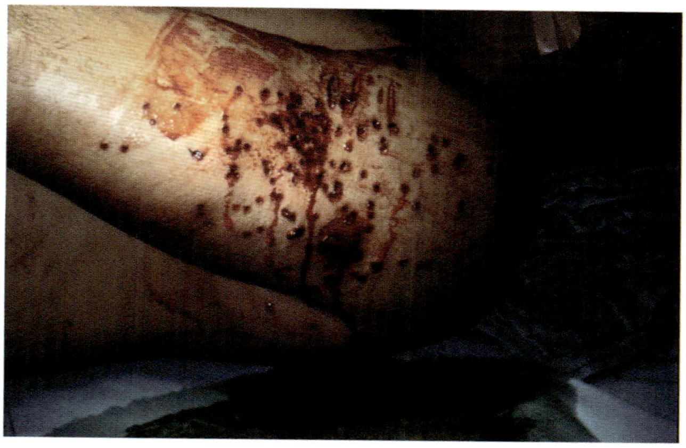

图 2　左上肢和腋之间的枪伤

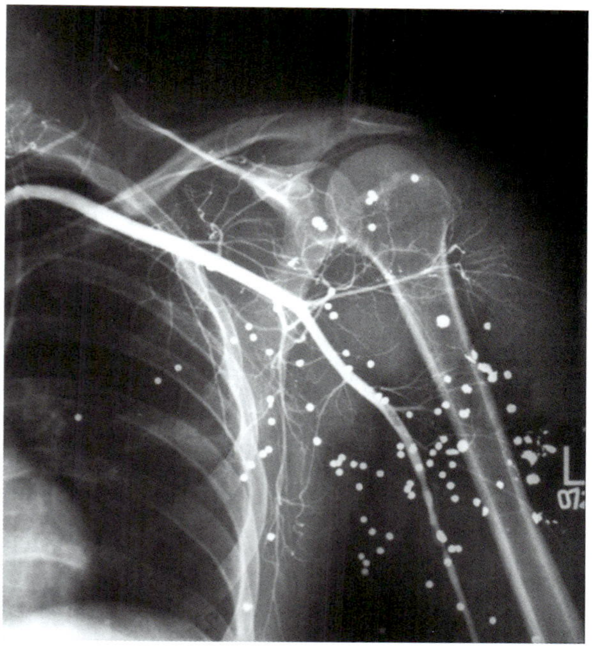

图 3　血管造影发现左腋动脉节段损伤

如弹片或其他异物存在，有时证实一个确切诊断是困难的。

外科治疗

血管损伤治疗的基本原则

一些关键性的手术手法是所有血管损伤的治疗标准，用于腋血管损伤的处理：

1. 直接压迫，控制活动性出血。
2. 术野中有人维持压力。
3. 选择恰当的手术显露和广泛显露损伤血管的

计划。

4. 鉴于合并损伤很常见，控制动脉和静脉的近端和远端。
5. 细致地解剖、分离损伤血管。
6. 受伤或非损伤血管的牵拉可以通过血管袢将其圈起或 Cushing 静脉拉钩操作。
7. 牵拉神经、轻柔解剖、放置 2 个血管袢在远侧点，以分散牵拉神经的力量。
8. 近端和远端控制后看准损伤位置直接进入。
9. 通过细致的解剖，尽可能广泛地显露损伤血管。操作可能须切断一些分支和侧支，注意尽可能多地保留血管。
10. 除非某些刺伤和裂伤血管可以直接修复或吻合，其他的损伤血管须切除适当长度，直到获得正常的近端和远端。在动脉，切除要注意避免掀起内膜瓣。
11. 检查动脉的横切边缘。如果有内膜瓣，重新切除。在有广泛内膜瓣的和进一步切除不可能的病例中，在内膜瓣内水平褥式 Halsted 缝合，从血管腔内侧进针，将结打在血管外，使用最细的聚丙烯单丝线缝合。
12. 用肝素盐水冲洗横断血管的近端和远端。检查远端回血情况，冲洗要频繁和轻柔。
13. 如果没有远端回血，轻柔地植入适当大小和长度的 Fogarty 导管，如果可能，在直视下取栓。球囊不要膨胀得过大，也不要送入过深，超过达到良好回血的深度可能增加内膜损伤的风险。如果没有动脉回血，可以注入罂粟碱解除血管痉挛。
14. 动脉损伤可以通过直接动脉缝合或端端吻合修复。也可能需要旁路术或间置逆行自体大隐静脉移植物或假体移植物。修复和旁路不要有张力，也不要过长以避免扭折。跨关节旁路术一定要考虑到活动范围（屈曲），留下适当的长度，避免扭折和移植物闭塞。全部吻合要用双针聚丙烯线，最好在开放的状态下。尽管通常认为直接吻合可能导致最终狭窄，情况并非如此。
15. 血管粗细不一致的时候可以通过竹片状或“鱼嘴样”移植物处理。小的端端血管吻合可以用全周聚丙烯线单纯间断缝合，困难的吻合可以用 Carrel 三点缝合技术。
16. 较小的血管的旁路手术，如远侧桡动脉和尺动脉可能能在远端做端侧吻合，从而增加吻合大小和血流。
17. 静脉损伤可以结扎或一期修复。对所有静脉损伤推荐丝线双重结扎。一期静脉缝合可以用细的聚丙烯单丝线缝合以防止修复的静脉狭窄。很少的情况下需要静脉转流。
18. 有指征的时候要及早行筋膜切开术。软组织损伤越多，耐受缺血时间越短。我们推荐用尸体皮肤移植物作为生物敷料。
19. 动脉修复或旁路术完成后应当用手指触摸检查脉搏或通过手持式多普勒探头探查旁路近端和远端吻合口、旁路本身和所有远侧血管。
20. 术后血管造影的应用应当个体化，但强烈推荐通过它发现可纠正的术中缺陷，以此避免血管或旁路失效。

腋血管损伤的特殊治疗

术前，外出血通过直接压迫伤口控制，而锁骨下血管的出血如果无法通过直接压迫控制的话很难控制。在这些患者用 Foley 导管球囊压塞可能有效。

术中患者呈仰卧位，上肢外展 90°，头偏向对侧。避免过度外展，因为会使解剖扭曲，使显露更加困难。在术野里的整个前胸、腹部和颈部都要术前准备和铺单，以应对可能的胸和颈探查。整个上肢要术前准备，以便重新定位、延长切口和触摸肱动脉、桡动脉和尺动脉搏动。

通过锁骨下路径显露腋动脉提供了良好的暴露（图 4）。切口起自锁骨中点下方，向外延伸到三角胸肌间沟。该切口可以向上肢近端延长到肱二头肌

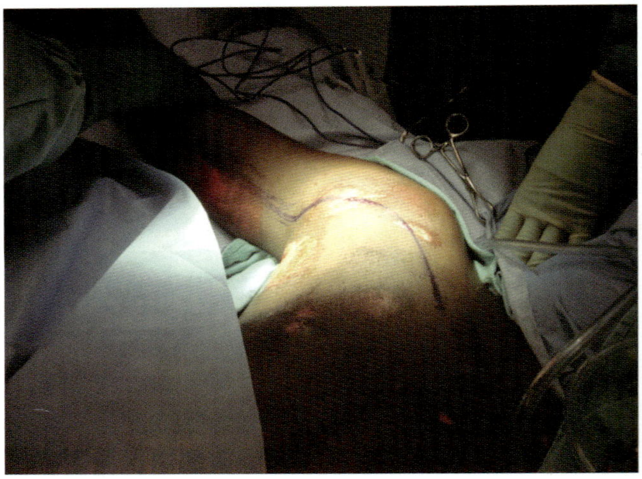

图 4　显露腋血管损伤的切口

内侧沟，以进一步显露腋动脉远端和肱动脉。如果须显露锁骨下动脉或对近端腋动脉加以控制，可以在胸锁关节做切口，延长至在锁骨中点越过内侧锁骨，向下经过三角胸肌间沟和锁骨下切口汇合。可以进一步分离和切除内侧锁骨，以得到近端腋动脉和锁骨下动脉的显露，特别是在出血患者。

显露腋血管须分离胸大肌纤维和牵拉下面的胸小肌。在活动性出血的情况下需要快速广泛的暴露，肌肉可以切开。胸大肌从其在肱骨的附着点切开2 cm，向下内侧牵拉。下面的胸小肌从其插入喙突的附着点切开，向下牵拉。这样腋血管就完全显露了。解剖过程中要全力保护侧支，避免医源性臂丛损伤。

在近端和远端控制后，损伤段的动脉应当仔细检查，以确定损伤程度。如果损伤接近无张力，可以简单动脉缝合。而在手术修复前损伤节段需要切除和清创。在修复损伤血管前，用Fogarty导管小心操作切除血栓，得到好的流动和回血。端端吻合在某些损伤是可能的，而在大多数枪伤中常用间置移植物的办法。移植物的选择——自体静脉还是人工移植物——依据个人喜好、可用性、患者一般情况而定（图5-7）。没有证据表明其中哪种更好。重症患者不能耐受决定性修复，结扎和使用Argyle转流管。暂时血管内转流是可行的损伤控制措施。而结扎急性损伤的腋动脉和9.0%～43.2%的截肢率有关。

腋静脉损伤可以简单静脉缝合，不要尝试更复杂的修复，包括静脉-静脉旁路或使用移植物，因为几乎所有患者对结扎静脉有良好耐受（图8）。而且，没有证据表明复杂的重建有更好的预后。腋静脉结扎后患者可能有一过性水肿，在几天内代偿。密切观察和有指征时的上肢筋膜切开提供了更安全

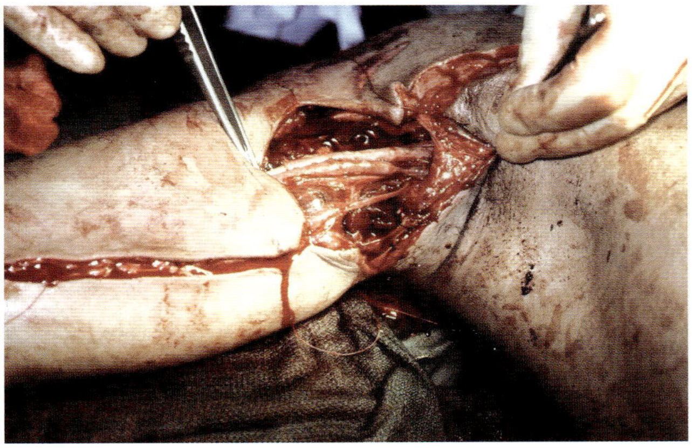

图5 逆行自体大隐静脉旁路移植物

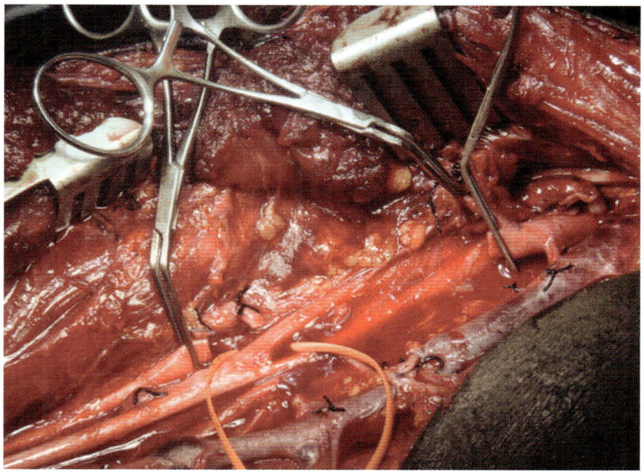

图6 枪伤后右腋动脉切除，计划行旁路术，注意腋静脉

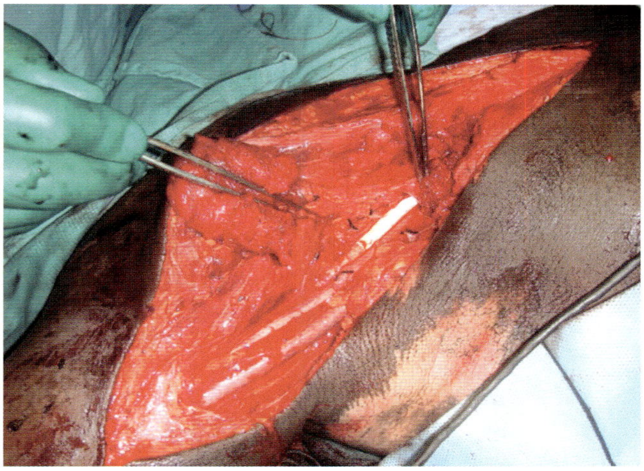

图7 6 mm聚四氟乙烯旁路移植物

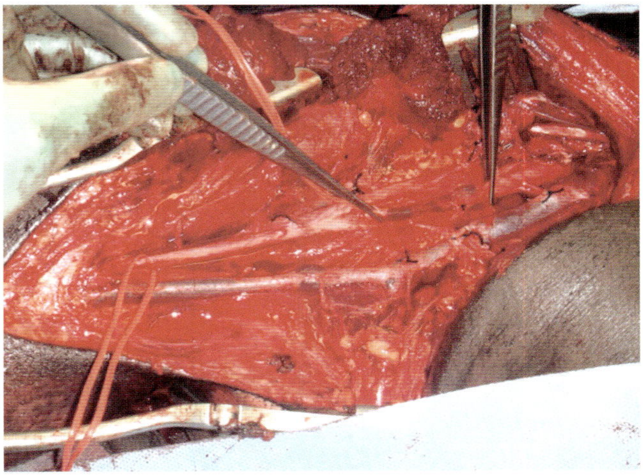

图8 结扎腋静脉

的方法。

预后和死亡率

近年平民系列研究中腋动脉损伤的截肢率为0～3%，和早期军事经验报告中的8.5%～43.2%相比已经很低了。相关的臂丛损伤仍是长期功能预后的主要限制因素。这些损伤的发生率为30.4%～35.4%。文献报告动脉修复后血栓形成的发生率为1.5%～10%，感染并发症发生率报告为0～21%。近年平民系列研究中的死亡率为3%～14.8%（表3）。

结论

虽然罕见，腋动脉损伤可以导致显著的并发症发生率、肢体缺失和死亡。早期诊断和及时修复动脉会产生好的预后。腋血管损伤处理中恰当的延长切口和恰当的动脉显露极为重要。

表3 近期平民系列腋动脉损伤的预后

作者（年份）	患者数量	治疗	截肢（%）	臂丛损伤（%）	死亡（死亡率）
Graham, 1982	65（动脉损伤31，静脉损伤14，动静脉复合损伤20）	动脉结扎，0 静脉结扎，9 动脉修复，51 静脉修复，25	2（3%）	23（35.4%）	2（3%）
Degiannis, 1995	32（腋动脉穿通伤）	修复，31 （修复前死亡，1）	0（0%）	11（34.4%）	2（6.3%）
Demetriades 和 Asensio, 1999	79（锁骨下和腋穿通伤；动脉损伤39，静脉损伤20，动静脉复合损伤20）	动脉结扎，0 静脉结扎，26 动脉修复，59 （血管内修复，1） 静脉修复，14 ED 血栓切除，18 （均死亡）	N/A	26（32.9%）	27（34.2%） 排除 ED 血栓切除 9（14.8%）
McKinley, 2000	260（近端腋动脉和锁骨下动脉损伤）	修复，236 结扎，5 非手术，19	N/A	79（30.4%）	10（11.5%）
Aksoy, 2005	38（腋动脉和锁骨下动脉损伤）	修复，33 结扎，5	1（2.6%）	12（31.5%）	2（5.2%）

ED，急诊科

肱血管损伤：高并发症发生率和低死亡率损伤

Juan A. Asensio, Patrizio Petrone, Alejandro Perez-Alonso,Parth Shah, Austin Person, Anthony M. Udekwu,John K. Bini 和 Ari Leppäniemi 著
张学民 译

来自平民和军事方面的动脉损伤的研究都报告肱动脉是最常损伤的血管，大约占全部周围动脉损伤的 25%～33%。在一些报告中肱动脉的损伤频率接近股浅动脉，两者都很长，位于各自肢体的脆弱部位。朝鲜战争和越南战争的经验都指出将近 30% 的动脉损伤累及肱动脉。

对肱动脉损伤而言，特定的解剖学特点非常重要。肱深动脉分支近端和远端损伤缺血程度明显不同。因此肱总动脉结扎的坏死风险大概是肱浅动脉结扎的 2 倍。

肱动脉被重要的周围神经包绕——正中神经、尺神经和桡神经——和肱骨和相关静脉平行。由于邻近这些组织结构，相关的神经和骨损伤也常见，这些神经损伤残余的神经病变经常是永久性残疾的主要来源。在下肢，承重是康复中很重要的方面；而在上肢，手的功能是最重要的预后因素。

历史回顾

1759 年，Hallowell 首次修复了肱动脉损伤，用“兽医缝合法或Farrier缝合法”取代先前的结扎技术，从而提供了治疗血管创伤的初始步骤。Torrance 在 1903 年成功缝合修复了一个钝伤导致的肱动脉损伤。Jones 在 1919 年报告了 2 例枪伤后患者肱动脉结扎 1 年的随访，两者都有残留的广泛上肢残疾。在那以后，产生了许多革新和革命性的进步。即便在这些早期报告中，结扎仍是在第一次和第二次世界大战期间的主要治疗措施，特别是在战斗中。转运时间长、缺乏抗生素、不当的液体复苏且这些都是需要截肢的非技术原因，这些患者的预后是不理想的，截肢率近 50%（表 1）。

发病率和损伤机制

肱动脉损伤是最常见的上肢动脉损伤。在大的军人和平民系列研究中，肱动脉损伤占全部周围动脉损伤的 15%～30%。损伤相对频率高的原因是肱动脉和其他周围动脉相比相对长、表浅、暴露。而且，上肢经常被用作杠杆、锤子和武器，也对躯干起保护或约束作用，这些都使肱动脉处于损伤的危险中。

全部的肢体血管损伤不常报告。最近的国家创伤数据库（National Trauma Database，NTDB）的医学记录回顾了 1 861 770 例患者，发现 1.6% 的患者有血管损伤，0.3% 的患者有上肢血管损伤，0.1% 的患者有肱动脉损伤。肱动脉损伤占全部上肢损伤的 28% 和全部周围血管损伤的 15.5%。97% 的肱动脉损伤是由于穿通伤导致的。一些研究报告不同的肱动脉损伤发生率，范围为 14%～50%。

军人系列研究报告血管相关的损伤占全部损伤的 3.8%～6.6%。肱动脉损伤占全部肢体血管损伤的 23% 和全部上肢血管损伤的 58%。军人和平民的损伤的平均年龄均报告为 27～31 岁。在平民中，男性患者占 90%，在军人中，男性患者比例接近 100%。

平民人群中，男性比女性占优势，几乎 90% 的肱动脉损伤者是男性。接近 100% 的肱动脉损伤的军人是男性。在这些损伤中最多数是穿通伤（94%），而钝伤少（6%）。

穿通性创伤仍是肱动脉损伤最常见原因。大多数损伤由枪伤、刀刺伤或碎玻璃切割伤或其他锯齿状物体导致，特别是平民创伤。Rich 在 1970 年进行的越南战争的大系列研究包含 283 例肱动脉损伤患者，其中 250 例患者有其他碎片或弹片导致的损伤。超过 50% 的肱动脉损伤继发于各种爆炸装置的碎片，将近 40% 的患者有枪伤。

最近，在大多数三级医疗中心，使用心导管诊断的数量增加，导致相应的肱动脉损伤数量增加，常伴随着血栓形成。与平民经验相反，在军事环境中，无论是在腋动脉还是在肱动脉中，血栓形成很少发生，少于 1%。穿通伤是最常见的损伤机制，大多数肱动脉损伤在术中发现是横断伤（60% ～84%），其次是裂伤（13%）、血栓形成（5% ～16%）、内膜瓣（3%）、假性动脉瘤（15.3%），AV 少见（3%）。有趣的是有相当数量的孤立肱动脉损伤，发生率为 22%。

肱动脉的钝性损伤发生较少，但值得重视，因为它的诊断很容易被忽视。对于肱骨髁上骨折，特别是前移位或肘关节脱位，创伤科医生应警惕潜在的肱动脉损伤的可能性。这导致 Volkmann 挛缩的缺血综合征。幸运的是由于对高风险损伤的认识和监测，这种现象很少发生。存在筋膜室综合征的症状时，应迅速血管修复和减压（表 2）。

表 1　肱动脉损伤的军事经验

冲突	作者（年份）	总动脉数	肱动脉	百分比
第一次世界大战	Makins (1919)	1 191	200	16.8
第二次世界大战	DeBakey 和 Simeone (1946)	2 471	601	24.3
朝鲜战争	Hughes (1958)	304	89	29.3
越南战争	Rich (1970)	1 000	283	28.3

表 2　肱动脉损伤的平民经验

城市	作者（年份）	总动脉数	肱动脉	百分比
Houston	Morris(1960)	220	55	25.0
Atlanta	Ferguson(1961)	200	29	14.5
Denver	Owens(1963)	70	14	20.0
Detroit	Smith(1963)	61	13	21.3
Dallas	Patman(1964)*	271	46	17.0
St. Louis	Dillard(1968)	85	26	30.6
New Orleans	Drapanas(1970)	226	39	17.3
Dallas	Perry(1971)	508	78	15.4
Memphis	Cheek(1975)	155	21	13.5
Denver	Kelly和 Eiseman(1975)	116	37	31.9
Jackson	Hardy(1975)	360	75	20.8
New York	Bole (1976)	126	14	11.1
Indianapolis	Cikrit(1990)	101	23	22.7
Johannesburg	Degiannis(1995)	170	37	21.8
Cape Town(SA)	Zellweger(2004)†	N/A	124	不详
Izmir(Turkey)	Ergunes(2006)†	N/A	58	不详
Tehran (Iran)	Rasouli(2009)	130	18	13.8
Chicago	Kim(2009)†	N/A	139	不详

* 连续系列。

† 系列中仅包含肱动脉损伤

解剖

肱动脉是腋动脉的延续，起自大圆肌下缘。出腋窝后，肱动脉是个相对表浅的结构，只被皮肤、皮下组织和深筋膜覆盖。向下，肱动脉走行在肱骨内侧，与正中神经（浅外侧）和尺神经、桡神经（内侧）伴行。向远端，肱动脉在肘窝内侧被正中神经跨越，后者移行到动脉内侧。在肘窝近端，肱动脉在尺骨内上髁后方，尺神经在动脉后方。肱动脉止于肘皮肤褶皱下大约 3 ~ 5 cm，在此它分为桡动脉和尺动脉。

肱动脉有 3 条主要分支，第一条（最近端）是肱深动脉，伴随桡神经向后在三头肌内侧头和长头之间走行。肱深动脉通过其旋肱后动脉分支提供与腋动脉的重要的侧支吻合。肱深动脉和桡侧返动脉也有侧支吻合。肱深动脉有 2 条分支：前分支和桡侧返动脉吻合，后分支和骨间返动脉吻合。2 条分支形成额外的重要的侧支路径。肱动脉的第二个主要分支是尺侧上副动脉，由尺神经伴行通过内上髁和尺侧后反动脉提供侧支吻合。第三条（最远的）主要分支是尺侧下副动脉，在肘部和尺动脉通过其前返支提供丰富的侧支吻合网络。

诊断

肱动脉损伤的诊断经常由临床表现得出。损伤硬体征包括无脉 / 脉弱、活动性（搏动性）出血、远侧缺血、扩大或搏动性血肿、震颤或杂音。损伤硬体征提示立即手术探查血管，除非患者有多系统损伤危及生命。

枪伤患者将硬体征作为手术指征的结果是 100% 的治疗探查率。损伤的软体征包括相关的骨损伤、邻近穿通伤、显著的出血已停止或失血性休克、神经功能缺损和血肿。在此情况下确认动脉损伤需要放射学评估。短绌脉在 43% ~ 89% 的肱动脉损伤患者中是最常见的表现。

要测量肱肱指数（如果另一侧肢体未受伤），它小于 0.9 是侵入性检查或手术探查的指征。作出诊断的其他有用方法包括非侵入性的研究，如多普勒超声（图 1-2）。血管造影仍为血管损伤诊断的金标准（图 3）；然而，CTA 有明显的优势，使其正取代标准血管造影。CTA 和血管造影比有更快、不依赖

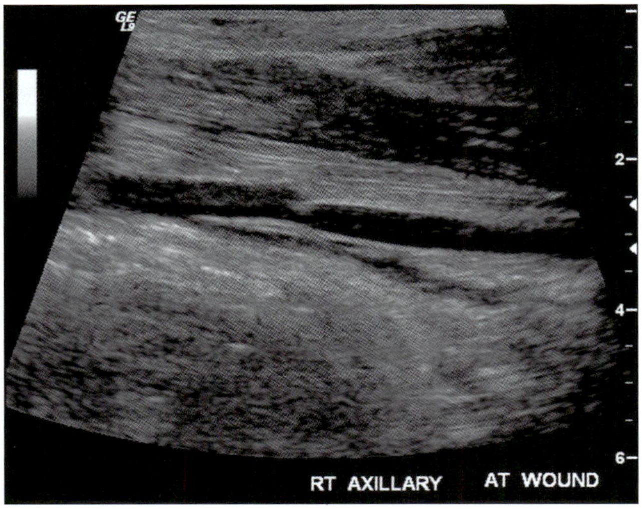

图 1　26 岁男性右侧肱动脉枪伤，伤及右腋区。灰阶超声图像证实肱动脉近侧 1/3 有内膜瓣

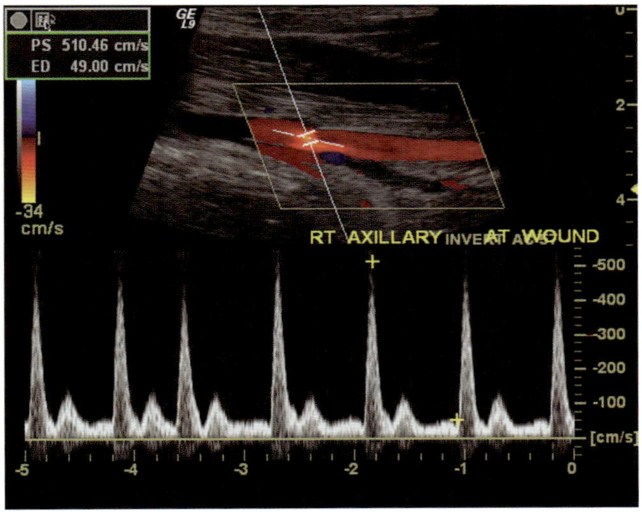

图 2　26 岁男性右侧肱动脉枪伤，伤及右腋区。彩色多普勒和波形谱表现收缩期流速局部高峰值，提示损伤处重度狭窄

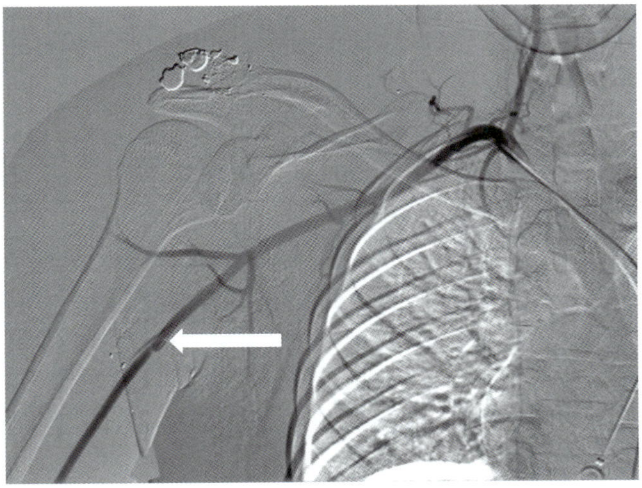

图 3　26 岁男性右侧肱动脉枪伤，伤及右腋区。血管造影确认肱动脉损伤（箭头），并显示肩锁关节处的弹片

操作者和更快速可及的优点。将近 10% 的患者需要血管造影。通常血管造影所见的肱动脉损伤表现有动脉闭塞、内膜撕裂和出现假性动脉瘤。

损伤的解剖学定位

肱动脉损伤在其全程包括近段、中段、远端分布概率是一样的，大概都是 1/3。

外科处理

在开放的伤口上直接压迫就可以控制出血。从不须在上肢盲法钳夹出血血管，否则有损伤伴随的正中神经、桡神经或尺神经的危险。对怀疑近端损伤的患者，应当像处理腋动脉损伤那样消毒铺单。对更远处的损伤，对手臂和手（到指尖）行手术准备，以便术中触摸桡动脉和尺动脉的脉搏。对对侧下肢行手术准备，以备静脉取材。上臂应放在可移动的平台上，铺单应当允许一个操作员在头部，另一个位于手臂支撑的尾部。

上肢大多数动脉通过在二头肌和三头肌之间的肌间沟纵切口显露，通过手臂外展二头肌易于分辨。一定要小心避免损伤浅层的贵要静脉，后者一旦分出很容易被牵拉。远侧，动脉扎入二头肌腱膜下，应切开以得到动脉的最大显露。在肘窝，做一个外侧起始的 S 形切口可以到达肱动脉分叉和避免关节挛缩。

血管显露的一般原则可用于治疗肱动脉损伤。包括近端 / 远端控制，显露损伤动脉段，清除失活血管和识别相关损伤（图 4）。可能的话，将肱动脉准备好。确切的修复方法取决于损伤的范围、周围组织的损伤数量和动脉破坏段长度。

逆行自体大隐静脉间置移植物是标准的修复长段损伤的方法（图 5）。用于军事和平民各种机制的损伤的修复已经得到详细阐述。在控制血管的近端和远端后同时获取自体大隐静脉，之后清理创伤血管，进行静脉或聚四氟乙烯（polytetrafluoroethylene，PTFE）人工血管端端旁路术（图 6-7）。

小损伤如果缺损小，可以清创后端端吻合或简单动脉缝合治疗。要注意，各种血管损伤修复步骤要确保动脉没有张力。

临时血管转流管的使用在军事和平民研究中都

已有报告。临时转流可以用于手术中损伤控制，或某些更复杂的复合伤和伴随骨折的损伤上肢（图8-11）。在一篇回顾严重创伤患者分流使用的文章中，保肢率为88%。如果有骨损伤，最常用的技术是放置暂时留置的转流管，以恢复动脉血流。在试图确切血管修复前，骨科医生要确保手臂的长度和稳定性。由于有明显的肢体缺失的风险，很少考虑结扎。如果患者在极端情况下有其他相关损伤，则通过沿动脉走行的纵切口快速显露肱动脉，需要的话近端跨腋窝和远端跨肘窝做S形延长切口。正中神经和贵要静脉和贵要动脉很近。可以快速放置临时转流管留置几日，而无需全身肝素化。

结扎可以用于有生命危险、严重伤害或无法修复的情况下。在结扎前无缺血体征的患者，常有明显的机会保存肢体和保留功能。

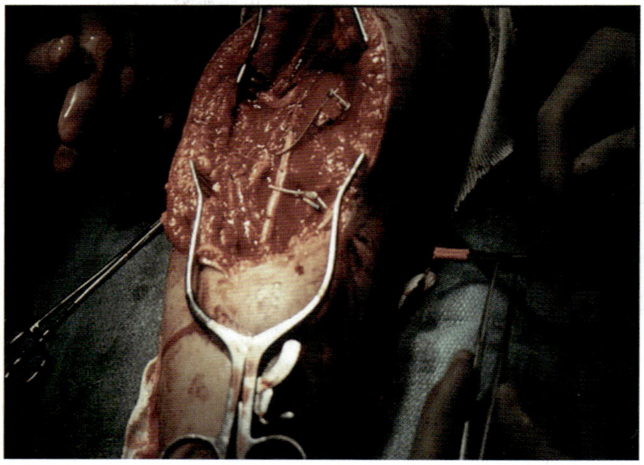

图4　远端肱动脉刺伤。注意近端和远端用 Dietrich 哈巴狗钳控制

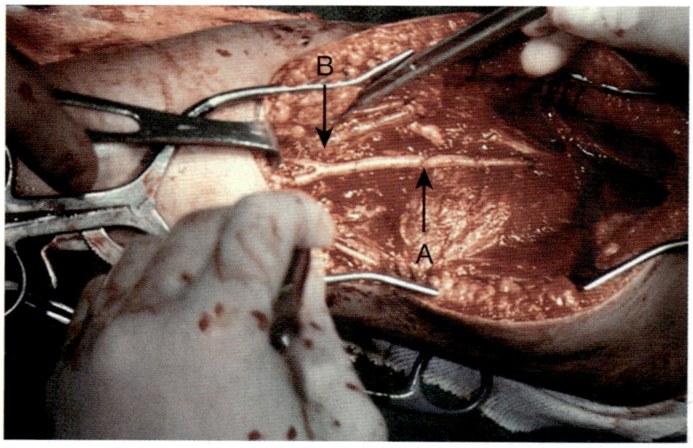

图5　远端肱动脉枪伤。用逆行自体大隐静脉移植物修复。远端吻合口（A）靠近肱动脉分叉（B）

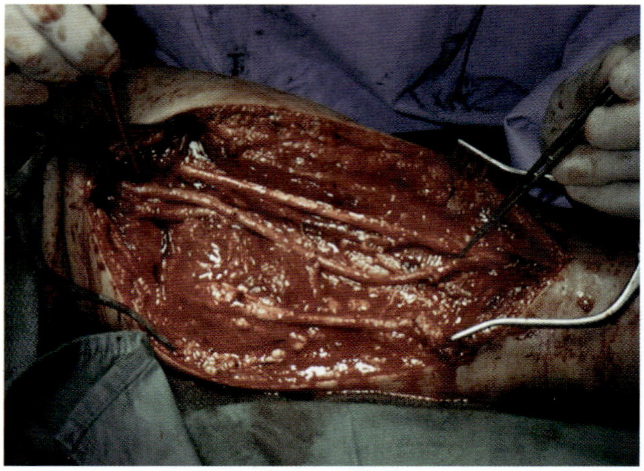

图6　肱动脉枪伤后节段切除，用逆行自体大隐静脉移植物肱肱旁路术。Gerald 镊指向近端和远端吻合口

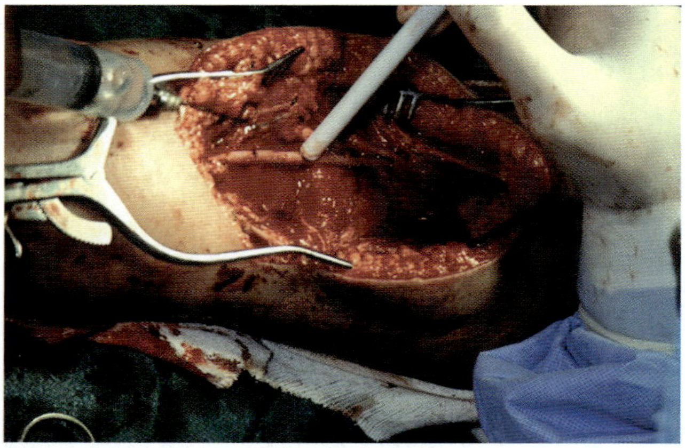

图7　修复后经常用多普勒探头评估三相血流信号和血流速度

如果最初没有实施筋膜切开术的话，往往有高达30%的病例需要（图12-15）。术中失血、动脉和静脉合并伤、开放性骨折是发生筋膜室综合征的独立危险因素（表3）。

预后和死亡率

早先的军人手术的主要技术包括结扎和随后的截肢。大多数患者在今天可以有更好的结果，如果他们的伤害不涉及大量组织破坏，可以及时修复。大系列研究报告肱动脉成功修复的一期通畅率为92%～98%。

Kim报告有7.2%的患者术中诊断为修复失败，Padayachy报告术后即刻诊断为修复失败者有4.4%。

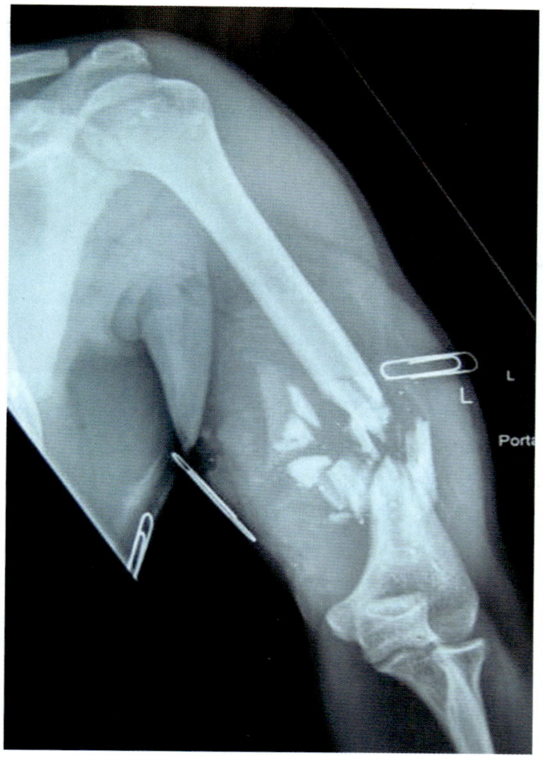

图 8　15 岁男性左上肢枪伤导致复杂的肱骨骨折和相关的肱动脉损伤

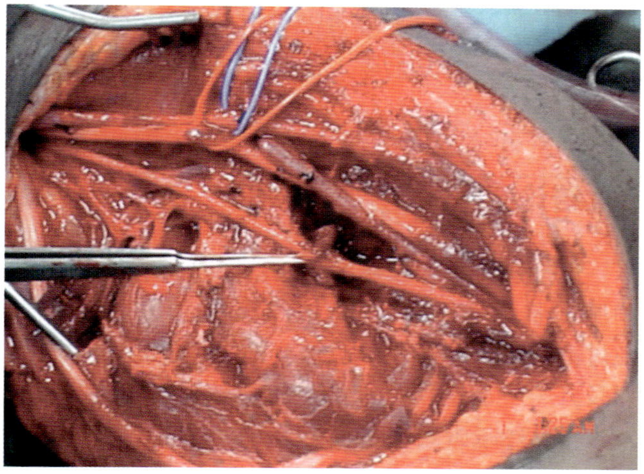

图 9　枪伤后血栓形成的左侧肱动脉节段。Jerrel 镊子指出这个非常小的血管的血栓节段。红色血管环牵拉左上的左正中神经

Klocker 和 Kim 报告有术后几天诊断为修复失败的病例。超过 10% 的战争相关损伤需要二次手术。移植物替代、血栓切除、筋膜切开、动脉结扎和罕见的截肢是这种情况下的手术选项。这类损伤的致死率很少，通常和即刻或后期损伤相关并发症有关。

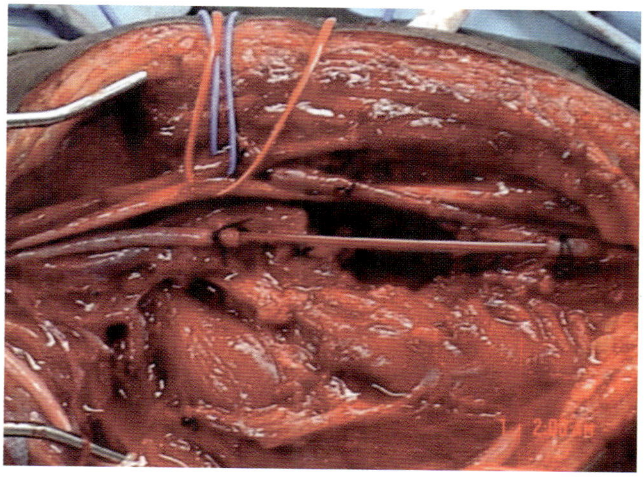

图 10　血栓形成的左肱动脉节段性切除。患者有明显的血管痉挛。在植入 8 号 Argyle 转流管以维持血流前，须用动脉内罂粟碱和使用 3.5 冠脉探针，以在确切性血管修复前切开复位和内固定

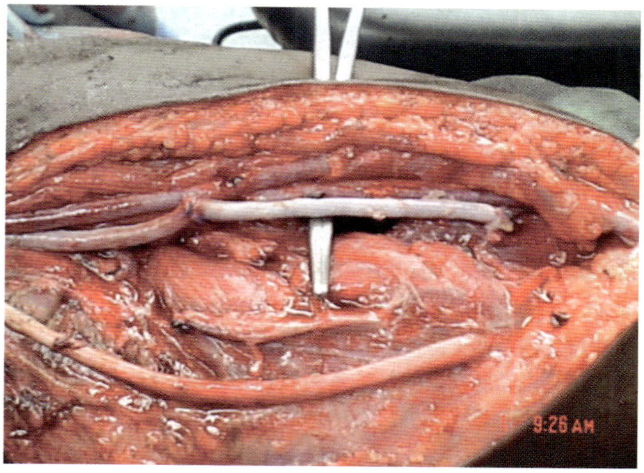

图 11　逆行自体大隐静脉移植物确切性血管修复。血管相当小，须 6-0 聚丙烯线用 Carrel 间断三点单层缝合修复，注意近端和远端鱼嘴样切口吻合以增大管腔。钳子通过整个伤口，图下缘可见正中神经

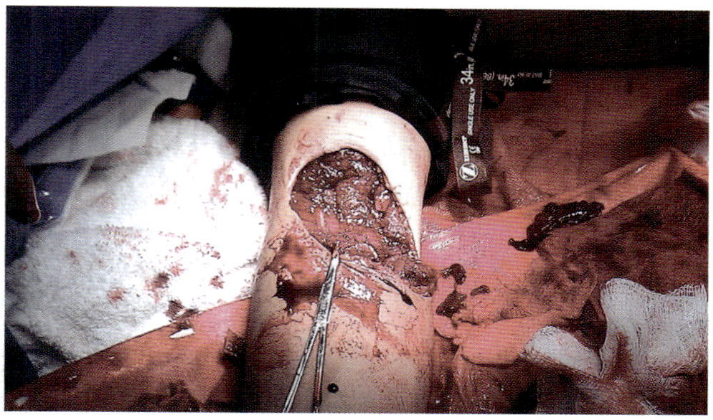

图 12　28 岁男性用碎玻璃自伤导致肱动脉横断伤。用止血带防止致命性出血。钳夹横断的贵要静脉

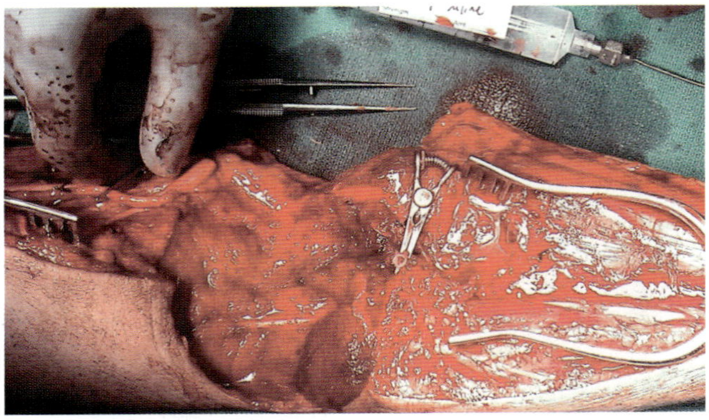

图 13 28 岁男性用碎玻璃自伤导致肱动脉横断伤。图示横断的肱动脉的近端和远端。远侧节段在分叉上方约 3 cm。用 Dietrich 哈巴狗钳控制血管。注意用肝素盐水冲洗

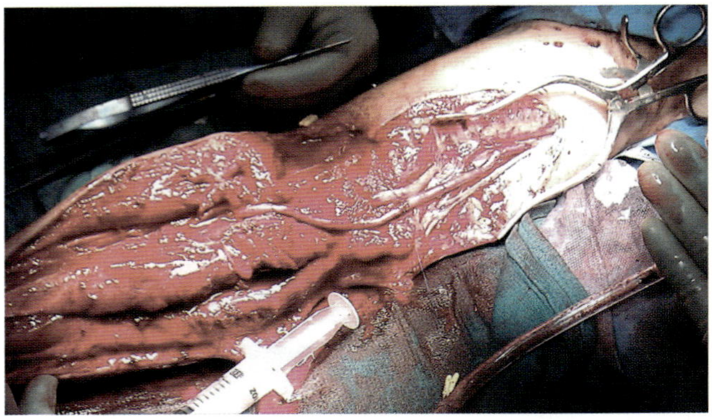

图 14 28 岁男性用碎玻璃自伤导致肱动脉横断伤。图示肱动脉用逆行自体大隐静脉移植物旁路修复，远侧延伸到分叉。患者还有桡动脉横断伤。注意用钛金 Castroviejo 镊和 6-0 聚丙烯线吻合。患者需要广泛的筋膜切开术和腕管松解术

并发症发生率

通常和动脉损伤相关的有神经损伤（62%）。按主要神经分层，正中神经为 79%，其次为尺神经

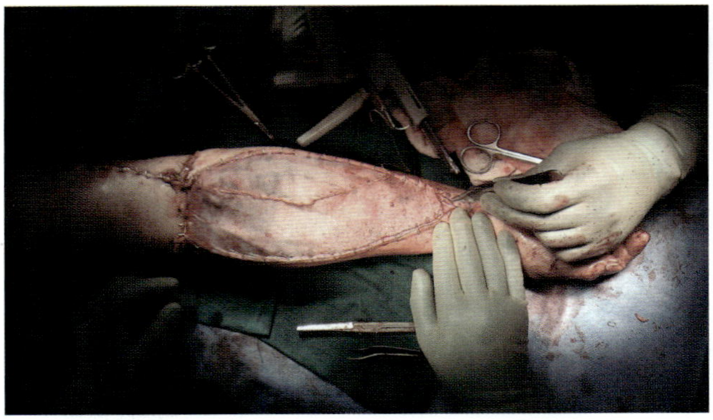

图 15 28 岁男性用碎玻璃自伤导致肱动脉横断伤。在用逆行自体大隐静脉移植物旁路修复肱动脉后，进行筋膜切开和用尸体皮肤覆盖，以期在损伤 5 天后用自体皮肤移植行确定性重建

（23%）、桡神经（12%）和肌皮神经（4%），多神经损伤略高于 10%。约 13% 的探查得不到损伤的证据，但不应被视为不必要或无指征。将患者送入手术室的标准必须低，以避免漏诊损伤。

即便做了成功的动脉修复，神经和骨损伤仍将损害患者上肢功能。大静脉损伤、骨折和广泛组织破坏也会影响肢体长期功能。一期和二期神经修复手术的有效性是争论要点。当上肢损伤包括神经损伤时功能丧失率为 27%～44%。

结论

肱动脉相关的发病率和死亡率取决于致伤原因、静脉或肌腱是否受损、肌肉骨骼和神经是否受损。在过去的 20 年，由于休克治疗的进步、抗生素应用，以及外科经验的增加，与上肢动脉损伤相关的截肢发生率已经减少到 3%。

表 3 用于治疗肱动脉损伤的外科技术：平民经验

作者（年份）	病例数	无修复	一期修复	大隐静脉间置	人工血管间置	结扎
联合系列（1984 — 1994）	223	5（2.2%）	121（54.2%）	87（39.0%）	0（0%）	3（1.3%）
Degiannis (1995)	37	0（0%）	13（35.1%）	24（64.8%）	0（0%）	0（0%）
Zellweger (2004)	124	0（0%）	47（21.1%）	74（59.7%）	2（1.6%）	2（1.6%）
Ergunes (2006)	58	0（0%）	40（70%）	18（30%）	0（0%）	0(0%）
Kim (2009)	139	0（0%）	46（33.1%）	82（60.0%）	8（57.6%）	1（0.7%）

髂血管损伤：困难的损伤和困难的问题处理

Juan A. Asensio, Patrizio Petrone, Alejandro Perez-Alonso,Richard Denney, Gerald Gracia, Michael Ksycki, Bradley S.Putty, James B. Sampson 和 Robert F. Wilson 著
张学民 译

髂血管损伤给所有创伤科医生带来了严重而令人沮丧的治疗困境。纵观平民和军事经验史，髂血管的损伤都是毁灭性的，因为它经常伴随着无法控制的出血和严重的伴随损伤。一般来说，患者表现为严重的继发于髂动、静脉严重出血或合并伤导致的严重出血的休克。相关的问题和伤害使治疗更为复杂，包括与小肠、大肠以及泌尿生殖道损伤有关的漏和污染。骨盆骨折在钝伤中常见，和髂内动脉和静脉及其分支的钝伤有关。即便经过努力实现近端和远端血管的控制，大部分患者会死于酸中毒、低血压、凝血异常和再灌注损伤的致命性影响。尽管 EMS 有很大进步、转运快速、创伤科医生进行了标准化培训和技术有所提高，髂血管损伤的并发症发生率和死亡率仍然很高，为 25%～40%。

历史展望

创伤外科领域的重大进展已经出现在军事和民用领域。已知最早的关于血管损伤的文献来自公元前 1600 年 Ebers 纸草，它报告了埃及人使用含有植物、硫酸铅和硫酸铜成分的药物止住出血。在公元前 1000 年，中国人首次使用加压包扎控制伤口出血，并结合使用止血药治疗出血。在整个中世纪，用沸油灼烫治疗血管损伤。1497 年，Brunswick 的 Jerome 发表结扎为枪伤出血的治疗手段的作品。Ambroise Paré 是第一个报告在截肢过程中使用结扎控制血管出血的。Paré 被认为发明了第一个止血剂，“le bec de corbin（乌鸦喙）”。血管重建的首次尝试是 Hallowell 在 1759 年报告用 Farrier 缝合法或兽医缝合法修补肱动脉。过了 127 年医生们才再次尝试血管修复。

在 19 世纪后期有这样的先驱者，如 Jassinowsky 和 Postemski 复兴了直接血管修复的想法。1883 年 Isreal 描述了首次成功地一期修复髂动脉裂伤。1897 年，芝加哥的 Murphy 首次成功地完成了股动脉端端吻合。1906 年，西班牙的 Goyanes 首次报告了使用自体静脉材料修补腘动脉。

巴尔干战争（1912–1913）期间出现了血管修复的尝试，Soubbotitch 报告了 77 例穿通伤造成的假性动脉瘤和动静脉瘘分别使用结扎治疗（45 例）、动脉修复（19 例）、静脉修复（13 例），还报告了 11 例动脉端端吻合及 4 例端端静脉吻合病例。在这个系列中有几例修复失败的报告，几乎全部手术都避免了感染。Carrel 1902 年报道的三重缝合和 Frouin1908 年用的四边形方法代表了血管吻合技术的进一步进展和改进。

在第一次世界大战期间德国外科医生尝试和成功地处理超过 100 个动脉损伤的多个血管，血管修复曙光初现。然而因高爆炸物引入一战的战场，冲突的方式将改变。一时间，创伤数量的增加加上疏散流程差，伴随高坏疽率，使德国军医的一开始的经验无法使用。同样地，那些成功治疗的患者随访不佳，导致许多人怀疑这些修复的长期通畅性。

尽管这些挫折存在，但仍有可喜的成果。Weglowski 呈献了他在俄罗斯军队服役及随后成为波兰军队总军医期间的一个包含 600 例患者的系列。在他的 1919 年报告中，他建议所有的动脉损伤和相关的创伤后动脉瘤在伤后立即修复，如果不行，1 个月后任何搏动性包块应修复。这包括所有的肢体损伤以及颈动脉、主动脉、锁骨下动脉和髂动脉损伤。1924 年他报告了 193 例血管修复的个人经验，包括侧壁修复 46 例，端端吻合 12 例，静脉移植 56 例。伤口感染迫使他为其余 79 例患者结扎。他的结果和数据很好，但不幸地被忽视了。

第二次世界大战期间，DeBakey 和 Simeone 报告的结果和第一次世界大战相比并不好。战时他们一共收集了 2 471 例动脉损伤。病例几乎全部选择结扎的方式，导致截肢率达 49%。81 例试图修复，其中 78 例需要侧壁缝合修复，只有 3 例做了端端吻合。作者总结他们的发现，声称结扎受损动脉是可行的，不须尝试其他的手术。“这不是一个选择的过程，这是一个为了根本的控制出血的目的的非常必要的步骤。”

尽管有这些发现，来自冲突双方的一些独立的尝试中有一些动脉修复的成功报告。这些不良结果的可能原因包括多种类型的高速武器造成的无法弥补的伤害；兵器的破坏力增大，导致伤亡人数较高；在运输中重大延误，造成不可逆的缺血；未能及时疏散到更高的外科中心和供应不足的战斗支援医院增加了结扎率和截肢率。

在朝鲜战争中可见动脉修复的巨大进步，这不仅基于外科技术在过去战争中的进步。其他因素包括麻醉改进、抗生素的出现和输血技术的发展，这些使血管修复的成功率提高。也许最重要的因素是伴随着直升机伤员迅速撤离的救护站的发展。由于接受和应用坏死组织清创、延期缝合和抗生素应用，伤口感染已经不那么猖獗了。1952 年，美国陆军成立专门研究小组，以改进血管损伤的治疗。1953 年，Jahnke 有显著发现，紧接着 Hughes 在 1955 年和 1958 有发现。在朝鲜战争中 Hughes 报告 304 例动脉损伤系列，其中 269 例修复，35 例结扎。总截肢率从第二次世界大战的 49% 显著减少到 13%。

在越南战争期间疏散和转运的进步，以及更多的受过训练的医生进行血管修复使预后得以改善。在 Walter Reed 军医中心的越南战争血管注册研究提供了有血管损伤的前 500 例患者的 718 个血管损伤，包括颈、锁骨下、腋、肱、主动脉、肾、髂、股和腘血管的更好的随访结果。Rich 在 1969 年报告越战期间的截肢率大约为 8%。这一数字随后被 Rich 和 Hughes 的 13% 证实，后者包括了在伤后第一个月做的截肢。在最初的报告中记录了 126 例端端吻合、127 例静脉移植、29 例侧壁缝合和 2 例人造血管移植。该注册研究又经过几次扩充了，包括了许多由其他军队治疗的患者，成为血管外科发展的宝贵的资源。

发病率

DeBakey 和 Simeone 报告了一共 2 471 例患者中的 43 例髂动脉损伤，发病率为 1.7%。髂动脉损伤率在朝鲜战争和越南战争中是相似的。1958 年 Hughes 报告朝鲜战争中髂动脉损伤的发病率为 2.3%，1970 年 Rich 报告其在越南战争中发病率为 2.6%。相当有趣的是，在许多不同的学院在过去几十年里报告髂血管损伤经验中，无论是发病率、并发症率和死亡率都非常相似（表 1 和 2）。

在城市创伤中心，平民髂血管损伤发生率由于暴力增加而增多。总体而言，髂血管损伤发生率中将近 10% 因穿通伤或枪伤引起，刺伤和刺穿占 2%。最不常见的是钝伤，在 Asensio 的包含 185 例髂血管损伤的系列中占 5%。髂内血管最常因钝伤受损；损伤的机制导致血管从骨性骨盆上牵扯，使内膜损伤和血栓形成。

髂血管损伤在大型军事冲突中的发生率是一样的。DeBakey 报告第二次世界大战中髂血管损伤的发生率为 1.7%，Hughes 报告朝鲜战争中为 2.3%，Rich 报告越南战争中为 2.6%。

解剖

后腹膜分为 3 个解剖区域。Ⅰ区是中后腹膜，从膈向下到腔静脉和主动脉分叉。Ⅱ区包括后腹膜的侧面和上方。Ⅲ区包括下后腹膜的正中和侧面与骨盆。腹主动脉在第 4 椎体左侧分为 2 个髂总动脉。每个大概 5 cm 长。它们从主动脉末端分开向下外侧走行，在最后的腰椎和骶骨之间的椎间盘层面分成 2 条分支，髂外动脉和髂内动脉。前者供应下肢，后者供应脏器和盆壁。

右髂总动脉比左侧长些，走行更斜、跨过最后 1 个腰椎椎体。在其前面是腹膜、小肠、交感神经分支，其分叉点是输尿管。后面，它和第 4 和第 5 椎体和中间纤维软骨分开，是 2 个髂总静脉的终点和下腔静脉的交汇点。外侧其解剖学关系有：上方为下腔静脉和右侧髂总静脉；下方为腰大肌，内侧上方是左髂总静脉。

左侧髂总动脉在前方与腹膜、小肠、交感神经分支和痔上动脉相邻，在其分叉点被输尿管跨越。它在第 4 和第 5 椎体和中间纤维软骨上。左髂总静脉部分位于动脉内侧，部分位于动脉后方。在外侧，动脉和腰大肌相邻。

髂总动脉分出小支到腹膜、腰大肌、输尿管和周围疏松组织，偶尔分出髂腰动脉或副动脉、肾动脉。起始点因主动脉分叉而不同。在 3/4 的病例中，主动脉分叉在第 4 腰椎上，或其与第 5 腰椎之间的纤维软骨上。1/9 的病例分叉点低于此点，1/11 的病例高于此点。大约 80% 的病例，主动脉分叉在髂骨嵴水平上下 1.25 cm，更多见的比上述位置低。

分叉点有很多变异。1 个大宗病例报告中，2/3 的病例的分叉点在最后一个腰椎和骶骨上缘之间，

表 1　战时髂血管损伤发生率

冲突	作者	年份	总血管损伤	髂血管损伤	发生率（%）
第一次世界大战	Makins	1919	1 191（单纯动脉）	6	0.5
第二次世界大战	DeBakey 和 Simeone	1946	2 471（单纯动脉）	44	1.7
朝鲜战争	Hughes	1958	304（单纯动脉）	7	2.3
越南战争	Rich	1970	1 000（单纯动脉）	26	2.6
伊拉克战争	Clouse	2007	408（301 例动脉和 107 例静脉）	14	3.4
伊拉克 - 阿富汗战争	White	2011	1 570（动脉和静脉）	61	3.8

表 2　平民髂血管损伤发生率

作者	年	总血管损伤	髂血管损伤			
			动脉	静脉	总计	发生率
Mattox†	1989	5 760	232	289	521	9.0
Bongard†	1990	478				10 ~ 15
Asensio*	2000	504	60	52	112	23.4
Davis*	2001	489	72	100	172	35.2
Tyburski*	2001	731	118	104	222	30.4
Paul*	2010	167	24	32	56	33.5
Clouse†	2007	408	9	5	14	3.4
White†	2011	1 570	19	17	61（25 例合并损伤）	3.8

* 报告腹部血管损伤的系列

† 报告心脏血管损伤的系列

1/8 的病例在上面，1/6 的病例在下面。左髂总动脉分叉比右侧低。

两个髂总动脉的相对长度也有所不同。在 63 例病例中，右髂总动脉更长，在 52 例中左侧更长，在 53 例中两者等长。动脉长度不同，在 5/7 的病例中为 3.5 ~ 7.5 cm。剩下的患者中大约一半动脉更长，另一半更短。最小长度小于 1.25 cm，最大为 11 cm。在罕见病例，右髂总动脉不存在，髂外动脉和髂内动脉直接从主动脉起源。

髂总动脉的侧支循环包括髂内动脉的痔分支和肠系膜下的痔上分支吻合，对侧子宫动脉、卵巢动脉和膀胱动脉的吻合，骶骨外侧和骶正中动脉的吻合，腹壁下动脉与内乳动脉、下肋间动脉和腰动脉的吻合，旋髂深动脉和腰动脉的吻合，最后方的腰动脉和髂腰动脉的吻合，闭孔动脉的耻骨支，与对侧的血管、腹壁下动脉的吻合。

临床表现

腹部、盆腔和臀部损伤，无论是枪伤或刺伤或刺穿伤都可能有腹部血管损伤。腹膨隆、失血性休克或下肢脉搏减弱或消失是主要表现。有关损伤也提示潜在的髂血管损伤。大量血尿提示肾或膀胱损伤，髂血管就在损伤路线中。直肠检查鲜血或大量鲜血便提示结肠或直肠损伤，髂血管就在损伤的潜在区域附近。

髂血管钝伤常和骨盆骨折有关。不稳定的骨盆出现下肢脉搏减弱或消失强烈提示髂血管损伤。在可能骨盆钝伤患者出现休克必须评估是否存在腹腔内出血。持续的髂内血管或分支出血是钝性骨盆损伤持续性低血压和休克的常见原因。这些患者体检时要注意保护不稳定的骨盆，有可疑骨折和骶髂关节破坏者，应立即通过影像学检查证实。用骨盆黏合剂通过压塞和减慢血肿扩散的速度使骨盆容量暂时复位，会导致骨盆出血减少。这些患者，没有其他来源的腹腔内出血，应进行血管造影评估，可能的话栓塞出血血管。不考虑损伤机制，稳定和复苏必须要迅速，若立即考虑进行手术干预的必要性，会对预后有积极影响。

诊断

存在穿通性腹部损伤和疑似腹部血管损伤的患者，除复苏和立即转运至手术室（operatirg room，OR）探查外，无需其他干预措施。诊断检查和射线照片评估不应延误将不稳定患者转运至 OR。血流动力学稳定的穿通伤患者垂直侧位射线照片对判断路径和子弹的位置是有益的，可以预测髂血管损伤。

FAST 检查可以提示骨盆内和损伤路径一致的髂血管损伤。在血流动力学稳定的患者中，钝伤可能需要更进一步的胸部、骨盆和受累下肢的射线照片检查。与髂血管损伤相关的发现包括骶髂关节破坏、双侧耻骨上下支骨折（“蝶形骨折”）和耻骨联合分离大于 2.5 cm。

先前提到的这些影像学表现应及时使用血管造影和外固定。腹部和骨盆 CT 的动脉增强造影已成为在血流动力学稳定的患者的一个可行的诊断方法。这是最有利于骨盆骨折诊断的基准骨盆片。造影剂溢出证实动脉损伤区域和可能的出血，其后血管造影和栓塞可以提供确切性治疗，尽管其使用受限。钝伤导致的骨盆骨折受益于其诊断能力和血管造影栓塞，阻止了髂内动脉及其分支的外渗。对于处理内膜撕裂、阻断髂外动脉或髂总动脉、终止活动性出血，用球囊阻断填塞直到手术干预是有益的。

手术处理

在对疑似髂血管损伤的剖腹探查术前，应备血以便在手术室中使用，另外应考虑应与机构签订大量输血协议。此外，要尽一切可能维持患者体温正常。在切开前要给予广谱抗生素，患者在常规消毒下准备和铺单，范围从胸骨切迹到双侧腋和膝。如果有继发于穿通伤的Ⅲ区出血，一定要探查。

通过压迫实现出血血管的初始控制，继而实现近端和远端控制。这可以通过 2 种方法实现：直接剥离到血管或将 Toldt 结肠旁腹膜的无血管线横断，将降结肠和乙状结肠向左翻、升结肠向右翻。必须注意在跨越髂总动脉分叉和动脉下方髂静脉时，不要损伤输尿管。

近端和远端阻断的水平取决于损伤区域，接近或处于髂总动脉或分叉的损伤的近端控制可以通过阻断主动脉实现。远端控制可以通过沿动脉逐步剥离实现，如果累及远端动脉，需要腹股沟切口，切开腹股沟韧带以控制近侧股动脉或远端髂外动脉。血管钳和代替的血管带可以用来阻断血流。近端和远端血管控制的一种替代方法包括用大口径 Fogarty 导管、小 Foley 导管或主动脉阻塞球囊。这一般不可行，因为大多数的髂血管损伤患者到达医院已休克，且多数其他相关损伤需要迅速控制。同样，绝大多数美国最繁忙的创伤中心缺乏混合手术室。

髂总动脉和髂外动脉撕裂伤或部分横断伤可用 4-0 或 5-0 聚丙烯线间断或连续缝合。无论选择哪个方法要注意避免将动脉缝窄。Fogarty 导管应大小适当，用以清除远端和近端动脉的潜在血栓，应在修复或吻合完成之前进行。任何损伤、破坏或失活组织都要清创，即使这使得一期修复不再是一个可行的选择。适当清创后只要有恰当长度可以做无张力修复就可以选择端端吻合。对半周损伤可以选择性使用聚四氟乙烯或静脉修复。再次，必须注意补片大小合适，不要使动脉狭窄或导致动脉瘤扩张。

当有明显的血管破坏和一期端端吻合不适合为间置移植物的指征。PTFE 是血管移植物的极佳选择，可以提供各种尺寸的移植物，且在感染方面有一定的抵抗力。大隐静脉很少有足够的尺寸，而且剥离静脉移植物对低血压患者太费时间，因此不推荐。

解剖外旁路包括腋股旁路，对可能有结肠损伤相关的大范围污染的患者是个有用的选择。文献中已描述几种形式的髂内动脉间置旁路，但都是耗时和技术困难的，特别是对于有低血压酸中毒和凝血功能障碍的患者。对于这些患者和多发伤患者，应尽早实施损伤控制。血管转流应及早使用。临时的 Argyle 血管转流管、儿童胸管和鼻胃管可提供临时的救命方法，可以置于动脉和静脉内。当面临缺血时间长或转流实现损伤控制的情况下，明智的做法是对大腿、小腿做筋膜切开。

对污染区域的 PTFE 旁路术和解剖外路径旁路术始终存在争议。Burch 对 233 例髂动脉穿通性损伤进行了回顾，一些损伤和胃肠道和尿道损伤有关。他指出污染的存在并不会影响移植物修复的手术决定或预后。然而，污染严重、解剖外旁路或更复杂的髂动脉转位应予考虑。这在面对多发伤和失血性休克时变得更加复杂。同样，找到合适大小的自体静脉对于这种大小的血管几乎是不可能的。

钝性动脉损伤与钝性创伤时骨盆带和脊柱之间的髂血管压迫有关。机动车碰撞和钝性力量直接作用在骨盆带上是常见原因。结果导致内膜损伤和血栓形成。手术需要损伤段切除和清创。随即用间置移植物（通常是 PTFE）修复。

静脉损伤的修复依赖几个因素，如损伤的部位、显露和静脉中断的大小和患者的稳定性。最好的结果是用 4-0 或 5-0 聚丙烯线直接缝合，小心不要造成管腔狭窄和限制。较少情况下可尝试获取一段大隐静脉用作补片，以 4-0 或 5-0 聚丙烯线缝合。如果血管损伤严重、一期修复不可能，结扎也可以，因为静脉损伤使用 PTFE 通畅率差。几个比较费时和技术难度大的方法包括颈静脉间置和大隐静脉板移植，据说有报道，但不推荐。另外，在多发伤不稳定的患者中，结扎可能是救命的选择（表 3，图 1-12）。

虽然可用生物补片如牛心包或其他抗生素浸泡移植物，有经验的创伤外科医生如 Asensio、Burch、Mattox、Bongard 和 Feliciano 在各自的研究中不推荐。Asensio 和 Burch 报告了全世界最大的系列。类似地，Mattox、Bongard 和 Feliciano 报告 PTFE 对感染有抵抗力。

腔内治疗的选择非常有限，就如 Asensio 的研

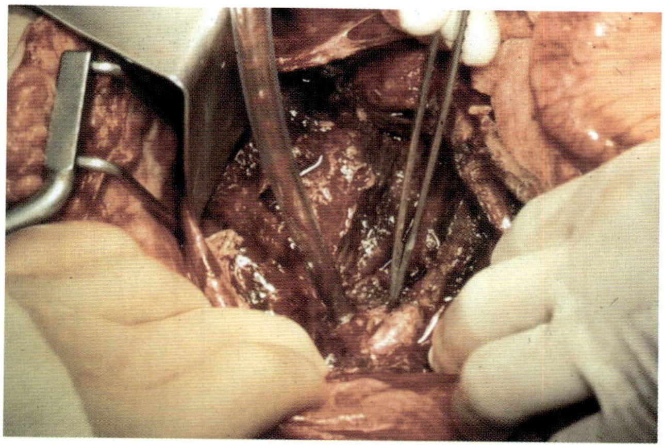

图 1　37 岁男性骨盆枪伤。他有右髂总动脉横断伤和右髂总静脉血栓形成。镊子提着横断的右髂总静脉随后结扎

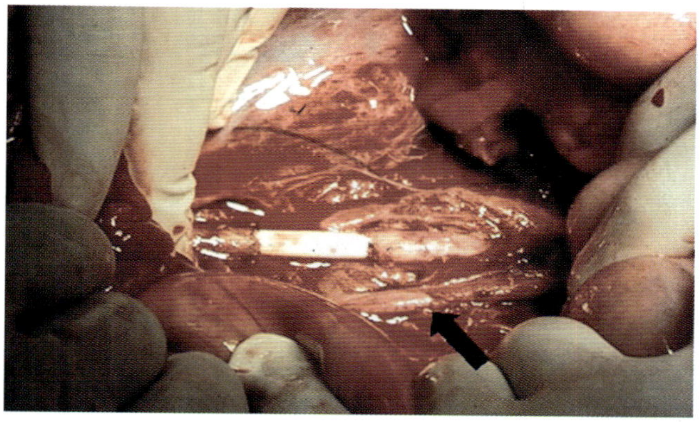

图 2　8 mmPTFE 聚四乙烯移植物端端吻合替代受损的右髂总动脉。注意右输尿管（箭头）

表 3　髂血管损伤的处理

作者		髂血管损伤总数	手术技术：动脉缝合	结扎	结扎和 EAB	端端吻合	PTFE	其他	无
Wilson (1990)	动脉								
	静脉	49	18(36.7%)	31(63.3%)					
Cushman (1997)	动脉	36	7(19.4%)	12(33.3%)	1(2.8%)	7(19.4%)	3(8.3%)	2(5.6%)	5(13.9%)
	静脉	56	17(30.3%)	33(58.9%)					5(8.9%)
Davis (2001)	动脉	72	29(40.3%)	25(34.7%)				10(13.9%)	8(11.1%)
	静脉	100	35(35%)	59(59%)					6(6%)
Asensio (2003)	动脉	72	57(79.2%)	1(1.4%)			14(19.4%)		
	静脉	113	12(10.6%)	101(89.4%)					
Haan (2003)	动脉	48	17(35.4%)	17(35.4%)	10(20.9%)			4(8.3%)	
	静脉	49	19(38.8%)	27(55.1%)				3(6.1%)	
Clouse (2007)	动脉	9	2(22.2%)	1(11.2%)			2(22.2%)	4(44.4%)	
	静脉	5	3(60%)					2(40%)	

EAB，解剖外路径旁路；PTFE，聚四氟乙烯

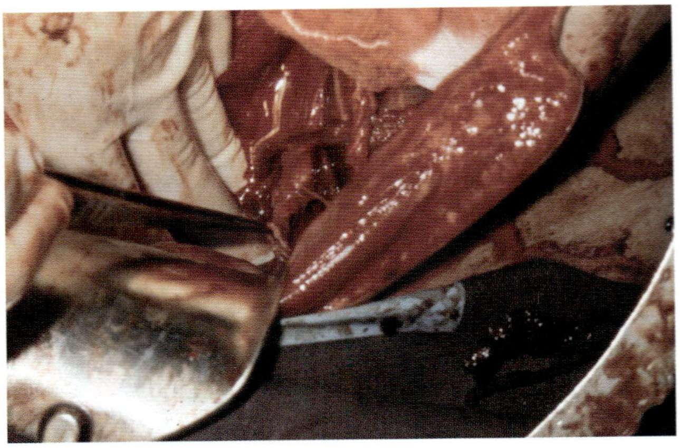

图 3　27 岁男性经骨盆的枪伤，入院时已休克。有左髂外动脉损伤，为控制出血已结扎。同时有乙状结肠的破坏性损伤、大量粪便污染和相关膀胱损伤尿液外渗。镊子提着结扎的左髂外动脉近端

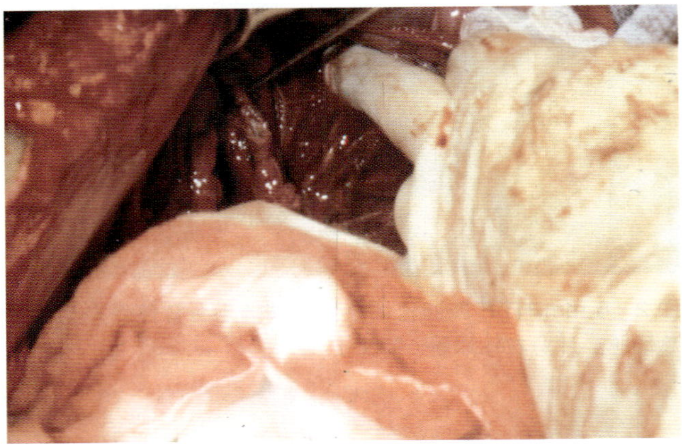

图 4　结扎左髂外动脉远端，它即将延续为股动脉

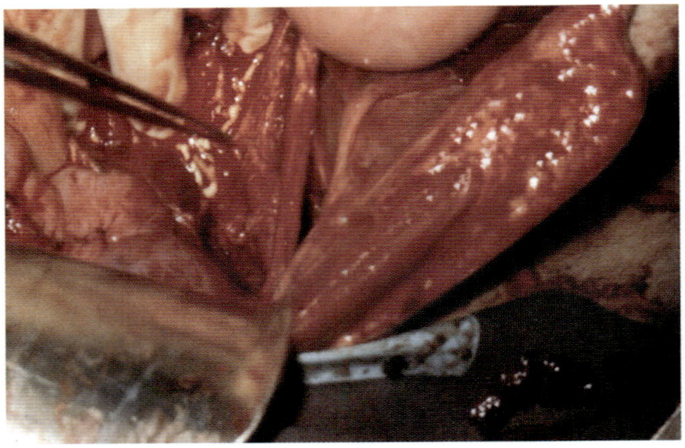

图 5　保留左输尿管

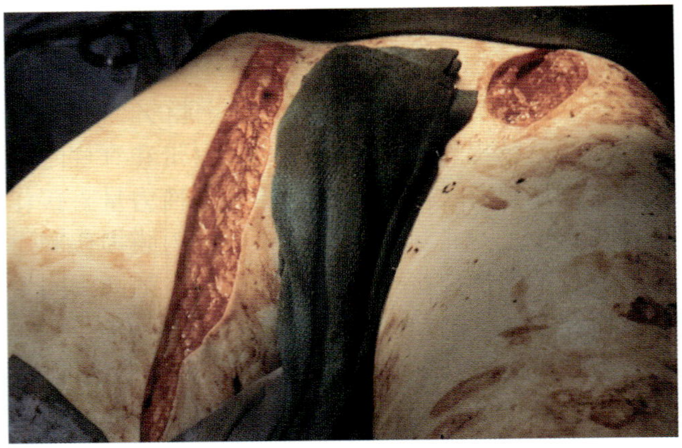

图 6　左腹股沟切口，左腹股沟韧带下方做隧道，用逆行大隐静脉从远端髂外动脉到近端股总动脉间置进行动脉重建。右腹股沟切口取大隐静脉。以资深作者对血管损伤的丰富治疗经验来说，这是唯一一个有足够大小的、合适的、用于间置移植物的大隐静脉的患者

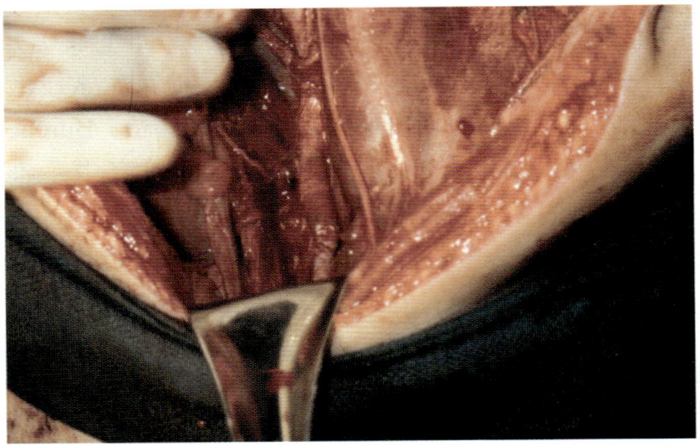

图 7　近端吻合口在远端左髂外动脉进入左腹股沟管前。注意髂腹股沟神经

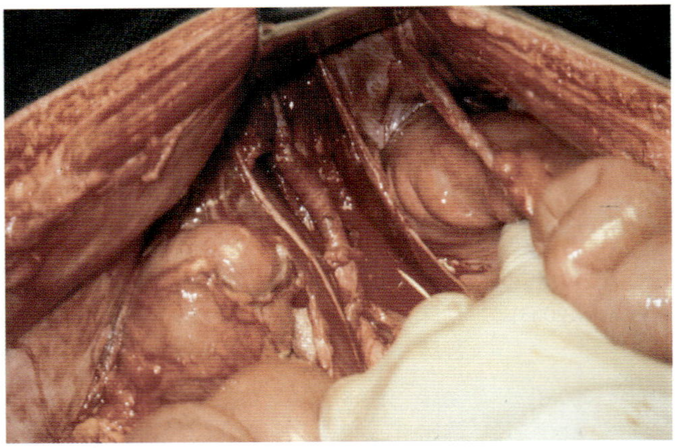

图 8　一个不同的视图显示移植物经过左腹股沟管。注意髂腹股沟神经

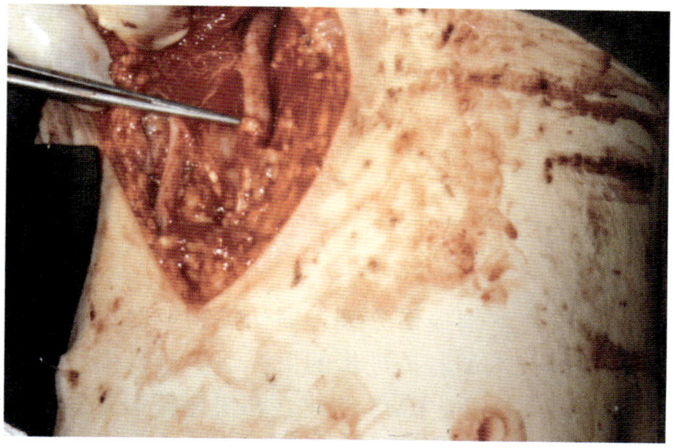

图 9 远端吻合口在股总动脉近端

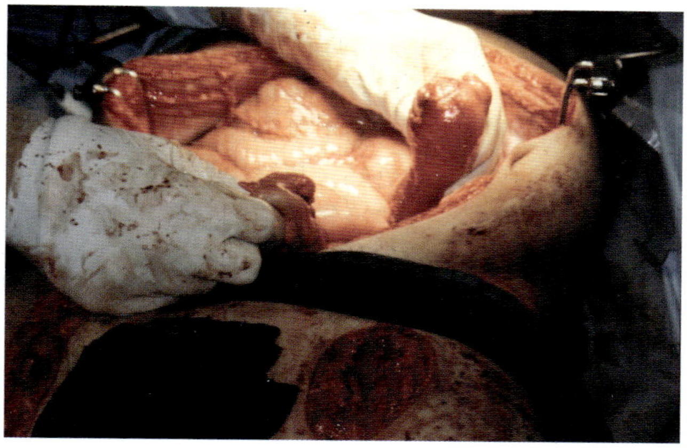

图 10 在破坏性损伤后乙状结肠部分切除。远端乙状结肠留在 Hartmann 袋，近端结肠左侧末端造口

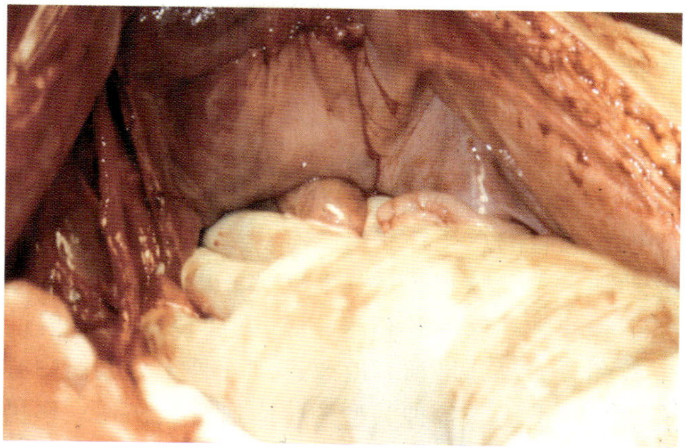

图 11 膀胱一期修复

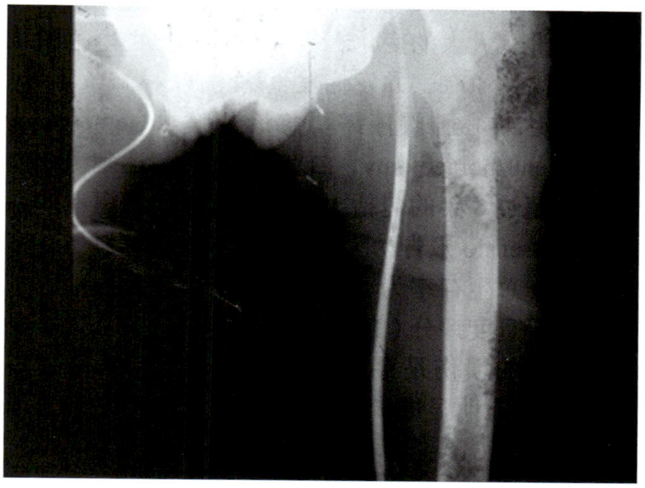

图 12 术后血管造影和在股总动脉水平的远侧吻合口

究中提到，绝大多数的患者可能是穿通伤，到院时已休克、血流动力学不稳定，不能转运去血管造影室。弹簧圈栓塞不适合，因为这种尺寸的血管，若没有缺血的影响是很难完全栓塞的。髂动脉钝伤非常罕见，会导致立即缺血、血栓明显延伸，由此排除了支架移植物的使用。但在 Asensio 的研究中也有支持性证据的描述，他报告了 8 例钝性髂动脉损伤，全都须间置移植物。虽然这是 185 例髂血管损伤中的 8 例患者，但就我们所知，这是髂血管钝伤的最大宗文献报告。大多数其他系列报告只有 1 ~ 2 例。

抗凝治疗对高流速、大直径血管不推荐，所以髂血管修复不推荐抗凝治疗。当动脉损伤邻近的静脉结扎，要考虑肢体筋膜切开以避免术后筋膜室综合征。

并发症发生率和死亡率

1997 年，Carrillo 等评估了他们学院髂血管损伤的结果，发现死亡率为 23%，和文献报告一致。一些关键点包括损伤控制和稳定后解剖外旁路维持下肢存活、静脉结扎后为保留肢体行筋膜切开和预防深静脉血栓（deep venous thrombosis，DVT），以及在面临肠道污染情况下使用 PTFE 人工血管。Haan 的学院的经验报告，单一血管损伤旁路术的死亡率为 25%，2 条血管都损伤的旁路术的死亡率为 83%。他们得出结论，休克对死亡率是明显的预后因素。

Lee 和 Bongard 报告他们中心的患者占腹部血管损伤患者的 10% 和全部血管损伤患者的 2%，髂血管损伤死亡率为 24% ~ 40%。Paul 等 2010 年评估他们之前腹部血管损伤的工作，并将结果同最近的经验相比。他们最早的系列是在 1970 — 1981 年间，包括 112 例腹部血管损伤的患者，其中有 17 例髂动脉损伤和 14 例髂静脉损伤，总死亡率是 32%。相比之下，他们的 1996 年 1 月至 2007 年 6 月的 242 例包含 24 例髂动脉损伤和 32 例髂静脉损伤的腹部血管损伤患者的总死亡率为 28%。最常损伤的动脉是髂动脉、主动脉和肠系膜上动脉，最常损伤的静脉是下腔静脉、髂静脉和门静脉。他们发现尽管院前急救和急诊复苏培训有所改进，并且 I 级创伤中心有更好的员工，各种类型的腹内血管损伤死亡率仍没有真正改善。

尽管在血管修复、损伤控制、重症监护的改进方面取得了进步，这些年髂血管并发症发生率和死亡率还没有太大的变化。最常引用的死亡率范围从 24% 到高达 40%，并发症发生率为 8% ~ 15% 不等。患者到达时心肺骤停需要急诊开胸术（emergency department thoracotomy，EDT），死亡率达到 100%。在一个超过 8 年的包括 185 例髂血管损伤患者的系列中，Asensio 报告动脉生存率为 57%，静脉生存率为 55%，总生存率为 51%。在这个研究系列中，平均损伤严重度评分（Inyury Severity Score，ISS）是 20，95% 的损伤是穿通伤，5% 是钝伤。Paul 发现尽管 EMS 有明显进步，I 级创伤中心的好的职工增加，但腹部血管损伤的并发症发生率和死亡率仍然超过 28%，髂动脉损伤的死亡率为 28%，髂静脉为 22%（表 4）。

结论

即使在解剖损伤分级、损伤控制上取得巨大进步，外科技术和监护进步的情况下髂血管损伤仍是一个艰巨的任务。EMS 的建立和快速转运并没有显著改变髂血管损伤的整体发病率和死亡率。血管移植物和手术设备的进步使修复这些损伤更容易和更快，而这些患者的迅速恶化和大量的相关损伤导致了大多数腹部血管损伤的损伤控制措施结合使用。在过去几十年，建立拥有受过训练的创伤外科医生和装备齐全的工作人员的 I 级创伤中心在血管急诊治疗中并没有表现得更好。和过去一样，髂血管损伤的高度怀疑和快速转运、迅速的外科出血污染控制仍然是治疗的支柱。当损伤控制启动，转流血管应伴随相关下肢的筋膜切开和恰当的 DVT 预防。尽管有在治疗方面和恰当的管理策略方面的各种进步，髂血管损伤的并发症发生率和死亡率还是很高，其治疗对当代创伤外科医生也提出了复杂的挑战。

表 4　髂动脉和髂静脉损伤的生存数据

		髂动脉			髂静脉		
作者	年份	患者数	生存数	生存率（%）	患者数	生存数	生存率（%）
Millikan	1981	19（6）*	9（5）*	47.4（83.3）*	16 (8)†	11 (8)†	68.8 (100.0)†
Ryan	1982	66 (17)*	41 (15)*	62.1 (88.2)*	97 (48)†	71 (45)†	73.2 (93.8)†
Sirinek	1983	21	15	71.4	28	23	82.1
Burch	1990	130（34）	80（26）*	61.5 (76.5)*	214 (81)†	153 (70)†	71.5 (86.4)†
Wilson	1990				49	24	48.9
Davis	2001	55	35	63.6	76	58	76.3
Tybusrki	2001	70	37	52.9	73	40	54.8
Asensio	2001				37 (22)†	23 (18)†	62.2 (81.8)†
Jasmeet	2009	39	11	71.8	36	8	77.8
White	2011	19			17		
总计		361 (57)*	217 (46)*	60.1 (80.7)*	590 (159)†	403 (141)†	68.3 (88.7)†

* 孤立髂动脉损伤

† 孤立髂静脉损伤

股血管损伤：高死亡率和低并发症发生率的损伤

Juan A. Asensio, Patrizio Petrone, Alejandro Perez-Alonso, Kulsoom Laeeq, Abhishek Sundaram, Mamoun Nabri, Brandon Propper 和 William G. Cioffi 著
张学民 译

股血管损伤在繁忙的创伤中心是最常见的血管损伤。暴力的演变和来自城市街道的城市战场的穿通性创伤的增加提高了股血管的损伤的发生率，它约占所有周围血管损伤的 70%。尽管这些损伤的死亡率相对较低，修复手术操作却需要较高的技术复杂性。因此，它们引起的死亡率低，但有高的并发症发生率。及时诊断和治疗是达到良好预后的关键，主要目标是管控缺血时间、恢复肢体灌注、完成保肢和尽快康复。

解剖

股动脉是髂外动脉的直接延续，在股三角中、腹股沟韧带后方。股动脉的近端部分叫股总动脉，在缝匠肌深部走行，在一个纤维鞘内股静脉与之伴行。股鞘包括 3 个部分：外侧部分内有股动脉，中间有股静脉，最内侧部分是股管。在一个短的节段后，股动脉在大腿内侧髂前上棘和耻骨结节连线中点的皮下可以触及，下行一小段分成股深动脉和股浅动脉。股深动脉向大腿肌肉深部穿行，是该区域的主要供血动脉。股浅动脉穿越几乎整个股骨长度，终于大收肌开口，就是 Hunter 管，在此成为腘动脉。股动脉主要分支是阴部动脉、腹壁浅动脉、旋髂动脉、大隐动脉和小隐动脉。

股静脉是腘静脉的直接延续。它和股动脉伴行，接受从股深静脉和大隐静脉回流的血液，后者在越过腹股沟韧带下方成为髂外静脉前，穿过股鞘的前方。

发病率

在军事背景下，创伤性股血管损伤约占所有血管损伤的 67%。最近，由于城市暴力的增加，平民股血管损伤的发生率增加。据报道穿通伤大约占 88%，通常继发于枪伤或由于刀或利器刺伤。钝伤不常见，占全部损伤的 12%。

在过去的一个世纪主要军事冲突中损伤的发生率有所不同，每个冲突中都略有增加。在第一次世界大战中，Makin（1919）经典教科书描述了英国医生报告的 31% 的发生率，而美国外科医生报告的股血管损伤率低至 22%。DeBakey 和 Simeone（1946）报告第二次世界大战中总共有 517 例股动脉损伤，发生率为 21%，截肢率却高达 53%。Hughes（1958）报告了朝鲜战争中略高的 31% 的股血管损伤发生率，Rich（1970）报告越南战争中 35% 的股血管损伤发生率。

历史视角与战争经验

最早的血管损伤记录在公元前 1600 年，Ebers-Papyrus 报道了埃及人已使用包含植物、硫酸铅和硫酸铜的物质控制出血。公元前 1000 年，中国首次使用加压包扎控制受影响的肢体出血，用止血药控制出血。

然而，在整个中世纪血管损伤治疗的选择主要是烧灼术。1497 年，Hieronymus Brunschwig，也被称为 Brunswick 的 Jerome，发表了他对继发于枪伤的血管损伤结扎治疗的工作。1552 年，Ambroise Paré 进一步革新了这项工作，促进了结扎控制出血的应用。Paré 还建议在分界线以上截肢以达到更好的预后，他还开发了第一个止血器，le bec de corbin（乌鸦嘴）。不过，Hallowell 是第一个尝试血管重建的人，他在 1759 年采用 Farrier 缝合法或兽医缝合法修复了一条肱动脉。

大约 127 年过去才重新有人尝试血管修复。19 世纪后半段的先驱 Jassinowsky 和 Postemski 促进了直接血管修复的理念。Isreal 在 1883 年描述首次成功一期修复髂动脉裂伤，1897 年来自芝加哥 Rush 医学院的 John B. Murphy 首次成功完成了股动脉端端吻合。随后 1906 年，西班牙的 Goyanes 首次用逆

行自体大隐静脉移植物修复腘动脉瘤。尽管 19 世纪末有了这些进步，血管修复再度系统性使用还要过将近 30 年。

第一次世界大战

在第一次世界大战的第一部分，血管损伤限于低速射弹的使用；而在第二部分可见高爆火炮和改进的高速弹药导致的血管损伤。军械的破坏力的变化导致人员伤亡人数的大量增加和伤员疏散人数的减少。损伤和确切的手术治疗之间的时间急剧增加，血管修复变得不切实际。尽管即刻修复的机会失去了，但在延迟基础上对假性动脉瘤和 AV 的后期处理增多了。

在第一次世界大战期间医学对股血管损伤的修复做了有限的尝试。Makins 报告 1 202 例患者中有 366 例为股动脉损伤，占 31%。美国外科医生也报告了 344 例患者中有 78 例为股血管损伤，占 22%。

第二次世界大战

第一次世界大战和第二次世界大战之间的时间呈现出破坏性装置和外科干预的发展不平衡。尽管血管损伤的严重程度增加，但血管手术似乎又退步了。DeBakey 和 Simeone 报告了 2 471 例来自欧洲战场的动脉损伤。不幸的是，几乎所有患者都采用了结扎，导致非常高的 49% 的截肢率。在这个研究中，DeBakey 和 Simeone 报告只有 81 例患者尝试修复，其中 78 例患者侧壁缝合修复 / 动脉缝合，只有 3 例端端吻合。在报告的 2 471 例血管损伤中，517 例是股血管损伤，发生率为 21%。

如此低的血管修复数量的主要影响因素是转运的延误、军医缺乏血管创伤训练和抗生素的相对缺乏。虽然青霉素和磺胺已经出现，供应量仍十分有限。其他因素包括恰当的缝合材料和血管仪器的缺乏。有趣的是，第一个血管夹是 Victor Satinsky 在第二次世界大战期间创造的。

朝鲜战争

在朝鲜战争期间，血管外科的跨越式发展得益与几个因素。麻醉的进步、抗生素的出现和输血的发展极大地增加了血管修复的成功率。可能最大的单一因素是前线救护站的发展和伴随的直升机转运伤员的快速疏散。类似的，如 Hughes、Jahnke、Spencer 和 Howard 等外科医生表现出对血管损伤修复技术发展的兴趣。

来自这个时期的一些综述表明血管一期修复得到了广泛接受。Jahnke 和 Seeley 报告了 14 例股动脉损伤，发生率为 19%。Hughes 随后报道了 304 例患者中的 95 例股血管损伤，血管损伤占 31%。这些都是最早的报告非常详细的治疗血管创伤的处理方法的文献。

越南战争

越南战争在疏散和伤员快速转运和大量血管外科医生技术培训的基础上建立，这些改善了患者的预后，且在战争结束后，将对更多的患者进行长期随访。Norman Rich 医生创办的越南血管注册体系和基于 Walter Reed 医院的体系使长期随访和继续评估所有源自越南战争的血管损伤成为可能。来自 1969 年的具有里程碑意义的报告显示，总共 1 000 例患者中有 351 例股动脉损伤，发生率为 35%。不幸的是，这场冲突中股静脉损伤没有数据。在战时文献中，结扎是标准的处理方法。

伊拉克和阿富汗战争

过去十年的大部分时间里，伊拉克和阿富汗的战役都对战斗伤亡的总体生存有了显著的改善。生存率的增加可以归因于广泛使用人体装甲（能够显著降低躯干损伤）、广泛使用院前急救止血带，并采用损伤控制技术和快速疏散到 Landstuhl Regional 医学中心和进而到美国本土实施确定性手术。

在这两场冲突中，创伤的特点明显不同于以往的战争。作为躯体盔甲广泛推广的结果，躯干损伤明显降低，但头部损伤和远侧肢体血管损伤大大增加。这些损伤模式的改变导致了从正规战到镇压暴乱战斗的飞跃，涉及反人类技术和杀伤性设备如简易爆炸装置（improvised explosive devices，IEDs）的使用。在这些 IEDs 中，高能爆炸物的使用导致非常高的各种严重肢体损伤的发生率，在一些病例中，会导致多肢体截肢。也有大量病例有血管损伤。

从战争登记处收集的数据表明各种血管损伤的概率总体增加，占总战斗伤亡的 4% ~ 9%。如果只计算肢体血管损伤，似乎大多数损伤血管在下肢。报告中股动脉损伤占 7%，孤立性股静脉损伤 3%，股血管合并伤占7%。广泛应用的处理血管损伤的损伤控制原则包括早期使用暂时血管转流管恢复血流、广泛使用筋膜切开、外固定开放性骨折和快速转运至地区医疗中心，使大量肢体得以挽救（资深作者个人经验）（表1）。

损伤机制

穿通性损伤仍是大部分股血管损伤的最主要的原因。这一点经过Cargile的研究证实，他报告了88%的穿通伤发生率和12 %的钝伤发生率。在Feliciano的研究中，穿通伤发生率为81%。Martin报告，105例股动脉损伤中104例是穿通伤。在Asensio的研究中，86%的患者因穿通伤入院，而28例（14%）为钝伤。

平民的流行病学

在平民损伤的文献中对股血管的发生率有明确描述。Feliciano报告了220例下肢血管损伤，其中142例为股动脉损伤，发生率为65%。Martin报告了188例下肢损伤，105例为股动脉损伤，占56%。Cargile报告Parkland医院超过17年的经验，233例患者总共有321个股血管损伤。在文章中他报告了112例孤立股动脉损伤（48%）、36例孤立股静脉损伤（15%）和85例合并损伤（36%）。股静脉损伤在Martin的研究中不常见，105例股血管损伤中仅有3例股动脉损伤。

Asensio报告了10年的204例患者的研究，其中含298个血管损伤。全部血管损伤的26%在这期间在他的研究院治疗（表2）。

临床表现

有股血管损伤的患者的临床表现可能为严重的血流动力学不稳定和心肺骤停需要EDT主动脉十字钳夹对血流动力学稳定住院并伴有经典的继发于远侧血流减少和缺血的血管损伤硬体征或那些存在血管损伤软体征的患者进行阻断和心肺复苏。

表1　股血管损伤的军事经验

冲突	作者（年）	总损伤数	股血管	发病率（%）
第一次世界大战	Makins (1919)	1 191	366	30.5
第二次世界大战	DeBakey 和 Simeone (1946)	2 471	517	20.9
朝鲜战争	Hughes (1958)	304	95	31
越南战争	Rich (1970)	1 000	351	35
伊拉克战争	Michael (2007)	192（仅动脉）	41	21.3
伊拉克和阿富汗战争	Jasmeet (2011)	1 570	268	17

表2　下肢血管损伤中股血管损伤的概率

			股损伤			
作者	年份	总下肢损伤	动脉	静脉	总计	发病率（%）
Feliciano (24)	1988	352	142	93	235	66.7
Timberlake (26)	1990	322		116（36%）		
Bongard (20)	1990					
Martin (16)	1994	188	105	21	126	67
Clouse (14)	2007	220	74	37	111	50.4
Randall (29)	2010	76	32（42.1%）			
Jasmeet (18)	2011	94	44（46.9%）		44	

Cargile 报告 87 例（37%）患者表现股血管损伤和收缩压低于 90 mmHg，其中 35 例（40%）表现有深度的休克。

Degiannis 报告 19 例股血管损伤患者到院时有低血压，收缩压低于 90 mmHg。81 例低血压患者中 37 例（46%）有孤立性肢体损伤，4 例入院时心肺骤停需要 EDT。在 Asensio 的报告中，11 例（5%）患者到院时心肺骤停，需要 EDT，其中 3 例（27%）最终存活。

不太常见地，股动脉裂伤或横断伤会回缩和形成血栓，导致远端肢体缺血。相关肌肉和骨损伤常合并穿通性损伤，因此长骨骨折时应精心护理。穿通性损伤导致的大量组织破坏可能表现为急性出血，须尽快根据损伤部位直接压迫或止血带控制。然而，如果股总动脉或股浅动脉近端受累，止血带可能无法使用。在这种情况下，直接压迫损伤部位尽快进行近端和远端手术控制。

在钝性损伤中，依受累相关结构不同，表现为失血伴随缺血疼痛和感觉、运动丧失。钝伤出血罕见，但可以继发于相关的骨科损伤功能导致血管部分或全部裂伤或横断。

在 Cargile 的研究中，233 例患者中 90 例（40%）有血管损伤硬体征须立即外科干预。尽管这些患者中有硬体征者数量很多，106 例患者术前做了造影。Degiannis 等更依靠临床检查，发现他们的患者中 70% 有肢体缺血表现。

在 Asensio 的研究中，大多数患者有血管损伤硬体征，48% 有远侧缺血，43% 为无脉或短细脉，29% 有扩张性血肿。在这个研究中，仅可靠的临床检查发现股血管损伤可减少术前造影至 15%。很少有患者表现血管损伤软体征：周围神经功能缺损占 10%，近端损伤占 7%。

诊断

在穿通伤中需要的诊断性检查有限，但通常在钝伤有临床混淆的表现时可以明确诊断。股总动脉和股浅动脉分叉足够表浅，可以通过视诊和触诊诊断。伴有组织破坏和活动性出血的穿通伤不需要诊断性检查。对没有活动性出血的疑似钝伤或穿通伤，完整的临床检查是有益的。股动脉、腘动脉、胫后动脉或足背动脉临床检查的改变或各自的脉搏和感觉或运动检查的改变可以提示血管损伤。紧张、疼痛的筋膜室和相关的骨损伤提示进一步探查。最容易和首选诊断试验是 ABI 检查。这项检查是通过测量踝部收缩压，然后除以肱动脉收缩压。差值小于 0.9 认为是疑似血管损伤，建议行进一步影像学检查，如 CT 血管造影或股动脉血管造影（表 3）。

表 3　住院时血管损伤的硬体征和软体征

硬体征
远端缺血体征
减弱的脉搏消失
血肿扩大
触及震颤
搏动性出血
杂音
软体征
毛细血管充盈时间 >3 s
周围神经缺损
近端损伤
中度出血（有限的）

外科处理

在进入手术室前备血。要尽一切努力防止低体温。广谱抗生素在手术开始前输入。由于手术可能涉及，手术准备应包括下腹部、双侧腹股沟和双下肢备皮和铺单。

先通过直接压迫控制出血的血管，紧接着近端和远端控制血管，它可能通过直接沿着从腹股沟韧带向远端到损伤区域的走行从纵切口切断股总动脉完成。更近端的控制可以通过开腹探查控制髂外动脉钳夹盆腔内的血管或切开腹股沟韧带在切口下象限分离肌肉到腹膜后腔达到。通过这个路径，可以不进入腹腔控制血管。股深动脉通过显露股总动脉的同一切口显露。向近端和后外侧股浅动脉可见股深动脉起始部。

控制近端流入道后，沿解剖学路径仔细分离减少对动脉的次损伤和避免接近血管继发性出血。血管钳、Silastic 血管套带和以放大眼镜的形式获得视觉放大的效果以确切控制损伤血管。仔细解剖股血管至关重要，特别是股静脉，它更薄、易出血，容易有医源性损伤。为实现近端和远端控制，我们推荐对股动脉和静脉使用 30°，45° 或 60° 的 DeBakey

钳。如果股浅静脉很容易侧壁缝合，可以使用部分阻断的 Cooley 或 Satinsky 钳（图 1）。股深动脉应当用特殊的深血管钳阻断。Argyle 转流管随时备用以恢复股总动脉或股浅动脉灌注和辅助损伤控制（图 1-2）。

最初的修复

可以用 4-0 或 5-0 聚丙烯单线连续或间断缝合动脉侧壁。无论哪种方法，注意避免动脉狭窄。选择恰当大小的 Fogarty 导管清除远端和近端股动脉的潜在栓子。这应当在完成修复或吻合前做。损伤或失活段的血管必须清创，即使这使得一期修复不再是一个可行的选项。端端吻合在合适的清创后是个选项，只要有足够的长度使修复无张力即可（图 3-22）。

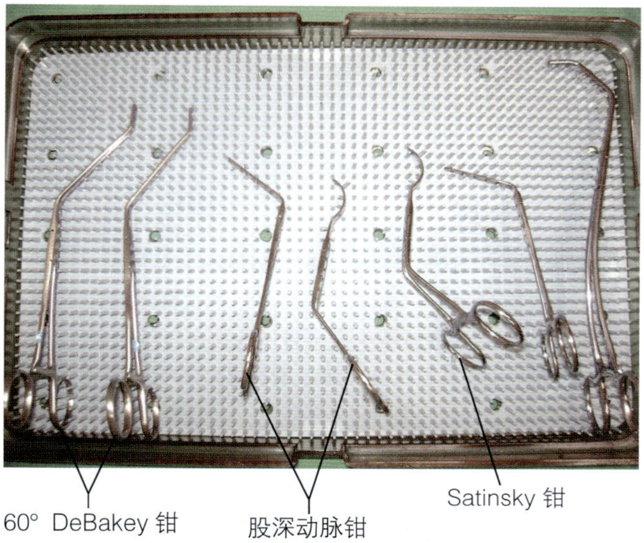

图 1　Asensio 教授的一个血管托盘。注意 60° 的 DeBakey 钳、股深动脉钳、Satinsky 钳

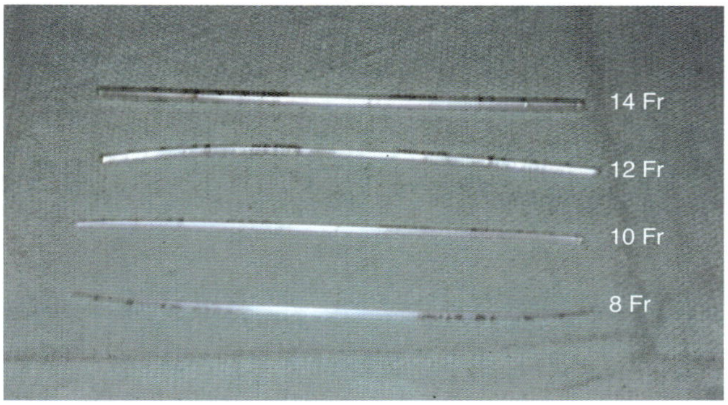

图 2　Argyle 转流管

移植物

当有明显的血管破坏和端端吻合不可能的时候一定要用间置移植物。聚四氟乙烯是个非常好的替代物选择，可以提供各种尺寸，在污染区域有不错

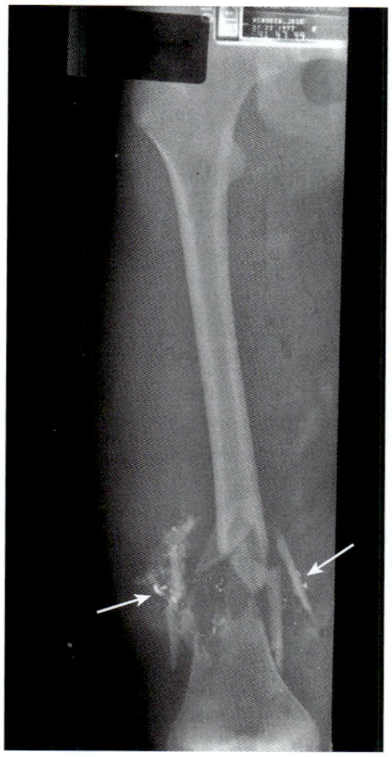

图 3　右股骨骨折相关远侧股动脉在 Hunter 管上方损伤的前后位片，注意伤口里的弹片（箭头）

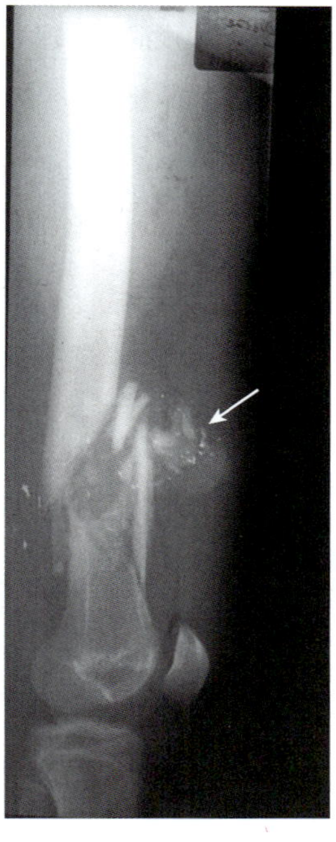

图 4　左股骨骨折相关股动脉和静脉损伤的侧位片，注意粉碎性的骨碎片经常扮演继发弹片的作用（箭头）

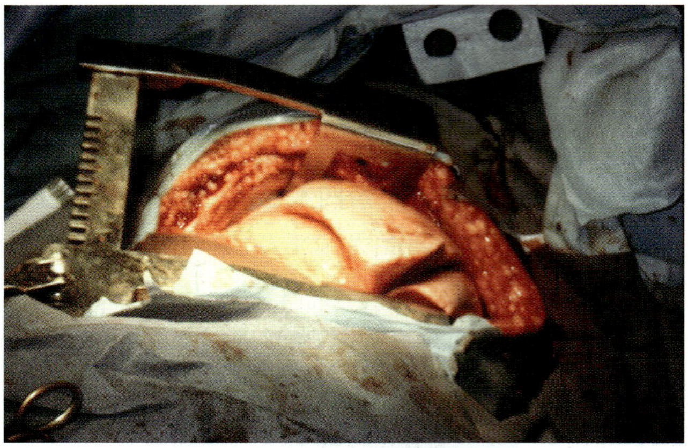

图 5　出血合并右股浅动脉和静脉枪伤的患者急诊室行复苏开胸术和主动脉十字钳断和开放心肺复苏

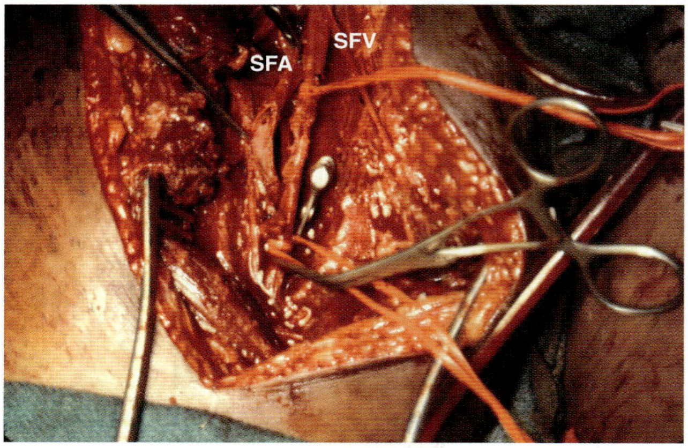

图 6　在急诊室成功开胸后患者转运手术室，用手指控制股血管，同时血管内输注晶体液、血液和血液制品，以更换内容物。图示右侧股浅动脉和股浅静脉的近端和远端控制

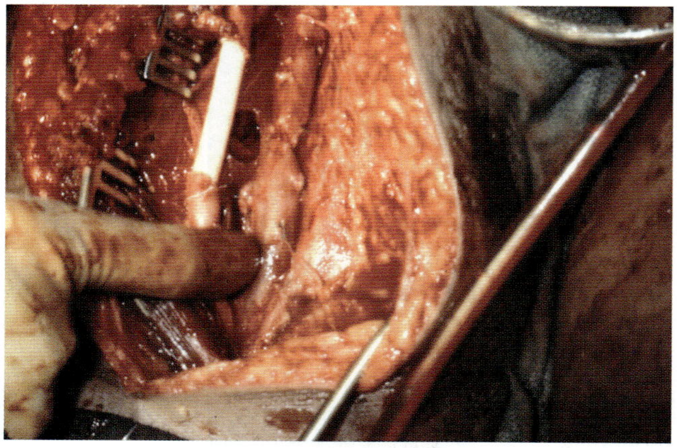

图 7　同一个患者用 8 mm 的聚四氟乙烯人工血管替代右股浅动脉和初步股浅静脉侧壁缝合。患者需要大腿和小腿四筋膜室筋膜切开，最初用尸体异种移植物覆盖，然后在术后第 5 天缝合

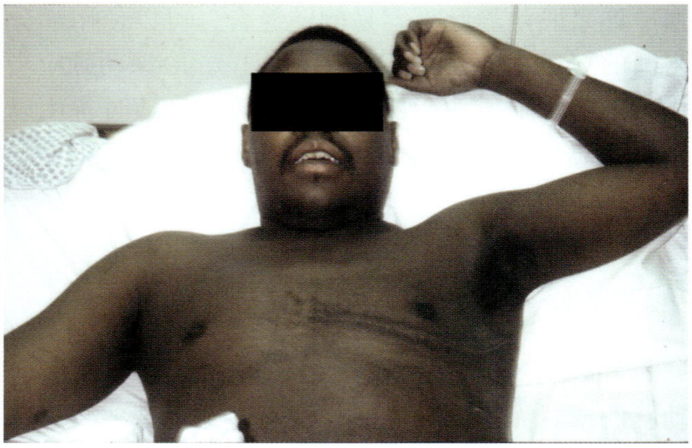

图 8　急诊室复苏开胸术后的患者

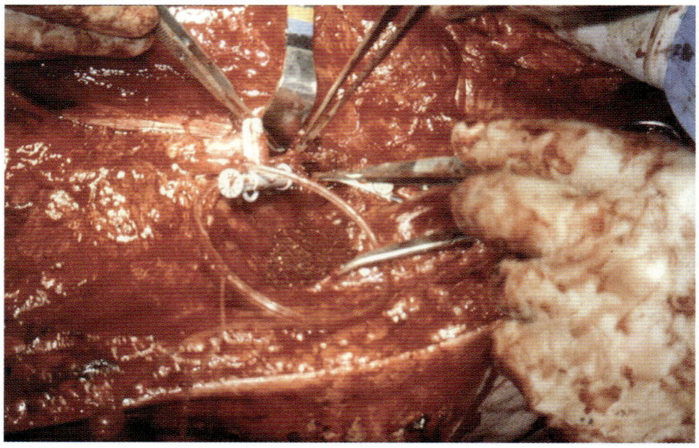

图 9　年轻男性继发于高速手枪子弹枪伤后的持续出血、右股浅动脉和右股浅静脉裂伤。患者迅速转运至手术室，用 10 号 Argyle 转流管迅速恢复血流。患者可疑右侧股骨粉碎性骨折

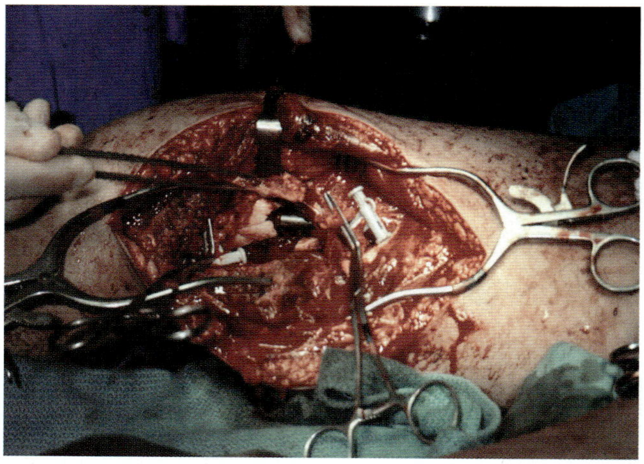

图 10　图 9 的同一个患者在移除转流管后，骨科医生对其实施开放减容和髓内针内固定。Fogarty 哈巴狗钳控制股浅静脉，用 45° 和 60°　DeBakey 钳控制股浅动脉

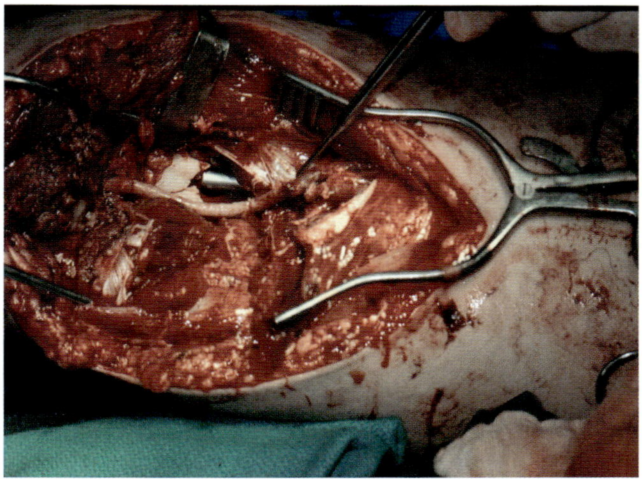

图 11　同一个患者（图 10）结扎股浅静脉后。患者用间置逆行自体大隐静脉移植物做股浅动脉端端吻合。注意股骨干桥接开放性股骨骨折

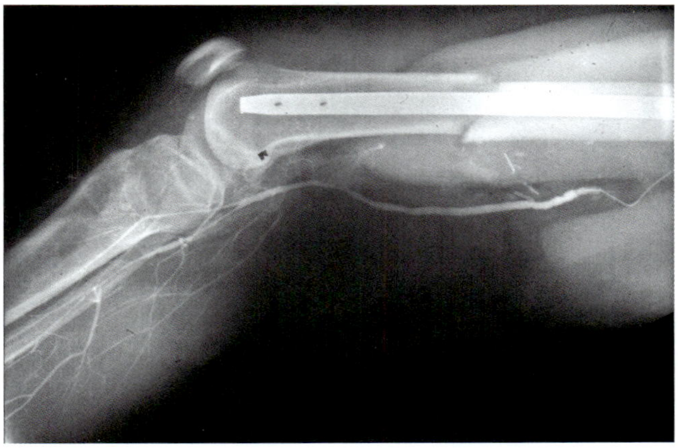

图 12　同一个患者（图 11）。术中动脉造影证实间置移植物通畅。注意股骨干远端没有锁定螺钉

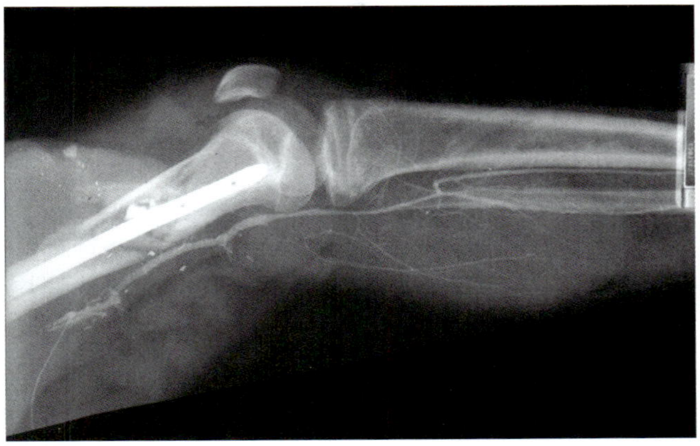

图 13　同一个患者（图 12）。术中动脉造影证实间置移植物血流好，胫腓干和小腿血管通畅。注意股骨干远端没有锁定螺钉

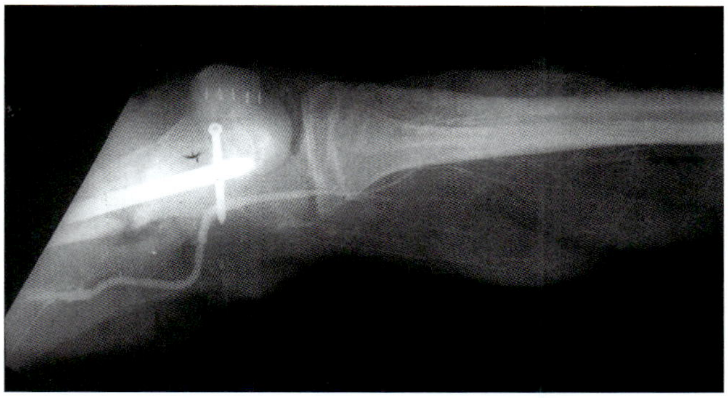

图 14　同一个患者（图 13）在骨科医生植入锁定螺钉后。注意在肢体适当对齐后，移植物一直呈 90°，这就须把原先的间置移植物拆掉

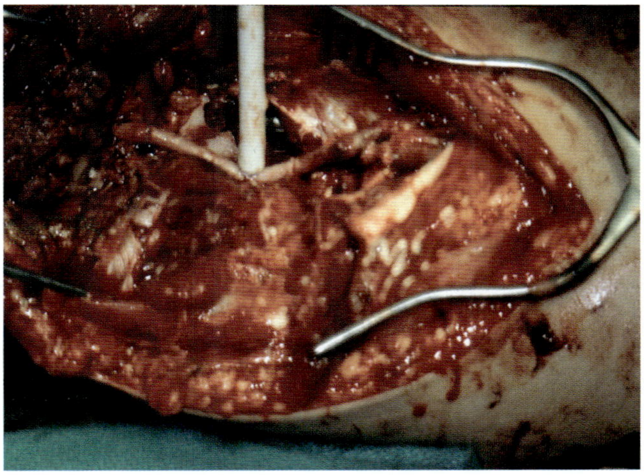

图 15　成角的间置移植物重做。多普勒探头探测移植物呈三相血流信号

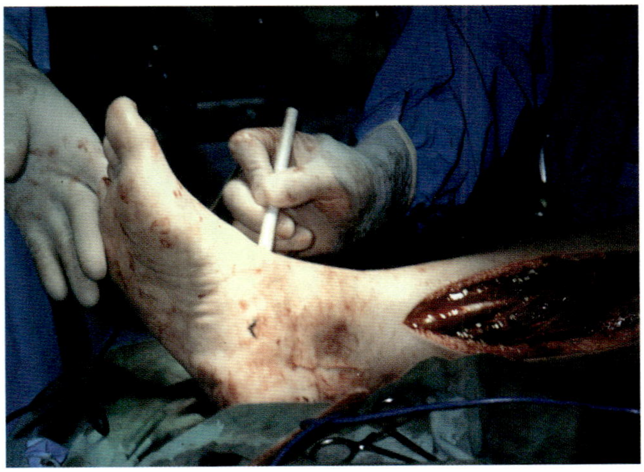

图 16　多普勒探头用于测量足背动脉在重做移植后的三相血流信号。注意小腿四筋膜室筋膜切开

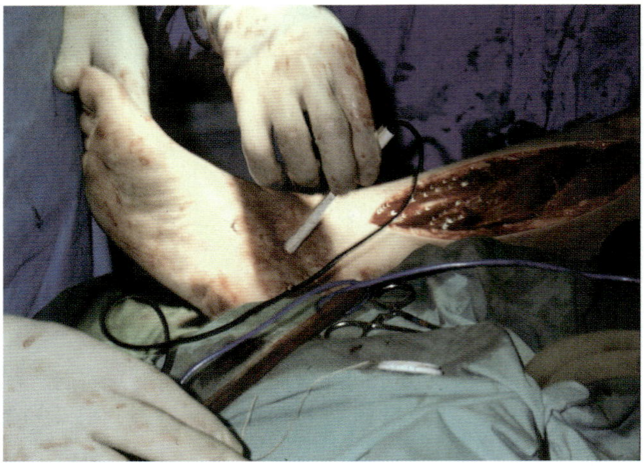

图 17　多普勒探头用于探测重做间置移植物后的胫后动脉的三相血流信号。注意小腿四筋膜室筋膜切开

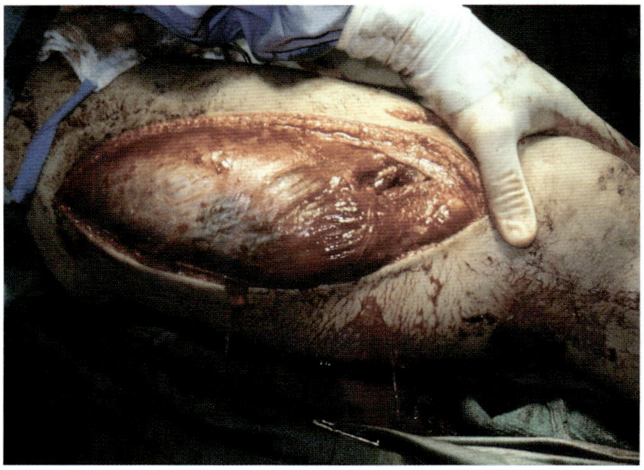

图 18　同一个患者 (图 17) 需要大腿和小腿的四筋膜室筋膜切开覆盖异种尸体移植物

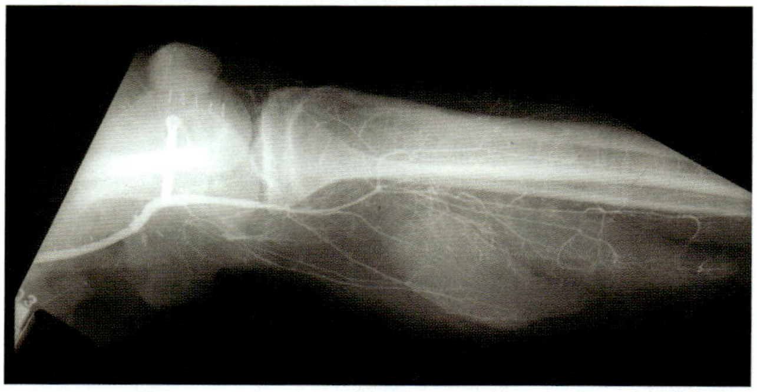

图 19　同一个患者 (图 18)，在矫正 90° 的移植物后。术中造影显示腘动脉、胫腓干和小腿血管有血流，有明显痉挛

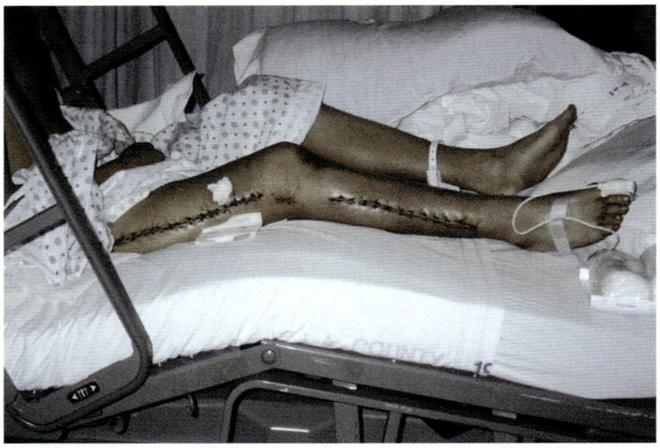

图 20　同一个患者 (19)，筋膜切开术关闭

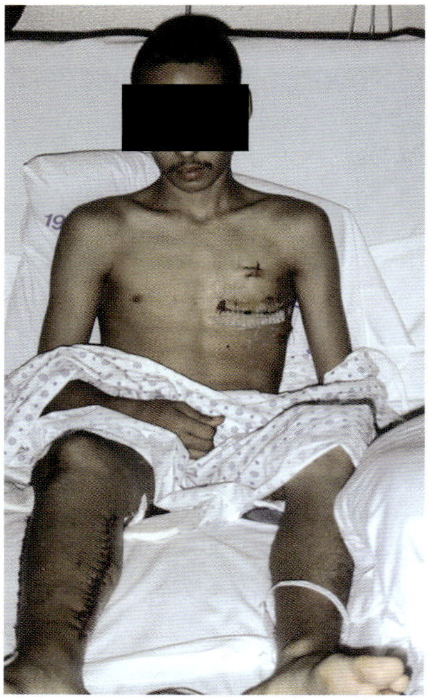

图 21　同一个患者 (图 20)。一期关闭的右小腿筋膜切口和愈合的左前外侧开胸切口

的抗感染能力。

逆行自体大隐静脉移植物因为其长期通畅性和抗感染能力，在传统上是推荐的。Feliciano 的使用 PTFE 的回顾性研究得出结论，其有良好的远期通畅率。Asensio 在其研究中报告使用 PTFE 与较高的死亡率有关，因为它常用于有严重损伤、有多个相关损伤和表现为休克的患者。他推荐将其用于低体温、凝血功能障碍、酸中毒和对血和血液制品需求增加的患者，因为其可用性高，且可以明显减少手术时间。

本章的高年资作者随后发展了带环的 PTFE 移植物的使用（图 3-22）。

筋膜切开和转流

肢体血管损伤的患者依缺血程度和相关组织损伤有发生筋膜室综合征的风险。漏诊此疾病的后果是可怕的，患者或失去整条肢体或失去整个肌肉筋膜室。即便在成功的血管再生后，再灌注综合征的全身并发症作用在肾，引起电解质和酸碱异常，会导致显著的死亡率。在血管再生的肢体上进行筋膜切开使肢体水肿、肿胀，而不会损失血管，由此可以保证保肢。筋膜室切开应当通过不同的切口（表 4）。应当完全切开筋膜，大腿筋膜切开，包括外侧和中部切口也是必需的（图 3-22）。

静脉损伤

股静脉损伤有生命危险但未到波及伴行动脉的程度，这些静脉通常在面临大的动脉出血时被结扎。结扎虽然是一个合理的办法，但结扎主要回流静脉有产生显著并发症的风险。静脉血栓形成使患者处

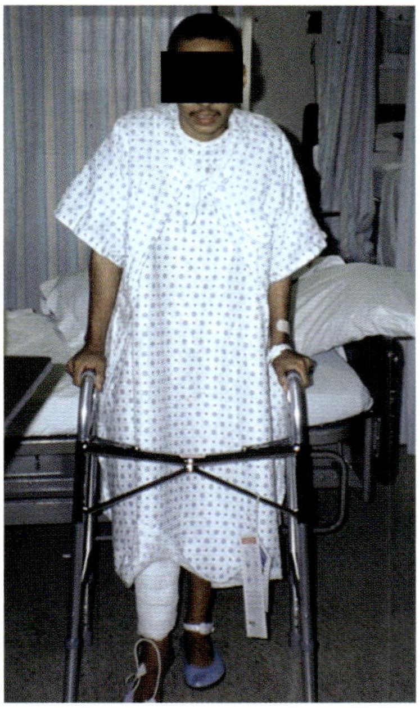

图 22　同一个患者（图 21）走动。物理治疗对这些患者是非常重要的

表 4　股血管损伤手术处理

作者（年）	血管	总股血管损伤	手术 侧壁缝合	结扎	端端吻合	自体血管	PTFE	静脉补片	其他	截肢
Phifer	动脉	25	7 (28%)	6 (24%)	8 (32%)	9 (36%)	1 (4%)			
(1984)	静脉	25	14 (56%)		2 (8%)	2 (8%)	1 (4%)			
Feliciano	动脉	142	10 (7%)	21 (14.8%)	40 (28.2%)		59 (41.5%)		6 (4.2%)	6
(1988)	静脉	93	49 (52.7)	19 (20.4%)	7 (7.5%)		18 (19.3%)			
Timberlake	动脉	116	45 (38.8%)	71 (61.2%)						
(1990)	静脉									
Cargile	动脉	190	34 (17.9%)	2 (1%)	81 (42.6%)	66 (34.7%)	1 (0.5%)	6 (3.2%)		11
(1992)	静脉	131	69 (52.7%)	12 (9.2%)	15 (11.4%)	22 (16.8%)	3 (2.3%)	70 (7.6%)		
Martin	动脉	105	25（23.8%）	6 (28.6%)		25 (23.8%)	55 (52.4%)			1
(1994)	静脉	21	10 (47%)			1 (4.8%)	4 (19%)			
Asensio	动脉	204	53（26%）	13（6.4%）		108（52.9%）	21 (10.3%)	9 (4.4%)		6
(2006)	静脉	94	41 (43.6%)	49 (52.1%)		4 (4.3%)				
Michael	动脉	44	8 (18.2%)	7 (15.9%)		23 (52.3%)		6 (13.6%)		
(2007)	静脉									
Clouse	动脉	74	14 (18.9%)	9 (12.2%)		46 (62.2%)	4 (5.4%)		1 (1.3%)	
(2007)	静脉	37	12 (32.4%)	11 (29.7%)		14 (37.9%)				

于栓子蔓延和潜在肺栓塞形成的危险境地，如果患者存活需要长期抗凝。静脉功能不全的发展可能会导致患者衰弱，增加整个手术后感染性并发症。下肢水肿对开始功能锻炼的患者可能是灾难性的。在适当的情况下，当患者的生存没有问题的时候，应鼓励修复股静脉。

一些研究，包括 Nypaver、Timberlake、Kerstein 和 Zamir 的研究赞成在可能的情况下要修复大静脉。Asensio 也推荐这样。手术修复静脉损伤取决于一些因素：保肢、患者安全和相关并发症。值得注意的是相关静脉损伤和动脉损伤极大地增加了肢体并发症。如果可能的话，静脉单纯裂伤应当首先用连续缝合的方法修复。如果有必要清创，无张力端端吻合是个好方法，尽管很少采用。当有广泛静脉系统损伤或重要静脉损伤（如股总静脉）时，可以放置转流管临时建立流出道，作为一个救命措施，并可以做静脉静脉旁路（图 23-26）。

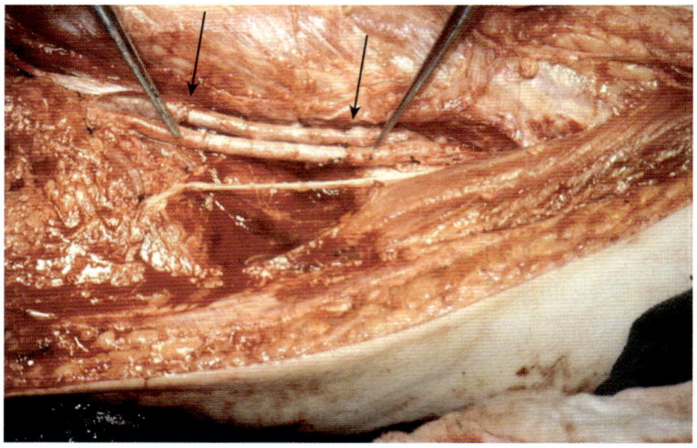

图 24　用 Gerald 镊指的是股浅动脉损伤间置逆行自体大隐静脉移植物。箭头指示的是股浅静脉间置逆行自体大隐静脉移植物

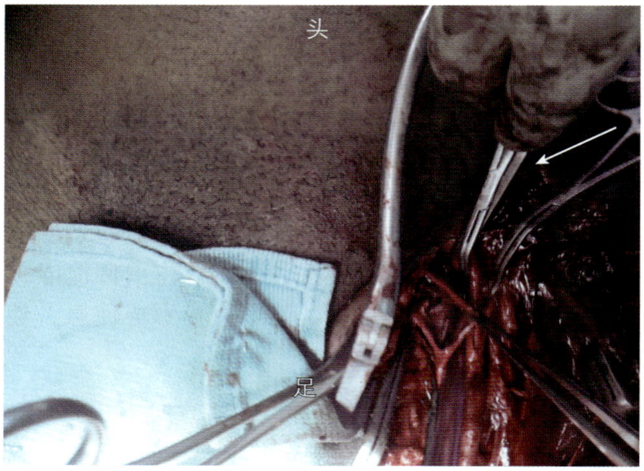

图 25　高速枪伤导致的左股浅动脉和股深动脉和股深静脉的合并动脉和静脉损伤。箭头指示股深动脉和股深静脉由股深动脉钳控制

预后和死亡率

如同 Asensio 所报告的，股动脉损伤技术和诊断的进步使生存率有了明显改进，接近 95%，伴有截肢数量下降和全身功能预后改善。尽管检查、手术技术和随访有了很大改进，并发病发生率还很高。Asensio 在他的包含 298 例股损伤病例、长达十年跨度的研究中鉴定和统计学验证了预后的预测因子。格拉斯哥昏迷等级评分（Glasgow Coma Scale，GCS）小于 8、需要急诊插管和需要 EDT，以及 ISS 超过 25 是显著的死亡预测因子。低血压、低体温、凝血功能异常和使用 PTFE 或相关腹部损伤或骨折，也和高死亡率和伤口脓毒症有关。除了及时发现、快速血管控制和良好的手术技巧，没有其他的措施可能会降低股血管损伤的并发症发生率和死亡率。

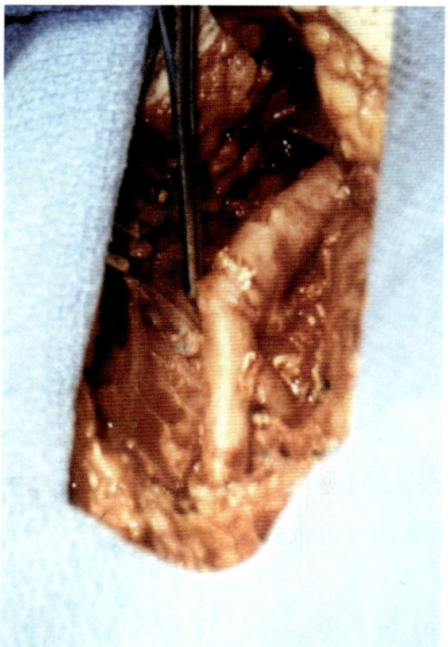

图 23　一例复杂的右股总静脉侧壁缝合。如果可能，右股总静脉要修复。结扎会导致严重的并发症和可能的肢体缺失

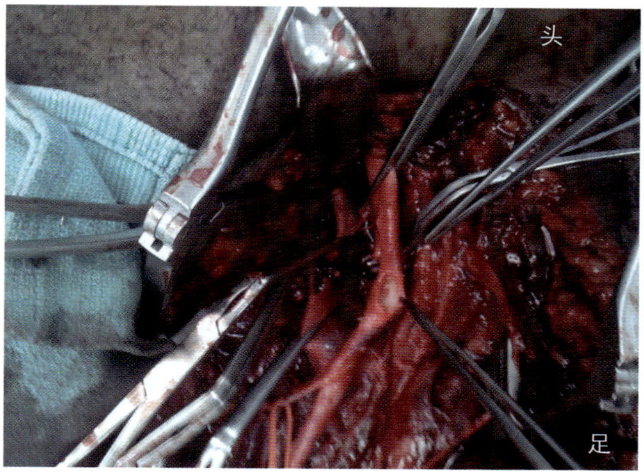

图 26 同一个患者（图 25）显示在大出血后控制股总动脉、股浅动脉和股深动脉。类似地左股总静脉和股浅静脉和股深静脉也控制住。患者到院时深度休克，收缩压为 60 mmHg，用手指控制出血，迅速转移到手术室。患者有酸中毒、低体温和凝血功能障碍。鉴于他有如此严重的血流动力学损伤的状态，我们首先进行损伤控制，但无法转流他的股总动脉。他须结扎股总动脉、股浅动脉和股深动脉作为保命措施。他也需要 8 mm 直径带环 PTFE CFA 到远侧股动脉，在 Hunter 管上方进行 SFA 间置移植物。不幸的是 PFA 损伤相对严重，不能和近端 CFA 吻合做股深动脉成形术。患者需要大腿和小腿筋膜切开、后期缝合。患者生存，并作为一个反恐小组的高级官员重回工作岗位

结论

股血管损伤是平民和军事领域最常见的周围血管损伤。纵观历史它们已经从罕见的高死亡率的损伤演变为常见低死亡率、高发病率的损伤。

临床评估对穿通伤经常是充分的；而对钝伤须结合临床和实验室检查，以明确损伤部位和类型。血管移植物和手术装备的进步使修复这些损伤血管更容易和快捷，但缺血时间延长导致相关的并发症发生率很高，静脉系统结扎造成的并发症还很多。对疑似病例，迅速转运和手术控制出血和恢复血流仍是主要的股血管损伤管理措施。当损伤控制开始后，血管转流应当伴随相关下肢的筋膜切开和恰当的深静脉血栓形成（deep venous thrombosis，DVT）的预防。随着迅速识别和快速外科干预和积极的术后护理的进步，对患者尽可能地采取预防措施，以降低由这些损伤的高并发症发生率，使他们能在这种情况下生存。

腘血管损伤：复杂的解剖和高截肢率

Juan A. Asensio, Patrizio Petrone, Alejandro Perez-Alonso, Mark Traynham, Ananth Srinivasan, Stephen Serio,Jeremy Cannon 和 John T. Owings 著
张学民 译

周围血管损伤占在大的城市创伤中心救治的全部创伤的 5%。腘血管损伤对创伤外科医生在术中和术后都是一个挑战。这些损伤根据损伤机制不同，可以和广泛软组织损伤、骨折、神经功能不全和其他致命损伤有关。无论在军事和平民经验中，腘血管损伤和显著的发病率和死亡率相关。历史上，这些损伤被证明有高的并发症发生率、截肢率和死亡率。而急诊应答系统的进步、积极的复苏、早期识别和迅速修复，使总并发症发生率和生存率有戏剧性的改善。

历史回顾

1906 年，来自西班牙的 José Goyanes 首次切除了损伤性腘动脉瘤，并用间置腘静脉移植物重建腘动脉。因此他被认为是第一个使用逆行自体大隐静脉移植物的人。

任何进一步的腘血管损伤的讨论都要从回顾战场损伤的救治获得的知识开始。这些教训已经被证明对治疗这些损伤非常宝贵的。绝大多数战伤包括了下肢和上肢。这些损伤是高速子弹、弹片和碎片、杀伤性装置导致的明显的软组织缺损、复杂骨折和神经损伤。

在战场和手术中心的任何延误都是有害的。在第二次世界大战结束末期，直到手术支持可以在未

来的冲突中前移到前线，疏散时间和手术准备才得以改进。在每一次冲突中，向前线引入手术小组被证明是个有价值的经验。然而，在早期的战争史中，下肢血管损伤比上肢有更高的并发症发生率。在英国从第一次世界大战得到的经验中，Makin 观察到腘损伤发生率为 12%，截肢率为 43%。在第二次世界大战中，DeBakey 和 Simeone 的综述证实有 502 例腘动脉损伤，总发生率为 20%。在那些患者中，499 例需要结扎，导致截肢率高达 72.5%。比较两次大战，高截肢率和武器装备的改变、明显的组织破坏、侧支循环的破坏和结扎作为首次外科干预（而不是修复）相关。

在朝鲜战争中，Hughes 报告了 79 例腘动脉损伤修复，其中 32.4% 的患者需要截肢。越南血管注册体系记录了将近 600 例腘血管损伤，包括识别出的 300 例腘动脉损伤，占全部患者的 18.3%。Rich 评估了这些完成全面随访的患者中的 150 例，发现 58.7% 例合并静脉损伤。此外，他们发现了 110 例单独的腘静脉损伤，没有任何相关的动脉损伤。结扎损伤静脉在早期战时血管损伤的治疗中也是一个可接受的方式。而在朝鲜战争中，相比于两次大战中经验性治疗（结扎）腘血管修复显示减少了截肢率。在越南和朝鲜战争中实行血管修复时，截肢率明显降低到 32% 和 33%。这些先前战时的努力明显为 21 世界的现代冲突提供了先进的血管创伤的经验。

在 Woodward 等的 Balad 血管注册数据库的分析中，在超过 32 个月中有 9 289 例战斗相关伤亡。其中 488 例患者诊断出 513 个血管损伤，包括 45 例腘血管损伤。单独的腘动脉损伤占 35.6%，合并腘静脉的动脉损伤占 62.2%。现代战时创伤和先前的历史冲突相比机制不同。IED 被伊拉克武装分子再次引进和使用，造成 27 例腘损伤，高速枪伤造成 18 例附加损伤。不管致伤机制如何，明显的软组织缺失和骨损伤是这些损伤的常见成分，由此需要多种外科干预和多学科的方法。

不幸的是，伊拉克战争中，血管损伤的发生率是越南战争的 2 倍。腘动脉损伤占血管损伤的 8.6%，幸存者中早期截肢率 14.3%。在 Fox 等的回顾性研究中，8 618 例伤亡者被送入巴格达战斗支援医院。所有损伤都来自枪伤或高能爆炸物，其中识别出 48 例腘动脉损伤，37% 合并静脉和动脉损伤。各种外科治疗被运用，包括逆行自体大隐静脉移植物（69%）、静脉补片（2%）、动脉侧壁缝合（19%）和端端吻合（2%）。任何明确的伴行静脉损伤需要结扎、修复或移植来治疗。总的保肢失败率为 29%，而并发症发生率还很高。

历史预后证实血管结扎导致血管损伤处理中的高截肢率。然而，外科修复的后期满意度明显改善。成功的现代战时血管外科源自这些历史冲突通过缩短疏散时间、改进复苏和改进外科经验来改良。疏散的改变和邻近外科护理的发展彻底减少了缺血延误，当结合积极的损伤控制和初始复苏，当代战时血管损伤有了更高的战伤存活率和保肢率（表 1）。

解剖

腘动脉起自股浅动脉在收肌管内行走，由缝匠肌和半膜肌、半腱肌所包围。随着其向腘窝后方行进，动脉和静脉以及胫神经由浅表皮下组织覆盖。腘动脉和腘静脉的解剖学位置在腓肠肌和腘肌内侧和外侧头之间。腘窝底部由膝关节囊、股骨腘面和腘肌筋膜构成。正是这样的位置使腘动脉受外伤后最易受骨损伤（如骨折或脱位）影响。在这个层面上，完整的侧支网络供应由腘动脉分出的膝支、腓肠肌支、肌支连接近端的股深动脉和远侧的胫动脉。在膝关节上，腘动脉分出上外侧膝动脉和上内侧膝动脉，在膝关节下，腘动脉分出下外侧膝动脉和下内侧膝动脉。腘动脉终末分支起自其分叉的层面，分为胫腓干和胫前动脉（图 1）。

表 1　腘血管损伤的战时经验

作者	冲突	年份	总动脉损伤	腘动脉损伤数	腘血管损伤率	总截肢	因腘损伤截肢
Makins	第一次世界大战	1919	1 202	144	12%	218（18%）	62（43%）
DeBakey 和 Simeone	第二次世界大战	1946	2 471	502	20.3%	995（40.3%）	364（72.5%）
Hughes	朝鲜战争	1958	304	79	26%	53（17.4%）	30（38%）
Rich	越南战争	1970	1 000	217	21.7%	128（13.5%）	64（29.5%）

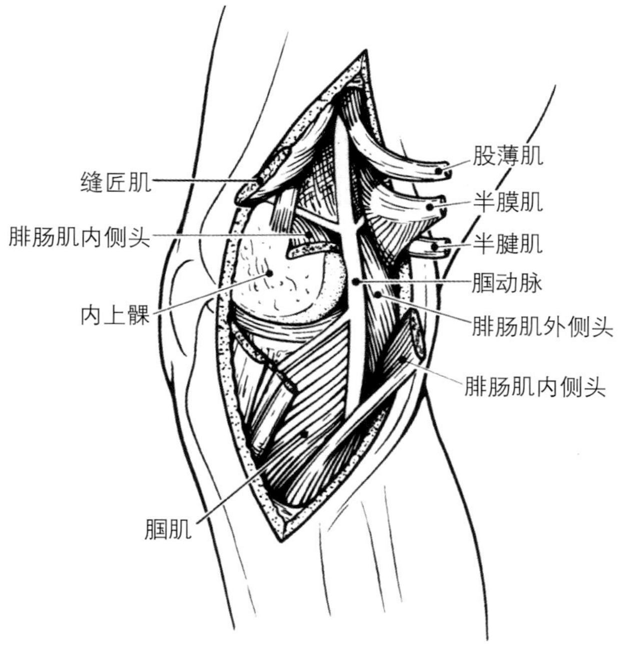

图 1　腘窝解剖 *(From Asensio JA, Demetriades D: Atlas of complex trauma surgical techniques, St. Louis, 2014, Elsevier.)*

理解“传统”腘动脉解剖学描述很重要，可以认识到成年人腘动脉和静脉血管网络在长度和分支模式上存在变异。最常见的腘动脉终末支的分布是胫前动脉、胫后动脉。一般在股骨髁远侧几厘米，后面是更远端的起自胫后动脉的分支动脉。“正常”腘动脉形式由 Bardsley 和 Staple 描述，占全部人群的 92.8%，其他一些公开发表的研究中也有类似的发现。腘静脉解剖的复杂变异由 Cross 报道的肢体解剖证实，它描述了不同的连接静脉的组成。这些解剖学描述描绘了各种腘窝内的可感知的血管变异，因此证明在可行时，手术修复的重要性。

发病率

在繁忙的城市创伤中心，平民腘血管损伤还是个令人生畏的艰巨任务。外科文献的大部分为学院回顾性数据综述。创伤机制和损伤特征基本一致。Mullenix 等分析了来自 NTDB 的 1 130 000 患者，明确了 1 395 例腘损伤，它的发生率低于 0.2%。在 Kauvar 等的 NTDB 综述中，651 个孤立的腹股沟韧带下动脉损伤被确认，腘动脉成为最主要的损伤血管，占 35.5%。国际文献报告，南非的有可比性的结果提示腘血管损伤的发生率为 30.7%（表 2）。

在大型Ⅰ级创伤中心，绝大多数下肢动脉损伤由穿通伤引起。在 Fabian 包括了 165 例腘动脉损伤的研究中，125 例损伤由穿通伤引起。其他创伤中心可以观察到创伤主要和钝性机制有关。Harrell 等评估了 38 例腘动脉损伤，都是由钝性机制直接造成。Frykberg 通过对 24 个研究的仔细分析，发现穿通性腘动脉损伤占 56%。总而言之，腘动脉钝伤的发生率在不同的城市创伤中心中为 20% ~ 84% 不等。

Hafez 的 10 年的综述回顾了 641 例下肢损伤，其中 30.7% 是腘动脉损伤。最高的肢体缺失率接近 25%，见于膝上腘动脉损伤。刺伤似乎较少导致截肢。肢体损伤的主要因素包括神经损伤和复合骨折。最常见的相关损伤是静脉，特别是静脉节段分支。几个回顾系列报告相关静脉损伤的发生率高达 34%。Franz 发现 25% 的腘动脉损伤有相关静脉损伤，Jaggers 发现 28% 的患者有动静脉合并损伤。

较早的系列比最近几十年的系列具有更高的截肢率。威胁肢体的血管损伤与导致膝关节脱位和复杂的骨损伤的高能钝性机制有关，高速枪伤也一样。平民腘血管损伤的截肢率为 6% ~ 37%。在特定的研究中，各种钝性挤压伤机制有高达 52.5% 的截肢率。

肢体缺血的处理是最紧要的，最重要的目标是迅速恢复循环。Patterson 报告了 18 例来自下肢评估项目研究的患者，它是一个多中心、回顾性、纵向研究。全部病例由钝性机械力和相关膝关节脱位和腘动脉损伤导致。16 例患者的两下肢至少有 1 个腘损伤修复，他们保留至最终随访；14 例患者的膝关节成功保住，4 例患者需要截肢。进一步回顾，膝关节脱位和相关血管损伤在大型创伤中心导致的截肢率高达 52%。

成年人创伤性血管损伤构成了大多数已发表的回顾性研究，对儿童创伤的关注最少。大多数儿童血管损伤是医源性的。然而，记录散发病例和穿通性、钝性损伤系列的综述文章虽然存在，但是非常罕见。Corneille 的回顾性研究历时 13 年，表明 116 例儿童创伤患者中有 138 个血管损伤。在这些系列中，有 29 例患者有下肢损伤，有 36 个血管损伤。腘静脉是最常损伤的静脉。而腘动脉，只占全部损伤的 19%，全部膝下血管损伤的 30.6%。不管怎样，非医源性血管损伤在儿童人群中是罕见的，当出现腘血管损伤且有表现的时候，早期识别和手术治疗有较高的保肢率。

表 2　下肢腘血管损伤的发生率

作者	年	下肢血管损伤	腘血管损伤（%）
Zorita	1990	11	45.4%（5）
Berga	1991	32	31.2%（10）
Martin	1994	188	21.2%（40）
Hafez	2001	641	37%（237）
Rozycki	2003	77	16.8%（13）
Yahya	2005	60	31.6%（19）
Tam	2006	57	70%（40）
Mäkitie	2006	38	21%（8）
Degiannis	2007	103	32%（33）
Henry	2010	19	26.3%（5）
Kauvar	2011	651	34.7%（226）
Franz	2011	75	21.3%（16）

表 3　腘血管损伤机制

作者	年	腘血管损伤数	穿通伤	钝伤
Jaggers	1982	61	49（80%）	12（20%）
Downs	1986	63	10（16%）	53（84%）
Krige	1987	28	16（57%）	12（43%）
Martin	1994	40	26（65%）	14（35%）
Fainzilber	1995	81	67（82.7%）	14（17.3%）
Melton	1997	102	62（61%）	40（39%）
Yahya	2005	19	6（31.6%）	1 395
Mullenix	2006	1 395	543（39%）	852（61%）
Moini	2007	40	8（20%）	32（80%）
Callcut	2009	36	34（94%）	2（6%）
Franz	2011	16	7（43.7%）	9（56.3%）

临床表现

急性下肢动脉损伤，不论是钝伤或穿通伤，都被认为是威胁肢体的，除非最终被证实不是（表 3）。创伤团队的第一反应是避免即刻的出血和迅速外科处理来恢复肢体灌注。大多数腘动脉损伤可以通过病史和体检诊断，而钝伤在其他相关胸腹部损伤存在的情况下可能难以诊断。Miranda 的前瞻性系列包括 35 例查体阴性的膝关节脱位报告，它得出结论，体检能可靠地识别出有血管损伤的患者。虽然对所有膝关节脱位患者行常规血管造影是不必要的。另一方面 Barnes 等做了 meta 分析，以确定体检对检测损伤是否敏感，并得出结论，其对损伤不敏感。

Frank 出血和其他血管损伤硬体征包括搏动性出血、血肿扩大、脉搏消失、有杂音或震颤和远侧缺血体征，须立即手术干预。临床缺血体征和发绀、神经功能缺失、温度改变的证据是在评估时得到的可靠线索。Wagner 发现全部肢体损伤的 55% 有可以在术前检测出的临床缺血，但毛细血管充盈被认为是对远端灌注的不可靠的测量方法。特定的患者在损伤后表现延迟超过 12 ~ 24 h，临床表现有假性动脉瘤坏疽或动静脉瘘时，需要迅速手术。在这些特定的病例，通过术前完成的血管造影画出血管。

如前所述，腘动脉损伤可能预示着广泛的软组织损伤及骨破坏。不幸的是，有这些复合伤的患者在院前转运过程中或到达急诊室前已经表现有低血容量性休克，应当早期院前使用止血带控制出血。这是一个改善可预防的死亡的措施。使用止血带的理论基础是任何孤立的下肢血管损伤致死都是因为出血。如果没有准备止血带，用局部的内源性止血剂有一些效果，就像最近在军事领域使用的。在平民钝性腘创伤患者中，使用临时转流管可以改善保肢率。

血管修复永远是第一位的，许多患者会有明显的复杂骨和神经损伤。相关的韧带损伤和软组织破坏影响膝关节稳定性。在最初检查的时候就应努力减少膝关节脱位或骨折。脉搏减弱或消失是个明确的腘窝内血管损伤体征，应当立即注意。Harrell 评估了 38 例膝关节后脱位患者，其中 90% 有相关血管损伤，做了腹部检查。当下肢出现创伤性血管损伤时，要想到需要四筋膜室筋膜切开。动脉静脉合并损伤的患者，缺血时间长，骨折和相关动脉或静脉损伤和筋膜室综合征的诊断延误都是最常见的四筋膜室筋膜切开的指征。Jaggers 回顾了 56 例腘动脉损伤，21 例在首次手术时需要筋膜切开，3 例需要延迟筋膜切开。

诊断

腘动脉损伤的诊断通常仅依靠体检就可以了。

大多数病例有硬体征的出现可作为清晰的临床血管损伤证据。在没有伴随生命危险的损伤和不复杂的下肢穿通性创伤中，这些硬体征中的一条或多条出现意味着需要立即手术探查。在体检中用这些硬体征表现作为手术指征被证明是安全和可靠的，治疗性探查率达到100%。任何进一步的影像学检查是不必要的，可能导致确定性修复的延迟和缺血延长。无症状非阻塞性的血管损伤是良性的，其中95%是时间自限性的。因为这些隐匿的损伤经常会自行缓解、无需修复，他们不须消耗检查资源。另外Fryberg表明那些没有表现为进展的隐匿的损伤可以修复，而无后遗症。当然也须注意哪些患者需要严密随访。

在特定条件下，动脉血管造影可能对确立腘动脉损伤的诊断有帮助。这些条件包括钝性损伤和下肢复杂损伤。这些损伤可能导致潜在的皮肤肌肉缺失和破坏性骨损伤。硬体征也可以潜在地由广泛损伤发展而来，甚至在没有血管损伤的情况下。在这种情况下推荐使用血管造影减少非治疗性探查。猎枪爆炸是另一种类型的伤害，成像是有价值的。这些损伤会导致多个解剖层次上的损伤，而在探查时可能遗漏。在这些病例的手术室血管造影可以减少诊断后开始修复的时间和减少截肢的可能性。如前所述，动脉造影在延迟成像(>12 h)的情况下也是有用的。时间不紧张的情况下，影像检查可以帮助制订确定性治疗方案（图2-4）。

如何应对软体征患者有些争议。软体征包括踝肱指数小于0.9、曾有明显出血后停止历史、非扩张性血肿和瘀斑的出现。动脉造影在历史上被证明是诊断临床明显损伤并有这些发现的患者的金标准。CT血管造影的应用表现出对检测临床明确的损伤的高灵敏度和特异度。

另一个非侵入性的诊断方法是多普勒超声。这个方法的灵敏度为50%～100%，特异度和准确性超过95%。这个技术的问题在于设备初始费用、要一个合格的超声医生24 h随叫随到，这潜在地限制了其使用，血管损伤的肢体在存在骨折、血肿、肿胀和笨重敷料的情况下准确性不确定。

处理

一旦诊断腘损伤，须立即转运到手术室。患者要备皮、铺单（包括损伤肢体和至少一个非损伤肢体作为获取自体静脉移植物的准备）。损伤的肢体的足应当留在术野内，以方便触摸脉搏。患者仰卧位，髋外展、外旋、膝轻微弯曲，且用折叠的布巾抬高。在急性损伤的情况下中线切口更为常用。

在股内侧肌和缝匠肌之间做一个充分的纵向切口，近端在远侧股骨后1 cm。切口典型地向下延伸至胫骨后缘的后方1 cm，直到达到适当的显露。大隐静脉在切口后皮瓣内，注意避免损伤。大隐静脉是下肢重要的流出血管，要非常小心不要损伤。分开缝匠肌、半膜肌和半腱肌。为减少术后残疾，这些肌肉术后要再近接缝合（图1）。

最初可以用手指控制出血，直到血管显露，用钳或环控制血管近、远端。失活段的动脉应当清创至大体上为有活力的血管。如果没有张力的话，端端吻合的一期修复是首选方法。如果血管缺失超过2 cm，此方法不可行。在大多数病例中，无法行无张力吻合，因此须取对侧大隐静脉，逆行作为间置移植物。人造移植物应当避免跨膝关节，因为在这个部位其通畅性不如静脉。如果相关损伤允许，在修复和术后要考虑全身肝素化。这会减少远端血栓风险，增加血管重建成功的可能性。修复前Fogarty血栓切除导管应当在远侧和近侧通过，以确认有好的向前和向后血流。肝素盐水应当注入远侧动脉，以防进一步血栓形成。

5-0或6-0单股聚丙烯线连续缝合修复腘动脉。如果损伤小于30%的血管周长，可以尝试侧壁修复。要小心避免狭窄。其他方法是切除损伤段，行一期吻合。在完成修复时可以做血管造影以帮助确认吻合口有无须修改的问题（图5-43）。

解剖外旁路只在特殊情况下考虑，包括伤口的修复是感染血管床或广泛软组织损伤或缺失的区域。在这种情况下，旁路可以从正常和无污染组织钻隧道通过。损伤血管应当移除，以防止假性动脉瘤形成，后者可以扩张、破裂或栓塞。

腘血管损伤有很高的导致下肢筋膜室综合征的风险。增加这种风险的因素包括缺血时间长（>4 h）、合并血管和骨损伤、血栓修复、合并动脉和静脉损伤、动脉或静脉结扎。临床上还要考虑四筋膜室切开的决定，一些研究推荐积极切开。涉及并存的骨损伤的损伤增加了治疗已经具有挑战性的血管损伤的复杂性。应当优先考虑血管重建。暂时再灌注通过使用腔内Argyle转流管完成。在骨骼稳定后再完成确切性修复。适用于股骨切开复位和内固定术。

早期截肢的情况仍是一个困难的决定，需要仔细判断。即便成功保肢，由于继发神经损伤和明显

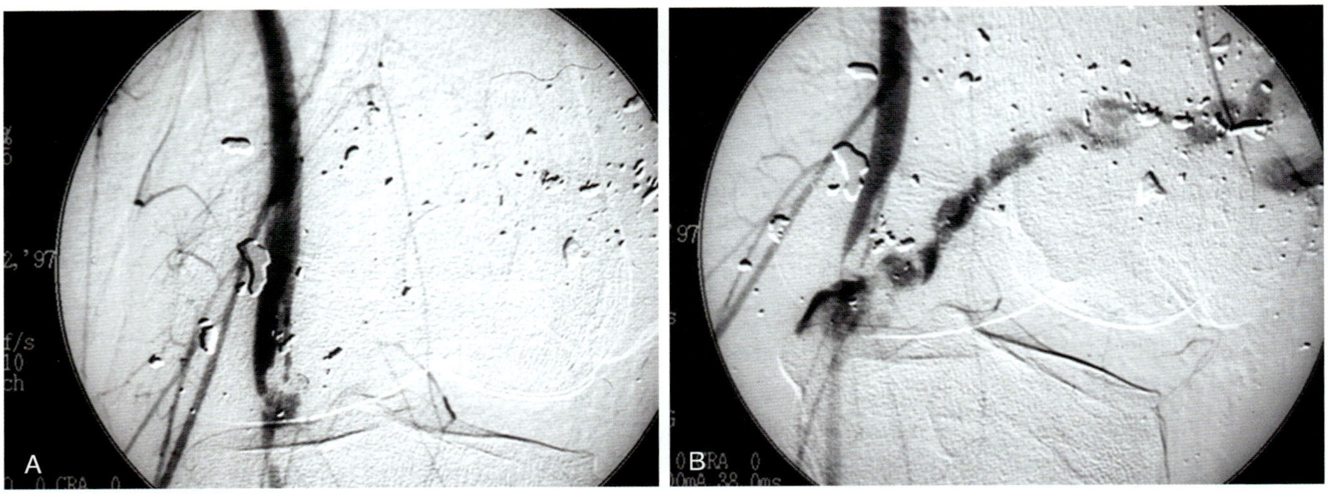

图 2 **A**，一个枪伤患者的血管造影，他到院时肢体无危险。**B**，同一个患者在血管造影室证实有活动性出血，患者被迅速转运到手术室

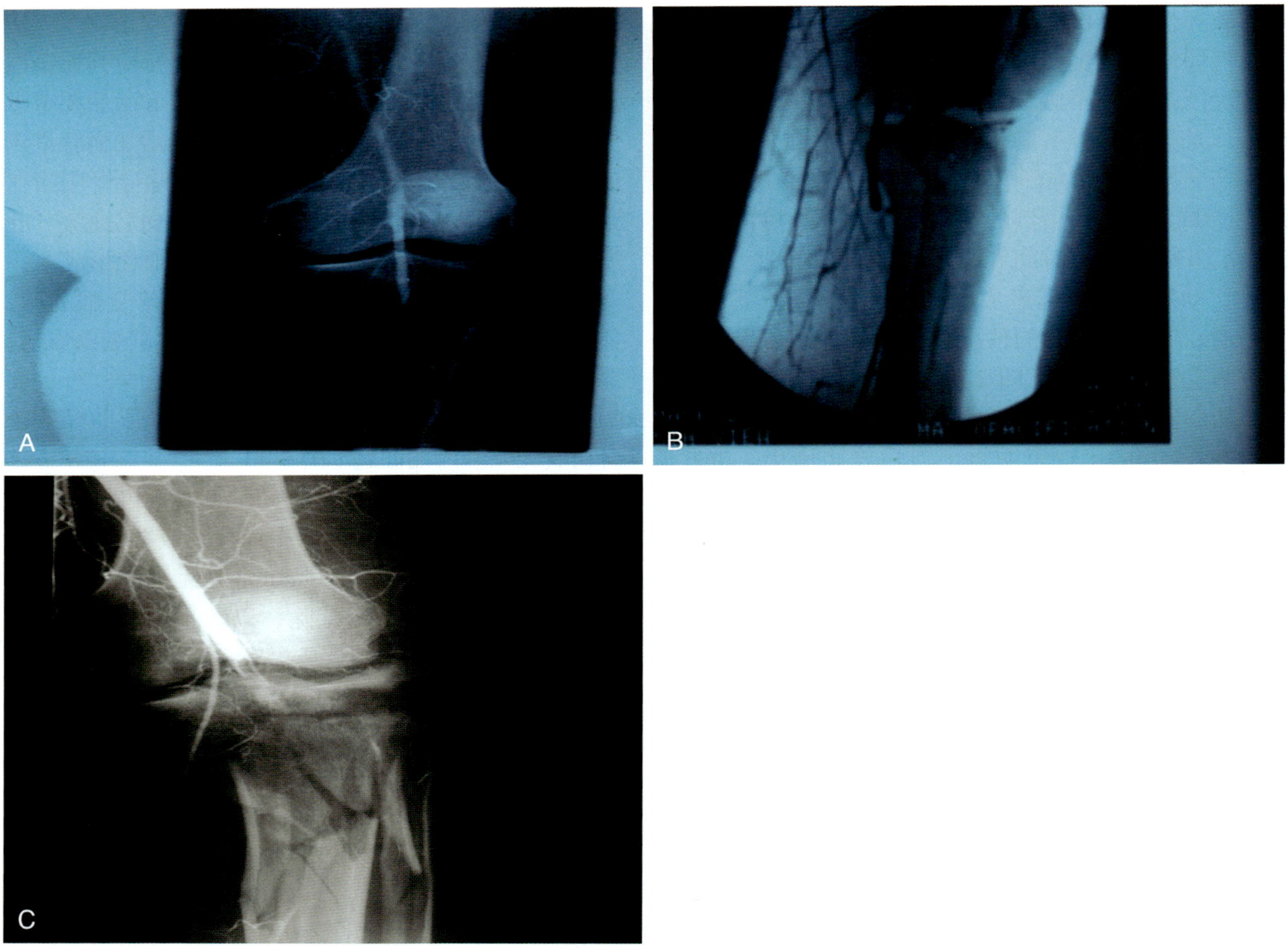

图 3 **A**，可疑膝关节脱位且腘动脉钝性阻断的患者的动脉造影。**B**，也是一个可疑膝关节脱位腘动脉钝性阻断的患者血管造影，注意侧支。**C**，严重胫骨近端骨折和腘动脉阻塞的患者的血管造影

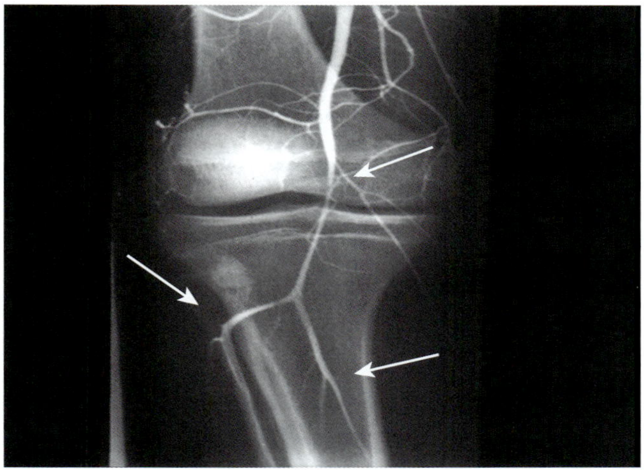

图 4　疑似腘窝枪伤、表现为踝肱指数降低的患者的血管造影，注意腘动脉膝后段狭窄。注意清晰地分出胫动脉、胫腓干及其分支的胫后动脉和腓动脉（箭头）

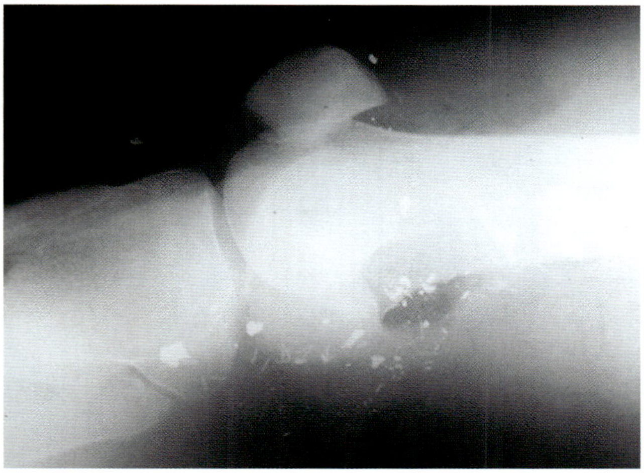

图 6　图 5 患者的 X 线片，注意多个组织碎片。患者被迅速转运至手术室

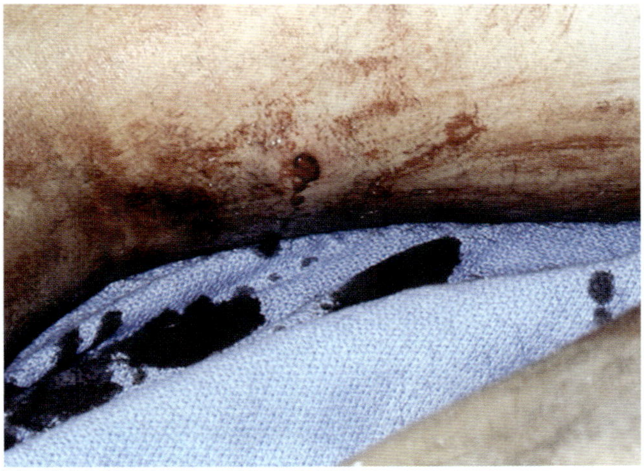

图 5　腘窝枪伤入院的患者

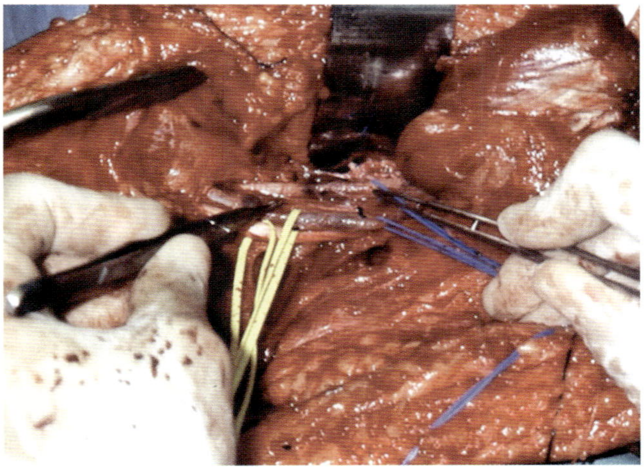

图 7　术中照片证实腘动脉裂伤。注意腘静脉用蓝色血管环环绕，胫神经用黄色血管环环绕

的肌肉和骨组织（包括整个筋膜室）功能缺失，预后可能不满意。损毁肢体严重度评分（Mangled Extremity Severity Score，MESS）用于挑选那些下肢损伤后需要截肢的患者。分值 7～10 作为挑选出那些很可能需要一期截肢的患者。最终的截肢决定一定要考虑个体基础，牢记患者的最佳利益。截肢的决定应当涉及多学科团队，如果可能应包括患者的意见。

如何治疗没有硬体征的非阻塞性损伤患者仍有争议。问题包括狭窄的血管、内膜瓣、小的假性动脉瘤和动静脉瘘。历史上，这些损伤常规使用手术探查。而 Frykberg 报告这些临床不明确的损伤大多有良性的自然史，可以安全地观察。在这种情况下，这些病变即使恶化到需要修复的程度，仍可以没有

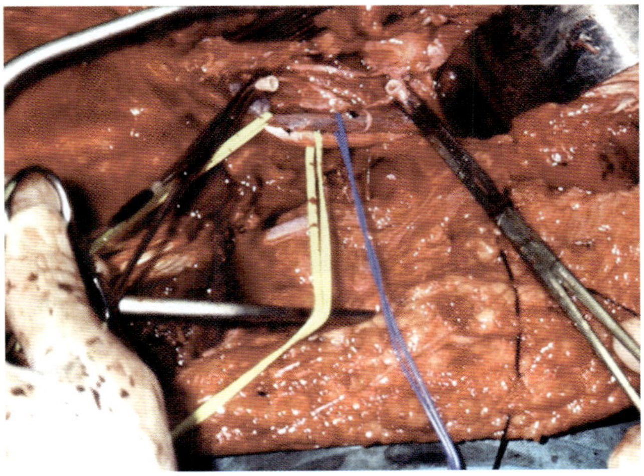

图 8　切除腘动脉

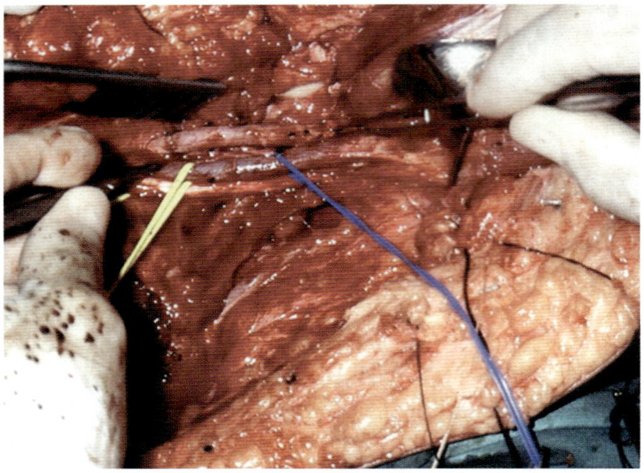

图 9　逆行自体大隐静脉间置移植物。注意腘静脉及其后方的胫神经

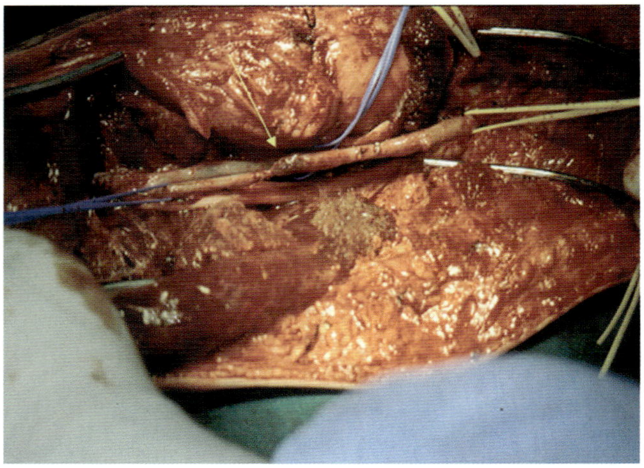

图 11　行人被车撞击，导致腘动脉钝性阻塞和血栓形成（箭头）

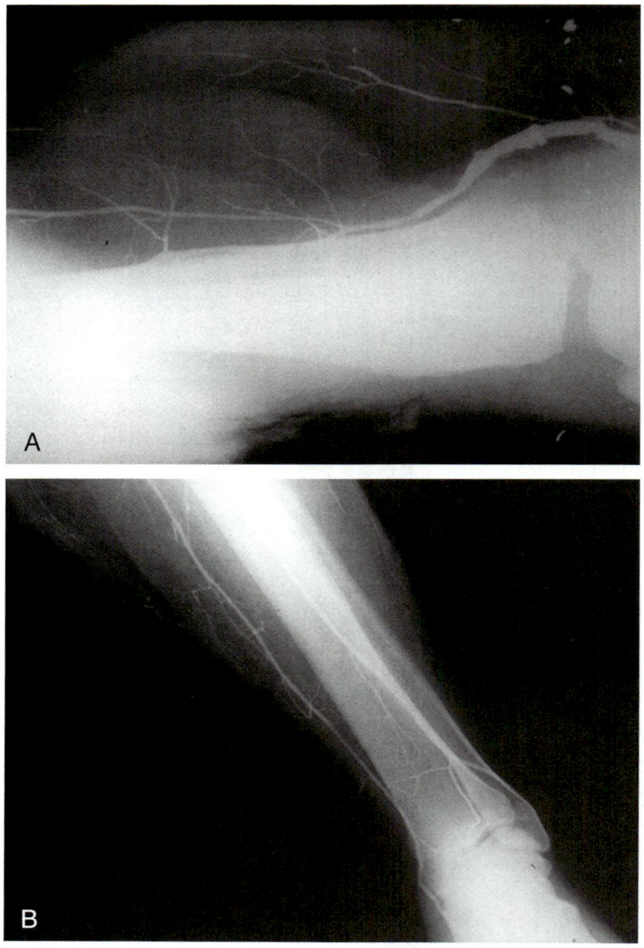

图 10　**A**，与图 9 为同一个患者，术后血管造影显示血管通畅。**B**，血管造影见胫前动脉和胫后动脉远侧血流

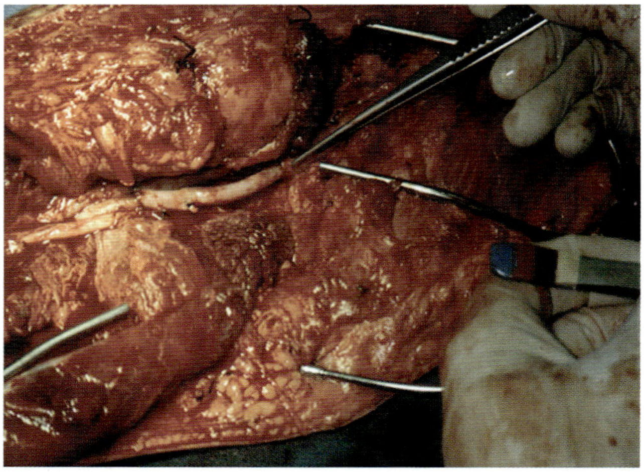

图 12　切除血栓的腘动脉用逆行自体大隐静脉修复

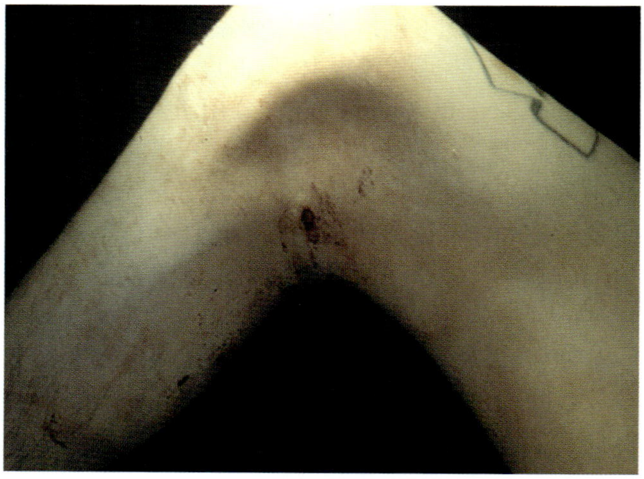

图 13　腘窝枪伤患者，多普勒探查脉搏显示双相血流信号。踝肱指数为 0.9。患者被送入手术室

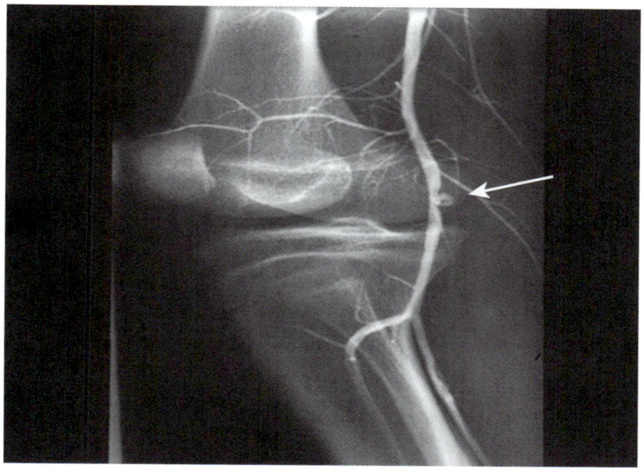

图 14　术中血管造影证实腘动脉的小的假性动脉瘤（箭头）。注意血管中度狭窄，远侧血流好

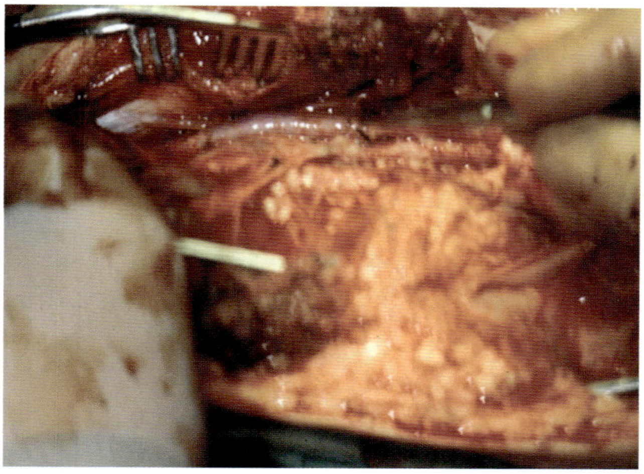

图 15　腘动脉和假性动脉瘤切除，动脉用逆行自体大隐静脉修复

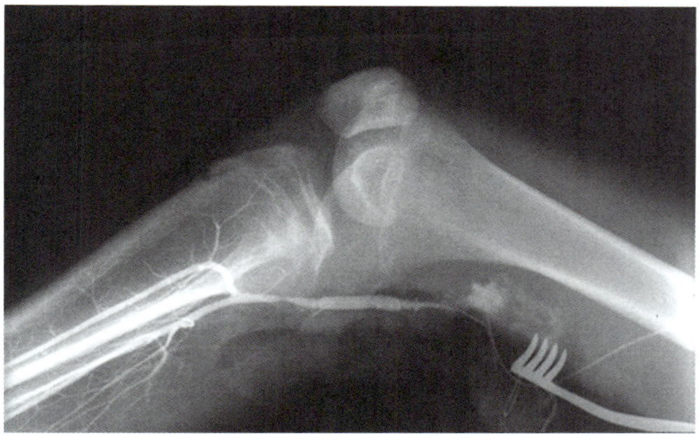

图 16　术中完成血管造影，见所有远侧小腿血管通畅

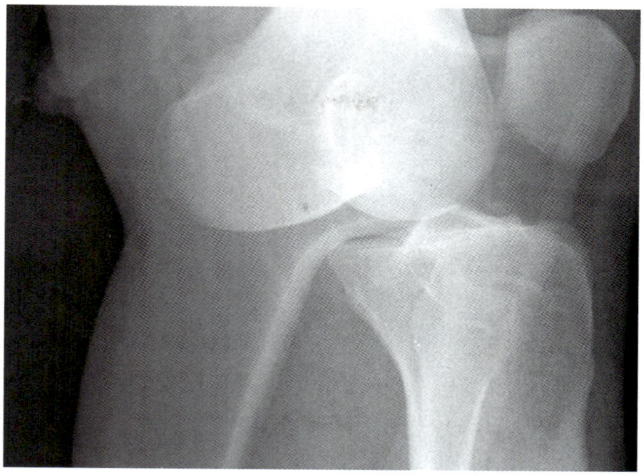

图 17　35 岁男性行人被撞导致双膝关节脱位，左腿缺血，右腿无缺血。患者可疑腹部钝伤，需要剖腹探查和广泛节段性小肠切除

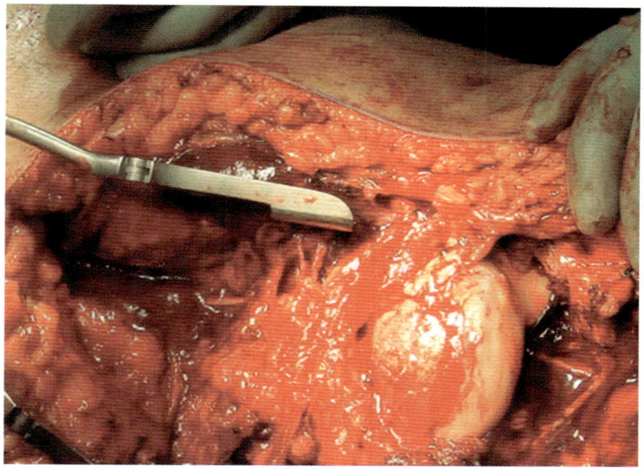

图 18　左膝显露，注意脱位以及关节囊和韧带破坏

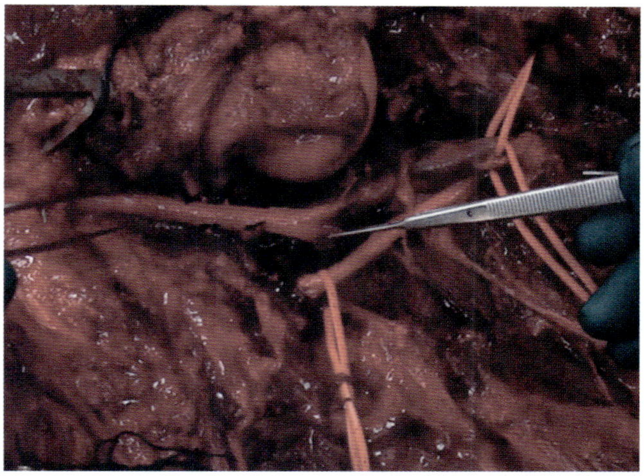

图 19　患者可疑右胫前动脉和胫腓干完全撕脱。Gerald 镊指着损伤部位

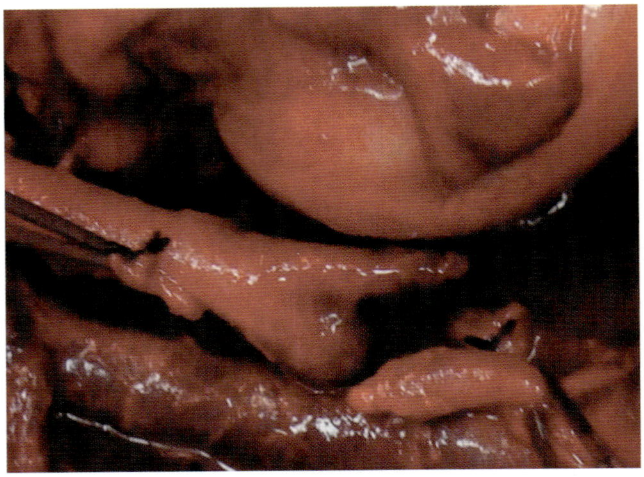

图 20 切断的胫前动脉和胫腓动脉的近端、远端血栓的近距离照片

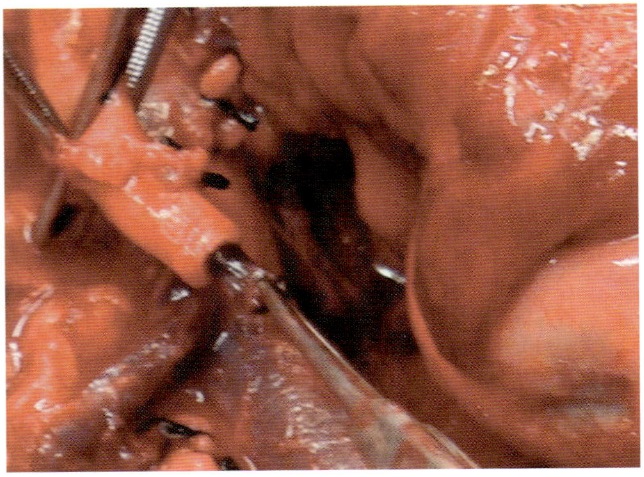

图 23 从近端取出的血栓

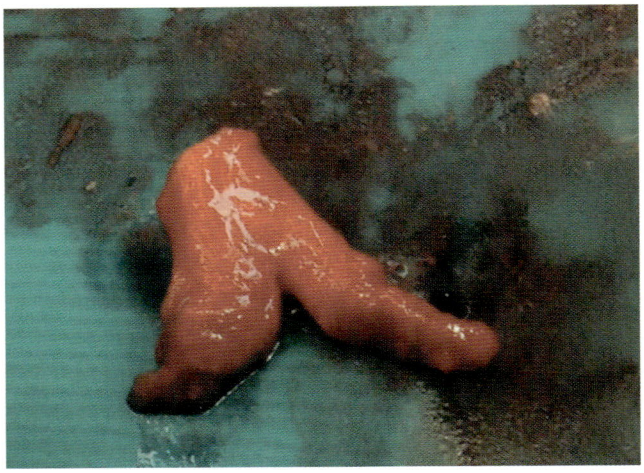

图 21 切除的标本

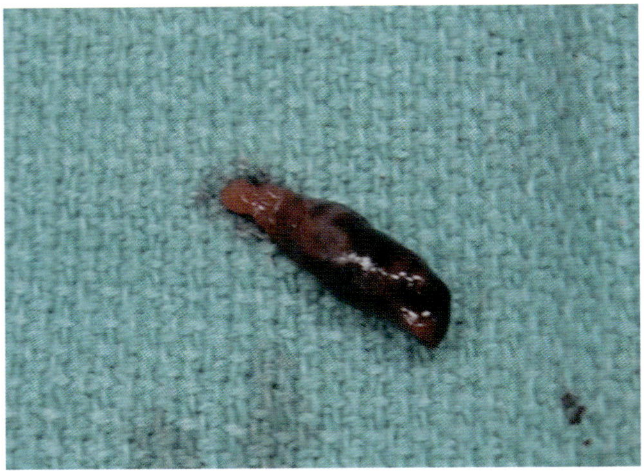

图 24 去除的血栓已经蔓延到近端腘动脉。取栓避免了近端血栓进一步蔓延

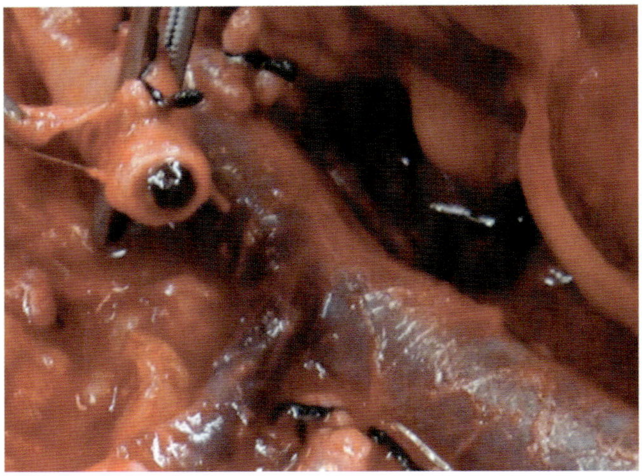

图 22 近端腘动脉的血栓，注意腘静脉

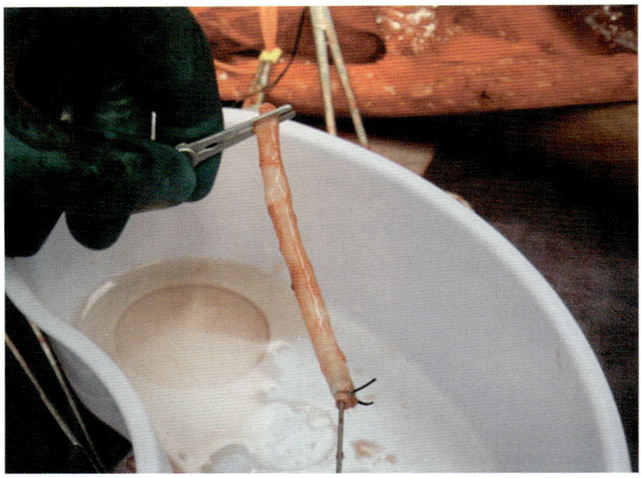

图 25 提取自体大隐静脉，用肝素盐水扩张制备

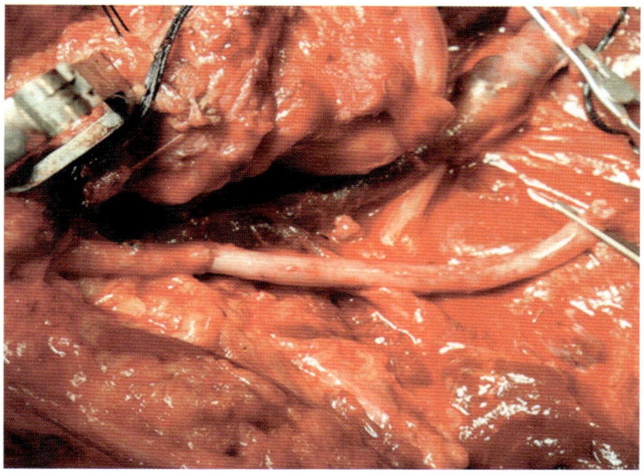

图 26　近端吻合完成

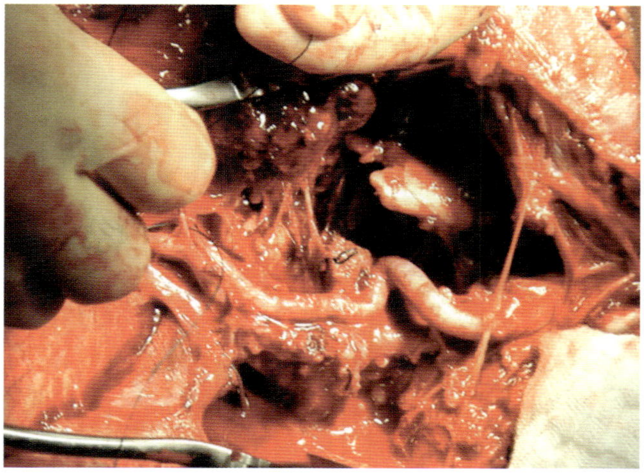

图 29　55 岁男性摩托车撞伤。患者可疑“浮动膝”和远端股骨粉碎性骨折和近端胫腓骨骨折。注意扭曲和有血栓的腘动脉和破坏的膝关节

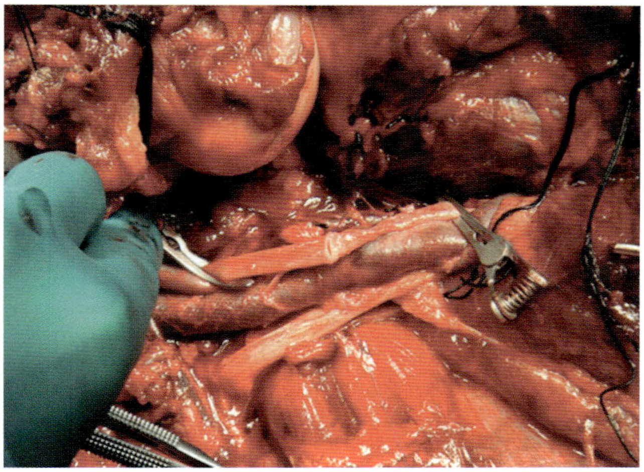

图 27　远端吻合基本完成，注意哈巴狗钳

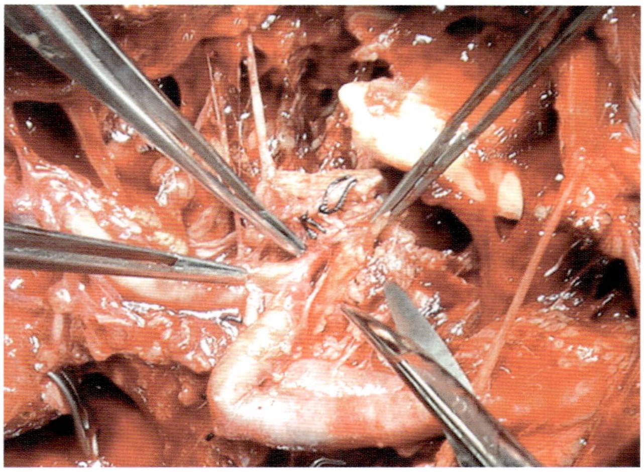

图 30　远侧动脉分离，注意骨碎片。镊子指着胫前动脉和胫腓动脉起始处

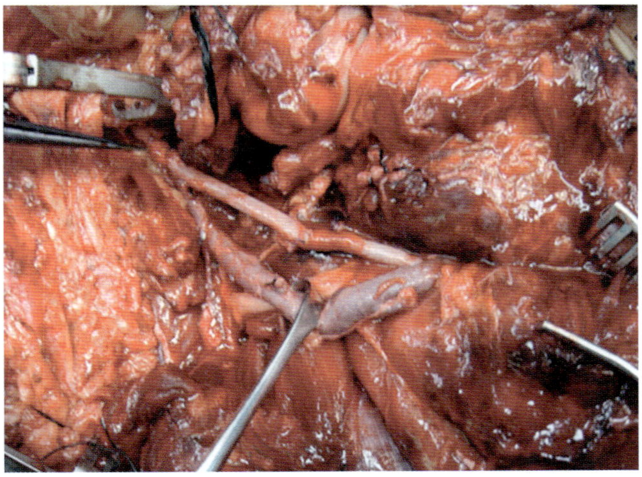

图 28　腘到胫腓干的逆行自体大隐静脉移植物显示 2 个吻合。胫前动脉结扎。注意腘静脉用 Cushing 静脉拉钩牵拉

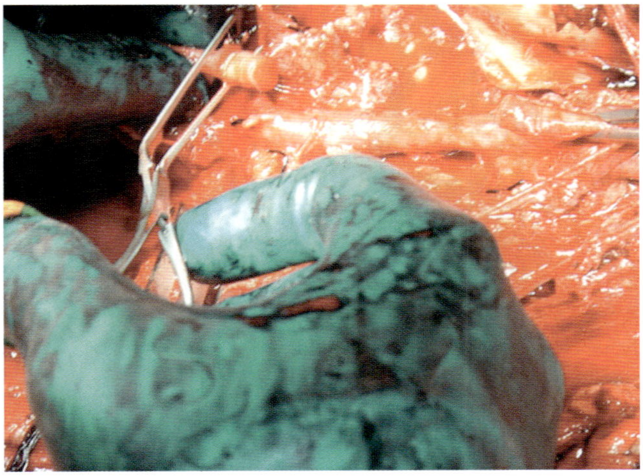

图 31　有血栓的腘动脉切除。远侧腘动脉未钳夹，注意 60° 的 DeBakey 钳

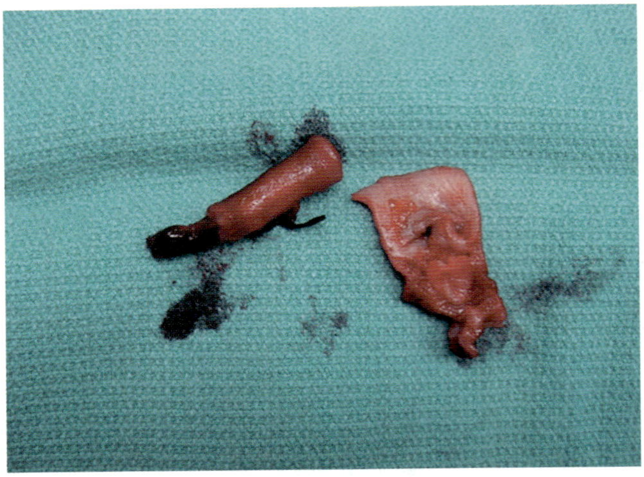

图 32 切除有血栓的腘动脉和内膜瓣

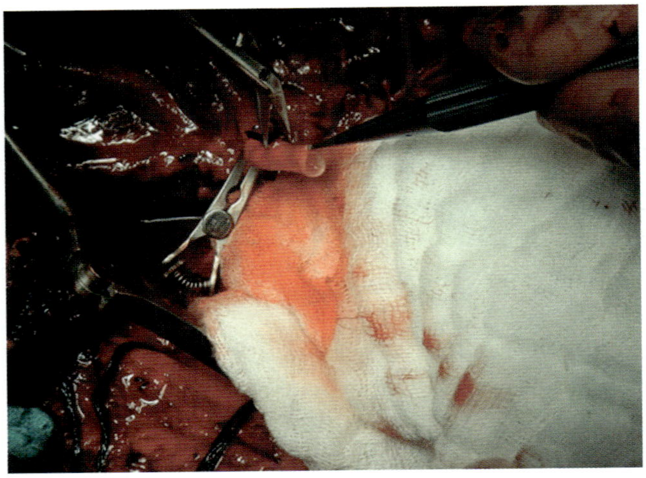

图 35 腘动脉再切除，准备吻合

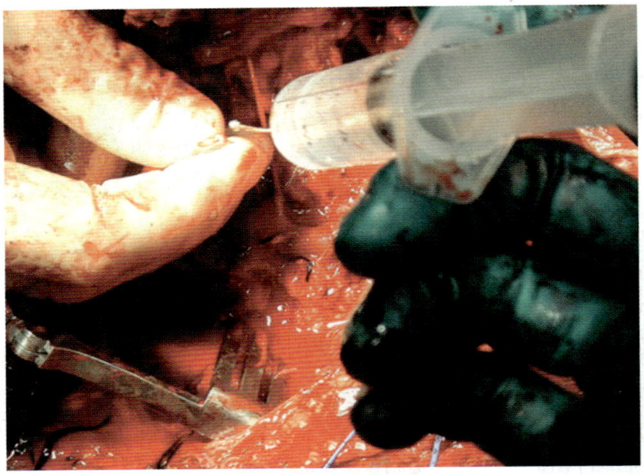

图 33 远侧腘动脉灌注肝素盐水

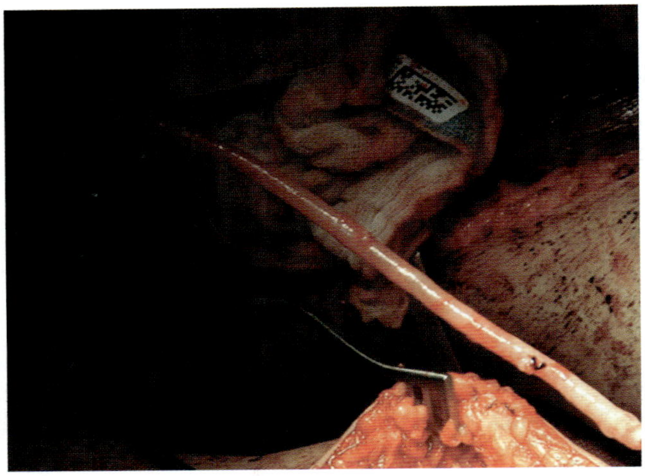

图 36 逆行自体大隐静脉移植物

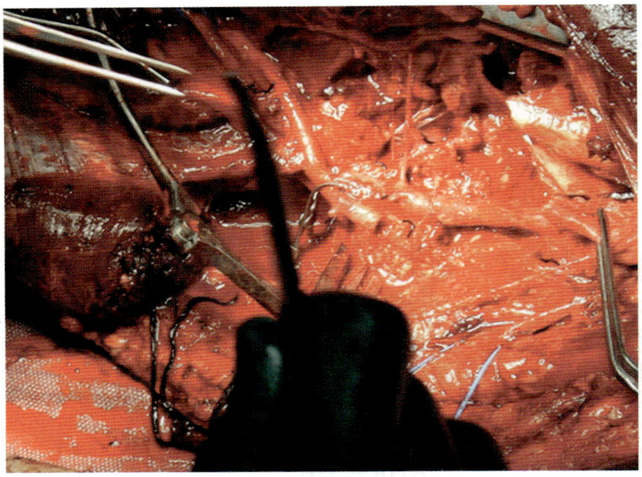

图 34 切除腘动脉

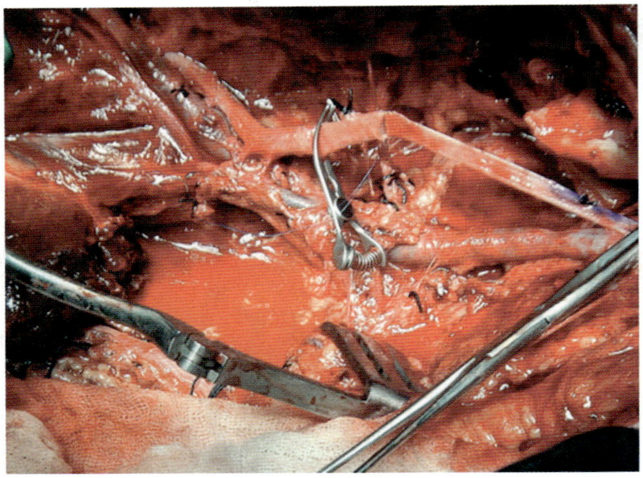

图 37 近端吻合基本完成。注意哈巴狗钳，标记静脉以保持位置

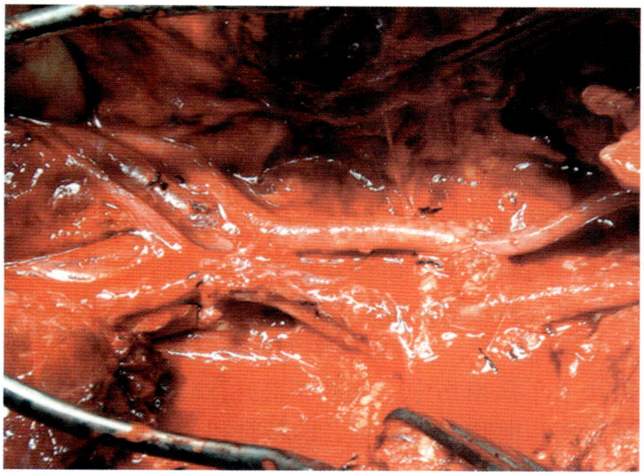

图 38　间置移植物完成

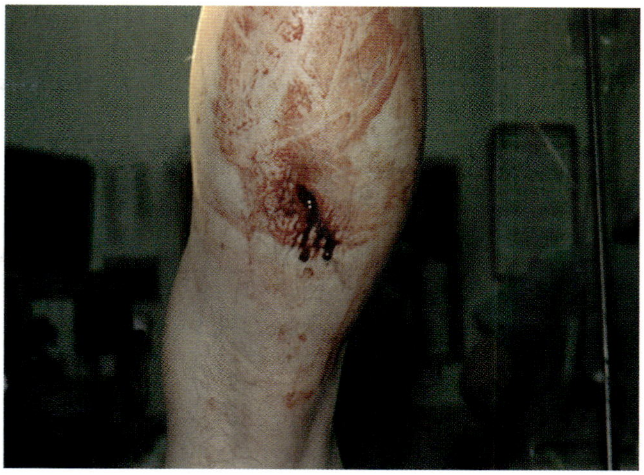

图 41　膝部枪伤患者，子弹出口提示腘动脉损伤

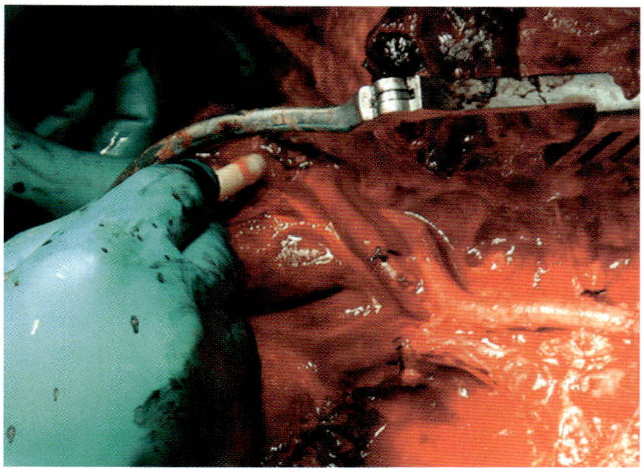

图 39　多普勒探头探查

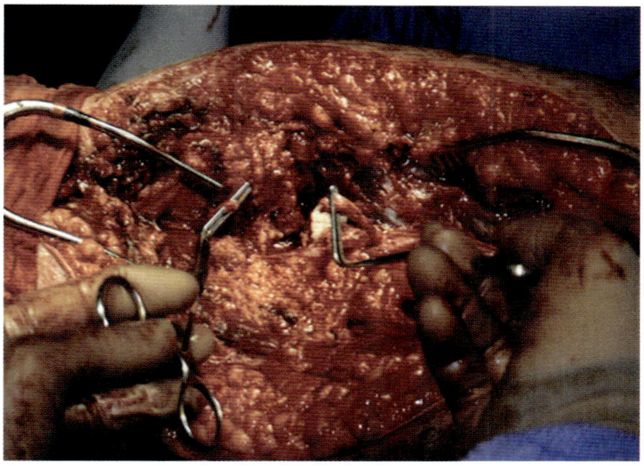

图 42　切除腘动脉

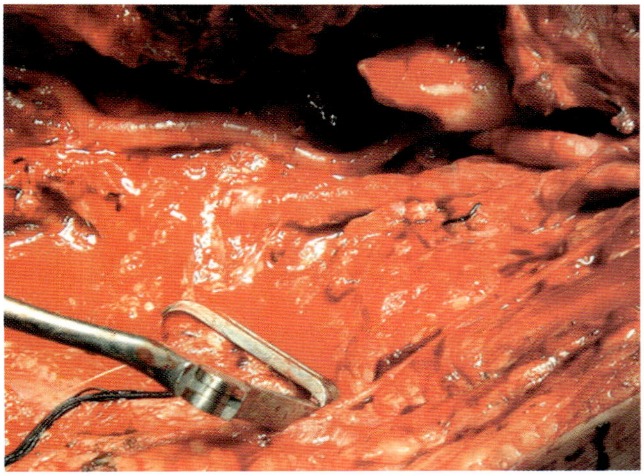

图 40　移植完成，注意骨碎片

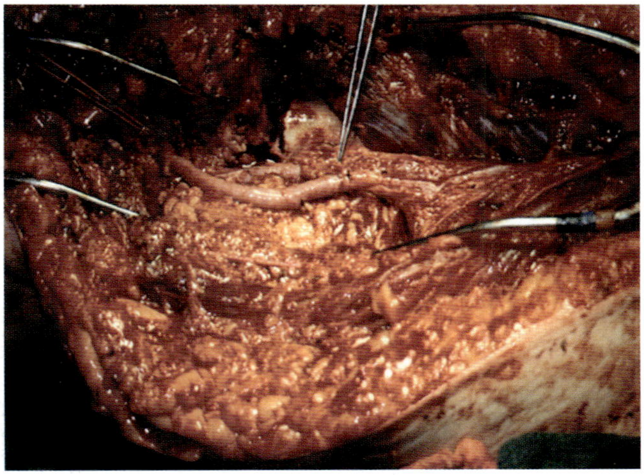

图 43　腘到腘逆行自体大隐静脉移植

任何不良后果。而这个研究患者数少，没有足够长的随访。本章的资深作者认为腘动脉是一种终末动脉，其分出的小分支具有低血流特征。此外，胫血管和腓动脉易产生严重的痉挛，这可能导致长时间缺血。因此推荐对所有腘动脉都必须行确切性修复（表 4）。

并发症发生率

腘动脉损伤的短期并发症包括急性血栓形成、远侧栓塞、出血、神经缺损和伤口感染。急性血栓形成有临床重要性，如果识别及时，能潜在逆转。术后早期应怀疑技术上的失误，必须立即手术处理。其他肢体并发症也由于非血管类型的损伤。在最初或随后的手术中失活组织的清创和异物去除是基本的。继发于修复破坏的血管的组织坏死和邻近伤口的感染可以导致致命出血。不幸的是，软组织覆盖是有限的。附加的外科皮瓣对保护修复的血管是必要的。

成功的肢体挽救和长期随访证实和腘血管损伤有关的残疾。出院的时候，患者已经接受了骨修复，需要广泛的康复，行走时需要机械装置的帮助。骨折不愈合、膝关节不稳定和骨髓炎也是众所周知的创伤中普遍存在的骨科并发症。神经缺损，如继发于会阴神经损伤的足下垂，无论是原发的还是继发于未治疗的筋膜室综合征，都需要支撑物的放置和积极的物理治疗。在 Melton 的研究中，20% 的成功挽救肢体的病例出院时有足下垂。Wagner 的回顾性综述，发现暂时性或永久性腓神经功能不全发生率分别为 63% 和 37%。

在早期战争中，保肢策略被证明可减少腘血管损伤的高截肢率。在过去几十年中，各种回顾性分析表明，腘动脉损伤有更好的预后和更低的截肢率。几个研究报告，平民截肢率为 6% ~ 37%。如前所述，钝伤或车祸损伤中，截肢率高达 52.5%。肢体筋膜室高压和保肢在外伤时、诊断时和住院时要重点考虑。关于筋膜切开的时机有持续的争论，而在筋膜室综合征的情况下，迅速的四筋膜室切开是可行的。在一些已发表的文章中，作为不积极筋膜切开的结果，肢体缺失风险是严峻的。在 Fainzilber 等的回顾性研究中，在最初血管修复的时候筋膜切开，可将截肢率降低到至 1/6。

历史上，腘静脉损伤有明显的与下肢有关的并发症，包括深度腿水肿、筋膜室综合征、血栓性静脉炎、慢性静脉功能不全和肺栓子。结扎导致的急性腘静脉中断的后果和后续静脉高压的发展以及腿水肿在 Rich 评估越南血管注册的研究中提及。腘静脉结扎有 51% 的明显水肿概率，而腘静脉修复只有 13%。这个观察明确证实无论何时，只要可能，修复静脉保护以流出道的重要性（表 5）。

表 4　腘动脉和腘静脉损伤的外科治疗

		腘损伤		静脉移植物		人工血管		一期修复		结扎		其他	
作者	年	动脉	静脉	动脉	静脉	动脉	静脉	动脉	静脉	动脉	静脉	动脉	静脉
Jaggers	1982	56	29	19.6%	13.8%	39.3%	6.9%	25%	70%		10.3%		
Downs	1986	58	17	60%		5%		34.5%	41.2				
Krige	1987	28	12	42.8%	25%	14.3%		35.7%	66.7%	1	8.3%		
Martin	1994	40	16	47.5%	56%	12.5%	18.7%	40%	25%				
Fainzilber	1995	73	42	41%	26.2%	15%	9.5%	19%	40.5%		23.8%	25%	
Melton	1997	90	28	51.1%	3.6%	2.2%	4.4%	43.3%	82%				
Hafez	2001	237		55.7%		6%		16.5%					
Yahya	2005	17	4	53%		6%		17.6%	50%				
Degiannis	2007	32				12.5%							
Callcut	2009	33	11	73%				27%					
Franz	2011	12				91.7%		8.3%					

表 5　腘血管损伤导致的截肢率

作者	年	总计	一期	二期	钝伤	穿通伤
Jaggers	1982			14.8%		
Downs	1986	28%	8%	22.4%	23%	20%
Krige	1987	10.7%			25%	0
Martin	1994	15%			43%	0
Fainzilber	1995	16.5%			47%	6.2%
Melton	1997	25%	11%	14%	36%	18%
Hafez	2001	27%	8.5%	18.5%		
Yahya	2005	26.3%	10.5%	15.5%	23%	33.3%
Mullerix	2006	14.5%			18%	9%
Degiannis	2007	18%	3%	15.6%		
Callcut	2009	14%	5.6%	8.3%	11.7%	50%
Kauvar	2011	9.7%				
Franz	2011	18.7%	6.2%	12.5%		

预后和死亡率

在城市创伤中心，表现为单独的腘血管损伤（排除相关的胸腹部和头部损伤）的患者中，与下肢血管创伤有关的死亡风险始终是低的。考虑到死亡可以预防，院前动脉大出血仍是一个因素，但在现场和在创伤中心积极使用止血带提高了生存率。2个系列的 NTDB 分析指出，总死亡率为 1.3%，而 Mullenix 等分析发现在院死亡率为 4.5%，不同的机械损伤间没有显著差别。在 Fabian 的研究中有 164 例腘损伤，13 例死于几种情况，包括头部损伤、肺栓塞、感染和术后出血。一些回顾性研究表明多发创伤性损伤有相似的预后，死亡率为 1% ~ 6%（表 6）。

表 6　腘血管损伤的生存率

作者	年	患者数	死亡数	生存率
Jaggers	1982	61	0	100%
Downs	1986	63	4	93.7%
Krige	1987	28	0	100%
Martin	1994	40	1	97.5%
Fainzilber	1995	80	3	96.25%
Melton	1997	102	5	95%
Mullerix	2006	1 395	63	95.5%
Callcut	2009	35	0	100%
Kauvar	2011	226	3	98.7%
Franz	2011	16	0	100%

结论

腘血管损伤无论在平民还是军事领域都有显著的并发症发生率。这些损伤本身是从入院到出院的一个严峻的挑战。虽然整体的发病率仍是低的，灾难性的后果如肢体缺失和永久的残疾是重大的风险。涉及保肢和生存率的成功的预后来源于早期诊断和迅速的外科干预。一个多学科原则的方法获得了巨大成功，包括创伤、骨科、整形外科的参与，这些仍然是腘血管损伤护理的一个特点。

临时血管分流

David V. Feliciano 著
张学民 译

大多数颈、躯干和周围血管损伤可以由普外科、创伤外科或血管外科医生用单一技术修复。而特定损伤部位和复合伤需要更多的显露的高级技术和革新的手术方法，以保全肢体甚至是生命。部分复合伤如下：在颅底的颈动脉损伤，颈动脉损伤合并食管、气管损伤，后部伤口或上纵隔或胸廓出口的动静脉瘘，腹部合并血管损伤，肝后下腔静脉损伤，来自肢体的伤口附近的出血，腹股沟枪伤，肢体血管损伤表面软组织缺失，GustiloⅢC肢体开放性骨折。虽然临时血管分流在选定的颈和躯干血管损伤中偶尔使用，列在这里的周围血管复合伤是很常用的指征。

定义

临时性血管分流定义为腔内成形管道用于临时维持动脉流入道 / 静脉流出道。

历史回顾

Alexis Carrel（1873–1944），1912 年的诺贝尔生理学或药学奖金得主，1911 年首次描述将表面涂石蜡的玻璃管插入狗的腹主动脉。在 1911 后，早期临床使用的血管分流管主要由 Walker 等描述。银管作为血管分流管在第一次世界大战期间由法国外科医生 Theodore Tuffier (1857–1929) 教授使用。皇家外科学院（英）前主席 George H. Makins 在他题为《*血管枪击伤，在 1914–1918 年世界大战中法国得到的发现和经验*》的一战后的教科书中充分描述了血管分流管的使用。

塑料分流管在第二次世界大战中由美国外科医生使用，希望随着分流管 / 导管栓塞，侧支循环得以建立。1950 年，Clatworthy 和 Varco 描述了使用“小孔聚乙烯分流管预防长时间钳夹阻断胸主动脉导致的机械休克”。1952 年，Creighton A. Hardin 发表了在创伤和选定的血管手术使用“聚乙烯分流管”的特别突出的临床和实验室报告。

1971 年，来自以色列 Beer-Seba 的 Eger、Golcman、Goldstein 和 Hirsch 首次描述了临时使用分流管。作者描述他们的分流管来自“合适直径和长度的常规的聚乙烯管”。有趣的是，他们在管道中间设置了一个三通适配器，可以往里面注射肝素。在 Eger 等的报告后，又有连续系列的文献报告在平民和军事中心使用临时血管分流。

临时血管分流的指征

7 个公认的临时血管分流指征如下：①颈内动脉在颈部Ⅲ区（从下颌角到颅底）的复杂的修复；②肢体 Gustilo ⅢC 开放性骨折；③当创伤后的复杂的血管再生需要灌注；④上肢再植前对离断部分灌注；⑤周围血管损伤出血患者“损伤控制”；⑥多发腹内损伤包括腹部血管损伤、复杂的腹部血管损伤或躯干血管损伤近端出血的“损伤控制”；⑦颈、躯干或周围血管损伤患者的“损伤控制”和有大量伤亡人数的手术团队或有限的资源和有限的血管损伤手术经验（军事线条图）（图 1）。

Ⅲ区需要复杂修复的颈内动脉并不常见。有许多方法控制继发于Ⅲ区穿通伤或颈部肿瘤切除术中的不幸事故的颈内动脉出血。这些方法包括经皮送入球囊导管做外部压塞、经颈路径送入球囊导管做内部压塞、植入血管内支架、手术结扎、手术修复。虽然球囊压塞或手术结扎是救命的，但将患者置于脑缺血或脑梗塞的风险中。血管内支架是一个吸引人的选项，取决于创伤团队暂时控制出血的能力、介入医生的经验和颈内动脉损伤的程度。如果用压迫或球囊压塞不能完全控制出血，就需要手术修复。动脉的显露需要强制性颞下颌关节的半脱位，在牙间用线或单皮质螺钉和金属线或使用垂直下颌支截骨术。由于血管控制延迟，在复杂修复（节段切除和端端吻合或放入间置移植物）前临时插入腔内分流，如果颈内动脉远端回血好可以做分流。

下肢 GustiloⅢC 开放性骨折定义为任何合并动脉损伤需要修复以保肢的开放骨折。有许多评分系统或流程以帮助决定是否试图保肢或立即截肢是适

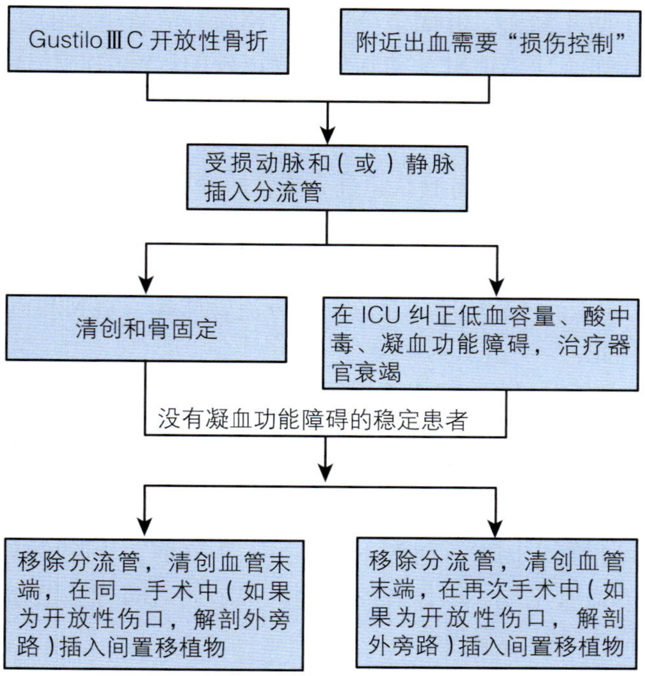

图 1　复杂骨折或需要“损伤控制”的患者使用分流管的流程图。ICU，重症监护室

当的。当试图保肢时，立即插入临时动脉，如果需要静脉分流以恢复足或手的血流的流入和流出。如此骨科创伤团队可以清创软组织和骨、稳定开放性骨折，无须考虑持续的缺血。在完成骨固定的情况下，依据患者的条件，创伤血管团队重新移除分流管，实施确定性的血管修复。

当肢体创伤后急性单一个复杂的血管重建，如解剖外旁路时，插入分流管对维持足或手的流入/流出血流是适当的。当使用确定性的移植物时，在近端和远端吻合口之间做适当的移植物隧道。

一个在手腕、前臂或上臂的“干净的”断肢可以通过再植术治疗。这种复杂修复的决心当然取决于患者整体的健康状况、其他损伤的大小、血流动力学状态的表现和专业知识。如果适合再植，在做清创和肢体缩短手术时，截肢部分可以用长的临时分流管连接受损肢体，提供灌注和引流。

周围血管损伤出血伴随低血压、酸中毒，如果在复苏过程中使用大量输血会产生一过性凝血功能障碍。深部低温（<35℃）、严重的代谢性酸中毒（动脉 pH<7.2）、凝血功能障碍（凝血实验 1.5× 正常值）推荐“损伤控制”的手术步骤。在出血控制的同时纠正这些代谢问题会需要几个小时，这时患者的生命仍处于危险中。无论是大的动脉或静脉损伤（股总血管、股血管、腘血管、胫腓血管），临时动脉和（或）静脉分流使保存受损肢体作为复苏（复温、输血或血成分）措施得以继续。

有多发腹内损伤的患者包括腹部血管损伤、单一复杂腹部血管损伤（如近端肠系膜上动脉接近受损的胰腺、髂总动脉或髂外动脉损伤邻近结肠损伤污染区），或躯干血管损伤附近出血，应插入临时动脉分流管替代正式修复。如前所述，真实的肠系膜上动脉或髂总动脉或髂外动脉损伤，因为结扎经常导致灾难性的术后并发症。在第二次世界大战中，DeBakey 和 Simeone 的经典的动脉结扎研究报告，髂总动脉或髂内动脉结扎分别导致 53.8% 和 46.7% 的截肢率。在损伤控制的剖腹探查后，患者在 ICU 中再次复温和复苏。在这期间，也应做好动脉重建（原位用大网膜覆盖或解剖外旁路）的计划。

今年由于前述原因，在伊拉克和阿富汗救护站（Echelon Ⅱ）的前线外科队用了大量的临时血管分流管。一旦受伤的士兵转运到合适的战斗支援医院（Echelon Ⅲ），将分流管移除，完成正式的血管修复。临时血管分流管不允许用于从阿富汗到德国法兰克福附近的地区医疗中心（Echelon Ⅳ）的航班上。

可用的分流管

虽然静脉内插管可以用作临时血管分流管，许多历史上用于颈动脉内膜切除术的患者现使用分流管，它成为平民创伤中心最常用的方法。Argyle 颈动脉分流管（Kendall、Mansfield、Mass.）是硬质的、有锥形头，可以切割到恰当的长度，可用的有 8～14 F 大小（图 2）。Argyle 胸廓造口术的导管有恰当的大小，可以作为肢体大静脉的临时分流管插入如股总静脉、股静脉和腘静脉。Javid 颈动脉分流管（Bard 周围血管，Tempe, Ariz.）是质软的、可弯曲的分流管，两端有扩张段，Javid 钳可以夹持。该分流管 17 F 大小，设计用来在颈动脉内膜切除术中放在术野外。Pruitt-Inahara 颈动脉分流管（LeMaitre Vascular, Inc., Burlington, Mass.）是质软、可弯曲的分流管，两端有可充盈球囊，以维持分流管位置。它有 7 F 大小，有 T 形部分，允许冲洗、动脉造影或注入抗凝药。Sundt 颈内和颈外动脉内膜切除术的分流管（Integra NeuroSciences, Plainsboro, N.J.）是质软、可弯曲的、不锈钢强化的管。它的两端有锥形的球防止漏血，可用于 3×4 mm 到 4×5 mm 直径的血管。临时保肢分流管（temporary limb salvage

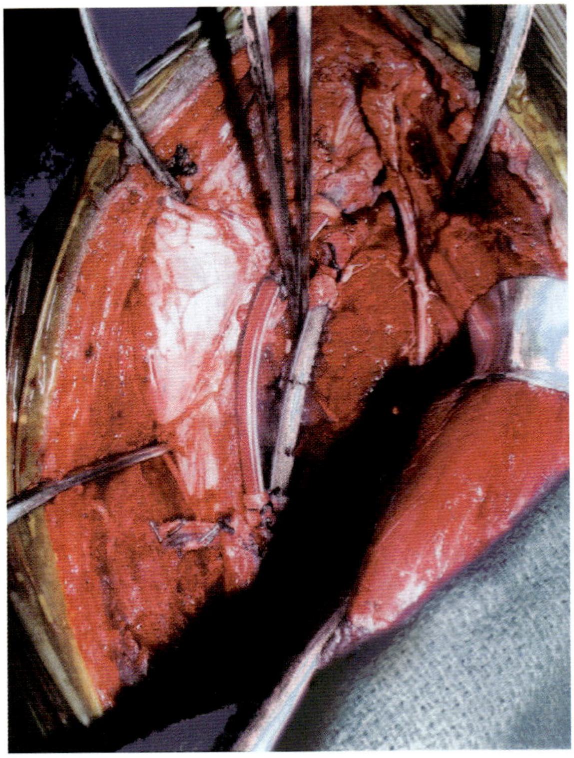

图 2 在左腘动脉和腘静脉的 Argyle 分流管（8F）

shunt，TLSS）(Vascutek Ltd., Renfrewshire, Scotland) 由 FDA（器械和放射健康中心）于 2007 年 2 月 9 日批准。这种分流管偶尔被美军军医使用，但目前在美国平民创伤中心不可用。

手术技术

近端和远端控制通过使用血管钳、哈巴狗钳或 Silastic 血管带控制损伤的血管。在血管的损伤节段或损伤末端清创至未损伤的内膜。如果硬质的 Argyle 分流管或胸腔闭式引流管插入，最大的尺寸要适应横断断端血管。分流之后在一端修剪，使整体长度比血管两端的间隙长度长 4 cm。2-0 丝线缠绕在特制的分流管的中点，并用止血钳在同一点阻断分流管。钝（修整的）端（比锥形段大的管腔）轻轻送入动脉近端或静脉远端约 1.5 cm。2-0 丝带缠绕在近端动脉或远端静脉，向下勒紧以防漏血，并固定分流管的末端。开放止血钳以确认动脉或静脉血流正常，并再次应用。分流管的远端平滑端轻轻送入动脉远端或静脉近端 1.5 cm。再一次，2-0 丝线用于防止漏血，并固定分流管。移除分流管中部的止血钳，应当能触及动脉分流管以外的远端的动脉搏动，多普勒在踝或腕能听到脉搏。当植入静脉分流管时，近端静脉扩张是分流管通畅的表现。可以用手持多普勒设备确认超过分流管的静脉回流。

如果用 Javid 分流管，Javid 前送到分流管末端，紧邻膨胀区域，以防漏血和稳定分流管。用 Pruitt-Inahara 分流管时，充盈末端分流管球囊，直到漏血停止。

一旦患者和肢体稳定，移除分流管，按 100U/kg 体重给予静脉内肝素（如果还没应用）。血管止血钳、哈巴狗钳或血管环用在血管末端分流管前，之后被移除。Argyle 分流管或胸腔闭式引流管用 2-0 丝带系牢固定。血管末端要进一步修剪，去除破碎的血管末端。以作者的经验，常须插入间置移植物而不是行端端吻合。

预后

至今美国已发表的最大平民研究中，在城市创伤中心，超过 10 年，将近 9% 的血管损伤患者插入了血管内分流管。7 例创伤当天死亡或第一次手术就截肢的患者被排除，66 例患者（8.4%）119 例血液分流（72 例动脉，47 例静脉）可用于综述。枪伤作为损伤机制的有 62%，钝伤 36%，刺伤（1 例）2%。插入分流管主要指征是“损伤控制”（47%）和“非损伤控制”（53%）（Gustilo ⅢC 骨折为 42%，需要临时分流者为 9%，需要肢体再植者为 2%，表 1）。正如预料的那样，“损伤控制”组有更糟的入院时的状况（-15.2 vs -7.2，P<0.001），需要更多的输血（15.2 vs 8.0 U，P=0.002），和更高的截肢率（23% vs. 11%，P=0.003）（表 1）。

60 例患者植入周围血管分流管，躯干或内脏损伤插入分流管者有 6 例（3 例髂外动脉，2 例肠系膜上动脉，1 例锁骨下动脉）。在插入分流管的患者中，最常插入的动脉位置在股浅动脉（21 例）、腘动脉（12 例）和肱动脉（10 例）。最常插入的静脉位置是腘静脉（15 例）和股静脉（12 例，表 2）。14 F 的 Argyle 分流管最常用，用于 18 例动脉损伤（17 例周围动脉，1 例躯干动脉）和 12 例周围静脉损伤（表 3）。

30 例患者（30/66=45%）插入 2 条临时血管内分流管，1 例患者在最初手术时有 3 条分流管。这

表 1 血管内临时分流指征

	损伤控制组			非损伤控制组					
	全部损伤控制	肢体	躯干	全部非损伤控制	Gustilo Ⅲc 开放性骨折	准备期间灌注	肢体再植	总计	*P* 值
患者数（%）	31（47%）	25（38%）	6（9%）	35（53%）	28（42%）	6（9%）	1(2%)	66(100%)	-
平均 BD	15.2+1.5	15.3±1.7	15.1±2.4	7.2±0.8	6.8±3.5	7.2±9.7	-	10.7±7.8	< 0.001
平均 ISS	18±1.7	18±2.0	17±3.1	13±1.3	13±1.6	11±1.8	9	15±1.1	0.016
平均 PRBCs (U)	15.2±2.2	12.6±1.8	26.0±7.3	7.9±0.7	8.0±4.4	10.7±7.7	18	11.8±9.7	.0002
筋膜切开率	86%	92%	67%	74%	68%	100%	100%	82%	0.19
平均“留管”时间（h）	23.5±2.8	23.0±3.2	25.7±6.6					23.5±2.8	
截肢率	23%	20%	33%	11%	14%	0%	0%	17%	0.003
分流血栓形成率	10%	4%	33%	0%	0%	0%	0%	5%	0.06
生存率	81%	84%	67%	94%	100%	67%	100%	88%	0.09

From Subramanian A, Vercruysse G, Dente C, et al: A decade's experience with temporary intravascular shunts at a civilian level I trauma center. *J Trauma* 65:316-326, 2008

BD, 碱缺失; ISS, 损伤严重度评分; PRBCs, 浓缩红细胞; prep, 准备

表 2 临时血管内分流的解剖学分布

分流管类型	n(%) SFA (*n*=21)	POA(*n*=21)	POV(*n*=15)	SFV(*n*=12)	BrA(*n*=10)
14F Argyle	9 (39%；全部为男性)	7 (33%;6 男，1 女)	7 (47%；全部为男性)	5 (42%；全部为男性)	
12F Argyle	5 (22%；4 男，1 女)	2 (10%；全部为女性)	3 (20%；2 男，1 女)		3 (30%；全部为男性)
10F Argyle		6 (29%;5 男，1 女)			3 (30%；全部为男性)
24F CT				2 (17%；全部为男性)	
20F CT			2 (13%；全部为男性)	1 (8%；女性)	
18F CT			1 (7%；女性)	1 (8%；男性)	
16F CT			1 (7%；女性)	2 (17%；全部为男性)	
9F P-I	7 (30%；全部为男性)	6 (29%;1 男，5 女)	1 (7%；男性)		3 (30%；全部为男性)
5F ped FT					1 (30%；男孩)

From Subramanian A, Vercruysse G, Dente C, et al: A decade's experience with temporary intravascular shunts at a civilian level I trauma center. *J Trauma* 65:316-326, 2008

Argyle, Argyle 分流管; BrA, 肱动脉; CT, 胸管; FT, 饲管; ped, 儿科; P-I, Pruitt-Inahara 分流管; POA, 腘动脉; POV, 腘静脉; SFA, 股浅动脉; SFV 股浅静脉

31 例患者第一次手术结束时在手术室留下 1 条或多条分流管，平均分流时间为 23.5 ±15.7 h。有趣的是，分流管在动脉留置的最长时间为 71 h，静脉为 35 h。

表 3 24 F Argyle 分流管的使用

受损血管	患者数（%）
SFA	9（30）
POA	7（23）
POV	7（23）
SFV	5（17）
EIA	1（3）
AxA	1（3）
总计	30（100）

From Subramanian A, Vercruysse G, Dente C, et al: A decade's experience with temporary intravascular shunts at a civilian level I trauma center. *J Trauma* 65:316-326, 2008.

AxA, 腋动脉；EIA, 髂外动脉；POA, 腘动脉；POV, 腘静脉；SFA, 股浅动脉；SFV, 股浅静脉

119 例受损血管中的 5 例（4.2%）在分流后有必要早期截肢或切除末端器官。3 例病例有无法挽救的肢体的指征，2 例分流管栓塞。在移除分流管后，其他 114 例血管损伤中，89 例间置移植物治疗（58 例大隐静脉，31 例人工血管），14 例端端吻合，11 例结扎。在此文章中，总生存率是 88%，保肢率是 74%，很少使用抗凝。这个研究的主要结论是适当直径的临时分流管保持原位很难移动。可维持手术部位的动脉流入 / 静脉流出。主要的分流指征是：①需要“损伤控制”的手术；②肢体 GustiloⅢC 骨折；③复杂血管损伤的患者在准备血管重建前须恢复灌注；④手、前臂或上肢再植。其他近期研究确认，在美国创伤中心中临时血管内分流管未被充分使用。

总结实践要点

1. 年轻患者伴随血管损伤的痉挛，可能须使用罂粟碱，轻轻扩张受损动脉远端，以插入最大的分流管。
2. 如果邻近的重要的大静脉被结扎，动脉分流管的通畅性会受损。套在结扎静脉上的带子应当移除并插入临时静脉分流管。以前未注意到的动脉分流管的血栓形成，不可避免地与远侧肌肉严重受损和缺乏适当的静脉回流有关。
3. 许多严重损伤患者需要损伤控制分流或 GustiloⅢC 开放性骨折分流。有一些术中和术后凝血功能障碍的要注意。在大量输血（“损伤控制复苏”）时，凝血功能障碍的发生率和程度大大降低。即便如此，由于患者损伤或相关损伤的严重程度，常在插入分流管后不敢用肝素抗凝。如前所述，没有前瞻性数据提示术后使用肝素会降低公开报道的分流管中等程度的血栓的发生率。
4. 肢体分流管经常用于术后暴露在 ICU 的污染环境中的开放性伤口。移除分流管的时候如果没有用健康的肌肉覆盖原位的间置移植物的话，强制性使用解剖外血管旁路。

第 11 章　肌肉骨骼系统、周围神经系统损伤

上肢骨折：骨科处理

Steven Kalandiak 和 Stephen M. Quinnan 著
王天兵 译

不同的上肢骨折和脱位有很大的区别，有的需要很轻微的干预，而有些为可能危及患肢甚至危及生命的急性事件。治疗计划须根据损伤类型（例如脱位）、损伤机制、软组织状态、是否累及血管和神经、是否合并其他损伤决定。本章主要讨论诊断过程的几个重要事件、具体损伤说明和相应的治疗方案。

开放性骨折

开放的软组织损伤使得骨折的治疗更加紧急。开放性骨折的定义是骨折或骨折端的血肿通过软组织的伤口与外界环境相通。开放性骨折可由骨折断端从软组织内向外穿透皮肤而致，也可能由外界向软组织内穿透至骨折断端所致。无论哪种情况，外界环境的污染会增加感染和骨折愈合并发症的风险。如果伤口位于骨折患肢的同一节段，这种骨折最初也当作开放性骨折对待，直到我们可以证实其并不是开放性骨折。表 1 所示为开放性骨折的分级系统。据报道，Ⅰ型、Ⅱ型和ⅢA 型开放性骨折的感染率通常比较低，约百分之几，但是ⅢB 型开放性骨折的感染率为 10%～50%，而ⅢC 型的感染率可达 25%～50%。

开放性骨折的治疗首先需要及时的抗生素治疗 / 预防破伤风、紧急灌洗并在手术室清创。虽然许多人仍然坚持清创时间在 6～8 h 内，但是一些具有专门骨创伤科室的医疗中心发现，夜间来院的开放性骨折患者，待治疗开放性骨折的医疗资源都更容易获得之后，延迟至次日早上再处理并不增加感染率。真正危及生命和患肢的急诊疾病，例如血管损伤、筋膜室综合征、严重挤压伤，是不适用于这些医疗中心的这种“新治疗原则”。并且，这些真正的急诊患者在一般情况足够稳定以接受急诊手术时，须尽快地送入手术室。

不管哪种情况，皮肤和筋膜层打开直到可以充分暴露内部全部损伤的范围。所有被污染的组织、坏死的肌肉和失活的骨干都须被仔细清除。尚没有确定是否已经失活的组织可以原位保留，并且须定期进行手术室清创，直到所有组织都有活性、失活组织彻底清除。进一步行骨折的初步固定或者确定性固定，并且须用适当的抗生素持续治疗。很显然，短期大剂量抗生素治疗对开放性骨折是有效的，不须在骨折愈合的整个过程使用抗生素治疗。指南推荐如下：

Ⅰ型和Ⅱ型开放性骨折（包括有软组织损伤的闭合性骨折）：入院时给予 1～2 g 的头孢类抗生素，然后每 6～8 h 应用 1 g 抗生素，持续 24～48 h。

Ⅲ型开放性骨折：加用覆盖革兰氏阳性菌和阴性菌的抗生素治疗——3～5 mg/kg · d 的氨基糖苷类抗生素，作为头孢类抗生素的补充治疗。如为肾衰竭患者，这个剂量须调整至肾毒性最小的剂量。严重挤压伤、发生在农场的损伤、泥土污染的损伤患者须加用 200～400 万单位青霉素 G，每 4 h 给药一次。

脱位

脱位也须及时地评估伤情、诊断、治疗。由脱位的定义我们可知：当关节表面不再有接触时即为脱位。关节脱位经常根据病史及查体来作出诊断。

急性的脱位一般会剧痛，伴有肌痉挛和活动受限。对于具体的脱位，肢体表现为固定位置的特征。例如，肩关节前脱位表现为手臂外旋、轻度外展，内旋和内收均受限，肩关节的正常轮廓消失，肱骨头明显前突，肩峰下有明显的沟。

在处理这类损伤时，须在尝试复位之前行X线片检查来评估是否存在骨折。未行检查可能导致骨折进一步移位，产生严重不良后果。

关节脱位是毋庸置疑的急诊，因为它会导致神经血管的损害或者神经血管随着脱位时间的增加而进行性的缺损而恶化。延长脱位时间也会增加骨坏死的风险，而这种骨坏死的风险更常见于下肢脱位。骨坏死被认为可能是由于脱位导致关节囊张力增高，从而破坏了关节囊的血供的结果。

表1 开放性骨折的分型

Ⅰ型：伤口<1 cm，伤口轻度污染或有轻微软组织损伤的低能量损伤。无或少量粉碎性骨折。
Ⅱ型：伤口>1 cm，无广泛的软组织损伤。中度污染、中等程度粉碎性骨折。
Ⅲ型：软组织损伤广泛，包括肌肉、皮肤及神经血管结构有严重污染。骨折粉碎程度较高。
ⅢA型：尽管有广泛的撕脱伤、皮瓣形成或高能量损伤，骨折处仍有适当的软组织覆盖。无论伤口大小，如有严重的粉碎性骨折或多段骨折也属于这一型。
ⅢB型：广泛的软组织损伤和丢失，伴有骨膜剥脱、严重的污染和严重的粉碎性骨折。清创之后局部需要游离皮瓣覆盖。
ⅢC型：开放性骨折伴有必须要修复的动脉损伤。

伴有神经或血管损伤的脱位和骨折需要尽快复位，以减少受影响的部位的潜在和不可逆损伤的风险。复位后，需多次复查，以确定神经血管的损伤是否已经缓解。

枪伤

枪伤导致的骨折应特别注意，因为这种类型的骨折很难分类为开放性或闭合性。这种骨折是开放性还是闭合性取决于致伤武器是高速还是低速的。精确的分类尚有些难度，但是依据卫生局长办公室的创伤弹道学手册，出膛速度大于2 500 ft/s（1 ft=30.48 cm）定义为“高速”。这一点很重要，因为子弹的动能与它速度的平方直接相关，与它的质量呈线性相关。枪伤一般被看做高能量损伤，尽管其出膛速度很慢，因为爆破可以产生高能量。

大部分低速武器所致的骨折可以用抗生素治疗，也可以被当做闭合性骨折治疗，感染风险并不高。这种类型的骨折许多可以用闭合性骨折的方法处理，如功能性支具或石膏固定。如果按照开放性骨折治疗，就会发现骨折粉碎的范围比我们在X线片上能预见到得更广。

相对低速枪伤来讲，高速枪伤所致的骨折最好按照开放性骨折治疗。由于高速子弹穿过肢体的时候，不仅造成严重的粉碎性骨折，子弹还会在其间存留。其冲击波可以穿透软组织，并且造成皮下空腔，同时伴有肌肉和神经血管损伤。在这种情况下，及时的清创非常必要，须清除坏死的骨和肌肉组织，并且须多次清创，直至所有组织都可以判定是否存活。

由于冲击波效应，最初的损伤可能会导致神经功能障碍。当损伤为低速枪伤时，子弹产生的冲击波通常会导致暂时的神经失用，而不伴有神经裂伤。这类损伤不须立即探查，因为大多数损伤可以通过观察解决。如果存在持续的神经损伤，可在3～6周行肌电图（electromyogram，EMG）检查来评价神经恢复情况。高速枪伤需要更积极的治疗。损伤所致的空腔可能会非常大，以至于破坏神经，甚至有节段性缺损。因为空腔伤口本身需要急诊清创，受损的神经应该同时进行探查。如果神经有裂伤，尽可能地修复神经。然而，大部分病例的冲击波所致的神经损伤无法在首次的探查中判断损伤范围，患者可能需要延期探查来判断神经缺损的范围，并施行分阶段的神经移植术来重建。

筋膜室综合征

在1881年，Volkmann首次描述了由缺血导致的前臂屈肌的永久性挛缩。他认为其病理生理学机制为动脉功能不全和由于石膏或绷带过紧导致的静脉回流受阻。近百年来，关注点主要都放在了动脉问题上。因此，临床上一些进展指出应把筋膜室切开，探查动脉损伤，并行动脉修复。

在20世纪70和80年代，大家对于筋膜室综合征的病理生理机制有了新的认识。任何可以增加闭合的筋膜室软组织压力的因素都会阻碍静脉回流。如果这个因素持续不缓解，压力将超过动脉压，它升高至某一点会使毛细血管床血流停止。这种情况通常发生在筋膜室内舒张压达到 30 mmHg 时。如果情况持续，内部的肌肉将开始缺血、坏死，甚至收缩。在上肢损伤中，前臂最容易发生筋膜室综合征。

筋膜室综合征的症状和体征包括被动手指运动疼痛、前臂张力增高或肿胀、手的感觉异常或感觉减退。筋膜室内部压力的测量对于判断疑似病例是非常有帮助的，但是一般情况下，都是基于临床依据来诊断的。一旦急性筋膜室综合征诊断成立，就须行前臂的急诊筋膜切开减压，以释放压力，防止肌肉坏死和因前臂屈肌坏死而继发的手指挛缩。

前臂的枪伤即使不伴有骨折也须特别注意，因为发展为前臂筋膜室综合征的风险很高。因为前臂相应筋膜室内空间有限，动脉损伤出血进入筋膜室会使压力升高，我们须观察患者至少 8 ~ 12 h 来监测前臂压力升高的临床证据。

相对于急性筋膜室综合征来说，晚期的筋膜室综合征或者“挤压”综合征不需要常规减压。最近有研究表明，这种损伤常见于地震受害者，例如海地和其他地震等。如果肢体受到严重挤压，肌肉会马上发生坏死。不是因为压力升高导致肌肉坏死，而是因为肌肉先发生坏死，然后压力才升高。一旦肌肉发生了坏死，筋膜切开也无法阻止肌肉继续坏死，而且切开会把坏死的肌肉组织暴露在污染环境中，从而导致感染和截肢的风险增高。

影像学检查

对于骨折和脱位来说，正确的影像学检查在确定治疗方案之前非常重要。从理论上讲，在拍摄与损伤骨相邻的关节的 X 线片时，损伤肢体的正、侧位片也须同时拍摄。肩胛带的损伤应该拍摄最少 3 张标准的创伤系列片。这个系列包括一张真正的正位片（称为“Grashey”片），一张肩胛骨 Y 轴片和一张腋位片。如果没有拍到足够的 X 线片，一些隐匿的损伤可能会被漏诊。图 1 所示，一个肩关节后脱位被漏诊，直到最初损伤后 6 个月拍 MRI 时才发现。

肩胛带和肱骨损伤

胸锁关节脱位

在人体的主要关节里面，胸锁关节是骨性稳定最不佳的关节。事实上，胸锁关节的完整性由其周围的韧带组成。胸锁关节脱位是最少见的关节脱位之一，发生率可能占肩胛带损伤的 3%，但是在大多数创伤中心也比较常见，每年也可以遇到 1 ~ 2 例。胸锁关节前、后脱位的比例不确定，因为大多数报告关注更少见的后脱位，但是显然前脱位更常见。

这类损伤很难行影像检查，因为胸锁关节在标准 X 线片上与脊柱和肋骨重叠。一张“偶然的”体位片，以胸骨为顶点，头倾 45° 的正位 X 线胸片，偶尔可以发现脱位。但是 CT 检查可以最明确地证实这种脱位（图 2）。

由于纵隔和它的大血管邻近胸锁关节，如果准备行开放性手术，我们一般建议在手术室中复位治疗，且须通知附近的创伤团队。虽然大多数前脱位

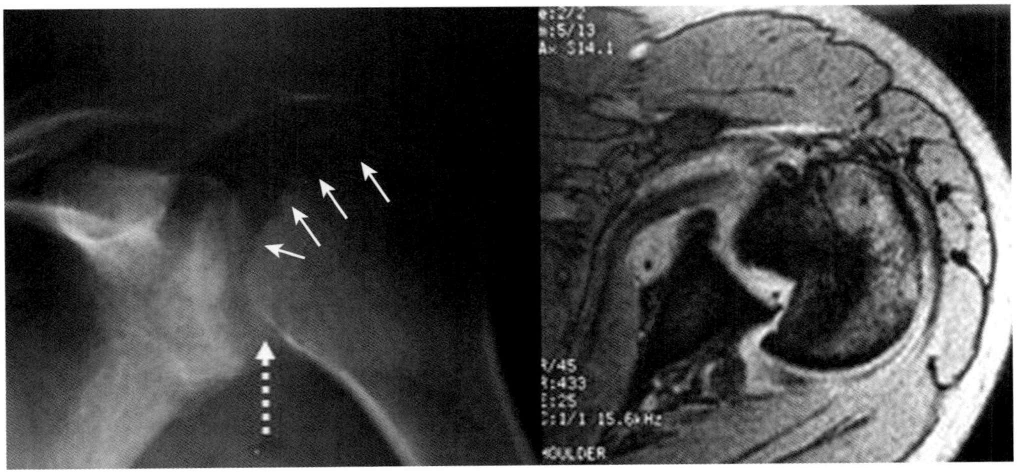

图 1　左图所示的正位片为一个漏诊的后脱位。肱骨头与关节盂部分重叠（白色虚线箭头），肱骨头有一个大的压缩骨折（白色箭头）。右图的磁共振检查清楚地显示了脱位和相关肱骨头的嵌入骨折

在闭合复位后并不稳定，但是我们仍然建议先尝试闭合复位。锁骨有时候也是如此复位，但是如果没有复位，患者通常可以接受这种畸形。因为胸锁关节前脱位一般没有症状，而且畸形相对于潜在的手术内固定的并发症来说，可以看作非常小的问题。

相对于前脱位，未复位的后脱位的并发症更多：胸廓出口综合征、血管损伤（包括锁骨下动脉的钝伤）、静脉损伤（包括静脉血栓）、锁骨近端进入胸锁关节后方重要的纵隔结构。急性胸锁关节后脱位通常可以闭合复位且比较稳定，一般需要全麻。但是如果后脱位无法复位或者复位后不稳定，就须行切开复位。依赖于精确的病理解剖学，无论切开复位修复韧带还是锁骨近端切除合并韧带重建都可以。

锁骨骨折

锁骨骨折是最常见的骨折之一，发生率占所有骨折的 4%，在肩部骨折中比例超过 1/3。锁骨近端 1/3 的骨折罕见，中段 1/3 的骨折发生率占 70%，远端 1/3 的骨折占 20% ~ 30%。尽管长期以来，大家广泛认为锁骨干骨折不需手术，且预后很好，但是最近有更详细的数据表明，事实并不是这样。

对锁骨骨折最初的研究表明非手术治疗的连接率大于 99%，手术治疗的骨不连率为 5% ~ 10% 或者更高。这些研究里缺少患者年龄、损伤的严重程度、选择手术治疗的骨折特点的信息。最近更多的研究把重点放在成年人锁骨骨折的自然史上。研究表明，所有骨折的骨不连率为 4% ~ 6%，严重移位的骨折骨不连率高达 15%。短缩超过 2 cm 的锁骨骨折愈合特别困难。

最近一项已发表的包含 2 144 例患者的系统性综述表明，移位的锁骨骨折骨不连率为 15%。当移位性骨折通过手术治疗后，骨不连的风险相对减少了 86%。最后，一项非手术治疗与钢板内固定的多中心随机对照试验表明，手术组患者可以更快、更容易、更完全地得以康复，并且医生和患者对于手术结果的评价在所有时间节点上都明显优于对照组，包括最后的结果。手术组的并发症主要与使用的植入物（钢板）有关。

最近的研究认为手术治疗的绝对适应证是短缩超过 20 mm、开放性损伤或皮肤受到波及、神经血管损伤、肩胛胸分离、病理性骨折移位。相对适应证是移位大于 20 mm、漂浮肩、多发伤、预计后期会长期卧床、患者无法耐受制动、双侧骨折、合并同侧上肢骨折。取得了患者的知情同意，并且患者愿意接受手术的风险，并希望更快速、更完全的康复，这种情况下，完全移位（在任何角度的 X 线片上主骨折块无骨皮质连接）也是相对适应证。

当锁骨骨折的患者选择保守治疗时，目前推荐悬吊制动，不需要骨折复位。当有内固定治疗指征时，用钢板和螺钉固定或髓内设备进行手术均可（图 3）。虽然两种技术均有支持者和反对者，但是并没

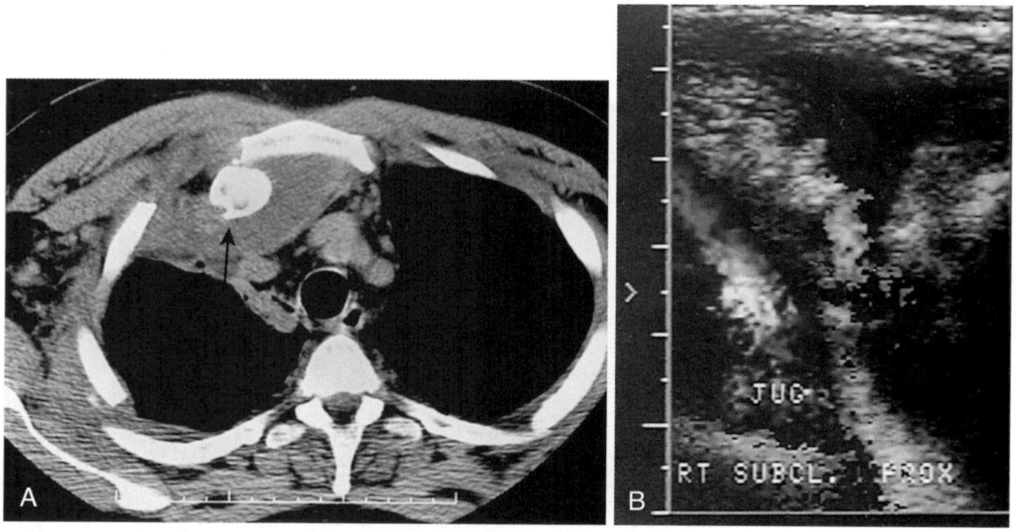

图 2 **A**，CT 显示胸锁关节的骨折 - 后脱位，伴有严重的软组织肿胀和肺门结构的损伤。**B**，多普勒超声检查显示右锁骨下动脉存在大的假性动脉瘤。注意颈部巨大的直径 1 cm 的假性动脉瘤（箭头处）(*From Bucholz RW, Heckman JD, editors:Rockwood and Green's fractures in adults, 5th ed, Philadelphia, 2001, Lippincott, Williams & Wilkins, p 1285.*)

有大规模的研究表明哪一种技术更占优势。

锁骨远端或外侧1/3骨折也非常普遍，大约占锁骨骨折的20%～30%。相对于中段骨折来说，Robinson很早就指出锁骨远端骨折更容易骨不连，骨不连率超过20%。虽然有些人指出其中很多骨不连的患者随着时间流逝已经没有症状了，而且建议非手术治疗，但是仍有一些专家推荐早期手术。

虽然锁骨远端骨折还没有像中段骨折研究的那么透彻，但是最近使用的新的手术技术的报告表明，手术患者可以获得良好的康复和功能，且并发症发生率很低。我们可以期待锁骨远端骨折治疗可能很快就会像锁骨中段骨折治疗一样——手术不是强制的，而是很可能会帮助患者更快、更容易地得到康复，得到比“平均水平”更好的结果。当选择手术固定时，虽然有很多方式，例如单独螺钉固定，但是钢板和螺钉固定可能是最常见的方法。

肩锁关节脱位（分离肩）

肩锁关节（acromioclavicular，AC）是一个牢固、稳定的关节，位于锁骨末端和肩峰之间。除了牢固的连接锁骨和肩峰的关节囊，从锁骨末端到肩胛骨之间还有一个很厚的喙锁（coracoclavicular，CC）韧带。在常见的关节脱位中，肩锁关节脱位是唯一一个不需要常规复位治疗的关节，虽然脱位的主要患者是从事碰撞类运动例如冰球或曲棍球的年轻男性，AC关节脱位也会发生在肩外侧持续受到直接击打的创伤患者。半脱位比完全脱位更常见，大部分患者可以采取保守治疗。

AC关节脱位可分为3型，最初是由Allman提出，然后Rockwood改进了分型，分为6型（图4）。Ⅰ型和Ⅱ型损伤（AC关节部分或完全破坏）事实上几乎不需要手术治疗，不需要复位。可以悬吊患肢，然后在此级别病情允许的情况下可以逐渐恢复患肢的活动。Ⅳ至Ⅵ型损伤很少见而且损伤比较重，通常都需要手术治疗来重建解剖、修复或者重建喙锁韧带。这种损伤的手术方式有很多，对于术式并没有统一的标准。Ⅲ型损伤（肩锁关节和喙锁韧带均完全破坏）的治疗存在争议。虽然一些人提倡Ⅲ型损伤须常规手术修复，但大多数美国肩关节外科医生仍采取保守治疗。保守治疗方法与Ⅰ型Ⅱ型损伤的治疗方法相同。对于Ⅲ型治疗的共识是，如果重体力劳动者损伤后在今后的工作中会出现问题，那么这种损伤就需要手术治疗。

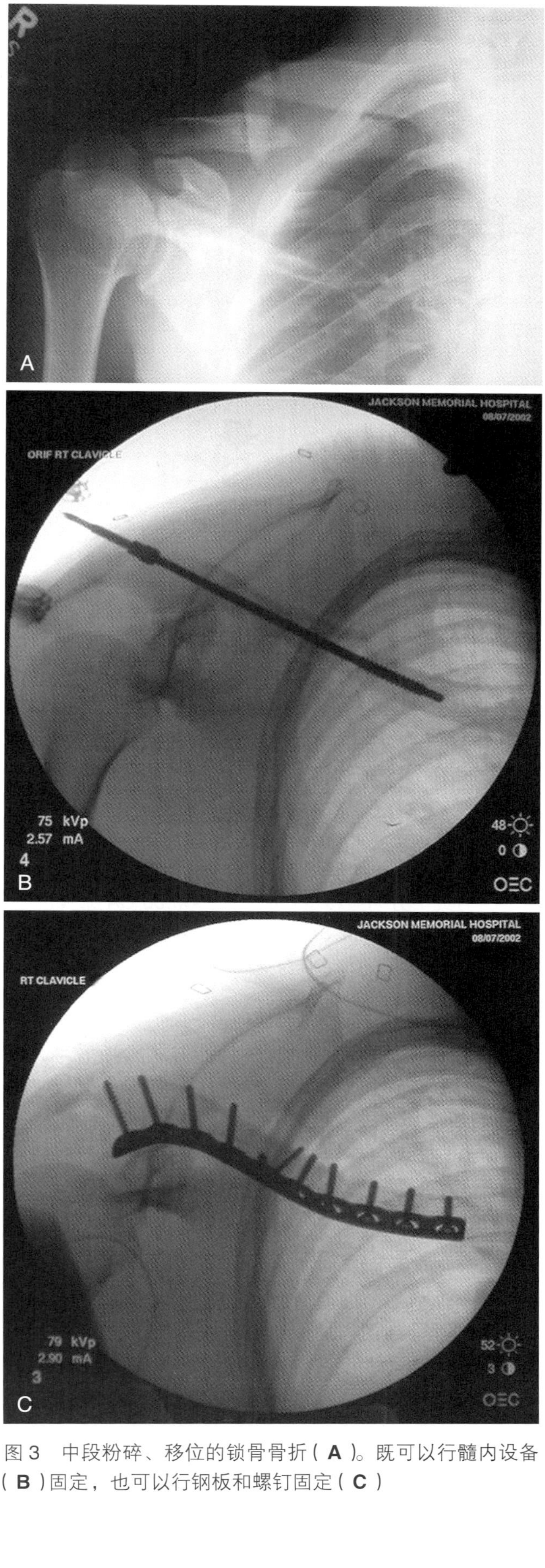

图3　中段粉碎、移位的锁骨骨折（**A**）。既可以行髓内设备（**B**）固定，也可以行钢板和螺钉固定（**C**）

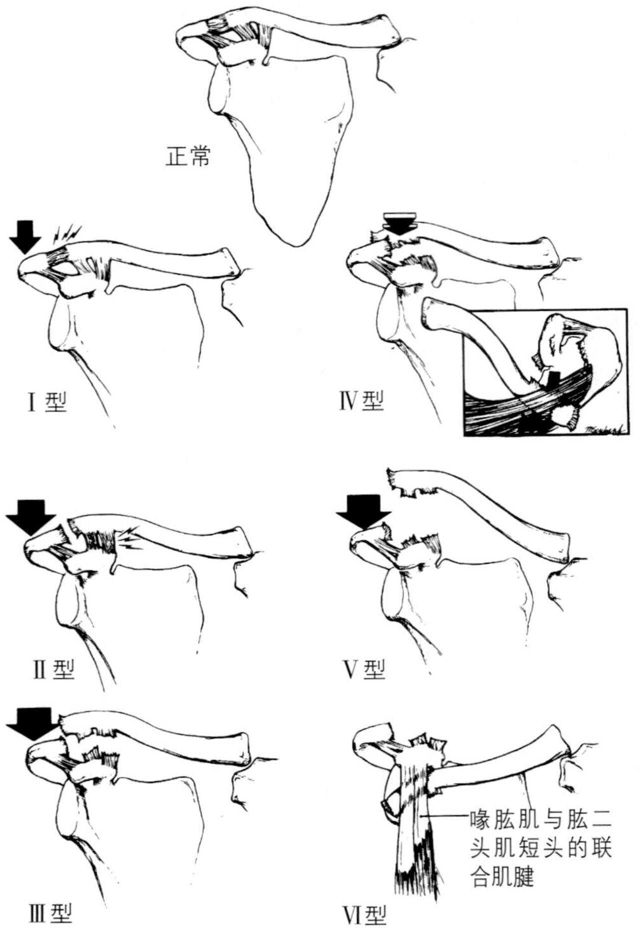

图4 肩锁关节脱位分型：Ⅰ型和Ⅱ型损伤的肩锁关节为部分或全部破坏。Ⅲ型损伤中，喙锁韧带也完全断裂。Ⅳ型、Ⅴ型和Ⅵ型损伤的关节破坏严重，锁骨远端分别向后方、上方或下方明显移位 *(From Rockwood CA Jr, Matsen FA, Wirth MA, Lippitt SB, editors:* The shoulder*, 3rd ed, Philadelphia, 2004, Saunders, Fig.12–14.)*

肩胛骨骨折

肩胛骨骨折相对比较少见，在肩胛带损伤中不到10%。通常它都是高能量创伤所致，这就可以解释为什么通常肩胛骨骨折都有生命危险，这种创伤比骨折本身要严重得多。在多发伤的患者中，肩胛骨骨折经常被漏诊，通常是在拍X线胸片或者做CT检查时偶然发现。

由于这种骨折通常为高能量损伤引起，合并损伤也是非常常见的。116个肩胛骨的148例骨折的研究显示，96%的肩胛骨骨折有合并损伤，其中上胸部肋骨骨折最多见。肺损伤也比较常见，总发生率为37%，29%存在血气胸，8%存在肺挫伤。34%的患者头部损伤，25%的患者有同侧锁骨骨折，12%的患者有颈椎损伤。

这类骨折一般选择非手术治疗，因为较厚的肩袖组织提供了丰富的血供，可以得到快速的恢复。肩袖还提供了一层衬垫来防止多数有症状的畸形愈合。当高能量损伤发生时，我们建议把患者收住院24 h，来评估其心肺状态。骨折的保守治疗为舒适的短时间的悬吊制动和随后的早期运动。大部分骨折临床上统一固定6周，然后可以开始加强功能锻炼。

明确的手术指证包括错位5 mm的关节盂内骨折、向关节内移位5 mm的喙突骨折、伴有持续或反复的盂肱关节不稳定的盂唇骨折。对于肩胛冈和肩胛盂颈的移位性骨折的适当治疗有更大的争议，一部分人倾向手术治疗，但是另一部分人提倡保守治疗。

称作“漂浮肩”的损伤类型应该特别注意。这种损伤可能称为上肩部悬吊复合体的“双侧破坏”更贴切。此复合体由骨性结构和软组织环构成，软组织环由关节盂及其周围组织组成。该软组织环悬吊于前方的锁骨和后方的肩胛骨间。单一悬吊结构的破坏通常是可以耐受的。然而，当前方、后方悬吊结构都被破坏时，肩胛带不稳定的潜在性增加。这种现象最常见于同侧锁骨和肩胛盂颈骨折。

漂浮肩的治疗存在争议。最初的非对照病例系列显示同时固定锁骨和肩胛骨以及单独固定锁骨都可以取得良好的临床疗效。然而，随后的研究表明，非手术治疗与之前手术治疗的数据相比，并未存在更多的优势。鉴于这些考虑，现在治疗的原则是分别评估锁骨和肩胛骨骨折，并根据各自的治疗指南对独立的骨折进行治疗。

肩胛胸分离

肩胛胸分离是一种少见但破坏性很强的损伤，它被认为是一种内部一侧的前半部的截断。它常由上肢强烈的牵拉引起，导致上肢在肩胛骨和它与胸的关节间发生明显的侧方移位。引起这种损伤所需的冲击力很大，以至于很多患者不能在胸腹损伤的最初阶段存活下来。根据Althausen等报道，88%的患者合并血管损伤，94%的患者合并严重的神经损伤以及臂丛和锁骨下血管的严重损伤。在这些患者中，52%的患者最终会四肢瘫痪，21%的患者需要早期截肢，10%的患者死亡。

临床上通过严重肿胀、虚弱、疼痛、压痛、脉搏减弱或消失这些症状来进行诊断。当出现无脉的情况时，不要简单地考虑为肢体远端的损伤，也须考虑到肩胛胸分离这种更近端的、危及生命的损伤也可能是病因。放射学检查，比如正位X线胸片可以显示肩胛骨的侧方移位。当与未受伤的对侧比较时，肩胛骨的内侧缘到棘突距离的增加，可以提示医生肩胛胸分离的可能性。此时可能合并也可能不合并胸锁关节脱位、肩锁关节脱位或者分离型锁骨骨折。

治疗方法目前是有争议的，但是合并动脉损伤须立即进行手术探查。在局部，可以同时进行臂丛神经探查。虽然没有必要全程探查臂丛神经至颈部，但是有时候在探查血管时可能发现臂丛神经从颈部或上肢完全撕脱。全臂丛神经撕脱恢复的预后较差，许多人认为这是立即进行肘部以上截肢的指征。如果没有发现全臂丛神经撕脱，应进行血管修复。骨性稳定可能是维持血管修复功能所必需的，但是内固定的作用并不清楚。因为操作和稳定骨性结构的过程可能损伤已经修复的血管，我们推荐的手术顺序是：①控制出血和分流血管损伤；②在需要的情况下，建立骨性稳定；③最后进行确定性血管修复。

肩关节脱位

由于缺乏骨性结构的约束，肩关节是身体中最容易出现脱位的关节。它并不是一个真正的球窝关节，而更像是高尔夫球在球座上待着。肩关节静态的稳定结构包含骨性结构，关节盂唇、关节囊和盂肱关节韧带，并且由肩袖组织提供额外的动态稳定性。

前脱位是最常见的肩关节脱位类型。通常在前臂处于伸展位时受到偏心力而引起，如排球运动员扣球时。肩关节屈曲、内收时受到向后的力量，或者患者阵挛、遭受电击时，肩关节内旋受到强力收缩时手臂弯曲，可以导致肩关节后脱位。

肩关节前脱位表现为上臂轻度外展、外旋或者位于身体侧面。肩关节正常的轮廓消失，在前面可以看到完整外观，在背面可以看肩峰下出现显著的“沟槽”征。肩部内收和内旋通常受限。相比之下，后脱位的患者其前臂保持在内收位置，前肩比正常情况更平坦，具有非常突出的喙突和前肩峰。

在复位之前，须进行彻底的神经学检查和X线片评估。神经损伤并非少见，发生率高达50%，腋神经最常受累。同时也应记录血管状态，因为血管损伤也可能发生。如前所述，标准的创伤系列X线片在评估相关关节盂损伤或肱骨近端骨折时非常有用。

镇静或者利多卡因关节内注射可以使关节复位更容易。缓慢的牵引可以复位大部分脱位。难复性关节脱位以及伴随肱骨骨折的脱位最好在手术室全身麻醉下进行。复位后照片可以确认盂肱关节是否复位。如果存在持续的肱骨近端骨折移位或明显的关节盂骨折，则须采取手术进行复位和骨折固定。否则，推荐使用一段时间的悬吊制动，这样可使患者舒适，然后推荐逐步进行肩关节功能锻炼。在大多数情况下，患者可以恢复以前的运动范围，不需要正式的物理治疗。

在年轻的患者中，骨骼损伤通常是盂唇和前下方的关节囊从关节盂边缘撕脱（Bankart 损伤）。最佳的自然史研究表明大约50%的年轻患者出现额外的脱位，其中大约一半发展为复发性不稳定并需要手术修复。非常年轻或活跃的患者，他们的工作或运动使他们发生复发性脱位的风险很高，可以考虑在首次脱位后进行韧带修复。但是一般来说，该损伤的初始治疗为非手术治疗，手术针对复发性脱位患者。

随着患者年龄的增长，韧带损伤和复发逐渐减少，但肩袖撕裂变得更加常见。到40岁时，肩袖撕裂变得比韧带损伤更常见，并且复发变得少见。复位之后须仔细查体，评估肩袖的力量。若没有肱骨近端骨折但患者有无力症状，须完善MRI，排除肩袖撕裂的可能性。肩关节脱位后急性肩袖撕裂通常是外科手术的指征。

肱骨近端骨折

肱骨近端骨折是常见的损伤，特别对老年人。大部分肱骨近端骨折移位较小或没有移位，可以进行非手术治疗。制订治疗方案时，须考虑患者的年龄、优势手、骨质量、骨折类型和骨折的位移。多发伤患者的合并损伤也是决定治疗方案的重要因素。

评估应包括彻底的神经血管检查以及创伤系列X线片。腋范围扩大或远端脉搏消失都与血管损伤有关。临床上明显的神经损伤发生在多达1/3的患者中，并且随着年龄增加更常见。当使用EMG检测它们时，神经损伤的发生率更高，发生在高达82%的移位性肱骨近端骨折中。如果存在神经损伤，可能需要几个月才能恢复，有时会出现功能恢复不完全的现象。

这些骨折常常根据Neer分型进行分类。Neer使用了Codman对肱骨近端的原始的4部分进行描述——关节节段、大转子、小转子、肱骨干，如果移位超过 1 cm 或成角大于 45° 定义为一部分。尽管观测者之间的可靠性相对较差，但这是迄今为止最常用的分类系统（图 5）。单纯的肱骨头骨折，或者在其内侧边缘的关节节段少于 8 mm，会影响至肱骨头的血供。这种情况须进行手术治疗，因为血供的破坏增加了肱骨头缺血性坏死的可能性。

肱骨近端骨折存在多种治疗方式，既有肩部骨折的非手术治疗（悬吊制动后逐渐活动），也有巨大移位性骨折的手术治疗或置换。非手术治疗：悬吊制动，然后逐渐进行肩关节功能锻炼。手术技术和手术方式的选择在外科医生之间差异很大，目前固定的方式包括钢板和螺钉、髓内钉、缝合线和经皮针固定（图 6）。肱骨头置换通常用于老年人的严重

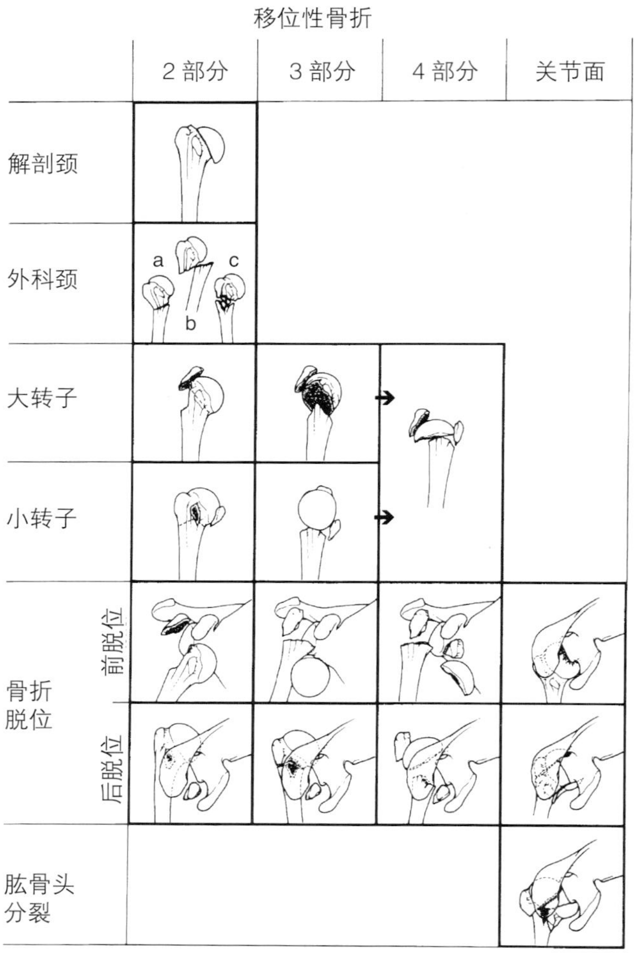

图 5 Neer 分型。肱骨近端 4 部分——关节节段。大转子、小转子和肱骨干，如果它们移位超过 1cm 或成角超过 45°，则被认为是有移位的。如果骨折没有移位，不能认为是一“部分”（*After Neer CS: Displaced proximal humeral fractures. Part I.Classification and evaluation.* J Bone Joint Surg Am *52:1077–1089, 1970.*）

骨折。肱骨头置换可以获得稳定的肩关节，并且缓解疼痛良好，但是肩关节的预后具有不可预测性。最近，我们对逆向肩置换治疗粉碎性肱骨近端骨折越来越感兴趣，因为它不依赖于假体周围肱骨大小转子的愈合，即可实现肩的功能。

肱骨干骨折

肱骨干骨折在 2 个年龄段高发：第一个是年轻人，主要由高能量机动车事故、高处坠落或枪伤引起；第一个是老年患者，主要由从站立姿势摔倒引起。

既往，这些骨折已经成功地用非手术治疗：起初使用夹板固定，然后在亚急性期使用功能支具固定。在一项研究中，922 名肱骨干骨折患者采用功能支具固定，只有 3% 的患者出现骨不连，98% 的

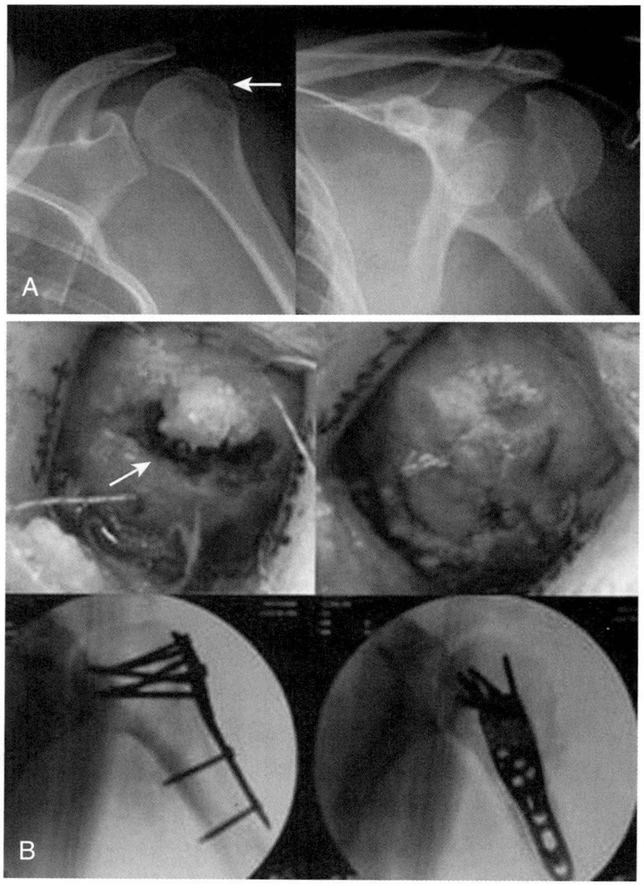

图 6 **A**，左侧是移位的肱骨大转子骨折（白色箭头），右侧是移位的解剖颈骨折。根据 Neer 分型，两者都被认为是“两部分骨折”。**B**，肱骨大转子骨折使用缝线固定的术中照片，以及使用解剖颈骨折切开复位内固定的术中荧光透视片

患者几乎完全恢复了肩部和肘部的运动。即使在严重移位或粉碎性骨折的患者中，如图 7 所示，功能支具固定也提供了一种治疗选择，可以使外科手术相关的风险最小化。然而，最近的研究比较了钢板固定和功能支具固定的疗效，结果显示钢板固定组骨不连、骨折畸形愈合发生率更低，而令人惊讶的是，手术组的患者出现桡神经麻痹的概率也更小。非手术组和手术组的感染率、骨折在 X 线片上的愈合时间或最终关节的活动范围没有显著差异。

骨折伴随相关神经损伤的治疗仍然是有争议的。报告显示肱骨干骨折伴桡神经麻痹的发生率为 1.8% ~ 24%。最常见的神经损伤是神经挫伤，伴随神经失用，大多数病例可以自行恢复。肱骨干中段 1/3 的横向骨折比远端 1/3 的螺旋型骨折更有可能出现神经失用。但是，越远端的骨折合并桡神经撕裂及长压的概率越高，如图 8 所示。对于急性神经损伤，尽管不常规推荐神经探查，但是在切开治疗骨折的时候可以一并探查神经，如开放性骨折或高能

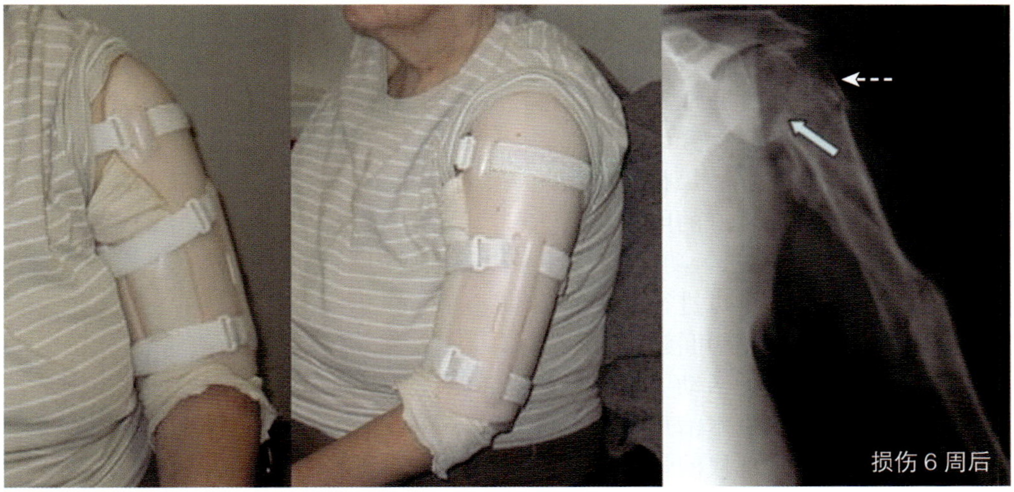

图 7　采用功能支具固定肱骨干骨折的临床照片。右侧的 X 线片显示复杂骨折在接受支具固定治疗 6 周后，所有部分的力学对线可以接受。大转子 (*虚线箭头*)，外科颈 (*实心箭头*) 及骨干碎片可形成早期骨痂 (*Courtesy Robin M. Gehrmann, MD*)

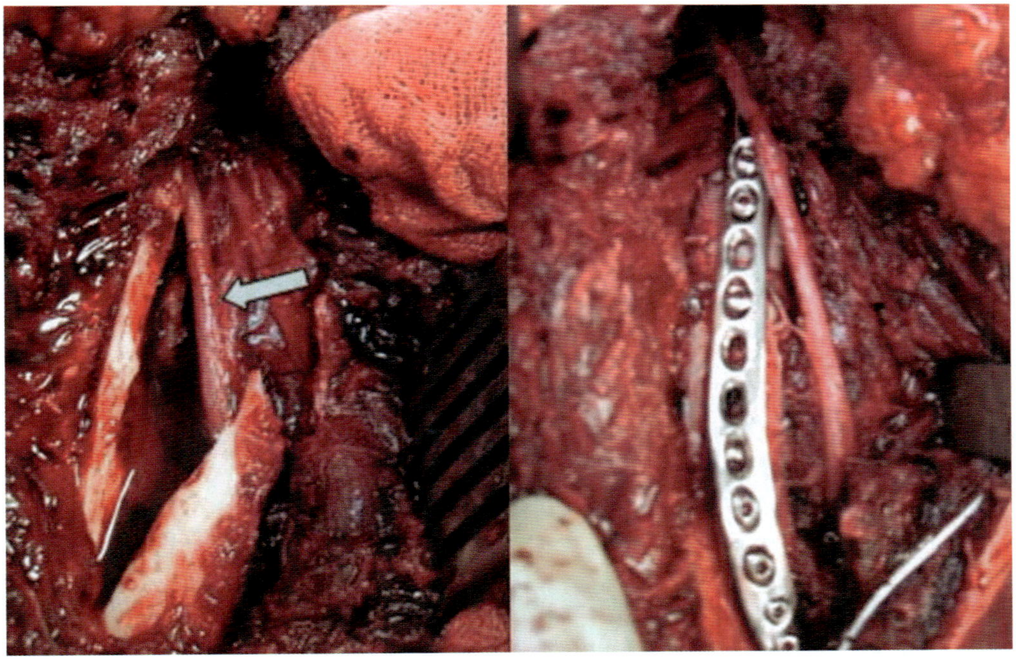

图 8　术中桡神经 (*白色箭头*) 被夹在肱骨远端 1/3 骨折碎片中 (*左*)。切开复位和内固定后桡神经越过近端钢板 (*右*)(*Courtesy Robin M. Gehrmann, MD*)

枪伤伴随的骨折。

标准的手术干预指征包括开放性骨折、高能枪伤所致骨折、骨折伴血管损伤、多发伤，以及无法使用夹板或功能支具对齐的患者，这一问题常见于肥胖患者和预期长时间卧床的患者。钢板和螺钉固定可以用于绝大多数肱骨干骨折内固定患者，但也有少部分患者存在髓内钉固定指征（图 9）

肘部

肱骨远端骨折

肱骨远端骨折较为少见，占所有成年人骨折非常小的一部分，无论手术治疗还是保守治疗，都因为疼痛、畸形、关节僵硬、骨不连、尺神经病而预后不佳。最有可能预示患者预后良好的因素包括达到关节面解剖学复位的能力和尽早进行功能锻炼。

无移位或移位程度较小的骨折可进行非手术治疗，进行短期的制动。如果一直保持可接受的位置，那么在几周内即可进行适当程度的活动。然而，如果存在移位性关节内骨折，那么手术治疗是唯一可以修复关节完整性的方式。使用现代的骨折治疗原则和修复设备，通常可以获得可接受的预后。

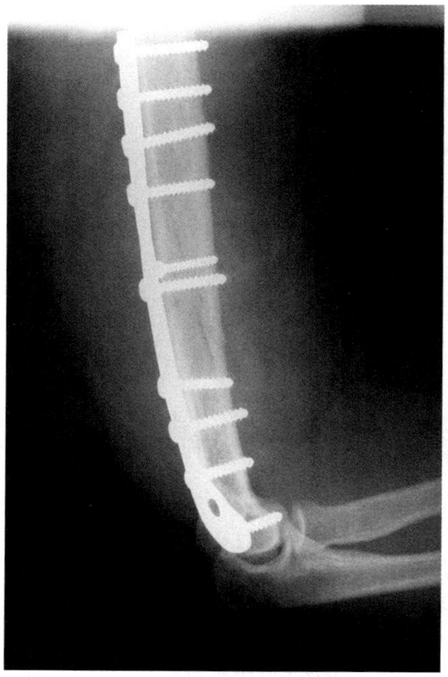

图 9　相似的骨折，采用内固定治疗

在成年人中，重建的目的在于修复关节面、重建肱骨内侧柱和外侧柱，并且稳定固定骨折部分，从而可以尽早活动（图 10）。通常需要尺骨鹰嘴截骨术才能充分显露关节面。必须识别和保护尺神经，有时在骨折修复后可能须行尺神经皮下前置术。骨折及手术修复的并发症包括关节挛缩、尺神经病、异位骨化，以及植入物突出。二次手术进行肘关节松解、切除异位骨化病灶、取出有问题的内固定物并不少见。

对于关节面严重粉碎的低需求老年患者，如果生活质量差，可以选择其他治疗方式，包括无固定的早期适当范围内活动（所谓“骨包”治疗）或者一期全肘关节置换。在实际操作中，前者只使用于最衰弱的患者，而肘关节置换逐渐增多。因为研究显示肘关节置换可以获得更早、更快的功能恢复。尽管老年患者肱骨远端骨折治疗的选择并不明确，对于无法获得稳定固定治疗的老年患者，肘关节置换逐渐成为治疗的一个选择。

肘关节脱位

肘关节脱位是第二常见的关节脱位（在肩之后），占所有关节脱位的 20%。肘关节的稳定接近一半归功于骨关节的匹配，而另一半靠其附属韧带的支持。内侧副韧带前束是稳定外翻应力的基础，而外侧副韧带复合体阻止了后外侧旋转的不稳定性。

肘关节脱位往往多发于青少年和年轻成年人，多数在肩部外展而肘部伸展时（上臂张开）摔倒引起。患者会出现肘部疼痛与无法移动，可能会有比

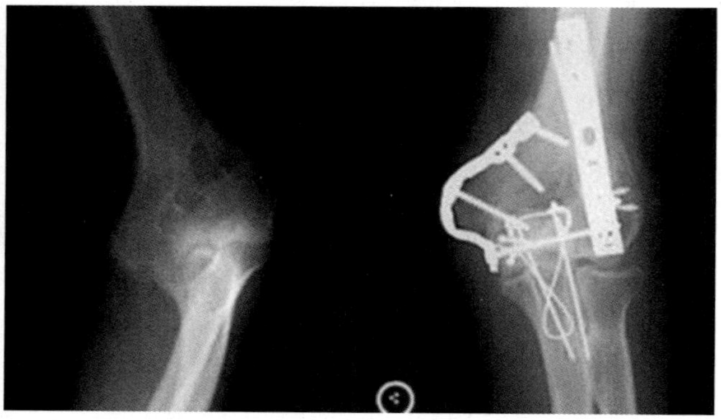

图 10　术前正位（AP）X 线片显示肱骨远端粉碎性关节内骨折（*左侧*）；术后 AP 片显示关节面、内侧柱、外侧柱已经恢复（*右侧*）（*Courtesy Robin M.Gehrmann，MD*）

较明显的畸形，但也会因为肿胀而被忽略。全面的神经血管检查是必要的，因为肘关节脱位伴随尺神经或者正中神经挫伤并不少见。此外，须仔细检查肩关节和腕关节，以除外相关的伴随损伤。前臂压痛或者远端桡尺关节（distal radioulnar joint，DRUJ）不稳定都应该视作存在骨间膜和 DRUJ 损伤（Essex-Lopresti 损伤）的可能。

确认肘关节脱位的诊断可用 X 线片检查。不涉及骨折的肘关节脱位是简单的脱位，并根据脱位的方向进行分类。合并有桡骨头颈或喙突骨折的肘关节脱位（如复杂脱位）必须完善影像学检查，因为此骨折有进行确定性治疗的指征。

急性肘关节脱位应即刻在足够的镇痛及肌肉松弛下进行闭合复位。通常在急诊室肌内注射或静脉给药下进行，几种闭合复位技巧如前文描述都涉及内外侧移位的纠正，伴随纵向牵引和前臂屈曲。通常在关节复位时闻及“咔啦”一声。

复位后，可通过检查活动范围及内翻外翻压力来评估肘关节的稳定性。如果没有骨折，被动伸展 30° 以内无不稳定，提示该复位是一个稳定的复位。待患者疼痛和不适症状好转之后，肘关节可以在几天内进行活动。如果复位后肘关节不稳定，那么应该将其弯曲 90° 后制动大约 1～2 周再开始活动。最近部分人认为早期弯曲运动可能对建立稳固的关节有益。

肘关节后脱位伴桡骨头及喙突骨折被称为“肘关节恐怖三联征”，因为这在治疗及护理上比较困难。复杂的肘关节脱位往往须进行确定性治疗，因为肘关节很不稳定，若治疗不恰当很容易出现并发症。手术治疗时，术者应当通过以下方式尝试修复肘关节不稳定：①通过修复或者置换假体重建肱骨与桡骨的接触；②修复附属韧带；③如果需要，则行喙突骨折内固定治疗，如图 11。

简单的肘关节脱位的非手术治疗预后往往十分好。出现制动的延长（通常大于 3 周）以及复原不充分为预后不佳。其他后遗症包括异位骨化和关节僵硬。另外，复杂脱位可出现肘关节不稳定反复发作、固定失败和创伤后关节炎。

桡骨头骨折

桡骨头骨折较为常见，约占肘部骨折的 1/3，并且通常伴有肘关节脱位，损伤机制通常是前臂旋前时受到轴向暴力。桡骨头骨折的患者常出现肘部伸展或前臂旋转时肘外侧疼痛。通常使用 Mason 分型。Ⅰ型骨折无移位，Ⅱ型骨折合并移位，Ⅲ型为粉碎性骨折。之后还包含了Ⅳ型骨折，指桡骨头骨折伴有肘关节脱位。

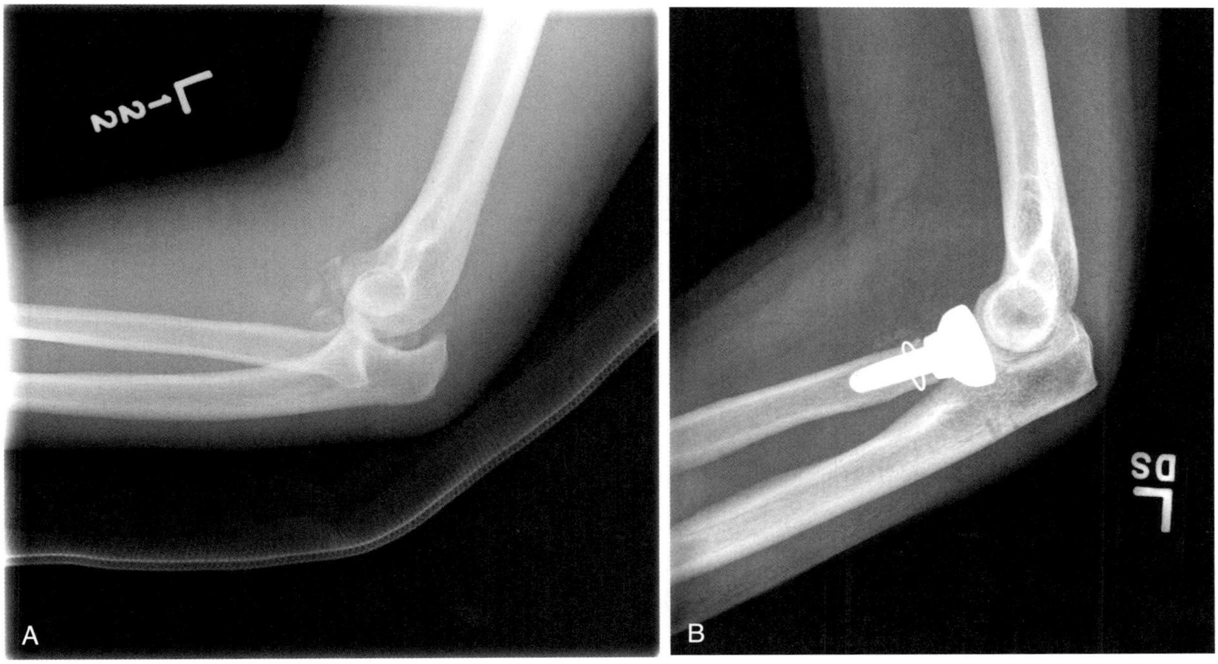

图 11　**A**，一位 40 岁男性肘关节脱位伴骨折。桡骨头粉碎性骨折无法修复。**B**，关节切开复位件桡骨头置换，并且修复侧副韧带达到肘关节稳定

无移位性骨折早期运动后预后良好。桡骨头骨折的手术指征包括移位大于 3 mm、前臂旋转时尺桡关节之间存在骨块、Essex-Lopresti 损伤（合并骨间膜损伤），以及肘关节不稳定。桡骨头骨折的手术方式包含括桡骨头切除、内固定或者假体置换。单纯桡骨头骨折而无肘关节不稳定，可安全切除桡骨头而不影响肘关节稳定性或其功能，尤其是老年患者。Ring 等指出，当桡骨头骨折的骨折块小于等于 3 块时，内固定是最好的选择。当无法做到稳定固定桡骨头时，可行桡骨头金属假体置换术，这在 Essex-Lopresti 损伤或 Mason Ⅲ或Ⅳ型骨折中尤为典型。

尺喙骨折

尺喙关节既为可防止肘关节后脱位的支持，也是内侧副韧带前束的附着点。因此它在肘关节稳定性方面有着重要的作用。尺喙骨折通常伴有肘关节脱位。最早有 3 种类型被明确定义，并且在肘关节侧位 X 线片上看得最清楚：Ⅰ型，尖端骨折；Ⅱ型，累及小于 50% 尺喙；Ⅲ型，累及大于 50% 尺喙。最近，尺喙前内侧冠状突斜形或垂直的骨折较为少见，但若不修复，可导致尺肱关节持续内翻不稳定和早期创伤后关节炎（图 12）。这类骨折最好完善肘关节 CT 检查。总而言之，Ⅰ型冠状突骨折可不固定骨块，而移位性Ⅱ型、Ⅲ型骨折及冠状突前内侧骨折，可引起肘关节不稳定。这 3 类骨折作为肘关节脱位手术处理的一部分，应行内固定治疗。

鹰嘴骨折

尺骨乙状大切迹是由鹰嘴和冠状突组成。鹰嘴构成了切迹的近端一半。涉及这个位置的骨折不会引起尺肱关节不稳定。鹰嘴骨折可以是直接暴力或来自肱三头肌的力量导致。微小移位性骨折（在屈肘 90° 摄片时间隙小于 2 mm）不常见，但是可以通过屈肘 30°～45° 位置的夹板固定治疗。更常见的情况是伴有移位的鹰嘴骨折，须进行切开复位内固定，恢复肱三头肌的机制和伸肘功能。固定鹰嘴骨折有多种方法，包括在克氏针或者螺钉辅助下的张力带技术、双皮质骨折块间或髓内的螺钉与钢板技术。粉碎性骨折最好采用背侧钢板固定。对于部分严重粉碎的病例，应切除骨折碎片，然后利用尚存在的尺骨近端重建肱三头肌止点。

鹰嘴内固定最常见的并发症是皮下植入物凸起，这可以在骨折愈合后移除钢板来处理。此外，肘关节僵硬、畸形愈合、骨不连和创伤后关节炎也会时有发生。

前臂

前臂骨折多因高能量损伤所致，经常伴随全身或其他骨骼肌肉的损伤。临床评估时须细致地检查患者的全身情况，而非仅仅关注四肢。当合并有开放伤、神经血管损伤、存在或即将有前臂筋膜室综合征时须尽快处理。射线照片检查须包括含有前臂、肘和腕部的 AP 及侧位片。事实上，除了无移位或仅累及尺骨干的微小移位性骨折，所有的成年人前臂骨折均需要切开复位。尽管髓内钉或者外固定术也偶有使用，但是加压钢板内固定依旧是金标准（图 13）。对于大多数病例来说，这允许其进行早期前臂的功能运动，这有助于骨折愈合和功能恢复。

蒙泰贾骨折

蒙泰贾骨折指的是尺骨近端骨折伴随桡骨头脱位。在前臂骨折中发生率约为 1%～2%。Bado 描述了 4 种损伤类型：Ⅰ型，尺骨任何水平的骨折，向前成角伴桡骨头前方脱位；Ⅱ型，尺骨干骨折，向后（背侧）成角伴桡骨头后方脱位；Ⅲ型，尺骨近端干骺端骨折，伴桡骨头外侧方脱位；Ⅳ型，尺骨近端和桡骨干骨折，合并桡骨头脱位（图 14）。成功治疗蒙泰贾骨折的关键是解剖复位和尺骨骨折的内固定。关于尺骨的复位，也需要桡骨头的稳定的重新置放。难以复位的桡骨头脱位往往与软组织卡压有关，须对肱桡关节切开复位。对于Ⅳ型损伤，尺桡骨的切开复位和内固定是必需的。

蒙泰贾骨折的并发症常常与未解剖复位或者尺骨骨折内固定失效有关，它们会导致桡骨头慢性的脱位或移位。不良结局也可能是由于异位骨化或者近端尺桡骨骨连接所致。

尺骨和桡骨干骨折

尺骨和桡骨干双骨折（前臂双骨折）在成年创伤人群中是一种常见的损伤。大多数医生倾向于对 2 处骨折分别切开行加压钢板内固定治疗。桡骨干的解剖弓必须保留，以保留前臂旋转功能。

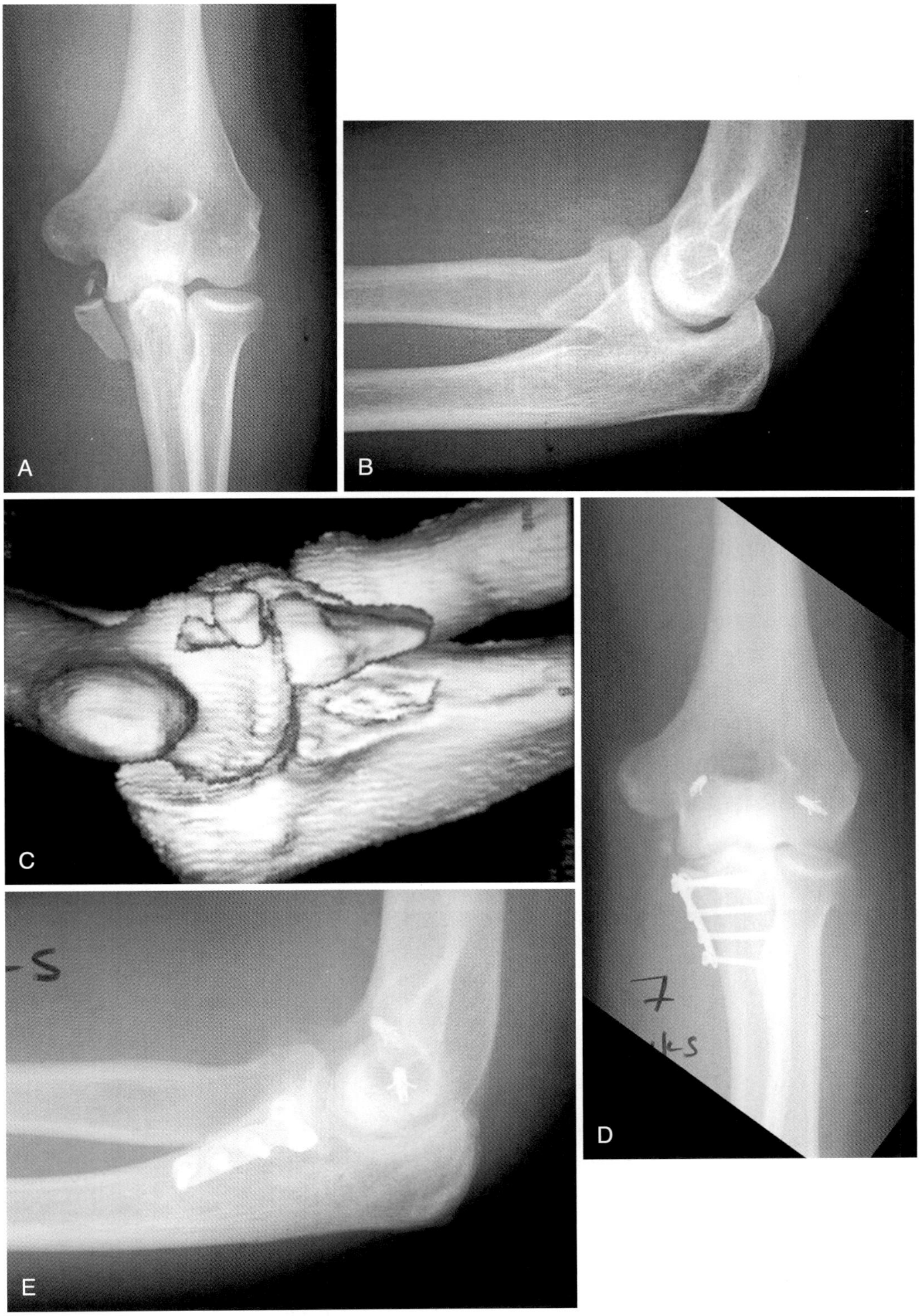

图 12　肘关节正位和侧位 X 线片（**A** 和 **B**）、三维 CT 片（**C**）提示冠状突前内侧骨折。此患者存在肘关节脱位，在拍片前已经予以轻柔的复位。**D**、**E**：该患者接下来进行了尺喙骨折切开复位内固定术，术中采用缝合锚钉修复了内、外侧副韧带 *(Courtesy of Virak Tan, MD.)*

单独的桡骨干骨折不常见，但也偶有发生。如果是移位性骨折，石膏固定效果不佳，因此大多采用内固定治疗。盖氏骨折指的是桡骨干骨折伴 DRUJ 脱位。其治疗可以采用桡骨解剖学复位加钢板内固定，然后保持 DRUJ 的位置稳定制动，或者复位、通过针临时固定 DRUJ。

单纯的尺骨干骨折也被称为“警棍骨折”。因为它常见于前臂遮挡警棍直接击打时发生。在现代，交通意外也是常见的原因之一。10° 以内的成角移位和 50% 以内的骨干移位可以采取保守治疗。钢板内固定则适用于超过上述范围的情况。

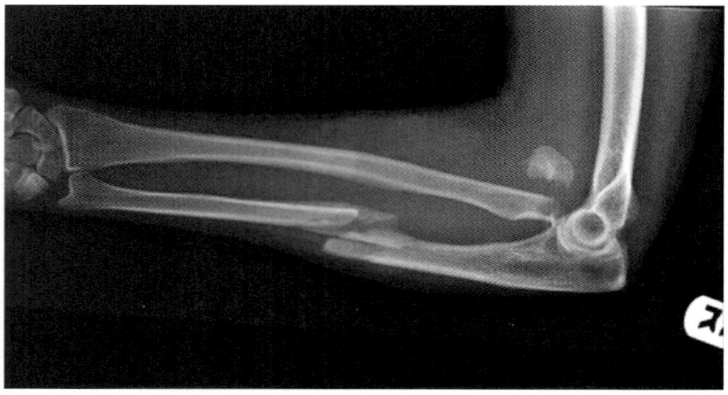

图 14 前臂骨折的前后位射线照片，提示 IV 型蒙泰贾骨折。尺骨中段和桡骨颈骨折伴桡骨头脱位 *(Courtesy of Virak Tan, MD.)*

盖氏骨折

盖氏骨折指的是桡骨远端骨折伴 DRUJ 的脱位或松弛。这是一种少见的骨折，在前臂骨折中发生率为 3% ~ 6% 之间。其创伤机制为直接击打腕部桡背侧，或者跌倒时前臂极度旋前、手伸直。盖氏骨折的 X 线片表现包括：尺骨茎突骨折、正位片 DRUJ 增宽、侧位片尺骨远端脱位和骨折部位桡骨缩短 5 mm 以上。

在成年人盖氏骨折中，手术治疗是必需的，因为封闭治疗有很高的失败率。在对桡骨进行解剖钢板固定后，需要检查 DRUJ 稳定性。如果前臂旋转时关节稳定，则可以不进一步制动。然而，如果 DRUJ 容易复位但不稳定，则手臂须保持在前臂旋转至 DRUJ 最大稳定性的位置（经典的是旋后位），或者使用螺钉将 DRUJ 固定在复位的位置。有时切开复位 DRUJ，并修复其软组织支撑结构也是需要的。盖氏骨折的并发症包括由于桡骨对齐不良导致的前臂旋转功能丢失和由于 DRUJ 不协调导致的前臂旋转功能受限或疼痛。

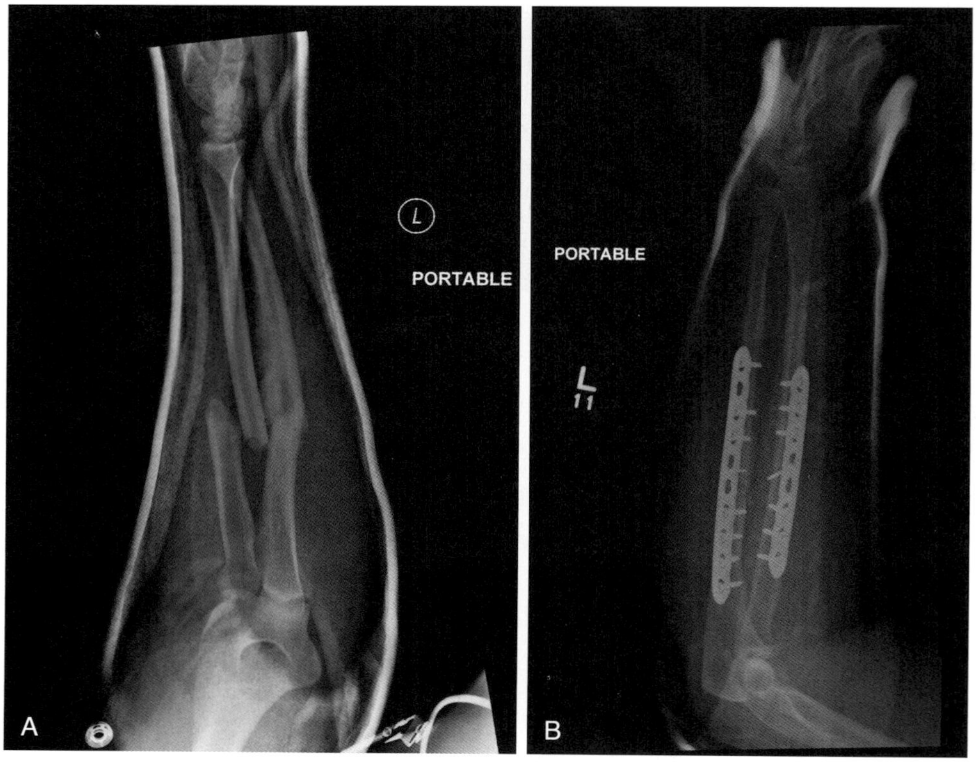

图 13 **A** 和 **B**，前臂双骨折均使用加压钢板内固定

下肢损伤和脱套伤

Peter G. Trafton, Herman P. Houin 和 Donald D. Trunkey 著
王天兵 译

下肢损伤可以是损毁性的（见此章节后的肢体损毁伤）和致命性的，也可以是轻微损伤，可以迅速恢复的。所有患者均须进行 ATLS 评估。病史（如果可以）须包括患者的受伤机制、急诊最初的体格检查和任何相关的医疗信息。治疗上应首先控制大出血，并进行夹板制动。

体格检查应包括疼痛点定位、脉搏、感觉、肤色、运动功能和成角或旋转畸形的评估。导致穿通伤的异物的入口或者出口、可能存在异物的位置须做好标记。

影像学评估

下肢损伤的影像学检查须包括受伤部位及上、下关节的正位及侧位片。穿通伤最好根据异物入口和出口位置而定。认真、仔细的临床评估可以减少血管造影的过度使用（其花费高且容易导致并发症）。然而，如果穿通伤中存在一处或多处肢体远端脉搏消失，则须进行血管造影检查或者 CT 动脉造影（CT arteriography，CTA），甚至是紧急手术。如果脉搏存在，则须测量踝肱指数（ankle brachial indices，ABI）。如果足背动脉或者胫后动脉的 ABI 达到或超过 1，则患者可以继续安全地观察其他损伤或者出院，然后 1 周后复查 ABI。如果足背动脉或胫后动脉的 ABI 小于 1，且远端有临床缺血的表现，或不能使用双功能超声扫描或者伤口在扩大，则须进行急诊的血管造影、CTA 或者手术（远端供血明显不足时）。如果临床上显示远端血供充足而 ABI 小于 1.0，则应选择性使用双功能超声扫描。如果检查呈阴性，或者显示仅有微小的损伤（微小的内膜损伤或者假性动脉瘤形成），则患者可以继续观察，1 周内复查 ABI。如果超声检查提示较大的损伤，如大的内膜缺损、较大的假性动脉瘤或腔内凝块，则应行血管造影或探查。

骨折

现在普遍认为，对于创伤患者的肌肉骨骼损伤进行积极的、恰当的早期治疗可以降低死亡率和花费，减少最终的医疗费用，对总体治疗有帮助，康复和最终的功能也更佳。这部分不是一个关于“如何”的讨论，而是建议应与一位有经验的骨科创伤专家进行快速和有效的合作。应注意的是，此时处理骨骼肌肉损伤仅仅是进行临时处理（因此要果断）。对于很多骨折，有多种可行的治疗方案。不同方案的选择当然也是不可避免的。

骨骼损伤不可能被孤立出来单独处理。医生处理时还应该同时考虑骨折本身及评估相关软组织损伤的情况、整个肢体的情况和患者整体的情况。其他损伤、年龄、预期活动水平、尚存的骨骼肌肉和有效的康复治疗计划也是须考虑的。处理骨折和关节损伤，取决于该损伤是独立损伤还是仅仅是患者多发损伤中的一个部分。治疗方案也受到医生可使用的医疗资源的影响。当缺乏良好装备的手术室、有效的影像学检查、有经验的外科医生团队时，进行现代的内固定技术很可能会失败。

骨骼肌肉损伤的早期治疗

肢体损伤可以是明显的，也可以是隐匿的。明显损伤的早期治疗包括活动性出血的加压包扎，不稳定损伤在可接受位置进行夹板外固定和动脉阻塞的紧急确认和治疗。

当紧急的复苏进展令人满意之后，须进行全身的、彻底的检查，以发现更多的隐匿的损伤。所有皮肤表面，从趾头到躯干都需要检查，以发现畸形、肿胀、瘀斑和撕裂伤的存在。皮肤擦伤也是很重要的。如果它们恰好在骨骼肌肉损伤的位置，任何手术都须恰当处理或者延期到擦伤愈合。应触诊检查各个骨头、关节的肿胀程度、畸形和压痛。人工施压检查确定各个骨头的稳定性。可活动各个关节以确认正常关节的被动活动度及反常活动的消失（不稳定）。当急诊医生也是患者创伤复苏或者早期治疗的人员时，在麻醉结束前应彻底检查肢体。明确有无周围血管脉搏。应获取不正常区域的所有 X 线片。

如果患者清醒且能够配合，应通过主动活动各个关节，以检查患者的运动神经和肌腱的完整性。检查主要的周围神经独立控制的感觉区以确定其感觉功能。对于从最开始就无法配合的重症患者，完成这些项目可能需要几天，但依旧需要彻底的检查以防漏诊。当多发伤患者须进行复苏时，可以将骨骼肌肉损伤的诊断和治疗滞后。很多损伤不能马上诊断。为获得更好的治疗效果，在恢复的早期应反复检查，以及时发现额外的损伤，使其得到及时治疗。

开放性骨折

辨认和分型

开放性骨折需要特殊的关注，以将破伤风杆菌感染和化脓性感染的风险最小化。治疗则须根据损伤的严重程度分级，该分级系统最主要的根据是软组织损伤的程度和污染程度（表1）。考虑软组织伤口是很重要的，而不是仅仅考虑开放的皮肤缺损。在严重的挤压伤中，小的皮肤撕裂伤可能存在广泛的挫伤或软组织坏死。

识别开放性骨折是早期处理的第一步。尽管大多数时候它们都很明显，但是开放性骨折依旧会因为不全面的检查而漏诊。须检查身体背侧的皮肤。看似表浅的伤口也有可能通过下方的损伤通达骨骼或关节。神经血管状态、肌腱功能和可能的多发损伤都应仔细检查。如果全面的检查和对于邻近骨折部位的伤口的治疗不能在急诊室开展，则假定骨折可能是开放性骨折。应到手术室去治疗，手术室有良好的麻醉、辅助设备、止血方法和灯光，有助于明确诊断和治疗。

表1 开放性骨折的分类

分型	临床发现
Ⅰ级	由低能量损伤导致的小伤口，有轻度的污染和软组织损伤（如有骨骼末端的皮肤撕裂伤或低速枪伤伤口）
Ⅱ级	伤口更长、更宽，无或有轻度的无血管或失活组织和轻微的污染
ⅢA级	由高能量创伤导致的明显的伤口，经常有广泛的软组织撕裂、软组织瓣。但尽管如此，在最终的清创后，还尚存足够的局部软组织覆盖，而且延迟关闭伤口是可行的。
ⅢB级	较大的伤口，含有明显的软组织失活、污染或两者皆有。骨折暴露于伤口，可能存在较大的骨膜撕裂。软组织覆盖有缺损，需要局部的或游离的带蒂微血管肌肉移植。
ⅢC级	开放性骨折伴有需要手术修复的动脉损伤。

一旦检查完肢体损伤，可以用无菌加压敷料控制出血，在去往放射科或手术室途中予以夹板外固定。如果患者来院前早已将开放性骨折覆盖好，伤口已经关闭，那敷料最好在手术室移除。对于创伤患者，对可疑区域进行影像学检查是必需的。不幸的是，急诊室的的条件相差巨大，而且重症患者在放射科时的监测不足和虚弱也是相当危险的。负责任的外科医生应随时准备，明确影像学检查是否已经是可能达到者中最佳的，及患者何时应该转送至手术室。胸部、骨盆和脊柱的X线片应首先进行。受伤的肢体也都须进行完整的检查。如果没有适当的影像学检查，骨科医生难以确诊骨折的程度，以及骨折是否为关节内损伤。当然，这些检查也可以当患者稳定后直接在手术室进行。

处理

强烈建议任何一个开放性骨折的治疗都在设备完善的手术室进行。术中拥有良好的麻醉，而且在生命安全保障的情况下，越快越好。

即刻的伤口治疗

外科伤口的处理原则从18世纪晚期被Desault首次提出以来几乎无改变，有效的药物辅助治疗是近期才使用的。要注意立即预防性注射破伤风抗毒素，开放性骨折在诊断后须马上静脉滴注抗生素。许多对照研究都已经证实了药物对手术的辅助作用。从进入急诊室到受伤后的48 h须连续输入抗生素，有效量为每8 h静脉输入1～2 g头孢唑林，不论这期间伤口还是不是开放性伤口。根据感染菌的来源和程度，对于革兰氏阴性菌推荐用氨基糖苷类抗生素。考虑到厌氧菌感染的需要，将青霉素类抗生素列入初期使用的抗生素之列，特别是在Ⅲ级开放性骨折时。其他可选择的抗生素可用于对上述药物过敏的患者。

一旦手术团队及器械准备完善，适当评估患者后就应该马上将其送到手术室。充分麻醉后，在处理其他须马上处置的外科情况的同时或之后着手处理开放性骨折。

开放性骨折的处理从再次全面评估患肢开始，这个过程可以与麻醉同时进行。须考虑是保肢还是必须一期截肢。如果有截肢的可能性，最好在术前将这种可能性告知患者及其家属。争得另一位术者的同意，在患者的同意书上注明截肢是最佳的治疗方式也是好的方法。

充气式止血带是需要的，但是仅在控制出血或者评估缺血后充血组织的活性时充气使用。原则上，当损伤肢体清洁后，应该能避免开放性骨折伤口的进一步感染。然而，当伤口上覆盖无菌封闭敷料时，是很难充分清洗患肢的。许多清洁剂和肥皂会损伤受损组织，所以应避免在伤口处使用清洁剂。将患肢放在无菌的防水一次性手术单上进行擦洗，10 min 内须换 2 次手术单。清洁剂的泡沫须冲洗干净，然后用无菌干毛巾擦干皮肤。这时，用聚维酮碘抗菌溶液消毒整个肢体包括伤口，然后再次铺上无菌的防水手术单。

冲洗和清创

接下来是冲洗和清创。必要时扩大伤口保证充分的检查和清洗。清创过程中须特别注意避免皮瓣失活和阻断浅表静脉（对于血供的恢复有重要作用）。手术切口应尽可能避免选择挫伤的皮肤处，保留有活性的组织皮瓣以覆盖骨折区域和植入的内固定装置区域。充分暴露伤口后，彻底清除所有的异物或者可疑的坏死组织。须保留神经、重要的血管，尽可能多的骨碎片。污染严重的骨面用咬骨钳咬除或刮匙刮除。所有贯穿关节的伤口必须打开关节，检查是否有碎片，包括软骨碎片。可以先将可能有活性的皮肤留下，它可以在损伤后几天快速评估。皮下脂肪、筋膜以及肌肉若失活或污染应予以积极切除，但注意不能过度剥离有活性的皮瓣。判断肌肉的活性时，检查肌肉的收缩性、连续性，这对于判断是否存在内生小血管出血可能比观察肌肉颜色更有效。

脉冲灌洗系统可更好地清洁损伤组织，但须注意轻柔使用，使软组织的损坏减少到最低程度。脉冲灌洗泵可允许使用小于 10 L 的冲洗液，但大于 10 L 的灌洗建议也常被采用。对于Ⅱ级开放性骨折，推荐使用 6 L 普通生理盐水或林格氏液。另一种辅助的杆菌肽溶液（50 000 U 加入 1 L 生理盐水，加入 2 安瓿碳酸氢钠碱化），作为最后灌洗的抗生素溶液，可用球形注射器应用。

清创过程中，对于损伤肢体须进一步做以下 2 个方面的决定：①稳定骨折；②闭合伤口。任一方面处理不当引起的并发症都会极大地延长肢体活动不便的时间，并会危害最终的手术结果。为了避免手术失败，外科医生必须使用完全熟悉的技术，并运用合适的清创设备。保证骨折足够稳定是重要的，外固定或内固定器械的运用可以减少感染风险，有助于整体管理。如果采用了内固定，或是Ⅱ级、Ⅲ级开放性伤口，须注意仔细清洗伤口，并延迟一期伤口闭合。

复位和固定

尽管关节处的骨折需要解剖学复位，但是关节外的骨折通常仅要求适当的角度恢复和旋转对齐，来维持肢体长度。至于如何稳定开放性骨折已经没有什么争议了。牵引、石膏支具、外骨骼固定和各种类型的内固定都可以应用，单独使用或联合使用均可。对于每一个骨折患者都应该重新审视 2 个问题：①怎样程度的稳定算是必需的，或者是可能的？②怎样的稳定方式能最大的获益，并付出最小的代价？很少有研究明确提出一种稳定方式比另一种更优越。除了最轻微的开放性骨折，其他骨折类型我们都推荐手术固定的方式，并多数情况下倾向于选用髓内钉或外固定而不是钢板固定。这是因为钢板固定用于开放性骨折引起的感染风险更高，也会面临更多的伤口愈合方面的问题。

对于骨折断端周围软组织损伤严重的患者，虽然内固定感染风险高，但内固定比外固定稳定性更好（如踝关节骨折、某些桡骨干骨折、股骨近端骨折），也更易于处理。邻近动脉吻合区域的骨折一期内固定时，不必保证血管的修复效果。

骨折外固定使用时必须同时注意伤口处理和骨移植。它能够保证开放性骨折的稳定性，是一种合适和强力的方式。它不会过度地暴露伤口，也不会阻断骨折端的血供，也没有石膏或牵引装置那么累赘。外固定器能迅速实施，而且出血最少，它适用于跨越不稳定的关节和复杂的骨折。它能临时稳定骨折部位，当患者能耐受复杂骨折固定的长时间麻醉和出血时，外固定方式被替换成更加稳定的内固定或外固定方式。外固定方式主要适用于那些不能忍受平卧的患者，保证他们一定的活动性，特别适用于不稳定的开放性骨盆骨折。这种骨折类型在没有强调积极复苏、骨盆稳定、伤口清创、开放性伤口护理、结肠造口术转流等处理之前，死亡率可达到 35%。

放置在预钻孔中的较大直径的螺纹针倾向用于骨干骨折固定。尽管环形外架有些麻烦，但是能更好地固定干骺端的骨折。用半穿刺骨针固定器跨越损伤关节提供临时固定，待患者生命体征更加稳定后，放置更加复杂的外固定装置。

对于单处开放性骨折，骨牵引是一种合适的临时或者最终固定方式。然而，相对于内固定和外固定，骨牵引因其长期强制性卧床，引起的全身并发症会更多，并且预后不佳。所以骨牵引往往仅在现代创伤中心临时使用，而且很少使用。

伤口覆盖

是否闭合开放性骨折伤口，以及何时、如何闭合的问题与保持骨折稳定性的问题一样具有争议。缝合感染伤口的皮肤的风险极大。当有内植物置入时，如果缝合，伤口感染风险增加，缝合伤口会致皮瓣张力增加，造成无效腔形成。尽管如此，处理开放性骨折的早期目标是将感染的开放性伤口变为清洁闭合性伤口。许多操作技术都支持这个原则，从二期愈合前一直保持伤口开放，如果单纯缝合不可行，则使用一些整形技术达到一期闭合伤口的改变。

除了最轻微的一些伤口，其他伤口特别是已经施行了内固定的开放性骨折，最好避免一期闭合伤口。当伤口保持开放时，运用抗生素珠袋技术仍然不失为好办法（该技术由 Henry 等开发）。它是由聚甲基丙酸甲酯骨水泥和 1.2 g 的妥布霉素粉剂混合而成。做成直径 5 mm 的球珠，然后塑形后用扭曲的不锈钢丝穿起来，并分成 3 ~ 4 mm 一段。虽然这可以由外科医生团队在手术室完成，但药剂科的人员通常会遵循 Henry 等描述的过程将之预加工，并对球链进行高压蒸汽灭菌，装入无菌分离的袋有利于在人体使用。这种球珠被放入伤口，用足够大的 Tegaderm 或 Opsite 覆盖伤口，密封伤口，保持伤口皮瓣恰当的张力，以防止皮瓣皱缩。

那些伤口更严重的患者须 1 ~ 2 天后返回手术室更换敷料，并根据须做进一步清创。当所有可疑的失活组织清理完后，应将伤口闭合。Ⅱ级和Ⅲ A 级伤口可在 5 ~ 7 天后缝合，但可能需要分层厚皮肤移植物（split-thickness skin grafts，STSG）。范围更大的伤口通常得益于带蒂肌瓣闭合，同周围组织或游离微血管一起转移。仔细选择皮瓣有一定帮助，但是其他组织的皮瓣用于严重受伤的肢体不一定有效。STSG 在任何时间用于健康伤口组织都有效，但是当其用于暴露的血管、肌腱及裸露的皮质骨时却不那么让人满意。用打孔装置在厚皮片上打出许多孔隙可减少 STSG 下的液体积蓄。

许多严重的开放性骨折不须通过复杂的整形手术也能处理。开放性骨折尽管有骨头和植入物暴露，但几个月后往往也能愈合好。

筋膜室综合征

由正常筋膜围绕骨骼肌群形成了“隔室”，多种损伤都能导致“隔室”内组织压力升高。一旦隔室内压力升高到足够高，阻碍了微血管的灌注，使肌肉、神经缺血，会导致相应的组织坏死。当隔室内压力降到正常水平后，肌肉和神经已坏死，这就是 Volkmann 挛缩的原因。

有效治疗的关键是早诊断。无论何时肢体被持续挤压或有严重挫伤，不管有没有骨折，都应该考虑是否可能有筋膜室综合征。清醒患者如果存在筋膜室综合征时会逐渐出现疼痛，隔室区域持续肿胀，然后隔室内的肌肉和神经很快就失去功能。此时，脉搏和皮肤的血流灌注往往正常。开放性骨折也可能出现筋膜室综合征，因此清创的伤口并不能提供足够大的手术切口。

对于严重创伤，每 2 h 必须检查患者是否出现难以忍受的疼痛、是否失去感觉、受伤肢体远端是否还能活动。当治疗可疑筋膜室综合征时，首先是松开过紧的绷带或拆除石膏，以便检查。还要避免外部对隔室加压，这能充分减少隔室压力，恢复组织灌注，阻止坏死。如果患者失去意识，或者有相关的神经受损，阻碍临床评估，则用市场上流通的组织压力测量装置（如 Stryker STIC，由聚乙烯制成窄芯导管，其末端多处纵向切开 1 mm 左右）。这种装置充满无菌生理盐水，连接变应计，用来测量压力，而后用大孔径的针将导管导入隔室中。令人满意的测量系统会对隔室的压力做出迅速反应，当外部压力解除后，间隔压力会迅速下降至可再生的水平。注意测量涉及区域的每个隔室的压力，如大腿，就须测量前部、外侧、后方深层和后方浅层区域；又如前臂，须在多个区域评估屈肌群和伸肌群。越靠近骨折区域，隔室压力往往越大。

如果发现患者神经肌肉正常，隔室压力却升高，必须临床监测压力变化或重复测量。如果患者肢体肌肉收缩的感觉受损，或者不能评估，隔室压力在

30～40 mmHg 时，须进行筋膜切开术。所有累及的隔室都要打开。对于腿，常使用 2 个切口。一个切口位于外侧，用于打开前部和外侧的隔室，须注意保护腓浅神经；另一个切口迅速从后部向内侧、胫骨干方向切开，打开深部和后部浅层隔室。皮肤切口长度为 8～10 cm，在肢体近端和远端盲法切开筋膜，可适当减压，但对于那些严重损伤的肢体，减压并不充分。对于这些肢体，最好是延长切口达隔室全长。皮肤切口应通过缝合或 STSG 延迟关闭。合并骨折时，在进行筋膜切开术的同时进行固定修复，可简化伤口的处理。固定骨折是用内固定还是外固定，取决于骨折结构和其他软组织需要分离的程度。

前臂筋膜室综合征可能会涉及前方（屈肌）群或后方（伸肌）群，须打开每一块相关肌肉的内在筋膜。须行扩大手术入路，比如 Henry 在 *Extensile Exposure* 一书中描述的 McConnell 联合暴露正中神经和尺神经入路。

任何下肢的开放性伤口均应该遵循开放性伤口的处理原则，负压辅助伤口闭合（vacuum-assisted wound closure，VAWC）技术已经成为处理这些伤口的常规手段。当伤口清洁冲洗后，聚氨酯泡沫塑料填充于伤口内，其上贴一层硅胶膜。然后在这层膜中央做一切口，转接器放置在此切口处，持续以 100～125 mmHg 负压抽吸伤口内积液。这种负压吸引装置可在病房更换，如果计划缝合伤口，则去手术室。当伤口水肿消退，肢体直径的扩张减少时可以考虑闭合伤口。这期间，患者会出现多尿的症状。通过这种技术，最终能彻底地闭合伤口。如果经过多次更换敷料，伤口缺损仍大，可使用 STSG。

定量组织活检是另一项帮助外科医生决定何时闭合伤口的手段。活检能区分伤口的定植菌或创面污染的侵入细菌。借助 VAWC 技术，可以帮助保持伤口干燥，减少细菌侵入伤口。

若组织高度坏死后才诊断筋膜室综合征，最好直接保持闭合而不要行筋膜切开术。因为手术会增加感染风险，而且对坏死组织减压后获益并不明显。

脱套伤

处理脱套伤必须仔细判断失活组织的范围、皮瓣的组织层、撕脱的方向（是从肢体远端向近端还是从近端向远端），还要全面评估受损组织的血供情况。

与肢体仍有连接的脱套的皮肤可作为皮瓣保持活性，它通过蒂获取血液中的营养，而不是皮下组织。彻底明白肌肉和筋膜与皮肤的关系，可帮助判断哪些皮瓣可以保留。远端带蒂或带有窄蒂的广泛的皮肤撕脱，带或不带表层皮下组织，且深层组织没有损伤，最好彻底分离出蒂，去除皮肤的脂肪，再将撕脱的皮肤作为全层厚皮瓣移植物。

如果伤口污染严重或水肿严重，撕脱的组织应该用脉冲式灌洗装置清洗，使组织无或有轻微张力，并在二次探查时进行处理。术中荧光素检查是一种可靠的判断组织活性的手段。如果动脉血流充分，可以进行软组织清创并闭合伤口，注意闭合伤口时减少张力。

脱套伤常因为静脉回流受阻而引起组织坏死。运用抗血栓药物治疗，如局部每 4 h 用 Dermaid 芦荟膏和每日应用 81 mg 阿司匹林，加上自由使用水蛭疗法，这些手段的综合运用提高了立即或延迟伤口闭合的组织生存率。刚开始时，每 4 h 使用一次水蛭疗法，一直持续到因静脉淤血导致的发绀缓解为止。大的皮瓣需要两只水蛭。水蛭可被放置在某处，不需要特别的处理，或者可以致电供应商，几小时内就能得到（供应商如 Leeches U.S.A, 1-800-645-3569）。当静脉血管再通时，可以适当减少水蛭的应用频率，多数情况下静脉再通 3 天后可停止使用。

肢体损毁伤：延迟截肢

理想情况下，普通外科医生或骨科医生须在评估完患者损毁的肢体后，做出理想的决策，决定是否立即截肢或尝试重建。不幸的是，并没有能够指导外科医生做出决定的文献，且大多数关于损毁伤的文献关注的都是下肢损伤。损毁伤的骨折被划分为Ⅲ C 级，且均为开放性骨折。一些有血管损失，一些没有。有的没有感觉，有的有感觉。

已开发了许多评分系统用来预测哪些患者需要立即截肢，哪些患者需要重建。Bonanni 等指出我们本身存在偏见，声称预测评分是徒劳的。他们在研究中发现，在运用毁损肢体综合征指数、预测保肢指数、毁损肢体严重度评分、保肢指数，这些评分系统时并没有表现出可靠的灵敏度和特异度。基于临床经验的外科判断仍然是金标准。

Bosse 等近期进行了一项研究，纳入 569 例严重的腿部损伤患者，分成重建组和截肢组，两组的疾病影响状态调查（sickess impact profile，SIP）并没有区别。他们的研究还提示如果患者出现以下情况，则这些患者的SIP得分差。再入院、严重并发症、受教育水平低、非白种人、贫穷、缺少个人医疗保险、社交支持网少、自我效能低、吸烟、涉及残疾赔偿诉讼。有意思的是，接受重建手术的患者再入院概率比接受截肢手术的患者高。返回工作的概率两组相似，这也揭示了外科医生做出的决策是正确的。

对于损毁伤，截肢的时间点是在早期还是后期，是有很大争议的。通常延迟截肢的原因包括如伤口缺少覆盖、骨不连引起感染、肢体无感觉、患肢反复出现溃疡、肢体营养不良、交感神经性营养不良、幻肢痛等。有的外科医生认为，相对于需要多次手术的保肢及重建手术，截肢手术恢复更快，花费更少。除了之前提到的Bosse等的研究，Pozo等研究了35例截肢的患者，他们均是在下肢的严重损伤治疗失败后接受的截肢术。其中7例是在损伤1个月后，局部缺血行截肢术，13例是因为受伤1个月至1年期间肢体出现感染，后出现组织缺少覆盖及骨不连的并发症，15例是在损伤1年后因为感染性骨不连接受截肢术的。后一个研究中，患者平均接受12次手术、长达50个月的治疗，其中平均住院时间为8个月。重建手术失败的主要原因有血管损伤、神经损伤、骨质损伤、肌肉损伤、皮肤覆盖和脓毒症。总之，研究者如果建议尝试行下肢重建手术，必须有两位专家一起进行早期评估，两位专家中一位来自创伤外科，一位来自骨科或整形外科，即使这样也不能完全避免失败。显然，这需要经验，且保肢手术的持续尝试比较困难。

另一项可能影响外科医生决策的研究来自Case Uhestern Reserve。该研究随访了34名患者，其中16名患者接受了保肢手术并取得成功，18名患者当时即行膝下截肢术（below knee amputation，BKA）。成功保肢的患者比截肢患者花费了更多的时间，来达到患肢正常负重，他们更不愿意或不能去工作，而且他们的住院费比早期BKA的患者高。此外，保肢患者会认为自己已经严重残疾，在工作和娱乐活动上比截肢患者面临的问题更多。这些生活质量的评估可能须纳入到之前提到的Bosse等的研究中去。

最后须提到的研究是Roessler等的研究。他们对80名患者进行了为期4年的随访，均询问了截肢的时间。他们得出神经、骨骼及组织的状态是影响是否立即行截肢手术的因素，但与后期的肢体缺失或死亡无关。有些令人惊讶的是，血液循环是至关重要的因素，血供可以通过触摸脉搏或者行多普勒超声检测出来。他们得出结论，在一些尝试保肢手术的病例中，如果患者有系统性损害，包括明显的体液正平衡等状况，必须在24 h内施行截肢术。他们还观察到，如果肢体末端无脉搏，最终截肢的概率会升高。

颈椎、胸椎、腰椎骨折

Nicholas Spoerke 和 Donald D. Trunkey 著
王天兵 译

脊柱损伤是创伤造成短期或长期疾病的主要来源。美国每年有超过10 000例脊柱损伤（spinal column injuries，SCI）患者，其中有超过一半是机动车碰撞导致的。其余原因包括坠落伤，含枪伤在内的穿通伤，运动损伤等。SCI中有超过一半发生在颈椎，其余的发生在胸椎和腰椎。

由于SCI大部分由高能量损伤和钝伤引起，因此大部分SCI患者是多发伤。几乎30%的SCI患者合并有脊柱外损伤，创伤性脑损伤较常见，另外，脊柱多发性骨折也很常见。

对于所有可能导致SCI的患者，在搬动、运输和初始评估期间应该适当地制动整个脊柱。这包括同轴的颈椎制动，通常用颈托或胶带和刚性背板实现。与其他中枢神经系统可疑损伤一样，最初的复苏工作应避免全身性低血压，并严格遵守ATLS指南。

脊髓综合征

损伤的位置和严重程度不同，SCI后引起的神经功能障碍差异较大。完全脊髓损伤指在损伤水平以下超过3个及以上节段的运动或感觉功能缺失。不完全SCI则是脊髓损伤部位对应的运动和感觉的缺失。外伤性损伤通常出现3种类型的不完全性脊髓损伤综合征：

*脊髓前综合征*通常由脊髓前部的血管损伤引起。所产生的神经损伤的特征是运动和感觉缺失的节段低于损伤水平节段，而本体感觉和位置感觉正常。这种综合征往往预后不良，只有10%的患者恢复运动功能。

*脊髓中央综合征*的特征主要是上肢无力的程度明显重于下肢。它通常在颈椎椎管狭窄时由颈椎过伸存在而引起，总体预后良好，超过75%的患者肢体出现功能恢复。

布朗-塞卡尔综合征，通常由穿通性创伤和脊髓半横断导致，典型表现是同侧运动和对侧感觉缺陷，这种综合征预后最好。

类固醇激素在脊髓损伤中的应用

开始时，神经细胞功能障碍由创伤性撞击产生的动能引起。继发性损伤则通过许多生物化学反应和细胞途径发生，这代表改善神经功能恢复的潜在干预区域。为了防止神经元的继发性损伤并促进神经系统恢复，许多研究一直致力于神经保护。避免低血压是预防继发性CNS损伤的重要初始步骤。在过去的30年中，已经对神经元细胞损伤和脂质过氧化的抑制进行了大量研究，包括了极具争议的国家急性脊髓损伤研究试验。虽然这一争议超出了本章的范围，但仍然没有对脊髓损伤中类固醇的最佳使用时间、剂量或适应证达成总体共识。目前建议应当在脊柱外科医生的陪同下，尽早使用甲基泼尼松龙（理想的是在损伤的3 h内，并且必须在损伤的8 h内）。甲基泼尼松龙也用于非穿通性脊髓损伤。研究显示，如果在损伤后8 h内静脉给予30 mg/kg剂量的，随后以5.4mg/kg · h的静脉滴注持续23 h，可以促进感觉和运动功能恢复。

颈椎损伤

颈椎相关解剖

颈椎总共有7块颈椎椎骨，通常分为C1、C2和轴下颈椎（C3-C7）。寰椎（C1）呈环形，由前后弓和2个侧块组成。C1与枕骨髁以及C2的齿状突和关节面形成复杂的高度专门化的运动关节，来维持头部旋转。齿状突仅独特地存在于枢椎（C2）上，其与C1的前弓连接，并且由横韧带固定。轴下颈椎（C3-C7）的椎骨形态较均匀，侧块保护成对的椎动脉（C6至C1）通过，关节面呈45°，首先允许颈部屈伸运动。与脊柱中的其他节段相对比，颈部脊髓在脊柱中的占有空间比相对较少，在C1处仅占椎管的33%。

颈椎损伤的模式和管理

疑似颈椎损伤的患者，应该在他们进行初次和二次检查时制动脊椎，且保持解剖力学对线。重点突出的神经系统检查应作为二次检查的一部分，并特别注意运动和感觉功能、疼痛和在触诊中线脊柱时的骨下移等情况。当存在压痛、神经功能缺陷或者患者感觉迟钝，以及患者处于不可检查的状态（如插管和化学麻醉）时，放射学检查应包括专用的脊椎CT。事实上，在脊椎损伤时CT已经取代了正位和过屈/过伸位X线。与CT比较，磁共振成像对软组织损伤更敏感，但不应该用作主要的影像检查，仅在CT检查上没有发现致阳性体征的原因时，为患者进行更详细的损伤评估。脊髓损伤最好根据美国脊髓损伤协会国际脊髓损伤神经和功能分类标准进行分类（图1）：

A= 完全性损害：S4-S5 无任何感觉、运动功能保留。
B= 不完全性损害：在神经平面以下，包括S4-S5，存在感觉功能，但无运动功能。
C= 不完全性损害：在神经平面以下存在运动功能，且平面以下至少一半以上关键肌肌力 <3 级。
D= 不完全性损害：在神经平面以下存在运动功能，且平面以下至少一半关键肌肌力 ≥ 3 级。
E 正常：感觉和运动功能正常。

图1 美国脊髓损伤协会损伤量表

枕骨髁骨折

枕骨髁骨折一般由解剖学上的敏感地区的高能量损伤引起，并且在涉及枕骨髁骨折的事故中，患者的死亡率相对较高。根据Anderson和Montesano分类（图2），这些骨折可以分为3种类型：

Ⅰ型：由轴向负荷引起的压缩性骨折（罕见）

Ⅱ型：颅底骨折延伸到枕骨髁

Ⅲ型：撕脱骨折（常见）

Ⅲ型骨折通常由通过分散的力导致的髁韧带撕脱引起。以上任何类型的骨折最好用颈托稳定。Ⅱ

型或Ⅲ型损伤，如果出现骨折移位，须使用 Halo 支架固定。不稳定的Ⅲ型骨折，须枕骨与 C2 进行融合，并且枕颈分离的发病率很高。

枕颈分离（寰枢椎分离）

造成枕颈分离的损伤很罕见，但往往是致命的。它们通常包括半脱位或有毁灭性脊髓损伤或横断分离。枕颈分离通常是不稳定的，并且进行对齐复位后，须通过外科手术将枕骨融合到 C2。常见的分型是：Ⅰ型（寰椎枕骨部的前移位），Ⅱ型（纵向关节面分离）和Ⅲ型（寰椎枕骨部的后移位）。

寰椎骨折

C1 骨折可涉及前弓、后弓、侧块或横突（图 3），很少引起神经功能损伤。爆裂骨折（也称为 Jefferson 骨折）包括前后弓的双侧骨折，通常是由轴向受力引起。侧块骨折应该更加注意有无椎动脉损伤，并结合颈椎 CT 血管造影进行评估，特别是涉及椎孔的时候更应谨慎。无横韧带破裂的稳定性骨折可以用颈托固定治疗。而有横韧带损伤伴移位的不稳定骨折，则须先进行温和牵引，然后行 Halo 支架固定。

齿状突骨折

齿状突骨折分为 3 种类型（图 4）。Ⅰ型骨折常由齿状突尖部韧带撕脱引起，通常是稳定的骨折，并且仅需要最简单的治疗或颈托固定。Ⅲ型骨折延伸到 C2 椎体，同样可以用颈托治疗 6～8 周。Ⅱ型骨折发生在齿状突的腰部，应根据患者的年龄、复合损伤、碎片移位程度和总体稳性来制订其治疗方案。年轻患者的移位小的稳定性骨折最好用 Halo 支架固定。手术复位的相关适应证包括骨折移位大于 6 mm、骨折向后成角、粉碎性骨折或患者年龄大于 50 岁。

Hangman 骨折

Hangman 骨折泛指双侧脊椎峡部发生的骨折（图 5）。它们由 Levine 和 Edwards 分类（表 1）。Ⅰ型损伤由 Halo 支架制动治疗，但Ⅱ和Ⅲ型损伤通常需要手术。

轴下颈椎骨折

C3-C7 椎骨的损伤归类为轴下颈椎损伤，由骨折、半脱位和分离的任意组合组成。棘突、椎板和横突的断裂较为常见，孤立性、关节面完好、没有成角移位或水平移位的骨折可以认为是稳定性骨折。更广泛的骨折分型是：①压缩性；②爆裂性；③泪滴形骨折。

压缩性骨折导致椎体的前部分楔入，但具有完整的椎体后部和椎管。当伴有较小成角（<11°）、较

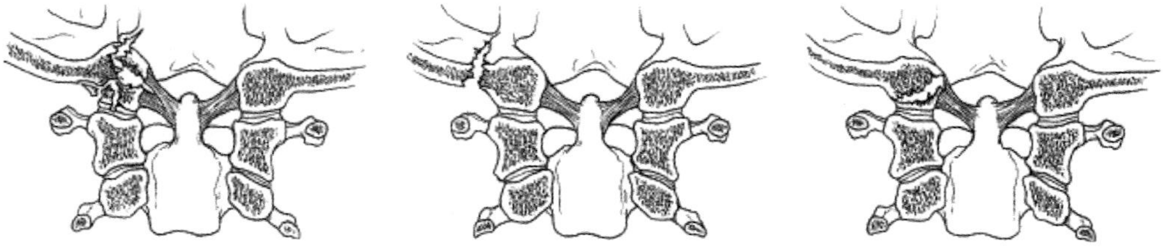

图 2 枕骨骨折的分型 (*From AndersonPA, Mirza SK, Chapman JR: Injuries tothe atlantooccipital articulation. InClark CR, Dvorak J, Ducker TB, et al,editors: The cervical spine, 4th ed,Philadelphia, 2005, Lippincott-Raven, p 594.*)

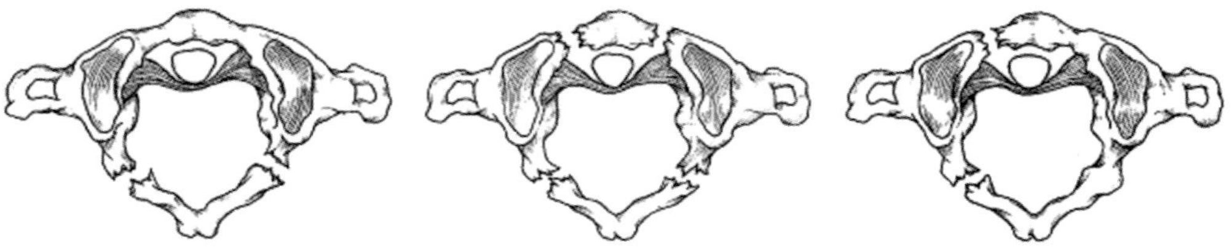

图 3 C1 骨折类型 (*From Hasharoni A, ErricoTJ: Fracture of the first cervical vertebra.In Clark CR, Dvorak J, Ducker TB, et al,editors: The cervical spine, 4th ed,Philadelphia, 2005, Lippincott-Raven, p 610.*)

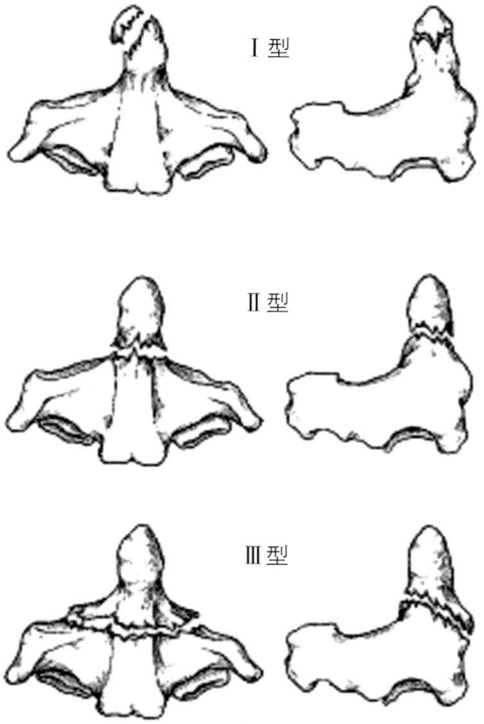

图 4　齿状突骨折类型 (*From Anderson LD, D'AlonzoRT: Fractures of the odontoid process of the axis. J Bone Joint Surg56:1663–1674, 1974*)

表 1　Hangman 骨折的分型

类型	临床表现
Ⅰ型	椎间移位小于 3 mm，没有因轴向挤压和过度伸展而出现成角
Ⅰ A 型	由于侧屈力导致过度伸展，具有较小程度的成角或移位的不对称骨折线
Ⅱ型	移位 >3 mm，成角明显
Ⅱ A 型	成角明显，无明显移位，因牵张 - 屈曲损伤导致
Ⅲ型	C2-C3 关节错位，因屈曲引起的过度伸展所致

小高度损失（<25%）和较小平移（<2.5 mm）时，可只进行简单的颈椎制动治疗。不稳定的骨折，包括那些椎体高度丢失大于 50%或椎体后部分散的患者，通常需要手术稳定和融合。

爆裂性骨折由轴向受力引起，其特征是脊柱前柱和中柱的破坏。如果前纵韧带和后纵韧带均出现损伤或者骨折不能进行复位、维持力学对线，则须进行手术治疗。如果没有神经损伤，可以采用 Halo 支架进行固定，再达到力学对线。

泪滴形骨折既可以位于前部也能位于后部。前部骨折通常是由过度伸展引起的撕脱伤引起，通常发生在 C2-C3 连接处，并且可用颈托进行治疗。后部骨折通常由屈曲 - 压缩机制引起，通常涉及脊柱的前、中、后 3 柱，伴随神经损伤。治疗通常需要急诊复位和手术固定。

胸椎和腰椎的损伤

由于肋骨和胸骨对脊柱的稳定支撑，胸椎的损伤相对少见。胸椎骨折通常由高能量机制引起，因此常常伴有基础损伤，例如肋骨骨折、肺挫伤和气胸，以及血管损伤。当损伤发生时，由于引起损伤的能量高、神经椎管空间相对狭小、胸段脊髓的血液供应不足等原因，可能会导致毁灭性的神经损伤。

胸椎和腰椎的相关解剖

由于胸椎两侧有肋骨连接、胸椎椎板呈重叠状，胸椎比颈椎或腰椎更难弯曲。这种相对僵直导致在 T1 和 T12 的过渡区域更容易出现骨折，并且这两个区域的部分也更容易出现损伤，这是脊柱第二常见的受伤区域。这些骨折的稳定性通常取决于脊柱是否能够维持生理负荷下的解剖学关系。通常使用 Denis 的三柱损伤模型来评估稳定性（图 6）。前柱

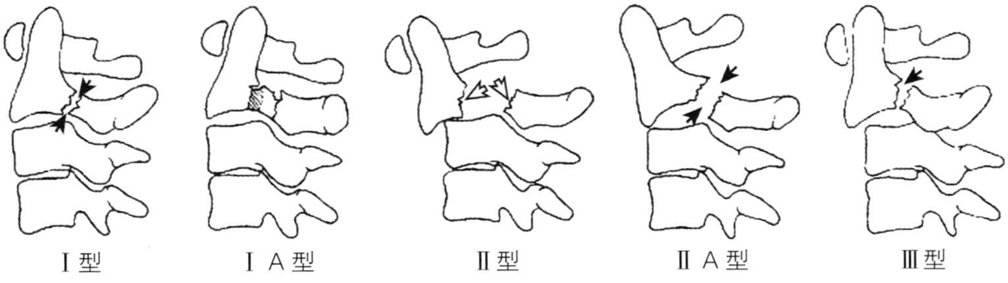

图 5　Hangman 骨折类型（*From Levine AM, EdwardsCC: The management of traumaticspondylolisthesis of the axis.* J Bone JointSurg *67:221–226, 1985.*）

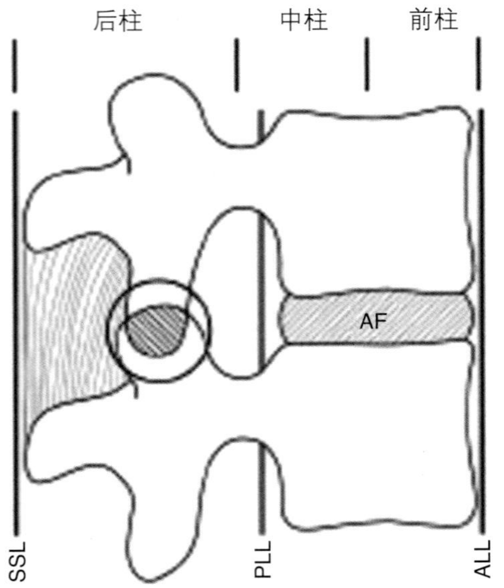

图 6 脊柱。AF，纤维环；ALL，前纵韧带；PLL，后纵韧带；SSL，脊柱前韧带 (*Modified from McAfee PC, Yuan HA, Fredrickson BE,Lubicky JP: The value of computed tomography in horacolumbar factures:an analysis of one hundred consecutive cases and a new classification.* J Bone Joint Surg *65:461–473, 1983.*)

由前纵韧带和椎体前半部组成。中柱由椎体的后半部和后纵韧带组成。后柱由黄韧带、棘上韧带、椎弓和关节面组成。根据定义，不稳定损伤是指涉及两个柱的损伤或者任何具有神经缺损的骨折。此外，椎体高度损失百分比和成角程度也用于评估稳定性。

胸椎和腰椎骨折

常见骨折类型分为：压缩性骨折、爆裂性骨折和屈曲分离性骨折。

*压缩性骨折*是胸腰段骨折最常见的类型。形态学上，压缩性骨折表现为椎体前部高度损失，而不累及脊柱中柱和后柱（图 7）。虽然这些骨折仅涉及一个柱，但椎体高度丢失大于 50% 或者存在大于 30° 的成角，这些骨折仍然可能是不稳定的。稳定性骨折可用支具治疗，但不稳定骨折则需要手术治疗。

*爆裂性骨折*同时破坏脊柱前柱和中柱，并具有较高的神经损伤风险（图 8）。不稳定损伤表现为椎体高度丢失大于 50%，成角大于 25% 或椎管变窄程度大于 50%，都需要手术固定。具有较小高度损失或成角的稳定性骨折通常可以用脊柱矫正治疗，密切监测以确保力学对线的维持。

*屈曲分离性损伤*既有骨折也有韧带部分损伤。这种损伤常发生于车祸中，机动车突然减速导致佩戴安全带的乘客发生此类损伤。前柱被压缩，中间柱和后柱过度拉伸（图 9）。原发性韧带损伤因愈合性差，通常须手术复位。这种在 T12-L2 椎体的损伤应该同时注意是否伴随有十二指肠、胰腺或腹膜后血管结构的损伤。

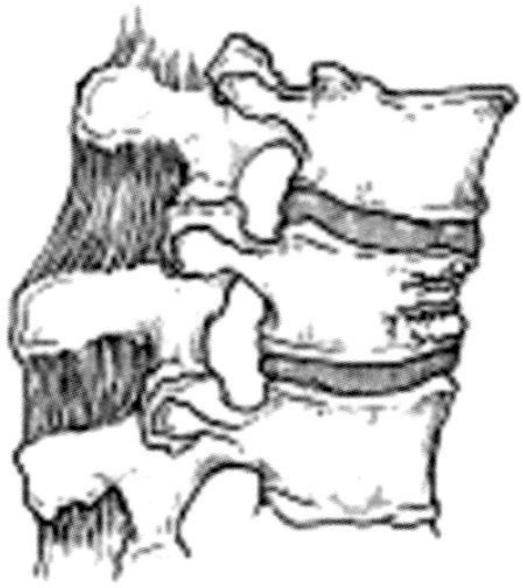

图 7 压缩性骨折 (*From Holdsworth FW: Fractures, dislocations and fracture-dislocations of the spine.* J Bone Joint Surg Br *52:1534–1551, 1970.*)

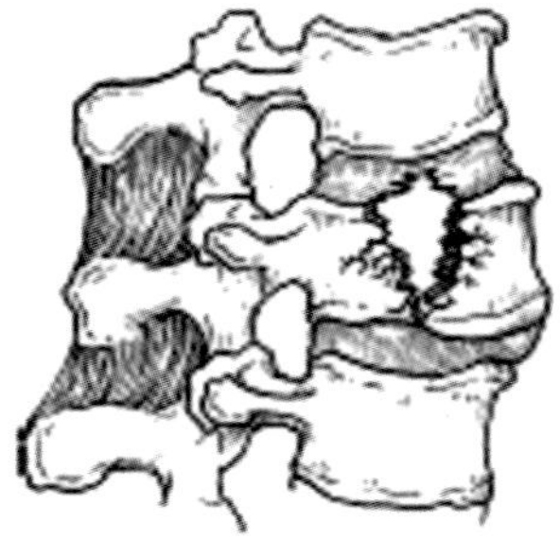

图 8 爆裂性骨折 (*From Holdsworth FW: Fractures, dislocations and fracture-dislocations of the spine.* J Bone Joint Surg Br *52:1534–1551, 1970.*)

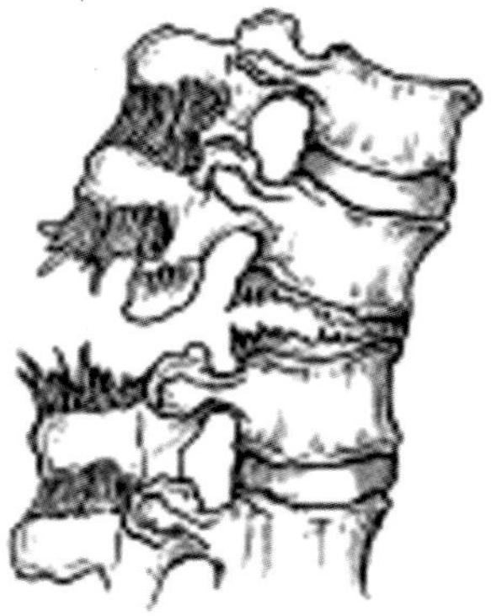

图 9 屈曲分离性骨折 (*From Holdsworth FW: Fractures, dislocations and fracture-dislocations of the spine.* J Bone Joint Surg Br *52:1534–1551, 1970.*)

骨盆骨折

Christopher H. Perkins 和 Stephen M. Quinnan 著
王天兵 译

骨盆骨折是相对少见的损伤，仅占所有骨折的2%。然而，20%的多发伤患者伴有骨盆骨折，其死亡率可达15%～20%。常见的损伤机制包括机动车事故、摩托车事故、汽车碰撞行人和高处跌落。骨盆骨折呈双峰分布，高能量不稳定性骨折常见于年轻男性，低能量稳定性骨折常见于中老年女性。12%～62%的骨盆骨折患者发生相关的损伤，其中最常见的是膀胱和尿路损伤（63%），其次是闭合性头部损伤（35%）、神经损伤（24%）、肠道损伤（20%）和胸部损伤（20%）。开放性骨盆骨折仅占骨盆骨折的2%～4%，但死亡率为25%～50%。骨盆骨折的死亡原因通常是由于盆腔内出血或相关腹部损伤导致的出血性休克。由于相关损伤的严重性和普遍性，需要协调的多学科方法来处理这些患者。已经在许多Ⅰ级创伤中心开发并实施了骨科创伤学家和介入放射科医生共同早期参与的治疗方案，以降低这些损伤的死亡率。

解剖

骨盆环包括骶骨和两侧髋骨，前方在耻骨联合处连接，后方在骶髂关节处连接。髋骨由坐骨、髂骨和耻骨在3个方向的软骨处融合形成。连接到骨盆环的韧带的强度决定了其稳定性的大小。其次，骨间韧带，前、后骶髂韧带为髂腰部提供主要支持，而骶结节韧带和骶棘韧带也发挥了部分作用。在前面，耻骨联合提供支持，并且作为支柱以防止坍塌。骨盆在承重时提供结构支撑，并保护、容纳在其内的器官和其他结构。骨盆环作为一个完整的环状结构而发挥作用。因此，骨盆环某一部分损伤有可能引起环的另一部分损伤。生物力学研究表明，耻骨联合切开后最多能分离2.5 cm。进一步切开前骶髂韧带则可以将骨盆打开，直至髂骨后上棘的骨性突起。同时离断后骶髂韧带将使骨盆失去垂直方向的稳定。

骨盆内还有许多重要血管，当骨折发生时可能使之损伤。主动脉在L5椎体水平处分出髂总动脉，并且在骶髂关节前进一步分成髂内动脉和髂外动脉。臀上动脉从髂内分出并通过坐骨切迹穿出骨盆，是骨盆骨折中最常见损伤的血管。骨盆内部可能受伤的其他分支包括骶外侧动脉、髂腰动脉、闭孔动脉、膀胱动脉和臀下动脉。多个静脉也在骨盆内穿行，并且也随之受到损伤。

影像学检查

对于怀疑骨盆骨折的患者应该在拍胸部和颈椎侧位X线片的同时拍骨盆平片，这是ATLS方案的关于创伤系列的一部分。大多数骨盆骨折可以通过单纯的正位X线片诊断，但入口和出口的X线片有助于进一步确定骨折形态特征。这些X线片在患者仰卧位拍摄，射束角度向头部45°为入口视角，向脚部45°为出口视角。入口视图显示骨折的前后和旋转移位，出口视图显示垂直位移和骶骨骨折。如果放置了底板并且初始X线片没有显示移位，则应在患者足够稳定后，在没有底板的情况下拍正位平片。CT扫描与重建有助于描述移位和骨折类型，是许多钝性创伤指南要求的一部分。对比创伤CT扫描具有60%～84%的灵敏度和95%的特异度，用于诊断与盆腔骨折相关的动脉损伤。它也有助于诊断并存的腹内和胸部损伤（图1-4）。

骨折分类

可依据损伤的机制或稳定性对骨盆骨折进行分类，这取决于所使用的系统。Young和Burgess开发的分类系统主要基于机制，是使用最广泛的。共有三种机制：前后压缩（anteroposterior compression，APC）、横向压缩（lateral compression，LC）和垂直剪切（vertical shear，VS）。APC损伤指伴有不同程度的后部损伤的前环损伤，损伤侧半骨盆外部随着受伤程度的增加而旋转。LC损伤指伴随有不同程度后部损伤的耻骨支骨折，损伤侧半骨盆内部随着受伤程度的增加而旋转。VS损伤指骶髂关节破坏以及伴有耻骨支或耻骨联合损伤的骶骨骨折，这种损伤

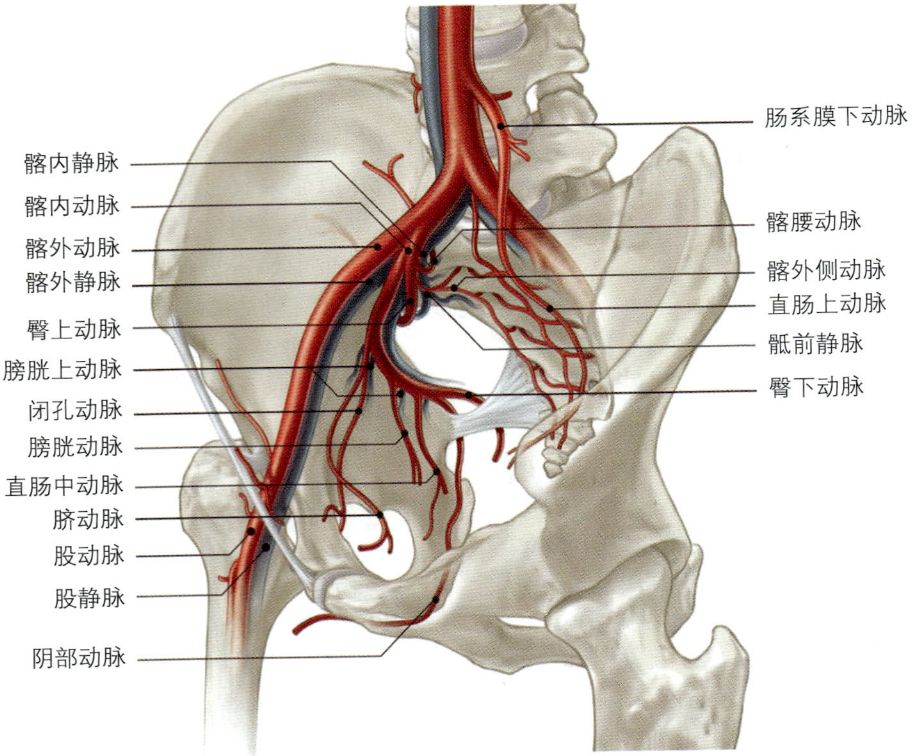

图 1 骨盆血管解剖 (*From Geeraerts T, Chhor V, Cheisson G, et al: Clinical review: initial management of blunt pelvic trauma patients withhaemodynamic instability.* Crit Care *11:204, 2007.*)

导致损伤侧的半个骨盆的垂直移位。因为损伤可以发生在多个力向量，故骨折分类可以允许联合机制损伤（combined mechanism injuries，CMI）。

Tile 开发的分类系统是基于稳定性的。骨盆以髋臼为界分为前弓和后弓，骨折分类主要基于后弓的稳定性。A 型骨折稳定；B 型骨折旋转不稳定，但垂直方向稳定；C 型骨折旋转和垂直均不稳定。

由骨科创伤协会制定的分类方法也基于稳定性。A 型骨折是稳定的骨盆骨折；B 型骨折部分稳定；C 型骨折是后弓完全破坏引起的不稳定性骨折。在该分类系统内有许多亚分组，其对于科学研究很有帮助，但不适合常规临床使用。

初步评估

骨盆骨折的院前管理是基于其损伤机制进行的。将患者救出并行气道评估后，若患者意识清楚且反应正常，急救人员可以通过询问病史以及行简单的临床检查对患者的骨盆骨折进行识别。出血可以将双腿内旋并绑定骨盆来控制。在该过程中应避免手动压缩骨盆，以及将患者翻动超过 15°。如果绑定骨盆是在院前进行的，那么在急诊部门进行适当的评估之前，不应该去除骨盆的绑定。

到达急诊室后，初始治疗应遵循 ATLS 协议，包括使用创伤系列 X 线片的初级和二级检查。FAST 可快速识别腹腔内损伤。然而，FAST 检查对于检测腹膜后血肿是不可靠的。即使 FAST 扫描阴性，25％的骨盆骨折患者仍会有腹腔内损伤。也可以使用诊断性腹膜灌洗（diagnostic peritoneal lavage，DPL），但应该在脐上切口，以避免由于骨盆骨折血肿导致的假阳性发现。CT 扫描是评估腹内和骨盆内损伤以及腹膜后血肿的最佳方式。泌尿生殖器损伤发生率占骨盆骨折的 15％～20％，前移位时损伤风险大大增加。逆行膀胱尿道造影可用于诊断泌尿生殖系统损伤。

骨盆的体格检查是对意识清楚患者，询问骨盆区域是否疼痛。骨盆损伤的典型特征是骨盆和会阴部的畸形、瘀斑或肿胀，耻骨联合分离征和双下肢不等长。骨盆上的伤口、直肠或阴道的出血可能提示开放性骨折。骨盆和直肠检查是必须进行的，以排除隐蔽的开放性骨折，并且高位前列腺可以提示

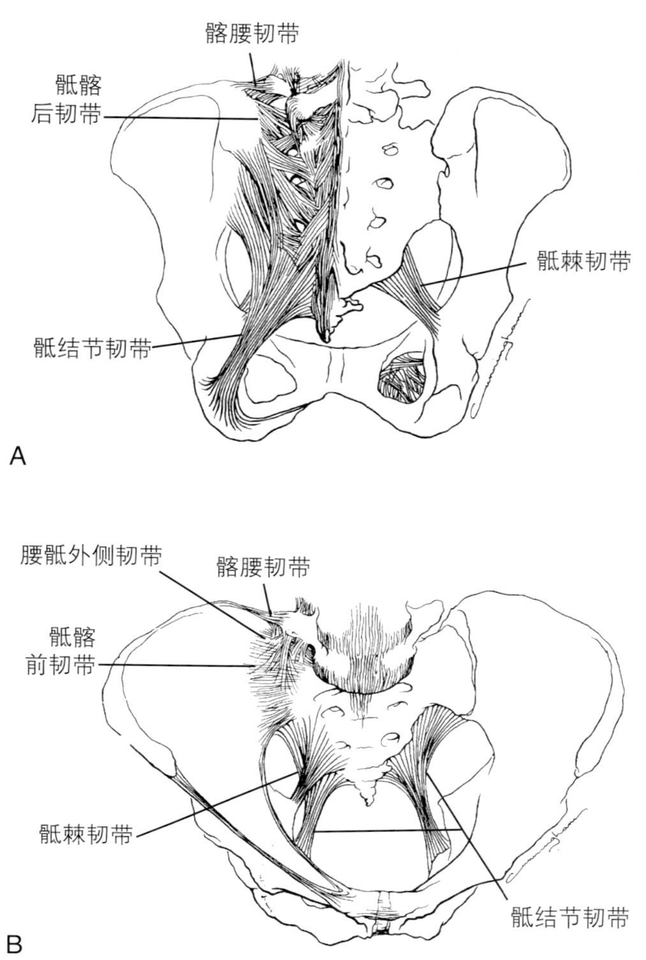

图 2 **A**，骨盆及其主要后方韧带；B，前位观 (*From Tile M, editor:* Fractures of the pelvis andacetabulum, *3rd ed, Baltimore, 2003, Williams& Wilkins.*)

男性尿路损伤。当患者的生命状态稳定时，也应进行完整的神经系统检查。是否行骨盆挤压和分离试验尚具有争议，因为它有引起更多的软组织损伤或血栓移动的可能。此外，它用于检测骨盆不稳定性时，其灵敏度仅为 71%，特异度仅为 59%，是不太可靠的。如果进行骨盆挤压试验，则应限于骨科创伤专家的单次尝试。

快速诊断骨盆骨折非常重要，因为有严重出血和导致死亡的危险。心动过速和周围血管收缩是出血的早期指标，低血压和低血细胞比容则出现较晚。初始液体和血液复苏应遵循公认的方案，如果存在凝血功能障碍，应进行纠正。碱缺失和乳酸水平可用于监测出血和复苏，尿量也是复苏和系统灌注的良好指标。骨盆骨折中的实质性出血来自出血的骨，以及髂内部分分布的动脉或静脉的损伤，血管破裂可导致大量腹膜后血肿。APC Ⅲ、VS 和 Tile C 骨盆骨折出血的风险最大。当骨折断端稳定时，在骨折部位骨出血减少。骨盆骨折中有 10% ~ 20% 的患者因动脉损伤导致血流动力学不稳定。尽管已经进行了充分的复苏，但对于明确骨盆骨折和血流动力学不稳定的患者，还应进一步使用技术手段控制出血和稳定骨盆。现代复苏和控制出血的技术将死亡率从 40% ~80%降至 20%（框 1，图 5）。

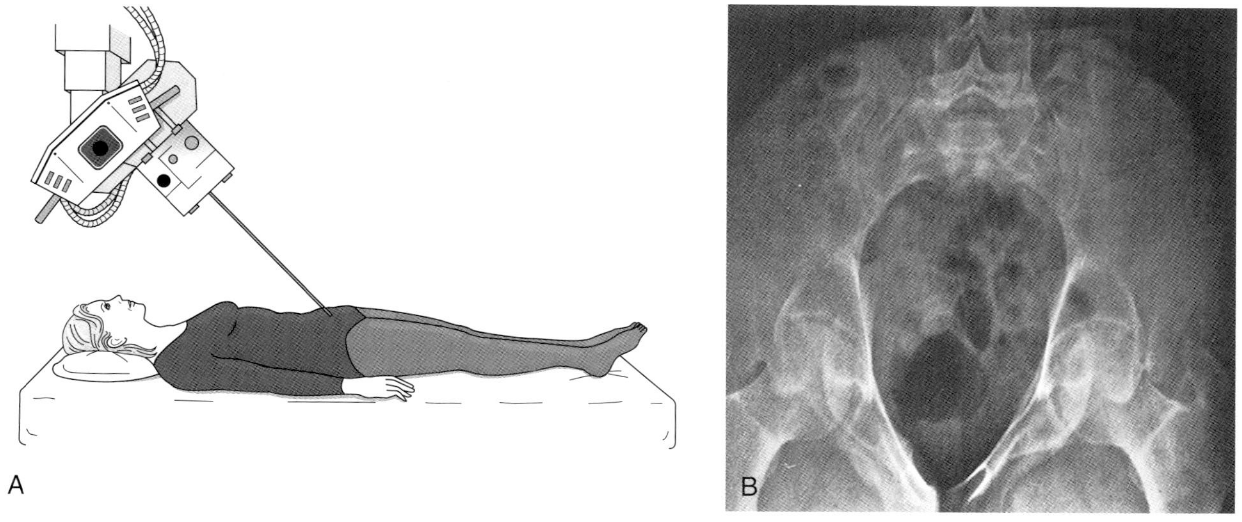

图 3 骨盆入口位。**A**，患者体位；**B**，X 线片表现 (*From Kellam JF, Browner BD: Fractures of the pelvic ring. In BrownerBD, Jupiter JB, Levine AM, et al, editors:* Skeletal trauma. *Philadelphia, 1992, WB Saunders, pp 849–897.*)

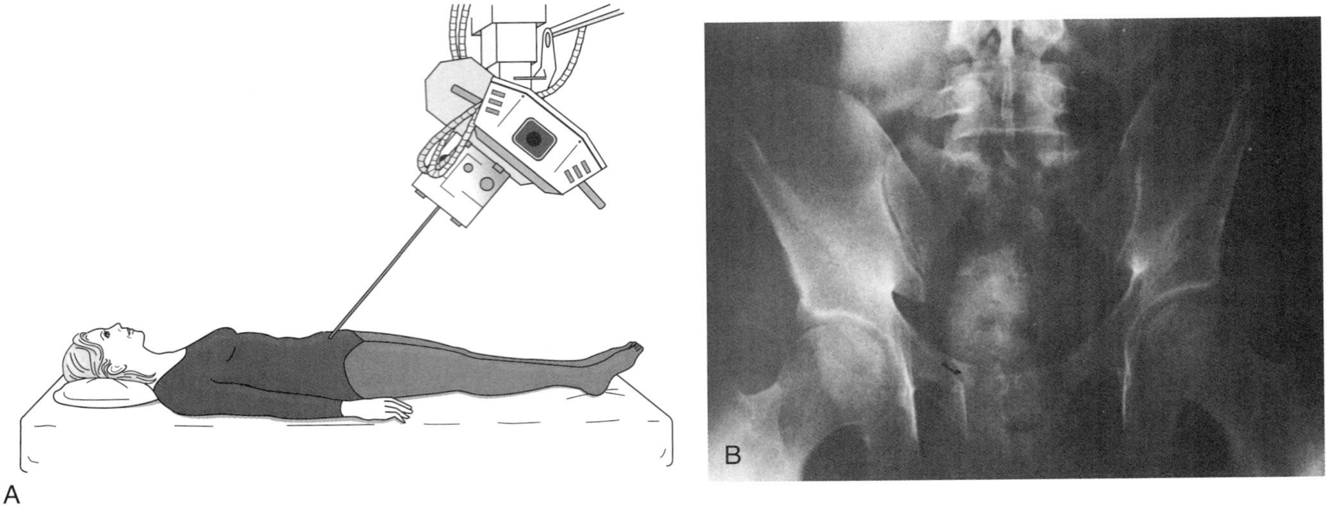

图 4 骨盆出口位。**A**，患者体位，**B**，X 线片表现 (*From Kellam JF, Browner BD: Fractures of the pelvic ring. In BrownerBD, Jupiter JB, Levine AM, et al, editors:* Skeletal trauma. *Philadelphia, 1992, WB Saunders, pp 849–897.*)

初步治疗

对于骨盆骨折患者，当通过查体和影像学检查发现骨盆容积增大时（APC 损伤），稳定和复位骨折的最简单方法是骨盆绑定。这可以用薄板或预制的固定物来实现。固定物放置在大转子水平并固定。最常见的错误是将固定物放在髂骨翼上。必须确保固定物位于大转子上，因为放置在骨盆边缘时，它不能减少出血和固定骨盆。使用这种技术，可以通过固定骨折部位减少出血，并且减少活动对已经形成的凝块的破坏。它还能有效减少静脉出血，但无法可靠地控制主要动脉的出血。骨盆绑定不应用于容积减小的骨盆骨折（LC 损伤）或经椎间孔骶骨骨折。此外，如果骨盆绑得太紧或保持在某个位置太长时间，可能发生皮肤坏死。有时，由于持续、严重的骨折不稳定，必须长时间保持黏合，但是必须认识到，用骨盆黏合维持骨盆稳定性的时间越长，皮肤坏死的风险越高。

另一种用于减少移位和稳定骨盆骨折的技术是气动防休克服。它们可以控制施加压力的大小，并且有效地减少腹膜后血肿。然而，气动防休克服具有体积庞大的缺点，并且可导致缺血和下肢筋膜室综合征。它们也难以进入腹部和会阴区。由于这些原因，气动防休克服没有广泛用于骨盆固定。

C 型的也可以用于减少和稳定骨盆骨折，但它在欧洲比在美国更受欢迎。它可以在手术室外迅速装配，能更直接地减少后环损伤。C 型钳经皮放置在与骶髂螺钉固定相同的位置，但与外固定相比仅是暂时的。然而，在手术室外装配时，这种技术还具有潜在的灾难性并发症的风险，特别是在粉碎性骶骨骨折中。

前部外固定是另一种用于稳定不稳定性骨盆骨折的技术手段。这项技术能有效地稳定骨盆骨折和减少出血。钉可以放置在髂前下棘（anterior inferior iliac spine，AIIS）或髂嵴。一般在手术室放置外固定架，但是带有髂嵴钉的固定架可以在急诊室中放置。髂嵴钉可以放置得更快，当需要时，他们可以在非荧光透视的条件下安全地放置。如果时间允许，在影像学引导下放置才是首选。AIIS 钉需要荧光透视检查以便安全放置，并且更耗时。但是，AIIS 钉具有更好的拔出强度、更强的硬度，为复位提供更好的轴。骨盆外固定架的放置通常与其他手术一起进行，例如治疗腹部损伤的剖腹术。钉的放置取决于多个变量，当患者处于危急状态时通常使用髂嵴针，用于“复苏框架”。当患者的生理状态允许时，优先使用 AIIS 钉，用“确定性治疗框架”。当存在垂直不稳定性时，单独的前部外固定不能完全控制后骨盆。对于垂直不稳定损伤（垂直剪切损伤），还须骨牵引协助维持骨盆复位。

骨盆骨折患者复苏之后，若血流动力学持续不稳定而骨盆暂时稳定的情况下应考虑进行血管造影。骨盆骨折出血 90% 来自静脉，10% 来自动脉，但是动脉损伤更易造成血流动力学不稳定。在血管造

框 1　骨盆骨折分型

Tile 分型

A 型（稳定型）

A1. 骨盆边缘骨折，不累及骨盆环，撕脱伤

A2. 稳定骨盆环有轻度移位

B 型（旋转不稳、垂直稳定型）

B1. 外旋损伤，开书样损伤

B2. LC 损伤或髋骨内旋不稳定，单侧损伤

B3. LC 损伤或双侧髋骨内旋不稳定（斗柄样损伤）

C 型（旋转和垂直不稳定型）

C1. 单侧伤

C2. 双侧伤，一侧旋转不稳，对侧正常

C3. 双侧伤，双侧旋转和垂直不稳定，或合并髋臼骨折

Young-Burgess 分型

横向挤压：侧方暴力引起暴力同侧或对侧耻骨支骨折

Ⅰ型：有影响的一侧骶骨压缩

Ⅱ型：有影响的一侧新月形髂骨翼骨折

Ⅲ型：有影响的一侧Ⅰ型或Ⅱ型损伤，对侧开书样（APC）损伤

前后压缩：耻骨联合分离或耻骨支纵向骨折

Ⅰ型：耻骨联合轻度分离（<2.5 cm）或骶髂关节前部轻度分离，骶髂韧带、骶结节韧带、骶棘韧带拉长但结构完整，骶髂后韧带完整

Ⅱ型：耻骨联合分离>2.5 cm或骶髂前关节增宽，骶髂前韧带、骶结节韧带、骶棘韧带受损，骶髂后韧带仍结构完整

Ⅱ型：骶髂关节完全破坏并横向移位，骶髂前韧带、骶结节韧带，骶棘韧带、骶髂后韧带均受损

垂直剪切：耻骨联合分离或向前后垂直位移，通常累及骶髂关节，偶尔累及髂骨环或骶骨

联合机制损伤（CMI）：损伤机制的联合，LC/VS 最常见

骨盆环骨折的骨科创伤协会分型

A 型：损伤少（后弓不移位）

1. 髋骨撕脱性骨折
2. 髋骨直接暴力骨折
3. 骶骨和尾骨的横向骨折

B 型：后弓不完全损伤，部分稳定型

1. 后弓外旋、部分单侧损伤（开书样损伤）
2. 后弓内旋、部分单侧损伤（LC 损伤）
3. 后弓部分双侧损伤

C 型：后弓完全损伤，不稳定型

1. 后弓完全单侧损伤
2. 双侧或暴力侧完全损伤或对侧损伤

From McCormack R, Strauss EJ, Alwattar BJ, Tejwani NC: Diagnosis and management of pelvic fractures. Bull NYU Hosp Joint Dis 68(4):281–291, 2010

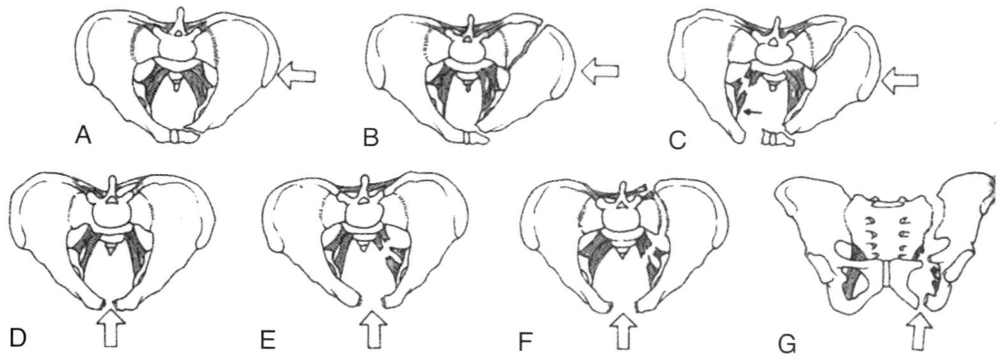

图 5　Young-Burgess 分型系统的图形描绘（*Repninted with permission Tornetta III P: Pelvis andacetabulum: trauma. In Beaty JH, editor:*Orthopaedic knowledge update, *ed 6, Rosemont, Ill., 1999, American Academy of Orthopaedic Surgeons, pp 427–439.*）

影中，大血管损伤的征象包括造影剂外溢、动脉缺损、血管壁不规则和在注射造影剂时静脉停滞。栓塞处理应该是有选择性和顺序的，应先解决仅动脉的损伤，并使剩余的血管保持完整，以保持血液供应到骨盆周围的结构。用格列酰脲进行非选择性栓塞，可以阻塞多种小出血。应该避免近端栓塞，因为有明显弥漫性缺血风险。据报道，血管造影的成功率为 80% ~100%。然而，为了使这种技术有效，必须每周 7 天，每天 24 h 有经验丰富的介入放射科医生值班。血管造影的并发症发生率大约为 5%，包括穿刺部位血肿、分离、血栓形成、下游组织坏死、造影剂过敏，以及血栓脱落风险增加。初次血管造影术后持续性出血患者可进行第二次血管造影。复发性出血的危险因素包括收缩压低于 90 mmHg，碱缺失大于 10 mEq/L 持续超过 6 h 以及无腹内出血性病变。

对于单纯的骨盆骨折患者，应该避免行剖腹探查手术，因为探查术可能会通过减压使腹膜后血肿再扩张，同时会增加深部感染的风险。据报道，对血流动力学不稳定的不稳定性骨盆环骨折患者行剖

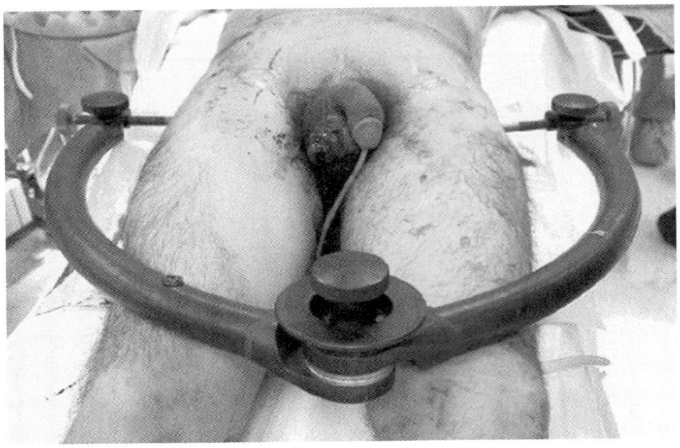

图 6 骨盆 C 型钳（*From Mohanty K, Musso D, Powell JN, et al: Emergent management of pelvic ring injuries: an update.* Can J Surg *48:49–56, 2005.*）

腹术来进行血管结扎，其死亡率达 66% ～83%。然而，剖腹手术适用于髂总动脉损伤或者髂外动脉损伤的患者。对于合并伤患者，建议在剖腹探查之前在骨盆前方放置外固定架。因为，对于骨盆前部而言，腹壁具有张力带作用，腹壁破坏可能导致开书样骨盆骨折加重。

骨盆填塞最近已经成为欧洲、美国的一些中心使用的治疗方案。这是一种损伤控制方式，用于等待动脉栓塞时恢复止血。它也可用于因其他原因需要立即手术干预的患者和血管造影术后残留血流动力学不稳定的患者。骨盆填塞时可以采用低位前正中切口或 Pfannenstiel 切口。填塞时将腹膜向上推移以增加填塞效果，然后用负压敷料暂时填充。与骨盆减压技术（如外固定）联合使用时效果最好。骨盆填塞物对动脉和静脉损伤有效，必须在 24～48 h 内更换。这种技术尚未在大量患者中进行使用，对开放性复位和内固定感染的影响也须重视（图 7）。

确定性治疗

到 20 世纪 70 年代中期，骨盆骨折通常使用加压装置、石膏和卧床休息进行非手术治疗。随着手术方式、经皮技术和内固定术的发展，现在大部分明显移位的骨盆骨折已经采用手术治疗。确定性重建手术是在充分的复苏和患者状况稳定之后进行的。骨盆环的稳定有利于患者的护理，包括允许早期活动、改善肺清洁功能和更利于护士护理。另外，解剖结构的重建可以降低骨盆环畸形愈合的发生，骨盆畸形一旦发生就很难纠正。固定方式的选择取决于骨折类型和移位程度。

骨盆后环的重建对于长期功能恢复是最关键的，因为可以防止双下肢不等长和坐位不稳。后环损伤的治疗可以选择经皮骶髂螺钉、钢板和螺钉或腰椎骨盆固定。如果可以闭合复位，优先选择经皮骶髂螺钉。如果不能闭合复位，或者骨折块不能使用单独的骶髂螺钉稳定，则采用其他方法。仅涉及髂骨翼的骨折不一定需要手术治疗，但是当需要时，通常使用切开复位、钢板螺钉固定。

前环损伤的治疗可以选择外固定架、钢板和螺钉、内部螺钉和杆结构。外固定可以允许经皮放置植入物，并且可以使用针操纵和复位骨盆。耻骨联合分离通常使用钢板和螺钉进行固定，其优点是没有外植入物。最近，已经研发出更加微创的治疗技术用于治疗前环损伤，如 AIIS 椎弓根螺钉和杆结构。这项技术具有一些优点，其对于耻骨支骨折最有用，

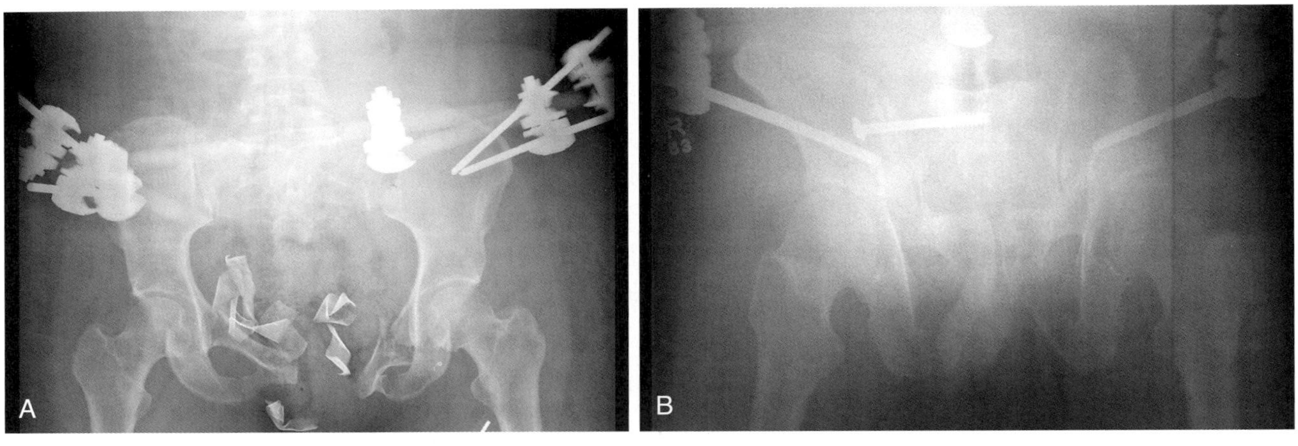

图 7 **A** 和 **B**，骨盆外固定架（左，髂嵴钉；右：髂前下棘钉）

这使得钢板或螺钉固定很困难，并且不需要广泛的复位。根据骨折类型以及固定的稳定程度决定术后负重情况。

泌尿生殖系统损伤在骨盆骨折中非常常见。这些患者的治疗通常须与泌尿科、妇科和创伤外科医生共同完成。这些损伤可导致长期并发症，如狭窄、失禁、勃起功能障碍、性交困难，以及自然分娩困难。成功解决这些方面的问题是处理骨盆肌肉骨骼损伤的重要组成部分（图 8）。

预后

关于骨盆骨折预后的文献中，很少有高质量的研究。非手术治疗时，骨盆骨折的愈合率为 83% ~100%，手术治疗时骨折的愈合率为93% ~100%。复位的好坏是关键，后环损伤固定的畸形愈合率最低。长期严重疼痛的发生与复位质量和畸形愈合相关。在开放复位内固定治疗的骨折中，感染率小于5%；但是在外固定架治疗的骨折中，感染发生率为 20%。大约 5%的患者也会出现复位和固定的失败。在手术干预治疗的患者中，术后步态异常发生率较低，也与复位的好坏有关。约 66% ~75%的患者能恢复工作，SF-36 评分在精神和身体方面均为 64 ~ 75，表明骨盆骨折的患者可能会存在遗留残疾。这最主要是与骨折造成的初始神经损伤严重程度相关。总的来说，研究表明创伤后畸形愈合和骨盆不稳定与持续性疼痛和功能受限相关。

总结

骨盆骨折在多发伤患者中很常见，是导致残疾和死亡的重要原因。初步评估和干预的主要目标是及时诊断、复苏和控制出血。了解机制和骨折类型有助于评估稳定性和潜在相关的软组织损伤。通过与血管造影相结合的多种方法使骨折稳定，降低了与这些损伤相关的死亡率。此外，确定性固定方式的进步改善了该患者群体的预后。对骨盆骨折患者进行多学科联合讨论治疗是很有必要的。

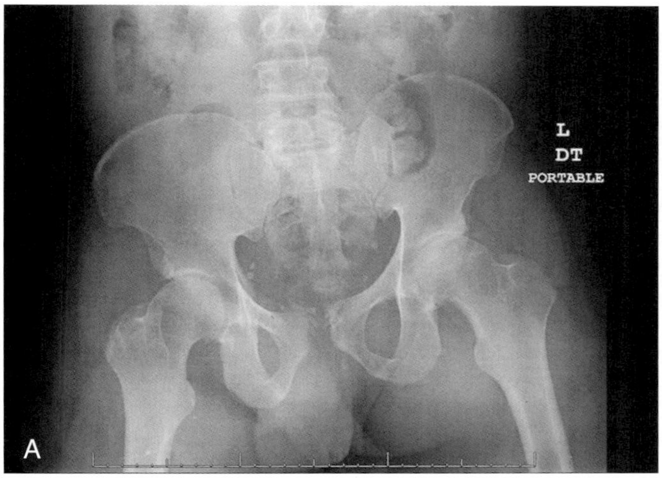

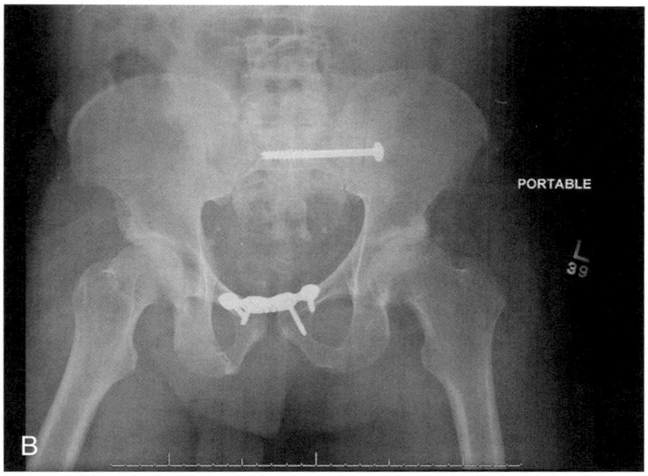

图 8 **A** 和 **B**，骨盆环损伤确定性固定

第 12 章　创伤处理中的特殊问题和情况

气道管理：每一位外科医生都应知道的创伤气道管理（麻醉师的观点）

Shawn M. Cantie 和 Edgar J. Pierre 著
王传林 译

急性气道创伤非常少见却能致命。大多数气道钝伤是由于机动车碰撞，其次由于运动及家暴相关性创伤。大多数气道穿通伤继发于枪伤或者刺伤。气道干预的主要目标是减轻或防止气道阻塞、确保无保护气道没有误吸、提供充足的气体交换，并且维持颈椎稳定。管理创伤气道是对医生的熟练度及临床能力的终极考验，因为医生必须要做好患者有大量胃内容物且合并颈椎不稳定的准备，这两种情况会使病情更加难以控制。管理创伤气道须具备处理继发于创伤本身及麻醉师干预后带来的危险的知识。

当伤者到达急诊室或复苏室，在最初的时刻应对其基本状况进行快速评价：稳定、不稳定、垂危或死亡。ATLS 的首次评估包括快速评估及稳定威胁生命的功能：气道通畅性、呼吸、保证循环及出血控制、用简单神经系统查体进行残疾评估、脱掉伤者衣物来完全暴露伤者。

医生必须在接触伤者的即刻留意到任何有关气道创伤的迹象，因为急性气道创伤管理最重要的步骤是识别这种状态。医生必须高度警惕颈前创伤。喉外伤时常出现如声音嘶哑、呼吸困难、吞咽困难、发声困难、发声疼痛的症状，然而捻发音、喘鸣、咯血、颈前水肿、瘀斑、撕裂伤常代表喉 - 气管损伤。对于喉 - 气管损伤的伤者，气道管理是急救基础，须尽可能快地完成。

手动轴线制动（manual in-line immobilization，MILI）的目的是为了给头颈足够的力量，以防止其因医疗干预措施，尤其是气道管理，而造成移位。MILI 一般是由助手完成，助手位于床头，或者位于担架侧面向床头。患者呈仰卧位，且颈在中间位置。助手用其手指按住患者双侧乳突，并且用其手掌托住患者枕骨（床头助手）或颈后和斜方肌（床侧助手）。适当 MILI 后，颈托的前半部分可以移除使嘴尽可能张大，以便进行气道干预。在喉镜检查过程中，助手巧妙地用力平衡术者在气管插管过程中产生的力，方向相反，以保持头颈在中间位置。

当患者有非常严重的韧带损伤且它导致脊柱不稳定时，进行 MILI 的操作时避免牵引力便特别重要。Lennarson 等发现当韧带完全损伤时，若进行牵引，不论是常规插管还是环甲膜切开术都能导致过度牵引。类似地，Kaufmann 等证实了在影像学评估中使用线性牵引导致了 4 名韧带断裂患者脊柱延长和分离。MILI 能有效减少气道操作时记录的整体脊柱运动，但在实际受伤位置的限制作用可能较小。这可能与脊柱的运动受到躯体下方的重量限制，但 MILI 的力量在颈椎的中点处没有受到限制有关。使用 MILI 期间施加牵引力可能会减少一些患者颈椎中部的运动，但牵引力也可能导致受伤处的移位。因此不鼓励在使用 MILI 时使用这种牵引力。

通过常规插管或环甲膜切开术可以控制受创伤的气道。大多数麻醉师非常适应直接或通过纤维喉镜进行插管，外科医生在建立手术气道上有更多的经验。最初认为，气管插管似乎是获得气道控制最有益和有效的好方法，但环甲膜切开术在某些情况下可以有更多获益。例如喉水平及以下的损伤，气管造口术提供了一个检查损伤部位的空间，可通过直接喉镜在气管造口处或其上进行检查。气管插管可能对后续损伤部位的检查带来困难，并且可能加重现有的喉损伤。颈部重要部位损伤的患者，行环甲膜切开术后发现有喉部气管分离风险时，应该通过环甲膜切开术建立手术气道。

合并面部及上呼吸道创伤会带来特别的难度。若不能识别面部或颈部损伤，可导致继发于肿胀和血肿的急性或亚急性气道阻塞。有严重面部损伤的患者，推荐在气道肿胀和水肿前早期行经口气管插管。

在此位置如果没有绝对禁忌证，应该允许和鼓励这些患者保持坐位，直到创伤团队决定开始进行气道管理。面部和咽部受伤的患者的某些表现（如筛状板损伤出现脑脊液漏等）也会提示某种特殊危险，而使得其他重要的损伤被忽视，如颈椎不稳定等。在气管插管过程中，应更加仔细地进行轴向牵引以稳定颈椎。

大多数面部受伤是显而易见的，并且可以通过出血、水肿、红斑、骨折、面部解剖学变形而识别。在少数情况下，主要是孤立的面部钝伤、水肿和红斑可能不会出现在极早期阶段。在这种情况下，出现触诊时，有捻发音、声音嘶哑、流涎、拒绝保持仰卧位时，应该警惕面部受伤和气道损伤。

因为这些情况非常紧急，在整个临床阶段都应该进行气道评估。须重点注意的表现包括焦虑、喘鸣、有无能力发声、通过口腔和鼻孔的气流量是否充足、气管是否存在偏移、呼吸肌的运动，以及膈的运动。

出现如口内出血、咽部红斑、下颌受伤和声音的变化都是早期插管的指征。双侧下颌骨折和咽部出血可能会导致上呼吸道阻塞，尤其是在患者呈仰卧位时。因此，发现患者呈坐位或俯卧位，且拒绝仰卧，是因为那是在进行麻醉诱导和气管插管前，保持气道通气的最好的体位。

虽然面部和咽损伤会给插管造成困难，但它并不是不可能完成。当务之急是在具备困难插管条件的环境中尝试插管。可能需要口咽或鼻咽通气道来暂时保持气道通畅，直到满足这些条件。快速贯序插管结合颈部轴线制动是创伤患者气管插管的首选方法。

然而，在气管插管上做太长时间的努力，会错过救治的黄金时间，影响患者的呼吸状态，并且增加患者颅内压。环甲膜切开术是一个非常有效的替代选择。也许是早期环甲膜切开，而不是多次重复气管插管，更能减少缺氧、改善患者的预后。由于操作时间长，并且会带来明显的并发症，紧急气管造口术并不被认为是一个恰当的方法，来紧急建立确定性气道。在 71 名有喉 - 气管损伤的患者中，有 39 名（54.9%）患者须紧急开放气道。48% 的患者最初接受了经口气管插管，然而各有 4% 的患者分别进行了气管造口术和环甲膜切开术。合并有喉气管钝伤的患者中有 78.9% 须紧急开放气道，然而那些合并穿通伤的 46 名患者中，只有 1 名（2%）须紧急开放气道。钝伤组的 15 名行气管插管的患者中，14 名插管成功；穿通伤组的 24 名行气管插管的患者中，20 名插管成功。

由于损伤显而易见，颈部穿通伤的诊断通常是简单的。相反，颈部钝伤的诊断取决于怀疑的程度。临床检查仍然是发现喉气管损伤体征最可靠的方法。唯一造成喉气管创伤诊断困难的情况是空气通过颈部伤口逃离，这通常给明确诊断造成困难。通过触诊脸、颈和上胸部出现捻发音，对快速识别皮下气肿也同样重要。患者颈部损伤时也可能出现呼吸困难、咯血、声音嘶哑、喘鸣、触诊时捻发音。患者损伤后出现的这些症状是继发于软组织肿胀，包括窒息感、呼吸困难、吞咽困难、声音嘶哑、喘鸣。受害者的音质（如声音嘶哑）是不可预测的。然而，除非证明并非如此，声音嘶哑才提示有大气道损伤。只有当患者清醒且与其当面确定这一点，我们才能假定患者声音嘶哑是出现在损伤之前。

创伤是一个病情变化很快的疾病，尤其是在急性期。患者的病情可以变化得非常快，频繁地再评估患者的状态是至关重要的。频繁地检查患者也有助于确定水肿和血肿的进展程度，以防出现潜在的气道阻塞。

颈部创伤最当务之急的是保护气道。最终目的应该是将一个位置适宜的经口腔气管导管与充气良好、密封性好的套囊，完全贯穿整个喉气管的远端。然而，气管插管可能是极其困难的，因为咽或颈部血肿可能遮住声带或改变了解剖学。盲目使用气管内导管是危险的，因为它可能沿着或产生错误的通道。在气道部分横断的实例中，一味推进气管内导管可能引起喉气管完全分离。

根据可能的危害，最明显的结论是避免对假定稳定的患者在现场或 ED 进行气管插管。更常见的颈部损伤如刺伤和低速枪伤不强制院前或急诊室插管。在这种情况下插管应该在手术室中，由具有经验的麻醉师，配备适当的工具，在具备手术气道的条件下执行。与之相反，高速枪伤和严重颈部钝伤应紧急进行气道控制。

传统上，快速序列气管插管仍是必要的。同时在适当的位置准备好光纤维支气管镜，也要准备好通过行环甲膜切开术以建立外科气道的准备。病情不稳定且合并喉割伤或者颈前大型撕裂伤的患者，可以通过伤口进行插管来挽救生命。如果患者不能等到到达医院后建立人工气道，这可能是紧急医疗服务人员唯一可行的替代方法。在过去，即使在医院，也可选择环甲膜切开术或气管造口术。

提示血管损伤的征象包括血肿、休克和持续的出血。血肿可以被限制而不危害气道。用抗凝剂治疗的患者更易出现出血和水肿。在这种情况下，可能会到达一个临界点，气道将会阻塞，患者病情会突然恶化。对于这类患者，在到达医院之前推迟气管插管是合理的，因为无法预测临床过程。然而，密切监测患者及其血肿的大小是至关重要的。如果血肿扩大或患者有气道损伤的生理体征，应行预防性气管插管。如果运输时间长，推荐对气管插管的指征降低。应有在院前、急诊室和手术室进行困难插管的预期，且相关的技术应被计划。

一旦保证了气道，便须开始细致检查，明确损伤的确切位置，并选择适当的手术治疗。这项工作主要包括咽、喉、气管和食管的纤维镜检查。

美国麻醉医师协会修订创伤困难气道管理

美国麻醉医师协会工作组为管理困难气道（difficalt airway，DA）提出了管理指南。这一指南为内科医生提供了一种在选择手术通气前，进行非手术通气的系统方法。这一方法通常只适用于创伤患者。非手术气道控制的时间并不是创伤患者的主要获益，因其经常存在出血性休克、误吸风险、头部创伤。的确，在严重创伤的情况下，紧急方法常常导致无法继续进行气道通气，这时在此情况发生之前会及时选择手术气道，这一方法也适用于其他类型的患者群体。最后，创伤患者的气道控制是以临床判断为指导的。

最近一项试验完成了对创伤的困难气道的管理的修改。将颌面部和颈部创伤归为疑似困难插管的类别。主要修改的部分如下：

1. 停止不再是创伤的一个选择。
2. 手术气道在一定条件下可以成为第一个或最好的选择。
3. 如果患者配合、稳定且有自主呼吸，清醒下气管插管技术应成为困难气道患者的一个选择。
4. 如果患者不合作或抵抗，可能须进行全身麻醉。如果有困难气道，应尽可能让患者保持自发通气（spontaneous ventilation，SV）。

修改后的困难气道管理指南将手术或经皮气管造口术和环甲膜切开术定义为气道的侵入性操作。值得一提的是，许多医生并不相信气管造口术是外科紧急气道控制的一个合适的选择（图 1-2）。

总结

气道穿通性损伤通常是明显的，但是钝伤存在时，应对此情况高度怀疑。必须要全面了解损伤的程度，以便在最佳时机以最适当的方法保护气道。如果气道稳定，建议在有经验丰富的麻醉师，且具备手术气道开放条件的手术室中进行气道控制。在任何条件下，只要怀疑困难气道，最好是保持自发通气。

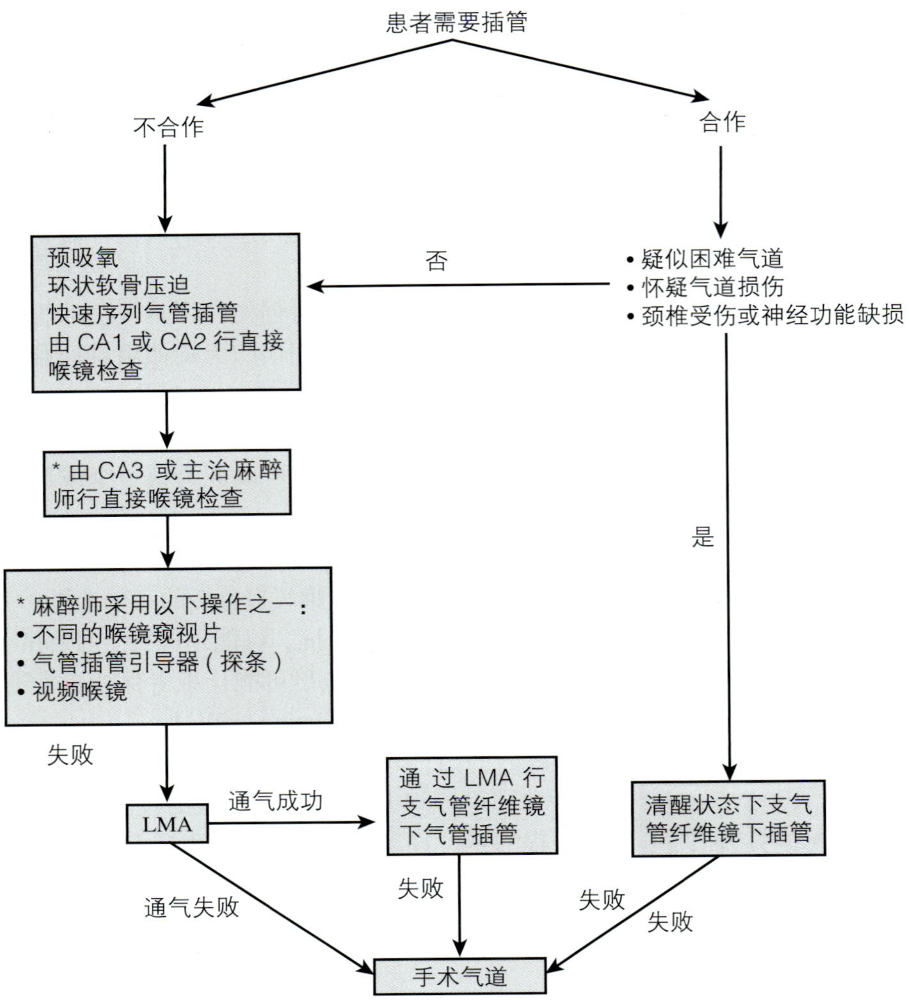

* 如果有以下情况之一进行球囊、瓣膜或面罩通气：

- 在呼吸暂停过程中有血氧不饱和的风险
- 创伤性脑损伤
- Spo_2 < 90%

DL，直接喉镜检查
CA1，临床麻醉学专业第一年住院医生（毕业后教育 2 年）
CA2，临床麻醉学专业第二年住院医生（毕业后教育 3 年）
CA3，临床麻醉学专业第三年住院医生（毕业后教育 4 年）

图 1　RTA，气道管理流程；C-spine，颈椎；LMA，喉罩气道

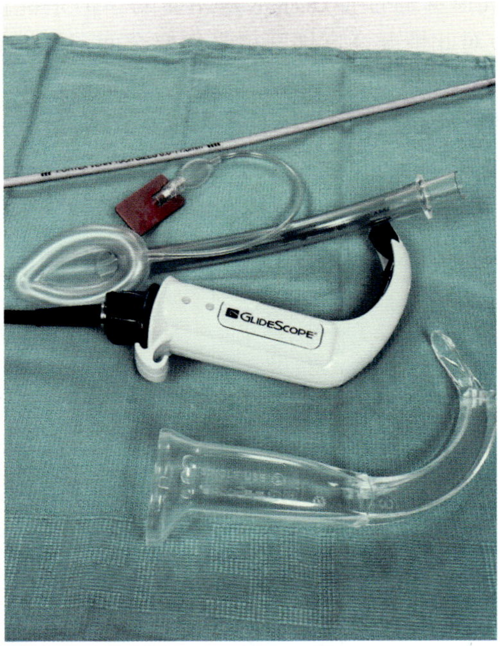

图 2　困难气道处理的 3 个工具：气管插管引导器、喉罩气道和 GlideScope

儿科创伤

David W. Tuggle 和 L.R. Tres Scherer 著
王传林 译

在美国，儿科创伤是导致儿童死亡的头号杀手，同时也是导致儿童终身残疾的主因。人们一贯认为儿童并不仅仅是小号成年人，这一观点在处理儿童创伤时尤为准确。尽管儿童外伤护理的原则与成年人相同，但在受伤儿童的最佳治疗上，护理需求存在差异。这一差异体现在需要更专业的知识、更细心的管理、更合适的医疗设备，以及要关注到儿童及青少年的独特的生理、心理。

儿科创伤的发生率

虽然新生儿和儿童的外科治疗的医疗技术已经取得了巨大的进步，但是意外伤害仍是19岁以下儿童的主要死亡原因。2009年，有9 143名儿童死亡，从2000 — 2009年，全年意外伤害死亡率下降了29%，从15.5/10万降至11.0/10万。在2009年，不同国家的儿童伤害死亡率差异很大，马萨诸塞州和新泽西州死亡率低于5/10万，而南达科他、蒙大拿和密西西比州死亡率高达23/10万。每有一名儿童因创伤死亡，就有25名儿童住院治疗，就有925名儿童需要紧急处理。

溺水是1 ~ 4岁儿童的头号死亡原因。机动车事故是导致1 ~ 4岁儿童创伤相关死亡的第二大原因。约半数死于机动车事故的4岁及以下儿童在坐车时无限制措施。住宅火灾导致伤害的人群中，5岁以下儿童占大多数。机动车事故是导致5 ~ 19岁儿童死亡的主要原因。溺水是导致5 ~ 14岁儿童创伤相关性死亡的第二大原因。15 ~ 19岁的儿童，自杀是导致其死亡的第二大原因。在车祸中死亡的骑自行车的人中有1/3是5 ~ 14岁的儿童。

儿科创伤机制

目前关于儿童受伤和死亡的机制的观点仍然非常一致。1 ~ 14岁的儿童，机动车辆事故相关性死亡仍是儿童最主要的死因，占各种死亡原因的46.5%（2009年）。溺水是第二大死因，其次为1岁以下儿童的窒息。一项关于死亡的详细数据分析结果提示，住宅是一个需要持续关注的地方，其他需要关注的地方包括摔伤和骑车相关的创伤，目前因全地形车祸导致的死亡和残疾的情况正在逐渐增多。（可见于美国消费品安全委员会2009年的报道，访问地址：http://www.cpsc. gov//PageFiles/108615/atv2009.pdf）

儿童创伤通常发生在能量突然变化时，或者突然加速，或者突然减速，或者是两者兼有。儿童的身体非常有弹性，因此能量可以转移，通过这一方式，可以带来内部创伤而没有明显的外部特点。由于儿童的重要器官相隔很近，与老年患者相比，儿童仅仅通过力量的传导便可造成多发损伤。在年纪小的儿童，穿通伤是比较少见的一种创伤形式，在儿科创伤中心，其所占的比例为1% ~ 10%。无论是哪种类型的创伤，医疗机构在对受伤儿童进行专业的评估和管理时，应该时刻记住这些重要区别。

受伤儿童的初步评估、稳定和管理

气道管理

大多数儿童没有先天性的肺部疾病，因此，如果在不吸氧时血氧饱和度大于90%，即可指示肺功能良好。如果呼吸困难，应该考虑到肺部有创伤、气胸或误吸。肺通气不足常见于头部受伤或者休克。如果存在任何这些情况，应考虑给予辅助通气及之后的高级气道技术。呼吸功能障碍且需要插管通常预示损伤严重。虽然没有一个明确的标准去决定是什么组成了儿童的“主要复苏”，插管和气道损伤已经证明了相比没有气道问题的创伤儿童，这一群体死亡率更高。和所有的患者一样，应该小心避免插管期间的颈椎移位。应该注意的是，在紧急情况下，经鼻支气管插管通常不用于小的儿童。

在许多情况下插管也便于评价和复苏。对于不合作的儿童应该快速评估其是否存在缺氧，虽然一个警觉、不合作的儿童也可能只有极小的创伤。体重/身高比例尺已经成为决定选择复苏设备重量、尺寸的标准，以及在复苏中药物剂量和滴定浓度的标准。

当合并有困难气道时，可能需要喉罩气道和支气管镜等高级气道技术。这种高级气道技术通常需要经验丰富的麻醉师或者特护医生。推荐使用弹性探条，因其可以使插管进入更加顺利，但是在儿童中应用受限。

气管插管后处理包括二次确认插管位置、胃肠减压和行 X 线胸片排除气胸和进行气管内定位。呼气末二氧化碳描记术或比色法应该被用来确认气道放置，但是不能定位。每一位患者都可能用鼻胃管或口胃管进行胃肠减压，因为胃膨胀会影响膈运动，导致儿童呼吸障碍。如果存在气胸，可行穿刺减压，但应该立即随后进行胸廓造口术置管。

血管通路

儿童血管的理想进针点是上肢的周围静脉，尤其是肘窝。如果这些血管不可行，可能从中央静脉获得通路（图 1）。这是一个高级且具有技术含量的操作。经股静脉置管，是另一个最好的选择，同时也是儿童在紧急情况下最常采用的方法。这一方法不用尝试切开，最好应用 Seldinger 技术。熟悉锁骨下静脉穿刺置管操作的外科医生可能选择这一方法作为另一种选择。对于熟练掌握儿童锁骨下穿刺这一技术的外科医生，并发症的发生是极少的。在紧急条件下，建立创伤儿童的骨内通路为最佳选择，禁忌证包括近端骨折和穿刺部位及周围的感染。胫骨近端前内侧表面是常用的进针点，距胫骨粗隆远端 2 ~ 4 cm。为注射进胫骨近端，针头在其下方以 45° 垂直进针。如果注射部位是胫骨远端，应该在其上方 45° 进针。在这两个例子中，操作时应注意避开生长面及关节区域。已经有专门用于此项操作技术的专业针了，包括动力骨内穿刺。应避免多次进入骨髓腔，因为多次尝试会导致渗漏，从而可能导致发生筋膜室综合征。

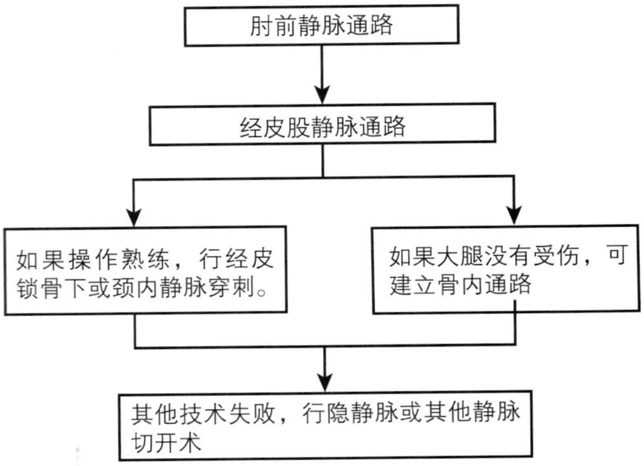

图 1　儿童静脉通道建立

循环管理

年龄相关性低血压是受伤儿童有无复苏必要性的指示（表 1）。全国儿科创伤注册机构的分析指出，报告的 38% 的死亡发生在收缩压低于 90 mmHg 的儿童中。这一组代表了 2.4% 的研究人群。决定儿童是否有年龄相关性低血压须知道正常儿童的血压。创伤儿童出现明显出血也可能表现为血压正常。通过增加心率及周围血管收缩，其他健康的儿童可以很快地代偿失去的血液。

因此，儿童的血压正常并不能代表循环稳定。血压评估更准确的判断方法包括监测心率和评估周围灌注。

低灌注的临床症状结合精神状态的改变是儿童

表 1　不同年龄组儿童的正常生命体征和体重

年龄	呼吸频率（次 / 分）	脉搏（次 / 分）	收缩压 (mm/Hg)	体重 (kg)	体重 (lb)
新生儿	30 ~ 50	120 ~ 160	50 ~ 70	2 ~ 4	4 ~ 7
1 ~ 12 个月	20 ~ 30	80 ~ 140	70 ~ 100	4 ~ 10	10 ~ 22
1 ~ 3 岁	20 ~ 30	80 ~ 130	80 ~ 110	10 ~ 15	22 ~ 33
3 ~ 5 岁	20 ~ 30	80 ~ 120	80 ~ 110	15 ~ 20	33 ~ 44
6 ~ 13 岁	20 ~ 30	70 ~ 110	80 ~ 120	20 ~ 45	44 ~ 99
14 岁及以上	12 ~ 20	55 ~ 90	90 ~ 120	45 及以上	99 及以上

低血容量性休克的典型表现。如果有上述表现，那么应立即给予 20 ml/kg 的等张晶体。如果还须再次补充这些总量的液体，并且症状没有得到明显改善，那么须立即开始输血（图 2）。必须要小心，因为过度复苏与复苏不足一样都会带来问题，尤其是合并有头外伤时。在某些情况下，积极补充晶体可以加重脑水肿。过度补充晶体治疗可能会导致血栓形成不良，这会加重出血状态，但可能对生存率没有影响。超常创伤复苏增加成年人腹腔隔室综合征的发生率，并且据报道，儿童也存在相同的问题。通常情况下，按体重 20 ml/kg 补充等张晶体是低血压的第一个治疗措施。如果有证据表明病情持续不稳定，可能再次给予这一剂量的液体。如果 2 次补入上述剂量晶体液后，患儿的生命体征仍不稳定，必须开始紧急输血。应输相应血型的浓缩红细胞或者在某些特殊情况下，必要时输注 O 型阴性血。如果在复苏时需要大量的血液，也考虑在早期复苏输入新鲜冰冻血浆和血小板。如果有意识水平下降而没有血容量不足表现，那么需要温和的液体复苏。

低体温是创伤儿童极其常见的一个表现。低体温可能发生在任何年龄的创伤儿童中，也可以发生在夏天。低体温反应时，机体会增加儿茶酚胺的释放和寒战，会导致耗氧量会增加及代谢性酸中毒。低体温及酸中毒会促进创伤后凝血功能障碍的发生。预防及治疗低体温须在对患儿进行最初评估时便注意到这些严重的并发症。一个温暖的房间、温暖的液体、空气加热毛毯或外部加热毛毯是复苏开始便需要的。复苏过程中，在急诊科时就应开始进行复温，并且在行放射相关检查时也应继续进行。有一些证据建议早期、仔细处理严重单纯头外伤儿童的低体温能带来益处，但这一治疗方案仍处于实验阶段。

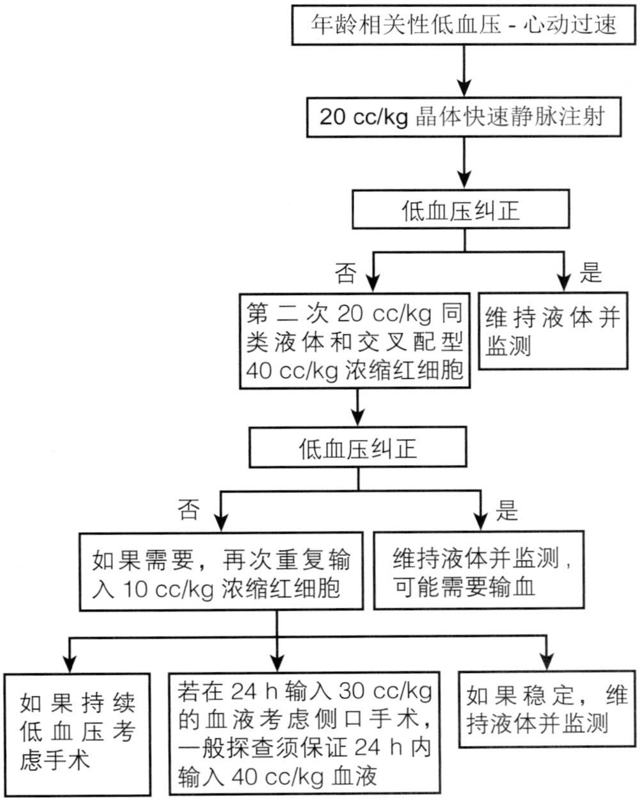

图 2　儿童液体和血液复苏的流程图。IV，静脉输液

诊断性评估

创伤管理的初步评估和复苏阶段开始进行受伤儿童的诊断性评估。体格检查是至关重要的第一步，因为这直接关系到其他评估方法的结果。最初的体格检查的结果也同时是患儿住院之后创伤小组对其进行体格检查的基线参照。体格检查做完之后，可能进行其他的辅助检查。

虽然患者在急诊科正在进行复苏，但创伤的诊断须借助常规射线照片。急诊科最经常须做的影像学检查包括胸部、腹部、骨盆、颈椎和四肢的 X 线片。当怀疑有神经损伤，或查体时发现脊柱有压痛点时，通常须做胸、腰椎 X 线片检查。检查是否有气胸、气腹、骨盆骨折或长骨骨折是创伤儿童初诊时的重要组成部分。颅骨的 X 线平片可能会发现骨折，但在头部创伤儿童的诊疗中并无价值，除非是穿通伤且怀疑为受虐儿童。

成年人和儿童创伤外科医生的一些研究试图确定创伤超声重点评估法（focused assessment with sonography in trauma，FAST）在评估受伤的孩子时的作用。最常见的 FAST 检查对心脏、腹部右上及左上象限和盆腔的积液进行检查（图 3）。一些外科医生还对胸部有无胸膜腔积液和气胸进行检查。

目前，无射线指导的超声检查应该与体格检查结果相结合，并且不应该认为其是一个诊断性结论。虽然它的灵敏度、特异度和准确性很高，但它只是个筛查工具，用来决定是否需要更深入的检查或侵入性评估。与青少年和成年人相比，大多数儿童皮下组织相对缺乏，这使得这一检查更易实行。FAST 检查法的明显益处包括它的可携带性，避免儿童行放射检查时的搬动、减少了儿童的放射线暴露。

疑似创伤可能危及生命时，CT 是绝大多数损伤儿童可选择的放射性诊断工具。无论何时，限制儿童 CT 扫描量是非常重要的。一般认为创伤时行

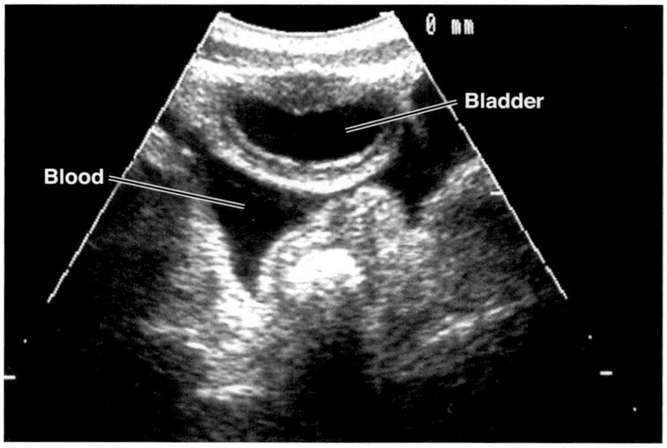

图 3　一个 4 岁 FAST 的阳性发现：盆腔积血

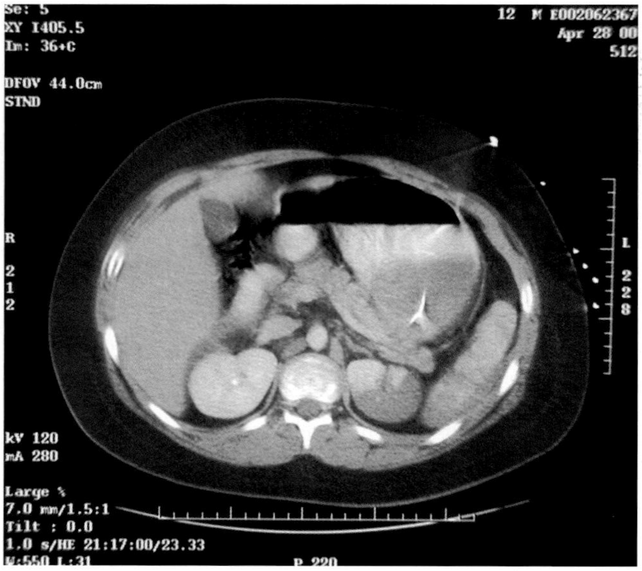

图 4　一个 CT 扫描阳性征象：一个 8 岁儿童的肾和脾创伤

CT 扫描是合适的，然而患儿经常被要求多次扫描。这种做法会导致潜在的医学影像导致的潜在的癌症风险。

一般认为成年人患者头至盆腔的平扫是标准医疗过程，但由于放射线的危险和其对损伤的低灵敏度，已经发展了另一项评估颈胸状态的替代技术。近期，加拿大创伤协会作出了一项关于最小化颈椎成像放射剂量的指南。几乎所有临床明显表现为胸部创伤的患者都经 X 线胸片明确诊断。大多数的怀疑合并腹内损伤的患儿，如果病情稳定，应在手术或非手术治疗前行 CT 扫描，除非有绝对手术适应证。在急诊室中，生理不稳定的儿童用其他的方法来评估，如诊断性腹腔灌洗术或超声。虽然 CT 平扫是评估病情稳定的创伤儿童的影像学技术，但是一般认为 CT 平扫的假阴性率非常高。只有 1/4 的患者表现有腹部 CT 异常（图 4）。对于极小部分合并有实质脏器损伤的患儿，CT 扫描的结果对其是否行手术治疗的决定有影响。CT 扫描上，能表明有腹腔内损伤而需要手术纠正的证据往往是细微的。游离的腹腔内或腹膜后气体、肠外有胃肠道造影剂、肠壁缺损、活动性出血的表现常常是明显的，并且与需要手术干预的肠道损伤有很高的相关性。然而，有的潜在的威胁生命的肠道损伤，仅表现为病变肠壁增厚或腹腔积液而没有实质脏器损伤。其他不典型的与肠道损伤相关的表现包括肠系膜索征、肠系膜根部积液、病灶血肿、肠系膜假动脉瘤、低灌注复合征。

其他评估创伤儿童的方法包括介入性放射技术、磁共振成像、侵入性和非侵入性血管检查。一般情况下，在急诊室所行的常规的实验室检查并未在儿童创伤群体的救治中体现出重要的价值。一些特殊的临床实验室检查，如碱缺失试验、尿液分析、动脉血气分析试验，可能在特定条件下具有一定的意义。多数情况下，在急诊室，进行评估和复苏时，实验室检测落后于临床决策过程。即时检测也并没有改变这一观点。存在头部创伤时，检测有无凝血功能障碍、血小板减少或高血糖可能有助于对后续决策建立一个基线参考，或可协助评估发病或死亡风险。在住院期间，只要存在特定的需要监测的指征，如非手术处理脾和胰腺损伤。接受机械通气患者的血气、头部创伤的患者，常规实验室检查是合适的。

特殊伤害的管理

应该注意的是，成年人与儿童所有器官创伤的标准是一样的——即美国创伤外科协会创伤后器官损伤标准。除非有适应证，儿童特定伤害的处理方法与成年人几乎相同。

头和中枢神经系统损伤

急性创伤性脑损伤是儿童最常见的死因和致残原因，在幸存患儿中，轻则造成可逆的缺陷，重则会导致严重残疾。儿童头部损伤的机制与年龄相关。婴儿最典型的是摔伤，如从桌子或照顾者手臂上摔下。故意伤害是 2 岁以下儿童死亡的常见原因。故意伤害，不论严重性，都会增加脑损伤儿童的死亡率。更大些的儿童，最常见头部损伤的原因是车辆相关的事故或娱乐活动。虽然儿童头部损伤生存率较成年人高，但并不意味着儿童在类似伤害中有较少的发病率。儿童神经元具有可塑性，这与髓鞘形成和神经元相互联系的建立有关。这使得儿童的大脑与发育成熟的大脑相比，受到损伤后能造成少一点的功能缺损。但是缺乏成熟同样也会使儿童更容易受到弥漫性损伤，并导致更大的认知障碍。

在对脑损伤儿童进行初步评估和复苏时，应小心避免由低血压和缺氧带来二次伤害。在这一期间，必须对颈椎进行控制。颈椎的临床和X线片评估对排除颈椎受伤是很重要的。格拉斯哥昏迷等级评分（Glasgow Coma Scale，GCS）可用于5岁以上儿童。而且一些修改后的GCS常用于5岁以下的儿童。如果确定评分小于9分，患者须进行气道管理、颅内压（intracranial pressure，ICP）的测定，并且须考虑治疗选择。评分小于8分表明患者昏迷。维持好的氧合和灌注在整个复苏过程中非常重要，这常常需要气管插管。注意保护颈椎，因为可能有未知的颈椎损伤。

初步评估患者，有继发脑损伤的因素，应立即行头部CT检查。如果有脑水肿的证据，提示应监测ICP，最好能通过可以完成脑脊液引流（如脑室造口术）的系统操作。避免发热非常重要，因为这可能造成继发性脑损伤。其他治疗技术包括甘露醇或高渗的盐溶液治疗。需要时可以镇静，用于维持较低的ICP。通常应避免过度通气。用高剂量的巴比妥酸盐使患者昏迷，已经被证实有一定的好处。目前开颅减压术在特定情况下被认为是脑外伤儿童进行外科手术的另一种选择。患儿脑外伤合并脑水肿和药物难以控制的颅内压时应予以考虑。这可能对有潜在的可恢复的脑外伤儿童有好处，但对已经遭受严重的继发性脑损伤或者GCS评分为3的儿童没有改变作用。营养支持、避免使用类固醇，需要时的外伤后癫痫发作治疗也是头部损伤患者治疗的重要部分。

胸部创伤

胸部创伤是儿童发病和死亡的一个重要原因，占儿童创伤的4%～25%，这些胸部损伤与其他系统的损伤相比死亡率更高。儿童表现有收缩压降低、呼吸次数升高、胸部体检发现异常（包括胸部听诊异常和股骨骨折），可以提示胸部创伤。

一般来说，儿童气道更容易有黏液堵塞和少量的气道水肿。儿童胸壁顺应性更好，用少量的肌肉保护软组织，这使得儿童在受伤时会有更大的能量传输到器官。纵隔在儿童患者中比在年长患者中更容易移动，特别是年幼的儿童。单侧胸腔压力的变化，如张力性气胸，可导致纵隔的摆动，在某种程度上能使静脉回心血量明显减少。它的病理生理影响类似于低血容量性休克。在这种典型的情况下，儿童的这种反应比成年人更加显著。

年幼儿童的肋骨骨折相对不常见，而在青少年较多见。虽然肋骨骨折不常见，肋骨下的脏器内部损伤十分常见，如肝或脾损伤和肺挫伤。肺挫伤是儿童最常见的胸部创伤之一。儿童胸壁在无肋骨骨折的情况下仍能发生肺挫伤。合并肺挫伤能导致肺顺应性降低、缺氧、肺通气不足、通气/灌注比值失调。在初步评估时行X线胸片检查可能显示有无肺挫伤。然而，胸部CT扫描能显示肺挫伤的区域，而X线胸片不能。治疗包括液体复苏、辅助供氧、疼痛管理和防止肺不张和肺炎的策略。儿童合并肺挫伤可能长时间有呼吸功能的改变和X线胸片显示的异常。

气胸和血胸在儿童中也并非是不常见的损伤。胸管治疗气胸是经典的治疗方式，胸管的型号应与患者匹配。胸廓造口术是血胸的治疗方式，通常选用最大的导管，以便进行插入置管引流。儿童胸腔内的快速失血达15 ml/kg或持续失血达2～3 ml/kg · h，且持续时间达3 h及以上，建议行胸部探查，控制出血。心脏创伤是极其罕见的，同样少见的还有气管支气管损伤和食管损伤。大血管的损伤常见于年龄稍大的、受到突然减速伤的儿童（平均年龄12岁，并且极少见于10岁以下儿童）。损伤的机制和胸部射线照片不正常的表现，如纵隔增宽、主动脉结或主动脉条消失、食管偏移或第1肋骨骨折都提示有损伤。胸部螺旋CT增强扫描的灵敏度很高，在正常时，可以提供准确的阴性预测。

腹部损伤

由于儿童的腹壁的相对薄弱，中等强度的力量可能会给腹部某个或多个脏器造成很大的伤害。由于脏器之间更加接近，一次击打可能造成多脏器损伤。评估腹部损伤首先应进行体格检查。检查可以显示擦伤、胎带痕迹或腹胀。体格检查应轻柔，且带有高度的怀疑性，并结合CT扫描的结果进行评估。应采用经口或经鼻胃管进行胃肠减压。

腹部创伤的常规非手术处理过程中，需要手术干预的创伤可能会被忽略很长一段时间。须注意的是延误诊断，虽然并非不常见，且与病死率的增加并不相关。然而，已经发现，在损伤超过24 h之后进行手术干预可能增加感染的并发症发生率。因此，住院后应对腹部检查不完全正常的儿童行相关系列检查。当腹部伤害发生在可疑情况下，应考虑儿童虐待的诊断。

钝性膈破裂并不常见，左侧较右侧多见，然而，也可在双侧发生。钝性膈破裂合并其他创伤的频率也非常高，尤其是肝、脾创伤。膈的钝性损伤可能有一些临床表现。异常的膈轮廓、膈高位或腹部脏器影重叠可能提示损伤。也应考虑疝气、鼻胃管位置异常或肠梗阻的诊断。CT用于明确这一诊断，但是在一些患者中CT扫描结果可能表现正常。很多膈破裂在创伤后的最初几天不能被发现，并且也可能在相当一段时期内不会被发现。急性膈破裂的修补术往往最好通过经腹的方式来完成。如果后期才做出膈破裂的诊断，最好考虑行经胸的修补术。

儿童合并十二指肠损伤常常表现有腹胀、胆汁性呕吐、气腹、腹膜炎，须行手术治疗。十二指肠血肿常常采用鼻胃管减压和全静脉营养的非手术治疗方式。这一治疗方法的成功率高，但是血肿吸收需要长达3周的时间。十二指肠血肿之后可能出现十二指肠穿孔，通常与并发症的增加相关，而与死亡率无关。

小肠、空肠和回肠，是儿童肠道损伤最常出现的部分。小肠损伤的机制是它位于可传导力量与脊柱之间。汽车内为成年人设计的安全带常常被用于保护儿童的安全，因此，增加儿童小肠损伤的风险。如果有安全带擦伤，那么合并有腹腔内损伤风险的可能性极高，因此需要高度怀疑。儿童由于钝伤导致小肠损伤，查体时都有异常表现。超声或CT扫描见到游离液体、腹部有压痛、没有实质脏器受损，几乎都要求行腹部肠损伤探查。即使在术中没有确诊穿孔，应当小心评估是否有肠系膜撕裂、血肿、腹膜后损伤。同样，腰椎压迫伤（机会性）也是常见的。并且一旦存在，患者常常因为疼痛须长时间住院。

结肠和直肠的损伤在儿童中并不常见。结肠和直肠损伤的偶然原因包括机动车碰撞，从而导致骨盆骨折、骨头碎片造成直肠穿通伤。虐待儿童造成的故意伤害也可以见到，通常见于钝器伤害。如果黏膜损伤或者损伤位于浅表，应当继续观察。在许多情况下，远端直肠全层损伤可以进行一期修补术。腹膜返折处以上，严重的结肠损伤须行暂时性结肠造口术。穿通伤往往可以行一期修补术，但面对复杂的特性时在修复时也可能需要转流。

脾损伤的儿童在没有任何干预措施的情况下几乎都会停止出血。非手术处理是标准治疗方案，并且任何潜在的手术干预的发生率是非常小的。当有经验丰富的儿科外科团队对患者进行管理时，手术干预的比例很可能会减少一半。须进行手术的是那些在受伤24 h内已经接受或很可能接受了相当于其自身血容量一半的输血量（40 ml/kg或在输入20 ml/kg的血流后仍然不稳定）的患儿。脾损伤的生理反应与脾损伤的分级相关。大多数需要手术干预的儿童将须行脾切除术。如果脾切除术必须要执行，应适度给予脾切除后免疫。如果5岁前行脾切除术，很多儿童须每日口服基础量的青霉素。如果怀疑免疫抑制，应该使用乙肝疫苗。

当仅有肝损伤，而没有涉及大血管或胆管损伤时，那么通过观察几乎均可以治疗成功的。对于合并孤立脏器损伤的患者，这一说法尤其正确。然而，肝损伤的死亡率可较脾损伤的死亡率稍高，这一点是有可能的。肝和脾联合损伤的并发症与高死亡率的关系非常明确。受伤程度越重，死亡率越高。与脾损伤时所提及的一样，若已输血量相当于血容量的一半，手术干预也是肝损伤有效的治疗方式。如果CT上看到有强化，生命体征不稳定的患者若在手术探查前，能立即行血管栓塞术，可能对治疗有利。栓塞并不是血流动力学稳定患者的合适的处理方法。早期手术干预作为一种提高生存率的手段，包括损伤控制性剖腹术，与血管栓塞术和早期再手术，已经卓有成效。儿童大量输血对生理及血液系统产生的作用，使得肝损伤行手术处理变得十分困难。

儿童胰腺损伤并不常见，并且大多数时候是源于钝伤。自行车相关性损伤也应该包括在这一分类中 。大多数儿童胰腺损伤可能通过非手术方式治疗成功，包括肠道休息、静脉内营养、间断抑制胰腺分泌药物治疗。儿童胰腺横断行保守治疗可能还有较多争议。应注意，即使延误了诊断，保留脾的胰腺切除术也能得到获益。当有能力行儿科内镜逆行胰胆管造影（endoscopic retrograde cholangiopancreatography，ERCP）时，导管支架可能带来显著获益。和我们的团队一样，其他外科医生已经能够在胰腺横断，且不能完成支架置入时，行腹腔镜保留脾的胰腺切除术。

钝伤是儿童肾损伤非常常见的机制。钝伤是最常见的损伤。肾损伤发生时血尿可以为阴性。大多数儿童肾损伤（Ⅰ至Ⅲ级）通过非手术治疗是安全的。大多数病例中，即使是Ⅳ级损伤，通过非手术治疗方案保留肾似乎也是成功的，但是Ⅴ级损伤时，通过手术保留肾似乎并不常见。患者合并肾集合系统损伤出现尿液泄漏，可能须行输尿管支架植入。极少数的情况下，大量失血的损伤可能须行肾切除术，应以 40 ml/kg 输血量输血来启动和实行。在某些情况下可以考虑行血管栓塞术，然而，大多数的患者并不需要紧急程序的干预。因为现今，大多数受伤儿童都做了腹部 CT 扫描，每一个儿童都应该考虑行膀胱增强 CT 评估有无膀胱损伤。大多数膀胱损伤可以通过尿管成功治疗，不需要额外的耻骨弓上的引流。

儿童血管损伤是不常见的。与成年人相比，儿童可以耐受四肢更大程度的血管完全闭塞。肢体血管损伤同样分为钝性和穿通性机制。保肢比例通常超过 95%。腹主动脉损伤可能发生于安全带受伤、自行车损伤和 ATV 相关性损伤。因为相关内部损伤，最佳的治疗方案是立即进行直接血管修复。并没有研究对血管内支架在儿童，尤其是生长发育阶段的儿童中的长期使用进行评估。

骨损伤是受伤儿童需要手术干预的最大原因。这些损伤通常非常明显，分散了儿童对其他部位的更严重的损伤注意力。因此，骨损伤也是受伤的儿童漏诊损伤的重要来源。损伤漏诊也是所有患儿进入医院后须行三级检查的重要原因。颈椎损伤经常被误诊，并且很多漏诊的损伤是由于正常的变异。

致谢

感谢 Paula · Milburn Miller 的支持（儿童医学研究所，儿童外科主席，俄克拉荷马市，俄克拉荷马州）。

妊娠期创伤

Amy C. Sisley 和 William C. Chiu 著
全传林 译

妊娠期创伤患者的救治是创伤外科医生的重大挑战。母亲在怀孕期间的生理变化是诊断和治疗的困境，而须同时治疗 2 个患者可能是创伤团队在临床和道德上面临的挑战。创伤使 7% ~ 8% 的妊娠变得复杂，是孕产妇非产科死亡的主要原因。

流行病学

妊娠期创伤患者对创伤外科医生提出了重大挑战。随着孕龄增加，孕产妇和胎儿损伤的发生率也显著增加，有略超过 50% 的伤害发生在妊娠晚期。

孕产妇受伤的最常见的机制是机动车碰撞（motor vehicle collision，MVCs），约占 55% ~ 70%，其次是钝性创伤攻击，占 12% ~ 22%，摔伤占 9% ~ 22%。

风险因素与不良胎儿结局包括损伤严重度评分（Injury Severity Score，ISS）大于 15，重要的头部受伤的 GSW 得分低于 8，头部、腹部、胸腔或下肢调整损伤得分高于 3。另外，骨盆骨折、孕产妇乳酸水平升高和 活跃的子宫收缩与胎儿死亡风险的增加有关。

来自美国外科医师学会国家创伤数据库的数据显示了有关妊娠患者迄今为止最大的研究（n = 1 195）。妊娠患者相比较于未怀孕的患者更年轻，更可能是非洲、美国和西班牙人。妊娠患者系安全带的概率会比未妊娠患者低。这种风险特性有利于设计防范策略来优化疗效。

受伤机制

钝性创伤

钝性创伤是孕妇和胎儿死亡的主要原因，通常是由 MVC、攻击或者坠落造成的。尽管孕妇和未怀孕者在受到钝性创伤时死亡率接近，但是在相同的 ISS 下，他们受到伤害的模式有本质上的差别。因 MVC

受伤的怀孕者比未怀孕者更能承受重大的腹部损伤和更少的头部损伤。脾、肝和腹膜后的损伤更频繁地发生在妊娠患者中，部分原因是怀孕引起的血管增多和子宫造成的腹内容物移位。多达 25% 的钝性创伤妊娠患者承受着严重的脾或肝的撕裂伤。胎儿受到直接的钝伤十分罕见（<1%）。钝伤导致胎儿死亡的最主要原因是产妇死亡，其次是胎盘早剥。因为子宫是有弹性的，而胎盘没有，一定的力量可以导致胎盘早剥，即使是在腹部外伤较轻的情况下。在腹部创伤较轻的情况下，胎盘早剥的概率是 2%～3%，当腹部创伤比较严重时，这一概率可达 40%。子宫破裂发生的可能性通常小于胎盘早剥，但其概率会随着胎龄的增加而增加。尽管子宫破裂威胁着母亲和胎儿的生命，考虑到可变因素和一些微妙的临床表现，诊断通常十分困难。临床医生必须要对任何腹部钝伤患者是胎盘早剥还是子宫破裂保持高度的怀疑，特别是在妊娠后期。

穿通性损伤

穿通性损伤通常是由于枪伤或刺伤所致。妊娠患者的这种类型的损伤通常是由配偶或亲密伴侣所造成的。实际上这类损伤的怀孕的患者比非妊娠患者死亡率低，因为母亲的妊娠子宫有保护作用。不幸的是，孕妇腹部受到枪伤和刺伤后，胎儿的死亡率分别是 71% 和 42%。还应该指出的是，由于妊娠期的子宫腹部内容物上升，上腹刺伤会带来很高的风险导致妊娠患者的小肠损伤。

亲密伴侣暴力

亲密伴侣暴力（intimate partner violence，IPV）在孕妇怀孕期间并不罕见。报道显示有 7.4%～21% 的妊娠患者受到过来自伴侣的暴力行为，并且超过 2/3 的患者在怀孕期受到的暴力会增加。身体受到虐待的孕妇相比正常孕妇有更高的概率会流产或者生出低体重的婴儿。相比普通的暴力行为，经常虐待孕妇者不仅仅只是使用暴力频率高，还有 3 倍的风险会成为一个杀人犯。因此，分娩期的重创是特殊暴力行为和潜在致命关系的标志。

妊娠期的生理变化

在正常怀孕期间发生的组织和生理上的改变取决于孕龄。在妊娠早期，早期的变化容易适应，所以生理功能的改变会很少。截至妊娠晚期，几乎所有的器官都经历了变化，来弥补扩大的子宫和生长的胎儿。最重要的是要记住，照顾受伤的妊娠患者时，胎儿的存在和孕妇腹部体积增大不是唯一要考虑到因素。

在早期妊娠期间，子宫大小足够小，所以它依然可以相对较好地受到骨盆保护。胎盘的存在导致了最早的生理变化。从胎盘分泌的激素，包括人绒毛膜促性腺激素、人胎盘催乳激素、孕激素、雌激素、促肾上腺皮质激素、促甲状腺激素。这些激素增加了孕妇的胰岛素抵抗性并促发了高血糖症。随后增加的胰岛素和葡萄糖转化为了胎儿增加的蛋白质合成。生殖激素也抑制了胃肠蠕动，这些因素使早在妊娠期 8～12 周，孕妇误吸的可能性增加。

雌性激素和孕激素，以及肾素和醛固酮的增加，导致钠的吸收和血浆容量扩充，这大约开始于妊娠的第 10 周。尽管心率、平均动脉压、中心静脉压尚未改变，但心排血量可能会增加 1～1.5 L/min（表 1）。从第 10 周的妊娠开始，孕激素还促进肾增大，导致受损胆囊收缩和胆汁淤滞。早期妊娠结束后，胆结石的形成可能会增加。

表 1 妊娠期心血管系统的变化

参数	妊娠期		
	早期	中期	晚期
心排血量	增加	增加	增加
每搏输出量	增加	增加	增加
心率	正常	正常	增加
MAP	正常	下降	正常
SVR	正常	下降	下降

MAP，平均动脉压；SVR，体循环血管阻力

妊娠中期

在妊娠中期，子宫开始上升超过骨盆，并且到第 20 周，它可能到达脐水平（图 1）。血压下降约 5～15 mmHg，到达妊娠期的最低点。在创伤产妇出血时，胎盘血流量优先减少，在出现休克体征前，产妇可能丢失了 30% 的血容量。“仰卧位低血压综合征”是由于妊娠子宫压迫下腔静脉，减少静脉血回流，从而减少前负荷和心排血量。在妊娠 20 周后，孕妇左侧卧位可增加 30% 心排血量。

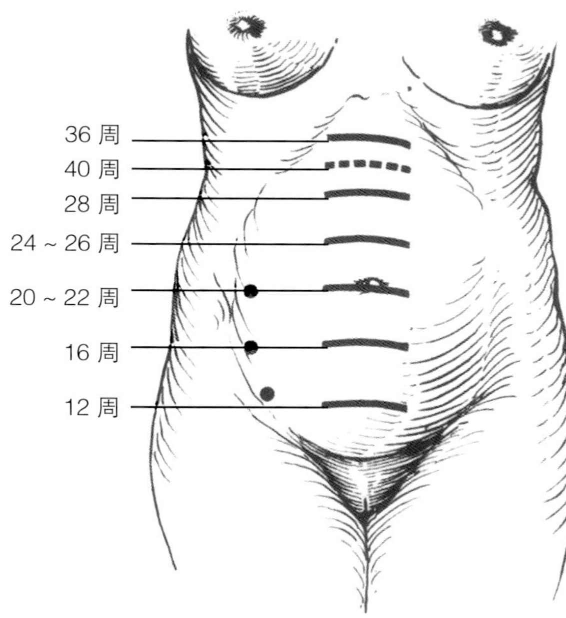

图 1 子宫底相对于腹壁的高度 (*Courtesy of David Gens, MD.*)

妊娠晚期

妊娠 7 个月时，耻骨联合和骶髂关节增宽。在大约妊娠 36 周时，子宫高度达到最大，靠近肋缘附近。腹腔内结构向头侧和外侧移位。

妊娠晚期期间，血压回归正常并且相较于非妊娠妇女，心率每分钟增加 20 次。当评估妊娠期创伤患者时应考虑到这一生理性心动过速。肺毛细血管楔压和左心室功能仍然正常，但体循环和肺血管阻力降低。

妊娠 30 周后，血浆容量增加了 40%，伴随着 15% 的红细胞重量的增加。这种差异导致了“生理性妊娠贫血”。因为血容量增加，人血白蛋白下降了 30%。良性的生理性心包积液非常普遍，并且使 FAST 变得复杂。胶体渗透压减少会增加肺水肿的风险。由于几乎所有的凝血因子、促凝素和纤维蛋白原的增加，以及纤维蛋白溶解活性的减少，可诱导出现高凝状态。

胸腔的解剖学变化包括膈约上升 4 cm，且胸腔的直径增加 2 cm。呼吸功能最重要的改变包括每分通气量的增加高达 50%，主要由于潮气量的增加（表 2）。功能余气量减少主要由于膈的上抬。代偿性呼吸性碱中毒导致慢性 $Paco_2$ 减少至大约 30 mmHg，碳酸氢根水平减少。2，3- 二磷酸甘油酸水平的增加也有利于胎儿氧气释放。这些变化使妊娠患者的氧储备和缓冲能力降低。

表 2 妊娠期呼吸系统的改变

参数	改变
Pco_2	降低
每分通气量	增加
潮气量	增加
功能余气量	减少
2, 3-DPG	增加

2, 3-DPG，2,3- 二磷酸甘油酸；Pco_2，二氧化碳分压

胃肠脏器向头侧移位与胃食管括约肌进入胸腔有关。胎盘释放胃泌素，促进胃酸分泌，使这一时期误吸的风险最大。

子宫压迫膀胱和输尿管导致代偿性肾盂积水。血容量的增加和心排血量增加使肾血流量增加 80%，肾小球滤过率增加 50%。血尿素氮和血清肌酐普遍降低，但尿量不显著改变。

诊断

初步评估

妊娠期创伤的初步评估如果条件允许应包括产科与新生儿的早期咨询（ > 妊娠 24 周）。创伤患者评估的一般原则也适用于妊娠患者，包括初始评估专注于评估和稳定孕产妇生命体征。这些包括对标准 ATLS 的评估，之后是对胎儿的活力做出快速和简单的评估。因为孕妇的子宫对下腔静脉的压力可能导致回心血量减少，孕妇应该努力使子宫偏向一侧。这可以通过倾靠在背板一侧或通过手动将子宫推向左侧完成。

妊娠期创伤患者插管的适应证与非妊娠期创伤患者相似，虽然怀孕期间误吸风险较高。然而，必须记住，胎儿与其母亲一样，不能耐受低氧血症。因此，所有妊娠期创伤患者都应该持续吸氧，并且监测血氧饱和度。

妊娠期间的生理变化，使得准确评估孕产妇血容量状态变得复杂。因为只要母体血容量有轻度减少，胎儿就会受到损伤。因此，应积极地进行容量补充。血管升压药和强心剂可以降低从母体流向胎儿的血流速度，因而在进行容量复苏时，不应该将

其用于缓解低血压。在母亲生命受到直接威胁时，可能偶尔须使用血管加压药或强心剂进行循环支持，但是必须要尽可能迅速、少量且间断的使用。

二次评估

二次评估按照 ATLS 的指南，但须说明的是，会阴的检查必须包括阴道和子宫颈的正式检查，以评估是否有出血。骨盆检查应尽可能由产科医生完成。

在妊娠期进行腹部查体是很困难的，因为腹部脏器从它们正常的位置发生了移位。此外，在妊娠晚期子宫使腹壁伸展，可能导致腹膜刺激征相对不敏感，导致通过临床查体诊断腹膜炎的难度加大。FAST 检查法代表了一种快速、无创地评估患者腹腔积液的手段。妊娠患者 FAST 检查法的灵敏度是 83%，比非妊娠人群的灵敏度稍低，然而两者的特异度相似，为 96%。虽然 FAST 检查法不能代替正式的胎儿超声，但它通过检测心率，可在复苏早期，快速获得胎儿的状态的大体情况。有报道指出，FAST 检查法也可检测在某些创伤患者中有无未知的怀孕，从而影响后续的治疗。使用超声不涉及电离辐射，并且对发育中的胎儿没有已知的危险。

胎儿的初步评估

胎儿的初步评估是二次评估的一部分，并且如果之前没有进行，可能包括超声、胎儿监测和产科咨询。正式的盆腔超声可以确定胎儿是否仍然存活，并且可以计算孕周。应该注意的是，在预测胎盘早剥时超声是不可靠的。

在妊娠晚期，心功能监测是胎儿评估最主要的方面。EAST 实践管理指南建议所有妊娠超过 20 周的胎儿都应进行至少 6 h 的监测。如果存在子宫收缩、胎儿心率异常、严重的孕产妇创伤时，建议延长监测时间。胎儿监测用来评估胎儿的状态和子宫收缩的存在及其频率，这是用于评估胎盘早剥的最可靠的工具。应该强调常规使用胎儿监测，甚至是在明的孕产妇轻度创伤的情况下。最近一项 13 家 Ⅰ 级和 Ⅱ 级创伤中心的多机构研究显示，只有 61% 的妊娠晚期创伤患者得到了胎儿监测。

诊断时的射线暴露

X 线片对评估妊娠期患者是必要的，这一必要性也总是使人们担忧射线暴露及其随后给胎儿带来的伤害。预测胎儿预后的最重要因素是孕产妇的结局，临床医生在治疗受伤的妊娠患者时应该毫不犹豫地获得诊断性 X 线片，因为这对于评估母亲的状态是必要的。这些诊断性检查仅应限于那些会影响产妇的结局，并且除此之外没有其他选择的患者。应禁止反复做这类检查，因此，如果知道患者将要行胸腹部 CT 扫描，那么就不须再行 X 线胸片、腹部平片和胸腰椎平片了。当胎儿在 CT 的视野之外时，辐射剂量是极低的。一般认为在怀孕的任何阶段，头、颈椎或四肢（不包括臀部和骨盆）的 CT 扫描是安全的。无论在何时，铅屏蔽可以使胎儿电离辐射的剂量进一步减少。

预测胎儿辐射导致的畸形是很困难的。然而，没有研究显示暴露剂量高于基线水平的 10 rad（100 mGy）。根据美国妇产科学会的关于妊娠期间辐射暴露的建议，暴露 5 rad（50 mGy）与任何流产或出生缺陷的风险增加无关。还应该记住致畸性与孕龄相关。胎儿在器官形成时期是最敏感的（怀孕后 2～8 周）。除了致畸性，胎儿辐射暴露的主要担忧是增加儿童癌症的风险。英国国家辐射防护委员会提出每有 100 rad 暴露，风险增加 6%。

大多数常规用于创伤患者评估的放射学检查，胎儿受到的辐射剂量为 1/100 rad 或更少（表 3）。其中例外的是腹部 CT，10 mm 层厚的腹部 CT，胎儿的辐射剂量为 2.60 rad。这仍然只是美国妇产科学会提出的安全剂量 5 rad 的约一半的剂量。然而，须记住新的多平面扫描仪可能有更高的辐射暴露。此外，未能考虑到不同患者的身体体质的区别，以及胎儿距产妇皮肤表面的深度，可能导致在估计胎儿的辐射剂量时发生重大错误。强烈建议在计划行放射学检查时向放射科进行咨询，以便将暴露的放射线最小化。

外科处理

大多数妊娠期创伤患者的治疗与非妊娠期创伤患者类似。一般来说，受伤需要手术干预的比例在妊娠期与非妊娠期患者中是一样的。对于妊娠患者须额外考虑的是全身麻醉和腹部手术可能造成早产。对子宫的直接伤害、产妇休克或胎儿窘迫，可能需要紧急剖宫产。

表3　胎儿暴露于放射照片的估计

过程	大约胎儿剂量 *（rad）
平片	
胸部（2个位置）	0.00002～0.00007
腹部	0.1
颈椎	0.002
骨盆	0.040
胸腰段脊柱	0.370
CT扫描 †	
头部CT	<0.05
胸部CT	<0.100
腹部CT	2.60

CT，计算机断层扫描

* 剂量因不同部位和使用习惯而不同

† 评估基于10 mm层厚

Modified from Barraco RD, Chiu WC, Clancy, et al: Practice management guidelines for the diagnosis and management of injury in the pregnant patient: the EAST Practice Management Guidelines Work Group. *J Trauma* 69(1):211–214, 2010; Eastern Association for the Surgery of Trauma, World Wide Web site, http://www.east.org/tpg/pregnancy. pdf; and Wakeford R, Little MP: Risk coefficients for childhood cancer after intrauterine irradiation: a review. *Int J Rad Biol* 79(5):293–299, 2003

钝性创伤

妊娠期间，只有0.6%的腹部钝伤的病例发生了子宫破裂。直接胎儿损伤也是非常罕见和复杂的，发生于不到1%的病例中。与非妊娠患者一样，非手术处理方案应该是血流动力学稳定的妊娠患者腹部实质脏器损伤的治疗选择。腹部创伤的非手术处理方案最大的区别是辅助血管造影治疗是不可取的，因为有潜在的巨大的辐射暴露。对于不稳定的患者，手术处理可能是改善母体和胎儿休克的最佳方式，剖腹术的手术适应证也类似于非妊娠患者。腹部钝的伤患者血流动力学不稳定，并且通过超声发现腹腔内有游离液体是紧急剖腹术的指征（图2）。在行剖腹术时，除非子宫有直接损伤，应保持子宫完整。

骨盆骨折会对妊娠患者造成一些严重的影响，而且在病例中有高达25%的胎儿死亡可能与此有关。有较大出血风险的骨盆骨折常有盆腔和腹膜后血管充血的表现。胎儿的受伤或死亡可能是因为胎盘直接损伤或产妇休克（图3）。盆腔动脉造影栓塞术应辅助用于威胁生命的盆腔出血，因为这一过程需要的辐射量超过胎儿的安全水平。

穿通伤

随着子宫扩大并且上升超过骨盆，其穿通伤发生风险也增加。子宫壁肌肉有弹性可以作为抵挡腹部低速刺伤的屏障，但对枪伤却并不足够。须行紧急剖腹术的患者是那些血流动力学不稳定、有明显经腹膜的穿透和通过超声发现腹腔有游离液体的患者。虽然可选择的检查方法与非妊娠患者相似，但是主要担心的是电离辐射的暴露。只要可能，就应谨慎地使用局部伤口探查评价浅表的刺伤。妊娠是诊断性腹腔灌洗（diagnostic peritoneal lavage，DPL）的相对禁忌证，特殊情况下可以考虑脐上DPL。

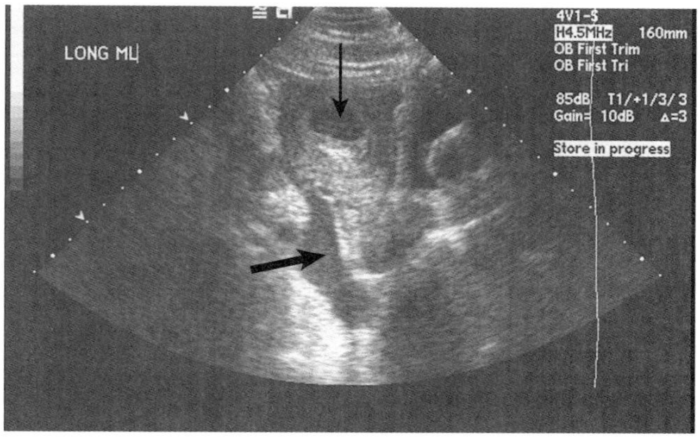

图2　车祸受害者的超声显示早期宫内孕（*细箭头*）和腹部游离液体（*大箭头*）

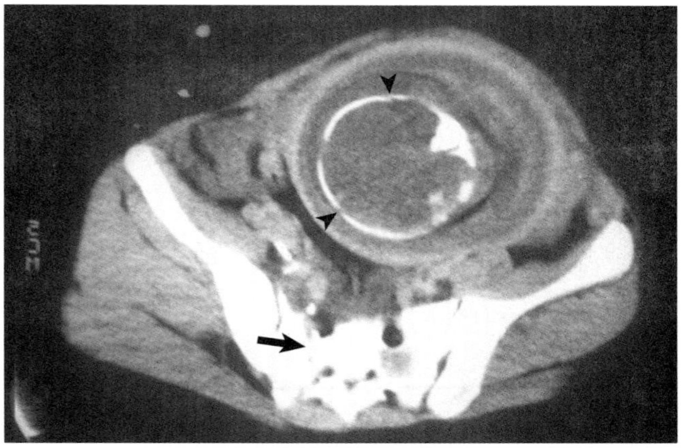

图3　CT显示孕产妇骨盆骨折（长箭头）伴随胎儿头骨骨折（*短箭头*）

CT 扫描在受到穿通伤的妊娠患者中的应用价值尚未得到充分的研究。在钝伤患者中，推荐进行腹盆腔 CT 扫描，以评估腹部创伤。在穿通伤患者中，必须考虑到选择的获益与风险。在非妊娠期患者躯干穿通伤时，腹盆腔三维重建 CT 能可靠地排除腹膜穿透，以避免不必要的剖腹手术。CT 扫描的风险包括胎儿暴露于电离辐射。也必须综合考虑到全身麻醉的风险和不必要的剖腹术的风险。没有明确证据和建议在躯干穿通伤时使用 CT 进行检查，应在紧急剖腹术和诊断性 CT 扫描中作出个体化的决定和判断。

剖宫产术

虽然紧急剖宫产术在胎儿抢救中的重要性是显而易见的，但是对死亡过程剖宫产术的适应证仍然有争议（表 4）。Morris 等的研究指出在妊娠大于 25 周的患者中，45% 的胎儿生存率与行紧急剖宫产术相关，并且有 60% 的婴儿死亡是因为胎儿窘迫的诊断延误。在这个多中心研究中，婴儿的幸存与母亲创伤无关，娩出时没有心音的胎儿均没有存活。

死亡过程剖宫产是指在产妇将要死亡的情况下紧急执行剖宫产术，无论是在产妇实际死亡之前或之后娩出。妊娠至少 24 周的濒死孕妇，如果胎儿心音仍然存在，应考虑行死亡过程剖宫产。当在孕产妇死亡之后执行时，胎儿的存活神经系统的预后和完全取决于孕产妇死亡和胎儿娩出之间的时间间隔。胎儿娩出必须在孕产妇死亡之后 20 min 内完成，但是最好在产妇心脏搏停后 4 min 内开始。当胎儿娩出在产妇死亡后 5 min 内完成时，胎儿的预期生存率高达 70%。

表 4　紧急和死亡过程剖宫产术的适应证

胎儿缺氧或窘迫
胎膜早破
子宫损伤或破裂
羊水栓塞
弥散性血管内凝血
妊娠后子宫并进行剖宫产术
孕产妇难治性休克或心脏搏停

疾病和并发症的处理

受伤的孕妇处于并发症的风险当中，特别是与怀孕和胎儿相关的并发症。怀孕带来的生理学和解剖学上的改变，可能将孕妇置于一个潜在的和妊娠没有直接关系的并发症的危险之中。

胎母输血综合征

高达 28% 的孕妇在创伤后会患胎母输血综合征。Rh 阳性血型胎儿对 Rh 阴性母亲的血液敏感数量是不确定的，但是大多数患者对 0.01 ml 的血液敏感。胎母输血综合征的程度和 Rh 同源免疫用 Kleihauer Betke 试验评估。这个试验用血红蛋白 F 标记在母体血液中的胎儿红细胞。胎儿和母体红细胞的比值可以被评估。要在产科咨询后尽早用 Rh 免疫球蛋白治疗，必须要在 72 h 之内。

早产

很多情况下，创伤之后轻微的子宫收缩会自然地解决。在实际的早产的例子当中，包含早产收缩和宫颈扩张的证据，可能须用药物安胎。几个药剂能有效地安胎，包括特布他林和硫酸镁，但只能通过产科咨询后才能使用。外伤、外科手术、全身麻醉会增加早产的危险。Drost 等在妊娠期的主要创伤的研究中，发现了子宫收缩松解术有 80% 的有效率。腹部钝伤可能造成胎膜早破，导致早产。

子痫和先兆子痫

体循环血压通常在妊娠中期开始减少。这些患者的任何高血压的情况都可能是子痫前期的标志，对妊娠高血压的控制作用能够有效防止子宫血管收缩和胎盘缺血。最初的治疗包括液体复苏的治疗方法，来扩张血管容量。这些患者可能还需要血管舒张药或正性肌力药来改善血流灌注。子痫前期通常在胎儿娩出后消失。

感觉器官发生变化、昏迷或癫痫的孕妇创伤患者可能有子痫。相关体征可能包括高血压、少尿、蛋白尿、肺水肿和 DIC。在治疗子痫前期时，液体复苏和血流动力学的支持是必要的。应给予硫酸镁，妊娠 28 周或更久的患者，应考虑剖宫产。

胎盘早剥

幸存的怀孕的创伤患者，胎儿死亡的最重要的原因是胎盘早剥，并且发生在30%～70%的严重受伤的患者之中。在腹部钝伤中，胎盘早剥的原因可能是产妇休克引起的子宫胎盘缺血或者减速力导致的机械剪切。子宫缺乏自动调整灌注的功能，所以对孕妇血压的变化很敏感。孕妇血容量减少或低血压导致子宫血管收缩和灌注不足。在怀孕后期，相对较小的钝伤可能导致胎盘早剥。

在受到创伤的情况下，胎盘早剥的体征是可能有微妙的隐匿性阴道出血和腹痛，或可能严重到足以导致休克或DIC。无阴道出血不排除胎盘早剥。高达25%的子宫胎盘分离可能导致阴道出血和早产。超过50%的子宫胎盘分离通常会导致胎儿死亡。有报道指出，发生迟发性胎盘早剥的最长时限为创伤后6天。

羊水栓塞

羊水栓塞是指羊水进入母体血循环。通常更多的发生在早产和产后即时，孕妇的死亡率高达80%。早产的怀孕创伤患者可能处于这样的危险之中，治疗方法大多根据临床体征来决定。临床表现包括呼吸困难、缺氧、低血压、感觉器官改变、痉挛，甚至可能心脏停搏。呼吸衰竭，如急性呼吸窘迫综合征，患者可能患有血小板减少或DIC。随着胎儿的娩出，这种情况下母体的治疗就会得到更大程度的支持。这些支持方法包括辅助供氧或者机械通气、液体复苏、正性肌力药、血管加压药和血液制剂替代。

静脉血栓栓塞

和怀孕相关的高凝状态的情况是由于凝血因子增加和抑制纤维蛋白溶解。神经损伤、骨盆或下肢骨折和重大疾病的患者，高凝状态使长期制动的情况恶化。推荐通过皮下注射低分子量肝素或者小剂量普通肝素来预防，结合下肢间歇性静脉气动压力设备治疗。胎盘屏障能防止肝素通过，肝素被认为在妊娠期是安全的。尽管华法林产品禁止在怀孕期间使用，但患者可能在产后能使用华法林产品。

急性深静脉血栓（deep vein thrombosis，DVT）应该用全部的肝素抗凝剂量来治疗。尽管普通肝素和低分子量肝素都被认为在怀孕期间安全有效，但能够连续注入的肝素对急性外伤和潜在的未计划的分娩有好处。

放射诊断肺栓塞的方法仍然是有争议的，Winer-Muram等研究表明，用胸部螺旋扫描肺栓塞胎儿平均暴露的电离辐射量比肺灌注扫描得更少，并且在孕期的3个阶段都是安全的。下腔静脉过滤器在肺栓塞的预防以及血栓溶解剂对于严重肺栓塞的患者的用途，还没有得到很好的研究。

腹腔内感染

尽管不必要的剖腹手术可能会让母体和胎儿冒着并发症的风险，被忽视的肠胃受损也可能导致较多的并发症。腹腔内感染对胎儿特别有害，应该考虑积极的手术或者介入治疗。应使用抗生素治疗传染性疾病，并且需要药物咨询，因为很多药物对胎儿有副作用。根据经验，抗生素的选择应该同时考虑到可能的病原生物和胎儿的安全。

死亡率

报道的胎儿死亡率因创伤程度不同而有所不同，但是严重创伤时高达61%，产妇休克时高达80%。即使是轻微的创伤，也与1%～5%的胎儿死亡率相关。随着妊娠时间的增加，孕妇和胎儿创伤的发生率也明显增加。有超过50%的创伤发生在妊娠晚期。胎儿死亡最常见的原因是孕产妇死亡，其次是胎盘早剥。与母亲和胎儿死亡相关的最常见的机制都是机动车碰撞。仅仅是这一机制已占到胎儿死亡原因的82%。应该注意的是，胎儿死亡率受母亲的年龄的影响，年龄在15～19岁之间的母亲，其胎儿死亡率最高。这可能反映了在这个年龄段的患者更倾向于参与冒险行为，如酒精和药物滥用，增加机动车碰撞和人际暴力的发生率。

推广使用安全带是减少孕妇死亡率一项最重要的措施。安全带的使用可使孕妇死亡显著降低，因此使胎儿的死亡率降低。有研究显示，与碰撞严重程度一样，有没有使用安全带是孕妇和胎儿预后的最佳预测指标。应使用安全带进行三点固定：骨盆下部、子宫底以下、肩带放置在乳房之间。

总结

妊娠期创伤患者的评估和治疗是创伤团队的重大挑战。结局依赖于对怀孕期间的生理变化的理解，以及对孕妇和胎儿必要评估策略的牢固掌握。在一开始必须对母亲开始治疗，因为挽救胎儿最好的办法是拯救母亲。在妊娠晚期，早期检测到早产迹象和胎儿窘迫而进行的胎儿监测是至关重要的。最后，包括早期产科咨询在内的多学科治疗是治疗成功的重要元素。

老年人创伤

Daniel J. Grabo, Benjamin M. Braslow 和 C. William Schwab 著
王传林 译

随着美国老年人口数量的增加，外科和内科医生了解年龄相关性结构和生理的变化规律是很重要的。除此以外，慢性疾病可以改变老年创伤患者的临床表现和处理方式。美国正经历着前所未有的老年人口的增长。老年人的定义为 65 岁及以上的人。随着一代婴儿潮人口的继续长大，卫生保健和预防医学的进步使预期寿命不断延长，美国老年人口的数量将在下个 25 年翻一番。至 2030 年，超过 65 岁的老年人的数量预期将会增加 7 000 万，而高龄老年人，那些年龄超过 80 岁的人，将会增加至近 2 000 万人。而我们“老年人”中更年轻的人群将会活得更久、更活跃、更健康。

随着年长的美国人继续变老，他们会经历常见的疾病情况，80% 的老年人至少患有一种慢性健康问题，50% 的人患有两种。此外，变老带来的后果如身体的稳定性、运动强度、协调性、视力、听力的下降，将会使老年人更容易受伤。尽管受伤的发生概率比 65 岁以下人群少，但美国老年人受伤后死亡率更高。创伤或意外伤害死亡是 55 ~ 64 岁美国人的第四大死亡原因，是 65 岁及以上美国人的第九大死亡原因。年轻和年长的美国人受伤的机制类似，如摔伤和机动车碰撞。然而损伤类型、影响和预后在这两个人群中差异显著。随着活动的减少，“高龄老年人”经历年龄相关性变化，使得他们的功能状态和能力受到限制。摔倒，尤其是地平面水平的摔倒，在急诊和住院人数的比例是巨大的。与年轻人相比，老年人创伤可导致病情加重，尽管 ISS 很低，但住院时间和死亡率增加。

随着美国老年人数量的增加，那些为他们提供的紧急治疗须重视，常见的损伤持续经常导致很高的发病率。理解与年龄相关的生理变化、常见的损伤机制和持续的特定器官损伤，很可能会带来更好的紧急治疗和改善这一特殊创伤群体的患者的治疗预后。此外，老年医学咨询服务与创伤团队联合也可评估跌倒风险、谵妄 / 痴呆和复方用药。另外，老年医学咨询可以援助创伤团队处理与严重受伤老年人相关的道德和临终问题。

生理变化

众所周知，老年人耐受手术、创伤和感染的能力减弱。这种变化是随着年龄增长、解剖和生理变化，所导致的必然结果，对每个器官系统都会产生影响。存在慢性疾病和服用某些药物（如抗凝药物和心血管药物）可以对老年创伤患者造成不良的影响。

老年人中枢神经系统（central nervous system，CNS）的功能受皮质萎缩和一些如淀粉样蛋白沉积和动脉硬化性脑血管疾病造成的病理变化的影响。临床上，这些通过感觉的钝化（视觉、听觉、触觉、疼痛和知觉）和认知的改变而被发现。这些变化除了改变小脑功能，还会改变步态和平衡，增加受伤的风险，尤其是摔倒。创伤和复方用药可以使受伤的老年人更容易焦虑、激越、谵妄。

心血管疾病是最常见的慢性病之一，存在于 80% 的八旬老年人中。逐渐减少的心肌细胞与代偿性肥大导致心脏代偿能力减弱和心功能不全。心脏自主神经组织的纤维化往往导致传导异常，出现心律失常和不同程度的心脏传导阻滞。动脉硬化性血管疾病容易损伤器官和组织的血流。老年人经常吃影响心血管系统的药物，如 β 受体阻断药、钙通道阻断药、降压药、利尿剂。由于老年性心血管系统的变化和常用的药物，对外源性压力和内源性儿茶

酚胺的反应往往无法改善老年人心脏的收缩力和心率。他们通常依赖前负荷，以此减少血容量。

随着年龄增加，胸壁顺应性、呼吸肌力量、肺弹性下降，导致呼吸功能下降。肺泡萎陷可以减少用于气体交换的表面积，导致动脉氧合减少。在受伤的情况下，由于年龄相关性肺顺应性改变、没有能力进行有效的咳嗽、气体交换功能受损，老年人可出现呼吸功能不全和呼吸衰竭。适当治疗损伤相关的躯体疼痛（特别是胸壁疼痛）是至关重要的，否则吸气用力不足、肺不张、肺炎可能会发展。硬膜外麻醉或镇痛已成为常用阿片类药物的辅助方法，通常通过患者自控镇痛的形式和非甾体抗炎药（nonsteroidal anti-inflammatory drugs，NSAIDs）来止痛。

随着年龄增加，肾的解剖和生理发生了变化。有效肾皮质质量下降，并且最终可以导致功能性皮质减少多达 25%。此外，肾小球滤过率（glomerular filtration rate，GFR）会降低，并且肾小管的重吸收和分泌功能也会受损。老年患者常常有溶质清除和液体平衡的问题。尽管肾功能明显下降由于瘦体重和肌酐生成量减少，血清肌酐水平能保持在正常范围内。肌酐清除率的计算应基于年龄和体重。

随着年龄的增加、肌肉体积、力量和反应性下降。骨密度也大大减低。骨折的频率和严重程度随着老年性骨质疏松症的程度的增加而增加。骨关节炎的患病率很高，与活动减少和疼痛有关。脊柱变得僵硬、缩短，导致呼吸力学改变。椎管狭窄、椎体骨赘可以是骨关节炎的结果，只要轻微创伤，即可诱发临床上重要的脊髓损伤。老年人的骨骼、关节、脊柱的这些结构改变也影响他们避免受伤的能力。增加活动被证明能增加肌肉体积和力量，因此减缓衰老过程。

一般认为年龄增加可以抑制老年人对感染和受伤产生适当的炎症反应。中性粒细胞是第一道抵抗感染的防线，并且，随着年龄增加，其功能也逐渐下降，如吞噬能力降低。自主神经系统（交感神经和副交感神经）的变化也对体内平衡和温度控制产生不良的影响。受体标志物（例如肿瘤坏死因子和白介素 6），在老年人中已被证明，在轻微的创伤、手术和感染时明显升高。老年创伤患者释放的这种细胞因子不成比例的增加，会导致全身炎症反应综合征（systemic inflammatory response syndrome，SIRS）。

老年人表现出对苯二氮䓬类、麻醉剂、阿片类药物和其他 CNS 活性药物的敏感性增强。心血管活性药物，如 β 受体阻断药，可以减弱反射，而儿茶酚胺可诱发心动过速。常见的药物，如抗生素、利尿剂和血管活性药物，可能会对肾功能产生有害的副作用。CT 是评估创伤患者常用的。尽管普遍担心，老年创伤患者使用静脉注射（intravenous, IV）造影剂并没有显示出急性肾损伤风险的不成比例的增加。

抗血小板药物、非甾体抗炎药和抗凝血剂（华法林）是常见的药物，用于慢性疾病情况的处理。阿司匹林和氯吡格雷不可逆地抑制血小板活性，血小板输注是首选的治疗血小板相关凝血功能障碍的方法。去氨加压素或 DDAVP 是替代血小板输注治疗尿毒症患者血小板相关性凝血功能障碍的方法。Cotton 等报道，一项全国创伤数据库的评估显示，华法林的使用正在增加，尤其是在年龄在 65 岁及以上的患者中。此外，华法林不仅在受伤患者中使用普遍，它的使用也是一个强力的死亡率的标志物。血浆（包含凝血因子）的输注被传统用来逆转华法林诱发的凝血功能障碍。老年患者的心肺储备能力通常有限，因此，常规用于逆转年轻患者的高 INR 所用的大量血浆（10～15 ml/kg，4～6 U，800～1 200 ml），通常可能导致老年人出现肺水肿。维生素 K（5～10 mg，静脉注射）可以作为血浆输注的辅助治疗。同时，维生素 K 依赖的凝血因子，包含从人血浆中提取的凝血酶原复合物，已被证明是有效缩短出血时间、逆转 INR 的方法，同时，通过这一方法，可能限制液体容量。重组凝血因子Ⅶa（rFⅦa）可以促进凝血酶生成，起了稳定的止血作用，已经被用于治疗创伤性脑损伤所致的中度凝血功能障碍，并且已被证明，其在老年群体中的应用既安全又有效。

损伤机制

钝伤是老年伤害的主要类型，摔倒是最常见的损伤机制，其次是机动车交通事故损害。据全国创伤数据库报道，在指定的创伤中心的年龄在 55 岁及以上的患者中有 148 382 次摔伤。老年女性往往比男性更频繁地摔倒，但是对于 55 岁及以上的患者，男性的死亡率明显高于女性。老年人往往从站立或坐姿摔倒，称为地平面摔倒（ground level falls，GLF），而年轻人更有可能从高处摔倒。尽管 GLF 的机制被认为是次要的，由于老年这一低能量的损伤可能造成超过预期的严重创伤本身是发病和死亡的潜在风险。有研究发现GLF患者，年龄在55岁以上是死亡的独立危险因素。多达6%的老年人摔倒，导致临床重要的骨折，其中有1%～2%为髋部骨折。年龄相关的变化，如步态障碍、本体感受减弱和周围神经病变，可能有助于摔倒的发生。频繁使用的药物，如β受体阻断药和镇静剂，可能引起直立性低血压或本体感受和认知的改变，也是摔倒的危险因素。慢性病情况可能导致晕厥发生和虚弱。摔倒干预的方法包括改善环境和药物的改善，并且已经显示当改善老年人居住设施后，可以使摔倒的发生率降低19%。此外，锻炼身体也可以成功地提高骨密度和整体健康，也能潜在减少摔倒。

根据美国国家公路交通安全管理局在2009年的报道，有187 000名65岁以上的人在机动车交通事故中受伤，并且有5 288名死亡。老年人占所有交通事故死亡人数的16%，占机动车交通事故伤害的8%。在2008年，有3 200万的注册老年司机，这个数字预计将随着人口老龄化而继续增加。年老的司机更有可能在白天、周末、好天气时发生车辆事故。同样，年龄相关的变化和慢性病情况，也会损害老年美国人的移动能力，会给他们的驾驶技能带来不利影响，如反应时间下降、视力下降等。然而与年轻人群相比，酒精中毒在老年人群相关机动车交通事故中起的作用很小。关于老年司机认知和身体能力的评估仍在讨论，但目前没有联邦或州执行驾驶限制令。

老年行人，被移动的车辆撞击的风险增加。视觉、听觉及步行速度的下降，以及认知和判断能力的降低，似乎是诱发因素。行人被撞是第三种最常见的损伤机制，并且导致了超过20%的汽车碰撞行人的死亡。年龄在创伤的分类和程度起到了关键作用。分配给行人穿越人行横道时间对许多步行速度缓慢的老年人可能不足。近1/3的65岁以上的行人死亡发生在人行横道。识别危险的十字路口和适当的安全措施，如求助于交通协管员，可能有助于减少老龄人群在人行道上的死亡率。

尽管老年人受到的主要伤害是钝伤，但穿通伤占老年人创伤相关死亡的比例超过50%。尽管在这个国家老年人占攻击受害者的一小部分，但他们的死亡率是年轻受害者的4倍。穿通伤的死亡率在年轻人群是稳定的（约10%），但是在55岁之后增加（14%～26%）。老年枪伤患者，GCS低、ISS为16及以上、低血压比年龄增加更能独立预测死亡率。力量和活动的减少是损害老年人自我保护能力的主要因素。认知和判断障碍可能影响老年人对事态的感知和决策的制定，使其受到攻击时出现更糟糕的结果。

体力和活动减少以及判断和认知受损导致家庭暴力的增加，也是老年人非意外创伤的重要原因。女性和年龄大于80岁更常与老年虐待相关。伤害经常发生在家里或公寓，由那些知道或者为受害者提供照顾的人造成。忽视往往先于暴力，并且财政困难和家庭地位的改变经常是虐待的原因。身体伤害与描述的受伤机制不符，并且有长期一般卫生条件不良的迹象时，应高度怀疑并调查，以防止即将发生的更糟糕暴力事件的可能性。

在美国，老年人的自杀率是14/10万，而且这个数字在城市地区甚至更高。在这个人群中，存在的慢性病、抑郁和疼痛是常见的自杀原因。近40%的枪伤老年人，被发现是自己造成的枪伤。

由于皮肤感觉下降和反应时间增加，老年人似乎特别容易受到热损伤。在法国马赛地区烧伤中心，有16%的烧伤入院患者年龄在65岁及以上，并且这一人群死亡率高达30%。烫伤，通常是浴缸里的水，似乎是老年人最常见的热损伤。死亡率高于伤害程度相近的年轻患者。烧伤面积超过总体表面积的50%是致命的，并且吸入性损伤也是非常不能耐受的。烧伤患者的处理中，复苏时所需要的大量液体会给心血管系统储备能力有限的老年患者带来有害的影响。

随着人们年龄增加，我们的老年人的活动水平将增加。老年人将会受到身体超负荷的缺点的影响，这大多数是由于老年人身体活动耐受能力受限。劳累型损伤常常是由于储备能力的减少。急性损伤常常会影响肌肉骨骼系统，并且常常是由于体育活动造成。有一些这种损伤会导致患者长期不能活动，并且需要很长一段时间去恢复。为了预防出现长期制动以及出现永久残疾的可能性，应积极处理这些损伤，且处理方式与年轻人相似。

预后

老年创伤患者与他们的同龄人相比在创伤后和其后相当长的时间内，花费更多。老年人创伤和创伤后续治疗过程中常常会出现并发症，如充血性心力衰竭、呼吸衰竭，急性肾损伤和感染。在最初受伤住院的5年内，老年创伤患者再次重伤或死亡的风险增加。合并有慢性病及慢性病的数量增加创伤相关死亡率。然而，如果 ISS＞15，那么慢性病与死亡率的关系不再那么明显。此外，ISS＞25，是老年人死亡率增加的独立相关因素。Perdue 等发现，当控制损伤严重度、合并症情况、并发症后，老年人群创伤后的死亡率是年轻人群的 5 倍。

在经验丰富的创伤外科医生的指导下，创伤小组的早期干预可以显著提高严重受伤的患者的生存率。生理学、损伤机制和解剖学位置是鉴定受伤患者是否会受益于成熟的创伤中心提供的高水平的治疗的经典方法。老年创伤患者的全因死亡率的范围为 15%～30%，而年轻创伤患者的死亡率不到 10%。评估老年创伤患者很困难，因为老年人对创伤和损伤的应激反应很迟钝。年龄相关性机体储备能力的减少、有一种或多种合并症以及慢性病药物治疗史，可能干扰正常机体对创伤的应激反应。例如，心动过速是血容量减少时的应激反应，而在使用 β 受体阻断药的老年人中，这一反应变得迟钝。此外，对于有高血压的患者，尽管有严重的出血，血压可能在正常范围内。经过创伤团队的救治，有 60% 以上的损伤程度严重（ISS>15）的老年人，和 25% 处于临界损伤（ISS>25）的老年人没有出现低血压（SBP<90 mm Hg）。通过早期复苏的努力和创伤团队的持续评估，以及随后在适当的时候进入 ICU，心血管功能衰竭、呼吸道功能恶化和许多并发症是可以阻止的。创伤团队的专业技能和 ICU 医务人员可以限制不必要的诊断性检查，提供一个快速和全面的损伤和生理功能紊乱的清单，加快治疗干预，而且准确地提供监测。早期识别休克并且限制灌注不足和缺氧，可以阻止多器官功能衰竭，提高生存率。

高龄老年人，年龄在 80 岁及以上，有 2 倍的可能性在受伤后的初始阶段死亡。如果他们在住院期间幸存，也很可能需要额外的医疗设备。当 ISS 相似时，年龄在 80 岁及以上的创伤患者与年轻患者相比（年龄 65～79 岁），死亡率显著增加。当无论是家庭有临终关怀想法还是意识到进一步的治疗是徒劳时，撤回高龄老年人的药物支持都会增加死亡率。

特定器官损伤的处理

老年创伤患者的初步评估和管理遵循美国外科医师协会委员会 ATLS 的年龄无关协议。然而，应早期关注先前存在的慢性病情况和慢性病治疗药物（如 β 受体阻断药和抗凝药物）和潜在的生理性反应迟钝。另外，虽然创伤团队主要在最初的诊断和复苏中起作用，但应该与患者家属或者看护人保持联系，以便了解药物信息，并且先进的指导对早期恶化很有用。传统的生命体征已经被证明并不能充分预测老年非神经系统钝伤患者是否发生休克。必须通过 CT、超声和心功能监测早期、全面地进行诊断性检查。虽然控制疼痛是至关重要的，但是对麻醉剂和其他镇静剂的剂量必须极其谨慎，因其可能改变药代动力学，常常造成不良的后果。

表 1　老年人的年龄相关性创伤治疗方法

年龄	注意事项
55～69 岁	假设有一些轻度的生理储备能力的减少。 怀疑年龄居中的人存在一些常见疾病（糖尿病、高血压）。 怀疑处方或非处方药物的使用 怀疑 TBI，并且有 LOC 病史或认知异常，行头部 CT。 进行标准的诊断和处理方案
70～80 岁	承认与年龄相关性和获得性生理变化的存在。 承认应用药物控制了获得性疾病 病史的判断能力，包括亲戚和私人医生 监测患者和控制生理参数，以优化心脏功能 存在认知改变，必须行颅脑影像学检查 进行标准的诊断和处理方案。 应做好早期、积极的手术治疗准备 应意识到结局并不理想，尤其是严重的中枢神经系统损伤 检查有无事先说明
80 岁及以上	过程如上述。 假设有中度严重的伤害，尤其是中枢神经系统或任何造成生理功能紊乱的伤害，预后很差。 进行积极的初始复苏和诊断之后，与患者及其家属讨论合适的治疗方式 尝试行人道主义关怀，认识其中所涉及的法律和伦理争议。 考虑早期伦理咨询和社会服务

Modified from Schwab CW, Kauder DR: Trauma in the geriatric patient

Arch Surg 127(6):701–706, 1992. Copyright 1992 American Medical Association. All rights reserved

CNS，中枢神经系统；CT，计算机断层扫描；LOC，意识丧失；TBI，创伤性脑损伤

表 1，老年人的年龄相关性创伤治疗方法，概述了这一患者人群的很多治疗原则。

老年人头部外伤的死亡率仍然是最高的［在头

部外伤简明损伤分级（abbreviated injury scale, AIS）3 级和更高的比例分别为 12% 和 19%]。老年创伤患者的脑外伤的评估非常困难，因为如果有潜在的痴呆，体格检查可能会产生误导。此外，当做精神状态的检查时，阿片类药物和镇静剂的使用可能会带来问题。高度怀疑并且早期行头部 CT 扫描对创伤性脑损伤的合理分类是非常重要的。脑组织实质重量的减少导致颅内容积丢失，并且增加血管剪切力损伤，这可能与频繁的颅内出血相关。此外，在颅内压（intracranial pressure，ICP）升高导致中线偏移及疝出前，有更多的颅内空间须被充满，如同图 1 所见。虽然老年患者合并创伤性脑损伤，其功能性预后非常糟是众所周知的，但不应该拒绝给高龄老年人使用医疗资源。当发现创伤性脑损伤时，与年轻人群相比，年龄在 80 岁及以上的老年创伤患者确实没有显示出更糟糕的结局。

先前存在的神经系统疾病，不论中枢性或周围性，都可以给老年创伤患者脊髓损伤的评估带来问题。退行性关节疾病可以体现在颈椎椎管狭窄和骨赘形成上。颈椎损伤主要集中在老年人中，齿突骨折是最常见的。与手术固定或通过坚硬的颈托进行的非手术处理相比，通过头胸支架处理老年人齿突骨折，与死亡率的增加和重要并发症（如肺炎）的发生相关。向前摔倒可以导致颈椎过伸、急性脊髓受压、脊髓的中心部位损伤。这一类型的损伤常导致中央型脊髓损伤综合征。老年人的预后不良，一般与呼吸衰竭相关，死亡率大约为 50%。死亡与颈椎固定后出现呼吸衰竭的并发症有关。诊断性影像学检查，如 CT 和 MRI，应该在怀疑脊髓损伤时早期获得。

躯干创伤是继创伤性脑损伤之后，老年创伤患者死亡的第二大原因。胸部钝伤是常见的，并且是发病，甚至死亡的最重要的原因。气胸、血胸和肺挫伤这些并发症的治疗与年轻患者相似。65 岁及以上患者，每有一根肋骨骨折，死亡率增加 19%，患肺炎的风险增加 27%。

老年创伤患者合并肋骨骨折、进入创伤中心、存在心功能衰竭、插管、年龄增加、ISS 分数增加都是明显的死亡预测因子。此外，合并肋骨骨折可以提示腹部实质脏器的损伤，如肝、脾损伤。连枷胸是指 3 个或以上连续的肋骨在 2 个或以上的部位骨折，与死亡率的明显升高有关。然而肋骨骨折的疼痛管理是必要的，呼吸衰竭可以迅速发生，特别是在看起来舒服的老年患者中。肋骨

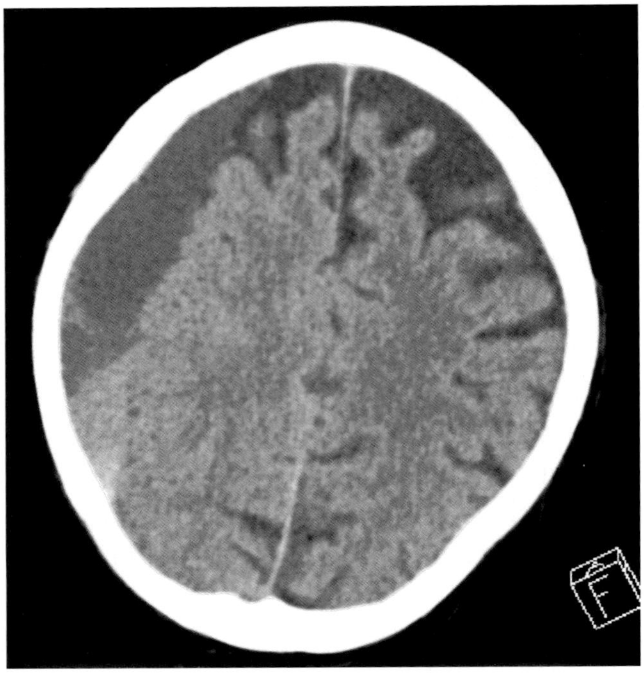

图 1　这是一个右侧额顶叶慢性硬膜下出血患者的典型的头颅 CT 平扫轴位图的影像表现。这个患者有摔倒史，并且格拉斯哥昏迷等级评分为 14 分，注意到在顶叶区域慢性硬脑膜下出血合并有急性硬膜下出血的分层。此外，有证据显示脑容量减少，这在老年人群中非常常见，并且使得颅内出血积聚而颅内压及质量最小限度的增加

骨折的疼痛管理是必要的，因为呼吸衰竭可以迅速发生，特别是在看起来舒服的老年患者。阿片类药物、非甾体抗炎药，以及硬膜外镇痛和麻醉的合理使用都是疼痛控制的重要方法。肋固定可以改善老年患者的结局。

创伤性主动脉损伤（traumatic aortic injury，TAI）由摔伤和机动车碰撞相关性快速减速伤引起，往往是致命的。那些受伤机制包括急性减速和 X 线胸片显示纵隔增宽的患者，应怀疑有 TAI。X 线胸片正常并不能排除 TAI，所以仍须高度怀疑主动脉损伤。胸部和主动脉 CT 是诊断 TAI 的首选方法。虽然 TAI 的处理与年轻人相似，但是老年人血管内修复术（endovascular repair，EVAR）使血管内移植物的稳定性减小了。年轻患者合并 2 型内漏也有越来越多的问题须关注。对于病情稳定的患者，药物治疗包括 β 受体阻断药治疗以及血管舒张剂，以减少受伤的主动脉壁的压力。外科修复是不稳定患者或最初复苏阶段之后的保留处理方式。为了计划血管内手术方案，常常延期进行手术，这大大取代了传统的开放性手术技术。血管内治疗对于有合并症

的老年创伤患者具有特殊益处，这些合并症可能使传统开放性手术的并发症发生率居高不下，但血管钙化和迂曲会使这项技术变得复杂。

腹部实质脏器钝伤管理的进展倾向于非手术方法，通过使用介入放射学的方法进行诊断和动脉栓塞治疗。这一处理方案仅仅适用于血流动力学稳定的，且没有腹膜炎表现的患者。如果采用这种治疗模式，可靠的检查是最重要的。那些由于一系列原因无法配合查体的老年患者、怀疑实质脏器损伤合并腹腔积血，以及血流动力学不稳定的患者仍推荐早期进行剖腹术。一项宾夕法尼亚州创伤系统基础数据库的评估显示，大多数合并脾钝伤的老年创伤患者（年龄 55 岁及以上）都已行非手术处理。年龄增加与非手术处理失败的比例相关。ISS 和脾损伤分级都是失败的预测因子。无论选择何种治疗方式，死亡率都很高，并且非手术处理的失败与医院和 ICU 治疗的时间相关。

随着年龄的增长，人体的解剖结构也发生改变，如骨质疏松症、摔倒，即使是很小的高度，都很可能造成骨盆骨折。这表明，即使是很小的力量也能造成老年人明显的创伤。在 Dechert 等的分析报告中，观察到死于骨盆骨折的老年人行介入血管造影或进行手术干预的比例很低。值得注意的是，骨盆骨折的老年人中有低血压表现的人数低于年轻人。并发症和死亡不仅仅是损伤初期的结果，也是损伤之后长期制动的结果。此外，骨盆骨折与住院时间的增加相关，也与更多资源的使用相关。

损伤控制外科原则和复苏策略改善了严重、威胁生命的创伤患者的结局。损伤控制性剖腹术（damage control laparotomy，DCL）已经显示出其在严重创伤的老年患者的治疗中的有效性。据报道，与年轻人相比，老年创伤患者进行 DCL 的死亡率增加（55～80 岁为 42.9% vs. 16～54 岁为 12.5%），并且死亡时间更早（9.8 天 vs. 26 天）。大多数的结果，如幸存者住院天数、ICU 治疗时间、呼吸机通气时间，在行 DCL 的老年患者与年轻患者之间无明显差异。虽然损伤的机制有很大不同，只有 14% 的老年人受到穿通伤，而年轻人受穿通伤的比例占到 60%。一般认为 DCL 在一般紧急手术和创伤手术时，都是对八旬老年人有益的。尽管总体并发症发生率为 62%，住院死亡率为 37%，对那些幸存的出院患者，这一人群的长期生存率可以增加。

总结

随着人群逐渐变老，我们的急诊科和创伤团队将面对越来越多的老年创伤患者。老年创伤患者会表现出生理的改变，甚至低速的损伤机制也会给他们带来严重的伤害，并且合并慢性病及相关药物使用也是老年人受伤的独特机制，且老年人对伤害反应迟钝。同样地，了解这些老年人固有的生理变化和独特的损伤机制，将有助于提高老年创伤患者的治疗水平，从而改善预后。必须要高度怀疑隐匿的休克和损伤，同样，也必须进行早期、全面的诊断性影像检查，尤其是脑损伤患者。此外，生理储备能力受限，不能耐受非手术治疗策略失败的老年创伤患者、应早期进行手术干预，包括损伤控制程序。增加老年医学咨询通常有助于评估创伤患者的年龄相关疾病和临终问题。

烧伤

John T. Schulz III，Kimberly A. Davis 和 Richard L. Gamelli 著
王传林 译

烧伤发生的频率和它随后带来的多系统的影响使得烧伤患者的治疗成为创伤和急救治疗的外科医生经常遇到的管理挑战。在烧伤初期治疗时，紧急外科处理包括液体复苏和通气支持，同时保护和恢复远端脏器功能。合适的复苏后，烧伤患者管理的重点是伤口护理和提供必要的代谢支持。烧伤伤口是否需要紧急或创伤外科处理，取决于伤口损伤的程度和深度，并且需要快速识别的这类患者，最好在烧伤中心进行治疗。

发病率

美国每年确切发生的烧伤数量并不清楚，因为 50 个州中仅有 21 个洲要求报告烧伤。

表 1 烧伤中心转介标准

部分全层烧伤累及超过体表总面积的 10%
任何年龄组的全层烧伤
烧伤累及面、手、足、生殖器、会阴部或主要关节
重要的电烧伤，包括闪电击伤
化学烧伤
吸入性损伤
烧伤患者在现有的医疗条件下，处理变得复杂，恢复时间延长或者影响生存率
烧伤较轻，伴随有足以改变结局的创伤 *
住院儿童任何程度的烧伤，没有合格的人员或照顾孩子的设备
需要特殊社会、心理干预或长期康复的患者的任何程度的烧伤

* 如果机械性创伤会立刻带来更大的风险，在转运到烧伤中心前应在创伤中心接受初步治疗维持稳定

Modified from American Burn Association: Stabilization, transfer and transport. In *Advanced life burn support course instructors manual*. Chicago, American Burn Association, 2001, Chap. 8, pp73–78

通过那些数据推算得到大致的烧伤的总人数。目前，在美国，估计每年有 125 万人发生了烧伤。其中 80% 的患者累及的烧伤面积少于体表总面积的 20%。估计每年，大约每 100 万人中有 150 ~ 170 人须在烧伤中心住院治疗。在每年需要住院治疗的烧伤人群中，有一小部分人，约 2 万人，如美国烧伤协会所定义的那样，最好在烧伤中心治疗。这一部分人包括每 100 万人中有 42 个严重的烧伤患者，还包括每 100 万人中有 40 个烧伤不严重但合并有复杂因素的患者。

损伤机制

某些特定人群是某种特殊创伤的高危因素，需要创伤外科或急诊外科的治疗。烫烧伤是烧伤损伤的最常见的形式，造成 58% 的烧伤损伤和每年超过 100 000 次的急诊就诊。65% 的 4 岁及以下的儿童须住院治疗烫烧伤，其中大部分造成烫烧伤的原因是接触热的食物和液体。通过调整热水加热器的温度设置或者安装特殊的水龙头阀门，以防止不安全水温的流出，可以最小化自来水烫伤意外的发生。因虐待儿童而发生的烫烧伤常常伴随着前后矛盾或者改变的病史，并且体格检查时也非常明显，可以立即被区分。这些伤害非常典型，累及足、腿后部、臀部（有时候是手部），并且常常是由于被看护人虐待而浸在滚烫的水中所导致。怀疑被虐待的儿童应该接受骨骼放射学调查。这对创伤和重症监护外科医生识别和报告虐待儿童是非常重要的。因为如果没有察觉到虐待儿童，儿童又会回到被虐待的环境，反复的虐待与高死亡率相关。

火和火焰源引起 34% 的烧伤，并且是成年人烧伤最常见的原因。1/5 ~ 1/4 的严重烧伤与职业相关。厨房工作人员烫伤的风险相对较高，而屋顶工和铺路工人热沥青烧伤的风险最大。参与电镀过程和制造肥料的工人受到强酸伤害的风险最大，而那些参与制造肥皂和使用炉灶清洁剂的人受到强烈的碱金属的伤害的风险最大。

电流每年导致约 1 000 人死亡。年幼儿童因家用电流导致电损伤的发生率最高，因其将物体插入电源插头与插座或者咬或吮吸电源插头与插座。成年人中有很高的高压电损伤风险者是公用事业公司的员工、电工、建筑工人（尤其是起重机人员）、移动灌溉管道的农民工、野外作业人员、卡车司机和安装天线的个体工。每年平均有 107 人死于雷击。绝大多数雷击相关死亡（92%）发生在夏季，在人们从事户外活动时，如高尔夫或钓鱼。

虐待是烧伤的一类特殊情况，影响儿童。通常是父母虐待儿童，但也可由兄弟姐妹和照顾者造成。儿童最常见的伤害是用故意点燃的香烟造成的。用热的熨斗烫伤手背是虐待儿童的另一种方式。正如前面所讨论的，烫烧伤非常常见。在近几年，看护或者家庭成员虐待老年人变得越来越常见。应该报道这些事件，并且保护受害者。

病理生理学

局部影响

烧伤造成的皮肤损伤与来源能量的温度和热容、暴露时长、累及的组织表面相关。当温度低于 45℃时，即使暴露时间很长，也不太可能发生组织损伤。当温度在 54℃时，成年人暴露 30 s 即会造成烫伤，但是儿童暴露 10 s 就会出现相同程度的烫伤。当温度上升至 60℃时，这是家用热水的常见温度，儿童暴露后不到 5 s 即可出现组织破坏。因此，当患者接触沸水或明火后会造成明显损伤。不管是有意还是

无意的烫伤经常导致诉讼。因此，供应商应该熟悉水温和致烫伤时间的关系，总结在表 2 中。

烫伤导致 3 种区域的损伤。中央位置是凝固或坏死的区域。在全层烫伤时，发生凝固的区域累及皮肤全层，延伸至真皮以下达到皮下组织。在部分全层烫伤时，这一区域仅仅延伸至真皮层，并且有幸存的上皮组织，最终能够修复创面。围绕着凝固区域的是非杀伤性细胞损伤区域，是静止的区域。在这一区域，血流发生了改变，但是当复苏有效时，随着时间会逐渐恢复。如果患者复苏不完全，会发生血栓，并且这一静止的区域会变成凝固的区域。最外面的区域是损伤程度最小的区域，是充血的区域，与没有损伤的区域相邻。充血的区域最常见于严重日晒而出现的表皮部分全层损伤的患者。这种液体聚集是由于经过毛细血管的流量导致的系统性变化，但过度的液体复苏可能会加重病情。

表 2　真皮损伤需要的水温和暴露时长

温度		
华氏温度（°）	摄氏温度（°）	时间
120	48.9	>5 min
125	51.7	1.5~2 min
130	54.4	30 s
135	57.2	10 s
140	60	<5 s
145	62.8	<3 s
150	65.6	1.5 s
155	68.3	1 s

随着创面血液供应的变化，烫伤组织会形成显著的水肿。创伤组织中产生的因子，成为局部介质，包括组胺、5- 羟色胺、缓激肽、前列腺素，白细胞三烯，IL-1、IL-6、IL-10，TNF-α，IL-17，这些都能改变局部组织的稳态，增加血管通透性。补体也被激活，可以进一步改变经毛细血管的血流量。这些变化的净效应是使血管内液体明显地进入血管外的液体腔室。在创伤后 24 h，水和蛋白的累积量达到最大，并且可以持续至少一周。另外，表面烫伤面积达到 20% ~ 25% 的患者，其未受伤的组织床也有相似的液体运动。

全身反应

机体对大的烧伤产生的生理反应能带来某些深远的改变，而患者对这些改变是能够耐受的。生理反应的大小与烧伤的大小是成比例的，当体表损伤面积超过 50% 时，反应达到最大值。改变持续的时间与创伤的存在相关，因此要解决伤口的问题。特定的器官反应与其他形式的创伤一样，都是最初是功能减退，即衰退阶段，接着是一个高动力性的“流动”阶段。

心血管系统的改变对烧伤患者最初的治疗和管理有重要和直接的影响。在烧伤后的即刻，有一个短暂的时期，心脏功能降低，并且周围血管阻力升高，如果容量复苏不充分，可能造成病情恶化。全身灌注不足可以导致全身血管阻力进一步增加以及血容量的再分配。未能充分复苏的烧伤患者心功能会更加恶化。相反，在 24 h 内充分复苏可以使心功能恢复正常，并且到第 2 个 24 h，这些功能会进一步增加至超常水平，而出现高动力学状态。随着创面的关闭，这一状态也会逐渐回归正常水平。

烧伤之后，由于发生了吸入性损伤，使肺实质受到了直接损伤，因此肺功能也会发生改变。没有发生吸入性损伤时，烧伤后出现的肺功能的变化是一般高动力学状态的反应。肺通气的增加与全身烧伤的体表总面积成比例，呼吸频率和潮气量均增加。没有发生烟雾吸入性损伤的烧伤患者，如果呼吸状态更差，提示有另外的情况发生，包括脓毒症、肺炎、隐匿性气胸、肺栓塞、充血性心力衰竭或急性腹腔内病变。没有这些情况的患者，肺气体交换功能是相对保持的，并且肺力学几乎没有变化。

肾对烧伤的反应很大程度上是取决于心血管系统的反应。在初期肾血流量是减少的，随着复苏，肾血流也逐渐恢复。如果患者正在进行复苏，那么肾灌注不足将持续下去，从而引起继发于肾缺血的早期的肾功能障碍。如果患者表现出肌红蛋白尿或血红蛋白尿（如高温性肌坏死、四肢筋隔室综合征或伴随的软组织创伤）可以加重肾功能障碍。这两种情况中的任意一种都能够造成直接肾小管损害。

烧伤能够影响胃肠蠕动和黏膜的完整性，通常是因为在复苏时导致的肠道灌注不足。相反，大量复苏的患者将会出现明显的腹膜后、肠系膜和肠壁的水肿，而导致麻痹性肠梗阻的出现。立即进行肠内营养，可能保留胃肠蠕动能力，保护黏膜的完整性，并且可以获得有效的营养输送。肠内营养延迟与肠梗阻的发病有关，当烧伤复苏变得复杂时，肠梗阻也可发生。

从神经内分泌的角度来看，烧伤导致激素和神经递质的反应升高，这与“战或逃”的反应程度相似。神经体液的反应时间会延长，并且在手术应激下会加剧。糖皮质激素和儿茶酚胺的增加是维持创伤患者应激反应所必需的。当应激激素反应不足时，一个不致命的损害可能也会变得致命。很多发生在烧伤之后的多系统的改变与儿茶酚胺的分泌改变相关，尤其是静息状态下的代谢不平衡的改变、底物的使用、心功能功能。一旦伤口完成修复，增加的神经体液反应消退，且合成代谢激素成为主导。

烧伤会影响造血系统，导致白细胞和红细胞的产生和功能失去平衡。总体表面积超过 20% 的烧伤与红细胞产生的改变相关，并且在皮肤血液循环层面增加红细胞的破坏，导致贫血。这种贫血可以因频繁的静脉切开、术中血液丢失、复苏时的血液稀释和红细胞膜完整性的短暂改变而进一步加剧。长期改变似乎与骨髓的红细胞祖细胞对促红细胞生成素的低反应性有关。通过适当的复苏，在早期复苏阶段，血小板数量减少、纤维蛋白原水平抑制、凝血因子改变至回归正常或接近正常。由于骨髓释放增加和去边界，白细胞数量很早就发生改变，伴随中性粒细胞的增加。简单的烧伤患者，保留了骨髓髓细胞生成功能。

除了骨髓会发生变化，免疫系统进一步出现显著的抑制。烧伤给机体的防御能力带来了全身性的损伤。体液免疫应答的改变包括 IgG 和 IgM 的分泌减少、纤维蛋白水平的减少和补体激活水平的增加。细胞免疫应答的改变包括 T 细胞反应性和细胞种群的改变，导致抗原呈递发生改变和延迟型超敏反应损害。白细胞功能也有不利影响，已注意到粒细胞趋化性受损、吞噬活动降低、抗体依赖细胞毒性减少，并且它们二次应答的能力也相对受损。这些发现的临床重要性在于，烧伤患者在烧伤后出现感染并发症的危险性相当高。

烧伤创面深度分级

损伤是组织破坏的后果，可能通过检查明显地发现。创面表浅、干燥、充血、容易漂白、无水疱表示一度烧伤。一度烧伤的损伤只达表皮，并且表皮的基底层与真皮并未分离。与一度烧伤不同，二度烧伤或三度烧伤，烧伤累及真皮层。浅二度烧伤（真皮层最小限度的破坏）与充血、水疱、感觉增加、触碰或与空气接触产生的剧痛感有关。创面充血、温暖、容易变白。深二度烧伤（更深层真皮层的坏死），其创面有完整或破裂的水疱，或可能会覆盖着一层薄薄的坏死真皮称为“焦痂”。查体最主要的发现是烧伤组织有感觉的存在，虽然感觉有减弱（表 3）。通过适当的处理，浅二度甚至深二度烧伤可以自己愈合，而不需要植皮。但是非常深的二度烧伤，完整的真皮和稳定上皮形成的表皮附属物太少，在功能上相当于三度烧伤。深二度烧伤的感染的风险是非常大的，并且如果一旦形成感染，会导致更深层皮肤的缺失（伤口转换）。全层伤口（三度）发生在皮肤全层都受到损伤，或者损伤延伸到皮下或更深的组织（四度）时。这些伤口将会出现苍白或呈蜡状、感觉缺失、干燥、没有弹性和包含形成血栓的血管。偶尔见于老年人、儿童和年轻女性。伤口最初可能表现为砖红色，因为从真皮层中红细胞破裂溢出的血红素。这种伤口将会有明显的水肿，没有弹性，也没有感觉。全层伤口很容易感染，因为皮肤不能再为机体提供任何防止生物入侵的屏障，并且如果不进行治疗，它将会迅速被病原体占领，而成为侵入性烧伤创面脓毒症的门户。

复苏的重点

液体管理

烧伤后应立即优先对引起的心血管系统的变化进行处理。所有创伤面积占到全身体表面积 20% 以上的患者以及烧伤面积较小，但生理指标提示须进行液体复苏的患者，应选择大小合适的周围血管行大静脉穿刺，最好是选择没有烧伤的皮肤。如果没有合适的周围血管存在，或患者准备插管而须多个静脉通道时，可以考虑中心静脉置管。乳酸林格氏液的使用方法为：成年人初始速度应为 1 L/h，而体重在 50 kg 或以下的儿童为 20 ml/kg · h。这一输液速度是根据烧伤后第一个 24 h 的液体需要量而调整过的。

复苏液体的需要量与烧伤的程度（将部分和全层烧伤的烧伤按体表总面积的百分比表示出来）成比，与体格（最常表达为体重）和年龄（儿童每单位体重的体表面积大于成年人）相关。入院患者应该

表 3　烧伤的临床特点

	部分全层烧伤		全层烧伤
特点	一度	二度	三度
病因	日光或低强度的光	高强度或更长时间暴露在强光下相对短暂地接触高温液体、火焰	高强度或更长时间暴露在强光下 长时间接触火焰或高温液体 接触蒸汽或热金属 高压电 化学药物
颜色	鲜红色	斑驳的红色	白色 半透明和羊皮纸般的 焦黑
创面	干燥 没有大疱	潮湿 有大疱	干燥、坚韧、僵硬 残余的烧伤皮肤 液化的组织
感觉	感觉过敏	针刺的痛感与损伤深度成反比	表面无感觉 深感觉仍存在
愈合	3~6 天	时间与烧伤深度成正比，10~35 天	需要植皮

From Pruitt BA Jr, Gamelli RL: Burns. In Britt LD, Trunkey DD, Organ CH, Feliciano DV, editors: *Acute care surgery*. New York, Springer, 2007, p128

称体重，并且通过标准的计算图表评估部分和全层烧伤的程度（图 1）。第一个 24 h 需要的液体量可以通过高级烧伤生命支持和高级创伤生命支持共识的公式进行估计（表 4）。虽然详细比较各种复苏公式已经超出了本章的范围，但所有以前描述过的烧伤复苏公式已经总结在表 5 中了。

由于儿童每单位体重的体表面积更大，儿童在复苏的第一个 24 h 需要的液体比成年人更多。在所有患者中，系统性毛细血管渗漏在前 8 h 内是很多的，继而，一半的估计量应在烧伤后的前 8 h 内输入。如果延误了最初的液体治疗，第一个 24 h 的估计输液量的一半应该在前 8 h 内（在创伤后的即刻计时，不是到达急诊科的时间）剩下的时间内完成。另外一半的液体应在接下来的 16 h 内输完。

儿童糖原储备能力有限，在烧伤时，可能被显著的应激激素反应而迅速地耗尽。应该监测烧伤儿童的血清葡萄糖水平，如果血清葡萄糖减少至低血糖的水平，5% 葡聚糖乳酸林格氏液是解决方案。在儿童烧伤范围较小时，估计的复苏液体体积可能不能满足日常代谢需要。对于这样的患者，维持体液应该添加到复苏方案中：所有体重小于 30 kg 者都应给予 5% 葡萄糖溶液以维持液体量。

输液速率根据患者损伤后的反应和复苏的方案进行调整。烧伤甚至非烧伤的肢体会形成严重水肿，常常使脉搏的速率、脉搏的轻重，甚至是血压的测量变得困难，使其作为评价复苏的充分性的指标并不可信。因此，应该使用每小时尿量来衡量复苏的充分性。应根据尿量来调整输液速度，成年人每小时尿量为 30 ml，体重小于 30 kg 的儿童每小时尿量应为按体重 1 mg/kg。只有在每小时尿量为 1/3 或更少，或者超过 25% 或更多时，才须相应地增加或减少液体量。非烧伤皮肤的毛细血管再充盈能反映内脏灌注，并且须保持和每小时检查一次。如果在成年人或儿童中，第一个 12 h 内输入的复苏液体将会导致第一个 24 h 每千克体重的每烧伤的体表面积的百分之一使用 6 ml 或更多的液体。应该输注稀释至生理浓度的人血白蛋白，晶体溶液的体积减少相当的量。

对液体复苏甚至在额外补充胶体后没有反应，提示应重新考虑受伤史：有没有可能有忽视了一个与出血相关的创伤？明显的，液体复苏并不能有效地解决持续的出血，出现严重的烧伤和有机械性创伤的病史的所有患者须进行彻底的评估，此外，对那些就诊时没有提供病史的患者，初期最安全的立场是，除非证明没有，那么患者是有创伤机制的。

此外，一些患者没有其他的伤害，也对液体复

年龄与部位的烧伤评估及图表

部位	出生至 1 岁	1～4 岁	5～9 岁	10～14 岁	15 岁	成年人	2°	3°	总计	备注
头	19	17	13	11	9	7				
颈	2	2	2	2	2	2				
前胸	13	13	13	13	13	13				
后背	13	13	13	13	13	13				
右臀	2 ½	2 ½	2 ½	2 ½	2 ½	2 ½				
左臀	2 ½	2 ½	2 ½	2 ½	2 ½	2 ½				
生殖器	1	1	1	1	1	1				
右上臂	4	4	4	4	4	4				
左上臂	4	4	4	4	4	4				
右前臂	3	3	3	3	3	3				
左前臂	3	3	3	3	3	3				
右手	2 ½	2 ½	2 ½	2 ½	2 ½	2 ½				
左手	2 ½	2 ½	2 ½	2 ½	2 ½	2 ½				
右大腿	5 ½	6 ½	8	8 ½	9	9 ½				
左大腿	5 ½	6 ½	8	8 ½	9	9 ½				
右小腿	5	5	5 ½	6	6 ½	7				
左小腿	5	5	5 ½	6	6 ½	7				
右足	3 ½	3 ½	3 ½	3 ½	3 ½	3 ½				
左足	3 ½	3 ½	3 ½	3 ½	3 ½	3 ½				
						总计				

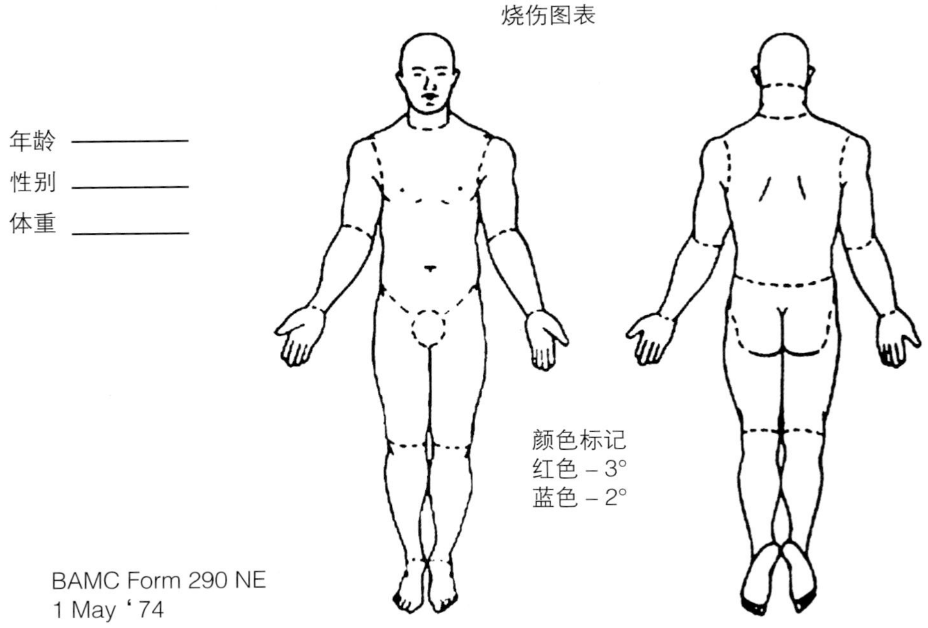

图 1 Lund-Browder 烧伤图用来描述烧伤的程度。图轮廓可以用蓝色和红色的铅笔填满，分别代表部分层和全层烧伤。注意每行显示出身体部位所占体表总面积的百分比是如何随时间变化的。*(From Martin RR, Becker WK, Cioffi WG, Pruitt BP Jr: Thermal injuries. In Wilson RF, Walt AJ, editors:* Mangement of trauma: pitfalls and practice*, 2nd ed. Baltimore, Williams & Wilkins, 1996, p 765.)*

表 4　烧伤后第一个 24 h 内需要的液体量

成年人：2 ~ 4 ml LR/%TBSAB/kg BW
儿童：3 ~ 4 ml LR/%TBSAB/kg BW + 维持量（体重小于 30 kg 的儿童）

BW，身体重量；LR，乳酸林格氏液；TBSAB，全身烧伤总面积

苏的反应不佳。当患者接受了 1.5 倍的经白蛋白调整过的（或 250 ml/kg）复苏容量，而没有任何迹象表明能够减少液体入量时，应该考虑加用血管加压药。当内源性抗利尿激素相对不足时有时会伴发严重炎症反应。为这些患者提供抗利尿激素可以迅速纠正他们对液体复苏的反应。另外，有些患者需要去甲肾上腺素。在复苏困难时，合理搭配液体和血管活性药物是具有挑战性的，须经验丰富的医生提供指导。

在或接近烧伤后 24 h 功能性毛细血管的完整性得到恢复。作为结果，在烧伤后的第二个 24 h，所需的液体量减少，并且可以输注包含胶体的溶液以减少容量负荷和盐负荷。稀释至生理浓度的人血白蛋白是包含胶体的溶液的首选。烧伤面积达 30% ~ 50% 体表总面积的患者，输注剂量是每千克体重、烧伤面积的百分比 0.3 ml；烧伤面积达 50% ~ 70% 体表总面积的患者，输注剂量是每千克体重、烧伤面积的百分比 0.4 ml。烧伤面积超过 70% 体表总面积的患者，输注剂量是每千克体重、烧伤面积的百分比 0.5 ml，也会给予一定量的 5% 的葡萄糖溶液，以维持足够的尿量。应根据相同的公式估算儿童含胶体的溶液注射量，但是应输入一半的生理盐水以维持尿量，并且避免因将大量无电解质的溶液输入血管和间质容量相对较小的儿童，而出现的明显的生理性低钠血症。在这一期间，也要开始适量减少液体输注，以进一步减少容量负荷。在被评估为已充分复苏的患者中，每小时输液量应该下降 25% ~ 50%。如果尿量下降至低于目标水平，应恢复之前的输液速度。如果尿量仍充足，那么在接下来的 3 h 内，应保持这一减少的速度。相同的时间内，减少的输液比例相似。这种递减过程将在烧伤后的第二天建立，并以最低输液速度保持足够的复苏。

表 5　烧伤的复苏公式，现在和过去

晶体公式：通常用乳酸林格氏液，尽管可以使用更新的等渗液体．	Parkland (Baxter) 公式：4 ml/kg · 烧伤占 TBSA 的比例，在最初的 8 h 内先给予一半，另一半在接下来的 16 h 内补足。根据尿量调整输液速度。在第二个 24 h，给予 20% ~ 60% 的计算后胶体（血浆）容量（关于第二个 24 h 的建议通常不采用）。 改良后的 Brooke 公式：2 ml/kg · 烧伤占 TBSA 的比例，在最初的 8 h 内先给予一半，另一半在接下来的 16 h 内补足。根据尿量调整输液速度。第二个 24 h，给予 0.33 ~ 0.5 ml/kg · 烧伤占 TBSA 的比例的胶体，将胶体加入 5% 葡萄糖溶液以维持尿量。
高渗公式：无胶体。	Monafo：250 mEq/L Na^+ + 150 mEq 乳酸 + 100 mEq Cl^-。根据尿量调整输液速度。在第二个 24 h，口服 1/3 的等渗盐。 Warden：乳酸林格氏液 + 50 mEq $NaHCO_3$（每升有 180 mEq 的 Na^+），在最初的 8 h（根据 Parkland 公式）。当 pH 值正常或在第 8h，可转为使用乳酸林格氏液。根据尿量调整输液速度。
胶体公式	F.D. Moore 的烧伤预算公式：1 000 ~ 4 000 ml 乳酸林格氏液 + 1 200 ml 0.5% 生理盐水 +7.5% 体重的胶体 + 1 500 ~ 5 000 ml 5% 的葡萄糖溶液。第二个 24 h，除了胶体量为 2.5% 的体重，使用相同的公式 Evans 公式：1 ml/kg · 烧伤占 TBSA 的比例的生理盐水 +1 ml/kg · 烧伤占 TBSA 的比例的胶体。第二个 24 h，给予第一个 24 h 的液体量的一半 +2 000 ml 5% 的葡萄糖溶液 Brooke 公式（原始）：1.5 ml/kg · 烧伤占 TBSA 的比例的 5% 的葡萄糖溶液 +0.5 ml/kg · 烧伤占 TBSA 的比例的胶体。第二个 24 h 改为 2 000 ml 的 5% 的葡萄糖溶液。 Slater 公式：2 000 ml 乳酸林格氏液 + 新鲜冰冻血浆 75 ml/kg · 24 h。根据尿量调整输液速度。 Haifa 公式：1.5 ml/kg· 烧伤占 TBSA 的比例的血浆 +1 ml/kg· 烧伤占 TBSA 的比例的乳酸林格氏液。根据尿量调整输液速度。 Demling 公式：右旋糖酐 40 溶于正常生理盐水，以 2 ml/kg · h 维持 8 h。在第 8 h 开始输注新鲜冰冻血浆 0.5 ml/kg · h。应该给予乳酸林格氏液以维持尿量。

TBSA，全身体表总面积

From Greenhalgh DG: Burn resuscitation. *J Burn Care Res* 28(4):555–565，2007

烧伤后的前 48 h 的液体管理应该予许排出一部分超负荷的水和盐，以达到复苏，防止脱水、电解质紊乱，并且使患者在烧伤后的 8 ~ 10 天体重恢复至烧伤前水平。为复苏输入大量的乳酸林格氏液常常会使体重增加 20% 或更多，使血清钠浓度减少至相当于乳酸林格氏液的水平，也就是说，130 mEq/L。通过烧伤伤口表面丢失大量的水，可以相对纠正低钠血症，这是复苏后的大量不显性失水增加的最主要组成部分。不显性失水补充不足，使高钠血症成为广泛烧伤患者复苏后最常见的水电解质紊乱的类型。这种高钠血症应该输注无电解质水处理，以增加全身钠量的排出，并且，可能防止血容量不足的程度上替代不显性失水。

电解质异常是烧伤后经常遇到的。血钾过高是其中经常遇到的，通常有一个实验室溶血的体征，但也可能有高压电击伤或深度烧伤导致肌肉破坏的体征。患者严重复苏不足，而出现高钾血症也可能与酸中毒有关。 患者受高压电击伤害且有重度高钾血症，应紧急透析，并且切除 / 截掉不能存活的组织或四肢，这是稳定血清钾和抢救患者所需要的。烧伤复苏后出现低磷酸盐血症也是很普遍的，这是因为长期肠外营养而未能提供足够的磷酸，以满足伤口愈合后的组织代谢的需要。通过适当的饮食补充磷酸可以预防和治疗低磷酸盐血症。

呼吸支持

烧伤患者初步评估的最关键的因素是评估其气道的开放性和气道功能，以便维护和保护气道。应当用标准方法来确定气道机械稳定的必要性。也要记住烧伤后的全身反应和气道损伤的局部反应，这可能导致气道进一步肿胀和水肿，削弱气流。躯干周围烧伤将会进一损害患者的呼吸功能。在气管插管和气道稳定前，允许气道处于危险的状态是不合适的。最安全的做法是当气道有风险时，尤其是需要转运治疗的患者，最好行早期插管。

患者遭受吸入性损伤和热灼伤时并发症的发生率明显增加，而且很可能死亡。虽然单纯的吸入性损伤的死亡率为 5% ~ 8%，但同时有热灼伤和吸入性损伤时，根据年龄和烧伤面积进行预测很容易计算出 20% 及以上的死亡率。呼吸道损伤是由于吸入燃烧产物的直接损害，引起炎症和水肿。口咽和上呼吸道损伤与吸入的热的内容物有关。相反，咽部的热交换能力充分，因此声门以下的损伤主要与包含在吸入内容物的烟、化学成分的颗粒物相关。潮潮的热气，常见于蒸汽，是干燥烟雾携热能力的 4 000 倍，并且能够引起支气管树更广泛的热损伤。

吸入损伤的症状和体征是喘鸣、缺氧和呼吸窘迫。患者遭受吸入性损伤的可能性与其在封闭的空间内发生头和颈部烧伤和一氧化碳水平升高程度相关。吸入性损伤的范围和严重程度与暴露的持续时间和烟雾包含的毒素类型直接相关，并且这些因素加剧了机体随后的炎性反应。激活的炎症级联反应的激活使中性粒细胞和巨噬细胞聚集，加重机体损伤。表面活性因子释放的改变使远端气道梗阻和塌陷。作为炎症反应的一部分，支气管动脉血流量明显、快速地增加，这与肺血管通透性的显著改变相关。广泛的破坏和炎症的净效应减少肺顺应性和损害气体交换，从而导致肺循环血量改变和通气 – 灌注不匹配。

吸入性呼吸道损伤患者的初始管理的一部分包括全面评估气道，包括支气管镜检查。吸入性损伤在支气管镜检查中的临床表现包括气道水肿，炎症，支气管分泌物增加，存在广泛分布在气道的含碳物质，黏膜溃疡和由于黏膜脱落、黏液堵塞、管型形成导致的管腔阻塞。胃内容物吸入的体征也很明显，重复支气管镜检查可以清除异物和管型，同时监测感染。

一氧化碳和氰化物气体存在于烟雾中，并且一旦吸入这些气体，它们会被迅速吸收并且引起全身毒性反应，同时也会影响氧的使用和释放。一氧化碳是没有气味、没有刺激性的气体，可以迅速在血液中扩散，并且其与血红蛋白的亲和力是氧气的 240 倍，因此很容易取代氧气。根据烧伤患者受伤的环境、体格检查、血碳氧血红蛋白的测量值的水平可做出一氧化碳中毒的诊断。注意到脉搏血氧测量值并不能区分碳氧血红蛋白和氧合血红蛋白，是非常重要的。患者有明显的一氧化碳中毒时也可有正常的氧饱和度，但是将不会有正常的血氧含量。当一氧化碳 - 血红蛋白（碳氧血红蛋白）的水平在 10% 或以下时，一氧化碳中毒的症状和体征是通常是轻微的或没有。当碳氧血红蛋白的水平在 10% ~ 30% 时，症状出现，通常表现为头痛和头晕。重度中毒见于碳氧血红蛋白水平高于 50% 的患者，这些患者会出现晕厥、癫痫、昏迷。一氧化碳中毒的主要治疗方法是提高氧气吸入水平。

氰化物中毒可以与一氧化碳中毒组合出现，通过与细胞色素氧化酶结合从而扰乱正常细胞的氧代谢，它是线粒体电子传递系统最末端的电子受体。

氧化磷酸化停止，导致细胞产生乳酸、细胞水平上的严重缺氧，并且生成有毒的活性氧自由基。氰化物的血液浓度高于 0.5 mg/L 即为中毒，治疗氰化物中毒包括吸氧和使用解毒剂（如亚硝酸异戊酯和硝酸钠）。这些化合物诱导高铁血红蛋白的形成，可以作为氰化物的清除剂。羟钴胺也是可选择的解毒剂。

吸入性损伤后机械通气的目标是提供充足的氧气交换，以最小化进一步的气道和肺实质的损伤。通过仔细的气道压力控制，可以很好地达到这一目标，从而限制通气诱导的气压伤。烧伤后出现的肺损伤不是均一性损伤而是分布不一致的，并且须使用 PEEP 以最大限度地复张气道，以避免通气诱导的肺损伤。在严重肺损伤时，机械通气可以导致肺泡剪切应力的增加和肺血流量的变化。高的充气压力可加剧这些问题，促进肺功能区损伤。这些损伤的发展与肺弹性减少和肺顺应性改变有关，可以导致进一步的肺损伤和通气 - 灌注异常。

对于支气管镜检查有吸入性肺损伤的患者，在初期使用支气管扩张剂和黏液溶解剂积极处理气道分泌物是有益的。早期行躯干焦痂切开术或者迅速治疗腹腔隔室综合征时，控制气道压力应该熟练、细致。应该保持中等气道压力，小于 32 ~ 34 cmH_2O，并且应使用化学镇静剂，给转换为压力控制通气一个低阈值，慢慢增加潮气量以减少呼吸机进一步诱导气压伤的风险。这可能须接受小于正常的潮气量，并且允许存在高碳酸血症。只要动脉血液 pH 值高于 7.26，并且患者的血流动力学稳定，高碳酸血症可以接受。气道压力释放通气（airway pressure release ventilation，APRV）是一个相对较新的通气模式。这一模式通过规律释放呼气压力使肺维持一个恒定的充气压力，这一模式也适用于有大的肺内分流比例的患者。

伤口的初步处理

最开始，伤口处理的重点是防止进一步的损伤。烧掉的衣服应该被移除，接触的金属物体可能保留热量，若只有熔融材料附着到皮肤表面，应冷却。不应该试图冷却烧伤伤口，因为局部血管收缩会削弱伤处血流，使损伤程度加深。同样，它也会使机体体温过低。准备转运或允许做特定治疗的患者应该使敷料无菌、清洁、干燥并保持温暖。在烧伤部位水肿前应去除衣物或珠宝，以防止出现进一步损伤循环。如果是化学损伤，应用大量的水冲洗化学物，除去污染的衣服，并且通过刷子移除看得见的粉状物质，防止进一步的损伤。不能试图去做中和反应，因为这一治疗会导致放热反应，进而造成额外的组织损伤。当处理化学损伤时，提供治疗的人操作时必须格外谨慎，以防止自身污染和个人受伤。

住院并且复苏治疗之后，烧伤伤口应该用温暖的液体、洗涤剂、消毒剂清洁，如葡萄糖酸氯己定，它有非常好的抗菌谱。在清洁的过程中，应避免低体温。紧密附着在伤口的物质，如蜡、焦油、塑料、金属，应该被轻轻地移除或允许其在下一次换药的过程中被分离。脱落的皮肤、失活的组织和破裂的水疱应该从伤口轻轻切除。在每次换药时，都应小心地进行伤口的清洁。如果需要，可以对失活组织行连续清创。应该监测伤口有无感染征象，以及与初步评估相比有无深度的变化。

受伤皮肤表面如果逐渐被感染，可以作为微生物入侵的门户。因为微生物的数量在伤口内增加可以达到每克组织中有 1 000 000 微生物的水平，可以出现侵入性伤口感染和全身性的脓毒症。局部应用可以穿透烧伤焦痂的抗生素药物，能够使其在伤口内到达有效的水平以控制微生物的增殖。应用全身性抗生素药物没有指征，因为它们不能充分渗透焦痂。局部的抗生素药物也用于烧伤的预防性治疗，并且是烧伤伤口感染处理的部分。局部用药不会治愈伤口，但是可以防止伤口局部的感染破坏伤口中有活力的组织的自愈能力。

磺胺嘧啶银是使用最广泛的药物，可以将其配成 1% 的水溶剂，呈乳状基质。乳膏使用简单，并且使用时几乎只造成一点点的疼痛或没有疼痛。乳膏可以作为连续的一层，直接在伤口上使用，并用敷料覆盖。在每一次换药时，乳膏应该完全被移除，而且不允许形成一个干酪样的层（术语“假痂皮”），因为这将会掩盖伤口床。磺胺嘧啶银最常见的毒副作用是短暂的白细胞减少，有 15% 的患者治疗后出现这一情况，可以自行缓解而不需要停药。磺胺嘧啶银的抗菌谱很广，包括金黄色葡萄球菌、大肠杆菌、克雷伯菌、很多但并不是所有的铜绿假单胞菌、变形杆菌属、白念珠菌。

醋酸磺胺米隆是用于烧伤伤口处理的最早的有效外用制剂药物之一。它最初是作为磺胺米隆烧伤膏，能够高效对抗革兰氏阳性和革兰氏阴性微生物，但是抗真菌活性几乎没有。醋酸磺胺米隆容易扩散到焦痂，因为它也能够穿透软骨，是耳朵烧伤首选的药物。醋酸磺胺米隆使用的缺点包括部分烧伤伤口在使用时的疼痛、对耐甲氧西林金黄色葡萄球菌的抗菌活性有限。醋酸磺胺米隆也抑制碳酸酐酶，可能引起自限性高氯性酸中毒。近期，可用5%醋酸磺胺米隆水溶液，这是一个很好的药物，可以用于新移植的创口，并且也不会带来醋酸磺胺米隆乳膏使用时存在的问题。

0.5%的硝酸银溶液对革兰氏阳性和革兰氏阴性微生物有效但不能穿透焦痂。硝酸银溶液能从伤口滤出钠、钾、氯、钙离子，这与穿透焦痂的水的吸收有关，进而导致电解质缺乏、碱中毒、水负荷。通过补充钠或其他电解质和调整液体治疗可以最小化那些副作用。这些问题和为有效使用硝酸银须做的努力限制了它的常规使用，并且大多数人认为磺胺嘧啶银盐可作为其有效替代。

近期银浸渍敷料也可供临床使用。当织物基底接触伤口渗液时，银不断释放，作为抗生素放置到伤口上。这样一个综合治疗的间隔可能会延长至几天，取决于敷料工艺设计，只须1周换药1或2次。这种膜敷料在治疗广泛的全层烧伤时的有效性治还未经证实，在目前，它被用来治疗部分全层二度烧伤。

在部分全层二度烧伤的创面，杆菌肽药膏也是另一个令人满意的选择，特别是对于一个已知的对磺胺类过敏患者。它可以用在开放性伤口中，尤其是浅表的面部烧伤，或者作为封闭式敷料的组成成分。在全世界，杆菌肽是一种最常用的外用制剂，但它不应大面积使用，因为当其被吸收后有显著的肾毒性。其他局部抗生素包括复合抗生素如三联抗生素软膏（新霉素、杆菌肽锌和多黏菌素B）和多链丝霉（杆菌肽锌和多黏菌素B）。如果是耐甲氧西林的葡萄球菌感染，莫匹罗星是一个有用的药物。

烧伤患者将被转移到烧伤中心，如果患者局部应用抗菌药物可能会妨碍生物膜敷料的使用，因为生物膜敷料必须贴在伤口表面才能有效发挥作用。此外，只要患者允许进入烧伤中心，之前使用的任何敷料都必须移除，以保证烧伤团队对烧伤的程度和深度做出精准的评估。除非距患者转运至烧伤中心还有相当长的时间，首选的初期处理须给患者放置一个干燥的敷料（最好是有一个不黏附的内衬的敷料），以保持患者温暖。

烧伤创面的切除和移植

对于全层烧伤的患者，须切除烧伤组织和植皮。这一治疗方法现在也被认为是混合深度伤口的最佳选择。有能力在受伤后2～3周内自然愈合的伤口可以按作者的期望处理，并且外观和功能结局也可以接受。需要切除和缝合的伤口应尽可能快地进行切除，因为这可以减少创伤组织功能障碍的时间和治疗的花费。在大面积烧伤的患者中，手术的时机和范围取决于患者相对稳定的生理功能和他耐受重大手术的能力。大面积烧伤的患者在早期进行烧伤组织的切除和缝合能缩短住院时间，减少住院费用，可能减弱过度的炎症反应，并且有利于减少烧伤的总死亡率。

伤口小而且呈线型可以行烧伤创面切除和伤口一期缝合的处理。这一处理对老年人上臂内侧烧伤、位于下垂乳房的烧伤、腹部烧伤、臀部烧伤、大腿烧伤很有用。当这些伤口在出现明显的微生物繁殖之前被早期切除时，这种方法显得更有效，因此每当能行此方法时就应该采用。

在某些情况下，截掉烧伤的部分可能是最合适的。在有明显的多系统创伤的患者中，迅速去除烧伤部分可能是患者存活的最好的选择。一个损毁的肢体，同时受到了严重的烧伤，并且确定没有救治的可能，应该进行早期截肢。并不须将截肢的范围扩大到可以允许非烧伤组织闭合的水平。如果在截肢水平附近存在有活力的肌肉，伤口床可以通过自体皮肤移植重新覆盖。移植后的截肢部位可以与现代假肢结合，它可持久地提供支撑。对于截瘫且下肢受到广泛、深度烧伤的患者，截肢是替代切除和移植的可行选择。对于烧伤前便存在明显的周围性血管疾病，使得肢体愈合和恢复功能的可能性非常小的患者，也可以考虑做出相似的选择。

不适合做一期缝合的伤口也需要切除和植皮。患者所能承受的扩大手术与患者的年龄和生理状态相关。这一方法需要经验丰富的治疗团队，一位须彻底理解大面积烧伤患者的独特情况的麻醉师和配备完善的手术室，能够随时获得的血液制品和术后护理。患者接受这一程度的手术在本质上承受了双倍面积的"损伤"，现在切除的和植皮的伤口（沿着二度烧伤伤口，由供体区提供）。患者烧伤面积较大（>30%体表总面积）或那些不能耐受一次手术达到伤口闭合的患者，可以采用分期切除烧伤组织，并且可以通过自体皮肤移植或者生物敷料来闭合伤口。

烧伤创面切除的技术取决于伤口的深度和需要被切除处的解剖学部位。最常见的切除方法是切线切除。通过切线技术将深的部分烧伤伤口切至真皮深层，直到具有均一性活性床的水平，并且立即以自体移植皮肤覆盖，可以使伤口迅速关闭，并且预后非常好。最好是能一 Weck 刀片下去便获得理想的创面床，其表现为弥漫性出血。经常出现的错误是对深度不合适的伤口进行这项技术的尝试，并且假定点状出血提示活性的创面床。这种伤口将会愈合很差，因为创面床包含少量的活性组织，并不能够支持自体移植皮肤的生长（尽管这类伤口有时出血量很大，但是是小动脉的出血，不是毛细血管的，对于移植物来说灌注不足）。在这一过程中，给烧伤肢体使用止血带或者用含肾上腺素的液体做焦痂下灌洗，可以血液的丢失最小。切线切除的替代方式是筋膜切除，这一方式涉及烧伤组织至筋膜或深层皮下组织的切除。筋膜切除的可行性应做仔细评估，并且，如果可行性遭到质疑，切除应转为移植前的下方肌肉。或者，在血管床的活性有质疑时，应该使用同种异体移植物，因为成年人皮下脂肪血管床的灌注相对差。同种异体移植物下的脂肪决定是否须做更深层的切除。

血液丢失发生在烧伤组织切除时，与烧伤后切除时间、切除面积、是否存在感染以及切除类型相关。供体区也可是血液丢失的一部分重要原因。血液丢失的量可以估算，波动为按切除的烧伤面积 0.45～1.25 ml/cm^2。可被用来控制出血的辅助措施包括抬高行切除术的肢体、在切除伤口和供体区局部应用凝血酶或者血管收缩药物、在移除前灌洗移植处皮肤或焦痂和应用止血带。纤维蛋白黏合剂喷雾的应用也可以减少止血带松开后伤口切除处的出血。在这一过程中，如果患者出现凝血功能紊乱、低体温或酸中毒，血液丢失将会加剧。有经验丰富的麻醉师的协助可以避免错误。必须要对严重烧伤患者的手术时机、程度和性质做出判断，记住获取自体移植物会增加患者伤口的负担以及代谢需求。

烧伤伤口的移植经常在切除后完成。然而，在一些情况下，建议分阶段完成皮肤移植。手术必须考虑到患者的整个术中状态，如果需要，中断手术。仅完成切除，分阶段完成移植可能是最好的。此外，如果怀疑创面床的活性，应该仅行切除术。可以用 5% 磺胺米隆敷料对伤口进行换药，或者用皮肤替代物覆盖，随后重新评估。分期进行创口闭合也是严重营养不良患者的合适选择。

存在一些皮肤替代物。2 种最常用的天然生物敷料是人类皮肤的同种异体移植物和猪皮肤的异种移植物。同种皮肤，可以血管化，在出现自体排斥反应前可以覆盖创面达 3～4 周。异种组织，不会出现血管化，可使用重组的网状猪真皮或新鲜或备好的全层皮肤。异种皮肤，本质上是一种惰性生物敷料，可以用来覆盖部分烧伤伤口或供体区，在异种移植物的下方会再次形成表皮。此外，各种合成膜也得到了发展，经伤口提供保护，并且可以提供蒸气和细菌屏障特性。例如生物膜（Dow-Hickham，Sugarland，Tex）可以和猪异种移植可以互换使用。Integra（Integra Life- Science Corporation，Plainsboro，N.J.），在另一方面，是一个再生的基质组织，包括交联胶原蛋白的真皮类似物、黏多糖和硅胶表皮类似物。它可以放在刚做完全层切除的伤口上，为伤口成纤维细胞提供创造模拟真皮类似物结构的原生蛋白质的新皮所需信息。只要真皮的类似物完全血管化（严重烧伤患者至少 2 周），硅胶表皮类似物就可以去除，并且血管化的新皮将会被薄薄的一层自体皮肤移植物覆盖。一个永久的皮肤替代物仍然是烧伤受害者的最佳选择，目前可给予在市场上流通的培养的自体移植表皮。但是其移植成活率不佳、皮肤表面脆弱、高费用（真皮或真皮等价物对维持表皮的稳定非常重要）限制了其使用。使用任何生物敷料都需要每天至少 1 次，仔细检查切除的伤口和使用的敷料。膜下化脓或出现感染必须去除敷料，用外科消毒剂溶液清洁伤口，甚至再次切除残留的失活伤口或出现的感染组织。

烧伤患者的伤口的合适的处理方式是非常重要的，它可以帮助患者达到最佳的美容和功能预后，并且及时恢复患者的活动。严重烧伤的患者，伤口必须适当处理和关闭，迅速减少因损伤带来的生理紊乱水平。如果不能做到，将导致有创性伤口感染、慢性炎症、瘦体重减少、进展性的功能缺陷甚至死亡。

特殊伤害：电烧伤

电损害组织的主要机制是通过将电能转换为热能。1 000 伏以上的电流被归类为高电压。一旦接触这样的电流，身体将作为一个容积导体。电流可能会诱发心肺骤停。在受伤后随时需要心肺复苏，还可能出现心律失常。在记录到最后一次心律失常后应至少再行心电监护至少 24 h。

高压电伤害的 2 个特征使患者的急性肾衰竭的发生率增加。首先，通常在未烧伤的肢体也有广泛的不明显的皮下组织损伤。有限的皮肤损伤可能导致对复苏液体的需要量的严重低估；其次，因电流导致的肌肉群受伤可能导致横纹肌溶解，从而造成肾小管的直接损伤。复苏液体量应该基于可见的烧伤的程度加上对患者的日常需求量的估计，根据患者的反应进行调整。如果尿液中含有血色素原（深红色），液体量应该调整，以获得 75～100 ml/h 的尿量，应在液体中添加碳酸氢钠以碱化尿液。如果血色素原不及时清除，或者患者仍然少尿，应以推注 25 g 的甘露醇，并将甘露醇按 12.5 g/L 的量加入到乳酸林格氏液中，直到色素清除。添加甘露醇，一个渗透性利尿剂，使得尿量作为复苏是否充分的监测指标变得不可靠，而须行中央静脉监测。

当身体功能作为一个体积导体，电流密度与涉及的身体的横截面积成反比。因此，破坏严重的组织可能发生在肢体横截面积相对较小的部位，而相对较少的组织损伤可能发生身体躯干。在高电压（大于 1 000 V）和高电流的情况下，有最高电阻的组织产热量也最大，这也是四肢骨周围软组织通常是受损伤最重的原因。肢体肌肉的损伤往往与损伤肌肉隔室中显著增加的压力有关，如果压力不能减轻，那么将进一步导致组织坏死。肢体隔室很难触到，要警惕有紧急手术探查的需要。有广泛的深层组织坏死的筋膜室综合征、持续或进行性的严重高钾血症时，应行手术干预和广泛的筋膜切开术。在探查时，广泛的破坏可能需要截肢，尤其是当无活性肌肉是持续的高钾血症原因时。清创术或截肢术后，伤口应开放性覆盖，患者在 24～36 h 内返回到手术室复查，必要时对无活性组织做进一步清创。当伤口内的所有组织均有活性时，可以确定性关闭。

低压电流或家用电流也可以使组织损伤。口角处的烧伤常见于年幼儿童，因为咬电线或吮吸带电的电线或者插座。病变可能有全层烧伤的特点，但是早期手术清创可能只会加重损伤，应尽量避免。这些损伤可以以最小的外观上的后遗症愈合，如果需要，后遗症可以有效地解决。对于严重的伤害，在完成一个可接受的美容重建时，经验是很重要的。

特殊伤害：化学损伤

各种化学试剂导致组织损伤是电子化学反应放热、蛋白质的凝固作用、脱水、去脂的结果。化学损伤的严重程度与化学试剂浓度、数量、与组织接触的持续时间相关。因此，应优先对化学伤害患者的伤口进行处理，去除或稀释刺激性试剂，刷掉干状物质，立即用大量的液体灌洗。发生了广泛的表面损伤的患者，灌洗液应该是温暖的，以防止体温过低。

化学试剂造成皮肤损伤其外观可以引起误导。例如患者受到强酸的损伤，损伤的皮肤表面可能有柔滑的质地和出现淡黄褐色的外观，这可能会被误认为是晒伤，而不是全层烧伤，而它确实是。石油馏出物引起脱脂作用，其造成的皮肤损伤可能是干燥的，显示很少的炎症反应，看起来似是没有损伤。然而，组织学检查却发现是全层烧伤。

特殊伤害：冻伤

继发于环境暴露的损伤可能导致局部损伤、冻疮或系统性低体温。冻疮的病理生理学机制是由于寒冷导致细胞外和细胞内液体形成晶体。冻疮患者的受伤部位会有冷的感觉，并且失去感觉和本体感受。初次检查时，四肢也会显得苍白、青紫或有从黄变白的变色过程。在 40℃ ～42℃的水中快速复温 15～30 min，皮肤会发生充血，继而出现疼痛、感觉异常、感觉缺失 ，当真正能确定损伤的深度和范围时，超过 1 周的时间过去了。受伤的肢体应该被抬高，以控制水肿，应被垫着以避免压力诱导性缺血而出现二次损伤。冻疮的伤口是破伤风易感伤口，因此，应基于患者的免疫状态，给予破伤风类毒素处理。

并发症发生率和并发症管理

早期并发症

随着复苏开始进行，肢体全层烧伤周围的非弹性焦痂下方水肿形成，下方血流量减少，远端非烧伤组织可能会受到损害。远端非烧伤组织发绀和感觉异常的加重，特别是持续的深层组织疼痛，是临床最可以信赖的临床上循环受损的征象，仅在相对较长时间后出现相对或绝对缺血才能作为证据。在肢体受到深度环状烧伤时，可以在没有麻醉的情况下行床旁焦痂切开术，因为全层烧伤是没有感觉的。焦痂切开术可以用手术刀或电力完成。在治疗时应不要损伤大的、开放的皮下静脉。由于焦痂和紧邻的浅表筋膜直接连接在极端情况下，焦痂切开术的切口选择在中线外侧（上肢的桡侧），并且必须能从上端延伸至烧伤处的最下端（图 2）。最后肢体的循环状态应该重新评估。如果焦痂切开术没有恢复远端血流，须再在患肢的中线内侧（上肢的尺侧）进行焦痂切开术。当患者肢体的循环恢复延迟，尤其是如果患者接受了大量的液体负荷时，可能须行筋膜切开术。

躯干全层烧伤伤口下方水肿的形成可以限制呼吸时胸壁的运动。如果胸壁运动的限制与缺氧和吸气压峰值升高有关，提示胸部焦痂切开术可以恢复胸壁运动、改善通气。这些焦痂切开术切口位于前腋窝线两侧，必须由横向焦痂切开术连接以充分释放胸部焦痂的压力。如果涉及整个躯干前部，横向的焦痂切开必须要在髂前上棘和胸骨切迹水平完成（图 2）。

及时进行充足的液体治疗，如前所述，对烧伤后消除急性肾衰竭是至关重要的。现在更为常见的是过度复苏的并发症，即筋膜室综合征和肺损伤。筋膜室综合征可以发生在筋膜下方的颅骨、肌肉隔室和腹腔。

过多的液体治疗也可能导致很多的腹水形成和腹部内容物水肿导致腹内高压。腹部筋膜室综合征表现为腹腔压力的逐渐升高直到出现器官功能障碍。包括心排血量减少从而出现低血压、气道压峰值增加、少尿、由于灌注不足出现的代谢性酸中毒的恶化。膀胱压力测量可作为一种间接测量腹部压力的方法。膀胱压力增加大于 25 mmHg 应该立即进行治疗干预，在刚开始时给予适当的镇静、减少输液速率、利尿和穿刺。如果有器官衰竭，提示进行剖腹术减压。

筋膜室综合征也可以出现在烧伤患者肢体筋膜下方的肌肉隔室，甚至是非烧伤肢体。通过触诊评估隔室压力。肌肉隔室很坚硬是不好的征兆，需要更直接的隔室间压力测量，肌肉间的压力达 25 mmHg 以上，须在手术室在全麻下执行累及隔室的筋膜切开术。

代谢和营养支持

烧伤改变营养物的分布和使用，同样改变代谢率，并且严重烧伤患者在他患病期间将会明显丢失肌肉量。当计划对代谢亢进的烧伤患者进行营养支持时，为使瘦体重丢失最小化、促进康复、恢复体能，所有的这些烧伤后代谢的改变都必须考虑到。尽管间接热量测定法是最准确的确定代谢率和营养需要量的方法，但是床边代谢治疗并不总是可行的。

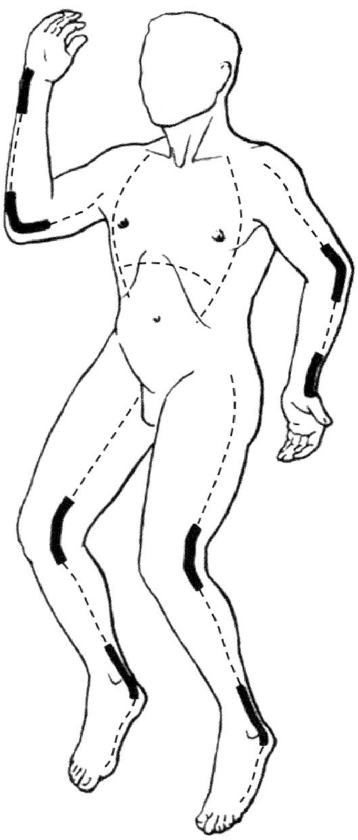

图 2 虚线提示焦痂切开术合适的切口位置：肢体（外侧中线和内侧中线）、胸部（腋前线和 肋弓下缘）和颈（外侧面）。肢体粗线部分强调切口跨关节时的重要性 *(From Martin RR, Becker WK, Cioffi WG, Pruitt BP Jr: Thermal injuries. In Wilson RF, Walt AJ, editors:* Management of trauma: pitfalls and practice*, 2nd ed. Baltimore, Williams & Wilkins, 1996, p 765.)*

初步估计烧伤面积超过 30% 体表总面积的患者需要 2 000 ~ 2 200 kcal 能量，而且每平方米的身体面积每天需要 12 ~ 18 g 营养（蛋白质 2.5 g/kg · d）。

在治疗的时候，患者应该有鼻胃管或鼻肠管放置。尽可能早地使用肠内营养是推荐的。当早期肠内营养时，在入院后 24 ~ 48 h 可能达到这一期望的代谢率。如果患者不能耐受肠内营养，那么可以使用甲氧氯普胺解决这一问题。如果患者对甲氧氯普胺的反应不好，可以尝试将导管直接送至十二指肠悬韧带。患者不能耐受肠内营养或者出现胃肠道并发症阻止肠内营养时，需要全肠外营养。

烧伤诱发胰岛素抵抗，可以导致高血糖，积极给予胰岛素补充使血糖维持在 120 mg/dl 以下可以给危重患者的预后带来好的影响。也必须给予钾和磷以满足患者的需求，尤其是当血糖大量升高后给予了很多外源性胰岛素时，这一需求常常会超过初期的评估。在患者治疗期间，随着开放性伤口减少和代谢亢进状态的缓慢改善，应调整营养负荷，使其维持代谢需要和使底物输送达到平衡，以防止过度喂养。促蛋白合成固醇显示可以增加烧伤患者净蛋白质保存量，而且氧雄龙常规用于严重烧伤患者以达到这一目的。重组人生长激素促进儿童的合成代谢，但是它在严重成年人烧伤患者中使用会增加死亡率。

运输和转移

烧伤受害者的治疗和管理取得了很多重要的进展。其中重要进展之一是明确了团队协作在严重烧伤患者治疗中的好处。美国外科医师学会和美国烧伤协会为提供烧伤治疗发表了最优化的标准，并且由烧伤中心验证了这一过程，认定这些表现和结果经历了同行评审的单位。患者具有烧伤和相关伤害和情况应转运至烧伤中心的条件在表 1 中列出。

一旦做了转运患者至烧伤中心的决定，关于患者的状态和转运需求应该做出医生与医生之间交流。这对患者转运前的稳定非常重要。在转运过程中，急救干预措施如气管插管或重新建立血管通路可能在相对不稳定和空间限制的急救车或直升机上非常难以完成。这一困难使得在航空或陆地转运前建立血流动力学和肺复苏，以达到稳定的状态变得很重要。必须放置一个安全的大直径静脉套管，以保证液体持续的复苏。患者应该给予 100% 氧气。如果关于气道的充分性有任何问题，应该建立气管插管和机械通气。每小时尿量应该监测，根据需要调整液体输注。所有患者应该禁食，并且烧伤体表面积大于 20% 者需要鼻胃管。烧伤伤口应该被洁净或无菌干燥片覆盖。禁止在转运之前应用局部抗生素药物，因为它们的影响必须在进入烧伤中心前去除。维持患者体温也是非常重要的，应该用热反射毛毯盖住患者，以热丢失最小化。烧伤伤口是破伤风易感伤口，需强制免疫，这与美国外科医师学会的推荐一致。

表 6 美国陆军中心烧伤患者死亡率的变化（1945—1991）年

年龄分组	导致 50% 死亡率的烧伤占体表面积的比例 (LA_{50}) 1945—1957	1987—1991
儿童 (0 ~ 14)	51	72*
青年 (15 ~ 40)	43	82†
		73‡
老年	23	46§

From Pruitt BA Jr, Gamelli RL: Burns. In Britt LD, Trunkey DD, Organ CH, Feliciano DV, editors: *Acute care surgery*. New York, Springer, 2006, p155

*5 年

†21 年

‡40 年

§60 年

死亡率

烧伤后早期肾衰竭是复苏延迟和复苏不足的后果，并且已经被消除。而吸入性损伤作为共病因素也已经被处理。侵入性烧伤创面脓毒症已经被控制，并且早期皮肤切除、移植和急救护理的总体改进减少了感染的发生率、消除了很多先前威胁生命的并发症、加速了烧伤患者的康复。不同年龄的死亡率和烧伤面积在表 6 中报告。不仅是生存率得到提高，而且很多先前威胁生命的并发症被消除了。伤口处理的进步甚至提高了那些广泛、严重热损伤患者的生存质量。但烧伤处理仍有挑战。虽然我们有能力恢复烧伤患者的表皮（一种对微生物热丢失、水丢失有效的障碍），我们仍然在恢复患者正常的社会属性上有非常大的不足。每当烧伤患者走进一个房间，明显的创伤使他们每个人成为“另类人”。这个世纪我们所面临的挑战是使患者的外观恢复审美“正常”，拯救他们的生活。

软组织感染

Sharon Henry 著
王传林 译

皮肤是人体最大的器官。有弹性而坚韧，作为微生物入侵的结构性屏障，皮肤和软组织感染可以无足轻重，也可以危及生命变化。这些感染可能包括表皮、真皮、皮下组织、深筋膜和肌肉。无论健康或损伤，它们都可以由多种原因导致。为了保证有效的治疗，应及时诊断。必须评估患者的疾病的严重程度和可能的病原体，选择特定的抗生素，以及适当时候进行及时手术治疗。无数的微生物能够产生软组织感染，并且感染有相当大的重叠的临床表现。

自古以来医学文章都对严重软组织感染进行过描述。在1世纪，摄氏度被认为是炎症的临床指征：红色的皮肤、疼痛、灼热和肿瘤。坏死性筋膜炎由希波克拉底在公元前5世纪提出，尽管Wilson在1952年创造了这个词。

我们关于软组织感染的治疗的许多知识一直是从军事冲突的经验中得到的。例如，在内战期间，Joseph jones首先描述了医院坏疽，他是邦联的外科医生。战场上感染的治疗影响了平民的医疗实践。

发生率

软组织感染经常发生，导致大约1 000例门诊患者中有43例。皮肤感染和软组织感染是医院最常见的感染。据估算，皮肤和软组织急性入院治疗的人数从2000年的675 000增加到2004年的869 800。等于增加了29%的入院人数，主要是治疗蜂窝织炎和脓肿的人，其中涉及儿童、青年、非裔美国人和群体他们都入住了安全系数较高的医院。住院患者当中有4.3%~10.5%是因为软组织感染引起的脓毒症发作。幸运的是，严重的软组织感染的发生率十分罕见。然而准确的发生率我们还不清楚。1994年，世界卫生组织指出大约每年有500~1 500例坏死性筋膜炎发生。尽管不常见，但也算不上罕见。疾病控制和预防中心能监控A组溶血性链球菌感染，大约每100 000人当中，有10~20人被感染。在加拿大的安大略，人口研究预测发病率为0.6/10万。

损伤机制

皮肤是身体最大的器官，能维持一个机械屏障，来保护人体不受微生物的侵害。除此之外皮肤还维持了体内温度的稳定，分泌电解质溶液、脂类和氨基酸，产生维生素D。它还是一个感觉器官，是一种不需要语言的交流方式。图1描述了皮肤的解剖学。

皮肤上有微生物定植，最常见的生物体包括棒状杆菌、葡萄球菌属、丙酸杆菌属和酵母。每体表面积生物体的数量变化很大，从干燥部位的几百，至潮湿部位的几千（如腋窝和腹股沟区）。最初的软组织感染最常发生在保护性皮肤屏障破坏之后。定植微生物可能防止病原微生物的生长。当皮肤损伤后，皮肤和软组织经常发生感染。这可以通过损伤、手术、咬伤（昆虫、蜘蛛、动物或人类）、烧伤、医疗注射或肠道外药物的使用而发生。当皮肤病变如皮炎存在时，也可继发感染。慢性溃疡（糖尿病性、静脉性或血管）或皮肤病皮肤损伤（如银屑病）也可成为继发性感染。当伴有胃肠道和泌尿生殖道的穿

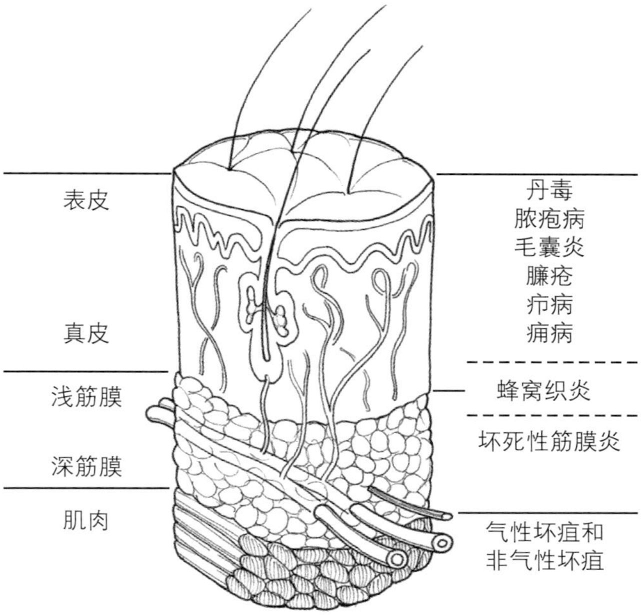

图1　皮肤的结构和相应的感染

孔时，从邻近结构直接扩散可以导致软组织感染。小的创伤组织可以成为细菌入侵的门户。这可能是脚癣、干燥病、用力搔抓后的皮肤擦伤所造成的不明显的皮肤磨损或毛囊和汗腺的刺激。经常不能确定病变的病因学。继发于血行播散的软组织感染并不常见，最常见于免疫抑制患者。静脉吸毒合并心内膜炎的人群通过这一机制出现皮肤软组织感染的风险也很高。

很多皮肤和软组织的感染由金黄色葡萄球菌，A 组、C 组和 G 组 β 型溶血性链球菌引起。糖尿病患者最常见的是 B 组 β 型溶血性链球菌。革兰氏阴性和厌氧病原体更可能见于涉及腹壁的手术后感染，或者肛周手术后感染。由革兰氏阴性和革兰氏阳性病原体导致的感染更易出现在有灌注损伤的患者中，尤其常见于糖尿病患者和动脉或静脉功能不全的患者。之前使用抗生素治疗的患者其菌群会发生改变，改变可能诱发致病微生物。因此，慢性感染经常是多重感染。因此抗生素的使用可导致微生物的耐药菌株的出现 。MRSA 已经达到流行的比例。在 1960 年 MRSA 被发现，最初这一问题局限于住院患者人群，在 1990 年代末，社区相关 MRSA（community associated-MRSA，CA-MRSA）出现在没有可识别危险因素的患者中。2007 年的一项研究指出，独立的 MRSA 导致软组织感染的发生率平均为 35.9%，在 2004 年，研究期间的最后一年，增加到 47.4%。表 1 列出了最常从皮肤和软组织感染组织中分离出的细菌病原体。

很多微生物产生内毒素和外毒素，有助于它们沿着筋膜进行扩散，并最终穿透筋膜。这些毒素可以使组织损伤、缺血和液化性坏死。在一些严重的病例中，它们可以以每小时 1 英寸的速度使感染迅速进展。梭状芽孢杆菌、葡萄球菌和链球菌是其中最出名的（表 2）。最重要的是这些毒素刺激巨噬细胞产生炎症细胞因子 TNF-α 白细胞介素 1、白细胞介素 6，这些细胞因子产生系统性炎症导致脓毒症、器官衰竭和死亡。中性粒细胞脱颗粒，释放过氧化物，产生内皮局部损伤。细菌产生的超抗原造成大量的 T 细胞刺激，放大炎症反应。它们也激活补体系统以及凝血级联反应，这种效应会导致小血管血栓形成，进一步造成组织缺血和损伤。

虽然是常见的经常发生的情况，其他不常见的病原体可以导致皮肤和软组织感染。这些微生物往往有特定风险因素，包括人类或动物咬伤或接触水（表 3）

表 1　只感染皮肤和软组织的最常见的十大细菌群

排名	生物体
1	金黄色葡萄球菌
2	铜绿假单胞菌
3	肠球菌
4	大肠杆菌
5	*肠杆菌*
6	克雷伯菌
7	ß- 溶血性链球菌
8	奇异变形菌
9	凝固酶阴性 葡萄球菌
10	沙雷菌属

表 2　细胞毒素和影响

微生物	毒性物质	影响
梭状芽胞杆菌	α 毒素	组织坏死 心功能衰竭
链球菌和葡萄球菌	M-1 和 M-3 蛋白质 外毒素 A、B 和 C 链球菌溶血素抗 O 超抗原	黏附和逃脱吞噬能力增加 内皮损伤，使微血管完整性破坏和组织水肿，并且使毛细学管血流受损 刺激 CD4 细胞和巨噬细胞 产生 TNF-α、IL-1、IL-6 刺激 T 细胞过度产生细胞因子 呕吐

IL，白细胞介素；TNF，肿瘤坏死因子

有人建议分类方案应简化对软组织感染的讨论和治疗的指导。出于对抗生素临床研究的目的，美国 FDA 使用简单与复杂的 2 个分类系统。（表 4）

简单非复杂性感染

表面的感染限于表皮和真皮结构。这些感染可以自发出现或继发于轻微的创伤。脓疱通常与破裂的水泡同时出现，产生厚厚的黄色外壳。这些病变通常位于面部、颈部和四肢。*金黄色葡萄球菌和化*

表 3 风险因素和相关病原体

风险因素	病原体
人咬伤	*侵蚀艾肯菌*
猫咬伤	*多杀性巴氏杆菌*
狗咬伤	*犬咬嗜二氧化碳细胞菌*
老鼠咬伤	*念珠状链杆菌* *小螺旋菌*
动物的皮毛	*炭疽杆菌* *土拉热弗朗西斯菌*
医用水蛭	*嗜水气单胞菌* *温和气单胞菌* *沙雷杆菌* *弗氏弧菌*
水接触	
盐水	*霍乱弧菌*
淡水	*嗜水气单胞菌*
热水浴缸	*铜绿假单胞菌*
鱼缸	*海分枝杆菌*
沙龙脚部按摩	*偶然分枝杆菌*
爬行动物接触	*沙门氏菌属*
注射药物使用	*肉毒梭菌、厌氧菌* *侵蚀艾肯菌*
旅行	*利什曼虫（利什曼病）* *巴西钩虫（幼虫移行症）* *蝇幼虫引起蝇蛆病* *噬人瘤蝇* *人肤皮蝇*
肝硬化	*胎儿弯曲菌、肺炎克雷伯菌、大肠杆菌，* *二氧化碳嗜纤维菌、其他革兰氏阴性杆菌、创伤弧菌*
中性粒细胞增多	*铜绿假单胞菌*

脓性链球菌是最常见的致病菌。大疱性脓疱病，如脓疱，通常是由金黄色葡萄球菌引起的。它的特点是小疱，汇集形成大疱。尽管它的确发生在年龄较大的儿童和成年人中，但发病高峰年龄在2~5岁的儿童。一般认为皮肤定植发生在感染进展之前，平均为10天。它最常发生在暴露的部位，如脸和四肢等。病变可能是在多个部位，但都是局限的。脓疮是脓疱病更深层次溃烂的形式。全身中毒症状不寻常。

毛囊炎是毛囊浅表的炎症。病变表现为脓疱或丘疹，常见于四肢、头皮、胡须，并且解剖学上位于表皮。漩涡浴池毛囊炎与氧化不充分的游泳池、浴池或热水浴缸有关，可见到弥散性脓疱。铜绿假单胞菌是典型的病原体。游泳者的疥癣是暴露于淡水引起的毛囊炎，在这个阶段温热、潮湿通常会促进流脓。

疖，更深层的炎性结节，当脓通过真皮延伸至皮下组织时，可以从毛囊炎发展而来。金黄色葡萄球菌是常见的病原体。痈是疖通过窦道相互连接而形成的。颈部是最常见的解剖学位置。金黄色葡萄球菌可经常被培养发现。疖、痈需要切开和排脓。当有周围蜂窝织炎或相关发热时，全身性抗生素应用是必要的。当发生耐药金黄色葡萄球菌感染复发时，应建议患者注意他们的个人卫生。那些可能滋生微生物的区域应该彻底清洗，并且使用抗菌肥皂和高温彻底清洁毛巾和床单可能是必要的。当有感染复发时，用莫匹罗星软膏清洁鼻子，每天2次，持续5~10天可能有用。

丹毒和蜂窝织炎是一个术语经常可以互换。它可能通过位于正常和病变皮肤之间的清晰界线而区分，并且通常高于皮肤表面。通常是由A组溶血性链球菌引起，但C组和G组也可以导致。

由金黄色葡萄球菌引起者少见。丹毒和蜂窝织炎最常见于儿童或老年人，经常累及下肢。在过去，面部是最常累及的部位，但现在下肢最常受累。

蜂窝织炎是皮下组织的炎症，因此病变较丹毒更深，有红斑、疼痛和不同程度的水肿。淋巴管炎和区域淋巴结肿大可能存在。毛囊周围水肿，而毛囊仍与真皮相连，而出现凹凸的外观，因此皮肤可以呈橘皮样改变。皮肤可能出现小疱和大疱。发炎的皮肤可能出现瘀点和瘀斑。细菌入侵的通道通常存在，它可以像干燥皮肤上的裂纹或脚癣一样。可以有系统性的症状，包括发烧、畏寒、萎靡、器官衰竭（很少）。链球菌（A组、B组、C组和G组）和葡萄球菌是常见的致病菌。有静脉或淋巴回流损害的部位容易导致这一感染，并且经常复发。盆腔放疗或淋巴结切除术、乳房切除术或静脉切除术使蜂窝织炎的发展更有可能。在特殊情况下其他传染性微生物可能引起蜂窝织炎（表3）

复杂感染

坏死性软组织感染

深部的感染更频繁地威胁生命和肢体。文献关于潜在的威胁生命的感染是混乱的。多个术语用来

表 4　皮肤、皮肤结构和软组织感染的分类

简单的皮肤和软组织感染		复杂性皮肤软组织感染	
浅表的	脓疱病 脓疮	病变的皮肤的继发感染 急性伤口感染	创伤性 咬伤相关 手术后的
更深层的	蜂窝织炎 / 丹毒	慢性伤口感染	糖尿病足 静脉曲张溃疡 压疮
毛囊相关	毛囊炎、疖	肛周的蜂窝织炎 / 脓肿	
脓肿	痈、其他皮肤脓肿	坏死性筋膜炎	Ⅰ型 Ⅱ型 Ⅲ型
		肌坏死	梭菌属 非梭菌属

描述相同的疾病，取决于它出现在临床的哪个部位。不管用哪一种术语来描述它，治疗是一样的。因此，解剖学分类更合理，也更容易让人记住。

在医学文章中，深部感染伪装在各种各样的化名之下。在这里使用“坏死性软组织感染”（necrotizing soft tissue infection，NSTI）这一术语。表 5 列出了一系列可能在医学文章中出现用描述这一感染的术语。

所有的术语都描述了累及皮下脂肪和筋膜的感染，而累及的皮肤是可变的。在一些严重病例中也可以累及肌肉。生物体的致感染能力取决于生物体的活力和抵抗机体的能力。在大约 80% 的病例中，感染从明显的损伤部位扩散。表 6 列出了潜在的感染部位。还有 20% 的患者并没有明显的感染源。这一疾病非常特殊，因为它可以影响受伤和未受伤的机体。多个研究确定多个风险因素与易感性增加有关。然而，有毒性的细菌，如 A 组链球菌，可以感染其他未损害组织。这些细菌产生外毒素，导致细胞因子的释放，导致强烈的系统反应。在细胞水平，毒素和酶（透明质酸酶和脂酶）促进细菌沿筋膜传播至皮下组织。浅筋膜和脂肪坏死通常产生一个稀疏的、水样的、难闻的液体（洗碗水样脓）。伴随这一感染，当皮肤营养血管形成血栓时，皮肤可以出现坏死。微观研究结果通常是严重的皮下脂肪坏死、严重的真皮和皮下脂肪的炎症、血管炎、动脉内膜炎、局部出血（图 2）。筋膜可以出现水肿和化脓，并且可能看见血管血栓形成。随着病情的进展，也可能出现肌坏死。

表 5　用于描述坏死性软组织感染的术语

Meleney's 协同性坏疽	医院坏疽
链球菌坏疽	富尼埃坏疽
气性坏疽	急性皮肤坏疽
化脓性筋膜炎	坏死性丹毒
崩蚀性溃疡	崩蚀性溃疡坏疽
“食肉的疾病”	坏死性筋膜炎
梭状芽胞杆菌性蜂窝织炎	

脓性肌炎

当肌群中有脓液时可以出现脓性肌炎。其临床表现通常有严重疼痛，在一开始常被认为是继发于肌劳损。因为治疗方法常是休息和非甾体抗炎药物，故常常使诊断延误，后疼痛症状加剧并且肌肉出现痉挛，如果不抑制，将出现发热。由于感染部位深，在早期，因感染在深部，异常不能被触及，当感染扩散，肌坏死可随之出现，脓肿的僵硬甚至膨胀可能是造成这一症状的原因。分离出的生物体通常是金黄色葡萄球菌。

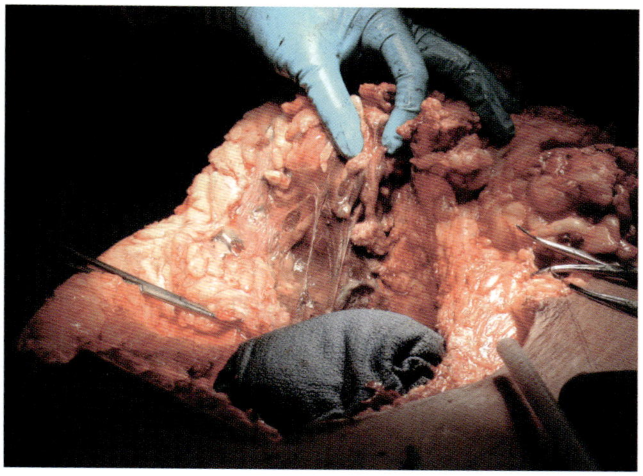

图 2 该患者为剖宫产术后引起的坏死性软组织感染，图示为浅筋膜和脂肪的液化坏死

表 6 坏死性软组织感染的潜在部位和原因

部位	原因
会阴	肛周脓肿
	前庭大腺脓肿
	泌尿生殖系统感染
	泌尿生殖道后方手术或插管
	肛后部手术
	大的新生物
四肢	糖尿病足部溃疡
	静脉曲张溃疡
	动脉缺血性溃疡
	静脉注射毒品
	创伤或骨折
	动物或人咬伤
	褥疮性溃疡
躯干	手术部位感染
	腹内来源的感染
	褥疮性溃疡
	绞窄性疝
头颈部	牙脓肿
	咽 / 扁桃体脓肿
	手术部位感染

手术部位感染

手术部位感染是住院患者的一种常见的不良事件。浅表感染只发生在皮下，并在术后 30 天内形成。至少有以下表现之一：

脓性引流

伤口液体或组织培养阳性

局部体征和疼痛、肿胀、压痛、红斑的症状

由主治外科或内科医生做出诊断

手术部位感染的定义是累及筋膜或肌肉，且在术后 30 天内形成的感染。

诊断

临床表现

坏死性软组织感染的体征和症状没有特异性（表 7），感染部位的疼痛、红斑、肿胀是最常见的表现。这些类似症状群往往出现在病情发展的早期阶段，单用抗生素治疗效果就非常明显。坏死性感染的确切表现包含张力性红斑、大疱、皮肤色素减退、捻发音和与检查不一致的疼痛、感染部位麻木感（图 3）。不幸的是，这些体征只有少数患者才有，且一旦发现这些体征，感染往往已经进展。

感染也会引起全身性表现，包括发热、心动过速、低血压和器官功能障碍，症状可以在数小时或数天内快速进展，或者在数天到数月内缓慢发展。通过部分治疗可以延缓症状出现的进程，表 8 中列出了考虑坏死性筋膜炎的几点临床特征。

这类患者的实验室检查同样没有特异性，在临床研究中已经观察到有白细胞增多、低钠血症、肌酸磷酸激酶升高，它们或许可以成为这类疾病的标志物。Wall 等在坏死性筋膜炎和非坏死性筋膜炎两组患者中匹配了 21 组研究对象，试图找出能够区分两组患者的变量。研究表明，白细胞计数大于 15.4×10^9/L，血清钠小于 135 mmol/L 是识别坏死性筋膜炎患者的最佳指标。它的灵敏度为 90%，特异度为 76%。在这个研究中，40% 的患者缺乏诊断坏

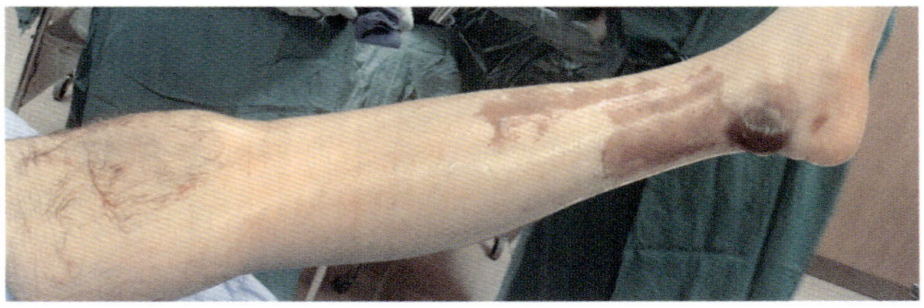

图 3 踝关节周围的出血性水疱

死性筋膜炎的确切表现。Wong 的团队制定了预测坏死性筋膜炎的实验室风险因子评分系统，该评分是通过回顾坏死性筋膜炎患者和其他严重软组织感染患者的特征得出的，包含白细胞计数、血红蛋白、血清钠、C 反应蛋白、肌酐和血糖，评分大于 6 分时，阳性预测值为 92%，阴性预测值为 96%。一项前瞻性的队列研究表明，该评分系统的阳性预测值为 40%，阴性预测值为 95%。肌酸磷酸激酶升高是一个团队在研究 A 组链球菌引起的坏死性筋膜炎和非 A 组链球菌引起的坏死性筋膜炎区别时发现的，在 A 组链球菌感染组，肌酸磷酸激酶大于 600 IU/L。对于生理方面异常的患者，检测乳酸水平和碱缺失情况可以指导复苏治疗。

表 7　坏死性软组织感染的临床体征出现的频率

作者	红斑 (%)	捻发音 (%)	水肿 (%)	出版年	研究对象（例数）
Callahan	77	3	20	1998	30
McHenry	72	12	75	1995	65
Brook	89	39	77	1995	83
Elliot	66	45	75	1996	197
Tang	50		58	2001	24
Theis	54			2002	13
Wong	100	13	92	2003	89

表 8　坏死性软组织感染的临床特征

1. 严重的持续性疼痛
2. 穿支血管阻塞导致的水肿
3. 皮肤坏死或坏死前瘀斑
4. 触诊或 X 线片发现组织积气
5. 红斑边缘水肿或硬结
6. 皮肤麻木
7. 全身毒性发热、白细胞增多、精神错乱、急性肾疾病
8. 应用抗生素后仍快速进展

诊断性影像学

对于诊断不确切或者表现不典型的患者，影像学检查很有意义。皮下组织积气是 NSTI 的一个特征，而气体可以通过多个影像学检查技术发现。只有 16% 患者的皮下积气可以通过 X 线平片发现。但是平片可以发现异物，这对于静脉注射药品的患者很有意义。在鉴别气体方面，超声检查、CT、MRI 的灵敏度比 X 线平片更高。这些检查还可以发现皮下组织间或肌肉间的积液。这有利于发现皮肤没有严重病变的患者的异常情况，有利于指导切口的选择、评估感染的程度。MRI 的另外一个优势是不须静脉注射对肾有毒性的造影剂，是合并肾功能异常患者的理想选择。但是对于全身状态不好的患者，不适合行 MRI 检查。对于大多数患者，诊断性检查也有可能仅仅提供证实性证据，很难直接确诊。抗生素治疗效果不佳、全身毒性反应或白细胞计数升高可以增加诊断的可能性。最近提出的一套 CT 评分系统可以区分坏死性与非坏死性软组织感染，它是根据回顾分析出院时诊断为坏死性筋膜炎、脓肿、蜂窝织炎的患者资料得出的，表 9 中列出了这些患者的 CT 表现。CT 评分大于等于 6 分，诊断坏死性软组织感染的灵敏度为 86.2%，特异度为 91.5%，阳性预测值为 63.3%，阴性预测值为 85%。

表 9　坏死性软组织感染的 CT 评分

发现	分值
筋膜间气体	5
肌肉 / 筋膜水肿	4
皮下间隙积液	3
淋巴结肿大	2
皮下水肿	1

Enron 等根据局部和全身感染的严重性以及其他合并疾病，制定了一个分型体系，主要用于指导入院和治疗（表 10）。坏死性软组织感染通常按病原菌分类，Ⅰ型为多种微生物感染，是最常见的类型，这型感染常见于有其他合并症的患者。革兰氏阴性肠杆菌、革兰氏阳性菌和厌氧菌均可发现。在患者身上已经培养出 15 种致病菌，每个患者平均培养出 5 种。Ⅱ型可能仅为 A 组链球菌感染，或者同时合并金黄色葡萄球菌感染。这种类型具有致命的病理变化过程，可以发生在年轻患者或健康患者身上。梭菌属感染在软组织中往往产气，然而，多种微生物感染导致的Ⅰ型患者也可以产气。当患者接触过贝壳或者淡水时，须警惕创伤弧菌和嗜水气单胞菌属引起的Ⅲ型感染。

一些学者认为应当按照疾病的临床进程进行分型，爆发型表现为患者急性发病，数小时内出现休

表 10　Eron 软组织感染分级

分级	患者情况	治疗	治疗场所
1	无发热、健康、无蜂窝织炎	必要时引流或口服抗生素	门诊
2	发热、病态，无不稳定的合并症	必要时引流或口服 / 静脉（Ⅳ）使用抗生素	门诊 / 短期住院观察
3	中毒表现或者至少一种不稳定合并症或者存在肢体感染	抗生素Ⅳ	住院
4	脓毒症综合征或威胁生命的感染	抗生素Ⅳ	重症监护病房 外科会诊

Eron LJ: Infections of skin and soft tissue: outcomes of a classification scheme. *Clin Infect Dis* 31:287, 2000

表 11　坏死性软组织感染的临床分型

类型	病程	之前 / 局部抗生素的使用	全身症状	器官衰竭	顽固的局部症状
Ⅰ、Ⅱ、Ⅲ	超急性		√	√	–/ √
Ⅰ、Ⅱ、Ⅲ	急性		√	√	–/ √
Ⅰ、Ⅱ	亚急性	√	–	–	√

克。急性型往往感染面积较大，病程持续数天。亚急性型持续数周，通常为局部表现（表 11）。利用蜂窝织炎或者小的脓肿区分病变进程很困难，在临床中，通过抗生素治疗未能改善或者全身毒性反应重往往提示这类疾病。

另外，Wong 的团队在 2003 年利用诊断为坏死性软组织感染的患者资料观察到了病变发展的过程。这些患者被诊断为坏死性筋膜炎，延误 96 h 以上的时间才进行外科手术。该团队将病变发展分为Ⅰ-Ⅲ个阶段（表 12）。

表 12　坏死性软组织感染的临床表现，阶段Ⅰ—Ⅲ

Ⅰ期：早期阶段
触诊压痛（延伸超过可见病变皮肤以外）
红斑
肿胀
灼热（皮肤温暖）
Ⅱ期：中期阶段
形成水疱或大疱（浆液）
Ⅲ期：晚期阶段
捻发音
皮肤麻木
皮肤坏死、色泽暗淡

外科治疗

软组织感染患者在治疗前，首先须评估全身生理状体。对于没有其他合并疾病的稳定、不复杂患者，仅仅通过口服抗生素或局部切开引流或许就能治愈。但是，对有器官衰竭表现、血流动力学不稳定的重症患者，须根据脓毒症指南（表 13）证据立刻行复苏治疗。

坏死性筋膜炎患者需要紧急手术治疗，主要的治疗方式为外科清创。这类手术往往不美观，须清除大面积皮肤组织、大量皮下脂肪、筋膜，必要时还会清除肌肉或骨。四肢的手术通常会选择较大的纵行切口。当感染范围很广泛时，肢体行筋膜切开术通常很有意义。切开必须够深，能够达到深筋膜，必须探查肌肉确认其活力（图 4）。对于有张力性水肿的患者，为了防止肌肉坏死，必须进行正式的筋膜切开。（图 5-6）

必须检查皮下脂肪或浅筋膜与深筋膜之间的组织平面的完整性，可以利用手指或者血管钳探查深筋膜（图 7）。对于发病早期的患者，以缺乏对探索的抵制为标志，打开伤口后可探查到组织内的液体。对于病变进展的患者，会发现坏死、化脓的物质。

表 13 脓毒症的简要指南

阶段	目标	干预
初始复苏 ≤6 h	CVP 8～12 mm Hg MAP≥65 mm Hg 尿量≥5 ml/kg·h MVo_2≥65%	液体复苏 如果 Hct <30% 或者应用多巴酚丁胺，输 PRBCs
诊断	若未延迟，在应用抗生素之前	2 次或多次血培养 其他部位的培养
抗菌治疗	在第 1 h 内诊断重症脓毒症或感染性休克	广谱抗生素 / 抗真菌治疗，确保对组织穿透力强 使用包含抗假单胞菌的 2 种药物 对中性粒细胞减少的患者联合用药
病因控制	≤6 h	脓肿引流、组织清创

CVP，中心静脉压；Hct，血细胞比容；MAP，平均动脉压；MVo_2，心肌耗氧量；PRBCs，浓缩红细胞

应当进行组织培养和革兰氏染色，包含有氧与无氧条件下的培养。对存在免疫抑制的患者，还应当进行分枝杆菌和真菌培养。广泛打开感染的组织，同时彻底清除失活的组织至关重要（图 8）。

当病变严重时，须最大限度地切开异常的皮肤组织，并且要切得足够深，到达异常组织（图 9—图 10）。对于广泛肛周感染的患者，行结肠造口术很有意义，可以避免大便持续漏出造成的污染。留置外科鼻饲管对于危重患者或大面积创伤需要长时间暴露的患者很有意义。

一定要在措施结束后制订好计划，以便 48 h 内重返手术室进行探查。在床旁很难充分评估那些深部伤口或者经常疼痛的创伤。目前有许多创伤敷料可以应用，伤口负压治疗技术（negative pressure wound therapy，NPWT）也是为此而设计的。它可以去除分泌物，进一步减少细菌数量，可以防止分泌物对周围组织的浸渍，保持患者身体及病床干燥。同时它也可以量化液体的流失量，补充这些流失的液体很重要。它可以评估伤口周围皮肤蜂窝织炎或者水肿的发生，也可以评估渗出液的性状。

仔细止血及纠正凝血功能障碍对于这类患者的伤口处理至关重要。医护人员必须关注患者引流液的量及性状。当无法提供这种敷料或者患者经济困难时，可以选择 Kerlix（Kendall Kerlix AMD）或含抗生素的纱布。有些材料具有细胞毒性，尽管如此，

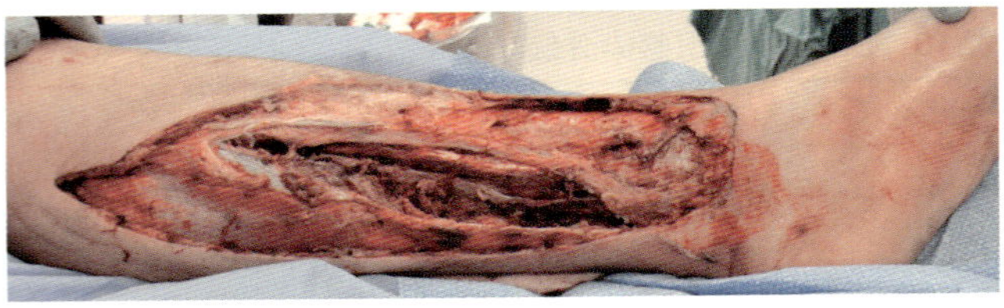

图 4 图 3 患者清创后的表现，坏死和化脓扩张至深筋膜，到达腓肠肌和比目鱼肌

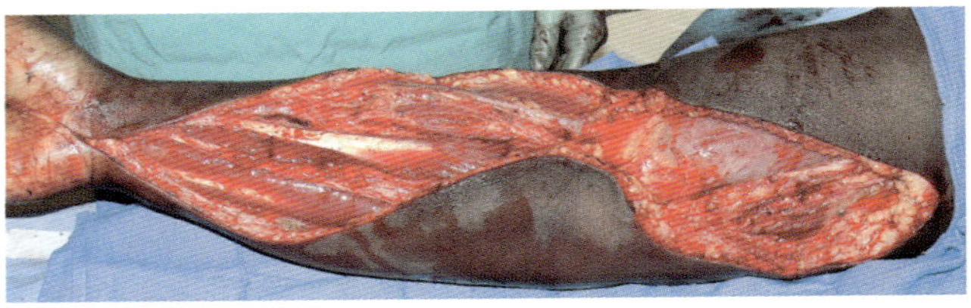

图 5 上肢筋膜切开减压

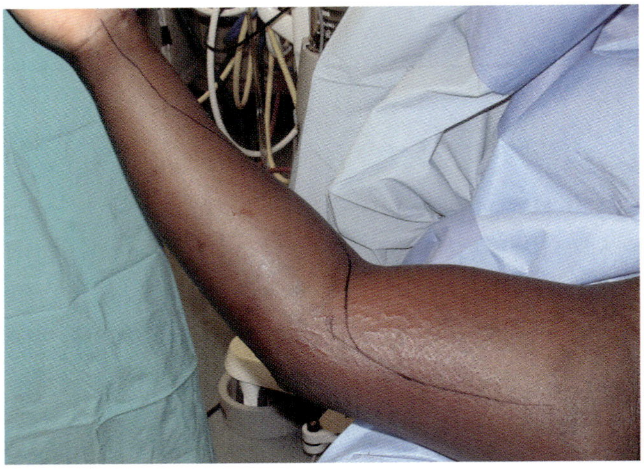

图 6 患者上臂和前臂严重肿胀，有红斑

考虑到它们的抗菌特性的优势比对正常组织的细胞毒性的劣势大，还是建议使用。当感染控制后可以选择非细胞毒性的产品，含银离子的产品就是很好的选择。

药物治疗

休克患者的初始治疗主要是复苏治疗，给予输注液体和血液制品以补充液体的缺失，纠正凝血功能异常。须强调的是，早期开始复苏治疗很重要，但在手术前不须完全纠正所有的功能障碍。因为术前、术中和术后许多功能障碍只有在充分处理好原因后才能纠正。对于重症患者，须使用升压药和类

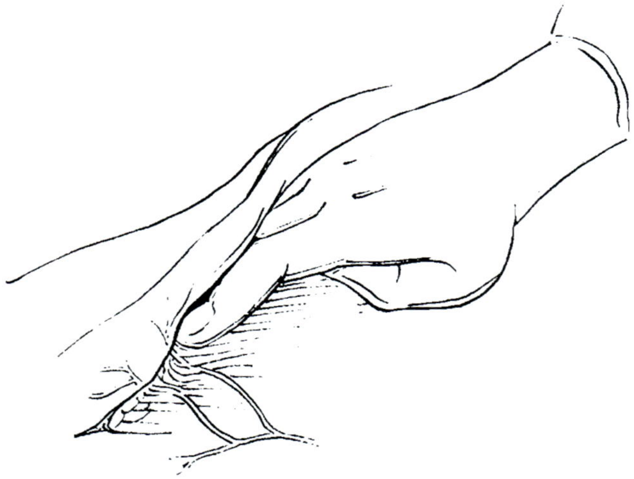

图 7　组织完整性丧失

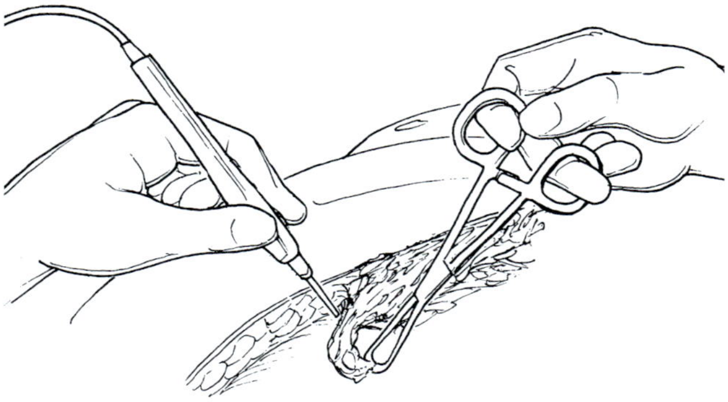

图 8　彻底的清创

固醇药物。当涉及 A 组链球菌感染时，可考虑给予静脉注射免疫球蛋白（intravenous immunoglobulin，IVIG）。早期应用广谱抗生素可覆盖大部分可能的致病菌（表 14）。超广谱青霉素是好的一线选择，疑似 A 组链球菌感染时可加用克林霉素。选择抗生素时须考虑到在社区存在甲氧西林耐药的问题。当在重症患者中怀疑出现耐药时，可考虑使用万古霉素或达托霉素，青霉素过敏的患者可考虑使用喹诺酮类抗生素，联合应用抗革兰氏阴性菌及厌氧菌的药物，或者使用碳青霉烯类抗生素。

高压氧治疗

高压氧（hyperbaric oxygen，HBO）疗法属于复苏治疗、外科清创治疗、广谱抗生素治疗以外的辅

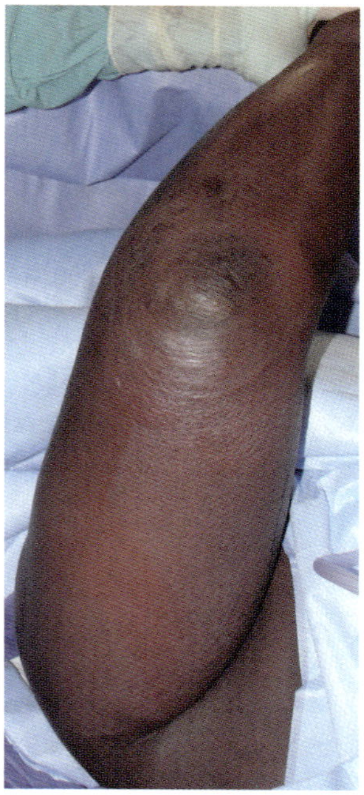

图 9　图 10 患者术前照片。注意肘部皮肤变色、有水疱、张力性水肿和红斑

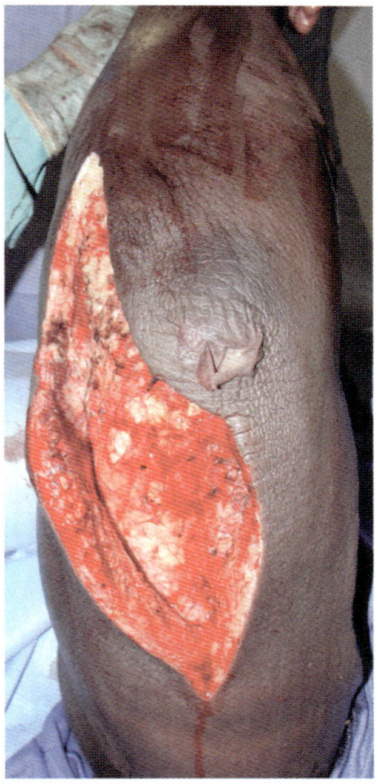

图 10　图 9 患者术后照片，是伤口清创前的表现。显示了浅筋膜及脂肪坏死延伸到肘部

助治疗手段。HBO 具有很多优势，有各种有益的影响（表 15）。但是目前尚无前瞻性随机对照研究系统地证实 HBO 的功效。许多回顾性研究表明 HBO 对于重症坏死性感染的患者治疗有益。一些研究表明，与其他对照组相比，使用了 HBO 疗法的患者死亡率

下降。其他研究表明，应用HBO疗法，可以增加组织保留面积，减少清创的数量，从而控制感染。然而，也有一些研究，质疑HBO疗法的功效。这些研究表明，接受HBO疗法的群组和仅仅接受外科清创术的群组相比，两组间在死亡率方面并没有统计学上的显著差异。HBO并不是国家的每个区域都可以获得，因此该疗法不是每个有此问题的患者的标准治疗手段。但如果有条件使用HBO，可以把它作为一种辅助治疗手段，因为此类疾病的死亡率和并发症发生率都很高。

死亡率、并发症发生率与并发症的管理

NSTI治疗过程中的发生率非常高，这些问题大多数源于感染导致的组织破坏。感染涉及的面积和清创的程度决定了病变恶化的程度。在清创过程中，对神经和组织的血液供应的医源性损伤会加重组织功能障碍，这是四肢感染治疗过程中最常见的问题。炎症反应、坏死或者之前的手术瘢痕会造成组织的改变，从而产生重要结构的功能改变。这部分组织对于解剖结构可能是至关重要的，患者可能会仅仅因为外科清创的程度导致重要功能的缺陷。有报道表明，极其严重软组织感染导致的截肢率为17%～33%。大面积的创伤会产生严重的疼痛，对于这部分患者，急性和慢性的疼痛管理都很有必要。

腹部感染的患者，清创时须处理腹壁，有发展为肠瘘的可能。肠瘘的早期治疗重点是处理外漏组织及提供充足的营养支持。

有报道称此类疾病的死亡率高达76%，同期的其他研究显示死亡率在8%～25%之间。死亡率与多种因素相关，患者的临床表现和外科处理的速度是两个最重要的决定性因素。延迟进行外科处理的患者死亡率更高，器官功能衰竭或者血清乳酸水平持续上升也会增加死亡率，合并其他疾病，如糖尿病、肾功能不全，以及高龄及清创范围大也可以增加死亡率。Anaya团队近期评估了大样本的严重软组织感染患者的数据库，提出了几个增加死亡率的预测因子，包含白细胞计数、血细胞比容、肌酐值、体温和心率。在此基础上，他们制订了对死亡分层的评分表（表16）。另外，针对NSQIP数据库的近期研究表明，出院诊断为坏死性筋膜炎的患者死亡率仅仅为12%，但是这类患者的住院时间是其他患者的平均住院时间的9倍。

总结

NSTI可以在各种临床状况下发生，可以发生在手术后、创伤后以及昆虫或动物咬伤后。中心必须与表面感染区分，以进行合适的治疗。对于没有接受恰当药物治疗的患者，或者表现为休克或器官功能衰竭的患者，常常会发展为深部感染。对于有些患者，如实验室检查表明白细胞增多、低钠血症、高血糖、肌酐值升高、C反应蛋白升高、肌酸磷酸激酶升高的患者，应积极给予评估，必要时进行放射学照相检查或手术探查。体格检查如果发现日益恶化的水肿、水疱、捻发音或者皮肤坏死，应当积极进行外科手术探查。图11描绘了合理的治疗流程，可以指导治疗，须强调的是，延误治疗会导致死亡率及并发症发生率的增加。

表 14　严重软组织感染抗生素的使用

抗生素	治疗的微生物	备注
青霉素 β- 内酰胺类抗生素抑制细菌细胞壁 X 耦联	链球菌 *梭菌* 消化链球菌	金黄色葡萄球菌高耐药率
克林霉素林克酰胺类抗生素抑制细菌蛋白质合成	*脆弱拟杆菌* *梭杆菌* *消化链球菌* MRSA，但可引起耐药	可与 GAS 一起抑制毒素产生，有抑菌作用
甲硝唑、硝基咪唑类抗生素使细菌酶失活	厌氧菌（上述）和*普里沃菌*	
万古霉素糖肽类抗生素 细菌细胞壁合成抑制剂	MRSA MSSA	青霉素敏感患者 红人综合征、血栓性静脉炎 必须监控药物浓度 为治疗 MRSA 引起的感染已注射非肠道药物
达托霉素脂肽类抗生素破坏细胞膜功能	MRSA 革兰氏阳性微生物	杀菌可引起肌病，不能治疗肺炎
利奈唑胺、恶唑烷酮类抗生素破坏细菌蛋白质的合成	MRSA VRE	长期使用与骨髓抑制 / 血小板减少、乳酸性酸中毒、周围神经病变有关
奎奴普丁 / 达福普丁、链霉杀阳菌素抑制蛋白质合成	MRSA VRE	每个单独的药物都为抑菌剂，但组合起来可引起杀菌、肌痛、恶心、呕吐
哌拉西林 / 他唑巴坦、超广谱青霉素	革兰氏阴性微生物，包括*假单胞菌* 革兰氏阳性微生物	
头孢噻肟、三代头孢菌素	革兰氏阴性微生物 无肠球菌活性	
环丙沙星、氟喹诺酮类抗生素 DNA、旋转酶抑制剂	革兰氏阳性微生物、革兰氏阴性微生物	许多药物有相互作用
亚胺培南、美罗培南、厄他培南、β - 内酰胺酶抵抗剂	需氧菌，包括*假单胞菌*；厌氧菌，不覆盖 MRSA	广谱有效，抑制需氧微生物释放内毒素

GAS，A 组链球菌；MSSA，甲氧西林敏感的金黄色葡萄球菌；MRSA，耐甲氧西林金黄色葡萄球菌；VRE，抗万古霉素肠道球菌

表 15　高压氧治疗的益处

抑制厌氧菌生长
减少梭菌毒素的产生
提高白细胞对细菌的杀伤能力
对多种病原体具有杀菌、抑菌作用
提高某些抗生素的功效
调节细胞因子水平
减少组织水肿
增加胶原形成

表 16　坏死性软组织感染患者死亡预测评分

变量（入院时）	分数
心率 >110 次 / 分钟	1
体温 <36 ℃	1
血肌酐 >1.5 mg/dl	1
年龄 >50 岁	3
白细胞计数 >40 000/μl	3
血细胞比容 >50%	3

分组	分值	死亡率（%）
1	0～2	6
2	3～5	24
3	≥6	88

复杂软组织感染管理流程

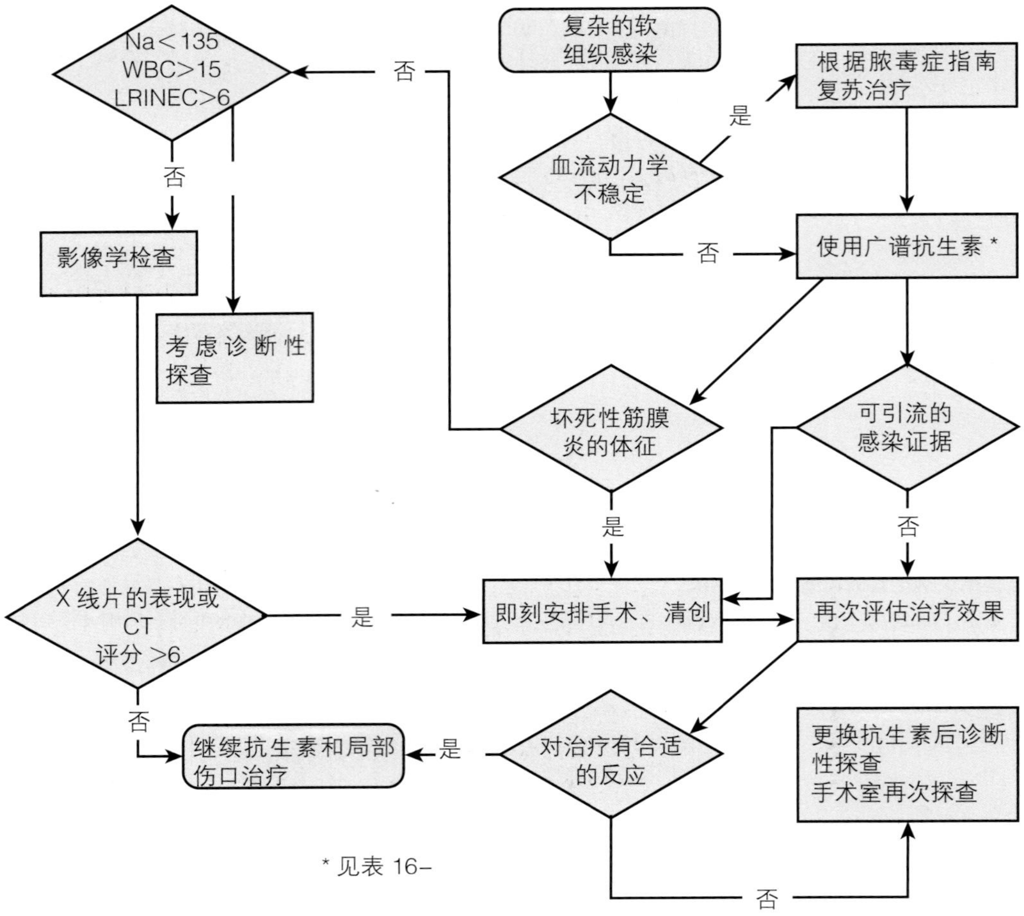

图 11 复杂软组织感染管理流程。CT，计算机断层扫描；LRINEC，预测坏死性筋膜炎风险的实验室指标；Na，钠；OR，手术室；WBC，白细胞

创伤救治中的常见错误

R. Stephen Smith，Allan S. Philp 和 Stepheny D. Berry 著
王传林 译

医学上经常发生处理错误的情况。最近医学研究所的一个报告估计，每年有 44 000 ~ 98 000 人死于医疗事故。这相当于美国每年因乳腺癌或获得性免疫缺陷综合征的死亡人数。这些错误大多发生在低强度的非急诊情况。显然，创伤护理不出现错误更难。必须要对受伤患者进行紧急护理。必须根据有限的信息迅速做出治疗决定。在许多情况下，必须在完成完整的临床和放射学评估之前进行干预。通常受伤的历史机制情况模糊不清，或受伤患者参与不为社会所接受的活动或犯罪活动，可能会误导创伤治疗团队成员。此外，受伤的患者经常没有反应、意识水平下降，或由于中毒而不配合治疗。严重受伤的患者经常表现为多处伤害，需要多学科团队。

通常，许多外科医生、外科专科医生、急救医学医生、住院医生必须准确地沟通和协调，以期获得最佳治疗后果。对于创伤治疗团队成员的住院医生，沟通、组织和监督方面的复杂性增加了。

创伤医疗错误的潜在原因非常多。因此，外科医生在创伤处理时必须特别注意导致错误的因素，并尽一切努力防止这些错误的发生。本章介绍了创伤患者处理过程中的一些常见错误，包括未发现膈损伤、未能发现肢体筋膜室综合征、未能防止或治疗的腹腔隔室综合征、延误损伤控制性剖腹术、未能识别的空腔脏器损伤、未进行三阶段调查，急诊科误行开胸，以及武断地进行结肠造口术。

未发现膈创伤

创伤性膈损伤在16世纪就已有描述，19世纪80年代和20世纪的文献分别引用过对穿通性和钝性膈损伤的修复手术。膈损伤的发病率因损伤机制而异，有报告指出，钝性创伤的发生率为0.5%～8%，穿通性创伤为3.4%～40%。只有1%～2%的患者会出现双侧膈损伤。双侧损伤患者的死亡率较高。穿通性和钝性膈创伤时，实质脏器和空腔脏器损伤常见。最初的诊断性评估中，高达66%的创伤可能会被漏诊，结果导致实质脏器和空腔脏器疝气、嵌顿、绞窄等。文献报道在膈损伤诊断延迟时，死亡率高达36%。

机动车事故的伤者腹内压（intraabdominal pressure，IAP）可明显增高，特别是如果伤者被束缚时。有人认为这种明显的压力梯度是导致钝性膈破裂的主要病理生理机制。此外，在吸气时胸腔负压可导致脏器疝入胸腔。减速损伤导致的膈破裂与主动脉横断有很强的相关性，高达10%的主动脉损伤患者也有膈创伤。膈损伤相关的其他损伤包括肝、脾裂伤，长骨骨折和创伤性脑损伤。穿通性胸腹创伤也常常导致膈损伤。因为这些损伤通常比钝性破裂损伤更小，即使进行了恰当的诊断性评估，可能也未能识别。

大多数膈损伤的体格检查结果不可靠。症状和体征往往不具有特异性，可包括胸膜炎性胸痛、腹痛、上腹压痛、胸部肠鸣音、血流动力学不稳定等。大的损伤造成张力性内脏疝入胸腔患者时可出现呼吸窘迫。诊断常规使用的创伤诊断方法包括X线胸片、FAST、CT，这些检查检出急性创伤患者存在的膈损伤的能力存在差异。膈损伤者中，高达50%的初始X线胸片评估结果正常。病例报告和小规模病例系列研究表明，FAST检查发现膈异常运动支持诊断，但这一技术尚未得到广泛认可。CT已将诊断的灵敏度和特异度提高至82%和99.7%，但是，这些结果并没有重复性。

尽管技术有所进步，手术（开腹、腹腔镜检查，开胸或胸腔镜评估）评估膈仍然是灵敏度、特异度和准确度最高的诊断工具。非治疗性手术并非没有风险。因此，在高度怀疑膈损伤时，应采用现有诊断技术来进行评估。成像研究结果模糊且高度怀疑时，须进一步审查。任何诊断工具诊断出膈创伤后，都须修复膈，以避免狭窄和穿孔风险。多数损伤可进行永久性缝合修复。一些大的缺损可能须人工修复加固。胸腔镜和腹腔镜修补膈损伤成功的报道也很多。应依据外科医生治疗这类创伤的专业知识和经验、患者的临床状况，以及是否存在相关损伤等，选用合适的手术方法。

未能发现肢体筋膜室综合征

上肢和下肢损伤患者经常发生筋膜室综合征。筋膜室综合征也可能发生在任何筋膜包裹的肌肉筋膜室，可包括手、肩、手臂、臀部、大腿和脚。一个普遍的误解是开放性骨折患者不会出现筋膜室综合征。约10%的开放性骨折患者会发生危及肢体的筋膜室综合征。筋膜室综合征要根据历史和体格检查结果，以及一些辅助评估工具进行诊断。提示筋膜室综合征的体检发现包括肢体紧张伴疼痛。感觉异常提示存在累及神经的晚期缺血。不能因为远端脉搏可触及，就错误地推定没有筋膜室综合征。事实上，无脉是筋膜室综合征晚期体征，可能只有发生不可逆的神经和肌肉损伤后才出现。

筋膜室综合征可发生在继发于多项因素的四肢损伤。筋膜室内出血和肌肉水肿可继发于骨折。由于筋膜室内压增加，筋膜室内压超过灌注压时，就会发生肌肉和神经缺血。另外，当筋膜室内压上升时，会出现静脉流出受阻。筋膜室综合征是电烧伤的一个已知的并发症。缺血再灌注也是一个已知的筋膜室综合征的原因。筋膜室综合征的医源性病因包括静脉导管错位进入筋膜室，造成液体进入筋膜室。长时间使用军用抗休克裤（military antishock trousers，MAST）也与筋膜室综合征的发生有关联。

筋膜室综合征的诊断依据的是临床评估和侵入性评估室内压。有一些技术可很容易检测出室内压。如果肌肉室内压大于30 mmHg，则必须考虑筋膜室综合征。一个更好的确定筋膜室综合征的方法是检测室内灌注压。将平均动脉压减去室内压即可计算出室内灌注压。如果室内灌注压小于 40 mmHg，则必须考虑筋膜室综合征。

筋膜室综合征的确定性治疗为筋膜切开术。上肢和下肢行筋膜切开术的技术很普及，可对累及的所有肢体筋膜室减压。

腹腔膈室综合征

腹腔膈室综合征（abdominal compartment syndrome，ACS）定义为由于腹内高压（intraabdominal hypertension，IAH）导致的病理生理过程和器官功能障碍。一般对肾、心血管和肺系统的影响最大。治疗方法为早期减压。然而，即使治疗得当，死亡率也接近 50%。

对 IAH 的不良影响的认识始于 19 世纪。Marey 和 Burt 证明 IAH 可影响呼吸功能。1890 年，Heinricius 观察到，猫和豚鼠的 IAP 从 27 增加至 46 cmH_2O 时，死亡率增加。

1911 年，Emerson 发现 IAH 和心血管不良影响有关。1913 年，Wendt 证明 IAH 与肾功能障碍有关。20 世纪后期，儿童外科医生开始意识到 IAH 的不良生理影响，并开发出一些技术来允许腹腔内容物扩张。1984 年，Kron 描述了一种测量 IAP 的技术，首先使用术语“腹腔隔室综合征”。

IAH 对心血管系统的影响一致、明确。胸腔内压力增加后，继发静脉回流减少，从而心排血量降低。在 IAP 大于 20 mmHg 时可发生这一现象，但静脉回流在 15 mmHg 时就已经受损。胸腔内压力升高也可导致心室顺应性降低，从而降低心肌收缩力。IAH 时发生的心排血量减少，可因低血容量和吸入麻醉药而加重。

IAH 对呼吸系统的作用是机械性的。由于膈移向头部，须增加气道压力以保持足够的换气。最终，这会导致通气 / 灌注不匹配，导致低氧和高碳酸血症。

ACS 导致肾衰竭的机制很多。肾灌注不足、心排血量降低可继发于灌注减少、肾静脉流出道阻塞，以及肾压缩都会促进与 IAP 升高相关的肾衰竭。大量研究证明，ACS 时发生的少尿和无尿可随腹腔压力减小而恢复。

很少有证据显示 ACS 可影响其他器官系统。然而，腹内压超过 40 mmHg 时，所有腹部器官血流均会减少。腹内压超过 20 mmHg 时，肝动脉、门静脉和微循环灌注减少。存在 IAH 时，腹腔减压可持续改善颅内高压和减少的脑灌注压的情况。

对于 ACS 存在许多原因。大量晶体液复苏在 ACS 的发展中具有突出和潜在性预防作用。任何腹腔内出血相关疾病均有 ACS 风险。这些疾病包括腹部创伤、腹主动脉瘤破裂、腹膜后出血、择期腹部手术、妊娠并发症、肝移植。除了血液外，其他腹腔积液也可能会导致 ACS 的发生。肠和腹膜后腔水肿、腹腔填塞、肠梗阻、腹水、休克时使用大容量液体复苏，以及腹部筋膜不当关闭均可增加 IAH 和 ACS 的危险。

ACS 的诊断基于临床参数和 IAP 检测结果。少尿（<0.5 ml/kg · h）、缺氧（氧输送<600 ml/min · m^2）气道压力增加（峰值大于 45 cmH_2O），全身血管阻力（systemic vascular resistance，SVR）大于 1 000 和腹膨隆均提示 ACS。两种 IAP 测量方法在临床可用于 ACS：①胃内检测；②膀胱检测，后者应用最广泛。Kron 等首先描述该技术，该技术须夹紧导尿管，之后将 50 ~ 100 ml 无菌生理盐水注入膀胱，然后将导管连接到压力计。

根据不同 IAP 水平的不良生理变化，有经验的外科医生认为，IAP 在 25 mmHg 以上时需要腹部减压，所有患者 IAP 在 35 mmHg 以上时均需减压。早期减压可在 ICU 进行，这可以逆转 ACS 的病理生理过程。为了避免减压过程中出现低血压，必须保证已经完成了充分的血管内容量复苏。腹部减压的并发症包括高钾血症、呼吸性碱中毒、出血、再灌注损伤。开腹减压的最后一步是临时腹腔关闭，以防 IAH 复发。其他问题包括感染、体液丢失、内脏取出、肠瘘和腹腔脏器暴露。许多方法可用于闭合，包括可吸收网、塑料静脉注射（Bogota）袋、负压辅助闭合。临时腹腔关闭产生的大的腹壁疝，经常须延期用不可吸收网片修补。即使减压，ACS 死亡率仍然接近 50%。如果不治疗，通常致命。早期临床高度怀疑的患者，应结合积极 IAP 检测，可以指导开展救命性减压。

神秘的强制性结肠造口术

北美人际暴力冲突仍然普遍存在。存在腹部穿通创伤、共存的损伤和伤口并发症时，结肠是第二常见的损伤器官（表 1）。当这些患者就诊时，外科医生必须决定是否一期修复结肠、切除、进行吻合术，或结肠造口术。穿通性结肠损伤的最佳治疗方案仍有争论。第一次世界大战期间，许多患者接受一期修复。由于广泛的损伤或左半结肠损伤结肠造口术保留。无论采用哪种方法，死亡率仍然很高。然而，这些令人沮丧的生存数据主要源于延迟治疗、复苏容量不足、输血不足或抗生素使用不足、缺乏重症监护支持。1943 年，美国陆军外科医生 W. H. Ogilvie 发表了一封公开信，要求为结肠损伤的患者行结肠造口术，之后，强制性结肠造口术就开始：

> 结肠损伤的治疗要依据已知的缝合和漏的风险。简单的缝合结肠伤口，无论多么小，都有风险。有从这样的手术中幸存的人，但也有人死于手术。如果他们被不那么乐观，且更有理智的外科医生救治的话，他们本可以幸存下来。损伤的节段要么必须被切除，要么行近端结肠造口术使其丧失功能。

表 1　美国创伤外科协会（AAST）结肠损伤分级

Ⅰ级	血肿或挫伤，血供没有中断
Ⅰ级	裂伤：部分全层损伤但无穿孔
Ⅱ级	裂伤 <50% 周长
Ⅲ级	裂伤 >50% 周长
Ⅳ级	结肠横断
Ⅴ级	结肠横断，伴节段性组织丢失

这个结论的依据有很少的证据，但是是应对死亡率超过 50% 的发布。根据 Ogilvie 自己的数据，一期修复患者死亡率为 50%，而结肠造口治疗死亡率为 59%。作为复员的军医，他们强化了对结肠损伤行结肠造口的教条式治疗。值得注意的是，早在 1951 年初，Woodhall 和 Ochsner 就报告指出，在普通民众中，一期修复比结肠造口术的死亡率要低（8.3% vs. 35%）。近几十年来，外科医生对结肠损伤行一期修复时更加放心，而过去则要转流治疗。对于右结肠损伤，无论修复或切除联合吻合术，许多医生都会比较放心，但左半结肠损伤的治疗则越来越少地使用结肠造口术。过去的几十年中，在结肠损伤行一期修复时，外科医生被强迫提供依据，但最近的数据改变了这个情况。1979 年，Stone 和 Fabian 发表了具有里程碑意义的前瞻性病例系列研究，表明许多损伤稳定的患者无须结肠造口治疗。1991 年，Chappuis 等报道了前瞻性、随机试验结果，在穿通性结肠损伤患者中比较一期修复和引流。不管损伤情况、污染、输血或休克状况如何，患者随机分组治疗。两组之间并发症发生率没有差异（17.9% vs 21.4%），结肠造口术组住院天数多 6 天。

1996 年 Gonzalez 进行的一项前瞻性、随机研究评估了穿通性结肠损伤的治疗效果，患者随机接受一期修复伴或不伴切除和强制性结肠造口术。随机化时未考虑合并损伤情况或其他危险因素。在一期修复组感染并发症发生率较低（20%vs.25%），但没有统计学意义。穿通性腹部创伤指数评分为 25 分以上的严重损伤患者，与结肠造口术组相比，一期修复组并发症发生率较低。虽然这些差异没有统计学意义，但这方面的经验表明，一期修复至少等同于强制性的结肠造口术，甚至可能优于结肠造口术。

一些作者（Cornwell 等）对下述患者行结肠修复或吻合术谨慎地提出了反对意见：高度破坏性损伤、需要大量输血（>6 单位 PRBCs）或伴污染的损伤时间较长（>6 h）。EAST1998 年的实践指南也敦促，休克、腹膜炎或有重大并存疾病和损伤的患者应谨慎。

几个随机试验似乎支持对这些患者行修复或吻合术。Gonzalez 等报道了他们在 6 年间对 181 例穿通性结肠损伤的治疗经验。不管其他损伤、严重粪便污染或低血压情况如何，这些患者随机进行一期修复或结肠造口术。在一期修复组，感染性并发症均发生率较低（18% vs 21%，$P<0.05$）。在血流动力学不稳定的患者中，一期修复组并发症的发生率也较低（26% vs. 50%）。两组患者中，并发症发生率随着时间的推移而下降，这可能是对创伤患者的整体护理改善的结果。

同样，Sasaki 等对 71 例穿通性结肠损伤患者进行的前瞻性随机对照研究，在随机化时没有采用排除标准。60% 的患者进行一期修复或切除联合吻合术。损伤分级无显著性差异。一期修复组并发症发生率为 19%（结肠和非结肠相关），而切除与吻合术组并发症发生率为 36%。穿通性腹部创伤指数评分大于 25 的患者一期修复组并发症发生率为 33%，而切除与吻合术组为 93%。过去一直争论是否要使用穿通性腹部创伤指数评分判断行强制性结肠造口术，但在这个研究及其他研究中，不管治疗方法如何，评分较高的患者并发症发生率也较高。作者报道在结肠造口术转流时，并发症发生率为 7%。Berne 等对 40 例创伤后结肠造口术转流时的情况进行了综述。他们发现，最初用结肠造口术治疗结肠损伤的患者中，55% 发生了并发症。

Ott 等对 174 例患者的综述显示在损伤控制性剖腹术后的开放式腹腔行吻合术时，漏的发生率增加 6 倍，提示医生要加倍小心。这说明腹腔关闭时延期修复或转流在某些情况下可能仍有一定的价值。

决定行转流结肠造口术理论上似乎很有依据，但当代创伤护理必须基于证据而不是直觉。多数病例并不能明确地显示有短期获益。转流结肠造口术患者需要后期手术再吻合，这将他们暴露于造口特异性的并发症风险之中，包括疝、造口狭窄或回缩、坏死和造口部位皮肤破裂，以及因造口管理而对生活方式的限制。根据目前的证据，穿通性结肠损伤不用必须行结肠造口术。任何结肠损伤在考虑行结肠造口术时，无论是否有共存损伤或疾病，必须在手术室内基于患者的生理判断。要意识到修复或吻合的安全性相同，在许多病例甚至修复的效果更好。

延迟损伤控制性剖腹手术

"损伤控制"这个术语源于美国海军对船舶吸收损伤和维持任务能力的定义，现在用于描述许多身体部位所用的外科策略。该术语描述了一种改进的手术顺序，其中抛弃了即刻修复所有的损伤的概念，而是采用分期方法。这种方法依据的是对危重患者生理性损伤的识别，以及病情在整个过程中不断恶化，这可能使损伤不可逆。简化剖腹术的概念源自 1908 年，当时 Pringle 描述了填塞和肝包扎控制门静脉出血的原则。这种做法在第二次世界大战后就不再流行，但 20 世纪 60 年代和 70 年代又出现了此治疗方法的报告，报告指出这种技术可改善治疗结局。1983 年 Stone 等介绍了现代的简化开腹术后复苏的概念，生理性恢复后隔断完成开腹术。1993 年 Rotondo 等推广使用术语"损伤控制"，该技术在创伤和急诊手术领域，迅速成为治疗生理参数不断恶化的危重患者的标准。

三阶段损伤控制最初是指控制出血和污染、持续复苏和随后的确定性损伤修复。第一阶段是在危及生命生理状况下行截断性剖腹手术。须腹腔内填塞控制出血，快速缝合、吻合或切除，控制肠道污染。本阶段的目的并不包括长血管修复，但可以临时分流。不用确定性重建肠道的连续性。过度填塞会增加 IAP 和继发 ACS 的风险。包扎不充分可能无法止血。填塞必须在重建破坏组织的平面内产生压力，但必须记住动脉损伤单纯通过填塞很难止血。如果不能进行快速修复、结扎或放置支架，那么应采用其他方法，如血管造影栓塞。胆道和胰腺损伤，在几乎所有急诊情况下都可以用外部导管引流处理。一旦完成简化剖腹术，用临时方法关闭腹腔。已有许多临时关闭技术，包括穿透毛巾钳夹闭、不行筋膜缝合而行皮肤缝合、使用附着于皮肤的静脉包（Bogota 包）和真空关闭装置。无论采用哪种方法，目标都一样：防止脏器取出，保护肠道，减少 IAH 和 ACS 的风险。因此，在这些情况下，无论是商业真空敷料或调整真空敷料都是主要敷料。

控制损伤的第二阶段须在 ICU 中持续复苏，逆转致死三联征：①低体温；②酸中毒；③凝血功能障碍。这些毁灭性的生理性并发症都对其他并发症具有复合作用。低体温定义为核心温度低于 35℃，可因长期暴露、灌注不足和急诊室或手术室不够温暖而加重。因创伤的剖腹术后，约半数损伤患者存在低体温现象，有液体复苏、血管加压药、强心药和输血的需求的增加。低体温为并发症发生率、器官功能障碍、凝血功能异常与死亡率增加的独立相关因素。在 ICU 中的环境、流通空气、静脉输液和血液产品都应该被加热。应积极使用热毛毯和强力空气加热器。出血继发的供氧不足可导致酸中毒，酸中毒又可导致无氧代谢和乳酸释放。酸中毒可加重凝血功能障碍，降低心肌收缩力，减少儿茶酚胺的收缩反应，并诱发心律失常。纠正酸中毒应改善氧输送和优化心排血量。一些病例系列发现，48 h 内不能纠正高乳酸水平或碱缺失时，死亡率接近 100%。凝血功能障碍可因低体温、酸中毒及大量晶体液复苏稀释凝血因子的综合影响而恶化。逆转低体温、酸中毒，以及用新鲜冰冻血浆、冷凝蛋白和血小板积极替换凝血因子，可纠正凝血功能障碍。其他辅助药物（氨甲环酸、重组因子Ⅶ a、凝血酶原复合物）可以帮助纠正凝血功能障碍，但正确的应用和生存获益仍在研究中。

损伤控制的第三阶段是指生理损伤逆转后，用确定性手术修复损伤。确定性修复的时间要基于生理参数正常化，而不是基于时间参数。可能须行一次以上的剖腹术，来修复所有的损伤。

损伤控制技术的最终选择取决于外科医生。因为一旦生理储备耗尽，即使最高质量的护理也无效。

因此如果能够充分发挥损伤控制技术的效益，应尽早进行损伤控制。损伤控制的适应证包括无法止血、不能接近出血源、严重多发损伤，对复苏反应差（通过温度、pH 值等生理参数的直接测量，以及生命体征判断）。损伤控制的并发症包括伤口感染、脓肿形成、肠瘘形成、裂开、胆汁漏、胰腺假性囊肿形成、肠坏死、ACS、多器官功能衰竭、ARDS 和死亡。

在选择的严重损伤患者中，损伤控制是一个可以挽救生命的手术方法。成功与否取决于早期应用、患者选择、迅速手术控制出血和污染、积极复苏，以及逆转致死三联征——低温、酸中毒和凝血功能障碍。

未能识别的空腔脏器损伤

在闭合性创伤中，对实质脏器损伤的非手术治疗措施使用增加，这时必须考虑未能识别的空腔脏器损伤的发生率，以及对它的及时诊断。所有创伤患者中的 1%、腹部闭合性创伤中的 15% 会发生空腔脏器损伤。机动车碰撞是最常见的致伤机制，小肠最常受累。即使影像诊断技术有了进展，在确定空腔脏器损伤方面也不如剖腹手术，因此诊断仍然面临困境。这些损伤中有一些在初始 CT 扫描的密切检查时显而易见，但其他损伤则不明显，直到数小时或数天之后才会显现。虽然 FAST 检测已证明对诊断腹腔积血有价值，但不能可靠地识别空腔脏器损伤。体格检查、DPL 和实验室检查同样都不可靠。

1999 年 Fang 等对延迟小肠损伤诊断的患者进行了研究。他们回顾性综述了 111 例钝性创伤的小肠损伤患者，发现在 24 h 内治疗时，死亡率没有差异。但如果诊断延误超过 4 h，则伤口感染、形成脓肿、肠瘘、伤口裂开和出现脓毒症的风险增加。那些损伤 24 h 后修复者的平均住院天数增加 20 天。Fakhry 等发现，小肠损伤诊断延迟时并发症发生率和死亡率均增加。伤后 8h 内治疗的死亡率为 2%，8 ~ 16 h 治疗为 9.1%，16 ~ 24 h 治疗为 16.7%，延误 24 h 以上为 30.8%。大型多中心 EAST 试验显示，如果手术干预延迟 24 h，死亡率由 5% 上升到 16%。

过去 20 年 CT 技术进展显著，但其识别实质脏器损伤的能力远优于空腔脏器损伤。Killeen 等研究了 150 位经 CT 扫描的钝性创伤的患者，并与手术发现进行了比较。螺旋 CT 扫描对肠道损伤的灵敏度为 94%，对肠系膜损伤的灵敏度为 96%。实质性脏器损伤的数量会影响空腔脏器损伤的诊断。有 1 个实质脏器损伤时，患者也存在 1 个空腔脏器损伤占 7.3%。2 个实质脏器损伤时，则发病率增加 1 倍（15.4%），3 个实质脏器损伤时，为 34.4%。Malhotra 等发现，以下 CT 发现可预测空腔脏器损伤：不明原因腹腔积液、气腹、肠壁增厚、肠系膜脂肪条纹，肠系膜血肿、腔内造影剂外渗、血管造影剂外渗。

漏诊损伤并非只见于钝性损伤。Sung 等对 607 例穿通性损伤患者的回顾性研究发现，最初手术时漏诊了 2% 的损伤。漏诊的患者中 42% 出现脓毒症，17% 出现肾衰竭，死亡率为 17%，显著高于 6.4%。

目前还不清楚评价存在空腔脏器损伤风险患者的最佳策略，因为没有一个特定的路径共识。Malhotra 等建议用 CT 成像，成像检查结果存在 1 个或多个重要发现时，进行 DPL 或手术干预。Mitsuhide 建议结合初步体格检查、CT 成像、诊断性腹腔镜检查，可以减少延误诊断和非治疗性剖腹探查的发生率。无论具体判断标准如何，肯定的是需要早期和专心的处理，这样可以防止延误诊断和确定性治疗并发症。

未进行三阶段调查

漏诊损伤，或政治上流行的术语“延误诊断”，对所有创伤中心都是个难题。ATLS 流程已成为危及生命的损伤者在初步评估期进行识别和治疗的金标准，该流程涉及一阶段和二阶段调查。然而，从发表的报告来看，虽然这个系统可有效地识别直接危及生命的情况，但不太能够有效地全面识别损伤。虽然对于漏诊损伤的具体标准没有共识，但通常是指初步评估时未发现的任何损伤。报告损伤的漏诊率由 2% ~ 50% 不等。大多数漏诊的损伤在临床上可能不显著，但有些可能致命。Buduhan 报道，他们漏诊的损伤中，15% 有临床意义，此人群中 2% 的死亡可以预防。即使是不太严重的损伤也会导致长期残疾、高额费用、痛苦，以及创伤团队和患者、家庭之间的关系恶化。导致漏诊的因素包括注意力集中在更为紧迫的优先治疗项目上、患者感觉改变、未重视体检结果、未适当开展或误解或没有审查影像学检查。漏诊在机动车碰撞事故患者、具有较高的 ISS 患者、有多处损伤的患者中更常见。另一个报告的可增加漏诊率的因素是医生治疗经验不足。

许多报告推荐使用三阶段调查来解决这个问题。第三阶段的调查是在入院后 24 h 内，对创伤患者进行彻底复查，并且在许多检查的限制性因素消除之后进行彻底复查。检查包括症状回顾、体检、审查或安排合适的放射学检查和实验室检查。由于治疗 24 h 后可能仍然存在血流动力学不稳定因素和感觉改变，当患者稳定和神经学上有功能时，要再次完成三阶段调查，因为诊断延迟可长达损伤后数周。许多医生建议影像学检查是第三阶段标准调查的一部分，因为原始的影像学检查可漏诊 25% 以上的损伤，它们应被三阶段调查纠正。Enderson 等报道，常规使用三阶段调查可确定额外 9% 的钝性损伤。Janjua 等发现在入院 24 h 内行第三阶段调查，可发现 56% 的早期漏诊和 90% 的有临床意义的漏诊。Biffl 等实施标准的三阶段调查策略后，漏诊率从 2.4% 下降到 1.5%。Soundappan 等在儿科患者中报告了相似的结果。最近 Lawson 等报告，按照创伤激活标准，对头部、颈部、躯干的常规 CT 检查，使得这些部位的损伤诊断延误率下降了 0.4%。但是，鉴于影像学检查的费用和对放射线的关注，这一操作尚未被确立为标准。

漏诊损伤的发生率令人失望的高，可引起潜在的显著的并发症发生和死亡。三阶段调查是一个全面的患者评估过程。从初始复苏期即开始评估，应包括彻底的体格检查、结合针对性的影像学检查（平片、超声或基于检查发现进行的 CT）。三阶段调查可降低对潜在的危及生命的损伤的诊断延误率，这表明三阶段调查应成为一个标准操作，并且应该是每个创伤患者护理的必要的特征性调查。

无效的开胸术

在创伤救治中最引人注目的一个措施是急诊开胸术。本操作在繁忙的环境中进行，但如果在适当选择的患者中进行，则可以挽救生命。不幸的是，这种技术经常在没有有效的指征，选择不当的患者中进行。毫无疑问，一个继发于右心室小刺伤的心包压塞——失去生命体征的患者可以借此挽救生命。但许多情况下，开胸术的适应证并不是很清晰。致命损伤的患者行无效开胸术也很常见。

Rhee 等回顾了 25 年多中心行开胸术的经验。钝伤患者接受急诊开胸术后的生存率为 1.4%。各创伤中心钝伤患者的生存率从 0～12.5% 不等。如果排除一个中心的 12.5% 的生存率，大多数中心的生存率小于 2%。许多钝性创伤、经历急诊开胸术后的“幸存者”，神经也不再完整。2004 年，Powell 等对他们 ED 开胸术治疗穿通性和钝性创伤，且需要院前心肺复苏（cardiopulmonary resuscitation，CPR）的经验进行了评估。他们发现有 4 个钝性创伤幸存者，他们都有严重的神经功能缺陷。即使是有心脏压塞的钝性创伤患者，急诊开胸术后也往往致命。对急诊开胸术患者进行的回顾性分析中，Grove 等报道 4 例钝性创伤伴心脏压塞的患者，在急诊开胸术后转入 ICU，9 天内全部死亡。显然，钝伤患者在伤害现场或到达创伤中心时，若没有生命体征应宣布死亡。钝伤患者在抵达急诊后不久就失去生命体征时，任何治疗手段的预后都不佳，我们认为不应该行开胸术。

一些穿通伤患者很显然会通过急诊开胸术受益。选择合适的有望挽救生命的患者是关键所在。Powell 等发现 CPR 的持续时间至关重要。所有急诊开胸术的幸存者中，CPR 时间都在 15 min 以内。任何穿通伤的患者，只要有长时间的 CPR（＞15 min），到达创伤中心时没有生命迹象，就应该宣布死亡。

如果院前 CPR 时间超过 5 min 几乎没有患者会生存。急诊开胸术是一个潜在的挽救生命的过程，但几乎没有幸存者。这种干预应限于穿通伤。那些非心脏损伤者的预后很差。FAST 检测可帮助了解可治疗的胸内损伤，有助于减少未来无效的急诊开胸术。

小结

创伤患者评估和治疗环境很有可能导致错误的发生。在多发性创伤时，诊断性评估和干预的延误是不可避免的。大量使用诊断性评估方法，并不能消除治疗的差异。然而，认识常见的错误、最小化错误发生频率，是所有救治创伤患者的医务人员义不容辞的责任。在给予最佳救治时，对于很难诊断的创伤，要保持高度警惕性。徒劳的抢救已经死亡的伤者昂贵又费时，应尽量减少。

战斗创伤护理：十年战争中吸取的教训

Colonel Matthew J. Martin 和 Colonel (retired) Brian Eastridge 著
王传林 译

现代运输创伤护理概述

现代战场是一个高度复杂和致命的竞技场，不断带动民间和军队创伤护理的创新和进步。在第一次世界大战前，多数战场上的并发症及死亡源于感染和其他医学疾病。之后医学和武器学方面的同时进步，导致创伤成为战地医疗的主要关注点。历史上民间医疗人员只有在战争时才被使用，部署于军队，但已经改变为全职专注于军事医疗服务、随时准备提供全面综合的战场创伤护理的人员。2001 年 9 月 11 日的恐怖袭击是越南战争以来第一次大规模和长期部署的军事医疗的应用。在这里不能广泛深入地充分说明从这些冲突中获得的创伤经验，但本章的目的是要突出过去十年中持续的战地医疗手术的一些主要经验教训（和再学习）。

虽然特定的单位类型和军队（陆军、海军、空军等）之间的配置和人力需求差别很大，但都遵循一些组织和能力的基本原则。这能够保证各种作战环境和条件下所需的灵活性和稳定性。战地医学总是从损伤出发，立即得到战友（“互救”）和医务兵或卫生员的救助。然后是一系列的级别的正式医疗服务，从 1 级到第 5 级，如表 1 所示。2 级设施能提供第一次外科护理，它主要专注于损伤控制和稳定患者。值得注意的是，我们得到的一个重要的教训是，严重受伤的患者应立即运送到最合适的级别的设施，这往往意味着须绕过 1 级甚至是 2 级设施，而直接到 3 级设施。

战场损伤

了解主要损伤机制、模式和伤口部位分布，对于充分利用和最大限度地提高战场医学资源至关重要。这些可能每个战区都具有独特性，甚至在战斗过程中可能差别很大。现代的伊拉克和阿富汗的战

表 1　持久自由行动和伊拉克自由行动期间军事战斗创伤管理的医疗系统分级

分级	例子	手术能力	其他能力	备注
1 级	营级救护站、休克创伤排	无	“营救包”，有限的物资供应，可能具备超声能力	医务人员和 PA 或初级保健 MD，无保留住院能力
2 级	陆军 / 空军：前方手术队（FST） 海军：前方复苏外科手术系统 (FRSS)	是，一般手术和骨科手术；维持 OR 24 ~ 48 h 的能力	损伤控制手术、基本实验室技术、基本影像学超声、供氧、有限的血液制品供应	专注于损伤控制和即刻转移到 3 级机构，团队可能会跟随手术单元或分开覆盖 2 个区域
3 级	军队：战斗支援医院 空军：战区医院 海军：船上医院	是，一般手术和骨科手术，手术、外科和医疗专家	多专业专家，高级实验室和血液制品支持、先进的影像学和 CT、物理治疗	损伤控制性外科手术和确定性管理，稳定和转移到 4 级机构
4 级	区域医疗中心 (Landstuhl, Germany)	广泛的、优秀的专科支持	主要医学中心能力	更确定性的外科干预，烧伤可直接绕过送至 Brooke 烧伤中心
5 级	CONUS 国立医疗中心 (Walter Reed, Bethesda, Balboa, Brooke)	全面的三级护理	全面康复和专科干预	执行延期最久的手术和重建护理

From Martin M, Beekley A, editors: Front line surgery, New York, 2010, Springer Publishing

CONUS, Continental U.S. Naval hospitals; CT, computed tomography; MEDEVAC, medical evacuation; OR, operating room; PA, physician assistant

地医疗中都有这种现象，初始入侵阶段和随后的叛乱和稳定阶段，损伤机制和致命性都有显著差异。不像平民创伤，战场创伤特点为以穿通伤为主，往往为高速致伤、严重多系统损伤、损毁伤和截肢。大多数损伤类型都需要某种类型的手术干预。目前作战行动的决定性因素之一是敌人广泛使用的武器的选择是 IED（图 1）。这些装置可以安装在几乎任何需要爆炸的源物体上，大小、触发机制，以及由此产生的爆炸力差异很大（图 2）。与以前的冲突相比，现代冲突中只有一小部分的创伤性伤口源自火器（25%），大多数源自爆炸装置（60%）。爆炸伤及相关的冲击、钝器伤和穿通碎片伤组合，常常造成严重而复杂的战伤，与真正的平民损伤完全不相同。

联合战区创伤登记详细、全面搜集的受伤、治疗以及预后资料，可以对战斗损伤的解剖学分布和严重程度进行分析，以用于对预防和治疗的实时改变。现代技术的发展，如先进的防弹衣、抗爆炸车辆，以及战中策略的变化，部分基于此数据的分析。图 3 显示了当前作战行动的复合战场损伤的解剖学部位分布，表 2 为现代和过去的冲突中伤口的解剖学分布对比。确切的分布情况和严重程度在很大程度上也取决于个人因素，如有无盔甲、车辆或翻车损伤，以及致伤机制。

战场死亡是一个特殊的研究主题，在过去十年的作战行动中曾进行过详细分析。对源自伊拉克自由行动和持久自由行动（Operation Iraqi Freedom/Operation Enduring Freedom，OIF / OEF）的解剖和临床数据进行的 2 个高质量分析，指出导致战场死

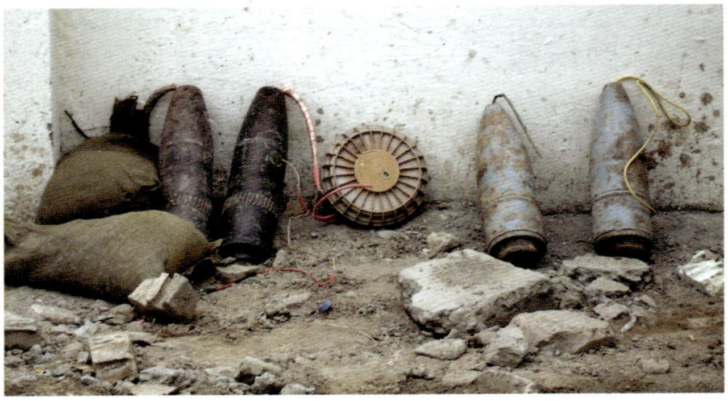

图 1　简易爆炸装置包括 4 个大炮弹和反坦克地雷（或“菊花链”）与导爆索连接在一起 (*Courtesy of U.S. Department of Defense*.)

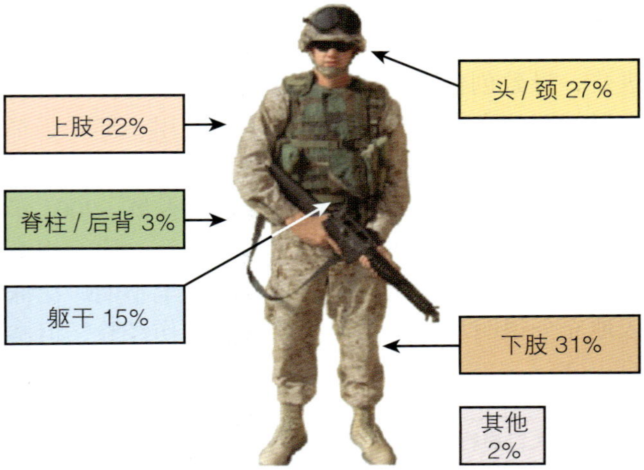

图 3　伊拉克和阿富汗战争时的战斗损伤分布
(Data from the Joint Theater Trauma Registry (JTTR) 2001–2009.)

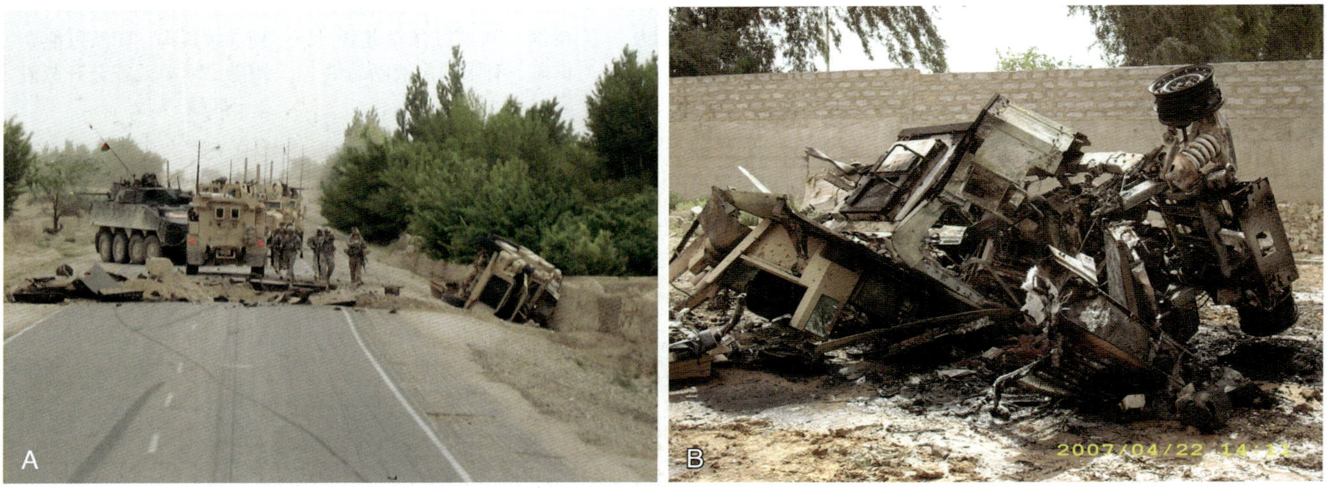

图 2　**A**，放置在主干道的 IED 爆炸导致的坑和翻倒的车。**B**，IED 摧毁的军用车辆（*Courtesy of U.S. Department of Defense*.）

亡的主导机制（爆炸和枪击）和损伤部位（头部和躯干）。令人感兴趣的是，高达 28% 的死亡是有望存活的，其中大多数（80%）死于出血。对这些数据进行的另一个分析表明，伊拉克 / 阿富汗冲突时，病死率（case fatality rate，CFR）是以前的冲突的大约一半（10.5% vs 20.2%），可能原因包括改善的防护设备、疏散能力和院前急救。然而，到达医疗机构后死于伤口（died of wounds，DOW）的比例却出现增加，第二次世界大战时为 3%，越南战争时高达 6%，阿富汗冲突时高达 8%。这个统计数字可能是更严重的伤员能够迅速后撤到医疗机构导致的，显示了前方医疗设施和人员应对这些高损伤情况的前瞻性准备。伊拉克的战斗支援医院对院内死亡进行了详细分析，强调了快速确定性干预的需求，大部分死亡发生在到达后第 1 h 内（78%），原因为出血（62%）。

表 2　伊拉克自由行动和持久自由行动中战斗创伤的身体区域分布及与以前的冲突对比

	体表区域 (%)	WW Ⅱ	朝鲜战争	越南战争	OIF/OEF
头 / 颈	12	21%	21%	16%	30%
胸部	16	14%	10%	13%	6%
腹部	11	8%	8%	9%	9%
四肢	61	58%	60%	61%	55%

Modified from Owens BD, Kragh JF Jr, Wenke JC, et al: Combat wounds in Operation Iraqi Freedom and Operation Enduring Freedom. *J Trauma* 64(2):295–299, 2008

OEF，持久自由行动；OIF，伊拉克自由行动；WW Ⅱ，第二次世界大战

院前和途中救护

当前作战行动和冲突中死亡率急剧下降，其原因很多，包括个人防护设备和车辆的改进，以及医疗护理的改善。为提高 IED 爆炸后的生存能力，最初的改进包括对现有军用车辆的改造，之后是专门设计车辆的配置（抗地雷伏击，mine-resistant ambush protected，MRAP），特别设计为可以承受较大的爆炸力（图 4）。虽然缺乏确定性的数据，但在 MRAP 车辆内的人 IED 相关死亡率似乎有显著下降（高达 90%）。可以说，在 OIF / OEF 战场上与改善生存同等重要的因素就是对装备和训练军队第一反应人员和医疗护送人员的大量投资（military first responders and medical evacuation，MEDEVAC）。战斗损伤护理技术（Tactical Combat Casualty Care，TCCC）课程是广泛应用的平民院前创伤护理课程在军队中的改编版，并提供旨在最大限度提高战场生存的现实性的和最新的培训和信息。与大多数平民机构不同，医务兵必须在恶劣的环境中提供初始的管理，并经常在直接或间接的敌军火力的攻击下进行。TCCC 课程概述了院前急救的 3 个原则和重点：①火力攻击下护理；②野战护理战术；③战术疏散护理，如表 3 所示。与平民创伤的 ABC（气道、呼吸、循环）相区分，培训医务兵时，优先事项是控制出血（C），然后才是气道和呼吸问题。

对战场上的死亡和可预防的死亡分析，可以指导快速培训，使军队第一反应人员有更多的信息。在冲突的早期阶段，最重要的措施之一是广泛

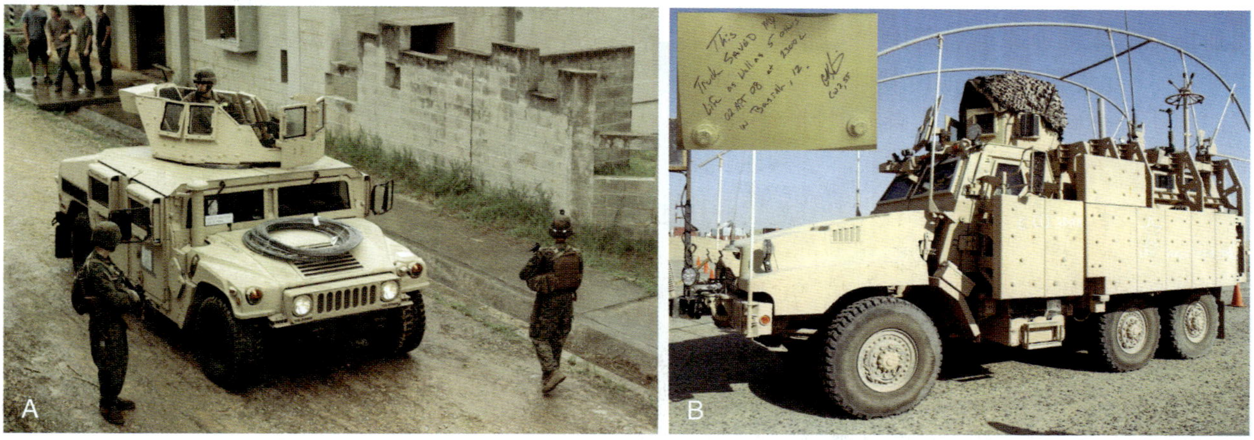

图 4　改进军用车辆，提高炸药爆炸生存率：**A**，增强（“装甲”）当前车辆，如高机动多用途轮式车辆（HMMWV 或“悍马”）。**B**，配备新设计的防地雷伏击车（MRAP）。插入物显示的是 MRAP 侧板写的题词，MRAP 受到简易爆炸装置袭击，但无乘客受伤（*Courtesy of U.S. Department of Defense.*）

配发人工四肢止血带，目前每名士兵都携带自己的止血带，随时可用，如果需要即可使用（图 5）。最近，用于控制“连接”部位出血（腋下和腹股沟）的设备已开发成功并配发。这些连接部位的止血带的早期研究结果显示其很有前景，特别是对腹股沟伤口或膝上截肢。战地医疗中，除了标准的纱布敷料外，医务兵还首次配备了先进的止血敷料产品，包括 HemCon 绷带（Hemcon 医疗科技公司，Portland，Ore.）、颗粒剂 QuikClot（Z 药物公司，Wallingford，Conn.）。随后，新一代的高岭土涂布纱布卷（作战纱布，Z 药物公司）得到了广泛应用，是当前 TCCC 推荐的止血敷料。除了作战纱布外，2014 年，另外有两个壳聚糖为基础的敷料也被批准使用。目前的研究重点是开发下一代止血敷料，包含活性凝血因子和先进的生物材料，甚至对严重中毒和凝血功能障碍者都有效。其他装备和变化包括应用较长的大孔针的胸廓造口术导管（3.25 英寸）、骨内通路设备、自主式低温预防和管理装备（hypothermia provention and management kits，HPMK）。根据当代战地医疗经验，院前复苏也有显著改变，重点是低容量初始复苏，避免大量晶体，对于有休克证据者早期使用血液制品。如果休克快速评估（精神状态和桡动脉脉搏）正常，则无须给予液体。如果异常，当前 TCCC 选择的液体治疗为静脉推注 500 ml Hextend（6% 羟乙基淀粉）。

虽然军方使用各种车辆运送一线伤员，伊拉克和阿富汗的绝大多数 MEDEVAC 由旋转翼飞机执行，通常使用黑鹰直升机（图 6）。虽然各个军事服务之间确切的医务人员和 MEDEVAC 人员培训的差别很大，但有共同的任务重点：患者快速评估、持续院前急救和复苏、尽快运送到 2 级或 3 级机构。在执行这些任务中常见的挑战包括敌军的火力袭击、热和噪声、肮脏、充满灰尘的环境、在低照明条件下或停电时进行手术（尤其是在夜间）、同时护理多个伤员、飞行时实施高级护理或手术。目前的措施正在寻找减轻这些限制性因素的方法，包括试点项目评估下述措施的影响：配备先进技术医务人员（重症护理护士、医生、外科医生）、配备复苏物品（血液制品，快速输液器），以及由 MEDEVAC 人员进行监督、“黄金时间”提供其他高级救助。

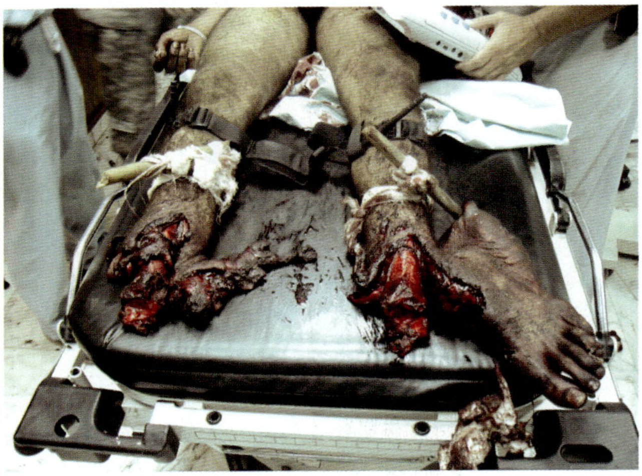

图 5　战地医疗中简易爆炸装置爆炸受伤后双腿应用止血带

表 3　战地创伤的院前护理和相关优先的三个阶段

火力攻击下护理	还击与掩护，如果可能，直接伤员还击 移动伤员至掩护处，如果伤员清醒、有反应则直接自救 撤离燃烧的车辆或建筑物 对危及生命的外部出血使用压力或止血带止血
野战护理战术	如果精神状态改变，解除伤亡人员武装 开放气道，如有必要，使用环甲膜切开术 用 3.25 英寸的导管对张力性气胸减压，包扎胸部开放性伤口 用止血带控制出血，如需要使用作战纱布 如果休克给予 500 ml Hextend，否则停止输液 镇痛、抗生素、局部覆盖敷料
战术疏散护理	如前所述评估气道和呼吸 如果胸腔穿刺术通气不足或预期需要长时间运送，建立胸管 评估控制出血、暴露情况和记录止血带使用时间 / 日期 如果持续休克，给予 500 ml Hextend，之后如果有血液制品，给予血液制品 通过除去湿衣物、应用低温防护设备，防止低温 如果需要，根据临床实践指南开始烧伤复苏 准备伤员运送，完成院前文档记录

分捡和立即治疗

战地医疗情况下，快速、准确、有组织的分流的重要性怎样强调都不为过，尤其是在大规模伤亡情况下（mass casualty，MASCAL）。前线战地医疗的标志是救助严重受限，因此资源和人员必须用在

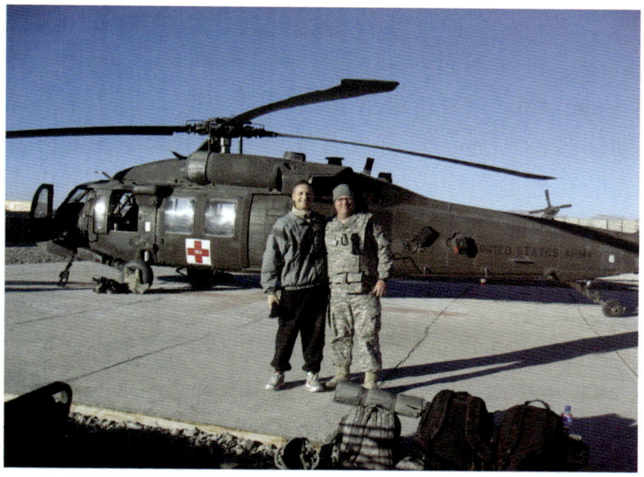

图 6　伊拉克和阿富汗黑鹰直升机用于承担大多数医疗疏散和患者运输任务（该章作者 Matthew Martin 和 Brian Eastridge 在阿富汗前方作战基地加兹尼）

表 4　战地医疗大量伤员救治政策

根据需要，分拣"干预备选伤员"至单独区域，提供舒适护理
首先控制出血，然后管理气道和呼吸
不要去除任何止血带，直到已排除其他危及生命的损伤
唯一一个紧急影像学检查通常是 X 线胸片，在完成所有 X 线胸片后才行四肢影像学检查
大多数实验室检测都没有必要，但在抵达时获得血型和交叉配型的资料很关键
优先考虑紧急 CT 扫描（通常为头部），推迟所有非紧急扫描
不稳定的伤者几乎都归于 OR，很少需要检查
在 MASCAL 时无紧急开胸手术，对有生命体征的伤者进行干预
准备分拣那些错误分拣的或临床恶化的伤者
MASCAL 后，所有相关人员开会进行事后回顾总结

CT，计算机断层扫描；ED，急诊科；MASCAL，大规模伤亡；OR，手术室

刀刃上，以期最优化患者的治疗效果和医疗单位持续救助的能力。在创伤医疗单位，高级分拣官员应该是一个经验丰富的人员，通常最好由外科医生或急救医生担任。一个经常被忽视的原则是，在分拣的第一步要评估当前的救治能力和供应情况，这将会大大影响分拣的决定。分拣是一个动态过程，涉及排序、分类和持续重新评估可用的资源，将需求和干预后伤员生存可能性进行平衡。那些低生存可能，或与分类为安全伤员相比需要更多资源者，应归类为干预备选伤员，其余则分拣为立即治疗或延迟救治。

并不仅仅在一开始时需要分拣，在 MASCAL 情况下，整个急性救治期间都要持续分拣。获取影像学和实验室研究结果通常会限制分拣速度，可以通过建立简单的方案和基本规则克服（表 4）。制订详细的 MASCAL 计划，结合演练，是减少和控制这些事件相关的不可避免的混乱的最佳方法。出血仍是前线医院早期死亡的最常见的原因，所以紧急救治的重点要始于控制持续出血、快速识别隐匿出血源，结合针对恢复止血系统以及器官灌注的复苏策略（见下一节）。

战场伤亡中可预防的死亡和疾病的最常见原因之一是手术干预延误，一般源自将标准的民用钝性创伤经验应用于这个独特的群体。战斗中可预防的源于出血的可预防的死亡中大约 2/3 是近端出血（腹股沟、腋下）或内出血（只能通过立即行综合手术治疗）。延误的常见原因包括制度层面的因素（运输时间、手术室可用性以及人员、行政流程）。这些可能无法改变，但更常见的原因是医生层面的因素，提示这些流程和质量可以作为目标加以改进。这些因素包括无法识别隐匿性出血部位或休克、不必要的和耗时的检验或程序、延误诊断和影像学检查、术前长时间复苏以"稳定"患者。这些措施大部分都没有必要或不紧急，可安全地推迟，而其余的（如气管插管、放置中心导管、输液）可以在手术室外科手术时进行。事实上，战斗时，院内死亡中 80% 是在抵达医院后 1 h 内发生的。因此早期和有效地对重点伤者排序、即刻给予救治十分关键。

损伤控制复苏和大量输血

过去对出血伤者标准的初始创伤复苏策略为早期给予大量晶体液，之后输注冷藏 PRBCs 产品。由于对这一战略的不良影响的认识增加，如容量负荷增加、免疫功能失衡、代谢紊乱、诱发或加重凝血功能障碍，促进医生开始搜寻更好的替代方案。过去十年中，战地创伤救治领域一个获得广泛称赞和讨论的进展一直是复苏策略的彻底改变，现在称为损伤控制复苏（damage control resuscitation，DCR）。这一策略的核心原则是用红细胞、血浆、血小板和凝血因子均衡复苏替代损失的血液。可用新鲜全血或成分血液治疗，包括 PRBCs、新鲜冰冻或解冻血浆和血小板。各类成分的最佳比例仍在研究和讨论，当前的实践操作中目标配比为 1∶1∶1，从最初救治持续到早期复苏期。虽然这一概念尚无 1 级证据，多个病例系列提示，DCR 在止血和总生存率方面有显著获益。DCR 已将战场损伤大量输血后的死亡率从 40% 降低到小于 20%。比成分的准确配比更重要的是，要坚持早期和积极地均衡止血复苏，结合避免大量输注晶体液和允许相对低血压，直到最终确定性出血得到控制。

唯一能常规和可靠地提供合格 DCR 的方法是，制订全面和机构特异的大量输血方案。通过自动提供输液包，而不是单成分进行初始复苏，使得坚持 1∶1∶1 的配比更容易操作。例如，在巴格达战斗支援医院，其方案为初始输液包包含 4 单位 PRBCs 和 4 单位新鲜冰冻血浆（fresh frozen plasma，FFP）。之后给予“大输液包”，各含 6 单位 FFP 和 PRBCs 和一个成分输血血小板包。此外，医疗人员已经越来越认识到长期储存血液产品相关的不良影响（“储存损伤”），最大限度地减少从采集和存储到使用的时间可能有临床效益。因此，目前战地指南推荐大量输血时使用存储时间最短的血液制品，也称为“后进先出法则”。然而，成分血液制品的可用性差异很大，很大程度上取决于部队作战地点和人员规模，以及供应链再次供应的可靠性。这会严重限制均衡复苏的能力，特别是在条件更差的地点或战斗早期。这些限制因素可通过建立“移动血库”来解决，当地预先筛查过的献血者库，可随需要而激活。我们的战地医疗经验提示，使用新鲜全血一直安全有效，可以延长 DCR 至更前方和更恶劣的环境，其效果相当于或优于标准成分血液治疗。

启动 DCR 和大量输血一直有很大争议，没有一个简单的规则或标准可以完全替代经验和临床判断。已经确定多个因素可以预测战斗中大量输血的需要，包括低血压、精神状态改变、碱缺失增加、异常凝血酶原时间、低血红蛋白、损伤模式识别，如多处损毁伤 / 截肢。如果存在以上因素之一，那么大多数情况下可以开始大量输血。我们发现的一个很有价值的简单规则是，在爆炸伤后避免复苏不充分或延迟的方法是，多处损毁伤 / 截肢者立即给予 4 单位 PRBCs 和 4 单位 FFP。

给予重组活化凝血因子Ⅶ（Novoseven，Novo Nordisk）在战地医疗救治的最初几年广泛用作大量输血的一种辅助手段，但之后由于没有有关疗效的数据以及有前期血栓形成的潜在安全问题，不再使用。目前对使用抗纤维蛋白溶解剂、氨甲环酸（tranexamic aeid，TXA）有浓厚兴趣，其已在平民创伤救治中显示具有死亡率方面的获益。2 个已发表的在战地医疗救治中使用 TXA 的分析（军事应用 TXA 的创伤急救复苏研究 1 和 2）显示，所有患者都有明显的死亡率获益，需要更大量血液制品的患者获益更大。现在联合战区创伤系统临床实践指南（Clinical Practice Guidelines，CPG）已经将 TXA 纳入 DCR 中（静脉推注 1 g 后静脉滴注 1 g，8 h），正在进行的研究将有助于澄清最佳适应证问题，以及应用时机和剂量问题。另一个正在进行的令人振奋的研究主题是“冰冻干”血浆的应用，简单稀释后即可应用。这可以克服目前的标准 FFP 储存和时间延迟问题。

战地手术

全面介绍战地创伤外科的原则和技术不是本章内容，但现在有一些优秀的书籍有这些内容的详细说明（见建议阅读书目列表）。虽然大多数战斗创伤中使用的外科技术与平民相同，如何以及何时应用的原则却是独一无二的。如同前面强调的，战场创伤患者多数会需要一些类型的手术治疗，接受多体腔和多系统手术比平民创伤更频繁。应尽一切努力减少严重伤者不必要的手术延误，某些情况下，患者最好采用“直接到手术室”的分捡，完全绕过典型的急诊部门评估。

往往不能进行专科咨询或患者转移，所以战地外科医生必须一开始就要精通从头到脚的初始手术管理。这包括一些救治程序，如紧急开颅术、复杂的面部重建、心脏或肺修复、骨折 / 截肢管理。在战地医疗救治以外的时间创伤外科医生很少或从来没有进行过这些操作。所有军事服务机构已经开始配备前培训，以提供普通创伤进修培训和专业技术的实际操作，如基本的颅骨切开术 / 颅骨切除术、骨折外固定、血管修复等。此外，军医已广泛应用先进技术，如视频会议和互联网教学，以提高他们的能力，提供远程“虚拟”专科咨询，甚至将服务提供至远至前线的医院。

外科手术的性质和类型在很大程度上取决于救治医院的位置和能力。如表 1 所述，一个前线的 2 级医院主要执行简单的损伤控制程序，以拯救生命和保存肢体，迅速转移到更强的医院。而3级医院有全面的人员配备和保留患者能力，能提供初始急诊手术以及更复杂的确定性手术或重建手术。在任何位置，处理急性创伤手术都适用同样的基本原则。损伤控制的方法应该是默认的，最好在酸中毒恶化、低体温、凝血功能障碍前就给予救治。初始手术的目标应至少包括：①控制出血；②控制任何的消化道漏出至呼吸道；③为污染或坏死组织提供初始清洗和清创术。之后快速临时关闭伤口或应用敷料，制订确定性手术计划。除了帮助达到生理稳定外，在有更多的伤亡人员等候时，这种方法可以减少无价的手术室占用时间、保留稀缺的资源（设备和人员）。

减少手术时间的目标常常与战地损伤的多系统性质和严重程度相冲突。在平民医院，这些患者通常由几组不同的外科医生共同管理，按顺序手术，这样患者的手术时间很长。在战地医院，如果资源许可，可以同时进行这些手术，多学科外科医生同时在不同身体部位手术（图7）。所有受累或受伤部位要准备并铺单到相同的手术视野，允许同时干预。这样可以观察所有受伤部位，避免术中的隐匿性出血。这种情况下，在60 min内3支团队同时完成损伤控制手术、损毁肢体的清创和固定和面部损伤的修复。在战场损伤控制中最重要的基本原则之一是将伤口暴露（躯干和四肢），避免初次手术时进行闭合。这样在高一级医院可以很容易再次手术和检查，对经常存在大量污染的伤口再次清创，避免感染或隔室综合征（特别是在长时间运送期间）。

战场创伤的另外一个独特因素，特别是爆炸或爆破伤，就是初始的伤口组织损伤和自然污染的程度。大量软组织丢失、损伤或随后的坏死可形成大而深的空洞，难以覆盖或闭合。此外，还有各种来源的显著的伤口污染，往往因爆炸力深入创面及邻近组织。通常包括灰尘、碎片、织物、子弹或来自爆炸装置和服装或制服和设备的金属碎片。较大的金属物体，如球轴承或螺母和螺栓一般见于爆炸装置组件（如“自杀背心”）或被IED袭击的车辆中的乘客。骨头碎片可出现于没有任何可识别表现的骨折中，可能是自杀式袭击者或附近受害者的组织碎片被冲击入伤口中（“生物弹片”）（图8A）。最后，所有战场的医务工作者必须要认识到在四肢或躯干伤口内未引爆的爆炸物的潜在问题（图8B和8C）。这些问题不仅给患者带来严重风险，而且对医护人员和其他附近的患者也构成了严重风险。一旦确定了这些患者，应将他们隔离开，必要的治疗人员应充分穿戴保护装备，并在爆炸专家和军械技师的帮助下，在受控条件下加快去除爆炸物。手术切除应包括避免金属设备与之接触，避免使用任何烧灼术和超声设备。

与平民创伤一样，战场创伤控制通常包括多阶段操作，按照设定的时间间隔处理。明显的差别是现代战争中，这些处理可在遍布三大洲的机构，由多个不同医生进行，通常在初始损伤后的48～72 h内完成。这就要求军事服务、医疗设施、医生和航空医疗运输之间的密切协调，需要大量努力才可成

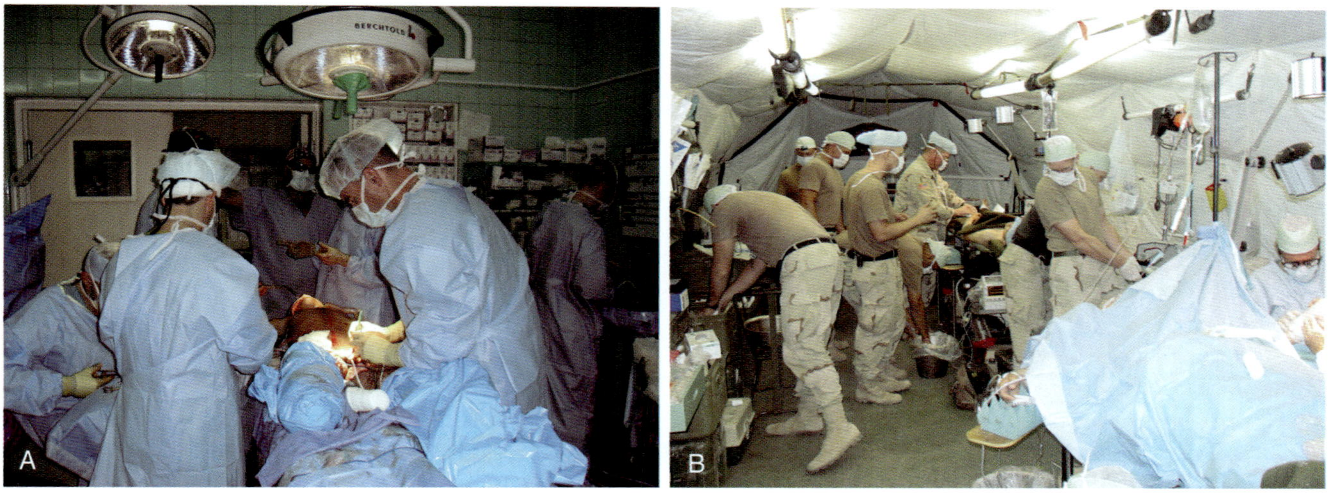

图7　战场创伤的团队管理方法。**A**，多个手术团队在战斗支援医院同时对受伤儿童的躯干、手臂和腿手术。**B**，一个前线外科手术团队手术台头对头并排，这样一个麻醉师可同时监测两台手术患者

功。因此，这些不同的元素，现在成为一个统一的系统。它们从战场上受伤地点开始，到最后在美国的恢复和康复，提供连续的高水平的手术和关键救治。

术后护理和运送

在管理战斗伤亡中，对于伤员转移和后续服务的计划的重要性怎样强调都不为过。由于床位空间和资源有限，任何延误伤员转移或转移过程出现的故障都可妨碍对患者救治的能力。必须要考虑到，这些医院不仅仅救治美国军人，也救治联盟军人、地方军人、承包商和平民伤亡，每一个都有自己的疏散或处置链。大多数医院的典型的患者中，至少有50%的患者是当地国家部队或平民，他们的处置将需要当地医疗设施和运送部门的密切协调。创造一些特定的职位、雇佣说双语的当地居民、进行一些医学培训以协调处置，会使这个过程变得非常流畅。

术后护理的重点通常集中在持续复苏、稳定和转移准备。与平民医院一样，军方已经认识到内科和外科重症护理人员来扩充战地医院的重要性。在快节奏手术时这特别重要，手术人员将忙于急诊、手术，不能充分重视术后ICU护理。然而，护理仍然是团队工作，需要基层外科医生和ICU之间的协调合作。大多数2级医院有非常有限的术后保留能力（1～2个病床）和ICU级别设备。3级医院一般有更强的能力，包括ICU、ICU护士和ICU人员、现代呼吸机、输液泵、压缩机等。一些先进的ICU治疗，如血液透析和部分通气模式［高频通气、体外膜肺氧合（extracorporeal membrane oxygenation，ECMO）］并非在手术室常规配备，因此出现这些治

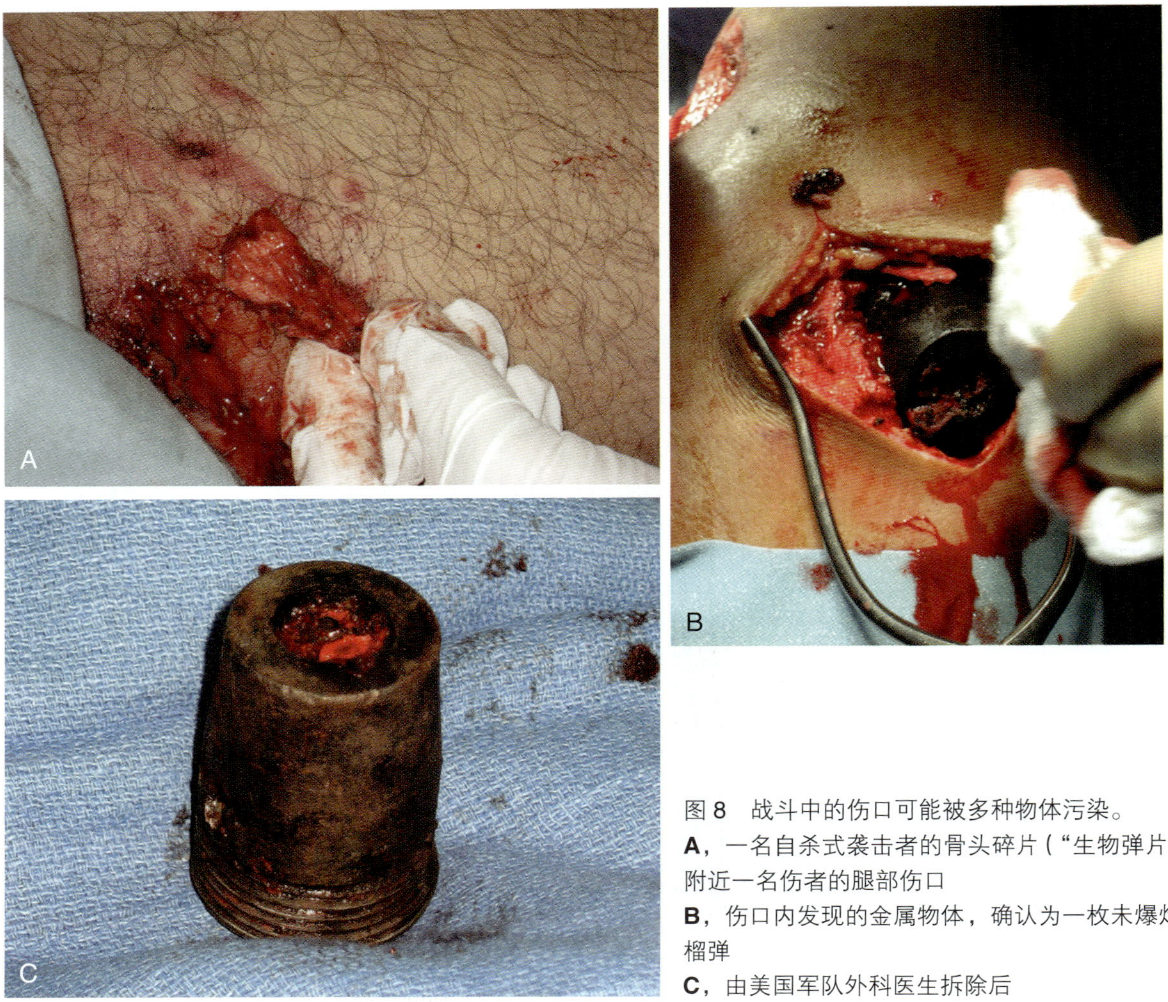

图8 战斗中的伤口可能被多种物体污染。

A，一名自杀式袭击者的骨头碎片（“生物弹片”）被冲击进入附近一名伤者的腿部伤口

B，伤口内发现的金属物体，确认为一枚未爆炸的火箭助推手榴弹

C，由美国军队外科医生拆除后

疗的任何适应证时，应立即安排转移。

将严重伤员疏散到高级别救治单位的准备往往难以决择，因为要考虑到疏散到高级别救治单位的运送过程中有潜在恶化可能性和其他问题。通常伤员在重大损伤控制手术后几个小时内进行疏散，并保持持续复苏。因此须制订伤员疏散准备的标准方案，包括飞行前医嘱和清单。此外，已经开发了针对机上人员，包括医学工作者、护士和内科医生的专业培训课程，以增强在旋转翼和固定翼飞机运送期间提供连续的、高水平护理的能力。转移患者前应彻底检查其生命体征、实验室结果，仔细检查所有手术部位和敷料。如果预期运送时间很长，则根据方案在撤离前最后冲洗或换敷料。最后一次换敷料或冲洗时间和日期都须记录在敷料上，所有现有的病历资料的完整复印件应与患者一起运送。现在由于互联网电子病历系统的应用，这一点得到了加强，大幅度改进了患者信息的流动和护理的协调。然而，有时前线最有效的病历是低技术条件下手写的笔记，带颜色标记（图 9）。

跨越长距离提供无缝高级创伤护理系统中的一个重要措施就是创立美国空军急救空运队（Critical Care Air Transport Team，CCATT）项目。CCATT 由内科医生领导，包括受过重症监护和空中救治培训的专科医生，能够在各种的固定翼飞机上手术。他们具备相应装备，接受过相应培训，可提供先进的呼吸机、监控和输液治疗，包括血液制品和压缩机。

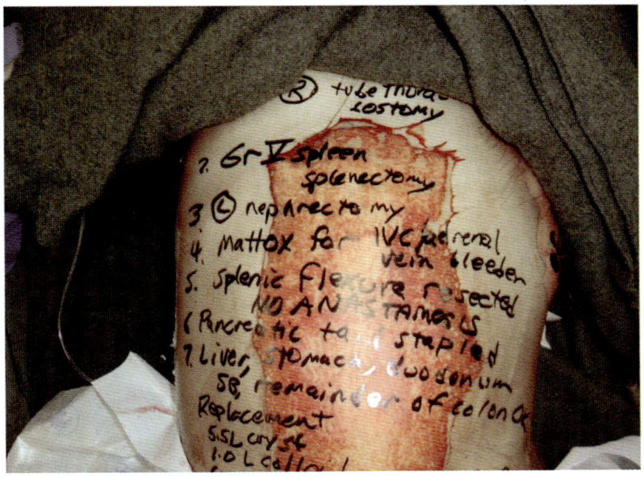

图 9　在前线外科手术机构（2 级）接受损伤控制性剖腹探查术的患者，腹部敷料上的手写手术报告，然后转移到伊拉克一个战斗支援医院（3 级）

特殊情况下，可以进一步扩大其救治范围，可实现先进的 ICU 治疗，如血液透析、高频通气，从战区 3 级医院至 4 级或 5 级医院进行确定性治疗的运送期间甚至可提供 ECMO。目前的冲突中，主要是从伊拉克（Balad）和阿富汗（Bagram）空军战区医院运送到德国 Landstuhl 地区医疗中心，然后运至美国。

协调与质量改进措施

行政监督和审查职能对完整和成熟的平民创伤系统至关重要，但在前线严苛、忙乱的战斗医疗单位往往不属于高优先级。现代冲突的一个标志是，已实现和民间 1 级创伤中心类似的系统流程和质量改进。JTTS 具有强大的数据收集能力，可将创伤救治的协调中心化，并全面实行质量改进措施。JTTS 主任一般由高级创伤外科医生担任，为轮岗制，负责全战区范围的外伤手术的监督。

创伤协调员护士由 JTTS 主任领导，已在所有前线 3 级医院配备。他们前瞻性搜集数据并录入 JTTR（目前含 25 000 多个美国军方病例数据），并监督相关医院的质量改进流程。目前有 48 个已经完成的专门的战地 JTTS CPGs，涵盖各种各样的临床主题，可协助部署医疗提供者（http://www.usaisr. amedd.army.mil/clinical_practice_guidelines.html）。已经在单位级别召开教育和有关疾病和死亡的会议，经常授予继续医学教育学分。整个系统中统一护理的最重要一方面是，鼓励 JTTS 工作人员主导每周视频会议，并通过它进行沟通和实时反馈。视频会议参会者来自各个级别的医院，从创伤地点到 5 级和康复机构。会议对每个患者进行审查，各级患者的救治情况由直接参与的人进行介绍。他们对所有感兴趣的患者的目前状态进行更新，积极讨论创伤护理的积极和消极内容。

数据收集和应用对于研究和质量改进项目都至关重要，因此创建了人员配备齐全的战场伤亡研究团队（Deployment Combat Casually Research Team，DCCRT），团队由科学家级别的医生担任主任，包括护理研究专家、科学顾问和行政支持人员。这些人员被配备到手术室，支持开展各方面的相关研究，包括促进制订和批准方案、协助数据收集、统计和分析咨询，保护人类研究对象的审查，并协助准备摘要或手稿以备报告。除了促进科学认识外，这一措施促进了战地医疗中由众多的实时数据驱动的改变与改进，这无疑对并发症发生率、病死率和战地医疗质量产生了巨大影响。

结论

涵盖现代军事医学各个方面的内容仅仅一章是难以涵盖的，所以我们试图对过去十年中战地医疗的一些关键点和发展进行了总结（图 10）。独特的致伤机制和各种严峻环境中手术时的问题都需要专业技能和知识基础。这是独立的学科，但又是标准平民创伤实践的补充。战争中少有的几个积极方面之一就是创伤护理相关的进步，我们必须继续最大化和应用这些在高额人力成本上产生的经验教训。

十大战地创伤经验教训

1. 患者死于 ER，和
2. 患者死于 CT 扫描机上；
3. 因此，低血压创伤患者应尽快手术。
4. 大部分爆炸伤或射击伤患者需要血液制品，而不是晶体液。
5. 对于血肉模糊的四肢和截肢，每个肢体给予一个红色编码（4 个 PRBCs + 4 个 FFP）。
6. 患者在极端情况下要在快速序列插管期间给予代码，尽可能在手术室准备插管并插管（不在 ER）。
7. 医院可以在数小时内病床就从空到占满，不要被缓慢的流程拖延。
8. 此流程不是连续护理，是吞吐式护理。如果 ICU 或病房已满，你就将伤者送入。
9. 对于 MASCAL 要妥善分拣、确定优先事项——由门口出发，包括进行 X 线片、实验室检查和处置。
10. 没有个人项目！这会阻塞系统、浪费资源、激怒其他人，见第 8 条

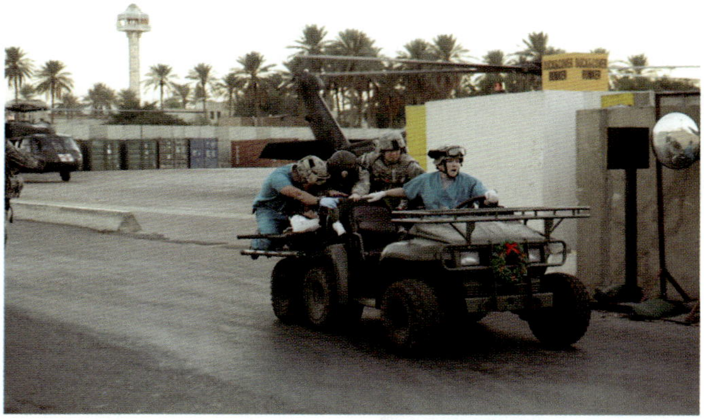

转自由伊拉克巴格达的 Ibn Sina 医院的美国陆军外科创伤医生团队撰写并不断更新的“*经验之谈*”（2008 年 1 月版本）

图 10 十大战场创伤经验教训。ASAP，尽快；CT；计算机断层扫描；ER，急诊室；FFP，新鲜冰冻血浆；IC，重症监护；MASCAL，大量伤亡；OR；手术室；PRBC。浓缩红细胞 *(From “The Volume of Experience” [January 2008 edition], a document written and continuously updated by U.S. Army trauma surgeons working at the Ibn Sina Hospital, Baghdad, Iraq.)*

第 13 章　重症监护Ⅰ：器官衰竭的处理与支持技术

心脏血流动力学：肺动脉导管及其读数意义

D. Dante Yeh, Mitchell J. Cohen 和 Robert C. Mackersie 著
朱凤雪　李　纾 译

肺动脉导管（pulmonary artery catheter，PAC）充满着神秘的色彩。自从 20 世纪 70 年代被发明以来，就饱受争议。它因能够提供通过其他方法难以获得的生理数据而受到称赞，同时，也有人认为它是一项无用的并具有潜在危害的有创性监测。很少的数据支持肺动脉导管的持续使用，同时部分数据支持避免应用它。尽管肺动脉导管的临床应用与安全性有很大的争议，但我们必须承认它是一项重要的 ICU 有创监测方法。本章节将回顾右心置管历史，检验置管的基本方法、数据的收集、解释以及故障的排除，探讨支持和反对肺动脉导管化的以及危重外科患者的复苏决定的临床证据。

历史争议

肺小动脉导管自 20 世纪 60 年代末诞生以来，很快在 1970 年被批准应用于临床，随之被纳入到重症监护医疗设备中。截止到 1999 年，美国每年大概平均卖出并使用 15 万根肺动脉导管。美国食品药品监督管理局（Food and Drug Administration，FDA）将其列为第 2 类设施，并严格控制以确保安全性及有效性。对其使用的争议和辩论仍在持续，其从未被认为是一项救命设施，从而它被免除许可，仍需要评估。

随着不断改进，肺动脉导管作为一种监测设施被更多地使用和认可。确实，肺动脉导管的普及与重症医学作为一项学科的出现是密不可分的，并作为重症监护医生的一项重要工具。随着几年的使用，我们发现只有很少的数据能够证实它的优点，因此，在 20 世纪 80 年代末，几篇论文提出了对其广泛应用和安全性的担忧。Gore 等对 3 000 名急性心肌梗死患者及其预后与肺动脉导管置入之间的关系进行了研究。报告指出对低血压患者进行 PAC 置入有较高的死亡率（42% vs.32%）。同样，在充血性心力衰竭小组中置管患者死亡率为 44%，而不置管患者死亡率 25%，置管组死亡率更高。须进一步指出的是，置管患者住院时间变长。随后，几项观察和回顾性研究很快也得出相似的结果。许多重症监护医生并不重视这些试验研究，因为病情越危重的患者，肺动脉置管越常见，这个因素与死亡率有关。在 1990 年，加拿大研究人员拟对置入 PAC 的重症监护患者进行前瞻性研究，该项研究是历史首次。由于 35% 的排除率以及许多临床医生拒绝对自己的患者进行随机研究，该项研究以失败告终。由于缺乏 PAC 临床共识，PAC 一直得以持续广泛使用直到 1996 年辩论再次燃起。Connors 等在 5 735 名 ICU 患者中对 PAC 使用进行调查研究，仔细比较置管组与对照组两组之间疾病的严重性以及其他混杂变量。最终，该项研究指出 PAC 置管增加了患者 30 天死亡率、平均费用以及 ICU 治疗时间。亚组分析不能明确指出某组患者从 PAC 置管中获益。

由于这些相似的研究结果以及美国医学协会杂志对此问题的关注，Bone 和 Dalen 要求国家心脏、肺和血液研究所对 PAC 的有效性、安全性进行前瞻性随机临床试验。他们再次引发了大的争议，以至于 FDA 发出停止使用 PAC 的通知直到一项合理的临床试验测定其安全性。为处理此次暂停呼吁，国

家心脏、肺和血液研究所与危重症医学学会共识会议在1997年举行。同年，在此次共识会议之后，发表了肺动脉导管共识声明。该声明引用足够的Ⅳ级证据支持PAC导管在心肌梗死和创伤患者组中的潜在优点，故不支持停止使用PAC，但承认需要合适的临床试验测定使用和安全性。NHLBI会议得出相似的结论。之后，虽然进行了很多试验，但由于有限的患者数目以及低随机化率，增加了试验Ⅱ型错误和选择性偏倚的可能性。此外，有良好证据支持的协议和治疗方案很少得到使用。

2003年加拿大一项研究小组发布了首次关于PAC的前瞻性随机研究，该项研究因所纳入患者数量大，故结果有很强的权威性和统计效能。在该项研究中，1 994名患者被随机分到PAC组和无PAC组。研究人员发现两组患者在住院期间生存率及6和12个月生存率上无差异。但是，肺栓塞事件的发生数量增多，PAC组8名，无PAC组0名。研究得出老年高危手术患者并未从PAC中获益的结论。尽管该项研究很重要，因为它是首次随机化一个较大的患者队列，但随机化率仍较低，仅为52%。此外，该项研究中纳入了不成比例的老年危重患者，并将年轻的创伤和脓毒症患者排除在外。其他试验得出相似的混合结果。最近Shah等对1985–2005年间13项随机临床试验研究进行了meta分析，该项研究使用随机效应模型对5 051名患者进行分析比较，结果PAC组与无PAC组在死亡、住院时长和收缩血管作用上无明显差异。

2006年Cochrane Collaboration对所有比较有（无）PAC治疗的成年人随机对照试验进行了meta分析。重要的是，12项被纳入的试验中，只有1项试验指出护理患者中的系统性差异与PAC存在与否无关。然而，研究者指出了每项研究的偏倚来源：分配偏倚、实施偏倚、随访偏倚以及测量偏倚。绝大多数手术试验组患者接受了常规大手术，大多数试验是单一的、小中心的。仅有1项试验具有权威性。最后得出结论没有证据表明患者可从PAC获益或受损。

同年，液体和导管治疗试验发表，在此试验中，ARDS试验人员随机使用PAC和中心静脉置管对1 000名急性肺损伤/急性呼吸窘迫综合征患者进行管理。此外，同时随机使用保守和自由液体管理策略对患者进行液体管理。创伤患者仅占总患者的不足10%。这个试验的优势就是详细的、明确的管理策略，确保36个中心的标准化治疗。此外，对所有人员进行了关于PAC所获得的数据的测量和解释的培训，同时对压力描记图也进行了集中审查。与其他试验类似，该研究的显著特点是低纳入率，91%的筛查患者被排除在外。该项研究发现，PAC引导下的治疗方案没有改善患者生存，同时导管相关并发症（主要是心律失常）发生率升高了1倍。PAC引起的严重并发症很少见，也没有发现置管相关的死亡。

截至目前，尚无随机前瞻性研究证实危重伤患者可从PA置管中整体获益。最近有些证据显示伤者可从PAC中获益，但仅限于创伤患者。一项来自国家创伤数据库的超过53 000名患者的回顾性研究显示PAC可降低老年患者和损伤严重度评分较高患者的死亡率。总的来讲，PAC可使碱缺失大于11的严重休克患者、损伤评分大于25分的患者，以及年龄大于61岁的患者受益。该项大规模非随机队列研究是首次也是唯一一次显示危重创伤患者可从PAC中获益。

对PAC的使用和研究造成混乱的偏倚是影响患者使用PAC的不同因素。2000年，Rapoport等对PAC使用特点进行了全方位的观察，该研究小组对10 217名来自美国34家的ICU患者进行回顾性研究，指出全职ICU员工与PAC使用的可能性降低有关。导管的使用与白人和私人保险有关。外科监护的患者留置PAC的可能性是其他患者的2倍。该项研究揭示了目前PAC缺少既定的协议和关于PAC放置的出版偏倚的存在。

另一个影响PAC研究的因素是没有质量控制措施以确保准确解释PAC所测得数据。一项对重症监护从业人员的研究显示，47%的医生不能从明确标出呼吸末期的压力描记图上准确确定肺动脉闭塞压（pulmonary artery occlusion pressure，PAOP）。更令人担忧的是，61%的患者竟不能识别明确的指示，此指示反映导管已经进入体循环中。另有研究指出"有经验的医生"通过波形分析预测PAOP摹图的准确性还不如扔一枚硬币。相似地，有研究指出仅有57.7%的重症监护护士可以准确的在清楚地压力描图上读出PAOP。鉴于逐渐增加的对不正确测量的担心、对数据不准确的解释、缺乏根据PAC数据指导操作的指南以及很少的PAC使患者受益的证据，人们对PAC使用的热衷逐渐消退并不惊奇。PAC使用率从1993年至2004年减少了65%。2004 — 2006年，PAC使用率降低超过了50%（图1-2）。使用率下降将会进一步扭曲风险/效益比，因为当前和以后的ICU医生会更容易在置管、解读以及合理应用PAC相关数据中犯错。

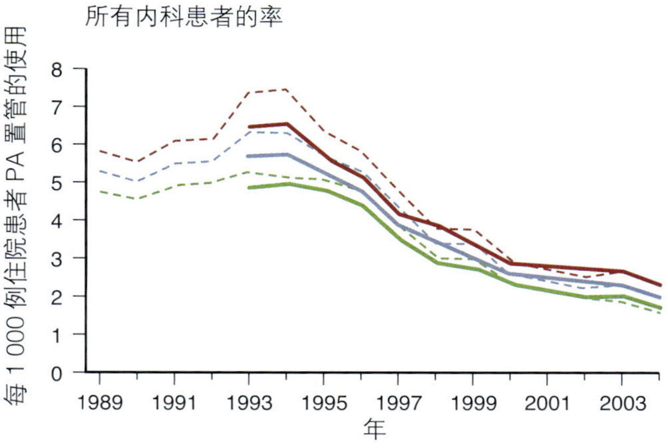

图 1 住院患者 PAC 使用率 *(From Wiener RS: Trends in the use of the pulmonary artery catheter in the United States, 1993-2004.* JAMA *298:423-429, 2007.)*

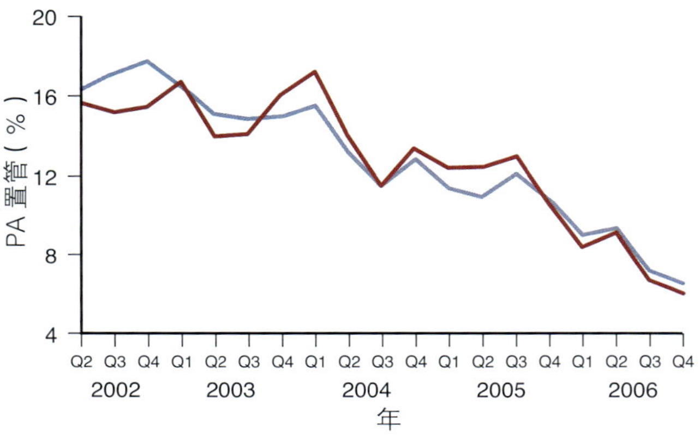

图 2 肺动脉置管率 *(From Koo KK, Sun JC, Zhou Q, et al: Pulmonary artery catheters: evolving rates and reasons for use.* Crit Care Med *39:1615–1618, 2011.)*

肺动脉导管使用和操作：构造及工作原理

PAC 全长 100 cm，外径为 7.5 F。通常 PAC 含有乳胶，因此对乳胶过敏的患者应多加留意，导管的外层有时会涂抹肝素或者抗生素涂层。外径 7.5 F 的导管内含有三腔。漂浮导管最顶端是肺动脉开口，用来测定肺动脉压力和抽吸混合静脉血。顶端附近有一个可容纳 1.5 ml 的气体的小球囊，它既可以促进漂浮导管使其进入肺动脉，又能阻塞肺动脉远端，测量 PAOP。另一开口位于距顶端 15 cm 处，可以用来滴注液体、血管活性物质及药物。在此开口附近是右心房 / 中心静脉压开口，该位置正好位于腔静脉与右心房连接处，用于测定中心静脉压。与附近的注射开口端类似，它也可作为液体和药物的滴注口。

PAC 在沿着开口进行测压及液体注入的同时，还结合了热线圈和远近端热敏电阻用来测定心排血量。通过测定近端与远端热敏电阻间的血液温度差来计算心排血量。传统上，我们向近端开口注入冷却液体，该液体的温度（已被血流缓慢加温）由导管顶端热敏电阻测得。使用本章节后面要讨论的公式，我们可以计算得出心排血量。现代的导管会在近端放置热线圈，它持续轻微加热血液，通过推测远近端温度差，持续对心排血量进行计算（我们会在此章节后面对心排血量监测进行更详细的讨论）。

置管的技巧和指南

导管置入时须通过 Cordis 导管的带垫圈的引导管导入。严格的无菌操作以减少感染发生率。我们通常在进行一次无菌准备及打开一次无菌装置后按顺序先后完成引导管和 PAC 的置入，这样可以防止引导管垫圈处的污染，预先放置引导管是必要的。然而，有时污染不可避免，并且 PAC 会沿着引导管的位置进行放置。在这样的情况下应对引导管及其周围的皮肤进行氯已定广泛洗浴消毒。任何情况下，我们都应行大范围的氯已定无菌准备和全面的无菌预防措施，包括衣物、帽子、口罩及无菌手套是必不可少的。很多研究已证实无菌操作中的任何疏忽会使感染率明显升高，操作前的预防措施已可使感染率降低甚至为零。另一个技巧是充分的准备。这些细节应着重强调，打开、准备和插入 PAC 导管会使导管、管道和转换器缓慢地穿过消毒和无菌的过渡区域。对大部分或全部病床进行无菌的准备可以方便操作并减少感染的发生。当引导管的管固定后，从准备包中取出肺动脉导管，护士或助手会对导管口进行连接并冲洗。此时，我们将对传感器进行连接、调零和测试。同时，对球囊也进行检查。放置导管鞘方便将来在非无菌条件下对导管进行进一步的调整。

操作者和助手间的不断沟通是非常必要的。当导管尖端通过引导管进入血管后，只有当球囊是膨胀的时候，才可以推送导管。相反，当球囊未充气时，才能撤回导管。俚语“浮动”的含义为导管随着血液流动漂浮前进。直接的推送可以导致血管损伤甚至穿孔。不断的交流如充气了和气瘪了，可以避免损伤，如血管、心脏和肺动脉破裂。

首先导管须插入 10 ~ 15 cm 长，这时允许球囊通过引导管。当导管尖顺利通过了引导管就可以把球囊充气，然后缓慢地推送导管，使导管在血管中变得松弛，进而可顺着血流向远端漂浮。成功放置 PAC 需要临床经验、插入长度合适以及对传感器监测的图像的仔细观察。当导管尖端进入血管后，首先测得的压力是中心静脉压（central venous pressure，CVP），这时导管深度至少有 15 ~ 25 cm，这与患者体型和穿刺点有密切关系。再前进 5 ~ 10 cm 时，导管进入右心房，这时传感器会记录特定的右心房波。当导管继续向前推送几厘米时，导管尖端通过三尖瓣（大约 30 cm），会监测到容易辨认的右心室压力峰。继续往前缓慢推送 5 ~ 10 cm，导管进入肺动脉内并很快被楔住，记录仪上检测到较扁的波形以及典型的楔形路径。

通常需要几次之后才能达到合适的楔入。当进入 35 ~ 45 cm 时，右心室波仍不明显或者当记录到心室波后前进 10 ~ 15 cm 后仍未测到楔形图像时，这时应抽瘪球囊把导管退至右心房或右心室。一旦测得可以明确导管位置的典型图像时，可以重新开始，再一次小心的插入和楔入。当导管插入肺动脉并被楔住时，便测得肺毛细血管楔压（pulmonary capillary wedge pressure，PCWP），此时球囊是压瘪的状态。导管固定在此位置，无菌罩前进包裹整个导管。通过 X 线胸片证实导管的位置。

在建立中心静脉通路、PAC 置管过程、球囊膨胀以及后续护理过程中会出现严重的并发症。建立中心静脉通路时的并发症（气胸、动脉穿刺）是所有置管过程中都会发生的，并不是 PAC 插入特有的。最常见的并发症是心律失常，通常出现在球囊膨胀、通过右心室的过程中，往往是一过性的、轻微的。其他更严重的并发症包括心脏穿孔、肺动脉破裂、心包压塞、持续右束支传导阻滞。导管打结是极其少见的（发生率低于 1%），尤其是在经验丰富的医生和现代的、柔软的导管情况下。血栓栓塞和导管感染也越来越少见，因为目前的导管是肝素化的，并且一旦无指征会及时拔出导管。

解释说明：它测量的是什么和它意味着什么？

初始警告和潜在的测量问题

虽然 PAC 提供了许多其他手段不可获得的数据，但是只有给予持续的关注和合适的解释才能使 PA 导管值得去冒险、投入时间和成本。如果没有合理的放置，所有获得的数据都是错误的，并且将导致错误的解释和不正确（可能有害）的干预。仔细注意 PAC 波形有助于确认导管放置。平均压下降和特征波形的出现证明进入了 PA。在进入 PA 时，看到三相波形，其反映心房和心室收缩。从 PA 中，导管的小心前进将楔住导管。

从 PAOP 和 CVP，我们开始压力 - 体积测量。一旦楔入或闭塞，膨胀的球囊防止来自右心室或近侧肺动脉的向前流动，并且仅允许转导导管尖端处的反向压。这个转导的楔压反映了从 PA 通过肺血管系统到左心房的连续流体柱。不受阻的血液继续通过二尖瓣进入（当打开时的）左心室，因此，

肺动脉 < 左心房 < 左心室 < 左心室舒张末期压

其中左心室舒张末期压为 LVEDP（left ventricle end-diastolic pressure）。需要重点关注的事情是只有当肺动脉和左心室之间存在连续的流体柱时，该关系才成立。对 PAOP 的不适当的解释常常发生在连续流体柱被中断或影响时。中断流体柱的实例包括二尖瓣疾病（狭窄或不全）和肺静脉阻塞。同时影响 PAOP 和左心室舒张末期容积（left ventricle end-diastolic volume，LVEDV）之间的关系是从压力测量外推体积的能力。由于肺毛细血管楔压（pulmonary capillary wedge pressure，PCWP）最终用来测量心室充盈（容积），因此须能够从压力可预测地外推容积，这仅在正常顺应性时才是可能的。实际上，LVEDP 仅在心、胸有正常顺应性时才近似 LVEDV。许多因素影响 PCWP 作为准确测量左心室充盈压力的能力。如前所述，LVEDP 和 LVEDV 之间的类比关系仅在心室通常是顺应性的情况下是准确的。在左心顺应性降低的情况下，例如心室肥大或缺血性心肌损伤，因与左心室压力 / 体积相联系，相应的 PCWP 将会升高，但是这是不准确的测量。虽然趋势分析可用于监测这些患者的液体复苏，但是创伤或脓毒症患者通常表现出快速变化的心脏顺应性，使得解释困难和可疑。实际上，多种动物模型显示了由损伤、复苏和炎症引起的心脏水肿的快速流动，所有这些都可以快速改变心室顺应性，并使 PAC 不能可靠地度量心脏充盈量。

除了适当楔入肺动脉和有正常顺应性的心脏，肺导管还必须放置在正确的肺区。为了使 PCWP 反映血管而不是肺泡压力，必须将导管放置在肺的西

区 3。这里 P_A>PV>PA，因此测量的肺静脉压反映血管压力而不是肺泡压力。如果导管在区域 1 中，P_A>PA>PV 或 $2P_A$>PA>PV，导管将反映肺泡压力而不是肺动脉压力。

来自通气（自发性或机械性）的不断变化的胸廓压力反映在 PAC 图形中。在正压通气患者中，应在呼气末当胸腔压力最接近 0 时测量 PCWP。如果患者自主呼吸，则是相反的。在自主呼吸的患者中，膨胀和吸入之间的压力是正常的，所以按照惯例，在吸气末时测量压力。直接监测和跟踪检查常常比依赖于自动收集显示的单个数字更好。在极端情况下，如在一个激越的患者或患者与呼吸机不同步的时候为获得一个有用的 PAWP 跟踪，短暂麻痹可能是必要的。

PEEP 也影响 PAC 图形，并且受内在或受外在 PEEP 影响的患者的 PCWP 的解释是很多推测和错误信息的主体。PEEP（内在和外在）引起透壁胸腔压力，这正向地影响 PAWP 测量。为了正确地确定 PAWP，PEEP 可以暂时断开（几秒钟或呼吸循环）。可替代地，内在或外在的 PEEP 的影响可以通过添加 2～3 cm 的 H_2O 到 5 cm 水柱使 PEEP>10 来估计。

心排血量（cardiac output，CO）通过热稀释测量。传统上，向近侧注射冷却的盐水团块，然后通过导管尖端处的热敏电阻测量团块的温度。通过确定曲线下面积并绘制积分来计算 CO。使用平均 3～5 次注射以使变化性最小。较新的导管通过集成热线圈来持续测量 CO，此热线圈轻轻地加热近端血液，测量导管尖端处的温度下降，并且使用类似的方法来计算 CO。在任一方法中，心内分流和三尖瓣反流将导致心排血量测量出现不可预测的误差。至少有一些学者建议通过绘制 Fick 曲线和外推 CO 来计算 CO，可以获得更高的可靠性。

压力，容积和做功测量

虽然现代 PAC 监测病房或 ICU 护士提供血流动力学参数的连续数据读取，但仍然有必要对 PAC 监测中涉及的生理原理和计算有一个基本的了解。实际测量参数以 CVP 开头。CVP 从导管的近端或 CVP 端口直接转导。如果在右心房和腔静脉之间没有阻塞，CVP 类似于右心房压力（right atrial pressure，RAP），又类似于右心室舒张末期压力（right ventricle end-diastolic pressure，RVEDP）和右心室舒张末期容积（right ventricle end-diastolic volume，RVEDV）。因此，

$$CVP \sim RAP < RVEDP < RVEDV$$

CVP 是右心室舒张末期容积或心脏预负荷的直接测量外推而来。正如 CVP 是右侧心脏充盈的测量一样，PCWP 测量左侧压力和体积。如前所述，当导管“楔入”在肺动脉中时，在 PA 和 LV 之间存在连续的流体柱。因此，

$$PCWP < LAP < LVEDP < LVEDV$$

CO 也通过前述热稀释直接测量。通过体表面积（body surface area，BSA）计算心排血量（cardiac output，CO）使得 CO 成为更规范化的心脏指数（cardiac index，CI）。BSA 源自高度和重量列线图，但也可以很容易地以 Mosteller 公式计算（其中 W 是以千克为单位的重量，H 是以厘米计的高度）：

$$BSA = \sqrt{\ } W \times H/60$$

一旦知道心排血量，则可以如下计算出每搏输出量（stroke volume，SV）：

$$SV = CO/HR$$

HR 是心率。

然后如下计算右侧射血分数（right-sided ejection fraction，RVEF）

$$RVEF = SU/RVEDV$$

RVEDV 的计算需要连续热敏电阻，其能够将 CI 分成收缩和舒张成分。知道 RVEF 能够计算 RVEDV：

$$RVEDV = SU/RVEF$$

右侧心脏工作估计心脏右侧做的功，因为它通过肺将血液泵送回左心室（left ventricular，LV）。右心室搏动功指数（right ventricle stroke work index，RVSWI）估计如下：

$$RVSWI = (PAP-CVP) \times SVI \times 0.0136$$

其中 PAP 是肺动脉压，SVI 是每搏指数

左侧的心脏体积和工作计算类似于右侧。左心室功是通过体循环循环的血液的功。计算公式如下：

$$LVSWI = (MAP-PCWP) \times SVI \times 0.0136$$

其中 LVSWI 是左心室搏动功指数，MAP 是平

均动脉压。

在 PAC 所有的测量指标中最有用的指标是肺血管阻力（pulmonary vascular resistance，PVR）和全身血管阻力（systemic vascular resistance，SVR）。分别估计跨肺或跨体循环系统的阻力，它们是血管紧张度的外推。SVR 是跨体循环中的压力降低乘以流量，并计算为：

$$SVR=(MAP-RAP)\times 80/CI$$

其中 RAP 是右心房压力。

PVR 是肺循环中的压力降低乘以右侧流量：

$$PVR=(PAP-PCWP)\times 80/CI$$

使用肺动脉导管的目标导向治疗

关于由正确放置和解释的PAC提供的大量数据，几乎没有分歧。所提供的数据是否带来更好的患者治疗结果才是大部分争论的根源。已经进行了许多临床研究以试图确定应当测量哪些 PAC- 衍生的生理参数和哪些是能够预测结果的参数。Shoemaker 等进行了对患者对创伤的生理反应定义和分组的初步工作。早在 1973 年，Shoemaker 和同事在几项研究中表明，测量的PAWP降低了CO。他们进一步表明，创伤后的死亡患者的特征是氧输送的减少以及周围血管阻力的增加。基于这些和其他类似的研究结果，为得到与生存回溯相关的生理值，许多研究团队将目标转向对严重创伤患者的复苏。在 Shoemaker 的初步研究十年后，他和同事们展示了达到正常生理值的患者的总生存收益。最后，该团队在存活患者中通过氧消耗（Vo_2）测量发现氧债更少。有趣的是，各组之间没有氧消耗的差异。在类似的研究中，Bishop 等检查了 90 名创伤患者的生理参数，发现在入院后 24 h 内实现更高水平的心脏指数（cardiac index，CI）、氧输送（Do_2）和氧消耗（Vo_2）的患者具有较低的 ARDS 发生率和降低的总死亡率。基于这些和类似的发现，几个团队随后将患者随机分为超常复苏和传统复苏组，目的是证明积极复苏的有创监测将实现超常生理学和更好的预后。这些研究提供了混合的结果。Bishop 组随机将患者进行超常复苏，使得与定义为实现正常尿量和 CVP 的传统复苏相比，CI 达到大于 4.5，Do_2 指数大于 670，Vo_2 指数大于 166。超常复苏组明显降低了死亡率和减少器官功能衰竭。有趣的是，在 70% 的研究组和 29% 的对照组中达到最佳参数。类似地，Fleming 等将超过 2 000 ml 的失血量的创伤患者随机分配到超常 CI、Do_2 和 Vo_2，并且发现实现这些目标后统计学显示：器官衰竭可能、ICU 天数、呼吸机使用天数，以及死亡率都有明显降低。

然而，其他研究指出，实现复苏比用何种工具实现复苏更重要，许多最近的研究没能发现监测或目标导向复苏的类似优点。Velmahos 等将严重受伤的患者随机分为超常复苏和传统血流动力学监测组。虽然两组患者的死亡率、器官衰竭发生率、脓毒症发生率、ICU 天数或住院时间没有差异，但他们发现 70% 的超常组和 40% 的传统组患者达到超常生理参数。这些最佳值同更好的预后密切相关，但与治疗方案无关。两组之间没有结果的差异。然而，在这项研究中，最有趣的是发现无应答者（即体积和变力性操作未能达到既定目标的人）的发病率明显比对照组差。这表明超常生理学的积极复苏对那些不能达到生理学指标的人是有害的，并且实际上这种尝试使他们的身体耗尽得更快。其他团队报告了类似的结果，这表明实现正常参数的能力与死亡率的提升相关，且最终它比为实现正常参数而设计的任何治疗更重要。综合起来，这些结果引起了对介入监测和复苏的有用性的怀疑。到目前为止，从未有团队进行过将“干预反应者”（其生理学指标低于目标，但对干预能作出反应）随机分为“继续治疗”和“停止治疗”组的研究。因此，基于 Vo_2 / Do_2/ CO 的干预，它们的最终效果从未被真正测试过。

许多人认为，应该在所有患者中进行过度复苏，而不须进行有创监测。其他人认为超生理复苏的的作用是有限的。一些数据表明 PAC 使用的结果较差。事实上，已经报道了过度复苏和 PAC 的有害后果。Hayes 等报道，用伴多巴酚丁胺和变力性增大的氧输送会增加死亡率。其他人报道超常复苏患者也会类似地增加死亡率。至少有一个团体声称 PAC 本身是一个发病率的预测因素，与方案驱动的复苏无关。Rhodes 等进行了 200 例患者的前瞻性随机试验，其中未进行方案驱动的复苏。在本研究中，根据 ICU 工作人员的临床判断，当患者复苏时，患者随机分为 PAC 和无 PAC 组。前瞻性地获得数据并回顾性地检查数据，发现 PAC 组在前 24 h 内接受明显更多的体液，并且发病率增加。在 Hayes 等的一项研究中发现 PAC 治疗的患者死亡率增加（54% vs. 34%），提供了 PAC 方案驱动的复苏是有害的证据。在这项研究中，为达到超常生理参数，进行了一个严格的目标导向尝试。为了实现这些目标，须使用过度液体复苏和变力性支持。

然而，这些不是良性的措施，因为过度给予液体的一个后果是腹内高压（intraabdominal hypertension，IAH）和腹腔隔室综合征（abdominal compartment syndrome，ACS）的发展。在其完整的临床表现中，ACS对每个主要器官系统都有不利影响，并且早期的描述报告几乎都有广泛的死亡率。这就解释了进行更积极的液体复苏的PAC产生负面结果的原因。随着意识的增强，ACS和IAH在早期阶段得到认可。预防措施使ACS的发病率下降，改善结果。

为了了解关于PAC和复苏终点的大量数据，Kern和Shoemaker对21项随机临床试验进行了meta分析，发现只有在脓毒症或器官功能障碍发作之前实现参数优化时，才能在早期血流动力学优化中显著降低死亡率。Heyland等分析了7项研究，发现通过实现优化的死亡率没有显著降低。最后，Poeze等的分析表明，生理优化使死亡率降低。在该分析中，得到有益处的均是围术期得到血流动力学优化的患者。在治疗之前具有确定的脓毒症或器官衰竭的患者不可能受益于“优化”。在接受紧急手术的创伤患者中，所有优化都发生在手术之后，因此，优化是否有益仍存在质疑。

其他人质疑实际PAC测量的准确性。Epstein等通过计算的反向Fick方法与间接热量测定法的直接测量相比来研究Vo_2测量的准确度，以试图确定PAC的氧消耗量的准确度。他们的研究表明存在41 ml/min·m^2的偏差，提示PAC措施并不足以对Vo_2进行测量。最后，Luchette等研究了连续CO测量的准确性，发现当患者温度高于38.5℃时，信噪比和精确度降低，导致对严重受伤或脓毒症患者中PAC测量的准确性的进一步质疑。

混合静脉饱和度：监测组织代谢

虽然超常复苏的结果是混杂的，但许多人认为PAC的最佳使用是作为组织灌注的测量。混合静脉饱和的PAC采样应作为组织水平灌注的辅助测量。即使对超常复苏的混杂数据仍然有争议，但是混合静脉血氧饱和度（$S\bar{V}o_2$）毫无疑问地可以提供有用的数据。不幸的是，虽然组织灌注的这种测量看起来可用作组织氧合和随后结果的测量，但是最终也没有显示作为复苏的目标终点的有效性。Gattinoni等发布了一项随机前瞻性试验，涉及56个ICU的762名患者，这些患者被随机分为传统复苏组或靶向目标心脏指数（CI）>4.5组或混合静脉血氧饱和度（$S\bar{V}o_2$）>70%组。三组之间的死亡率或器官功能障碍没有差异。与前面讨论的研究一样，亚组分析显示，实现血流动力学目标的患者具有与随机分组无关的类似的死亡率。

右心室舒张末期压力作为心脏指数和心脏功能的测量

正如Starling曲线所预测的，舒张末期容积是前负荷的最佳预测因子。不幸的是，如前所述的PAC压力测量在内在心室顺应性和外在PEEP改变的环境中被混淆。RVEDV监测提供了前负荷的第一个实际测量值。RVEDV使用具有快速热敏电阻的PAC来提供直接测量的体积，而不是作为体积的压力替代物。为了尝试找到作为心脏功能的量度的PAOP的替代方案，Cheatham等发现CI与RVEDVI的相关性比PAOP与RVEDVI相关性更好。相同的团队之后研究了64名呼吸衰竭和高PEEP需求的患者，并提示在所有PEEP水平上，RVEDVI都比PAOP能更好地对CI进行测量。在PEEP水平超过15后，CI与PCWP呈负相关。总之，这些发现使得该团队得出以下结论，即应该使用RVEDVI代替PAOP作为心脏功能的量度。

尽管最初保守地认为数学耦合可以解释RVEDV和CI之间的密切相关性，几个团队已经表明，直接测量体积优于压力（CVP和PAWP）测量的外推。Chang等发现，RVEDV预测的内脏灌注不良比PCWP更好，反过来RVEDV这与多器官功能障碍综合征（multiple-organ dysfunction syndrome，MODS）和死亡率有关。这些团队也已报道了RVEDV、组织灌注和结果之间的其他相关性。最后，Kincaid等提供的数据显示可以为每个个体患者计算最佳RVEDV。总之，这些数据支持使用RVEDV作为心脏功能和目标导向复苏的优良测量方式。

对准确获得和解释的PAC数据的合理应用的证据也是缺乏的。通过对重症监护护理从业者使用真实生活的低复杂度的病例场景进行模拟调查，专家认为超过15%的受访者可能进行了有害的治疗。这个现象在各个国家、地区或专业上没有区别。根据观察到的反馈，作者指出，在前瞻性随机研究中，不适当的应用PAC数据可能导致PAC对死亡率的潜在有益效果减少30%。

肺动脉导管的替代方案

新世纪以来，我们逐渐将注意力转向发展和验证无创性监测，旨在为医生提供有用的血流动力学参数，协助制定重要的临床策略。无创性监测包括经食管心脏超声、经胸超声心动图，以及脉搏轮廓分析。

经食管心脏超声技术可对胸降主动脉进行血流速度、纠正血流时间和主动脉直径的测量。近期，一项目的导向性的临床随机试验证实经食管心脏超声指导创伤患者复苏有显著的效果。此项技术的缺点是操作人员需要专业的技能培训和数据解读，同时很难保证长时间的准确定位。

动态血容量测定替代了静态测定，例如 CVP、PAOP 以及 RVEDI。动态测定包括每搏量变异度（stroke volume variation，SVV）、收缩压变异（systolic pressure variation，SPV）和脉压变异（pulse pressure variation，PPV）。SVV 可通过计算速度时间积分与流出跟踪区域的乘积获得。这两项数据由食管多普勒超声测得，还可通过计算脉冲轮廓分析获得。PPV 可从动脉压力追踪仪中直接获得。SVV 和 PVV 均不需要肺动脉插管。两种方法均依赖机械通气过程中的心肺相互作用。因此正压通气替代了流入左房和左室的肺循环血液，导致吸气相早期左室前负荷增加以及心搏量和收缩压也随之增加。同时，右心室前负荷减少（通过减少回心血量），后负荷增加（通过增加跨肺压）。右心射血分数减少使左心前负荷降低，结果导致吸气末左心心搏量减少。血容量减少的患者，血压下降是 PPV 的主要组成部分，但心力衰竭的患者恰是相反的，血压升高是主要症状。这些影响因素可以在 Frank-Starling 曲线的陡峭部分明显地显示出来，因此可以用来预测容量反应性。尽管早期研究时所用的潮气量是 8～12 ml/kg，但是即使在低潮气量以及高呼气末正压的呼吸机条件下，PPV 仍有很高的特异性。最近的系统回顾总结动态测定较传统的静态测定在预测流体反应性上更准确。虽然动态无创监测很具吸引力，但不要忘记它们不能提供有关心室功能的任何信息。此外，动态测定只能在完全机械通气和无心律失常的情况下，对患者进行准确测定。不能重蹈盲目崇拜和接受新技术的覆辙。

总结

从一开始，PAC 就是重症监护医生的一项得出数据的工具。正如看到的那样，详细的文献回顾、小样本前瞻性研究，以及结论性数据均支持 PAC 的应用。然而，同时有些文献和临床支持对重症患者行早期目标导向性复苏。但是，对创伤患者的适当复苏目标仍有待确定。由于他们的损伤和机制，创伤患者的病情往往难以预估。PAC 很难进行准确的测量，也无法对已收集数据进行解读。在许多 PAC 复苏试验中所收集的数据是否真实反映人体情况以及数据如何解读，我们无从得知。然而在争议中，要明确 PAC 不是药物或者治疗干预是很重要的，因此不能直接评价它的使用效果。PAC 已经受到严格审查，且其他诊断和监测设施，例如经食管超声、X 线胸片、动脉线和脉搏血氧计被广泛接受。Ⅰ类证据还没有明确证实 PAC 的生存益处。PAC 的有效性取决于其他很多因素，其中许多在临床研究中不能得到测量和评估，包括适应证和风险的评估、适当的位置和降低风险的措施、科学性使用和解读以及前后关联性和 PAC 所测得数据的使用。

由于从监测中能获得混杂因素和有力数据，我们支持继续选择性地谨慎使用 PAC，PAC 可以作为危重病患者适当复苏的工具。尽管复苏参数和目标尚不能完全明确，以及患者病情随时都在变化，通过临床判断滤出的数据应该有利于患者护理。然而，正确使用的前提是安全、合适的放置和使用前评估以确保正确地使用。在这时，不断的数据收集及监测同患者实际情况互为佐证尤为关键。对生理变化进行间歇监测是远远不够的。的确，某一时间点下患者生理情况以及随后可预测的结果是大量可测与非可测变量的总和和这些类型的变量相互综合相互作用的结果。当技术足够先进以至于可以识别许多变量时，每一项测量应该增加并得到解释。基于某些未能发现这些数据用途的研究而否定来自 PAC 所测得数据是目光短浅的，并且忽视了其他测量方法不能测得的数据。事实上，尽管多项研究证实 PAC 联合其他监测方法可使患者受益，同时，临床医生也在临床工作中持续使用 PAC，但它们可能无法在大样本临床试验中进行研究。也就是说，PAC 的应用需要不断观察、监测以及干预，我们相信关于 PAC 的大部分的质疑及否定的数据来自对 PAC 数据粗略的观察（一般不关心它们的准确度）而没有对患者状态的持续变化予以仔细研究。否定 PAC 是愚蠢至极的，临床医生可通过自身学习和努力让该项工具更好地发挥它的作用。

氧的运输

Patricio Polanco, Juan Carlos Puyana, Mitchell Fink 和 Andrew B. Peitzman 著
朱凤雪 李 纾 译

心肺系统的最主要的功能是运送足够的氧气满足新陈代谢需要、维持组织有氧呼吸，以及消除多余的二氧化碳，以达到机体的稳态。运送至组织或器官的氧量与有氧新陈代谢所需氧量间的平衡决定组织的适当氧合。

单细胞生物已进化到通过使用氧作为电子受体来充分氧化有机分子（尤其是葡萄糖）而获取大量能量。在这个过程中，化学能转化为腺苷三磷酸（adenosine triphosphate，ATP）高能分子同时产生二氧化碳。氧气不能储存在机体细胞中，因此，通过有氧酵解产能完全由氧气供应决定。没有氧气，生物（氧消耗）将迅速死亡。

在单细胞生物中，所需的氧气和产生的二氧化碳可通过扩散迅速穿过细胞膜。这在多细胞生物中，如人类中，是不能发生的。相反的是，复杂的氧气运送机制及二氧化碳清除维持有氧代谢。因此，我们完全依赖呼吸、循环和血液系统间的相互协调来维持能量产生。

在分子 - 细胞水平，休克被定义为一种病理状态，发生于氧供成为机体产能的限制步骤时。在氧输送（Do_2）少于组织氧消耗（Vo_2）的情况下会出现细胞水平低灌注状态。氧气的输送是血液流动（心排血量）和动脉氧含量的乘积。休克期间氧供与氧使用之间的差异可以被测定。我们通过这些变量来监测治疗的有效性。本章节介绍氧输送和氧消耗的计算方法。

细胞产能

葡萄糖分解成二氧化碳、水和能量的过程是机体产能的主要方式，尽管其他分子如氨基酸和脂肪酸也可以在不同的阶段参与产能的过程。

糖酵解（葡萄糖代谢过程的第一步）将葡萄糖分解成 2 分子丙酮酸。这一步反应普遍发生在所有哺乳动物细胞的细胞质中，同时产生 2 分子 ATP。这只占葡萄糖可释放能量的 5.2%。在缺氧的状况下，丙酮酸在乳酸脱氢酶的作用下代谢为乳酸。在厌氧的状况下，正如我们在剧烈活动或者休克状态下看到的一样，乳酸会在循环中迅速积累。乳酸吸收和葡萄糖再生发生在肝中。血液中正常乳酸浓度应低于 2 mmol/L。乳酸产量增加、清除率下降以及乳酸在血浆内积累反映厌氧代谢增加以及休克状态。血浆乳酸增加程度是一个反应预后的可靠指标，所以成功的休克治疗后应在血浆中进行乳酸水平的正常化。乳酸清除不足或延迟与创伤死亡率增加紧密相关。

在氧气存在的状况下，丙酮酸被氧化并最终代谢成二氧化碳和水。葡萄糖代谢的有氧阶段也被称为呼吸，完全发生在线粒体内。丙酮酸产能涉及 3 个阶段。第一阶段是产生乙酰辅酶 A，该过程不可逆。第二阶段，乙酰辅酶 A 经过 8 个步骤的酶促氧化反应（柠檬酸循环）产生二氧化碳和储存在烟酰胺腺嘌呤（nicotinamide adenine dinucleotide，NADH）以及黄素腺嘌呤二核苷酸（flavin adenine dinucleotide，$FADH_2$）中的能量。最后一个阶段（电子传递链），NADH 和 $FADH_2$ 被氧化，并将电子最终传递给氧气。

在葡萄糖代谢的有氧阶段，产生了 36 分子的 ATP，因此，细胞有氧呼吸产能是无氧酵解的 18 倍。机体中绝大多数细胞都通过有氧呼吸产能并最终生存。葡萄糖不是唯一的能够产生丙酮酸的有机分子，如某些氨基酸和脂肪酸分子同样能够产生丙酮酸。因此，氧气而不是丙酮酸成为患者产能的限速步骤。

涉及异常线粒体使用氧气的病理状态可在各种临床过程中观察到。例如，电子传递链中的氰化物中毒将导致快速发展的能量耗竭、乳酸积累和死亡。更常见的是，感染性休克被认为导致线粒体疾病，使得这些细胞器无法有效地使用氧气生成能量。

微循环和氧气运输

氧气扩散进入细胞受细胞本身与氧源间距离的限制，并且仅限于 100 ~ 200 μm。机体存在高度复杂的毛细血管网（微循环）以将氧气分布到细胞和组织中。微循环的表面积远超过血容量，因此在给定时间内，所有血管床都打开将会导致低血容量状态。为避免这种状况发生，选择性地分配血流到各血管床以满足氧的需求。

感染性休克时微循环的氧气分布调解能力崩溃，因此，感染性休克是一种分布式休克。一氧化氮是一种血管扩张剂，它的过量积累被认为在脓毒症恶性缺氧过程中起重要作用。此外，缺氧所致的组织水肿增加了毛细血管与细胞间的距离，更进一步使氧气扩散变得更差。毛细血管流量的分布不均也是脓毒症的重要组成部分。因此，贫乏的氧摄取是脓毒症的特征。

血红蛋白，终极氧载体

氧气在血中以 2 种方式携带：溶解型和血红蛋白结合型。大约 98% 的氧气与血红蛋白结合，2% 的氧气以溶解的方式在血中进行运输。血红蛋白作为一种独特的氧载体从肺泡中捕获氧气，通过微循环分布运输，最终在细胞周围环境中将氧气释放。成年人血红蛋白由 2 个 α 和 2 个 β 多肽组成，各自与一个分子的携带 1 分子的氧气的血红素基团结合。每克血红蛋白能够携带 1.34 ml 氧气。因为 Hb 浓度容易测量，所以每 100 ml 血液中携带的氧气含量可以计算如下：

1.34（ml/g）× Hb（g/dl）× 氧饱和度（Sa 氧气，分数 1）= 氧含量 /100 ml

例如：

$$1.34 \times 15 \times 0.98 = 19.7\ \text{ml}/100\ \text{ml}$$

测定 Hb 氧饱和度的光的分光光度吸收仪（脉搏血氧计）是重症监护中广泛使用的工具。血红蛋白氧饱和度呈高度非线性，大致如 S 型曲线（图 1）。这可以确保 Hb 在生理状态下能够轻松地携氧和释氧。当血氧饱和度低于 90% 时，血氧饱和度小幅度的下降将反应氧分压大幅度的变化。粗略地，90% 的血氧浓度对应 60 mmHg 氧分压。血氧饱和度曲线会跟随 pH、温度和 2, 3- 二磷酸甘油酸浓度的变化而变化。

一小部分血浆携带的氧气，它可以通过 Po_2 计算。该浓度约为

0.003 ml/100 ml（血浆）/（Po_2）mmHg。

因此，我们可以计算给定的血液动脉氧含量（arterial oxygen content，Cao_2）中所含的总氧气量如下：

1.34（Hb）× Sa 氧气 +0.003（Po_2）=Cao_2

基于此公式，我们推测通过输血增加血清中血红蛋白量可以增加动脉氧含量及氧输送。这在理论上是正确的，但是尝试让重症患者达到正常的血红蛋白水平并不是有益的。Hebert 等的重症监护输血适应证试验显示，用自由输血策略的患者（当 Hb 低于 10 g/dl 时，就予以输血）死亡率较使用限制性输血策略（维持 Hb 在 7 ~ 9 g/dl）的患者高。然而，该研究没有测定氧消耗与氧输送。此外，有证据显示给脓毒症患者输注红细胞会增加氧输送，但通常氧消耗并没有增加。

已经对开发基于血红蛋白的氧载体（hemoglobin-based oxygen carriers，HBOC）投入了相当大的兴趣和努力。HBOC 的潜在益处包括普遍兼容性、有效的血管半衰期、无感染性物质和同红细胞相比更长的储存时间。虽然这些产品在氧输送和微循环

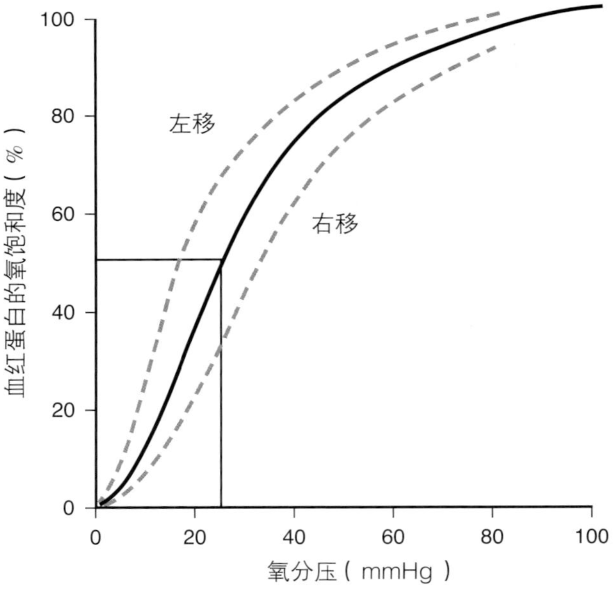

图 1　氧合解离曲线。实线代表成年人正常血红蛋白的氧合解离曲线。右移或左移的曲线代表在给定氧分压时，增加或者降低血红蛋白载氧能力时曲线的左、右变化

上有很好的前景，但仍需要进一步研究。最近的一项 meta 分析报告说给予手术、中风和创伤患者 HBOCs，他们发生心肌梗死和死亡的风险会提高。

心脏——氧的输送泵

最终向细胞输送多少氧（Do_2）由心脏泵送的血液的量（心排血量）决定，使得心脏性能成为分析需氧细胞能量产生的一个重要方面。心排血量（Q）可通过几种方法在床边计算。虽然使用的 Swan-Ganz 导管已被质疑，但它仍然是测定 Do_2 最实用的工具：

$$Q \times Cao_2 = Do_2\ (ml/min \cdot m^2)$$

心排血量由前负荷（血管内容积）、收缩性、后负荷（血管阻力）和心率决定。不当的心脏功能将快速导致休克。因此，在心肌梗死后观察到的收缩性不足导致氧输送不足，这种状态被称为心源性休克。7% 的心肌梗死患者会出现心源性休克，这也是心肌梗死患者早期死亡的最常见原因。导致心源性休克的心肌梗死的其他并发症包括乳头肌破裂伴急性二尖瓣功能不全、心室壁破裂与心包压塞。

总结：测量患者机体细胞氧消耗和摄取

我们可以使用先前开发的函数简单地量化整个有机体中消耗的氧的量。细胞耗氧量（Vo_2）是关于心排血量（Q）与动脉（Cao_2）和静脉（Cvo_2）血氧含量差异的函数。使用与测量动脉血氧含量相同的方法计算 Cvo_2，在中心循环（右心房或心室）中测量静脉血氧饱和度（Svo_2）：

$$Q \times (Cao_2 - Cvo_2) = (Vo_2)$$

并非所有输送到细胞周围的氧气均被消耗或摄取。实际上，通常仅约有 25% 的所输送的氧气被摄取，虽然不同器官有着很大的变化。消耗的氧气除以输送的氧气可计算氧摄取率（oxygen extraction ratio，O_2ER）：

$$Vo_2/Do_2 = O_2ER$$

组织摄取的氧气量可以在生理条件下显著增加，以满足细胞需要。这便提供了关键的缓冲区，它允许在组织需求增加的时间内维持组织足够的氧消耗。此外，当氧输送减少时，氧摄取可允许组织维持足够的氧消耗。

一些作者已经描述了使用氧输送和 Svo_2 作为复苏的有效终点，这已被定义为早期目标导向治疗（early goal-directed therapy，EGDT）。尽管其广泛使用，Svo_2 作为监测复苏的工具的有效性仍有争议。Shoemaker 报道当高风险手术患者被治疗至心脏指数（≥4.5 $L/min/m^2$）和氧输送（≥600 $mL/min/m^2$）达超常值时，患者死亡率下降。Gattinoni 等和 Hayes 等发现与传统的复苏治疗相比，使用心脏指数、氧输送和 Svo_2 测量没有改善预后。相比之下，Rivers 等发现，在感染休克患者中，使用中心静脉血氧饱和度的恒定测量代替肺动脉导管（定义为 $Scvo_2$）的 EGDT 与接受标准治疗的患者（46.5%）相比有较低的死亡率（30.5%）。人们对有创性血流动力学监测的作用如使用肺动脉导管获得心脏指数、Svo_2，计算休克复苏的 Do_2 仍有争议。之前已经叙述了，如果不把这些单独测量的参数与本身改善结果的治疗方案结合起来，那么这些参数的测量是徒劳的。

病理状态下氧消耗和氧输送的关系

在生理状态下，氧输送超过氧消耗，因此据说氧气消耗与输送无关（图 2）。在实验模型中，氧输送的逐渐减少与 O_2ER 的增加和正常有氧代谢的维持相关。当氧消耗开始依赖于氧输送以及有氧呼吸产能失败时，达到 Do_2 中的临界点（cDo_2）。结果，乳酸在血液中堆积。毫不奇怪，测量氧气输送和消耗状态的变量是临床预后的良好预测因子。

血清中乳酸和碱缺失的水平已被用来作为描述组织灌注和细胞氧使用的间接指标。一些作者确定血清乳酸和碱缺失与出血性休克结果之间有很强的相关性。Broder 和 Weil 于 1964 年，以及随后的 Vincent 等和 Dunham 等在临床研究和动物模型中均证实了前述的结果。

确定给定患者中的 cDo_2 将有助于临床医生确认患者是否存在休克。然而，使用常规技术不容易确定 cDo_2。cDo_2 因患者而异，并且根据病理状态而不同。此外，Vo_2 和 Do_2 共享几个变量，包括 Hb 和心脏功能。改变这些共享变量中的一个或多个将改变 Vo_2 和 Do_2，这种现象被称为“数学耦合”。

尽管有这些限制，测量氧输送和消耗仍然是临床医生治疗休克状态的重要工具。对氧变量的有效测量允许对复苏过程进行“微调”——优化氧输送

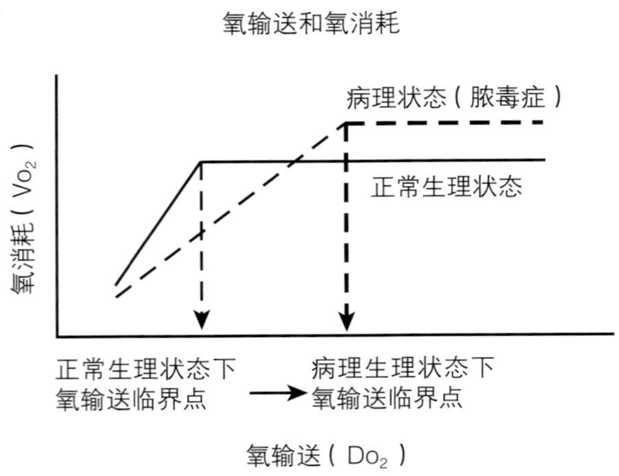

图 2 氧输送（Do_2）和氧消耗（Vo_2）。实线表示正常状态下，Vo_2 始终保持不变，当 Do_2 逐渐减少直到氧输送的临界点（cDo_2）。虚线表示病理状态（脓毒症）下，由于氧利用损伤，Vo_2 及 cDo_2 升高

和心脏功能，并使生理性消耗最小化。临床医生常规控制的变量数组包括增加氧饱和度、增加 Hb 浓度、优化前负荷和心肌收缩力、改变后负荷和减少细胞氧消耗。在给定患者中这些变量如何改变在很大程度上取决于存在的休克类型。

休克状态下氧输送变量的特征

出血性休克

出血性休克的特征在于血液丢失（Hb 减少），从而降低氧携带能力，血容量减少负向影响前负荷。因此，在出血休克时，由于 Hb 和心排血量减少，Do_2 减少，O_2ER 相应增加。治疗出血性休克最好的方法是早期控制出血部位和尽快恢复血容量和 Hb 含量。早期出血部位的控制和氧债的快速偿还对于改善预后至关重要。新鲜全血，虽然通常不可获得，但是治疗严重出血性休克的理想方案。应提供足够的容量以恢复心排血量和血红蛋白含量。

心源性休克

心源性休克的特征是心肌收缩力降低，常常由心肌梗死所致。心源性休克的其他不常见的原因包括急性心肌炎、持续性心律失常、急性瓣膜性疾病，以及由多种原因引起的终末期心肌病失代偿。心源性休克的特征是在肺毛细血管楔压（>15 mmHg）升高和 O_2 ER 增加情况下的低血压和低心排血量及低心脏指数（<2.2 L/min/m^2）。

感染性休克

在足够容量复苏的情况下，脓毒症休克通常导致高血流动力状态，其特征是心排血量增高、氧输送增加，以及后负荷或全身血管阻力降低。脓毒症导致微血管停流增加。在感染性休克中毛细血管血流分布不均导致氧输送和氧需求不匹配。氧消耗增加，但周围组织的氧摄取能力受损导致乳酸酸中毒。线粒体功能障碍和 ATP 生成减少可导致器官衰竭和脓毒症死亡。这种器官功能障碍的基本发病机制仍不清楚，组织缺氧和线粒体功能障碍导致的氧使用受损似乎与此有关。O_2ER 减少，因此观察到特征性升高的 Svo_2。

神经源性休克

在高段脊髓受到损伤后可观察到神经性休克，此类休克的特征是正常的心排血量，无反应性心动过速和后负荷下降。神经性休克是一种归因于脊髓内自主神经通路遭受破坏的分布型休克。低血压是由于全身血管阻力减少导致血液在缺乏交感神经张力的四肢内汇集而发生。

总结

哺乳动物细胞中使用氧气进行有氧代谢对生产足够多的能量是必需的。氧必须被运输到细胞周围的环境中，因为它在组织中仅能扩散一小段距离。复杂的毛细血管网络使得由 Hb 运输的氧得到充分传递。Hb 是主要的氧载体，并且增加其浓度可增加氧输送，但不增加氧消耗；因此，不推荐自由输血策略。不同的疾病过程、不同的心肺功能障碍和各种类型的休克，都具有其各自氧输送变量的特点。对氧输送和氧消耗的系统评估能够提供重要的预后信息，进而协助调整治疗各类休克的治疗方法。

心力衰竭的药物支持

John W. Mah 和 Orlando C. Kirton 著
朱凤雪　李　纾 译

根据美国心脏协会在2008年的统计，心血管疾病影响超过8 200万人，大约570万成年美国人受到充血性心力衰竭的影响。虽然心力衰竭的生存率已经改善，但死亡的风险仍较高，诊断后5年生存率约为50%。急性失代偿性心力衰竭（acute decompensated heart failure，ADHF）的入院通常由预先存在的疾病加剧引起或者发生在其他一些事件之后，包括急性心肌梗死、瓣膜疾病和心律失常。此外，现今的患者年龄较大，病情更重，可能正在进行心脏和非心脏手术，以及发展其他原因引起的急性心力衰竭，如脓毒症或肺栓塞。ADHF的患者通常被分诊到医院的ICU中去。然而，这些患者可能正在面临着紧急性和选择性手术。无论患者呈现出的是急性还是慢性心脏病，这类严重的人群对于外科医生来说是越来越困难的挑战。诊断和治疗原发病因是势在必行的，治疗的主要方法是最佳的药物血流动力学处理。

病理生理学

必须明确导致ADHF的病理生理学机制以及药物治疗的目的，以便成功治疗ADHF患者。了解每个特定疾病过程的复杂性及其生理反应对于改善功能和结果至关重要。心力衰竭通常是多个生理因素紊乱的结果，包括前负荷、后负荷、收缩力、心率和心律。

前负荷增加在ADHF中比较常见，并且通常继发于体液潴留，但也可以伴随心肌缺血和瓣膜功能障碍发生。身体的自然代偿反应是通过增加心室壁上的应力（在Frank-Starling曲线上向上移动）来增加充盈压力以改善心肌收缩力。心力衰竭通常导致肾血流量减少，随后激活肾素-血管紧张素醛固酮轴（renin-angiotensinabdosterone axis，RAAA）。这些代偿机制的最终结果是血管紧张素Ⅱ致使血管收缩增加肾血流量；醛固酮释放，其增加钠吸收以换取钾；促进心室肥大、纤维化和重塑，最终致心室僵硬度增加。

心脏后负荷增加常见于围术期，是由于多种原因导致，例如预先存在的高血压、儿茶酚胺激增、术后高血压，以及细胞因子和炎症介质的释放。此外，肺动脉压升高也是由于相似的原因，但是也可以通过相对缺氧的血管收缩和酸中毒加剧。在心力衰竭时，交感神经系统（sympathetic nervous system，SNS）被刺激，调动全身反应进而增加全身血管阻力（systemic vascular resistance，SVR），以保持对重要器官的正常灌注。心力衰竭进一步加重，因为它试图增加心排血量抵抗更高的流出压力。增加的交感神经紧张还刺激肾素的释放，进一步激活RAAA及其在心力衰竭发生机制中本身的作用。随后，心肌需氧量增加，钠水潴留恶化，致命性心律失常加剧的可能性增加。此外，血浆中较高的循环儿茶酚胺水平与较差的预后相关。

心肌收缩主要受SNS刺激的影响。肾上腺素能剂增加细胞内环腺苷一磷酸，这反过来增加钙流入并加强收缩。然而，随着慢性增加的交感神经张力，心脏变得对循环儿茶酚胺的反应较小，似乎是在保护肌细胞免受过量的儿茶酚胺及其导致的变性和变时驱动的干扰。这种抑制反应是由持续在充血性心力衰竭中的心肌对长期升高的儿茶酚胺水平的敏感性降低和心肌的β-受体下调导致的。心肌的收缩力下降并且对生理需求以及作用于β-肾上腺素能受体的药理学试剂的反应较差。此外，心力衰竭时心肌对体容量过载的反应不足。Frank-Starling机制变得迟钝，并且前负荷的显著增加是很难耐受的，这进一步加剧了充血性症状。

越来越多人认为RV衰竭是ICU中发病和死亡的重要原因。右心室壁较薄，顺应性比LV好，并且被设计成在低压、低阻力的环境中起作用。收缩发生在3个阶段：①乳头肌收缩；②RV朝向室间隔运动；③RV的扭转的LV收缩。在等容性收缩和松弛中花费的时间最少，导致血液几乎连续不断地流向肺。右心室主要受右冠状动脉（right coronary artery，RCA）灌注，只要低压系统保持完整，灌注发生在收缩期和舒张期。RV容易受到肺血管阻力升高的影响，这将增加在等容性收缩和舒张中花费的时间，减少总体正向血流量。两个心室都依赖室间隔的运动，其可以朝向RV或LV移动，这两者都可能损害充分的充盈和增加舒张末期压力。

在心脏手术后，即使在术前具有正常心室功能的患者，心室功能也会暂时受损。这是由几个因素导致的，包括主动脉十字钳夹、不足的心肌保护、低体温和心搏停止和再灌注损伤，以及围术期中过度的正性肌力药。心室功能的恢复有双相模式，在从心肺旁路术（cardiopulmonary bypass，CPB）停止后到最初恢复，心室功能最低点约持续 3～6 h，然后在 8～24 h 内完全恢复。这种模式显然可能由于术前心室功能不良而延迟。药物支持通常是必要的，直到适当的功能恢复。

治疗

支持急性失代偿性心脏的一般药理学目标是减轻后负荷，优化前负荷和心肌功能，同时调节心肌耗氧，并使神经激素的进一步活化级联最小化。通常需要额外的支持以维持足够的平均动脉血压，以确保足够的冠状动脉血流。

利尿剂

利尿剂是治疗 ADHF 的主要药物，因为容量过载是最常见的情况。但是，没有随机临床试验证明利尿剂可以改善 ADHF 的生存率。尽管如此，利尿剂仍然是治疗容量过载的有效药物。此类药物的作用是降低前负荷和血管内容量，缓解呼吸困难和肺充血症状。此外，血容量过多常见于先前存在充血性心力衰竭的手术患者中，往往由对创伤、脓毒症、大手术或围术期液体管理患者进行容量复苏而导致。通常使用袢利尿剂如呋塞米，更有效的替代品如布美他尼或托拉塞米对利尿药耐药患者有用。静脉内推注或连续输注都是可以的。虽然许多较小的研究发现“温和”的利尿药使用连续输注的用法，药物毒性更小，甚至更有效。但最近更多的证据表明，在对全身和肾功能的影响上，推注给药和连续输注之间没有差异。应该对容量状态进行临床管理，必要时可以行有创监测，因为对血容量正常的患者进行过度或正常利尿可能会导致低血压或器官低灌注。在处理下面这些情况时利尿剂可能是有害的，如急性心肌梗死、其他器官功能障碍，以及在术后早期出现毛细血管渗漏和第三间隙液体隔离的患者。其他问题包括大剂量使用利尿剂会激活 RAAA 和 SNS，以及各自有长期不良反应。

血管扩张剂

硝酸甘油（nitroglycerin，NTG）是用于快速治疗心源性肺水肿和 ADHF 的有效药物，并且症状迅速缓解。NTG 的主要作用是扩张静脉，但血管扩张只有在高于 30 μg/min 的较高剂量下发生。NTG 对心脏和骨骼肌的静脉具有较小的影响，并且主要引起平滑肌内静脉松弛，使血管容量增加。该类药物有效地和快速地降低心室充盈压（前负荷），减轻心室壁应力，更重要的是，减少心肌需氧量。此外，NTG 通过降低冠状动脉阻力和延长舒张期来改善冠状动脉血流。NTG 的半衰期短、持续时间短、起效迅速，同时很快失效，但它较易地发生快速耐受并且通常须持续增加剂量。其他副作用包括与强大的血管舒张相关的头痛和腹痛。用药前应确定容量状态，并且利尿剂可以有助于消除机体对硝酸盐增加的耐药性。

硝普钠诱导动脉和静脉系统相对平衡的扩张，与给药剂量无关。静脉张力降低，使得前负荷降低。此外，硝普钠导致后负荷显著降低，进而改善心排血量、SU，降低 LV 充盈压和心室壁应力，并最终降低心肌需氧量。它在 ADHF 中特别有用，因为它可以在急性二尖瓣或急性主动脉瓣反流的情况下迅速减轻后负荷。硝普钠还可使冠状动脉血管舒张，并且在心室舒张压降低超过主动脉舒张压降低时，改善心肌灌注。然而，冠状动脉疾病患者有发展“冠状动脉窃血”的潜力，将血流从缺血心肌转移到非缺血心肌。应用此药物时应特别注意的是血压急剧下降以及氰化物和硫氰酸盐毒性。

奈司立肽是人脑类型利尿钠肽的重组形式，其与血管和内皮受体结合以增加细胞内环鸟苷酸的水平。这导致平滑肌松弛和主要的动脉以及静脉舒张。虽然被认为是“利尿钠”，利尿并未是其主要的效果。然而，它可以加强其他利尿剂的效果。奈司立肽已经用于控制充血性心力衰竭的症状和降低 PCWP。因为可能发生症状性低血压，随后限制其用于体液不足、低血压或灌注不足等情况。此外，研究人员在随机对照试验（randomized controlled trail，RCT）的汇总分析中揭示了奈司立肽可增加肾衰的发生率以及短期死亡风险，并建议仅当利尿剂和 NTG 的组合的传统治疗失败时方可使用奈司立肽。事实上，最近对 7 141 例急性心力衰竭患者进行的大型随机对照研究表明，奈司立肽在控制症状方面似乎优于安慰剂，然而在死亡率或再入院率上没有变化。

强心剂和血管加压剂

好的强心剂可以增加心肌收缩力而不增加心率、后负荷、前负荷或者心机耗氧量。这些受体介导的激动剂可以通过 α_1，α_2，β_1，β_2 受体或者多巴胺受体激动系统发挥它们的作用。而磷酸二酯酶（phosphodiesterase，PDE）Ⅲ抑制剂则可以通过增加细胞内 cAMP 的浓度来增强心肌收缩力（表 1）。血管加压剂虽然本身具有内在正性肌力的效果，但常被用来治疗低血压和保持适宜的动脉血压，保证足够的冠脉血流量。

正性肌力药

多巴酚丁胺是人工合成的儿茶酚胺类物质，主要有占主要地位的 β_1 受体活性和弱 β_2 受体活性，也有弱 α_1 受体活性。它的主要功能是增加心肌收缩力和增快心率，增加心排血量和 SV（表 2）。在多巴酚丁胺的 β_2 受体活性激动之后，会产生舒张全身血管的效果，体循环和肺循环都会受到影响。尽管多巴酚丁胺可以增加心肌氧消耗，但它也可以通过扩张冠状动脉来增加心肌氧供。然而只有当有害的心率增快得以避免的时候，多巴酚丁胺的这一优势才得以显现。多巴酚丁胺禁用于由左心室和主动脉间压力增加所引起的特发性低肥厚性主动脉瓣下狭窄。多巴酚丁胺具有致心律失常的药理作用，所以用于心房颤动或心房扑动的患者的时候应格外小心。当患者已经长期服用 β 受体阻断药或者已经患有慢性心力衰竭时，应禁用多巴酚丁胺，因为这些患者需要更高剂量的药物才能起效。在这种情况下，联合应用 PDE 抑制剂往往有效。

肾上腺素主要作用于 α_1、β_1、和 β_2 受体，当低剂量使用时（0.02 μg/kg · min），药物的 β 效应占主导地位。此时它对心脏的作用是最有利的，心肌收缩性会随着周围血管扩张和心率的增加而改善。在患者血容量正常的情况下，心排血量和心肌收缩力增加，舒张压、系统血管阻力和肺血管阻力（pulmonary vascular resistance，PVR）降低。事实上，在心脏旁路术后低剂量的肾上腺素可以产生等量的多巴胺和多巴酚丁胺，不产生显著的增加心率的作用。但高剂量的肾上腺素会增加心律失常的发生率，这时应主张寻求替代性的正性肌力的支持。

表 2　血流动力学反应及应用剂量

药物	CO	心排血量	收缩口	全身因管阻力	用药速率
多巴酚丁胺	↑↑	↑↑	↑↑	↑↓	2~40 μg/kg · min
肾上腺素	↑↑	↑↑	↑	↑	1~4 μg/min
	↑	↑↑	↑↑	↑↑	4~7 μg/min
	↑↓	↑↑	↑↑	↑↑↑	>7 μg/min
米力农	↑↑	↑↑↑	↑↓	↑↓	50 μg/kg 的推注，然后 0.375~0.75 μg/kg · min
去甲肾上腺素	↑↓	↑	↓	↑↑↑	0.01~0.1 μg/kg · min
多巴胺	↑↓			↑↓	0.5~2 μg/kg · min
		↑		↑↓	2~5 μg/kg · min
	↑↓	↑↑	↑↑↑	↑↑	5~10 μg/kg · min
去氧肾上腺素	↓		↓	↑↑	20~400 μg/min

CO, Cardiac output; HR, heart rate; SVR, systemic vascular resistance

PDE 抑制剂是一种在心肌和血管平滑肌细胞中发现的可以特异性抑制 PDE Ⅲ酶的一类药物，可以导致细胞内 cAMP 水平升高。这种较高水平的细胞内 cAMP 导致心肌收缩力的增加和心肌、血管平滑肌的舒张。全身血管舒张功能也得到了增强，周围血管阻力（peripheral vascular resistance，PVR）和

表 1　肾上腺素受体位点的儿茶酚胺活性

儿茶酚胺	多巴胺受体	β_1 受体	β_2 受体	α 受体
多巴胺	+++	++	+	+++
多巴酚丁胺	0	+++	++	+
去甲肾上腺素	0	+++	0	++
肾上腺素	0	+++	++	+++

0, 无活性；+, 轻度活性；++, 中度活性；+++, 强度活性

SVR 均显著降低。平均动脉压可降低，但其对心肌耗氧量和心率有轻度的影响。在 β 受体下调所致脱敏的条件下，这种独特的作用机制可以有效改善心肌收缩力。PDE 抑制剂事实上可能和 β 受体激动剂有协同作用，从而降低了这些药物的最低起效浓度，并减少了药物的有害的副作用。小剂量 PDE 抑制剂的加入可以对心脏指数产生较大的影响，而不增加收缩压。PDE 抑制剂已被证明对由心肌收缩能力和肺血管舒张功能下降（RV 后负荷下降）所致的 RV 衰竭有效。PDE 抑制剂比大多数强心药物半衰期长但起效快速。米力农由于其改进的安全性能和功效已基本上取代氨力农在临床的应用。米力农的药效是这是氨力农的 20 倍，可在 2 min 内达到峰浓度，半衰期约为 2 ~ 4 h。其半衰期明显长于肾上腺素能药物，因此在使用前必须考虑系统性低血压的风险。它和多巴酚丁胺相比，在引起近似的心排血量增加的条件下，PDE 可以导致更明显的血管扩张。此外，在充血性心力衰竭或肾功能不全的患者身上，由于清除率下降，药物的半衰期会进一步延长。其他的使用注意事项包括警惕室性和室上性心律失常、低血压、头痛和血小板减少（较少见）的发生。

血管加压剂

多巴胺是一种天然存在的配体，根据血清浓度不同，刺激不同的受体。至少它的作用有一部分是通过心肌细胞内神经末梢释放的去甲肾上腺素完成的。多巴胺通常是伴有低血压的急性心力衰竭（也被认为是心源性休克）的首选药物。在低剂量（高达 3 μg/kg · min）条件下，多巴胺主要表现为多巴胺受体的激动剂。当给药速率提高到 5 ~ 10 μg/kg · min 时，它作用于 β_1 受体。正是在这一范围内，心肌收缩力增加，而心率、血压和全身血管阻力的增加最小。更高剂量导致 α_1 受体受到的刺激增加。因为多巴胺没有 β_2 肾上腺素能效应，结果是全身以及冠状动脉强烈收缩。高剂量的多巴胺的应用常常受限于其导致的心动过速、心律失常和冠状动脉收缩的副作用。因此，在心力衰竭患者中使用多巴胺最好用中、低剂量。

去甲肾上腺素在治疗急性心力衰竭中价值不大，仅在其他药物无效时使用。它的主要功能是作用于 α 受体，只有轻微的 β_1 受体激动活性。任何 β 受体的活动通常都会受到血管强烈收缩以及后负荷增加的调节，进而补偿肌心肌氧气的供需比。然而它是用于感染性休克或其他原因引起的明显的血管舒张性休克的一线药物，用于治疗心力衰竭患者，如在心源性休克时，它维持动脉血压、保证足够的冠状动脉血流灌注。

精氨酸血管加压素（arginine vasopressin，AVP）是垂体后叶通释放的一种内源性激素，可以对血流量、血压以及血浆渗透压做出反应。它在治疗急性心力衰竭时作用有限，但它最近被发现可以用于难治性感染性休克患者的治疗。在休克早期，AVP 的含量高，紧接着循环系统中 AVP 含量相对枯竭，出现 36 h 的血管麻痹状态。把低剂量的 AVP 调节至生理水平已经被证明可以恢复血管正常的张力水平，提供反常的血管扩张，使其他器官血流量增加。AVP 结合儿茶酚胺（V_1）受体和、肾（V_2）受体，使肾有一些保护性潜能，还可能具有使肺血管舒张和终末肺血管收缩的作用。不管怎样，应用小剂量的 AVP（0.01 ~ 0.04 U/min）可以恢复儿茶酚胺抵抗的状态，从而降低额外的一线血管加压药的高使用剂量及其伴随的不良反应的增加。

其他药物

甲状腺激素已用于改善器官移植捐献者的心脏功能。病态甲状腺综合征是最常见的诊断，在危重病患者中其他非甲状腺疾病也较常见。甲状腺激素的替代治疗被建议用于改善心脏功能和增强缺血性事件后心室功能的恢复。在心脏病患者中，三碘甲状腺原氨酸（T_3）激素水平已被证明随着 CPB 后显著降低，而与血液稀释或使用肝素无关。这些激素水平在 12 ~ 24 h后恢复正常。虽然有一些证据表明，使用 T_3 可以改善心脏功能，但是关于是否可以给围术期虚弱的 CPB 患者使用 T_3 还存在争议。虽然没有在 T_3 不足的患者中使用甲状腺激素导致不良反应的报道，它的使用尚未得到明确支持，仍然存在争议。

亚甲基蓝在难治性休克中具有潜在的应用价值，但尚缺乏强有力的循证研究。它因其独特的和未被研究的在脓毒症中的作用机制或在其他全身炎症反应综合征（systemic inflammatory response syndrome，SIRS）导致的休克的作用机制而被提到。SIRS 状态下一氧化氮产生增加，平滑肌内的 cGMP 导致低血压，机体对儿茶酚胺的反应性降低，心肌处于抑制状态。亚甲基蓝能抑制 NO 和 cGMP 产生、增加动脉血压、改善心肌功能和维持氧的运输，并已在少量的小型研究中被证明对难治性感染性休克有效，可以减少患者对肾上腺素能药物的需求。曾经有报道说被给予亚甲基蓝的患者由于明显的肺血管收缩，出现了表现为恶化性缺氧的急性肺损伤。这一副作用似乎随着减少剂量和连续输注而得到改善。

特殊情况

感染性休克伴心力衰竭

多因素导致的低血压状态和相对心力衰竭与感染性休克相关。虽然脓毒症通常会导致心脏高输出状态，然而，心肌收缩功能的下降往往不能满足组织代谢需求。左、右心室的收缩力直接受损。前负荷由于SVR的显著下降和因毛细血管漏液使血量减少而减少，静脉回流受损。内源性血管加压素虽然最初分泌增加，但因为垂体长期受到紧张刺激，储备很快耗竭。尽管多巴胺、去甲肾上腺素、去氧肾上腺素和血管加压素已被证明可以提高感染性休克患者血压，多巴胺和去甲肾上腺素是经积极液体复苏后维持正常血压的一线药物。但值得注意的是，当治疗感染性休克时，多巴胺与去甲肾上腺素相比，发生心律失常的概率较高。

尽管通常用作二线药物，但添加低剂量的血管加压素并未降低死亡率，同时，它不比单独使用去甲肾上腺素更有效。脓毒症时可出现心肌收缩力明显下降，因而需要变力性支持。多巴酚丁胺可有效使心排血量保持在正常范围，并随后增加Svo_2。一般来说，可被接受的复苏终点包括建立至少65 mmHg平均动脉血压，使CVP维持在在8～12 mmHg（如果需要机械通气则为12～15 mmHg），$Scvo_2$≥70%。

右心室衰竭

目前，急性RV衰竭在ICU中一直是被忽视的。据报道，RV衰竭的发生率与LV衰竭的发生率相似，并且在多种临床背景中可以发生，包括心脏或肺移植、ARDS、植入左室辅助装置（LV assist device，LVAD）、右室梗死、正压机械通气或显著的肺栓塞。右心室前负荷、右心室后负荷或左心室的任何功能损害都可能导致右心室功能被破坏。右心室对后负荷的增加非常敏感。如果肺血管阻力持续升高，它可能进展为右心室扩张、三尖瓣反流、心肌耗氧量增加，并且使右心室输出量明显减少，引发RV衰竭的恶性循环。此外，RV的RCA灌注（其通常持续整个心脏的收缩和舒张期）在存在显著肺动脉高压的情况下退化为仅舒张期灌注。增加的右心室舒张末期容量也可以对左心室功能产生不良影响，如果这个不良影响足够大的话将导致室间隔的偏移，进而损害左心室充盈。在LVAD植入的前几天内，因为左心室负荷不足，室间隔向左移位，所以右心室出现功能不全。

如果右心室的收缩力、PVR和室间隔功能正常，则保持较高的充盈压力就可以恢复正常的血流动力。然而，如果平均肺动脉压已经大于30 mmHg，则容量负荷的增加可能反而会产生反作用。多巴酚丁胺和PDE抑制剂（如米力农）可增加右心室心肌收缩力，同时舒张肺（和全身）血管，并通过增加右向左的血液分流增加左心室的充盈。肾上腺素和异丙肾上腺素也是改善右室心肌收缩力的有效药物。有实验表明血管加压素可以增加动脉血压，并改善冠状动脉血流灌注。与其他α肾上腺素能药物相比，去甲肾上腺素被推荐用于低血压患者，以增加RCA灌注。NO可以有效减少PVR，改善氧合，并且随后由于其选择性舒张肺血管和改善通气灌注（V/Q）匹配从而改善右心室功能。其吸入途径避免了对全身血压的显著影响。然而，对预后的研究缺乏，对死亡率的影响还没有得到很好的研究。其他刺激性选择性肺血管扩张剂，例如吸入性前列环素联用或不联用吸入性的PDE，已经在临床上使用，并证明有效，它们拥有类似的肺选择性，可避免全身性低血压，并且比吸入NO更便宜，但这些策略都很需要人力。不管采用何种药物治疗，诊断必须明确，并且必须纠正潜在的病因以恢复右心室功能。肺动脉监测和超声心动图非常有助于建立正确的诊断，并可能有助于增强治疗。

钝性心脏损伤

钝性心脏损伤（blunt cardiac injury，BCI）极少须使用正性肌力支持，除非患者先前就存在的心脏疾病。钝性心脏损伤常由胸部直接受到打击、减速型损伤或脊柱和胸骨之间的压缩性损伤导致。目前尚没有标准治疗指南可供参考，因此必须根据损伤模式和临床实际情况提供护理和支持。医生必须熟悉所有潜在的心脏衰竭诱因，并相应分别处理。钝性心脏损伤是一个广泛的术语，它包括所有类型的损伤。术语“心肌振荡”用于文献中，并且可在组织学检查或影像学研究中不存在可识别的损伤时发生。这是最常见的低影响事件，例如在接触运动中发生。然而，当心搏停止在T波波峰引起心室颤动前15～30 ms时或冲击发生在QRS期时，会导致完全性心脏传导阻滞。挫伤意味着心肌损伤，由于解剖学位置靠前常常涉及右心室和隔膜损伤。当发生ARDS、PEEP较高或有严重的胸部创伤和肺挫伤时，RV后负荷增加，进而会发生右心室功能障碍，因为右心室对后负荷增加较为敏感。有创监测和超声心动图可以帮助指导低血压患者、老年人和先前存在心脏病的患者的治疗。还有关于围术期问题的报道，包括全身性低血压、心律失常和心搏停止的发生风险增加，并已表明上述问题在损伤后持续至少1个月。治疗主要是支持性的，确保足够的前负荷和变力性支持。右心室挫伤常见，故首先应怀疑是否存在右心功能障碍。必须解决右心室后负荷增加的问题，包括纠正酸中毒、缺氧和肺动脉高压，同时避免常规机械通气和高PEEP。

总结

ADHF是外科ICU中的常见事件，其中紧急手术问题由于预先存在的心力衰竭或心脏损害逐渐变得更复杂。这些患者给外科手术带来了额外的挑战。尽管ADHF的病理生理学机制都相同，但附加的、同时出现的围术期病理生理学使外科患者的治疗变得越来越复杂。识别诊断和适宜的药物支持可以改善ADHF中的患者预后，并使他们获得从早期损伤中恢复的机会。

心律失常的诊断与治疗

Kareem R. AbdelFattah 和 Joseph P. Minei 著
朱凤雪　李　纾 译

对与其外科疾病无关的多种并发症的患者的治疗已经成为当今外科医生的常见问题。在复杂手术后，外科医生在治疗住院患者时须对大多数主要医疗问题及其潜在后果有普遍的认识。鉴于大多数接受大手术的患者将被置于支持连续监测技术的环境中，快速鉴别和治疗心律失常已经成为外科重症监护病房（surgrcal intensive care unit，SICU）的常见做法。术后出现心律失常可能有几种原因，其中一些最常见的原因包括缺氧、心肌缺血、儿茶酚胺过量、常规药物和电解质异常。

心律失常可以通过集中体格检查、标准的12导联心电图（electrocardiogram，ECG）以及从对特定操作或药物治疗的反应来诊断。大多数心律失常的紧急治疗取决于患者的稳定性、心律失常的准确分类，以及对引起心律失常的机制的理解。治疗可以涵盖简单的药理学干预到急性不稳定的患者中的心脏复律，并且有时可能须经皮或经静脉起搏、通路消融或植入起搏器或除颤器。

风险因素以及发病率

心律失常的发生率从没有明显心脏病史的非心脏手术患者的9%到心脏手术患者的超过40%波动。在ICU接受心脏治疗、非心脏治疗和医疗急救患者中进行的一项研究发现，平均20%的住院患者在住院期间经历了心律失常。除了窦性心动过速之外，最常见的心律失常是心房颤动（atrial fibrillation，AF），在心脏手术患者中接近一半的患者群体中看到。高达15%的下壁心肌梗死（myocardial infarction，MI）的患者将呈现房室传导障碍或完全性心脏传导阻滞。本身患有心脏或肺部疾病的患者的心律失常的风险增加，在进行非心脏手术、存在创伤或危重疾病时将十分复杂。血管加压素的需求与由心脏组织上儿茶酚胺的致心律失常性质引起的心律失常风险增加有关。只有10%的心律失常是缓慢性心律失常。心律失常的来源在心房和心室之间平均分布，AF和室性心动过速（ventricular tachycardia，VT）是最常见的。患有心律失常的患者已被证明ICU住院的时间更长，并且在几项研究中显示出较低的生存率，这表明心律失常可能是更严重的危重疾病的标志。

许多回顾性研究已经检测了心律失常进展的危险因素。在接受心脏手术的患者中，危险因素包括高龄、所进行手术的类型［例如，瓣膜置换术联

表 1　NYHA 心功能分级基线特征 *

特点	NYHA Ⅰ级 (n=10 592)	NYHA Ⅱ级 (n=3242)	NYHA Ⅲ级 (n=869)	*P*
男性	8 702 (82)	2 517 (78)	651 (75)	<.001
年龄（0, 年）	60 ± 7	61 ± 7	60 ± 7	<.001
目前吸烟	1 092 (10)	353 (11)	109 (13)	0.04
高血压	3 336 (32)	1185 (37)	318 (37)	<.001
糖尿病	1 860 (18)	718 (22)	216 (25)	<.001
既往心肌梗死	7 749 (73)	2 222 (69)	605(70)	<.001
心绞痛	5 285 (50)	2 913 (90)	799 (92)	<.001
外用血管疾病	326 (3)	168 (5)	65 (8)	<.001
体重指数（均值 ± 标准差，kg/m^2)	26.6 ± 3.4	26.9 ± 3.7	27.3 ± 3.9	<.001
葡萄糖（均值 ± 标准差，mg/dL)	112 ± 44	118 ± 49	123 ± 56	<.001
总胆固醇（均值 ± 标准差，mg/dL)	224 ± 39	225 ± 41 ± 225 ± 43	0.24	
高密度脂蛋白（均值 ± 标准差，mg/dL)	37.9 ± 10	37.7 ± 10.6	37.1 ± 10.2	0.07
三酰甘油（均值 ± 标准差，mg/dL)	155 ± 86	164 ± 100	167 ± 94	<.001
低密度脂蛋白（均值 ± 标准差，mg/dL)	156 ± 34	155 ± 35	156 ± 38	0.92
高密度脂蛋白占总胆固醇的百分比（0）	17.3 ± 5.0	17.1 ± 5.1	16.9 ± 5.0	0.03
高血压药物	8 024 (76)	2 782 (86)	768 (88)	<.001
糖尿病药物	1 082 (10)	451 (14)	140 (16)	<.001
抗血小板药物	6 497 (61)	1 706 (53)	458 (53)	<.001

From Koren-Morag N, Goldbourt U, Tanne D: Poor functional status based on the New York Heart Association classification exposes the coronary patient to an elevated risk of ischemic stroke. Am Heart J 155(3):515–520, 2008, pp 515-520.

HDL, High-density lipoprotein; LDL, low-density lipoprotein; NYHA, New York Heart Association; SD, standard deviation.

*Data are presented as number (percent in parentheses) unless otherwise indicated

合冠状动脉旁路移植（coronary artery bypass graft，CABG）较单独进行 CABG 的患者的心律失常发生率更高］、放置起搏器的需求、手术期间的任何正向肌力支持，纽约心脏协会分类表 1 的评分的增加以及心肺旁路的复杂脱机经历。其他风险因素包括肥胖、手术期间的积极流体平衡和代谢综合征。最后，一些群体已经将某些患者群体术后的心律失常指向是由遗传倾向导致的。

缓慢性心律失常

虽然不像快速性心律失常那样常见，但缓慢性心律失常是潜在危及生命的疾病。它们可以根据起源的节点，即 AV 或窦房（sinoatrial，SA）节点来分类。缓慢性心律失常可能由外在因素或心脏传导系统中的内源性疾病引起。外在原因包括药物、心肌缺血、代谢异常、迷走神经张力的增加和急性呼吸衰竭。缓慢性心律失常的进一步分类取决于节律的可逆性，患者是否由于节律而出现症状，以及特定节律将发展或复发的可能性。治疗选择可以如消除一个异常起搏点一样简单，也可以如放置一个永久起搏器一样复杂。

窦房结

正常心跳起源于 SA 节点，其在正常条件下作为心脏的起搏器。由 SA 节点功能障碍引起的心动过缓起因于冲动生成或传导的失败。之前被称为“病态窦房结综合征”，用于描述反映这些功能障碍的一系列状态。目前，由 SA 节点引起的缓慢性心律失常被描述为以下情况之一：不适当的窦性心动过缓、窦性间歇或停搏、窦性传出阻滞和心动过缓 – 心动过速综合征。

窦性心动过缓定义为每分钟心跳低于 60 次（bpm）的心率。单独的这样的表现并不能代表 SA 节功能障碍，因为心率低于40 bpm可以是无症状的，并且在训练有素的运动员中被认为是正常的。当患者出现症状（如晕厥）或在活动期间无法适当增加心率时，窦性心动过缓被认为是病态的。当 SA 节暂时不能自发性发生冲动时，会发生窦性间歇或停搏。同样，窦道传出阻滞导致窦性间歇，但是 SA 节不会触发。冲动传导被延迟或不能传导至 SA 节会导致心房去极化的失败。心动过缓 – 心动过速综合征是指伴有心动过缓和心动过速的 SA 结功能障碍。比较典型的是心动过缓发作紧随心动过速的终止，并且可以与晕厥前期或晕厥的临床症状相关。处理十分具有挑战性，因为用于快节律的药物治疗通常使患者倾向于心动过缓，反之亦然。通常，心动过缓须植入起搏器，并须结合心动过速的药物治疗。

SA 节功能障碍的治疗取决于患者的临床状态和假定的病因。如果心动过缓是暂时性的，并且与血流动力学损害无关，则不需要治疗。调查心动过缓的原因应该包括纠正代谢和电解质异常；最大限度地减少可能增加迷走神经张力增加的操作；停止或减少潜在的违规药物剂量，如 β 阻断药，钙通道拮抗剂和锂的剂量。如果心动过缓持续或严重到足以导致血流动力学不稳定，应该考虑用抗毒蕈碱剂例如阿托品或 β- 激动剂（异丙肾上腺素）进行治疗。在急性环境中的一些患者可能需要经皮或经静脉起搏，并且可以进行旁路术直到给患者放入永久起搏器。血流动力学稳定但有症状的窦房结功能障碍的患者几乎总是需要永久起搏器。

房室结

传导在房室结或希氏 - 浦肯野束系统受阻被称为房室传导阻滞。房室传导阻滞可以是暂时的或永久的，这取决于延迟传导的原因。在成年人中，最常见的原因是药物中毒、冠状动脉疾病和传导系统的退行性疾病。许多其他病症，例如电解质紊乱、心肌炎、结节病、硬皮病和高迷走神经反应，也可引起房室传导阻滞。PR 间期反映的是传导通过 AV 结和希氏束的时间。当 PR 间期延长（大于 210 ms）时，则患有一度房室传导阻滞。当传至心室的传导冲动发生间断，传导失败时，即出现二度房室传导阻滞。莫氏 Ⅰ 型，二度房室传导阻滞表现为 PR 间期的逐渐延长，直到发生传至心室的冲动传导失败（图 1）。然后，在脱落的搏动后 PR 间期缩短。这种传导失败源于房室结本身，并且 QRS 波群窄。在莫氏 Ⅱ 型二度房室传导阻滞中，到达心室的传导间歇性失败，其与 PR 间期的进行性延长无关。在脱落的搏动后没有缩短的 PR 间期。这种传导失败被认为是“节下的”，源于希氏 - 浦肯野系统。QRS 波群可能延长，并且这种类型的房室传导阻滞更令人担忧。因为此型传导阻滞存在显著进展至完全性心脏传导阻滞的可能性，并伴随心室反应不足。三度或完全的心脏传导阻滞导致所有冲动通过 AV 结或者浦肯野系统失败，导致房室分离。心室依赖于它们的自主节律性，其产生典型的宽大的 QRS 逸搏心律，节律在 40 ~ 50 bpm 之间。而心房率通常更快，产生与心室 QRS 波群无关的多个 P 波（图 2）。

房室传导阻滞的治疗取决于患者的血流循环稳定、心律失常的瞬时性质，以及阻滞部位源自传导系统内部的位置。急性药物治疗依赖阿托品和异丙肾上腺素。但应该避免在缺血性心脏病患者中使用异丙肾上腺素，因为此药物会使心肌需氧量增加。没有针对房室传导阻滞的治疗的长期的药物，当发生房室传导阻滞时应该首先去除目前正在使用的常见的阻断传导的药物，例如洋地黄或 β 受体阻断药。临时起搏可用于循环血流不稳定的患者，莫氏 Ⅱ 型，

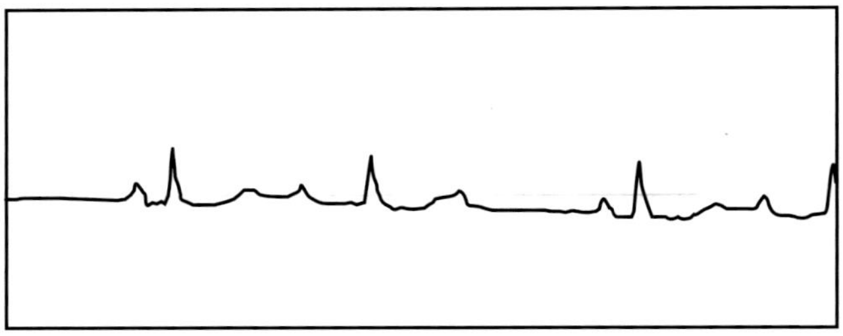

图 1 莫氏 Ⅰ 型二度房室传导阻滞心电图特征：节奏显示 PR 间期逐渐延长直到 QRS 波丢失

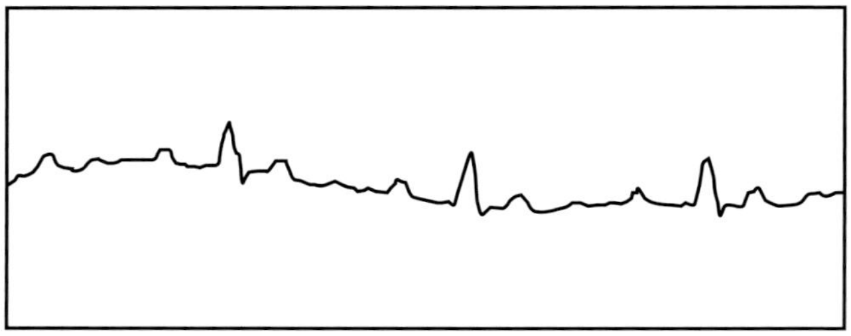

图 2 三度房室传导阻滞心电图特征：心房与心室按各自节律跳动，心房 P 波与心室 QRS 波群之间无关系

二度房室传导阻滞和三度房室传导阻滞通常需要永久起搏。应该注意的是，美国心脏协会的 2010 年指南建议使用变时性的药物治疗作为起搏的替代方法，因为已经证明当使用阿托品无效时，此类药物与外部起搏一样有效。

快速性心律失常

根据快速性心律失常起搏点与房室结的解剖学关系对其进行分类，因此，任何快速性心律失常治疗的第一步都要确定心律失常是源于窦房结［室上性快速性心律失常或室上性心动过速（supra ventricular tachycardia，SVT］之上，还是窦房结［室性快速性心律失常或室性心动过速（ventricular tachycardia，VT）］之下。这些也可以被认为是在 ECG 上产生窄的 QRS 波群（SVT）或者宽的 QRS 波群（VT）。窄波心动过速包括窦性心动过速，AV 结内折返性心动过速（AV nodal reentrant tochycardia，AVNRT，有时称为阵发性 SVT）、来自辅助途径的 AV 折返（沃 - 帕 - 怀综合征，也称为 AVRT，房室折返性心动过速）、AF 和心房扑动。相比之下，室性快速性心律失常起源于房室结以下，并且包括室性心动过速和心室颤动（ventricular fibrillation，VF）。快速性心律失常的恶性潜能的重要决定因素是持续时间、血流动力学后果和严重结构性心脏病的存在。急性处理取决于对机制的基本理解、药物干预的选择（表 2）和每种情况的紧急心脏复律的适应证。介入技术，如异常通路消融和植入起搏器和除颤器，大大改善了患者离开 ICU 后的长期预后，并且显著增加了我们治疗心律失常的医疗设施。

快速性心律失常发生的机制被分类为：①异常自律性，②触发活动；③折返。当正常传导系统外的细胞发生自发冲动形成时，便产生异常自动性。在“后去极化”期间发生触发活动，其导致膜电位早期达到阈值并产生异常冲动。折返是最常见的机制，当冲动可以沿着由不易兴奋组织区域分开的两个路径行进时发生。其中一个途径含有单向阻断，使传导减慢，使得恢复和进一步激发可以随后发生。这定义了可以自我传播的心脏组织，并且因此成为产生快速性心律失常的焦点（图 3）。

应用增加迷走神经张力的方法有助于对 12 导联心电图上观察到的快速性心律失常进行分类。通过颈动脉按摩或腺苷给药，房室结传导时间减慢并且不应性增加。这可以向临床医生证明 P 波在 ECG 上的存在，或者可以中断返折路径。对这种操纵的反应，通常可以帮助临床医生判断正在处理的快速性心律失常的类型（表 3）。

窦性心动过速

窦性心动过速不应该被认为是真正的心律失常，

表 2 抗心律失常药物分类

分类	例子	作用机制	是否延长 QT 间期
Ⅰ A Ⅰ B Ⅰ C	奎尼丁、普鲁卡因胺、丙吡胺 利多卡因、美西律 氟卡尼、普罗帕酮	钠离子通道阻滞 对延长动作电位时间以及钠通道解离有不同影响	是
Ⅱ类	美托洛尔、艾司洛尔	阻断 β 肾上腺素受体 阻断交感神经	否
Ⅲ类	胺碘酮、溴苄胺、索他洛尔	阻滞、延迟钾电流 显著延长动作电位	是
Ⅳ类	维拉帕米、地尔硫卓	阻滞钙离子通道 减慢 AV 结传导	否
其他	腺苷、地高辛	激活向内的电流 K^+ 和短暂抑制钙离子通道 极短的作用，主要在 AV 结 阻断钠 – 钾 ATP 酶，并增加细胞内钙 起效缓慢，中毒很常见	否

Modified from Brunton L, editor: *Goodman & Gilman's the pharmacological basis of therapeutics,* 11th ed, New York, 2005, McGraw-Hill.
ATPase, Adenosine triphosphatase; AV, atrioventricular

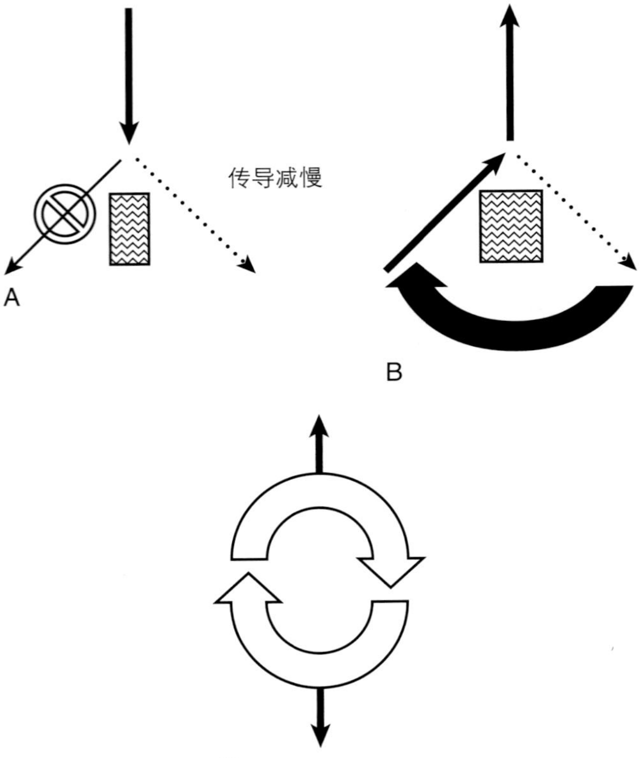

图3 A，折返形成的条件：2条传导通路被不易兴奋的组织分开、单向阻滞、传导减慢。B，启动因子允许在之前阻滞的通路上逆行向上传导。C，折返回路形成

表3 提高迷走神经张力对各种心律失常的影响

心律失常	对迷走神经张力提高的反应
窦性心动过速	暂时减慢，稍后恢复心动过速
房室结内折返性心动过速	突然心搏停止或者暂时心率减慢
心房颤动 或者心房扑动	增加房室结阻滞以及减慢心室反应率
多源性房性心动过速	增加房室结阻滞以及减慢心室反应率
室性心动过速	无反应

Modified from Tarditi DJ, Hollenberg SM: Cardiac arrhythmias in the intensive care unit. *Semin Respir Crit Care Med* 27(3):221–229, 2006

而是一种与氧需求增加相关的生理反射，因此，它是必须寻找原因的重要体征。发热、血容量不足和贫血都适当地增加心率，以至少维持或增加心排血量。在未明确原因时使用药物钝化这种反射可能是危险的。较不常见的原因包括甲状腺毒症、嗜铬细胞瘤或拟交感神经药物的副作用，它也引起窦性心动过速而不考虑反射机制。处理窦性心动过速的主要目标是找到和适当地处理混杂条件。窦性心动过速将通过对这个刺激过程的解决而得到解决。

阵发性室上性心动过速

术语“阵发性室上性心动过速”实际上描述了一组不同的快速性心律失常，通常称为室上性心动过速，最常见的是AVNRT。AVNRT在女性中比男性更常见，并且可以在任何年龄出现。潜在的病理状况由双传导途径组成，每个具有不同的传导速率。如前所述，这便允许出现折返的可能性和自传播性快速性心律失常聚焦的可能性。在AVNRT中，2个途径在房室结本身或周围。顺向传导通常通过较慢的路径发生，并且逆向传导通过更快的途径。140 ~ 220 bpm的心率是常见的，并且在ECG上不能看到P波，因为逆向心房激动和顺向心室激动同时发生。QRS波群通常很窄，因为向心室的顺向性传导通过正常的房室结和希氏 - 浦肯野纤维系统。

AVRT中存在类似的系统。相比之下，AVRT也具有2个传导通路，但是附加通路远离房室结并位于房室沟中，通常被称为“辅助通路”。顺向传导通过房室结和希氏 - 浦肯野系统，逆向传导则通过辅助路径发生。AVRT的QRS波群也很窄，并且因为辅助路径仅进行逆向传导，所以在ECG上不可见，并且被认为是“隐匿性的”。通过房室结的顺向传导与通过辅助路径的逆向传导结合，有时称为“正向性”心动过速。相比之下，电传导可以以相反的配置（即通过辅助路径的顺向冲动和通过AV结的逆向冲动）进行，被称为“顺向”心动过速。这种形式的折返性心动过速在心电图上的特征是宽大复杂的QRS波群，并且比正向形式更不常见。

紧急处理措施取决于阵发性SVT患者的稳定性。当出现心肌缺血、急性心力衰竭或低血压时，常需要紧急的直流心脏电复律。在血流动力学稳定的患者中，旨在减缓或打破房室结传导的药物干预是治疗的主要手段。静脉注射用腺苷是首选的药物，因为其对房室结传导有有效而短暂的抑制作用。腺苷能成功终止超过90%的用于AVNRT和AVRT导致的快速性心律失常（表3）。钙通道阻断剂或β受体阻断药（维拉帕米 / 地尔硫或美托洛尔）也是有用的，特别是当腺苷无效时，然而由于它们可能会产生低血压和心动过缓的作用，应谨慎使用。

沃－帕－怀综合征

辅助路径（Kent 束）允许顺行和逆行传导时，沃-帕-怀综合征出现，并且通常在早期 QRS 波群中可以看到 δ 波或预激综合征（图 4）。这种综合征发生在人群中的比例为 0.1%～0.3%，通常出现在成年早期，并且初始表现可以是 VF。在这些患者中，辅助路径传导发生顺行的患者的治疗与前面描述的狭波 AVRT（房室折返性心动过速）的治疗不同。腺苷仅在通过房室结发生顺行传导时才有效。否则一旦它激发 AF，当这些患者存在顺行辅助路径时，可导致 VF 的退化。这种退化继发于心房冲动传导与心室传导的比例为 1∶1。作为该病自然病史的一部分，每年有 0.1% 的患者诊断患有沃-帕-怀综合征。钙通道阻断药和地高辛已被禁用，因为它们会减缓房室结的传导，并通过旁路通路增强传导。Ⅰ类和Ⅲ类抗心律失常药，包括氟卡尼、普鲁卡因胺和伊布利特，能够抑制辅助路径的传导，降低心室率，并可能终止广泛的 QRS 快速性心律失常。直流电心脏复律用于血流动力学不稳定或抗心律失常治疗失败的患者。最终，对这些患者的治疗的选择将需要辅助路径的消融。

多源性房性心动过速

多源性房性心动过速被认为是由于自律性异常引起，通常与慢性呼吸系统疾病、充血性心力衰竭和肺部栓子有关。它具有不规则的速率和节律，其特征在于在 ECG 上存在 3 种或更多形态学上不同的 P 波，并且速率为 110～140 bpm（图 5）。如果 P 波在节律中不突出，它很容易与 AF 混淆。一线治疗包括治疗基础疾病、高碳酸血症或矫正缺氧，以及补充电解质。钙通道阻断药通常可以提供速率控制，但 β 受体阻断药应谨慎用于阻塞性肺疾病患者。胺碘酮可以有助于难治患者的一线治疗。

心房扑动

心房扑动是由于来自心房组织内的折返环路引起，并且与心房增大有关。由于类似的相关原因和类似的治疗方案，它通常与 AF 分为一组。典型的心房速率为 250～350 bpm。房室结不应期只允许这些心房搏动的一部分传递到心室，通常是 2∶1 的比例。当心室脉搏率测量为 150 bpm 时，应考虑心房扑动。通过用腺苷或 β 受体阻断药增加房室结的不应性，通常在 ECG 上可以看到特征为锯齿状外观的心房“颤动波”，并且最常见于下壁导联（图 6）。腺苷可用于诊断，但是与 AF 一样，它很少将节律转换回窦性。β 受体阻断药和钙通道阻断药允许为长期治疗控制心室率，但是如果异常节律持续存在，将需要更为常见的抗心律失常药物治疗或电复律。在血流动力学不稳定的患者中，使用 50 J 的直流电同步（DC 同步）心脏复律，具有非常高的成功率。现在已经投入使用的药物包括伊布利特、索他洛尔和普鲁卡因胺，但在急性环境中转化率较低。

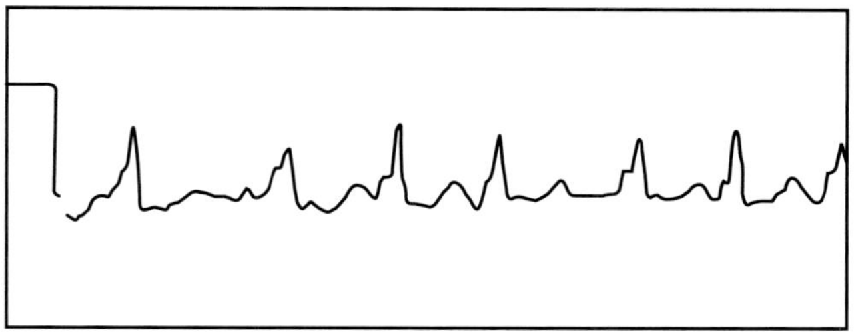

图 5 多源性房性心动过速的心电图特征：波形显示不规则的心动过速，含有 3 种及以上的形态学不同的 P 波

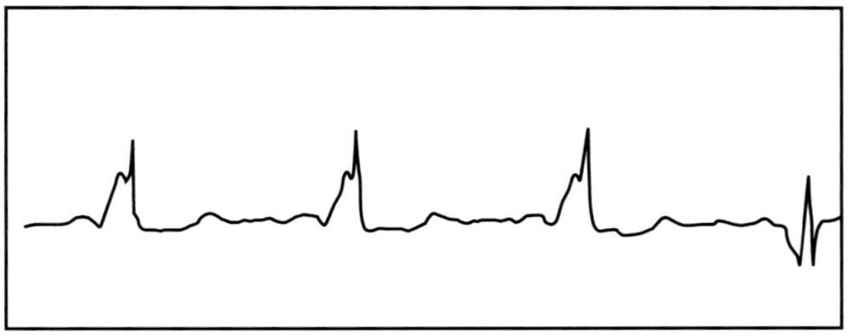

图 4 心电图 II 导联上可以看到与沃-帕-怀综合征诊断相一致的明显的 δ 波

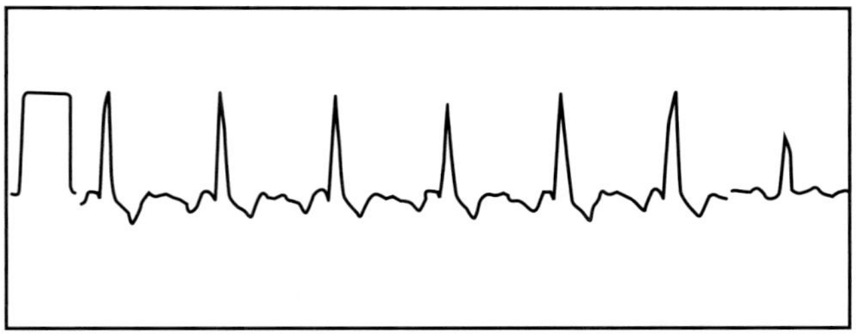

图 6 该心电图中的导联 II 可见心房扑动的特征：“锯齿”状颤动波及 2∶1 的传导。心率大约为 150 bpm

心房颤动

AF 是在 ICU 中最常被识别的 SVT（VT 是最常见的），并且可以有许多负面的后遗症。AF 和心房扑动在非心脏外科手术患者中占 SVT 的 60%以上，并且可以影响心脏手术后 40%的患者。AF 通常与左心房扩张有关，包括急性体液转移还是结构性心脏病继发的慢性扩张。必须排除的其他相关因素包括电解质失衡、心肌缺血、心包炎、糖尿病、甲状腺功能亢进、缺氧 / 高碳酸血症、肺栓塞，以及肺炎。在一般人群中鉴定的风险因素包括慢性高血压、瓣膜病和左心室肥大。ECG 上没有 P 波，且是一种“不定期的不规则”节律（图 7）。这是由多个移位的重入回路引起的，其以多个脉冲冲击房室结，使得其中一部分开始进行心室收缩，频率为 110 ~ 190 bpm。没有器质性心脏病的患者耐受心室充盈性较好的心房部分的损失。然而，在已知器质性心脏病变的患者中，心房颤动可以加重高血压、急性充血性衰竭和心肌缺血。另一个与之相关的结果是附壁血栓形成的可能以及来自于不收缩的左心房的相关栓塞风险。血栓在新发心房颤动持续时间超过 3 天的患者中的发生率高达 10%。

治疗的总体目标包括控制心室率、恢复和维持窦性心律，以及预防栓塞事件。如果患者在血流动力学上不稳定、有急性心力衰竭或者心律失常导致心肌损伤时，则应当进行直流电心脏复律。这在近期 AF 患者中恢复窦性心律的成功率达到 90%，但如果没有进行抗凝，可能导致 7%的卒中风险。2010 年 ACLS 指南推荐双相能量转换剂量为 120 ~ 200 J。在血流动力学稳定的患者中，控制心室率应是主要优先事项。钙通道阻断药、β 受体阻断药、胺碘酮和地高辛都显示出在不应期中增强房室结的功能。β 受体阻断药已显示在静息和运动期间能提供比钙通道阻断药更有效的心率控制。继发性低血压是常见的副作用，其可能需要伴随的体液管理和钙输注。地高辛与低血压无关，但是当静脉内给药时，其发挥作用需要约 30 min，因此限制了它在 ICU 环境中的用处。

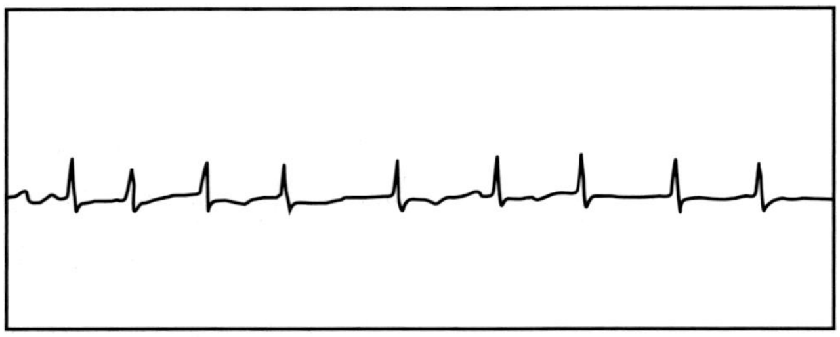

图 7　心房颤动心电图特征：波形显示 P 波消失，QRS 波形正常，但节律明显不齐

可以使用多种治疗方法来终止 AF 并恢复窦性心律。常见的选择包括单独使用抗心律失常药物或与心电复律联合使用，但这些药物必须针对每种个案进行调整。已经证实，如果在发病后 7 天内，对患者单独进行Ⅲ类抗心律失常药物治疗，如胺碘酮、伊布利特和普罗帕酮或与电复律联合使用，有 30% ~ 80% 的患者的 AF 终止。使用抗心律失常药物治疗时必须记住这类药物的副作用情况，包括药物诱导的尖端扭转型室速、VT 和其他严重的节律障碍。关于在药物或心电复律至窦性心律的过程中，应该强调什么仍存在争议。心房颤动节律处理的随访研究（一项多中心试验检查老年高危患者）的结果显示，那些用心室率控制治疗者与节律控制治疗者相比，长期预后没有差异。尽管存在这些争议，在围术期，高达 1/3 的新发房颤患者自发转换为窦性心律，未进行抗心律失常性治疗。在那些房颤持续不减弱的情况下，选择药物或电复律，或者单独控制心室率。目前，Ⅰ级证据支持 β 受体阻断药作为一线治疗药物，用于术后患者的心率控制和向窦性心律的转化。在血流动力学不稳定或已知的射血分数（ejection fraction，EF）<40%的患者中，胺碘酮可被用于一线治疗。

心房血栓和栓子的风险在 AF 中随着时间的变化变得更加引人关注，并且如果在 48 h 后没有转化为窦性心律，则应当考虑抗凝治疗。美国胸科医师学会建议在这些患者中，除非有复律需要，否则应在复律前和复查后 4 周继续进行抗凝治疗。在一些情况下，使用经食管超声心动图（transesophageal echocardiogram，TEE）来识别血栓的存在或不存在，可以用于允许立即心脏复律以及同时肝素化。抗凝的潜在好处必须与术后出血的风险进行权衡。当从 AF 到窦性心律转变时，栓塞风险增加，反之亦然。如果 TEE 显示心房血栓存在，则抗凝应当持续 4 ~ 6 周，并且在选择性复律之前应该证实血栓已经溶解。

室性心动过速

新诊断的 VT 的适当处理取决于精确的节律分类和患者风险因素分层，以便及时提供适当的治疗。

严重的 VT 发生在不到 2% 的心脏手术后的患者中。在非心脏手术中，它们最常见的是与后期心肌缺血和明显的器质性心脏病有关。应该经常评估血管内植入物的位置，因为移位可能与机械诱导的心律失常相关。在心肌缺血和外源性或内源性儿茶酚胺过量的条件下代谢、酸碱和氧合紊乱都涉及促进触发活动、异常自主性和在心室组织中的折返现象。重要结构性心脏病的存在是未来恶性 VT 和突发性心脏病死亡的最重要的预测因子。典型的 ECG 将显示 QRS 波群心动过速，其可以来自室上，或者更常见地由 VT 引起。如果不能进行区分，则较宽波的心动过速可当做 VT 进行治疗。注意考虑 QT 间期，因为不考虑 QT 间期延长的治疗可能会造成严重的后果。大多数（不是全部）抗心律失常药物本身是“致心律失常”的。尖端扭转型室性心律失常（见后文）占这些药物诱发的 VT 的大部分，因此最有效的是使用单一抗心律失常药物治疗，并避免联合治疗的致心律失常效应。VF 是一种固有的不稳定性节律，关于 ACLS 的详细讨论不是本章的重点。更重要的是对具有退化成 VF 的倾向的节律的理解，以及以适当的方式干预以防止这种情况发生的能力。

VT 分为单型和多态亚型。单形 VT 被认为源于单个心室异常起搏点并且具有较宽的 QRS 波，具有相似的形态学外观（图 8）。相比之下，多形性 VT 的特征在于不规则的起伏的外观，在 QRS 形态外观上具有显著变化。区分疾病类型是很重要的，因为多形性 VT 通常退化为 VF。进一步的分类由节律的持续性决定。与持续 VT 相比，非持续性 VT 通常持续小于 30 s 并自发终止。在对 60 ~ 85 岁的患者超过 10 年的研究中，非持续性 VT 无法预测冠状动脉事件。即便在心肌梗死后 1 周内发作，心源性猝死的风险仍增加了 1 倍。

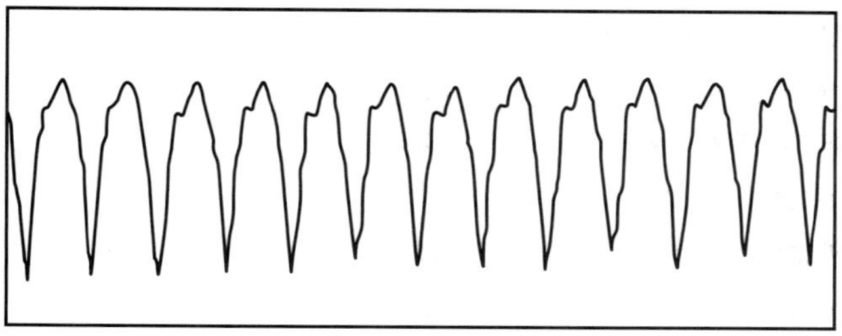

图 8　持续性单形性室性心动过速的心电图特征是经典的宽大畸形的 QRS 波群且具有相似的形态外观

室性期前收缩

室性期前收缩（premature ventricular contractions，PVCs）在术后临床护理患者中很常见。它们可以是单一的，也可以相连或以二联律形式出现。它们与许多电解质失衡和代谢异常有关，例如低钾血症、低镁血症、碱中毒、缺氧和儿茶酚胺过量。纠正这些异常并使用 β 受体阻断药，通常可以消除大多数 PVC。在没有器质性心脏病的无症状患者中，很少需要进一步治疗或抑制 PVC，并且没有相关的短期或长期后果。在有冠状动脉疾病、MI 病史或左室功能受损（EF<40%）的患者中，PVC 可能是产生更多的恶性心律失常的预示。应首先对包括心肌缺血在内的可医治的危险因素进行校正，然后尝试减少血管加压药或正性肌力支持。对于在多种 PVC 的情况下不产生足够的搏出量的症状性患者，用抗心律失常药物进行暂时性抑制可能对危重患者有益。

单形性室性心动过速

非持续性单形性 VT 可以被认为是 PVC 的延长版本。节律与促进或引发触发活动、异常自律性或折返机制的相似电解质和代谢异常相关。β 阻断效应和任何前述的激化因子的逆转，将降低这种节律的频率和持续时间。仅须对表现出症状或血流动力学损害的患者使用抗心律失常药物治疗或电复律。与非持续性单形性 VT 相关的长期预后再次取决于器质性心脏病的存在。在冠状动脉疾病和左心室功能不全的患者中，心源性猝死的风险总体增加（EF<40%）。由于这种关联，患有器质性心脏病的患者应参考电生理（electrophysiologic，EP）测试。在 EP 测试时发现具有诱导节律的患者将受益于植入式心脏复转除颤器（implantable cardioverter-defibrillator，ICD）的放置。在没有器质性心脏病的患者中，非持续性单形性 VT 不会增加长期风险。

引起持续单形性 VT 的最常见的机制是折返。这种节律最常见的是由于先前 MI 的愈合瘢痕，其允许折返回路发生。这通常意味着预后不良，手术后院内死亡率超过 40%，最初存活的患者复发率超过 30%。高达 20% 的从医院出院的患者将在 24 个月内死于心脏性死亡。因为用于维持单态 VT 的基质（例如瘢痕）的持续存在，那些在急性疾病中幸存的患者推荐 EP 测试和随后放置 ICD。

单形性VT的急性处理取决于患者的血流动力学状态。直流电同步复律（单相或双相波形心脏复律，起始于100 J）是治疗那些有症状或不稳定的单形性VT的主要手段。电复律是高度有效的，也推荐对血流动力学稳定的VT结合足够的短期麻醉进行治疗。在那些稳定的患者中，或当电复律不合适或不可用时，静脉注射的普鲁卡因胺、索他洛尔或胺碘酮是目前推荐的抗心律失常药物。胺碘酮是那些心脏功能受损患者的首选药物。美国心脏协会2010年对ACLS的更新还建议，腺苷可以被考虑用于评价和治疗未分化、常规、广泛、复杂的单形性快速性心律失常。抗心动过速起搏也是已放置静脉或内部起搏器的患者的一种选择，尽管存在心动过速加速的可能性，如果要尝试使用这种方法，应将除颤器放置在床边。

多形性室性心动过速

多形性VT应被认为是具有明显恶化为VF倾向的缺血性节律。非持续和持续的作用区别较小，因为这种节律的短暂爆发通常会演变成持续多形性VT。这种节律是持续不变的症状，需要及时的直流电复律。一旦患者的情况变得更加稳定，这时最重要的步骤就是通过ECG分析确定QT间期。在没有QT间期延长的患者中，最可能的病因是急性心肌缺血和相关的严重左心室功能障碍。应该开始进行任何相关的电解质和代谢异常的纠正，最小化外源儿茶酚胺的支持和使用β受体阻断药。在那些患有严重冠状动脉血管疾病的患者中，须进行血管的重建，并且可能须使用主动脉内球囊泵来桥接患者，直到可以血管再生为止。静脉注射胺碘酮、普鲁卡因或索他洛尔的抗心律失常药物治疗可促进窦性心律的维持，但重点应放在治疗潜在的心脏病上。预后取决于患者的血流动力学状态，而不是VT是否存在。在那些急性恢复的患者中，放置ICD已被证明可以改善长期结果。

多形性VT在QT间期延长（QT>460 ms）的条件下通常称为尖端扭转型综合征或“扭转点”。ECG显示广泛的QRS心动过速，其表现为周围的ECG基线扭曲。这种综合征需要不同的处理办法，因为该机制归因于继发于早期去极化之后的触发活动而不是折返。获得性QT延长可由许多电解质异常和多种药物引起（表4）。ICU中常见的原因包括低钾血症、低镁血症、特定抗生素和精神药物，最重要的是Ⅰ和Ⅲ类抗心律失常药。在尖端扭转型室性心动过速的处理中最重要的是识别和去除违禁药剂和纠正所有电解质异常。直流电心脏复律用于血流动力学不稳定时，重点是不能给予任何的可以进一步延长QT间期的药物。应该给所有疑似扭转的患者静脉注射镁。因为QT间期的长度与RR间隔（每次搏动之间的时间）成比例，所以患者可以受益于使用异丙肾上腺素进行超速起搏或经静脉起搏。在冠状动脉血管疾病患者中应谨慎使用异丙肾上腺素。可以使用不延长QT间期的抗心律失常药，包括利多卡因和苯妥英。长期治疗依赖于避免使用延长QT间期的药物。总体预后一般良好，通常不推荐长期治疗。

表4 可导致尖端扭转性室性心动过速的ICU常用药物

药物分类	例子
抗心律失常药	普鲁卡因胺、奎尼丁、胺碘酮、索他洛尔、伊布利特
抗菌药	红霉素、甲氧苄啶－磺胺甲恶唑
精神药物	氟哌啶醇、锂、水合氯醛、三环抗抑郁药
其他药物	他克莫司、血管加压素

Modified from Parrillo J, Dellinger R, editors: *Critical care medicine: principles of diagnosis and management in the adult*, 2nd ed, St. Louis, 2001, Mosby

总结

心脏节律障碍的诊断和处理依赖于准确的节律分类、潜在机制的知识，以及对适当治疗方案的透彻理解。旨在预防促进这些节律障碍的电解质和代谢紊乱的措施不得被忽视。抗心律失常药物的使用必须限于有症状或血液动力不稳定的患者，以限制其诱导心律失常状态的潜力。对于血流动力不稳定的患者和具有恶化为VF倾向的患者，应该毫不犹豫地使用直流电复律。特别强调的是更常见的心律失常的诊断，包括沃－帕－怀综合征和尖端扭转型室性心律失常，因为以下标准治疗方法可能导致灾难性后果。与心脏病学团队的磋商对于疾病的长期处理、患者风险分层和介入治疗过程是至关重要的，可以改善患有心律失常的患者的急性和长期预后。体检、心电图解释和经验是适当控制节律障碍所必需的工具。几乎在每个ICU设施中，这些工具都可以被敏锐化和微调，以便最终使患者获得最大的好处。

机械通气的基础

Soumitra R. Eachempati, Jerry A. Rubano, Jared M. Huston, Philip S. Barie 和 Marc J. Shapiro 著
朱凤雪 李 纾 译

要点

- 新型技术提供了更多的通气方式，可更好地改善气体交换，使患者更舒适，缩短机械通气时间。
- 对于清醒且可以配合治疗的或通气的处于氧合状态边缘患者，无创通气（noninvasive ventilation，NIV）能有效地避免插管或再插管的发生。
- 目前，基本的通气模式有辅助-控制通气（assist -control ventilation，ACV），间歇指令通气（intermittent mandatory ventilation，IMV）和压力支持通气（pressure support ventilation，PSV）。
- 应用低潮气量（6 ml/kg）机械通气（mechanical ventilation，MV）策略可以降低 ALI 和 ARDS 患者的发病率和病死率。
- 谨慎使用镇静药物，并每日施行镇静中断，以及时评估是否满足脱机条件。
- 应用“通气集束化管理”（如预防压力相关的胃黏膜出血、静脉血栓疾病，在没有禁忌证的情况下始终保持床头抬高 30°，每日镇静中断，口腔护理及应用氯己定）可减少 MV 时间，降低 VAP 的发生。

对于创伤患者及重症患者，机械通气是经常需要的，包括进行气道保护、全麻时的管理，对急性呼吸衰竭（acute respiratory failure，ARF）患者的处理（表 1）。目前，新的机械通气技术提供了更多的通气方式，能更好地改善患者的气体交换、使患者更舒适，并缩短机械通气时间。此外，无创正压通气的使用使一部分 ARF 患者避免插入人工气管道内气道，降低有边际储量的患者拔管后再插管的可能。几乎所有的通气都包括两方面设置考虑：即要保证对患者给予充分的支持，也要使患者有锻炼的时间。然而，实际应用时，机械通气参数的设置大多都是依据医生的喜好设定（表 2）。控制性通气在很大程度上抑制了患者的自主呼吸，导致呼吸肌肉的快速萎缩。因此，推荐使用辅助通气模式，即由患者自身吸气努力触发呼吸机送气。基本的辅助通气模式包括 ACV、同步间歇指令通气（synchronized intermittent mandatory ventilation，SIMV）和 PSV。

表 1　机械通气适应证

气道管理或气道保护
气道阻塞
常规吸入麻醉
血流动力学不稳定
低氧血症
代谢性酸中毒
气道分泌物管理（分泌物过多）

大部分 ARF 患者会使用机械通气治疗，触发呼吸机送气所做的功为原来的 4～6 倍。因此，进行机械通气的目的是一定程度地降低患者的呼吸功。此外，机械通气还有一些潜在优势，可以改善患者的气体交换，且在提供的支持力度与患者的需求之间达到最大程度的协调。它可以缓解呼吸肌疲劳并预防肺功能恶化，且可以预防医源性肺损伤的发生，促进肺损伤的愈合。然而，如果不能按照患者呼吸中枢驱动的实际情况精准选择呼吸机参数使它与之同步，MV 反而会造成呼吸功增加。但不论应用何种 MV 模式，所有的 MV 都是气道正压通气的转变形式，是患者与机械通气支持的相互作用。

无创通气

NIV 即在未建立气管内气道的情况下进行的通气支持。先前 NIV 通常是间歇负压通气，但随着技术的进步，目前主要是指通过鼻导管或者面罩进行的正压通气，已被广泛应用于急、慢性呼吸衰竭和部分心力衰竭的患者。

NIV 可以给患者带来很多益处，主要因为其避免了因气管插管的并发症。它保留了患者吞咽、进食、讲话、咳嗽，以及和鼻–口咽部的生理气道的

表 2 机械通气相关专业术语

控制：调节气体流速
容量控制——气道压力不恒定（容量限制，容量目标） **压力控制**——输送的气体量不恒定（压力限制，压力目标） **双重控制**——较少应用［容量目标（保证），压力限制］
切换：通气转换
时间切换——例如，压力控制通气 **流速切换**——例如，压力支持通气 **容量切换**——例如，容量控制通气
触发：引发呼吸机开始循环吸入
时间触发——呼吸机按照预设的取决于控制频率的呼吸频率送气 **压力触发**——呼吸机感受到患者吸气导致的气道压力的下降。 **流量触发**——呼吸机在整个呼吸周期都存在一定量持续的基础气流。患者在吸气时，会造成气流的改变被呼吸机检测到从而触发送气。流量触发与压力触发相比，可以降低患者的吸气做功
呼吸：使呼吸机从吸气到呼气的循环
指令（控制）通气——由呼吸频率决定 **辅助通气**——例如辅助控制、同步间歇指令通气、压力支持 **自主通气**——没有任何额外的辅助，例如 CPAP
流速形态：恒定波、减速波或正弦波
正弦波——例如自主呼吸和 CPAP **恒定波**——在吸气过程中始终保持流速恒定至达到预设潮气量；较少应用 **减速波**——吸气初期以较快流速使肺泡压力上升；例如压力目标通气、容量目标通气，它相对于持续恒定流速可以降低气道压峰值
模式（呼吸形式）
医疗控制通气——控制通气指不允许任何自主呼吸，用于麻醉患者通气 **辅助控制**——控制通气——辅助呼吸模拟控制通气 **间隙指令通气**——控制通气及自主呼吸结合，可具有同步性避免“堆叠”发生 **压力支持**——除气道压力限制，患者自主掌握呼吸频率及形态

加温、湿化能力。未建立人工气道的患者可以更有效地沟通，避免或减少镇静药物的使用，使患者主观感受更为舒适。另外，此类患者往往可以经口进食。它较有创通气而言，避免了一些并发症的发生，如导管插入造成的创伤、黏膜溃疡、误吸、感染（如肺炎、鼻窦炎）及拔管后吞咽困难。

Auriant 等的一项前瞻性、随机试验，对 48 名肺叶切除后急性低氧性呼吸功能不全患者随机分为有创 MV 和经鼻罩 NIV 两组进行对比，结果发现 NIV 组患者再插管率和死亡率明显降低。同样，Squadrone 等对 209 名主要腹部手术后在麻醉恢复室发生呼吸衰竭的患者，随机使用单纯氧疗或经面罩持续气道正压通气（continuous positive airway pressure，CPAP）氧疗，发现联合 CPAP 氧疗组患者气管插管率明显降低，同时降低了肺炎、感染和脓毒症的发生率。

无创通气禁忌证

无创通气成功的关键是患者保持清醒、配合且有一定自主呼吸能力。当患者存在气道问题、心电图明显异常或血流动力学不稳定时，对 NIV 使用存疑。使用时还需要患者有完整有效的咳嗽反射及气道清洁分泌物的能力，它们是导致失败的常见理由。NIV 的相对禁忌证还包括无法合适地适应或封闭面罩、无咳嗽反射、发生呕吐时自己不能摘除面罩。若患者近期接受过胃肠手术或存在胃肠道胀气，也是 NIV 使用的假设禁忌证。应尽量保持通气压力在 30 mmHg 以下，即不超过食管括约肌的闭合压力，避免吞气症的发生。此外，病态性肥胖由于身体状态和仰卧位时腹部脏器和胸壁的重量，会明显增加通气压力支持的需求，也是 NIV 的相对禁忌证之一。

无创通气并发症

NIV 最主要的并发症是皮肤的局部坏死，以鼻梁最为常见，颧骨处也较常见。在使用全脸面罩行 NIV 患者中的发病率为 7%～10%。其他可能发生的并发症（发生率 1%～2%）包括胃胀气、误吸及气胸。理论上与胃扩张有关的是随后的呕吐、误吸和肺炎。由于面罩近眼部周围漏气可能会造成 2% 的患者出现结膜炎。

然而最严重的并发症是医务工作者未能及时发现 NIV 不能保证气道通畅、不能满足患者通气及氧合的需求。人工气道建立的延迟或失败，会导致患者病情持续恶化甚至死亡。

压力支持通气

压力支持通气是对通气患者自主呼吸提供部分或全部的辅助。患者自主控制除压力限制以外的其他呼吸状态。当患者触发呼吸机后，呼吸机输送一定流速的气体以达到预设的压力（例如 10 cmH_2O），此压力的设定以满足患者每分通气量（V_E）的需求。当最大吸气量下降到某一比例时（通常为 25%）切断气流循环。潮气量（V_T）可能有变化，正如自主呼吸时一样。

使用呼气末正压（positive end-expiratory pressure，PEEP，亦称 CPAP）可以恢复患者的功能残气量（functional residual capacity，FRC）至正常。对于肺顺应性差、需要较高胸腔压以使肺扩张达到目标 V_T 的患者，亦应使用 CPAP。添加压力支持可上移患者的压力 - 容积曲线（在一定的施加压力下造成容积明显的改变）。因此，压力支持通气就是将压力支持与 PEEP（或 CPAP）相结合。压力支持通气常用于自主呼吸的患者，也可用于 SIMV 中辅助自主通气。在脱机过程中联合使用这两种方式，开始断开 SIMV，后续使用压力支持。

氦氧混合气

氦气比空气或氮气的密度低，用氦气代替氮气可以降低气体密度，它与混合气体的数量成正比。吸入氦氧混合气体（临床上应用的范围为氦氧比 80：20～60：40）更容易产生层流，降低气道阻力，减少呼吸功。通常用于气道阻力较高的患者，如哮喘、急性加重的慢性支气管炎或慢性阻塞性肺疾病、其他原因造成的支气管痉挛，以及上呼吸道阻塞伴有喘鸣的情况。患者对吸入氦氧混合气体的耐受性较高，且没有明显副作用。但不足之处是价格昂贵且当患者需要较高的吸入氧分数（FIO_2）时不能使用。如果氦氧混合气体直接通过呼吸机而非由喷雾器（常规方法）引入时，则必须对呼吸机进行重新校准，以确保呼吸机对气流的正常测定。

机械通气模式

辅助－控制通气

在内科及外科重症监护病区，ACV 是最常用的机械通气模式。此模式须设置的参数包括吸气流速、频率（f）及 V_T。呼吸机按预设频率及 V_T 进行通气。吸气（I）、呼气（E）时间及 I：E 由 V_T 及流速决定。平台压或肺泡压与 V_T 及呼吸系统顺应性相关。患者通过努力吸气，当超过预设的触发级别时便会触发额外的呼吸。即通常都会为给定的 V_T 设定一个通气频率，但当患者的呼吸频率明显高于预设频率时，则可触发全部的呼吸。在这种模式下，如果患者没有触发呼吸，呼吸机依然可以提供充足的通气。在送气过程中，如果患者仍保持很强的吸气努力，则会造成触发叠加呼吸。如果提高触发阈值或降低 V_T 设定，则可能导致患者吸气努力增加。

同步间歇指令通气

在被动呼吸患者中，SIMV 与 ACV 并无太大差异，通气由设定的呼吸频率及潮气量决定。然而，当患者并非完全被动接受通气时，在指令呼吸期间可有呼吸系统的工作。另外，患者可能通过自主呼吸触发了额外的呼吸如果触发发生在触发窗内，定义为下一次控制通气前的一个短暂时间窗，则呼吸机提前进行指令通气与患者触发同步。若患者在同步窗外开始呼吸，则为自主呼吸而非控制通气，V_T、流量、I：E 都由患者自身努力和呼吸系统机制决定，而不是呼吸机设置。这些自主呼吸可能导致低 V_T 及每次呼吸间差异很大的情况发生。SIMV 这种模式通常用于增加患者呼吸功，常采用降低控制通

气频率及 V_T 设定，迫使患者增加呼吸频率以保证充足的 V_E。因此临床上常联合 PSV 使用，可增加一定的“叹气”作用减少肺不张。较单纯的 PSV 模式，SIMV+PSV 模式保证了一些备份的 V_E，尤其适用于由呼吸中枢驱动的恶化的高危患者，并被广泛应用于辅助脱机的过程。

呼气末正压

所有机械通气模式几乎都会涉及 PEEP。虽然 PEEP 称为呼气末正压，但正压却贯穿整个呼吸循环，更准确的应称为 CPAP。PEEP 的应用主要有 3 个目标：①重建 ALI 及肺不张的患者中下降的 FRC，避免肺泡去复张；②在肺泡开放闭合造成肺损伤时，保护肺膨胀不全区肺组织；③通过调节胸腔内压，辅助心力衰竭状态下的心功能。

FRC（functional residual capacity）是肺部的生理储备量。当胸壁或肺组织顺应性（单位压力下所导致的容量变化率）降低时，FRC 减少。FRC 指正常呼吸末时，呼气末残留在肺内的气量（～2.5 L）；肺内气体充分交换开始。在 FRC 时，肺部萎陷与胸壁向外扩张的趋势相等。此时存在一个气压稍高的内部负压有助于维持此平衡。当发生气胸时，此负压消失，平衡被打破。

FRC 受肺及胸廓顺应性的影响。任何限制胸廓扩张的原因会使其顺应性降低，同样，任何原因导致的肺容量降低都会造成肺顺应性降低。FRC 包括 2 部分体积：补呼气量（expiratory reserve volume，ERV）和残气量（residual volume，RV）。在 FRC 以下的呼气是主动的，须压缩肺组织将气体呼出。在 RV 位时（～-1L，成年人），即使再施加更大的压力也不会造成气体呼出，此时肺泡压力超过大气压，气道的压力梯度为逆向的。肺泡中充满气体且表面附有表面活性剂，因此很难压缩，但气道却可以被压缩。当胸腔内压超过小气道内压力时，会导致气体陷闭在肺泡内，造成“动态气道塌陷”。气道塌陷进一步造成呼吸功增加，使通气 - 灌注比（V/Q）不匹配、且这些塌陷的气道较难复张，进一步导致呼吸功及氧消耗的增加。

在 PEEP 后的观念为增加 FRC，根本上是使肺泡在最容易保持膨胀的地点上放气（为压力 – 容积曲线的低位拐点）。我们须给患者设定足够的 PEEP 以防止肺泡去复张。但是过高的 PEEP 可能会造成肺泡过度膨胀，肺泡微循环不足导致无效腔通气（V_{DS}）。同时 PEEP 还会降低右室前负荷、右室输出量及最终心排血量，导致低血压的发生。

auto–PEEP 是由于呼气末期发生的气体陷闭而造成的，增加患者呼吸功。存在气道阻塞性疾病的患者通常会伴有吸气和（或）呼吸阻力的增加。缩短 E 时间（如小气道疾病、痰液阻塞、压力控制通气时 I : E 为反比等）可以导致呼气末气体陷闭，造成肺过度膨胀，增加胸腔内压，破坏气道内原有的压力梯度。然而，我们可以通过延长 E 时间，缩短 I 时间或降低呼吸频率来改善 auto–PEEP。

最佳 PEEP 目前仍存在很大争议（表 3）。普遍认为，应用 PEEP 行肺复张，即应用较高的压力打开萎陷的肺泡，它同时可以防止绝大部分肺泡去复张，并避免肺泡过度膨胀发生。应用 PEEP 将肺单元的大部分与 P-V 曲线的有利部分重合可以降低气体交换和过度膨胀，但是实践有难度，因为其低位拐点有时是模糊的。由于肺泡表面存在肺泡表面活性物质而导致的迟滞性现象，使得在呼气时肺扩张的趋势大于吸气，在呼气时膨胀的体积比吸气时更大。

机械通气患者的“集束化”管理策略

对于机械通气患者的管理，不仅仅是单纯提供通气、改善氧合。因为这些患者通常病情危重，发生各种并发症的风险高，与 ARF 及 MV 直接相关的并发症仅是其中一部分。因此，临床上应格外关注机械通气患者的各方面情况。此类患者可能面临长期卧床、神经失调、静脉血栓相关并发症，以及压疮出现的风险。损伤或镇静 / 镇痛药物的应用可能会影响患者的感觉中枢，导致自身气道保护能力的下降，胃内容物误吸的风险增加。过度镇静是也导致 MV 的可能因素之一，且它是 VAP 发生的确定危险因素。需要长期 MV（超过 48 h）提示患者病情危重，发生胃部应激性出血的风险增加，这不常发生但死亡率可达 50%，且预示着重症患者预后不良。

在循证医学的指导下，临床上对一些“最佳实践方法”进行组合，拟定了机械通气的“集束化”管理策略，以最大程度优化 MV 的预后。这个策略最初为 4 项，现在包括 5 项：①在没有禁忌证的情况下始终保持床头抬高 30°；②预防静脉血栓疾病；③预防应激相关性胃黏膜出血；④实施每日镇静中断，通过自主呼吸试验的评估考虑是否可以脱机。新增项是⑤局部应用氯己定进行口腔护理。临床上应谨慎采用并依从以上所有要求，并联合其他方法，如坚持感染控制原则，以降低 VAP 发生风险。

常规设置

呼吸机的通气设置是按患者的理想公斤体重和医疗情况所决定的。长时间暴露在 FIO_2>60% 中，便有可能发生氧中毒。因此，临床上应在动脉血充分氧化［动脉氧分压（PaO_2）为 60 mmHg 或动脉血氧饱和度（SaO_2>88%）］的情况下使用尽可能低的 FIO_2（表 3）。

对于肺部正常的患者（如全麻患者），V_T 设定为 8～12 mL/kg 可保证长时间安全通气。以前认为 ALI/ARDS 的危重患者应按理想体重将 V_T 设为 10～15 mL/kg，现在认为这样是不恰当的，会造成肺泡的过度膨胀，使肺泡上皮细胞、内皮细胞及基底膜损伤。这与微血管的渗透性增加，医源性（呼吸机诱发）的肺损伤（ventilator-induced lung injury，VILI）有关。临床上，直接监测肺泡容积不可行，一个合理的替代方法是通过平台压力估算峰值肺泡压力。测量时须保证患者放松，在吸气末期短暂阻塞呼吸环路，监测此时的平台压（Pplat）。对于有肺功能障碍的患者，临床上可减低 V_T 至 4～6 ml/kg 或更低，以保证 Pplat≤35 cmH_2O。当 Pplat 高时，VILI 的发生率明显增加。而应用低 V_T 通气时可能会造成 $PaCO_2$ 升高。为了控制肺泡压力，我们允许 CO_2 浓度增长，这就是所谓的允许性高碳酸血症。在实施过程中，一定要密切关注 pH 值而非 $PaCO_2$。一旦 pH<7.25 应立即增加 V_E 或应用 $NaHCO_3$。

呼吸频率的设定与选择的模式有关。ACV 时，

表 3 ALI/ARDS 患者机械通气策略

呼吸机初始设置
最初应用容量控制通气以保证潮气量
V_T 初始设置为 8 ml/kg，随后每 2 h 减少 1 ml/kg，最终达到 6 ml/kg。V_T 的下限为 4 ml/kg
呼吸频率设为 12～20 次 / 分，上限为 35 次 / 分
根据动脉 pH（7.25～7.45、通气频率）和吸气末平台压（Pplat）（<30 cmH_2O；VT）的目标调节呼吸机设置
从转入 ICU 起每天早晨测量动脉 pH，在调整呼吸频率或 V_T 设定后 15 min 测量动脉 pH
碱中毒时，至少降低呼吸频率 2 次 / 分
轻度酸中毒（pH 7.15～7.25）时，应增加通气频率直至 pH>7.25 或 $PaCO_2$<25 mmHg，呼吸频率最高不超过 35 次 / 分。如果通气频率为 35 次 / 分或 $PaCO_2$<25 mmHg，则应给予碳酸氢盐
重度酸中毒（pH<7.15）时，须增加通气频率至 35 次 / 分。若通气频率为 35 次 / 分、pH<7.15，给予碳酸氢盐，以 1 ml/kg 的增长速度来提高 V_T 直至 pH>7.15。在这种情况下，允许一定范围内超过目标 Pplat
维持 Pplat<30 cm H_2O：至少每 8 h 测量一次 Pplat。每次调节 PEEP 或 V_T 后 5 min，当存在肺顺应性改变可能时应增加测量频率。为保证 P_{plat} 准确，应保证测量时患者静止且无呛咳发生
当存在漏气时，P_{plat} 无法准确测量，可用吸气压峰值替代
氧合的目标是 PaO_2 为 55～80 mmHg 或 SaO_2>88%，可以自由组合 PEEP 及 FIO_2。通常当 FIO_2>0.45 时，须保证 FIO_2：PEEP≤5
当 PEEP 超过 10 cm H_2O 时，对 PEEP 的调整应按照每次 2～5 cmH_2O 的幅度增加，最高为 35 cmH_2O，直到达到目标 PaO_2 状态。如果并不能使 PaO_2 提高大于 5 cmH_2O 或由于心排血量的下降造成氧输送结果的恶化，则应降低 PEEP 至原有水平
至少每 4 h，通过动脉血气测定或血氧定量法评估动脉氧合状况
如果动脉氧合状况没有达到目标范围，可逐步增加 FIO_2（最高为 1）和 PEEP（在 30 min 内，最高为 35 cmH_2O），且每次调整后 15 min 后须进行评估，直至达到目标。可以允许 5 min 以内的 SaO_2<88% 的情况发生。在存在动脉稀释或进行吸痰或纤维支气管镜检查时，允许暂时性（<10 min）FIO_2=1.0
ALI，急性肺损伤；ARDS，急性呼吸窘迫综合征；ICU，重症监护病区；PEEP，呼气末正压。

Modified from Nathens AB, Johnson JL, Mine JP, et al; Inflammation and the Host Response to Injury Investigators: inflammation and the host response to injury, a large-scale collaborative project: patient-oriented research core—standard operating procedures for clinical care. I. Guidelines for mechanical ventilation of the trauma patient. J Trauma 59:764-769, 2005.

ALI, Acute lung injury; ARDS, acute respiratory distress syndrome; ICU, intensive care unit; PEEP, positive end-expiratory pressure

设定的频率应低于患者自主呼吸频率4次，以保证当患者自主呼吸能力迅速降低时提供充足的V_E。在SIMV中，最初呼吸频率的设置通常较高，耐受性逐渐降低至患者状况一致。

在ACV及SIMV模式中，通常设定流速为60 L/min。而COPD患者，通常将流速提高至100 L/min，以提高E，使陷闭气体能够排空，改善气体交换。若设定的流量不能满足患者的需求，患者会对抗自身肺阻抗和呼吸机阻抗，会增加自主呼吸功。

在ACV、SIMV、压力控制通气模式（将在高级机械通气支持技术章节中介绍）中，患者须使气道压力下降至低于一个预先设定的数值（通常为1～2 cmH_2O），以触发呼吸机输送潮气呼吸。大多数情况下这是很直接的，触发灵敏度越低，就需要患者更多的呼吸功触发。当auto-PEEP存在时，患者必须降低同水平的肺泡内压力，才能影响气道开放压，进而触发呼吸开始，这使得患者呼吸功显著增加。流量触发系统可用于降低触发做功，相比于其他触发方法，即患者须打开阀门以获得协助，持续流量系统可始终提供高的持续流量。当患者开始呼吸时，增大的流量更大。因此，流量触发较其他方式可一定程度降低呼吸功，但并不解决呼吸重叠时的触发问题。

镇静

大部分需要MV的患者都需要镇静，但仅少部分（～10%）须联合使用神经肌肉阻断药。大部分药物有双重作用（表4），因此在选择药物时要慎重，个体化治疗，避免过度镇静及药物滥用。应用时对患者药物用量进行滴定，维持患者舒适、保证Ramasy或Riker评分3～4分（表5）。目前认为，间断镇静优于持续镇静，并尽可能地减少镇静药物的使用。对神经肌肉阻断药的应用，应严格把握适应证。

长期镇静或过度镇静都会延长MV时间、增加气管造口术的风险。相反实施每日镇静中断并行自主呼吸试验（详见后文），可明显缩短MV时间，降低VAP及其他并发症的发生。

监测

血气

血气分析所得到的诸多参数中，仅氧分压（Po_2）、二氧化碳分压（Pco_2）及血pH是直接测定的。动脉血氧饱和度（Sao_2）是根据测定的Po_2及氧合血红蛋白解离曲线计算而来，且假定P_{50}（当Sao_2为50%时，Po_2为26.6 mmHg）、血红蛋白结构功能正常。一些血气分析结合血氧计共同使用的方法，可以直接测定各种形态的血红蛋白，包括氧合血红蛋白、总血红蛋白、二氧化碳结合血红蛋白及高铁血红蛋白。而实际HCO_3^-、标准HCO_3^-以及碱剩余是根据pH和Pco_2推算得出。

对血气标本的采集有着严格的要求，必须是新鲜、经适当肝素化且不含气泡的动脉血。由于肝素本身呈酸性，一旦过量则会造成Pco_2、HCO_3^-测量值偏低。若采样后不能及时分析，应保存在冰袋中，最长不超过1 h，否则会因红细胞的代谢继续进行而造成pH、Po_2的下降及Pco_2的升高。而混入气泡则会造成Pco_2下降及Po_2的升高。

血气分析中，包括CO_2及O_2在内的所有气体，在血中的溶解都会随温度的降低而增加。因此，低体温会造成Po_2和P_{CO_2}的降低及pH值的增加。如测量时患者体温过低并没有进行温度矫正（37℃）将会造成结果偏高，但此误差在临床上可以忽略。

脉搏血氧测定法

通过脉搏血氧测定法计算Sao_2，是通过监测氧合血红蛋白和非氧合血红蛋白对红光（660 nm）和近红外（940 nm）光谱的特定吸收而精确计算得出。但保证数据准确的前提是必须检测到血液的搏动。可用于监测的部位有很多，如手指、耳垂甚至额头，且测量结果具有一致性。当Sao_2在70%～100%范围内，脉搏血氧饱和度的度差异不大（±2%），但当Sao_2低于70%时，精确度较低。

但在实际临床应用时，脉搏血氧饱和度的确受很多技术、操作和患者生理因素影响。当无法检测到搏动的血流、显示的波形明显衰减时，估测并不可靠。因此，当患者存在低体温、低血压、低血容量、周围动脉病变以及接受血管活性药物治疗（如去甲肾上腺素）时都会干扰脉氧饱和度监测的精确性。由于二氧化碳结合血红蛋与氧合血红蛋白可吸

表 4　ICU 中镇痛、麻醉、镇静处方的选择

药品	初始静脉剂量	备注
诱导药物		
依托咪酯	0.3mg/kg	维持 CO、BP。能在维持 CPP 的同时降低 ICP。$T_{1/2}$ 短，须持续输注。可能会影响肾上腺功能
氯胺酮	1 ~ 2 mg/kg	起效快、持续时间短，通常用于麻醉诱导。可持续输注，在低剂量时仅有镇静，而无麻醉作用。可出现 BP、HR 一过性增高，ICP 和眼压升高。一般不抑制自主呼吸。新生儿、儿童及孕妇可安全使用。联合使用麻醉药或巴比妥类药物可能会导致代谢延迟。会出现焦虑、定向障碍、烦躁不安，甚至产生幻觉，一旦发生，可应用短效苯二氮䓬类药物缓解。联合使用阿托品进行预处理，可以有效减少分泌物，但同时会增加躁动的发生。经肝代谢。
丙泊酚	1.5 ~ 2.5 mg/kg	无镇痛作用，有较强遗忘作用。可造成呼吸暂停或呕吐反射消失。造成低 BP。长期镇静时维持剂量为 0.05 ~ 0.3 mg/kg · min。能最大程度减少蓄积，促进药物排泄（肝功能不全者）。用于营养处方时，约合 1 kcal/ml（脂质输注）。一瓶药物持续使用超过 12 h，将明显增加感染风险。此药物的儿童使用安全仍存在很大争议
静脉、镇痛药		
咪达唑仑	0.5 ~ 4mg	$T_{1/2}$ 短，但由于代谢产物仍存在活性，可能导致蓄积。仅苯二氮䓬类有强效的遗忘作用。可造成 BP 下降、呼吸抑制。主要应用于 ICU 患者的短期镇静。经肾排泄
劳拉西泮	1 ~ 4 mg	有效的抗焦虑药物。给予一定初始剂量（1 mg/h）后可持续输注。可出现 BP 下降，尤其是对存在低血容量可能或反常躁动患者应用。经肝代谢
吗啡	2 ~ 10 mg	具有镇痛、镇静效果。可引起 BP、CO 降低，甚至发生窒息。长期应用可产生耐受性及停药有戒断症状。可 IV 输注或通过 PCA 给药，提高机械通气及脱机时的耐受性及护理质量。经肝代谢
双氢吗啡酮	0.5 ~ 2.0 mg	是吗啡的半合成衍生物，与吗啡在用法及注意事项上相似，但药效为吗啡的 8 倍。经肝代谢
芬太尼	50 ~ 100 μ g	药效是吗啡的近 50 倍，且常规应用时，较少引起低 BP 的发生（组胺释放减少）。在 ICU 可选择 IV、硬膜外输注或 PCA。与传统麻醉相比，硬膜外麻醉或达到消除手术应激反应的作用可应用更少的药物。可能造成躯干强直，无法手动通气而窒息（须联合使用神经肌肉阻断药以完成插管）。经肝代谢
神经肌肉阻断药		
琥珀酰胆碱	0.75 ~ 1.5 mg/kg	为去极化型 NMBA（与 Ach 受体结合）。起效快、单次剂量作用时间仅为 10 min。可能会导致高钾血症、恶性高热的发生，使 ICP 及眼压升高。药品禁忌证为 TBI、脊髓损伤、神经肌肉疾病的患者。药物须通过胆碱酯酶代谢，当酶缺乏时（比较常见）可使麻痹时间延长
阿曲库铵 顺阿曲库铵	0.2 ~ 0.5 mg/kg	短效非去极化型 NMBAs（竞争性抑制 ACh）。相对起效慢。与其他药物作用相似，但能引起组胺释放、导致 HR 增快、BP 降低。目前，临床上顺阿曲库铵为首选。由于为短效药物，可通过 IV 注射延长药效。低钾血症会增加药效。与许多药物有相互作用。通过霍夫曼降解 / 酯水解代谢，可应用于肝 / 肾功能不全的患者
泮库溴铵	0.05 ~ 0.1 mg	起效快、作用时间长。可导致 BP 升高、HR 增快。用于诱导神经肌肉阻滞，但完成诱导后应更换药物，如顺阿曲库铵以维持效果。经肝 / 肾代谢，当合并器官功能障碍时可造成蓄积
维库溴铵	0.08 ~ 0.10 mg/kg	非去极化型 NMBA，起效快、作用时间短。有较弱的促进组胺释放的能力。可造成恶性高热的发生。经肝代谢
其他药物		
右美托咪定	负荷量 1 μ g/kg 维持量设定为 0.2 ~ 0.7 μ g/kg/h	中枢性选择性 α_2- 受体激动剂，可作为短效（<24 h）镇静药。具有交感神经阻滞作用，可降低 AR 和 BP。可以达到轻度镇定，无呼吸抑制作用，并可用于药物 / 酒精戒断以及脱机过程。但价格相对昂贵
氟哌啶醇	2 ~ 5 mg	通常用于抗焦虑（优于劳拉西泮），尤其当须避免呼吸抑制发生时。临床上常 IV 输注，但给药途径并未获得 FDA 批准。帕金森患者严禁使用抗多巴胺能类药物，可引发锥体外系症状。经肝代谢

表 4　ICU 中镇痛、麻醉、镇静处方的选择（续表）

药品	初始静脉剂量	备注
酮咯酸	15 ~ 30 mg q6h	注射用 NSAID 类药，用于替代阿片类药物或与吗啡联合应用以减少用量。造成不可逆的血小板功能障碍；可能导致伤口或 GI 出血和急性肾衰竭。术后使用应严格限制在 5 天内
逆转剂		
氟马西尼	0.1 ~ 0.2 mg	苯二氮䓬拮抗剂。起效快、作用时间短。停药后副作用便可逐渐消失。短时间内重复使用计量最高不超过 0.8mg。长期用药后突然出现拮抗作用可能会发生癫痫。
纳洛酮	最高 0.4 mg	阿片受体拮抗剂。起效快、作用时间短。通常稀释为 0.4 mg/ml，在 0.04 ~ 0.08mg 范围内滴定，已满足在不发生副作用的前提下达到最佳镇痛效果。可使用最高为 0.4mg 的重复计量或使用连续 IV 输注。突然停药会造成高血压、HR 增快、肺水肿或心肌梗死
依酚氯铵与阿托品	0.5 ~ 1.0 mg/kg，0.1 mg q5 ~ 15 min 最多 4 剂	具有抗心率失常作用的抗胆碱酯酶抑制剂。起效快，作用时间短。常联合阿托品，以减少分泌增加、HR 降低及支气管痉挛的发生。不能逆转由于去极化引起的神经肌肉阻滞。经肝和肾代谢（依酚氯铵）。阿托品可引起发热
新斯的明与格隆溴铵	0.5 ~ 2.0 mg 0.1 ~ 0.2 mg	新斯的明经肾代谢，可导致唾液分泌增加和严重心率过缓的发生。引发喉痉挛或支气管痉挛。经肾代谢。不能逆转由于去极化所引起的神经肌肉阻滞。因可能造成心动过缓，通常使用相同剂量的格隆溴铵（或有时联合阿托品）。格隆溴铵在避免此副作用的同时可导致心率增加，亦可导致发热。新生儿和 GI 绞痛 / 梗阻是格隆溴铵使用的禁忌证。

ACh，乙酰胆碱；BP，血压；CO，心排血量；CPP，脑灌注压；FDA，美国食品及药物管理局；GI，胃肠道；HR，心率；ICP，颅内压；ICU，重症监护病区；IV，静脉注射；NMBA，神经肌肉阻断药；NSAID，非甾体抗炎药；PCA，患者 - 控制镇痛；$T_{1/2}$，消除半衰期；TBI，创伤性脑损伤；Vo_2，氧消耗

收相同的光谱，此外，二氧化碳血红蛋白含量的增高会导致 Sao_2 值错误地升高。周围环境的光、移动的伪影在内的诸多因素都会造成测量偏差。

二氧化碳图

二氧化碳图是监测整个通气周期中呼气时 CO_2 的浓度变化，是机械通气患者最简便、最可靠的方法。其原理是通过质谱分析或红外吸收法检测 CO_2 的存在。可通过主流或侧流方法收集气体进行检测，且后者更为常用，具有轻量级分析器的优点。然而，侧流取样监测时可能会在管道里产生冷凝水。在 ICU 中当呼吸气体为湿化的，采用主流取样的方法监测是更可取的。

CO_2 浓度峰值在呼气末出现，通常被称为“呼气末 CO_2”（$ETCO_2$），此时 $ETCO_2$ 接近肺泡内气体浓度。二氧化碳图是用来评估气管造口术及气管内导管放置位置是否合理，评估脱机、复苏的最有效方法。在脱机时能及时发现高碳酸血症，且可减少连续的血气测量等操作。同时联合脉搏血氧测定法，大部分患者可成功脱机，有效避免过多的血气检查或有创血流动力学监测。

此外，通过二氧化碳图还可以获得其他信息。如创伤患者复苏后 $ETCO_2$ 与 $Paco_2$ 的差值与预后有一定相关性，大于 13 mmHg 则可增加死亡率。若 $ETCO_2$ 下降明显或监测不出，可能预示有潜在重大疾病或事件的发生，如低心排血量、呼吸机管路断开或肺血栓栓塞的发生。而 $ETCO_2$ 逐渐上升，则提示通气不足；反之亦然。除此外，低血容量也可导致 $ETCO_2$ 降低。

有创血流动力学监测

动脉导管置入

动脉压监测是用来评估血流动力学最简便且重复可行的方法之一。自动化血压袖带装置是准确的（误差 ±2%），但只能实现定期测量。如果血流动力学波动明显，需要频繁监测，则须通过动脉留置导管监测。临床上，留置动脉导管的指征为预计手术时间或 MV 时间较长（超过 24 h）、血流动力血不稳定、大量失血、需要频繁抽血采样、需要精确血压控制（如神经外科患者、体外转流的患者）。但留置和拔除导管甚至置管时的反复穿刺可能会带来一定的并发症，因此，临床应用时，尤其对“相对稳定”

表 5 常用镇静评分

评分方法	分值	临床表现
Ramsey 镇静评分		
清醒评分 1～3	1	焦虑、躁动或不安
	2	合作、可定向活动、安静
	3	可配合指令
非清醒评分 4～6	4	刺激反应灵敏
	5	刺激反应迟缓
	6	对刺激没有反应
Riker 镇静躁动分级		
危险躁动	7	拉拽并试图拔除各种导管，攻击医护人员
非常躁动	6	需要保护性束缚并反复语言劝阻无效
躁动	5	焦虑，语言提示劝阻可安静
安静合作	4	安静、容易唤醒、服从命令
镇静	3	对刺激有反应
非常镇静	2	对刺激有反应，但不能服从命令
不能唤醒	1	对强刺激反应弱或无

Modified from Ramsay M, Savege T, Simpson B, et al: Controlled sedation with alphaxalon-alphadolone. *BMJ* 2:656–659, 1974; and Riker RR, Picard JT, Fraser GL: Prospective evaluation of the Sedation-Agitation Scale for adult critically ill patients. *Crit Care Med* 27:1325–1329, 1999

* 刺激：指轻压眉眶或常规声音刺激

的患者，临床医生须认真权衡利弊。

动脉导管可以放置的位置很多。目前动脉导管采用比较特殊的专用薄壁导管，以保证波形监测的真实性，且尽可能同时保证血管通畅。动脉导管不可与静脉导管混用。临床上最常选择的位置是桡动脉，尽管尺动脉直径更大，但由于其经皮难以接近，所以不常规选择。切记在桡动脉放置导管前，一定要评估手部的侧支循环状况，以避免由于动脉阻塞或栓塞造成的组织缺血。新生儿可通过脐动脉置管，极少数会造成肠道缺血。腋动脉，因其形成动脉粥样斑块的风险低、在肩部侧支供应较多，且易于经皮置管，亦是不错的选择。浅表的股动脉也可置管，但并不是首选，因为此处易造成血小板堆积（理论上形成血栓风险较高）且感染风险较高。颞浅动脉由于较细且曲折，置管相对困难。若患者存在周围血管病变，应尽量避免使用。此外，如周围侧支循环差，肱动脉置管导致手部或前臂缺血风险极高，应尽量避免。当应用血管活性药物且导致的末梢血管强烈收缩时，应选用更长的导管且放置在中央位置（如腋窝、股动脉），以最大程度减少副作用的发生。院内动脉导管相关感染发生率较低，发生后应按相关感染控制原则积极干预，并尽量避免股动脉置管。应注意留置动脉导管造成出血、血肿及假性动脉瘤等并发症的发生。

中心静脉压监测

CVP 是综合反映循环血容量、静脉张力和右心室功能的参数，通过测量右心室的充盈压以评估血容量状况。可以通过贵要静脉、股静脉、颈内静脉、颈外静脉或锁骨下静脉置管。在 ICU，置管静脉首选颈内静脉，其次为锁骨下和股静脉。因颈内静脉容易辨识，置管成功率较高且并发症少。但使用过程中，较难固定且发生感染的概率较锁骨下静脉置管高。锁骨下穿刺需要较高的技术水平，且气胸发生率较高（1.5%～3%），但感染发生率最低。虽然股静脉置管操作难度最低，但通常是最后的选择，在心肺复苏或紧急插管时才予以考虑，这两者可以同时发生。因为较颈内静脉及锁骨下静脉而言，股静脉置管更易发生感染、有误穿刺到动脉的风险（9%～15%），且发生静脉血栓栓塞的风险也较高。总之，股静脉置管发生并发症的风险（13%～19%）高于颈内静脉或锁骨下静脉置管（6%～12%）。颈内静脉置管时颈动脉穿刺的发生率（6%～9%）明显高于锁骨下静脉置管时锁骨下动脉穿刺的发生率（3%～5%）。

肺动脉导管置入

PAC 是经中心静脉置入，通过血流对导管尖端球囊的推动经过右心，最终到达 PA。PACs 主要监测心排血量（Q）、前负荷，临床上常用肺动脉闭塞压（PA occlusion pressure，PAOP）或“楔压”衡量。PA 舒张与 PAOP 有良好的相关性。当肺血管阻力增高（如肺间质纤维化、肺动脉高压）时，舒张压超过 PAOP。

正常情况下，PAOP 接近左房压可以反应 LVEDP，且本身可反映 LVEDV。LVEDV 反应前负荷，是临床上的实际目标参数。实际测量中，很多因素都会导致 PAOP 不能准确地反应 LVEDV，例如二尖瓣狭窄、应用高 PEEP（超过 10 cm H_2O），以及右室顺应性改变（发生心肌梗死、心包积液或后负荷增加）。此外，球囊充气过度、导管位置不当、肺泡压力超过肺静脉压力（MV 时应用 PEEP），或者严重的肺动脉高压（PAOP 测量风险高）时，都会影响测量结果。PAOP 升高可见于左心衰的患者，而降低常见于低血容量或前负荷降低的患者。

理论上，理想的 PA 置管可以测定中心静脉血氧饱和度（$S\bar{V}o_2$）。尽管存在争议，对通过中心静脉导管获取上腔静脉内血样本可以提供可比数据。标准的混合静脉血氧饱和度是通过 PAC 导管获取上腔静脉、下腔静脉，且在右心房内混合的血标本进行血气分析得出。目前，某些导管有内置光导纤维感应器，可以直接测量 $S\bar{V}o_2$。当合并贫血、肺部疾病、一氧化碳中毒、低 Q 或组织氧需求增加时，会造成 $S\bar{V}o_2$ 降低。Sao_2 :（Sao_2 － $S\bar{V}o_2$）反应氧输送（Do_2）是否充足。理想状态下，$P\bar{V}o_2$ 为 35～40 mmHg，Sao_2 为 70%，Sao_2 低于 30 mmHg 即视为非常低的值。

肺动脉导管的临床应用

临床上有很多 PAC 的应用指征，但并没有研究证明应用 PAC 可以降低发病率或死亡率。尽管如此，PAC 对心肌病、各种原因导致的休克、怀疑有肺动脉高压、对常规液体治疗无反应或反应差的患者还是很有帮助的。研究发现，对接受液体复苏并联合使用正性肌力药的重症患者进行 PAC 监测，可能有一定的临床获益。而近期的 ARDSnet 研究表示，对 ALI/ARDS 患者进行 PAC 或 CVP 监测，两组患者预后并无差别。

经食管超声心动图是评估 Q 的相对无创的方法，且近年在 ICU 的使用率有所增加。生物阻抗和生物电阻抗法是测量心排血量和其他血流动力学参数，如每搏输出量和心脏指数的无创方法。生物阻抗法是监测胸腔内容量变化，即由于左室收缩血液进入胸主动脉，所导致的电流改变。胸主动脉内血容量的增加会导致胸腔内阻力的变化。可通过在患者胸部放置电极，监测电压变化来评估阻抗的变化。本质上，生物阻抗的测量是跟踪胸腔电压变化的振幅，而生物电阻抗跟踪的是电子的相位电流在胸腔内传导的过程。每搏输出量越高，这一阶段内监测的信号越多。

此技术进步与无线电中振幅调制（amplitude modulation，AM）和调频调制（frequency modulation，FM）的发展类似。FM 无线电是通过监测不同波形的频率而非幅度发现并分析无线电信号的，并能最大程度的降低噪音干扰以达到保真效果。在监测过程中，当存在血流动力学不稳定、患者情绪波动大或电极位置不牢固以及胸腔内流量改变时，高信号 / 噪音比可以提高准确性。

机械通气的脱机

尽量采取可行的战略及积极的措施，使机械通气患者尽早脱机。因为，通过建立人工气道（如气管插管或气管造口插管）进行 MV 的患者，往往须应用镇静药物，而此又会造成脱机延迟，增加 VAP 的风险，导致更加长时间地需要 MV。

临床上，疾病或治疗相关因素会导致部分患者延迟脱机。通常认为脱机失败是由多方面的因素共同作用导致的结果，其中以呼吸肌疲劳，即呼吸系统超负荷最为常见（表 6）。呼吸负荷的增加可能是由于 V_E 的需求或呼吸功的增加所导致的。当 CO_2 产生增加、V_D 通气增加或呼吸驱动增强都会使 V_E 增加。而 CO_2 产生增加可能是由于分解代谢或营养支持过程中过多碳水化合物的摄入。V_D（有通气但无或低组织灌注）的增加则可能是由于 Q 减少、肺动脉栓塞、肺动脉高压、严重的 ALI 或应用正压通气的医源性问题所致。当存在呼吸肌疲劳或衰竭、刺激肺 J 受体（通常发生在肺部存在炎性或有肺实质出血时）或存在中枢神经系统病变时，都可能会造成呼吸驱动的增强。心理应激也是非常重要的影响因素，可导致呼吸急促、低氧血症、躁动及谵妄的发生。然而重症患者往往因没有给予充分的镇痛或镇静以及未及时处理的谵妄造成了应激。此外，急性酒精或药物戒断症状也是部分患者的主要影响因素。

表 6　呼吸系统的负荷

每分钟通气需求增加	二氧化碳产生增加 无效腔通气量增加 呼吸驱动增加
呼吸功增加	气道阻塞 呼吸系统顺应性降低
呼吸系统功能降低	呼吸的中枢神经驱动受损 膈神经传导系统完整性受损 呼吸肌肌力受损

增加气流阻力或降低胸廓顺应性都会增加呼吸功。气道阻塞的原因可能是小气道可逆性病变（支

气管痉挛）、气道狭窄、气管软化、声门水肿或功能障碍、痰液阻塞，以及肌无力或疲劳。呼吸肌功能障碍可能是由于营养或代谢不均衡导致（包括低钙血症、低钾血症、低磷酸盐血症）。危重病性多发性神经病的发病机制尚未明确，但与脓毒症及多器官功能障碍综合征有着密切的关系，通常须根据肌电图的特异表现做出诊断。此外，低氧血症、高碳酸血症，甚至贫血等其他潜在因素，都可能会导致肌衰竭或无力。

患者与呼吸机“打架”称为人与呼吸机不同步的综合征。造成此问题的原因有很多，在临床工作中必须及时发现并处理。但如果在未明确原因并纠正前，加深对患者镇静程度（或应用神经肌肉阻断药）是极其错误的，可能会由于气道的不稳定而造成灾难性的后果。因此，需要一个系统的评估方法，来评估人机是否协调，并具体区分是因呼吸机设置还是患者自身原因导致的。问题可能出自任何环节，从电源接头到气源到肺泡，必须系统地寻找（表 7）。但通常首先应确定患者插管位置正确、气道通畅。

短期带机患者的脱机比较容易。但仍有近 25% 的患者会经历呼吸窘迫须重新通气。且 ARF 恢复期的、伴有 VAP 坏死或主要躯体创伤的患者的脱机也具有挑战性。如果患者不能耐受脱机，则在自主呼吸试验时有一些特征性表现，其中最直接的是呼吸频率增加以及 V_T 的降低。通常整个自主呼吸试验持续 30 ~ 60 min，较正常的呼吸相比增加 4 ~ 7 倍。患者氧需求增加时机体会增加氧摄取，最终导致 Do_2 下降、动脉低氧血症。肺顺应性降低及延长 I：E 造成气体陷闭都会造成 auto-PEEP。浅快呼吸时 V_E 虽然有所提高，但无效腔通气明显增加，反而会导致 CO_2 蓄积。同样还要考虑心血管系统的压力，因患者躁动导致胸腔内压力骤变，造成肺循环及体循环高血压及两心室后负荷增加。

脱机的时机非常重要；不必要的延迟脱机会增加呼吸机相关性并发症发生的风险。但如果过早拔管则可能会导致心肺功能失代偿，并延长 MV 时间。通常，在心肺功能不稳定或 Fio_2 为 0.6 及以上但 Pao_2 低于 60 mmHg 时，不考虑脱机。当然，良好的氧合状况并不能作为预示脱机成功的可靠指标。重要的是要评估呼吸肌肉是否可以耐受呼吸功的增加，但完全基于临床而做出的判断并不一定准确。即使是综合传统指标评估，如最大吸气负压、肺活量、V_E 等。目前认为自主呼吸试验 30 min 后评估 1 min 内的 f/V_T（浅快呼吸指数或 Tobin 指数），且 f/V_T 低于 80 是相对更可靠的预测指标（95% 成功率）。计算 PSV 中的 f/V_T，准确度会比较低

脱机时，首先应考虑患者的状态是否适合（表 8）。须仔细评估患者血流动力学是否稳定、精神状态能否合作、呼吸肌力量、意识状态是否清醒、是否能处理气道分泌物、营养状态、酸碱平衡及电解质水平是否正常，以及人工气道型号是否合适等。对于既往有慢性疾病（如 COPD）的患者，应允许

表 7 逆转通气失败的治疗

改善肌肉功能
治疗脓毒症——避免使用氨基糖苷类药物
营养支持，但避免过度喂养（通过间接热量学指导治疗）
维持电解质正常
在患者可耐受范围内锻炼，保证休息
严格控制神经肌肉阻断药的使用
避免过度镇静
发现并纠正甲状腺功能减退
降低呼吸负荷
气道阻力
确保气道始终保持通畅、气道宽度足够
顺应性（弹性）
治疗肺炎
纠正肺水肿
识别并尽量降低内源性 PEEP（auto-PEEP）
充分引流胸腔积液
排空气胸
治疗肠梗阻（应用胃肠动力药物）
胃肠减压、治疗腹腔隔室综合征
保持患者抬头 30°
每分通气量
治疗脓毒症
降低体温（T ＞40℃）
避免过度喂养
纠正代谢性酸中毒
识别并尽量降低内源性 PEEP（auto-PEEP）
支气管扩张
维持最小的可能的 PEEP
纠正休克 / 纠正低血容量
识别并治疗肺栓塞

PEEP，呼气末正压通气

表 8　Cornell 机械通气脱机流程

筛选（每天至少进行 1 次，通常在清晨，依据当地流程，由呼吸治疗师、护士或医生执行）
潜在疾病得到缓解 无血管加压药或镇静药物的持续使用（除外丙泊酚及右美托咪定） 无神经肌肉阻断药的使用 允许间断使用镇静药物 近期没有心肌缺血或心律失常的发生 V_E<15 L/min 在 F_{IO_2}<0.55 时，Pa_{O_2}：F_{IO_2}>120 Pa_{CO_2}<50 mmHg pH 值在正常范围内（7.35~7.45） PEEP < 8 cmH_2O 压力支持 < 8 cmH_2O 咳嗽反射存在且有效 / 有良好的气道自洁能力
是 / 否 → 重新评估 ↓
进行自主呼吸试验，并暂停肠内营养，密切监测血糖变化，尤其是在持续泵入胰岛素时
自主呼吸试验 评估 RSBI；目标值应低于 105 ↓
是 / 否 → 重新评估，治疗以降低呼吸负荷 ↓
继续进行自主呼吸试验
应用流量触发的 CPAP 模式，并保证 CPAP 及 F_{IO_2} 不变，试验维持 1 h 提示失败的指标 RR > 35 次 / 分，持续 5 min 以上 Sa_{O_2} < 90%，持续 30 s 以上 HR > 140 次 / 分，或△ >20% BP_{syst} > 180 mmHg 或 <90 mmHg 患者出现明显焦虑、躁动及出汗 ↓
通过 / 失败 → 重新监测 ↓
每天需吸痰次数少于 4 次 有足够的气道保护能力（咳嗽、呕吐反射存在） 之前的 48 h 内没有上气道梗阻的征象 之前的 48 h 内没有因分泌物过多而发生再插管 ↓
T 形管试验（可选） ↓
拔管

BP，血压；CPAP，持续气道正压通气；HR，心率；RR，呼吸频率；RSBI，浅快呼吸指数

一定程度的高碳酸血症，并避免新发代谢性酸中毒。最后，还应注意影响肌肉功能的电解质水平（如钙、磷、钾），并保证其维持在正常水平。如果上述条件都满足，则可以尝试脱机。

有 4 种脱机方式。最简单的是每天通过 T 形回路管给氧进行自主呼吸试验。并由最初短暂锻炼（5 ~ 10 min）开始，逐渐增加时间及频率，直至患者可以耐受自主呼吸数小时。另一种方法是单用 T 形回路管并单日维持最多 2 h，如果患者可以耐受，则可以脱机；如果失败，则第二天再进行重新评估。目前，越来越多的患者使用 SIMV、PSV 模式，尤其是将二者联合。通过逐渐降低 f 或压力，降低通气辅助。当使用联合模式时，应先逐步降低 f 直至较低时再降低压力水平。通常，压力支持降至 5 ~ 8 cmH_2O 时停止，一般认为此压力正好用于补偿呼吸机管路所造成的阻力增加。如果患者能在此条件下呼吸则可以考虑脱机，但实际上目前并没有准确规定压力降低的最低值。有随机对照研究表明：脱机过程中应用 IMV 模式而非实施自主呼吸试验，会导致脱机时间延长 3 倍，并可能预示患者存在较严重的疾病。亚组分析中发现，近 10% ~ 20% 的患者需要再插管，且死亡率较其他患者增高 6 倍。再插管的发生提示患者病情重、预后差。脱机拔管后使用 NIV，在一定程度上可以提高成功拔管的可能性。

其他特殊情况

意外拔管

意外拔管（通常为患者自行拔除）是一件严肃的事件，在 MV 患者中发生率大约为 10%。高危因素包括慢性呼吸衰竭、气道固定不牢固、经口气管插管（患者舒适度低），以及不充分的镇静。其相关并发症为二次插管（约 50%）、肺炎、声带损伤，少数患者会产生呼吸道缺损以及心血管或神经系统并发症。通常再插管的原因为紧急情况插管、精神状态差、意外拔管或 Pa_{O_2}：F_{IO_2} 低于 200。临床上可通过给予合理且充分的镇静、注意患者的动作及床头的位置、牢固固定人工气道，以及每天日常巡视及评估患者能否脱机，以减少意外拔管的发生。

再插管

即使患者按照流程并满足所有脱机指标，仍有近20% 的患者需要再插管。当然不同机构的发生率有很大差异。例如，某些单元脱机拔管相对不够积极，致使再插管率极低；某些单元大部分患者都是神经损伤患者，即脱机失败风险极高的患者，而导致再插管率极高。有趣的是，脱机流程本意仅是为了使患者尽快脱离 MV，但在实践过程中还起到了降低再插管发生的作用。临床上，再插管可以作为疾病严重程度较重的一个标志物，是发生肺炎及死亡率增加的危险因素。而导致再插管的原因可能是气道狭窄或肺 / 胸壁呼吸力学受损或衰竭（脱机失败）。

气管造口术

准确判断患者是否能成功脱离呼吸机具有一定的挑战性。可能的影响因素包括：气道阻塞、患者焦虑不安或躁动（需要大剂量镇静药物）、吸入综合征、碱中毒、支气管痉挛 / 喘鸣、COPD、危重病性多发性神经病或其他神经肌肉疾病、电解质异常、心脏病、甲状腺功能减退、病态肥胖、营养（过度喂养或喂养不足）、使用阿片类药物、过度镇静、胸腔积液（大量）、肺水肿和脓毒症。

气管造口术的时机仍存在争议。并没有相应的共识准确定义“早”（带机超过 12 天？）和“晚”（带机超过 21 天？）。但目前通常提倡尽早进行气管造口术，增加患者舒适度，减少镇静药物使用，降低 VAP 的发生风险，有利于脱机的进行。气管造口术导管长度较插管明显缩短，可以大幅度降低气道阻力，减少呼吸功，有利于气道清洁。此外，经皮气管造口术大大降低了常规气管造口术的并发症的发生，且插管所用的高容低压球囊已可保证经喉插管几周内的放置相对安全。但当患者血流动力学不稳定、凝血功能障碍或 PEEP 水平较高时，则不建议在病情未稳定前实施气管造口术。

高级机械通气技术

Jared M. Huston, Marc J. Shapiro, Soumitra R. Eachempati 和 Philip S. Barie 著
朱凤雪　李　纾 译

要点

- 机械通气（mechanical ventilation，MV）必须在保证气体交换的同时提高人机同步性，最大程度避免压力过高导致肺损伤的发生。
- 低潮气量保护性通气策略，可明显降低 ALI 及 ADRS 的发病率及死亡率。
- 压力控制通气（pressure-controlled ventilation，PCV）时产生的潮气量是由预先设定的压力和患者自身呼吸状况共同决定的。
- 气道压力释放通气（airway pressure release ventilation，APRV）时患者可有或无自主呼吸，此模式可提高人机同步性，降低患者呼吸功。
- 允许性高碳酸血症是指为避免气道压力过高，防止发生气压伤，采取减少潮气量、允许 CO_2 浓度在一定范围内增高的通气策略。
- 成比例辅助通气监测患者通气需求的变化调整气体流速，是一种同步部分辅助通气（闭环通气模式）。
- 神经辅助调节通气是通过监测膈电活动（electrical activity of the diaphragm，EAdi），按患者呼吸驱动进行成比例支持。
- 应用吸入性 NO 或表面活性剂，理论上可以改善氧气交换，但除新生儿外应用较少。
- 其他能使患者受益的通气方式包括：体外膜肺氧合（extracorporeal membrane oxygenation，ECMO）、高频振荡通气（high-frequency oscillatory ventilation，HFOV）、PEEP 及俯卧位通气。

50 多年前现代正压 MV 正式应用于临床。主要目标是辅助患者维持肺泡气腔与毛细血管间氧及二氧化碳的充分交换。在临床上 MV 的首要目的是改善气体交换，但避免较高的气道正压导致的 VILI 同样重要。无创通气技术如双相气道正压通气（bilevel positive airway pressure，BiPAP）的广泛应用，很大程度上减少了气管插管的应用。

近年来随着通气技术的快速发展，使得很多患者可以通过仪器辅助获得更充分的支持，极大程度地避免了由于人力物力条件有限导致的死亡。本章节将重点介绍一些可使 ALI 或 ARDS 继发急性呼吸衰竭（acute respiratory failure，ARF）患者获益的先进通气支持方式及新技术。

急性肺损伤导致的氧合作用障碍

ALI（Pao_2：FIo_2<300）或 ARDS（Pao_2：FIo_2<200）的患者由于气道反应、肺水肿及炎症，导致氧合难以维持。病理上可见肺泡毛细血管通透性增加、中性粒细胞迁移加速。ALI 及 ARDS 时肺水肿及炎性反应为异质性的，不同肺组织间通气血流比例（V/Q）不同。并且目前已意识到机械通气可能会加重肺部炎症反应、加重组织损伤及导致发病率及死亡率增加。

呼吸机诱导的肺损伤

VILI 通常是由于潮气量（tidal volumes，V_T）过大或气道高压而造成肺泡过度膨胀，产生过高的应力而造成肺损伤。肺泡过度膨胀可诱发肺泡局部和全身的促炎细胞因子反应。而限制肺泡过度膨胀及减少肺泡周期性去复张肺萎陷可降低炎症反应。体外研究及临床数据都建议采用低 V_T 保护性通气策略，预防由 VILI 造成的促炎性反应。新型 MV 模式的设计正是利用这一原理，最大程度地降低医源性损伤（表 1）。

肺泡过度膨胀一般是由于高气道压或高 V_T 导致的，即气压伤或容积伤。因此，在 MV 时气道平台压、气值压峰值及 V_T 是很重要的监测参数。急性呼吸窘迫综合征网络工作组的研究是具有里程碑意义的，再一次强调了高 V_T 及高气道压给患者带来的严重后果。在此项多中心随机对照研究中，将 ALI 患者分为传统通气组（V_T 为 12 ml/kg、限制平台压≤50 cmH_2O）和低潮气量通气组（V_T 为 6 ml/kg、限制平台压≤30 cmH_2O）进行对比，发现小 V_T 组患者生存率显著改善，而提前终止了研究。

ARD 网络工作组研究发现低潮气量通气策略，不仅可以改善 ALI/ARDS 患者的预后，而且可以降低循环、凝血紊乱及肾衰竭的发生，而且对降低血浆中白介素 -6 的浓度，减少由 VILI 导致的全身炎性反应有一定的帮助。

表 1　机械通气模式

通气模式 / 策略	优点	缺点
容量控制通气	预设呼吸频率及潮气量	气压伤
低潮气量通气	气道压低，死亡率降低	通气不足、低氧血症
压力控制通气	预设气道压力	通气不足、低氧血症
反比通气	增加肺泡复张	auto-PEEP、气压伤
气道压力释放通气	预设气道压力，允许自主呼吸	通气不足
允许性高碳酸血症	控制低潮气量及气道压力	增加 ICP、心律失常
成比例辅助通气	改善人机同步性，适应患者呼吸力学	不预设潮气量，须监测呼吸驱动
适应性支持通气	预设每分通气量	潮气量高
神经调节辅助通气	改善人机同步性	须进行有创操作监测膈的电活动
分钟指令通气	预设每分通气量，允许自主呼吸	肺不张、气道压力可变
体外膜肺氧合	避免肺机械应力产生	须建立体外心肺循环
高频振荡通气	控制低潮气量	平均气道压高、需深度镇静
俯卧位通气	改善 V/Q	须增加镇静深度、压疮

ICP，颅内压；PEEP，呼气末正压

非传统机械通气模式

压力控制通气

大部分传统 MV 都是容量周期的，按照设定的呼吸机 V_T 进行通气。因此气道压受送气量及患者呼吸力学影响。而 PCV 模式则是预先设定吸气压力，所以最终输送的 V_T 受患者的气道阻力及肺顺应性影响。吸气循环初期吸气压力明显增高，并在整个送气过程中维持。吸气流速是以指数方式递减，以保证维持预设值恒定，且递减模式可更好地改善气体交换，这也是 PCV 的优势所在。PCV 不是一个自主呼吸模式，患者不须主动参与呼吸，最主要的缺点是 V_T 依赖于气道压力和肺的力学特性。例如，当气道压峰值恒定时，气道阻力增加或肺顺应性降低，V_T 明显降低。因此在使用 PCV 时潮气量是不恒定的。因此当患者存在 ARDS 或肺损伤、肺无顺应性时，可能会导致低通气或低氧血症的发生。

最近一项随机对照研究，对 20 名 ARDS 患者按不同通气策略即严格限制气道压（平台压 $<30\ cmH_2O$）以及按 ARD 网络工作组（低 V_T）的控制通气策略进行分组比较。发现两组带机时间、ICU 治疗时间、住院时间并没有显著差别。但限制通气组患者全身促炎因子浓度明显降低，且在一定程度上降低了后续的器官损害。但仍需大的临床研究来证实并评估通气策略是否可以影响死亡率。

开放肺通气

“开放肺”通气策略可预防由于往复的开放闭合导致的剪切伤，并预防肺萎陷、降低相关促炎因子的释放、最大程度地改善气体交换。肺不张通常发生在气体呼出时。因此，在呼气时应用一定的压力（即 PEEP）可以预防肺泡的萎陷。近期，有较多在 ALI 及 ARDS 患者 PCV 联合低潮气量通气“开放肺”通气、肺复张通气策略对预后影响的研究。Villar 等进行的一项多中心、随机对照试验，对比应用高 PEEP、低 V_T 与传统 V_T（9～11 ml/kg）通气对患者的影响。结果发现高 PEEP 及低 V_T 组患者带机时间、住 ICU 及住院期间死亡率明显降低。但这并不能区分患者具体是因为高 PEEP 还是低 V_T，或因为二者的共同作用而获益的。为了进一步明确，Meade 等随后进行了一项多中心、随机、对照研究，对比了 ALI 和 ARDS 患者应用低 V_T 通气联合高 PEEP、低 PEEP 和肺复张操作的差异。结果发现患者的全因死亡率并没有太大的差异，但研究组难治性低氧血症的发生率及因此而致死的概率显著降低。但低 V_T 通气时联合“开放肺”所产生的益处仍需进一步评估。

反比通气

反比通气（inverse-ratio ventilation，IRV）即调整吸气时间（I）与呼气时间（E）的比值为反比，通常与 PCV 模式联合（称 PC-IRV），为常规 MV 失败后的首选考虑（图 1）。正常的 I∶E 为 1∶4。降低吸气流速可使 I 时间延长、I∶E 缩短至 2∶1。甚至是 4∶1。增加 I 可以减少肺泡萎陷，复张肺泡。研究显示 ARDS 患者应用 PC-IRV 可明显改善氧合。尽早应用 PC-IRV 可使吸入氧分数（fractions of inspired oxygen，FIO_2）、高的 PEEP 水平及吸气压峰值（peak inspiratory pressures，PIPs）逐渐降低。但有潜在发生呼吸重叠（auto-PEEP）、肺泡过度膨胀及气道压高、气压伤的风险。auto-PEEP 的出现会使胸腔内压增高，进一步导致静脉回心血量的减少，心排血量（Q）降低。目前，并没有研究比较传统通气方式与 IRV 对患者死亡率影响的差异。

气道压力释放通气

气道压力释放通气（airway pressure release ventilation，APRV）是有压力限制、时间周期且合并“开放肺”策略的通气模式。类似于 CPAP，在此基础上定时、短暂、间歇性地降低气道压力以促进气体呼出。此模式的整个呼吸周期都允许患者自主呼吸，也可用于需要较强通气支持的窒息患者。应用 APRV 可降低气道压峰值、胸腔内压，减少对静脉回流及心排血量的影响，改善 V/Q。对存在自主呼吸患者应用，可以改善人机同步性，减少镇静药物用量，避免神经肌肉阻断药的使用。APRV 通过改善呼气可使支气管痉挛及存在小气道疾病的患者获益。APRV 也可在脱机过程中应用。但此模式的缺点与 PCV 相似，对气道及循环阻力的影响较大，可造成跨肺压降低及对自主呼吸的潜在干扰。

APRV 相关术语与其他通气模式有所不同。可调节的参数包括高压（P_{high}）、低压（P_{low}）、高压时间（T_{high}）、低压时间（T_{low}）。P_{high} 即基础气道压力，亦称 CPAP、膨胀压力或 P1 压力。P_{low} 即压力释放后的

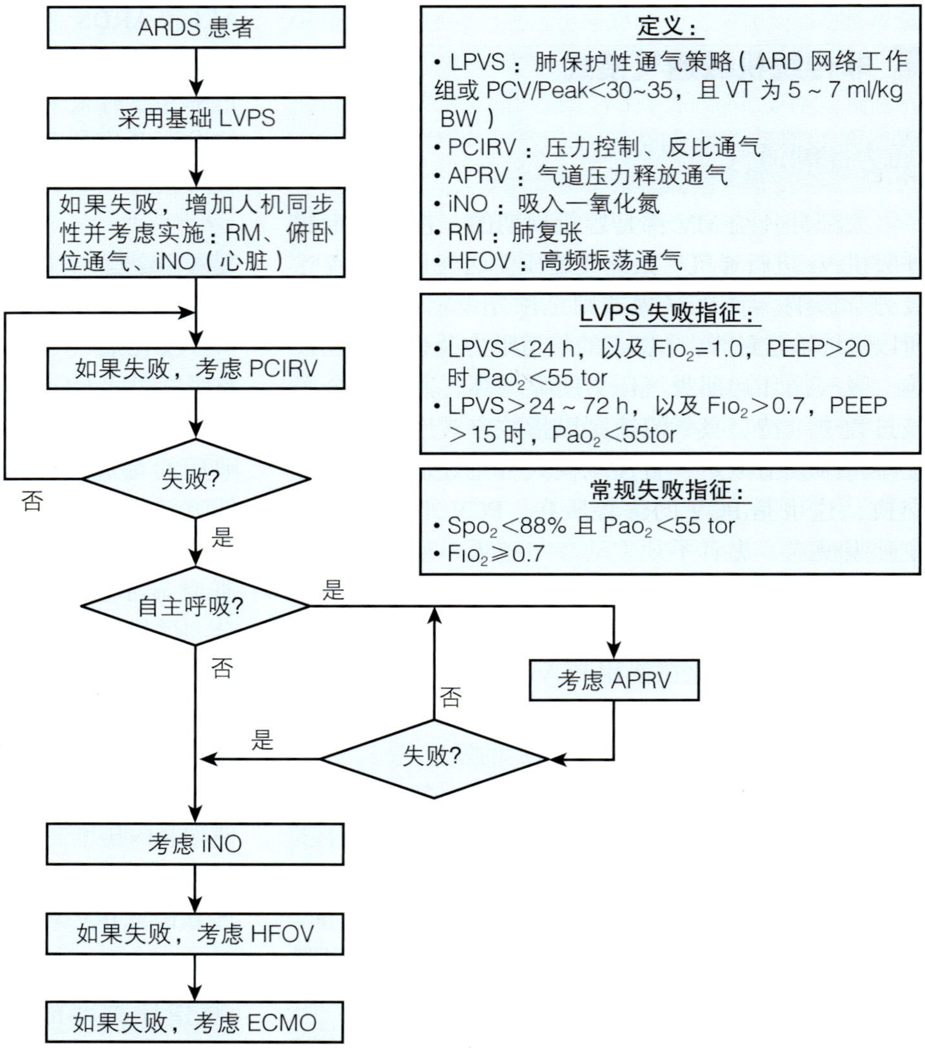

图 1 ARDS 患者的分层通气管理。ECMO，体外膜肺氧合；PBW，预测体重；PCV，压力控制通气；PEEP，呼吸末正压；VT，潮气量 (*Modified from Haas CF, Bauser KA: Advanced ventilator modes and techniques. Crit Care Nurs Q 35:27–38, 2012.*)

气道压（亦称 PEEP、释放压力或 P2）。T_{high} 是 P_{high} 维持的时间（T1），而 T_{low} 是 P_{low} 维持的时间（T2）。平均气道压力可以通过以下公式计算：

$$\frac{(P1 \times T1)+(P2 \times T2)}{T2+T1}$$

由传统通气转化为 APRV 时，并没有标准化的操作指导。通常，压力设定是依据传统通气时的值而设定的。例如，P_{high} 可以按照传统通气时的平台压（P_{plat}）（前提是不超过 35 cmH_2O）设定，维持目标 V_E 为 2 ~ 3 L/min（较传统通气低）。P_{low} 初始设为 0 cmH_2O。T_{high} 至少为 4 s，T_{low} 可以设为 0.8 s（0.5 ~ 1.0 s）。若患者顺应性较低（如病态肥胖、腹部膨隆），则须提高 P_{high} 的设定至 40 ~ 45 cmH_2O。患者呼吸力学改善时，可以按每次 1 ~ 2 s 的速度延长 T_{high} 时间至 12 ~ 15 s。延长的 T_{high} 时间，可以减少由于气道及肺泡周期性的开放闭合所造成的 VILI 发生。T_{low} 的最佳设定是使呼气流量维持在 20% ~ 50% 呼气流量峰值。在整个通气过程中始终允许患者自主呼吸。

转变为 APRV 后患者的临床状况并不能立即改善，研究认为大约 8 ~ 16 h 后氧合改善最为明显。使用 APRV 脱机也须按照一般脱机原则进行，逐步调节 P_{high}、T_{high} 的设定。P_{high} 每次降低 2 cmH_2O 直至 15 cmH_2O 左右，并按 1 ~ 2 s 的增幅逐渐延长 T_{high} 至 12 ~ 15 s。监测每分通气量判断是否存在通气不足的状况。目标是过渡到单纯 CPAP 为 6 ~ 12 cmH_2O，并判断患者患者是否可以耐受拔管。

目前，并没有随机对照试验研究 APRV 与低潮气量通气策略对 ALI 和 ARDS 患者的影响。仅在回顾性研究中发现APRV可减低ALI和ARDS患者的气道压峰值并改善氧合。Maxwell等进行了一项前瞻性随机研究，比较了多发创伤后MV超过72 h的重症患者应用APRV及肺保护性通气策略的差异。参与研究的近45%的APRV组的患者及近34%肺保护性通气组的患者存在ALI或ARDS。发现APRV组患者机械通气时间、ICU治疗时间明显延长，并发生呼吸机相关性肺炎的比例明显增高，但须注意的是两者患者急性生理和慢性健康评分Ⅱ（Acute Physiology and Chronic Health Evaluation，APACHE Ⅱ）的基线存在差异，APRV组较高，这可能是导致此不良结果的一个原因。如果想把APRV作为ALI或ARDS患者的标准化通气模式，还须进行更多的研究。

允许性高碳酸血症

允许性高碳酸血症是一项ARF患者的辅助性肺保护性通气策略，目的是通过严格限制气道压力在30～35 cmH_2O，防止气压伤发生。研究证实，气压伤的发生可进一步刺激炎性介质的释放，并加重MODS。而对肺顺应性不好的患者，PCV可导致肺换气不足及高碳酸血症。正是应用这种策略允许$Paco_2$一定程度地增高，发生一定程度的高碳酸血症。Hickling等对比了允许性高碳酸血症通气策略与低V_T同步间歇指令通气（synchronized intermittent mandatory ventilation，SIMV）的辅助性益处，结果显示限制PIPs在30～40 cmH_2O，并允许$Paco_2$在正常浓度上适当增高，使ARDS患者的预期死亡率有所降低。Amato等的对照研究也得出相似的结果：应用保护性通气策略与允许性高碳酸血症策略都可以改善患者28天生存率，但两组院内生存率并没有显著差异。

尽管一些研究证实了ARDS患者应用允许性高碳酸血症可以获益，但仍然须考虑由于生理上导致的高碳酸血症带来的相关问题，如神经系统、心血管系统、肾系统等。允许性高碳酸血症是有生理上限的（如$Paco_2$不超过80 mmHg，动脉pH不低于7.20），一般不会达到，且目前并没有具体的$Paco_2$及呼吸性酸中毒的安全范围规定。此外还须关注可能造成的肺不张及V/Q失调加重的问题，允许性高碳酸血症的禁忌证包括颅内压增高、脑水肿、心脏功能不全、心律失常、肺血管阻力增加及代谢性酸中毒并导致生化功能紊乱。

成比例辅助通气

成比例辅助通气（proportional assist ventilation，PAV）是一种部分同步通气支持形式，它不预设容量或压力，而是根据患者的吸气努力程度同步部分呼吸支持，增大气流量。PAV是一种新型闭环通气模式，用患者的固有的呼吸驱动来决定机械支持水平。它完全由患者触发送气，并决定通气深度及频率，而不是由呼吸机。理论上闭环通气可通过反馈机制，保证患者通气充足，改善患者的舒适度，极大程度地减少人机对抗。应用PAV可以降低气道压峰值、避免过度通气及肺泡过度膨胀、改善呼吸驱动，以及提高负压通气的效率。

为保证PAV的有效性必须要充分了解患者的呼吸力学情况，尤其是须监测患者的气道阻力、顺应性及内源性PEEP（auto-PEEP），以确定通气负荷及须提供的通气支持。Younes等提出了一项创新技术，可以应用于PAV期间无创测量被动弹性的情况。一旦测定出弹性及气道阻力，便须逐个调节PAV参数，包括PEEP、限制气道峰压在30 cmH_2O以内、容量辅助为弹性的8%，并监测患者的通气状况、呼吸形态及气道峰压。但总体上此模式临床应用相对有限，且PAV对ALI及ARDS患者的有效性并不明确。

适应性支持通气

适应性支持通气（adaptive support ventilation，ASV）是一种新型通气方式，可提供低V_T肺保护性通气策略及适当的频率。须预设目标V_E，通气时可自动调节最适V_T以保证患者呼吸功最低。理论上当肺顺应性降低时，呼吸机会选择低V_T并增加呼吸频率。当患者合并阻塞性肺疾病时，呼吸机会增加V_T，并降低呼吸频率，最大程度地减少气体陷闭的发生。在临床工作中时刻保持高度警惕并频繁地手动调整呼吸及参数并不现实，如果一个呼吸机模式可以根据患者的实际呼吸力学自主调节吸气容量，则会使肺损伤的发生明显降低。Dongelmans等对346名心脏术后患者进行分析，应用ASV（n=262）或PCV/PS（n=84）维持V_T接近6 ml/kg。结果发现ASV组平均V_T为8.3 ml/kg而PCV/PS组为7.3 ml/kg。且在ASV组中55%的患者V_T超过8 ml/kg，还有近12%的患者超过10 ml/kg。

神经调节辅助通气

神经调节辅助通气（neutrally adjusted ventilator assist，NAVA）也是闭环通气，通过监测固有吸气作用，调节呼吸机支持力度及时间。此外，部分辅助通气最主要的目标是尽最大可能保证人机同步性，包括自主呼吸开始和结束时停止呼吸机辅助。NAVA是通过食管在膈水平放置电极，测量EAdi，对EAdi进行处理，控制调节MV。理论上应用EAdi指导通气可以最大程度地改善人机同步性。

目前有关NAVA的临床研究十分有限。Spahija等的一项前瞻对照交叉研究，对14名未接受镇静药物治疗的重症患者（其中12名患者合并慢性阻塞性肺疾病）分组，进行NAVA或标准PSV通气比较。发现尽管NAVA组患者延迟触发及延迟循环的发生显著降低，但两组患者的动脉血气结果并没有显著差距。Terzid等对内科ICU中的11名由于肺疾病导致ARDS的患者进行了一项前瞻性干预研究，发现当患者存在自主呼吸时，使用NAVA较PSV可明显降低人机对抗的发生。

分钟指令通气

分钟指令通气（mandatory minute ventilation，MMV）会给予患者较大的通气支持，仅须患者保持最低的V_E水平。如果患者自主呼吸不能达到预设的V_E，则呼吸机会提供一定的压力支持以弥补。如果患者的自主呼吸超过目标V_E，呼吸机则不给予任何帮助。MMV也是闭环通气的一种，通过监测患者的通气需求，反馈调节设置参数。尤其适用于患有严重神经肌肉相关疾病、药物过量或深度镇静的患者。但MMV可能会造成患者肺泡通气与呼出V_E不匹配，造成闭合容积减少以及肺不张的发生。在MMV与其他闭环通气模式广泛应用于临床前，都须进行更严格的评估与测试。

高频振荡通气

高频振荡通气（high-frequency oscillatory ventilation，HFOV）在新生儿和小儿中的应用较为成熟。是应用较低的V_T（通常低于解剖无效腔量）及高呼吸频率（2.5～3.0 Hz）。HFOV可从多方面达到肺保护性通气目的，如减少肺泡萎陷及过度膨胀的发生。在成年人，HFOV仅常用于复杂胸科手术（如单肺通气或离体肺通气）、纤维支气管镜操作时的通气支持及支气管胸膜瘘的辅助治疗。目前有限的相关研究发现HFOV较常规V_T通气可以更快地改善氧合，但维持时间较短，且并不能改善患者30天生存率。近期发表的一篇文章，对8个ARDS患者（包括成年人及儿童）的随机对照研究进行meta分析，发现HFOV可明显降低死亡率，明显提高治疗的有效性（难治性低氧血症、高碳酸血症、低血压或气压伤）。此外，目前仍进行的一项较大的多中心研究，旨在进一步确定HFOV治疗较其他治疗，尤其是低V_T保护性通气策略，是否存在明显的有效性。

药物治疗

应用表面活性剂

ALI是由于肺及内皮细胞的炎性而造成的肺水肿、V/Q不匹配的低氧血症、肺动脉高压及纤维化、表面活性物质的合成的损伤和破坏其合成，共同作用导致肺的顺应性进一步降低，加重肺不张的疾病。气管内应用肺表面活性物质可能具有改善呼吸力学及气体交换的潜力的作用。目前仅批准应用于新生儿ARDS。既往成年人相关研究并未发现应用天然或合成表面活性物质有任何益处。近期对5项ARDS患者接受充足表面活性蛋白-C（rSP-C）的多中心研究进行汇总分析。在亚组的析因分析中发现，由于肺炎或误吸导致的ARDS患者应用rSP-C可显著降低死亡率，但此组患者仍包括了部分创伤及脓毒症患者。因此，在被作为标准化治疗方案应用于临床前，须进行更多的临床研究且保证研究对象的同质性。

吸入一氧化氮

NO作用于肺泡内皮细胞，选择性扩张肺血管，以保证通气良好的肺单位产生区域性血管舒张。通常吸入一氧化氮（inhaled nitric oxide，iNO）的剂量为40 ppm，可明显改善ALI及ARDS患者的V/Q不匹配、低氧血症、肺动脉高压。相比之下，系统应用血管舒张药物可同时增加通气不良区域的血流灌注，使V/Q不匹配继续恶化，加重低氧血症，并进一步加剧血管收缩。NO还具有扩张支气管及一定的抗炎作用，这可能使肺移植患者从中受益。iNO最终会弥散入血，并通过肾快速代谢并排泄，以减少全身副作用。近期的一项meta分析，收集了14个随机对照研究，发现iNO对患者的全因死亡率、带机时间、住院及ICU治疗时间没有明显的改善，反而可增加肾损伤的风险，但可在最初的24 h治疗时明显改善氧合。因此，目前并不推荐ALI及ARDS患者常规应用iNO。

非常规通气方式

体外膜肺氧合技术

ECMO通过体外循环改善氧合、清除CO_2。因此，在应用ECMO治疗可逆性心肺衰竭患者时，须建立体外心肺旁路。ECMO在保证充分气体交换的前提下，尽可能地降低正压通气水平。理论上，可使由于严重炎性反应及重度肺损伤的ARF患者的肺休息和愈合，而不是让其忍受为达到合适气体交换而采用的高级别呼吸机支持产生的机械压力。早在19世纪70年代，就有成年人重症创伤患者成功应用ECMO的报道。1979年，美国国立卫生研究院组织了一项有关ECMO的随机、多机构研究，但并未发现患者有明显的生存获益。Cordell-Smith等在2006发表了一项回顾性研究，指出ECMO的使用使得大部分合并严重肺部损伤的成年人重症创伤患者得以存活。在2010年，Arit等报道一项有关合并心肺功能衰竭合并失血性休克的重症创伤患者的通气方式研究，结果显示应用ECMO较传统通气有较明显的优势，但由于它并非随机对照研究，证据力度较低。有趣的是，近期一项meta分析，收集了8项有关成年人及儿童ARDS患者通气方式应用的随机对照试验，结果发现HFOV可明显降低死亡率，治疗的有效性明显提高（难治性低氧血症、高碳酸血症、低血压或气压伤）。

目前认为，当成年人ARDS患者其他治疗失败的情况下，可考虑接受ECMO，此推荐是矛盾的。因为ECMO越早建立效果越显著，且ARF的死亡率与在ECMO前接受机械通气时常成正相关，即带机时间越长，死亡风险越高。但目前，随着技术的发展，ECMO的生物相容性已明显提高，操作相关并发症的发生也在逐渐减少，使得我们应重新评估ECMO对ARDS患者的应用价值。

俯卧位

俯卧位是采用特殊的翻身床和仪器，使患者定期（如每12 h）从俯卧位转换为仰卧位。通气肺段倾向存在于非依赖区肺组织，而灌注肺段（或高肺血管压力和肺水肿）则存在于依赖区肺组织。正压通气会使这种分布不均加重。俯卧位通气则可以通过降低V/Q失调改善由于氧合。俯卧位是逆转依赖的肺组织。新的依赖区肺通气良好，可接受灌注，直到重力和正压通气在几小时后调整原先的V/Q不平衡。此外，俯卧位也可以使肺及呼吸道分泌物的引流便利。Gattinoni等的一项大规模、随机、多中心对照研究发现，俯卧位通气可以明显改善患者10天生存率，但并不能持续影响转出ICU后的预后。一项近期的meta分析对7个包括ALI及ARDS患者的随机对照研究进行分析，发现俯卧位并不能改善患者在ICU期间的死亡率。但近期相关研究严格限制研究对象为ARDS患者，则明显发现回顾性研究中提到的俯卧位通气的优势。尽管俯卧位并不增加主要气道并发症（如导管移位或脱出）的发生，俯卧位自身的并发症包括翻转过程中保证气道通畅或重建气道的难度增加，且长期俯卧位可导致压疮、对镇静药物的需要增加、面部水肿的发生。呼吸衰竭的患者是否能从中获益，仍须进行更多研究进行评估。

展望

MV是现代急危重症医疗的一个重要组成部分。目前提倡建立保护性低V_T通气策略，最大程度地降低气压伤及肺萎陷伤的发生风险。随着微处理技术的发展，出现了许多新型、复杂的通气模式。因缺乏严格的科学评价，这些模式的精确作用并不十分明确，需要更多的研究发现来帮助将这些快速发展的应用于临床。

肾衰竭的管理：肾替代治疗和透析

Joseph M. Gutmann, Christopher McFarren, Lewis M. Flint 和 Rodney Durham 著
朱凤雪 李 纾 译

急性肾衰竭（acute renal failure，ARF）是常见且危急的临床难题，它会导致重症患者住院时间延长和病死率上升。虽然肾替代治疗（renal replacement therapy，RRT）是 ARF 的一种有效的治疗手段，然而它并不是最理想的选择，最好的治疗方法是预防它的发生。

肾主要参与调节机体容量和内部液体环境的构成，并促进代谢产物排出。肾衰竭会导致其调节功能损害，出现含氮代谢废物堆积，以及水、电解液、酸碱平衡紊乱。ICU 患者的肾损伤是一个渐进的过程，通常开始于肾前性的损害，进而发展到严重的肾损伤。同时其他系统的问题也会加重肾的损害。

重症患者的 ARF 是一个日益严重的临床问题。RRT 通常可以选择经典的、以弥散原理为代表的、间歇血液透析治疗或选择以对流原理为代表的、持续血液滤过治疗。对于具体方式的选择要根据患者的需求而定。当前和未来的相关研究对于改善其疗效至关重要。

发病率

ARF 是指突然和持续的肾小球滤过率（glomerular filtration rate，GFR）下降，导致含氮代谢废物和尿毒素蓄积。在重症患者中，超过 90% 的 ARF 是由于急性肾小管坏死（acute tubular necrosis，ATN）所致，而急性肾小管坏死多是由于缺血、肾素性原因或两者的共同作用所引起的。约 5% 的住院患者和 15% 的重症患者会出现 ARF。正如很多其他疾病的诊治现状一样，目前 ARF 也没有诊断的金标准、特定的病理证据以及统一的临床表现。

ARF 若作为独立事件，其死亡率大约为 10%～15%。而在 ICU 中，ARF 患者合并多器官功能障碍时，其死亡率大大升高，在文献中为 40%～90%。

在某些情况下，先前的情况可能会更加恶化。肾衰竭有可能加速如脓毒症、呼吸衰竭等新出现的并发症。需要 RRT 的 ARF 往往具有较高的死亡率，也有证据显示不需要 RRT 的病情相对缓和的 ARF 患者具有更好的预后。

外科疾病的许多方面及其护理可能会导致肾实质的毒性损害以及肾灌注的减少（或两者均有），从而增加了肾功能损害的潜在风险。危重患者 ARF 的预防包括最大限度地减少肾毒性作用和确保充足的血供。避免肾功能的损害优于任何其他治疗措施。因此，临床上应严密监测肾功能的变化，这样使肾损害的不利因素被限制。

鉴于 ARF 对死亡率的影响，因此对于 ARF 的预防，即使是最轻的 ARF，尽快合理的处置就显得至关重要。ARF 综合征预防性策略的目的是保护肾功能，避免急性肾衰竭相关并发症（容量过负荷，酸碱平衡紊乱，以及电解质异常）、长期透析治疗（使不良反应最小化）以及死亡的发生。

本章着重探讨 ARF 的预防策略、主要挑战和关键问题。患者是否可进行保守治疗？ RRT 是否必要？如果必须进行 RRT，如何选择最合理的 RRT 方案？

损伤 / 病因学机制

诊断

如氮代谢产物、尿素和肌酐等机体的水溶性代谢产物以及尿量等参数是重症监护病房评估肾衰竭易获得的常规指标。为进一步理解肾衰竭，我们还须先从肾的生理方面进行探讨。

水和液体平衡

由于体液是细胞体液渗透压的主要决定因素，根据体液质相对于体液是否过量或不足，体液稳态失衡可以分为低渗性紊乱和高渗 性紊乱。循环血容量任何变化的最终结果是肾钠排泄的改变，它由交感神经系统激活、肾素、血管紧张素－醛固酮和尿钠肽的释放或抑制引起的。

肾功能评估

血清中血尿素氮（blood urea nitrogen，BUN）和肌酐的浓度是评估肾功能最常用的标志物。尿素是蛋白质和氨基酸分解代谢的最终产物。在正常条件下，80%～90%的含氮代谢废物由肾排泄。肌酐是肌肉中肌酸和磷酸肌酸的非酶降解产物，主要由肾小球滤过排泄。仅一小部分肌酐主动分泌到肾小球滤液中，被肾小管重吸收的肌酐含量可以忽略不计。

循环中肌酐和尿素氮的水平不仅由肾排泄功能的效率所决定，还受其生成速度的影响。尿素的形成取决于蛋白质和氨基酸分解代谢的数量。高蛋白饮食、血肿的重吸收和消化道出血的消化均会增加尿素氮的含量，而饥饿会使其含量下降。即使肾功能完好，以上因素均可改变尿素氮的水平。肌酐的生成量反映了肌肉质量，其含量在短期内应保持恒定。肌肉质量随着年龄增长而降低，内在肾功能也如此，当肌肉减少时肌酐生成的水平也会逐步下降。因此，通常血清肌酐的水平相对保持稳定。

肌酐清除率

肌酐清除率（creatinine clearance，Ccr）的测定是衡量肾功能的指标。肾对肌酐的分泌和重吸收可以忽略不计。清除率是指在一段时间内可通过肾清除的血浆或血清体积。具体计算方法如下：

$$Ccr(ml/minute) = (Ucr \times V)/Pcr$$

Ucr，尿肌酐；Pcr，血清肌酐；V，容量。

GFR是一定时间内通过肾滤过的血清量，清除率反映了GFR的净效应。最常用的估计肌酐清除率的方法是Cockcroft-Gault评估法：

Ccr_{men}=GFR（ml/min）=（140－年龄）×［理想体重（kg）/72×血清肌酐（mg/dl］

$Ccr_{women}=Ccr_{men} \times 0.85$

正常的GFR是125±15 ml/min·1.73m^{2}体表面积（body snrface area，BSA）

钠离子在细胞外液的所有阳离子中浓度最高。钠离子的转运必须伴随着水的转运。肾钠清除是细胞外液容量调节的一个重要机制。醛固酮促进肾小管对钠的重吸收，从而影响肾小球小动脉静水压力的变化。如果肾血流量或压力下降，肾小管对钠的重吸收将会上升，从而保证细胞外液的容量相对稳定。钠消除率与Ccr的比值为钠排泄分数（fractional excretion of sodium，FENa）。

$$FENa=[(Una \times Pcr/Ucr \times Pna)] \times 100$$

在这里，Una和Ucr是尿钠和尿肌酐浓度，Pna和Pcr是血钠和血肌酐浓度。如果FENa很低（≤1%），可能提示肾小动脉压力不足。这可能说明由于肾小球动脉压力低而非肾自身因素导致临床上出现肾功能不全。

尿液的生成和排泄

肾功能的最终结果是尿液的生成。定量测量尿量对肾功能的评估至关重要。尿量对肾血流量高度敏感，它是评估肾功能和反映全身血管灌注情况的关键指标（表1）。

表1　充足的尿量

年龄	尿量（ml/kg·min）
婴儿（＜10 kg）	2.0
幼儿（10～20 kg）	1.5
儿童（20～50 kg）	1.0
成年人（20～50 kg）	0.5

患者处理

保守治疗

尽管医疗技术不断进步，ICU中ARF患者的并发症发生率和死亡率仍居高不下。防止ARF的主要策略包括充足的水化、保持大于60 mmHg的平均动脉压，以及尽量减少有潜在肾毒性的药物的使用。虽然水化作用被证明是有益的，但在水化治疗中应用不同液体类型的选择上仍然存有争议。

考虑低成本、低毒性等相关因素的影响，有学者认为N-乙酰半胱氨酸的静脉水化应用被认为可以降低高危患者的肾病患病率。值得注意的是能否把NAC作为常规治疗目前存在争议，还未被充分研究。

预防急性肾衰竭的非药物治疗方法

预防ARF的非药物治疗方法包括保证充足的水

化（限制脱水）。维护足够的平均动脉压力，以及尽量减少肾损药物的使用。以下 4 种特殊治疗方法值得回顾：①液体；②氨基糖苷类；③两性霉素脂溶性准备；④非离子型造影剂。

液体治疗

充足的水化是肾衰竭防治的基础。一项随机对照试验（n=1 620），比较应用 0.9% 生理盐水和 0.45% 葡萄糖盐水的水化治疗方案，用于预防接受冠状动脉造影后放射造影剂诱导的肾病的发生。应用 0.9% 生理盐水的水化治疗方案，与应用 0.45% 葡萄糖盐水的治疗方案相比，可显著降低造影剂肾病的发生率（0.7% vs. 2%，P=0.04）。这种效果在女性、糖尿病和接受大剂量造影剂（大于 250 ml）的患者中更为显著。最近一项单中心随机对照试验，比较碳酸氢钠和 0.9% 生理盐水用于预防造影剂肾病的发生的功效。这项研究共纳入 119 名接受造影剂（碘帕醇）的患者，其血清肌酐至少维持在 1.1 mg/dl 以上。患者在注射造影剂之前或之后被随机分配到生理盐水输注组（n=60）和碳酸氢盐输注组（n=59）。造影剂肾病定义为在应用造影剂 48 h 后肌酐上升水平超过其基线水平的 25%。研究发现碳酸氢盐输注组的 59 例患者中，仅 1 例出现造影剂肾病（1.7%），生理盐水输注组的 60 例患者中，有 8 例出现造影剂肾病（13.3%），两组差异具有统计学意义（P=0.02）。

肾毒性药物的使用

最小化暴露于潜在肾毒性药物是 ICU 中预防 ARF 的重要措施。ICU 中经常应用放射造影剂、氨基糖苷类抗生素、两性霉素和其他抗生素它们是肾毒性药物。一项研究系统回顾了接受氨基糖苷类抗生素治疗的中性粒细胞减少性发热患者，分别采用每日 1 次和每日 3 次的给药方式，两者的药效和肾毒性没有统计学差异。

使用两性霉素 B 脂质形式，相比标准的两性霉素 B，会产生更少的肾毒性损害，而对于远期药物安全性的直接比较尚缺乏证据支持。一项由 31 个随机对照试验构成，共涉及 5 146 例患者的系统性回顾研究，比较了低渗造影剂与标准造影剂，发现二者对于 ARF 的发展影响以及透析需求并无差异。

急性肾衰竭的药物预防

髓袢利尿剂

多个小型临床试验用于探讨髓袢利尿剂对预防 ARF 的功效，所得结论存在不一致。这些试验是低效的，并非随机对照试验，方法上也存在缺陷。一项系统综述，在各种原因导致 ARF 高危的患者中分别进行体液治疗和利尿剂治疗并进行比较，发现应用利尿剂治疗并未改善由各种原因有 ARF 风险患者的 ARF 的发病率、透析需求以及患者死亡率。

N– 乙酰半胱氨酸

系统性综述发现相对单独水化治疗而言，N-2 酰半胱氨酸（N-acetylcysteine，NAC）联合水化治疗可明显降低有基线肾损害和接受放射研究的患者造影剂肾病的发生率。然而最近的一项研究发现，NAC 可以单独降低血清肌酐水平，但不影响 GFR，CGFR 的评估是根据其他代谢产物如血清胱抑素（水平得出）。因此应用 NAC 预防造影剂使用后的血清肌酐水平降低，其结论和意义仍需进一步探讨。

急性肾衰竭肾替代治疗的指征

慢性肾病，细胞外液容量和体液成分紊乱是 ARF 需 RRT 的客观指征（表 2）。这些客观指征具体包括容量超负荷、高钾血症、严重代谢性酸中毒、尿毒症、氮质血症。

表 2 肾替代治疗的指征

容量超负荷
高钾血症
代谢性酸中毒
尿毒症
氮质血症

容量超负荷

容量超负荷一般是公认的 ARF 患者的 RRT 指征。RRT 的所有模式均可有效地减少血管内容量。须开始 RRT 的主观标准包括由于肺淤血或肺损伤导致的心肺功能障碍或由于周围性血肿导致的皮肤完整性受损和伤口愈合延迟。

Mehta 等进行了一项回顾性研究，数据来自 522

例 ARF 重症患者。其中 59% 的患者曾使用过利尿剂治疗。在调整相关协变量和利尿剂使用的倾向后研究观察到患者应用利尿剂会显著增加死亡率以及肾功能不可逆损害的发生率（OR = 1.77，95% CI 为 1.14～2.76）。他们在此基础上得出结论，应用利尿剂治疗 ARF 具有潜在的危害性。但他们也指出，上述风险的增加也能反映出对肾损伤程度更重的患者的筛选。

高钾血症

具有心肌毒性证据的高钾血症是 ARF 患者血液透析治疗的早期指征之一。高钾血症是公认的 ARF 并发症，如不及时处理可能会迅速导致患者死亡。大多数治疗高钾血症的临时措施包括静脉注射钙离子，以直接对抗高钾对心肌细胞膜的影响；静脉注射葡萄糖 / 胰岛素或吸入 β 受体激动剂，从而使钾离子转移至细胞内。3 个可以有效减低全身钾负担的方法：①利尿剂治疗；②肠道内钾离子黏附交换树脂；③透析治疗。

严重肾衰竭的患者应用利尿剂治疗通常是无效的，因为此类患者缺乏对利尿剂的反应。尽管聚磺苯乙烯可以提高粪便钾的排出，但其使用受到近期腹内或胃肠道手术、肠梗阻和肠道缺血等因素的限制。血液透析是降低血清钾浓度的最快方法。然而，由于研究设计的多变性以及透析技术的演变，单次的血液透析治疗很难达到预期的降钾效果。

更多钾离子的清除可能须通过使用渗透性更好的人造血液透析膜和更大的血液流速来实现。然而，血钾清除的速率最终还会受到血浆和透析液之间浓度梯度迅速下降的限制。与容量负荷评估类似，一个特定的血清钾离子阈值水平也不能作为开始 RRT 的指征。当血清钾浓度小于 6.5 mmol/ L 时，高钾血症的心肌毒性并不常见。因此，关于控制高钾血症起始治疗的决策必须考虑到血钾的浓度、血钾的上升速度、患者的整体状况和药物治疗可能产生的效果。

代谢性酸中毒

在处理代谢性酸中毒，尤其是乳酸酸中毒时，是否应用碱性药物治疗存在争议。相比碱性药物而言，使用 RRT 处理代谢性酸中毒，可以避免由于积极使用碱替代、容量超负荷以及高钠血症所导致的一系列有害作用。尽管进行性加重的代谢性酸中毒是 RRT 的公认指征，但有关血清 pH 值阈值、血清碳酸氢浓度以及证明可改善患者预后的临床试验还未进行。

其他电解质紊乱

在发生 ARF 时，肾替代治疗也可用于纠正各种其他类型的电解质紊乱。其中包括严重的低钠血症、高钠血症、高磷血症、低钙血症、高钙血症和高镁血症。在纠正低钠血症时，必须警惕由于低钠血症纠正过快所导致的渗透性脱髓鞘综合征。为快速降低血清磷酸盐和尿酸水平以及控制酸血症，对肿瘤溶解综合征患者使用 RRT 来支持肾功能恢复是有必要的。

尿毒症

ARF 患者尿毒症相关症状或体征的恶化是开始 RRT 的显著指征。早期尿毒症表现为厌食、恶心、呕吐和瘙痒。这些都是非特异性表现，很难在重症患者中与其他合并症情况相区别。精神状态的变化可能是由于尿毒症脑病引起，但这种改变在危重患者中也很难与其他原因导致的谵妄相区别。尿毒症心包炎是一种常见的晚期并发症，当有心包出血和心包压塞的高风险时，须紧急开始 RRT。正如 40 年前 Teschan 等强调过的，最佳 RRT 时机应选择在严重的尿毒症症状出现前开展。

氮质血症

许多 ARF 患者在缺乏尿毒症或其他肾支持治疗指征时，进展性的氮质血症可能是唯一开始 RRT 的指征。但是关于须开始进行 RRT 的氮质血症的严重程度，目前并没有达成共识。一项多中心研究用以评估合并 ARF 的危重症患者进行 RRT 的时机选择。研究发现多个独立研究机构以及某些尚未公开发表数据的研究机构的调查显示，具体尿素氮水平应升高到何种程度才应开始进行 RRT 并未达成共识。许多的肾学专家认为重症患者只要尿素氮≥60 mg/dL 即应开始 RRT。

肾替代治疗开始时间

从 Paul Teschan 等的研究开始，到朝鲜战争之后大量研究都在尝试定义 ARF 患者须开始进行 RRT 的具体临床标准。这些研究试图去平衡三大竞争风险，分别是：① RRT 延误所导致的内部风险；② RRT 损害导致的潜在风险，如 RRT 的相关并发症和由于透析治疗导致的 ARF 的病程延长；③过早进行 RRT 的风险。此类患者通过保守治疗，而无需肾替代治疗，肾功能便可以自行恢复。

Teschan 等进行了一项前瞻性非对照研究，这是一个标志性的报告，共涉及 15 例接受预防性血液透析治疗的少尿 ARF 患者。预防性血液透析治疗定义为在尿素氮达到 100 mg/dl 前即开始进行透析治疗。患者每日接受透析（平均持续时间 6 h）：使用双线圈管纤维素透析器，血流速度为 75～250 ml/min，以保持透析前尿素氮＜75 mg/dl。患者不限制热量和蛋白质的摄入。所有患者的全因死亡率为 33%，因出血或脓毒症导致的死亡率为 20%。尽管本项研究没有设置对照组，研究人员发现与过去使用的经验性透析指征相比（直到有常见指征出现才开始治疗），预防性透析治疗疗效具有显著差异性。

急性肾衰患者肾替代治疗的模式

ARF 是危重患者的常见并发症，其相关死亡率＞50%。多达 70% 的患者需要 RRT，这使得 RRT 成为 ICU 中处理 ARF 的重要组成部分。理想情况下，RRT 可以控制容量、纠正酸碱失衡、通过清除毒素而改善尿毒症、促进肾功能恢复、提高生存率，且并不导致并发症（如凝血功能障碍和低血压）。可用的 RRT 的模式包括间歇性血液透析（intermittent hemodialysis，IHD）、连续 RRT（continuous RRT，CRRT）和持续低效透析（sustained low-efficiency dialysis，SLED）。目前没有足够的证据来确定哪种形式的 RRT 最适合 ARF 的重症患者。对于接受 RRT 的患者而言，存在一个共识，即使用低血流量、低血液清除速率模式会降低心血管事件发生率和死亡率。因此可见 RRT 模式的选择并不影响患者的死亡率。正确理解各种透析模式的优势和局限性，是 ICU 中合理选择 RRT 模式的基础。

肾替代治疗的原则

所有形式的肾替代治疗都依赖于水和溶质通过半透膜运输并丢弃废物的原则。超滤是水通过半透膜运输的过程。扩散和对流是溶质通过膜转运所依靠的 2 个过程。肾替代治疗可应用超滤来清除液体，并利用弥散、对流或联合弥散对流来清除溶质。

超滤是通过液体驱动半透膜两侧的压力梯度来实现清除体内液体。这种压力梯度被称为跨膜压力梯度，它是血浆渗透压和静水压力之间的差。超滤率的决定因素包括膜的表面积、膜的透水性和跨膜压力梯度。

弥散是指溶质通过半透膜从溶质高浓度一侧向溶质低浓度一侧移动。透析液逆血流方向经过半透膜，从而使浓度梯度达到最大化。透析液是一种电解质溶液，通常包含钠、碳酸氢、氯、镁、钙等溶质。血液中高浓度的溶质（如钾离子和尿素），通过膜时会降低其溶质浓度梯度，接着会进入透析隔室中。相反，透析液中高浓度溶质（如碳酸氢盐）也会弥散到血液中。在血液和透析液中若溶质浓度相近时（如钠和氯），则很少出现溶质在半透膜两侧的移动。因为小分子溶质（如尿素和肌酐）比大分子溶质弥散更快，所以小分子量分子（分子量小于 500 dalton）相比大分子能更有效地被清除。溶质弥散的速率取决于血流速率、透析液流量、透析时间、膜两侧的浓度梯度、半透膜的表面积和半透膜的孔隙大小。

对流发生在超滤过程中，跨膜压梯度驱动水穿过半透膜，与此同时小分子物质（如尿素氮、肌酐和钾离子）和大分子物质（如菊糖、β_2 微球蛋白、肿瘤坏死因子、维生素 B_{12}）也被随着水分一并拉出。半透膜孔径的大小限制了可通过半透膜的溶质分子大小。增加跨膜压可以使更多的液体和溶质被拉出膜外。由于溶质清除的效率主要取决于超滤率，通常至少须每小时有 1 L 的液体通过半透膜。提高超滤率以提供溶质的对流清除的过程称为血液滤过。超滤率是由跨膜压力、膜的水通透性、膜的表面积以及孔隙大小所决定。

肾替代治疗的分类

ARF 的 RRT 基于治疗的持续时间可以分为间歇性和连续性。间歇性治疗的持续治疗时间小于 24 h，而连续治疗的持续治疗时间至少为 24 h。间歇治疗包括 IHD 和 SLED。连续治疗包括腹膜透析和 CRRT。腹膜透析很少在紧急情况应用，因为对于重症分解代谢异常患者而言，这种方式的溶质清除效率低下，会增加发生腹膜炎的风险。另外，腹膜透析由于阻碍膈移动而影响呼吸功能。因此，对于腹部手术或腹部脓毒症患者而言，腹膜透析均禁止使用。

间歇性血液透析

对于 ARF 患者而言，传统方式是肾内科医生经验性地给予每周 6 次、一次 3 ~ 4 h 的 IHD。每次透析血流速率控制在 200 ~ 350 ml/min，透析液流动速率控制在 500 ~ 800 ml/min。在 IHD 时，溶质的清除主要通过弥散来完成，液体的清除通过超滤来实现。溶质清除的程度，也称为“透析剂量”，很大程度上依赖于血液的流速。通常增加血流量可以增加溶质清除率。关于透析时间和频率的选择取决于患者的代谢状态、容量状态和血流动力学的不稳定程度。

IHD 的优点是快速移除溶质和液体，从而在数小时内快速纠正电解质紊乱以及快速清除致命中毒者体内的药物或其他物质。与其他类型的 RRT 相比，IHD 由于具有更高的血流速率以及更短的治疗时间，因而可以减少对抗凝药物的依赖。

IHD 的主要缺点是由于快速电解质改变和液体清除而引起的全身性低血压风险。血液透析治疗过程中，大约 20% ~ 30% 的患者发生低血压。在 IHD 时可通过钠建模，给透析液降温、增加透析液钙离子浓度、静脉注射白蛋白、应用间歇性超滤治疗等方法来改善其血流动力学的稳定性。尽管如此，仍有约 10% 的 ARF 患者因血流动力学不稳定，而不能耐受 IHD。全身性低血压会影响 IHD 的效率，从而导致溶质清除率下降，无法充分纠正酸碱平衡紊乱以及容量负荷过重。因为仅仅在 4 h 的透析时间里，很难达到和维持循环稳定的超滤率。

快速清除血管内的溶质会导致脑水肿和颅内压增加。合并头外伤或肝性脑病的 ARF 患者，脑水肿风险较大，甚至可能形成脑疝。由于不能用终末期肾病患者尿素氮的代谢速率来推测 ARF 的代谢水平，所以对于急性肾衰患者如何评估溶质清除认（透析剂量）以及适合的剂量构成，临床上缺乏统一共识。

尽管一些研究结果显示每日血液透析方案优于传统的 IHD 方案。目前尚不清楚是可以通过增加每次透析剂量来更好地控制尿毒症，还是可以通过减少每次透析过程中清除的液体量，以此来减少血流动力学不稳定的发生，从而改善患者预后。

连续性肾替代治疗

尽管大家公认的标准 RRT 方案是 IHD 治疗。对于血流动力学不稳定的 ARF 患者而言，CRRT 是一个更可行的方案。连续治疗使用双腔静脉，利用泵驱动系统建立体外循环，它依靠动脉通路和血压维持血液流动。由于存在溶质清除效果差、动脉置管并发症等问题，持续动静脉血液滤过（continuous arteriovenous hemofiltration，CAVH）现在已很少在 CRRT 中使用。与 IHD 不同，CRRT 一般是 24 h 不间断的连续治疗。如果使用弥散的 CRRT 模式，其血流速率通常为 100 ~ 200 ml/min，透析液流动速率通常为 17 ~ 40 ml/min。CRRT 可以选择弥散模式、对流模式或弥散对流联合模式来清除溶质。

所有类型的 CRRT 使用的半透膜对水分子和低分子量溶质均具有较高的渗透性。CRRT 根据溶质清除的不同方法进行分类。现在的标准模式是采用静脉静脉循环，CRRT 根据溶质清除的机制划分不同类型的静脉静脉替代治疗模式。4 个提高复杂度的主要模式是：缓慢连续超滤、持续静脉静脉血液滤过（continuous venovenous hemofiltration，CVVH）、持续静脉静脉血液透析（continuous venovenous hemodialysis，CVVHD）和持续静脉血液透析滤过（continuous venovenous hemodiafiltration，CVVHDF）。

在缓慢连续超滤时，低容量超滤速度控制在 100 ~ 300 ml/h，从而维持液体平衡，不会出现严重的对流溶质清除。无论是否存在肾衰竭，缓慢连续超滤的目的仅仅是处理容量超负荷，其适应证是对利尿剂无效的充血性心力衰竭所导致的容量超负荷。

在 CVVH 时，溶质通过对流方式被清除。通过液压引导的超滤清除血液中的溶质。此过程中可以不使用透析液。所有分子量在一定范围内能渗透膜的溶质，其清除率相似。对流的清除效果由超滤率决定。超滤率是由跨膜压力、渗透性、半透膜孔隙大小、膜表面积和膜厚度所决定。通常情况下，超滤率维持在 1 ~ 2 L/h 就可以满足溶质清除的目的。当超滤率高时，会快速地引起机体容量减少、低血压和电解质的迅速丢失。静脉体液替换是在清除过多的自身体液后，补充机体所需的溶质和液体。替换液可以通过滤器前或滤器后的管路补充回体内。

在 CVVHD 时，透析液是逆着血流方向流动，其速度为 1 ~ 2.5 L/h。溶质通过弥散方式被清除。与 IHD 不同，透析液流动速率要远远低于血流速率，使得小分子溶质在血液和透析液之间达到完全平衡。超滤用于容量控制，但可以允许一些高速率对流清除的存在。CVVHDF结合了CVVH的对流溶质清除和CVVHD的弥散溶质清除两种模式。正如在CVVH的过程中，较高的超滤率有助于采用对流的方式清除溶质，同时需要替换液的及时静脉补充。

替换液可以通过滤器前或滤器后的方式给予。滤器后替换的方式容易导致滤器中的血液浓缩，增加凝血的风险。尤其是当滤过分数>30%时，此类风险更容易出现。滤过分数的计算公式是超滤率与血浆流动速率的比值，其数值有赖于血流速率和血细胞比容。滤器前替换的方式可以在滤器前稀释血流，从而减少滤器栓形成血的发生。但滤器前溶质的稀释会产生较低的弥散驱动力和对流浓度，从而减少了高达15%的溶质的清除速率。

优点和缺点

CRRT的优点是由于其缓慢的超滤率从而达到血流动力学的耐受。逐渐的连续容量清除更易于控制容量状态，并且可以不用过度关注容量超负荷问题，允许药物治疗和营养支持。因为它是一个连续模式，可以减少溶质浓度的波动，并更好地控制氮质血症和电解质酸碱平衡状态。血流动力学的稳定可能与肾灌注血流的下降减少、肾缺血的发生减少、肾功能的快速恢复有关。Mehta等开展了一项涉及166名ICU的ARF患者并随机分组为IHD组或CRRT组的前瞻性随机对照研究。此研究发现，相比IHD，接受CRRT的患者，存活的患者的肾功能更容易恢复。因为CRRT不会引起溶质的快速转移，所以这种模式也不会像IHD那样，增加患者的颅内压。

CRRT的累积溶质清除远大于IHD。Ronco等提供了一个令人信服的证据，对于伴有ARF的重症患者而言，CRRT可以增加溶质清除率，并改善患者预后。在一项前瞻性随机对照试验中，425例CRF的重症患者应用CVVH。根据其超滤率的不同分为3组，超滤率分别为20 ml/kg · h（组1）、35 ml/kg · h（组2）和45 ml/kg · h（组3）。在研究时，超滤率20 ml/kg · h是建立在相关文献报道的临床实践中总结出来的平均速率上。血液流速的范围是120～240 ml/min，使用滤器后置换。主要研究的预后是终止CVVH15天后的生存。次要预后是肾功能的恢复以及CVVH相关并发症的发生。在终止CVVH后，1、2、3组的生存率分别为41%、57%、58%。1组的生存率明显低于2组（P=0.007）和3组（P=0.01），说明通过CVVH治疗的具有生存率优势的患者其超滤率至少为35 ml/kg · h。然而，目前尚不清楚仅清除小分子溶质或清除小分子和中分子溶质是否会减少患者死亡率。

间歇性血液透析对比连续性肾替代治疗：预后

很少有前瞻性研究比较IHD与CRRT的结果。这些结果包括死亡率和肾功能恢复等。Mehta等随机选取166例患者接受CRRT（CVVH或CVVHDF）或IHD。单因素治疗意向分析结果显示接受CRRT的患者死亡率更高。随机分配到CRRT的患者具有更高的APACHE Ⅲ评分和较高的肝功能衰竭发病率，以上因素将混杂试 验结果。多因素分析显示无论哪种RRT，对于患者的全因死亡率和肾功能的恢复均无影响。相反，疾病严重程度的相关评分（如APACHEIII评分和衰竭器官的数量），对于患者的预后影响更为重要。研究表明由于缺乏随机对照试验和各类偏倚及混杂因素的影响，故尚无充足的数据来导出可靠性的结论。

持续低效透析或延长的每日透析

SLED和延长的每日透析是更缓慢的血液透析模式，它们都是使用传统的血液透析机器，通过调整血流和透析液的流速，来延长血液透析时间。通常，SLED和延长的每日透析使用通常为200 ml/min的低流速血泵，低透析液流速为300 ml/min，每天进行6～12 h。SLED和延长的每日透析结合了CRRT和IHD的各自优点。这两种模式如同CRRT一样，通过逐步清除溶质和体液，从而改善患者血流动力学的稳定。与此同时，它们如同IHD一样，能够提供高的溶质清除率，并避免了CRRT的昂贵的机器、定制的解决方案和培训员工的费用。

因为SLED和延长的每日透析可以根据患者的需要间断进行，故其可以避免此类患者需要的各种诊断和治疗程序的干扰。在加州大学戴维斯医疗中心，Kumar等进行了前瞻性研究，入组患者中25例进行延长的每日透析，17例进行CVVH。两组的平均动脉压和强心剂的需求情况无显著差异。延长的每日透析组的死亡率更高（84% vs. 65%）。然而在开始治疗时，延长的每日透析组 APACHE Ⅱ分数更高。作者认为延长的每日透析治疗由于无需持续的透析设备监测也可以减少护理的工作量，故成本效益更好。

总结

重症患者伴 ARF 是一个重要的临床问题。此类患者的 RRT 选择包括对流和弥散两种方式。肾替代治疗可以是间歇性的治疗模式（如经典的血液透析）或连续性的治疗模式。RRT 需求根据不同患者的具体需求来决定。未来仍需进一步的研究去探讨肾替代治疗的相关准则。

鉴于 ARF 对死亡率的影响，重要的是避免或减少 ARF 即使是最轻微的发生。临床主要目标是预防 ARF 综合征的出现。其预防策略是保护肾功能、避免慢性透析的发生、使 RRT 的相关副作用降到最小、防止相关并发症的发生。这些并发症具体包括容量超负荷、酸碱平衡紊乱和电解质异常。

在这一章，我们讨论了 ARF 的预防策略和不同的治疗选择。近年来 RRT 的进步为 ICU 患者 ARF 的治疗提供了多种 RRT 方案。CRRT 应用静脉静脉模式为广大患者所接受。对于血流动力学不稳定患者而言，其具有优势。目前几乎没有数据支持具体哪种 RRT 方式最佳。也很少有相关的随机对照试验，大多数存在的研究均为回顾性、非对照性试验。研究中还有许多混杂因素存在，例如疾病的严重程度和肾衰竭的原因等。这些因素可能是影响 ICU 急性肾衰患者预后最重要的因素。一些最近的研究也表明，高剂量的透析预示着一定的生存优势。

透析方式的选择应根据个体患者的具体需求来决定。IHD 最适合那些须快速进行代谢控制的患者（例如高钾血症患者）。而容量超负荷最有效的治疗方法是 CRRT。血流动不稳定或颅内压增加的患者最好的治疗手段也是 CRRT。对于有抗凝禁忌的患者而言，除进行枸橼酸抗凝的 CRRT，也可行 IHD。CRRT 由于其巨大花费，较高的护理时间要求以及长时间的患者活动受限等问题，往往限制了它的使用。从理论上讲，肾替代治疗的选择要根据潜在疾病和 ARF 的原因来决定。实践中模式的选择还应基于患者具体的临床状态和医疗机构能提供的资源来共同决定。

重症监护病房凝血功能障碍的处理

Christopher P. Michetti 和 Samir M. Fakhry 著
朱凤雪 李 纾 译

外科医生在诊治患者的过程中常会遇到凝血功能障碍。尤其是对于严重外伤以及经历手术或从手术中恢复的患者而言，凝血功能障碍更容易出现。众所周知，出血是人类一开始就已清楚了解的一种状态，随着我们对复杂凝血和纤维蛋白溶解机制的进一步研究，对于出血和凝血的病理生理学过程的理解也在不断深入，并进一步帮助我们改进有效的治疗方法。在 1900 年，Karl Landsteiner 发现 A、B、O 血型，以及在 1902 年，Decastello 和 Adriano Sturli 发现 AB 血型之后，我们才有能力开始有效地治疗出血。

自从 1937 年美国开始建立第一个血库至今已有 40 余年的历史。由于塑料储血袋、血浆去除术设备的问世，从而促进了交叉配型、抗凝、血液贮存技术的发展，最终使得成分输血成为了可能。凝血途径的发现和可靠的凝血试验技术的进步使得我们治疗不同类型的凝血功能障碍成为了可能。这些疾病也包括了通过输注血液制品以及外科干预止血从而纠正的凝血功能障碍。

在现代外科手术和创伤处理的过程中，替换丢失的血液至关重要。另外，为需要个体化血液成分的患者提供有效的治疗也同样重要。目前人们对于血液及其相关产品的需要在不断增加，而血液制品的供给不足的问题却持续存在，因而我们应更珍惜并有效利用这种宝贵资源。本章的目的是帮助外科医生熟悉危重及创伤患者的凝血功能障碍类型，了解凝血功能障碍的诊断思路，并知晓这些疾病有效的治疗策略。

发病率和发病机制

先天性出血性疾病

血管性血友病

血管性血友病（Von Willebrand disease，vWD）是最常见的遗传性出血性疾病，发生率为1/100～1/1 000，为常染色体遗传病。这种疾病是由于血管性血友病因子（von Willebrand factor，vWF）缺乏或功能障碍导致的。vWF可以促进血小板黏附于受损的血管内皮，并稳定Ⅷ因子活性。血管性血友病分为3种类型，了解其具体类型对于我们指导临床治疗非常重要。1型是vWF缺乏，3型是vWF缺失。2型主要分为2 a和2 b两个亚型，其共同特点是vWF功能缺损。

部分促凝血酶原时间（partial thromboplastin time，PTT）有助于诊断血管性血友病。1型和3型血管性血友病vWF抗原水平降低。血管性血友病患者的Ⅷ因子活力可能下降，出血时间或其他血小板功能试验也可能出现异常。瑞斯托菌素辅因子测定可以用于评估vWF诱导的血小板聚集功能。

1-脱氨基-8-D-精氨酸血管加压素（1-deamino-8-D-arginine vasopressin，DDAVP）可用于激活vWF产生，增加1型和2型血管性血友病患者的Ⅷ因子水平。然而，对3型血管性血友病而言，DDAVP是无效的。2b型血管性血友病患者禁用此类药物，因为DDAVP会导致血小板减少，增加出血的风险。病毒灭活的vWF Ⅷ因子的浓缩物通常被用于治疗2型和3型血管性血友病，同时也可用于对DDAVP无反应的1型血管性血友病。包含Ⅷ因子和vWF的冷凝蛋白质可用于治疗所有类型的血管性血友病。然而这种冷凝蛋白质是汇集的，且并非是病毒灭活的，通常只被推荐作为三线治疗。抗纤维蛋白溶解的氨基酸，例如氨基己酸和氨甲环酸，可以用作所有先前提到的血管性血友病类型的辅助治疗。

甲型血友病

甲型血友病是一种由于Ⅷ因子缺乏导致的先天性出血性疾病。由于其为X染色体遗传，故在男性中为表型表达，而对于女性中表现为携带者状态。出血倾向与Ⅷ因子水平负相关。通常在Ⅷ因子水平低于正常的30%时（轻度血友病），临床上才会出现明显的凝血功能障碍。当Ⅷ因子水平不到5%（中度血友病）时会有自发出血的风险。当Ⅷ因子水平不到1%（严重的血友病）时，自发性出血的风险尤其严重。凝血试验表现为延长的PTT，正常的凝血酶原时间（prothrombin time，PT）和较低的Ⅷ因子水平。

临床上严重出血或经历手术的患者应该接受Ⅷ因子浓缩物治疗，最好是其重组产品。DDAVP可提高内源性Ⅷ因子水平，可用于轻度患者。多达20%的患者在使用因子Ⅷ后会产生IgG抗体，从而使得未来的治疗无效。在这种情况下，重组激活因子VIIa（rF Ⅶ）可用于诱导止血。这一点在后面的内容将做进一步阐述。相比Ⅷ因子浓缩物而言，Ⅷ因子冷凝蛋白质中Ⅷ因子的浓度偏低。但Ⅷ因子避免了病毒感染的风险。目前输注Ⅷ因子浓缩物导致病毒感染的发生率较低，并且使用重组因子可以进一步减少病毒感染的发生。

乙型血友病

乙型血友病（圣诞节病）是Ⅸ因子缺乏导致的凝血功能障碍。临床上类似于甲型血友病，凝血试验提示PTT延长、PT正常以及Ⅸ因子水平低下。重组Ⅸ因子浓缩物可以获得，汇集捐献浓缩物也是。相比甲型血友病而言，乙型血友病患者出现抑制剂的发生率不高（1%）。在治疗严重的出血时，也可以应用rFⅦa。在这种情况下，应在血液科专科医生指导下进行联合治疗。

获得性出血性疾病

出血性休克的凝血功能障碍

出血性休克是由多种因素引起的复杂的凝血功能障碍，通常这一过程被误解为弥散性血管内凝血（disseminated intravascular coagulation，DIC）或简单的稀释性凝血功能障碍，从而误导了临床治疗。出血性休克、失血和组织灌注减少会导致机体出现无氧代谢，导致乳酸生成增加，最终出现酸中毒的表现。由于组织缺氧使得三磷酸腺苷生成减少，导致无法维持核心体温。此时患者无法保证机体正常的核心温度，从而引起凝血功能障碍，出现严重出血和无法纠正的出血性恶性循环。使用室温液体进行复苏治疗，反而对低体温患者有害。大规模出血性休克的复苏中，其凝血因子的稀释程度各不相同。

最近的研究表明，出血性休克会导致复杂的凝血功能障碍，这包括了损伤后的早期凝血功能障碍。

休克引起的细胞缺血和组织因子的暴露共同导致了早期的凝血功能障碍。低体温、酸中毒是导致出血性休克患者出现凝血功能障碍的主要原因。在手术室和ICU中，多种治疗方法同时联合应用是非常常见的。然而，对于出血性休克，首先须做的是阻止出血，同时应使用晶体液和血液制品来纠正缺血和酸中毒，并避免及治疗低体温。因为低体温和酸中毒的巨大影响，凝血功能障碍主要表现为无效的血栓形成。这一点与DIC不同，DIC表现为凝血系统过度激活，从而导致不受控的广泛微血管栓内血形成。

凝血因子的稀释可以导致大出血，过去往往使用液体复苏治疗。当凝血因子浓度低至正常的30%以及纤维蛋白原水平大于75 mg/dl时，机体仍可以充分止血。即使人体全部血容量都替换了，机体仍会保留大约1/3的正常凝血因子浓度。这可能是导致稀释性凝血功能障碍的最小输液体积。虽然凝血因子的稀释可能导致凝血（如PT和PTT）试验结果出现异常，但这些改变并不一定影响机体的凝血功能。此外，失血量也不能准确预测血小板的计数。更新的出血性休克复苏技术提示在输注红细胞的同时给予高比例的凝血因子，这可以在一定程度上缓解稀释性凝血功能障碍的发生。最近的报告表明，在输注红细胞的同时配合输注更高比例的血浆有助于提高患者的生存率。如美国血库协会（American Association of Blood Banks，AABB）等国际组织的当前指南都给情况的变化性留了很多空间，许多中心在输注红细胞的同时，给予高比例的血浆输注。了解更多相关信息，请参见休克复苏章节。

低体温

如同SIRS、脓毒症、休克等问题一样，低体温通常也常在重症监护环境出现。它们降低机体耗氧量，会阻碍核心体温的维持。低体温通常伴随着大手术导致的出血性休克的出现，它会加剧凝血功能障碍，应该使用“损伤控制”策略。另外，输注室温的血液制品和液体中和了出血导致的机体热量的丢失。在创伤患者中，若体温低于32℃，其死亡率接近100%。

低体温会降低凝血的蛋白水解酶的反应速率，导致止血功能受损。对创伤患者而言，体温低于34℃会影响其凝血酶活性以及血小板功能。血小板功能障碍是多种原因造成的，他们会导致血栓素生成的减少以及血小板黏附和聚集功能的下降。

及时而有效的复温对于外科低体温性凝血功能障碍患者至关重要。虽然控制性低体温在诸如心搏停止等情况下被证明是有益的，但没有充分的证据表明其对创伤或外科手术患者是否也有益处。最应优先考虑的治疗是处理原发病问题，例如停止手术相关的活动性出血、排空未引流的脓肿、治疗感染，以及时清除坏死组织。外部复温方法尽管缓慢而低效，但仍有助于防止进一步的热量丢失。应提高室内环境温度，给予患者热空气毯子和液体垫（包括头部）。核心复温技术远比外部复温技术更有效。至少，所有液体和血液制品在输注前均应加热，通过机械通气给予加温、加湿空气。有条件的情况下，也可以考虑使用积极的、快速的持续动静脉复温技术。一项前瞻性随机对照研究表明，与其他较慢的复温方法相比，使用此种快速复温技术可以提高患者早期生存率和减少液体复苏的需要。

酸中毒

代谢性酸中毒一直以来被认为会导致患者凝血功能障碍，也会因凝血功能障碍产生。然而酸中毒导致凝血功能异常的具体原理尚未明确。动物实验的数据表明，低体温会延缓凝血酶的生成，而酸中毒会降低凝血酶的生成速率。伴有严重酸中毒（$pH<7.1$）、低血压和低体温的重症创伤患者，会发生威胁生命的凝血功能障碍。治疗不仅仅是纠正pH值，更应关注导致酸中毒病因的处理。在处理突发事件的同时，应给予积极的体液复苏，来优化组织灌注，从而纠正乳酸酸中毒。临床上可以根据乳酸和碱缺失水平来指导具体治疗。在乳酸酸中毒时，不合理的使用碳酸氢钠往往是无效的，有时甚至是有害的，不推荐使用。

血小板减少

血小板减少通常被定义为血小板计数低于100 000/mm^3，当血小板计数为50 000/mm^3 ~ 100 000/mm^{3}时，手术或严重创伤的出血风险增大。当血小板计数低于10 000/mm^3 ~ 20 000/mm^{3}时，自发性出血的风险大大增加。在ICU中，血小板减少的鉴别诊断较为耗时，但其原因可以大致分为3个类别：血小板生成减少、血小板消耗或隔离以及血小板被稀释。恶性肿瘤或化疗可能影响血小板生成，大量输血和液体复苏会导致全血小板计数的稀释。危重外科患者的脓毒症会导致消耗性凝血反应，其最严重的形式表现为DIC。免疫机制也可以导致血小板的消耗（血小板糖蛋白抗体），尤其是机体对某些药物的反应。这些药物包括肝素、H_2受体阻止剂、磺胺类、利福平、奎尼丁、降糖类药物、氯金酸钠等。

肝素相关的血小板减少十分少见。但在疾病状态下，患者血栓形成风险通常会增大。由于储存血中血小板的含量较低，故大量输血时容易出现稀释性血小板减少。然而，血小板计数的下降与血液制品的输注量不成正比。因此，简单的稀释并不是血小板计数下降的唯一决定因素。脾和骨髓会释放血小板，可以解释此变化。由于有凝血因子的存在，单独的稀释性血小板减少并不会导致微血管出血。关于治疗和输血指南将在本章后面讨论。

弥散性血管内凝血

DIC是在具体的临床情况下发生的弥散性系统性高凝和纤维蛋白溶解的综合征。外科ICU所涉及DIC的原因包括脓毒症、创伤、重症胰腺炎、恶性肿瘤、暴发性肝衰竭，以及输血反应等。DIC综合征包括微血管系统中过度纤维蛋白沉积、血小板聚集和微血管血栓的形成。DIC的病理生理学过程涉及炎性级联和组织因子途径，具体情况在其他地方介绍。情况包括亚临床血管内血栓形成加速、纤维蛋白溶解亢进以及明显的病理性出血的发生。暴发性DIC甚至会导致多器官功能障碍和死亡。

DIC诊断有赖于一些实验室检查结果，确诊前须排除其他原因导致的凝血功能障碍。一些评分系统和计算方法有助于临床对DIC的诊断。鉴于DIC的非特异性特点，在临床诊断DIC时设定诊断阈值是不必要的，然而其阈值设定标准仍需治疗性的研究和试验。此外，DIC通常发生在接受了大量输血和体液复苏的患者身上，而他们的凝血功能障碍常源于其他更常见的可逆原因。临床上观察到创伤的DIC患者血栓形成和纤维蛋白溶解过程也不同于通常的创伤止血反应。

DIC是一个广泛的凝血功能障碍和临床微血管出血的过程。实验室检查结果包括低的血小板计数、PT和PTT延长、纤维蛋白裂解产物（fibrin split products，FSPs）增加。94%诊断为DIC的患者具有D-二聚体水平的上升，D-二聚体试验是此情况其最敏感的试验。除了严重的DIC之外，纤维蛋白原水平一般可维持。

治疗DIC的核心是处理原发疾病过程，移除该综合征的促炎刺激。止血才是临床目的。血小板计数、PT/PTT可用于对治疗的反应性进行指导，但它们并不是临床治疗的终点。FFP和血小板往往被用于活动性出血的患者和在手术后常常会出现实验室检查紊乱的患者。如果纤维蛋白原水平低于100 mg/dl，且FFP输注无法纠正时，可选用冷凝蛋白质取代纤维蛋白原进行治疗。

许多其他治疗药物也在进行研究，但迄今为止仍没有特定的治疗被证明在改善DIC患者预后上具有明确效果。抗凝被用来试图缓解DIC的高凝状态，尽管某些实验室参数的改进已被报道，但没有足够的证据表明应用低分子量肝素（low-molecular-weight heparin，LMWH）、凝血酶抑制剂或抗纤维蛋白溶解药物会提高DIC患者的生存率。

严重脓毒症

近年来，相继有研究表明炎症反应过程和凝血机制有着复杂的相互关系。最初两者之间的关系会导致机体出现高凝状态。脓毒症的炎症反应会导致循环中单核细胞、组织巨噬细胞和内皮细胞表面组织因子的表达，并抑制纤维蛋白溶解。当纤维蛋白溶解受损时，纤维蛋白沉积于血管系统的过程不再受到抑制。此外，大多数严重脓毒症患者有低水平的天然抗凝蛋白C和抗凝血酶Ⅲ。弥漫的血栓形成会导致组织缺血和MODS的发生。

脓毒症的凝血功能障碍是多因素导致的。脓毒症诱导的凝血功能障碍通过免疫机制介导、激活的内皮细胞对血小板的隔离，以及DIC对血小板的消耗等途径发生。大量凝血酶的生成消耗凝血因子，纤维蛋白原通常也会减少。（虽然由于急性期反应可能会使机体促凝相关产物增加，从而使凝血因子和纤维蛋白原保持在正常水平）病理性出血可能是由于循环中缺乏凝血因子以及血小板的消耗，但这种情况的发生相对少见。一般认为严重的脓毒症患者估计有15%～30%会有发展为出现DIC的风险。但最近也有一项研究显示，仅有5%的患者出现了严重的出血。

存在活动性出血或出血高危因素的脓毒症患者有FFP或血小板输注的指征。如前所述，输注凝血因子和血小板通常只会有短暂的效果，因为微脉管系统内凝血因子和血小板在持续不断的消耗。然而面对活动性出血，积极控制出血是必需的。与此同时，也应尽一切努力来积极治疗和移除脓毒症的病因。

创伤性脑损伤

TBI与凝血系统的改变有关，一般认为是因为脑内高浓度组织因子的释放（促凝血酶原激酶）。组织因子的暴露会导致机体处于高凝状态，随后出现纤维蛋白溶解，此过程类似于无TBI创伤患者的改变。虽然应用实验室检查可以反应很多患者的凝血及纤维蛋白溶解状态，但临床表现的严重度范围从消耗性凝血功能障碍到临床上无法检测到的偶发性病理性出血。钝性和穿通性TBI患者若伴有凝血功能障碍，其死亡率会增加，但相关机制尚不清楚。

止血变化的重要性在于它可以通过脑血管微血栓形成，促进继发性脑损伤。这种继发性脑损伤会进一步加重脑缺血。目前尚不清楚是否应进行目标止血治疗，以防止脑损伤患者的进一步出血发生，或阻断凝血途径，从而避免脑内微血栓的形成以及脑缺血的出现。在人们对凝血相关的病理生理学有更进一步的理解之前，治疗目标应直接导向临床治疗的终点，并保证机体具有止血所需的血小板和凝血因子（在本章其他部分概述）。

维生素K缺乏

维生素K是凝血因子Ⅱ、Ⅶ、Ⅸ、Ⅹ酶反应过程中的必需辅助因子。蛋白质C，蛋白质S被称之为维生素K依赖性凝血因子。维生素K缺乏会损伤钙结合作用，导致相关凝血因子的活性降低。这些因素构成了传统的凝血级联反应的外源部分，这些凝血因子的功能可以通过国际标准化比率（international normalized ratio，INR）或PT试验来测量。临床上可导致机体维生素K缺乏的原因包括：饮食摄入不足、营养吸收不良、抗生素破坏产生维生素K的肠道细菌、肠外营养补充不足、肾功能不全和肝功能障碍。维生素K可以通过口服或肠外方式给予，用于纠正凝血功能障碍或阻断华法林的抗凝效果，在后文有详细的讨论。

抗凝药

抗凝药物的止血效果广泛而迅速。此类药物会影响血小板功能和纤维蛋白溶解，并且没有特效药。但是有一些凝血酶抑制剂和糖蛋白Ⅱb/Ⅲa半衰期短，且能够被血液透析所清除。阿司匹林和其他抗血小板药物导致的严重出血，可能通过输注血小板而部分改善。但在血小板输注前应进行功能性血小板计数或血小板功能试验来评估血小板病的水平。肝素、华法林无疑是外科ICU最常见的导致出血并发症的药物。最近一组新型口服抗凝药物已被证实可用于多种指征，其中包括非瓣膜性心房颤动。新型口服抗凝药物包括直接凝血酶抑制剂和Xa因子抑制剂，此类药物目前尚无特效的药来有效地逆转其效果。关于此类药物的具体使用将在以后的章节中讨论。

肝硬化和终末期肝病

严重肝疾病多伴随着凝血功能异常。肝病变导致其合成凝血因子的能力下降，在终末期肝病（end-stage liver disease，ESLD）和肝硬化失代偿期，纤维蛋白原水平处于较低水平，但由于急性期炎症反应，可能导致此项指标仍正常。肝合成的血小板生成素减少，血小板破坏或隔离，可导致血小板减少。循环中过多血小板抑制剂聚集，如一氧化二氮等的出现，也会导致血小板功能的改变。肝对纤维溶解酶的清除能力下降，也会导致系统性纤维蛋白溶解的发生。ESLD患者存在一个基线级别低的DIC，有较高的风险转化为明显DIC。DIC的发生频率和严重度通常与肝疾病的进展程度相关。

需要手术治疗的肝硬化患者对于外科医生是一个重大的挑战。此类患者的发病率和死亡率明显增加，尤其是对于急诊手术而言，其死亡率可高达50%。在一项研究中，合并肝硬化的剖腹手术患者死亡率为45%，明显高于非肝硬化的对照组中24%的死亡率。且合并肝硬化的试验组的术后ICU治疗时间也明显延长。ESLD患者接受手术治疗，可能会使组织纤溶酶原激活物（tissue plasminogen activator，tPA）和其他相关因子释放增加，最终导致纤维溶解反应亢进，妨碍稳定的血栓形成。ESLD患者一方面凝血功能障碍，出血风险较大；另一方面，此类患者多合并有腹腔内和腹壁的静脉曲张。因此，对于此类患者，腹部手术本身也是一项艰巨的任务。鉴于此，对于ESLD或肝硬化患者而言，任何有创操作都应权衡利弊，谨慎进行。

凝血功能障碍的ESLD患者的治疗目标是临床止血，而不是使所有化验指标完全恢复正常（这通常是不可能的）。凝血相关实验室指标的轻度改变是很常见的，通常不会引起出血。FFP常用作凝血因子和纤维蛋白原的替代品，但如果纤维蛋白原水平低于100 mg/dl时，则可选择冷凝蛋白质。有时临床上甚至允许FFP的连续输注，直到达到临床目标为止。在危及生命的出血或急诊手术时，可以应用

rFⅦa 因子用来纠正 INR。然而 rFⅦa 因子的半衰期较短，仅能维持几个小时的止血效果，故必要时可以重复使用。血小板减少的输血指南在本章也有相同描述。然而脾大患者可能破坏所输注血小板，使得血小板计数上升的趋势低于临床预期。含有正常血小板计数的微血管出血患者可能存在血小板功能障碍，应考虑加做血小板功能试验。但是这些情况下，输血可能仅出现短暂止血或完全没有改善患者的凝血功能，除非血小板病的根本原因得到纠正。临床上也可尝试应用 DDAVP，但其具体功效如何尚未得到明确证实。

尽管患者存在凝血功能障碍，但仍有血栓形成的风险。肝硬化患者不应被认为是天然的抗凝保护状态。事实上，肝静脉和门静脉血栓形成在此类患者中也很常见，尤其在进展期患者。对于终末期肝病患者而言，往往会伴有 INR 的增高。因而 INR 没有必要调整到一般患者常规接受华法林治疗的指标水平。若此类患者仍然按照常规 INR 指标指导治疗，往往会误导我们的诊治。由于Ⅶ因子半衰期较短，若Ⅶ因子合成不足，可能会出现实验室测量指标异常，但临床上并不会出现凝血异常的表现。除非到后期阶段，维护正常的纤维蛋白原水平通常已足够满足凝血的需要。

肾衰竭

肾衰竭和尿毒症会导致血小板功能异常，从而影响机体凝血。这种血小板功能异常主要表现为血小板黏附和聚集功能的下降。但是确切机制尚不清楚。尿毒症毒素会导致血小板功能障碍。这些毒素包括尿素、肌酐、醛酸和胍基琥珀酸。血液透析可能是治疗尿毒症引起的血小板功能障碍的最有效的方法。然而血液透析一般不单独用于纠正凝血功能障碍。如果出现活动性出血，可以尝试应用 DDAVP，通常剂量为 0.3 μg/kg。DDAVP 可以减少肾衰竭患者的出血风险。冷凝蛋白质和结合雌激素是目前的二线治疗药物。尽管肾衰竭患者伴有血小板功能缺陷，但行透析治疗的慢性肾衰竭患者由于存在纤维溶解功能障碍，故也可能发生血栓性的并发症。

肝损伤

肝损伤可间接导致凝血功能障碍。如前所述，严重的肝创伤可能导致出血性休克和凝血功能障碍的伴随病因。当肝有广泛的直接损伤时，肝自身会有相当大的代偿能力。因此，一小部分正常的肝实质就可以产生足够的凝血因子，并有效清除循环中的致纤溶作用的物质。当肝切除范围高达 75% 时仍可以维持机体正常的肝功能，此时的肝实质损害也不会导致机体凝血功能异常。

诊断

临床评估

危重症患者的出血应进行系统性评估，用以明确导致出血的原因并及时指导止血治疗（图 1）。外科 ICU 中，对于出血患者的首要任务是区分手术出血与非手术凝血功能障碍性微血管出血。这可能是外科医生面临的最困难的问题之一。对于凝血功能障碍患者而言，一个非治疗性手术也可能使凝血功能恶化。但有些情况若不及时采取手术方式止血，往往又是致命的。

对患者的评价应从病史的细节着手，尤其应注意手术及介入性操作的具体操作过程。体格检查有助于发现手术创伤或导管、引流管的出血，这些的发现可以提示是否进行再手术。相反，多处或小的出血（如静脉导管位置）常常提示凝血功能障碍。除了回顾患者病史之外，还应关注患者近期治疗过程中所有可能影响止血的用药。

术后出血广义上可以分为手术无法止血和凝血功能障碍。手术无法止血通常是手术部位的出血，其原因可能是由于结扎线滑脱或手术操作止血不充分等外科相关技术问题导致。在手术期间，血管收缩可以防止可见的出血，但体温的增加和复苏可能使出血再次发生。手术止血失败通常需要再次手术，以确定性控制出血。术后手术出血可能伴随着从血容量减少到出血性休克等相关的症状和体征。医生应在休克早期的体征的基础上进行干预，而不是等到严重休克发生后。这些休克早期体征包括心动过速、不安、焦虑、皮肤苍白和少尿。对于术后患者焦虑或不安的处理，应在给予止痛药或镇静药前，首先应评估其灌注和氧合状态。低血压是出血的晚期表现，往往提示非常严重的容量不足。

影响凝血功能的因素可分为主要因素（初始血小板栓的形成）和次要因素（凝血因子和凝血级联反应）。临床也可以将凝血功能障碍分为定性缺陷（如血小板功能异常、肝素对因子的抑制作用等）和定

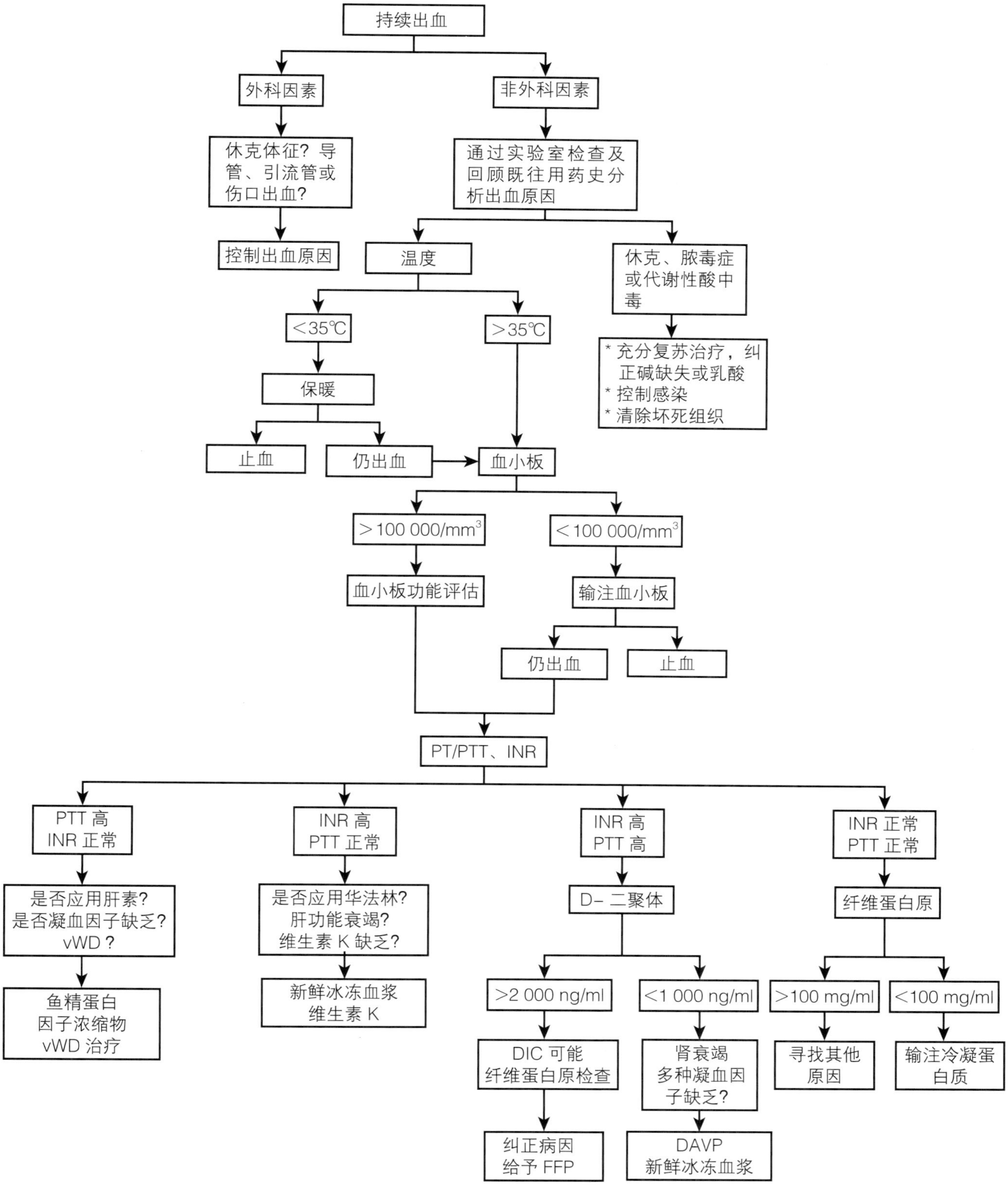

图1 出血患者分析处理流程。DDAVP，1-脱氨基-8-D-精氨酸血管加压素；DIC，弥散性血管内凝血；INR，国际标准化比率；PT，凝血酶原时间；PPT，部分促凝血酶原时间；VWD，血管性血友病

* INR，PT/PTT，血小板计数、碱缺失或乳酸的动脉血气，考虑血小板功能试验和血栓描记图

量缺陷（如血小板减少和凝血因子缺陷等）。此外还可以按照先天性或获得性因素对患者进行划分。图1以系统性方法为例，此方法对于大多数外科患者的治疗有帮助，甚至是凝血功能障碍原因不明的外科患者。但此方法应用于ICU患者的快速评估和启动治疗，而不是用于具体的出血性疾病的诊断。

一些基本的实验室检查有助于凝血功能障碍的诊断和治疗。这里值得重申的是，临床主要治疗目标是止血，而不是使得凝血功能各项参数完全变得正常。血小板计数、PT、INR、PTT都是最基本的实验室检查，有助于区分主要或次要止血因素的问题。应核对患者的血细胞比容水平，并牢记急性出血并不会影响血细胞比容的变化。直到液体输注使得血管内容量增加，血液被稀释，血细胞比容才会相应地改变。血栓弹力图（thromboelastography，TEG）是一种全球性的凝血功能的监测方法，此方法有助于判断凝血功能障碍的原因。纤维蛋白降解产物、D-二聚体和纤维蛋白原水平并非是确诊由于凝血功能障碍导致的出血性休克的必要条件。但这3项指标可能有助于确诊DIC。在接下来的章节中，相关具体试验将被详述。

凝血功能实验室检查

PT：这个测试通过添加包括组织因子、磷脂和钙的促凝血酶原激酶到富含枸橼酸的血浆中，以秒为单位测量纤维蛋白的凝固时间。PT可以评估外源性凝血途径（Ⅶ因子）和共同凝血途径（纤维蛋白原，Ⅱ、Ⅸ和Ⅹ因子）的活性。PT通常用于华法林治疗的监测评估，并且PT也受到维生素K依赖性凝血因子的影响。维生素K依赖性凝血因子包括Ⅱ、Ⅶ、Ⅸ、Ⅹ因子以及蛋白C和蛋白S。

INR：INR是利用PT值通过一系列换算得出，用于校准各自实验室PT测量差异的指标。目前INR已被广泛用于监测华法林的抗凝效果。

PTT：通过将部分促凝血酶原激酶（磷脂类的混合物）、活性物质和氯化钙添加到含有柠檬酸的血浆中，从而计算出PTT的具体数值。PTT用于测量内源性凝血途径和共同凝血途径的活性。内源性凝血途径包括高分子量（high-molecular-weight，HMW）激肽原、前激肽释放酶、Ⅷ因子、Ⅸ因子、Ⅺ因子和Ⅻ因子。共同途径包括纤维蛋白原、Ⅱ因子、Ⅸ因子和Ⅹ因子。仅仅Ⅶ因子活性无法通过PTT来测量。

出血时间（bleeding time，BT）：评估血小板功能和止血效果的主要检查。然而由于实验室检查的差异性，导致其灵敏度和特异度较低，并不能确切反映血小板功能，也不能准确预测外科出血情况。

血小板功能试验：临床上可以通过多项实验室检查和快速检查手段来判断血小板功能。作者所在的医院已经不再使用出血时间而利用PFA-100（血小板功能分析方法，Dade-Behring）来评估血小板功能。PFA-100通过在高剪切应力情况下在全血流动的在滤器上封闭一个孔来判断血小板功能。这是一个被广泛应用的止血试验，通过此试验可以判断血小板功能障碍的具体原因。引起血小板功能障碍的原因包括确定的药物和疾病因素和某些先天性疾病。其他试验还包括测量正常功能的血小板的比例来判断功能血小板的具体计数，此方法经常用于心脏手术。另外还有一些即时检查，可以通过使用阿司匹林或GPⅡb/Ⅲa抑制剂等药物，观察血小板抑制的效果。血小板聚集试验应用不同浓度的受体激动剂去诱导富含血小板的血浆的凝固，并揭示其定量或定性上的不足。此试验是临床上的评价金标准，但须花费数小时才能完成此试验，因而此试验在急性凝血功能障碍的管理中很少应用。

TEG：TEG是全血样本形成时的图像表现（图2）。TEG是基于几个因素所构成的，它们包括凝块

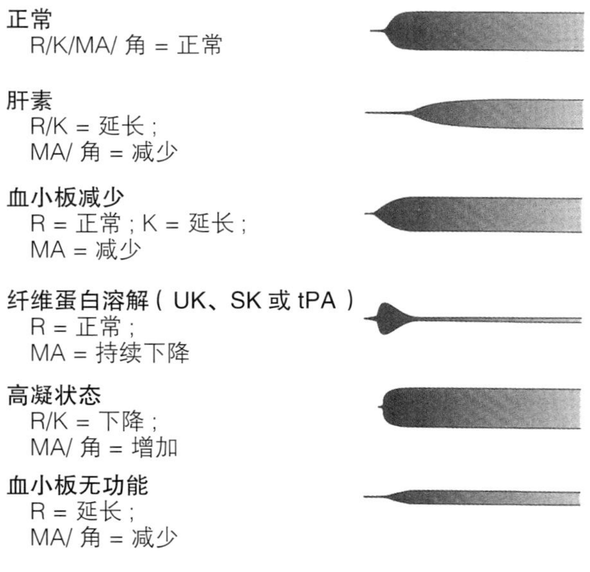

图2 血栓弹力图。DIC，弥散性血管内凝血；K，动力学；MA，最大振幅；R，反应时间；SK，链激酶；tPA，组织纤溶酶原激活物；UK，尿激酶（*Modified from Kaufmann CR, Dwyer KM, Crews JD, et al: Usefulness of thromboelastography in assessment of trauma patient coagulation.* J Trauma *42:716, 1997.*）

形成的速度、纤维蛋白的交联和血小板纤维蛋白的相互作用。通过测量图像的各种参数，TEG 可以用于评估血小板功能、凝血酶活性和凝血功能的整体水平。TEG 还可以区别原发性纤维蛋白溶解、消耗性凝血功能障碍、抗凝治疗和低体温的影响。由于 TEG 的快速可用性，并能以一种综合的方式评估凝固的成分，因而 TEG 现已被广泛用于体外循环、肝移植手术和 ICU。TEG 和 ROTEM 等不断更新的凝血试验技术已被用于指导复苏治疗和凝血功能障碍的成分输血治疗。并且这类试验有助于提高复苏成功率和成分输血的治疗效率。

凝血酶时间（trombin time，TT）：TT 是通过添加凝血酶（添加或不添加无钙）到含有柠檬酸的血浆中而测得。TT 是测量纤维蛋白原转化成纤维蛋白的时间，这个过程由凝血酶诱导而实现。临床上会导致 TT 延长的因素包括：纤维蛋白原缺乏（<100 mg/dl）或异常、循环中存在肝素等抗凝剂（包括纤维蛋白裂解产物和肝素）和在纤维蛋白溶解过度期间。由于 TT 对如肝素等外源性抗凝剂的高敏感性，限制了其在住院患者身上的使用。但是 TT 可用于循环中肝素低水平状态下的监测，因为此种低水平状态下 PTT 并不改变。

纤维蛋白原：纤维蛋白原是一种大分子蛋白质，它是纤维蛋白在凝血酶作用下裂解产生的纤维蛋白单体。在消耗性凝血功能障碍或使用溶栓剂导致抗凝过度时过多的凝块产生，纤维蛋白原水平可能会下降。纤维蛋白原同时也是一种急性期反应物，其升高也可能是生理应激的反映。

纤维蛋白裂解产物（fibrin split product，FSPs）：FSPs 是纤维蛋白分子的碎片，它由血浆纤维蛋白裂解而成。FSPs 并非特异性试验，但其升高可提示纤维蛋白溶解和临床上消耗性凝血功能障碍。D- 二聚体是 FSP 的一种特殊形式，它通常与 DIC 相关。

凝血因子测定：凝血因子水平测定可以帮助临床确诊凝血因子缺陷导致的相关疾病。临床上常见的凝血因子缺陷导致的疾病包括Ⅷ因子缺乏导致的甲型血友病以及Ⅸ因子缺乏导致的乙型血友病。另外，还可以通过此方法来进一步判断Ⅴ因子、Ⅶ因子、Ⅹ因子、Ⅺ因子、Ⅻ因子（Hageman 因子）、前激肽释放酶和高分子量激肽原的缺乏。这些物质的缺乏在临床上相对比较少见。在 ICU 中并不常规测定凝血因子水平。

处理

血液制品输注

新鲜冰冻血浆

FFP 是从人体血液中的非细胞成分中提取出来的产物，并以冰冻方式储存。每 250～300 ml FFP 中包含所有的凝血因子和大约 400 mg 的纤维蛋白原。它将会提升 3% 的凝血因子水平。在应用 FFP 治疗时，可利用 PT 和 PTT 来测量其输注效果。

外科 ICU 使用 FFP 的适应证相对较少。适应证包括伴有临床出血的凝血功能障碍、测量或怀疑凝血因子缺陷导致 PT 或 PTT 延长超过 1.5 倍，以及由于华法林使用不当导致的获得性凝血功能障碍、肝疾病以及 DIC。FFP 不应用于扩容、促进伤口愈合或治疗低白蛋白血症。FFP 可以在大量输血或按一定比例的预设公式的红细胞输注时应用。同时临床上也应避免不必要的 FFP 输注。这有助于减少输血反应风险、细菌感染和输血相关的急性肺损伤的发生，并有效地控制成本。FFP 的具体用量应以使患者凝血因子浓度达到正常值的 30% 以上，以及实现临床止血的目的。实际上，10～15 ml/kg 的 FFP 即可达到这一目的。在逆转华法林的抗凝效果时，常应用低剂量的 FFP（5～8 ml/kg）来纠其正凝血功能。

血小板

血小板减少或血小板功能障碍的治疗重点在于纠正其根本原因和改善患者的临床症状。当没有活动性出血或急诊手术时，若患者血小板计数大于 10 000/mm^3，无需额外处理。但当血小板低于 10 000/mm^3，应给予血小板输注，以避免自发性出血的发生。微血管出血和血小板减少的患者在排除低体温后可从输注血小板的治疗中获益，因为低温状态下，输注的血小板无法发挥正常功能。对于血小板计数在 50 000～100 000/mm^3 的外科手术患者，目前缺乏基于指南的证据指导治疗。其治疗要根据患者的自身条件、出血风险、手术，以及高风险有创操作来决定。一般而言，在脑部、脊柱及眼科手术前，须输注血小板，使其达到 100 000/mm^3 以上，而对于其他主要操作，血小板也应保持在 50 000/mm^3 以上。

一般来说，血小板在此水平下若没有微血管出血，无须给予血小板输注。消耗性凝血功能障碍的患者应用输注血小板治疗的效果欠佳，因为机体也会以同样的方式消耗新输注的血小板。然而，对于脓毒症或DIC的微血管出血，通常须给予输注血小板治疗。如果血小板计数低的和有消耗性过程的患者有手术或有创操作的必要，应在其操作前或操作中输注血小板，以使得循环中的血小板数量足以达到止血的效果。

不同的血小板浓缩物是可以接受的。传统的“六袋”来自于随机捐赠者的浓缩物，其血小板来自不同个体，相当于6单位的血小板浓缩物。单独采集捐献者1单位的血小板，又称之为单采血小板，其所包含的血小板的容量与6个随机供体的单位所得到的血小板容量相同。但单采血小板由于仅来自独立的捐献者，因此仅对一组抗原暴露了受体。一般而言，每输注6单位随机供体血小板或1单位单采血小板，其血小板计数会上升30 000/mm^3。反复输注血小板可能会导致一些患者出现抗体，这将给之后的血小板输注带来困难。在上述情况下可能须进行人类白细胞抗原匹配或血小板交叉配血试验。单采血小板输注已被多家机构所采纳，此方法可以减少抗体形成，以尽量延长血小板输注治疗时间。

冷凝蛋白质

冷凝蛋白质提取自温度为1～6℃的FFP，然后移除并再次冷冻其不溶解的沉淀物。每一袋冷凝蛋白质中含有15 ml液体，大约包含有150～250 mg纤维蛋白原、80～100单位Ⅷ因子，以及其他成分（如纤连蛋白和vWF）。它通常为一个大约8～10袋的混合产品，相当于为患者补充1 200～2 000 mg的纤维蛋白原。虽然并没有给予病毒灭活的处理，它对病毒彻底筛查过，使其病毒传播的风险相对较低。冷凝蛋白质通常用于治疗甲型血友病、vWD、低纤维蛋白原血症、血浆纤维蛋白原低于100 mg/dl的DIC患者，以及因前面提到的因素须被替换为低体积的液体的患者。在治疗出血性休克的凝血功能障碍时，冷凝蛋白质的重要性已经逐渐减少，由于体积已不是问题，纤维蛋白原很少需要替换，只需新鲜冰冻血浆就足以完成凝血因子的替换。

对华法林的逆转

随着年龄的增加，受伤患者使用华法林的比例逐渐升高。此类药物对于创伤患者的发病率和死亡率的影响是变化的，但具体的影响程度尚不明确。须紧急进行华法林拮抗的情况包括创伤性脑损伤和伴随出血的严重损伤。无须紧急进行华法林拮抗的情况包括由于创伤或围术期状态导致出血风险增加的患者。在开始治疗之前，临床还应考虑一些因素，包括紧急逆转华法林，至下一次抗凝治疗的期望时间间隔，以及患者的心功能（如容量负荷的耐受性）。

华法林的逆转效果需要INR来评价，它被标准化的循证指南推荐为最佳。维生素K是INR过高的非紧急治疗首选，通常起效时间需要8～12 h。然而，由于华法林有较长的半衰期，如果预计在接下来的几天内须应用华法林持续抗凝，应避免一次性给予过高剂量或重复剂量。口服维生素K是非紧急情况下逆转华法林药效的首选治疗方案，然而皮下途径并不推荐，因为此种给药方式吸收效率很低。静脉输注维生素K应有持续心脏监测，因为此途径给药有过敏风险。FFP是伴有INR过高的严重出血或须进行有创操作的患者标准治疗手段。

许多使用华法林治疗的老年患者常伴有心脏疾病，临床上应关注此类情况，避免由于强烈的容量超载导致的充血性心力衰竭。在临床实验室中，INR＞2时，很难通过输注1～2单位FFP来成功纠正凝血问题。另外，患者因素也须考虑在内，这些因素变化很大，可能导致无法达到预期效果以及有非线性剂量反应关系。当出现紧急情况（如创伤性脑损伤或危及生命的出血）时，通常须紧急纠正抗凝状态，临床上通常会使用rFⅦa因子。rFⅦa因子的半衰期只是反映华法林的部分抗凝效果，因此应使用FFP和维生素K来保持正常的凝血功能。在2014年，美国可使用4因子凝血酶原复合物（prothrombin complex concentrate，PCC-4）。其相关凝血因子包括Ⅱ、Ⅶ、Ⅸ和Ⅹ因子，它们通常能在低容量液体（大约150 ml）时，迅速有效地拮抗华法林作用。当须逆转危及生命的出血或需要紧急手术时，PCC-4管理也是一个可行的逆转方案。美国麻醉医师协会在2015年指南中提出，在给予华法林拮抗治疗时，应考虑到患者的这些具体情况。表1展示了应用华法林导致INR升高和出血风险的患者的管理方案。

对肝素的逆转

普通肝素（unfractionated heparin，UFH）和LMWH通常用于外科ICU静脉血栓的预防或其他情况的治疗。尽管使用预防剂量肝素的出血风险较低，

表 1 华法林抗凝和出血风险的管理

临床情况	治疗选择
INR<5，没有明显活动性出血	继续应用华法林抗凝
INR>5，没有明显活动性出血	口服 1～5 mg 维生素 K
INR>1.5，出血或存在出血高危因素，非急性出血	给予输注新鲜冰冻血浆 2～4 U，每输注 1 U 血浆复测 INR 直至出血停止或 INR＜1.5 口服 5 mg 维生素 K
INR>1.5，危及生命的出血或需要急性手术或有创操作	给予输注新鲜冰冻血浆 4 U，每输注 1 U 血浆复测 INR，并缓慢静脉注射 10 mg 维生素 K 4 因子凝血酶原复合物： INR＞2,且INR＜4 时，予 25 U/kg INR 为 4～6 时，予 35 U/kg INR>6 时，予 50 U/kg 给予输注Ⅶ a 因子（如仍持续出血，可每隔 2～3 h 重复输注）

INR，国际标准化比率

但足量的抗凝可能会增加出血风险。当应用肝素治疗的患者出现非手术出血时，逆转药物的作用很重要。普通肝素的半衰期是 1 h，因此大多数治疗剂量的肝素输注可以维持药效达 6 h 左右。如果须紧急进行肝素的逆转，可以尝试应用鱼精蛋白。鱼精蛋白可以结合肝素，从而中和它的效果。1 mg 的鱼精蛋白可以中和 100 U 的肝素。当估算鱼精蛋白的使用剂量时，也必须充分考虑肝素半衰期的问题。例如，给予肝素治疗后，其剂量每过 1 h 会减半一次。如果采用肝素连续输注的方式，则须评估累计剂量。使用鱼精蛋白有导致低血压的风险，临床上可以通过超过 10 min 的减慢输注速度的方式来避免。对于过去曾经应用过鱼精蛋白或 NPH 的患者，出现过敏反应的概率约为 1%。

低分子量肝素的半衰期各有不同，但大多数保持在 2～5 h。低分子量肝素只能部分被鱼精蛋白中和，它能逆转大多数抗Ⅱ a 因子（凝血酶）的活性，但仅仅能部分逆转抗Ⅹ a 因子的活性。逆转作用基于抗 Xa 因子活力的水平，通常 1 mg 鱼精蛋白可以中和 100 U 抗Ⅹ a 因子。

新型口服抗凝药的逆转

几年来，新一代口服抗凝血药已经获得美国FDA 的批准，并应用于心房颤动和静脉血栓栓塞的治疗。这些药物有无须在治疗过程中反复进行实验室监测的优点，但也有尚缺乏有效的拮抗剂的缺点。

达比加群是此类药物的典型代表，它是直接的凝血酶抑制剂。达比加群发挥凝血作用却不影响促凝血酶原时间，目前仅能通过检测蝰蛇毒凝血时间来评估抗凝疗效。PT、PTT 和 INR 等常规凝血实验室指标在用于监测其疗效时不可靠。利伐沙班和阿匹沙班是Ⅹa 因子抑制剂，它们的疗效可通过 PT 进行监测。应用此类药物的患者若 PT 正常，可能无须进行逆转。然而 PT 正常也不能保证完全的药物清除。

由于缺乏特殊的拮抗剂，因此应用此类药物的出血管理成为使用这些药物者的主要挑战。近期各类其拮抗剂疗效的临床数据十分有限，即便有些药物有效，也仅能部分恢复其凝血功能。这是一个正在进步的领域，研究者采用了多学科的方法来解决此问题。以下是具体方法举例。达比加群和利伐沙班在被摄取的 2 h 内或阿匹沙班被摄取的 6 h 内，均可以应用活性炭来清除。血液透析是清除达比加群的最有效方法。对于一些危及生命的出血，可以尝试应用Ⅷ因子抑制物旁路活性剂（factor Ⅷ inhibitor bypassing activity，FEIBA）和重组活化Ⅶ因子（rFⅦa）。FEIBA 包含Ⅱ、Ⅸ和Ⅹ因子（通常未激活）和活化的Ⅶ因子。临床上也可以尝试应用 4 因子 PCC（既往曾用于拮抗华法林）来逆转利伐沙班和阿匹沙班的抗凝作用。

在非紧急情况或择期手术的情况下，直接凝血酶抑制剂或Ⅹa因子抑制剂可能会通过正常代谢，在一定时间内被中断或清除。这些药物的半衰期取决于其具体药剂，达比加群和利伐沙班主要取决于患者的肌酐清除率。当肌酐清除率（creatinine clearance，Crcl）为 50 ml/min 时，择期手术应该在停用达比加群和利伐沙班 24 h 或停用阿匹沙班 48 h 后进行。针对如心脏手术、神经外科手术、较大的腹部手术，以及矫形手术等出血风险较大的手术而言，临床上应在停用达比加群和利伐沙班 2 天或停用阿匹沙班 2～3 天后进行。对于 Crcl 下降导致药物半衰期延长的患者，其建议观察时间也需要相应的延长。在这种情况下，咨询药剂师是有益的。

重组活化 Ⅶ 因子

rFⅦa 是人工合成的Ⅶ因子，它可以促进血液凝固。rFⅦa 是 FDA 推荐的用于处理血友病活动性出血的药物，但同时它也可以用于其他各种类型的凝血功能障碍。其主要机制仍然在讨论和分析中。当绑定于内皮下暴露的组织因子时，rFⅦa能够活化X因子和Ⅸ因子，这2个凝血因子会促进血栓的形成。这个机制可以用于解释为何此类因子只在损伤部位被激活和表达。其他的试验数据显示高剂量的rFⅦa可以不依靠组织因子，通过激活血小板表面的Xa因子，直接促进血栓的形成。

多个动物实验证实，失血性休克凝血功能障碍时应用rFⅦa可以减少出血和提高生存率。根治性前列腺癌的人体试验也证实，应用rFⅦa可以明显减少出血和缩短手术时间。rFⅦa可以避免钝性创伤患者的大量液体或血液的输注。然而对于穿通伤患者而言，并不能从应用rF Ⅶa中明显获益。有一项关于钝性创伤导致严重出血的随机对照试验，观察在创伤后的12 h内分别给予3剂量的rFⅦa和安慰剂。rFⅦa的首剂剂量为200 mcg/kg，并在之后的1 h和3 h分别再给予100 mcg/kg的剂量。此试验由于有两组总体死亡率均较低的结果而被迫终止。rFⅦa组相比对照组需要更少的红细胞输注，但在死亡率上两组无明显统计学差异，并且最初的关于rFⅦa组会增加血栓的风险的猜想也并未证实。许多研究表明在人体和动物实验中，rF Ⅶ a并不会增加循环血栓和血栓相关并发症的风险。

外科患者应用rFⅦa的合理剂量目前尚无定论。在多个临床试验中，rFⅦa的剂量范围从20～200 μg/kg不等。由于rFⅦa半衰期较短，如果在严重凝血功能障碍的情况下，在积极处理其他出血原因的同时，在初始剂量维持止血的最初的几小时内须再给予2次或3次药。由于在应用rFⅦa的多个随机试验中均缺乏生存率的获益情况，所以对于创伤导致的出血性休克患者并不常规推荐应用rFⅦa。

结论

重症或创伤患者的凝血功能障碍十分常见。当遇到出血时，首先要控制出血，并应用晶体和血液进行复苏治疗。当然临床诊治时也要考虑到先天性凝血功能障碍的可能，同时还应评估患者是否存在由于药物导致的获得性凝血功能障碍。凝血功能障碍常常伴随大量出血和复苏治疗，导致这种凝血功能障碍的原因可能是多方面的。虽然凝血功能障碍的病理生理过程常常涉及稀释，但低体温、酸中毒、休克在凝血功能障碍中也扮演重要角色。最新的复苏策略认为在输注红细胞的同时应增加血浆和血小板的输注比例，在帮助止血上更有效。

血液成分的具体应用要根据临床症状和实验室数据所见的凝血功能障碍的客观证据来决定，而不是基于公式的使用。选择性地给予成分输血，尤其是血小板的输注，将更加安全和高效。本领域研究的持续进步使患者的凝血功能得到了更有效的改善，使血液成分治疗的使用更加明智。此领域的持续进步可以给凝血治疗提供新的机遇，但临床还是应遵循患者出血的基本处理原则：迅速控制出血、对于休克患者给予迅速的复苏治疗、积极调控体温，以及动态监测凝血功能异常的实验室检查。

外科监护病房内分泌功能紊乱的处理

Anthony Falvo 和 Mathilda Horst 著
朱凤雪 李 纾 译

外科要点

1. 伴有尿量明显增多的头部损伤患者应警惕尿崩症（diabetes insipidus，DI）的发生。
2. 由于脑耗盐综合征或抗利尿激素分泌失调综合征（syndrome of inappropriate of antidiuretic hormone，SIADH）导致高钠血症，其治疗措施完全不同。
3. SIADH可引起容量增加，而脑耗盐会引起容量减少。
4. 发热患者的鉴别诊断应考虑到甲状腺危象可能。
5. 甲状腺危象须及时治疗，不可延误，无须等待实验室检查结果。
6. 许多常用的ICU用药会影响甲状腺激素和抗利尿激素（antidiuretic hormone，ADH）水平。
7. 当出现对血管活性药物和体液复苏无反应的低血压，应考虑肾上腺皮质功能不全的可能。
8. 应用糖皮质激素治疗的肾上腺皮质功能不全患

者具有更好的预后。

9. 内分泌功能异常的患者常伴有相关的临床症状和体征的先兆。

10. 严格的血糖控制会改善患者预后。

内分泌系统是神经内分泌轴的一部分，临床通常称之为下丘脑 - 垂体 - 肾上腺轴。内分泌系统紊乱会改变创伤和应激的生理反应。已确诊为内分泌系统问题的重症患者应给予及时的替代治疗，但未认识到的内分泌系统紊乱患者通常处理起来相对棘手，且死亡率偏高。内分泌功能紊乱可以发生在由于原始疾病和继发性疾病、药物或终末期器官衰竭导致的神经内分泌轴功能障碍的任何阶段。

人体神经内分泌轴由下丘脑、垂体、自主神经系统所支配，负责应激反应。压力感受器对血管内容量的反应、组织损伤导致的交感神经兴奋和组织创伤导致的炎性物质释放都会激活神经内分泌系统。损伤反应释放的激素与细胞表面受体或细胞内受体结合，并产生一系列的细胞反应和反馈过程，从而维持细胞过程。本章重点讨论内分泌系统功能紊乱对危重患者的影响（图 1）。

脑部问题：下丘脑 / 垂体反应异常

损伤会干扰垂体、下丘脑对激素的产生。脑外伤、脑部手术、渗透性疾病以及大病灶、脑血管损伤、脑缺氧损害、颅内感染均会使垂体激素分泌障碍导致单一或复合的异常。脑水肿和颅内压增高被认为会限制下丘脑和垂体区血流量。临床通常会遇到的相关临床疾病是 DT、SIADH 和脑耗盐综合征。这些综合征均是由于水电解质平衡异常所致。评估容量状态、血液和尿液中钠浓度以及渗透压可有助于决定综合征是否存在，并进一步指导合理治疗。（表 1）

表 1　水钠异常的原因比较

特征	尿崩症	脑耗盐	SIADH
血钠	↑	↓	↓
血浆渗透压（mOsm/kg）	＞290	＜280	＜280
尿渗透压（mOsm/kg）	＜300	＞100	＞100
尿钠（mEq/L）	不确定	＞20	＞20
容量减少	是	是	否
治疗	DDAVP，补充水分	生理盐水	限制容量

DDAVP，1- 脱氨基 -8-D- 精氨酸血管加压素；SIADH，抗利尿激素分泌失调综合征

图 1　神经内分泌轴。E，肾上腺素；NE，去甲肾上腺素

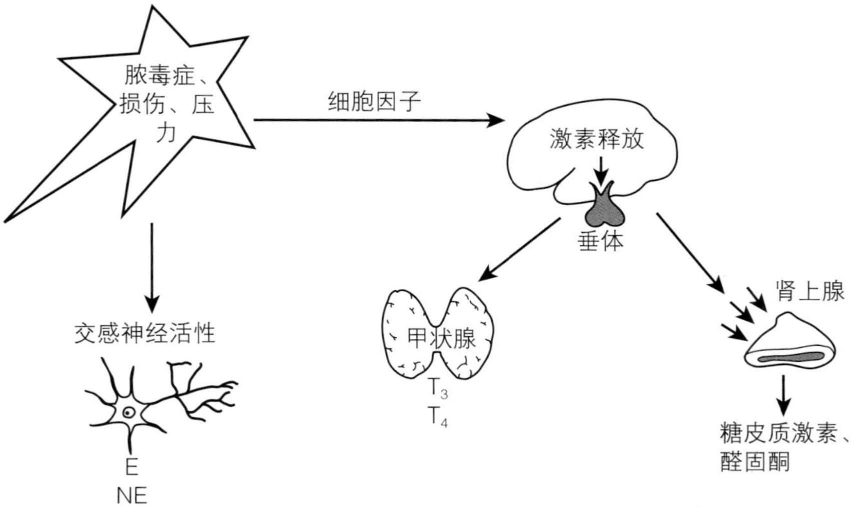

下丘脑：释放激素
- 促肾上腺皮质激素释放激素：刺激促肾上腺皮质激素（ACTH）释放
- 促甲状腺激素释放激素（TRH）：刺激促甲状腺激素（TSH）释放
- 抗利尿激素（ADH）/ 血管加压素：由下丘脑产生，并垂体后叶释放

垂体：刺激激素
- ACTH：刺激肾上腺
- TSH：刺激甲状腺
- ADH/ 血管加压素：包括血管和肾等多个脏器系统均会受到影响

尿崩症

中枢性尿崩症是由于血管加压素（抗利尿激素）缺乏所致，它会导致尿量超过 3 L/d、脱水和高钠血症。患者出现尿液稀释、尿渗透压低于 300 mOsm/kg，以及尿比重低于 1.005。尿渗透压高于 800 mOsm/kg 可除外尿崩症。当持续 2 h 以上稀释尿量超过 200 ml/h，临床可以诊断为尿崩症。此类 ICU 患者中，除非有积极的液体替换治疗，否则其血清钠水平会急剧上升。神经外科手术患者尿崩症的发生率高达 3.7%，而死亡率更高达 70%。尿崩症通常见于严重脑损伤和脑疝患者。有效的治疗措施包括液体再水化、血管加压素替代治疗，以及静脉应用 DDAVP 治疗。应频繁监测电解质水平和中心静脉压。临床还可以计算失水量并缓慢替换治疗。当出现严重高钠血症时，应在 24 h 内补充所需要液体量的一半，从而避免脱髓鞘病变（表 2）。

表 2　水分丢失量计算公式

水分丢失量 =0.6* ×（Wt kg）× [（Na/140）-1]

* 女性为 0.5

抗利尿激素分泌失调综合征和脑耗盐综合征

脑损伤可导致 SIADH 和脑耗盐的发生，其结果会出现低渗性低钠血症。脑耗盐通常见于蛛网膜下隙出血患者，但 SIADH 却常因为脑损伤、脑肿瘤以及药物因素的影响而产生（表 3）。SIADH 的原因是抗利尿激素的过度释放，导致水的潴留增加以及细胞外液容量增加。容量增加会促进肾的排钠功能，并导致低钠血症发生。脑耗盐综合征被认为是中枢神经系统紊乱使肾排钠增多，或中枢性利钠因子分泌过度所致。钠离子通过肾排出，导致细胞外容量下降并刺激 ADH 的分泌。低钠血症随着细胞外体积的减少而发展。

以上两种疾病的诊断均开始于血钠浓度低于 135 mmol/L,并且两者血浆渗透压均低于 280 mOsm/kg，两者的尿渗透压均高于 100 mOsm/kg。两者的区别点在于有效血容量（effective blood volume， CVP），SIADH 患者通常具有正常的血容量， 而脑耗盐综合征的患者往往伴随有效血容量的降低。 有效血容量降低通常会导致直立性低血压、 心动过速、 CVP 降低、 尿钠减少以及 BUN 的上升。 两者的尿酸水平均较低。 当低血钠被及时纠正时， SIADH 患者的尿酸水平基本正常， 而脑耗盐综合征患者的尿酸水平通常不会恢复正常。 抗利尿激素分泌失调综合征的治疗是体液的限制， 通常要保持在 800 ~ 1000 ml/d 以上，偶尔也会用高渗的生理盐水。 地美环素、 苯妥英钠以及锂可用于治疗慢性 SIADH。 脑耗盐综合征目前可给予正常生理盐水替换治疗， 从而提高细胞外液体含量。

甲状腺功能异常

对于危重患者而言，没有及时发现和处理甲状腺问题可能会危及其生命。甲状腺激素可控制所有组织的基础代谢率。重症疾病可通过影响促甲状腺激素的释放和周围基础代谢率改变，或结合蛋白的改变，从而改变其甲状腺激素的产生。细胞刺激因子和 ICU 常用药物均会影响患者的甲状腺功能（表 3）。

上述内容描述了重症患者的非甲状腺疾病。甲状腺功能异常导致的症状和体征是一个连续的演变过程，此过程通常从甲状腺功能亢进开始，逐步过渡到甲状腺危象和甲状腺功能减退，并最终发展成黏液性水肿昏迷。

甲状腺激素过量

Graves 病、甲状腺肿和甲状腺腺瘤的门诊患者约有 3% 会出现甲状腺功能亢进（甲亢）表现。使用胺碘酮治疗甚至会增加高达 9% 的发病率。甲状腺危象（严重的甲状腺功能亢进）第一次被临床医生所认识是发生在未经术前准备的甲状腺切除患者身上。目前在所有住院患者中，甲状腺功能亢进的发生率仍为 1% ~ 2%，死亡率高达 20% ~ 30%。当发生手术、创伤、分娩、重症疾病、甲状腺药物应用过量、碘剂治疗或造影剂应用等特殊情况时，可能会诱发甲状腺危象的发生。甲状腺危象的典型症状包括发热、心血管功能异常、精神状态改变。心动过速的频率超过了由于发热因素对心率的影响。发热时体温超过 106°F 是此类疾病的典型标准。甲状腺功能亢进所致的高排血量性心力衰竭会导致洪脉、双肺出现啰音、肝大、甲状腺杂音等临床表现。对于老年甲亢患者而言，常常会伴随心房颤动和充血性心力衰竭的表现，往往不表现出发热症状（甲状腺心脏危象）。甲亢危象还可以表现出从焦虑到昏迷等各种类型的精神状态改变。另外，Graves 病可以出现非特异性消化道症状。

临床可以通过症状和体征来辨识这种综合征。等待实验室结果回报的时间长，治疗应在临床怀疑的基础上开始。实验室检查通常会出现 T_3 和 T_4 增高、T_3 明显高于 T_4、TSH 无法测得。同时患者还会出现白细胞、血钙、血糖和肝功能的上升。此类患者的治疗包括减少甲状腺激素的产生和释放、阻断其对相应效应器官的作用、提供优质的护理服务，以及处理原发病（表 4）。

甲状腺激素不足

甲状腺功能减退多发生于 50 岁以上的患者，此年龄段约有 8% 的女性以及 2% 的男性会出现甲状腺功能减退。手术史、放射和自身免疫性疾病都是此病的常见原因。黏液性水肿昏迷是重症甲状腺功能减退的表现。黏液性水肿昏迷十分少见，但其死亡率却高达 60%。创伤导致的生理应激、手术、烧伤、感染心血管事件、低温，以及甲状腺相关药物使用不当均会促使黏液性水肿昏迷的发生。药物可以减少激素的产生和降低其功能（表 3）。甲状腺功能减退患者可出现基础代谢率下降、氧消耗下降、低体温、心动过缓、低血压、通气不足以及精神状态改变。精神状态改变包括从昏睡到昏迷的各种表现，并且精神状态改变的程度往往与深反射的减弱程度相关。由于心肌收缩力下降可导致患者心排血量下降，伴左心衰或右心衰。同时患者还会出现慢性便秘和肠梗阻等消化道症状。皮肤、指甲和头发的变化与甲状腺功能减退有关。黏液性水肿名词来源于粘多糖的皮肤浸润。有助于黏液性水肿昏迷诊断的实验室指标包括 TSH 上升，T_4 和血钠明显下降，低血糖、肌酸磷酸激酶上升，Pao_2 降低以及 $Paco_2$ 升高。甲状腺功能减退其有特征性的心电图改变（表 5）。

黏液性水肿昏迷的治疗包括 ICU 监护支持性治疗以及甲状腺激素的替代治疗。ICU 监护治疗管理

表 3　干扰甲状腺激素和抗利尿激素的药物

导致 SIADH 的药物
ADH 衍生物：血管加压素、催产素、去氨加压素
刺激抗利尿激素释放的药物：鸦片、阿片类药物、巴比妥类药物、尼古丁、噻嗪类、异丙肾上腺素、抗抑郁药、MAO 抑制剂、氟哌啶醇、利培酮、乙酰胆碱
增加肾敏感性的药物：非甾体抗炎药、对乙酰氨基酚
刺激抗利尿激素释放和增加肾敏感性的药物：氯磺丙脲、甲苯磺丁脲、环磷酰胺、苯丁酸氮芥
磷酸二酯酶抑制：茶碱
其他：胺碘酮、ACE 抑制剂、袢利尿剂、噻嗪类利尿剂、全身麻醉
影响甲状腺功能的药物
影响其转化能力的药物：糖皮质激素、β 受体阻断药、造影剂、胺碘酮、丙硫氧嘧啶
增加 TSH 的药物：甲腈咪胺、多巴胺拮抗剂、氟哌啶醇、碘化物、锂、造影剂、甲氧氯普胺
减少 TSH 的药物：肾上腺素能受体激动剂、多巴胺、类固醇、鸦片、苯妥英钠、酚妥拉明
增加结合能力的药物：雌激素、美沙酮、氟尿嘧啶（5-Fu）、海洛因、他莫西芬
减少结合能力的药物：类固醇、雄激素、肝素、水杨酸盐、治疗癫痫发作的药物、呋塞米

ACE，血管紧张素转化酶；ADH，抗利尿激素；MAO，单胺氧化酶；NSAID，非甾体抗炎药；TSH，促甲状腺激素

表 4　甲状腺危象的治疗

抑制激素合成： 口服丙硫氧嘧啶负荷剂量 1 000 mg，然后每 6 h 300 mg。
减少激素对靶器官的影响： 静脉注射普萘洛尔 1 ~ 10 mg，然后每 6 h 口服 20 ~ 120 mg。或静脉注射艾司洛尔 250 μg/kg，注射时间大于 1 min。然后 50 μg/kg · min 持续静脉给药
阻止激素释放：口服碘化钠 500 mg 或每 8 h 静脉注射一次。
阻止周围组织转化：普萘洛尔或每 8 h 静脉注射氢化可的松 50 ~ 100 mg
补充容量
处理疾病突发事件
支持治疗： ICU 监护 充血性心力衰竭的处理 应用冰毯或对乙酰氨基酚降温治疗

CHF，充血性心力衰竭；ICU，重症监护病房；IV，静脉输注

表 5　甲状腺功能减退的心电图表现

窦性心动过缓
QRS 波群压低
T 波低平或倒置
PR、QRS 和 QT 间期延长
心脏传导阻滞

包括心电图监测、心脏起搏器、动脉血管监测、外复温设备（包括毯子）的应用，以及含葡萄糖液体的输注、温度的监测和神经系统检查。第一天可静脉给予 300 ~ 500 ug 的 T_4，之后每天给予 50 ~ 100 μg 的维持剂量，直到过渡到口服药物治疗。肾上腺功能不全的患者应迅速进行 ACTH 水平检查，并每 8 h 经静脉给予一次 100 mg 的氢化可的松。

甲状腺病态综合征

甲状腺病态表现或非甲状腺的疾病在 ICU 患者中非常常见。目前尚不清楚这种综合征是否是重症疾病的一种适应性的病理生理过程。甲状腺功能异常导致的疾病按严重程度分为3种类型：①T_3下降；② T_3 和 T_4 下降；③ T_3、T_4 以及 TSH 下降（表 6）。患者若仅为 T_3 下降，通常只会有轻度或中度的临床症状。而仅 T_3 下降往往是甲状腺病态综合征最常见的类型。此类患者在周围组织中 T_4 向 T_3 的转换也会下降。此类型主要由药物引起（表 3）。此类疾病主要是由于药物影响血清中 T_4 转换或增加综合水平血清 T_4 水平在急性疾病早期会有所升高。而随着疾病的进展，T_4 又会逐步回到正常水平。此种类型的甲状腺病态综合征通常发生在老年患者以及存在精神疾病的患者身上。甲状腺病态综合征最严重的类型是 T_3、T_4，以及 TSH 均明显下降，而游离 T_4 可能下降、正常或升高。此种类型的患者除了存在 T_4 向 T_3 的转换问题，其结合蛋白也非常低。T_4 下降水平与患者预后相关。当 T_4 水平下降至 4 μg/dl 或以下时，其死亡率明显上升。并且当 T_4 水平下降至 2 ug/dl 时，其死亡率甚至高达 80%。

表 6　甲状腺功能异常

激素	黏液性水肿昏迷	甲状腺危象	甲状腺病态综合征		
			轻度	中度	重度
促甲状腺激素	↑	↓	—	—	↓
T_3	↓	↑	↓	↓	↓
T_4	↓	↑	—	↓	↓

TSH, 促甲状腺激素

此种综合征的诊断有赖于甲状腺功能测验。这些测验仅可作为疾病严重程度的判断依据，不可用于评价其是否可以治疗。目前甲状腺病态综合征的治疗方案尚不明确。临床上可予甲状腺替代治疗或不予特殊处理。动物实验证实了甲状腺替代治疗的效果，但相关人体试验并未得出相同的阳性结论，所以目前无治疗建议。

肾上腺功能异常

肾上腺是神经内分泌轴的重要组成部分。肾上腺可以产生儿茶酚胺类物质、糖皮质激素、盐皮质激素和性激素。临床问题通常表现为肾上腺激素产生过度或分泌不足。人体各类细胞功能的维持均需要皮质醇激素。重症患者的肾上腺皮质醇激素水平缺乏，会导致肾上腺功能异常发病率和死亡率的上升。儿茶酚胺类物质是由肾上腺髓质产生，它的合成需要皮质醇。通常情况下重症患者的性激素不会恢复到正常水平。并且机体有一些对盐皮质激素活性减退的补偿机制。下面将分别讨论嗜铬细胞瘤和肾上腺功能不全。

嗜铬细胞瘤

嗜铬细胞瘤产生儿茶酚胺类物质，这类肿瘤有以下特点：① 10% 的嗜铬细胞瘤为恶性；② 10% 的嗜铬细胞瘤为肾上腺外的；③ 10% 的嗜铬细胞瘤患者是通过放射性检查才偶然发现；④ 10% 的患者为多发性嗜铬细胞瘤。低于 0.2% 的高血压患者在诊断时会发现嗜铬细胞瘤。嗜铬细胞瘤通常不会在 ICU 病房诊断，但伴有高血压危象或处于围术期或需 ICU 处理的患者应警惕此类疾病的可能。患者通常具有典型的头痛、多汗、心动过速或心悸。至少 50% 的嗜铬细胞瘤患者会出现每周周期性发作的高血压，其原因是某些诱因导致的儿茶酚胺类物质大量迅速释放。其他症状还包括视物模糊、直立性低血压、体重下降、多饮和烦渴等。

临床怀疑嗜铬细胞瘤患者可进行血、尿的儿茶酚胺类物质及其代谢产物的测定。约有 95% 的嗜铬细胞瘤患者可以通过这些实验室检查来确诊。对于采用以上相关实验室检查仍无法确诊的患者，临床可以应用可乐定抑制试验。试验要求在停止降压药使用 12 h 后，口服可乐定 0.3 mg，并观察其效果。试验同时要求受试者不能使用 β 受体阻断药、利尿剂，以及三环类抗抑郁药。α 受体阻断药对于试验结果无明显影响。如果患者没有嗜铬细胞瘤，在应用可乐定后，其血浆儿茶酚胺浓度应下降 500 pg/ml。

嗜铬细胞瘤可以通过 CT 或 MRI 等影像学检查来发现其具体定位。应用造影剂的 CT 检查可能会使高血压症状恶化。如果 CT 或 MRI 仍无法定位肿瘤部位时，可以应用间碘苯甲胍扫描、奥曲肽试验、全身 MRI 扫描等方法来进一步明确诊断。

急性高血压危象须及时给予硝普钠或酚妥拉明。酚妥拉明首剂给予静脉团块注射 2.5 ~ 5 mg，之后每 5 min 重复给药，直至血压控制为止。硝普钠可以以 0.5 ~ 10 μg/kg · min 持续泵入。

外科手术前应使用 α 受体阻断药，起始剂量为每日口服 10 mg，并逐步加量至血压和症状控制。在应用 α 受体阻断药后，可再给予 β 受体阻断药来控制心动过速。手术通常在用药 10 ~ 14 天后进行。患者术后仍然要给予生命体征的严格监测，并给予适度的体液复苏。α 受体阻断药可持续给予。

肾上腺功能不全

对于 ICU 患者的肾上腺功能不全的诊断和治疗一直存在争议。在普通人群中肾上腺功能不全的发生率不足 0.01%。而对于重症患者而言，肾上腺功能不全的发生率高达 28%，死亡率高达 25%。若能早期及时发现，其死亡率可以下降至 6% ~ 11%。重症患者为应对急性炎症反应和保持血管舒缩功能稳定也需要一定数量的皮质醇。皮质醇具有促进新陈代谢、抗炎和维持血管活性的作用。肾上腺功能不全最常见的原因是由于使用类固醇药物导致肾上腺功能受到抑制。对于使用类固醇药物的患者，这种抑制作用可能会延续 1 年以上。感染、出血、系统性炎症等情况均可导致 ICU 患者出现肾上腺的破坏。但更常见的原因并非肾上腺解剖学结构上的破坏，而是重症疾病所导致的皮质醇浓度降低。第二常见的导致肾上腺功能不全的原因是脓毒症。

重症患者肾上腺功能不全的症状和体征并不明显。这类重症患者虽然给予体液复苏和应用血管活性药物，但血流动力学仍无法保持平稳。肾上腺功能不全患者应及时评估皮质醇水平和治疗效果。最常见的 ICU 患者肾上腺功能不全的异常表现见表 7。先前有肾上腺功能不全的患者可出现劳累、体重下降、恶心、腹痛、关节痛、晕厥、皮肤色素沉着、白癜风、厌食，以及性欲减退等临床表现。

重症患者肾上腺功能不全的诊断和治疗在不断更新。有人可能说，这使得我们对其的理解更加困惑。临床上怀疑有肾上腺功能不全的患者可进行随机的总体皮质醇水平检查。如果总体皮质醇少于 10 μg/dl，则提示存在肾上腺功能不全。临床可以通过静脉注射 250 μg 合成促肾上腺皮质激素（adrenocorticotropic hormone，ACTH）的方式进行相关激发试验。在注射 ACTH 的即刻、30 min 和 60 min 时分别观察皮质醇水平。如果皮质醇水平改变 9 μg/dl 以上，肾上腺皮质功能不全的诊断几乎不成立。如果皮质醇水平改变小于 9 μg/dl，则诊断肾上腺功能不全的可能性很大，此时需要治疗。

表 7 ICU 内肾上腺功能不全患者的异常表现

血管加压药和体液复苏无效的低血压
腹痛
恶心、呕吐
近期使用过类固醇药物
心动过速
发热
低血糖
低钠血症
高钾血症
嗜酸性粒细胞增多症

临床上无需肾上腺不全的相关实验室检查结果，便可开始相应的治疗。对于充足的体液复苏后仍需要血管加压药支持的感染性休克患者、对血管加压药无反应的感染性休克患者以及治疗进行 48 h 后的 ARDS 患者而言，可以在没有实验室诊断的情况下酌情开始糖皮质激素治疗。如果之前已确诊或可通过实验室检查结果证实的肾上腺功能不全患者，也应及时采取相应的治疗措施。可每日给予 200 ~ 300 mg 氢化可的松，最常见的给药方案为每 6 h 给予 50 mg 或每 8 h 给予 100 mg，也可见持续给药。激素治疗时间一般须维持 1 周左右，通常无须给予氟氢可的松。若是 ARDS 患者，治疗时间往往须延长到 2 周左右。如果患者在治疗完成后临床情况变差，可考虑再次给予初始剂量的激素治疗。

2008 年 1 月新英格兰医学杂志发表的关于感染性休克患者皮质类固醇治疗的研究，是一个多中心、随机、双盲、对照研究。试验组每 6 h 静脉给予 50 mg 氢化可的松，并以此方案持续治疗 5 天。之后观察对促肾上腺皮质激素无反应的患者 6 天内的死亡转归情况。研究发现，氢化可的松并没有提高感染性休克患者的生存率，但确实有助于休克的恢复。

高血糖的问题

大多数重症患者均会发生高血糖。已确诊和尚未确诊的糖尿病会进一步促进高血糖的出现。然而，交感神经的活性的增加以及相关细胞因子的级联激活是重症患者出现高血糖的主要原因。有些药物制剂也会促使高血糖的发生，包括全肠外营养、β受体阻断药、环孢素、儿茶酚胺类物质和糖皮质激素。如低钾血症等电解质紊乱会导致胰岛素释放减少，从而导致高血糖发生。压力同样可以诱导交感神经兴奋，从而增加肝糖原分解、肝糖原异生和外周胰岛素抵抗，最终导致血糖水平增高。炎症反应过程会促进细胞因子的产生，这会导致胰岛素抵抗，并激活下丘脑 - 垂体 - 肾上腺轴。所有这些因素共同作用于重症患者，从而引起糖的产生和摄取失衡，最终导致高血糖的发生。

除了以上高血糖的发生机制外，心血管系统、脑血管系统、神经肌肉系统和免疫系统均会出现器官系统功能障碍。关于高血糖对于心血管系统的影响已被广泛研究。高血糖会增加心梗患者的住院死亡率。胰岛素缺陷或抵抗与机体游离脂肪酸的增加有关。游离脂肪酸对心肌细胞具有毒性，会导致心律失常。高血糖也会导致渗透性利尿，导致有效循环容量下降，从而增加心脏收缩力和氧消耗。

对比血糖正常患者而言，伴有缺血性脑卒中和脑损伤的高血糖患者预后更差。伴随着血糖水平的升高，缺血性脑卒中的非糖尿病患者的入院死亡率也会相应的增加。持续性高血糖是梗死区增大的独立预测因素，同时也与缺血性脑卒中的差的功能性预后具有一定的相关性。脑损伤患者的 GCS 评分和死亡率也与患者的血糖水平具有相关性。对于已经发展为重症相关神经病变的患者，临床上也可以快速的判断和处理。

由于脑组织缺血导致血糖进行无氧代谢，从而出现酸中毒的表现。乳酸酸中毒会促使自由基的产生和蓄积，导致线粒体活性下降。这种影响在神经元梗死灶的边缘最为显著。很多动物实验表明伴有高血糖的实验动物脑梗死的面积会增加。血脑屏障的破坏以及出血性脑梗死的发生均提示脑功能的进一步恶化。

重症患者多发性神经病与血糖水平升高也具有相关性。Van den Berghe 等研究发现严格控制血糖的多发性神经病的重症患者发生重大疾病神经病变的可能性较低。那些发展为重大疾病神经病变的患者也能快速恢复。并且血糖升高的水平与多发性神经病呈直线正相关。关于重症多发性神经病及其与高血糖的作用机制目前尚不明确。

高血糖会增加患者术后创伤感染、肺炎、泌尿系统感染和菌血症的发生率。高血糖也会通过白细胞的活性影响机体的免疫系统。多形核细胞会影响趋化作用、吞噬作用和细胞氧化途径。巨噬细胞损害细胞吞噬功能，降低补体黏附能力。胶原蛋白沉积受损，粒细胞黏附不规则，杀菌能力下降。

越来越多的临床试验证明，积极控制重症患者的血糖水平可以改善其预后。2 项大型临床试验表明，将心胸外科手术患者的血糖控制在 200 mg/dl 以下可明显降低深部伤口的感染。心肌梗死后给予积极的血糖控制也有助于提高患者的生存率。目前尚缺乏积极的血糖控制是否会改善神经病学预后的证据。Van den Berghe 等研究表明，相比传统的血糖控制方案（血糖维持在 180 ~ 200 mg/dl）而言，严格的血糖控制方案（血糖维持在 80 ~ 100mg/dl）有助于改善外科 ICU 患者的发病率和死亡率（图 2）。另一

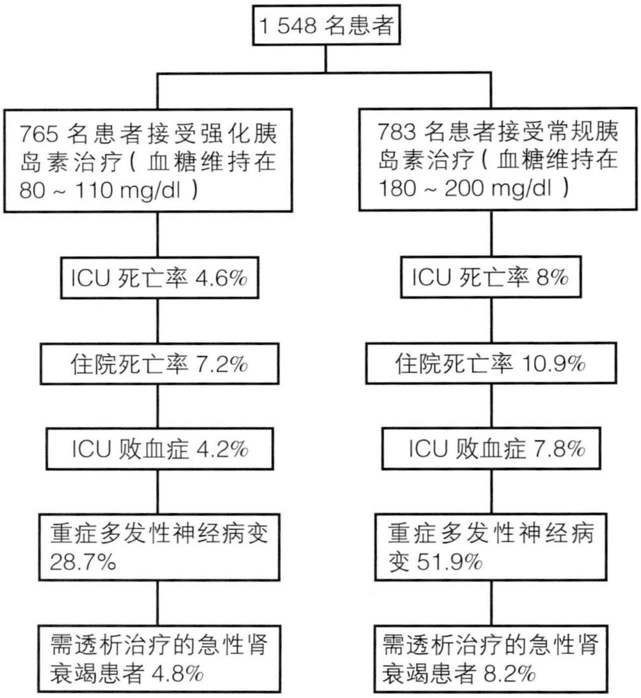

图 2　强化血糖控制的结果。ICU，重症监护病房（*Data from Van Den Berghe G, Wouters P, Weekers F, et al: Intensive insulin therapy in critically ill patients.* N Engl J Med *345:1359 - 1367, 2001.*）

项 NICE-SUGAR 研究也进一步表明目标血糖应控制在 180 mg/dl 以下。相比之下，严格的血糖控制可以降低 ICU 内患者死亡率以及 90 天内的患者死亡率，同时可以减少低血糖的发生。但严格的血糖控制并不会改善患者 ICU 和普通病房的住院时间、器官功能衰竭的发生率、机械通气时间和肾替代治疗时间。

高血糖应及时给予静脉注射胰岛素来积极控制，并使血糖维持在 180 mg/dl 以下（表 8）。临床上可应用胰岛素持续泵入来迅速控制血糖。肾衰竭、肝功能衰竭 / 切除、肾移植患者更容易出现高血糖。

其他内分泌激素：降钙素原

降钙素原是血清降钙素的激素原。人体甲状腺可以产生降钙素原，另外肺和肠道的神经内分泌细胞也会生成降钙素原。虽然降钙素会影响钙的平衡，但降钙素原已作为判断细菌感染的标志之一。相比实验室检查而言，近期的文献越来越将降钙素原与其他临床和实验室感染的指标作为评估抗生素应用时间的指南。

临床上现已开始逐步推荐降钙素原的使用。第一，降钙素原连续测量可用于确定下降水平来辅助判断抗生素治疗的停止时间。第二，降钙素原可用于指导经验性抗感染治疗。降钙素原可帮助判断是否存在急性感染，并指导抗感染治疗时长。第三，降钙素原的水平与重症脓毒症患者的死亡率具有相关性。第四，降钙素原有助于判断抗感染治疗是否成功。当感染得到控制后（手术治疗或化学治疗），降钙素原的水平会相应下降。

降钙素原对感染的监测有一些使用限制。当出现肝硬化、肠缺血、心源性休克、失血性休克、严重烧伤和严重创伤时，降钙素原的水平也会上升。其原因可能是细菌移位，但此原因分析尚未得到进一步证实。在病毒感染时，降钙素原的水平不会上升。

非感染患者的降钙素原浓度维持在 0.033 ~ 0.003 ng/ml。若判断患者为非感染状态，其降钙素原浓度至少应低于 0.1 ng/ml。当降钙素原浓度在 0.25 ~ 0.5 ng/ml 时，往往提示细菌感染，且需要及时治疗。当降钙素原浓度小于 0.25 ng/ml 时提示患者可能仅出现局部感染，且感染并不严重。降钙素原水平通常在感染 2 h 后上升，并在 24 h 达峰。而 C 反应蛋白上升较慢，且 48 h 才能达峰。

2010 年出版的法国的一项多中心随机对照研究，主要探讨应用降钙素原缩短抗生素的使用时间。此研究名为 PRORATA（降钙素原改善急性患者的抗生素治疗），试验组应用降钙素原判断是否应开始进行抗生素治疗，以及何时应停止抗生素使用。当降钙素原超过 0.5 μg/L 时，应开始进行抗生素治疗。当降钙素原水平下降到峰值 80% 以下或浓度小于 0.5 μg/L 时停止抗生素应用。对比对照组而言，试验组的抗生素治疗时间显著缩短，平均缩短约 2.7 天。

2010 年在重症医学杂志刊登了一篇 meta 分析，该研究涵盖 7 项 ICU 中应用降钙素原指导抗生素治疗的随机对照观察试验，共涉及患者 1 010 人。研究发现 ICU 中使用降钙素原指导抗感染治疗能够在不影响临床预后的情况下减少抗生素的使用。机体内分泌系统通过降钙素原的指标有助于临床对危重患者的诊治。

总结

尽管神经内分泌轴对于保持机体内环境的稳态有着至关重要的作用，危重疾病通常会有患者的激素水平异常。诊断此类异常需要临床早期的积极治疗，可有助于改善此类疾病的发生率和死亡率。

表 8　美国密歇根州，底特律市，Henry Ford 医院，外科 ICU 病房强化血糖控制方案

开始胰岛素治疗		
血糖	181 ~ 219 mg/dl	>220 mg/dl
开始胰岛素治疗	静脉推注 2 U 胰岛素，然后 2 U/h 持续输注。如果是肾衰竭（肌酐＞2 mg/dl）、肝功能衰竭、肝移植、肾移植患者，胰岛素可从 1 U/h 开始输注。	静脉推注 4 U 胰岛素，然后 4 U/h 持续输注。如果是肾衰竭（肌酐＞2 mg/dl）、肝功能衰竭、肝移植、肾移植患者胰岛素可从 1 U/h 开始输注。
维持胰岛素治疗		
血糖水平	胰岛素输注速度 1 ~ 3 U/h	胰岛素输注速度＞3 U/h
＜41 mg/dl	核实血糖检查结果，停止胰岛素输注，给予 1 安瓿的 50% 葡萄糖，并通知医生。每小时监测血糖，直到血糖高于 80 mg/dl 后，改为每 2 h 监测一次血糖。当血糖达到 139 mg/dl，重新给予 0.5 U/h 的胰岛素输注。当血糖高于 80 mg/dl 时通知医生。	核实血糖检查结果，停止胰岛素输注，给予 1 安瓿的 50% 葡萄糖，并通知医生。每小时监测血糖，直到血糖高于 80 mg/dl 后，改为每 2 h 监测一次血糖。当血糖达到 139 mg/dl，重新给予 0.5 U/h 的胰岛素输注。当血糖高于 80 mg/dl 时通知医生。
41 ~ 60 mg/dl	停止胰岛素输注，给予 1/2 安瓿的 50% 葡萄糖，并通知医生。每小时监测血糖，直到血糖高于 80 mg/dl 后改为每 2 h 监测一次血糖。当血糖达到 139 mg/dl，重新给予 0.5 U/h 的胰岛素输注。当血糖高于 80 mg/dl 时通知医生。	停止胰岛素输注，给予 1/2 安瓿的 50% 葡萄糖，并通知医生。每小时监测血糖，直到血糖高于 80 mg/dl 后改为每 2 h 监测一次血糖。当血糖达到 139 mg/dl，重新给予 0.5U/h 的胰岛素输注。当血糖高于 80 mg/dl 时通知医生。
	胰岛素输注速度 1 ~ 3 U/h	胰岛素输注速度＞3 U/h
61 ~ 139 mg/dl	停止胰岛素输注，每小时监测血糖，使血糖维持在 61 ~ 80 mg/dl；或每 2 h 监测一次血糖，使血糖维持在 81 ~ 139 mg/dl。当血糖超过 139 mg/dl 时，重新给予 1 U/h 胰岛素输注。	停止胰岛素输注，每小时监测血糖，使血糖维持在 61 ~ 80 mg/dl；或每 2 小时监测一次血糖，使血糖维持在 81 ~ 139 mg/dl。当血糖超过 139 mg/dl 时，重新启动胰岛素输注，其输注速度减少至既往输注速度的 50%。
当血糖低于 140 mg/dl（最好大于 60 mg/dl）若要停止胰岛素滴注，须每小时监测血糖变化，直到血糖大于 80 mg/dl 后可，每 2 h 监测一次血糖。若连续 3 次每 2 h 检测血糖均低于 140 mg/dl，则须重启最初的血糖控制方案。对于血糖大于 180 mg/dl 的患者，应开始胰岛素治疗并每 4 h 检测一次血糖。		
	胰岛素输注速度 1 ~ 3 U/h	胰岛素输注速度＞3 U/h
140 ~ 180 mg/dl	无须改变治疗方案，除非对比之前的血糖水平，下降超过 40 mg/dl，可以减少 1 U/h 的胰岛素输注（如果现在剂量为 1 U/h，则不改变）。	无须改变治疗方案，除非对比之前的血糖水平，下降超过 40 mg/dl，可酌情减少胰岛素用量。 先前输注速度　降低幅度 4 ~ 7 U/h　1 U/h 8 ~ 12 U/h　2 U/h 13 ~ 17 U/h　3 U/h 18 ~ 22 U/h　4 U/h >22 U/h　5 U/h
血糖	胰岛素剂量：其他情况	胰岛素剂量：肾衰竭（肌酐＞2）、肝功能衰竭、肾移植、肝移植或血糖＜61 mg/dl
181 ~ 216 mg/dl	给予 2 U 胰岛素静脉注射，提升胰岛素输注速度 1 U/h。如果对比之前的血糖水平，已下降超过 30 mg/dl，可维持胰岛素输注速度不变。	给予 2 U 胰岛素静脉注射，提升胰岛素输注速度 0.5 U/h。如果对比之前的血糖水平，已下降超过 30 mg/dl，可维持胰岛素输注速度不变。
217 ~ 25 mg/dl	给予 4 U 胰岛素静脉注射，提升胰岛素输注速度 1 U/h。如果对比之前的血糖水平，已下降超过 30 mg/dl，可维持胰岛素输注速度不变。	给予 2 U 胰岛素静脉注射，提升胰岛素输注速度 0.5 U/h。如果对比之前的血糖水平，已下降超过 30 mg/dl，可维持胰岛素输注速度不变。
253 ~ 400 mg/dl	给予 6 U 胰岛素静脉注射，提升胰岛素输注速度 2 U/h。如果对比之前的血糖水平，已下降超过 50 mg/dl，可维持胰岛素输注速度不变。	给予 6 U 胰岛素静脉注射，提升胰岛素输注速度 1 U/h。如果对比之前的血糖水平，已下降超过 50 mg/dl，可维持胰岛素输注速度不变。
＞400 mg/dl	核实血糖检查结果，若血糖水平已超出常规调控范围，应及时请内分泌专科会诊。	核实血糖检查结果，若血糖水平已超出常规调控范围，应及时请内分泌专科会诊。

D/C，停止；IVP，静脉推注

输血：创伤中的血液以及血液制品管理

Lena M. Napolitano　著
朱凤雪　李　纾　译

在美国，大约15%的输血会用于持续性创伤患者的护理上。输血对于失血性休克对于晶体液复苏没有反应的患者来说是救命的。另外，输血伴随着迅速止血也是至关重要。失血性休克患者表现出急性创伤性凝血功能障碍（acute coagulopathy of trauma，ACOT），早期输血以及接近全血（止血复苏，损伤控制复苏时的）比例的血液制品（血浆、血小板、冷凝蛋白质、纤维蛋白原）有纠正ACOT的作用，与一些前瞻性以及回顾性群组研究的积极结果相一致。目前正在进行随机试验以证实这些非对照临床试验的初步结果。

在很多研究中，创伤后输血也被认为是MOF、SIRS、创伤后感染，以及死亡率增加的独立危险因素。输血的累积风险与输入的浓缩红细胞单位数、输注血液的存放时间以及可能供体的白细胞数呈正相关。对血流动力学稳定的严重疾病的患者的红细胞注输无效也被记录。因此，一旦在急性创伤中出血控制被使用，治疗创伤患者无症状性贫血时就应尽量减少输血。

创伤中可能调节副反应与输血相关的一些潜在机制已经被证明，包括全身炎症反应增加、免疫调节、红细胞变性造成的微循环障碍、通过游离血红蛋白增加一氧化氮结合、血管收缩，以及其他一些机制。这些数据得出了在可能的条件下受伤患者应尽量减少输血的结论。

发生率：哪些创伤患者需要输血?

大多数可能避免的早期创伤因为出血（包括不可止住的躯体出血）而死亡。失血性休克的创伤患者在等渗晶体液复苏没有效果、有持续性明显出血并且表现出慢性休克的生理体征（低血压、心动过速、少尿、乳酸性酸中毒，异常碱缺失）的情况下绝对有理由进行PRBCs输血——表明氧消耗依赖于血红蛋白浓度（重要氧气输送来源）。对于这些患者来说尝试快速输注PRBCs和血液制品，并结合快速止血措施才能挽救生命。

表现出代谢性酸中毒以及碱缺失的失血性休克患者已经被证明需要血液以及血浆的输注（表1）。一个单机构的研究表明8%（479/5 645）的急性创伤患者接受了PRBCs输血，使用了5 219单位。大多数患者（62%）的输血是在治疗的前24 h进行的。只有3%的患者（n=147）接受了10单位以上的PRBCs输血，并且为了应对已经发生的或潜在的稀释性凝血功能障碍，这些患者也接受了血浆以及血小板的输注。需要输血的创伤患者比例高，为27%～39%。

大量输血

大量输血被定义为在24 h内完全替换患者的血液容量或24 h内输入10单位以上的PRBCs。更新的定义包括大于150 ml/min的持续性失血，或3 h之内替换50%的循环血液容量。这些新的定义对早期发现大量出血，并为有效预防失血性休克，以及对其他大量出血和输血并发症进行有效干预是极其有益的。

治疗失血性休克的大量输血（massive transfusion，MT）须遵照表2列出的基本要求的一个协调而详细的方法。缺少预定义的MT的参照流程，获取适当的血液制品（以及充足的血液制品容

表1　创伤患者的输血要求和入院碱缺失

入院碱剩余	说明	在第一个24 h内的PRBCs单位	总的PRBCs单位	总的FFP单位
≥-2	正常	0～1	1～2	0～1
-3～-5	轻度碱缺失	1～2	2～3	0～1
-6～-9	中度碱缺失	3～4	5～6	1～2
≤-10	重度碱缺失	8～9	9～10	3～4

Davis JW, Parks SN, Kaups KL, et al: Admission base deficit predicts transfusion requirements and risk of complications. J Trauma 41:769–774, 1996

FFP, 新鲜冰冻血浆；PRBCs, 浓缩红细胞

表 2　失血性休克大量输血的处理

提供充足的通风和氧气
加快出血源的控制
恢复循环血量 减少或停止晶体液复苏 低血压复苏，收缩压为 80～100 mmHg
开始血液成分疗法：RBC、FFP、Plt、Cryo 启动大规模输血程序 预测和治疗凝血功能障碍、血小板减少
维持或恢复正常体温
评估治疗反应 检测凝血功能障碍、血小板减少和 DIC 考虑 TEG 或 ROTEM
了解并执行处理大规模输血物流需求的具体程序

Cryo，冷凝蛋白质；DIC，弥散性血管内凝血；FFP，新鲜冰冻血浆；Plts，血小板；RBCs，红细胞；ROTEM，旋转血栓弹性检测；TEG，血栓弹力图

量）可能会被显著地延误。没有这些血液制品的有效替代品，凝血情况可能会更糟，失血也会继续。事实上，在创伤患者中处理出血时“大量输血准则”的有效贯彻对于患者预后以及减少血液制品用量来说都是有益的。研究表明，使用这样一个大量输血参照流程可以增加失血患者的生存率（16%～45%）。表 3 列出了应对急性大量失血的指南。为应对战伤救护中的损伤控制复苏的《联合战区创伤系统临床实践指南》是一个证据确凿的、提供大量输血参照流程模板的、基于证据的极好的指南资源（表 4）。我们大学的密歇根创伤大量输血参照流程为市民大量输血提供了模板（图 1）。

为了检测 2004–2009 年的康复策略，一项大的多中心的队列研究评估了钝器损伤导致的失血性休克的成年人的预后，结果表明这些年来需要大量输血的患者越来越少。在研究周期内，对于接受大量输血的患者（n=526）来说，最初的碱缺失以及入院时的 INR 并没有变化，但是 ISS 显著上升。在大量输血患者中，6 h、12 h 以及 24 h 的 FFP ：PRBC 和 Plt ：PRBCs（血小板 PRBCs）的输注比例没有显著性变化。在近期，亚大量输血患者（n=344）6 h 后 FFP ：PRBCs 的比例显著上升，并且 6 h、12 h 以及 24 h Plt ：PRBCs 的比例显著上升。6 h、24 h 输注 FFP 以及 Plt 总百分数在近期也显著上升（FFP：54%vs.70%，P=0.004；Plt：46%vs.61%，P=0.048）。这个研究表明在需要大量输血的严重受伤的患者队列中，FFP ：PRBCs 以及 Plt ：PRBCs 的比例不会随着时间变化，然而大量输血的比例显著下降。在近期（2007 年 12 月以后），亚大量输血群组的输血比例显著增加，伴随着 6 h、24 h 输注 FFP 以及血小板比例的显著上升，那些低于 PRBCs 输注阈值的患者被定义为 MT。这些数据表明过早地、过强烈地使用高比例血液制品输入可能会降低大量输血的要求并且可能改变全血需求至低于现今定义的大量输血要求的状态。这些结论需要进一步的证据证实。

需要大量输血的创伤患者的识别

开始止血以及损伤控制复苏被认为和改善大量输血患者的预后相关。早期识别创伤后需要大量输血的先兆可以避免创伤患者最后不得不选择大量输血的治疗方法。一项近期研究使用多个机构对于主要创伤后输血的前瞻性观察性研究验证了诱发因素。这个研究前瞻性地检测了独立的需要输血诱发因素研究以及血液消耗评价给出的独立诱发因素对于迅速识别需要大量输血患者的预测能力，以上两种标准都被证明在平民中使用简单有效，且可以预测 MT 的使用。需要输血诱发因素研究给出的诱发因素是以前军事上使用的诱发因素改良而来，包括 SBP<90 mmHg、血红蛋白水平低于 11g/dl、体温低于 35.5 ℃、INR>1.5、BD≥6。ABC 包括 SBP<90 mmHg、HR≥120 次 / 分（bpm）、FAST 的阳性结果，以及损伤渗透机制。CITT 和 ABC 研究包括了 8 项独立的诱发因素。在 297 名接受大量输血的患者中，除了损伤渗透机制以及心率为独立的需要大量输血的诱发因素以外，INR 是最有预测价值的（调整 OR 为 2.5；95% CI 为 1.7～3.7，表 5）。

血液成分输注

红细胞

对于严重出血性休克患者，由于即时可用性可以输注未交叉配型的 O 型血。ATLS 鼓励在使用 2 L 晶体溶液无法实现血流动力学稳定性后，立即转换使用红细胞制品。因为紧急输注是在确认患者血型之前常规应用的，通常使用非交叉配型 RBC。Rh 阳性血通常在男性创伤患者中使用，其发生输注相关综合征的概率最低，Rh 阴性患者中有低的血清转

表 3　急性失血过多：指南模板

目标	过程	评价
止血	及时停止出血 手术干预 介入性放射学 血管造影栓塞术	所有尝试在早期出血停止时应启动，可能包括多种模式
恢复循环血量 复苏至一定程度恢复或保持重要器官灌注，直到采取了明确措施来控制出血，再尝试恢复至正常血压	插入大口径周围静脉管 给予适当体积的热晶体液、胶体、血液 目的是维持适当平均动脉压和尿量（0.5 ml/kg · h）	使用 14 号或更大的管 血液丢失经常被低估 参考 ATLS 指南 保持患者温暖
需要实验室测试	PT、PTT、INR、CBC、血库样品血型和交叉配型、DIC 监测 确定正确的样品血型 每隔 4 h，每次 1/3 的血液替换后进行重复检测 成分输注后进行重复试验	取入院时初始样本 血型误认是最常见的输血风险 如果有凝血功能障碍 / 出血的临床证据，在凝血检测起效之前给予 FFP 和血小板
需要红细胞	出血严重程度决定了选择 迫切需要：RhD 阴性 O 型血 15 ~ 60 min 内需要：当明确血型后，将提供未交叉匹配的特异的 ABO 型血 60 min 或更久需要：充分交叉配型血液 如果时间允许，使用更温暖的血液和快速的输血装置 如果有效且适当的话，使用的血液进行回收（即污染最小化）	如果患者是男性或绝经后女性，则 Rh D 阳性血液的紧急使用是可接受的 实验室将在问题完成后进行交叉配型 补充一个血容量（8 ~ 10 单位 PRBCs）之后不需要进一步交叉配型 较温暖的血液表明如果大量迅速输血可以防止低体温 伤口严重污染是保治疗的禁忌征
需要血小板 用于新生儿 / 儿童的剂量为按体重 10 ml/kg 一个成年人的治疗剂量	可能延迟运输时间 替换 2 个血容量之后预期血小板计数 <50 × 10^9/L 在血小板输注后在 10 min 和 1 h 重复进行血小板计数评估疗效	目标血小板计数：>100 × 10^9/L（多发伤 / 中枢神经系统创伤或血小板功能异常）；其他情况 50 × 10^9/L 可能在实验室结果可用之前使用血小板（血小板输注前取样）
需要 FFP 用于成人的剂量为按体重 15 ml/kg 或 4 单位（1 L）	1.5 个血容量丢失后预测凝血因子缺陷 针对 PT 和 PTT<1.5 进行控制 允许解冻 30 min（如果医院没有已解冻的 FFP）	PT 和 PTT>1.5 × 与手术出血增加相关的控制 在实验室结果可用之前可能须使用 FFP（FFP 输注之前取样）
需要冷凝蛋白质	代替纤维蛋白原和凝血因子Ⅷ 针对纤维蛋白原 >1 g/L 允许运输和 30 min 解冻时间	纤维蛋白原 <0.8 g/L 与微血管出血密切相关 当出血后输注血浆 PRBCs 时，纤维蛋白原缺乏症早期进一步发展
怀疑 DIC	如果可能的话治疗潜在诱因	休克、低体温和酸中毒导致 DIC 的风险 DIC 的死亡率很高

Modified from Stainsby D, Maclennan S, Hamilton PJ: Management of massive blood loss: a template guideline. Br J Anaesth 85:487–491, 2000 ; and McClelland DBL: Clinical use of blood products. In McClelland DBL, editor: The handbook of transfusion medicine, 3rd ed, London, 2001, The Stationery Office, p 79.

CBC，全血细胞计数；CNS，中枢神经系统；DIC，弥散性血管内凝血；FFP，新鲜冰冻血浆；INR，国际标准化比率；PRBCs，浓缩红细胞；PT，凝血酶原时间；PTT，部分促凝血酶原时间

换率。

Rh 阴性血应该尽可能在女性育龄期使用。尽快完成至应用特定血型的转换（ABO，Rh 匹配，特定类型的红细胞大约需要 10 min），继续使用以上血型血液制品直到完全交叉配型的血液可以使用（完全交叉配型大约需要 30 ~ 40 min）。一旦创伤患者输注

表 4　联合战区创伤系统损伤控制复苏临床实践指南

USCENTCOM Ⅲ级设备的大量输血过程的范例
使用大量输血的考虑：在 ED、OR 和 ICU 使用的一套灵活的程序，可以由定点的医疗服务提供者启动或停止。当在特定的地点时，取决于患者口述的需求。它由组成如下，组成物不尽相同，但都倾向 PRBCs、FFP、血小板和冷凝蛋白质 1∶1∶1∶1 的比例。注：1 单位单采血小板大约相当于 6 单位随机供体血小板，因此每 6 单位 PRBCs 应给予 1 单位单采血小板，给予比例约 1∶1∶1 的复苏。
如果患者接受 4 单位 PRBCs / 4 单位 FFP 紧急释放血液制品，则启动 MT 程序。
包裹一：4 单位 PRBC，4 单位 FFP，1 单位单采血小板，1 包 10 单位冷凝蛋白质。务必考虑早期使用 TXA：在输注血液和血液制品的同时独立静脉输注 1 g 溶解于 100 ml 0.9% 生理盐水中的氨甲环酸 10 min 以上。（据报道，更快速的注射会引起低血压）。应避免使用人造血浆溶液作为流体载体。8 h 后再次静脉输注 0.9%生理盐水作为 1g 的氨甲环酸的载体。
包裹二：4 单位 PRBCs 和 4 单位 FFP
包裹三：4 单位 PRBCs、4 单位 FFP、1 单位单采血小板，1 包 10 单位的冷凝蛋白质和 +/-F Ⅶ a（从药房获得）
包裹四：4 单位 PRBCs 和 4 单位 FFP
包裹五：4 单位 PRBCs、4 单位 FFP、1 单位单采血小板和 1 包 10 单位的冷凝蛋白质
应当在医疗服务提供者护理患者时重新评估复苏、止血的进展，以及是否须继续大量输血。

From Joint Theater Trauma System Clinical Practice Guidelines, Approved 2/1/13. Available at http://www.usaisr.amedd.army.mil/assets/cpgs/Damage%20Control%20Resuscitation%20-%201%20Feb%202013. pdf. Accessed December 2014.

FFP，新鲜冰冻血浆；IV，静脉注射；NS，生理盐水；PRBC，浓缩红细胞

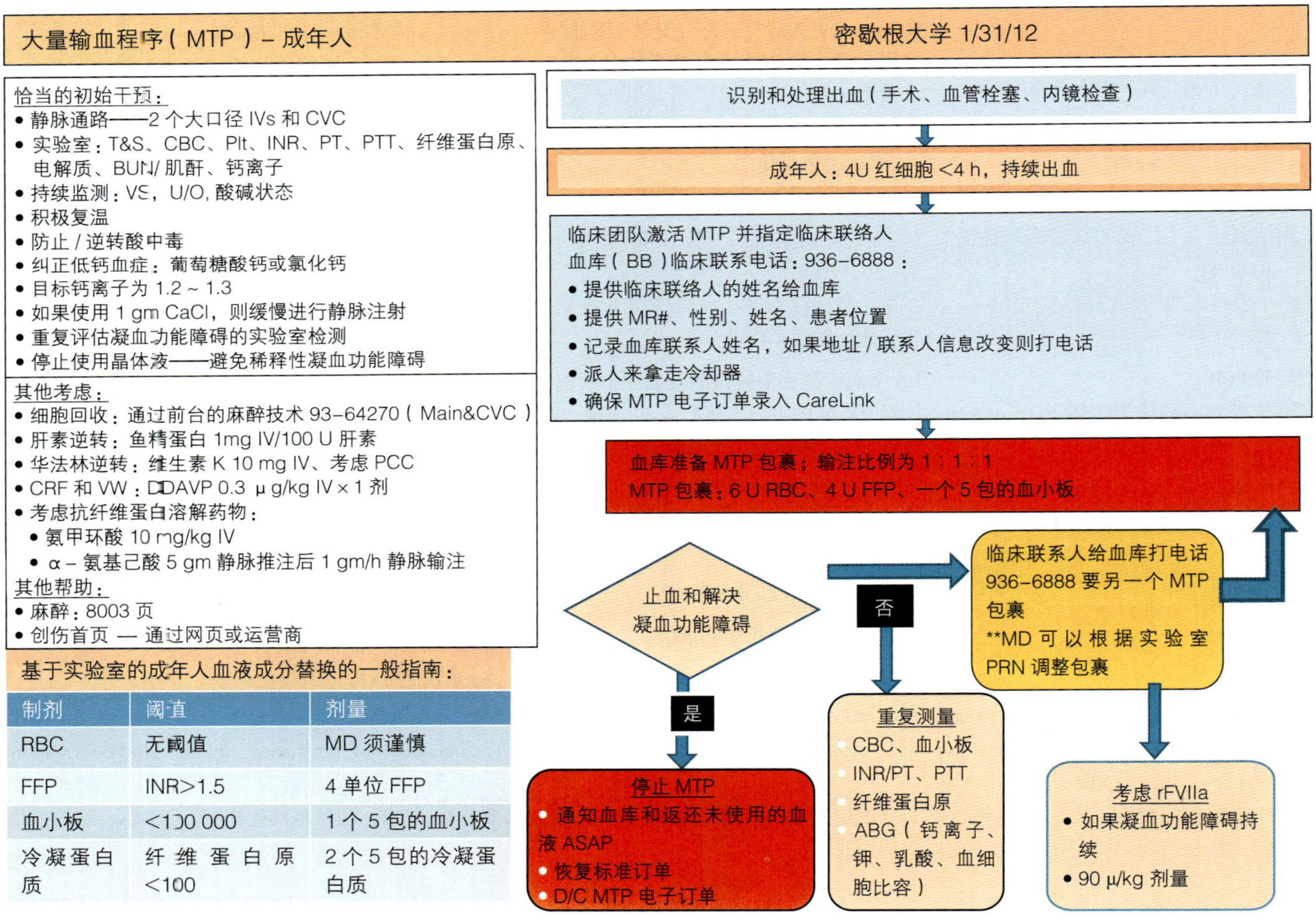

图 1　大量输血流程。ABG，动脉血气；ASAP，尽可能快；BUN，血尿素氮；CBC，全血计数；CRF，慢性肾衰竭；CVC，中心静脉导管；FFP，新鲜冰冻血浆；INR，国际标准化比率；IV，静脉注射；PCC，凝血酶原复合物浓缩物；Plts，血小板；PRN，如所需；PT，凝血酶原时间；PTT，部分促凝血酶原时间；RBCs，红细胞；T&S，类型和监测；U/O，尿量；VS，重要体征；VW，血管性血友病（*Coartesy of the University of Michigan.*）

表 5　大量输血和平均 RBC 输注体积达到创伤中个人输血诱发因素的可能性

诱发因素	有效数据 n=pts	有效数据 %pts	输入红细胞平均单位 有诱发因素	输入红细胞平均单位 无诱发因素	输入红细胞平均单位 *P* 值	MT 可能性（OR，95%CI） MT 24 h	MT 可能性（OR，95%CI） MT 24 h+	MT 可能性（OR，95%CI） MT6 h+	如果达到诱发因素 MT%（PPV） MT 24 h	如果达到诱发因素 MT%（PPV） MT 24 h+	如果达到诱发因素 MT%（PPV） MT6 h+
INR >1.5	1 081	87%	13.5 ± 1.0	6.6 ± 0.3	$P<0.0001$	3.4（2.5 ~ 4.7）	4.0（2.9 ~ 5.5）	5.8（4.0 ~ 8.2）	43%	49%	40%
SBP <90 mmHg	1 213	97%	11.2 ± 0.7	6.5 ± 0.3	$P<0.0001$	2.6（1.9 ~ 3.4）	2.5（1.9 ~ 3.3）	2.4（1.7 ~ 3.3）	36%	37%	25%
Hb <11 g/dl	1 198	96%	10.3 ± 0.6	6.8 ± 0.3	$P<0.0001$	2.4（1.9 ~ 3.2）	2.6（2.0 ~ 3.4）	3.5（2.6 ~ 4.8）	34%	37%	28%
BD ⩾6	960	77%	10.5 ± 0.6	5.5 ± 0.3	$P<0.0001$	2.8（2.0 ~ 3.9）	3.0（2.2 ~ 4.2）	4.5（3.0 ~ 6.9）	32%	35%	25%
dFAST（+）	1 245	100%	12.0 ± 0.7	7.0 ± 0.3	$P<0.0001$	2.4（1.8 ~ 3.2）	2.4（1.8 ~ 3.2）	2.9（2.1 ~ 3.9）	37%	40%	30%
HR ⩾120bpm	1 218	98%	9.9 ± 0.6	7.3 ± 0.3	$P<0.0001$	1.5（1.2 ~ 2.0）	1.6（1.2 ~ 2.1）	1.8（1.3 ~ 2.4）	29%	31%	23%
渗透压	1 242	100%	9.0 ± 0.6	7.7 ± 0.3	$P=0.04$	1.0（0.8 ~ 1.4）	1.1（0.8 ~ 1.4）	1.5（1.1 ~ 2.0）	24%	26%	21%
体温 <35.5℃	630	51%	7.7 ± 0.8	6.4 ± 0.4	$P=0.11$	.5（0.9 ~ 2.4）	1.6（1.0 ~ 2.5）	1.5（0.9 ~ 2.6）	22%	28%	28%

Modified from Callcut RA, Cotton BA, Muskat P, et al ; PROMMTT Study Group: Defining when to initiate massive transfusion: a validation study of individual massive transfusion triggers in PROMMTT patients. J Trauma Acute Care Surg 74（1）:59–65, 67–68 ; discussion 66–67, 2013.

BD，碱缺失；bpm, 每分钟心跳次数；CI，置信区间；FAST，创伤重点超声评估；g/dl，克每分升；Hb，血红蛋白；HR, 心率；INR，国际标准化比率；MT，大量输血；OR，比值比；PPV, 阳性预测值；RBC，红细胞；SBP，收缩压；temp，体温 .

*MT 24 h，24 h 内 10+ 单位红细胞；MT 24 h+，24 h 内 10+ 单位红细胞再加上 24 h 内出血性死亡；MT6h+，6 h 内 10+ 单位红细胞再加上 6 h 内出血性死亡 .

一个容量以上的血，初始抗体检测阴性，除了 ABO 匹配外没必要再进行兼容性测试。

新鲜冰冻血浆

FFP 在创伤患者失血时使用来尝试纠正 ACOT。系统性地回顾 37 个观察性试验数据，发现在使用 MT 的患者中，用 MT 高 FFP：红细胞比例与死亡率的显著降低（OR＝0.38；95% CI 为 0.24～0.60）和多器官衰竭有关（OR＝0.40；95% CI 为 0.26～0.60）。然而，这些证据的质量由于重要的无法解释的异质性和一些其他因素的原因很低。在经历外科手术而无 MT 的患者中，血浆输注与死亡率提高相关（OR＝1.22；95% CI 为 0.73～.03）。血浆输注与急性肺损伤的风险升高有关（OR＝2.92；95% CI 为 1.99～4.29）。研究的结论是很少有证据表明对于使用 MT 的创伤患者来说 FFP 输注与降低死亡和多器官衰竭的风险有关，但是会将急性肺损伤的风险提高 3 倍。因此我们仍在急诊在创伤的复苏时应用解冻的血浆来止血损伤控制复苏。

尽管 FFP 作为纤维蛋白原的潜在资源应用广泛，但是它有着许多的不足，如应用时间长、输注相关并发症和有限的效率。操作需要血液配型和因为 FFP 存放在 -20℃，使用前需要解冻。尽管人与人之间有很大的差异，FFP 中纤维蛋白原的平均浓度为 2.5 g/L。FFP 中纤维蛋白原的低浓度限制了纤维蛋白原水平的提高。FFP 中的病毒比较活跃，所以有病毒传染的风险。不幸的是，用甲基蓝或者溶剂洗涤剂治疗会在血浆成品中降低纤维蛋白原的水平（尤其是在用甲基蓝，会减少约 30% 的水平）。最后，许多文献记录了使用 FFP 输注后发生的严重的不良事件，包括容量超负荷和输血相关的急性肺损伤（transfusion-related acute lung injury，TRALI）。

血小板

血小板输注被早期应用，同红细胞和 FFP 一起作为止血 / 控制损伤复苏的一部分。特别是在需要 MT 的患者，血小板应该输注给出血的创伤患者使他们的血小板数量高于 100 000，来建立稳定的凝块。

血小板输注对接受 MT 的创伤患者的影响由单一机构的回顾性研究评估。对获得 MT 的受伤患者来说，单采 Plt：RBC 比例提高，可导致生存率的逐步提高。同样地在最近出版的军事数据中，输注 Plt：RBC 比例为 1：1 与早期与晚期生存率的提高、失血性死亡率的降低和相伴随的在大的多中心回顾性研究中 MOF 相关死亡率的提高有关。基于这些数据，提高和早期使用血小板是合乎情理的，直到在前瞻性的创伤随机输血试验得出结论为止。

同样地，在 RBC 输注的数据中，血小板储存时间的增加与不良结局相关。在一个有 380 例危重创伤患者接受血小板输注的研究中，使用储存时间久的血小板，患者的不良反应，尤其是脓毒症在逐步增加。进一步评估潜在的机制和方法，来减少暴露于长时间储存的血小板是必要的，因为我们须更进一步前瞻性地评估血小板输注在需要大量输血患者中所起的作用。

冷凝蛋白质

冷凝蛋白质包括与 FFP 相比更高浓度的纤维蛋白原，常规在 15 g/L 左右，然而，它有着许多同 FFP 一样的缺点。病毒传染的风险与 FFP 相同，但事实上每份冷凝蛋白质包含着多个捐献者的血浆，所以其风险是增高的。不过在血库有内部质量控制条例，纤维蛋白原的浓度是不一样的，还须进行血型匹配。最后解冻冷凝蛋白质也需要时间。几年前，出于安全的考虑，在大多数欧洲国家，冷凝蛋白质被召回，尽管它仍在斯堪的纳维亚、美国和英国使用。冷凝蛋白质不适用于减少病原体的步骤处理，但是它能从经过处理的血浆中提取。

纤维蛋白原浓缩物

最近的治疗是补充通过 FFP、冷凝蛋白质和浓缩纤维蛋白原（fibrinogen concentrate，FC）来补充血浆纤维蛋白原。FC 最近针对有先天性纤维蛋白原缺乏的患者，包括纤维蛋白原缺乏血症和纤维蛋白原过少，用来治疗急性出血。FC 在有出血性休克的严重创伤患者中使用率增加，但是关于它的作用有着巨大的争议。第一个检测 FC 在创伤性出血中的作用的庞大的多中心研究是来自德国创伤登记处的回顾性研究。2 个队列的配对分析用来比较接受 FC 治疗的患者和没有接受的患者（每组 n=294）。创伤患者有严重损伤（平均 ISS 为 37±14）、低血压（SBP≤90 mmHg）者为 50%，入院时碱剩余为 -7.5±6 mmol/L，并且他们接受了大约 12±12 单位的 PRBCs。总体的住院死亡率分别是 28.6% 和

25.5%（P=0.40）。早期使用 FC 与 6 h 死亡率的明显降低[10.5% vs. 16.7%（P=0.03）]、生命的延长[7.5 ± 14.6 vs. 4.7 ± 8.6 天（P=.006）]相关，但是 MOF 的发生率也提高了。没有在接受 FC 治疗的患者身上观察到所有住院患者死亡率降低。

在一个包含 128 例失血创伤患者的研究中，以 FC 和凝血酶原复合物浓缩物作为一线治疗一起使用，来调节凝血系统，针对此措施进行回顾性综述。观察的死亡率明显低于创伤和损伤严重度评分和修正的损伤严重度分类评分所推测的死亡率。Stiager 报道了在军队作战支持医院中 252 名获得 MT 的受伤士兵的纤维蛋白原和死亡的关联。每个患者所输注的纤维蛋白原总量（通过血浆和冷凝蛋白质）被登记下来，纤维蛋白原：RBC 被计算。提高的纤维蛋白原：RBC 比例与增加的生存率有独立的关联性。

系统性综述比较在创伤或围术期患者中使用 FFP 和 FC 的功效。证据不足以支持 FFP 用于外科和严重创伤的患者有很好的临床功效，同时也不足以提出它是有害的。在围术期，FC 通常作为改善患者结局的措施，尽管在确切的结论提出之前还需要更多高质量前瞻性的研究。

TEG 功能性纤维蛋白原试验研究表明纤维蛋白原在创伤后纠正异常的凝血功能有着关键的作用。体外研究显示，添加 FC 会导致功能性纤维蛋白原、血凝块强度的增加，纤维蛋白原的百分比对凝块强度有影响。这些数据表明纤维蛋白原要早期给表现出 ACOT 的创伤患者输注，但是还需要额外的其他研究，来确定输注的时间和剂量。

血液制品疗法：新鲜冰冻血浆、血小板和冷凝蛋白质

给予血液成分治疗时必须进行稀释（图 2）。使用一单位的 PRBCs、FFB 和血小板不会被重组入一单位全血的凝血因子中。因此，稀释性凝血功能障碍和稀释性血小板减少在早期积极输入血液制品的患者中很常见，特别是在获得大量输血的患者中，即使止血 / 损伤控制需要 RBC：FFP：Plt 比例为 1：1：1 的血液成分复苏。

应用 RBC、血浆和血小板的早期平衡复苏的治疗（止血复苏、损伤控制复苏）已经在大量的回顾性研究中被证明，对需要大量输血的患者有改善死亡率的作用。越来越多的证据证明高的 FFP：PRBC 和 Plt：PRBCs 的输注比例能够阻止或减少使 MT 变得复杂的早期凝血功能障碍的发生。尽管研究提出了在严重损伤的患者中进行止血 / 损伤控制复苏的好处，但是要能够在损伤的早期就简单地判断谁最可能从这个疗法中获益仍然十分困难。

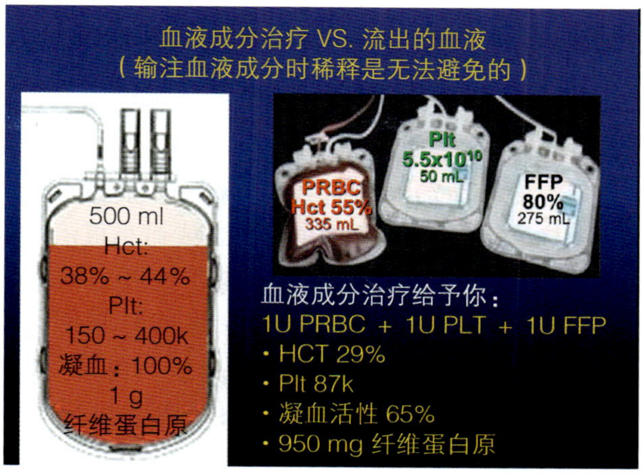

图 2 全血与血液成分治疗。注意输注贮存血液成分不可避免会被稀释。FFP, 新鲜冰冻血浆；Plt, 血小板；RBC, 红细胞.（*Data from Armand R, Hess JR: Treating coagulopathy in trauma patients.* Transfus Med Rev *17:223–231, 2003, pp 223–231.*）

凝血功能障碍和血小板减少在创伤复苏中很常见，并且出血是导致创伤性死亡的主要原因之一。目前应用的凝血因子替代物各不相同，而且有些是不充分的。最近的一个药代动力学模型被运用于模仿出血时的凝血功能障碍的稀释成分，并与不同的 FFP 输注策略进行比较，用于稀释性凝血障碍的预防或纠正或两者兼有。这个研究表明，一旦发生了凝血因子的严重缺乏或不可抑制的出血，每输入 1 单位的 PRBCs，必须输入 1 ~ 1.5 单位的 FFP。如果在血浆因子浓度降至正常值的 50% 以下之前就输入 FFP，那么 1：1 的 FFP 和 PRBCs 的输注比例可以预防远期稀释的发生。他们得出结论：对大的创伤患者进行复苏时，输注全血可以阻止或预防稀释性凝血功能障碍的发生。

所以，对稀释性或消耗性凝血功能障碍和血小板减少的患者的额外的血液制品的输注治疗必须在血液凝血检测的指导下进行，即对血红蛋白、血小板计数、PT、PTT 和纤维蛋白水平的常规监测（表 3），并且要考虑应用 TEG 和 ROTEM 对 ACOT 进行更详细的分析。

前瞻性观测性多中心的重大创伤的输血的研究

PROMMTT，第一个关于出血性创伤患者（n=1 245，入院的 6 h 内接受至少 1 单位的 RBC）的活动性复苏的输血治疗的研究，测试了 905 位在 24 h 内至少接受了 3 单位的 RBC、FFP 或血小板治疗的患者。在第 1 个 24 h 内血清：RBC 和 Plt：RBC 的比例并不是恒定的。在一个多变量的时间依赖的 Cox 模型中，当出血性死亡占上风时，血浆：RBC（调整 HR 为 0.31；95%CI 为 0.16～0.58）和 Plt：RBC（调整 HR 为 0.58；95%CI 为 0.31～0.98）的比例的增加与 6 h 内死亡率的降低有独立相关性。在最初的 6 h 内，输注比例小于 1：2 的血液制品的患者死亡的可能性是比例为 1：1 或更高的患者的 3～4 倍。24 h 后，当非出血性的因素为主时，血浆和血小板的比例与死亡率无关。第一个前瞻性研究表明，在入院后最初的 24 h 内接受了至少 3 单位的血液制品的治疗的患者中，血浆和血小板所占比例的提高与死亡率的降低有关。损伤 24 h 后的幸存者中，后续 30 天的危险因素与血浆和血小板所占比例无关。

随机最佳血小板和血浆比例试验

PROPPR 试验是一个在美国和加拿大的 I 级创伤中心进行的Ⅲ期试验。PROPPR 是为了了解在最初 24 h 内接受了至少 10 单位的 RBC（这可预测患者可能接受 MT）的创伤患者中，24 h 死亡率和 30 天死亡率的差异。PROPPR 的目的是为了增加医生在选择严重出血患者的输血方案时的依据。PROPPR 是一个复苏预后共同体（Resuscitation Outcomes Consortium，ROC）方案，由国家心肺血液学会、美国国防部和加拿大国防研究与发展部门建立。第一组随机接受 1：1：1 的血浆、血小板和红细胞。第二组随机接受 1：1：2 的血浆、血小板和红细胞。PROPPR 试验的纳入标准是：①在每个参与的创伤中心中为最高级别救助队的活动；②大于等于 15 岁，或在年龄不详的情况下大于等于 50 kg；③直接从受伤环境中收治；④在到达医院或转运至医院的过程中的最初 1 h 内输注了至少 1 单位的血液制品；⑤根据 ABC 评分或创伤主治医生的判断标准，超过了阈值，预计会接受大量输血的患者。这项重要研究的结果，将必定会帮助决定出血的创伤患者的复苏策略的最佳血液成分。

创伤中的限制性输血策略

一旦出血被控制，患者完全从出血性休克中恢复，尽力限制创伤中红细胞的输注是明智的。贫血是危重的创伤患者的常见症状，并且在危重疾病中持续存在，这被一组来源于美国的一项多中心队列研究中针对创伤患者（n =576）的析因分析结果证实。ICU 中，319 名（55.4%）创伤患者共接受 1 858 单位血液（平均每人 5.8 ± 5.5 单位血液）。绝大多数（87.1%，n =278）需要输血的 ICU 创伤患者，在住院前 4 天内得到输血治疗，其输血量几乎占 ICU 总输血量的一半。然而，5%～10% 的患者 4 天后继续接受输血治疗。重要的是，这项研究记录了当血红蛋白浓度大于 10 g/dl，患者要使用大量输血治疗。

国际指南关于输血的指标不同，比如美国麻醉协会推荐维持 Hb 高于 6 g/dl，而国际健康协会推荐危重患者 Hb 应维持在大于 7g/dl。一项 Cochrane 数据库系统性综述总结了有限的已发布的证据（10 个试验，n =1 780 位患者），支持在没有心脏疾病的患者中使用限制性输血触发因素（当 Hb<7 g/dl，RBC 输注）。来源于关键医疗社会、EAST、美国血库协会的 2 项最近的指南，宣布了限制性输血的策略（当 Hb<7 g/dl,RBC输注）。

一项来源于前瞻性多中心随机控制试验（重症监护的输血要求）的分析，比较了在危重创伤患者（n=203）苏醒时使用限制性输血（只有在 Hb<7 g/dl 时输血）和无限制性输血（只有在 Hb<10 g/dl 时输血）的输注策略。平均血红蛋白浓度（8.3 ± 0.62 g/dl vs. 10.4 ± 1.2 g/dl，P <0.0001）和每个患者输注的红细胞单位量（2.3 ± 4.4 vs.5.4 ± 4.3，P<0.0001），限制组明显低于非限制组。在死亡率、多器官功能障碍、ICU 治疗时间和住院时间上没有显著的区别，这说明限制性输血策略对于危重的创伤患者，在没有出血和血流动力学不稳定的情况下是安全的。

输血的风险

美国的血液供给从来没像如今这样安全。在过去的几十年里，输血传播的临床上严重的感染的风险有了巨大的降低。

尽管在最近的几十年间，输血传播感染性疾病的风险减少至万分之一，但输血的非感染风险并没有减少。英国和爱尔兰的一项关于 366 例自然报告死亡和输血发生主要不良反应的病例的分析表明，这些不良事件发生大多数（53%）和不正确的输注血液成分有关（如办事员或人为错误）。作为结果，人们输血所承受的非感染性的严重伤害超过感染性伤害的100～1000倍（表6）。

表6 输血相关风险

风险类型	发生率
非感染性风险	
红细胞生成抑制	普遍的
容量超载、肺水肿	10%～40%
发热反应	1/10～1/100
荨麻疹反应	1/33～1/100
输血相关的急性肺损伤（TRALI）	1/1 120～1/5 000
延迟溶血性输血反应	1/2 500
溶血性输血反应	1/38 000～1/70 000
致命的溶血性输血反应	1/600 000
过敏性休克	1/500 000
免疫抑制	未知
移植物抗宿主疾病	1/400～1/10 000
同种异体免疫（RBCs）	1/100
同种异体免疫（血小板）	1/10
ABO-Rh 错误配型发生率 死亡率	1/6 000～1/20 000 1/100 000～1/600 000
感染性风险	
巨细胞病毒转化	7%
Epstein-Barr 病毒	0.5%
细菌污染（PRBCs+ 血小板）	1/2 000
乙型肝炎传播	1/220 000
PRBCs 相关细菌脓毒症	1/500 000～1/786 000
甲型肝炎传播	1/1 000 000
西尼罗病毒传播	1/1 400 000
丙型肝炎病毒传播	1/1 600 000
HIV 传播	1/1 800 000

Modified from Klein HG: Allogenic transfusion risks in the surgical patient. Am J Surg 170；6A:21S–26S, 1995；Silliman CC, Moore EE, Johnson JL, et al: Transfusion in the injured patient: proceed with caution. Shock 21（4）:291–299, 2004；Busch MP, Kleinman SH, Nemo GJ: Current and emerging infectious risks of blood transfusions. JAMA 289（8）:959–962, 2003；and Spiess BD: Risk of transfusion: outcome focus. Transfusion 44:4S–14S, 2004
HIV, 人免疫缺陷病毒；PRBCs, 浓缩红细胞；RBC, 红细胞

输血出现的风险包括通过输血渠道传播西尼罗病毒（West Nile virus，WNV）。在2002年8月至2003年1月，有23例来自14个献血者的确诊的输血相关WNV感染的病例。2003年7月试验性的WNV核酸扩增检验在献血者中施行。2003年9月的报告阐述了在4 137份已知的WNV感染报告给CDC的期间，用前述检验从250万单位供体的血液中识别了超过600单位感染的血液。尽管捐献血液的核酸扩增检验防止了数以百计的WNV的感染，但它不能识别低病毒血症程度的血液单位——这些血液的抗体是阴性的，并且有感染性。这些数据支持在WNV高流行区域使用个人捐献血液靶向核酸扩增检验，在2004年该策略被成功实施。

关于红细胞储存负向影响病情结局的证据越来越多。在多中心、双盲、前瞻性血液的年龄评估研究中，进入ICU的成年患者随机接受储存少于7天的去白细胞型红细胞或者接受标准程序化的血液（平均储存时间为19天）。此研究初期的终点是90天的全因死亡率。患者的目标数目是2 510（在初期的终点中预期的增长率大于5%）。患者的招募在2013年1月完成，长期随访正在进行中。

尽管我们的血液供给是安全的，最近20年出现的数据阐述了输注红细胞的严重风险，包括死亡率和并发症发生率的增加（SIRS、TRALI、感染、MOF）。关于危重患者中红细胞输注效用的最大的系统性综述包括45个观测到的队列，包含272 596位患者。45个研究中的42研究发现，中输注红细胞的风险超过益处；2项研究发现，风险与益处持平，1项研究中的1个小组发现益处大于风险（年老的有急性心肌梗死和血细胞比容少于30%的患者）。18项研究中的17项论述了红细胞输注是一个死亡的独立预测因素，汇总OR值（12项研究）是1.7（95%CI为1.4～1.9）。22项研究检验出红细胞输注与院内感染的关系，在所有的研究中红细胞输注是感染的独立危险因素。发生感染的不良反应的汇总OR值（9项研究）为1.8（95% CI为1.5～2.2）。红细胞输注同样提高了发生多器官功能障碍综合征（3项研究）和ARDS（6项研究）的风险。发生ARDS的汇总OR值为2.5（95%CI为1.6～3.3）。除了队列研究分析时固有的限制以外，这项分析指出在成年人、ICU、创伤和手术患者中红细胞输注与并发症发生率和死亡率的提高有关，因此现在进行输血治疗时需要重新评价。在每个患者输血前应该评估红细胞输注为患者所带来的风险和益处。

输血相关急性肺损伤

TRALI 是输血中一项危及生命的不良反应。TRALI 是如今输血相关死亡的首要因素，尽管这一观点仍然被低估和没有被诊断。NIH 国家心肺血液学会召集了一个关于 TRALI 的工作组，并且建立了通用的定义：输血后 6 h 内新发的急性肺损伤。TRALI，类似 ARDS，可能是 2 个事件的现象——有接受者的倾向性，血液单位的储存因素发挥着巨大的作用。血液细胞成分输注中，TRALI 报道的总患病率为 1/1120。

一项近期的前瞻性的队列研究指出输血总量与出现 ARDS 和院内死亡有着重要的独立的关联。在疾病严重性、创伤类型、种族、性别和 BD 的多变量 logistic 回归模型中，输血总量与出现 ARDS 的关联仍然显著。一项涵盖 5 260 位钝性创伤患者的研究指出，无论伤害的严重性，延迟输血（在入院的前 48 h 未接受输血）与呼吸机相关性肺炎、ARDS，创伤患者的死亡都有着独立的关联。同样地，一项监测 ARDS 临床预后的补充研究证实了 PRBCs 输注是提高 ARDS 发生风险和提高 ARDS 患者死亡率的独立危险因素。以上这些研究帮助制定了在创伤复苏过程中合理的输血策略，强调了对安全有效的血液替代品和输血方案的需求。

输血和损伤后多器官衰竭

输血在一项历时 3 年的意图找出损伤后预测模型的单一机构的前瞻性队列研究（n=394）中，被首次确认为是 MOF 独立危险因素。ISS 大于 15 和存活超过 24 h 的创伤患者接受了测试。以下变量作为 MOF 早期独立相关因素被识别出：年龄超过 55 岁、ISS 不低于 25、入院后首个 12 h 内输血超过 6 单位。此外，在获得这些测量值的患者亚组中，BD＞8 mEq/L（0～12 h）和乳酸＞2.5 mmol/L（12～24 h）是 MOF 的独立预测因子。在这项研究中，输血是否仅仅是出血性休克严重程度的替代指标还有待进一步探索。

该小组随后的前瞻性研究证实，输血是损伤后 MOF 的独立危险因素，控制包括 BD 和乳酸盐在内的其他休克指数。这项研究有类似的试验性设计，513 例 ISS 大于 15 的创伤患者进入 ICU，存活时间超过 48 h。已经确定了早期输血和损伤后 MOF 之间的剂量反应关系，并且所测试的 15 个多因素回归模型中的 13 个确认输血为独立的危险因素。OR 值很高，特别是在早期的 MOF 模型中。

最近，该小组发现尽管 MOF 风险增加，但是在过去的 12 年中，损伤后 MOF 的发生率、严重程度以及随之而来的死亡风险已经降低。这样的进展与创伤和重症监护的改善以及复苏期间输血的使用减少有关。

输血和全身炎症反应综合征 / 死亡率

创伤中的输血（在前 24 h 内）与在单一机构中研究纳入的 7 602 名创伤患者的全身炎症反应综合征（systemic inflammatory response syndrome，SIRS）（定义为 SIRS 评分≥2）的发病率的增加有关。在最初的 24 h 内对 954 名患者进行输血，占全部研究人群的 10%。通过 ISS、格拉斯哥昏迷等级评分和年龄的分层后，进行多元 Logistic 回归分析，发现输血总量的增加是创伤患者 SIRS、入住 ICU 和死亡率的明显的独立预测因子。接受输血的创伤患者的 SIRS 发病率增加了 2～6 倍（$P<0.0001$），并且入住 ICU 的概率（OR=4.62）和死亡率（OR=4.23，$P<0.0001$）增加了 4 倍以上，并且相较于未输血的创伤患者 ICU 和医院 LOS 明显延长。

最近的一项前瞻性研究证实，在整个住院期间，创伤患者都输入同种异体血液，并在输血前有相对较高的血红蛋白水平（平均值为 9 g/dl）的情况下进行输血。104 例患者（87%）接受了 324 次输血，其中 20 例（6%）在急诊室给予，186 例（57%）在外科 ICU，22 例（7%）在 SICU 出来后，以及 96 例（30%）在手术室。每位患者输血的平均体积为 3 144 ml（±2 622ml）。输注超过 4 单位的血液是 SIRS 发生的独立危险因素。限制输血的策略应该在群体中进行研究。

输血与死亡率

随访研究评估了损伤后最初 24 h 内输血对更大样本量（n＝15 534，3 年研究，1998–2000）的创伤患者预后的影响。该研究控制入院时所有潜在的混杂的休克变量[包括 BD，血清乳酸和休克指数（HR/SBP）]，以及年龄、性别、种族 / 民族、格拉斯哥昏迷等级评分和 ISS 的分层。当按照休克指标进行分层时（BD、血清乳酸、休克指数和贫血），输血是死亡率（OR=2.83，95% CI 为

1.82～4.40，$P<0.001$）、入住 ICU（OR=3.27，95% CI 为 2.69～3.99，$P<0.001$）、ICU LOS（$P<0.001$），以及医院 LOS（系数为 4.37，95% CI 为 2.79～5.94，$P<0.001$）的强独立预测因子经历输血的患者的死亡率几乎是未输血患者的 3 倍。因此，ICU 入院、ICU LOS 和医院 LOS 在通过入院 BD、乳酸、休克指数和贫血控制休克严重程度后，在损伤后（前 24 h 内）的输血被证实是死亡率的独立预测因子。

我们还检查了输血和创伤的预后，这取决于患者是否在损伤后 24 h 内或后输血。这项回顾性研究证实了我们的血库的创伤登记数据，并描述了输血和死亡之间的关系。当患者在损伤后早期（24 h 之内）输血时，输血和死亡的相关性更高（OR=4.13 vs. OR=3.10）。

一篇 4 年的单一机构回顾性综述，对所有接受Ⅰ级创伤中心治疗的钝性肝或脾损伤的成年人进行输血检查作为预后的独立风险因子。在 316 例呈现钝性肝或脾损伤的患者中，143 例（45%）在前 24 h 内接受输血。总共有 230 名患者（72.8%）被选择进行非手术治疗，其中 75 名（33%）在前 24 h 需要输血。输血在控制休克和损伤严重程度的指标后是所有患者（OR=4.75，95% CI 为 1.37～16.4，$P=0.014$）和所有的非手术治疗组患者（OR=8.45，95% CI 为 1.95～36.53，$P=0.0043$）死亡率的独立预测因子。每单位的 PRBCs 输注都会使死亡风险增加（每单位 OR=1.16，95% CI 为 1.10～1.24，$P<0.0001$）。输血也是医院 LOS 增加的独立预测因子（系数为 5.45，95% CI 为 1.64～9.25，$P=0.005$）。输血相关的死亡风险在非手术治疗的患者亚组中最高。作者建议在对钝性肝和脾损伤的治疗中，输血的前瞻性检查是有必要的。

另一项单一机构研究检查了老年患者是否受到创伤后输血的与输血量不相符的影响。为了确定年龄，PRBCs 输注量和损伤后死亡风险之间可能的相互作用，在损伤后的最初 24 h 内接受输血的成年患者的 6 年回顾性综述（1995 年 1 月至 2000 年 12 月）已完成。在受伤后 24 h 内接受 PRBCs 的 1 312 例患者中，1 028 例（78%）年龄在 55 岁及以下，284 例（22%）年龄在 55 岁以上，总死亡率为 21.2%。年龄、ISS、格拉斯哥昏迷等级评分和 PRBCs 输注量为死亡的独立预测因素。老年幸存者的平均 PRBCs 输注量（4.6 单位）明显低于较年轻的幸存者（6.7 单位）。没有 75 岁以上的 PRBCs 输注体积大于 12 单位的患者存活。作者得出结论，年龄和 PRBCs 输注量独立而非合作地作用于增加损伤后的死亡率。

最近，一项 5 年的单一机构的研究证实，低血红蛋白、异常凝血酶原和 PTT，以及休克的生理体征（低 SBP 和升高的 BD）是创伤死亡的独立预测因素。目前，治疗低血红蛋白和具有出血性休克体征的创伤患者的唯一有效的方法是输注储存的红细胞。在 2 项大型前瞻性多中心研究中，在确定危重患者贫血发生率和红细胞输血的使用的关系时，发现输血也与增加的死亡率相关。

输血和感染

免疫抑制是人类同种异体输血的结果，并且与潜在的根治性手术后癌症复发率的风险增加以及术后细菌感染的频率增加相关。meta 分析检查了同种异体输血与术后细菌感染的关系。1986–2000 年发表的 20 篇同行评议文章被纳入一个 meta 分析中。纳入标准包括有明确定义的对照组（未输血）与治疗组（输血）的对比和包括多元 Logistic 回归在内的对累计数据进行的统计分析。此外，仅包括创伤性损伤患者的出版物的一个亚组也被包括在单独的 meta 分析中。

该 meta 分析中纳入的受试者总数为 13 152 例（输血组 5 215 例，非输血组 7 937 例）。在本次 meta 分析评估的同种异体 RBC 输血与术后细菌感染发生率的关系的所有文章中，总 OR 为 3.45（范围为 1.43～15.15），20 项研究中有 17 项的统计结果为 $P=0.05$。这些结果提供了压倒性的证据：同种异体 RBC 输血与手术患者术后细菌感染的风险显著增加相关。

创伤患者亚组的总 OR 为 5.263（范围为 5.03～5.43），所有研究显示 $P<0.05$（范围为 0.005～0.0001）。这些结果表明，当与选择性手术期间或之后接受同种异体红细胞输血的那些患者相比，同种异体红细胞输血与创伤患者术后细菌感染的风险增加相关。

单一机构的研究记录发现，输血（入院前 28 h 内）以剂量依赖的方式与创伤患者的感染相关。它研究了从 1996 年 11 月至 1999 年 12 月接受Ⅰ级创伤中心的创伤服务的所有成年患者（n=1 593）。其中，12.6% 患者至少出现 1 种感染。总输血率为 19.4%。接受至少 1 次输血的患者（33%）的感染率明显更高（$P<0.0001$），而 7.6% 的患者没有输血。每位患者

的输血量范围为 0 ~ 46 单位。接受 0 ~ 15 次输血的患者感染风险与输血次数之间存在明显的指数关系（$R^2 = 0.757$）。多元 Logistic 回归分析，用于识别感染进展的危险因素，证实输注的 PRBCs 是感染的独立危险因素（OR = 1.084，95% CI 为 1.028 ~ 1.142，$P = 0.0028$）。本研究记录了 PRBCs 输血和创伤患者感染发展之间的明显剂量依赖性相关性。类似地，危重患者的研究证明，根据患者疾病严重程度和年龄分层后，输血患者的院内感染相较于未输血患者比例明显增加。

输血相关的不良预后的潜在机制

已经描述了许多关于输血的不良作用的潜在机制，包括血液储存时间的增加，RBC 变形性降低导致微循环灌注的减少，炎症反应、免疫抑制与微嵌合的增加（与非白细胞减少血液中供体白细胞相关）和一氧化氮结合的游离血红蛋白增加。对这些潜在机制的讨论超出了本章的范围。

最近一篇关于危重病患者输血的综述总结如下：① RBC 输血不能改善危重患者整体或微循环水平的组织氧消耗；② RBC 输血与危重患者临床预后的改善无关，且可能导致一些患者的预后更差；③ RBC 输血能改善情况的患者的特定因素的识别是很困难的；④ RBC 输血失效可能与储存时间、储存的 RBC 的内皮黏附、储存的血液中的一氧化氮被游离血红蛋白结合、供体白细胞、宿主炎症反应和 RBC 变形性降低相关。

红细胞储存损伤

在储存 35 天的血液中分析红细胞聚集参数、变形性和形状描述。RBC 变形性与新鲜样品相比降低 5%。Hovav 等报道，血液储存诱导 RBC 的变化与其聚集性的持续增加相关（图 3）。另一个最近的研究表明，人类 RBC 变形性在储存 4 周后下降了 34%。另一项调查中发现储存期间红细胞转变为棘状细胞的过程具有时间依赖性。这种转化增加了高、低剪切速率下的悬浮液黏度。这些研究者还证实，储存前白细胞消耗可以减少这些影响。

创伤性损伤也伴随着 RBC 变形性的降低。通过扫描电子显微镜检查 43 例多系统创伤患者的 RBC 形状。在入院时和之后每 24 h 取血样，持续 4 ~ 10 天。入院时观察两组患者，相较于志愿者组两组患者的盘状红细胞的百分比显著降低（$P<0.01$）。不可逆性改变的 RBC（鞘脂瘤细胞、球状细胞）的百分比在存活者中较低（12.9 ± 2.0% vs.20.3 ± 9.4%，$P<0.01$）。这项研究证实 RBC 形状改变出现在创伤后的最初几小时内，并持续至少 7 ~ 10 天（图 4），这些变化在继发感染并发症的患者中更严重。

输血相关并发症的处理

大量输血治疗的目的是恢复足够的血量、支持

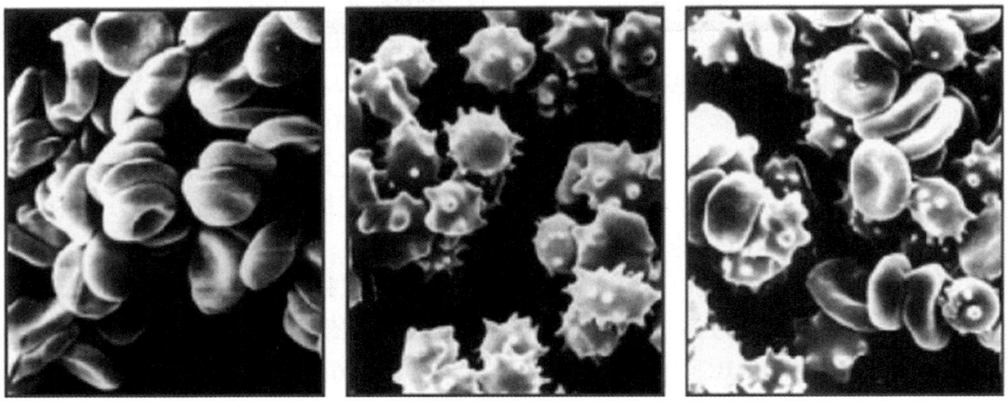

第 1 天　　第 21 天　　第 35 天

图 3　使用扫描电子显微镜观察储存红细胞的形状改变。在储存过程中，红细胞形态逐渐由正常扁平状变成棘状。分类计数显示 3 周后棘状细胞 RBC 占细胞群体的 80%，在储存期的终期其超过 95%（*FromHovavT, YedgarS, MannyN, BarshsteinG: Alterationofredcellaggregabilityandshapeduringblood storage.* Transfusion *39[3]: 277–281, 1999.*）

止血、维持血液携氧能力、恢复或维持胶体渗透压。虽然创伤中大量输血的患者生存率已经改善，但是他们可能发生与输血相关的许多并发症。照顾需要大量输血的患者的医生必须预测、识别和快速治疗这些并发症，以确保患者有最佳的治疗效果。

血小板减少

大量输血后，稀释性血小板减少是不可避免的，因为血小板功能在储存几天后下降到零。至少 1.5 倍的血液体积必须被替换已经成为了一个临床问题。然而，如果发生 DIC 或存在预先存在的血小板减少，则在少量输血后可发生血小板减少。

凝血因子消耗

储存的血液含有除Ⅴ和Ⅷ之外的所有凝血因子。这些因子的产生由于对创伤的应激反应而增加。因此，输血只引起凝血功能的轻微变化，随之出现的 DIC 更可能是造成止血失控的原因。DIC 是延迟或不充分复苏的结果，并且是与输血体积不成比例的异常凝血指数的普遍原因。

低血钙

每单位的血液含有约 3 g 柠檬酸盐，它与钙离子结合。健康的成年人的肝将每 5 min 代谢 3 g 柠檬酸。因此，输血速度大于每 5 min 1 单位或肝功能受损可能导致柠檬酸中毒和低钙血症。低钙血症在临床上对凝血功能没有明显的作用，但是患者可能表现出短暂性的痉挛和低血压。只有在有低钙血症的生化、临床或心电图证据的情况下才应给予钙。

低钾血症和高钾血症

储存的血液中的血浆钾浓度在储存期间增加并且可能大于 30 mmol/L。高钾血症通常不成问题，除非患者快速输注大量的血液。相反，低钾血症更常见，因为红细胞开始活跃代谢，并且钾的细胞内摄取重新开始。

酸碱紊乱

血包中的乳酸水平使储存的血液的酸负荷高达

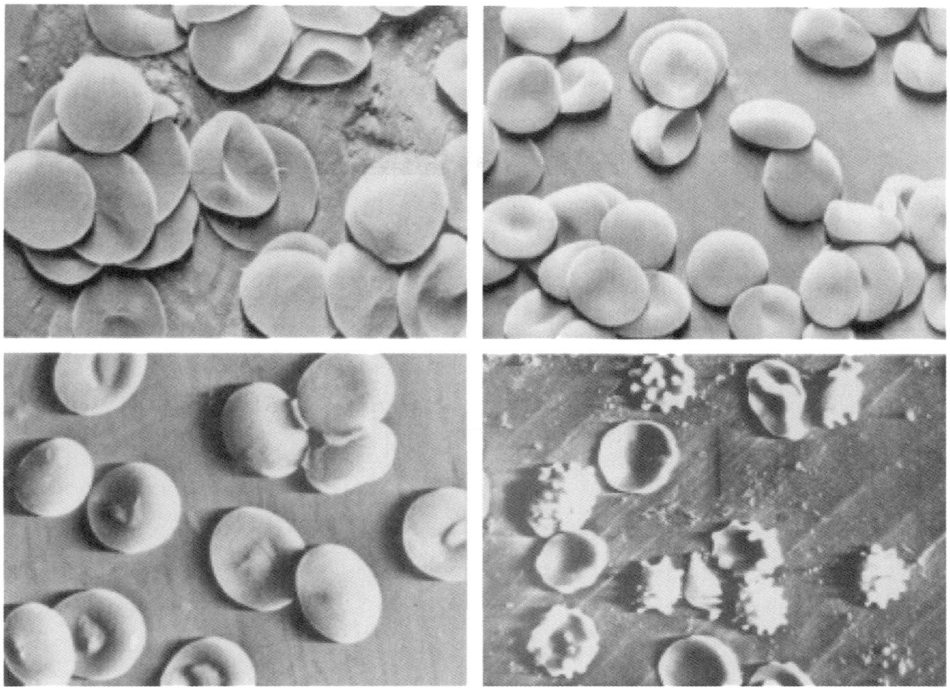

图 4　创伤患者内源性红细胞形状和变形性的改变。上面 2 张图片是幸存者损伤后第 3 天（左）和第 7～10 天（右）。底部 2 张图片是死亡患者损伤后第 3 天（左）和第 7～10 天（右）。创伤死亡患者显示出了更高比例的有不可逆性改变的红细胞（*From Berezina TL, Zaets SB, Machiedo GW: Alterations of red blood cell shape in patients with severe trauma.* J Trauma *57[1]:82–87, 2004.*）

30～40 mmol/L。它和柠檬酸通常能一起被快速地代谢。事实上，柠檬酸被代谢为碳酸氢盐，并且可能出现严重的代谢性碱中毒。输血者体内的酸碱状态通常更为重要，最终的酸碱状态取决于组织灌注、输注速率和柠檬酸代谢。

低温

低温导致柠檬酸和乳酸代谢减少（导致低钙血症和代谢性酸中毒），增加血红蛋白对氧的亲和力、损害红细胞变形性、使血小板功能障碍、使患者有增加的心律失常倾向。

总结

用储存的 PRBCs 给损伤的患者输血，须在损伤后的急性抢救与恢复阶段保持谨慎观察。目前，输血是治疗严重出血性休克的唯一选择，可以挽救生命。止血或损伤控制复苏时，RBC：FFP：Plt 的血液成分比例约为 1：1：1，与生存率的增加有关，但血浆输注过多也伴有急性肺损伤风险的增加。MTP 应该用于大量输血存在高风险的出血性休克患者，促进其快速的血液成分复苏。然而，在过去二十年中，出现了安全性问题，数据记录了接受输血的患者的明显增加的并发症发生率和死亡率。因此，一旦出血得到控制，应当在具有稳定无症状性贫血的创伤患者中使用更保守的输血方法。发展输血公共协议（图 5）以促进在血流动力学稳定的创伤患者中用限制性的方法恰当地使用这种稀缺资源。输血的决定应个体化，基于个人的生理和血红蛋白值来决定。为了最大程度减少不良反应、免疫抑制和过度炎症反应，所有试图减少创伤患者输血的方法都有必要进行尝试。

A　创伤患者输血指南

损伤的炎症和宿主反应

1. 根据血红蛋白 <7 gm/dl（或 Hct < 21%），可识别危重患者。
2. 如果血红蛋白 <7 gm/dl 输注 PRBCs 是合适的。
   a. 严重心血管疾病的患者，输血阈值较高可能是适当的。
3. 如果血红蛋白 >7 gm/dl，评估患者血容量不足。
   a. 如果患者血容量不足，给予静脉输液以达到正常血容量。
   b. 如果患者无血容量不足，确定是否有证据表明氧气输送受损（低 Svo_2、持续 / 恶化的碱缺失、存在 / 恶化的乳酸酸中毒）。
4. 如果存在氧气输送受损，考虑肺动脉导管放置，测量心排血量，并使氧气输送最优化。
5. 如果不存在氧气输送受损，则如临床指示监测血红蛋白。

* 该方案假定急性出血已被控制，初始复苏已经完成，并且患者在 ICU 中稳定，没有进行性出血。

B　创伤患者输血指南（不包括快速复苏）

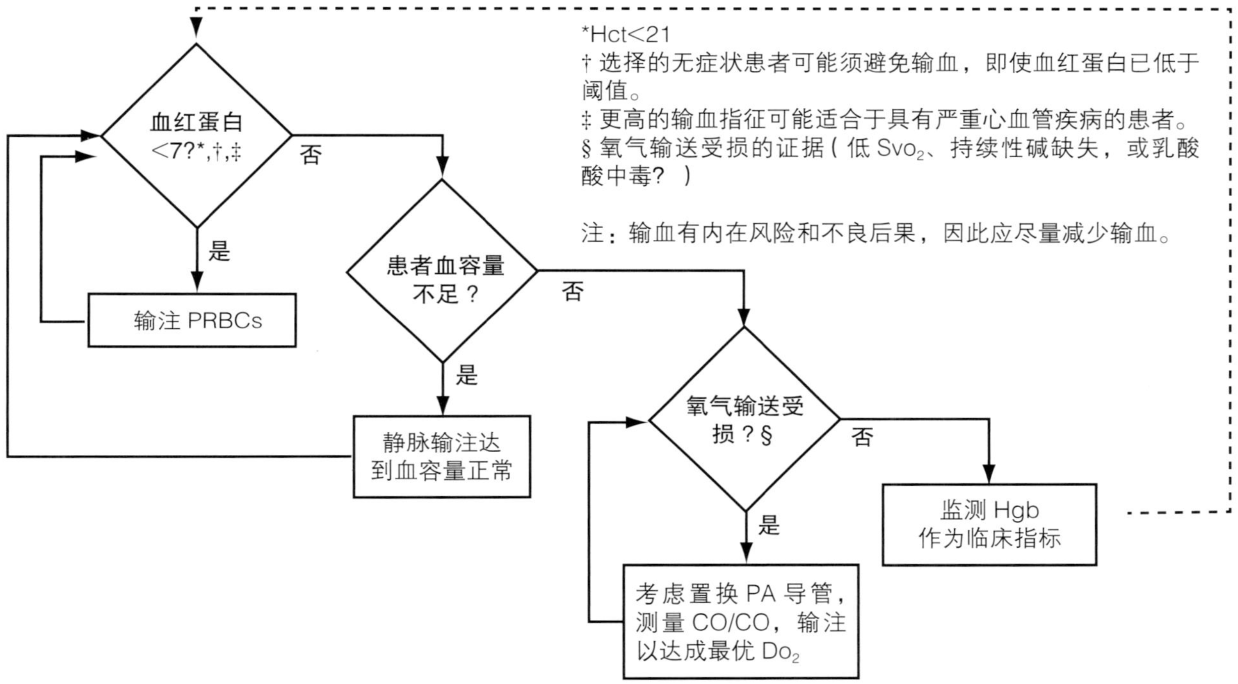

图 5　创伤输血指南。床边使用方案概述。IV, 静脉输液；PA, 肺动脉；PRBCs, 浓缩红细胞；Pt, 患者（*From West MA, Shapiro MB, Nathens AB, et al:Inflammation and the host response to injury, a large-scale collaborative project: Patient-oriented research core-standard operating procedures for clinical care. IV. Guidelines for transfusion in the trauma patient.* J Trauma *61[2]: 436–439, 2006.*）

第 14 章 重症监护Ⅱ:特殊问题和治疗

急性呼吸窘迫综合征

Matthew C. Bozeman, Keith R. Miller, Nicholas A. Nash 和 Jorge L. Rodríguez 著
吕 杰 译

随着机械通气的出现和现代危重症医学的开始，许多话题曾被大家激烈地讨论和研究。40 年前，一名叫 Asbaugh 的外科医生首先报道了 ARDS 这一话题。尽管针对 ARDS 进行了许多试验和治疗策略的尝试，但是这种疾病仍然伴随着较宽的死亡率范围。ARDS 是大量疾病的最终共同途径，比如钝性胸部创伤、输液介导的肺损伤导致的脓毒症等，并常发展至多系统器官功能衰竭（multiple systems organ failure，MSOF）。目前 ARDS 的治疗取得了一定进展，近期在机械通气策略、早期诊断和病理生理的理解方面取得的进步，可以帮助我们改善肺内气体的弥散，并减少医源性肺损伤的发生，这都是 ARDS 治疗的关键。这几项进展，已经将 ARDS 的死亡率从 20 年前 60% 减少至目前报道的 30%～35%。

定义、表现及临床诊断

自从越南战争以来，相关文献已经对急性肺损伤（acute lung injury，ALI）和 ARDS 进行了描述，民间医生注意到这是一种以双肺渗出、缺氧、中心性及周围性发绀为特征的疾病。对于 ARDS 广泛适用的定义在早期的 20 多年里并未确立，这大大阻碍了对该疾病流行病学及治疗的研究。1988 年 ARDS 的新定义被制定，之后 1994 年，欧美 ARDS 联合会议对其进行了改进，确立了 ALI/ARDS 诊断所需的特定临床标准。

ALI 以及 ARDS 被定义为左心房压力未提高（≤18mmHg），肺毛细血管楔压（pulmonary capillary wedge pressure，PCWP）监测的情况下，双肺出现急性的浸润及水肿。

将 ALI 和 ARDS 的低氧血症按动脉氧张力与吸入氧分数的比例（Pao_2/Fio_2）的不同进行了区分。ARDS 的 $Pao_2/Fio_2 < 200$，ALI 的 $Pao_2/Fio_2 < 300$（表 1）。

应该指出的是，当计算 Pao_2/Fio_2 比例的时候不应使用呼吸末气道正压（positive end-expiratory pressure，PEEP）；而有证据建议使用 PEEP/Fio_2 比例更有助于及早诊断 ARDS。ALI 和 ARDS 之间低氧程度的差别是很重要的，因为符合标准的患者大部分需要机械通气。对于缺氧的诊断往往通过动脉血样进行判断，但是有些患者不具备采集动脉血的条件。这些情况下，合理的方法是以脉搏血氧计测得血氧饱和度（Spo_2）与 Fio_2 之比来替代。

ARDS 的患者早期往往合并呼吸道损害和刺激性事件。超过 60 种疾病都与 ARDS 的触发有关系，但只有一小部分原因可以被识别出来。脓毒症、肺炎、肺挫伤、多次输血、误吸是常见的病因。肺挫伤和输血相关的急性肺损伤（transfusion-related acute lung injury，TRALI）经常与创伤相关。

呼吸困难、呼吸急促和低氧血症往往是早期症状，有些在数小时内即可发生，但多数还是出现在 72 h 内。早期出现的急性加重也很典型，往往需要机械插管。实验室检查提示代谢性碱中毒、低氧血症以及继发于肺血流分流的肺泡 - 动脉血氧分压差增大。其他的检查异常通常继发于基础疾病。如前所述，X 线胸片显示弥漫性双肺渗出性病变，它在病程上是急性发生的。渗出的程度和多少与诊断无关。与肺水肿程度相关的标志物目前尚未发现。疾

病早期的胸部 CT 扫描可见重力依赖区域肺实变并伴有肺不张。

ALI/ARDS 的临床特征与其他疾病具有相当大的重叠，这使 ARDS 的诊断成为一种排除性诊断。诊断 ARDS 必须除外心源性肺水肿和其他引起低氧性呼吸衰竭的因素。心源性肺水肿非常难与 ARDS 鉴别，因为二者的临床表现可以是相同的。除了对液体平衡的评估，心功能检查经常也是必须的。测定 B 型钠尿肽（B-type natriuretic peptide，BNP）水平以及经胸或者经食管超声心动图可以评估心脏功能，然而超声心动对于肾衰竭或者液体超负荷的患者意义有限。多项研究显示，使用肺动脉导管（pulmonary artery catheter，PAC）对于 ARDS 的诊断和管理并无益处。然而，右心导管插入在其他检查无法将 ARDS 和心源性肺水肿区分开来的时候，仍然可以考虑使用。

表 1　定义 ARDS 和 ALI

特征	ARDS	ALI
低氧血症	Pao_2/Fio_2 比例 <200	200<Pao_2/Fio_2 比例 <300
急性弥漫性双肺浸润	有	有
左心房压力	≤18 mmhg	≤18 mmhg

ALI，急性肺损伤；ARDS，急性呼吸窘迫综合征

其他导致低氧性呼吸衰竭的原因有：不同类型的肺炎、癌症、粟粒性肺结核、肺泡出血以及肺挫伤。这些都可以通过病史、临床以及实验室检查、支气管镜检查以及开放肺活检（部分筛选后的患者适用）进行区别。

流行病学

ARDS 的发病率在多个研究都有提及，首先在 1972 年曾报告其发病率为 75/100 000 人年。这与每年 150 000 例的发病人数基本相符。其他研究表明，ARDS 发病率已增加至 190 000 例 / 年，与其相对应的是每年 360 万住院日。高达 20% 的机械通气患者以及 10% 的 ICU 住院患者达到了 ARDS 的临床标准。

ARDS 导致的死亡多数不与低氧血症直接相关。早期充足的氧合是有益的，但是由 Fio_2/Pao_2 判断的低氧血症的程度与最终的死亡率并不相关。对于死亡率的预测应考虑到患者特异性、疾病特异性与治疗特异性。大于 85 岁的老年人预后较年轻人更差。疾病特异性包括肺血管功能障碍、肺无效腔、感染、多器官功能障碍、急性损伤事件，并且越来越多的证据表明生物标志物以及基因多态性与 ARDS 的预后和易感性相关。治疗上须注意的是限制输血、避免液体过负荷、早期识别传染源，还有一些其他的策略将在后文进行讨论。

早期的死亡多继发于急性损伤事件，而继发于肺部感染的脓毒症是导致晚期死亡的首要原因。

病理生理学

正常、健康的肺有助于整个机体维持稳态的各种过程，包括氧吸收、二氧化碳释放和酸碱平衡，以及其他功能。特别是气体交换，依赖于干燥的肺泡和正常毛细血管床的开放。与其他半渗透性组织相似，肺的液体平衡依赖于 Starling 方程描述的渗透梯度。跨过血管及间质组织的液体流动，取决于静水压及渗透压（包括细胞内蛋白）。这种平衡允许少量的液体流出毛细血管，并有 3 个主要机制防止肺泡水肿的形成和气体交换中断。这些机制包括维持肺泡上皮细胞之间紧密的连接、细胞内蛋白质促进重吸收、间质淋巴管收集丢失的体液回流入循环。

ALI / ARDS 是一种肺泡表面被破坏的病理过程，包括肺泡细胞膜的破坏，结果导致肺泡重吸收能力的丧失及富含炎症因子的体液丢失到肺实质里。无论是直接的肺损伤（肺炎、误吸、肺挫伤、手术）还是间接的肺损伤（脓毒症、休克、输血或其他疾病，如急性胰腺炎），这个过程都是动态发展的。

ALI/ARDS 是由肺泡上皮的丧失引起的。局部损伤引起的促炎细胞因子聚集，如组织坏死因子（tissue necrosis factor，TNF）、白细胞介素（interleukin，IL）-1、IL-6 和 IL-8。这些细胞因子对中性粒细胞和巨噬细胞的吸引起着重要的作用，并促进这些聚集的细胞激活和释放，如蛋白酶、弹性蛋白酶及活性氧代谢产物等有毒介质，引起细胞损伤。一旦毛细血管内皮细胞和肺泡上皮细胞被这些物质包围，造成的细胞损伤将导致原来细胞内蛋白质释放，并破坏胶体渗透压梯度驱动的液体重吸收。一些证据表明这些病理变化还导致了淋巴管重吸收的降低。肺泡上皮的破坏伴随液体超负荷，导致了 ALI/ARDS 发生时肺顺应性的降低。

根据临床表现可将 ALI/ARDS 分为组织学上 3 个不同的阶段。分别为渗出期、增生期和纤维化期。在病程早期，渗出期阶段，中性粒细胞和巨噬细胞使局部肺泡损伤和Ⅰ型肺泡上皮细胞的缺失变得普遍。低氧血症、气体交换障碍通常可在这个早期阶段看到。一般这种渗出期约持续 1～10 天，然后转入增生期。增生期显著的组织学变化是Ⅰ型肺泡上皮细胞被Ⅱ型肺泡上皮细胞所替换、胶原蛋白沉积，成纤维细胞浸润间质、鳞状上皮化生。肺泡表面活性物质的产量增加，肺水肿开始缓解。第二阶段，患者的临床病程往往不同，其原因目前仍然知之甚少。一些患者病情开始缓解，另外一些迅速恶化并死亡，还有一些继续进展为纤维化期，此阶段特点为肺泡闭塞、间充质细胞替代正常肺组织、弥漫性纤维化，以及导管形成。组织学上，这个阶段似乎表现为纤维性肺泡炎，并预示着一个糟糕的预后。

治疗和支持性措施

ARDS 的管理可广泛地分为治疗策略和支持策略。治疗策略方面，导致肺损伤的促炎症反应的特性被广泛地研究。支持策略方面，通过成功的通气策略，保证氧合和通气，为病情的缓解争取时间。不幸的是，到目前为止，治疗策略方面的进展结果为令人失望的，治疗仍多为支持性的。ARDS 的原因有很多（创伤、脓毒症、胰腺炎、肺炎等），原发病因必须以一个快速有效的方式解决。这类似于感染性休克中的感染源控制的概念，但不应过分强调。由于疾病是经不同阶段进展而来，对于患者的支持措施和通气策略应该随时调整，以适应患者不同的反应。最终，顽固性低氧血症和高碳酸血症代表疾病发展的终点，并会导致多器官功能衰竭和死亡。

液体复苏与管理

液体复苏和整体容量状态的评估是所有重症患者管理的基础，ARDS 的患者亦是如此。从理论上讲，在潜在的肺灌注损伤时，最大限度地降低容量超负荷对肺部弥散障碍的恢复是有利的。反过来讲，液体复苏不足也会增加患者发病率，应当避免。为了精确的液体复苏，无创及有创血流动力学监测是基本的措施。一个析因分析研究 ARDS 协作网（ARDSnet）的 244 例发生 ARDS 的外科患者，将他们分为两组，比较保守组（中心静脉压<4 mmHg，肺动脉闭塞压<8 mmHg）和积极组（中心静脉压为 10～14 mmHg，肺动脉闭塞压为 14～18 mmHg）液体复苏策略的效果。用一根肺动脉导管或者中心静脉导管用于评估患者的容量状态。这个试验证明以保守策略为目标导向的液体处理虽然没有减少死亡率，但是减少了患者的插管时间和 ICU 治疗时间。应用肺动脉导管同样对死亡率没有显著影响，但是其患者较使用中心静脉导管的患者接受了更多的液体，同时插管时间和 ICU 治疗时间都更长。

无创机械通气 vs 有创机械通气

医生在最初的评估时就应决定 ARDS 的患者是否须接受有创机械通气或是创伤较小的治疗措施。治疗重症 ARDS 患者时，机械通气仍是医生们最可靠的措施。用于评估其他重症患者气管插管的标准同样适用于 ARDS 的患者。在治疗其他原因导致的危重症过程中，越来越多的患者使用无创通气（noninvasive ventilator，NIV）技术解决了问题，对 ARDS 患者使用 NIV 策略让我们产生了疑问。零星的个案报道了无创连续气道正压通气的成功，但一项关于所有类型呼吸衰竭的多中心研究显示，ARDS 所致的所有呼吸衰竭中，使用无创通气经常是失败的独立预测因素。一个由 Ding 等进行的前瞻性队列研究显示，无创通气使超过 70% 的患者成功避免了插管，另外最终仍需插管的患者往往病情在最初几个小时就急剧恶化。这些有限的证据表明，无创通气对于非明确需要插管的患者是一个不错的尝试。然而，该策略增加了临床医生对于最初数小时内使用 NIV 无明显效果的患者的临床警惕，以及弃用 NIV 的想法。

机械通气技术

大多数中至重度 ARDS 患者最终将需要机械通气（mechanical ventilation，MV）。MV 的目的是保证充足的通气和氧合，并避免医源性肺损伤。MV 并不是一个温和的支持措施，在过去的 20 多年里，这一点得到越来越多的证实，正压通气可以导致显著的肺损伤。呼吸机相关性肺损伤（ventilator-induced lung injury，VILI）是多种因素导致的，包括容量伤（容积）、气压伤（压力）、剪切伤（循环复张 / 萎陷），以及生物伤（全身炎性介质）。无论是胸部还是肺周期性的顺应性变化，在疾病进展或缓解过程中，需要临床医生的持续关注，以防止进一步的损伤发生。此外，尽管肺血管通透性发生均匀的变化，肺部不同区域力学仍然有显著的异质性。从实践的角度来讲，肺功能的3个不同分区的概念，在理论上是有用的。这些区域包括有功能区、无功能但可复张的实质区，以及无功能也无法复张的实质区。这一原则强调有功能区适当通气、复张有顺应性的区域、避免不可复张区域的VILI。

因为较高的死亡率以及临床复杂性，ARDS成为了许多针对危重症患者进行确定性的随机对照试验的主题。对于ARDS患者而言，没有一种呼吸机模式是比其他所有模式都优越的。传统的呼吸机模式包括同步间歇指令通气（synchronized intermittent mandatory ventilation，SIMV）和辅助控制通气（assist-control ventilation，ACV），可以满足大部分患者，但是模式的选择由机构的喜好决定。对于适当潮气量下平均气道压仍不断升高的患者，常使用压力控制通气技术。更先进的呼吸机模式，比如气道压力释放通气（airway pressure release ventilation，APRV）和高频振荡通气（high-forequency oscillatory ventilation，HFOV）应用于传统通气模式无效的患者。尽管尚无证据表明使用不同的呼吸机模式对患者的预后有何影响，呼气末正压（positive end-expiratory pressure，PEEP）、潮气量和平均气道压这3个参数仍然是许多随机对照试验关注的焦点，并被认为可能改变预后。另外，调整参数最大化以减少医源性损伤，相较于处理基础疾病，起到了更重要的作用。

一项具有里程碑意义的描述最佳通气处理的试验将ARDS患者分为小潮气量组（6 ml/kg，平台压＜30 cm H_2O）和大潮气量组（12 ml/kg，平台压＜50 cm H_2O），并证实了小潮气量可以降低损伤风险。这项精心设计的研究共纳入800多例患者，并在死亡率、不使用呼吸机天数和非肺的器官功能衰竭等方面发现了显著差异，即证明了小潮气量通气的优势后提前停止了试验。小潮气量通气已经成为ARDS患者的标准治疗措施，传统的大容量通气多数情况下已经被淘汰了。一项研究使用动态CT技术证实，持续PEEP通气时，使用12ml/kg通气的患者较6 ml/kg者，可以获得更好的呼气末通气，但是增加了循环复张和萎陷。小肺泡重复的打开和关闭导致了肺泡受到剪切力影响而正常形态破坏，最终引起功能的损害，周期性肺复张及萎陷被认为是造成肺塌陷伤的关键因素。动物实验中，低潮气量和高PEEP联合用于防治剪切伤，其中PEEP似乎是两者中更重要的因素。一项使用支气管肺泡灌洗和血清试验的研究显示炎症标志物的变化并不大，证实这似乎是一个力学现象，而不涉及生物损伤。尽管有明确的证据支持小潮气量通气，但适当的或“最佳”的PEEP仍然存在一些争论。提出保持FiO_2/PEEP比例为5∶1，这样可以在ARDSnet的实验中与PEEP表一致。提到潮气量，先前讨论的疾病进程的异质性导致了显著的通气的区域差异，顺应性正常的肺组织被过度充气，而顺应性不足区域充气不足。这可能是小潮气量通气的一个优势，使“正常肺组织”部分不被损伤并保证充分的通气与氧合，并使受损的肺组织逐渐恢复。在ARDSnet研究中，气道平台压目标为小于30 cmH_2O，分别调整呼吸频率和PEEP，以获得更好的氧合和通气。这种策略下，通气常为限制因素，为获得充足的每分通气量须增加呼吸频率。允许性高碳酸血症的概念提出70 mmHg的二氧化碳分压常被良好地耐受，但这也有一些局限性。高碳酸血症是否应被允许，生理作用，包括其对于患者个体的心肌收缩力的损伤和颅内压的影响，须考虑进来。

目前适用于ARDS的循证指南是从大量人群中获得的，对于医生来讲是很有意义的。但是许多策略对于急性情况的个别患者是不适用的，须医生根据患者情况不断评估。

其他治疗

吸入性一氧化亚氮（inhaled nitric oxide，INO）疗法在20世纪90年代早期就已经应用于ARDS患者。其作用分为两方面：① INO作为一种强效的选择性血管扩张剂作用于肺组织，增加了通气区域肺组织灌注（改善了V/Q不匹配），提高了氧合，降低了肺动脉高压。② INO具有抗炎性的特性，减慢了ARDS的进展。常规的治疗浓度为1/100万～40/100万。尽管一些研究显示INO治疗早期可改善氧合，但其对住院死亡率、通气时间、不使用呼吸机天数并无显著影响。此外，似乎INO的剂量-反应曲线在ARDS中随时间变化。因此，既往研究中NO的给药方案，可能导致一氧化亚氮中毒，致使患者病情恶化。而基于Gerlach等的研究，新的给药策略可能取得更好的临床结果。INO治疗的不良反应包括肾功能不全、高铁血红蛋白血症。

自从 2001 年 Gattinoni 等提出俯卧位通气对于改善 ARDS 患者的氧合有利后，俯卧位通气，显示出其潜力。俯卧位通气通过重力影响肺泡的复张而改善患者通气 / 血流不匹配，还可以减少纵隔器官对肺的挤压。最近的一项 RCT 的 meta 分析表明，区别于 ALI（Pao_2/Fio_2 为 201～300）的患者，真正的 ARDS（$Pao_2/Fio_2<200$）患者，应用俯卧位通气时，死亡率显著降低。因此，特定的人群包括严重低氧血症（尤其 $Pao_2/Fio_2<100$）者，俯卧位通气是一种有效的治疗措施，并应当尽早实施。俯卧位通气的不良反应包括患者身上必要的插管、引流管和导管的意外脱落，压疮的发生，以及护理这种特殊情况所需要的人力。

HFOV 是另一种可以改善氧合的治疗方式，尤其在最初使用的 24 h 内。这种呼吸机模式通过小潮气量（1～5 ml/kg）、高频率（300～900 次 / 分钟）送气，可以取得持续较高的平均气道压，防止肺泡的周期性萎陷，以及减少容量伤。不幸的是，一项最大型的随机对照试验［MOAT 试验（ARDS 多中心振荡通气试验）］并没有显示出其对于死亡率有改善作用。在这一领域正在进行许多研究试验，未来 HFOV 可能会被证明有更多的益处，尤其是在早期应用于难治性低氧血症的 ARDS 患者。

部分液体通气是一种已经不在再被大家重视的非常规的 ARDS 治疗方式，但是为了文章的完整性还是囊括在这里。这种方式是利用氟碳混合物较高的氧亲和力，将其滴注入肺内尤其无通气部分来提高气体交换。这种治疗在动物实验中显示有效，但目前还没有任何人类的 RCT 显示有效。另外，与传统通气方式相比有更高的气胸、缺氧发作、低血压发生率。所以目前没有将其作为 ARDS 推荐的治疗方式。

体外膜肺氧合（extracoporeal membrane oxygenation，ECMO）是一种再度被重视的治疗方式，最初在 1990 年因为一项 RCT 显示其对死亡率无改善，它曾淡出人们视线。但是近年来科技上的进步提高了这项技术的应用，包括静脉 - 静脉通路的建立、肝素涂层的管道、低剂量肝素策略（降低出血风险），以及通气策略的改善。驱动泵将血液从股静脉泵出，通过机械膜氧合器进行气体交换，并将血液通过颈内静脉泵回体内。这种体外氧合装置允许受损肺组织以更低的潮气量和气道压来维持通气。在英国进行的 CESAR（常规机械通气 vs. 体外膜肺氧合治疗成年人重度呼吸衰竭）试验是到目前为止最具说服力的，它显示体外膜组 6 个月的无残疾生存率明显更高。ECMO 的并发症分为机械相关的和患者相关的。机械相关的并发症包括机械膜氧合器失灵、管道 / 循环中断，驱动泵或者热交换器故障，以及套管移位或者脱落。患者相关的并发症包括出血、神经系统并发症、多脏器功能衰竭、气压伤，感染，以及代谢紊乱。这种治疗需要人力，而且只能在特定的中心进行，但是对于其他治疗无效的患者确实有一定作用。

考虑到表面活性物质在新生儿 ARDS 中的益处，它对于 ARDS 患者也应有一定作用。但是，关于外源性表面活性物质的随机对照试验和 meta 分析显示其对患者的生存率或者不使用呼吸机天数并无明显改善，还证实了这种表面活性物质的治疗方法的不一致性。这可以用多种表面能活性物质制剂、剂量方案、用药方式，以及治疗时机的不同来解释。针对于最佳用药时机和患者个体化用药策略的研究将会进一步改进这种治疗，但目前还没有应用于成年人 ARDS 患者。

类固醇用于 ARDS 治疗仍是有争议的。阻断炎症级联反应一直是 ARDS 治疗的目标。用于 ARDS 的类固醇分为高剂量和低剂量两种策略，似乎是基于 ARDSnet 研究 2006 年的结果。低剂量的甲泼尼龙（2mg/kg）逐渐减量（共治疗 25 天，最后 4 天逐渐减少剂量）的方式可以取得最好效果。结果显示这种策略提高氧合、肺顺应性、不使用呼吸机天数和非休克天数，并减少血管加压药用量。不增加感染风险，但使神经肌肉无力的发生率增高。另外，类固醇没有增加 60 天或 180 天死亡率，但在 ARDS 开始后 14 天的死亡率明显升高。最近一个相关 meta 分析的作者提倡低剂量甲泼尼龙应用于 ALI 和 ARDS，因为其可改善死亡率和并发症发生率，并且没有增加明显的不良反应。

总结

ARDS 仍然是充满挑战的一个难题，有多相的病因。目前的规范治疗应该基于对于病因的识别和处理，使用小潮气量通气策略避免医源性肺损伤，为了严重疾病患者继续健全对于这类疾病的 ICU 护理措施。可以使用俯卧位通气以及类固醇阻断炎症级联反应，尤其对于通气和氧合困难的患者。APRV 和 HFOV 通气策略仅用于传统通气无效的患者，直到确切证据证明它们比目前传统策略更有效。ARDS治愈的患者可以获得很好的恢复和生存，关于这一难治性疾病仍需进一步研究，以改善难治疾病的并发症发生率和生存率。

全身炎症反应综合征和多器官功能障碍综合征：定义、诊断和处理

Gregory Tiesi, Leonard Mason, Benjamin Chandler,Anthony Watkins, David Palange 和 Edwin A. Deitch 著
吕 杰 译

1973 年，Tilney 等描述了 18 位腹主动脉瘤破裂术后发生“序贯性系统衰竭”的患者。就在这一时期，严重生理损伤可以导致多器官功能衰竭（multiple-organ failure，MOF）的概念被建立起来。几十年后，MOF［或多器官功能障碍综合征（multiple-organ dysfunction syndrome，MODS）］仍是外科监护病房（surgical intensive care units，SICUs）中主要的死亡原因和伤后致病来源。虽然这种综合征的发病机制尚未完全明确，但显然脓毒症、SIRS、ARDS、MODS是与其密切相关的。因此，本章的目的是回顾 SIRS 和 MODS，主要是关于如何诊断、治疗，以及（最重要的）预防这些综合征的策略。

发病率

创伤死亡有 3 个主要原因（出血、颅脑损伤、脓毒症 / 器官衰竭）。MODS 是晚期创伤死亡最常见因素，是研究的重点。有一些危险因素可以预测 MODS 的可能性，包括年龄、ISS，输血次数，以及乳酸或者 BD 水平。在最近的几十年，高危创伤患者 MODS 的发生率似乎在降低，因为医生对这些危险因素，包括对于休克和创伤引发的免疫炎症反应的认识提高了。例如，一项耗时 12 年的前瞻性研究，入组了 1 344 例创伤患者，得出 MODS 的发病率是 25%，比预测的要低。

这位作者总结，这种疾病的发病率降低是因为非正规输血的下降，这是 MODS、SIRS 以及死亡率的一个独立危险因素。不仅 MODS 的发病率下降了，其死亡率也下降（一项 25 年内 MODS 相关钝器多发创伤后患者死亡率的回顾性研究发现）。这项研究发现，MODS 相关的死亡率从 29% 降至 14%，下降了一半。这篇文章后边也会讨论，一些治疗上的进步促使其死亡率下降，以及器官功能障碍发生率降低。尽管有所进步，一旦确立 MODS 的诊断，其死亡风险还是很高的——患者的预后和发生衰竭的器官数量这一因素最为密切相关，包括引起 MODS 的潜在过程。

发病机制

MODS 的临床表现是由一系列炎性反应决定的，常常是感染、不能控制的炎症和严重创伤所导致的。几个不同的、相互矛盾的假说被提出来解释 MODS 潜在的机制。MODS 被看作是一种系统过程，涉及由循环因子介导的某些炎症反应的过度刺激。所述循环因子导致损伤或障碍的作用与开始的损伤无关。很多时候 MODS 中的级联事件，是通过相同的因素导致的。实际上，宿主对于损伤或者感染导致的炎性反应，相比微生物或者初始损害因素，在 SIRS、ARDS 和 MODS 中扮演了更重要的角色。这样，对于治疗和预防这种综合征而言，了解炎性反应的过程是至关重要的。

最早，伤后 MODS 报道大约一半的病例源自隐匿性腹腔内感染。然而，后来发现 50%～70% 的 MODS 患者并没有合并感染，这说明感染不是导致 MODS 的普遍原因。这个早期的工作使我们认识到，只有一小部分有脓毒症表现的患者是被感染的，患者自己对于组织损伤或者休克的反应会引起非感染性脓毒症状态。反过来我们认识到，微生物感染、组织损伤、组织坏死或者休克导致免疫炎症反应，产生的细胞因子类的免疫细胞产物促进了 MODS 的发展。

总体的假设基于过度的免疫炎症反应概念，激活的巨噬细胞和其他免疫细胞导致细胞因子介导的组织损伤，导致了 SIRS 和 MODS 的发展。这个假设基于一些实验和临床观察。例如，创伤患者的细胞因子水平增加，对人类使用肿瘤坏死因子 α

（TNF-α）引发类似SIRS的临床反应，而临床前动物实验证明TNF-α中和作用提高了这些接受致死剂量内毒素的动物的生存率。然而事情并没有这么简单，这从许多抗炎物质相关临床试验的失败和一些复杂临床前动物实验的结果可以看出。实际上，现在我们认识到，细胞因子有许多有益的功能，如控制感染。细胞因子水平升高更多地是宿主反应的预测因素或标志物而不是MODS的诱导物。

另外一种机制，失血性休克或者创伤导致的MODS是通过缺血-再灌注损伤或者微循环损伤导致的。因为休克是一种全身缺血-再灌注损伤，并且微循环损伤容易由缺血-再灌注介导，这个过程称为MODS的微循环假说。生理学上讲，循环性休克可以因总体氧输送的不足、缺血-再灌注现象或者内皮细胞-白细胞相互作用引起MODS。

尽管长时间的组织缺氧会导致腺苷三磷酸产生不足以及潜在的不可逆细胞损伤，临床上许多休克时间不够长，不足以导致这种情况的发生。临床上大多数缺血后组织损伤因获得再灌注而减轻，而这种损伤是由再灌注释放的氧自由基和促炎症反应因素（如氧化剂、氧化亚氮，趋化因子、细胞因子）引起的。实际上，研究显示再灌注诱导氧化亚氮和超氧阴离子，通过产生过氧硝酸盐（一种长期存在并强效的氧化剂，通过脂质过氧化作用造成细胞的直接伤害）协同增加细胞的损伤。增加的氧化亚氮在MODS的发病机制中发挥重要作用，这被许多临床研究证实，研究中血清硝酸盐含量（一个体内氧化亚氮水平的指数）和MODS患者的病情评分有很高的相关性。最近，缺血-再灌注损伤的研究发现损伤或者死亡细胞的产物，如高迁移率族蛋白B1（high-mobilty group box，HMGB1）以及其他再灌注损伤介导的宿主来源的分子，也可以引起细胞以及组织损伤，并加剧炎性反应。这些宿主来源的促炎症反应和组织损害分子被命名为“危险信号”或者“警报素”，是目前研究的热点。

白细胞-内皮细胞相互作用导致组织损伤，也是理解SIRS、ARDS和MODS的发病机制的关键。许多因素与休克和组织损伤有关，包括细胞因子、坏死组织、内毒素和氧化剂，可将内皮细胞从静止状态转化为促炎症及促凝的状态，并可激活中性粒细胞。这些内皮细胞表型的变化和中性粒细胞的激活，被证实共同导致了中性粒细胞粘连微循环内皮，并促进了中性粒细胞介导的血管损伤。实验证明，阻止中性粒细胞-内皮细胞的相互作用可以限制休克以及脓毒症对包括肺在内的多数脏器的损伤。另外，创伤患者的中性粒细胞激活预示着SIRS、ARDS和MODS病情的进展。由休克、脓毒症或者扩大的炎性反应引起的内皮细胞-中性粒细胞的相互作用，似乎在ARDS和MODS的发生发展中扮演重要角色。

肠道假说被用来解释30%不能确定感染部位的但死于MODS的菌血症患者的感染。很多的试验和临床研究支持这一点。例如，临床研究显示主要热损伤或者创伤后导致脓毒症的患者其肠道通透性增加，以及肠道屏障功能的丧失与发生全身感染、ARDS和MODS相关。尽管临床和试验研究表明肠道损伤和菌群易位发生于SIRS和MODS，但Moore等的一项研究开始怀疑菌群易位的临床意义。

这些研究没有在严重创伤患者，包括一个发展至MODS的亚组的患者的门脉血液内发现细菌或者内毒素。一个可能的解释是这些导致SIRS、ARDS和MODS的肠源性致病因子通过淋巴系统离开肠道。研究证明，在啮齿类动物和灵长类动物的创伤失血性休克模型中非细菌性因素离开缺血性肠道，导致ARDS、MODS、中性粒细胞激活，以及内皮细胞损伤/活化，这一理论使肠道-淋巴假说产生。此MODS的肠道淋巴假说提出由受损肠道释放出的非细菌性、非细胞因子性因素，通过淋巴系统激活中性粒细胞和内皮细胞，导致了器官功能障碍。过去的几年里肠道假说已经被扩展，不仅局限于菌群易位，也代表肠源性非细菌性促炎症反应和组织损伤因子在SIRS、ARDS和MODS发病机制中的重要作用。

尽管每一种MODS的假说都是被单独提出，对于患者来讲，许多假说是重叠的，每一种假说在发展中都会牵动其他假说的发生。例如，严重细菌感染激活了免疫炎症反应，后者又导致了微循环障碍和肠道缺血。这样，肠源性非细菌性因素导致了中性粒细胞激活，加重了炎性反应和微循环障碍。休克状态与微循环衰竭、肠道损伤、炎性反应的诱导，以及白细胞-内皮细胞的相互作用有关。另外，许多发生MODS的患者并无一个明确的主要事件，而与多个小的损害有关。

这个临床观察提出了MODS的“二次打击”学说，即温和的临床初期事件刺激了患者，导致患者对后续的继发事件的反应放大，最终引起SIRS、ARDS和MODS。此外，休克后的免疫抑制状态，称为代偿性抗炎症反应综合征（compensatory anti-inflammatory response syndrome，CARS）。CARS造成重症患者感染的增加。尽管二次打击理论还需要进一步研究，但很容易理解，创伤或者烧伤如何将非致命的感染或者低氧血症变成非常致命的损伤。实际上，图 1 很清楚地解释了寻救有效预防和治疗 MODS 的困难在于被创伤和休克激活的多个系统的重叠效应，以及一个系统引起其他系统的更严重的继发性生理效应。但是，这些研究获得的炎症和 MODS 相关的知识对治疗的理解产生了非常重要的影响，如重视充足和及时的容量复苏和微循环血流以阻止器官低灌注、早期切除不可再生组织、限制全身炎症，以及保护肠道屏障和限制难以控制的炎症。

诊断

治疗一种疾病的关键是诊断。为此召开了许多会议，为了 SIRS、ARDS 和 MODS 的诊断，提出各种分类方案。SIRS 是对于各种严重的临床损害产生的全身炎性反应，对它的诊断应符合所列的 4 个条件中的 2 个及以上（表 1）。尽管这些 SIRS 的诊断标准被认为过于灵敏而不够特异，但 SIRS 应被视为一种发展的动态过程，并且反应宿主在大多数情况下且适应生活的价值。它是身体对伤害或外部威胁如细菌感染的反应。然而，如果这种保护性的炎症反应变得失控或者过度，会对患者自身组织造成损伤，产生适应不良的影响。

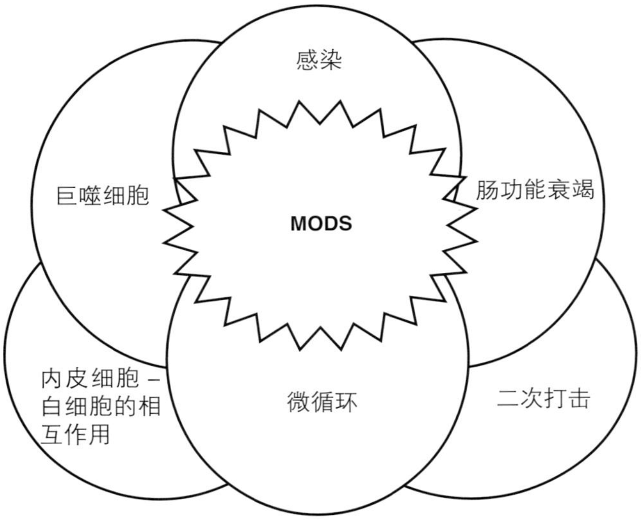

图 1 多重假设的重叠作用被认为是导致 MODS 的原因

术语“MODS”源自于美国胸内科医师学会（American College of Chest Physicians，ACCP）和美国重症医学协会（Society of Critical Care Medicine，SCCM）1991 年的联合会议。在那之前，这种疾病有许多称号，包括序贯性器官功能障碍综合征与多器官功能衰竭综合征。一些 MODS 评分系统建立起来，对 MODS 的严重程度分级，强调疾病过程中存在从轻度到完全功能障碍的不同程度，在一些患者中，它们与死亡率和发生率有关（表 2）。

这些系统，就像 Vincent 等制订的序贯性器官衰竭评分，通过分配不同的数值尺度来评估器官衰竭，某器官功能障碍越重，分配的分数越高。这些分数可以每天计算，来评估病情的恶化或改善和器官功能障碍的进展或者缓解。虽然不能预测个体患者的

表 1 全身炎性反应综合征定义

体温＞38 ℃或者＜36 ℃
心率＞90 次 / 分
呼吸频率＞20 或者 $Paco_2$＜32 mmHg（＜4.3 KPa）
白细胞计数＞12 × 10^9/L 或者 ＜4 × 10^9/L；未成熟细胞＞10%

bpm，次 / 分；RR，呼吸频率；WBC，白细胞

表 2 多器官功能障碍评分的对比

系统	Brussels 评分	MODS 评分	LOD 评分	SOFA 评分
呼吸系统	Pao_2/Fio_2	Pao_2/Fio_2	Pao_2/Fio_2	Pao_2/Fio_2
心血管系统	动脉压对液体的反应性酸中毒	与血压适应的心率	动脉压 心率	动脉压 血管活性药物
肾功能	肌酐	肌酐	肌酐、尿素、尿量	肌酐、尿量
血液系统	血小板	血小板	血小板、白细胞	血小板
肝功能	胆红素	胆红素	胆红素、PT	胆红素
神经系统	GCS	GCS	GCS	GCS

GCS，格拉斯哥昏迷等级评分；LOD，逻辑器官功能障碍；MODS，多器官功能障碍综合征；PT，凝血酶原时间；SOFA，序贯性器官衰竭评分；UO，尿量

病死率，但这类评分系统对于评估危重患者的病情和治疗是有帮助的。这些帮助包括每天对患者治疗反应性的评估、对流行病学研究的帮助、对临床试验中新疗法的评估。虽然这些评分系统使用略微不同的参数来分级器官衰竭，但大多数研究发现，这些评分系统的临床应用是有可比性的。

处理

目前，对于MODS的治疗主要是对症治疗和对于衰竭器官的支持。因为MODS没有“治愈”的方法，所以一旦MODS出现——特别是由于出现MODS的患者死亡率很高——预防就成为高风险的创伤患者的关键。因此，理解和使用某些可以减少MODS发生风险的策略和方法是很重要的。创伤患者应快速转运至医疗机构，预防应开始于现场，并贯穿于整个复苏、手术和ICU治疗期间（表3）。因为在患者护理的不同阶段使用的方法和策略可能有所不同，故每个阶段单独讨论，但在实际临床实践中这些阶段往往会发生重叠。

表3 器官功能衰竭的预防

复苏阶段
休克复苏
碱剩余和乳酸监测
限制性输血策略
手术阶段
警惕损伤遗漏
损伤控制性剖腹术
早期固定骨折
ICU阶段
感染相关问题
早期营养支持和血糖控制
特殊器官支持
认识腹腔隔室综合征
药物治疗

ICU，重症监护病房

复苏阶段

复苏阶段的中心目标是有效血容量的恢复、微循环血流量的优化（因此优化组织灌注）和预防/限制缺血-再灌注损伤。随着认识到休克会导致一个全身性的缺血再灌注损伤以及直接和间接导致细胞和器官损伤，充分的容量复苏以及更有效的复苏液体得到越来越多的重视。然而，复苏的主要终点仍然存在争议。碱剩余和乳酸水平、氧输送、胃粘膜pH、肺动脉导管无创监测都被用来尝试优化容量复苏。

血压和尿量可能不能准确地反映严重创伤患者容量复苏的水平，而动脉碱剩余和血清乳酸水平被证明是监测复苏的重要标志物。碱剩余或血清乳酸水平的升高与持续失血或容量复苏不足相关，这些参数的改善提示容量复苏是充分的。因为在严重受伤的患者，容量复苏阶段可能持续48 h，连续测量很重要。一些前瞻性试验表明，48 h内清除患者的碱剩余和乳酸，可以降低ARDS和MODS的发病率，并提高生存率，复苏的目标应该是降低并控制碱剩余低于–2 mmol/L，血清乳酸含量低于1.5 mEq/L。

随着对乳酸林格氏液会加剧促炎症反应并导致休克状态时器官损伤加重的认识，复苏液体的选择成为一个比较有争议的话题。鉴于这些问题，加上近年来认识到大量使用晶体液进行容量复苏与ACS的发生发展有关，创伤患者早期复苏时，葡聚糖、高渗盐水和胶体等其他替代品重新进入人们的视野。目前，由于缺乏临床试验，没有足够的数据来确定哪种液体更适用于创伤患者的容量复苏。另一种方法是使用含有抗氧化剂的复苏液体，共有3项临床试验，包括一项前瞻性随机试验，表明抗氧化治疗有助于创伤患者预防MODS。随着对新型复苏液体药理学（即肠道保护、免疫调节）研究的继续，患者早期复苏液体由乳酸林格氏液发展为其他液体类型是可能的。

基于临床试验，创伤患者的输血也在临床研究的基础上被不断地重新评估，输血会导致免疫抑制，并且是MODS的独立危险因素，尤其是输注超过2周的陈旧血。鉴于这些，加上ICU患者和创伤患者在血红蛋白水平在7 g/dl以上的处理都是相对安全的，导致选择性输血策略的出现，其中贫血患者预防性输血不再作为常规。事实上，重症监护中的输血需求（Transfusion Requirements in Critical Care，TRICC）研究证实，在重症监护室中血红蛋白浓度低于7 g/dl时再行输血，可以减轻新的器官功能障碍。因此，基于临床上贫血患者预防性输注RBC治疗的临床疗效的现有的文献，可以得到2个结论：①预防性输注红细胞，将血红蛋白提高至高于 7 g/dl，并不能改善危重患者的组织氧消耗，无论是在全身水平或微循环水平；②预防性输注红细胞，不能改善危重患者的临床预后，并可能导致一些亚组患者的预后更差。最后，在患者大出血时，自由地输血并使用大量输血策略（massive transfusion protocol，MTPs）来输注大量的血液制品对患者的临床预后有利。进一步深入探讨见章节“输血：创伤救治中血液和血液制品的管理”。

手术干预

在 MODS 的一篇早期里程碑式的文章中，Eiseman 等描述了 42 例发生 MODS 的外科患者，其中 24 例由于术中或术后管理不当发展为 MODS。这项研究强调了创伤患者围术期护理的重要的一点：创伤患者常发生损伤的漏诊，而且这是发展为 SIRS、MODS 和死亡的重要危险因素。虽然创伤患者手术监护的细节覆盖了很多方面，但其中某些方面对于 MODS 是非常重要的。其中一个例子是损伤控制性剖腹术（damage-control laparotomy，DCL）的使用可以限制急性和延迟性 MODS 的发生。尽管 2010 年的 Cochrane 对于 DCL 的综述发现，没有随机对照试验比较腹部创伤患者 DCL 和即刻确定性手术。目前的标准治疗是，对于不稳定的患者，为避免复杂手术操作，可在 ICU 成功复苏后行再次分期手术。在一些研究中，避免“致死三联征”的酸中毒、低温、凝血功能障碍，防止不可逆的生理损伤和随后的 MODS 的发生发展，可使患者获得明显的生存获益。

另一个可以减少 ARDS 和 MODS 发生率的例子是长骨骨折的早期固定手术。大量的前瞻性和回顾性临床研究报道了所谓的“骨科损伤控制”，发现早期固定长骨骨折比晚期固定骨折，可以改善患者的早期活动、提高肺的清洁能力、降低全身炎症反应及血栓形成事件的发生率、降低患者并发症发生率和死亡率，以及减少医院资源的消耗。尽管固定手术会使患者暴露于再次损害，可能会增加胸部创伤患者 ARDS 的发生率或加重疑似脑损伤患者的病情。但是即使对于这些高危患者，早期确定性固定术的并发症发生率相比延期固定术患者，也是低的。

ICU 处理阶段

术后及外伤后 MODS 可以通过某些策略来阻止，如持续复苏、感染相关并发症的管理，早期营养和特定器官的支持治疗。虽然有些器官（如肺系统）有随机的前瞻性数据支持某些治疗，以改善临床结果，但其他系统（如肝系统）很少需要具体的治疗。这部分，我们关注研究预防和治疗策略以期减少 MODS 的发病率或者改善 MODS 患者的预后（表 3 和表 4）。

因为感染会加快 MODS 的发展，增加患者死亡率，故我们应谨记一些关键的措施来阻止感染相关的 MODS。对怀疑肺炎的患者早期经验性应用抗生素很重要，因为已经证明早期足量应用抗生素可以降低肺炎相关的死亡率。第二种方法是预防性应用抗生素方案，涉及选择性肠道去污（selective digestive decontamination，SDD）和选择性口咽去污（selective oropharyngeal decontamination，SOD）。SDD 过程包括口咽部应用不被吸收的抗菌膏和口服不被吸收的抗生素进入胃肠道，并全身使用针对革兰氏阳性菌的抗生素。而相较于 SDD，SOD 不涉及全身抗生素的应用。尽管两者在美国的应用都不是非常普遍，但是这两种方案都能减少创伤和外科重症患者的感染发生率和病死率。口咽部和肠道细菌是引起肺炎和菌血症的主要细菌来源，这是这 2 种杀菌方式的理论基础。通过控制口咽部和胃肠道细菌的过度生长，感染的发生率和病死率均会降低。一项大型随机多中心的研究证实，应用 SOD 和 SDD 会提高生存率，并降低 ICU 获得性菌血症的发生。SOD 更易被接受，因其不须全身应用抗生素。这种方式并没有被广泛应用的原因是因其非常耗费人力，并且近期才被证明可以提高生存率。

表 4　ICU 中降低病死率和减轻器官功能障碍的干预

目标	干预
复苏	早期目标导向性复苏
预防	SDD/SOD
ICU 支持治疗	限制性输血策略 小潮气量通气策略 每日唤醒 血糖控制 肠内营养 补硒
调节靶向治疗	活化蛋白 C 低剂量类固醇治疗（+/-）

ICU，重症监护病房；SDD，选择性肠道去污；SOD，选择性口咽去污

术后或创伤后发生MODS，应仔细搜寻感染源，尤其注意伤口、切口、以前的损伤或手术部位、静脉导管部位，因为隐匿性感染引起ARDS和MODS并不少见。尽管对于严重脓毒症的各种药物治疗的研究非常多，但除了活化蛋白C外，其他免疫调节剂的相关试验结果都是不乐观的。一项前瞻性随机试验表明，重组形式的活化蛋白C提高了患者28天的生存率，并促进严重脓毒症患者的心血管、呼吸和血液功能障碍更迅速地恢复。活化蛋白C有效的原因是，它同时具有抗凝血和抗炎活性，可以保护微循环并限制炎症反应，这可能是其他药剂不具备的。最后，当脓毒症休克患者对于血管加压药和液体治疗不敏感时，长期低剂量类固醇治疗仍是维持血压的一个有效的手段。早期的研究表明这种方法可以提高生存率，但这还没有被最近的前瞻性临床研究验证。因此，虽然低剂量类固醇治疗继续应用于难治性感染性休克患者，但其最终对总体生存率的影响可能是有限的。除了感染问题，其他非器官特异的治疗似乎也是有益的，包括早期肠内营养、血糖控制，床头抬高，并对机械通气镇静的患者实施每日唤醒。早期肠内营养的概念是基于限制肠源性脓毒症的概念，因为恢复喂养的肠道更能耐受肠道诱导的损伤，并且肠外营养与肠道黏膜萎缩、通透性增加和屏障功能的丧失密切相关。多个前瞻性随机对照试验证实，早期肠内营养可以有效减少感染相关的并发症，缩短ICU治疗时间和总住院天数，虽然它似乎并没有提高生存率。因此，为进一步提高肠内营养的作用，一系列免疫增强型肠内营养配方出现，并在创伤和ICU的患者中试用。一些研究比较了免疫增强型肠内营养和普通类型的产品，发现免疫增强型肠内营养可以减少感染相关并发症。当对饮食和饮食补充剂的确切成分进行分析时，可提出一些临床建议。随机临床研究显示，这些营养策略改善高危患者的死亡率和并发症发生率。这些临床策略包括静脉使用硒（400～1000 μg/d）含或不含维生素C（1.5～3 g/d）和维生素E（50 mg/d，口服），肠外谷氨酰胺，如丙氨酰胺谷氨酸胺（0.50 g/kg·d），并使用静脉ω-3脂肪酸或口服含有较高ω-3脂肪酸水平的肠内饮食。虽然这些营养物质提高患者生存率的相关机制仍有待确定，但已经证明它们可以减少氧化剂介导的组织损伤并支持免疫系统。因此，早期肠内营养加硒、维生素C、维生素E、静脉谷氨酰胺和ω-3脂肪酸似乎是限制MODS发展的一种成功的方法。

代谢方面很重要的另一点是严格控制血糖，使用胰岛素以保持血糖水平低于120 mg/dl。自从最初的前瞻性随机对照研究显示，严格的血糖控制（120 mg/dl）与更宽松的血糖控制方案（<215 mg/dl）相比，患者在存活上有优势。之后其他的研究，包括几个系统综述和meta分析得出，使用强化胰岛素治疗严格控制血糖的、与之前研究不同的结论。最近，一项最大的随机的国际多中心试验显示，使用强化胰岛素方案会增加患者90天死亡率和严重低血糖的发生率。因此，保持严格的正常血糖的概念（81～108 mg/dl）可能不像以前认为的那样，对危重患者是有益的。基于这些最新的研究结果，考虑到严格控制血糖的不利影响，建议使用更宽松的血糖控制目标（180 mg/dl）。

其他易于实施的ICU治疗也已被证明可以减少相关并发症。例如，在机械通气的危重患者中每天中断镇静治疗，可降低ICU住院时间和并发症发生率，而将机械通气患者的床头抬高，可以降低肺炎的发生率并有助于保护患者的肺功能。

除了床头抬高和每日镇静中断治疗外，在过去的几年里，呼吸衰竭患者的其他护理措施也取得了一定进展。其中最重要的是认识到高潮气量和气道压力增加，通过诱导肺部炎症会引起肺损伤，而不是预防肺损伤，这个过程被称为呼吸机相关性肺损伤（ventilator-induced lung injury，VILI）。与这种生理概念一致，多中心随机对照试验证实，ARDS以及急性肺损伤的机械通气患者，较低的潮气量（即6 mg/kg）比之传统潮气量通气方案能更少地引起促炎症反应介质的局部和全身释放，并降低患者死亡率。此外，进一步的临床试验证实，当保持气道平台压小于30 cmH_2O时，无论是较低还是较高的PEEP水平，在急性肺损伤和ARDS患者的临床试验当中，结果是近似的。

尽管在小潮气量通气和允许性高碳酸血症的情况下可以维持患者氧合，而且CO_2的升高是以降低通气为代价，但这些似乎也是无害的。使用小潮气量通气并维持气道平台压小于30 cmH_2O，可以预防及治疗急性肺损伤和ARDS。很多通气策略（吸入氧化亚氮和HFOV）证明了它们可以提高ARDS患者的氧合，然而这些并没有提高患者的生存率。最近的一个meta分析证明，俯卧位通气对于ALI和严重低氧血症患者来说，可以显著提高他们的生存率。因此，俯卧位通气被建议用于难治性低氧血症的患者，尤其对于使用其他特殊治疗手段受限的一些中心。

肾替代治疗通过调节容量和电解质平衡，对于治疗 MODS 是有效的。肾替代治疗还可以清除患者体内毒素和循环的炎性介质。一些支持肾功能的方法，如预防性应用小剂量多巴胺，未被证明是有效的。目前预防肾衰竭最好的办法是避免低容量复苏以及对于感染性并发症的快速诊断和治疗。一旦肾衰竭已经发生，持续静脉静脉血液透析似乎优于动脉静脉血液透析，因为它不需要全身抗凝，并且不易引起衰弱患者的低血压事件。

近期认识到对于 MODS 很重要的一个措施是治疗 ACS。ACS 可以看作 MODS 中一个可逆的过程，是腹内压增高引起的。随着腹内压增高，腹腔内脏灌注降低、通气受损、心排血量下降。临床上，ACS 表现为尿量减少、通气不足和气道压峰值升高和低血压。ACS 风险最高的是那些患有多发创伤、大出血、大容量复苏伴长时间手术，以及腹腔内填塞以控制出血的患者。

ACS 也发生在严重出血性休克的患者，即使没有腹部或者腹膜后的损伤也会发生，这种现象被认为是继发 ACS。继发 ACS 是休克患者毛细血管渗漏并接受了大量晶体液复苏，而导致的内脏和腹膜水肿所引起的。ACS 的诊断是通过膀胱内置入 Foley 导管来测量腹腔压力来确定的，当压力大于 25 mm Hg，发生渐进性器官功能障碍（进行复苏的前提下，尿量少于 0.5ml/kg · h 或 Pao_2/Fio_2＜150 或气道压峰值大于 45 cmH_2O 或心脏指数小于 3 L/min · m^2），并且外科腹腔减压术可以改善脏器功能，可被认为是 ACS。外科治疗，包括持续性腹腔开放，大多数情况下可以快速并彻底地纠正这种病理状态。如果不治疗，ACS 的致死性极高，死亡率接近 100%。

总结和原则

SIRS 和 MODS 对于创伤患者而言是很常见的。随着对免疫炎症系统和发病机制研究的深入，现在已经出现了一些有效的治疗和预防措施。这些进一步降低了 MODS 的发病率，并提高了 MODS 患者的生存率。用来达到这些目的的策略，包括预防和治疗，应在复苏阶段开始并贯穿于整个手术和 ICU 阶段中（图 2）。

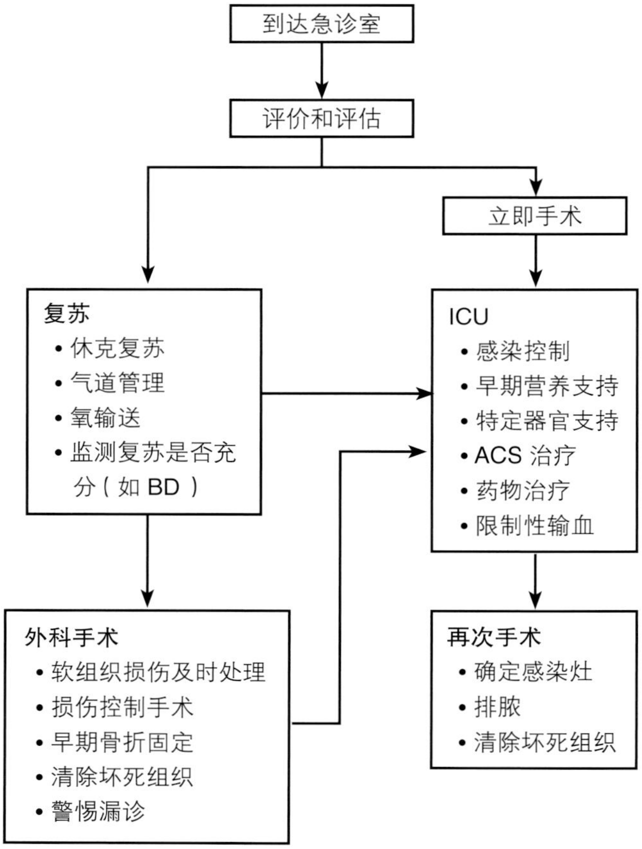

图 2　预防和治疗多器官功能障碍的流程。ACS: 腹腔隔室综合征；BD：碱缺失；ICU：重症监护病区

脓毒症、感染性休克及其治疗

Corrado Paolo Marini, Gary Lombardo, Anthony Policastro 和 Dimitryi Karev 著
吕　杰 译

在美国，每年大约有 750 000 例菌血症，造成约 275 000 例严重脓毒症和感染性休克，造成的死亡率为 20%～30%。脓毒症仍是 ICU 死亡的首要原因，不幸的是，脓毒症的发生原因正在增加，包括人口老龄化、脓毒症患者合并症增加、细胞毒性和免疫抑制药物的使用，更重要的是，耐药菌的出现。创伤患者的严重脓毒症和感染性休克的发病率增加，是由于一些危险因素的增多，包括高龄创伤患者术后合并症增多，而且随着治疗的进步，更多创伤患者存活下来继而其发生感染的概率也相应升高。另外，创伤患者发生严重脓毒症和感染性休克越来越多地是因为中枢神经系统损伤、钝性胸部外伤后的肺挫伤、术前休克、频繁输血，以及其带来的免疫抑制效应。

感染性休克是一系列事件的最后阶段，从感染到菌血症、脓毒症、严重脓毒症，最终是感染性休克。这一连续过程的特点是与全身炎性反应综合征（systemic inflammatory response syndrome，SIRS）相关的一些特征——体温高于 38℃或低于 36℃，心率＞90 次 / 分，呼吸频率＞20 次 / 分或者 $Paco_2$＜32 mmHg，白细胞计数大于 12 000 个 / 立方毫米或者小于 4000 个 / 立方毫米或者占总细胞的比例大于 10%——会发生器官功能障碍、低血压和灌注不足，并可根据乳酸水平升高、尿量减少以及精神状态变化来判断。最后，患者经过充足的液体复苏仍表现出持续性低血压（SBP＜90 mmHg），或者是需要强心剂和血管加压药才能维持正常血压。从 SIRS 转化为严重脓毒症以及感染性休克是由于氧供需平衡的失衡和它导致的不同器官灌注不足的程度不同，最后导致全身组织缺氧、乳酸水平升高。脓毒症的氧代谢在病理生理学中的新概念正在形成。

尽管只有 4% 的患者由 SIRS 发展到感染性休克，但 71% 的培养阳性的感染性休克患者从开始就已经确诊，只是处于疾病进程中相对比较温和的阶段。由于这个原因，识别可能发展为严重脓毒症和感染性休克的患者的早期轻型的脓毒症是非常重要的。但还不清楚的是，患者发展为严重脓毒症和感染性休克时，哪种生物标志物具有最佳的预测值，并可以对这些患者的区分起到帮助，以进行早期目标导向性治疗（early goal -directed therapy，EGDT），来阻止晚期成熟的分布性休克。一旦发展到这种情况，我们认为多数时候很难成功救治。

至少有 3 种类型的疾病，如果早期诊断并实施及时的治疗会对整体死亡率和患者的功能预后有益处，它们是心肌梗死、脑卒中和创伤。有一点是有目共睹的，那就是及时的治疗是治疗策略中最重要的。与严重脓毒症和感染性休克患者有关的一个重要问题是：是否有证据表明他们的治疗应遵循类似于心肌梗死和卒中患者的时效性治疗的方法，以及是否在细胞和分子水平有充足的证据以支持 Rivers 等关于 EGDT 的作用的发现。EGDT 是否影响了炎性反应而与抗感染治疗无关？通过利用静脉血氧饱和度（Svo_2）和乳酸等反应氧输送和心排血量变化的相关指标进行治疗，以使细胞质和线粒体获得氧是否是严重脓毒症和感染性休克患者治疗成功的关键？我们的意见是脓毒症患者应接受及时的治疗，这与治疗脑卒中、心肌梗死和创伤的特点没什么不同。尽管对于这 3 种疾病来讲，前两者治疗的时间窗已经被明确界定，而脓毒症患者并没有。这一章，我们将重点集中在识别脓毒症患者（可能发展为严重脓毒症和感染性休克者，且不一定是创伤患者）在细胞和分子水平研究脓毒症患者时，使用时效性很窄的方法证实 EGDT 的效果和有适用于所有脓毒症患者的专门的治疗流程。

诊断

对于创伤患者而言，诊断感染、严重脓毒症和感染性休克是很困难的，因为多数时候在未感染创伤患者出现 SIRS 的体征也很普遍。引起创伤患者产生脓毒症的常见原因包括：机械通气时间过长导致的呼吸机相关性肺炎、导管相关血流感染，以及胃肠道损伤或者实质脏器损伤的患者接受剖腹术后导致的腹腔感染。对于可能感染和发生脓毒症的患者而言，有一个重要问题，那就是低血压是否是组织灌注不足的一个足够敏感的监测指标？它是否可

以区分患者是感染还是脓毒症，严重脓毒症还是感染性休克？许多研究认为乳酸水平较低血压等一些其他指标更好，因为它对于区分患者从脓毒症到严重脓毒症及感染性休克的发展阶段和预测脓毒症相关病死率更有优势。尽管阴离子间隙和碱剩余也常用于对创伤患者进行危险分层，但已经证实它们不够敏感。当平均乳酸水平为 4 或 7 mmol/L 时，分别有 22% 或 25% 的患者阴离子间隙和碱剩余表现为正常值。似乎当乳酸水平超过 10 mmol/L 时，阴离子间隙、碱剩余和乳酸之间的差异会消失。乳酸是独立于血压之外的一个对于预测组织缺氧和疾病严重程度非常有效的临床指标。以前有研究证明，符合 SIRS 标准的患者，乳酸水平大于 4 mmol/L 时，血压正常患者的 ICU 住院率和死亡率显著增加。在 ICU 中，乳酸可以像在急诊一样，2 min 测一次，并且当止血带使用时间较短时，静脉乳酸水平可以代替动脉乳酸水平。所以动脉或者静脉乳酸水平应该在脓毒症患者中进行检测，以区分须进行 EGDT 的脓毒症，来阻止其发展为 MODS。

持续升高的乳酸水平对于预测死亡率而言，比氧运输相关变量（氧输送、氧消耗，氧摄取比）更优。Bakker 等将“乳酸时间”定义为乳酸保持在 2 mmol/L 以上的时间，并且发现乳酸酸中毒的持续时间可预测器官衰竭和患者生存水平。乳酸水平 24 h 内恢复正常的患者（乳酸时间大于 24 h），患者生存率可达 100%，而乳酸升高超过 6 h 则提示患者死亡率增高。另外，术后血流动力学稳定的患者，乳酸浓度升高大于 48 h 也会有较高的死亡率。以我们的经验而言，乳酸清除时间延长与外科患者死亡率增加有关。实际上，如果患者不能将乳酸降至正常水平，死亡率将达 100%。当怀疑患者感染时，应在培养皿中培养，比如尿培养、体液培养、痰培养、脑脊液培养，包括两组血培养，并且测量动脉或者静脉乳酸。如果乳酸水平升高，应想到患者有从感染到严重脓毒症和感染性休克进展的风险。因此，在经验性广谱抗感染治疗前，EGDT 应尽早开展来尽量缩短“乳酸时间”。

脓毒症中乳酸的产生

要理解应用乳酸对脓毒症患者进行危险分层并监测对治疗的反应，以及脓毒症患者血乳酸升高的致病机制，就必须先了解乳酸产生的生化途径。在正常情况下，胞质内的氧分压达 6 mmHg 和线粒体氧分压达 1.2 mmHg 时，会产生正常的有氧糖酵解。来自无氧糖酵解的丙酮酸盐，进一步氧化分解生成乙酰辅酶 A，在线粒体中进入 Krebs 循环（三羧酸循环）。未发生脓毒症时，微循环通过多种机制调节，包括机体毛细血管密度和器官供氧量 / 需氧量的匹配。

如图 1 所示，无氧糖酵解期间有 3 个耗能、限速的步骤。它们分别与葡萄糖外激酶、磷酸果糖激酶和丙酮酸激酶有关。磷酸果糖激酶是无氧糖酵解的“起搏器”，因为它发挥了最主要的限速作用。它是糖酵解途径中第一个不可逆反应，被称之为关键步骤。这个过程主要是将 6- 磷酸果糖磷酸化为 1,6- 二磷酸果糖。这样，磷酸果糖激酶成为无氧糖酵解的主要控制点或起搏器。它的作用受到细胞能量水平（腺苷三磷酸的水平）、细胞液 pH 值、可用的柠檬酸含量、热休克蛋白、内毒素和特殊基因的影响。尽管脓毒症患者中乳酸水平升高是因为缺氧，还是因为活跃的糖酵解产生了过多的丙酮酸，超过了丙酮酸脱氢酶产生乙酰辅酶 A 的能力，进而使丙酮酸转化为乳酸这个问题还存在争论。但最终的结果就是丙酮酸不能储存而转化为乳酸，使得乳酸产物增多。图 2 是另外 2 种的更有效丙酮酸转化途径：①丙酮酸通过乳酸脱氢酶转化为等摩尔的乳酸，同时乳酸在肝和肾皮质通过 Cori 循环转化为葡萄糖；②丙酮酸接受一个氨基，通过转氨基作用转化为丙氨酸，这样它们就可以进入 Krebs 循环。通常成比例的丙酮酸转化为乳酸不会改变细胞质 pH，导致细胞酸中毒。然而了解乳酸过量伴有或不伴有酸中毒的区别是非常重要的（图 3）。

乳酸是一种低 pKa（3.86）的弱酸，在水中部分解离，产生乳酸离子和 H^+。与环境 pH 值有关，乳酸在低 pH 条件下呈非解离状态，在高 pH 条件下呈离子状态。在生理情况下，pH 值一般高于 pKa，所以人体内的大部分乳酸都以游离的形式存在。目前认为乳酸 / 丙酮酸（L/P）的比值反映了 NADH/NAD 的比值，NAD 即烟酰胺腺嘌呤二核苷酸。正常情况下，细胞能量水平在正常状态，也就是说 NADH/NAD 比值是正常的，L/P 的比值小于 20。当乳酸水平与丙酮酸成比例增加，且比例小于 20 时，有足够的能量保证腺苷二磷酸、无机磷酸盐和氢离子来合成 ATP。这样细胞内液内氢离子和 pH 就没有发生变化。相反，当 L/P 的比值＞20 时，细胞能量水平损伤。ATP 水解为腺苷二磷酸、无机磷酸盐，氢离子浓度增加，导致细胞酸中毒。随后，ADP 水解为腺苷一磷酸，然后腺苷会导致毛细血管前括约肌松

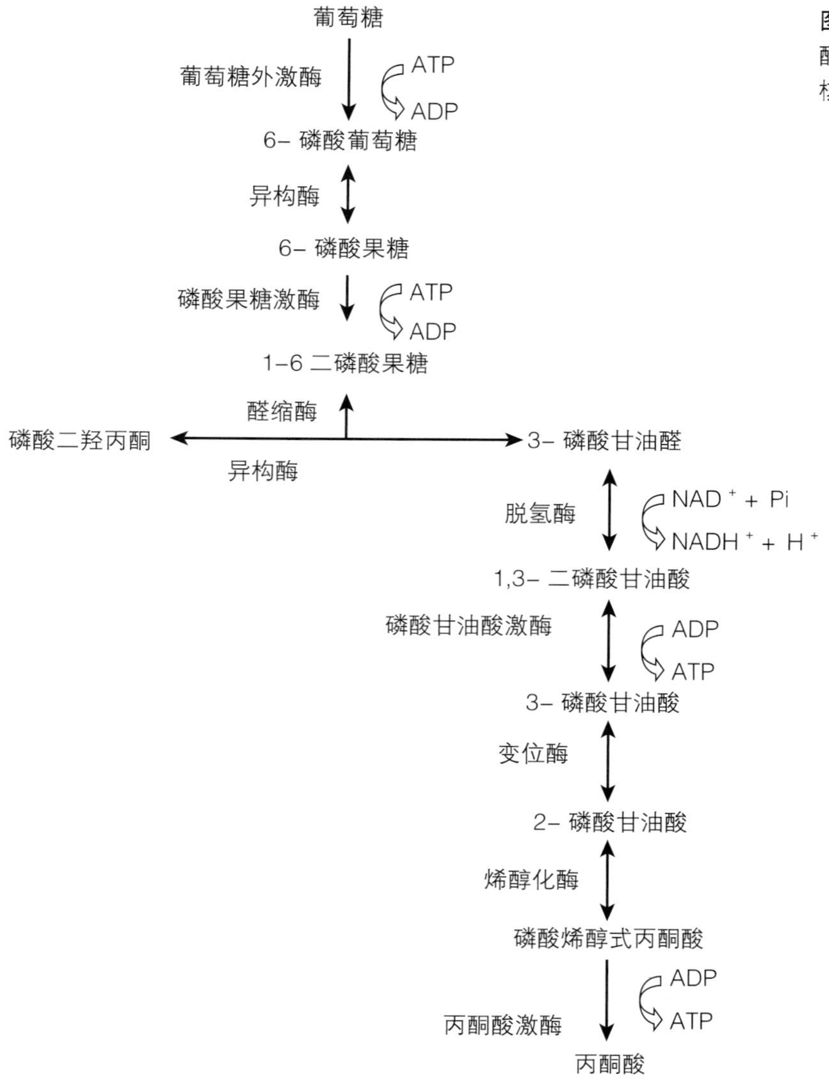

图 1　糖酵解途径及限速环节。ADP，腺苷二磷酸；ATP，腺苷三磷酸；NAD，烟酰胺腺嘌呤二核苷酸；NADH，还原型烟酰胺腺嘌呤二核苷酸

弛、增加功能毛细血管密度、使局部血流和氧气能恢复氧化还原电位和细胞 pH 值。

图 4 展示了氧输送、氧摄取和氧消耗的关系。正常情况下，当氧输送降低时氧消耗可以通过提高氧摄取而保持不变。然而，当氧摄取比例达到 60% 即无氧阈，氧输送和氧消耗成线性相关，患者处于供应依赖性氧消耗状态，并产生乳酸。氧输送的进一步增加或减少将伴随着氧消耗的增加或减少。虽然当氧摄取率达到 60%，达到无氧阈，产生乳酸，但这并不是机体最大的摄取比例（80%）。Do_2/Vo_2 曲线的斜率在脓毒症患者中会不会改变，使氧输送临界水平右移，这个问题已经被讨论了很多年，仍没有结果。在重症患者中使氧摄取比例正常化的必要性一直存在争议。如图 4 所示，供应依赖性氧消耗在氧摄取率达到 60% 以前都可以维持。增加氧摄取比例使其达到供应依赖性状态氧消耗的患者相较于通过治疗，使氧摄取比例恢复正常状态的患者更容易发展为 MODS？高氧摄取比的脏器，如心脏，可以通过提高血流保持氧消耗供应。低氧摄取比例的器官，如肾，可以通过增加氧摄取比例保持正常氧耗。总体氧摄取比例的增加，导致器官氧供需的不平衡，是否会激活炎性反应导致 MODS？

正常摄取比例和乳酸升高

当微循环水平（容易产生乳酸的区域）的氧供需平衡被打破，脓毒症开始的时候，氧摄取比例正常而乳酸水平升高的现象可以出现。在脓毒症晚期可以见到这种分布异常：其特点为高动力的血液动力循环状态下，需氧量小的区域获得较多的氧输送，而需氧量较大的区域只有较少的氧输送。正常的摄取比例通常不会发生乳酸升高，因为25%的氧摄取比例低于产生乳酸的无氧阈值。然而，尽管总体摄取率可能是正常的，局部器官的摄取比例可能已经达到了无氧阈值，而产生乳酸。所以，当氧摄取率正常而乳酸水平升高时，临床医生必须判断，在Svo_2和氧摄取比例正常的情况下，躯体的哪部分正在发生缺氧。低剂量、短半衰期血管舒张剂，比如前列腺素类（PGI_2、PGE_2），或者硝酸甘油可以通过改变微循环的功能性毛细血管密度来揭示正在加重的氧债，重新调整器官的氧供需平衡。有反应的患者，氧摄取比例增加，乳酸水平下降。反应不佳者，乳酸会继续升高，静脉血氧饱和度不变，预示着线粒体水平的氧使用存在着不可逆的损伤。

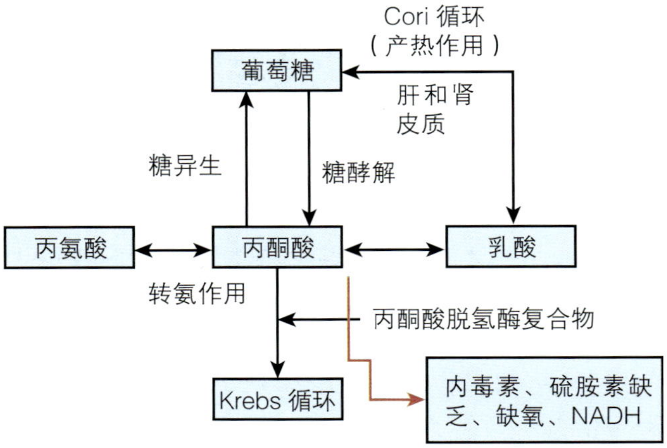

图2 丙酮酸代谢途径。如果丙酮酸脱氢（PDH）复合物被内毒素、硫胺素缺乏或者细胞缺氧所限制，丙酮酸的产生将增加。这一点独立于其诱发原因，将激活不同的转化机制，因为它不能被储存。丙酮酸可以通过乳酸脱氢酶转化为乳酸，乳酸在肝内和肾皮质内会通过Cori循环转化为葡萄糖。这个生化反应不使用或产生能量，但必然产生热量。通常情况下，丙酮酸与乳酸的成比例的转换不会导致细胞质内pH的变化。另一种用于转化丙酮酸的机制是通过转氨作用利用氨基酸以氨基的形式形成丙氨酸，以便进入Krebs循环。ATP：腺苷三磷酸；NAD：烟酰胺腺嘌呤二核苷酸；NADH：还原型NAD

缺氧的化学转换和炎症上调

是否有具体的病理生理机制，可以解释EGDT对于特定的氧输送变量终点产生有益效果的问题，仍然没有答案。然而，如果认为氧分子在细胞水平可作为细胞因子应答的主要调节剂，那么，在某些微循环区域，氧供需之间的不平衡通过激活细胞质内的促炎质反应机制实现炎症反应的上调也是有可能的。无论是在动物模型还是人类，是否有直接或间接的临床或实验室证据显示，是否达到特定氧输送终点、获得适当的细胞氧张力，与细胞因子反应的降低或升高，有无关系？

人类有对缺氧的应答机制，帮助我们适应缺氧。在用于感知氧气的机制中，有一种缺氧诱导转录因子（hypoxia-inducible transcription factor，HIF）。HIF是一种异二聚体，由HIF-1β亚基和α亚基组成，α亚基根据氧依赖性和转录活性的不相同，分为3种，被认为促进了对缺氧适应的促进。在含氧量正常的情况下，HIF-1α亚基持续产生，但是并不会累积，它们会被脯氨酰4-羟化酶（prolyl 4-hydroxylases，PHDs）缺氧诱导转录因子的抑制因子（factor inhibiting HIF，FIH）羟化并被泛素连接酶von Hippel- Lindau蛋白俘获并降解，目的是蛋白酸降解或呈现转录不活跃（图5）。相反，缺氧时，PHDs酶的活性明显降低，因为它的底物α-酮

图3 乳酸过量伴或不伴有酸中毒。ADP，腺苷二磷酸；AMP，腺苷一磷酸；ATP，腺苷三磷酸；L/P，乳酸/丙酮酸；NAD，烟酰胺腺嘌呤二核苷酸；NADH，还原型NAD；Pi，无机磷酸盐

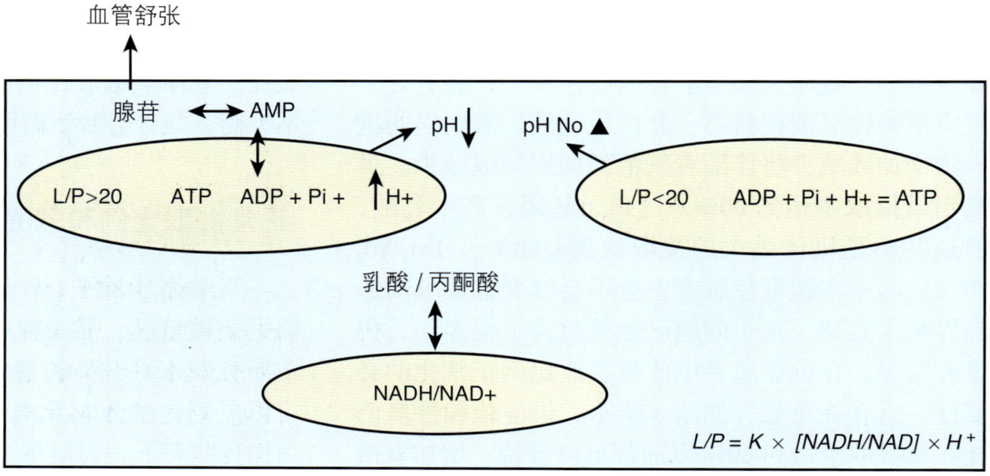

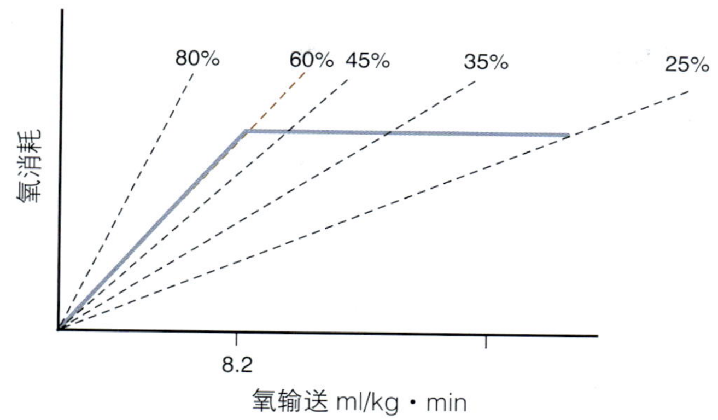

图 4　氧输送、氧摄取和氧消耗之间的关系。正常情况下，当氧输送降低时氧消耗可以通过提高氧摄取而独立供应。然而，当氧摄取比例达到 60% 即无氧阈，出现于氧输送为 8.2 ml/kg · min 时，氧输送和氧消耗成线性相关，患者处于供应依赖性氧消耗状态，并产生乳酸。氧输送的进一步增加或减少将伴随着氧消耗的增加或减少

戊二酸，因线粒体呼吸链损伤导致 Krebs 循环限制而减少。这样，HIF-1α 和 HIF-1β 亚基累积并进入细胞核，形成异二聚体的缺氧反应元件（hypoxia response element，HRE），促进基因转录例如核转录因子 κB（NF-κB）和 toll 样受体（toll-like receptor，TLRs）等（图 6）。缺氧通过提高 TLRs 的表达，活化 NF-κβ 通路，同时也增加了细胞因子和炎症的产生。小鼠短暂地暴露于低氧浓度后，发生血管渗漏、各器官白细胞聚集，血清细胞因子升高。已经知道促炎细胞因子水平也会升高，如 IL-6、IL-6 受体和 C 反应蛋白在人体内可升高至 3 400m 以上。缺氧仅 2～4 h，巨噬细胞中的 TLR4 的表达就会通过 HIF-1 的作用上调，促进对细菌感染炎性反应的放大，也使得患者对可能导致 MODS 的发展的长期炎性反应得到一定的适应。有充足的证据表明，在提高脓毒症患者的炎性反应过程中，细胞缺氧扮演了一个重要角色。所以 EGDT 最重要的一个目的就是通过给予患者最佳的容量水平，阻止细胞的缺氧。仅通过扩容使胞质 / 线粒体获得更多可用的氧气，对于促反应炎症或者抗炎症反应可以起到作用吗？如果这之间存在关系，那么它是时间敏感的吗？有一项志愿者应用大肠杆菌内毒素的试验证据表明，试验组患者在预水化后以对照组 2 倍的速率继续水化，它相比于对照组，降低了症状评分并使肿瘤坏死因子（α tumer necrosis factor，TNF-α）下调但不影响 IL-10，使细胞因子反应向抗炎症反应的方面变动，而对血压和心率没有影响。基于这些证据，我们建议脓毒症患者应尽早接受充分的液体复苏，以调节炎性反应的缺氧的上调。液体复苏最好在脓毒症诊断后的 2～6 h 内完成。

图 5　正常氧条件下缺氧诱导转录因子和核转录因子 β（NF-κB）的作用途径。正常氧条件下，缺氧诱导转录因子（HIF）-1α 亚基持续产生，但是并不会累积，它们会被脯氨酰 4- 羟化酶和缺氧诱导因子抑制因子（FIH）羟化。泛素连接酶 von Hippel- Lindau 蛋白（vHL）俘获之后的目的是进行蛋白酶降解，或呈现转录不活跃。HRE，缺氧反应元件；IKK，IκB 激酶；OH：羟基；TLR，toll 样受体

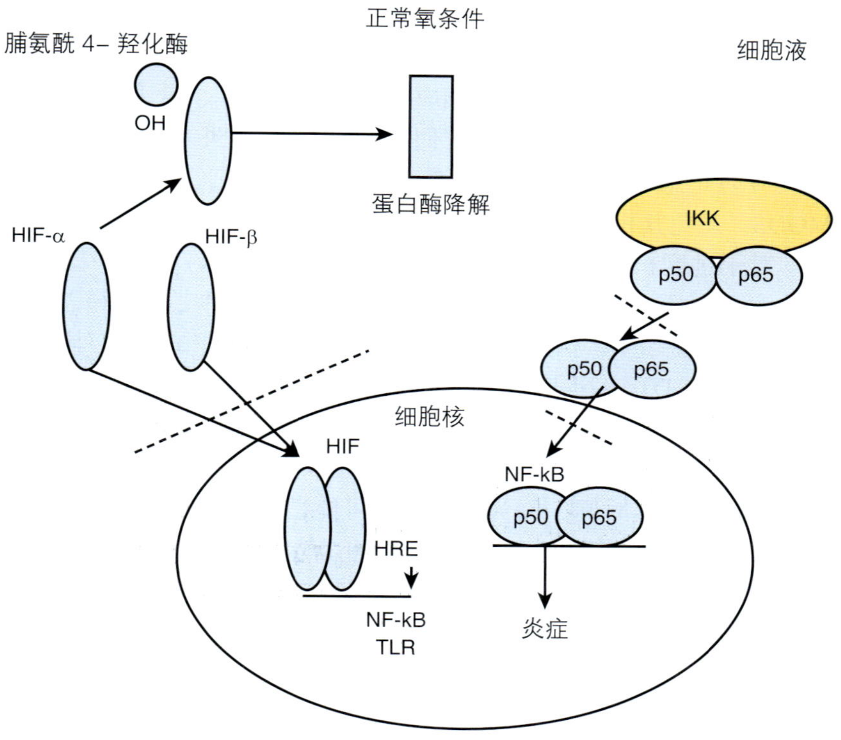

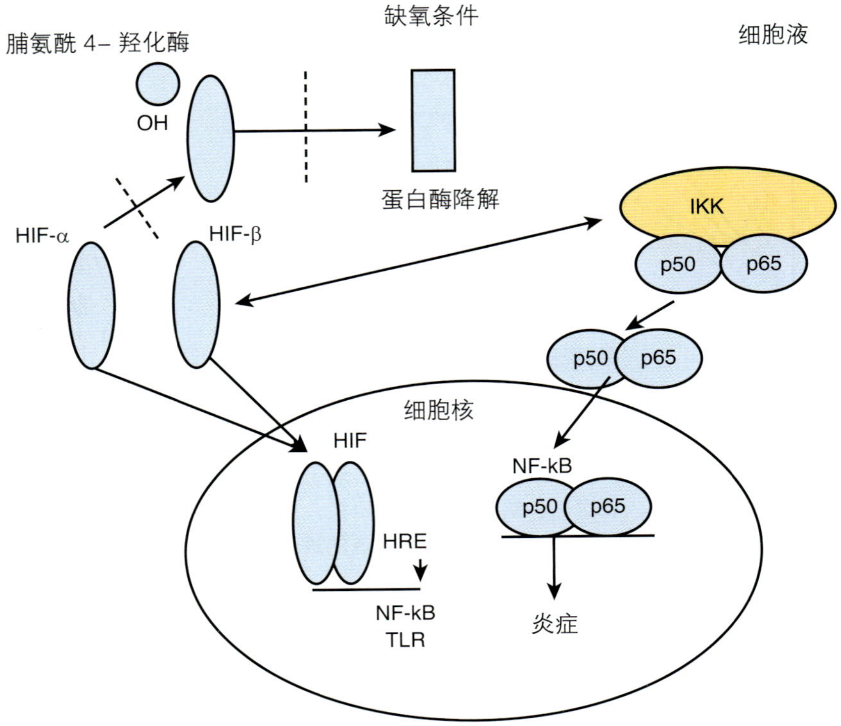

图 6　缺氧条件下缺氧诱导转录因子和核转录因子（NF-κB）的作用途径。缺氧激活缺氧诱导转录因子（HIF）和 NF-κB 途径，尽管它对 HIF 和 NF-κB 通路的调节存在差异。在不同水平生成的两通路有交差。脯氨酰 4-羟化酶（PHDs）的活性明显降低，因为它的底物 α- 酮戊二酸，因线粒体呼吸链损伤导致 Krebs 循环受阻而减少。这样，HIF-1α 和 HIF-1β 亚基累积并进入细胞核，形成异二聚体的缺氧反应元件（HRE），促进基因转录，例如核转录因子 κB（NF-κB）和 toll 样受体（TLRs）等。NF-κB 通路的缺氧敏感成分是 IKK（IκB 激酶）复合物水平。OH，羟基

治疗

越来越多的证据表明，治疗脓毒症应与时间赛跑，这与卒中、心肌梗死和创伤患者的治疗没有什么不同。如 Rivers 等所展示的，脓毒症最初的 6 h 对于治疗来说是最重要的。由于积极的目标导向性治疗和促炎性细胞因子的减少之间存在联系，似乎早期积极的液体容量复苏以达到相应的终点，如 Svo_2、乳酸正常化，控制感染源。它们可以通过调节炎症反应防止患者发展为严重脓毒症、感染性休克、MODS，避免其相关的高死亡率。

对于过度积极的液体治疗所导致的潜在的肺部并发症，包括机械通气时间增加、腹内压增高、神经系统状态恶化，应结合主要以扩容为基础的对时间敏感的 EGDT 治疗。它可以降低脓毒症患者病死率。开始于脓毒症发生后的 24～48 h 内，积极的液体治疗相较于相同时间点的保守的疗法，会导致更长的机械通气时间，因为这时患者可能已经出现 ALI。然而，在脓毒症诊断 2 h 内，以获得正常的乳酸水平和正常的氧摄取比例（复苏阶段）为目标的积极的液体复苏策略，将可能限制感染源引起的炎症反应和随后 ALI、急性呼吸窘迫综合征 ARDS、肠壁和第三间隙水肿引起的腹内高压，以及器官功能障碍。这和以前研究中观察到的不利后果无关。

显然，一旦脓毒症的诊断确定，必须对患者逐步地实施复苏。治疗策略应是渐进的。首先应实施积极的液体复苏，并应用广谱抗生素。如果必要的话，及时地对感染源实施外科干预或者穿刺引流。我们相信，一旦脓毒症诊断确立，应将患者转入 ICU，置入动脉导管（桡动脉优先），监测血压和中心静脉血氧状态。我们不建议使用无创血压监测，即使患者没有明显的休克（收缩压小于 90mmHg），主要原因是有一些患者存在代偿性休克。我们赞同不使用静态的中心静脉压（central venous pressure，CVP）评估容量并指导液体治疗，取而代之的是使用一些更准确的动态指标，比如超声测量下腔静脉直径、脉压变异（pulse pressure variation，PPV），或心搏量变异（stroke volume variation，SVV）。因为 PPV 和 SVV 依赖于正压通气引起的周期性变化的胸内压，对于有自主呼吸的患者它们并不适用。当治疗有自主呼吸的患者时，液体治疗应该以使 Svo_2 恢复正常为目标。而对于机械通气的患者，我们更倾向于使用 SVV 指导液体治疗。

关于对严重脓毒症和感染性休克患者仅使用 10% 乳酸清除率和将乳酸盐正常化而不是使 $Scvo_2$ 正常化作为目标，如 Jones 等在关于乳酸清除率对中心静脉血氧饱和度的非劣效性试验所示。作为早

期脓毒症治疗的目标。我们倾向于使用 $Scvo_2$ 监测而不是单独使用乳酸监测，它可以更快速地实现血流动力学的调整。治疗的目的是通过调整心血管系统功能来提供足够的氧输送，以达到组织水平的氧消耗的最佳状态（通过 $Scvo_2 \geq 70\%$ 时，乳酸水平的正常化间接测得）。

液体复苏

液体选择仍是复苏中一个有争议的话题，因为一些对比了晶体和胶体的多中心试验得出的结果并不一致。一些研究显示使用胶体（白蛋白）患者死亡率更高，而另一些研究却显示其存在一些潜在的益处。实际上，一项关于 SAFE（生理盐水 vs. 白蛋白）试验中，严重脓毒症患者的亚组分析显示，以 28 天死亡风险为终点来看，白蛋白复苏效果比生理盐水更佳。603 例严重脓毒症患者使用白蛋白复苏，186 例死亡（30.7%）；而 615 例患者使用生理盐水复苏，217 例死亡（35.3%）（RR＝0.87；95% CI 为 0.74～1.02；P=0.09）。基于目前的研究证据，我们不建议使用羟乙基淀粉进行液体复苏，因为其有导致急性肾衰竭和需要肾替代治疗的风险。在我们看来，晶体液性价比更高，但同时也必须承认，胶体液可以用量更少地达到同样的血流动力学目标，且需要的时间更短，这有一定优势。关于使用生理盐水（normal saline，NS）还是乳酸林格氏（lactated Ringer's，LR）液，尽管我们承认 LR 会带来一些免疫问题，我们仍然优先选择 LR 而不是 NS 进行复苏，以避免大量使用 NS 后的高氯性酸中毒。对于机械通气且潮气量大于 7 ml/kg 的患者，应从一开始就监测 SVV，输注 LR 直到 SVV 小于 13%，并监测 $Scvo_2$ 和动脉乳酸水平。准确实施容量复苏相比于使用正性肌力药或者血管加压药，可以使心肌耗氧量减少，并且不会造成肾上腺素带来的全身氧消耗增加。

正性肌力药和血管加压药的使用

如果患者接受 SVV 指导下的容量复苏没有达到治疗终点，我们会为患者置入肺动脉导管实施血氧饱和度及心排血量连续监测，优化心血管系统功能，指导正性肌力药和血管加压药的使用。目前正性肌力药和血管加压药，主要包括多巴胺、多巴酚丁胺、米力农、肾上腺素、去甲肾上腺素、去氧肾上腺素和血管加压素等。对于轻体重患者（60～80 kg），用去甲肾上腺素，来治疗经适度复苏后血压仍低的、全身血管阻力降低的患者。它通过将有效的左心室收缩末期心肌弹性优化在 1.5～2 mmHg/ml 之间和增加心脏后负荷，匹配小于 50% 的心肌收缩力。对于输注去甲肾上腺素无效的低血压患者，若动脉血气 pH 大于 7.3，应给与氢化可的松 50 mg，每 6 h 一次，来保证体内皮质醇水平。如果皮质醇水平大于 25 μg/dl，不再使用氢化可的松；相反，如果皮质醇水平小于 25 μg/dl，使用氢化可的松 7 天，之后以 3 天为期进行药物逐渐减量。对于近期行胃肠吻合的患者，在我们的机构中，我们不使用血管加压素，因为其会导致内脏缺血，继而对胃肠伤口愈合产生不利影响。最近的研究显示，血管加压素与去甲肾上腺素合用，对于脓毒症患者并未带来有益的临床效果。对于血压正常的已经有过容量复苏的患者，如果须增加心排血量，我们优先使用起始剂量为 7.5 μg/kg · min 的多巴酚丁胺而不是肾上腺素来达到治疗目标。相反，在需要正性肌力药的低血压患者，我们使用肾上腺素而不是多巴酚丁胺。对于右心后负荷过重导致的右心功能下降者，我们加用米力农。

输血治疗

我们没有足够的证据来证实输入的浓缩红细胞可以增加氧输送、提高脓毒症患者 $Scvo_2$，除非使用新鲜血液。实际上，因为多种原因，包括增加感染风险、ARDS 风险及危重患者的死亡，我们相信输注浓缩红细胞（通常储存时间为大于 14 天，使用时多在 21～24 天），不应作为常规治疗流程中的一部分，除非是使用新鲜血液。众所周知，储存红细胞的 p50 非常低，一般为 6 mmHg，而非一般情况下的 27 mmHg。这样的红细胞对氧的负荷能力下降。储存红细胞变形能力变差，在像内脏这样的低剪切率区域会损伤微循环血流，造成组织缺氧。乳酸产生增加。另外，储存血倾向于促炎质反应和血栓形成。输注浓缩红细胞的脓毒症患者，会损伤微循环血液、损伤组织氧合。如果使用新鲜血液，我们认为，血细胞比容为 30%～35% 对于恢复氧摄取效果最佳。

总结

脓毒症，严重脓毒症和感染性休克的病因多

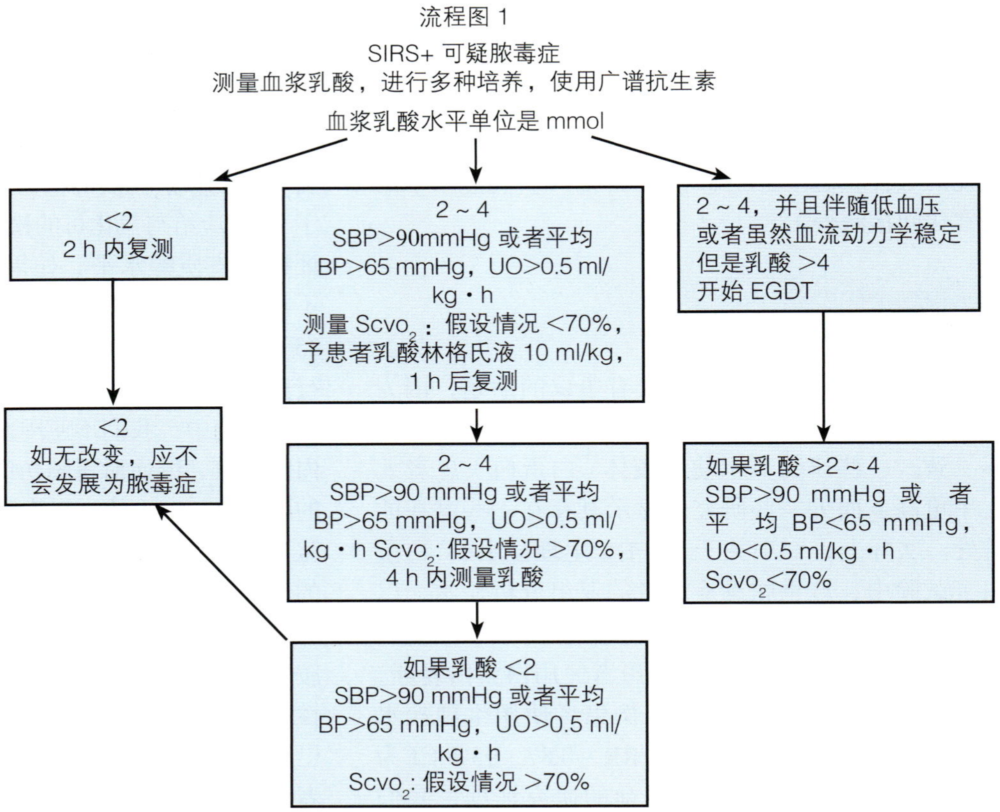

图 7 全身炎性反应综合征（SIRS）+ 可疑脓毒症的处理流程。BP，血压；EGDT，早期目标导向性治疗；LR，乳酸林格氏液；SBP，收缩压；UO，尿量

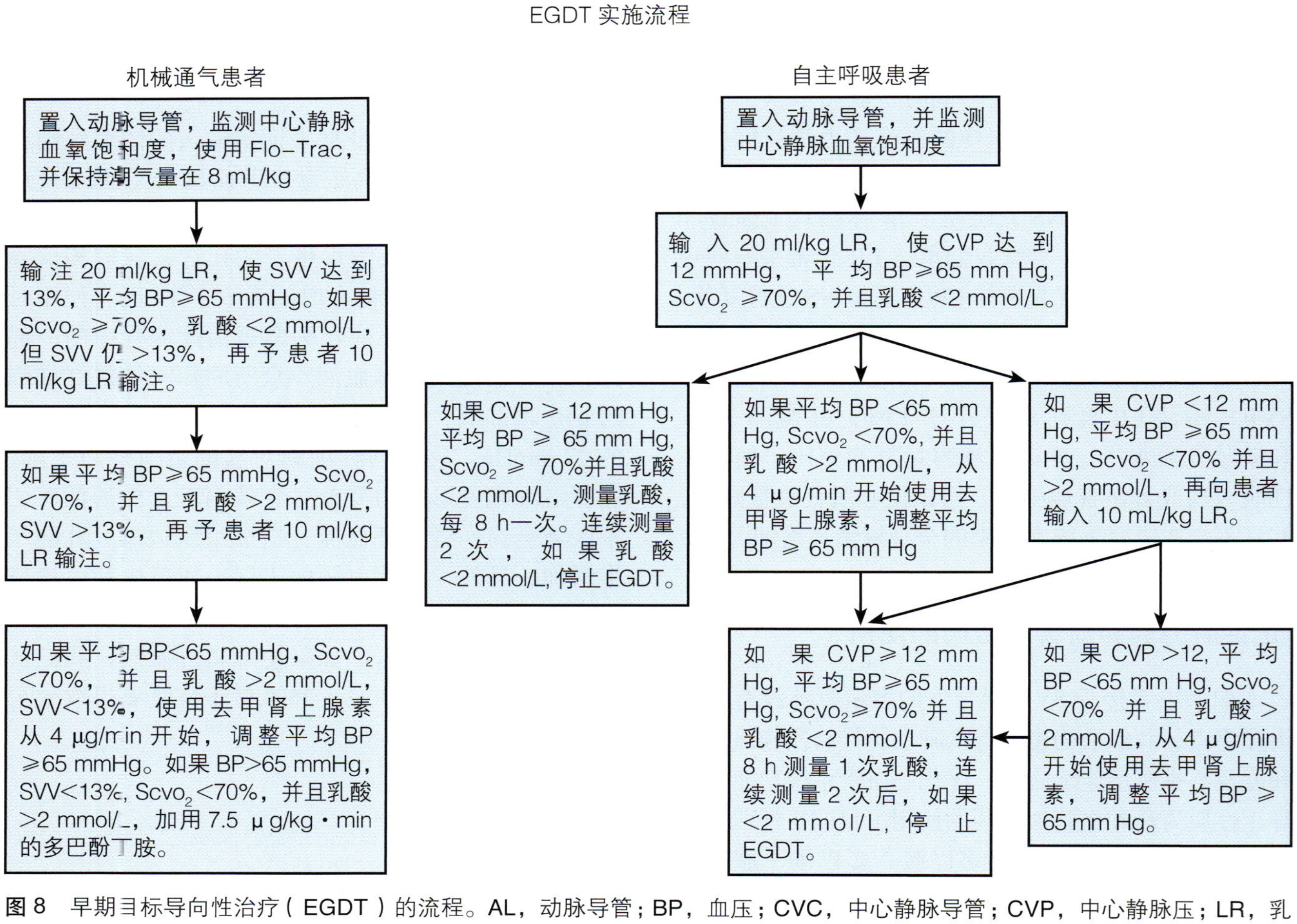

图 8 早期目标导向性治疗（EGDT）的流程。AL，动脉导管；BP，血压；CVC，中心静脉导管；CVP，中心静脉压；LR，乳酸林格氏液；SVV，心搏量变异；TV，潮气量

种多样，患者死亡率高，大约为 20%～30%，合并 MODS 时可高达 80%。减少死亡率最好的治疗方法应该是理解它的治疗，这与治疗卒中、心肌梗死和创伤患者没什么区别。早期诊断、快速开始使用抗生素、控制感染源，早期目标导向性治疗，应尽早实施，以使混合静脉血氧饱和度和乳酸水平正常化（图 7）。EGDT 的标志是恢复患者血容量，使患者心血管功能最佳化来提供充足的氧输送来满足氧需求，以防止患者从脓毒症发展至严重脓毒症和感染性休克，并改善脓毒症患者的总体死亡率（图 8）。

创伤免疫学

Christine S. Cocanour 和 S. Rob Todd 著
吕 杰 译

对于创伤的免疫反应是由先天性免疫系统和后天性免疫系统介导的。先天性免疫是非特异的，包括多形核白细胞（polymorphonuclear leukocyte，PMNLs）、嗜酸性粒细胞、自然杀伤细胞（natural killer，NK）和补体。后天性免疫系统是抗原抗体特异的，由 T 细胞与 B 细胞介导。原始的模式识别受体（pattern recognition receptors，PRRs）识别并结合称为病原体相关分子模式（pathogen-associated molecular patterns，PAMPs）的保守微生物组分。PAMPs 允许感染性和非感染性抗原之间的分化。

通常，免疫反应被认为是基于自我和非我的相互作用，但由于这个概念不能充分解释其他免疫情况，如肿瘤、自身免疫性疾病或肿瘤，另一个模型被 Matzinger 等提出。危险模式理论，提出是“危险”，而不是“外来者”启动了免疫应答。细胞死亡的机制决定了免疫反应是否启动。通常，发生凋亡的细胞都会被清除而不会发生免疫反应。当创伤或者感染导致细胞损伤（裂解或细胞凋亡释放胞内物质），先天性免疫和后天性反应都会启动。这些内源性控制信号称为警报素。它们是应激或者损伤组织释放的预警信号。PAMPs（对外源性信号的响应）和警报素（对内源性信号的响应）都有相似的保守的疏水性部分，可以引发同样的 PRRs 和可比的炎症反应。因为它们的相似性，PAMPS 和警报素同被分类为危险相关（或者有时损伤相关）分子模式（danger-associated molecular patterns，DAMPs）。

创伤引起的免疫反应与微生物感染引起的免疫反应相似（图 1）。创伤和感染引起的 PAMPs/DAMPs，通过相似的 PRRs，如 TLR 家族，引发自身炎症性免疫反应。TLRs 是链接组织损伤、感染和炎症的关键分子链。TLRs 是膜结合受体，可以激活炎症反应的 2 个不同的信号转导途径。第一个是髓样分化因子 88 依赖的途径，是由除 TLR3 外的所有 TLRs 所激活。这个信号级联通过大量 IL-1 受体 - 相关激酶和随后快速激活的核因子 κB（NF-κB）细胞和丝裂原活化蛋白激酶（mitogen-activated protein kinase，MAPK）传导放大，并导致促炎细胞因子产生［IL-1α/β、IL-6、IL-8、巨噬细胞炎

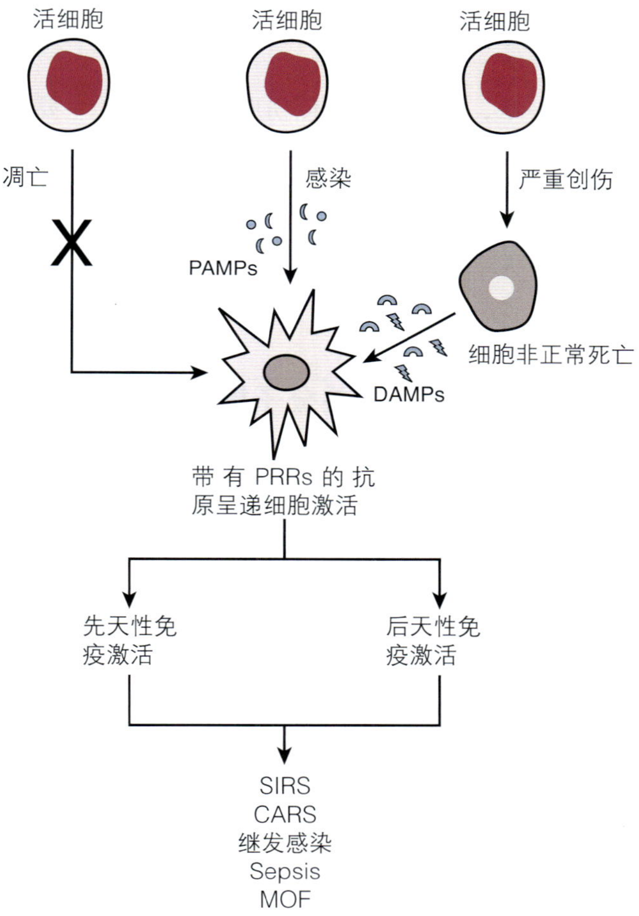

图 1 感染和创伤免疫应答的相似性。CARS，代偿性抗炎反应综合征；DAMPs，损伤相关分子模式；MOF，多器官功能衰竭；PAMPs，病原体相关分子模式，PRRs，模式识别受体；SIRS，全身炎症反应综合征

性蛋白（macrophage inflammatory protein，MIP）-1α/β、肿瘤坏死因子（tumor necrosis factor，TNF）-α］。第二个信号通路是非髓样分化因子 88 依赖性途径，是通过 TLR3 和 TLR4 结合激活。这一途径通过干扰素诱导而达到高峰。

因为有大量的 TLRs（目前 12 种人类 TLRs 被发现），每一种 PAMPs/DAMPs 有其不同的作用机制，功能性反应的不同取决于不同的 TLR 信号通路的激活。创伤、组织损伤、缺氧、低血压，以及继发性损伤（如缺血 / 再灌注、筋膜室综合征、手术干预和感染），通过 Toll 样受体引起反应，特点是有加剧局部和全身促炎细胞因子、花生四烯酸代谢产物的释放，补体因子激活，激肽、凝血因子以及激素介质的释放。临床上，这就是 SIRS。同时也发生了一种抗炎反应，称为代偿性抗炎反应综合征（compensatory anti-inflammatory response syndrome，CARS）。为了愈合和恢复，受伤的患者，必须找到 SIRS 和 CARS 之间的平衡。当这些过程难以平衡时，患者就有感染和发生多器官功能衰竭易感性增大的可能（图 2）。

这一章，我们将讨论创伤后免疫反应的主要组成部分，包括特异性 DAMPs：细胞因子反应、白细胞招募集、蛋白酶和活性氧类、补体、激肽和凝血作用、急性期反应产物、SIRS、CARS 和二次打击模型。

危险（损伤）相关分子模式

许多被认为是 DAMPS 的分子是损伤后由细胞释放的蛋白质。细胞内蛋白包括 HMGB1 和热休克蛋白（heat shock proteins，HSPs）；细胞外基质蛋白包括透明质酸片段。非蛋白 DAMPs 包括脱氧核糖核酸（deoxyribonucleic aid，DNA）、腺苷三磷酸（adenosine 5'-triphosphate，ATP）和尿酸。2 种 DAMPs 会在后面进行讨论。

高迁移率族蛋白 1

HMGB1 是一种核内非组蛋白染色体 DNA 结合蛋白，是一种 DNA 转录调控和基因表达的结构辅因子。当从损伤或者坏死的细胞释放到细胞外，它会刺激先天性和后天性免疫反应。它带动并增强促炎症反应介质的起始和增强作用，包括细胞介导反应［1 型 T 辅助细胞（T helper，T_H）］，并可以作为未成熟的树突状细胞的趋化因子。在凋亡细胞，HMGB1 不可逆地结合在染色质，并不刺激免疫反应。如果大量凋亡细胞被巨噬细胞清除，HMGB1 会被动释放。HMGB1 分泌于许多类型炎性刺激后的细胞，增强创伤、烧伤和感染后的炎性反应，同时引起组织再生。

热休克蛋白

HSPs 是高度保守的细胞内蛋白，具有分子伴侣的功能，促进蛋白质的合成和折叠。在非生理条件下，如热休克、pH 偏移或缺氧，它们的表达增加，稳定未折叠蛋白，并允许细胞修复或合成替换蛋白来保护细胞。当热休克蛋白大量产生，会被释放到细胞外。这是一种危险信号，可以引起免疫反应，其中有一些是通过与 TLRs 的相互作用介导的。

细胞因子反应

一旦免疫反应启动，会释放大量的介质。细胞

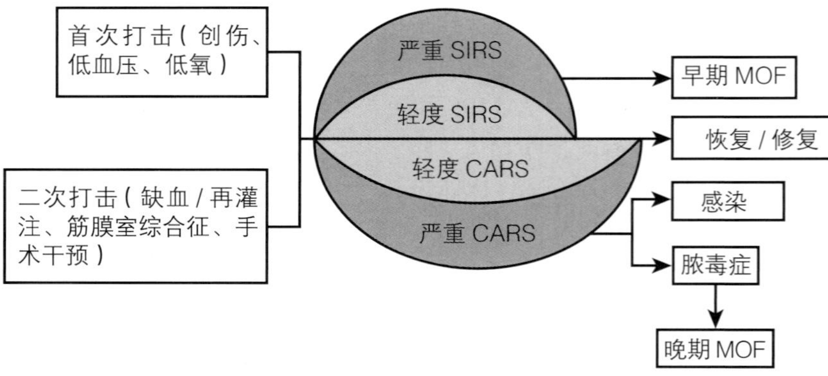

图 2 伤后多器官功能衰竭（MOF）作为功能性炎症失调的结果出现。CARS，代偿性抗炎反应综合征；SIRS，全身炎症反应综合征

因子以旁分泌和自分泌两种形式发挥作用。促炎细胞因子 TNF-α 和 IL-1β 在 1～2 h 内释放。继发性促炎细胞因子以亚急性的形式释放，包括 IL-6、IL-8、巨噬细胞迁移因子（macrophage migratory factor，MMF）、IL-12 和 IL-18。临床上，IL-6 水平与 ISS、多器官功能衰竭的发展、ARDS、脓毒症有关。

IL-6 作为一种免疫调节因子，通过刺激释放抗炎症反应介质如 IL-1 受体拮抗剂和肿瘤坏死因子受体（与循环促炎细胞因子结合）发挥作用。IL-6 也触发巨噬细胞释放前列腺素 E_2（PGE_2）。PGE_2 可能是最有效的内源性抑制剂。它不仅抑制 T 细胞和巨噬细胞反应，并诱导 IL-10 的释放。这是一个强有力的抗炎细胞因子，可以使单核细胞活性下降。血清 IL-10 水平与 ISS 以及创伤后并发症的发展相关。

外伤后，IL-12 分泌减少，有利于刺激 Th2 细胞的移位和后续抗炎介质 IL-4、IL-13、IL-10 和转化生长因子 β（transforming growth factor，TGF-β）的产生。IL-12 的减少和 Th2 细胞相应的升高与临床不良预后相关。表 1 和表 2 中有促炎症反应介质和抗炎症反应介质的列表。

细胞介导的反应

创伤改变脾、腹膜和肺泡的巨噬细胞释放 IL-1、IL-6、TNF-α 的能力，导致这些促炎细胞因子水平的降低。Kupffer 细胞，一种产生促炎细胞因子能力很强的细胞。细胞介导的免疫不仅需要功能性巨噬细胞和 T 细胞，而且还需要完整的巨噬细胞 - T 细胞相互作用。受伤后，人类白细胞抗原（human leukocyte antigen，HLA-DR）受体表达减少，导致细胞抗原呈递能力下降和肿瘤坏死因子 -α 产生减少。PGE2、IL-10 和 TGF-β，都促进这种“免疫麻痹”。

辅助性 T 细胞分化为 T_H1 或 T_H2 淋巴细胞。T_H1 细胞通过释放 IL-2、IFN- γ 和 TNF-β 促进炎症级联反应，T_H2 细胞产生抗炎症反应介质。单核细胞 / 巨噬细胞，通过释放 IL-12，刺激辅助性 T 细胞分化为 T_H1 细胞。创伤由于抑制 IL-12 的产生，促进 T_H2 细胞的比例增加，这与不良的临床预后有关。

白细胞黏附到内皮细胞，是由于黏附分子的上调介导的。选择素如白细胞黏附分子 -1（leukocyte adhesion molecule，LAM-1）、内皮白细胞黏附分子 -1（endothelial leukocyte adhesion molecule，ELAM-1）和 P- 选择素负责多形核白细胞的“滚动”。整合素如 CD11/18 复合物或细胞间黏附分子 -1

表 1　促炎症反应介质

介质	作用
IL-1	IL-1 是多效性的。在局部，它刺激 T 细胞的细胞因子和细胞因子受体的产生，并刺激 B 细胞增殖。在全身，IL-1 调节内分泌系统，并诱导急性期反应。
IL-6	IL-6 诱导肝细胞内的急性期反应物，在 B 细胞最终分化为免疫球蛋白分泌细胞的过程中起着至关重要的作用。此外，IL-6 具有抗炎症反应特性。
IL-8	IL-8 是炎症反应的一种主要介质。它是一种趋化因子，同时也是一种有效的血管生成因子。
IL-12	IL-12 调节 T 细胞向 T_H1 细胞的分化。刺激 T 细胞生长和各项功能，并改变细胞凋亡的正常周期。
TNF-α	TNF-α 是多效的。如前所述，TNF-α 和 IL-1 单独或共同诱导全身炎症反应。TNF-α 也趋化中性粒细胞和单核细胞，并增加中性粒细胞的活性。
MIF	MIF 是联系免疫和神经内分泌系统之间的一个关键环节。它提高 IL-1 和 TNF-α 的分泌。

IL, 白细胞介素；Ig, 免疫球蛋白；MIF, 移动抑制因子；T_H1, 辅助性 T 淋巴细胞；TNF, 肿瘤坏死因子

表 2　抗炎介质

介质	作用
IL-4	IL-4、IL-5、IL-13、IL-3 和 CSF2 形成染色体 5q 的细胞因子基因簇，这个基因尤其接近 IL-13。
IL-10	IL-10 对于免疫调节和炎症有多种效应。下调 T_H1 细胞因子、MHC Ⅱ类抗原、巨噬细胞共刺激分子的表达。它也增强 B 细胞的存活、增殖和抗体的产生。此外，它可以阻断 NF-κB 活性，并参与 JAK-STAT 信号通路的调控。
IL-11	IL-11 刺激 T 细胞依赖的 B 细胞产生免疫球蛋白。它也支持造血干细胞和巨核细胞祖细胞增殖。
IL-13	IL-13 参与 B 细胞成熟和分化的几个阶段。上调 CD23 和 MHC Ⅱ类抗原表达，促进 B 细胞分泌的 IgE 同型转换。它能抑制巨噬细胞的活性，从而抑制促炎细胞因子和趋化因子的产生。
IFN-α	IFN-α 增强和修饰免疫应答。
TGF-β	TGF-β 调节细胞分化、增殖、伤口愈合和血管再生。
α-MSH	α-MSH 通过 3 个机制调节炎症：①对于周围炎症细胞的直接作用；②作用于脑的炎症细胞调节局部反应；③间接激活下行神经抗炎通路，控制周围组织炎症。

CSF, 集落刺激因子；IFN, 干扰素；Ig, 免疫球蛋白；IL, 白细胞介素；JAK-STAT, Janus 激酶 / 信号转导与转录激活因子；MHC, 主要组织相容性复合体；MSH, 促黑色素；TGF, 转化生长因子；T_H, 辅助性 T 细胞

（intercellular adhesion molecular，ICAM-1）的表达上调负责 PMNLs 附着于血管内皮细胞。多形核白细胞的迁移、积累和活化是由如趋化因子的化学诱导物和补体过敏毒素所介导的。集落刺激因子（colony-stimulating factor，CSF）刺激单核细胞和粒细胞的生成，并减少 SIRS 中多形核白细胞的凋亡。中性粒细胞凋亡的减少是由其他炎症介质介导的，从而导致局部破坏组织的 PMNLs 的积累。

白细胞募集

炎性细胞因子促进 PMNLs 募集，增强吞噬细胞的活性，并促进 PMNLs 释放蛋白酶和氧自由基。这种聚集的白细胞虽然可能引起二次组织损伤的发展，但其代表宿主创伤后防御的一个关键因素。它是涉及白细胞移位的一个复杂的级联反应，最终使细胞发挥其作用。首先是捕获和黏附，由以 L- 选择素为代表的过度表达的白细胞选择素介导。L- 选择素通过识别白细胞上的糖蛋白配体和激活细胞因子活化的内皮细胞的上调发挥作用。

捕获和黏附后，内皮中的 E- 选择素、P- 选择素协助白细胞滚动成减慢速度。P- 选择素是在内皮细胞的存储颗粒中发现（Weibel-Palade 小体）。颗粒分泌后，P- 选择素与白细胞上 P- 选择素糖蛋白配体（P-selectin glycoprotein ligand，PSGL-1）呈递多糖结合。与此相反，E- 选择素不被储存，但它是炎性细胞因子存在时重新合成的。这些选择素导致白细胞在活化的内皮上滚动，从而使白细胞的二次捕获通过同型细胞的相互作用实现。

白细胞募集的第三步是牢固黏着，这是细胞膜上表达的 β_1- 和 β_2- 整合素介导的。整合素与细胞间的相互作用，最终导致细胞信号转导。这一步是稳定的抗剪切 - 黏着形成的关键，从而使白细胞移位。

随着上述整合素和免疫球蛋白超家族成员的结合，白细胞转移，这也就是白细胞聚集的最后一步。捕获的白细胞跨过内皮细胞层，发生白细胞的转移。这一过程由血小板内皮细胞黏附分子（platelet-endothelial cell adhesion molecules，PECAM）介导。

蛋白酶和活性氧类

多形核淋巴细胞和巨噬细胞不仅负责微生物和细胞碎片的吞噬作用，同时也可能通过脱颗粒释放的胞外蛋白酶和形成活性氧类或呼吸爆发，造成组织和器官的二次损伤。弹性蛋白酶和金属蛋白酶对于结构蛋白和细胞外基质蛋白的降解，导致创伤后其深度的增加。中性粒细胞弹性蛋白酶同时诱导促炎症细胞因子的释放。

活性氧类由膜相关的烟酰胺腺嘌呤二核苷酸磷酸氧化酶产生，由炎性细胞因子、花生四烯酸代谢产物、补体因子和细菌产物激活。超氧化物阴离子在 Haber-Weiss 反应中，被存在于细胞质，线粒体和细胞膜中的超氧化物歧化酶还原成过氧化氢。盐酸通过髓过氧化物酶由 H_2O_2 形成，同时 Fenton 反应将 H_2O_2 转化为氢氧根离子。这些自由的活性氧类导致内皮细胞和实质细胞的脂质过氧化、细胞膜解体和 DNA 损伤。氧自由基诱导 PMNLs 释放蛋白酶和胶原酶以及灭活蛋白酶抑制剂。

活性氮类引起创伤后的额外组织损伤。一氧化氮是由在 PMNLs 或血管平滑肌细胞内的诱导型一氧化氮合酶和内皮细胞中的内皮型一氧化氮合酶催化 L- 精氨酸产生的。NO 诱导血管舒张。iNOS 是通过细胞因子和毒素刺激产生，而 eNOS 通过机械剪切应力刺激产生。由活性氧类和活性氮类产生的损伤导致全身水肿和毛细血管渗漏综合征。

补体、激肽、凝血

补体、激肽系统和凝血级联密切参与创伤后的免疫反应。它们通过促炎症反应介质、内源性内毒素和组织损伤被激活。补体激活的经典途径通常是通过抗原抗体复合物［免疫球蛋白（immuno globulin，Ig）M 或 G］或活化的凝血因子Ⅻ（FⅫ）实现。替代途径被细菌产物如脂多糖激活。创伤后补体活化最有可能来自于蛋白水解酶释放、内皮细胞破坏和组织缺血。补体活化程度与损伤严重程度相关。C3 和 C5 裂解导致调理素、过敏毒素和膜攻击复合物（membrane attack complex，MAC）的形成。调理素 C3b 和 C4b 通过调理作用增强细胞碎片和细菌的吞噬。过敏毒素 C3a 和 C5a 通过募集和激活吞噬细胞（如单核细胞、中性粒细胞和巨噬细胞），增强肝急性期反应和释放血管活性介质（如组胺）加剧炎症反应。它们也增强白细胞与内皮细胞的黏附，从而增加血管通透性和水肿。C5a 通过其受体和 MAC 的相互作用诱导细胞凋亡和细胞裂解。

此外，C3a 和 C5a 激活修复机制。C1 抑制剂抑制 C1s 和 C1r，从而调节补体经典途径。然而，在炎症过程中，通过多形核细胞弹性蛋白酶降解，血清 C1 抑制物水平降低。

血浆激肽释放酶 - 激肽系统，是一种补体和凝血级联反应相关的血浆蛋白酶的接触系统。它由血浆蛋白 FⅫ、前激肽释放酶、激肽原和因子Ⅺ（FⅪ）组成。FⅫ和前激肽释放酶的激活是通过接触内皮损伤时暴露的基底膜。FⅫ激活形成因子Ⅻa（FⅫa），从而通过经典途径启动补体级联。而前激肽释放酶激活形成激肽释放酶，它可以通过刺激纤维蛋白溶解酶原转化为纤溶酶，或者刺激尿激酶型纤维蛋白溶解酶原激活剂（urokinase-like plasminogen activaton，uPA）从而促进纤维蛋白溶解。组织型纤维蛋白溶解酶原激活剂（tissue plasminogen activator，tPA）是一种辅因子。此外，激肽释放酶促进激肽原和缓激肽的转化。缓激肽的形成通过组织激肽释放酶 - 激肽系统的活化发生，最有可能通过器官损伤诱发，因为许多器官和组织中都存在着激肽释放酶 - 激肽系统，包括胰腺、肾、肠和唾液腺。激肽是强有力的血管扩张剂。它们还增加血管通透性和抑制血小板的功能。

内源性凝血级联与接触激活系统有关，通过由因子Ⅺa（FⅪa）转化来的Ⅸa 因子（FⅨa）的形成而实现。它的形成导致 FⅫ、前激肽释放酶、FⅪ、血浆酶抑制剂复合物水平升高。这些化合物包括 FⅫa-C1 抑制剂和激肽释放酶 -C1 抑制剂。C1 抑制剂和 α1 蛋白酶抑制剂是内源性凝血途径的抑制剂。

尽管内源性凝血途径可以为激活凝血级联提供刺激，但是创伤导致的凝血途径激活主要是外源性的。内皮细胞和单核细胞的组织因子（tissue factor，TF）表达增加，由促炎细胞因子 TNF-α 和 IL-1β 诱导发生。因子Ⅶ（FⅦ）-TF 复合物刺激形成Ⅹa（FⅩa），最终形成凝血酶（FⅡA）。凝血酶激活因子Ⅴ（FⅤ）、因子Ⅷ（FⅧ）和 FⅪ导致凝血酶形成增加。接着凝血酶促使纤维蛋白原的裂解，形成纤维蛋白单体，单体聚合，从而形成稳定的纤维蛋白凝块。凝血因子的消耗是通过肝细胞形成抗凝血酶（antithrombin，AT）Ⅲ控制的。凝血酶 - 抗凝血酶复合物抑制凝血酶 FⅪa、FⅩa、FⅪa、FⅫa。其他抑制剂包括 TF 途径抑制物（TF pathway inhibitor，TFPI）和与游离蛋白 S 结合的活化蛋白 C。游离蛋白 S 在炎症过程中由于和 C4b 结合蛋白结合而下降。

弥散性血管内凝血（disseminated intravascular coagulation，DIC）可能发生在创伤后。最初的阶段过后，可以观察到血管内和血管外纤维蛋白凝块。缺氧诱导的细胞损伤是形成血管内纤维蛋白凝块的原因。同样，细胞损伤也增加了内皮细胞和白细胞之间的相互作用。临床上，凝血因子消耗和血小板功能障碍是弥漫性出血的主要原因。通过纤溶酶作用下纤维蛋白凝块水解为纤维蛋白片段，凝血因子的消耗进一步增加。

急性期反应

急性期反应描述了创伤后的早期全身反应和其他损伤状态。在这个阶段，肝的生物合成显著发生改变。在正常情况下，肝在稳定状态时，合成一系列的血浆蛋白。然而，在急性期反应中，肝细胞对炎症过程中必不可少的正性急性期蛋白的合成增加［即 C 反应蛋白（C-reactive protein，CRP）、血清淀粉样 A 蛋白（serum amyloid A，SAA）、补体蛋白、凝血蛋白、蛋白酶抑制剂、金属结合蛋白和其他蛋白质］，同时伴有负性急性期蛋白的消耗。急性期蛋白列于表 3。

表 3　急性期蛋白

蛋白簇	单个蛋白质
正性急性期蛋白	
主要的急性期蛋白	C 反应蛋白、血清淀粉样 A 蛋白
补体蛋白	C2、C3、C4、C5、C9、B、C1 抑制剂，C4 结合蛋白
凝血蛋白	纤维蛋白原、凝血酶原、von Willebrand 因子
蛋白酶蛋白质	α1- 抗胰蛋白酶、α1- 抗胰凝乳蛋白酶、α_2- 抗纤维蛋白溶酶、肝素辅因子Ⅱ、纤溶酶原激活物抑制物Ⅰ
金属结合蛋白	触珠蛋白、血红素结合蛋白、铜蓝蛋白、锰超氧化物歧化酶
其他蛋白质	α_1- 酸性糖蛋白、血红素化氧酶、甘露糖结合蛋白、白细胞蛋白Ⅰ、脂蛋白（a）、脂多糖结合蛋白
负性急性期蛋白	白蛋白、前白蛋白、转铁蛋白、载脂蛋白 AⅠ、载脂蛋白 AⅡ、α_2-Heremans-Schmid 糖蛋白、间 α- 胰蛋白酶抑制剂、富组氨酸糖蛋白、蛋白 C、蛋白 S、抗凝血酶Ⅲ、高密度脂蛋白

正性急性期蛋白在急性期反应中增加，负性急性期蛋白在急性期反应中减少

急性期反应是由肝的 Kupffer 细胞和炎性细胞因子的释放引发的。IL-1、IL-6、IL-8 和 TNF-α 是刺激性的细胞因子。急性期反应通常持续 24～48 h。

IL-4、IL-10、糖皮质激素和其他激素的刺激作用，可以抑制急性期反应的促炎症介质。这种调节是至关重要的。在慢性或复发性炎症的情况下，异常急性期反应可能会导致组织损伤加剧。

主要的急性期蛋白包括 CRP 和 SAA，其作用机制目前知之甚少。CRP 如此命名是因为其有将 C- 多糖结合于肺炎球菌的能力。在炎症过程中，CRP 水平可能会在几个小时内增加高达 1 000 倍，取决于外界刺激和损伤的严重程度。它可视为细菌、寄生虫、和免疫复合物的调理素，通过经典途径激活补体，并结合染色质。结合染色质可以减少自身免疫反应，通过处理组织碎片部位的核抗原来实现。临床上，CRP 水平是相对非特异性的，并不能预测创伤后的相关并发症。尽管如此，对它的连续测定对评估患者的病情发展是有帮助的。

SAA 与高密度脂蛋白（high-density lipoprotein，HDL3）相互作用，从而成为在急性炎症中的主要载脂蛋白。这会增强巨噬细胞与 HDL3 的结合，可将胆固醇和脂质碎片吞噬。多余的胆固醇，用于组织修复或排泄。此外，SAA 抑制凝血酶诱导的血小板活化和中性粒细胞的氧化激发，有防止氧化组织破坏的潜力。

全身炎症反应综合征

介质释放导致了我们所说的 SIRS。1991 年，美国胸科医师学会和美国重症监护医学会的会议共识定义 SIRS：它是各种感染性和非感染性事件引起的全身炎症反应。他们通过会议建立了一些临床参数。表 4 总结了 SIRS 的诊断标准。诊断 SIRS 必须满足 4 个条件中的至少 2 个。须注意的是，这个定义强调炎症过程，而不是有无感染。脓毒症是发生 SIRS 时存在或者怀疑感染。随后的研究已经证实这些标准对于 ICU 患者死亡风险的增加有一定的预测作用。符合标准的条数越多，死亡风险越高。

SIRS 的特点是局部和全身产生并释放多种介质，包括促炎症细胞因子、补体因子、接触相蛋白和凝血系统、急性期蛋白、神经内分泌介质，并在组织损伤的局部激活免疫活性细胞。创伤的严重程度、刺激持续时间、遗传因素和个人的一般情况决定了促炎症细胞因子和磷脂的局部和全身的释放。

表 4　全身炎症反应综合征的临床参数

1. 心率＞90 次 / 分
2. 呼吸频率＞20 次 / 分，或者 $Paco_2$＜32 mm Hg
3. 体温＞38℃或者＜36℃
4. 白细胞＞12 000/mm^3 或者＜4 000/mm^3，或者幼粒细胞＞10%

$Paco_2$：动脉二氧化碳分压

代偿性抗炎反应综合征

创伤不仅刺激促炎症反应介质的释放，同时也释放抗炎症反应介质。这种代偿性抗炎反应是与 SIRS 同时存在的（图 2）。当这两个对立的反应达到适度的平衡，创伤患者可以有效地治愈损伤，而不会因自身免疫反应而造成二次损伤。然而，过度的 CARS 会导致创伤后免疫抑制，这会导致发生感染和脓毒症的概率增加。SIRS 逐渐停止，而 CARS 成为主要存在。

二次打击模型

在二次打击模型中，损伤刺激引起全身炎症反应（图 3）。“首次打击”对免疫系统继发性的刺激引起了过度的，甚至致命的炎症反应（“二次打击”），而首次打击其本身可能是不致命的。这种二次刺激可以是内源性的，也可以是外源性的。内源性二次打击，包括心血管不稳定、呼吸窘迫、代谢紊乱与缺血 / 再灌注损伤。与此相反，外源性二次打击包括手术干预、血液制品输注和漏诊。二次打击模型提出了二次打击引起破坏性

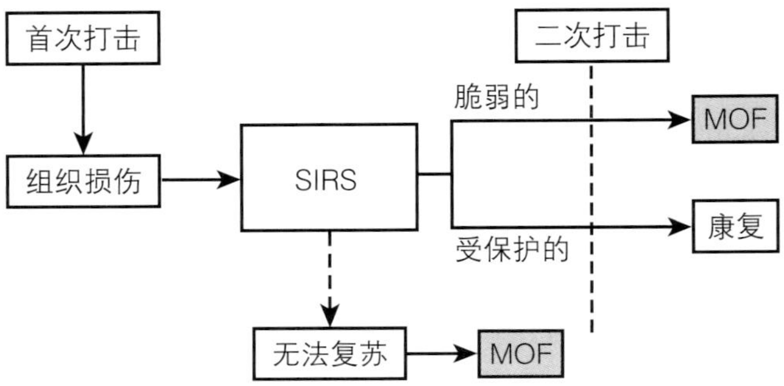

图 3　伤后多器官衰竭的发病机制

炎症，导致 MOF 和潜在的死亡结果。这种模式被 Moore 等支持，他们将创伤后机会性感染与 SIRS 和 MOF 联系在一起。

总结

创伤触发一个极其复杂的反应，涉及众多的系统。个体的免疫系统必须平衡炎症反应，这是清除损伤组织所必需的。同时通过必要的炎性过程的下调，避免引起过度的内源性损伤，为机体提供一个炎症反应最小化的内环境，以满足愈合所需要的细胞增殖和组织重塑。这种平衡的丧失会通过免疫反应引起额外的组织损伤或使个体容易感染和发生脓毒症。随着我们对创伤后免疫反应认识的增加，我们能够有效地监测和治疗创伤危重患者，有望改善患者的预后。

创伤患者感染性疾病的概述

Donald E. Fry 著
吕 杰 译

对于创伤后第一个 24 h 因复苏或其他干预措施成功存活的大多数严重创伤患者，感染是这些患者之后面临的主要威胁。感染风险可能来自于损伤环境的污染参与损伤过程，也可能来自于患者体内紊乱的器官结构的内源性菌群感染。当然，感染可能使损伤修复手术更为复杂。严重创伤患者在 ICU 中接受大量的护理。每位创伤患者在 ICU 中都有多个侵入性管道和监测装置，然而这每一个管道都是微生物入侵和危及生命的感染的途径。从损伤到恢复，创伤患者都暴露在损伤部位的病原体中，并且病原体在治疗过程中有可能经手传播至全身各处。

创伤患者不仅面临着很大的感染风险，而且还面临着严重的免疫抑制反应。基本上每一种目前可测量的固有免疫或获得性免疫应答的组分都被抑制。这种创伤后的免疫抑制虽然很难在进化论中找到合理的解释，但是通过调控大量组织损伤激活固有免疫，进而激活全身免疫反应这一通路，对创伤发生的主体是有保护作用的。遗憾的是，数千年的进化并没有预料到积极复苏、外科手术和 ICU 等因素的出现。然而，目前在严重的多系统损伤情况下得以存活，并恢复的宿主类似于是人体培养皿。ICU 成为所有创伤 / 危重患者经历免疫抑制和感染风险的地方。并非所有严重的创伤患者都会因感染而死亡，这本身就是一个奇迹。

本概述将简要讨论在创伤患者的护理中引起感染的常见临床问题。因为在其他章节对感染的解剖学部位、病原体以及抗生素的选择有详细讨论，此处不在对此问题进行详细讨论。本章节将突出阐述与创伤患者重要感染相关的共同特征，并将通过对特定感染和特定病原体举例，来强调这些特征。本概述有望阐述许多须继续关注和研究的领域的概况。

感染的决定因素

并不是所有损伤和所有患者都有相同的感染风险，感染作为病原体和宿主的许多变量复杂相互作用的结果而发生（图 1）。

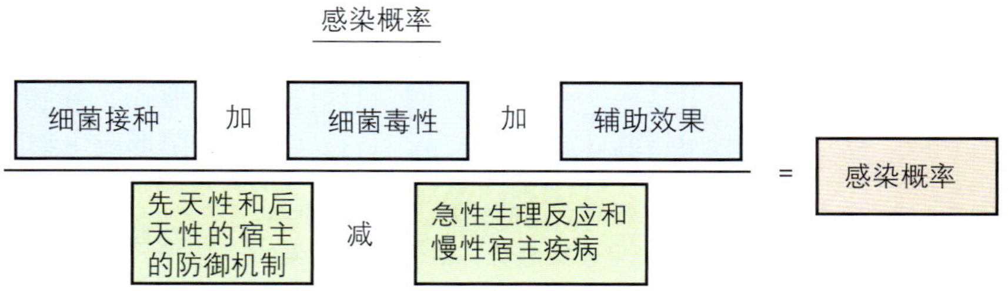

图 1 该示意图表示预测创伤患者感染的变量的假设方程。“分子”表示在创伤患者的感染发展中具有累加甚至协同作用的 3 个主要变量组。宿主防御的“分母”抵消分子的促感染事件。急性生理反应和慢性疾病可损害宿主的反应，提高发生感染的概率

微生物接种

一个污染（解剖学）部位的微生物数量以及感染发生所需的临界阈值是感染问题中最常见的研究问题之一。所有受伤部位、手术切口和侵入性医疗装置在进行细菌培养时都可培养出细菌。我们的环境不是无菌的，人类比真核细胞具有更多的微生物菌落。检出存在细菌并不一定都能确诊感染，但是单位重量的组织或单位表面积组织的细菌数量可预测感染发生情况。

经典的实验室和临床关于伤口的研究已经确立了伤口组织中，平均每克组织中有 10^5 个微生物为发生感染的微生物阈值。10^5 的阈值作为尿路感染定义中的标准。10^4 被认为是 ICU 肺泡分泌物的支气管肺泡灌洗液的细菌的确定界限。难辨梭菌芽孢有一定的界限，在被摄取后可产生结肠炎综合征。尽管在 10^5 的阈值附近存在一些生物学变异，但是支持性研究已经清楚地限定了可控污染大小的界限。这种可控污染可以在每个解剖学部位处理，避免感染的发生（图 2）。

微生物的毒性

细菌具有毒性特征的个体化差异。微生物的毒性因子包括细菌细胞的结构组分（例如内毒素）、细菌分泌的可损伤组织或特异性阻滞吞噬细胞功能的蛋白质，以及损害治疗策略有效性的抗菌素耐药性

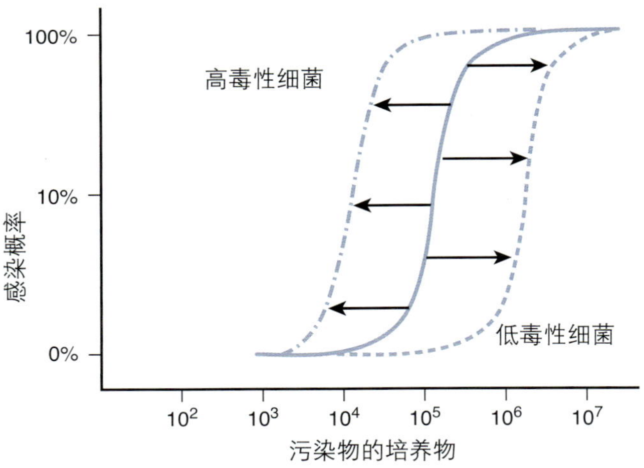

图 2 感染细菌培养物与感染概率之间的关系。常规病原体，细菌数 >每克10^5 个时，感染呈聚集趋势，对于毒性更强的细菌，曲线向左移动。毒性较低的细菌曲线移向右移动，即毒性较弱的细菌须有更大密度（或受损的宿主）才可引起感染

因素。革兰氏阴性菌内毒素中的脂质 A、产气荚膜梭菌产生的强效外毒素、化脓性链球菌的超级抗原和金黄色葡萄球菌的凝固酶都意味着更大的发生感染性疾病的风险。这意味着导致感染所需的微生物数量比传统观点中的每克 10^5 个的细菌数量更少。

相反，许多种类的细菌缺乏有效的毒性因素，但仍然存在感染风险。铜绿假单胞菌、表皮葡萄球菌、肠球菌和白念珠菌是在试验模型中表现出低毒性特征的微生物，但在临床工作中已被证明是许多感染患者的病原体。它们具有对许多药物都耐药的能力，并且在免疫抑制的重症监护患者中，在已有治疗消除常见的或可疑细菌病原体时，这些细菌就会成为他们出现感染的主要病因。本质上低毒性的微生物由于其结构及分泌产物的耐药性也可以在危重患者发生的感染中扮演重要角色。在重症监护室中，几乎任何微生物都可以在消除竞争性微生物菌群后，发挥作为病原体的作用，并抑制宿主反应。

辅助因素

据说，巴斯德在辉煌的科学生涯结束时曾说：“微生物什么都不是，环境就是一切。”此种说法虽然近乎夸张，但足以见巴斯德对微生物所在局部环境的重视。他认为微生物是否能在创伤患者身上致病，此因素是最重要的。创伤或手术部位血红蛋白和血肿为微生物生长提供了丰富的营养物质和关键数量的铁元素。坏死组织为细菌增殖提供了一个宿主吞噬细胞难以接近的避难所。

异物以一个感染发展的辅助变量，在所有外科手术患者的感染发展中起着重要的作用，在损伤患者中这种作用表现得更为突出。创伤可能会导致损伤途径中的许多外来的碎片物质，也可能使充满微生物的粪便从破裂的结肠溢出，以上情况都会促进感染的出现。手术部位会有缝合材料，有研究已经证实这些缝合材料可降低感染发生所需微生物数量的阈值。气管插管、尿管、引流管和血管内留置的装置为细菌定植提供了附着面，并且成为感染的孵育地。细菌的生物膜屏障是细菌的一种独特的毒力形式，异物表面可降低宿主的吞噬功能，同时为细菌形成生物膜生产提供了表面。

各种留置装置不仅损害宿主功能，它们还可能直接损伤患者的非特异性的上皮和内皮屏障。气管插管不仅破坏声门的正常屏障，还为外部环境进入下呼吸道提供了直接通路。尿管不仅为微生物提供

了入侵途径，还侵蚀膀胱内部保护性移行细胞。类似地，血管内留置装置为治疗提供了通路，但是入口部位的凝块和内皮损伤必然在感染中起作用。

宿主防御

在创伤和危重患者中，宿主受损的防御系统可能是感染产生的最重要的决定因素。每个患者都具有独特的、固有的遗传基因编码和适应性免疫应答。每个患者都有因感染而死亡的遗传脆弱性。不同的患者之间，宿主对感染反应的内在多态性差异难以量化，所有患者在消除软组织污染方面没有相同的效率，对待感染的生理反应也不尽相同。

获得性免疫对创伤患者具有重要意义。受伤患者的全身波动已被良好地记录，免疫效应也被广泛接受。出血、休克、低氧血症和广泛的软组织损伤对宿主的反应性具有深远的影响。低温和高血糖也是宿主免疫反应减弱的因素。既往存在糖尿病、慢性肾衰竭、营养不良和长期应用药物（如皮质类固醇）可影响免疫功能。受伤患者使用的治疗手段（如输血）可能会产生不利的宿主反应。很有可能这些获得性的外界因素对免疫效应的影响比个体遗传变异性在临床上与免疫效应更相关。

因此，我们可以为创伤患者建立一个预测感染事件的通用模型。无论是在软组织、腹膜或胸膜间隙、肺、尿道的感染，还是艰难梭菌感染，感染的决定因素是相同的。感染发生的风险是进入解剖学部位的细菌数量，微生物感染物的毒性特征和微环境因素的生物因素的总和。这些潜在的感染变量又被宿主的特异性及非特异性防御机制所抵消，之后宿主的反应性可受急性和慢性疾病的影响。目前我们对创伤患者发生的感染的预防和治疗就是尽量避免人为操作带来的感染，提高机体防御的有效性（图1）。

感染预防

感染预防在创伤疾病介绍的时候已经提及。复苏和手术治疗期间感染预防策略的失败将带来长期的感染发生的风险。尽管创伤最初的24 h护理及治疗的直接目的是保证患者的急性期生存，但是如果在开始到之后几天的治疗中，贯穿高度警觉的预防感染意识，将会对以后的治疗及患者的预后有利。

微生物接种数量的减少

感染预防从复苏室的衣服和手套开始。在实现止血后使用封闭敷料，以避免开放性伤口的进一步污染。留置的血管留置针可以合理地放置，但是一旦初次留置的导管的应用减少，这些留置针都应在适当的感染控制条件下进行更换。更换中心静脉导管应遵循公认的指南标准。Foley导管在这些患者的处理中可带来感染风险，应当在适当消毒后放置。从急性期到后期重症监护室的护理，必须避免对留置导管和输液管的不必要污染。一旦这些留置针、导管、引流管的主要功能完成，尽早及时将其拔除。

尿管留置时间过长是创伤患者护理中普遍重复出现的事件。细菌可以进入尿路内导管周围的空间并进入膀胱。虽然我们为保持会阴清洁已做出一定努力，但是人类的现实情况就是必然存在大量的微生物定植，并且感染的概率将随着导管留置时间的增加而增加。虽然保持引流系统的封闭性和用锚定方法避免尿管运动引起的“水坑”效应很重要，但是在创伤患者中尽早拔除尿管是预防尿路感染的最佳手段。

在对危及生命的问题进行即刻治疗之后，应对软组织创伤进行治疗。来自机械损伤的环境污染须清除坏死组织和去除异物，精确的清创术将减少微生物负担，并将微生物的培养基——坏死组织去除。盐水的脉冲灌洗可以除去存在于这些损伤中的细菌负载的纤维蛋白剥离物，适当应用封闭敷料以避免继发性污染。干燥可以使坏死组织增加，故而长期的开放性软组织伤口须应用湿敷料。大多数局部抗生素的使用可能会损伤软组织，故而应该避免使用。局部抗生素的应用在预防创伤性伤口感染方面没有价值。预防特别大的伤口的感染可以适当考虑应用局部烧伤的治疗剂，如醋酸磺胺米隆或磺胺嘧啶银，直到皮肤移植或皮瓣闭合。

预防外科手术部位的感染是一个重要目标。手术室环境的所有常规预防策略在创伤患者中仍然十分重要。用电动剪刀去除毛发。备皮尚未被证明可以降低感染率，故而在特定的患者中，可以不去除手术部位毛发。对于开颅手术和对于多毛患者来说，脱毛显然是必要的。防腐剂的擦洗可以使建议手术部位清洁皮肤的局部消毒剂的制备可减少伤口的污染，拟进行手术的部位应用抗菌剂消毒，并且最好用氯己定消毒。

预防性应用抗生素已经成为预防手术部位感染

的重要措施。虽然没有安慰剂对照临床试验证明预防应用抗生素使创伤患者的手术部位感染（surgical site infection，SSI）减少，但在许多其他领域有大量证据来证实这些患者术前应该适当使用抗生素。对于切开皮肤前给药和使用适合于可疑病原体的抗生素的重要性已有文献报道。抗生素必须在污染时即存在于组织中，如果抗生素在污染后起效将不改变 SSI 的发生率。对于手术部位以外的其他部位，来源于严重软组织损伤或肠破裂的组织污染已经发生。然而清创和损伤部位的处理意味着解剖和打开新鲜的组织平面，因此很有理由相信软组织修复或肠损伤处理时，组织中的抗生素将起到积极的作用。

应根据手术部位可能遇到的病原体来选择抗生素，对于整形外科、神经外科和胸外科的手术，患者皮肤上的定植菌和手术室环境中的细菌是污染切口的主要来源。建议术前应用头孢唑啉（静脉注射 1～2 g）覆盖金黄色葡萄球菌，在农场损伤或切口靠近会阴时，抗生素应覆盖革兰氏阴性菌和厌氧菌。创伤患者剖腹术的术前用药应覆盖肠革兰氏阴性杆菌（大肠杆菌）和肠道厌氧菌（如脆弱拟杆菌）。美国 FDA 不提供创伤环境中抗生素预防性应用的具体适应证。抗生素在创伤环境中的应用被 FDA 认为是假想治疗，并且在剖腹术中的预防性药物就是治疗腹腔内感染的药物。药物预防的选择的研究在表 1 中列举。应该注意的是，自 2000 年以来没有可以确定腹部创伤中的预防性抗生素的随机临床试验。

在主要创伤中心经常观察到软组织或腹部切口的大量污染。在清创术后或控制感染源的胃肠损伤处理后，外科医生留下有大量细菌的创伤性伤口或外科手术部位，感染似乎是肯定会发生的一个事件。这种情况下，延期一期或二期关闭是传统外科处理的一个重要选择，清洁伤口保持开放，用封闭敷料覆盖，并每天换药。外用醋酸磺胺米隆或磺胺嘧啶银是一种较好的局部治疗。特定的伤口可能适合延迟缝合。负压处理一直是治疗这些开放性伤口的重要补充措施。开放性软组织损伤可能需要皮肤移植或皮瓣封闭，腹部切口处理通常是次要目的。持续全身应用抗生素不是预防开放性软组织或外科伤口感染的恰当选择。

创伤患者在长期护理中须时刻保持警觉，以避免患者在 ICU 暴露于病原微生物。必须将预防的感染作为目标。耐甲氧西林金黄色葡萄球菌、耐药革兰

表 1　创伤患者剖腹探查的随机临床试验特点 *

作者（年份）	患者人群	抗生素	患者人数	感染人数（感染率）	总结
Kirton, 2000	剖腹术 穿通伤	氨苄西林舒巴坦：5 天 氨苄西林舒巴坦：1 天	159 158	16（10%） 13（8%）	延长抗生素应用超过 24 h 没有益处
Cornwell,1999	剖腹术 穿通伤	头孢西丁：1 天 头孢西丁：5 天	31 32	6（19%） 12（38）	低效度研究，但较长疗程的抗生素治疗没有优势
Schmidt-Matthiesen，1999	穿通伤 创伤	头孢曲松：1 剂 头孢西丁：3 天	97 98	4（4%） 5（5%）	治疗不同种类的损伤，长期应用抗生素没有益处
Bozorgzadeh, 1999	穿通伤 腹部损伤	头孢西丁：1 天 头孢西丁：5 天	148 152	24（16%） 26（17%）	长期应用抗生素没有益处
Tyburski, 1998	穿通伤 腹部损伤	环丙沙星 / 甲硝唑 庆大霉素 / 甲硝唑	35 33	7（20%） 5（15%）	胃或小肠损伤推荐使用抗生素，结肠损伤推荐使用 4 天；低效度研究
Sims, 1997	穿通伤 腹部损伤	头孢哌酮 头孢曲松 / 甲硝唑 庆大霉素 / 氨苄西林 / 甲硝唑	101 95 95	6（6%） 2（2%） 5（5%）	给药持续时间随损伤严重程度而变化；多种抗生素联合无益处
Fabian, 1994	穿通伤 腹部损伤	氨曲南 / 克林霉素 庆大霉素 / 克林霉素	37 36	1（3%） 7（19%）	$P<0.03$，氨曲南 / 克林霉素更有效；低效度研究
Weigelt, 1993	腹部损伤的剖腹术	头孢西丁 氨苄西林 - 舒巴坦	309 283	22（7%） 6（2%）	$P<0.004$，氨苄西林 - 舒巴坦更有效

* 所提供的药物、结果和评论。在过去的十年中还没有进行新的抗生素的临床试验

氏阴性菌和艰难梭菌芽孢，可以由于治疗过程中的失误，导致污染从一个患者传播到另一个患者。每个医生接触患者时手套和隔离衣必不可少。洗手在避免耐药细菌和艰难梭菌芽孢的传播上十分重要，标准洗手法洗手是避免微生物传播的最佳策略。依赖呼吸机的患者的吸痰以及所有留置管的操作在感染控制上仍然十分重要。在拔除体内的留置针、导管及引流管保持警觉仍然是最好的预防策略。

选择性肠道去污（selective gut decontamination，SGD）是一种用于减少创伤和危重疾病患者感染的方法。胃肠道被认为是许多院内感染的来源，所以SGD的概念是给予吸收较差的患者口服抗生素，以减少病原菌的微生物储量。需氧细菌是清除目标，努力保持厌氧菌定植和维持定植抗性。大多数研究已经证明这种方法可以减少一些感染的发生，但是创伤患者的死亡率并没有受到这种方法的影响。

微生物毒性的管理

显然，外科医生不能控制可能有污染的患者感染的病原体的毒性特性。然而，如果我们认为微生物的耐药性是微生物毒性的重要组成部分，那么，抗生素的应用就可以影响微生物毒性。

直到损伤后期，仍全身应用预防性抗生素，对创伤患者预防感染是目前最有问题的一种方式。术后再预防性应用抗生素，将不能预防手术部位的感染、医院获得性肺炎、血管内装置感染、导管相关尿路感染和艰难梭菌感染。后期继续应用抗生素来“覆盖”留置的引流管、导管或开放性伤口的观点缺乏证据。长期全身性应用抗生素保证后期的院内感染与预防用药耐药的病原体有关。

开放性骨折患者的处理就是一个例子。毫无疑问，对开放性骨折患者感染的担忧是有意义的。这些感染可以增加并发症发生率，并带来潜在的肢体缺失的风险。医生应该在清创时全身使用适当的抗生素，并且应用脉冲式的灌洗，以进一步减少微生物定植。在开放性伤口的管理过程中进行适当的感染控制，当临床证据表明可以安全关闭伤口时，再关闭伤口。毕竟骨折是一种夹杂着碎骨片的软组织损伤。开放性骨折伤口中使用预防性抗生素的理念在治疗其他软组织伤口的感染时同样适用。长期全身性应用抗生素可以导致耐药微生物定植，耐药微生物不仅可以感染开放性骨折伤口，它们还可以在其他解剖学部位定植，造成感染。

艰难梭菌感染的全国流行影响了创伤患者，这种流行在很大程度上是由抗生素的滥用造成的。全身性抗生素的应用对人类结肠的生态有不良影响，影响正常的厌氧微生物，并促使依附性的艰难梭菌芽孢转变为有活性的生物体。有活性的革兰氏阳性杆菌黏附于结肠上皮细胞，并产生外毒素A和外毒素B，可以造成损伤性小肠结肠炎。此外，分离出的高毒性艰难梭菌菌株可产生20倍的肠毒素的量，引起可能会导致中毒性巨结肠和需要外科结肠切除术的暴发性感染。预防这种小肠结肠炎综合征须倡导遵守洗手规范，进而减少患者之间的芽孢传播。基于乙醇的洗手比传统的肥皂洗手和清水洗手效果差。必须增强总体感染控制策略，尤其是在重症监护病房中。正如在研究中看到的，减少不必要的抗生素使用以及延长术后预防性用药，对于预防感染同样重要。

创伤患者院内获得性感染的耐药病原体逐渐增加。耐甲氧西林金黄色葡萄球菌（methicillin-resistant Staphylococcus aureus，MRSA）、耐万古霉素肠球菌、产生超广谱β-内酰胺酶（extened-spectrum β-lactamases，ESBL）的革兰氏阴性杆菌和革兰氏阴性菌中耐碳青霉烯酶肺炎克雷伯杆菌已经变得非常普遍，这些耐药菌的产生都是由于抗生素的滥用。首先，预防细菌出现耐药性，要求抗生素治疗以适当的剂量覆盖所确定的病原体，低治疗剂量是细菌耐药性产生的原因。显然抗生素的联合应用将在病原学培养证据之前开始，但一旦培养结果出来后，可以将抗生素治疗逐渐降级。遗憾的是，当培养证据表明可以使用较少的药物或低毒性（或昂贵）的替代品时，多余或不必要的抗生素治疗仍会持续使用。我们没有理由培养病原体，却忽略结果。最后，有记录表明短疗程的抗感染治疗与长疗程的抗感染治疗无疗效差别。肺炎和腹腔内感染的短疗程抗感染同样有效。当使用过量的抗生素时，会对接受治疗的患者造成更大的医疗负担。

辅助因素的管理

消除感染的辅助因素，须在患者护理时选择恰当的治疗技术，做出恰当的判断。清除血肿、引流胸腔积血或积液、有效地止血避免随后的组织血液积聚都是有效手段。此外，清除坏死组织、有选择性地应用电刀可以减少伤口内烧焦的坏死组织，这些坏死组织都可能成为微生物在伤口内的培养基。

在整体使用的缝合材料上，减少整体使用缝合材料、避免编织材料和更多使用单丝纤维值得鼓励。

在创伤患者中留置异物，对于临床监测、治疗干预和减少无效腔是十分必要的。所有导管、留置针和引流管都是使伤口或体腔对外部环境开放的双向通路。异物的表面促进微生物的生长。所有留置管、针都应该遵守感染控制原则，并在留置目的完成后尽快移除。尽管已经提出了留置装置用抗生素和银浸渍，但是这些导管抗感染的有效性仍未得到证实，并且它们相对于普通留置装置价位更高。最好的感染预防措施是及时移除。

宿主的强化

尽管在增强或调节宿主对感染的反应方面的许多努力不是很成功，但是优化宿主的正常生理状态可以增加预防感染的有效性，这一学说已经取得了相当大的进展。氧是细胞内杀死病原体这一白细胞功能所必需的。相当多的试验证据为优化氧输送，以防止感染提供了强有力的证据。此外，一些选择性手术的经验也为这一观点提供了支持证据。宿主防御无疑受益于充足的组织氧供。这可能也不会导致超常氧浓度的情况。

长期以来，我们认为创伤患者维持核心体温以避免可预防的凝血功能障碍十分重要。试验证据表明在轻度低温时，生物反应速度减慢，白细胞向受损或感染的组织迁移的功能受损。结肠的择期手术经验已经证明维持核心温度是有利的。在患者管理的早期阶段，如复苏，手术期间和早期在 ICU 的患者管理，都须应用各种机械加热装置支持核心体温，但是最佳的温度控制方法仍有待确定。

支持宿主防御功能方面一个有争议的问题是血糖控制。一项大型临床试验表明严格血糖控制（80 ~ 110 mg/dl）在外科危重患者中可以降低多器官功能障碍的发生率和死亡率。最近，更多的临床研究对这种血糖控制的程度提出了异议，并且指出了低血糖发作对患者的负面影响。损伤和脓毒症可以出现高代谢反应，多余的外源性葡萄糖的管理以及糖异生加快是其中的特征。由于葡萄糖耐受不良，高血糖成为创伤患者的实际状态。适当的血糖控制可能有益于创伤患者，但管理程度仍不确定。心脏外科手术的预防策略表明血糖控制以 200 mg/dl 为上限是恰当的。实时血糖监测将是一项亟待发展的技术，有望解决葡萄糖处理中血糖限制标准的问题。

常规建议对创伤患者进行营养支持以防止蛋白质消耗和预防感染。常规推荐有效蛋白质补充（1.5 g/kg · d），适当应用非蛋白质卡路里（蛋白质 100 ~ 150 cal/g）。有证据支持使用谷氨酰胺、精氨酸、核苷酸、ω-3 脂肪酸、抗氧化剂和微量矿物质的特定组分。这种营养支持应尽可能由消化道输送。

最后，在治疗过程中要提高警惕，一些治疗方法可能抑制宿主反应性。输血是必要的，但是会有免疫抑制，故而大多数情况下有必要重新评估输血需求。抗组胺阻断药和质子泵抑制剂通常用于危重创伤患者，以预防应激性黏膜出血。然而，胃酸是公认的非特异性防御机制，胃酸抑制与医院获得性肺炎和艰难梭菌感染相关。类似的，非甾体抗炎药物与艰难梭菌感染相关。

感染的诊断

感染诊断的传统方法是识别特异的症状和体征，并通过培养病原体，来诊断并指导治疗。伤口和切口的炎症、硬结和脓性分泌物是感染的典型症状。发热和白细胞增多虽然不是感染的特异性表现，但通常是有价值的。X 线胸片和 CT 是公认的临床感染部位的影像学方法。渗出物、血液、血管内导管和尿液的培养物是诊断的金标准。粪便中毒素的检测是艰难梭菌感染的诊断方法。然而，对于感染的诊断仍然存在一些问题。

感染部位不适当的标本取样可能误导医生对病原体的判断。感染伤口的浅表拭子可能错过发现深层病原体的可能，特别是在软组织的多重感染中，这种现象更为明显。更深层组织的活检取样的培养结果将给出更可靠的诊断。脓液和腹腔感染须快速培养以发现厌氧菌和兼性厌氧微生物，并且在采样时直接接种到培养基中可以最好地分离这些病原体。气管吸出物不同于支气管肺泡取样，培养结果也许不是病原体，而是定植菌。

创伤患者留取血培养非常常见，但是培养出单独的病原体的概率较低。软组织和腹腔中的许多感染是多重感染和化脓性感染，很少与菌血症相关。相似地，肺部感染通常不与菌血症相关。但是，血管内装置感染以菌血症为其标志，当怀疑导管相关性感染时，血培养有较大价值。若创伤患者中出现的金黄色葡萄球菌的阳性血培养结果，首先考虑血管内装置感染，除非证明有其他来源。

导管相关的尿路感染仍然是创伤患者一个目前有许多问题的领域。传统意义上尿中培养出微生物每毫升多于 10^5 个可诊断为尿路感染，然而这个诊断指标源自社区获得性膀胱炎患者，研究对象不是带有尿管的患者。微生物可以沿着尿管表面生长，也可脱落进入尿液。细菌尿可能并不能直接说明有侵入性感染或异物效应。进一步的研究表明，尿培养阳性并不一定是创伤患者发热的原因。针对有导管的患者的尿路感染诊断的进一步研究是必要的。

感染的治疗

发生感染时，创伤患者针对感染须在感染部位进行机械干预，包括控制污染、充分引流和清创。感染的伤口必须打开、清除坏死组织、去除异物、引流脓液。必须从感染的软组织损伤和手术切口中清除纤维蛋白/炎性碎片，包括腹腔内的穿孔以及缝合线泄漏所造成的病原体。脓肿及脓胸必须充分引流。必须清理支气管脓性分泌物及潜在气道栓子。必须去除感染的留置在血管内装置。化脓性血栓性静脉炎必须切除。只有当感染的原发灶用物理手段处理并控制之后，后续的抗感染手段才能成功。

支持措施是创伤患者发生感染后所必需的，使用也很广泛，此问题在别处已详细描述。“拯救脓毒症策略”已经提供了针对严重感染患者的良好的支持措施。脓毒症患者临床治疗重点是通过所有必要的支持方法和药物干预来维持有效的氧合和组织灌注。通过脉搏、呼吸、血氧饱和度和尿量的简单测量，来监测患者的反应，已被证明是一种评估支持性护理的简单、有效的方法。对于多系统损伤，必须尽早有效地启动营养支持，以避免损伤和侵袭性感染后的强烈分解代谢反应。

抗生素治疗是创伤患者治疗中的双刃剑。当在受伤早期（3～5天）出现感染时，治疗应针对受伤组织的可疑病原体。钝性软组织损伤对革兰氏阳性球菌易感。农业事故将涉及多种微生物：革兰氏阳性微生物、革兰氏阴性微生物和肠道厌氧菌。导弹和穿通性武器受伤之后的感染将对应于受伤的组织。在创伤患者的腹腔内感染中，临床推定此病原体为肠道革兰氏阴性菌和肠道厌氧菌，在得到培养证据之前，针对它们进行治疗（表2）。

艰难梭菌感染必须及时治疗，如果可能，应口服适当的抗生素（表3）。当艰难梭菌感染的患者出现急腹症、严重的全身炎症反应综合征和结肠积气，有必要进行腹腔探查术和结肠次全切除术。万古霉素灌肠加回肠造口术最近被报道为一种创新的干预手段，可以避免对结肠切除术的需求。

如果感染在进入ICU5天后出现，那么感染可能是医院获得性病原体感染。在培养获得结果之前，抗生素覆盖面须与目前ICU的病原体抗菌谱一致。当确认了病原体后，抗生素的经验性应用应降阶梯为针对确定病原体的抗生素。特定抗生素用于治疗重新出现的单独菌株的敏感性会在其他章节中提到。

要点

创伤患者发生感染后抗生素应用及其他问题的要点如下：

- SSIs在无周围蜂窝织炎或伤口坏死的证据时很少须全身应用抗生素，有效的局部引流和清创才是治疗的关键措施。
- 开放性手术伤口和开放性创伤伤口都将可能出现微生物培养阳性，但如果经过充分引流和清创，通常不会出现感染。抗生素应该用于治疗感染，而不是清除定植菌。
- 腹腔内脓肿和引流管、尿管处的积脓，抗生素应用后的细菌培养结果将有医院获得性病原体。抗生素对分离的病原体的敏感性是至关重要的。
- 抗生素使用的剂量应该是充分的治疗量。感染的创伤患者具有更大的分布体积和高动力循环。更频繁地给予更大剂量的抗生素是确保在已确定的感染中充足的药物输送的最佳方式。在危重的创伤患者中，未来须考虑抗生素的药物动力学给药剂量的扩展方案（图3）。
- 站在患者的立场，应用抗生素时间越短越有利。如果它们在7天内无疗效，那么有可能须引流脓液，或者你必须重新评估诊断或病原体。
- 除非有其他病原学证据腹泻基本都是艰难梭菌感染，当在ICU中发生腹泻时，不要使用抑制肠道蠕动的药物。抑制肠道蠕动的药物可引起中毒性巨结肠和结肠坏死。新的艰难梭菌的高毒性菌株快速产生大量毒素，甚至在没有腹泻的情况下可导致快速发展的疾病（中毒性巨结肠）。ICU的高龄的创伤患者和进行性腹部膨胀者都要考虑艰难梭菌感染。
- 肠道微生态学的破坏是艰难梭菌和念珠菌属感染的基础。如果可能，应停止针对这两种微生物的抗生素之外的其他抗生素。此外，肠道是微生物易位、内毒素释放和细胞因子从肠相关淋巴组织播散的可能储存地，它成为成果反应和器官功能障碍的驱动。

- 不要一味将损伤后发热和白细胞增多归因于尿路感染，特别是对于排尿通畅的尿路，此时常有其他部位的感染。
- 当发生菌血症，或者有推测来自血管内留置装置的葡萄球菌感染时，须更换所有管路、静脉抗葡萄球菌的抗生素治疗应延长到 14 天，以避免出现心内膜炎的并发症。
- 尽管万古霉素在治疗感染中已经被证实是有效的，但是也有证据证明在甲氧西林敏感的金黄色葡萄球菌（methicillin-sensitive S. aureus，MSSA）中，万古霉素用于预防和治疗是疗效不佳的。早期应用β- 内酰胺仍然是 MSSA 的

表 2 抗生素的选择、生物清除半衰期、剂量选择、创伤患者腹腔感染治疗选择的评论 *

抗生素	半衰期（$t_{1/2}$）	成人剂量	腹腔内感染的评论
哌拉西林 - 三唑巴坦	1 h	3.375 g/6 h	最受欢迎，可覆盖需氧菌和厌氧菌，单药治疗
头孢唑啉	1.7 h	1 ~ 2 g/8 h	必须与甲硝唑联合治疗，通常用于外伤患者的感染预防
头孢西丁	0.75 h	2 g/6 h	短半衰期，已使用 30 年，可以覆盖需氧菌和厌氧菌，但耐药性是个问题
头孢替坦	4 h	1 ~ 2 g/12 h	有需氧菌和厌氧菌活性，但革兰阴性菌的耐药性是个问题
头孢呋辛	2 h	1.5 g/8 h	必须与甲硝唑联合治疗，此种情境下应用较少
头孢噻肟	1 h	1 ~ 2 g/6 ~ 8 h	不与甲硝唑连用时对厌氧菌作用弱，代谢产物有生物活性
头孢他啶	2 h	2 g/8 h	必须与甲硝唑联合治疗，最常用于革兰氏阴性杆菌感染
头孢曲松	7 ~ 8 h	1 g/12 h	长半衰期，抗厌氧菌活性弱，常与甲硝唑联合治疗，最常用于社区获得性肺炎
头孢吡肟	2 h	2 g/8 ~ 12 h	不覆盖厌氧菌，必须与甲硝唑联合治疗，最常用于革兰氏阴性菌、医院获得性感染
环丙沙星	4 h	400 mg/12 h	不覆盖厌氧菌，必须与甲硝唑联合治疗
左氧氟沙星	6 ~ 8 h	750 mg/24 h	不覆盖厌氧菌，必须与甲硝唑联合治疗
莫西沙星	12 h	400 mg/24 h	只有喹诺酮类有厌氧菌活性，可作为单剂使用
甲硝唑	8 h	500 mg/8 h	专门治疗厌氧菌的药剂，必须联合使用才可以覆盖肠道革兰氏阴性菌
庆大霉素	2 h	1 mg/kg/8 h，5 ~ 7 mg/kg/24 h	抗革兰氏阴性菌作用强，需要药代动力学剂量，必须与甲硝唑联合治疗
妥布霉素	2 h	1 mg/kg/8 h，5 ~ 7 mg/kg/24 h	抗革兰氏阴性菌作用强，需要药代动力学剂量，必须与甲硝唑联合治疗
阿米卡星	2 h	7.5 mg/kg/12 h，15 ~ 20 mg/24 h	抗革兰氏阴性菌作用强，需要药代动力学剂量，必须与甲硝唑联合治疗
多尼培南	1 h	500 mg/8 h	综合覆盖需氧菌和厌氧菌，更常用于医院获得性感染
厄他培南	4 h	1 g/24 h	综合覆盖肠道需氧菌和厌氧菌，碳青霉烯类有长半衰期
亚胺培南 - 西司他丁	2 h	500 mg/6 h，1 g/8 h	综合覆盖需氧菌和厌氧菌，更常用于医院获得性感染
美罗培南	1 h	1 g/8 h	综合覆盖需氧菌和厌氧菌，更常用于医院获得性感染
氨曲南	1.7 h	1 ~ 2 g/6 ~ 8 h	覆盖厌氧菌，必须与甲硝唑联合治疗
替吉环素	40 h	50 mg/12 h	全面覆盖需氧菌和厌氧菌

* 所有剂量均为静脉给药剂量。药物的选择应针对革兰氏阴性菌和肠道厌氧菌（脆弱拟杆菌）。对于再次手术和抗生素前期治疗时的感染细菌培养是非常重要的，因为在这种情况下病原体中可能混有耐药菌。当之前就使用引流管时，耐甲氧西林金黄色葡萄球菌将出现在再次手术或经皮引流患者的培养结果中

表 3　针对艰难梭菌感染的当前的药物选择

抗生素	剂量	评论
甲硝唑	250 ~ 500 mg，一天 4 次，连用 10 天；或者 500 ~ 750 mg，一天 3 次，连用 10 天	治疗轻中度感染的患者首选
万古霉素	250 ~ 500 mg，一天 4 次，连用 10 天	推荐用于治疗重症病例
非达霉素	200 mg，一天 4 次，连用 10 天	FDA 批准治疗初始感染
利福平	300 mg，一天 4 次，连用 10 天	与甲硝唑联用治疗复发性感染的昂贵药剂
杆菌肽	25 000 单位，一天 4 次，连用 10 天	不易吸收、良好的体外活性、昂贵，且不容易获得
夫西地酸	250 mg，一天 3 次，连用 7 ~ 10 天	临床经验有限，全身吸收显著
替吉环素	静脉注射 50 mg，一天 2 次，直到临床其他决断	仅用于难治性病例

* 甲硝唑和万古霉素仍然是初始感染的选择。非达霉素于 2011 年 5 月获得批准。其他选择仅考虑初始治疗难治的感染或复发性感染患者。所有药物均口服给药，除了替吉环素

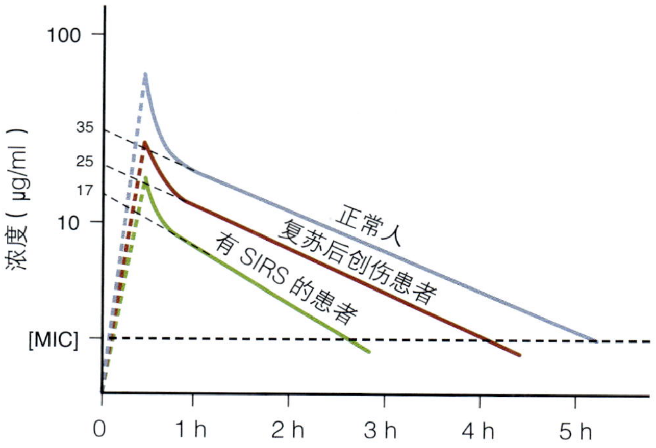

图 3　该图说明了在“正常患者”中具有约 6 h 的半衰期（$t_{1/2}$）的假定抗生素的血清清除率。给药剂量为静脉内 1g，最小抑菌浓度（MIC）的目标示为 1 μg/ ml，峰浓度为约 60 μg/ mL，平衡的时间零点（t_0）浓度为 35 μg/ ml（y 轴上的截距）。在复苏后创伤患者中，分布体积扩大，并由 25 μg/ ml 的 t_0 浓度的下降证明。抗生素浓度高于 MIC 的持续时间减少 1 h。在全身炎症反应综合征（SIRS）的创伤患者中，分布体积比正常患者进一步扩大 2 倍（t_0 浓度 =17 μg/ ml），并且 $t_{1/2}$ 由于高动力循环和更快的药物消除，到达临界 MIC 的时间小于 3 h。在复苏后或感染的创伤患者中，抗生素必须使用更大的药物剂量或更频繁的给药频率

合适选择（萘夫西林、头孢唑啉）。

■ 发热是宿主的积极反应，在创伤患者应用解热药是一个误区，须积极治疗感染而不是发热。

总结

创伤患者的感染将继续是未来的挑战。最近 40 年，我们目睹了细菌的毒性特性和微生物的耐药性的惊人的变化，这些趋势很可能会继续。此外，整体治疗手段的提高，导致那些过去无法存活的患者得以存活。因此，在严重免疫抑制的宿主中将遇到更强毒性和更强耐药性的细菌。

在未来几十年，这些患者的处理的变化将是什么？抗生素研究是否会继续产生具有针对新一代病原体活性的新药剂？用于治疗革兰氏阴性菌感染的新抗生素的数量很少。毫无疑问金黄色葡萄球菌将继续产生新的耐药模式和新的致病因子。革兰氏阴性耐药菌在过去 20 年中不断变异，并且没有停止变异的证据。令人惊讶的是，在过去十年中针对新抗生素的随机试验数量下降。抗生素时代可能即将结束。

治疗创伤患者的感染的新策略集中于对抗细菌毒性上，包括中和特异性毒素、干扰附着机制和调节毒性基因的抗体治疗。现已证明控制离子环境可以调节微生物毒性，这将是另一个潜在的新治疗战略。也许益生菌治疗将通过恢复宿主正常的定植环境和通过竞争性抑制消除病原体、中和微生物毒性。在开发新的治疗手段之前，预防和处理创伤患者的感染将继续在改善感染控制的手段、感染发生时消除病原体、增强宿主反应方面进行努力。

医院获得性肺炎

Paul M. Maggio and David A. Spain 著
吕 杰 译

肺炎可以分为是社区获得性肺炎（commmunty-acquired pneumonia，CAP）和医院获得性肺炎两大类。医院获得性肺炎包括医院获得性肺炎（hospital-acquired pneumonia，HAP）、呼吸机相关性肺炎（ventilator-associated pneumonia，VAP）和医疗机构相关性肺炎（health care-associated pneumonia，HCAP）。HAP 是指患者入院时不存在、也不处于感染潜伏期，而于入院 48 h 后发生的肺炎。如果在患者进行插管和机械通气超过 48 h 后发生感染，则该病症称为 VAP。HCAP 可以在医院内部或外部发生，并且指在因为先前的医疗行为，暴露于多重耐药（multidrug-resistant，MDR）病原体的高风险患者的肺炎。VAP 是在危重患者或受伤的手术患者中常见和严重的感染，与医院死亡率和资源使用（即机械通气天数、ICU 治疗时间和成本）的显著增加相关。因此，预防是最好的策略。

发生率、并发症发生率和死亡率

肺炎仍是 ICU 中最常见的院内感染，是 HAP 引起死亡的主要原因。HAP 占所有医院感染的 25% ~48%，死亡率为 20% ~50%。VAP 的发生率根据危险因素、患者人群和诊断方法而变化。在美国，VAP 的发生率在 ICU 患者中为每机械通气 1 000 天 2.2 例，对于创伤或烧伤 ICU 患者为每机械通气 1 000 天中 8.1 例和 10.7 例。其中外科手术、多次输血、脊髓损伤和高级设备使用影响感染发生的风险。机械通气仍然是发生 VAP 的最重要的风险因素，每天机械通气发生 VAP 的累积相关风险约为 1%。在机械通气的最初 5 天（每天 3%）风险最大，然后稳定下降。患有 HAP 的患者具有更高的死亡率、更长的 ICU 治疗时间和住院时间、更高的医疗成本。HAP 使总住院时间增加约 9 ~ 12 天，对于危重患者，ICU 治疗时间增加 4 ~ 6 天。

危险因素及预防措施

可改变的和不可改变的危险因素

虽然 VAP 的最大危险因素是机械通气的持续时间，但还有许多其他危险因素（表 1），这些与 VAP 的发病机制直接相关。由于下呼吸道在正常情况下是无菌的，所以将病原体引入肺中和损害传统宿主防御（在局部和全身水平）是引起感染所必需的。越来越多的证据表明，口咽或胃肠道的病原体定植或污染可导致下呼吸道感染。气管插管本身的细菌定植也可能导致在吸痰或支气管镜检查期间发生肺泡感染。其他较不常见的来源包括菌血症和感染性气溶胶吸入或血行扩散。

机械通气

机械通气是 HAP 的最大的独立危险因素，并且可使肺部的感染风险增加 6 ~ 20 倍。气管插管本身增加了肺炎发生的风险，因为其在操作过程中可能直接将病原体接种到肺中。因此，在临床情况允许的条件下应尽可能避免插管，使用无创正压通气。无创通气与机械通气的前瞻性研究显示，在校正疾病严重程度后，使用无创通气的患者 VAP 和院内感染的风险通常会降低。其他侵入性操作如气管造口术、支气管镜检、留置鼻胃（nasogastric，NG）管和胸廓造口术置管也可增加感染风险。胸部创伤和胸部手术会导致 VAP 不成比例的更高的发生率。

在创伤或手术过程中，大多数患者应用机械通气是因为胸部损伤或术后呼吸衰竭。我们最好通过每日评估镇静需求和评估脱机和拔管可能性来努力减少镇静和努力使患者术后尽早脱机。在不同患者群体中的许多研究已经证明，在患者的诊疗过程中使用这种方法，患者使用呼吸机的时间会显著减少。

对于插管患者，口咽分泌物积聚在气管内的皱襞部位，之后可泄漏到下呼吸道，这是下呼吸道感染的一个潜在来源。特别设计的气管内导管可以在通气间歇时进行吸痰。最近对 5 项研究（896 名患者）进行 meta 分析发现，在预期需要 72 h 机械通气的患者中吸引声门下分泌物将早发性 VAP 的发生率降低近一半（RR＝0.51,95% CI 为 0.37 ~ 0.71）。然而，

表 1　呼吸机相关性肺炎的危险因素

不可改变的	可改变的
年龄≥60 岁	机械通气≥3 天
男性	意外拔管
有 COPD 病史	二次插管
有严重合并情况	气管造口
使用皮质类固醇	支气管镜检查
诊断烧伤	鼻胃管
诊断创伤	气管内皱襞压力为 20 cmH_2O
头部损伤和其他 CNS 疾病	仰卧位
	抗酸药、H2 受体拮抗剂
突发事件或现场插管	胃液 pH 值升高
急诊手术	误吸
	使用镇静药物
	GCS≤9
	感染性休克
	贫血
	入住 ICU 前 48 h 未使用抗生素
	患者转运出 ICU
	血液透析
	输血
	APACHE Ⅱ评分

APACHE，急性生理和慢性健康评分；CNS，中枢神经系统；COPD。慢性阻塞性肺疾病；GCS，格拉斯哥昏迷等级评分；ICU，重症医学病房

它们似乎在预防迟发性 VAP 方面效果较差，并且存在黏膜损伤的风险，还有吸引腔经常闭塞。因此，使用声门下气管插管吸引进入临床实践进展缓慢。

呼吸机管路也可能被冷凝水和患者分泌物污染，应及时清除这些污染物，以免吸入的发生 VAP。常规呼吸机管路更换可能会导致误吸和提高发生 VAP 的风险，故管路更换只应在呼吸机管路损坏或明显污染时进行。气管插管在皱襞处的压力也应该保持在 20 cm H_2O，以防止皱襞周围的病原微生物进入下呼吸道。应当监测皱襞压力，25 cmH_2O 或更大的皱襞压力可以引起气管黏膜血流量的减少，导致气管损伤。最近引入了改良的气管内导管（例如银涂层的气管内导管）以帮助抵抗感染。虽然早期有些令人鼓舞的研究依据，但常规使用尚未建立。

宿主防御的损伤

损伤宿主防御的始作俑者，如年龄的增加、肺部疾病和其他合并情况的存在（包括脓毒症、皮质类固醇激素的使用、一次或多次输血史），都已被证明是危险因素。有这些危险因素的患者应严格监测预防措施的实施，以防止肺炎发生。

口咽部定植

虽然口咽部通常没有肠道革兰氏阴性菌定植，但这种定植在入院 48 h 内的 ICU 群体中有 75% 的发生率。口咽定植可以通过口腔卫生护理和使用口腔抗菌的氯己定而减少，此外还应该定期进行口腔检查、刷牙和行口腔拭子检查。多项随机试验显示，使用氯己定的术后患者，VAP 发病率降低了 60%，但大多数研究证明，VAP 发病率可降低，但降低幅度没有这么大。

误吸

一些因素可以增加误吸风险，如持续镇静、低格拉斯哥昏迷等级评分（Glasgow Coma Scale，GCS）评分、麻醉剂的使用和仰卧位，同时这些因素均已显示增加 VAP 的风险。我们应尽一切努力减少胃和口咽内容物的吸入。仰卧位相比于半卧位，可以增加误吸和 VAP 风险。因此，患者应该半卧位，床头尽可能提高到 30°～45°。这是一个简单、低成本的操作，可以显著降低 VAP 的风险，应该定期实施。对于确诊或疑似脊柱损伤的患者，可以使用反 Trendelenburg 体位。ICU 患者的连续横向旋转也显示出保护效果，但是因为它需要专门的床，此方法更昂贵。可能由于转运期间的仰卧位，将患者从 ICU 运出进行手术也增加了 VAP 的风险。因此，患者应尽可能在转运期间保持半卧位。

虽然由于误吸，推测肠内营养与肠外营养相比，将增加 VAP 发生率，然而证据表明事实并非如此。只要保持初始速率适度在 48～72 h（约一半），然后 72～96 h 增加至目标速率，即可优先在半卧位进行喂养。其他数据表明较小型号的鼻胃管以及幽门或小肠喂养的益处，然而，这些技术都没有被证明可持续降低 VAP 的风险。

胃肠道细菌过度生长

抑酸剂和 H_2 受体拮抗剂使胃肠道易于发生细菌过度生长，并且与 VAP 的发生风险增加相关，究其原因可能是由于误吸。尽管硫糖铝对 VAP 的影响有争议，但最新的大型随机试验表明，虽然硫糖铝与

雷尼替丁和抑酸药相比，硫糖铝所致 VAP 的发生率显著降低，但硫糖铝可使胃肠道出血的发病率增加。因此，并没有哪种应激性溃疡的预防方法具有明显优势。

SDD 可能会有效降低 VAP 的发生率。它试图减少需氧型革兰氏阴性杆菌和念珠菌在口咽和胃的定植，而不影响厌氧菌群。大多数方案包括联合使用氨基糖苷类、两性霉素 B 或制霉素，与不可吸收的抗生素，例如多粘菌素。在许多试验中也添加了全身性应用抗生素。多项随机对照试验显示 SDD 可使 VAP 的发生率降低、住院死亡率降低、MDR 感染降低。然而，这些预防作用与研究质量成反比，且在具有高水平耐药菌的医院中更不明显。最后，最近的数据表明，长期使用SDD导致细菌耐药性增加。因此，SDD 不推荐常规使用，特别是对于那些有耐药病原体感染的患者。目前推测 SDD 静脉应用的抗生素组分是改善存活的主要原因，然而，目前不推荐静脉抗生素的预防性使用。

耐药微生物

最近，耐药微生物引起了 VAP 发病率的增加。特别地，MRSA 引起的 VAP 可以占 15% ~27%。耐药菌感染的危险因素包括近期使用抗生素、住院 5 天或更长时间、来自相关卫生机构的转院、免疫抑制疾病或免疫抑制治疗、存在严重的慢性合并症、该特定医院或社区中频频出现细菌耐药。另一项最近的研究还表明，误吸、紧急插管和 GCS≤9 是耐药菌引起早发性 VAP 的特定危险因素。

综合所有危险因素

创伤后 VAP 的发病率可以用公式计算：

VAP 发生概率 $=e^{f(x)}/(1+e^{f(x)})$

f（x）=–3.08–1.56（损伤机制为穿通伤 =1，为钝伤 =0）-0.12（GCS 分数）+1.37（脊髓损伤，是 =1，否 =0）+0.30（胸部简明损伤分级）+1.87（紧急剖腹手术，是 =1，否 =0）+0.67（抢救室输血）+0.05（损伤严重度评分）+0.66（现场或抢救室插管，是 =1，否 =0）。这个公式对后续发展出现 VAP 的预测的准确率为 95%。

一般预防

最大限度地执行手卫生规范对预防和防止医院内感染的发生和传播至关重要。通过引入乙醇泡沫和凝胶，执行手卫生规范的程度已大幅提高。与彻底的洗手相比，这些产品具有改良的功效，并且花费时间明显更少。卫生保健人员应在与机械通气患者接触前后使用这些产品。在任何可能受到呼吸道分泌物或其他体液污染的情况下，还应适当使用隔离衣和手套。

有效的预防措施——“集束化”

越来越多的证据表明，旨在预防 VAP 的各种常规规范和各种预防措施的联合应用在预防 VAP 方面是有效的。“集束”是指将一组有循证证据表明可改善患者治疗的实践行为一起来执行，若正确实行，它对患者的预后是有益的。一个机构表明，经过培训将床头抬高≥30°、适当使用镇静剂、注意常规口腔卫生和呼吸设备管理之后，VAP 的患病率降低了 51%。由于 VAP 可以导致住院时间增加，因此导致成本增加，该计划非常具有成本效益，预计节省超过 40 万美元。

诊断

当患者出现肺部感染的临床症状（即发热、白细胞增多、脓痰、呼吸窘迫和氧合状态恶化），X 线胸片出现新的浸润影或肺浸润影进行性发展（图 1）时，须怀疑肺炎（表 2）。值得注意的是，在诊断为 ARDS 的患者中，肺炎需要高度怀疑。几项研究已经注意到 ARDS 患者中肺炎的发病率较高。例如，一项研究显示 ARDS 患者的肺炎发病率为 55%，而没有 ARDS 的患者的肺炎发病率为 28%。另一项研究指出严重 ARDS（Pao_2/Fio_2 比值小于 150 mm Hg）患者的肺炎发病率为 60%。

诊断策略

创伤患者从气管插管内所吸出的痰的革兰氏染色，对疑似肺炎的诊断或治疗几乎没有作用。接受机械通气的 ICU 创伤患者在没有肺炎的情况下在 X 线胸片常常有肺浸润影，以及发热和黏稠的呼吸道

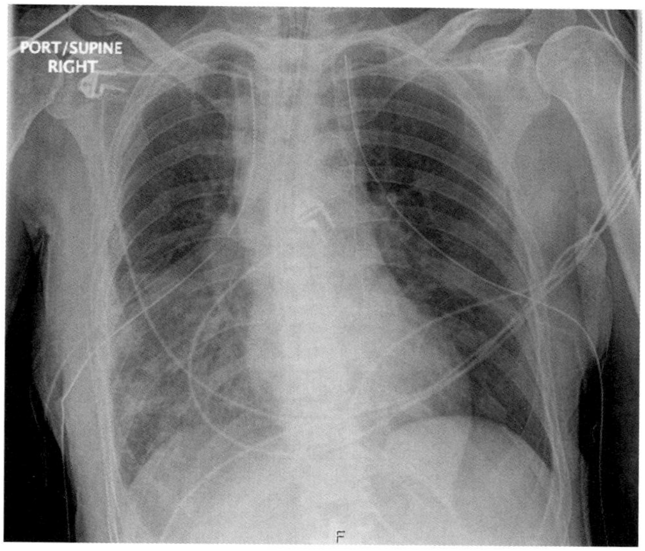

图 1 右下叶实变的 X 线胸片

分泌物。对于肺炎的诊断和致病微生物的判定，微生物的革兰氏染色结果并不可靠。为了评估单独的临床诊断标准对 VAP 的诊断效果，一项研究回顾了在使用机械通气时死亡的 25 名患者，应用肺组织学发现加定量肺组织培养作为肺炎的标准。影像学的胸部浸润影加上 3 个临床症状中的 2 个（白细胞增多、脓性分泌物、发热）的灵敏度为 69%，特异度为 75%。因此，重要的是获得痰培养以确认 VAP 的诊断，此外鉴定病原体，有助于选择合适的抗生素。

一项对于经历机械通气并显示肺炎症状的 43 名创伤患者的研究，说明了获得痰培养的意义（发热、白细胞增多、脓痰和 X 线胸片上浸润影的改变）。在该组中，20 个患者具有大于或等于 10^5 个集落形成单位（colony-forming units，CFU）/ 毫升的阳性培养结果。在其他 23 例患者中停用抗生素，65% 的患者在停止抗生素后显示改善。总体而言，两组之间的死亡率没有差异。

获得痰培养标本的方法

可以通过无创方法获得痰培养标本，也可以通过大气道吸痰、侵入性支气管镜检查、支气管肺泡灌洗（bronchoalveolar lavage，BAL）或受保护的样本刷（protected sample brush，PSB）获得。可以因为一些气管定植菌而出现痰培养阳性，导致对肺炎率的高估。侵入性方法所得痰培养标本在诊断肺炎方面更准确。在一项多中心随机试验中，接受侵入性支气管镜治疗的患者虽然 28 天的死亡率没有降低，但在 14 天时死亡率较低，在第 3 天和第 7 天时平均脓毒症相关器官功能衰竭评分较低。在 28 天时，侵入性治疗组具有明显更多的不使用抗生素天数（11.6vs.7.7）。多变量分析显示死亡率有显著差异（HR＝1.54，95 % CI 为 1.10～2.16）。BAL 和 PSB 都具有大于 80% 的灵敏度和特异度。研究表明，这两种技术有相似的结果（表 3）。大多数涉及 BAL

表 2 疾病控制和预防中心定义医院获得性肺炎的标准

影像学	症状 / 体征	实验室检查
2 个或 2 个以上影像学检查中至少出现一个以下表现： 新发的或者持续存在的或者进展性的浸润影 实变 空洞 小于 1 岁的肺囊肿患者注意：没有潜在的肺或心脏疾病（例如，呼吸窘迫综合征、支气管肺发育不良、肺水肿或慢性阻塞性肺疾病），此时 1 个最终的 X 线胸片是可接受的。	至少有下列之一： 发热（＞38℃或＞100.4° F），无其他原因 白细胞减少（＜4 000/ml） 或白细胞增多（>12 000/ml） ≥70 岁老年人、精神状态改变，没有其他原因 同时 至少有下列之一： 新发脓痰或痰液性质改变或气道分泌物增加，或吸痰需求增加 新发的或加重的咳嗽、呼吸困难、呼吸急促 啰音或支气管呼吸音 恶化的气体交换［例如，氧合下降（如 Pao_2/ FIO_2 比例＜240），增加的氧需求或增加的通气需求］	至少有下列之一： 与其他感染源无关的阳性血培养结果 胸腔积液培养结果阳性 低污染样品的阳性培养结果（例如 BAL 或 PSB） ≥5% BAL 获得的细胞在直接显微镜检查中含有细胞内细菌 （例如革兰氏染色） 组织病理学检查显示至少有一种以下肺炎证据： 脓肿形成或在细支气管和肺泡中大量的 PMN 的脓肿形成或实变病灶 肺实质定量培养 真菌菌丝或假菌丝侵入肺实质的证据

BAL，支气管肺泡灌洗；PMN，多形核白细胞；PSB，受保护的样本刷；WBC，白细胞

表 3 呼吸机相关性肺炎的下呼吸道分泌物定量培养和显微镜检查

诊断技术	灵敏度	特异度	阳性预测值	阴性预测值
PSB 细菌培养（$>10^3$ CFUs/ml）	82	89	90	89
BAL 细菌培养（$>10^4$ CFUs/ml）	91	78	83	87
BAL 液体显微镜检查（>5% 胞内微生物）	91	89	91	89

BAL，支气管肺泡灌洗；CFU，集落形成单位；PSB，受保护的样本刷

的研究使用 10^4CFU/ml 或 10^5CFU/ml 作为培养阳性的阈值。细胞内微生物的可以通过革兰氏染色检测，因为它提供具有高预测价值的快速结果（表 3）。如果不能立即获得支气管镜采样，非支气管镜技术也可以可靠地获得下呼吸道定量培养物。盲法支气管取样、迷你 BAL 和盲法 PSB 都是将导管盲插到远端支气管，并获得标本，这些技术的灵敏度和特异度类似于纤维支气管镜检查的那些技术。除了支气管采样技术，当高度怀疑肺炎或患者临床不稳定或有脓毒症时，无论是否从远端呼吸管道检测到细菌都应立即启动抗生素治疗。

创伤患者临床肺部感染评分的价值

临床肺部感染评分（clinical pulmonary infeetion score，CPIS）试图通过汇集几个肺炎的临床指标来优化无创诊断方法（表 4）。CPIS>6 高度暗示肺炎，并且与来自侵袭性培养标本的细菌的高浓度相关。CPIS 主要不足之处是所有组成因素权重相同，即使一些组成因素有更强的肺炎预测意义，且一些因素是主观的（例如 X 线胸片的解释）。此外，CPIS 的大多数组成指标都受创伤影响，因此可以简单地反映 SIRS。对创伤患者最近的研究发现，由 BAL 诊断的 VAP 的 CPIS 平均分为 6.9，BAL 阴性的患者中 CPIS 平均为 6.8。 CPIS>6 对于诊断 VAP 的灵敏度和特异度分别仅为 61% 和 43%。

表 4 临床肺部感染评分的计算

变量	结果	评分
体温（℃）	>36.5 和≤38.4	0
	>38.5 和≤38.9	1
	>39 或 <36	2
血中白细胞（n/ml）	>4 000 和≤11 000	0
	≤4 000 或 >11 000	1
	异形细胞 >50%	+1
气道分泌物	无	0
	非脓性分泌物	1
	脓性分泌物	2
氧合作用（Pao_2/Fio_2）	≥240 或 ARDS*	0
	<240 且没有 ARDS	2
肺部影像学	无浸润	0
	弥漫性（或片状）浸润	1
	局部浸润	2
进展的肺浸润	无放射学进展	0
	有放射学进展（排除 CHF 和 ARDS 后）	2
气管分泌物培养	致病菌极低或低量生长，或不生长	0
	致病菌中或大量生长	1
	部分致病菌革兰氏染色阴性	+1

注：ARDS，急性呼吸窘迫综合征；CHF，充血性心力衰竭；Fio_2，吸入氧分数；Pao_2，动脉血氧分压；PAWP，肺动脉楔压

* 定义为 Pao_2/ Fio_2≥200 和肺动脉楔压≥18 mmHg，伴有急性双侧肺浸润

处理

充足的初始抗生素治疗

HAP 的有效治疗取决于快速制订适当的抗生素治疗方案，当初始方案选择的抗生素治疗不充分时，死亡率几乎翻倍。初始抗生素覆盖范围必须足够宽，以覆盖最可能的微生物。如果患者接受适当的初始抗生素治疗时间，较指南推荐时间推迟超过 24 h，VAP 的归因死亡率为 39%，而接受及时抗生素治疗的患者 VAP 的归因死亡率为 11%。

MDR 肺炎的常见风险是住院 5 天或更长时间、最近使用抗生素或最近接受治疗（表 5）。在确定微生物耐药的可能性之后，选择适当的初始治疗。如果耐药性的可能性低，抗生素有几种可以选择（表 6）。如果患者具有 MDR 肺炎的危险因素，初始抗生素应覆盖革兰氏阴性微生物和 MRSA。双重覆盖

表 5 多重耐药病原体感染的医院获得性肺炎和呼吸机相关性肺炎的危险因素

已经接受 90 天的抗感染治疗
住院 >5 天
社区或特定医院耐药菌的高发
最近接受治疗
90 天内有大于 2 天的住院治疗
在疗养院或护理机构居住
家庭输液疗法（包括抗生素）
30 天内的慢性透析
家庭伤口护理
感染多重耐药病原体的患者的家人
免疫抑制疾病和（或）免疫抑制治疗

表 6 对于无多重耐药菌感染危险因素的医院获得性肺炎或呼吸机相关性肺炎患者初始经验性抗生素选择

潜在病原体	推荐的初始抗生素
肺炎链球菌 流感嗜血杆菌 甲氧西林敏感的金黄色葡萄球菌 肠道革兰氏阴性杆菌 大肠杆菌 肺炎克雷伯杆菌 肠杆菌属 变形杆菌属 沙雷杆菌	头孢曲松 或 左氧氟沙星或莫西沙星 或 氨苄青霉素 / 舒巴坦 或 厄他培南

表 7 对有迟发性疾病或有多重耐药病原体感染危险因素的医院获得性肺炎或呼吸机相关性肺炎患者的初始经验性治疗

潜在病原体	抗生素联合治疗
表 6 中列出的病原体或多重耐药病原体	抗假单胞菌的头孢菌素（头孢吡肟、头孢他啶）
铜绿假单胞菌	或
肺炎克雷伯广谱 β- 内酰胺酶杆菌（ESBL +）*	抗假单胞菌的碳青霉烯类（亚胺培南、美罗培南）
	或
不动杆菌属 *	β- 内酰胺 /β- 内酰胺酶抑制剂（哌拉西林 - 他唑巴坦）
	加
	抗假单胞菌的氟喹诺酮（环丙沙星或左氧氟沙星）
	或
	氨基糖苷类（阿卡米星、庆大霉素、妥布霉素）
	加
耐甲氧西林	利奈唑胺或万古霉素
耐甲氧西林金黄色葡萄球菌（MRSA）	
嗜肺军团菌 †	

* 如果怀疑是 ESBL + 菌株，如肺炎克雷伯杆菌或不动杆菌，碳青霉烯是一个可靠的选择

† 如果怀疑为嗜肺军团菌，则抗生素联用方案应包括大环内酯类（例如阿奇霉素）或氟喹诺酮（例如环丙沙星或左氧氟沙星），而不是氨基糖苷类

革兰氏阴性菌是否必要，存在争议，并且对多种抗生素协同作用是否有效的证据不一致。双重覆盖一个潜在的优势就是增加治疗概率，至少有一种药物会对疑似耐药菌有作用。对于 MRSA 覆盖，重要的是记住万古霉素在肺部的药物分布浓度较低，应当监测血清药物水平以确保有效的血药浓度。达托霉素与肺表面活性物质强力结合，因此不能用于治疗肺炎。MDR 肺炎治疗的另一种选择是利奈唑胺。2 个研究回顾性分析了万古霉素与利奈唑胺治疗 MRSA 院内肺炎的结果，显示使用利奈唑胺治疗 MDR 肺炎可以改善生存率和提高临床治愈率（表 7）。

恰当和快速针对最可能的致病生物体应用广谱抗生素，对于 VAP 的临床治疗至关重要。对于任何临床情况，都有许多抗生素治疗方案，可以作为第一选择。医院特异性耐药或 ICU 特异性耐药情况在指导抗生素选择中十分重要。

已经使用抗生素对诊断和治疗的影响

已经接受抗生素治疗可能影响获得准确的培养结果，这种影响主要取决于抗生素使用的持续时间。开始使用抗生素 24 h，就可降低获得阳性痰培养标本的概率。不过这种影响相比于其他方法，对于 BAL 的影响更小。然而，在接受抗生素超过 72 h 的患者中，BAL 和 PSB 的灵敏度和特异度基本上不受影响，因此这两种方法仍然可用于抗生素治疗过程肺炎的诊断。此外，这两种方法还能帮助辨认那些已经有足够的抗生素覆盖面，但仍然治疗失败的危重患者。

抗生素降阶梯治疗

虽然VAP有必要应用广谱抗生素，以确保足够的覆盖，但是治疗期间不适合常规使用这些广谱抗生素。在诊断时应该有下呼吸道痰培养结果，然后根据培养结果及药敏结果（36～48 h）使用合适的抗生素治疗方案，所有最终决定都应该基于培养结果。然而问题是，如果痰培养是阴性的，如何制定抗生素治疗方案。痰培养阴性的患者通常分为两组：经过治疗临床改善的患者和病情恶化或缺乏改善的患者。在前者中你可能治疗了一些还没有诊断的其他感染；在后者中，只能说明治疗不充分。在任何一种情况下，都应努力寻找脓毒症的其他来源。如果没有发现，则应停用抗生素，并在24～36 h内对患者重新进行临床评估。

治疗时间

为了帮助确定治疗的最佳持续时间，一项前瞻性随机临床试验研究了401例VAP患者。该研究中，无论患者的病情如何，抗生素都在治疗8或15天后停止，除非有明确的肺炎复发的情况。结果显示，两组患者在不需要呼吸机的天数、住院时间和60天死亡率方面有相似的结果。较短疗程的唯一明显缺点是非发酵性革兰氏阴性杆菌（如铜绿假单胞菌）有较高复发率，除此以外肺炎复发率在两组之间是相似的。总之，对于大多数患者，抗生素疗程应为8天。

抗生素治疗方案

当怀疑一个严重创伤患者或者危重患者患有VAP时：

1. 怀疑有VAP时，应开始广谱抗生素覆盖。抗生素选择应主要根据患者特征（住院时间、先前抗生素暴露史）和单位特异性的微生物耐药特征。原则是对最可能的生物体有足够的初始抗生素覆盖。
2. 诊断后立即从下呼吸道取痰培养标本（基本上与抗生素的启动同时）。标本取样可以使用多种技术，但最有特点的是来自下呼吸道的痰标本。
3. 应在36～48 h内检查培养结果，根据所得培养结果有针对性地应用覆盖病原体的抗生素，实现抗生素的合适的治疗。
4. 对大多数患者，抗生素治疗时间应该是8天。对于非发酵性革兰氏阴性菌（例如铜绿假单胞菌）感染的患者，应该考虑治疗时间为15天。

预防性应用抗生素胸廓造口术置管

EAST实践小组建议胸腔闭式引流术后24 h内使用第一代头孢菌素治疗，预防肺部感染所需要治疗的数量为6。放置胸腔闭式引流是已知的VAP发生的危险因素，这样的预防治疗可以很好地降低VAP的发病率，同时可以降低脓胸的发病率，并且这种预防感染的措施应该定期进行。

ICU中抗生素的应用：过去和现在？

Philip S. Barie 著
吕　杰 译

不仅外科医生进行各种侵入性手段来控制严重感染（如复杂腹腔感染和严重的皮肤或软组织感染），手术患者更是医院获得性感染的易感人群。因此，外科医生必须关注可能会影响手术患者的相关感染的预防及治疗措施，包括手术部位感染（surgical site infections，SSI）、中心静脉导管相关性血流感染（central line-associated blood-stream infections，CLABSI）、尿路感染（urinary tract infections，UTI）和HAP/VAP等。创伤患者的伤口组织特别容易发生感染，他们还会发生院内环境因素相关的感染（如低体温）、宿主免疫抑制（如血糖控制不良）和干预相关的感染（如多个切口和导管、输血）等。

充分认识并且以最小的风险对上述感染做出最积极的诊断与治疗至关重要。感染在某种程度上是可以预防的，每一个危重治疗医生必须做出最大的努力来预防感染。制定一个系统的策略来预防感染是非常必要的，因为包括预防性应用抗生素在内，没有一个方法是独立有效的。感染控制是至关重要的。正如许多重症患者，很多外科疾病和损伤会引起免疫抑制。手术切口和创伤伤口必须小心处理并每日检查，必要时用严格无菌的敷料覆盖。引流管和导管应尽量避免使用，如果病情允许，须尽早移除。无论是经验性还是针对性治疗一个已知的感染，无论是预防性还是治疗性使用应尽量选择最优的方法，以减少多重耐药菌导致的抗生素选择压力。

药代动力学和药效动力学

药物代谢动力学（pharmacokinetics，PK）描述的是药物的吸收、分布和代谢的规律。剂量、给药间隔和给药途径可影响剂量反应关系。吸收、分布和消除通过影响药物代谢和排泄从而影响血浆和组织的药物浓度。药物效应动力学（pharmacodynamic，PD）原理可描述局部药物浓度和效应的关系（见接下来的相关讨论）。

生物利用度是口服后到达体循环的药物剂量的百分比，其影响因素为吸收、肠道转运时间和肝代谢。半衰期（$t_{½}$）是指血清药物浓度减少一半所需的时间，它既反映清除率，也反映分布容积（volume of distribution，V_D）。分布容积用于评估定量给药后血浆的药物浓度。分布容积根据病理生理学的变化而变化，分布容积值的减少会引起血浆药物浓度的升高，反之液体潴留和低蛋白血症（减少药物结合）增加分布容积值，使剂量变得更复杂。

清除率是指不管何种清除方式，在单位时间完全清除药物的液体容量（如代谢、分泌和透析）。药物清除率对于维持稳定的药物浓度所需的药物剂量非常重要（图1）。大多数药物是由肝代谢为极性化合物，最终通过滤过或主动、被动运输由肾排泄。一般来说，如果40%或更多的活性药物（包括活性代谢物）在尿中以本体形式被清除，则在肾功能降低时就须调整剂量。

因为药物-患者、药物-微生物及微生物-患者之间的互相作用，所以药效学对于抗生素的治疗是独一无二的。必须考虑到微生物的生理学、培养液的特性（即大小、群体效应、装置相关菌膜的生成）、微生物增长阶段、耐药机制、微环境（如局部pH值）及宿主反应。如果没有达到足够的剂量或浓度，由于微生物的耐药性，仅仅是"正确"的用药并不能够杀菌。如果使细菌被抑制的药物浓度在临床不能实现，体外结果是无用的。

抗生素的PD参数由实验室分析决定，包括最小抑菌浓度（minimal inhibitory concentration，MIC）、抑制细菌生长的最低血清药物浓度（MIC_{90}指90%抑制）（图2）。然而，一些抗生素在亚抑菌浓度时也许会抑制细菌生长（抗生素后效应，postantibiotic effect，PAE）。使用PK及PD的复杂的原理分析，例如通过测定血清峰值浓度/最小抑菌浓度的比值、血浆浓度保持在MIC之上的时间（fT>MIC）。血浆浓度时间曲线大于MIC的曲线下面积（area under the curve，AUC）（图3）。因此，氨基糖苷类药物展示了浓度依赖的杀菌，而β内酰胺类药物通过高于MIC的时间表现出有效性。尽管延长β内酰胺类药物的给药间隔可能使药效相同，也为其他药物留出使用空间。但对于短$t_{1/2}$的β内酰胺类抗生素，持续

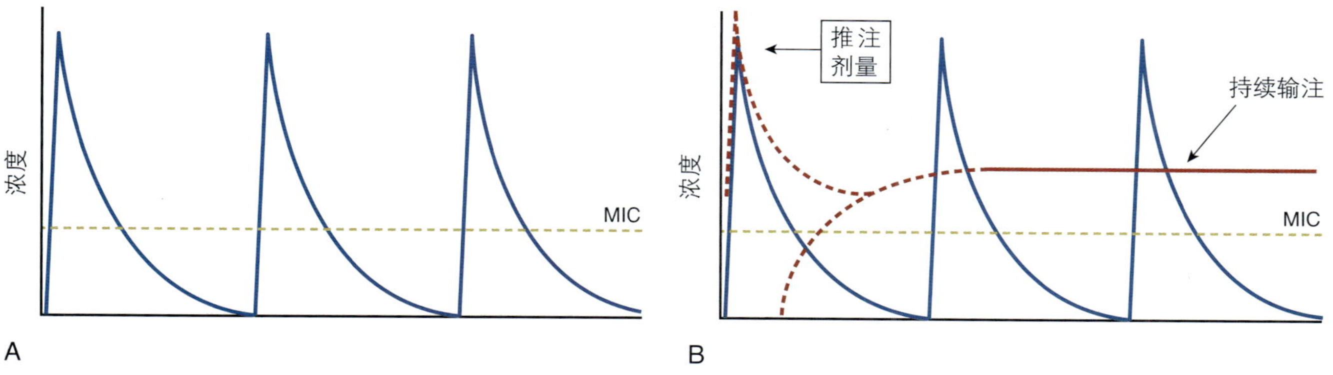

图1　A，抗生素每间隔6 h，静脉注射30 min的消除曲线。在大部分的病例中，高于MIC的浓度的时间的比例超过40%才有抑菌活性。如果MIC数值小，药物的常规剂量即可实现；但若微生物的MIC较高，则不容易实现。**B**，在初始负荷量（推注与否，虚线）后，持续输入抗生素。不仅fT/MIC更高，而且抗生素对高MIC的微生物更有效，这也取决于持续输入的速率。治疗低MIC的细菌，抗生素每日的总剂量也会减少。对于有时间依赖性的杀菌活性的药物（如β-内酰胺类抗生素），如果血管通路充分，这就是理想的用药模型

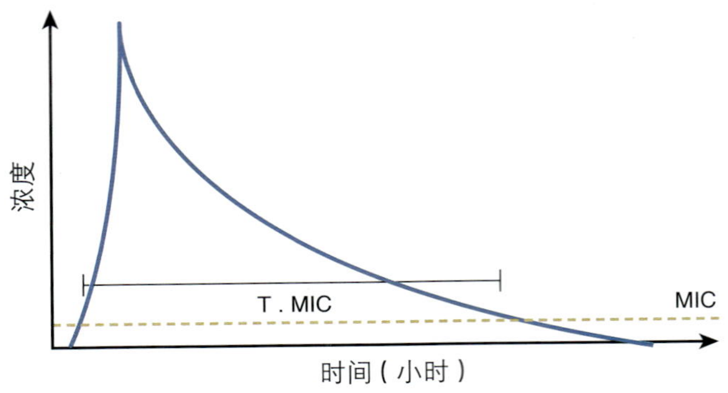

图 2 消除曲线展示了静脉用药的单次静脉推注剂量。一些药物（氨基糖苷类）展现出浓度依赖性杀菌活性，血清峰值浓度 /MIC 比例超过 10，显示最佳杀菌效果。β- 内酰胺类药物展现出时间依赖性杀菌活性，高于 MIC 的时间至少大于 40% 才有最佳杀菌效果。其他药物（万古霉素、氟喹诺酮类）的效果通过曲线下面积（AUC）体现。药物生物利用度的测量方法是频繁地间断测量血药浓度。AUC 与患者血液中未代谢的药物总量成比例。AUC/MIC 的比例超过 125 表明抗菌效果最佳和耐药性最小

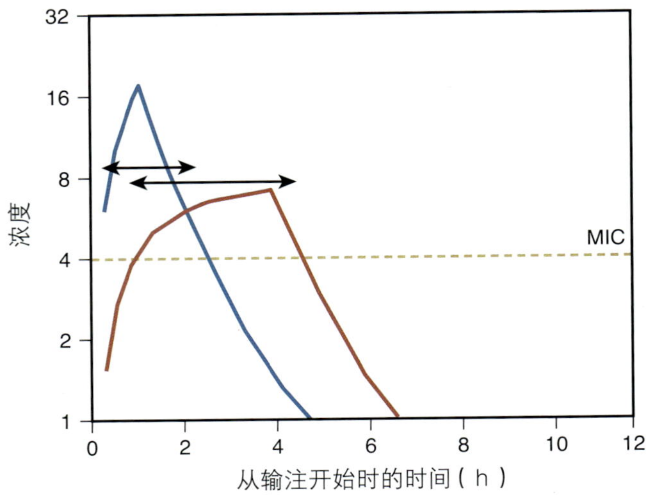

图 3 每隔 6 h 静脉注射 30 min 常规剂量的抗生素，与 4 h 注射相同剂量药物相对比。fT/MIC 增加了 2 倍（对比长短两个双箭头的长度），但对高 MIC 的微生物仍然能够起作用。在用药间歇可以静脉输入液体或其他药物，而不影响杀菌作用

输注可能效果更好。一些药物（如氟喹诺酮、万古霉素）展示了双重特性，随着药物浓度增加至饱和点，杀菌性也是增加的，饱和点之后药效就没有浓度依赖性了。24 h 的 AUC/MIC 的比值大于 125 与最佳效果相关。

抗生素的预防性治疗

预防性应用抗生素是已经明确有益的，并且最常用的用来预防手术部位感染的治疗方式。但是如果使用不当，抗生素的预防性应用不仅无效甚至是有害的。但抗生素的预防性应用并不能预防术后患者的院内感染，实际上长期预防性治疗后，患者发生感染的概率会增加。因为当患者真正发生感染时，之前的长期预防性治疗会导致更多耐药病原体的出现。

指导预防应用抗菌药物的 4 项原则：①安全；②一个合适的窄谱可覆盖相关病原体的药物；③很少或没有治疗性使用的抗生素；④切开之前及时给药和切开之后短暂的一段时间（不超过 24 h，心脏手术时间不超过 48 h，理想情况下，单剂量给药）应用。最佳给药时间是切开之前 1 h 以内。药物给予得更早或在切口关闭之后是无效的。在长期或出血的操作中，短半衰期抗生素（超过 2 h，如头孢唑林、头孢西丁）应该每 3 h（头孢西丁）或 4 h（头孢唑啉）输注一次。

革兰氏阳性球菌造成大部分的手术部位的感染，因此在清洁病例和高危清洁 - 污染的上腹部手术中，预防主要应该针对葡萄球菌。在大多数情况下，第一代头孢菌素是首选的，克林霉素用于青霉素过敏的患者。如果须覆盖革兰氏阴性菌或厌氧菌（如腹部穿通伤），首选的治疗方案是头孢西丁 / 头孢唑啉加甲硝唑治疗。除了 MRSA 发生感染风险高（MRSA 占手术区域感染的 20% 以上）的患者以外，万古霉素一般不建议预防性应用。

污染或肮脏的切口部位的皮肤缝合增加了手术部位感染的风险，但是目前缺乏很好的研究来评估外科医生伤口缝合的多种方式的优劣。外伤或严重的腹膜炎的治疗越来越多地采用临时腹腔关闭的“开放式腹部”技术。尽管无法证实传统的关腹方式是否与院内感染（肺炎、血行感染和手术部位的感染）及住院时间延长、住院费用持续增加等有关，但患者的死亡率并未明显升高。所以在剖腹手术中预防性应用抗生素仍不推荐。

对于创伤患者来说，伤口的手术处理或预防感染须预防性应用抗生素。此外，许多外科手术相关的创伤可能会在一个被污染的领域操作（如穿通性损伤、开放性骨折的切开复位内固定）。对于穿通性腹部创伤，甚至是结肠损伤患者，在 24 h 内预防性应用第二代头孢菌素的建议，证据是充足的。同样，尽管大多数创伤伤口会存在伤口污染，当污染加重时，患者发生感染的可能性会增加，但这并不是长

期的抗生素预防性应用的适应证。

抗生素的治疗原则

抗微生物治疗是治疗感染的中流砥柱，但普遍的过度使用和滥用抗生素导致多重耐药病原体以惊人的速度增加（表1）。新的药物和现有的抗生素的创新使用方法可能会缩短治疗疗程，这对于节约成本和微生物生态学是有益的。没有毒性的有效治疗须快速仔细寻找感染源和准确了解药物的PK（见之前的讨论）。

可能存在的感染的评估

发热通常引发感染存在的评估（因此，"发热检查"）。然而一些感染的患者无明显发热，甚至可能是体温过低的，例如老年患者、开放的腹部伤口、终末期肝疾病或慢性肾疾病等患者，以及服用抗炎、退热的药物等的患者。除了发热，以下任何的临床症状如低血压、心动过速、呼吸急促、意识错乱、寒战、皮肤损伤、低氧血症、少尿、乳酸酸中毒、白细胞增多、白细胞减少、未成熟中性粒细胞（例如杆状核粒细胞比例大于10%）等均表明须进行感染评估和即刻的经验性抗感染治疗。在术后早期（术后4天以内）的发热通常是非感染因素引起，因此并不等同于感染（表2）。此外，非感染和感染性发热

表2　非感染性发热的其他原因

无结石胆囊炎
急性心肌梗死
急性呼吸窘迫综合征（纤维增生阶段）
肾上腺功能不全
细胞因子释放综合征
脂肪栓塞
痛风
血肿
异位骨化
免疫重建炎症综合征（IRIS）
存在梗死组织
颅内出血（创伤或血管原因）
心肌梗死
胰腺炎
心包炎
肺梗死
卒中
甲状腺危象
输血或血液制品
移植排斥
肿瘤溶解综合征
静脉血栓性疾病
戒断症状（如药物、酒精）

表1　抗生素选择相关的细菌耐药的起因与影响

初始治疗药物	耐药细菌	耐药细菌的治疗
氟喹诺酮类	MRSA	万古霉素、其他
	多重耐药革兰氏阴性杆菌	碳青霉烯或多黏菌素或替吉环素（不适用假单胞菌）
	艰难梭菌	万古霉素、甲硝唑、非达霉素
万古霉素、达托霉素	VRE	替吉环素、利奈唑胺
	VISA	头孢洛林、替吉环素、利奈唑胺、达托霉素
头孢菌素、达托霉素	VRE	替吉环素、利奈唑胺
	多重耐药革兰氏阴性杆菌	碳青霉烯或多黏菌素或替吉环素（不适用假单胞菌）
	艰难梭菌	万古霉素、甲硝唑、非达霉素
碳青霉稀类	多重耐药革兰氏阴性杆菌	碳青霉烯或多黏菌素或替吉环素（不适用假单胞菌）
	嗜麦芽窄食单胞菌	甲氧苄啶/磺胺甲异噁唑
	艰难梭菌	万古霉素、甲硝唑、非达霉素

MRSA：耐甲氧西林金黄色葡萄球菌；VISA：中度耐万古霉素金黄色葡萄球菌；VRE：耐万古霉素肠球菌。多重耐药革兰氏阴性杆菌包括超广谱β-内酰胺酶、金属β-内酰胺酶碳青霉烯酶这几个种类

可能共存，感染的患者可能有多种离散的感染并存。

我们必须在抗生素使用前进行评估，包括培养样本的收集。因此，评估必须迅速，延迟抗生素的使用与死亡风险增加相关。一定要检查所有的伤口。如果打开一个伤口进行细菌培养，须收集、培养深部组织，而不是简单地擦拭开放性伤口或收集引流管的引流液（有较高的定植可能性）。除非机械通气、体格检查、血气分析异常或气道分泌物等提示感染，那么 X 线胸片才可作为患者术后发热的评估手段。除非通过询问病史或化验检查怀疑有尿路感染，术后早期的尿液检查/尿液培养不是必需的。然而，术后第 4 天之后患者院内感染的概率增加，我们需要更加全面的评估，经验性治疗的门槛也相应降低。

经验性抗生素治疗

经验性抗生素治疗必须是明确和迅速的。不规范的随意治疗可能导致已有感染的处理不当，无菌炎症的不必要治疗或某些细菌的定植。随意性治疗对患者可能是有害的。不恰当的治疗（如延迟超过 1 h、对常见病原体的错误治疗、治疗多重耐药病原体的失败等）必然会导致患者死亡率的升高。

抗生素的选择基于几个相互关联的因素（表 3）。最重要的是抗菌药物对明确的或很有可能的（经验性治疗）病原菌有效，能够区分可疑感染与微生物定植，最好应用有效的窄谱抗生素。重要的因素包括严密监测疾病进程、确定感染是否是卫生医疗相关或社区或医院获得性相关，以及多重耐药菌是否存在或可能存在。了解局部抗生素耐药情况是非常重要的。患者重要的个体因素包括年龄、衰弱、内在器官功能状态、是否存在免疫抑制、之前的过敏或其他不良反应及近期的抗生素治疗等。制度的重要因素包括指南、处方的可行性、多重耐药菌引起的感染的暴发和抗生素的控制程序。

抗生素的选择

有许多可用于治疗的药物（表 4）。药物的选择除了之前的各种因素，还要基于抗菌谱是广泛的还是有针对性的（抗铜绿假单胞菌、抗厌氧菌）。如果怀疑是院内革兰氏阳性菌（如伤口或 SSI、CLABSI、HAP/VAP）或 MRSA 流行，恰当的治疗方式是经验性使用万古霉素（或利奈唑胺）。一些专家建议治疗严重的假单胞菌感染使用双重覆盖抗生素（即抗铜绿假单胞菌的 β- 内酰胺药物 + 氨基糖苷类），但有

表 3 抗生素选择的影响因素

对已知或怀疑的病原体有效
可引起疾病
区分感染和定植
窄谱抗生素最有可能覆盖
抗菌素耐药性的模式
发病之前的环境：在家 vs. 医疗单位
近期的抗生素治疗
疾病的严重性
年龄
免疫抑制
器官功能障碍
过敏
机构的指南/限制条件：须机构预批准
处方药物
策略：起始、剂量、给药间隔，单次或多次给药
输液时间和治疗疗程

关疗效的证据不太明确。无论如何选择，任何由革兰氏阳性菌或革兰氏阴性菌（HAP/VAP、医院获得性腹腔内感染）引起的感染的经验性治疗，必须对所有可能的病原体有效。

优化治疗

传统的抗生素剂量可能不适用于危重或受伤患者。当出现多重耐药菌、细胞外容量增加、血清白蛋白浓度降低或肾小球滤过率增加时，抗生素剂量须增加（如烧伤、创伤性脑损伤、多发性创伤）。低于有效剂量的抗生素使用是在治疗和治疗失败时产生耐药性的主要因素。相反，当发生多器官功能障碍综合征、急性肾损伤、慢性肾疾病时可能需要较低剂量的抗生素。通过测定血清中药物浓度来监测万古霉素和氨基糖苷类药物的使用剂量。

连续或长期输注 β- 内酰胺药物可能是使用这些药物的最佳方法。延长药物大于 MIC 的 fT，尤其是治疗 MIC 较高的微生物时，会增加治疗成功率，使耐药性的产生最小化。延长输注时间也可以减少耐药性产生，并且不会单独占用一条静脉通路。可以持续输注万古霉素，但目前并不推荐使用。

万古霉素已经成为治疗危重患者感染的主要药物，但万古霉素对耐甲氧西林金黄色葡萄球菌的

表 4 抗菌药物的经验性应用

抗铜绿假单胞菌
哌拉西林—三唑巴坦
头孢吡肟、头孢他啶
亚胺培南—西司他丁、美罗培南、多利培南
环丙沙星、左氧氟沙星（取决于当地的易感性模式）
氨基糖苷类
多黏菌素［多黏菌素 B、黏菌素（多黏菌素 E）］
特定菌谱药物
革兰阳性细菌
糖肽类（万古霉素、特拉万星）
脂肽类抗生素（达托霉素，不可在已知 / 疑似肺炎使用）
恶唑烷酮（利奈唑胺）
革兰氏阴性菌
第三代头孢菌素（非头孢曲松）
单环 β- 内酰胺类抗生素
多黏菌素［多黏菌素 B、黏菌素（多黏菌素 E）］
广谱抗菌药物
哌拉西林钠—他唑巴坦
碳青霉烯类
氟喹诺酮类(取决于局部感染种类）
替吉环素（加抗铜绿假单胞菌药剂）
复方新诺明（首先用于 CA-MRSA、嗜麦芽窄食单胞菌）
抗厌氧菌药物
甲硝唑
碳青霉烯类
β- 内酰胺类 /β- 内酰胺酶复合物
替吉环素
抗 MRSA 药物
头孢洛林
达托霉素（不针对肺炎）
米诺环素
利奈唑胺
特拉万星
替吉环素（怀孕和 8 岁以下儿童禁用）
万古霉素

CA-MRSA, 社区获得性耐甲氧西林金黄色葡萄球菌；MRSA：耐甲氧西林金黄色葡萄球菌

MIC 已增加，但还在易受影响范围内。最终，金黄色葡萄球菌耐药的 MIC 临界点已经下调，以减少无效治疗，尽管可能增加肾毒性的风险，但仍然推荐更高剂量的万古霉素。单独使用万古霉素治疗 MIC 是 1 和 2 mg/ml 的 MRSA 引起的感染患者时，应该谨慎进行。足够的治疗浓度可能无法成功治疗 MIC 大于 2 μg/ml 的金黄色葡萄球菌时，我们应该考虑其他治疗方法。利奈唑胺一般效果较好，但已经有对达托霉素耐药的报道。

虽然使用的经验治疗方案仍然争论不休，但由于产生 ESBL 和碳青霉烯酶的菌株的概率升高，导致多重耐药菌药物的选择有限，所以氨基糖苷类药物治疗重新被重视。氨基糖苷类的单日剂量确保血清浓度峰值 /MIC 比值＞10，治疗才会达到最佳治疗效果。庆大霉素和妥布霉素（7 mg/kg）或阿米卡星（20 mg/kg）的剂量输入体内，在给药后 23 h 出现谷浓度（一些草案呼吁一个在给药后 16 h 的中间的数值，以便可以更精确地描绘消除曲线）。庆大霉素和妥布霉素的谷浓度的目标为 0.5 ~ 2 μg/ml，而阿米卡星的理想谷浓度是 5 ~ 10 μg/ml。在毒性降低方面，此结果与常规剂量相比，相似或更好。单一剂量氨基糖苷类治疗效果在一些人群尚未明确，如儿童、怀孕期间、烧伤、年龄超过 70 岁的患者，或对细菌性心内膜炎进行的治疗。

高度耐药（“泛耐药”）的革兰氏阴性杆菌的感染是一个大问题。碳青霉烯、替吉环素和多黏菌素（见后）对产 ESBL 的微生物仍然有效。多重耐药的非发酵性革兰氏阴性杆菌（如铜绿假单胞菌、不动杆菌、嗜麦芽窄食单胞菌）和产碳青霉烯酶的肠杆菌属的治疗可能需要多黏菌素、长期输入大剂量碳青霉烯或非常规的在体外有协同作用，但临床疗效尚未明确的药物组合。

治疗持续时间

停止使用抗生素的指征仍未明确，因为此方面的数据较少。如果培养是阴性的，在之后的 48 ~ 72 h，大部分病例的经验性抗生素治疗应该停止。不必要的抗生素治疗会增加多重耐药菌感染的风险，因此培养阴性的病例长期抗生素治疗通常是不合理的。抗生素治疗的并发症还包括过敏反应、院内重复感染（真菌、肠球菌、艰难梭菌相关感染）、器官毒性、随后培养产物减少、维生素 K 缺乏凝血功能障碍或华法林的效果增强。

如果感染是确定的，临床上应持续治疗，但须进行微生物培养，以提示抗生素是否可以降阶梯治

疗（如选择窄谱抗生素，由多种药物改为单一药物治疗）。如果抗菌素经验性治疗得当，很少须升级治疗（如选择一个更广谱药物，把单一用药改为多种药物治疗，增加抗真菌治疗）。

一旦开始使用抗生素，药物持续时间的问题也会伴随而来。超出预期时间的继续治疗的理由必须很充分。有效药物的反应就是快速消灭细菌，但是宿主反应没有那么迅速。因此，患者的临床反应不应该是唯一的决定因素。越来越多的人相信抗生素的短程治疗会产生更少的副作用，治疗方案应提前制订好，到达治疗时间之后应及时停止。

降钙素原作为生物标志物指导抗生素治疗的持续时间，已被广泛评估（11 个前瞻性随机试验：启动治疗——3 个试验、结束治疗——4 个试验和作为指南——4 个试验）。毫无例外，临床预后没有变化（9 个试验）或住院时间减少（2 个试验）。另外，降钙素原监测能够节省抗生素的使用，在 3 个临床试验中将抗生素处方减少了 32% ~ 72%，并且在 8 个临床试验中减少治疗持续时间 1.7 ~ 7.1 天。

很少有数据和临床指南指导我们如何处理抗菌治疗失败的患者。甚至没有一个对什么是失败的明确的定义。如果患者的全身性炎症反应持续 3 天、5 天或 7 天，这叫失败吗？什么时间应该更换抗生素？是选择了适当的抗生素，但是患者已经无法控制感染，必须进行手术（或再次手术）时吗？如果在预期的治疗结束时，患者仍然有全身炎症反应综合征，与单纯继续治疗或无证据的更换抗生素相比，更有用的是停止治疗再重新评估持续或新发的感染、多重耐药病原体和 SIRS 的非感染性原因。

抗生素的抗菌谱

在严重感染的患者治疗方面，微生物的药敏试验是非常必要的（包括所有的院内感染）。本章将集中讨论最有效的严重 / 院内感染的治疗药物，不是每个药物都将被提到。对于特定微生物的推荐药物仅作为指导，因为体外药物敏感性可能与临床疗效不一致。

针对细胞壁的药物

β– 内酰胺抗生素

β- 内酰胺类抗生素包括青霉素、头孢菌素、单环 β- 内酰胺类和碳青霉烯类。在这些药物中，几种药物结合 β- 内酰胺酶抑制剂来扩大抗菌范围。抗生素在组内分为几个亚组，尤其是耐青霉素酶的青霉素和几“代”的头孢菌素。

青霉素类

耐青霉素酶的半合成青霉素包括甲氧西林、苯唑西林、萘夫西林。这些药物用于治疗葡萄球菌敏感菌株，因为有较多情况是耐甲氧西林金黄色葡萄球菌，所以经验性用药时较少选择。实际上几乎所有肠球菌都是耐药的。

除了羧基青霉素和脲基青霉素，青霉素对革兰氏阴性杆菌几乎没有活性。羧基青霉素（替卡西林和羧苄西林）和脲基青霉素（阿洛西林、美洛西林和哌拉西林，有时被称为酰脲类青霉素）如果没有和 β- 内酰胺酶抑制剂结合（如他唑巴坦、克拉维酸、舒巴坦），就不会被使用。它能够提高 β- 内酰胺亲代的有效性（哌拉西林 > 替卡西林 > 氨苄西林）和较少的抑制剂的有效性（他唑巴坦 > 克拉维酸和舒巴坦）。哌拉西林 - 他唑巴坦对革兰氏阴性菌具有最广泛的抗菌活性，对铜绿假单胞菌强力有效。氨苄西林 - 舒巴坦对大肠杆菌和克雷伯杆菌效果不佳（耐药率为 50%），但由于舒巴坦，所以它对一些不动杆菌有效。所有结合 β- 内酰胺酶抑制剂的药物都有很好的抗厌氧菌活性。

头孢菌素

二十多种头孢菌素药物的差别很大，因此临床医生应该广泛熟知这些药物。第一和第二代头孢菌素的使用只针对预防、简单的感染或知道药敏结果后的降阶梯治疗。“第三代”头孢菌素增强了抗革兰氏阴性杆菌的效果（一些有特定的抗铜绿假单胞菌的效果），但只有头孢曲松对革兰氏阳性球菌有效（但对 MRSA 无效），也没有药物对厌氧菌是有效。“第四代”头孢菌素，头孢吡肟对铜绿假单胞菌和大多数革兰氏阳性球菌有效，但对 MRSA 无效。头孢洛林（常规剂量，每 12 h 静脉注射 600 mg）没有分类。但与一代头孢菌素相比，其在抗革兰氏阴性杆菌有效的同时，对 MRSA 也有效。没有头孢类药物对肠球菌有效。第三代头孢菌素，尤其是头孢他啶在肠杆菌属中的应用与诱导 ESBL 的产生相关。

对于诱导 ESBL 产生，头孢吡肟少于头孢他啶，但头孢吡肟也对肠道球菌和肠道厌氧菌无效。头孢吡肟在本质上更耐 β- 内酰胺酶的水解，但不足以消灭产 ESBL 的细菌。

单环 β- 内酰胺类

这一类的单剂氨曲南与第三代头孢菌素相比，对革兰氏阴性杆菌更有效，但对革兰氏阳性菌或厌氧菌无效。氨曲南诱导 β- 内酰胺酶能力不强。尽管对氨曲南耐药普遍存在，但因为药物交叉反应率很低，所以氨曲南对敏感菌株的治疗和青霉素过敏的患者仍然有效。

碳青霉烯类

亚胺培南 - 西司他丁、美罗培南、多利培南和厄他培南均在美国可以使用。亚胺培南 - 西司他丁、美罗培南、多利培南（和一般抗生素相比）有最大的抗菌谱，包括对需氧和厌氧链球菌、对甲氧西林敏感的葡萄球菌和除了不动杆菌、军团菌、洋葱假单胞菌和嗜麦芽窄食单胞菌之外的几乎所有的革兰氏阴性杆菌有效。所有碳青霉烯类对厌氧菌均有效，因此无须把碳青霉烯与甲硝唑结合使用。由于亚胺培南 - 西司他丁在肾功能正常时的高剂量应用或肾功能不全时的低剂量应用时，有可能出现罕见的肌阵挛或癫痫大发作（约 0.5%），所以中枢神经系统（脊髓除外）疾病或损伤时禁用该药物。美罗培南与多利培南比亚胺培南 - 西司他丁有更小的神经毒性。厄他培南对假单胞菌、不动杆菌、肠杆菌或耐甲氧西林金黄色葡萄球菌效果不佳，但长半衰期允许其一天只用一次给药。厄他培南对产 ESBL 的肠杆菌有效，其潜在的神经毒性较低。对于所有的碳青霉烯类药物，它们对宿主菌群的损害可能会导致重复感染（如真菌、艰难梭菌、单胞菌和耐药肠球菌）。

脂糖肽类

万古霉素是可溶性脂糖肽类，有杀菌作用，但组织渗透性差，限制了其有效性（表 5）。虽然金黄色葡萄球菌的 MIC 值增加，需要更高的万古霉素使用剂量，而且在一些报告中，临床失败率超过 50%，但金黄色葡萄球菌和表皮葡萄球菌通常对万古霉素还是敏感的。化脓性链球菌、B 型链球菌、肺炎链球菌（包括耐青霉素肺炎链球菌）和艰难梭菌都对它敏感。万古霉素的浓度对大部分的粪便肠球菌的作用是抑制而不是消灭，现在粪肠球菌对万古霉素的耐药性也在增加。

万古霉素衍生物特拉万星只被批准用来治疗复杂性皮肤软组织感染（complicated skin/soft tissue infections，cSSTI）。特拉万星具有双重的作用机制，包括破坏细胞膜和抑制细胞壁合成。特拉万星对耐甲氧西林金黄色葡萄球菌、敏感的耐青霉素肺炎球菌和对万古霉素易感、MIC 低于 1 μg/mL 的肠球菌有效。特拉万星最常见的副作用是味觉障碍、恶心、呕吐和头痛。而且可能会增加急性肾损伤的风险。特拉万星最常用的剂量是 10 mg/kg，静脉输注须超过 60 min，每 24 h 一次，疗程 7 ~ 14 天，当患者肾功能不全时剂量须减少。当患者进行肾替代治疗时，暂无相关用药剂量信息。

表 5　不推荐使用万古霉素的情况

没有危及生命的对 β- 内酰胺类抗生素过敏的常规外科手术的预防性用药
缺乏革兰氏阳性菌感染的证据，对发热性中性粒细胞减少的经验性治疗
当微生物检测证明治疗合理时，继续进行经验性治疗
血管内留置导管的全身性或局部预防用药（导管冲洗）
选择性消化道去污
耐甲氧西林葡萄球菌定植的根除
艰难梭菌导致抗生素相关结肠炎的治疗
血液透析或连续腹膜透析患者的常规预防性用药
局部灌洗或应用

环脂肽类

达托霉素对大部分革兰氏阳性菌有快速强力的杀菌作用。杀菌作用机制是膜的快速去极化，钾外流，阻止 DNA、RNA 和蛋白质的合成，最终导致细胞死亡。达托霉素表现为浓度依赖性的杀菌作用，有较长的 $t_{1/2}$（8 h）。当患者发生 cSSTI 时，达托霉素推荐的剂量是 4 mg/kg，而当患者发生菌血症时，剂量为 6 mg/kg · d。当患者肌酐清除率小于 30 ml/min 时，给药间隔应该增加到 48 h。达托霉素对大部分的需氧和厌氧革兰氏阳性菌有效，包括消化链球菌属、产气荚膜梭菌、艰难梭菌和耐甲氧西林金黄色葡萄球菌、耐甲氧西林表皮葡萄球菌和耐万古霉素肠球菌（vancomycin-resistant Enterococcus，VRE）。已经有报道 MRSA 和 VRE 对达托霉素耐药。重要的是，因为达托霉素穿透肺组织能力弱，肺表面活性物质可使其灭活，所以达托霉素不得用于肺炎治疗或肺炎未确定时的经验性治疗，即使是由敏感微生物引起的也不推荐。

多黏菌素类

多黏菌素是环状的、有脂肪酸残基的阳离子多肽；多黏菌素 B 和 E（多黏菌素 E= 黏菌素甲磺酸盐或黏菌素）用于临床。多黏菌素与阴离子细菌外膜结合，破坏细胞膜的完整性，导致洗涤剂效应。脂多糖的一半紧紧结合脂质 A，会产生一个内毒素中和效果。多黏菌素 B 的剂型是标准化的，但黏菌素甲磺酸盐（临床上应用的毒性更少的黏菌素前体药物）不是标准化的，所以使用剂量取决于药品提供规格。大多数报告均报道了黏菌素甲磺酸的使用，但药物在治疗上是等价的。

多黏菌素 B 的剂量是每天 1.5 ~ 2.5 mg/kg（15 000 ~ 25 000 U/kg）并分次给药，而黏菌素甲磺酸盐（多黏菌素 E）剂量范围为每天 2.5 ~ 6 mg/kg，也是分次给药。药物应用需要大容量稀释，故每天给予大量液体输注。尽管多重耐药菌广泛出现，但该药仍然保持较好的抗菌活性。多黏菌素的 PK 的数据很少，但药物表现出浓度依赖性，且具有广谱的抗革兰氏阴性杆菌活性，包括大部分的大肠杆菌、克雷伯杆菌、肠杆菌、铜绿假单胞菌、嗜麦芽窄食单孢菌和不动杆菌。多黏菌素和利福平结合使用表现出体外的协同作用。多黏菌素组织吸收性差，但鞘内注射和吸入是可行的。

多黏菌素最初由于肾毒性和神经毒性遭到弃用，但多重耐药菌的出现已经使该药物恢复使用。黏菌素甲磺酸盐治疗的患者的急性肾损伤的发生率是 40%，多黏菌素 B 治疗的患者的发生率是 5% ~ 15%。两者的神经毒性（5% ~ 7%）通常会表现为肌肉无力或多神经病。

蛋白合成抑制剂

氨基糖苷类

由于新抗生素的耐药，氨基糖苷类的使用开始复苏了（尤其是第三代头孢菌素和氟喹诺酮类药物）。庆大霉素、妥布霉素和阿米卡星仍在使用。氨基糖苷类与细菌 30 S 核糖体亚单位结合，从而抑制蛋白质合成。庆大霉素对革兰氏阳性球菌有一定效果，药物的活性谱几乎是相同的。处方应该基于药物毒性和局部的耐药情况。由于氨基糖苷类潜在的毒性，除了协同治疗严重的铜绿假单胞菌感染、肠球菌引起的心内膜炎或多重耐药革兰氏阴性杆菌引起的感染，氨基糖苷类很少用于一线治疗。氨基糖苷类抗生素对不动杆菌疗效不大，对洋葱假单胞菌、气单孢菌属及嗜麦芽窄食单胞菌的作用有限。

氨基苷类抗生素最有效的杀菌浓度的峰值 /MIC 大于 10，因此负荷剂量和血清药物浓度监测是必要的。肾功能不全的患者须降低剂量，但每次血液透析治疗后，药物被滤过，须给予一定的维持剂量。

四环素

四环素不可逆转地结合到 30 S 核糖体亚单位上，但它们只有抑制细菌作用。在医院大范围的耐药限制了四环素的使用（除了多西环素、米诺环素和只能静脉注射的替吉环素）。四环素对厌氧菌是有效的，也可以成功治疗放线菌。由于四环素对牙齿的毒性，在怀孕妇女和 8 岁以下儿童中禁用。

替吉环素属于甘氨酰环素类抗生素的一个新种类，甘氨酰环素类抗生素制剂是米诺环素的衍生物。除了假单胞菌和变形杆菌，替吉环素的抗菌谱很广，包括许多多重耐药的革兰氏阳性菌和革兰氏阴性菌，其中有 MRSA、VRE、产 ESBL 的菌株和不动杆菌。替吉环素的抗厌氧菌效果也较好。

最近在包括未注册试验的三、四期临床试验中，析因分析发现应用替吉环素治疗患者的死亡率更高，这引起了较大关注。替吉环素和对照药物之间，基于试验比重分层的随机效应模型试验的死亡率的调整风险差异为 0.6%（95%CI 为 0.1 ~ 1.2），但是试验中应用哪种药物是未知的。在 8 篇发表的随机对照试验（4 651 名患者）的独立 meta 分析中，没有发现上述临床试验中这样的生存率差异。总的来说，无论是临床结果（OR = 0.92，95% CI 为 0.76 ~ 1.12），还是微生物评估结果（OR = 0.86，95% CI 为 0.69 ~ 1.07），2 组药物之间没有明显差异。

恶唑烷酮类

唯一商业化的药物利奈唑胺与核糖体 50 S 亚单位结合，防止络合 30 S 亚单位，从而阻止 mRNA 翻译和阻断蛋白质合成的起始复合物的装配。利奈唑胺对敏感细菌起到抑制作用（肺炎双球菌除外）。有一个小例外，因为药物从细菌通过外排泵细胞分泌，所以革兰氏阴性细菌对利奈唑胺耐药。

MRSA、对万古霉素敏感或者耐药的肠球菌，对青霉素敏感或耐药的肺炎双球菌，这些菌群对利奈唑胺均敏感。它也对拟杆菌属有效。其组织渗透性较好，肾功能不全的患者不须减少利奈唑胺的剂量。meta 分析表明在治疗 HAP/VAP 时用万古霉素等同于利奈唑胺，但是临床医生相信利奈唑胺应该取代万古霉素，作为治疗革兰氏阳性球菌所致的严重感染的一线用药。

大环内酯类－林可胺类－链霉菌素类

克林霉素

用于外科中的唯一有效的林可酰胺类药物是克林霉素，其也与核糖体 50 S 亚单位结合。克林霉素有一定的抗厌氧菌活性，对敏感的革兰氏阳性球菌有较好的活性（不是 MRSA 或 VRE）。克林霉素体外抑制外毒素的产生，比青霉素更优先考虑作为一线治疗药物治疗侵袭性化脓性链球菌感染。克林霉素偶尔用于厌氧菌感染和在青霉素过敏的患者清洁手术中预防感染，且优于万古霉素。

干扰核酸的药物

氟喹诺酮

氟喹诺酮类药物通过抑制 DNA 旋转酶抑制细菌的 DNA 合成，DNA 旋转酶将 DNA 复制之前折叠成为一个超螺旋。氟喹诺酮类有较好的口服生物利用度、逐渐缩小的抗菌谱和各种毒性［如光敏性、软骨（特别是儿童）和肌腱损伤、QT 间期延长］。这些药物有诱导耐药的倾向。环丙沙星、左氧氟沙星和莫西沙星（有一定的抗厌氧菌活性）有静脉与口服两种剂型。

氟喹诺酮类药物对肠道革兰氏阴性菌有一定活性，特别是肠杆菌科和嗜血杆菌。有一些药物对铜绿假单胞菌、嗜麦芽窄食单胞菌和革兰氏阴性球菌有效。氟喹诺酮类药物对敏感的革兰氏阳性球菌的有效性是不同的，莫西沙星效果最差，环丙沙星效果最好。然而，滥用氟喹诺酮类药物短时间内易形成耐药，从而减少其对包括大肠杆菌、克雷伯杆菌、铜绿假单胞菌和 MRSA 的疗效。氟喹诺酮类药物可能会延长 QT 间期和促发心室节律障碍导致尖端扭转型室性心动过速。所以在氟喹诺酮类药物治疗前和治疗期间，使用心电图测量 QT 间期是很重要的。同时，氟喹诺酮类药物与华法林交叉使用会导致国际标准化比率快速、显著延长。所以在氟喹诺酮类药物治疗期间，必须密切监测华法林的抗凝治疗。

细胞毒性抗生素

甲硝唑

尽管甲硝唑对放射菌是无效的，但其对几乎所有的厌氧菌和寄生于人类的原生生物都有强力的杀菌活性。其耐药性仍较为罕见，甚至在临床中可以忽略不计。甲硝唑的硝基在细胞内还原，从而引起 DNA 损伤。药物能很好地穿透包括神经组织在内的几乎所有组织，治疗深部感染和防止细菌迅速地增加。口服或直肠给药后，甲硝唑快速且几乎全部吸收。由于羟基代谢物的活性，甲硝唑的半衰期是 8 h。通常静脉注射甲硝唑是每 8～12 h 一次，但每日一次的用量也是有可能的。肾功能不全的患者不须减少剂量，但药物可被透析排除，所以甲硝唑须在透析后使用。肝功能不全的患者，建议甲硝唑的剂量减少 50%。

复方新诺明

磺胺类药通过干扰细菌 DNA 合成所必需的叶酸的合成发挥抑菌活性。它的耐药非常广泛，限制了该药物的使用。磺胺甲恶唑和甲氧苄啶的合剂通过影响二氢叶酸还原酶的作用阻断二氢叶酸转化为四氢叶酸，加强甲氧苄啶的作用。

复方新诺明（trimtehoprim-sulfamethoxazole，TMP-SMX）对金黄色葡萄球菌、化脓性链球菌、肺炎链球菌、大肠杆菌、奇异变形杆菌、沙门氏菌和志贺杆菌、小肠结肠炎耶尔森菌、嗜麦芽窄食单胞菌、单核细胞性李斯特菌和耶氏肺孢子菌是有效的。嗜麦芽窄食单胞菌的感染和由社区相关性耐甲氧西林金黄色葡萄球菌（community associated MRSA，CA-MRSA）引起门诊患者（或住院患者）的感染，复方新诺明都是一个不错的选择。

TMP-SMX 可供注射用的固定剂量组合的比例为 1∶5。标准口服配方是 80 mg/ 400 mg，更小和更大的剂量都是可行的。TMP-SMX 口服吸收迅速，生物利用度近 100%，有较好的组织渗透性。10 ml 注射配方含有 160 mg/800 mg 药物。如果肌酐清除率超过 30 ml/min，药物可足量给予（150～300 mg 甲氧苄啶，3～4 次），如果肌酐清除率小于 15 ml/min，则不推荐该使用药物。

抗生素的毒性

β- 内酰胺类药物的过敏反应

β- 内酰胺类抗生素最常见的毒性表现是过敏反应。在青霉素的治疗过程中，过敏反应发生率约为 7 ~ 40/1 000 次治疗，在静脉输注治疗中的发生率更高。大部分严重的反应发生在没有过敏史的患者。之前发生过过敏反应的患者发生另一个过敏反应的概率是一般人群的 4 ~ 6 倍，但是随着时间的延长，风险降低，如在 2 个月时皮肤反应的发生率为 80% ~ 90%，而 10 年后则降低为 20%。青霉素和其他 β- 内酰胺类抗生素之间交叉反应的风险（碳青霉烯和头孢菌素）大约是 5%，最高的为一代头孢菌素。青霉素与单环 β- 内酰胺类的交叉过敏反应可以忽略不计。

红人综合征

万古霉素静脉治疗后出现面部、颈部及胸部的潮红、刺痛，但较发热、寒战或局部静脉炎来说并不常见。红人综合征是由于局部高渗状态，释放组胺而发生。红人综合征与过快输注万古霉素有关（1 h 以内输入 1 g，或 1.5 ~ 2 h 以内输入更大剂量），而不是真正的过敏。万古霉素输注过快也会导致低血压。过敏造成的斑丘疹发生率大约为 5%。

肾毒性

所有氨基糖苷类抗生素几乎没有区别，均为肾毒性。氨基糖苷类不会引发炎症，因此任何氨基糖苷类的毒性表现中没有过敏反应。肾毒性是由于肾近端小管细胞缺血导致。肾损伤表现为肾小球滤过率降低和肌酐清除率下降，但通常是可逆的，很少需要肾替代治疗。加重氨基糖苷类肾毒性的因素有频繁用药、高龄、钠或者容量不足、酸血症、低钾血症、低镁血症和同时患有肝疾病。如果每日使用单剂给药可以降低风险。如果肾功能恶化，除非治疗危及生命的感染，否则建议停止抗生素使用。

如果高剂量使用万古霉素和联合其他肾毒性药物使用，会导致万古霉素的肾毒性增加。多黏菌素的肾毒性可能是不可避免的，当需要的替代药物很少或没有时，我们就须使用一种潜在肾毒性的药物治疗由多重耐药革兰氏阴性杆菌引起的严重感染。

耳毒性

氨基糖苷类抗生素引起不可逆的耳蜗和前庭的损害，而且停止治疗后可能仍会进展。重复使用导致风险累计增加。大多数患者可能发生耳蜗损害，也可能发生前庭病变，但损害很少同时出现。耳蜗毒性很微小，因此很少的患者有基线听力图，而且更少的患者接受正规的筛查。少数患者抱怨听力损伤，但当我们进一步检查时发现耳蜗损害的发生率可能会超过 60%。临床听力损失可能发生在 5% ~ 15% 的患者中。当万古霉素和另一种耳毒性的药物（如氨基糖苷类、呋塞米）合用时，万古霉素导致的耳毒性是尤为常见的。使用可导致耳毒性和肾毒性的药物（氨基糖苷类、万古霉素）时，这些药物导致的耳毒性和肾毒性之间没有互相的联系。

避免毒性：抗生素剂量调整

肝功能不全

肝代谢和排除亲脂性药物，然后经肾排泄。细胞色素 -450（基因大家族超过 300 种不同的酶）把亲脂性的化合物氧化成水溶性物质。氧化是受影响的，特别是当肝功能受损时，更是如此。其他酶调节与糖类、氨基酸、硫酸、醋酸酯的结合，促进胆汁或肾排泄。

结合粗略的临床肝功能评估（表 6）以及依据损伤程度改变代谢（如解决胆汁淤积），肝功能不全的药物剂量的调整是复杂的。肾功能改变伴随肝功能进行性恶化极大地增加了药物治疗的难度。一般来说，如果肝代谢只剩 40% 或更少，而肾功能是正常的，那么剂量减少最多至常规剂量的 25%。如果药物长期使用，治疗指数较小、蛋白质结合率明显降低或药物经肾排泄和肾功能严重受损，那么药量须减少达 50%。

肾功能不全

肾对药物的清除取决于肾小球的滤过、肾小管的分泌和重吸收，当任何方面改变时就会发生肾功能障碍。肾疾病或急性肾损伤可能会影响肝和肾的药物代谢途径。患者肾功能不全时也可能损害肝代谢的药物包括氨曲南、青霉素、一些头孢菌素、大环内酯类、碳青霉烯等（表 7）。

在轻度到中度肾功能障碍患者中，准确地评估

表 6　肝病患者所需的抗生素剂量减少

氨曲南
头孢哌酮
氯霉素
克林霉素
红霉素
异烟肼
甲硝唑
萘夫西林
奎奴普丁 / 达福普汀
利福平
替吉环素

肾功能很重要，因为许多药物通过肾替代治疗的方式清除使给药更加方便。影响药物血液滤过清除的因素包括分子大小、水溶性、血浆蛋白结合率、血浆和组织之间的平衡动力学和表面的维生素 D。在肾替代疗法治疗期间或之后患者对药物的剂量要求一定要记住（表 8）。在连续肾替代治疗期间，除了患者的内生肌酐清除率，估计肌酐清除率大约是 15 ~ 25 ml/min。持续低效血液透析（sustained low-efficiency dialysis，SLED）可能会使肌酐清除率达到 60 ~ 100 ml/min。在头孢洛克、头孢哌酮、头孢曲松、氯霉素、克林霉素、氯唑西林和双氯西林、多西环素、红霉素、利奈唑胺、甲氧西林 / 萘夫西林 / 苯唑西林、甲硝唑、利福平和替吉环素的治疗中，肾衰患者无须减少剂量。延长 β- 内酰胺类抗菌药物的输注时间是可以的。

表 7　肾功能不全抗生素剂量减少

药物 常规剂量	肌酐清除率 (10 ~ 50 ml/min)	肌酐清除率 (<10 ml/min)	滤出 与否
氨基糖苷类	个体需要	个体需要	是
氨苄西林 （1 ~ 2 g, q4 h）	0.5 ~ 1 g，q6 h	0.5 ~ 1 g，q12 h	是
氨曲南 （1 g，q8 h）	0.5 g，q8 h	0.5 g，q12 h	仅 HD
头孢孟多 （1 ~ 2 g, q6 h）	1 ~ 2 g，q8 ~ 12 h	1 ~ 2 g，q8 ~ 24 h	HD/ CAVHD
头孢唑啉 （1 g，q8 h）	1 g，q12 ~ 24 h	1 g，q48 h	仅 HD
头孢吡肟 （2 g，q12 h）	1 g，q12 h	1 g，q24 h	是
头孢噻肟 （1 g，q6 h）	1 g，q8 ~ 12 h	1 g，q24 h	仅 HD
头孢替坦 （1 g，q12 h）	1 g，q24 h	0.5 ~ 1 g，q24 h	否
头孢西丁 （1 ~ 2 g, q6 h）	1 ~ 2 g，q8 ~ 12 h	1 ~ 2 g，q24 h	HD/ CAVHD
头孢他啶 （1 g q8 h）	1 g，q24 h	1 g，q48 h	是
头孢唑肟 （1 g q8 h）	1 g，q12 ~ 24 h	1 g，q48 h	仅 HD
环丙沙星 （0.4 g q8 ~ 12 h）	0.4 g，q8 h	0.4 g，q16 h	否
亚胺培南 / 西司他丁（0.5 g q6h）	0.25 ~ 0.5 g，q6 ~ 8 h	0.25 ~ 0.5 g，q12h	仅 HD
左氧氟沙星 （0.5 ~ 0.75 gq12 h）	0.5 g，q24 h	0.5 g，q24 h	仅 CAVHD
哌拉西林 （2 ~ 4 g q4 h）	2 ~ 4 g，q6 h	2–3 g，q8 h	HD/ CAFHD
万古霉素 （1 g q12 h）	个体需要	个体需要	高流量 HD

CAVHD，持续的动脉静脉或静脉静脉血液透析；Ccr，肌酐清除率；HD，血液透析，PD，腹膜透析

计算肌酐清除率的公式（Ccr）：140- 年龄 ×［1（男）或 0.85（女）］× 体重（kg）

Ccr（ml/min）= 血清肌酐浓度（mg/dl）× 72

表 8 透析后静脉应用抗生素剂量的选择

抗生素	剂量
阿米卡星	2.5 ~ 3.75 mg/kg
氨苄西林	1 g
阿洛西林	3 g
氨曲南	0.125 g
头孢孟多	0.5 ~ 1 g
头孢吡肟	0.5 g
头孢西丁	1 g
头孢他啶	1 g
头孢唑肟	1 ~ 3 g
头孢呋辛	0.75 g
氯霉素	1 g
庆大霉素	1.0 ~ 1.7 mg/kg
亚胺培南 / 西司他丁	0.25 ~ 0.5 g
美罗培南	0.5 g
美洛西林	2 ~ 3 g
奈替米星	2 mg/kg
哌拉西林	2 g
哌拉西林 / 他唑巴坦	2.25 g
替卡西林	3 g
替卡西林 / 克拉维酸	3.1 g
妥布霉素	1.0 ~ 1.7 mg/kg
甲氧苄啶 / 磺胺甲异噁唑	5 mg/kg 甲氧苄氨嘧啶
万古霉素	如果用聚砜透析膜，则为 0.5 g，否则不用补充

重症患者真菌的定植与感染

Marc J. Shapiro, Eduardo Smith-Singares, Soumitra R.Eachempati, Jared M. Huston 和 Philip S. Barie 著
吕 杰 译

要点

1. 院内感染患者中，真菌感染的比重越来越大，特别是在重症监护病房的患者。
2. 造成真菌感染的危险因素包括糖尿病、免疫抑制、之前使用抗生素、ICU 住院时间延长、恶性肿瘤、肠外营养、中性粒细胞减少、长期的中心静脉导管留置。
3. 虽然白念珠菌感染是最常见的真菌感染，但其他真菌感染包括其他念珠菌属亚群（如光滑念珠菌和克鲁斯念珠菌）和曲霉菌属等均对早期的鉴别和治疗提出了挑战。
4. 有许多可用的抗真菌药物种类。选择恰当的药物，关键须熟悉他们的敏感和耐药情况。

历史与流行病学

侵袭性真菌感染已成为影响住院手术患者并发症发生率与死亡率的主要原因。据估计，在美国院内念珠菌血症的发病率大约是 8/10 万，每年卫生保健额外支出大约 10 亿美元。每名念珠菌血症患者大约花费联邦医疗保险 34 123 美元及商业保险 44 536 美元。在美国，念珠菌在导管相关性感染中位居第 4 位。在一个最近的前瞻性观察性研究中，在外科重症监护病房中，每 1 万人中就会有 10 人发生真菌血症，未调整死亡率为 25% ~ 50%。在美国，真菌血症在脓毒症中排在第 4 位，每年大约发现 20 种新的机会致病性真菌。美国以外的研究报告显示，念珠菌血症和其他形式的念珠菌感染正在增加。在 EPIC Ⅱ（重症监护病房中广泛感染的流行研究）的研究中，针对 75 个国家的 7 087 名感染患者进行研究。在培养出的最常见的几种微生物中，念珠菌菌株以 17% 排在第 3 位。自 1991 年以来，单独的念珠菌菌株有所增加，现在在单一医疗机构中，其占所有血培养的 6%。一般来说，欧洲医院报道的百分数是略低于北美的。然而，在台湾国立大学医院，念珠菌是自 1993 年以来最常见的一种医院血行感染的菌属。在一个用氟康唑预防的随机、安慰剂对照

试验的 meta 分析中，真菌感染率明显减少，但是患者的生存率并没有明显提升，因此提出了真菌预防性治疗的必要性问题。第 1 次临床描述念珠菌感染要追溯到希波克拉底和鹦鹉，直到那时才意识到真菌感染与患者疾病的严重程度有关。Lagenbeck 揭示了真菌可能是感染源，Berg 通过把“物质膜”接种到健康婴儿上，建立了在微生物和鹅口疮之间的因果关系。然而直到 1923 年，白念珠菌才由 Berkout 命名，但早在 1861 年，Zenker 已经第一次描述了白念珠菌引起的深部感染。另一方面，在 1729 年，Michaeli 第一次描述了曲霉菌属，并且在 19 世纪中叶，有人描述了人患曲霉病的病例。随着抗生素和 ICU 的引入，机会致病性真菌感染的病例开始出现。免疫抑制剂的使用、器官移植、植入性治疗技术和人类免疫缺陷病毒从根本上改变了真菌致病的状况。

真菌是处处可见的异养真核生物，环境适应能力很强，能够在极端环境中繁殖。真菌既属于假菌界也属于真菌界。为了容易识别，病原的分类是根据孢子产生的方法，在分子生物学技术的帮助下（rRNA 和 rDNA），进一步完善真菌种系，在群组之间建立新的联系。最重要的引起人类真菌感染的病原体是酵母菌和霉菌（从挪威引入，有绒毛的）。自从上个世纪有了双重命名法，已经证实了真菌繁殖的两种模式（有性繁殖和无性繁殖）。

真菌感染的预测因素

国家医疗安全网络在 2005 年开始收集志愿者的相关报告数据。第一份报告显示，在所有与健康相关的感染（healthcare associated infections，HAI）的病例中的菌株，念珠菌属排在第 4 位。在中心导管相关的感染中，念珠菌属排第 3 位，在尿道相关的感染中排第 2 位。此外，在重症患者中，患者本身的身体状况及疾病自身的情况可作为侵袭性真菌并发症的独立危险因素（通过使用多元 logistic 回归分析）。通过单变量 logistic 回归分析，患者的疾病严重程度及机械通气时间是患者死亡的独立危险因素，但是念珠菌感染不是这样。同患者的疾病严重程度、免疫状态的改变、医疗设备应用的数量等相关，念珠菌感染可影响患者的 ICU 治疗时间。中性粒细胞减少、糖尿病、新开始的血液透析、全肠外营养（total parenteral nutrition，TPN）、使用广谱抗生素、膀胱插管、氮质血症、腹泻、使用糖皮质激素和细胞毒性药物均与念珠菌血症有关。

糖尿病

糖尿病是黏膜念珠菌病、侵袭性念珠菌病和曲霉菌病等的独立预测因素。未受控制的糖尿病和酮症酸中毒与鼻脑毛霉菌（由接合菌产生）和其他非典型真菌感染有很强的相关性，而高血糖是肝移植和心脏旁路术后发生念珠菌血症的最强的预测因素。有假设分析，高血糖改变了宿主对感染的反应，增加了真菌的毒力。已经有些假设提出，高血糖会导致正常人体对感染的反应有所改变，同时也改变真菌本身，使其毒性更强。一些模型研究涉及促使真菌结合，随后内吞并使靶细胞坏死的糖基化过程、调理素的糖基化（使调理素不能识别真菌病原体）、糖尿病血清结合铁的能力下降（使得病原体可以获得更多的铁）。模型还改变了 T_H1 淋巴细胞对真菌的识别（损害 γ 干扰素的产生），以及念珠菌属过度表达会促使真菌黏附内皮和黏膜表面的类 C3 样受体蛋白的证据。假定树突状细胞和其他的抗原呈递细胞在对真菌的细胞调节反应的诱导中发挥重要作用，在糖尿病患者接种疫苗的研究中显示抗原与 T 细胞的相互作用受到破坏。

中性粒细胞减少

中性粒细胞减少的程度和侵袭性真菌感染进展的风险之间有直接的相关性。尽管在美国，中性粒细胞减少的癌症患者常规进行预防或预先治疗，但最近的 meta 分析得出结论，上述患者并没有从中获益。对于经历过化疗或骨髓移植并且伴有发热症状的严重中性粒细胞减少的患者，经验性的抗真菌治疗是标准化治疗。当患者有严重的中性粒细胞减少时，发生彻底的念珠菌菌血症的危险性更高，病原体对于伏立康唑（或其他抗真菌药物）的反应降低。对于中性粒细胞减少并伴有浸润性真菌感染的患者来说，新的治疗方法包括粒细胞输注和干扰素 γ 注入等。

器官移植和免疫抑制的药物处理

器官移植患者最常见的两种机会性真菌感染是念珠菌属（胃肠道来源）和曲霉菌属（吸入来源）。有趣的是除非因排异反应需要强化免疫抑制方案，那么移植后 6 个月后患者发生真菌感染的风险就减小了。实质器官接受者，移植物常常受到影响。在肝移植手术，随着手术持续时间的延长和输血需求的增加，菌血症发生的风险也相应增加。其他危险因素包括胆管吻合的类型（Roux-en-Y）、组织缺血、巨细胞病毒（cytomegalovirus，CMV）感染、移植物抗宿主病等。在肺移植患者中最常见的是曲霉菌感染导致的支气管炎。它最易发生在支气管吻合处，吻合处定植感染既是破坏或出血的危险因素，也是排异反应和移植后患者生存率降低的预测因素。在这种情况下，建议使用支气管镜进行监测。曲霉菌属是在心脏移植术后主要的真菌血症病原体，仅次于术后1个月内引起肺炎的巨细胞病毒。

感染相关的并发症是影响胰腺移植和胰腺肾联合移植患者并发症发生率及死亡率的主要原因。革兰氏阳性球菌是最常见的微生物，其次是革兰氏阴性杆菌和念珠菌。真菌感染的危险因素包括膀胱引流和使用OKT-3进行抑制治疗。所有实质器官移植中，肾移植的感染相关并发症最少。在纽约长老会医院的SICU中，只在实质器官受体中将氟康唑作为预防性应用。

恶性实体肿瘤和血液病

癌症患者容易发生机会性感染。癌症和化疗造成3种类型的免疫功能障碍的影响，从而使患者容易受到机会性感染：①中性粒细胞减少（之前提到过）；②淋巴细胞免疫调节缺损（如霍奇金病和皮质类固醇治疗期间）；③体液免疫缺陷（如多发性骨髓瘤、瓦氏巨球蛋白血症、脾切除术后）。前两种类型最容易感染真菌。恶性肿瘤化疗后发生的伴发热症状的中性粒细胞减少患者中高达1/3是由于侵入性真菌血症（见后文治疗部分）。

尽管T_H1类型反应（TNF-α、干扰素-γ和IL-12）提供保护、抑制真菌感染，T_H2（IL-4和IL-10）与疾病的进展相关，但淋巴细胞减少的类型和淋巴细胞计数的最低点同样重要。由于糖皮质激素对各种转录因子，尤其是核因子κB（NF-κB）的活性有抑制作用，所以糖皮质激素有抗炎的特性。在小鼠模型中，类固醇的治疗为应对真菌的损伤而增加了IL-10的产生，并降低了单核细胞向感染区域的聚集。然而，抑制了中性粒细胞向炎症区域的聚集（IL-8介导）。

长时间应用中心静脉导管

众多研究已经表明，真菌血症与导管相关的实例即使不是占大多数，数量也是非常多的。最大的前瞻性真菌血症治疗研究中，72%的真菌血症感染是与导管相关的。从血液培养分离出的近平滑念珠菌与中心静脉导管感染、静脉营养液输注、假体设备等相关。中性粒细胞减少的患者的真菌感染源与非中性粒细胞减少的患者的感染源是不同的。在非中性粒细胞减少的患者中最常见的因导管引起污染（随后出现感染）的途径是在放置导管时、处理留置导管周围皮肤和通过工作人员的手交叉传播到ICU患者中。其他的导管定植可能来源包括污染了的静脉营养液、通过导管的不合理多重用药，以及应用其他医疗设备等。血管内导管和其他与血液直接接触的异体设备，如心脏起搏器、心脏瓣膜、骨科关节等作为二次污染途径是通过胃肠道的菌群易位出现的。但这在中性粒细胞减少和其他免疫抑制的患者中是最常见的途径。一旦导管污染，一系列事情将会发生：酵母菌粘连到导管的表面，然后生成菌丝合成多糖的基质和蛋白，以增加它们的大小并形成立三维立体骨架。这就是所谓的菌膜，是通过感染医疗装置形成真菌二次感染的主要原因。菌膜帮助抵抗抗真菌的药物和保护性的免疫反应。

一般来说，移除所有中心静脉导管意味着接下来须进行全身真菌感染和真菌血症的诊断。在感染胃肠道源性真菌的中性粒细胞减少的患者中，可能没有必要移除相关导管。在导管移除后或排除念珠菌在眼内的播散（见于眼内炎后）之后，抗真菌治疗仍要继续。

念珠菌的定植

来自多个部位的无临床症状的念珠菌的过度生长和复苏高度提示念珠菌感染，这两种情况下患者死亡的累计风险相似。念珠菌定植生长的危险因素包括之前用过抗生素或因细菌感染进入ICU、ICU治疗时间延长和复杂性胃肠道手术。直到20世纪80年代，绝大多数真菌感染为白念珠菌。然而，目前真菌感染的一半是由于北美和大部分的欧洲第二高发的光滑念珠菌等非白念珠菌属。光滑念珠菌的致死率更高，部分原因是由于其对氟康唑的耐药率为10%～15%，以及细菌培养需要5天的时间才可以鉴别诊断。在ICU有6个鉴别光滑念珠菌的独立危险因素：年龄超过60岁、近期腹部手术病史、从进入ICU到第1次血培养达到或超过7天、近期应用头孢类抗生素、存在实体性肿瘤、无糖尿病。同样，近平滑念珠菌的发病率也在逐年上升。菌落定植后的全身念珠菌病的爆发大部分是来源于胃肠道。

因为重症患者发生念珠菌的定植不是一个好的信号，我们需要在侵袭性念珠菌病的危险性方面来鉴别和进一步筛查可能发生念珠菌感染的高危患者。在ICU患者中，筛查技术包括常规培养监测。最初由Pittet提出的改良方法（改良定植指数）已经在手术患者中得到验证。尽管很多专家认为在这种情况下存在多个念珠菌分离株，但在重症患者的经验型抗真菌治疗的最初阶段仍应该把0.4作为阈值指数（见后文治疗部分）。

广谱抗菌药物的应用

尽管对于真菌的过度生长和侵袭性感染，广谱抗生素的使用是最有说服力的危险因素，但这种风险的精确机制并不完全清楚。当我们思考使用抗生素的影响时，必须首先考虑到在人体内细菌和真菌的复杂的相互关系。

为了调查和描述细菌和真菌病原体之间可能的相互作用，已经至少创建了3个实验模型。一个小鼠模型中，替卡西林-克拉维酸和头孢曲松（抗厌氧菌治疗）的应用与肠道的酵母菌群大量增长是相关的。另一方面，抗厌氧效果差的抗生素（如头孢他啶和氨曲南）不会出现这种影响。临床综述对使用此种抗生素的免疫功能低下的患者粪便定植菌的数量是确定的。然而，在真菌的过度生长和厌氧菌抑制之间的相互作用与大肠杆菌和脆弱拟杆菌导致的腹腔脓肿的模型不相同。Sawyer等的研究显示，白念珠菌诱发细菌移位到脓肿，但这种关系是菌群直接的能力，而并非协同或合作产生。这个过程与白念珠菌和金黄色葡萄球菌、黏质沙雷菌和粪肠球菌的扩增作用不同。许多免疫调节和免疫抑制病毒已被证实能够促进机会性真菌的重复感染，最著名的例子是巨细胞病毒和人类疱疹病毒-6，因为它们诱导免疫抑制细胞因子的产生。在免疫功能低下的情况下白念珠菌可以大量生长，在特定的情况下增加了已经存在的细菌感染的毒性和致命性。这一点从临床观察中已经证实，在单独使用抗菌素治疗后加用抗真菌治疗也不会增加太多的治疗效果。

因此，抗生素尤其是抗厌氧菌的抗生素的使用（3种或以上）构成了真菌定植和过度生长的危险因素，从而反过来预测可能发生全身真菌感染。这一现象的精确机制是未知的，但跟真菌-微生物的毒力和相互的生长抑制也许是相关的。念珠菌可能提高特定而不是所有的细菌的致病性，两者之间的相互作用仍有待阐明。

念珠菌腹膜炎

几乎可以在20%的腹部手术术后患者的样本中找到念珠菌，它们主要集中在上消化道穿孔和院内感染的病例中。存在的危险因素包括急性生理和慢性健康评分（Acute Physiology and Chronic Health Evaluation，APACHE Ⅱ）超过17分、入院时存在呼吸衰竭、上消化道腹膜炎和腹水中检测出念珠菌等，患者的死亡率是明显升高的。因此，在严重脓毒症或感染性休克和腹膜炎的情况下，留取标本的酵母菌阳性提示需要抗酵母菌的全身治疗。

ICU住院期与机械通气是相关的：机械通气管道的长度与流行病学观察相关所需要的重症监护数量与全身真菌感染和真菌定植相关。

包括全身念珠菌病的发病机制和易感性的其他因素是：TPN、H_2受体阻断药的应用、获得性免疫缺陷综合征、放射治疗、发生过菌血症、腹部手术、血液透析、年龄过大或过小、黏膜与皮肤的念珠菌的复发和心肺旁路术时间超过120 min。

病原微生物

白念珠菌

不管是在美国还是在其他国家，最常见的真菌病原体和被视为ICU脓毒症最常见的病原体来源之一，白念珠菌是在人类疾病经常出现的罪魁祸首。白念珠菌占念珠菌属的59%，其次是占真菌感染15%～25%的光滑念珠菌。没有任何播散迹象的单发部位的菌群存在的证据，定植就已经发生了。侵袭性念珠菌病可以呈多发病灶或播散样。多发病灶的念珠菌病是念珠菌在2个或更多的下列部位同时出现：呼吸系统、消化系统、泌尿系统、伤口或引流管等。侵袭性念珠菌病通常是从脑脊髓、胸膜、心包、腹膜等正常无菌部位的液体中发现菌群，或来自深部器官的组织学标本，或眼内炎的诊断，或导管尖端培养阴性的念珠菌菌血症的微生物学证据。在过去的 30 年中念珠菌菌血症的发病率已经明显升高，而在一些报道中患者的死亡率高达 80%。疾控中心的 NNIS 系统发现 1993 年的美国，念珠菌属占了所有院内血行感染的 8%～15%，被认为是第四大最常见的血行感染的独立病原体。

已经证实，从酵母到菌丝的形成，白念珠菌的形态的改变是其播散的重要决定因素，因为菌丝状态有致病性。宿主及病原体在念珠菌的播散中均发挥作用。在真菌菌丝的产生过程中会生成一些目前重点研究的蛋白质。巯基特异性抗氧化剂 1（thiol-specific antioxidant，TSA1）在由宿主细胞产生的抗氧化环境里，可增强其生存能力。宿主识别分子（黏附分子），分泌的天门冬氨酰蛋白酶和磷脂酶，伴随着抗原表达改变的表型转换、菌落形态改变和组织亲和力是其他可识别的毒力因子。诱导机制和引发这种变化的多重刺激因子目前尚未知。

从宿主方面来看，吲哚胺 2,3 - 二氧化酶（indoleamine 2,3-dioxygenase，IDO）与阻止菌丝形成的抗真菌的防御机制有关。干扰素 - γ 在感染部位和树突细胞诱导该酶的生成。所以干扰素在白念珠菌侵入的免疫中发挥重要作用。其他阻止菌丝形成的免疫机制包括唾液组氨酸、其他胃肠道抑制肽、常驻的树突细胞。双态的变化导致了易感宿主的侵袭性念珠菌病（被称为肝脾念珠菌病）和特定终末器官的参与。在这些转移的感染灶中，从临床角度来看，最有趣的点就是真菌性眼内炎。

类似于其他微生物感染，侵袭性念珠菌病和真菌血症可以导致感染性休克。研究表明在易感个体双态的变化过程中会发生休克和终末器官的衰竭，这些情况不依赖于 TNF-α。作为引起脓毒症的原因，真菌血症的诊断依赖于强烈的临床怀疑。只有 50% 的侵袭性念珠菌病的血培养呈阳性，细菌病原体可能会干扰念珠菌的痊愈。没有可靠的实验室检查来区分念珠菌的定植和侵袭性念珠菌病。在预测患者有发生全身感染可能的方面，没有任何一个部位的定植比其他部位有更大的可能发生全身感染。真菌血症的诊断标准是组织培养阳性（包括烧伤切除培养和腹膜的培养）、眼内炎、骨髓炎及念珠菌尿等。爆发性紫癜和无法解释的肌痛提示有念珠菌病病史。3 个或更多的定植部位或 2 个至少间隔 24 h 的血培养阳性，其中一个是在移除中心导管后的结果，高度提示真菌血症。尽管尿中存在念珠菌，但机体没有症状时，一般不需要治疗，但出现症状、中性粒细胞减少的肾移植患者和仪器使用后则需要治疗。至少拔除或更换尿管后需要治疗。

真菌眼内炎通常是由全身真菌血症血行播散导致的。尽管曲霉菌、隐球菌、镰刀菌、丝孢菌属等已报告均可导致眼内炎，但念珠菌属是最常见的病原体。在所有念珠菌感染的患者中，视网膜病变的诊断率为 28%～45%，也许会是临床上未被发现的真菌感染的首发症状。对于深部组织真菌感染的系统性治疗，早期内生真菌感染眼内炎的发病率会明显减少。对于全身念珠菌病和真菌血症的患者应强制性进行正规眼科评估，来排除眼部病变。一个典型的三维视网膜玻璃体炎症的检查可作为念珠菌属感染的内源性眼内炎的诊断。

治疗包括积极的静脉内抗真菌治疗，也许须眼内注射两性霉素 B、卡泊芬净或伏立康唑等。如果感染扩展到玻璃体或部分前段感染较明显，需要外科清创或玻璃体切除。延迟治疗将会导致患者失明。

非白念珠酵母菌

最近几年非白念珠菌的真菌血症和全身性感染综合征的发病率在逐渐升高。成年人 ICU 感染，占所有非白念真菌感染的一半。原因可能是多因素的。毫无疑问，对于光滑念珠菌和克柔念珠菌出现的解释是通过抗真菌药物的使用，导致不敏感种类被筛选出来。其他种类的真菌是与特殊事件相关，例如中心导管的存在与近平滑念珠菌。在肿瘤患者中，热带念珠菌的发病率升高是继发于微生物侵入性的增长，尤其是胃肠道黏膜受损。这种感染的临床特征与白念珠菌并无区别。

曲霉菌

非侵袭性的曲霉菌病包括过敏性支气管肺曲霉病（哮喘患者的一种超敏反应）和曲霉肿。没有组织的侵入，通常不需要抗真菌治疗。在过去的十年里侵袭性曲霉病发病率明显升高，已成为血液恶性肿瘤患者死亡的主要原因。尽管通常吸入孢子是发生侵袭性曲霉菌感染的原因，但食物（如胡椒、花草茶、水果、玉米和水稻）中也常常存在真菌。曲霉菌耐热的孢子和其他真菌存在形式很难消灭，免疫功能低下的患者成为其入侵渠道。肺泡中巨噬细胞不能够清除的孢子在肺泡表面生长，以菌丝的形式侵入肺组织，并随之侵犯血管和早期播散（图 1-3）。

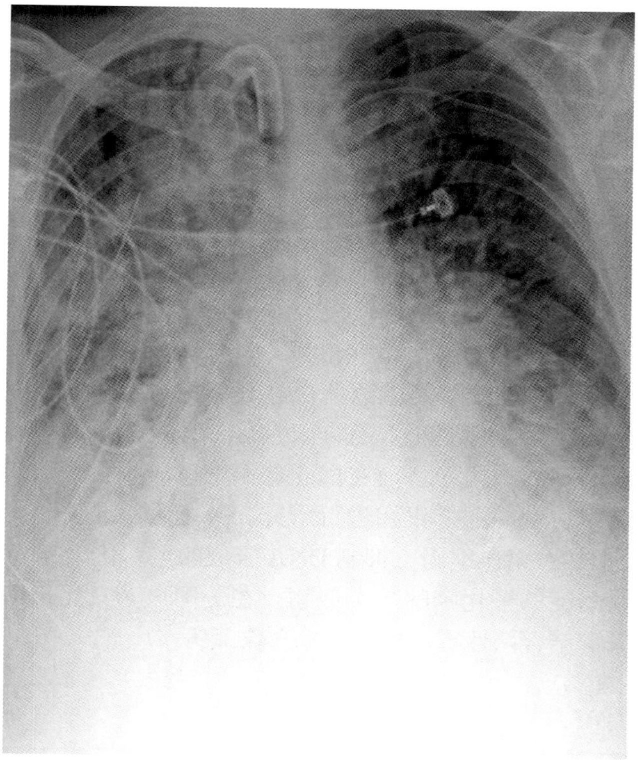

图 1. 侵袭性曲霉菌感染肺炎的患者的 X 线胸片。图像的表现与急性呼吸窘迫综合征是相同的 (*Courtesy of E. Smith-Singares, P.S. Barie,and S.R. Eachempati, The Anne and Max A. Cohen Surgical Intensive Care Unit,New York–Presbyterian Hospital, Weill Cornell Medical College, New York.*)

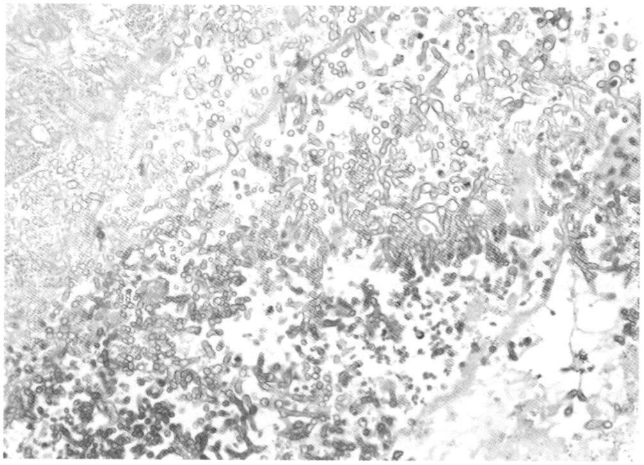

图 2. 图 1 中患者侵袭性曲霉菌感染的肺部显微镜下照片 (*Courtesy of C.R. Minick, E. Loyd, and B. Amin, Department of Pathology and Laboratory Medicine, New York Hospital, Weill Cornell Medical College, New York.*)

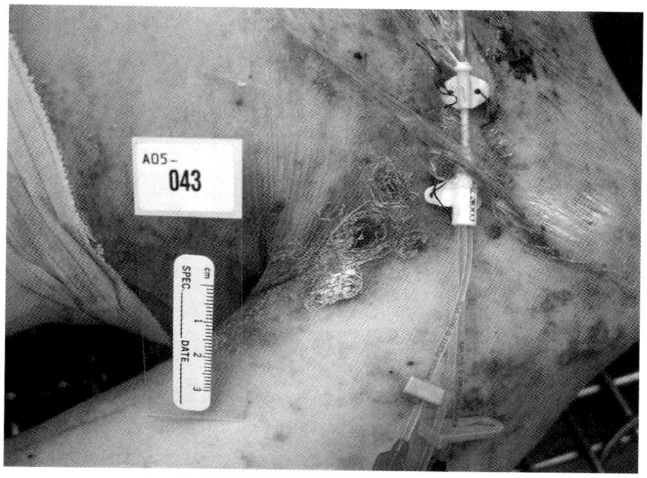

图 3. 肝脾念珠菌感染患者的爆发性紫癜 (*Courtesy of C.R. Minick, E. Loyd, and B. Amin, Department of Pathology and Laboratory Medicine, New York Hospital, Weill Cornell Medical College, New York.*)

其他新出现的真菌病原体

在 ICU 患者中接合菌（毛霉菌）正变得越来越重要。尽管已经有经皮暴露（外科手术或创伤和烧伤）的报道，但免疫力低下患者的感染途径通常是雾化吸入和耐热孢子的吸入。这些孢子的来源通常是在土壤中腐烂的有机物，但它们可以在医院食物中找到，如水果、面包、甜点、花草茶和胡椒等。毛霉菌病的主要危险因素是糖尿病酮症酸中毒、中性粒细胞减少、铁过载、去铁胺治疗和蛋白质热量营养不良。治疗方式取决于疾病的严重程度，必要时行外科清创术。

治疗原则

尽管关于抗真菌药物的列表已经有了两性霉素低毒性剂型、改良的三唑类、棘球白素的发展，还有一个英国研究中报道的作用在真菌胞壁的药物。ICU 和真菌治疗表明目前大部分真菌没有已记录的治疗方案，而是在很低的阈值简单地经验性给予患者抗真菌治疗。通过 Flanagan 和 Barnes 的描述，ICU 中治疗真菌感染有 4 个不同的方案：预防、预先、经验性和确定性治疗。一些研究数据表明，对已经感染念珠菌病的非中性粒细胞减少的外科手术患者，进行预防性的侵袭性真菌感染治疗是逐渐减少的。其他数据表明在未经选择的 SICU 患者中预防性使用抗念珠菌治疗方案会增加患者死亡率，延长患者的住院时间，出现抗真菌药物的耐药更能使ICU的成本增加。在SICU中预防性应用氟康唑可导致高达80%的耐药率及继发性真菌感染。表1、表2、图4和图5显示一个在纽约长老会医院的SICU中使用抗真菌药物的模式。不考虑真菌的种类，氟康唑的耐药性使患者的死亡率增加了一倍。Pittet等和Ostrosky-Zeichner发明的定植指数已经被证实，它们支持高危患者是指在ICU住院时间超过4天并且有中心静脉置管或使用抗生素，并且包含下面中的2项的人：全肠外营养、透析、近期大手术、胰腺炎诊断和使用皮质固醇类或其他免疫抑制剂的治疗等。该研究已经证实，未选择的外伤和ICU患者使用氟康唑治疗没有益处，甚至在念珠菌菌血症患者的致死率方面，其作用已经超过了年龄和疾病严重程度。

表3提供了一个目前可用的抗真菌的药物列表。两性霉素B是一种天然多烯大环内酯类药物，其主要结合麦角固醇——真菌细胞膜上的甾醇化合物，导致离子通道及细胞凋亡。两性霉素也会产生氧自由基。其可对抗大部分真菌，包括在脑脊液中也有效。由于其较高的蛋白结合率，药物含量不会受到血液透析的影响。在高达73%的患者中，首次输入两性霉素即会发生输液反应，它在接下来的治疗中逐渐消失。虽然快速输液会发生急性钾释放并导致心搏停止，但两性霉素相关的肾毒性导致的氮血症和低钾血症更常见。两性霉素B脂配方可用的剂量更高，肾毒性更小。制霉菌素是一种类似于两性霉素的多烯结构，目前在白念珠菌的感染中使用。当前注射用的配方正在进行研究。氟胞嘧啶是一种可使RNA错误编码、抑制DNA合成的可转化为5-氟尿嘧啶的氟化嘧啶的类似物。在美国该药只用于口服，结合两性霉素用于治疗念珠菌病。

表1　念珠菌属对抗真菌药的敏感性

念珠菌属	氟康唑	伊曲康唑	伏立康唑（非标准化）	两性霉素B	卡泊芬净（非标准化）
白念珠菌	S	S	S	S	S
热带念珠菌	S	S	S	S	S
近平滑念珠菌	S	S	S	S	S ~ I（R?）
光滑念珠菌	S-DD ~ R	S-DD ~ R	S ~ I	S ~ I	S
克柔念珠菌	R	S-DD ~ R	S ~ I	S ~ I	S
酵母念珠菌	S	S	S	S ~ R	S

I: 中效；R: 耐药；S: 敏感；S-DD: 敏感-剂量依赖（通过更高的剂量提高最小抑菌浓度，如氟康唑12 mg/kg · d）

表2　抗真菌药物每日大约的费用，2005

抗菌药物	每次用药大约花费/剂量	通常成年人的剂量	每天用药大约花费/剂量
氟康唑，400 mg，IV	$ 14	400 mg，IV，每天	$ 14
氟康唑，400 mg，PO	$ 1	400 mg，PO，每天	$ 1
依曲康唑，200 mg，PO 溶液	$ 43	200 mg，PO，一天2次	$ 86
伏立康唑，400 mg，IV	$ 230	400 mg，IV，一天2次（负荷量）	$ 460
卡泊芬净，70 mg，IV	$ 421	70 mg，IV，每天（负荷量）	$ 421
卡泊芬净，50 mg，IV	$ 405	50 mg，IV，每天（维持量）	$ 405
两性霉素B，常规70 mg，IV	$ 12	70 mg，IV，每天	$ 12
两性霉素B，脂质（脂质复合体）	$ 300	350 mg，IV，每天	$ 300

Courtesy Marc R. McDowell, PharmD, Advocate Christ Medical Center, Oak Lawn, Ill

IV, 静脉输注；PO, 口服

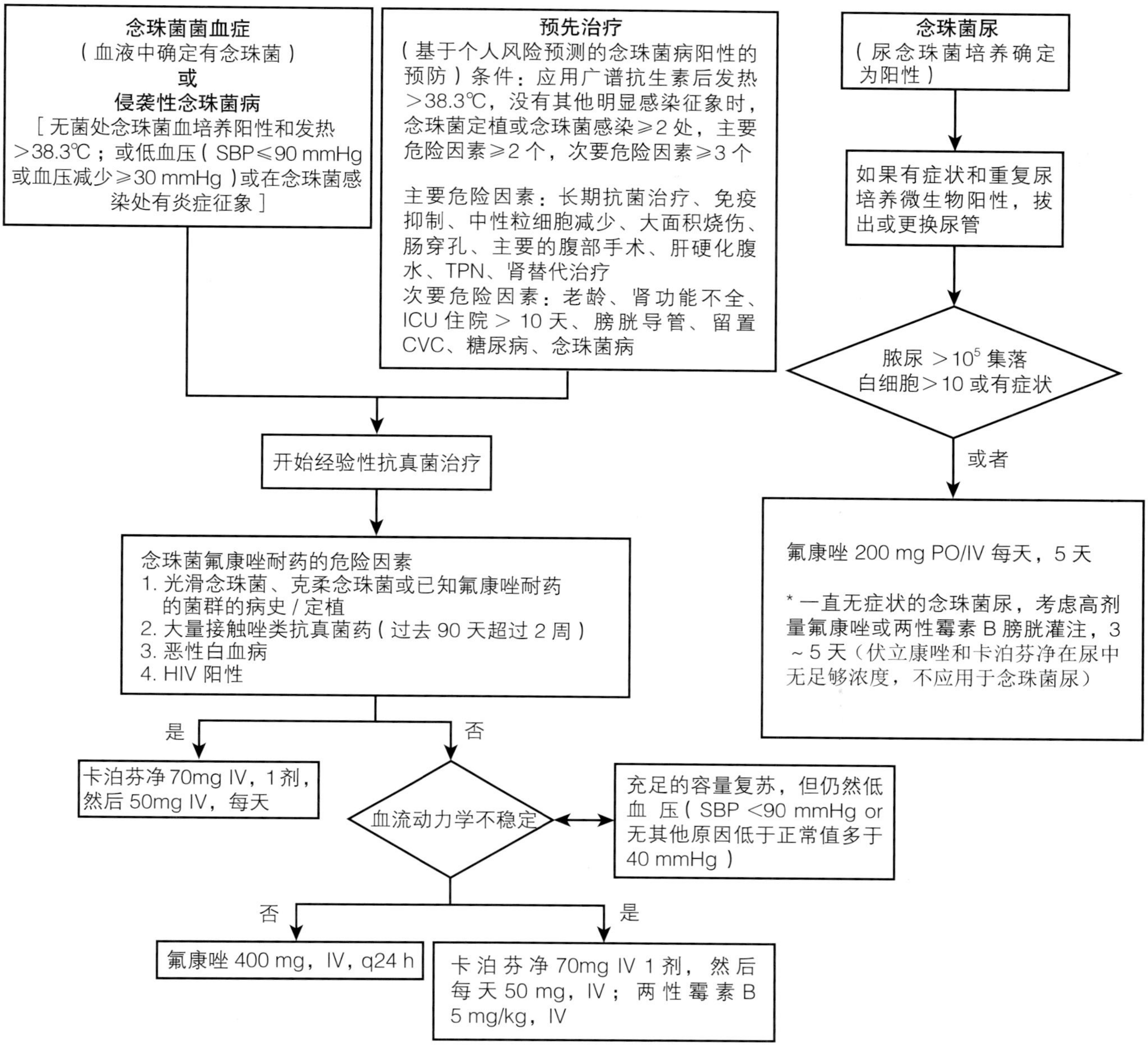

图 4　念珠菌引起的成年人感染的抗真菌药物的治疗。CVC，中央静脉导管；HIV，人类免疫缺陷病毒；PO，口服；SBP，收缩压；TPN，全静脉营养；WBC，白细胞

唑类可抑制细胞色素 P–450 依赖的酶，改变真菌的细胞膜。酮康唑只有片剂形式，用来治疗念珠菌病、鹅口疮和念珠菌尿等。氟康唑和伊曲康唑对除了克柔念珠菌和镰刀菌的其他念珠菌群均有效。伊曲康唑对曲霉菌是有效的。如前所述，光滑念珠菌和克柔念珠菌对氟康唑是耐药的，而氟康唑对隐球菌和球孢子菌病脑膜炎是有效的。氟康唑和伊曲康唑也受到许多药物如抗酸药、H_2 受体阻断药、异烟肼、苯妥英钠和苯巴比妥的影响。

第二代三唑类抗真菌药物包括泊沙康唑、雷夫康唑、伏立康唑。这些抗真菌药物的有效范畴包括念珠菌、对氟康唑耐药的真菌、曲霉菌等。

棘白菌素类包括卡泊芬净是治疗侵袭性曲霉菌的三线药物。由于其独特的作用机制，棘白菌素可用于更多的规范抗真菌药物的联合使用。美国传染病学会支持棘白菌素类主要用于治疗中重度念珠菌菌血症的患者。

非中性粒细胞减少患者发生侵袭性真菌感染需要治疗的情况为以下几点：除了黏膜，针吸活检的组织学和细胞病理学检测显示酵母细胞或假菌丝；除了尿液、鼻窦、黏膜，从无菌的临床或放射学异常的感染部位培养出阳性结果，或临床症状、体征

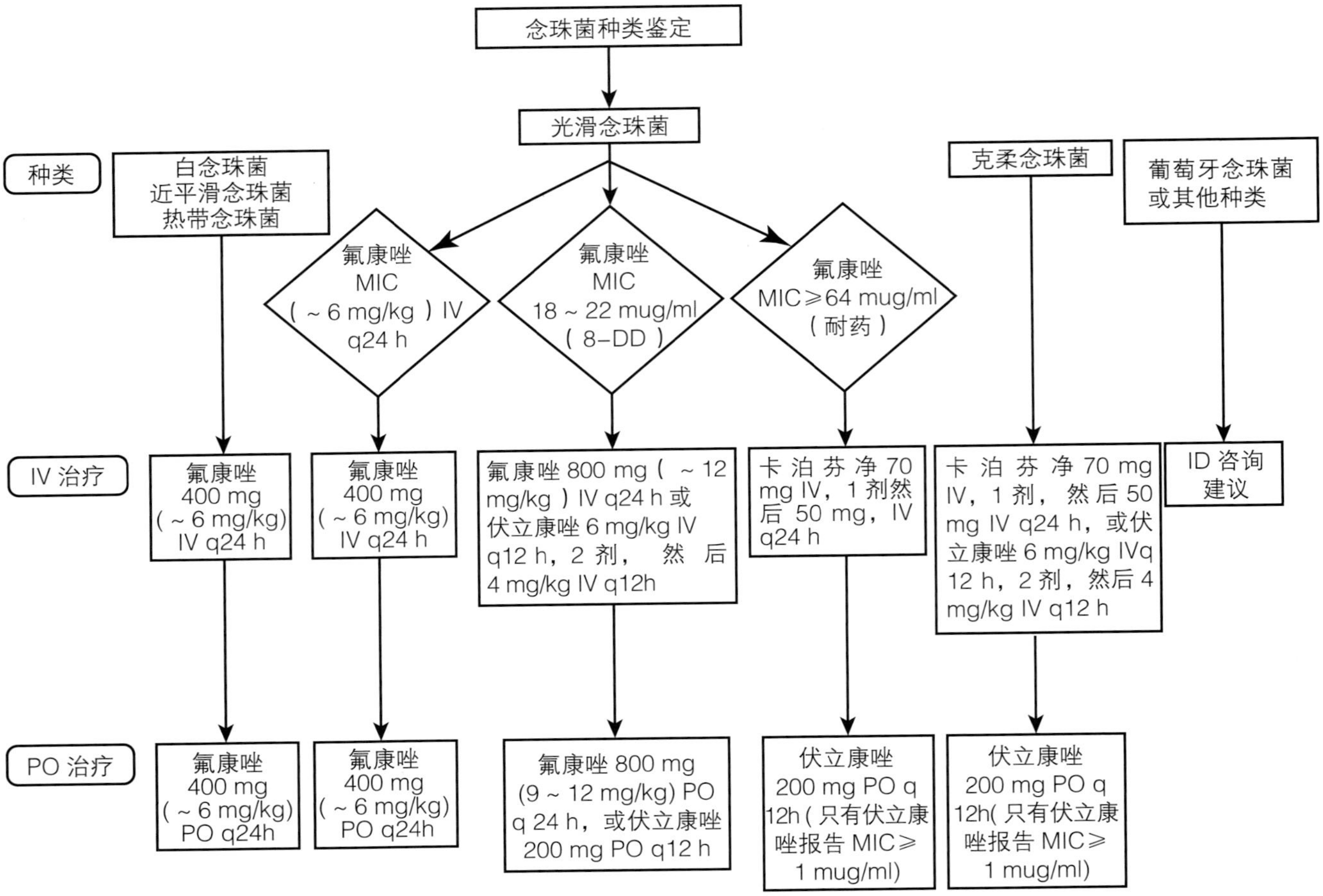

图 5 当念珠菌感染确定后，治疗的计算方式。ID，传染疾病；IV，静脉输注；MIC，最小抑菌浓度；PO，口服；q，每

表 3 抗真菌药物

抗真菌药物	微生物	常规剂量
两性霉素 B	白念珠菌（>95%） 光滑念珠菌（>95%） 近平滑念珠菌（>95%） 克柔念珠菌（>95%） 热带念珠菌（>99%） 季也蒙念珠菌 酵母念珠菌 活性不定：曲霉菌、贝吉尔毛孢子菌、镰刀菌、皮炎芽生菌	IV：0.3～1 mg/kg·d，超过 2～6 h 口服：1 ml 混悬剂，一天 4 次，使用 2 周
两性霉素 B 脂质（较少肾毒性）	白念珠菌（>95%） 光滑念珠菌（>95%） 近平滑念珠菌（>95%） 克柔念珠菌（>95%） 热带念珠菌（>99%） 季也蒙念珠菌 葡萄牙念珠菌 活性不定：曲霉菌	IV：3～5 mg/kg·d

表 3 抗真菌药物（续表）

抗真菌药物	微生物	常规剂量
两性霉素 B 胶态分散（更多用来静脉滴注）	白念珠菌（>95%） 光滑念珠菌（>95%） 近平滑念珠菌（>95%） 克柔念珠菌（>95%） 热带念珠菌（>99%） 季也蒙念珠菌 酵母念珠菌 活性不定：曲霉菌	IV：3 ~ 4 mg/kg · d
两性霉素 B 脂质复合物	白念珠菌（>95%） 光滑念珠菌（>95%） 近平滑念珠菌（>95%） 克柔念珠菌（>95%） 热带念珠菌（>99%） 季也蒙念珠菌 酵母念珠菌 活性不定：曲霉菌	IV：3 ~ 5 mg/kg · d
酮康唑	白念珠菌	PO：200 ~ 400 mg/d
伏立康唑	曲霉菌、镰刀菌 白念珠菌（>99%） 光滑念珠菌（>99%） 近平滑念珠菌（>99%） 克柔念珠菌（>99%） 热带念珠菌（>99%） 季也蒙念珠菌（>95%） 酵母念珠菌（>95%）	IV： 6 mg/kg q12 h × 2， 然后 4 mg/kg， IV，q12 h PO：>40 kg，200 mg，q12 h； <40 kg，100 mg，q12 h
氟康唑	白念珠菌（>97%） 光滑念珠菌（85 ~ 90% 耐药 / 中间物） 近平滑念珠菌（>99%） 热带念珠菌（>98%） 克柔念珠菌（>5%） 抑制真菌的曲霉菌	念珠菌病： 预防（IV 或口服）：200 ~ 400 mg/d 大剂量：400 ~ 800 mg/d 口咽的：第一天 200 mg，然后每天 100 mg，2 周
伊曲康唑	曲霉菌，白念珠菌（>93%） 光滑念珠菌（>50%） 近平滑念珠菌（>45%） 热带念珠菌（>58%） 克柔念珠菌（>69%） 季也蒙念珠菌、葡萄牙念珠菌 芽生菌病、组织胞浆菌病、色素性真菌病	IV：负荷量 200 mg IV，每天 2 次，4 剂量；然后 200 mg，每天 4 次，最多 14 天 PO：每天 200 mg 或 q12 h 重症患者：负荷量为 600 ~ 800/d，3 ~ 5 天，然后 400 ~ 600 mg/d
卡泊芬净	白念珠菌、光滑念珠菌、近平滑念珠菌、热带念珠菌、克柔念珠菌、季也蒙念珠菌、酵母念珠菌	IV：70 mg，然后每天 50 mg
氟胞嘧啶	对克柔念珠菌无效 白念珠菌、热带念珠菌、近平滑念珠菌、酵母念珠菌	PO：50 ~ 150 mg/kg · d，q 6 h
制霉菌素	白念珠菌	100 000 U，一天 4 次，吞服
克霉唑	鹅口疮	口服片剂，每天 5 片，14 天

IV，静脉输注；PO，口服；q，每天；qid，一天 4 次

与相关微生物特征一致的患者经皮穿刺血培养阳性。

中性粒细胞减少的患者和预先治疗

在没有表现出全身念珠菌病的临床特征前给予患者抗真菌治疗的新方法就是预先治疗。不只是语义差异，预防性治疗被定义为一种危险分层触发的治疗（指的是患者“可能”感染真菌）。但是抢先治疗是针对确定有感染，但还没有症状患者的早期治疗，通常是通过检测指标或其他非血液培养的方式检测出来的。预先治疗的优势在于理论上结合了真菌预防的证据和早期治疗的益处，以及针对性治疗的信心，也没有批评者指出的增加真菌耐药性和耐药菌株的恢复。因为有证据表明预防性使用氟康唑在治疗非发热性的中性粒细胞减少患者中并没有获益，所以药物应用的频繁监测和筛查（而不是治疗）的新规范的提高是势在必行的。

实质器官移植受者预防性抗真菌治疗

在实质器官移植受者中，侵袭性真菌感染仍然是一个最常见的并发症。在移植术后早期，患者的感染风险更高，手术 6 个月后风险会降低。肝移植患者真菌感染风险最高，紧随其后的是心脏和肺移植。已经确定的其他的危险因素包括肝和肾功能障碍、二次移植、排斥反应、手术相关并发症和巨细胞病毒感染等。最近最有力的证据表明，氟康唑可以有效地预防侵袭性真菌感染，但并不能减少患者的死亡率。在肝移植患者中，鉴于目前 10% 的发病率，为了预防 1 例感染，需要治疗的患者例数是 14 例。meta 分析得出结论，对于感染风险低的受者来说（如肾移植受体），需要治疗的患者例数增加到 28 例。预防性治疗应该留给那些风险等级更高的和真菌并发症更普遍的患者。对于那些非念珠菌真菌感染的免疫抑制患者，延长的抗真菌治疗可能需要，以防复发。

获得性免疫缺陷综合征和经验性抗真菌治疗

侵袭性念珠菌病的发病率很低，但当考虑到感染人类获得性免疫缺陷病毒的患者来说，无处不在的念珠菌性黏膜与皮肤感染的事实令人费解。这说明宿主用来抵御皮肤黏膜念珠菌感染和侵袭性念珠菌感染的防御机制是不同的。因此，发展成获得性免疫缺陷综合征和相关的念珠菌感染的患者经常有额外的风险因素，如全肠外营养、导管置入、广谱抗生素，以及人类获得性免疫缺陷相关的淋巴瘤或细胞毒性治疗导致的中性粒细胞减少。对这些患者经验性使用氟康唑不符合成本效益，不应当鼓励使用。

针对特定的危险因素和有可能感染的微生物的治疗

纽约长老会医院基于流行病学方面的研究，已经制定出抗真菌药物的使用剂量和指南（表 1-2 和图 4-5）。表 3 列出了在美国最常使用的抗真菌药物。几项研究已经表明，因为唑类抗真菌药物干扰中性粒细胞和淋巴细胞的功能，故唑类抗真菌药物有免疫抑制作用，酮康唑类似于血栓素 A_2 合成酶抑制剂，可能用来试图减少 ARDS 在高危患者中的发生率。伊曲康唑和咪康唑是 5- 脂氧合酶强有力的抑制剂。对血浆血栓素和白三烯水平无影响的氟康唑已被证明在动物和离体实验中增强了中性粒细胞的杀菌活性，在治疗脓毒症患者中显示出积极的作用。

真菌的附带效应

重症医学的最新进展已经使很多之前可能因为原发疾病面临死亡的严重患者能够存活下来。在患者幸存方面的改善已经超过（在部分病例中相等）真菌定植的爆发性生长和 ICU 患者的感染及抗菌药物治疗的有效性。随着抗生素的种类越来越复杂，随即导致耐药性的产生，同样地，真菌感染的复杂性也导致多学科综合治疗的扩大化。虽然有这样的观点，侵袭性真菌感染会增加患者的死亡率、发病率及延长住院时间（ICU 和医院），但感染造成的患者的精确死亡率仍然存在争议。尽管在预防真菌定植和侵袭性感染方面已进行提前预防性治疗，但这并没有改变患者的死亡率，这是比较麻烦的。在住院天数方面，数据仍然是矛盾的。尽管局部真菌感染和真菌定植在 APACHE 评分更高的重症患者中作为预测真菌感染的指标，但根据疾病的严重程度，局部真菌感染和真菌定植有不同的自然病程。

总结

ICU 患者的真菌感染越来越普遍。最常见的真菌致病菌是白念珠菌、其他念珠菌属种和曲霉属。治疗应针对具体的危险因素，但在非中性粒细胞减少的患者和血培养阴性的患者中，不鼓励抗真菌治疗。

术前和术后的营养支持：肠内和肠外营养的治疗策略

Patricia Marie Byers, S. Morad Hameed 和 Stanley J. Dudrick 著
吕 杰 译

营养支持是创伤和重症护理管理的一个重要组成部分，它的作用在二十世纪的最后二十年里经历了巨大的演变。这些变化是因为我们在处理手术应激的过程中，对复杂炎症和代谢途径有了更好、更全面的理解。目前，对手术应激反应以及其固有的分解代谢反应的研究，已经成为新兴营养疗法的主要焦点。

营养不良

营养不良可以被定义为一种损害宿主防御能力，并且会增加并发症和死亡风险的相对营养缺乏和代谢紊乱的状态。多年来，蛋白质—热量营养不良都被认为具有体重减轻、低蛋白血症、骨骼肌减少、脂肪储存减少，总淋巴细胞计数减少这些特点。1936 年，Hiram O. Studley 首次把术前营养不良作为消化性溃疡病患者的特有的手术风险因素。他指出，失去了超过 20％的体重的患者的死亡率增加了 10 倍，同时他也提出是否可以想办法在术前解决营养不良的问题，从而提高患者的生存率。自此之后进行的多项研究已经证实，营养不良可导致伤口愈合不良、感染率增加、术后肠梗阻时间延长、住院时间延长、死亡率增加。

代谢应激

受伤或接受了大范围复杂手术的患者，对组织损伤、再灌注和血流动力学紊乱表现出明显的急性期反应。儿茶酚胺和皮质醇代谢的增加引起能量消耗及蛋白质周转的增加。随之而来，患者会产生胰岛素抵抗，这会引起葡萄糖的外周使用减少以及脂肪分解和蛋白质水解的速率提高，从而提供更多的氨基酸和脂肪酸作为人体能量合成的原料。通过糖异生作用将外周动员的氨基酸（主要是丙氨酸）转化为葡萄糖，且它并不会被高血糖病或在这种条件下输注葡萄糖溶液所抑制。因为支链氨基酸优先用作骨骼肌中的能量来源，氨基酸池中的必需氨基酸会被迅速耗尽，而大量的必需氨基酸，如谷氨酰胺，对于代谢过程是必需的，特别是在肠黏膜中。骨骼肌和胃肠道中蛋白质合成的减少伴随着蛋白质分解的增加，新分解出的氨基酸会转移到肺、心脏、肝和脾组织，以更好地维持蛋白质合成。由于这种分解代谢过程是通过细胞因子激活而维持的，故而危重患者和受伤的患者会一直保持分解代谢并且迅速消耗骨骼和内脏肌肉以及脂肪储备。所有这些干扰都可以消耗重要的微量元素和维生素，它们的缺乏可能与最终的器官功能障碍有关。

在应激状态下，营养不良可能表现为器官系统功能的恶化以及伤口愈合不良或伤口裂开。呼吸肌无力可引起肺不张、肺炎和长时间的呼吸机依赖。此外，免疫应答的所有方面都可能由于营养不良而受损。当细胞生长和更新减少时，宿主屏障功能、细胞介导以及体液免疫都会受到损害。

术前营养

有 2 个值得注意的情况，在这两种情况下，术前营养支持应高度优先。第一种情况涉及需要大手术干预，但不能立即进行手术的患者，并且可能会有超过 5 天的长时间禁食。另一种情况是患者必须从显著的营养缺乏状态恢复，故而延迟手术干预，如果营养状态不改善或纠正，可能增加术后并发症的发生率（图 1）。

在术前患者中，对饥饿的反应与来自周围组织

的底物流的再分布相关，以满足代谢需求。胰岛素水平的下降促进脂肪酸和氨基酸从脂肪组织和骨骼肌释放。虽然大多数周围组织可以使用脂肪酸作为能量来源，但需要蛋白质水解，继续促进糖异生，以支持葡萄糖依赖组织的能量需求（图 2）。随着时间的推移，对饥饿的适应发生。此时脑代谢适应了使用酮作为其 50%的能量需求。随着来自脂肪的能量来源更多地被使用，对蛋白质分解代谢的依赖性从 85%降低到 35%（图 2-3）。

上消化道恶性肿瘤患者蛋白质 - 热量营养不良发生率最高，超过 30%的患者表现出显著的营养缺乏。术前化学治疗和放射治疗，结合癌症恶病质、梗阻、营养物质损失增加和底物代谢异常，都会增加营养风险。

前瞻性研究显示，延迟手术并且对严重营养不良的患者进行术前肠外营养支持后，主要并发症例如吻合口漏和伤口破坏有所减少。然而，当给营养良好或仅轻度营养不良的患者施用术前肠外营养时，感染性并发症有所增加且并没有明显的临床益处。因此，精确地定义营养不良很重要，这样才能更好地选择适合的患者。

严重营养不良的诊断可以使用临床营养评价工具来建立，例如主观全面评估。在 1982 年，Baker 证实，基于更客观的实验室检查所做的评估，临床评估的效果好。在这种评估中，临床医生会询问近期食物摄取或无意的体重减轻相关的历史信息，并检查患者营养缺乏的体征。患有多重或严重的营养不良体征或在 6 个月内体重下降超过 15%的患者将被认为存在严重营养缺乏。然而，在活检证实的癌症患者中，6 个月中体重减轻仅为 10%的患者也归于高风险组，他们从术前营养支持过程中获益的可能性也比较高。

在选择术前营养的患者之后，须选择适当的配方和治疗方式。尽管治疗的最佳疗程尚未确定，但术前 7 ~ 15 天的营养治疗是标准的。总的非蛋白质卡路里应为基础能量消耗的 150%。基础能量消耗使用间接量热法测量或从 Harris-Benedict 方程式导出（表 1）。对于严重营养不良和饥饿的患者，在最初几天的营养计划应该以基础能量消耗率补充，以防止发生再喂养综合征，然后再将营养支持增加到目标水平。一般在 3 天后，支持可以增加到基础需求的 125%，然后增加到在密切代谢监测下能耐受

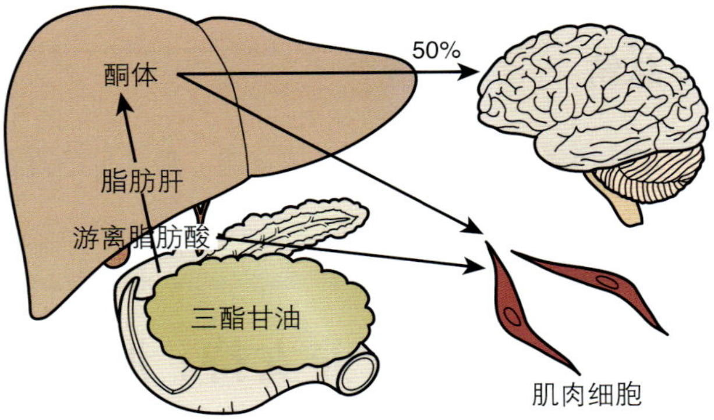

图 3 随着时间的推移，适应饥饿的大脑就能够把酮作为 50% 的能量需求。由于来源于脂肪的能量资源越来越多，依赖蛋白质的分解代谢从 85% 降至 35%

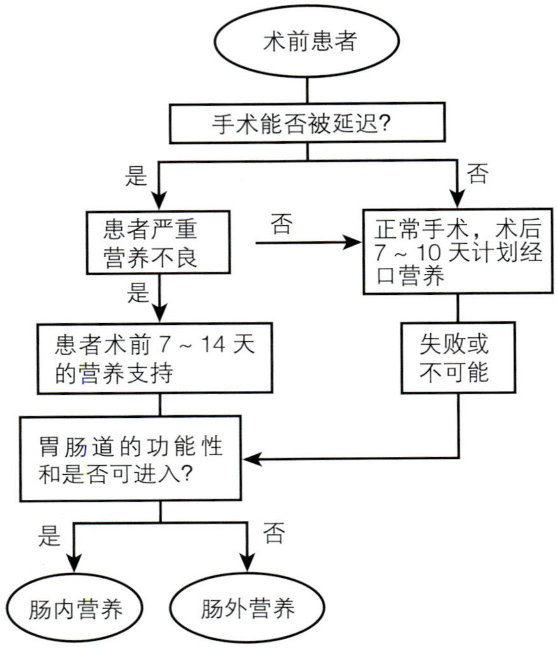

图 1 术前营养支持的流程

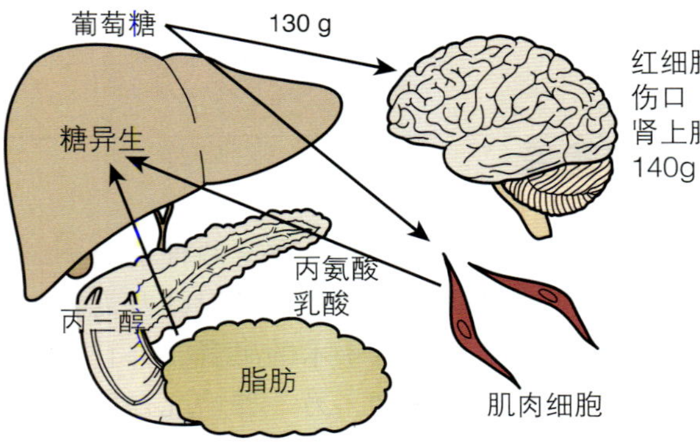

图 2 胰岛素的水平下降促进脂肪酸和氨基酸从脂肪组织和骨骼肌的释放。尽管大多数周围组织可以利用脂肪酸提供能量，但为了满足依赖糖的组织的需求，蛋白质水解通过糖异生来提供葡萄糖

的目标。

表 1　Harris–Benedict 方程

BEE 女性 =655 +[9.6 × 体重(kg)]+[1.7 × 身高(cm)-[4.7 × 年龄（岁）]
BEE 男性 =66 +[13.7 × 体重(kg)]+[5 × 身高(cm)]-[6.8 × 年龄（岁）]

BBE，基础能量消耗

术前全肠外营养

全肠外营养（total parenteral nutrition，TPN）应该用于严重营养不良且胃肠道损伤或无功能的患者。葡萄糖和脂肪乳液配方用于提供非蛋白质热量，通常以 70：30 的比例配比。TPN 底物的热值可以在表 2 中找到。使用的葡萄糖的量应当在 4 ~ 6 mg/kg · min 之间。然而，在患有慢性阻塞性肺疾病或糖尿病的患者中，建议将葡萄糖使用值维持在 4mg/kg · min 或更低。必须监测血糖水平，并严格控制在 100 ~ 140 mg/dl 之间。

表 2　肠外营养和肠内营养物质的热值

营养成分	肠外（kcal/g）	肠内（kcal/g）
碳水化合物	3.4	4.0
脂肪	9.0	9.0
蛋白	3.4	4.0

脂肪乳液可用于补充非蛋白质热量，然而，数据表明术前静脉内脂质治疗应限制在总热量的 30% 以下。脂质通常应用 20% 的乳液，并且根据热量需要，每天可以给予 100 ~ 250 ml 的量。

蛋白质通过游离氨基酸溶液以每天 1.5 g/kg 的剂量使用，以促进蛋白质合成代谢，并且不应作为热量来源计算。必须使用足够的非蛋白质热量，以支持蛋白质合成，通常为 150：1 的热量与氮的比例。此外，多种维生素和微量元素作为综合营养方案的一部分。

虽然，有时须为胃肠功能障碍患者提供术前肠外营养，但是考虑特定患者的液体需求同样重要。在具有大量液体缺乏或损失的患者中可能需要更稀释、高容量的液体补充，但是对于有心力衰竭、肾衰竭或肝功能不全而需要容量限制的患者则需要更浓缩、更低体积的液体补充。

对于蛋白质 - 热量营养不良，钾、镁和磷的细胞内损失与钠和水的潴留同时发生。在不恰当的再喂养过程中，钠平衡可能更容易达到，并导致水潴留。在营养支持开始时，钾、磷和镁的血浆水平可能急剧下降，因为这些离子与注入的大量常量营养物和微量营养素一起向细胞内转运。所以仔细监测电解质和液体平衡非常重要，以避免再喂养综合征发生的风险。此外，如果合成代谢开始增加，则必须纠正钾、磷和镁缺乏（表 3）。

微量矿物质是无机化合物，维生素是调节代谢过程的复杂的有机化合物（表 4）。这些微量营养素中的大多数作为辅酶或作为调节碳水化合物、蛋白质和脂肪的生物转化的酶复合物的必需元素成分。已知铁、锌、铜、铬、硒、碘和钴对于人类的健康和正常的功能是必需的。此外，在营养不良和严重疾病的患者中，必须特别评估锌和硒的需求，在必要时给予补充。

如果患者的液体和电解质状态在肠外支持期间稳定，并且血糖水平在良好控制下，患者就可以在等待手术的同时回家，一日之内连续喂养以维持营养治疗的连续性。肠外营养周期逐渐地从 24 h 降

表 3　不正常电解液需求、分布和后遗症

电解质	每日需求	体液分布	过量的影响	不足的影响
钠（Na^+）	60 ~ 120 mEq	细胞外	黏膜干燥、躁狂行为	癫痫、精神状态改变
钾（K^+）	40 ~ 120 mEq	细胞内	心博停止、T 波高尖、心电图宽 QRS 波群	心律失常、肌无力
镁（Mg^{2+}）	10 ~ 20 mmol	细胞内	心律失常、张力减退	低血钾、低血钙、癫痫
磷（PO_4^{2-}）	14 ~ 20 mmol	细胞内	磷酸氢钙盐沉积	精神状态改变、肌无力、溶血作用、感觉异常
钙（Ca^{2+}）	5 mg	细胞内	嗜睡、便秘	强直、反射亢进、癫痫、心律失常

表 4 日常膳食中对维生素和无机物的需求

维生素或无机物	功能	每天需要量
生物素	羧化酶的辅酶	60 μg
铬	胰岛素的使用	10 ~ 20 μg
铜	酶系统和血浆铜蓝蛋白	0.1 ~ 0.5 μg
叶酸	核酸合成	600 μg
铁	卟啉类化合物、酶、线粒体	0 ~ 2 mg
烟酸	烟酰胺腺嘌呤二核苷酸的组分和其磷酸基	50 mg
泛酸盐	辅酶 A 的组成部分	15 mg
维生素 B_6	氨基酸代谢的辅酶	5 mg
维生素 B_2	氧化还原系统中的辅酶	5 mg
硒	谷胱甘肽过氧化物酶的组成部分	20 ~ 200 μg
硫胺素（维生素 B_1）	辅羧酶系统	5 mg
维生素 A	上皮表面、视网膜色素	2 500 IU
维生素 B_{12}	核酸合成	15 μg
维生素 C	氧化还原反应、胶原蛋白、免疫功能	1 000 mg
维生素 D	骨代谢	25 ~ 100 mcg
维生素 E	膜磷脂	50 IU
维生素 K	凝血因子、骨骼健康	1 ~ 2 mg
锌	酶系统	1 ~ 15 μg

至每天 18 h，对于能够耐受的患者，可以降至每天 14 ~ 16 h，以允许患者在输注营养间期有一些自由。永久性中心静脉通路通常用于最大限度的、安全和有效的家庭肠外营养。

术前肠内营养

肠内营养支持是将营养物质输送到胃肠道中，其可能须临时或永久地留置饲管。肠内喂养是营养支持的首选途径，应尽可能使用。手术患者应用肠内营养可以获得诸多益处，如肠相关淋巴组织（gut-associated lymphoid tissue，GALT）的维持，黏膜血流的增强和黏膜屏障的维持。

最初的胃肠屏障功能由含有乳铁蛋白和溶菌酶的黏液提供，两者都是有效的微生物生长的非特异性抑制剂。通常情况下，未受干扰的细菌菌群也发挥类似的效果。上皮紧密连接形成下一层非特异性防御，其中连接的完整性是能量依赖性的，并且至少部分依赖于管腔内能量底物的存在。特异性肠免疫受 GALT 控制。派尔集合淋巴结中的诱导位点提供抗原呈递细胞和循环淋巴细胞之间的接口。一些动物研究已显示与肠外营养组相比，肠内营养组的免疫力有所改善，但是迄今为止在前瞻性的、随机对照的人类研究中尚未统一或明确地证实这一发现。

患者的食欲或胃肠功能可能会不足，以致单独口服摄入并不能维持最佳营养。肠内喂养已经被成功地应用，以满足这些患有各种各样的外科问题（包括癌症、炎性肠病和胰腺疾病）的患者的营养需要。然而，其在诸如肠梗阻、持续喂养不耐受、血流动力学不稳定、消化道大出血和不能有效和安全地建立喂养通路这些情况下，使用是禁忌的。

一旦决定使用肠内营养，必须选择最佳类型的喂养途径。决定喂养途径选择的因素包括胃肠道的哪些组分可用、肠内营养计划持续时间、患者是否存在吸入的风险，以及患者的营养状况。如果可以的话，通常优选经胃的喂养途径。若患者存在早期饱胀感、胃病或误吸风险的情况，可以短期采用经十二指肠或空肠喂养。由于其易于放置、低成本和低并发症发生率，推荐使用鼻胃管和鼻肠管用于短期喂养。经皮内镜胃造口术，已经成为放置胃造口管以用于长期喂养的最常见方法之一。放射介入的方式也可以将饲管经皮放入胃以及空肠中。如果这些微创技术不成功，可以通过开放或腹腔镜技术放置饲管。然而，这种方法在具有严重营养不良的术前患者中不太适用。

肠内营养配方的正确选择须知道每种常量营养素的消化和吸收的生理机制。在肠内营养配方中存在的碳水化合物的来源包括从单糖到复杂淀粉。较大分子量的淀粉在肠腔中产生较小的渗透压，不太甜，并且在吸收之前需要更多的消化时间。不同的肠内配方含有不同量的碳水化合物，其范围可以是总热量的 28% ~ 70%。患有糖尿病或者由于慢性阻塞性肺疾病而有二氧化碳潴留的患者应该给予具有较低百分比的碳水化合物热量的配方（参见“术前全肠外营养”部分）。

许多肠内营养配方现在含有纤维，可能是可溶的或不溶的。不溶性纤维改善结肠功能和肠通过时间，但没有其他的营养益处或需求。相比之下，可溶性纤维结合胆固醇和胆汁盐，因此可以降低血清胆固醇水平。此外，结肠细菌可消化可溶性纤维，从而产生可被结肠细胞用作燃料来源的短链脂肪酸。

肠内配方含有通常来自玉米、大豆和红花油的脂肪。脂质提供浓缩的能量源，并且在改善肠内营养配方风味的同时，不增加渗透压。脂溶性维生素的吸收须每天摄入最少 15 ~ 25 g 的脂质。同时须补充亚油酸或亚麻酸，以防止必需脂肪酸缺乏。ω-6 脂肪酸由于产生炎性产物，而显示具有免疫抑制作用。因此，可以抵抗这些作用的 ω-3 脂肪酸已经加入到一些肠内营养产品中。中链三酰甘油也可以作为脂肪吸收不良患者较好的热量来源，因为它们不须被胰脂肪酶水解，在十二指肠和上段空肠中被吸收到门静脉循环中而没有微泡形成，并且不须肉碱运输进入线粒体。

肠蛋白可以以完整蛋白的形式提供，例如酪蛋白，部分水解的寡肽或结晶的 L- 氨基酸。完整的蛋白质和蛋白质水解产物须通过胰腺和刷状缘蛋白酶进一步消化成短链肽和氨基酸。然后这些营养物被肠细胞自由吸收，主要发生在近端小肠。吸收不良的患者可以以短肽和游离氨基酸的形式受益于肠内蛋白质。术前，应给予患者每天 1.5 g/kg 蛋白质，以支持蛋白质合成。

目前，超过 100 种肠内产品在市场上流通，并且大多数配方具有 1 ~ 2 kcal/ml 之间的热量密度，不含乳糖，并且在每天少于 2 L 的配方中可以提供维生素和矿物质。大多数患者可以耐受标准肠内营养配方，然而，在吸收不良的患者中可能需要单体的（元素）配方。通过围术期使用免疫增强的肠内营养配方能够很好地改善免疫功能和手术结果。其他疾病相关制剂已经为患有肝病、肾衰竭、肺功能不全和糖尿病的患者所使用。肝病和肝性脑病患者的配方含有较高百分比的支链氨基酸蛋白质，几乎没有芳香族氨基酸。肾衰竭患者的配方含有较高百分比的必需氨基酸和非常低水平的钾和磷。然而，值得注意的是，肝和肾疾病相关配方均具有非常低的总蛋白含量。晚期肺部疾病患者须应用脂肪来提供大部分的热量需求，以减少二氧化碳的产生。糖尿病患者的配方还含有脂肪来提供额外的热量，但也含有可溶性纤维以降低血糖水平。值得注意的是，所有这些特殊配方是非常昂贵的，应当仅在具有适当营养素特征的标准制剂不能为患者提供最佳营养支持时使用。

监测患者接受肠内喂养的营养状况改善、胃肠道耐受性以及液体和电解质平衡是重要的。当经胃喂养时，重要的是自觉地监测胃残留量，因为增加的残留量可导致呕吐、误吸、肺炎、延长的住院时间甚至导致死亡。在营养不良的患者中可能发生的另一种并发症是腹泻，其可能导致或加重液体和电解质异常，这可能由是药物、配方的组成或感染造成的。如果感染和药物的原因被排除并且没有其他可疑药物，则配方应该改变为单体（元素）的配方以增加吸收。如果需要，可以增加抑制胃肠蠕动的药物的剂量，以减缓肠内转运。

因为大多数营养配方仅含有 65% 的水，所以可能须间断补充低渗的肠内营养液，以达到较好的液体和电解质平衡。应当监测电解质水平以及血浆渗透压，以避免高渗状态的出现，并在喂养过程中补充和平衡钾、磷和镁的血清水平。否则，患者可能会出现液体潴留和电解质紊乱，从而导致危及生命的心律失常。血糖水平必须仔细监测，高血糖应进行有效治疗，以避免增加感染和高渗状态的风险。

大量研究表明，术前肠内喂养与对照组相比，术后并发症发生率可降低 10% ~ 15%，但是在现实中，这一优势所需的治疗时间仍存在争论。有文献支持，应在在手术前 5 ~ 20 天的进行肠内喂养。最近，免疫增强配方被指出可能更有优势，它可以单独作为术前补充，或与术后支持组合使用，但这还未被证实。

术后营养

当制订术后营养计划时，重要的是预测患者可能需要通气支持或经历肠梗阻的时间。必须评估患者的病前的营养状况，以及高代谢和分解代谢的状态，以及在术中决定最好的肠内喂养途径（图 4）。然而，这种类型的详细评估，对于紧急手术的患者或具有急性创伤性损伤的患者，估计不可能实现。为了简化这些评估，一种专用于创伤患者的模型被开发出来（图 5）。这种适用于紧急手术的简单流程和 ISS，在筛选适用于早期营养支持的创伤患者时，具有 88% 的准确度。在我们的一系列研究中发现 80% 的 ICU 的创伤患者，符合创伤后的营养支持标准。

虽然稳定的成年患者的蛋白质需求仅为 0.6g/kg · d，但在病情危重期间增加的分解代谢所需的蛋白质的量更多，以维持平衡。随着大多数术后患者的蛋白质合成增加，氮平衡会得到改善，这时，须提供 25 ~ 30 kcal/kg 的总热量以及每天 1.5 ~ 2.0 g/kg 的蛋白质。碳水化合物应以每千克体

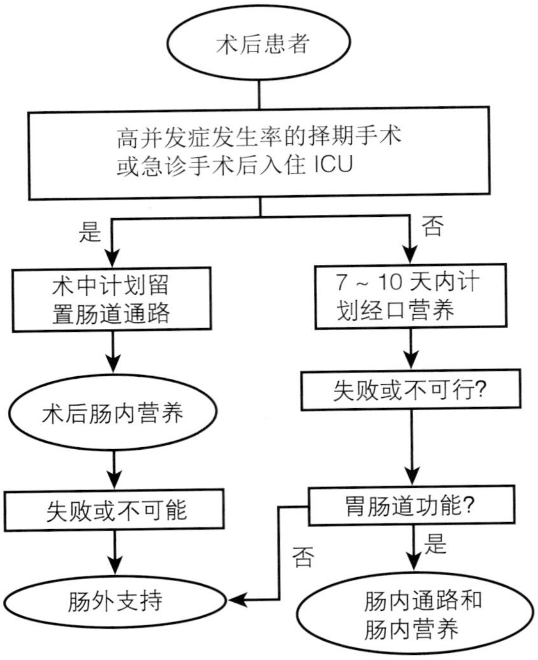

图 4 术后营养支持的流程

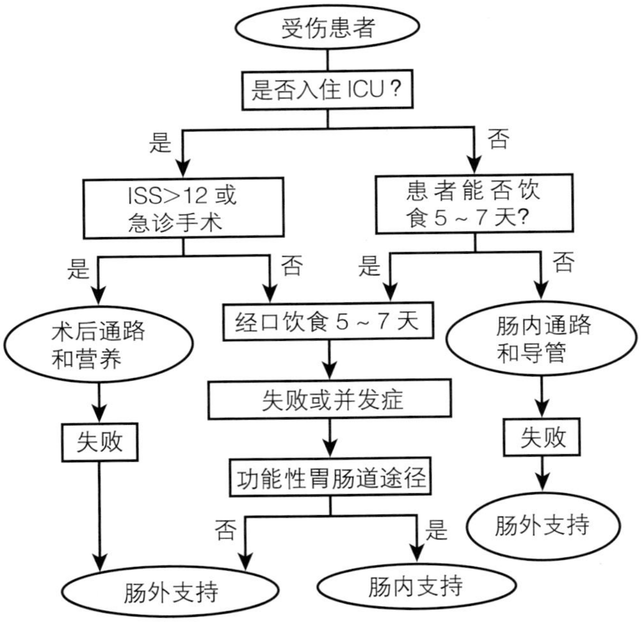

图 5 创伤患者护理营养支持的流程。ISS，创伤严重度评分；ICU，重症监护病房（*Modified from Byers P, Block E, Albornoz J, et al: The need for aggressive nutritional intervention in the injured patient: the development of a predictive model. J Trauma 39:1103, 1995.*）

重，每分钟 4～6mg 葡萄糖的最大速率应用，以维持血清或血糖水平在 100～140 mg/dl 之间。脂肪不应超过总热量的 30%。如果可以使用间接热量测定法，则应该使用它来测量热量需求，以避免过度喂养。肠内谷氨酰胺的补充量应为 0.5 g/kg · d，配以多种维生素和微量矿物质（包括锌和硒）。

除了监测血糖水平、电解质和液体平衡之外，还应监测患者接受术后营养的疗效。具有短半衰期的血清蛋白标志物在测量内脏蛋白质组分的改善方面最有效（表 5）。如果通过这些标志物水平未能发现有所改善，应当注意对过去几天使用的营养物的评估，同时寻找未治疗的感染或炎症。可以进行氮平衡研究，其中根据在尿、粪便和伤口引流中损失的氮量来评估所使用的蛋白质的量（表 6）。危重患者应保持在中性氮平衡，而合成代谢患者应保持在轻微正氮平衡。治疗的目标应包括内脏蛋白标志物趋于正常和每日物理治疗能够改善体细胞肌肉量。

表 5 内脏蛋白标志物

蛋白标志物	正常值	半衰期（天）
白蛋白	>3.5 g/dl	20
转铁蛋白	>200 mg/dl	8.5
前白蛋白	20～30 mg/dl	1.3
视黄醇结合蛋白	4～5 mg/dl	0.4

表 6 氮平衡

氮（N）平衡 =N（摄入）-N（排出）
氮（摄入）= 蛋白 /6.25（g/d）
氮（排出）= 总尿氮 *（g/d）+ 胃肠道丢失（2～4 g/d）+ 皮肤损失（0～4 g/d）

* 总尿氮直接测量或通过尿液中的氮含量除以 0.8 估算出来

术后肠外营养

因为大多数营养良好的患者在术后 7～10 天内可以耐受营养缺乏，因此在这些患者中使用常规的术后肠外营养是不合理的（图 4）。另一方面，营养充足的严重应激患者和术前过度消耗的患者，如果预计 7～10 天会出现营养摄入不足，应尽早接受术后营养。同样需要术后肠外营养的是那些已经用术前肠外营养治疗，但是不能耐受或吸收足够的术后肠内营养的患者，以及那些因出现并发症而禁止使用胃肠道的患者。此外，肠外营养可以在具有高输出近端肠道皮肤瘘、广泛小肠切除术和末端空肠造口综合征的这些情况下挽救患者的生命。

必须建立具有用于肠外营养的指定的中心静脉

通路。对于不需要液体限制的患者，葡萄糖浓度可以保持在12%～18%之间，同时，氨基酸溶液浓度在5%～6%。脂质应限制在总热量的20%。

某些新的模式可以增加术后肠外营养的功效。已显示添加生长激素可改善烧伤患者的伤口愈合，但也已显示它在危重的外科手术患者中是有害的，因此不能常规使用。静脉营养添加谷氨酰胺和抗氧化剂也显示一定的效果，并且在将来，两者可能会成为危重患者的营养配方的一部分。虽然科学研究证明了这些模式的潜在益处，但需要更多的临床研究来说明其安全性和有效性，从而为其在增加费用的前提下常规应用来提供证据。

术后肠内营养

大量的研究数据支持择期和紧急手术后患者的术后营养首选肠道喂养途径，这同样也是遭受创伤和热损伤患者的选择。通过肠道途径输送营养物减弱对应激的代谢反应，可以稳定地控制血糖，减少临床感染的发生率，并且可能增加肠吻合口的强度。

在接受剖腹手术的患者中，在术中可以选择最佳的肠内喂养途径（图4-5）。术后肠内营养支持应在手术或损伤后12～72 h开始。然而，应始终首先保证血流动力学稳定，以避免肠系膜循环出现低灌注状态和继发性的缺血性肠坏死。连续管饲的速度通常以10～20 ml/h开始，并且可以根据临床情况和患者耐受性，每8～24 h增加相同的喂养速度。出现腹胀时应使管饲速度立即降低一半，如果仍然腹胀明显，应停止喂养。也可以给予每2～6 h 200～300 ml的推注式喂养。即使有会中断喂养的日常护理和诊断测试，它可以帮助保持足够的饲喂量。应该注意，在患者能够口服足量饮食之前，连续的肠内喂养是重要的。

正常的食物可以混入，通过口服或通过管饲直接进入胃[鼻胃管、经皮内镜胃造口术（percutaneous endoscopic gastrostomy，PEG）、胃造口术]，以提供营养。或者可以使用聚合物溶液，该溶液是整蛋白、三酰甘油和碳水化合物3个组分整合在一起的常量营养素的制剂，其设计目的是通过胃进行完全营养。单体元素溶液中，蛋白质是以肽和氨基酸的混合物形式存在。脂肪为长链甘油三酯（long-chaintrig lycerides，LCT），或LCT和中链甘油三酯（medium-chain triglycerides，MCT）的组合。碳水化合物为部分水解的淀粉麦芽糖糊精和葡萄糖寡糖，并且主要设计用于在十二指肠下进入空肠的管饲，或者用于消化或吸收功能异常的患者。

针对特殊代谢患者的营养液也是可用的，该类营养设计用于有独特代谢需求的患者，这些患者的营养需求可能与肾衰竭、肝功能衰竭、心力衰竭、肺功能不全和创伤相关或继发于这些疾病（参见“术前肠内营养”下的讨论）。这些特殊营养素的应用的一些实例包括对于具有多器官衰竭、应激和脓毒症的一些患者应用大量的支链氨基酸。应用由ω-3脂肪酸、RNA和精氨酸组成的免疫调节溶液，该溶液已经被证明可以减少炎症、创伤并发症，以及住院时间，这可能是由于炎症的减少，以及随之而来的多器官功能障碍发展的趋势下降的缘故。已被确定为免疫调节营养液的潜在重要组分的其他营养素包括肉碱、牛磺酸、谷氨酰胺、N-乙酰半胱氨酸、抗氧化剂维生素和微量元素。促进伤口愈合的配方已显示对烧伤患者效果较好，并含有较高水平的锌、维生素C和维生素A。虽然一些研究已经证明使用免疫营养减少了感染的发生率和住院时间，但对患者死亡率的影响并不明确（见下文“营养支持挑战和争议”）。

营养支持挑战和争议

研究提供最佳安全和有效的营养支持的这个领域，非常热门，已经产生了数千个基础和临床研究，以及相应的报道。然而，兴趣还是主要集中在3个最重要的动态领域：①严密血糖控制的角色、理由和结果；②免疫营养；③最适合危重患者的目标营养所需要的喂养途径、频次和喂养的组合。

在ICU中的高血糖治疗对营养支持的使用具有重要影响，并且它是在过去和现在各种有争议的临床试验的焦点。一个新兴的数据表明，实际上不可能将强化胰岛素治疗与ICU中的最佳营养处理分开。然而，这个最重要的问题在文献、培训计划、临床实践或研究工作中没有得到足够的重视。血糖控制在几种类型的患者当然很重要，但让患者得到充分的喂养可能也同样重要。在最近的临床营养指南的版本中，美国肠外和肠内营养学会和重症医学学会没有对能量补充给予足够的重视，这种遗漏实际上可能会无意中导致常规喂养不足的营养不良增加。事实上，营养不良仍然是ICU患者的主要威胁，早期肠内和肠外营养结合的营养支持似乎是这个问题的合理答案。考虑到现有数据和我们对ICU患者生理学的理解，致力于严格的血糖控制同时让患者存在喂养不足是不明智的，并且可以解释在最初Leuven试验的后续研究中，严格的血糖控制组的死亡率会增加。尽管避免这两种情况都很重要，但是最近重要性已经远远从过度喂养摆向喂养不足，并且必须做出更大的努力，以实现最佳或理想的位于这两个极端之间的喂养目标。

在重大创伤和外科手术后，从营养支持早期开始，免疫功能已经改变。最近，已经通过T细胞增殖、皮肤无变应性、IL-2和干扰素-γ的产生减少，以及T细胞受体复合物的异常，证明了获得性免疫损害的存在。免疫营养是一种营养治疗方法，其中先天性和获得性免疫的这些病理性改变，据称可以通过补充含有免疫增强或免疫调节功能的营养素的配方，产生优于常规喂养的配方。

多个临床研究已经证实了各种"免疫配方"在手术患者中的效果。然而，它并不适用于所有的人群。在对高风险的，须接受上消化道和下消化道外科手术治疗的，且存在营养不良的癌症患者的研究中观察到较好的反应，其中包括感染性伤口并发症减少和住院时间缩短。

使用免疫营养的大部分不确定性在于其在危重患者中的应用，在这类人群中进行了许多的研究，结果不尽相同。事实上，2个最大规模的控制良好的研究显示，在感染性并发症方面得到了完全不同的结果（一个阳性和一个没有效果）。通过meta分析解决免疫营养争议的尝试尚未有明确的结论。报道指出，虽然这种治疗可以降低感染率，但它不会降低全因死亡率。目前的研究进展显示，应该避免对重症患者，特别是那些脓毒症患者给予免疫营养。试图调节这些患者中的免疫系统可能须使用更强的治疗形式，例如阻断细胞因子产生或作用的药理学试剂或抗体。因此，正是对于具有潜在营养不良和较少危及生命的疾病的免疫脆弱的患者，营养支持（包括免疫营养）最可能获益。免疫营养支持的真正要义应该是这个问题的什么部分尚未令人满意地解决。或许许多ICU患者病情太严重或代谢损害太严重，而不能受益于免疫营养处理。需要额外的前瞻性、强有力的、随机对照的试验来确定免疫营养喂养的组成、时间和使用。这一重要领域的演变将不可避免地继续进步和发展，以确定其使用和有效性的问题。

最后，随着世界各地的研究数据的积累，对"肠道营养总是优选的，并且优于肠外营养"这一论断持续评估和调整，结果表明积极使用早期肠内喂养可能会改善患者的预后，而且在保证最大耐受性的前提下，结合早期肠内喂养和足够的早期肠外营养补充，从而精确和充分地满足患者的营养需要，是对危重患者来说最佳的，也是最理性、实用和有效的方法。

早期肠内营养仍是ICU患者推荐的喂养途径，然而，它通常不能完全满足营养需求。因此，如果肠内营养不可行或不足以满足需求时，则推荐使用肠外营养（无论是单独使用还是与肠内营养组合使用）。大多数重症监护营养师旨在提供25 kcal/kg · d的热量，通过鼻胃管、胃造口或空肠造口实施肠内营养。文献中有大量证据表明，仅通过肠内营养实现营养目标是困难的，特别是在进入ICU之后的早期阶段。这些研究进一步强调，早期无法提供足够的营养与最终增加的发病率和死亡率相关联。研究者列出了在提供早期最佳营养方面的困难，其与许多因素相关，包括胃肠功能障碍（例如呕吐和腹泻）、导致肠内喂养中断的二次手术和外科手术、饲管的移位、护理程序导致肠内喂养实施延迟或过早撤除肠内营养支持。

在14家加拿大的合作医院中，ICU患者的存活得到改善，这得益于其认真地遵循有证据的营养指南和坚持不懈的充足的营养供给。其他研究报道，只有58%的使用肠内营养方案的ICU患者实现了他们的营养目标。另一方面，当对肠内营养方案能够良好依从时，到开始营养后的第3天才达到超过80%的营养处方量。尽管近年来提出了几个改进的措施，但对ICU患者单独的肠内营养仍然与营养缺乏相关，营养缺乏最终与短期和长期临床预后有关。因此，尽管已知重症患者的营养不良与更高的ICU住院率和死亡率有关，尽管喂养不充分被认为是增加ICU住院率的因素，但是接受肠内营养的大量ICU患者仍然未能达到其预想的营养目标。当单独肠内营养不能达到既定目标时，应考虑补充肠外营养以达到能量和蛋白质目标。然而，这样的组合营养支持是否可以为整体临床结果提供额外的帮助，仍然要在未来的前瞻性研究中被证明。

肠外及肠内营养通路的技术

中心静脉通路

中心静脉通路导管的插入应由有经验的操作者在完成无菌预防措施后进行（包括抗菌洗手后，佩戴手术衣、手套、面罩、帽子）。这些抗微生物导管可以在床边临时置入，也可在手术室进行永久性置入术。另外，导管可直接经中心静脉置入，也可通过周围静脉间接置入中心静脉。静脉多普勒装置的常规使用已经被证明可以减少与静脉穿刺相关的并发症。常规应用静脉多普勒超声引导被证实可以降低静脉穿刺相关的并发症。经周围静脉插入中心静脉导管（peripherally inserted central venous catheters，PICC）可以由训练有素的临床专家进行。这些导管可以由硅树脂或聚氨酯制成，并且有单腔或双腔两种，规格大小为 16 ~ 23。在市售试套装中提供易弯曲的管心针或导丝，以帮助使用具有剥离髓鞘的 Seldinger 技术或使用针上套管这两种技术进行操作。通常在肘前空间或下面的静脉进行静脉穿刺。推荐患者为仰卧位，并且手臂与身体呈 90°。如果导管置入遇到任何阻力，则应立即停止。操作完成后，须拍摄 X 线胸片，以确定导管尖端在中心静脉系统中的位置是否合适。

股静脉插管相对安全，并且不一定会增加感染风险。然而，由于对血栓形成的易感性增加及其相关并发症和并发症发生率，其不是长期静脉导管通路的优选部位。可以获得上腔静脉通路，如果可以耐受，应该将患者摆在 Trendelenburg 体位下进行，以最大限度地扩张穿刺的目标静脉。颈内静脉是建立短期中心静脉通路的优选部位，特别是在麻醉师或其他急性情况下使用的时候，可以使用 3 种不同的入路：胸锁乳突肌前、胸锁乳突肌的两个肌腹之间的中点，或胸锁乳突肌后。也可以使用外颈静脉。然而，通过该通路成功插入上腔静脉的概率只有 50% 或更少。由于解剖可靠性和位置的稳定性，锁骨下静脉通路，尽管可能最危险，但是是用于长期中心静脉通路的优选位置，使用于留置中心静脉通路的具有皮下隧道导管和输注端口导管。锁骨下通路应当仅由熟练、经验丰富且经过认证的临床医生尝试。这些临床医生已经接受过训练并且严格遵守既定的技术、无菌和抗菌原理，以及操作规范，从而可以保证患者的最大安全性和有效性。

胃肠通路

在具有足够胃排空的患者中，通过小直径、灵活的、惰性、加重的鼻胃管输送营养是足够的。这些管的直径为 5 ~ 8 F，通常由聚氨酯制成，并且通常设置有用于插入的导丝。在插入之前，导管应该润滑，并且患者应该在鼻孔中应用局部麻醉剂。导管通过鼻孔插入，并通过鼻咽、咽和食管推进大约 50 cm 的距离。接下来，轻轻地注入 50 ~ 100 ml 的空气，随后管沿着胃大弯朝向幽门进一步前进。在开始喂养之前，应该拍摄腹部 X 线片以确认导管的位置。

通过一些修改，这种技术也可以用于幽门后导管放置。首先，在手术之前给患者静脉注射甲氧氯普胺。第二，将管沿着胃大弯进一步前进，直到在幽门处达到阻力点。第三，在管上保持轻微的压力，直到幽门打开，管进入十二指肠，并且应该拍摄腹部 X 线片，以确认管在十二指肠中的位置。

如果须长期留置胃肠通路，则需要更具侵入性的方法。内镜指引下经皮胃造口术置管现在是标准的方法，并且可以在 ICU 床旁进行。如果采取特别的预防措施，这个技术也可以安全地用在之前有腹部手术史的患者中。当然前提是要知道是否先前的手术导致了胃肠道解剖结构的变化。获得腹部影像学资料和回顾之前的扫描很重要，以确保胃是否可以安全通过腹壁窗口。在内镜检查期间，应该可在接近管放置的区域，经腹外观察到明亮的光。导丝应当通过腹壁插入胃中，以确保当注射器抽吸空气时，针在胃腔中被内镜看到。胃造口术置管可以使用推入或牵拉技术，并且应当具有在插入之后将它们固定在位的垫片。组合管可用于具有胃造口术置管的内部空肠造口术部分，其可以经幽门放置。这些管也可以通过专门培训后的放射介入团队留置。值得注意的是，在荧光透视的引导下经腹壁放置导管、穿刺和进入胃，并不像开放性手术置管那样的牢靠。当使用放射学方法时，建议在幽门后置管，并向远端输注，以防止胃胀和漏液，直到管周围形成通道（通常在穿刺后大约 5 ~ 7 天后）。

只要预期术后需要营养支持，患者就应当在主要的腹部手术期间建立肠内营养通路（图 4-5）。建立通路的方式取决于进行的主要外科手术和预期的胃肠功能。当残胃的尺寸足够时，胃造口术可以较为容易地在左上象限中进行。应用 Stamm 缝合将胃固定到腹壁上。如果须进行幽门后喂养，同时进行近端胃引流，可以使用内部的空肠造口术置管空肠。单独的空肠造口术置管也可以直接放置在空肠中，但可能会引起肠扭转或潜在的肠扭转。而且须注意的是，肠道喂养后所发生的空肠坏死的所有病例都与此种空肠通路有关。为了避免这种风险，建议在可能的情况下通过胃置入长的胃空肠造口术应用的导管进入空肠。

并发症的发生率和处理

代谢并发症

一些并发症的发生，可能直接与不慎重的外源性底物管理有关。营养不良的患者在进食过度时可能引发电解质紊乱和充血性心力衰竭。这可以通过限液和限钠，并且仔细监测血清磷、钾和镁的水平，同时最初喂养时给予低热量喂养来避免。此外，摄入过量的碳水化合物剂量可导致继发性糖尿的高血糖、渗透性利尿、电解质紊乱、脱水，以及感染性并发症的发生率增加。呼吸功能受损的患者可能出现高碳酸血症和继发于过量碳水化合物负荷的呼吸衰竭。

肠外营养的并发症

值得注意的是，留置中心静脉导管输注肠外营养时可能发生并发症。如果没有足够的细心和观察，空气栓塞可能会发生，并伴发严重的血流动力学紊乱。如果发生或怀疑有空气栓塞，患者应立即置于完全 Trendelenburg 位，右侧朝上。如果可能，可以尝试通过导管从右心房抽吸空气。在尝试进行中心静脉导管插入之前，通过给患者补液，以填充静脉隔室，身体上部在 Trendelenburg 位置时产生静脉高压，可以使这种并发症最小化。并且通过确保输注管线的从输液袋到留置导管的所有连接固定妥当，以最小化或防止意外的断开，从而防止空气在整个治疗过程中进入系统。邻近锁骨下静脉的解剖学结构可能受伤。锁骨下静脉和颈内静脉的导管放置可导致血胸或气胸，这是由于血管或肺损伤导致的。左侧的置管可能导致胸导管损伤，从而使插入部位流出淋巴液或乳糜胸形成。在拔去导管后，必须行胸腔引流，直到淋巴外漏停止。导管误入胸膜腔或纵隔也是可能发生的并发症，会导致纵隔积液或胸腔积液。导管尖端误入入心房可能导致心律失常、损伤或感染性血栓形成，而且可能最终导致心房穿孔和心包压塞。所有导管并发症都是技术性的，并且通过充分的培训、积累的经验和遵守既定的原则和操作规范是可预防的。

导管脓毒症是留置中心静脉导管的最常见的并发症，并且须移除导管。原发性导管感染通常以发热、流感样症状和血培养阳性为特征。在菌血症存在的情况下，应当移除导管，但是如果对诊断有怀疑，则可以通过导丝留取导管的皮内部分进行半定量培养。当有 15 个或更多个菌落单位出现时，半定量培养则具有诊断价值。通常，导管的移除可以缓解症状。但是，如果是链球菌性导管脓毒症，或与其他生物体并存的菌血症，静脉内抗生素治疗可能要长达 2 周。

留置中心静脉导管的另一常见并发症是静脉血栓形成，其可能表现为血栓性静脉炎和肢体水肿。这通常可以通过导管移除和肢体抬高来治疗。锁骨下静脉血栓形成时，患者发生非致死性肺栓塞的风险高达 30%，应接受抗凝治疗。导管血栓形成是另一种潜在的并发症，并且可以通过滴注溶栓剂成功治疗。

肠内营养的并发症

值得注意的是要知道肠内营养是把双刃剑，在使患者受益的同时也可能会引起并发症。在 ICU 中，鼻肠管脱落的发生率达 45%。经皮置入肠道的导管，从肠腔进入腹膜的移位是更严重的并发症，并且可能与严重的腹膜污染、腹膜炎和死亡相关。应当通过 X 线片，以确认导管放置或重置后的位置，以帮助避免这种并发症发生。胃肠导管可能发生的另一个问题是导管闭塞。这些导管的护理必须包括经常用水冲洗以保持导管的畅通。长期保持原位的肠内饲管可能漏液，并导致皮肤损害。放置较小的导管，并在 1 天或 2 天内减少输注量，通常将使得导管出口部位在替换导管周围收缩，这样可以解决在原导管周围发生的漏的问题。

由于内脏灌注减少、损伤内脏相关的操作，交感神经张力损伤，炎症反应和高剂量阿片类药物的使用，术后患者可能发生无动力性肠梗阻。胃肠道运动障碍也可导致误吸和肺炎。临床实践中通过保持床头和患者的头部升高 30°，可以使误吸发生的风险降到最小。

当内脏灌注严重受低血流状态损害时，可发生非梗阻性肠坏死（参见“胃肠通路”下的讨论）。最常见的症状包括心动过速、发热、白细胞增多和腹部膨隆。可以通过尽量少用阿片类药物、使用硬膜外麻醉来钝化交感神经系统活动和使用胃肠动力药来增加管饲的耐受性。尽管如此，腹胀必须通过降低输注速率或停止喂养来解决。当发生肠坏死时，对于这种潜在高致死性并发症的早期干预和及时的手术治疗可使患者有约56%的生存率。

由于各种原因频繁中断管饲显然损害了营养支持的充分性，并导致营养不良。在一系列研究中发现，只有52%的喂养目标能够在24 h内完成。喂养通常由于并发过程、诊断性测试和护理操作而停止。新的高级营养泵允许护理人员记录在每个周期期间使用的精确的喂养量，使得该问题能够被及时发现，并且被治疗或纠正。

总结和原则

术前肠外营养应该提供给严重营养不良并且须进行大手术干预的患者。这类患者在术后恢复中可能出现并发症的风险大，且长时间的肠内营养又不能实现，7～15天的支持一般认为是安全和可行的（图1）。术后肠外营养应当在以下几种情况下使用：①术后或损伤后没有足够或可行的口服或肠内营养，且预计超过7～10天；②患者接受了术前营养准备，但并不适合在术后进行肠内喂养；③手术并发症在术后时期发生，并且与胃肠功能障碍相关。精确的血清葡萄糖控制对最大功效，且并发症最小地使用肠外营养至关重要。肠内喂养是向胃肠道有功能的患者提供营养物的优选方法，不过须专业地、审慎地计算喂养目标，这对于大多数患者是可行的，特别是存在专门的营养支持团队时候。肠内喂养可以保持肠的结构和功能，并且会减少感染和代谢并发症的发生（图4）。最后，危重的外科患者喂养是一个动态的和不断变化的过程，使用过程必须是经过深思熟虑的、有计划的、认真的，且由胜任者操作，并且针对不同患者制订不同的个体化营养方案。喂养必须有多重且复杂的营养支持技术和理论的专业应用、修改、调整和改进，同时喂养要提供最有效的营养物，保证患者最好的身体代谢和预后。

要点

- 肠内喂养应在进入ICU 24 h内，复苏完成并且血流动力学稳定后开始。
- 对于损伤或手术后10天内的所有患者，如果预测其不可能耐受肠内喂养，TPN应该在严格控制血糖的基础上开始实施。
- 对于危重患者和受伤患者，在损伤期间，25 kcal/kg和1.5～2 g/kg的蛋白质通常是足够的。如果50%的营养可以通过肠内喂养，则可能获益更多。
- 对于能量缺乏的患者，液体不平衡以及镁、钾和磷的缺乏必须积极治疗，以避免再喂养综合征的发生。
- 在接受小于4 mg/kg · min的碳水化合物营养的患者中，CO_2潴留一般不会发生。
- 肾衰竭是一种分解代谢状态，蛋白质不应该被限制。患者需要充分、平衡的营养支持和积极的透析治疗。
- 支气管和肺误吸最经常发生在肠内营养患者的转运期间。
- 谷氨酰胺是应激代谢环境中的条件性必需氨基酸。
- 伴随肠萎缩发生的腹泻应该对单体元素营养配方产生反应。如果没有，则必须考虑和治疗艰难梭菌的肠道感染。

静脉血栓形成：诊断和治疗

Susan Evans 和 Ronald Sing 著
吕 杰 译

静脉血栓形成（venous thromboembolism，VTE）是治疗受伤患者的一个挑战。患者诊疗的主线在于对预防、诊断和治疗做出深思后的决策，所有这些决策都存在风险。因此，许多机构已经转为使用流程，对特定患者群体做出决策。然而，创伤群体的风险耐受性尤其具有差异性（例如制动、出血、颅内出血），这使得一般的流程难以应用。考虑到存在这种差异性，我们将提供这样一种方法，它在提供基本框架的同时，又允许灵活的应用，以解决每个患者的具体情况。最终，重要的是确定哪些患者适合于哪种评估途径，以及哪些患者需要多学科团队来制订治疗计划。

发病率

静脉血栓形成在不接受预防的受伤患者中发生的概率达 58%，并且大多数这些血栓形成（98%）最初是无症状的。VTE 发生率在以下患者中最高，下肢骨折（69%），脊髓损伤（62%）和创伤性脑损伤（54%）。此外，其他因素，如年龄较大（OR = 1.05）、输血（OR = 1.74）和手术（OR = 2.3）都会增加 VTE 的风险。国家创伤数据库 2004 年的综述显示，所有损伤患者的 VTE 和肺栓塞（pulmonary embolism，PE）发生率分别为 0.36% 和 0.13%。尤其重要的是，VTE 可以在损伤后早期发生，6% 的 PE 在损伤的 24 h 内发生，25% 在伤后的前 3 天发生。虽然血栓预防在过去 20 年中已经使得 VTE 有所减少，患者管理的其他方面，例如尽早活动及手术时间缩短，也改善了患者的总体预后，以及 VTE 的发生率。

病理学

创伤会导致 Virchow 三联征的 3 个方面（血液淤滞、内皮损伤、高凝状态）均有发生，这可以解释 VTE 在损伤后的发生率。患者整体或四肢受伤导致不能移动会引起静脉系统内的血液淤滞。血液淤滞在 ICU 中经常发生，特别是在需要神经肌肉阻滞的患者中。这也是为什么间歇气动压迫（intermittent pneumatic compression，IPC）装置被创造出来的原因，尽管它们对纤维蛋白溶解的作用超过它们的局部效应。静脉系统的直接损伤可以伴有或不伴有出血。血管损伤的患者累及内皮系统，引起组织因子的释放。冲击造成的拉伸、压缩和挤压伤害、骨折，以及由枪伤的空化引起的剪应力，都会可能导致静脉系统的内膜损伤，但不会破坏静脉。然而，直接静脉损伤并不会增加受伤患者血栓形成的风险。创伤后外伤性细胞因子释放，在一个远处的区域导致促凝血因子的活化、抗凝血因子的减少和相对的高凝状态。当身体认识到需要止血时，血栓即开始形成，并且 VTE 可以在创伤后几分钟内形成。事实上，在没有血管损伤的 200 名重伤患者中，26 名患者中超过 1/3 的患者在 1 周内发生深静脉血栓（deep venous thromboses，DVTs），其中 10% 在第一天就发生了。

诊断

DVT 的诊断是使用双功能超声（duplex ultrasound，DUS）进行的，其取代静脉造影作为该疾病的诊断工具。DUS 应该在出现血栓的体征时进行（单侧肢体水肿）。美国胸科医师学会（American College of Chest Physicians，ACCP）或 EAST 不支持无症状患者进行常规筛查。然而，ACCP 和 EAST 支持对处于最高风险，并且预防不足的患者进行筛查。值得注意的是 DUS 不足以诊断骨盆血管中的 VTE。因此，如果怀疑有中央型血栓形成，静脉的 CT 血管造影是可以选择的诊断方式，并且在大多数机构中也已经成功实现了静脉造影。CT 血管造影也已替代常规血管造影和通气灌注扫描用于 PE 的诊断。虽然 CT 血管造影在具有低肌酐清除率或静脉造影剂过敏的患者中，受到相对禁忌证的限制，但在这些条件下仍然没有其他检查方式可以替代它。在这些患者中，决定使用静脉造影剂进行 CT 血管造影，须对检查的风险和利益进行分析，来决定研究须提供的信息。此外，造影剂过敏的患者可以在检查之前使用药物预防。

治疗

风险评估

不是所有诊断损伤的患者 VTE 发生的风险都会增加。这可以通过回顾国家创伤数据库的数据来证明，VTE 的发生率是极低的。虽然低发病率是由于使用了预防 VTE 的措施，但大部分低发生率可归因于损伤极小的患者人群，这些患者发生 VTE 的风险等于未受伤人群。因此，为 VTE 发生风险增加的受伤患者建立评估体系是有帮助的。虽然这样的评估公式不可行，但某些损伤和情况与 VTE 的风险增加有关（表 1）。因此，应考虑对这些损伤的患者进行血栓预防。

预防

预防是 VTE 治疗的重中之重，但同时也是疾病最具争议的地方。具体地说，低分子肝素（依诺肝素 30 mg，皮下注射每日 2 次）和低剂量普通肝素（每 8 h 皮下注射 5 000 单位）是减少 DVT 发生的最有效的干预，但对于存在出血风险的患者则会增加其出血的风险。ACCP 指南支持使用肝素（低分子肝素或低剂量普通肝素），它表示，“对于多数创伤患者来说，我们建议应用低分子肝素抗凝（2C 级别），尤其配合应用 IPC（2C）预防 VTE 发生”。同时 EAST 指南也是支持的，它表示，“对于 ISS 评分超过 9 分的创伤患者来说，如果能够接受抗凝治疗，应该首先考虑应用低分子肝素作为预防 VTE 的手段（Ⅲ级证据）”。重要的是，尽管低剂量普通肝素（low-dose unfractionated heparin，LDUH）以前被认为在创伤患者中，不如低分子肝素（low-molecular-weight heparin，LMWH），但是当前版本的 ACCP 指南认为它们的效果是相等的。在肌酐清除率低（小于 20 ~ 30 ml/min）的患者中禁止使用 LMWH，LDUH 是更优的选择。此外，在第 9 版 ACCP 指南出版后已说明，达肝素（表 2）是在 VTE 预防和治疗中有效的 LMWH。

对于有临时限制，不能使用 VTE 药物预防的患者（例如患有实质器官损伤、长骨骨折出血、TBI 的患者），应使用机械预防。这包括 IPC 和 A 级压缩袜。此外，足泵对于带有外部固定器或铸件的患者，可以用作 IPC 的替代品。ACCP 指南指出，“对有 LMWH 和 LDUH 禁忌证的创伤患者，我们建议进行机械预防，最好应用下肢静脉循环泵，在没有预防禁忌的下肢损伤中应用（2C）。在出血风险去除或无肝素应用禁忌的情况下，我们建议增加药物预防 VTE（2C）”。显而易见的问题是，出血的风险何时去除？确定活动性出血程度评估的参数有助于建立治疗的模式。在作者的病房中，在 4 h 内血红蛋白减少小于 1 g/dl 被认为是出血停止，并可启动药物预防血栓。这种做法不适用于中枢神经系统损伤的患者，特别是 TBI、脊柱骨折和脊髓损伤。在这一群体中开始药物预防须更加谨慎。相对小的活动性出血进入脑或脊髓，可对预后产生严重的影响。

表 1　创伤患者的 VTE 的危险因素

脊髓损伤 *
下肢或骨盆骨折
需要手术
静脉损伤 / 静脉导管插入
高龄 *
长时间制动
血栓预防延迟

* 与 meta 分析是一致的

表 2　低分子肝素

肝素	剂量	适应证	禁忌证
伊诺肝素	预防：30 mg SC bid 或 40U SC 每天 * 治疗：1 mg/kg SC bid	VTE 的预防，治疗不稳定型心绞痛和心肌梗死	出血风险高 在脊髓和硬膜外麻醉中的每日推荐剂量
达肝素（法安明）	预防：5 000 U SC 每天 治疗：抗Ⅹa 因子 100 U/kg SC bid	VTE 的预防，治疗不稳定型心绞痛和心肌梗死	出血风险高

VTE：静脉血栓形成；SC：皮下；bid：一天 2 次
* 当患者体重 >150 kg 时，把剂量增加至 40 mg，一天 2 次，皮下注射

持续时间

受伤患者所需的血栓预防的持续时间尚未确定。在整个住院和康复期间持续进行药物预防是合理的。ACCP 和 EAST 指南都支持这种做法。很可能一些长期不动的患者即使在出院后仍然处于发展为 VTE 的高风险中。尽管没有数据可以为延长 VTE 的预防提供指导，但是可以考虑延长 LMWH 或维生素 K 拮抗剂（vitamin K antagonist，VKA，如华法林）的使用，直到患者可以活动。

抗凝治疗

当 VTE 发生时，除非存在抗凝禁忌，否则应给予低分子肝素抗凝（每日 2 mg/kg 或 1 mg/ kg，每日 2 次皮下注射），磺达肝素（见表 2），通过静脉注射 LDUH（控制活化部分促凝血酶原时间为 50 ~ 80 s）。此外，这些药物应该在中度或高度疑似 VTE 的患者中开始使用，同时等待检查，以确诊 VTE。静脉抗凝应持续到开始 VKA 治疗后至少 5 天，直到国际标准化比率（international normalized ratio，INR）达到 2.0，并持续治疗 3 个月。与以前的建议不同，目前的 ACCP 指南指出，在这种创伤后的情况中，3 个月的疗程对于 DVT 和 PE 都适合。此外，如果存在严重的症状或存在血栓继续延伸的高度风险，远端（膝下）血栓形成的治疗应等同于近端血栓形成。

溶栓治疗和血栓切除术

对于 PE 症状严重的患者，应考虑采取干预措施以解决凝块负荷，选择侵入性由低到高的治疗方式。具体地，如果患者出现低血压［例如，收缩压（systolic blood pressure，SBP）$<$90 mmHg］，ACCP 建议“全身给药溶栓治疗（2C），在 2 h 内通过周围静脉输注（2C）。此外，他们建议在以下 3 种情况下给予导管辅助清除血栓：①患者有溶栓禁忌证；②溶栓失败；③休克并可能在全身溶栓治疗前就引起患者死亡（2C）。在导管辅助的栓子切除术困难或休克快速进展难以进行溶栓治疗时，建议行手术肺栓子切除术（2C）”。ACCP 强烈建议，侵入性操作只能在出血风险小的患者中进行，并且需要适当的外科专业知识和资源（2C）。此外，这些操作应该只在除 VTE 外，具有良好的全身功能状态和预后的患者中应用。无论是在溶栓治疗还是血栓切除术后，后续的抗凝治疗仍然是必需的，且方式和持续时间与没有接受溶栓治疗 / 血栓切除术的患者相同。

腔静脉滤器

常规适用于腔静脉过滤器（vena cava filter，VCFs）的情况包括：①近端（腘静脉或以上）DVT 或具有对治疗性抗凝有禁忌证的 PE，②尽管给予足量抗凝，但仍然复发的 PE。适应证在过去几十年中已经有所演变，其包括以下情况：①髂静脉或下腔静脉中的大的游离血栓；②大块 PE 之后，栓塞复发可能会致命；③在手术栓子切除术期间 / 之后。在溶栓期间关于 VCF 的应用时机存在争议。然而，大多数介入医生会在药物机械溶栓后留置 VCF。

创伤患者中 VCF 的留置仍有争议。Rogers 等在 20 世纪 90 年代中期证明了，选择高风险创伤患者“预防性”留置 VCF，是有益处的。使用术语“预防性”，因为这些患者没有诊断 DVT 或 PE 就留置了 VCF。自从这些早期报告以来，许多其他试验（Ⅱ级和Ⅲ级证据）也显示对高风险创伤患者留置 VCF 可能获益，这也是 EAST 指南中 VTE 对 VCF 留置给予谨慎推荐的原因。脊髓损伤联合会支持在 72 h 内应用预防剂量的抗凝治疗不安全时，考虑使用 VCF。与之相反，ACCP 指南第 9 版指出：“对于外伤患者，我们建议下腔静脉滤器不用于 VTE 的初始预防（2C）。”重要的是定义与 VCF 相关的术语“预防性”。事实上，所有 VCF 都是预防性的，因为它们对 DVT 或 PE 没有治疗作用，它们只是阻止血栓栓塞到心脏和肺部。因此，VCF 不是专门用于预防 DVT。然而，对有 VTE 药物预防明显禁忌证的高危患者，VCF 可至少降低 PE 这一 VTE 致命并发症的发生率。EAST 对这些难以治疗的患者提供了一些指导，“一个预防性下腔静脉滤器置入，对很多无法接受抗凝治疗的高风险创伤患者来说非常必要，抗凝会增加出血的风险，主要包括以下损伤类型：严重闭合性头部损伤（GCS 评分小于 8）、伴有对侧或四肢瘫痪的不完全脊髓损伤，伴有长骨骨折的复杂骨盆骨折，四肢长骨多发性骨折（Ⅲ级）。”类似地，脊髓损伤联合会建议“考虑放置下腔静脉滤器只在预计有活动性出血，且可能持续超过 72 h 的患者中进行，并且须尽快恢复抗凝治疗（等级Ⅲ / Ⅳ C）。”在常规或扩展的适应证之外使用 VCF 应基于对每个患者的风险 / 益处分析。在我们的临床实践中，这通常是关于 PE 风险和预防性抗凝风险的多专业讨论。

法国的 PREPIC 试验，是唯一一项对 VCF 的随机对照研究，对其有很多讨论。在该试验中，在有 DVT 和适当抗凝的患者中，放置了 VCF 的患者（除了 VTE 抗凝），死亡率和 DVT 的增加率没有差异。该试验的结果经常被引用，并且可能已经影响了在美国使用 VCF。然而，仔细回顾该报告则发现多缺陷和误解。首先，随机化（有过滤器或无过滤器）的患者都是有抗凝治疗的。在美国，可以抗凝的患者留置 VCF 不是推荐的做法。因为 DVT 和 PE 在抗凝治疗后的死亡率很低，所以不能期望 VCF 为死亡率带来多大益处。在这项试验中，最常用的 VCF 是 B.Braun Vena Tech LGM，其已经报道 IVC 血栓形成率高达 25%。使用的另一种装置是 Bard Cardial 过滤器，还未被批准在美国使用。此外，PREPIC 试验中的所有 VCF 都是永久性置入的，因此，无法评估在 PE 风险解决后过滤器回收的优点。由于这些原因，PREPIC 试验不适用于当前的设备、标准和实践。

腔静脉过滤器置入术

在过去几年中，围绕 VCF 的置入和回收的技术已经发生了很大的变化。最初通过剖腹手术和静脉切开术放置，VCF 现在使用各种装置经皮置入，其中一些装置仅使用小至 6 F 的插入鞘。为了在 IVC 中放置过滤器而开发的这种技术的进步，现在已被诸如介入放射学和介入心脏病学的其他学科采用。这些学科的术者在手术室外、在心脏导管室或放射介入室进行置入和回收操作。更有甚者，由于 VCF 经皮置入和回收技术的简便，使得它甚至可以方便地在 ICU 床旁操作。

VCF 插入对设备的需要相当简单。无菌技术用于个人保护，包括帽子、眼睛保护、无菌长袍和手套。大多数 VCF 通常与使用扩张器的插入鞘一起包装，该扩张器用作腔静脉成像的注射导管。这些导管具有多个侧端口，以增强造影剂与血液的混合。预测量的不透射线标志物来帮助测量 IVC 直径（图 1）。根据置入方式（类似于中心静脉导管插入术），患者将行范围较广的消毒与铺单。静脉通路最常选择的是右股静脉，但也可以使用颈静脉。一些小型装置可以使用其他静脉插入，如锁骨下静脉、腋静脉、甚至肘前静脉和腘静脉。 通路的选择应避免有已知 DVT 的静脉。需要造影术来安全地置入 VCF。在我们的实践中，成像是用荧光透视法完成的，因此，必须对躯干和甲状腺进行适当的铅屏蔽保护。

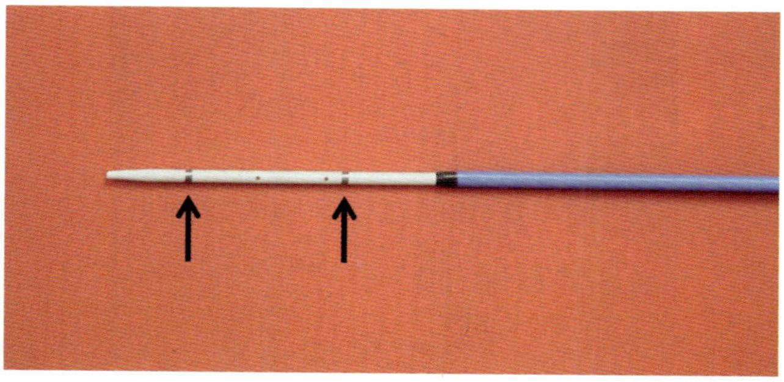

图 1　腔静脉过滤器扩张器的插入鞘展示了不透射线的标记辅助线和侧孔（箭头）

其他操作者已经证明了血管内超声（intravascular ultrasound，IVUS）和 DUS 的安全性和有效性。ICU 中的床旁插入中使用荧光透视法，需要具有荧光透视条件的床。腔静脉的路径图或成像是标准的操作，并且已经被证明可以大大减少插入的并发症。在荧光透视时，须使用造影剂，包括碘化造影剂、钆或二氧化碳气体。二氧化碳气体不会导致过敏，且没有肾毒性，有一定的优势，但是需要数字减影，并且图像质量受到肥胖和肠内气体的不良影响。值得注意的是，荧光透视中使用的 CO_2 与腹腔镜手术中使用的 CO_2 不同：腹腔镜使用的 CO_2 纯度为 99.90%，而血管级别的 CO_2 纯度为 99.99%。

一旦获得静脉通路，将长导丝［通常 150 cm 或更大（长度），0.035 in（宽度）］推进下腔静脉（inferior vena cava，IVC）。进行 IVC 的造影，以确定 IVC 的解剖结构和置入位置，并测量 IVC 直径（图 2）。我们通常使用 30 ml 非离子碘化造影剂，使用压力注射器在 2 s 内注射。肾下位置是首选的，但如果该区域存在解剖异常或血栓，则可能须选择肾上腺的位置。一般制造的 VCF 会有最大直径的范围，大多数是 28 ~ 30 mm，因此测量腔静脉直径是重要的。应当注意，在美国没有可选的（可回收）直径大于 30 mm 的 VCFs 被批准使用。一旦确定 IVC 解剖结构和直径，则插入保护鞘被推进到适当位置以用于在 IVC 中放置。为了防止穿孔，重要的是不能将保护鞘或扩张器在没有导丝的情况下置入。我们通常将保护鞘插入超出计划的放置的位置，并将保护鞘回撤到正确的位置。过滤器的实际释放 / 布置可以因设备不同而不同，但是，在原理上，它们都是使用“拔出鞘”技术而不是“推出”到 IVC 中的方式。之后通过手动注射造影剂经插入的保护鞘进行完整的造影，以记录过滤器的方向和放置。在手术

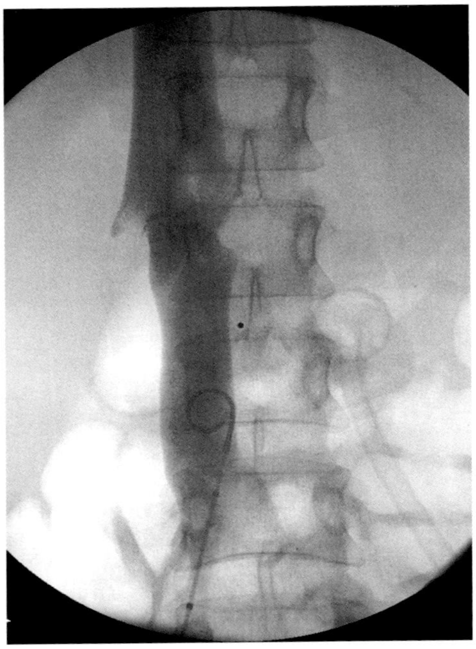

图 2　IVC 的对比造影

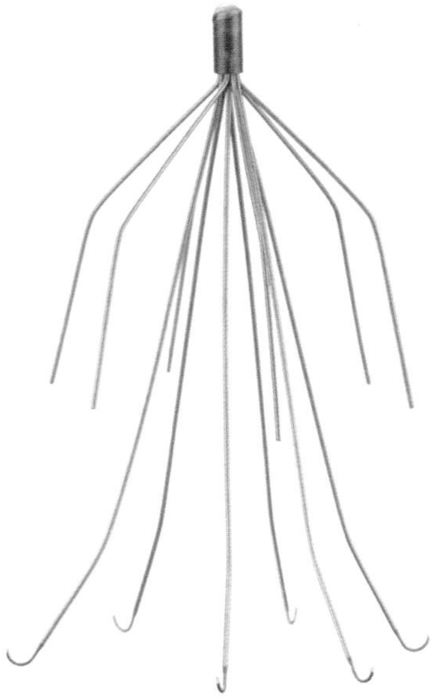

图 3　Bard Recovery 腔静脉过滤器

之前和手术期间，我们用盐水冲洗所有导管、扩张器和管路，以避免导管内形成血栓，并避免出现空气栓塞。移除插入的保护鞘，并给予适当压力压迫 10 min（如果患者为抗凝状态，则要压 15 min），之后将黏性敷料贴在该部位。

在床旁置入 VCF 的过程中，特别是当使用荧光透视法时，须考虑几个注意事项。首先，辐射安全最重要。在满足辐射安全的 3 个原则（时间、距离和屏蔽）后，这个手术才可以在床旁安全地进行。荧光透视时间应保持最小（通常小于 60 s）。任何未直接参与的人员应与患者保持至少 3 m 的距离，散射暴露才可忽略不计。那些参与手术的人应该对躯干和甲状腺做适当的铅屏蔽。床旁 VCF 置入的第二个注意事项是不要降低床侧栏杆，因为对于导管、注射器等，无菌窗帘可以形成“谷”，防止其掉落。此外，升高的栏杆可以保持患者不滚落到地板上。

腔静脉过滤器回收程序

在 2003 年，美国 FDA 批准的第一个回收装置是 Bard Recovery IVC 过滤器（图 3）。使用专用的锥体回收器回收滤网。从那时起，许多其他“可选”设备陆续也得到批准（图 4）。这些设备都在头部或尾部末端有一个钩子，允许它们可以用血管内圈套套上。

大多数回收手术可以在门诊进行，给予一定的时间使 PE 的风险下降。已经接受抗凝治疗的患者，一旦在 7 天内没有出血的证据，可以考虑移除 VCF。在术前 72 h 内，应进行下肢 DUS 检查，以确定已知 DVT 的稳定性或检查有无新的 DVT 出现。显然，除非患者处于抗凝状态，否则对于无抗凝且出现新发 DVT 的患者，过滤网是不能回收的。

麻醉基于患者的偏好和耐受程度。在我们的大多数手术时，在回收保护鞘的点选择局部麻醉，然后持续镇静。长时间（超过 12 个月）置入的 VCF 在脱离 IVC 时会更不舒服，在这些情况下，我们倾向于使用更深的镇静或全身麻醉。我们还对脑损伤患者使用全身麻醉，因为他们往往多动，且无法通过安慰来保持体位。

通过使用鹅颈管或多环血管内圈套器，在过滤器上“锁定”钩子来完成回收。大多数当前使用的可回收装置通过颈静脉系统回收，除了 OptEase（Cordis Endovascular），其通过股静脉系统回收，和 Crux（Volcano Corp），其可以通过颈静脉或股静脉系统回收。一旦进入静脉通路，将 5F 注射导管尾部置于 VCF 附近。在正位和侧位投影中进行对比腔内成像，以确定 IVC 内过滤器的定位，同时确定过滤器内是否存在血栓。在无抗凝患者中，若过滤器内存在血栓则应该终止该手术，然后让患者开始进行抗凝治疗，以便稍后尝试再次回收。如果患者处于抗凝状态，可以将过滤器和小的凝块一起回收（小于孔的

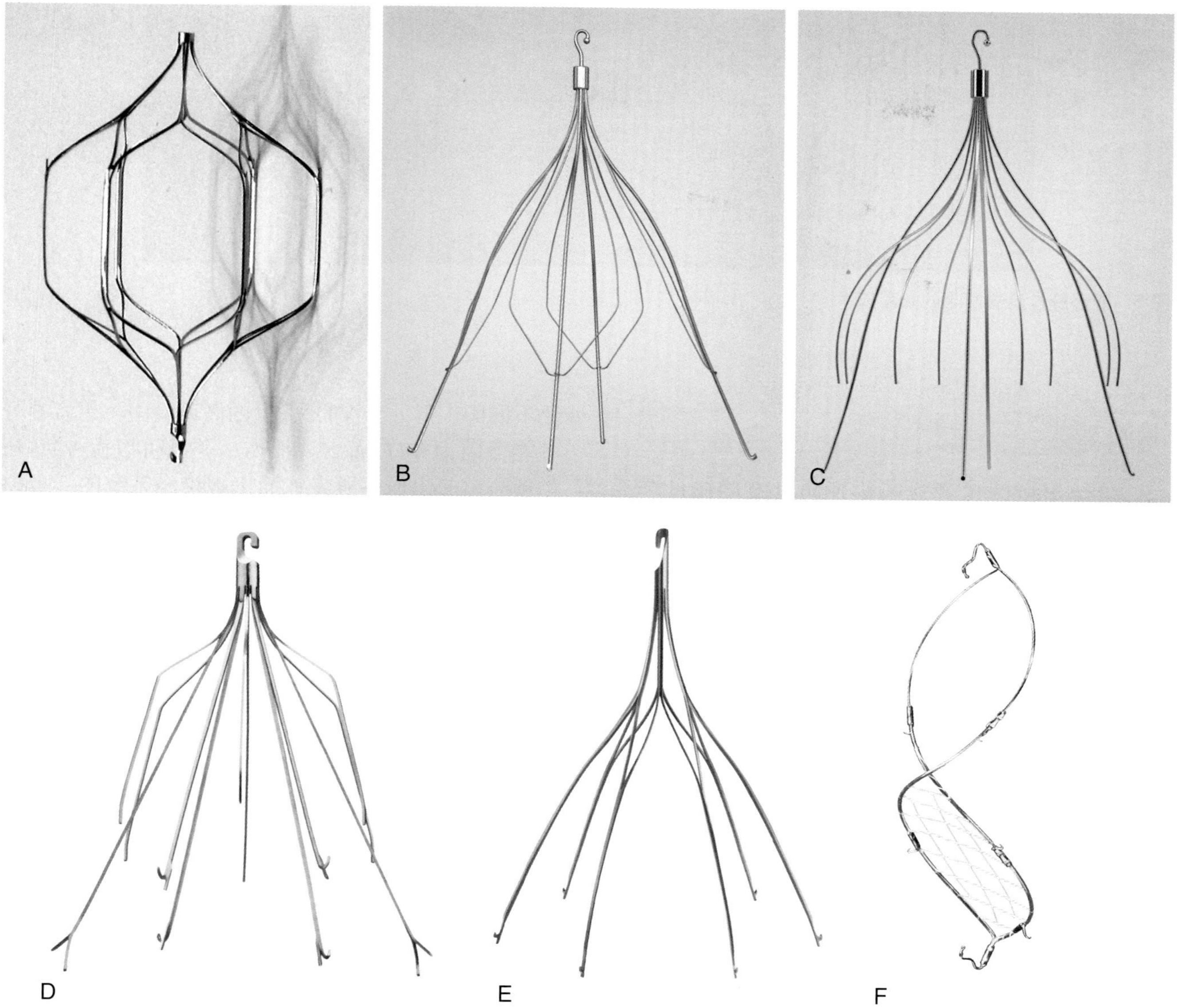

图 4　几个可选的腔静脉滤器。**A**，OptEase（Cordis Endovascular）**B**，Tulip（Cook Medrcal）**C**，Celect（Cook Medrcal）**D**，Denali（© 2015 C.R. Bard, Inc Vsed wrth permission）**E**，Option Elite（Argon Medical）**F**，Crux（Volcano Medical）

深度的 25%）。腔静脉检查之后，通过导丝移除注射导管，并且插入大的保护鞘。我们使用双鞘系统，12 F 外鞘在 9 F 内鞘上。一旦保护鞘就位，插入圈套以“套住”钩子。VCF 的钩被套住后，内鞘在过滤器的尖端上前进，同时将过滤器拉入保护鞘并保持之前与圈套的张力（图 5）。将过滤器撤回到内鞘中，并且为了避免将过滤器拖过保护鞘，我们直接移除整个内鞘（图 5）。不同的设备可能回收技术略有不同，通常需要短的牵引杆把支撑架从 IVC 的壁上剥离。VCF 被拿出后在桌上记录过滤器是否完整。注射导管被重新插入，并且进行腔静脉造影以记录 IVC 无外渗和结构完整。在移除保护鞘后保持穿刺点压迫 10 min（如果患者处于抗凝状态，则最少压迫 15 min）。没有必要为了回收而纠正 INR。患者在观察 2 h 后离开恢复室。

指南的局限性

尽管预防和管理 VTE 的建议对一部分人群有帮助，但许多受伤患者的状态使他们并不适用于这些建议。通常这些都是危重患者，医疗决策在许多方面具有挑战性。我们在下面的章节讨论这些患者。

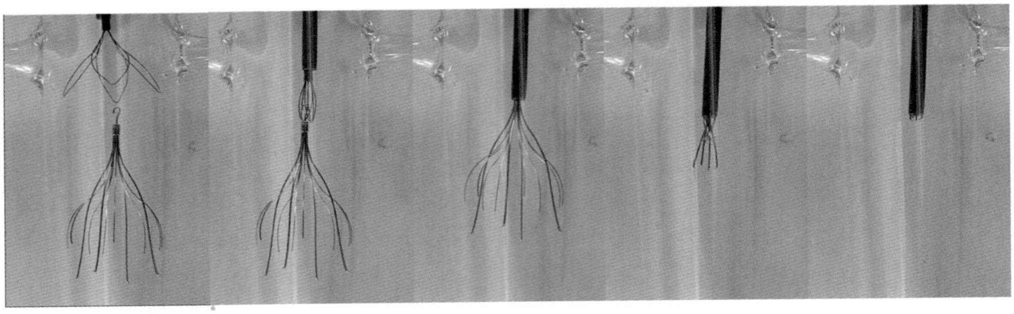

图 5 腔静脉过滤器回收的圈套技术

出血患者

持续出血的患者对药物预防具有明确的禁忌证。有趣的是，相关的凝血功能异常并不能避免出血患者出现 VTE。出血控制至关重要。在出血时，下肢静脉泵是 VTE 预防的合理选择。当出血被控制时，可以开始药物预防。生理参数如血红蛋白变化趋势是出血是否停止的重要表现。如前所述，诸如在 24 h 内小于 1g/dl 的 Hb 降低，可以被认为是出血停止和开始药物预防的标志之一。

多发伤伴随血红蛋白波动

创伤后患者的常见临床情况是多发性损伤、无活动性出血，但血红蛋白水平会波动。这通常可以持续许多天，取决于损伤的数量、稳定的时间（例如脾栓塞、长骨骨折的固定），营养状态和患者的分解代谢状态。通常这些患者在随后的几天中 Hb 降低近 1 g/dl。虽然每日小的 Hb 减少不是药物预防的禁忌证，但累积的变化可能会需要输血，如果患者不稳定可能会导致手术的延迟，故而不愿意启动药物预防。另外，下肢静脉泵的使用可能因为夹板、石膏或牵引而不能使用。

在这些患者中，常常须确定 VTE 药物预防增加患者需要输血的风险是否可以接受。如果不能接受，并且不使用药物预防，可以考虑置入 VCF。重要的是，多发性损伤的患者是发生 VTE 风险最高的人群，并且对这种损伤的耐受力最差。

创伤性脑损伤

创伤性脑损伤的患者可能是关于 VTE 预防的最有争议的患者群体。这是可以理解的，因为这种广泛不同的人群处于 VTE 发生的高风险中。患者本身可能会因为 VTE 而出现损伤，并且可以由 VTE 药物预防引起出血性并发症而出现神经系统的严重损害。有趣的是，建议预防 VTE 的机构对 TBI 患者几乎没有任何指导。ACCP 没有推荐，EAST 表示“低分子肝素尚未在头部损伤伴颅内出血的患者中有充分的研究来证明它的使用（Ⅲ级）。并且颅脑损伤协会也认为，目前没有可靠的数据来支持何时开始药物抗凝是安全的（Ⅲ级证据）。最近一项前瞻性观察性研究的作者建议，在入院后 48 h 内开始使用依诺肝素是安全的，并强烈鼓励其用于 TBI 患者和有其他高风险的创伤性损伤的患者。然而，1.1%的患者在使用依诺肝素后出现临床上显著的脑出血表现，且一个患者因为脑出血的进展而死亡，这与依诺肝素的使用直接相关。此外，许多脑损伤患者（例如，脑内血肿或直径超过 2 cm 的挫伤、脑内一个区域内的多发小挫伤、硬膜下或硬膜外血肿超过 8 mm，持续性颅内压大于 20 mmHg、在 24 h 随访 CT 扫描中脑损伤的大小或数目增加，以及神经外科医生或创伤外科医生不愿意启动预防）被排除。这一高度具体的排除标准大大限制了可适用这项建议的人群。

与从腹腔内出血的患者相比，对于保护免受 VTE 的益处来说，脑损伤的出血的处理显然不是可接受的“折中”。这个患者群体中的注意应该集中在预防出血，而不是预防 VTE。对 TBI 患者的决策应权衡初始损伤的程度、进展的风险和 VTE 危害的风险。例如，具有几个点状前额挫伤和 GCS 为 15 的患者，同具有 2 cm 额叶挫伤和 GCS 评分为 6 的患者相比，具有不同的 VTE 和出血风险。类似地，具有蛛网膜下隙出血的清醒患者，与具有需要引流的 1 cm 蛛网膜下隙出血的昏迷患者相比，具有较低的出血风险。开始 VTE 预防应该是一个多专业讨论的结果。决策组应包括神经外科医生、创伤外科医生，以及（根据机构）处理患者的特护医生。为了确定在开始预防之前出血的稳定性，诸如复查 CT 扫描之类的措施都是有用的方式。

脊髓损伤

脊髓损伤患者是另一个独特的患者群体。无论是否使用药物预防，他们发生 VTE 的风险都最高，并且因为他们长时间不能动，他们的风险比大多数患者持续时间都长。ACCP、EAST 和脊髓损伤联合会都推荐早期进行药物预防。然而，在脊柱血肿的患者中，药物预防应当延迟，直到出血已经明确止住。

肥胖

肥胖导致许多护理方面的并发症增加。关于 VTE，总体风险仅仅是由于肥胖，给药剂量并不明确，并且 VCF 置入在肥胖患者也异常困难。由于 VTE 的风险增加，所有损伤的肥胖患者，即使仅为轻微的损伤，也应该被当做高风险人群来治疗。此外，常规剂量的预防和治疗性 LMWH 和 LUFH 可能不足以用于肥胖患者。最近使用抗凝血因子Ⅹa 解决 LMWH 安全性的研究表明，大多数患者的给药方案剂量不足，而肥胖患者最常发生剂量不足的问题。ACCP 建议："对住院接受减肥手术的患者，我们建议应用比普通非肥胖患者更高剂量的低分子肝素或依诺肝素进行抗凝。"虽然这项建议是不明确的，但它与常规剂量不足所关注的问题是一致的。如果能够确定合适的剂量，抗凝血因子Ⅹa 水平可能是治疗中最有帮助的指导。将依诺肝素剂量增加至 60 mg，每日 2 次或 0.5 mg/kg · d 是一个合理的选择。

广泛的制动

虽然广泛的制动常常与脊髓损伤相关，但它通常也可能与多个下肢骨折有关，需要超过 12 周的负重限制。对于这些患者，在住院期间开始的血栓预防，理想情况下应该在出院后以某种形式继续。虽然没有随机对照试验来指导这种治疗，但从当前的 ACCP 和 EAST 指南，我们可以推断，VTE 预防应该在制动期间继续进行。在这种情况下，VKA 优于 LMWH。

硬膜外导管

唯一提出有关硬膜外导管建议的组织是 EAST，其中指出"低分子肝素不应在硬膜外导管放置或取出时应用（Ⅲ级）。"然而，当符合特定标准时，许多麻醉学会已经接受了 LMWH 与硬膜外导管的联合使用。来自多个国家麻醉组织（包括美国区域麻醉和疼痛医学学会）的指南联合提供了关于 LMWH 与硬膜外导管的使用的建议（表 3）。

表 3　硬膜外导管和低分子肝素

低分子肝素每日应使用 1 次。
只适用于预防使用
在插入或移除导管前，至少 10 ~ 12 h 应用一次低分子肝素
在插入或移除导管后，至少 2 ~ 4 h 应用一次低分子肝素

肝素诱导的血小板减少

血小板减少是创伤和手术后的常见表现。常见原因包括由于出血导致的血小板消耗和由营养不良和急性疾病引起的血小板生成缺乏。然而，对于接受肝素（肝素或低分子肝素）的那些患者，当出现血小板减少时，肝素诱导的血小板减少（heparin-induced thrombocytopenia，HIT）必须被要被考虑到。对于由肝素以外的原因引起血小板减少的患者，肝素给药仍然是 VTE 较好的预防方式。因此，鉴别那些由于肝素给药而导致血小板减少的患者是至关重要的。HIT 的常见表现包括，在 5 ~ 14 天之间，患者使用初始肝素剂量而血小板计数减少 50%，但高于 20 000/ml 的血小板的最低值。或者，患者最近（过去 30 天）暴露于肝素，肝素抗体可能先前已经形成，并且可能促使血小板计数立即减少。

HIT 可以分为 2 种类型。Ⅰ型 HIT 患者血小板计数低于 150 000 × 10^9/L，但高于 100 000 × 10^9/L，并且与免疫反应无关。虽然Ⅰ型 HIT 导致血小板减少可能因为其他原因继续恶化，但并不须停止肝素的使用。相比之下，Ⅱ型 HIT 与血小板因子 4（platelet factor 4，PF4）的 IgG 抗体的形成相关，导致血小板、肝素免疫复合物形成和局部血栓形成。Ⅱ型 HIT 存在于 5% 接受肝素治疗的患者中，并且可导致更显著的血小板减少（血小板计数为 10 000 × 10^9/L ~ 200 000 × 10^9/L）以及严重的并发症，甚至血栓形成而死亡。此外，血小板减少可以加重活动性出血。Ⅱ型 HIT 的确诊，须通过酶联免疫吸附测定（enzyme-linked immunosorbent assay，ELISA）和流式细胞计量术鉴定肝素 PF4 抗体的存在。肝素给药必须停止，以允许解决免疫活化和血小板浓度恢复的问题。此外，必须使用其他可以预防血栓的措施，以限制血栓形成。阿加曲班和重组水蛭素是 2 种 FDA 批准的用于治疗 HIT 患者的药物（表 4）。由美国血液学协会与 ACCP 联合创建的、关于疑似肝素诱导血小板减少的成年人的评估和治疗的临床实践指南，提供了关于外科和非外科患者中，HIT 的诊断和处理的有用信息。

上肢 / 胸部深静脉血栓形成和浅静脉血栓形成

上肢和胸部 DVT 的治疗基本上与下肢 DVT 相同。上肢和胸腔的深静脉包括腋静脉、锁骨下静脉、颈内静脉和无名静脉。对于与中心静脉导管相关的上肢 DVT，ACCP 建议“当导管是有功能的或者持续被需要时，不能拔除中心静脉导管（2C）。”抗凝应持续 3 个月（1B）或与导管留置期限相同（1C）。

至少 5 cm 长的下肢浅静脉血栓形成（superficial venous thrombose，SVTs）应该治疗，通常使用预防剂量的磺达肝素（每日 2.5 mg）或 LMWH 治疗 45 天（2B）。目前没有对上肢的 SVT 的建议。

并发症发生率和并发症的处理

VTE 的并发症取决于血栓的位置。在末端，长期血栓导致静脉淤滞，静脉瓣完整性丧失、血管扩张和肢端水肿。这可能最终导致皮肤变化和伤口愈合不良。虽然大多数静脉淤滞不会产生急性病症，但可导致终生迁延的并发症。

PE 的发生往往是非常剧烈的，而且是急性发作。低氧血症，甚至血流动力学不稳定须立即干预，给予生理支持和进行血栓切除。

结论和评估

所有受伤患者应进行 VTE 风险评估。由于应用下肢静脉泵的风险低，因此在所有患者中都应考虑应用这些装置。分级为中或高风险类别的 VTE 患者，在住院期间或直到其活动正常化之前，应接受 LMWH 治疗。对于存在 LMWH 禁忌证的患者，在损伤后 72 h 以上，可以考虑 VCF 置入。禁忌证的确定应该是多学科专家讨论得到的。图 6 中的评估原则可以作为这些具有挑战性和关键性的决定的指南。

低体温和创伤

表 4 肝素诱发的血小板减少可选择的抗凝剂

药物	剂量	检测	注释
阿加曲班	推注：没有 注入：2 μg /kg · min	目标 aPTT =1.5 ~ 3.0 × 基线	肝功能衰竭的患者剂量减少
比伐卢定	推注：没有 注入：0.15 mg /kg · h	目标 aPTT =1.5 ~ 2.5 × 基线	
磺达肝素	<50 kg: 5 mg，SC，每天 50 ~ 100 kg: 7.5 mg，SC，每天 >100 kg: 10 mg，SC，每天	调整至 1.5 U/ml 的药物的抗凝血因子 Xa 活性峰值	在肾功能损害患者中有限制或禁忌
重组水蛭素 *（Refludan）	推注：0.4 mg/kg 注入：0.15 mg /kg · h	目标 aPTT =1.5 ~ 2.5 × 基线 无血栓时，不使用推注目标；aPTT =1.5 ~ 2.0 × 基线	肾衰竭患者中剂量减少

aPTT：活化部分促凝血酶原时间；SC：皮下

* 目前美国已经停止使用

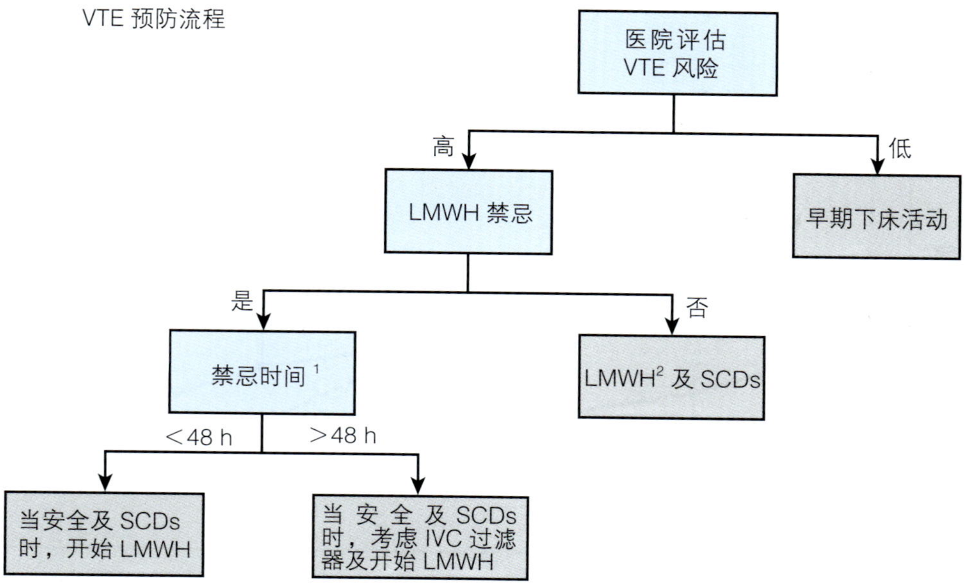

图 6 VTE 预防流程。1. 低分子肝素禁忌证：a. 血红蛋白不稳定；b. 实质脏器损伤。当患者在超过 24 h 血红蛋白减少小于 1g/dl 而无其他禁忌证时，开始使用低分子肝素。c. 颅内出血和脊髓损伤。VTE 中的神经损伤发生率很高，且与将来出血发生率有关。低分子肝素使用须尽快由神经外科医生决定。d. 凝血功能障碍定义为血小板计数低于 $5\,000 \times 10^9/mm^3$ 或 INR 或 aPTT 超过正常的 1.5 倍。e. 肌酐高于 1.6。如果没有其他药物预防的禁忌证，这些患者应该皮下每 8 h 使用 5 000 单位肝素。低分子肝素每 12 h 给予 30 mg。如果患者体重超过 150 kg，剂量每 12 h 增加至 40 mg VTE，静脉血栓形成；IVC，下腔静脉；SCD，下肢静脉泵；LMWH，低分子肝素

低体温的有害影响

Larry M. Gentilello 和 R. Lawrence Reed II 著
吕 杰 译

人类作为恒温动物，体温保持在核心温度 37℃ 的狭窄范围内。低体温与创伤患者死亡率增加相关。然而，由于创伤越严重，低体温越容易出现，所以死亡率的增加是否由于低体温本身，还是潜在的创伤的严重程度引起，目前仍然不能确定。有人提出，在休克患者中，体温降低是具有保护性的。当严重创伤或其他危险因素出现时，致死率没有因为低体温变得更高。然而，最近的前瞻性研究已经证实了低体温对创伤患者预后与既往研究相反的影响，及加以积极处理可显著提高患者复苏成功的可能性。

对凝血的影响

低体温最严重的影响也许是凝血功能（图 1）。由于有潜在的多种因素可引起凝血功能受损，所以低体温引起的损害程度通常被低估。这些患者通常有酸中毒、组织创伤、休克、循环血容量的稀释、凝血因子浓度的降低。正常的凝血功能需要充足的血小板计数和功能，以及充足的凝血因子水平和活性。理论上，低体温会影响血液凝固的每个环节。

血小板计数和功能的影响

在狗的实验研究已经证实了一项与全身低体温相关的可逆性的血小板减少。然而，该疾病仅发生在低体温水平，远低于一般创伤的温度（＜30℃）。

血小板在低温期间被可逆性地抑制，部分通过

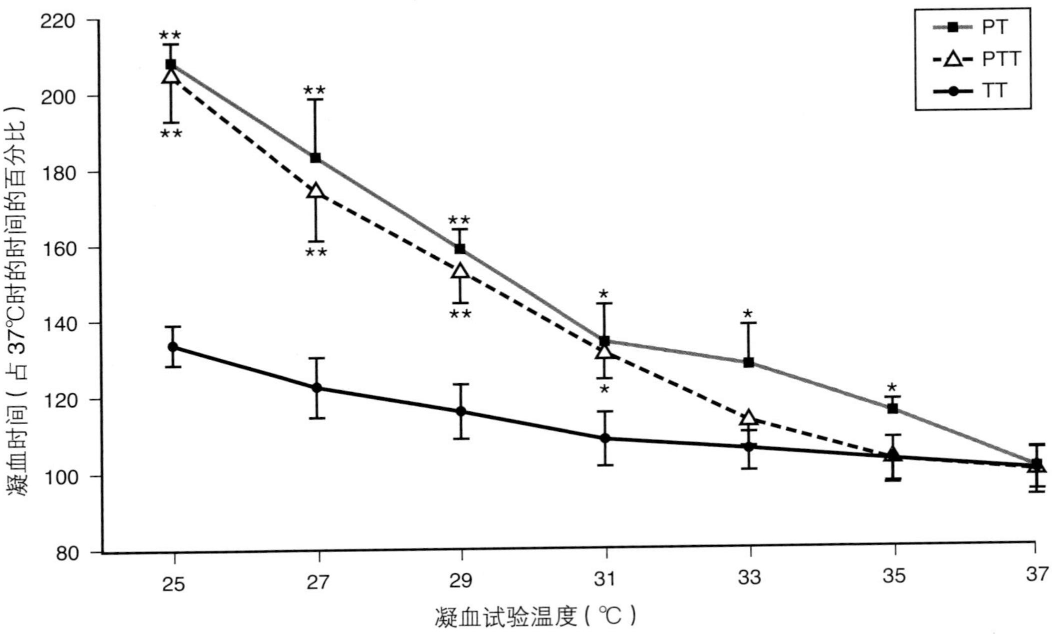

图 1 对比不同程度的低温对凝血试验影响。以标准血浆浓度来进行凝血时间检测，通过调节控制温度，用纤维蛋白检测法测量当时温度的凝血时间。PT：凝血酶原时间；PTT：部分促凝血酶原时间；TT：凝血酶时间。$^*P<0.001$：与凝血酶时间延长相比。$^{**}P<0.0001$：与凝血酶时间延长相比 (*Modified from Reed R, Bracey A, Hudson J, et al: Hypothermia and blood coagulation: dissociation between enzyme activity and clotting factor levels. Circ Shock 32:141–152, 1990.*)

血栓素 B_2 进行温度依赖性调节，血栓素 B_2 是一个强有力的血管收缩剂，以刺激血小板聚集。Valeri 等通过狒狒做实验，验证了低体温的作用。他们通过使用加热毯和辐射加热器来保持对照组处于常温状态。同时，测量体温正常与体温降低组的出血时间分别是 2.4 min 和 5.8 min。由于低体温影响血小板的功能，在未行有效的复温前，给予低体温患者输血对于减少血液丢失也许是无效的。

凝血因子水平和功能的影响

研究显示，只有温度低于 33℃，凝血因子活性才会改变。但是，临床经验并不支持这种观点。Reed 等在低体温患者的凝血因子功能的动力学效应研究中发现了明显的不同。医院标准的血液凝集分子纤维蛋白检测法的标准温度是 37℃，并没有在患者实际核心温度下测量凝血时间。在这项研究中，一个外接数字温控连接器接到一个加热装置中，能够测量出创伤患者低体温范围下的凝血时间。

从 25℃到 37℃，把含有正常凝血因子的人血浆进行测量，得到凝血酶原时间、部分凝血活酶时间、凝血酶时间。随着 3 个凝血试验时间延长，凝血因子功能显著降低，程度与低温程度是一致的。随后有研究证实，即使体温降低程度不严重，或者凝血因子没有实际的缺乏，低体温仍可以导致功能性凝血功能障碍，这相当于严重凝血因子缺乏（图 2）。

Gubler 等用改进了的方法证实了这些结果：在稀释性凝血功能障碍患者中，温度降低产生了进一步的影响（图 3）。最近的研究分析表明，与凝血因子相比，在 33℃ ~37℃，轻度体温下降过程中，虽然凝血因子功能障碍随着温度的降低变得更加严重。但对血小板活性和聚集影响更大，它们更能导致低体温相关性的凝血功能障碍。

总之，低体温很少影响血小板和凝血因子水平，但会影响凝血成分的功能。

对其他器官的影响

最常受低温影响的器官系统包括循环、免疫、神经、凝血系统。体温过低通常会诱发心脏发生心动过缓，当核心温度低于 28℃ ~30℃时，通常会发生心室颤动。机体由于恢复正常体温时会发生寒战，

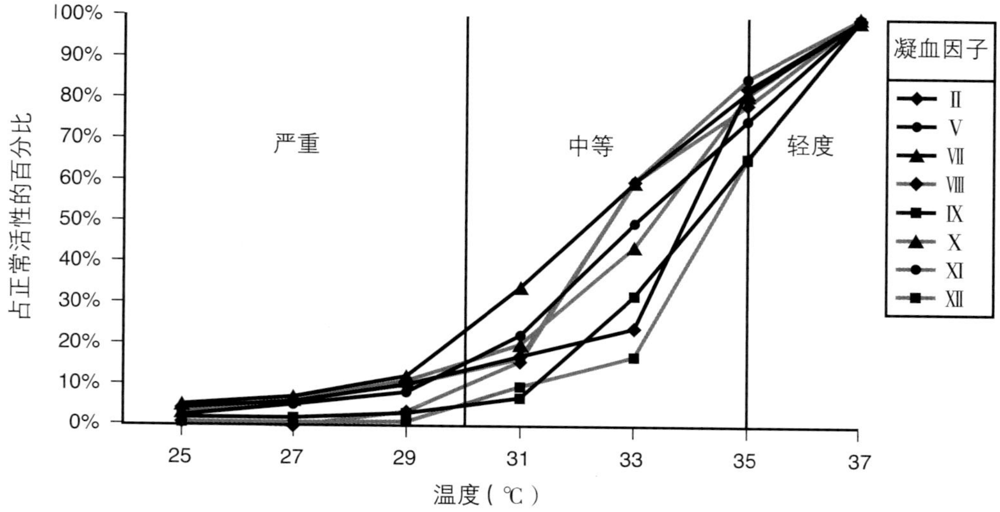

图 2　在不同温度的环境下，相关凝血因子活性占正常凝血因子活性的百分比（*Data from Johnston T, Chen Y, Reed R: Functional equivalence of hypothermia to specific clotting factor deficiencies. J Trauma 37:413–417, 1994.*）

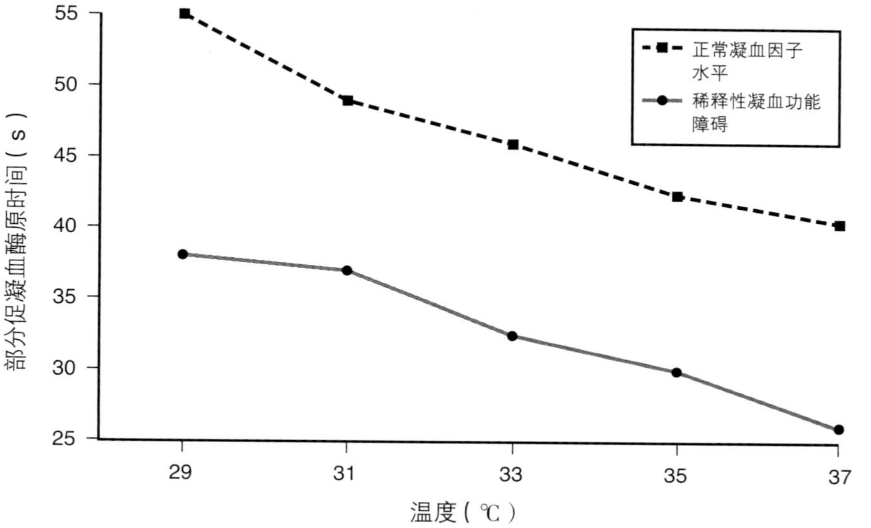

图 3　正常凝血因子水平和稀释凝血因子水平的血液样本的冷却均会导致部分促凝血酶原时间（PTT）的延长（*Data from Gubler K, Gentilello L, Hassantash S, Maier R: The impact of hypothermia on dilutional coagulopathy. J Trauma 36:847–851, 1994.*）

可导致机体氧消耗明显增加，从而加剧了主要器官供氧不足的程度，增加老年人心脏疾病的发生风险。

低体温对于免疫学的潜在影响已经被广泛的研究证实。因为大多数具有免疫功能的酶的特性，低体温肯定会抑制酶的功能。此外，我们的免疫系统也经常在非恒温下抵抗细菌，所以在如此低温环境下也不会出现严重功能障碍。但有临床研究提供可信证据，轻度的体温降低增加了手术部位感染的风险。

从神经系统方面来说，当体温降低到33℃以下时，患者会产生精神状态的改变，说明低体温是有害的。在体温降低的早期阶段，呼吸驱动力是增加的，但当体温低于33℃时，就会出现呼吸的抑制，导致每分通气量下降。血压降低和心排血量减少降低了肾小球滤过率，但由于肾小管对 Na^+ 的重吸收（冷利尿）功能的损伤，机体仍可以维持一定的尿量。血管收缩也会导致回心血容量的增加，导致患者出现多尿。

处理

人体通过氧消耗即氧化作用产热此为氧消耗的副产品。从治疗的角度来看，低体温的潜在机制非常重要。体温正常的人掉入冷水或陷入冷的环境中，才导致最初的偶然性的低体温。患者由于寒战使产热增加，但冷刺激的程度超出了温度保护的能力。

多种原因均可导致创伤患者发生低体温，也可以称为继发性低体温。休克的定义是氧输送的减少导致机体正常氧消耗不能维持。产热的减少使患者对轻度冷刺激敏感，如发生在急诊室或手术室环境的低体温。由于这个机制，所有由于严重创伤引起休克的患者均属于发生低体温的高危人群。

被动复温

人体的比热是 0.83 kcal/kg · ℃。这意味着每千克体重升高 1℃需要 0.83 kcal。因此，一个体重 70 kg 的患者升高 1℃，需要能量 58.1 kcal。因为基础热量的产生是大约为 1 kcal/kg · h，如果没有进一步的热损失，那么一个 70 kg 的患者内生热复温大约是 1.2℃ /h（图 4）。

对比患者内生热的产生，大多数复温方法不会增加额外的热能。临床观察到的复温通常是患者自身产热的结果，同时使用隔热技术以防止进一步的热损失。在治疗低体温时，最重要的原则是纠正潜在的休克，因为纠正休克可以把氧消耗和产热恢复至正常水平，同时积极预防热量的进一步损失。

积极体外复温

热力学定律（熵）是指热量从温度较高的区域传递至较低温度区域。因为皮肤的温度通常比血管中心处的温度低 10℃。低体温的患者，必须先把皮肤温度加热至高于中心温度，这样热量才会传递至中心区域。因为体外复温不会立即起效，所以体外复温不会作为主要的复温方法。

空气对流复温器提供较大的热交换面积。然而，空气密度低，包含的热能也少。例如，一个人可以在 150°F 的桑拿中忍受 10 min，但是如果把一只手放到 150°F 的热水里，10 s 就会导致严重的烫伤。

低载热能力的空气意味着有很少的热量是通过吹热空气传递给患者的。然而，热力学定律的推论是当两个物体相互接触时，热量总是从温度较高的区域流向温度较低的区域。对流复温器是形成环绕在患者周围高于皮温的空气层。尽管很少有热能通过对流热传递给患者，但热力学定律显示，它可以防止热量通过皮肤损失（出汗除外）。

尽管这些设备把热损失减小到最低，但在治疗低体温方面效果不佳，大部分的温度升高是患者自身产热的原因。在一项随机对照研究中，对流加热毯并没有比标准棉花毯的复温效率高。

铝制太空毯是由救生衣内里为材料做成的，并旨在通过反射回发射的光子，从而把患者热损失减少到最小。发射和反射面的距离是影响效果的重要因素。正确的使用方法是用毯子紧密地包住患者，并在太空毯上额外放置一个标准毯子来减小潜在的空气流动。由于患者体温降低时，头皮部血管不收缩，颈部以上的部位会损失大量的热量。用反射帽包裹或覆盖头部可以预防头部热量的损失。

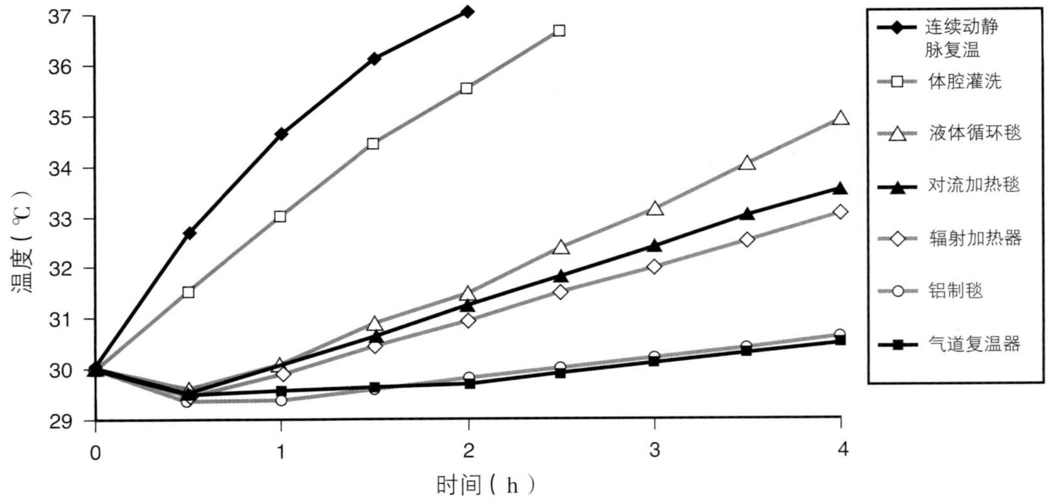

图 4 计算机模拟各种临床技术的复温速率（*Modified from Gentilello LM, Moujaes S: Treatment of hypothermia in trauma victims: thermodynamic considerations. J Intensive Care Med 10:5–14, 1995.*）

积极核心复温

最常用的复温方式是使用 41 ℃的潮湿空气。1 L 41 ℃的完全饱和的空气可以容纳 0.05 ml 水。1 L30 ℃的空气只有 0.03 ml 水。如果一位 30 ℃的患者吸入了 1 L 饱和的 41℃的空气，当它在肺内冷却至 30℃时，会有 0.02 ml 的水凝结出。因此，当每分通气量是 10 L 时，每小时会凝结出 12 ml 的水。当水凝结时，热量从蒸汽中释放出的情况是 0.58 kcal/ml（汽化的潜在热量）。因此，此情况下气道复温的最大热量是 7 kcal/h（0.58 kcal/ml × 12 ml/h）。还会有通过吸入空气所产生的 1～2 kcal 的热量，该热量的传递不依赖水的凝结。由于 70 kg 的患者通过外部复温技术需要 58 kcal 的热量才增加 1℃核心温度，所以气道复温作用有限。

当患者低体温导致出现病情不稳定时，我们会考虑进行胸腔或腹腔灌洗。热量转移取决于进入和流出水温度之间的差异以及水的流量。由于水的比热是 1 kcal/kg · ℃，那么如果 1 L 42℃水注入到体腔，流出时是 35℃，传递至机体的热量是 7 kcal。然而，为了通过开放的腹腔灌入温水，从而延长手术时间只会产生不良效果，因为水的大部分热量没有传递给患者，而是散发至 21℃的手术室环境中。

由于水的比热容较高，在给患者输入液体前加热是非常重要的。因为患者须产生 16 kcal 的热量，才能把 1L 晶体溶液的温度由室温 21 ℃提高至正常体温。患者在麻醉状态下时，他们的代谢率是相对固定的。如果他们不能增加代谢率来产生额外的热量，那么一个 70 kg 的患者会因为损失 16 kcal 的热量而降低 0.28℃，这足以引起患者剧烈的寒战。

由于血液制品在 4℃的条件下冷冻储存，明显需要有效的复温方式须加热后再输入体内。血液的比热容接近于水。因此，注入 1 L 4℃的血液就足以使体温降低 0.56℃。在休克或麻醉状态下的创伤患者体温降低的主要原因是输入了未加热的静脉液体和血液制品。

当患者需要大容量液体复苏时，简单的复温方式就是充足加热的静脉液体输注。注入体内的液体在调节温度的过程中释放热量。1 L 40℃的晶体溶液输入到 32℃患者体内，实际相当于输入 8 kcal 的热量。因为低体温的创伤患者经常需要大量的液体复苏，根据身体和输入液体之间的温差，通过加热静脉输注的液体来提供大量的热量。

死亡率

目前对于创伤患者的救治要求严格预防低体温的发生，一旦发生进行积极治疗以逆转。一些建议基于一些临床研究，这些临床研究证实，一旦发生体温降低，患者的死亡率会明显升高。一项研究通过用 ISS 评分、有无休克和液体或血液制品的需求来对创伤进行分级。在相同损伤程度的患者中，发生体温降低者比体温正常的患者的死亡率更高。如果机体核心体温降至 32℃，即使损伤较轻，死亡率也为 100%。

通过研究分析国家创伤数据库的数据，运用逐步 logistic 回归（OR = 1.54，95%CI 为 1.40 ～1.71）（图 5），发现低体温是创伤患者死亡率的独立预测因素。一个长达 8 年的国家创伤数据库的分析把低体温和常温患者根据 ISS 和休克进行分级，并使用 Logistic 回归来控制多个潜在混杂因素，包括年龄，性别，受伤机制，头部、胸部、腹部损伤的严重度，格拉斯哥昏迷等级评分分数和碱缺失。尽管创伤越严重，低体温越常见，但低体温仍然是与创伤患者死亡率关系最密切的、独立的危险因素（OR = 1.19，95% CI 为 1.05～1.35）。

一个前瞻性研究对比了历时 10 个月的低体温患者（<35℃）的死亡率，一组患者使用的治疗方式是结合气道复温、液体循环毯或电热毯、一个铝制头部覆盖物，以及静脉液体加热输入等多种方式，另一组患者用连续动静脉复温（continuous arteriovenous rewarming，CAVR）。以温度大于 35 ℃为目标，标准复温技术的复温时间是 3.23 h，而 CAVR 是 39 min。CAVR 的快速复温导致血液制

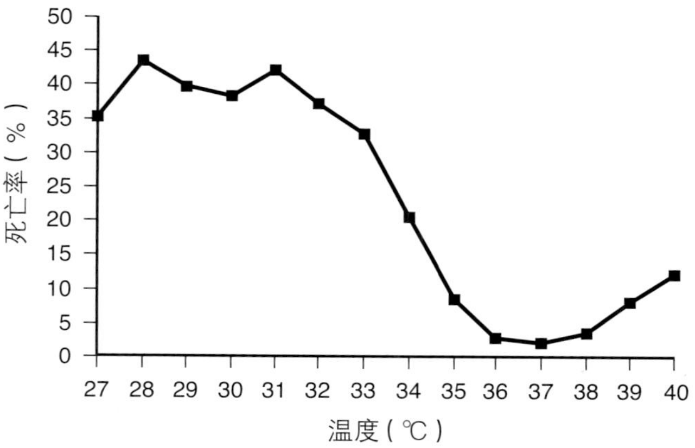

图 5　来自国家创伤数据库的体温改变和死亡率的关系

品需求下降 57%，而晶体溶液的需求下降 67%，同时创伤患者的死亡率也随之下降（图 6）。

在一个前瞻性随机临床试验中，把缓慢和快速复温重伤患者的结果进行比较可以得出结论，CAVR 组能够成功复苏更多患者（$P<0.01$）。

诱导低体温

在不同的临床背景中，通过诱导低体温来减少缺血损伤已经有很长时间了。最初的实验室研究表明，创伤性脑损伤后的低体温治疗初现成效，被证实有保护神经的效果。然而，为了治疗创伤患者而故意诱导低体温，会导致一些亚组人群没有任何保护效果，但并发症和伤害却不断增加。

Clifton 进行了北美急性脑损伤研究，该研究是由美国国立卫生研究院进行的一项随机、多中心临床研究。该试验共招募 392 名患者，在诱导创伤患者低温方面是最大型的研究。由于 2 组有 56% 的患者预后不良，以及有相似的死亡率（28% 和 27%），所以研究提前终止。低体温组患者的并发症更多，包括低血压发作和感染。低体温的不良结果更常见于大于 45 岁的患者（88% vs. 69%，P=0.08）。

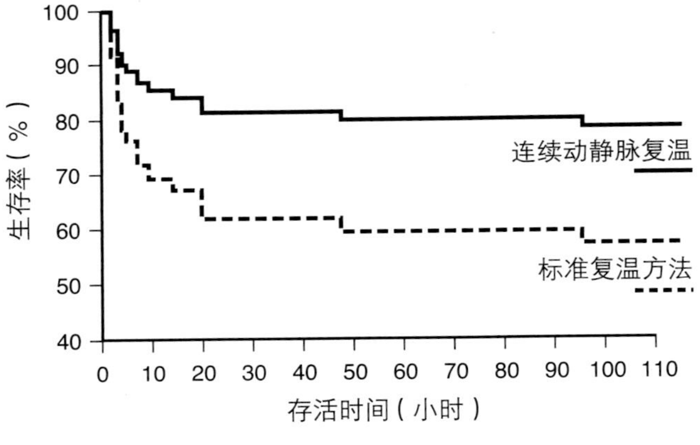

图 6 对比标准复温（SR）和连续动静脉复温（CAVR）2 种复温方式的累计生存曲线（Kaplan-Meier）。CAVR 是一种体外复温技术，导管放置于患者的股动静脉处，然后利用血压使血液流经液体加热装置，创造一个瘘。CAVR 明显更快（$P<0.001$）。死亡率的差异主要发生在复苏期间（P=0.047）（*From Gentilello LM, Jurkovich GJ, Stark MS, et al: Is Hypothermia in the major trauma victim protective or harmful? A randomized, prospective study. Ann Surg 226:439- 449, 1997.*）

研究人员还进行了北美急性脑伤研究Ⅱ，这是一个与之前类似的随机试验，低体温进行得更早，降温也更积极。尽管快速诱导低体温，但结果仍然不理想：52 位低体温患者中有 31 位出现预后不良（60%），死亡 12 位；而 45 位对照组患者中仅有 25 位出现预后不良（55%），死亡 8 位。本研究最终也因无价值，被迫终止。研究人员得出结论，但并没有进一步的基础来支持低体温能在脑弥漫性损伤后起保护作用的观点，需要更多的研究来确定它是否可以保护有血肿的患者。

低体温的损害对于儿童来说更加严重。在低体温的多中心试验中，共有 225 名颅脑损伤的儿童（1 ~ 17 岁）低体温组的不良预后率为 31%，而正常体温组为 22%（P=0.08）。7 岁及以上的患者低体温时出现不良预后的风险更大（RR = 1.71，95% CI 为 0.96 ~ 3.06，P=0.06）。在颅内压正常的患者中，低体温组的死亡率明显更高（RR = 2.12，95% CI 为 1.07 ~ 4.19；P=0.03）。

已经有关于在穿通性损伤后出现心搏停止，应用心肺旁路术快速诱导低温的研究。动物模型已经展示了其可行性。然而，在开始临床试验之前仍存在伦理问题。在创伤患者中诱导低体温的方法仍然没有潜在获益。

应用低温治疗导致的并发症包括：反跳性颅内高压、感染、低血压、经常需要血管加压药、心动过缓、由于应用血管收缩药物导致的褥疮、肠梗阻、低钾血症、酸碱平衡紊乱及其他电解质相关的并发症。

结论

人体的比热容相对较高，使得低体温极难治疗。出血的快速控制及休克的纠正可恢复机体正常产热，加上之前所说的热损失机制，是最好的治疗方式。基于目前的数据分析来看，低体温对预后有很多不利影响，一旦发生，应用各种方法试图积极纠正。